PATHOLOGY AND INTERVENTION IN MUSCULOSKELETAL REHABILITATION

PATHOLOGY AND INTERVENTION IN MUSCULOSKELETAL REHABILITATION

SECOND EDITION

David J. Magee
PT, PhD, CM
Professor
Department of Physical Therapy
Faculty of Rehabilitation Medicine
University of Alberta
Edmonton, Alberta, Canada

James E. Zachazewski
PT, DPT, SCS, ATC
Clinical Director
Department of Physical
and Occupational Therapy
Clinical Content Lead
Health Professions, Partners eCare
Massachusetts General Hospital
Adjunct Assistant Professor
MGH Institute of Health Professions
Boston, Massachusetts

William S. Quillen
PT, DPT, PhD, FACSM
Associate Dean
Morsani College of Medicine
Professor and Director
School of Physical Therapy
and Rehabilitation Sciences
University of South Florida
Tampa, Florida

Robert C. Manske
PT, DPT, MEd, SCS, ATC, CSCS
Professor and Chair
Department of Physical Therapy
Wichita State University
Physical Therapist
Via Christi Health
Wichita, Kansas

EDITORIAL CONSULTANT
Bev Evjen
Swift Current, Saskatchewan, Canada

ELSEVIER

ELSEVIER

3251 Riverport Lane
Maryland Heights, Missouri 63043

PATHOLOGY AND INTERVENTION IN MUSCULOSKELETAL
REHABILITATION, SECOND EDITION

ISBN: 978-0-323-31072-7

Notice

Knowledge and best practice in this field are constantly changing. As new research and experience broaden our knowledge, changes in practice, treatment, and drug therapy may become necessary or appropriate. Readers are advised to check the most current information provided (i) on procedures featured or (ii) by the manufacturer of each product to be administered, to verify the recommended dose or formula, the method, and duration of administration, and contraindications. It is the responsibility of the practitioner, relying on their own experience and knowledge of the patient, to make diagnoses, to determine dosages and the best treatment for each individual patient, and to take all appropriate safety precautions. To the fullest extent of the law, neither the Publisher nor the Editor assumes any liability for any injury and/or damage to persons or property arising out of or related to any use of the material contained in this book.

The Publisher

International Standard Book Number: 978-0-323-31072-7

Executive Content Strategist: Kathy Falk
Senior Content Development Specialist: Courtney Sprehe
Publishing Services Manager: Julie Eddy
Senior Project Manager: Richard Barber
Design Direction: Reneé Duenow

Printed in the United States of America

Last digit is the print number: 9 8 7 6 5 4

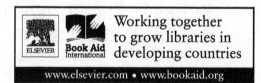

Working together
to grow libraries in
developing countries

www.elsevier.com • www.bookaid.org

Contributors

Omar El Abd, MD
Newton Wellesley Interventional Spine, LLC
Wellesley, Massachusetts

Jeanna Allegrone, DPT
Physical Therapist
Newton-Wellesley Hospital
Newton, Massachusetts

C. Dain Allred, MD
Chief, Sports Medicine
Orthopedic Surgeon
U.S. Air Force Academy
Colorado Springs, Colorado

Christine Alvero, PT, DPT, ATC
Manager, Rehabilitation Services
Moffitt Cancer Center
Tampa, Florida

Joao Eduardo Daud Amadera, MD, PhD
Head and Director of Research - Spine Center, HCor
São Paulo - Brazil Interventional Physiatry
University of São Paulo
São Paulo, Brazil

Susan L. Armijo-Olivo, BSc PT, MScPT, PhD
Adjunct Professor
Faculty of Rehabilitation Medicine
University of Alberta
Edmonton, Alberta

Christopher A. Arrigo, MS, PT
Owner/Physical Therapist
Advanced Rehabilitation
Tampa, Florida

Peter Asnis, MD
Instructor, Harvard Medical School
Mass General Hospital Sports Medicine Service
Department of Orthopaedic Surgery
Massachusetts General Hospital
Boston, Massachusetts

Steven A. Aviles, MD
Iowa Ortho
Des Moines, Iowa

Oladapo M. Babatunde, MD
Sports Medicine Fellow, Orthopaedic Surgery
Stanford University
Redwood City, California

Mary F. Barbe, PhD
Professor, Anatomy and Cell Biology
School of Medicine
Temple University
Philadelphia, Pennsylvania

Helen E. Bateman, MD, CCD
Rheumatology Section
Chief James A. Haley VA Medical Center
Associate Professor
USF Health Morsani College of Medicine
University of South Florida
Tampa, Florida

Eric M. Berkson, MD
Instructor, Harvard Medical School
Mass General Hospital Sports Medicine Service
Department of Orthopaedic Surgery
Massachusetts General Hospital
Foxborough, Massachusetts

Jennifer Bessire, PT, PhD
Assistant Professor
Physical Therapy Department
Center for Health Sciences Education
St. Ambrose University
Davenport, Iowa

Odion Binitie, MD
Assistant Member
Moffitt Cancer Center
Tampa, Florida

Mark D. Bishop, PT, PhD, CSCS
Associate Professor
Department of Physical Therapy
College of Public Health and Health Professions
University of Florida
Gainesville, Florida

Joanne Borg-Stein, MD
Associate Professor
Department of Physical Medicine and Rehabilitation
Harvard Medical School
Director, Harvard/Spaulding Sports Medicine Fellowship
Boston, Massachusetts
Medical Director, Spine Center and Chief of Physical
    Medicine and Rehabilitation
Newton-Wellesley Hospital
Newton, Massachusetts

Martin J. Bouliane, MD, FRCS(C)
Division of Orthopaedic Surgery
Faculty of Medicine and Dentistry
University of Alberta
Edmonton, Alberta, Canada

**Peter D. Brukner, OMA, MBBS, DRCOG, FACSP,
    FASMF, FACSM**
Associate Professor
Centre for Health, Exercise, and Sports Medicine
The University of Melbourne
Director
Olympic Park Sports Medicine Centre
Melbourne, Victoria, Australia

David B. Burr, PhD
Professor, Department of Anatomy and Cell Biology
Professor, Department of Orthopaedic Surgery
Indiana University School of Medicine
Professor of Biomedical Engineering
Indiana University-Purdue University, Indianapolis
Indianapolis, Indiana

Nancy N. Byl, PT, MPH, PhD, FAPTA
Professor and Chair Emeritus
University of California, San Francisco
San Francisco, California

Carolyn Byl Dolan, PT, MS, DPT, Cert MDT
Spine Orthopedic Active Rehab
Reno, Nevada

Judy C. Chepeha, MScPT, PhD
Assistant Professor
Department of Physical Therapy
Faculty of Rehabilitation Medicine
University of Alberta
Edmonton, Alberta, Canada

Melissa Colbert, MD
Chief Resident Physician
Department of Physical Medicine and Rehabilitation
Harvard Medical School
Spaulding Rehabilitation Hospital
Charlestown, Massachusetts

Marie B. Corkery, PT, DPT, MHS, FAAOMPT
Associate Clinical Professor
Department of Physical Therapy, Movement, and
    Rehabilitation Sciences
Bouvé College of Health Sciences
Northeastern University
Boston, Massachusetts

Elias Dakwar, MD
Assistant Professor
Department of Neurosurgery and Brain Repair
Morsani College of Medicine
University of South Florida
Tampa, Florida

Armen Deukmedjian, MD
Assistant Professor
Department of Neurosurgery and Brain Repair
Morsani College of Medicine
University of South Florida
Tampa, Florida

Charles Deveikas, OTR/L, CHT
Occupational/Certified Hand Therapist
Owner, Upper Hand Therapy and Training
Arlington, Massachusetts

Joanne G. Draghetti, MS, OTR, CHT
Occupational Therapy
Bedford, New Hampshire

Caroline Drye Taylor, MS, PT, OCS, FAAOMPT
Taylor & Thornburg Physical Therapy, Inc.
Oakland, California

Eric O. Eisemon, MD
Massachusetts General Hospital
Boston, Massachusetts

Rafael Escamilla, PhD, PT, CSCS, FACSM
Professor
Director of Biomechanics Laboratory
Department of Physical Therapy
California State University
Sacramento, California

Timothy L. Fagerson, DPT
President
SOSPT, Inc. (Spine Orthopaedic Sport Physical Therapy)
Wellesley, Massachusetts

Manuela L. Ferreira, BPT (Honours), MSc, PhD
Senior Research Fellow
Musculoskeletal Division
The George Institute for Global Health/Sydney Medical
    School
The University of Sydney
Sydney, New South Wales, Australia

Paulo H. Ferreira, BPT (Honours), MSc, PhD
Senior Lecturer, Physiotherapy
Faculty of Health Sciences
The University of Sydney
Sydney, New South Wales, Australia

Kristina Fleming, PT, DPT, CSCS
Sports Physical Therapy Resident
Department of Physical Therapy, Movement, and
    Rehabilitation Sciences
Northeastern University
Boston, Massachusetts
Massachusetts General Hospital
Sports Physical Therapy Service
Charlestown, Massachusetts

Walter R. Frontera, MD, PhD
Chair, Department of Physical Medicine and
    Rehabilitation
Professor of Physical Medicine and Rehabilitation
Medical Director, Rehabilitation Services
School of Medicine
Vanderbilt University
Nashville, Tennessee

John P. Fulkerson, MD
Orthopedic Associates of Hartford
Farmington, Connecticut

Inae C. Gadotti, PT, MSc, PhD
Assistant Professor
Department of Physical Therapy
Nicole Wertheim College of Nursing & Health Sciences
Physical Therapy Department
Florida International University
Miami, Florida

Steven Z. George, PT, PhD
Associate Professor and Assistant Department Chair
Department of Physical Therapy
College of Public Health & Health Professions
University of Florida
Gainesville, Florida

Thomas J. Gill IV, MD
Associate Professor of Orthopedic Surgery
Department Orthopedic Surgery
Massachusetts General Hospital
Boston, Massachusetts

Grant Glass, MPT, CIMT, OCS, CAFS, GPS
Galena Sport Physical Therapy
Reno, Nevada

James Green II, PT, DPT
Physical Therapist
Newton-Wellesley Hospital
Newton, Massachusetts

Jennifer B. Green, MD
Hand and Upper Extremity Surgeon
Mt. Auburn Hospital
ProSports Orthopedics
Cambridge, Massachusetts

Lindsay C. Groat, PA-C
Syracuse Orthopedic Specialists
Syracuse, New York

Sanaz Hariri, MD
Orthopedic Surgeon
Los Gatos, California

Diane M. Heislein, PT, DPT, OCS
Physical Therapist
Massachusetts General Hospital
Boston, Massachusetts
Clinical Associate Professor
Sargent College of Health and Rehabilitation
    Sciences
Boston University
Boston, Massachusetts

Jay Hertel, PhD, ATC, FACSM
Joe H. Gieck Professor of Sports Medicine
Professor of Kinesiology
Department of Human Services
Curry School of Education
University of Virginia
Charlottesville, Virginia

Carole High Gross, PT, MS
Central Bucks Physical Therapy, LLC
Doylestown, Pennsylvania

Thomas F. Hobson, DPT
Physical Therapist
Scarsdale, New York

Paul W. Hodges, PhD, MedDr, BPhty(Hons)
Director, NHMRC Centre for Clinical
    Research Excellence in Spinal Pain, Injury
    and Health
Professor, School of Health and Rehab
    Sciences
The University of Queensland
Brisbane, Queensland, Australia

Jamie Holloway, PT, DPT, PCS
University of Alabama at Birmingham
Departments of Physical and Occupational Therapy
Birmingham, Alabama

Christopher D. Ingersoll, PHD, AT, ATC, FACSM, FNATA, FASAHP
Dean, College of Health Sciences
Professor, Athletic Training
College of Health Sciences
The University of Toledo
Toledo, Ohio

Maura Daly Iversen, PT, DPT, SD, MPH
Professor and Chair
Department of Physical Therapy
Northeastern University
Boston, Massachusetts

Jaeson Kawadler, DPT, CSCS
Brigham and Women's Department of Rehabilitation Services
Mansfield, Massachusetts

Hollie Kirwan, MSc
Clinical Research Coordinator
Sports Performance Biomechanics
Massachusetts General Orthopaedics Sports Performance Center
Massachusetts General Hospital
Foxborough, Massachusetts

Diane Lee, BSR, FCAMT, CGIMS
Physiotherapist, Owner, Educator and Director
Diane Lee & Associates
Surrey, British Columbia
Professional Associate
School of Rehabilitation
McMaster University
Hamilton, Ontario, Canada

Linda-Joy (LJ) Lee, PhD, BSc, BSc(PT), FCAMPT, CGIMS, MCPA, MAPA
Director and Lead Instructor, Discover Physio
Founder, Synergy Physio
North Vancouver, British Columbia, Canada

Trevor A. Lentz, MPT, CSCS
Rehabilitation Sciences Doctoral Program
College of Public Health and Health Professions
University of Florida
Gainesville, Florida

Bruce M. Leslie, MD
Newton Wellesley Orthopedic Associates
Newton, Massachusetts

G. Douglas Letson, MD
Site Director, Professor of Orthopaedic Oncology
Department of Orthopaedics and Sports Medicine
Morsani College of Medicine
University of South Florida
Executive Vice President and Physician-in-Chief
Moffitt Cancer Center
Tampa, Florida

Toby Long, PhD, PT, FAPTA
Georgetown University
Center for Child and Human Development
Washington, DC

David J. Magee, PT, PhD, CM
Professor
Department of Physical Therapy
Faculty of Rehabilitation Medicine
University of Alberta
Edmonton, Alberta, Canada

Robert C. Manske, PT, DPT, MEd, SCS, ATC, CSCS
Professor and Chair
Department of Physical Therapy
Wichita State University
Physical Therapist
Via Christi Health
Wichita, Kansas

Ronald R. Mattison, BPE, BScPT
Allan McGavin Sports Medicine
University of British Columbia
Vancouver, British Columbia, Canada

David J. Mayman, MD
Associate Professor in Orthopaedic Surgery, Weill Cornell Medical College
Associate Attending Orthopaedic Surgeon and Clinical Co-Director of Computer Assisted Surgery Center, Hospital for Special Surgery
Associate Attending Orthopedic Surgeon, New York-Presbyterian Hospital
New York, New York

Owen P. McGonigle, MD
Orthopedic Surgery
Tufts Medical Center Orthopedics
Boston, Massachusetts

Jim Meadows, BScPT, MCPA, FCAMT
Owner, Swodeam Institute
Strathmore, Alberta, Canada

Donna L. Merkel, PT, MS, SCS, CSCS
Bryn Mawr Rehab Hospital
Exton, Pennsylvania

Joseph T. Molony, Jr., PT, MS, SCS, CSCS
Board Certified Sports Clinical Specialist
Certified Strength and Conditioning Specialist
Sports Performance and Rehabilitation
King of Prussia, Pennsylvania

David P. Newman, PT, DPT, OCS
Tampa, Florida

Stephen J. Nicholas, MD
Director
Nicholas Institute of Sports Medicine and Athletic
    Trauma (NISMAT)
New York, New York

David Nicoloro, PT, MS
Supervisor, Rehabilitation Services
Newton-Wellesley Hospital
Newton, Massachusetts

David Nolan, PT, DPT, MS, OCS, SCS, CSCS
Associate Clinical Professor
Department of Physical Therapy, Movement, and
    Rehabilitation Sciences
Northeastern University
Clinical Specialist
Massachusetts General Hospital Sports Physical Therapy
    Service
Boston, Massachusetts

Sabrina Paganoni, MD, PhD
MGH Physical Medicine and Rehabilitation Service
Massachusetts General Hospital
Neuromuscular Diagnostic Center
Boston, Massachusetts

Alex Petruska, PT, SCS, LAT
Senior Sports Physical Therapist and Athletic
    Trainer
Sports Physical Therapy Service
Department of Orthopedic Surgery
Massachusetts General Hospital
Boston, Massachusetts

Rose Pignataro, PT, PhD, DPT, CWS
Assistant Professor
Department of Physical Therapy and Human
    Performance
Florida Gulf Coast University
Fort Myers, Florida

Daniel Camargo Pimentel, MD, PhD
Department of Pathology
School of Medicine
University of São Paulo
São Paulo, Brazil

Andrew Porter, DO, FAAFP
Via Christi Sports Medicine
Wichita, Kansas

Christopher M. Powers, PT, PhD, FACSM, FAPTA
Associate Professor
Director, Program in Biokinesiology
Co-Director, Musculoskeletal Biomechanics Research Lab
USC Division of Biokinesiology & Physical Therapy
Los Angeles, California

Daniel Quillin, DPT, ATC
Sports and Orthopedic Physical Therapist
Via Christi Health
Wichita, Kansas

Alejandro Ramirez, MD
Endocrinology, Diabetes, and Metabolism
Assistant Professor of Medicine
James A. Haley V Medical Center
University of South Florida
Tampa, Florida

Helen E. Ranger, PT, MS, CHT
Newton-Wellesley Hospital
Newton, Massachusetts

Glenn R. Rechtine II, MD
Orthopaedic Surgeon
Rochester, New York

Yoav Ritter, DO
Assistant Professor
Department of Neurosurgery and Brain Repair
USF Health Morsani College of Medicine
University of South Florida
Tampa, Florida

Neil S. Roth, MD
Founder and Director
New York Sports Medicine Institute
New York, New York
White Plains, New York

Harry E. Rubash, MD
Edith M. Ashley Professor of Orthopedic Surgery
Harvard Medical School
Head of the Department of Orthopedic Surgery
Massachusetts General Hospital
Boston, Massachusetts

Marc R. Safran, MD
Professor, Orthopaedic Surgery
Associate Director, Sports Medicine
Stanford University
Redwood City, California

Edgar T. Savidge, PT, DPT
Rehabilitation Manager
Newton-Wellesley Ambulatory Care Center
Newton-Wellesley Hospital
Newton, Massachusetts

Evan D. Schumer, MD
Assistant Clinical Professor
Department of Orthopedic Surgery
School of Medicine
Tufts University
Boston, Massachusetts
Newton Wellesley Orthopedic Associates
Newton, Massachusetts

Keiba L. Shaw, PT, MPT, MA, EdD
Associate Professor
Physical Therapy
College of Health Care Sciences
Nova Southeastern University
Tampa, Florida

David M. Sheps, MD, MSc, FRCS(C)
Assistant Clinical Professor
Division of Orthopaedic Surgery
Faculty of Medicine and Dentistry
University of Alberta
Edmonton, Alberta, Canada

Richard B. Souza, PhD, PT, ATC, CSCS
Associate Professor
UCSF School of Medicine
University of California
San Francisco, California

Robert Spang, MD
Resident
Department of Orthopaedic Surgery
Massachusetts General Hospital
Boston, Massachusetts

Ashley G. Sterrett, MD, CCD
Rheumatology Section
James A. Haley VA Medical Center
Associate Professor
USF Health Morsani College of Medicine
University of South Florida
Tampa, Florida

Anne-Marie Thomas, MD, PT
Assistant Professor
Department of Physical Medicine and Rehabilitation at
    Spalding Hospital
Harvard Medical School
Boston, Massachusetts

Timothy F. Tyler, MS, PT, ATC
Research Consultant
Nicholas Institute of Sports Medicine and Athletic
    Trauma (NISMAT)
New York, New York

Stuart J. Warden, PhD, PT, FACSM
Associate Dean for Research
Associate Professor, Department of Physical Therapy
Indiana University School of Health and Rehabilitation
    Sciences
Associate Professor (adjunct), Department of Anatomy
    and Cell Biology
Indiana University School of Medicine
Associate Professor (adjunct), Department of Biomedical
    Engineering
Purdue School of Engineering and Technology
Director, Center for Translational Musculoskeletal
    Research
Indiana University-Purdue University Indianapolis
Indianapolis, Indiana

Kevin E. Wilk, PT, DPT, FAPTA
Champion Sports Medicine
Birmingham, Alabama

D.S. Blaise Williams III, PhD, MPT
Director, VCU RUN LAB
Department of Physical Therapy
Virginia Commonwealth University
Richmond, Virginia

Jeff Wong, MD
Mass General Hospital Sports Medicine Service
Department of Orthopaedic Surgery
Massachusetts General Hospital
Boston, Massachusetts

James E. Zachazewski, PT, DPT, SCS, ATC
Clinical Director, Department of Physical and
    Occupational Therapy
Clinical Content Lead, Health Professions, Partners
    eCare
Massachusetts General Hospital
Adjunct Assistant Professor, MGH Institute of Health
    Professions
Boston, Massachusetts

"TO TEACH IS TO LEARN TWICE"

*To those who invested in us that we might, in turn, pass on
their knowledge and wisdom to future generations of colleagues and students.*

Preface
Musculoskeletal Rehabilitation Series

Musculoskeletal conditions have an enormous impact on society. Today, musculoskeletal conditions have become the most common cause of disability and severe long-term pain in the industrialized world. The knowledge and skill required by the community of health care providers involved in managing the impairments and functional limitations resulting from acute or chronic musculoskeletal injury/illness have grown exponentially as the frequency of visits to practitioners' offices for musculoskeletal system complaints has risen.

The art and science of musculoskeletal rehabilitation began as a consequence of the injuries suffered on the battlefields of Europe during World War I. Since that time, numerous textbooks have been published regarding musculoskeletal rehabilitation. These texts have encompassed the areas of basic science, evaluation, and treatment. However, these books have most often been developed and written in professional "isolation" (i.e., from a single discipline's perspective). As a consequence, topics have either been covered in great depth but with a very narrow focus or with great breadth with very little depth. Our goal in the development and production of this musculoskeletal rehabilitation series was to develop a series of four textbooks that complement and build on one another, providing the reader with the needed depth and breadth of information for this critical area of health care.

Volume I of the series is the 6th edition of David Magee's *Orthopedic Physical Assessment*. This now classic text provides the clinician with the most comprehensive musculoskeletal assessment text available on this topic. First published in 1987, it has withstood the test of time and is the most widely used text in this area. In 1996, three of the editors developed and published *Athletic Injuries and Rehabilitation*. Based upon feedback from both students and clinicians, we decided to expand and broaden the scope of *Athletic Injuries and Rehabilitation* into three new volumes. *Volume II, Scientific Foundations and Principles of Practice in Musculoskeletal Rehabilitation*, provides clinicians with currently available science regarding musculoskeletal issues and principles of practice that should guide clinicians regarding therapeutic intervention. In this *Volume III, Pathology and Intervention in Musculoskeletal Rehabilitation*, now in its second edition, we have attempted to provide readers with a comprehensive text containing information on the most common musculoskeletal pathologies seen and the best evidence behind contemporary interventions directed towards the treatment of impairments and limitations associated with acute, chronic, and congenital musculoskeletal conditions, which occur across the lifespan. *Volume IV, Athletic and Sport Issues in Musculoskeletal Rehabilitation*, covers those topics edited by the original editors plus a new editor, Robert Manske, updated and expanded the sports related topics from the original text and provided information to clinicians interested in treating high-level athletes.

International contributors have provided their unique perspectives on current diagnostic methodologies, clinical techniques, and rehabilitative concerns. We hope that our continued use of interdisciplinary author teams has in some small way broken down the professional "territorial turf" barriers that have existed in past decades of health care. Health care professionals involved in the contemporary care of musculoskeletal conditions must continue to share and learn from one another to advance the provision of the most time- and cost-efficient care possible in twenty-first century society.

Each volume in our series is liberally illustrated. Key concepts in each chapter are highlighted in text boxes, which serve to reinforce those concepts for the reader, and numerous tables summarize chapter information for easy reference. Because of the comprehensive nature of this multi-volume series, each text, although complete in itself, has been edited to build and integrate with related chapter materials from the other volumes in the series. It is the editors' hope that this series will find its way into use by faculty as a basis for formal coursework as well as a friendly companion and frequently consulted reference by students and those on the front lines of clinical care.

As with our previous collaborations, we look forward to the feedback that only you, our colleagues, can provide, so that we may continue the development and improvement of the *Musculoskeletal Rehabilitation Series.*

David J. Magee
James E. Zachazewski
William S. Quillen
Robert C. Manske

Preface
Pathology and Intervention, 2nd edition

Pathology and Intervention is the third book in the *Musculoskeletal Rehabilitation Series* dedicated to providing students and practicing clinicians with a comprehensive integrated musculoskeletal resource to consult regarding the most common area of practice for most clinicians involved in musculoskeletal rehabilitation. In this text, we have assembled an exceptional multidisciplinary group of clinicians to present the best evidence behind contemporary interventions directed toward the treatment of the impairments and functional limitations associated with acute, chronic, and congenital musculoskeletal conditions occurring across the lifespan. In this second edition, we have added chapters on skin and wound healing, rotator cuff pathology, and musculoskeletal bone and soft tissue tumors.

In an effort to maximize the volume of information presented on specific pathologies and methods of interventions, and to minimize the duplication of information, we have asked the authors, and edited the text, to refer readers to *Volume I, Orthopedic Physical Assessment,* and to *Volume II, Scientific Foundations and Principles of Practice,* for basic science information regarding inflammation, healing, tissue deformation, and the development of muscular strength and endurance. This has allowed the authors to provide the reader with as much information as possible on the specific pathologies most often seen in the clinic and the best methods of treatment intervention.

We have again asked the authors to concentrate on answering the key questions of who?, what?, when?, where?, why?, and how?. **Who** usually suffers from the types of injuries and conditions described? **What** are the best methods of intervention for these conditions? **When** should intervention be initiated? **Where** does the practicing clinician find the information on which the authors base their recommended methods of intervention? **Why** should the reader utilize the author's recommendations? **How** should the clinician progress the patient toward full recovery? We believe that the authors have effectively answered these questions, giving the reader a textbook that will prove valuable for years to come.

Finally, we would like to thank those authors who contributed to the first edition of this book but decided, for various reasons, not to be involved in the second edition. We would especially like to thank the previous authors and new authors who contributed to the second edition. Your expertise and taking the time to update and add new information to chapters and to add new chapters have been a great contribution to the book. Thank you!

David J. Magee
James E. Zachazewski
William S. Quillen
Robert C. Manske

Contents

Patient Education, Motivation, Compliance, and Adherence to Physical Activity, Exercise, and Rehabilitation

KEIBA L. SHAW

INTRODUCTION

The importance of physical activity and engagement in structured and planned activities through exercise has been considered to be one of the main determinants that influence the aging process as well as health-related quality of life. This concept of health-related quality of life exploded in 1996 with the Surgeon General's Report on Physical Activity and Health that brought forth the importance of engaging in an active lifestyle to prevent the onset of chronic disease and illness,[1] followed by the National Blueprint in 2001 that stressed the importance of physical activity in adults aged 50 years and older[2] and the U.S. Department of Health and Human Services (HHS) 2008 Physical Activity Guidelines for Americans document that provided "science-based guidance to help Americans aged 6 and older improve their health through appropriate physical activity" (p. vi).[3] The Centers for Disease Control and Prevention (CDC) issued a State Indicator Report on Physical Activity in 2014, presenting state-level information on physical activity behaviors and environmental and policy supports for physical activity. In this report, physical activity among adults and high school students was found to be higher in some states than others (e.g., Colorado >25% versus Mississippi <15%) and that overall most states have environmental and policy strategies that encouraged physical activity.[4] This is good news, but more work needs to be done. It can be safely said that being sedentary is one of the most important health problems of our time and increasing activity levels is often devalued by a large portion of the population

as well as health care providers who perhaps believe that there is a "magic pill" that will reduce health care risks. Physicians and other clinicians are more likely to measure cholesterol, blood pressure, and body mass index (BMI) than measure parameters that assess fitness levels, such as a maximal exercise test or at the very least a questionnaire examining physical activity or exercise history.[5]

THE PROFESSIONAL'S ROLE IN MOTIVATION ADHERENCE

What is Meant by Motivation, Adherence, and Compliance?

Motivation is literally the desire to do things. It is the critical element in setting and attaining goals—and research shows that one can influence one's own levels of motivation and self-control. The word motivation is derived from the Latin term *movere*, meaning "to move."[6] In essence the term *motivation* attempts to capture the "how" and "what" that moves a person to make certain choices, engage in action, expend effort, and therefore persist in action. Although this definition captures the essence of motivation, there is considerable debate on what this term actually means to individuals and at times to a population as a whole. Motivation has a range of influences on human behavior, and because of this there is no one motivational theory in existence that gives a comprehensive and integrative account of this concept. Nonetheless, a discussion of some of the more prominent and pertinent motivational theories is warranted to help explain or rather hypothesize why individuals think and behave as they do. Motivation to perform an action typically comes about through a gradual awakening of complex mental processes that takes initiative, planning, goal setting, intention formation, task generation, action implementation, action control, and outcome evaluation.

Obtaining a desired reward or experiencing pleasant sensations or escaping undesired, unpleasant consequences is often the impetus for engaging or not engaging in a behavior. Behavioral needs will often inspire individuals to act so as to avoid unwanted consequences or pursue desired responses. Socially, individuals will strive to be valued members of a group, thereby being able to imitate the positive (or negative) behaviors of others within the group. As biological beings, individuals strive to increase or decrease stimulation or arousal while seeking to maximize pleasurable sensations that affect our five senses (i.e., sight, touch, taste, smell, and hearing). In addition, individuals strive to minimize those unpleasant sensations, such as thirst, hunger, and anything that makes one uncomfortable, seeking to maintain homeostasis and balance as a system in the long term. At the cognitive level, individuals are inspired to maintain an attention to things that one deems interesting or threatening, while seeking to develop meaning and understanding to those things with which one is unfamiliar. Again, one strives to increase equilibrium while eliminating anything that one may see as a danger to his or her survival. In the affective domain, motivation plays a large role in order to decrease emotional dissonance. There is a drive to feel good and a need to increase one's sense of well-being and self-esteem. Security in one's surroundings and within oneself is sought after, and the individual strives to maintain adequate levels of optimism and enthusiasm to obtain it. Optimism is a cognitive construct (e.g., expectancies regarding future outcomes) that relates to motivation. People who are optimistic exert effort, whereas pessimistic people disengage from effort.[7] Evidence suggests that individuals who are pessimistic do not fare as well as those who are more optimistic with exercise participation. In a study assessing the relationship between optimism and indices of healthy aging, it was concluded that dispositional optimism was associated with healthy aging.[7] The relationship between optimism and healthy aging was assessed across three dimensions of health behavior: smoking, alcohol consumption, and physical activity. It was found that higher optimism was positively related to healthy behavior choices.[8]

Motivational Theories

In both the psychology and sport psychology literature, motivation has been classified as either being intrinsic (internal) or extrinsic (external). In addition, individuals will act to satisfy or meet basic needs (Figure 1-1).[9,10] In fact, people will satisfy a need or want by engaging or

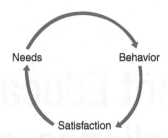

Figure 1-1 The basis of motivational theories.

not engaging in certain behaviors. These needs can be classified as behavioral or external and social, biological, cognitive, affective, conative, or spiritual.[11]

Behavioral needs will often inspire individuals to act to avoid unwanted consequences or pursue desired responses. We strive to be valued members of a group and therefore will imitate the positive and/or negative behaviors of others within the group. As biological beings, we strive to maximize sensations that engage our five senses and are pleasurable while striving to minimize sensations that we find to be unpleasant (e.g., thirst, hunger). In this way, we seek to maintain homeostasis and balance in the long term. Cognitively, individuals maintain attention to things that are of interest or that they feel are a threat while seeking to construct meaning and to understand those things with which one is unfamiliar. This again serves to achieve equilibrium while eliminating things that may be seen as threat or danger to one's survival.

> Research has shown that individuals who are pessimistic do not fare as well with exercise participation as those who are more optimistic.

Decreasing emotional dissonance is accomplished in part by how much one is motivated to feel good and to increase one's self-esteem. Individuals strive to increase feelings of security in their surroundings as well as within themselves. Seeking to maintain adequate levels of optimism and enthusiasm helps to secure this feeling. Research has shown that individuals who are pessimistic do not fare as well as those who are more optimistic with exercise participation.[12]

The framework surrounding the most popular theories on motivation revolves around three major areas: social cognition, humanistic, and multidimensional.

> Taking control, developing and maintaining self-efficacy, and meeting individually developed goals are additional aspects of motivation. Individuals have personal dreams and needs related to fulfilling those dreams.

Social Cognitive Theory

Social cognitive theory, as developed and postulated by Albert Bandura, proposed reciprocal determinism as a leading factor in motivation.[13] Individuals act as

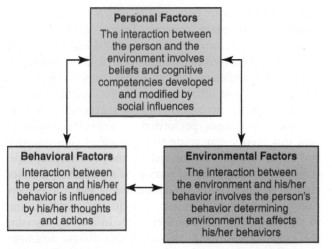

Figure 1-2 Social cognitive theory. (Redrawn from Kosling A, Heppner C, Elliott S: Motivation-project, wikispaces.com. Available at: http://motivation-project.wikispaces.com/Socio-cognitive+Theories+of+Motivation. Accessed December 5, 2014.)

contributors to their own motivation, behavior, and development. In addition, the environment interacts with the individual's behavior and characteristics in order to produce engagement or disengagement in an activity. Simply stated, human development is a back-and-forth interaction between the individual (his or her interpretation and retention of specific information), his or her behaviors, and the environment (Figure 1-2).

In addition, Bandura suggested that self-efficacy, which is the belief that a particular action is possible and can be accomplished, along with the ability to self-regulate, was the primary mediator in producing a change in behavior. He advocated that self-efficacy was a good predictor of intention. Self-efficacy and the mediating effect of cognition are seen as a circular process by which an increase in self-efficacy in turn produces success, thereby contributing to an increase in self-efficacy and the thought that one can indeed be triumphant in his or her actions. In turn, failures undermine self-efficacy, especially if failure occurs before one has developed a strong sense of self-efficacy. For example, a person who has successfully rehabilitated from an injury in the past will have the same belief that, if injured, he or she will be able to successfully recover from that injury and return to his or her accustomed activities. The more experience that one has in successfully overcoming the obstacles (i.e., multiple successes within the same area, in the example, injury recovery), the more one will believe that he or she has the "tools" with which to cope with other challenges to come. Bandura theorized that the best way to create a strong sense of efficacy was through mastery, whereby successes served as a base for development of the individual's personal efficacy. It is in this way that further mastery will promote repeat performances and improve adherence to physical activity, exercise, and rehabilitation.[14]

Self-determination Theory: An Empirical Framework for Understanding Health Behavior Change

Self-determination theory (SDT)[11] is a broad psychological theory of motivation particularly suited to understanding health behavior.[15] One of its basic tenets is that human motivation varies in the extent to which it is *autonomous* (i.e., when an individual engages in a behavior with a full sense of volition and choice) or *controlled* (i.e., when an individual engages in a behavior while experiencing internal or external pressure) along a continuum. *Identified regulation* (i.e., engaging in an activity because it is perceived as personally important and useful), *integrated regulation* (i.e., engaging in an activity because it is perceived as coherent with his or her values and identity), and *intrinsic motivation* (i.e., engaging in an activity because of the inherent satisfaction it conveys) represent increasingly autonomous forms of motivation. In contrast, *introjected regulation* (i.e., engaging in an activity to avoid negative emotions, such as anxiety or guilt) and *external regulation* (i.e., engaging in an activity to obtain a tangible reward, to avoid a punishment, or to comply with an external authority) represent increasingly controlled forms of motivation. In addition to autonomous and controlled forms of motivation, SDT also considers *amotivation* (i.e., individuals see no relationship between behavior and outcomes), which represents the absence of motivation.[11]

While the differentiation between autonomous versus controlled motivation is central to SDT, *perceived competence* (i.e., individuals' feeling of efficacy with respect to the behavior) is an important variable of the theory presumed to facilitate autonomous motivation.[11] Furthermore, SDT suggests that the social context—in particular the degree of autonomy support provided by health care supervisors (i.e., active listening, collaboration, respect, and thorough support)—may improve patients' autonomous motivation, perceived competence, and health-relevant behaviors.[16] Research has shown that perceived *autonomy support*, *autonomous forms of motivation*, and *perceived competence* are related to positive health outcomes,[15] such as a reduction in BMI[17] and an increase in physical activity among obese or overweight patients.[17,18] In a study[19] evaluating the effect of a motivational interview (MI)-based intervention as an addition to a standard weight loss program on physical activity practice in obese adolescents over a 6-month period, the standard weight loss group with MI intervention had a greater BMI decrease and a greater physical activity practice increase over time. This group also reported greater autonomy support from medical staff at the end of the program, greater increase in integrated and identified regulations, and a decrease in amotivation. The determination was made that MI is an efficient counseling method as an addition to a standard weight loss program to promote physical activity in the context of pediatric obesity.[19]

A subtheory within the SDT is *cognitive evaluation theory* (CET), which, simply put, means that people engage in activities to satisfy certain inherent needs as well as to gain intrinsic rewards and satisfaction. CET also proposes that if an individual who was previously intrinsically motivated to meet certain psychological needs but was then given extrinsic rewards for their behavior, by the very nature of the process (i.e., through cognitive rethinking), the individual would lose his or her "locus of causality" and move to being more extrinsically motivated.[20,21] Events or actions that occur and are affected by feedback, communication, and rewards and that elicit a sense of competence during the action will serve to enhance intrinsic motivation for those events or actions.[21] In this way, external sources may serve to either increase or decrease intrinsic motivation for action.

SDT suggests that humans have psychological needs for competence, relatedness, and autonomy that must be satisfied in a way that fosters immediate well-being and strengthens inner resources contributing to subsequent resilience. *Competence* pertains to the mastery and a need to control desirable outcomes. In this sense it is related to self-efficacy or the confidence in one's ability to achieve a certain outcome.[13] Goal setting and action planning are avenues that can serve to increase feelings of competence.

Relatedness refers to the universal need to feel connected to and experience caring from others. It is the need to be understood by important others in our lives.[22] Feelings of relatedness can influence motivation if one does not feel as if he or she is heard or if there is conflict within a social setting. For example, relatedness and thus motivation are enhanced via the empathetic listening of clinicians and during social interactions, such as during exercise group sessions.[22]

Autonomy or independence is the universal urge to act in harmony with and to be in control of one's own life. As clinicians it is essential not to impose one's thoughts or ideas but rather to incorporate clients/patients into important goals and decisions regarding their lives. Vansteenkiste and Ryan have noted that if these needs are not satisfied, subsequent feelings of frustration will heighten vulnerabilities and trigger defense mechanisms.[23]

Health Belief and Health Promotion Models: Theories of Reasoned Action and Planned Behavior

The health belief model includes the motivational, attitudinal, and self-efficacy components of various theories. The *theory of reasoned action* (TRA) and *theory of planned behavior* (TPB) as developed by Ajzen and Fishbein[20] and Ajzen[21] take into account the individual's attitude and social norms as well as the individual's perceived control as accurate predictors of behavioral intentions. TRA is most successful when applied to behaviors that are under an individual's voluntary control. If behaviors are not fully under voluntary control, even though individuals may be highly motivated by their own attitudes and subjective norms, they may not actually perform the behavior due to intervening environmental conditions. The TPB was developed to predict behaviors in which individuals have incomplete voluntary control. Taking self-esteem and self-efficacy into consideration, the TPB expands on the concept of perceived behavioral control. *Perceived behavioral control* indicates that an individual's motivation is influenced by how difficult the behaviors are perceived to be, as well as the perception of how successfully the individual can (or cannot) perform the activity. It is easy to see how this theory may relate to the concept of motivation and adherence to physical activity and/or exercise, especially in the rehabilitation setting. If a patient's perceived control or self-efficacy or self-esteem is low, the perception and belief that he or she can influence own behaviors in a positive manner is undermined. In a study assessing risk behavior following coronary heart disease diagnosis, planned behavior was found to be the main factor in predicting self-reported exercise and observed fitness levels.[24] When exercise intention and behavior were assessed in a sample of 225 older women aged 65 years and older, significant predictors of exercise intention were behavioral beliefs, normative beliefs, and perceived control beliefs.[25] In other words these women were more likely to exercise if they perceived more positive than negative consequences of performing the behavior (i.e., behavior beliefs), if they believed that people close or important to them approved versus disapproved of their behavior (i.e., normative beliefs), and, lastly, if they believed the difficulty of the task was manageable by them (i.e., perceived control belief).[25]

Humanistic Theory: Maslow's Hierarchy of Needs

This theory, as proposed by Abraham Maslow,[9] is one of the most popular theories of motivation. According to the theory, humans are driven to achieve their maximum potential and will always do so unless obstacles are placed in their way. This theory states that specific needs must be met in order to achieve ones' potential, which Maslow termed *self-actualization*, or a complete understanding of oneself and those around us. In essence, self-actualization includes focusing on problems, incorporating a continuous appreciation for life, concern about personal growth, and the ability to have peak and meaningful experiences. Needless to say, there are few, if any, individuals who have reached this level. Illustrated is Maslow's pyramid of needs (Figure 1-3).[26]

According to Maslow the obstacles put in our paths are reflective of basic needs, such as hunger, thirst, financial problems, safety, and time constraints, essentially anything that detracts from our pursuit of maximum growth. In this theory it is not possible to focus on the higher levels without first obtaining some mastery of the lower levels. Indeed, how can one concentrate on transcendence and actualization if basic needs for food, comfort, sleep, and safety are unmet? In the same vein, one can ask the question: How can one focus on the maintenance or improvement of one's health through physical activity and exercise if basic needs go unfulfilled?

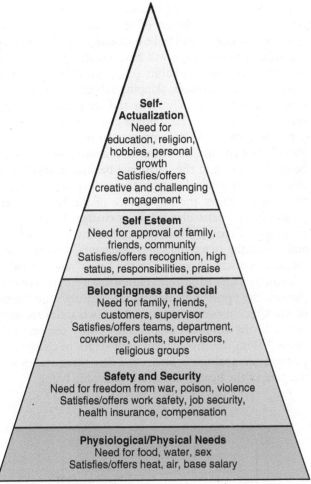

Figure 1-3 Maslow's hierarchy of needs. (Data from Maslow A: *Motivation and personality*, ed 2, New York, 1970, Harper.)

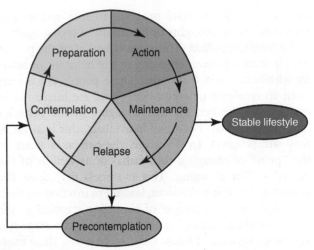

Figure 1-4 Transtheoretical model. (Redrawn from Donovan D, McDowell I, Hunter D, editors: *AFMC Primer on population health*, The Association of Faculties of Medicine of Canada. Available at: http://phprimer.afmc.ca/. Accessed December 5, 2014.)

Multidimensional Model: Transtheoretical Model and Stages of Change

The transtheoretical model (TTM) was first introduced by Prochaska and DiClemente[27] as a theoretical model of behavior change related to smoking cessation. This model has since been used for developing effective interventions to promote health behavior change across a variety of settings and individuals of varying ages. The TTM is an integrative model of behavioral change that incorporates a decisional balance, temptation, and self-efficacy scales.[27-30] The model describes stages of change, including precontemplation, contemplation, preparation, action, maintenance, and relapse (Figure 1-4; Table 1-1).

Precontemplation Stage. The hallmark of this stage is the person's lack of intention to take action. Individuals will have a variety of reasons for not being engaged in an activity. These reasons range from being uninformed or underinformed about the benefits of participation to having attempted the behavior previously and not being successful. The latter may often prove to be demoralizing to the individual attempting the behavioral change. For example, an obese patient may have tried unsuccessfully

TABLE **1-1**

Stages of Change Model

Stage	Characteristics
Precon-templation	Identified with individuals who do not intend to take action regarding the specific behavior (e.g., "I don't exercise, and I don't intend to start.")
Contemplation	Identified with individuals who intend to change their behavior within the next 6 months (e.g., "I don't exercise, but I'm thinking about starting.")
Preparation	Identified with individuals who intend to take action in the immediate future (e.g., "I exercise once in a while but not regularly.")
Action	Identified with individuals who have made specific and explicit changes in their behaviors and lifestyle within the past 6 months (e.g., "I exercise regularly and have done so for the past 6 months.")
Maintenance	Identified with individuals who are actively working to prevent relapse into previous behaviors and habits (e.g., "I exercise regularly and have done so for longer than 6 months.")
Relapse	There is a resumption of old behaviors (e.g., "fall from grace"): • Evaluate trigger for relapse • Reassess motivation and barriers • Plan stronger coping strategies

to engage in an exercise program to lose weight and therefore has no thoughts or intentions of trying again.

Contemplation Stage. This stage is typical of the person who is thinking about engaging in the behavior or activity within the next 6 months. These people are usually open to receiving new knowledge and are interested in listening to the benefits that engaging in the behavior might accomplish. For some individuals, this is as far as they will progress. In this stage, the person is aware of the "pros" of changing their behavior as well as of the "cons" of not changing. This awareness may cause the person to become ambivalent, leading to inaction on their part, and there is a danger of becoming stagnant in the "information gathering" mode. Patients in this stage will say things such as, "I know I should be doing these exercises, but I don't have the _____ (e.g., time, money, equipment)."

Preparation Stage. Individuals in this stage are intending to take action within the immediate future (i.e., within 30 days) and are typified by both intentional and behavioral components. These individuals have taken some concrete action toward the behavior change. In essence, they have a plan of action that they have begun to implement. For example, they may have made an appointment with the clinician, or they have bought appropriate workout shoes.

Action Stage. Individuals are actively engaged in the behaviors and/or lifestyle changes that will promote improved health. Individuals within this stage are encouraged and taught relapse prevention strategies because the changes they have made are considered new and therefore tenuous. In this stage, relapse prevention is critical and there are criteria that have been established that qualify the change in behavior as sufficient for reducing the risk of disease. These strategies include making sure the individual is aware of occasional "slips" in commitment to routine. The person needs to be made aware that missing an occasional workout session or rehabilitation appointment does not doom one to failure or that "cheating" on diet does not mean that one cannot get back on task. Shifting the focus from failure to successes (e.g., "You did it for 6 days; what made that work?") promotes problem solving and offers encouragement.

Maintenance Stage. Engagement in the behavioral change for more than 6 months will classify individuals in this stage. Prevention against boredom and changing focus is essential during this stage. This can be accomplished through the establishment of creative, new supporting behaviors. Supportive behaviors include the continual addressing of barriers as they arise, reformulation of the rules of their lives as related to the behavior change, and acquisition of new skills (e.g., problem-solving and coping mechanisms) to deal with life and avoid relapses. Anticipating situations in which a relapse could occur and preparing coping strategies in advance should be emphasized to individuals who are in this stage.

Being patient with themselves and recognizing that it often takes a while to let go of old behavior patterns and practice new ones needs to be encouraged and reinforced. Individuals in this stage will have recurring thoughts of returning to their old habits (e.g., not exercising, making poor dietary choices, skipping rehabilitation appointments), but they usually resist the temptation and stay on track because they have noted progress. As mentioned previously, the TTM encompasses an integrative schema for behavior change, including an examination of cost and benefits inherent in the decisional balance model. Using this model, individuals weigh the relative importance of the "cons" against the importance of the "pros" of engaging in any particular behavior change. In examining the stages of change in relation to healthy (e.g., exercise) and unhealthy (e.g., smoking) behaviors, Velicer et al.[31] found a predictable pattern in the "pros" and "cons" in relation to stages of change (Figure 1-5).[32] In precontemplation, the "pros" of smoking far outweigh the "cons" of smoking. In contemplation, these two scales are more equal. In the advanced stages, the "cons" outweigh the "pros." With healthy behavior and stages of change, the patterns are analogous across the first three stages with the pros of the healthy behavior remaining high.

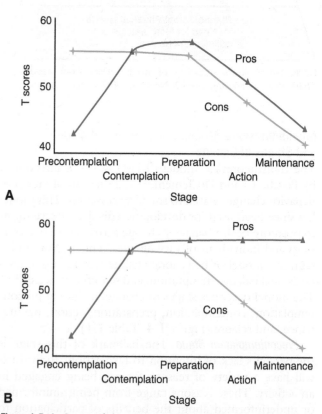

Figure 1-5 A, Stages of change and smoking. **B,** Stages of change and exercise. (From Velicer WF, Prochaska JO, Fava JL, et al: Using the transtheoretical model for population-based approaches to health promotion and disease prevention, *Homeostasis in Health and Disease* 40:174-195, 2000.)

Relapse Stage. Relapse is considered an important stage in the change process and commonly occurs during lifestyle changes. Relapse should be used as an opportunity to learn about sustaining maintenance of the behavior change over time. Clinicians can help to encourage their clients/patients by explaining that even though a relapse has occurred, the patient has learned something new about oneself and about the process of changing or maintaining the changed behavior.[33] For example, patients who have started an exercise program recognize that if they do not do it at a set time each day, they may not get it done at all. Patients with diabetes may learn that they can be successful in adhering to their diet if they order from a menu rather than going to an all-you-can-eat buffet. Discouragement over occasional "slips" may halt the change process and result in the patient giving up. However, most patients find themselves "recycling" through the stages of change several times before the change becomes truly established.[33]

Focusing on the successful part of the plan (e.g., "You did it for 6 days; what made that work?") shifts the focus from failure, promotes problem solving, offers encouragement, and allows the client/patient to get back on the "proverbial horse." The goal is to offer support and help clients/patients to renew and reengage their efforts in the change process. They should be left with a sense of realistic goals to prevent discouragement, and their positive steps toward behavior change should be acknowledged.[34]

Advocates of using the stage of change model have cited its advantages as a model to predict and promote healthy behavior. One advantage of using this model is that it is able to match the stage that each individual is in with the proper intervention. For instance, if a person has purchased a pair of gym shoes and has joined the local gym, it can be stated according to the stage of change model that the individual is in the preparation stage. Interventions can then be focused on providing positive support and encouragement in facilitating the individual to move into the action stage. Another advantage of this model is that it helps the health and exercise professional to identify individuals who are indeed ready to change their behavior, thereby saving time and resources that could be better used elsewhere. Both the clinician and the patient should anticipate recycling *through the stages.* Many patients will recycle several times through the stages before achieving long-term maintenance as progression through the stages is circular rather than linear. Professionals, patients, and programs that expect people to progress linearly through the stages of change are likely to gather disappointing results. Clinicians should, as mentioned previously, be prepared to help their clients/patient by including relapse prevention as part of the treatment, anticipate the probability of recycling for patients, and try to minimize guilt and patient shame over recycling through the various stages.[35]

In a study examining barriers to physical activity by general practitioners and practice nurses, results indicated that general practitioners in the action or maintenance stage of behavioral change were 3 times more likely to regularly promote the same behavior in their patients than those in other stages.[9] In a critical review of the literature examining activity promotion interventions in a variety of populations based on the TTM, 26 studies using written material, counseling, or both were found.[36] Based on the review the authors found some evidence of short-term benefit in terms of activity levels or stage of activity change. Longer term effects were harder to achieve and maintain. In 73% of the short-term studies, a positive effect of TTM-based interventions over control conditions was seen. This is in contrast to longer term studies that showed only a 29% increase or positive effect of TTM-based interventions over the control. The numbers are encouraging, however, as the review seems to suggest that even a brief intervention using the TTM will have an effect on behavior change and should be encouraged in other settings and studies. In a study assessing motivational readiness to change, aerobic capacity and reported participation in leisure activities were higher for men and women in the stages of contemplation, preparation, action, and maintenance. Additionally, men in the contemplation stage had a higher BMI and a greater percentage of body fat compared with men in the maintenance and action stages. Likewise, men who were randomized to an exercise intervention group and who were initially in the contemplation and preparation stages had a 14% and 15% increase, respectively, in aerobic capacity at follow-up, whereas men in the action and maintenance stages had a 5% increase in aerobic capacity. For women, those in the contemplation, preparation and action stages had a 16%, 14% and 10% increase, respectively, in aerobic capacity. This study also examined the baseline stage of motivational readiness for exercise and found that over a 9-month intervention period, there were no differences in baseline stages of motivational readiness for exercise for the subjects reporting an increase in activity. Of the men in this study who participated in the exercise intervention and met their exercise goals, 54% were in the contemplation stage, 69% were in the preparation stage, and 68% were in the action and maintenance stages. For women, 35% initially in the contemplation stage met their intervention goals, whereas 67% and 24% who were initially classified in the preparation and action stages met their goals. This surprising finding revealed that adherence did not differ by baseline exercise motivational readiness stage as was often found in other studies.[37] The most reliably predicted stage of change for exercise were maintenance (90.2%), precontemplation (73.8%), and contemplation (70.8) stages in a study assessing factors influencing exercise behavior in adults with physical disabilities.[36] As previously mentioned, the primary role of clinicians in the maintenance stage is to help to prevent the relapse in their clients. This can be done by helping clients to reengage in their efforts in the change process by focusing on successes and promoting realistic goal setting to prevent discouragement and to help them to continue to uphold their positive steps toward the changed behavior. Clinicians attempting to help clients who are in the precontemplation stage should be empathetic while attempting to engage their clients in questions that require thoughtful insight into the behavior requiring change. Instilling hope and the identification of incongruities between goals and statements can play a large part in inducing change in individuals in this stage. For individuals in the contemplation stage, clinicians should attempt to develop and maintain a positive relationship with their patients. This can come in the form of helping the individuals personalize risk factors while posing questions that provoke thoughts about the risk factors and potentially negative outcomes if they indeed do not change their behavior.

Multidimensional Model: Socioecological Model

The socioecological model serves as a framework for understanding the multiple levels that influence behavior. Ecological models assume not only that multiple levels of influence exist but also that these levels are interactive and reinforcing. These models vary from individual behavioral and cognitive models that do not offer a thorough explanation of how and why behavioral change occurs.[38] What the socioecological model offers is a consideration of the far reaching influences on behavior that consists of both internal and external factors ranging on an individual level to a more global or societal level and the interaction of each upon one another (Figure 1-6).

> Ecological models assume not only that multiple levels of influence exist but also that these levels are interactive and reinforcing.

There are several assumptions made by the socioecological model. The first is that behavior is influenced by a multitude of factors at several levels, including biological, individual, interpersonal, community, environmental, policy, and global. The second assumption revolves around the understanding that the human environment is complex, meaning that we do not pay attention to only the physical or actual environment but also to the social attributes and the perceived qualities of the environment.[39] A third assumption of this model is that those who are active participants within the environment are, like the environment, complex and should be observed on multiple levels from the individual to small groups to larger organizations and the broader population.[40] The key of this assumption is that the focus should not be on any one element but on a coordinated effort to address multiple elements. A fourth assumption of the socioecological model is that there are factors in any individual's environment that can encourage or encumber participation in healthy behaviors. This simply means that once a person makes a choice, it is independently influenced more or

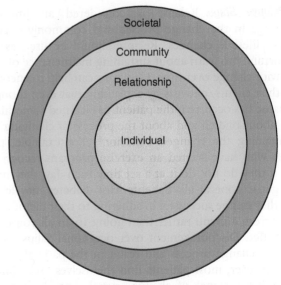

Figure 1-6 Socioecological model. (Redrawn from CDC: *The social-ecological model: a framework for prevention*, Centers for Disease Control and Prevention, National Center for Injury Prevention and Control, Division of Violence Prevention. Available at: http://www.cdc.gov/violenceprevention/overview/social-ecologicalmodel.html. Accessed December 5, 2014.)

less, positively or negatively, by the social and environmental situation in which the person lives and works.[39]

A fifth assumption is that behavioral responses will vary from one person to the next even when viewed within a similar environmental context. Given two people within similar circumstance, the influence of familial norms, culture context, and emphasis as well as the influence of the physical environment (e.g., perceived safety, access) will play a role in whether either person engages in a behavior change.

The last assumption reflects that behavior as well as the environment is dynamic and fluid. Behavioral choices will be made in response to the ever changing environment. To put it another way, because the environment is not stable, behavioral choices will not always be the same; therefore flexibility on the individual's part is required.

THE PROFESSIONAL'S ROLE IN PHYSICAL ACTIVITY AND EXERCISE ADHERENCE

It is important to discuss the health care professional's role in motivating individuals to participate in physical activity and exercise. The importance of this role is particularly significant to the older adult population. In one study examining older adults who were frail and obese, lifestyle interventions associated with weight loss improved insulin sensitivity and other cardiac and metabolic risk factors, but continued improvement in insulin sensitivity was only achieved when exercise training was added to weight loss.[41] A study done by Schutzer and Graves[42] showed that individuals who were older or chronically ill saw their physician at least once a year and preferred to receive advice about exercise from their physician or personal health care provider. Forty percent of older individuals on Medicare surveyed revealed participation in an exercise program was the result of their physician's advice.[43] In a study assessing long-term exercise adherence after rehabilitation for chronic low back pain, results revealed that physicians' and physical therapists' conveyance of the patient's capacity to perform the recommended exercises in spite of pain symptoms went a long way in reinforcing self-efficacy in the patient's ability to complete the exercises.[8] In assessing barriers to physical activity promotion for general practitioners and nurses, McKenna et al.[44] found that general practitioners in the action or maintenance stage of changing their own physical activity level were 3 times more likely to regularly promote the same behavior in their patients. It is in this way that professionals who exercise on a regular basis and "practice what they preach" will transfer these same beliefs, attitudes, behaviors, and action to their patients. In a study examining socioenvironmental exercise preferences among older adults,[45] results suggest that the perception of the exercise instructor as qualified, advice of the medical doctor to begin exercising, and evaluation by a health professional to monitor the physical effects of exercise were rated as most important in 320 adults 74 to 85 years of age living independently within the community. In addition, the health professional's ability to evaluate and demonstrate appropriate exercises and their ability to evaluate and monitor the physical effects of exercise were rated as very important. The latter finding is especially relevant to clinicians who treat older adults and who would like to encourage them to be active participants in their rehabilitation programs.

Dorflinger et al.[46] found that patients benefited from a biopsychosocial and patient-centered approach in the care of their low back pain. They found that patients were more likely to fully disclose when providers responded in an empathetic way. Sluijs et al.[47] found a relationship between positive feedback given to the patients by their physical therapists and noncompliance. It was inferred that if physical therapists did not give positive feedback to their patients, compliance to the rehabilitation program was decreased. The question remains, however, whether it was the positive feedback that facilitated compliance or compliance that facilitated the physical therapist to give positive feedback. It is presumed that it would be beneficial to give positive feedback so as to increase the likelihood that adherence to the rehabilitation program was obtained. Exercise professionals have the most influence over program factors when designing a plan for increasing client retention. Remembering to keep clients involved in designing their exercise programs is necessary because it will increase feelings of self-efficacy and greatly affect choice of exercise.

The author of a physical therapy blog quoted Albert Einstein stating "the definition of insanity is doing the same thing over and over and expecting different results." He also implied that even with this sage saying, clinicians continue to follow the same routine of creating patient exercise programs with diagrams and pictures of varying quality and expect them to go home and complete them without ensuring the exercises are understood and done correctly. He points out that practitioners do not change the routine when the patient does not comply with their directives. "We know that the majority of our patients aren't doing their exercises at home, and we aren't implementing strategies that affect change." He hypothesized that the reason clinicians do not do anything was because they believed that they did not have the capability to improve their patients' adherence. In turn, clinicians' low self-efficacy and perception of barriers translated into their patients having low self-efficacy and perceived barriers.[48]

Adherence

Adherence is defined by the World Health Organization (WHO) as the extent to which a person's behavior—taking medication, following a diet, participating in an exercise regimen, and/or executing lifestyle changes—corresponds to the recommendations of a health care provider.[49] *Exercise adherence* is the extent to which a patient acts in accordance with the advised interval, exercise dose, and exercise dosing regimen. The unit of measure for adherence is performed exercise doses per defined period of time reported as a proportion of prescribed exercise doses undergone at the prescribed time interval. *Exercise persistence* is the accumulation of time from initiation to discontinuation of therapy, measured by time metric (e.g., number of weeks or months to discontinuation). According to the WHO, adherence is simultaneously influenced by several factors, such as patient-related factors, social and economic factors, factors related to the health care team or system, condition-related factors, and therapy-related factors.[49]

Adherence can be assessed by subjective or objective methods or both. The subjective methods include physical activity questionnaires and diaries filled in by patients. Objective methods include the recording of data from pedometers, accelerometers, pulsometers (heart rate monitoring), and electrocardiogram (ECG) telemonitoring.[50]

FACTORS ASSOCIATED WITH MOTIVATION AND ADHERENCE TO PHYSICAL ACTIVITY, EXERCISE, AND REHABILITATION

As the reader has probably concluded, motivation and how it relates to adherence to physical activity and exercise is not an easy concept to explain. There are factors that have been identified and shown to be associated with increased or decreased motivation and adherence to physical activity, exercise, and rehabilitation. Forkan et al.[51] found that exercise adherence following discharge from a physical therapy program was poor among older adults. It was also concluded that barriers, not motivators, were predictors of adherence across all factors associated with motivation and adherence to activity and exercise (Table 1-2).

Personal Factors

Characteristics that are considered inherent to the individual's personality fall into the category of personal factors that influence motivation and adherence. According to Whaley and Schrider,[52] how people view themselves from past experiences to current reality will greatly influence their choice for physical activity. A person's sense of self-perception plays a major role in whether one will start an exercise program. So even if, for medical reasons, one has been encouraged to exercise, the person's own self-perception may impede this from happening. These characteristics are referred to as being stable and representative dispositions of an individual's persona. These include concepts such as self-motivation, biomedical status, education, socioeconomic status (SES), age, ethnicity, and gender.

Various studies have examined these concepts and how they relate to adherence and compliance in a variety of populations and as they relate to physical activity or exercise and rehabilitation adherence. The sport psychology literature covers other personal concepts, such as pain tolerance, task and ego involvement, and trait anxiety, as they influence rehabilitation adherence in the athletic population.

Personal Factors that Influence Motivation and Adherence

- Self-motivation
- Biomedical status
- Socioeconomic status
- Age
- Ethnicity
- Gender
- Marital status
- Education
- Smoking status

Self-Motivation

Self-motivation is the ability to persist in behaviors in spite of situational or environmental reinforcements[53] and has been found to be most consistently correlated with

TABLE **1-2**

Characteristics Associated with Motivation and Adherence to Physical Activity, Exercise, and Rehabilitation

Factors	Description
Personal factors	Considered inherent individual's personality; stable and representative of the individual's persona
Self-motivation	Ability to persist in behaviors despite situational or environmental reinforcements
Biomedical status	Poorer health tends to lead to decreased adherence
Socioeconomic status	The individual's income bracket tends to influence the ability to access medical care as well as exercise equipment and venues
Age	In various studies, older individuals tend to adhere to exercise programs more than younger individuals
Ethnicity	Caucasians tend to participate in more physical activities than other racial or ethnic groups
Gender	Males tend to adhere to cardiac rehabilitation programs more than females; men report greater levels of total and vigorous activity than women
Marital status	Singles tend to have lower rates of adherence to physical activity and exercise than married couples
Education	Individuals with higher levels of education adhere to exercise programs more than those who are uneducated
Smoking status	Cigarette smokers tend to show less adherence to exercise programs
Situational and environmental factors	Social and physical environment in which the individual interacts will influence the positive or negative perception of the individual
Cognitive factors	What a person thinks about a situation or action influences the individual's emotional and behavioral responses
Behavioral factors	These factors are influenced by cognitive appraisal and by the person's belief that he or she can or cannot change his or her behavior

adherence to rehabilitation in athletes who have sustained a sport injury.[54,55] It stands to reason that individuals who are highly self-motivated will be more inclined to adhere to self-monitored exercise programs longer than those who are not as highly motivated. This being the case, increasing self-motivation would be advantageous for promoting adherence to various rehabilitation programs. Clinicians can help to improve one's ability to be self-motivated by assisting the person in building a history of success. For example, starting an individual with a task or exercise that is easily accomplished by the person and gradually increasing the level of difficulty will promote confidence and thereby inspire continued motivation to reach a particular goal. Allowing the individual to focus on successes rather than failures that may prevent the person from trying again is beneficial. To promote adherence to a self-pain management approach from a biopsychosocial perspective as well as a patient-centered approach has been successful.[46]

Biomedical Status

When a panel of geriatric exercise experts were asked to assess personal characteristics in regards to exercise behavior in older adults, biomedical status was rated as the most important factor in determining whether the older adult would initiate and adhere to exercise.[56] In other words, the determination of exercise participation is based on whether one perceives himself or herself to be in good health or not. This is important because health care providers can offer physical screens that would serve to reassure the individual that it is indeed safe and beneficial to exercise. This same panel also found that past exercise history and socioeconomic level were important for adherence in this population. Incorporating the individual's past exercise history will help identify strategies that will optimize future exercise behavior. This includes inquiring about what activities the individual liked or disliked in addition to soliciting information about perceived and real barriers and rewards.[43]

Questions to Ask to Determine Likelihood of Compliance with Exercise or Rehabilitation Programs

- Have you exercised or participated in a rehabilitation program in the past?
- What are some barriers that might prevent you from engaging in exercise and rehabilitation?
- What are some things that might help you to "stick" with the program?
- When you exercise, do you exercise alone or with others?
- Do you prefer to exercise alone or with others?
- What kind of activities and exercise do you like to do?
- What are your goals for participating in an exercise and rehabilitation program?

Socioeconomic Status

Interestingly, SES was found to be extremely relevant in the older population in promoting exercise adherence. As the income levels of individuals decrease or were fixed, the ability to pay for exercise advice, equipment, and an exercise facility became limited. For individuals who can no longer afford these expenses, adherence tended to decrease. Therefore it is essential for the health care provider to seek out information regarding income in order to best suit the needs of their clients and to increase the probability of adherence to an exercise and/or rehabilitation program.

Age

Age is another personal factor that has been found to be correlated with adherence to exercise and rehabilitation. In a group of church-going African Americans, older individuals tended to adhere to an exercise program more than younger individuals participating in an exercise intervention.[57] The researchers did note in this study that the exercise intervention was timed and coordinated to accommodate the schedules and needs of the older subjects, thereby potentially biasing the results. In a study assessing training levels and adherence in coronary heart disease patients between the ages of 30 and 67 years, it was found that older patients were more likely to sustain an exercise attendance schedule necessary to recoup therapeutic benefits.[58] In yet another study, participation and adherence to a physical activity program decreased in older individuals.[59] This decrease in participation might be attributed to an assortment of reasons, including poor health, lack of time, fear, and unsafe environment. In a more recent study, middle-aged women (40 to 62 years of age) stated that the most common barrier interfering with adherence to regular exercise was attributable to the demands inherently placed on them at this life stage, meaning demands at home and with others that led to lack of time to engage in regular exercise and menopausal symptoms associated with this life stage.[60]

Ethnicity

It has been found in the literature that Caucasians participate in more physical activities than other racial and ethnic groups regardless of age.[61] In a sample of African Americans, a 27% attendance rate to a church-based exercise program was noted, providing some support for the notion that minorities tend to adhere less to physical activity and exercise programs. In a study examining adherence to the Dietary Approaches to Stop Hypertension (DASH) diet, it was found that African Americans were less likely to be adherent to the dietary eating plan than Caucasians.[62] In a pilot study assessing irrational health beliefs as a predictor to cardiac rehabilitation adherence, it was found that adherence was lower among African Americans than Caucasians.[63]

Gender

Men have been found to be more engaged and adherent to physical activity or exercise and cardiac phase II rehabilitation programs than women.[64] In a study examining the effects of a 6-month home physical activity program on adherence, it was found that retention rates and adherence were higher for men than women.[65] In assessing the effect of tailored interventions on exercise adherence, Keele-Smith and Leon[61] found women to be more inactive than men and that more men than women were reported to have engaged in vigorous physical activity. When demographic and other variables were examined, assessing participation in American College of Sports Medicine and Center for Disease Control exercise guidelines in a cohort of adults 18 years and older, women were less likely to meet the guidelines as recommended by these groups. In addition, men reported greater levels of total and vigorous activity with women reporting engagement in low to moderate activities.[66] In a sample of college students, 92% of males versus 63% of females reported engaging in regular exercise.[67]

Marital Status

Another personal factor that may play an important part in determining level of motivation for physical activity or exercise and rehabilitation participation is marital status; those who were unmarried tended to have lower adherence,[61] which may be directly related to social support, which will be discussed later. A meta-analysis of the general medical literature concluded that adherence to medical recommendations was higher in married patients.[68]

Education and Smoking Status

Other personal factors include education, in which individuals who were not as educated adhered less to health-related programs,[56,61] and smoking status, in which cigarette smokers tended to be less committed to making healthy lifestyle changes[45] and were less able to maintain a consistent exercise program.[58]

Situational or Environmental Factors

Situational factors are representative of the social and physical environment in which the individual interacts. Therefore the presence of other people, including the health care or exercise specialist and other patients or clients, will influence whether the individual has a positive or negative perception and experience with physical activity, exercise, or rehabilitation.[69] Seguin et al.[69] emphasized that there was a significant relationship in a client/patient's exercise adherence with his or her personal trainer's leadership style. It was found that exercise leaders who were perceived to have a high mastery of exercise favorably influenced client exercise adherence. Thus exercise professionals may be esteemed role models for their clients.

Situationally, convenience of location of exercise facilities and convenience of exercise opportunities (e.g., research solicitations) will often facilitate adherence to exercise programs. In addition, the quality of the patient/client–practitioner interaction will either help or deter the quality of the participation on the individual's part.

Environmentally, the characteristics of the actual exercise or rehabilitation setting and time of day also are important to individuals and can, in part, determine adherence. Individuals have a preferred time of day and setting in which they will feel the most comfortable and be the most likely to follow through with established exercise and/or rehabilitation protocols. Therefore it is critical for the practitioner to establish an environment and situation to best suit the individual's need to best ensure adherence.

Cognitive Factors

What a person thinks about a situation or action will mediate emotional and behavioral responses to an event. If one perceives something to be out of one's control, then one will either not attempt to perform the behavior or will expect to fail in that behavior. This is especially relevant when trying to elicit changes in health behaviors. If individuals do not believe they will be successful in the tasks set forth by the exercise and physical activity guidelines, they may be more apt not to engage in the activity. It is in this sense that education is helpful in facilitating cognitive reappraisals and the belief that individuals can engage in behaviors conducive to positively affecting health.

Behavioral Factors

Whether individuals engage in behaviors is reflective, as stated previously, on the cognitive appraisal of the situational context. In rehabilitation, one's cognitive belief that he or she will not only be able to cope with the injury but also cope well will determine if he or she will exhibit behaviors conducive to recovery. Changing behaviors, especially health-related behavior, has proven to be difficult. Strategies in the form of behavioral modification (also known as behavioral interventions) are practiced in psychology and rehabilitation in order to encourage the desired change in individuals. For example, encouraging the individual to make a commitment in private by choosing and committing, and then later going public by announcing to others the decision to change is a powerful step toward behavior change. The public commitment is more powerful than the private decision. Another way to encourage behavior change is to have an individual sign a written contract. This contract is an agreement made between themselves and the clinician to engage in specific steps in order to reach mutually established goals.

BARRIERS ASSOCIATED WITH DECREASED MOTIVATION AND ADHERENCE, OR COMPLIANCE TO PHYSICAL ACTIVITY, EXERCISE, AND REHABILITATION

The factors discussed pertaining to motivation, adherence, and compliance to exercise and rehabilitation, although reflective of mainly theoretical manifestations of personality, situation, and cognition, do not adequately identify the perceived and real issue of individuals who are most at risk for health-related decline as a result of nonparticipation or inadequate participation. The following discussion will include an identification of barriers (Table 1-3), both perceived and real, and how health care providers and exercise specialists can help individuals overcome them.

Knowledge regarding patients' barriers for nonadherence and reasons for drop-out from cardiac rehabilitation programs may provide guidance for designing successful strategies to increase participation. The main barriers identified in a study examining adherence to exercise rehabilitation in patients with congestive heart failure ranged from patient-related (e.g., older age, low level of education, low SES, minority status, anxiety and depression, and lack of motivation, insight, and time) to

TABLE 1-3

Barriers Associated with Decreased Motivation and Adherence or Compliance to Physical Activity, Exercise, and Rehabilitation

Barrier	Overview
Environment	Includes physical obstacles, access to and cost of health clubs and rehabilitation centers, and climate
Health	Includes unhealthy behaviors, such as smoking, perception of poor health, and individuals suffering from chronic illness
Supervision and direction	Lack of supervision and guidance for exercise has been a deterrent in initiation of and compliance to exercise
Time	Lack of time for exercise; exercise programs taking too much time
Family	Family responsibilities and obligations may take priority over rehabilitation and exercise
Occupation	Responsibilities and obligations of work may take priority over rehabilitation and exercise

health care system or team barriers (e.g., lack of expertise, lack of referrals) and condition-related barriers (e.g., severity of symptoms, level of disability, rate of disease progression, impact of co-morbidities). This same study also cited therapy-related barriers, such as lack of exercise relevance and difficulty of incorporating exercise into the patients' daily life.[70] There were several barriers to adherence that were found in a systematic review by Jack et al.[71] In this review there was strong supporting evidence that poor treatment adherence to outpatient physical therapy was associated with low levels of physical activity at baseline, low in-treatment adherence with exercise, low self-efficacy, depression, anxiety, helplessness, poor social support or activity, greater perceived number of barriers to exercise, and increased pain levels during exercise. An exploration of many of these barriers and possible strategies to overcome them follows.

Environment

The physical environment can be a detriment to some individuals when deciding if they should commit to an exercise and/or rehabilitative program. This is true across the lifespan, from the young to the older persons who would be well advised to change their exercise behavior. In a sample of African American women (18 to 64 years of age) with physical disabilities, the cost of joining a fitness center, lack of transportation, and being afraid to leave their home were ranked 1 through 3, respectively, as barriers to exercise.[72] When examining ways to overcome exercise barriers in older adults, identified environmental barriers included physician advice, access to and cost of health clubs and rehabilitation centers, and climate.[73] As mentioned previously, if physicians did not inquire about diet and exercise, the perception that they were not important on the part of the patient was high. In addition, lack of follow-up to monitor progress or goal achievement and busy schedules on the part of the health care provider and/or exercise specialist will often promote nonadherence in individual patients.

When one considers access and cost, many individuals, especially those living in low income areas and the elderly, do not have the monetary funds to join an area gym. Although there are some areas that will provide free access to fitness and recreational equipment, individuals may not be able to afford the transportation to these facilities. Similarly, walking may not be an option because some patients may live in dangerous neighborhoods where crime is high.[42,74] Finding a safe environment for patients and clients to exercise should be a priority for the health care provider and other exercise specialists.[75] It has been shown that older adults who do not live in the vicinity of recreational facilities often do not participate in regular exercise and are more sedentary.[75] For individuals living in the northern climates, weather conditions may not be conducive to engaging regularly in outdoor activities.[42] In the same sense, individuals living in warmer climates may be impeded by high humidity and/or heat. In either case, extremes in the weather often will preclude individuals for up to 6 months from participating in a regular exercise routine.[73] In the rehabilitation environment, patients with physical disabilities often point to lack of adaptive space and/or accessible equipment, along with poor equipment maintenance, as barriers.[72] These individuals also revealed that they perceived fitness and recreational facilities to be unfriendly to individuals with physical disabilities.

Health

Unhealthy behaviors, such as smoking and leading a sedentary lifestyle, are contributors to both acute and chronic diseases in the general population. Abolishing or at the very least reducing these practices ideally should promote increased quality of life. Facilitating exercise and adherence to exercise programs is often encumbered by the individual's perception that poor health is limiting the ability to participate in exercise and rehabilitation programs. Older adults in particular will often cite poor health as the leading barrier to physical activity and exercise.[76] In a group of cardiac rehabilitation patients, gender and barrier efficacy were related to overcoming health barriers, such as fear of having another cardiac event, medication side effects, and angina or chest pain.[64] These investigators also found that men more than women tended to have higher barrier efficacy (i.e., they felt more capable of engaging the cardiac program without experiencing detrimental effects to their health). During the initiation and adherence stage of a study examining exercise behavior in older adults, biomedical status was implicated as the most important determinant of exercise adherence.[43] A panel of experts agreed that initiation and adherence to an exercise program in the older adult depended on their state of health.[56] When examining factors associated with physical activity participation in older adults in the population (≥ 65 years old), the most commonly reported barrier to increasing physical activity was health problems.[77] Sluijs et al.[47] reported in their review of the literature that characteristics associated with certain illnesses related to compliance: "When the illness causes more disabilities and handicaps and patients perceive the illness as very serious, they appear to be more compliant (with rehabilitation) than patients with less serious illness" (p. 772). They also reported that patients with chronic illnesses seemed to be less compliant than those with acute illnesses, suggesting that recovery from the illness is an incentive within itself to participate in the exercise regimen as dictated by their rehabilitation. In a group of middle-aged and older women participating in the Sedentary Women Exercise Adherence Trial (SWEAT), the most common reason stated for withdrawal from an exercise program was illness or injury.[78] Add to this, fear of injury or reinjury, and compliance to rehabilitation and other exercise programs decreases.[73]

Supervision and Direction

Individuals have reported that a lack of supervision and guidelines for exercise have been a deterrent in initiating and adhering to exercise. It is not unreasonable to think that those who have not had training in exercise prescription would want some assistance with the planning and implementation of an exercise program. This is especially relevant for some older adults and other individuals who may have significant health-related issues. It is also essential to monitor participants in any exercise program for excessive effort. If the activity is too intense for their comfort, they are more likely to drop out or sustain an injury. When examining exercise preferences in older adults, researchers found that those older individuals who had higher levels of reported pain were more likely to feel that their exercise should be monitored and evaluated by a qualified professional.[76] This finding is in alignment with other research that has reported a higher degree of noncompliance to exercise and rehabilitation in older individuals who have significant health problems and pain.[78] The literature supports the finding that adherence to exercise protocols is best established when the protocols are supervised. Morey et al.[79] conducted a study that investigated whether a supervised exercise program could predict adherence in the same group of individuals when transitioned over to a home-based program. They found that adherence to weekend home-based exercise as a preparation to transition to the home-based program during the supervised portion of the study was the strongest predictor of adherence to the home-based program. Of interest in this study was the fact that individuals who were assessed and determined to be adherers versus those determined to be nonadherers remained so throughout the study. It can then be surmised that adherence to exercise can be predicted at an early stage, say, for example, using the "stage of change model" of behavioral change.

Studies have indicated that marital status plays an important part in exercise preference and supervision. Cohen-Mansfield et al.[45] reported that unmarried participants rated supervision by an authority figure (i.e., providing advice, monitoring, and/or evaluation of the exercise program) to be highly important, suggesting that encouragement and direction were relevant for these individuals to initiate and adhere to the exercise program.

Time, Family, and Occupation

Time is often perceived as a barrier to engaging in physical activity, exercise, and rehabilitation. Cohen-Mansfield et al.[76] found that older individuals (74 to 85 years of age) preferred to exercise between 9 AM and 12 PM, with the oldest group preferring to exercise between 12 PM and

3 PM. Interestingly, these researchers also found that the group that had a preference for early exercise (between 9 AM and 12 PM) were healthier than the group that preferred exercise later in the day.[76] College-aged students regularly listed exercise taking too much time as a barrier.[67] Physical therapy patients also indicated that exercise in the form of rehabilitation required extra time that they did not have.[76] In a sample of Australian subjects (18 to 78 years of age), lack of time was cited as a barrier to exercise participation most frequently.[80]

For individuals with children and who work, child care and the responsibilities of the work environment may be prohibitive to incorporating exercise and physical activity into their daily or weekly routine. Accomplishment of work goals and tasks may be made a priority over participating in rehabilitation, physical activity, or exercise. If one is retired, other activities (such as volunteering and spending time with grandchildren) may supercede exercise or rehabilitation participation.[73,75]

As can be implied from these findings, rehabilitation and exercise specialists need to be flexible in scheduling patient/client appointments to increase the likelihood of these individuals participating in an exercise or rehabilitation program. In addition, physical therapy clinics, gyms, fitness centers, and other recreational environments should vary their hours of operation in order to accommodate individual's preferences and conflicts of other activities.

Psychological

As alluded to earlier, there are psychological factors that influence motivation to exercise and rehabilitation. Depression, anxiety, and helplessness have been found to significantly contribute to decreased adherence to rehabilitation.[71] A study examining adherence to exercise in older veterans found that participants with both depression and/or posttraumatic stress disorder (PTSD) had lower 1-month and 11-week exercise adherence rates compared with participants without these conditions. It was also found that veterans who were screened and found to have both depression and PTSD had the lowest rates of exercise adherence compared with those with only depression or those with neither PTSD nor depression.[81]

In another study looking at the effects of depression and anxiety on cardiac rehabilitation, it was found that individuals with the highest dropout rates also had higher depression and anxiety scores and lower quality of life.[82] It was also found that younger, female patients had higher dropout rates and that women had higher psychological distress, lower quality of life, and less distance walked than men.[82] In another study looking at the effects of depression and anxiety, improvement in adherence to medication, and health behaviors in acute depressed cardiac patients, it was found that improvement in depression was consistently and independently associated with superior self-reported adherence to medications and secondary

prevention behaviors across a 6-month span, whereas improvement in anxiety was not.[71] Another study by Zen et al.[83] found that among patients with heart disease, those with PTSD were more likely to report physical inactivity, medication nonadherence, and smoking.

OVERVIEW OF ADHERENCE TO REHABILITATION IN THE CLINICAL POPULATION

Rehabilitation specialists, such as physical therapists, occupational therapists, speech language pathologists, and athletic trainers, use exercise as one component of their intervention in order to effectively treat their patients. Having a thorough understanding of the pathology of the injury and physiological demands of the exercise is presumed. However, when confronted with the unique physical impairments and disabilities that the injury may cause, the psychological or motivational impact, although intuitively important to the success of the exercise program, is often ignored.

In rehabilitation, successful outcome is often linked to attending clinic appointments and compliance with therapist-developed exercise programs.[70,80,84,85] This, however, is not always the case. Brewer et al.[54] found that outcomes in rehabilitation after anterior cruciate ligament reconstruction were not mediated by adherence to rehabilitation. Even so, encouraging individuals to actively participate in rehabilitation is important to increase the probability of recovery from injury. In a position paper introduced by a study group of the Heart Failure Association of the European Society of Cardiology examining exercise training adherence in persons with heart failure, it was found that increasing adherence to exercise often led to positive health benefits.[86]

In a study examining perceived barriers and motivators to exercise in patients who were receiving hemodialysis, adherence to exercise among these patients was low, with 38% stating that in a typical week, exercise did not reach 15 minutes.[87] The results also suggested that it was not health-related impairments that stopped these individuals from exercising but lack of motivation and barriers (see Table 1-3).

In a sample of African American women with physical disabilities as rated by the Americans with Disabilities Act (ADA), adherence to regular physical activity was found to be directly related to the number of barriers that existed in the individual's life.[72] These barriers included (in rank order) cost of the exercise program (84.2%), lack of energy (65.8%), transportation (60.5%), and not knowing where to exercise (57.9%). These have some implications regarding what strategies rehabilitation and exercise specialists will use to encourage these individuals to engage in habitual exercise and/or rehabilitation.

Short-term adherence to a pelvic floor muscle exercise program significantly predicted long-term adherence (i.e., 1 year post program) to the same program in a clinical population of women with urinary incontinence.[88]

This may be directly related to the severity of symptoms each individual experienced (i.e., the number of incontinence episodes on a weekly basis). It appeared that individuals with more frequent episodes were more adherent to the program and tended to maintain their adherence 1 year post program.[88] This may also be due to the social stigma and embarrassment that individuals may feel with this health problem.

A major health concern today, cardiovascular disease, results in the loss of independence and quality of life for individuals who have sustained a cardiac event. Because of this, cardiac rehabilitation programs have been developed to provide exercise, education, and assistance in a medically supervised environment to assist in behavioral changes, so as to enhance quality of life.[66] Facilitation of adherence to these programs by health care professionals is essential to help to bring about the behavioral changes needed to maximize function in these individuals. A few studies have examined adherence and motivation to participate in cardiac rehabilitation programs.[89,90] In a review of the literature, Beswick et al.[90] identified several themes that improved recruitment, adherence, and professional compliance to cardiac rehabilitation.

Identified themes that increased patient adherence to cardiac rehabilitation included (1) formal patient commitment via written contract, (2) spouse or familial involvement, (3) strategies to aid self-management, (4) educational intervention, and (5) psychological intervention via group psychotherapy. The themes identified had varying levels of success in improving adherence to the cardiac program and will be discussed later in this chapter. In yet another study, personal factors, such as health and work status, significantly impacted adherence to the cardiac program.[91] It was noted that individuals who were not working and categorized in the "high risk" group for health were found to have the lowest mean physical activity scores (i.e., participation) in the cardiac rehabilitation program at baseline and the conclusion of the study one year later.[91] When motivation in conjunction with health-promoting lifestyle was examined after a 12-week cardiac rehabilitation exercise program, it was found that individuals who participated in the program had higher motivation for a healthy lifestyle than those who did not participate. In addition, perceived benefits of exercise, barriers, and self-efficacy, as well as emotional well-being and health improved in the exercise group versus those in the comparison group.[92] A review of the U.S. National Exercise and Heart Disease Project[93] found that participation in a cardiac rehabilitation program had a compliance rate of 79.6% after 2 months of continuous, monitored training but that adherence decreased to 13% at 36 months.[94] In a study by Blanchard et al.,[89] barrier self-efficacy was shown to be associated with compliance in a phase II cardiac rehabilitation program. In essence, individuals who believed that they had sufficient abilities to overcome specific cardiac related barriers had better adherence to the rehabilitation program. Bray and Cowan[95]

found that proxy efficacy had an effect on predicting exercise self-efficacy and post-program intentions in cardiac rehabilitation. Simply stated, proxy efficacy means the confidence that individuals had in their clinicians' communication, teaching, and motivating capabilities was predictive of exercise self-efficacy and post-program participation in cardiac rehabilitation. Considering that the research performed correlating increased physical activity and exercise with positive outcomes after a coronary event, the impetus to increase compliance and adherence in this population is great.

Methods of Increasing Patient Compliance

- Formal written contract
- Spousal or family involvement
- Strategies to aid self-management
- Educational intervention
- Group psychotherapy

Another clinical population that would warrant the benefits of an exercise program is the chronic obstructive pulmonary disease (COPD) population. This disease is the fourth leading cause of death in the United States for people ages 65 to 84 years and is the fifth leading cause of death for people ages 45 to 64 and those aged 85 and older.[96] In addition, COPD is a primary cause of disability among older adults.[74] There are many psychological as well as physical benefits to participation in an exercise program for individuals who have COPD. Major benefits as detailed in the literature include increased physical capacity, decreased anxiety about dyspnea, greater independence in activities of daily living, reduced fatigued, and improved overall quality of life.[97] Emery et al.[98] conducted a study examining cognitive and psychological outcomes in patients with COPD after 1 year and found that adherence to a regular exercise program in patients in COPD was associated with increased physical and cognitive performance and greater emotional well-being. Those who did not adhere to the program were found to have a decrease in both physical and psychological constructs.[98] The danger of noncompliance in any of these clinical populations, but with COPD most specifically, is that any benefits gained will diminish over time,[99] which makes increasing the likelihood of exercise participation and maintenance over time warranted.

INCREASING ADHERENCE AND MOTIVATION TO EXERCISE AND REHABILITATION

Theoretical approaches, models, and barriers notwithstanding, increasing motivation and subsequently adherence to exercise and/or rehabilitation is the goal of health care professionals, exercise specialists, patients, and clients in a variety of settings with a variety of health-related

TABLE 1-4

Examples of Strategies That Increase Compliance

Strategy	Effect
Solicit social support from family, significant others, children, friends	Family support is the most important type of social reinforcement. If possible, have the family participate in the exercise or take part in the patient's rehabilitation. Suggest fitness routines with children
Make the activity fun and enjoyable	In conjunction with the individual, target activities that he or she has enjoyed in the past and incorporate them into his or her exercise or rehabilitation routine
Increase the individual's knowledge about the activity and/or injury	Teach the patient about the benefits of exercise or rehabilitation and the dangers of not engaging in the suggested activities
Make the physical environment pleasant and appealing	Remove clutter; ensure décor is bright and cheery
Address perceived and real barriers	Compile a list of potential barriers and help the individual solve problems by identifying realistic alternatives

TABLE 1-5

Factors That Increase Motivation

Factor	Effect
Social support	High self-efficacy
Establishment of therapeutic rapport	Individual involvement in planning aspects of the exercise or rehabilitation program
Decreased perception of discomfort	Individual engagement in planning and establishing goals
Positive reinforcement by clinician	Increased knowledge about benefits of engaging in a regular exercise or rehabilitation program

issues. Based on this, there have been several factors identified across the rehabilitation, sport psychology, psychology, and sociology literature that have sought to identify ways to increase motivation and adherence to exercise and rehabilitation (Tables 1-4 and 1-5). Some of these strategies have been identified previously (e.g., behavior written contract, spouse or familial involvement, strategies to aid self-management, educational intervention,

and psychological intervention via group psychotherapy). Others include self-efficacy, social support, education, and client–practitioner interaction.

Self-Efficacy

Self-efficacy can be defined as an "individual's beliefs in his or her abilities to execute necessary courses of action to satisfy situational demands" (p. 236).[100] It is often hypothesized to be a strong influence on behavior because higher levels of self-efficacy are related to a propensity to undertake more challenging tasks, expend more effort in pursuit of goals, and demonstrate greater resilience in the face of adverse stimuli.[101] Human motivation, well-being, and sense of personal accomplishment are based on self-efficacy beliefs. Unless people believe that their actions can produce the outcomes they desire, they have little incentive to act or to persevere in the face of difficulties. Therefore it is presumed that the development of self-efficacy will promote action to initiate and complete various tasks. The development of self-efficacy occurs through mastery of tasks or performance experience, vicarious or observational experiences of others successfully completing the task, verbal persuasion from a voice of authority (e.g., physician, physical therapist), emotional desire to perform the task (i.e., motivation), and physiological states (e.g., reduction in physical discomfort, such as pain or fatigue).[42,102] In a study examining self-efficacy and motivation in the prediction of short- and long-term adherence to exercise among patients with coronary heart disease, both self-efficacy and motivation significantly predicted exercise behavior at 6 months.[103] It has been determined that self-efficacy can be developed through supervised exercise training, peer support, and seeing peers undertake exercise, realistic goal setting, and support from family and friends.[104,105]

Self-efficacy may be increased through the following:

- Mastery of tasks
- Performance experience
- Vicarious or observational experience of successful task completion
- Verbal persuasion from a voice of authority (e.g., physical therapist)
- Emotional desire to perform the task (motivation)
- Physiological states (reduction of discomfort)

When individuals master a task(s), their success will contribute to their sense of personal efficacy. In the same sense, failure to master a specific task(s)—in this case, exercise—will undermine self-efficacy, especially if failures outweigh the successes.[106] In the general adult population, self-efficacy is often a strong indicator of physical activity engagement.[107,108] In populations with acute or chronic illness, improved self-efficacy has been predictive of long-term exercise compliance.[102]

In the health care setting, clinicians have often used the successful experience of patients to engage other patients to increase participation in rehabilitation. The rehabilitation environment may be set up in such a way as to help patients view and translate the positive experiences of other patients with similar injuries or diagnoses, thereby increasing self-efficacy and facilitating positive outcomes for themselves.

Social Support

Whether in the beginning, middle, or end stage of an exercise or rehabilitation program, individuals have stated that social support from family, friends, significant others, peers, and/or health care providers is desired. Indeed not having the support of important persons in their lives has been cited as a barrier to participation or maintenance to exercise and rehabilitation programs. Studies have found that married individuals tend to adhere longer to physical activity and exercise programs than individuals who are not married[109] and that unmarried individuals were more likely to participate in exercise programs if there were social opportunities available,[45] thereby implying that the support provided by their spouse was important to them. In a study examining the role of social support and group cohesion on exercise compliance, Fraser and Spink[110] found group cohesion and social support to be contributory to the prediction of exercise session attendance. Social support was identified as a main motivator in a group of southern women participating in a walking intervention.[110] These women reported spouses, significant others, friends, coworkers, neighbors, as well as children, siblings, parents, and extended family members as sources of exercise support. Of interest was the finding of differences in support plans for people in different income groups. Nies et al.[111] found that high income women appeared to incorporate significant others (spouses, boyfriends, partners) and pets into their walking schedule more than women in a low income group. This is in contrast to a study assessing attendance to a community-based exercise program for an African American church congregation that reported increased adherence in those individuals who had a high sense of community affiliation.[57] In an attempt to predict long-term maintenance of physical activity in older adults, McAuley et al.[112] examined the role of social, behavioral, and cognitive factors and found an indirect correlation between increased levels of social support for exercise and pleasant effects mediated by high levels of self-efficacy at the end of the program. Scores on the social support subscale of the exercise motivation questionnaire (EMQ), although not statistically significantly, differentiated between individuals who exercised regularly and those who did not. Regular exercisers tended to have higher than average scores on this subscale.[112] Increased adherence to home-based rehabilitation programs may in part be due to the familiarity of the environment as well as the increased likelihood of support from family members, significant others, friends, neighbors, and/or peers.

As stated previously, significant others may play an important role in encouraging patients to increase daily physical activity and to reinforce the changes. Support interventions that focus on changing physical activity behavior through building, strengthening, and maintaining social networks that provide supportive relationships for behavior change (e.g., setting up a buddy system, making contracts with others to complete specified levels of physical activity, or setting up walking groups or other groups to provide friendship and support).[113] Higher social interaction either with family members or with others has been shown to have a positive impact on motivation and adherence to cardiac rehabilitation.[114,115] Although heart failure patients do not always have a strong social support system, they might be motivated to be active in an exercise group or with family members in order to be less isolated.[116] Recognizing the important role that social support plays in exercise and rehabilitation should inspire health care providers and other specialists to include people of importance in their patients' and clients' lives.

Education

Intuitively, the more knowledge one has about a topic, the more comfortable and confident he or she will feel in making a decision regarding that topic. This is also true for exercise. It has been suggested that education should be an integral part of any exercise or rehabilitation program.[56] When a panel of experts was asked to examine personal characteristics that may have an influence on exercise behavior in older adults, educational level was rated as the third most important determinant of whether older adults would initiate an exercise regimen.[56] In a sample of women experiencing urinary incontinence, the lack of information regarding sex was a significant predictor of long-term adherence to a regimen of pelvic floor muscle exercises given to them by a physical therapist.[88] This study found that women who did not have sex education in school and who attended school for fewer years tended not to adhere to their prescribed exercise program. Given the findings of these studies, delivery of information on what constitutes good exercise habits, parameters, and benefits is necessary.

Delivery of educational information about exercise and rehabilitation may be done through a variety of verbal and nonverbal interactions on the part of the health care professional or exercise specialist. Interactions can come in the form of telephone counseling, written materials, direct conversation between the therapist/exercise specialist and patient/client, as well as through committee liaisons.

The educational component should be composed of explanations regarding the impact or benefits engaging in exercise and physical rehabilitation will have on the individual's health status and symptoms. It should also include a general explanation on the major concepts of exercise based on the individual's past and current exercise behavior, health status, and baseline physical functioning. Relevant information to include is target heart rate, perceived exertion, and body composition, as well as written handouts with pictures and that are appropriate for the educational level of the individual.

Other areas that need to be included in the educational component, especially for those individuals in rehabilitation, include an accurate explanation of the nature of the injury, treatment approach and rationale, and what constitutes realistic expectations for recovery.[85,117] In addition, delivery of the information, whether done verbally or nonverbally, should occur through a health care or exercise professional that the patient or client trusts and perceives to have a strong knowledge about exercise.

Patient/Client–Practitioner Interaction

Development of rapport between a patient and health care provider and effective communication is necessary for the promotion of motivation and adherence to rehabilitation.[118] Patients who were found to have effective communication with their physical therapists also were found to attend scheduled physical therapy appointments and comply with established rehabilitation activities during the sessions.[118] In the athletic population, it has been suggested that those athletes who felt that medical professionals who were honest, interested in their well-being, and showed an awareness of psychological symptoms relating to their injuries may be more likely to adhere to their rehabilitation program.[119] Having open lines of communication and fostering a collaborative atmosphere more often than not has a positive influence on adherence to treatment.[120] In addition, enhanced communication between the client and the health care practitioner will help to bring to light and resolve any issues that may affect adherence. Building a sound therapeutic relationship plays a major role in adherence, and both the clinician and patient must communicate in partnership in order to build trust.[121]

Another essential component to exercise and rehabilitation adherence is feedback. The health care and exercise professional should provide positive feedback to their patients and clients so as to improve adherence to any rehabilitation and exercise program. Studies have found that positive reinforcement increases the likelihood and maintenance of the activity.[122] Monitoring and supervision by a qualified health care professional has also been shown to improve compliance to exercise and rehabilitation programs.[47] In studying correlates of exercise compliance in physical therapy, Sluijs et al.[47] found that compliance was significantly related to the amount of positive feedback that the patients received. In addition, patients who perceived that their therapist were satisfied with how they were exercising were more compliant than those patients who were not aware of their clinician's feelings regarding their exercise. In the same study, patients who were more compliant with their exercises had therapists who frequently asked them to participate in establishing the exercise regimen and supervised them more often throughout its implementation. The findings from the previous studies again strengthen the association between the development of trust, communication, and caring as some of the most important factors in establishing a therapeutic relationship that fosters patient adherence.

MOTIVATIONAL INTERVIEWING (MI)

Ambivalence is often at the core of why people struggle to embark upon change. Patients faced with recommendations to make behavioral changes will often experience ambivalence, the simultaneous holding of contradictory feelings or attitudes, in other words, having both the desire to change and not change at the same time. When patients are ambivalent about making recommended changes (such as taking a prescribed medication, stopping smoking, or modifying their diet or physical activity level), clinicians may try to persuade them via the use of logic, problem solving, an emphasis on the importance of making the change as well through advice giving as to how the change might be implemented. When recommendations are not followed, as is frequently the case, clinicians may react in one of several ways. One reaction may be to state that their clients/patients are noncompliant and that helping to motivate their clients/patients toward behavior change is impossible. This assumes that patients will only make recommended behavioral changes when they are ready. Another reaction by clinicians may be to increase their advice-giving and problem-solving strategies by reiterating the importance of following the recommendations. This approach will typically not be successful and will serve to have the client/patient "tune out" or not return to the clinic. Yet another way may be to confront patients out of concern or frustration. These providers may simply present patients with a brief description of what is to be done and then hope for the best. Neither of these approaches is ideal and is ineffective in encouraging the client/patient toward behavior change.

Some important questions to be asked and answered are: How can clinicians help their clients/patients find motivation to progress toward their goals? Why are methods of persuasion and confrontation not useful for promoting change? Why is the threat of poor health not enough to persuade a patient to quit smoking, begin exercising, change his or her diet, or take medication? Is there a more effective way to evoke behavioral change?[123]

MI offers an alternative response to ambivalence. The approach is grounded in the assumptions that struggles with ambivalence are a normal part of the process of change. MI allows for a "collaborative, person centered form of guiding to elicit and strengthen motivation for change" (p. 137).[124] The MI approach was initially developed by Miller and Rollnick[125] to help problem drinkers reduce or abstain from alcohol use. Many of its principals and the techniques of MI are founded in the client-centered approach of psychologists Carl Rogers and Robert Carkauff,[124,126–128] although MI is perhaps more goal driven than classic Rogerian client-centered therapy.

MI has evolved into helping individuals commit to making positive behavior changes in a variety of areas, including health. In contrast to delivering simple advice, a practitioner using the MI approach helps the patient discuss the "pros" and "cons" of the target behavior; in turn, resolving the patient's ambivalence about the behavior. In a meta-analysis examining the effectiveness and applicability of MI as a treatment, it was found that MI was 10% to 20% more effective than no treatment and equal to other viable treatments for a wide variety of problems ranging from substance use (i.e., alcohol, marijuana, tobacco, and other drugs) in reducing risky behaviors and increasing client engagement in treatment.[129,130]

In patients with congestive heart failure it was found that in the short term (≤6 months), MI and other strategies that enhanced patient self-efficacy for exercise were successful in increasing exercise in intervention groups by 25% to 30% compared with the control groups.[70] For positive healthy behavior change to occur, there are an innumerable amount of things that need to happen. For instance, a discussion should ensue about the behavior in question that needs to change. The patient needs to be queried about lifestyle, for example, whether they require the use of an assistive device, other aids and/or medications, and if they are physically active. In this regard, patients are often ambivalent or unmotivated to change, and as clinicians, the response is to impart knowledge and advice as to what positive behavioral changes need to be made and how to approach making them. It is in this instance that clinicians may make a mistake and lose the therapeutic rapport that had been established with the patient. Advice giving using a directive style may generate resistance or passivity on the part of the patient. A way to reengage or prevent this disconnection from happening is to use an approach that has been developed to engage and encourage behavior change across a variety of settings.[131] MI is an alternative approach to discussing behavior change that fosters a constructive provider–patient relationship that leads to better outcomes for the patient because it allows for patients to say why and how they might change and is based upon a guiding style as opposed to a directing one.[132,133] In one systematic review that included 72 studies, it was found that using MI with its guiding style outperformed traditional advice giving in 80% of studies.[134] Meta-analyses show that MI is equivalent to or better than other treatments, such as cognitive behavioral therapy (CBT) or pharmacotherapy, and superior to placebo and nontreatment controls for decreasing alcohol and drug use in adults and adolescents.[135–137] MI has also been shown to be effective in health conditions, such as diabetes management.[138] Additional studies support the applicability of MI to human immunodeficiency virus (HIV) care, such as improving adherence to antiretroviral therapy.[139] Given the evidence, MI has been shown to be an important therapeutic intervention that has wide applicability within health care settings in motivating people to change.

Motivational Interviewing (MI) Framework

Prochaska and DiClemente[27] proposed readiness for change as a vital mediator of behavioral change. Their TTM of behavior change (stages of change) describes readiness to change as a dynamic process, in which the "pros" and "cons" of changing generate ambivalence. Ambivalence is a conflicted state in which opposing attitudes or feelings coexist in an individual who is stuck between simultaneously wanting to change and not wanting to change. Ambivalence is particularly evident in situations in which there is conflict between an immediate reward and longer term adverse consequences (e.g., substance abuse, weight management). For example, the patient who presents with serious health problems as a result of heavy drinking, shows genuine concern about the impact of alcohol on his health, and in spite of advice from his practitioner to cut back his drinking, continues to drink at harmful levels embodies this phenomenon.

It is important to note that MI is *not* based upon the transtheoretical stages of change. Both TTM and MI refrain from blaming the client or patient and do not accuse them of being unmotivated and instead focus on the clinician's role in helping to enhance motivation for change.[124] The stages of change model provided a rational way to think about the clinical role of MI, and MI in turn, provided a clear example of how clinicians could help people to move from precontemplation and contemplation to preparation and action. Miller and Rollnick noted that "TTM is intended to provide a comprehensive conceptual model of how and why changes occur, whereas MI is a specific clinical method to enhance personal motivation for change" (p. 131).[124] They stated that explaining the TTM stage of change model is not necessary when engaging in MI, but many practitioners have found it helpful in their work with clients and patients to change their behaviors because it helps to determine how ready these people are to make a change.[124]

Research globally supports the view that MI provides a promising framework for enhancing adherence to health behaviors. Meta-analyses report medium-to-large effects of MI on treatment adherence and small-to-medium effects on treatment outcomes (e.g., drug consumption, psychological well-being).[130,136] Regarding weight loss, MI has also been recognized as an efficient approach among adults to improve adherence to physical activity routines.[140] It has also been shown to be an effective treatment technique for weight loss in people who are obese.[141] A core theoretical assumption of MI is having the knowledge that people will often modify their behavior as a result of their interaction with others. Related to the previous assumption is having the knowledge that health professionals possess critical counseling skills that can help facilitate personal change in their clients and patients.[142]

Principals of Motivational Interviewing (MI)

Expressing empathy (i.e., the counselor's attitude of acceptance), developing discrepancy (i.e., amplifying discrepancy between the patient's present behavior and his or her important goals), avoiding argumentation (i.e., assuming that the patient is responsible for change), rolling with resistance (i.e., acknowledging and exploring the patient's arguments against changing), and supporting self-efficacy (i.e., helping the patient to find resources to implement new behaviors and overcome barriers) are the general principles upon which MI is based.[132,142] It is thought that if the clinician can get the client/patient to do anything toward changing his or her behavior for the better, the greater the chances are for continued forward movement and success. This is a major tenet in social psychology on which Rollnick and Miller base MI.[143] For example, the question that clinicians should ask themselves, according to Miller and Rollnick,[132] is how can I get my client/patient to take action on his or her own behalf? Another major tenet of social psychology relates to when one takes a position and defends it verbally, such as what occurs in a debate; that person then becomes committed to that position (whether he or she still believes it). As such, an MI principle, rolling with resistance, advocates for a nonconfrontational approach because people are more likely to grow and change in a positive direction if they are not engaged in a battle of wills with their clinician.

Principles of Motivational Interviewing

- Expressing empathy—the counselor's attitude of acceptance
- Developing discrepancy—amplify discrepancy between the patient's present behavior and his or her important goals
- Avoiding argumentation—assumption that the patient is responsible for change
- Rolling with resistance—acknowledgment and exploration of the patient's arguments against changing
- Supporting self-efficacy—helping the patient to find resources to implement new behaviors and overcome barriers

---

Key Strategies in Motivational Interviewing (MI)

The essence of MI lies in its spirit, and for a true understanding of MI to be had, it is vital to distinguish between the *spirit* of MI and the *techniques* that are used to manifest that spirit. Clinicians who become too focused on matters of technique may lose sight of the spirit and style that are central to MI.[143] There are four key strategies that are discussed that help the clinicians remain true to the spirit that is MI (Figure 1-7). They include (1) resisting the "righting" reflex, (2) understanding the patient's own motivations, (3) listening with empathy, and (4) empowering the patient.

Resisting the "Righting" Reflex

The "righting" reflex in the context of motivation describes the tendency of health professionals to advise patients about the right path for good health. This can often have a paradoxical effect in practice, inadvertently reinforcing the argument to maintain the status quo. Most people resist persuasion when they are ambivalent to change and will respond by recalling their reasons for maintaining the behavior. MI requires clinicians to suppress the initial "righting" reflex so that they can explore the patient's motivations for change. It is essential for the clinician to refrain from responding to the client/patient with questions or unsolicited advice. Questions can be biased by what the clinician may be most inclined to hearing, flavored by their worldview or prior experience, rather than by what the client wants or needs to explore to facilitate the change. Unsolicited advice can evoke resistance on the part of the client/patient. It is best that the direction of the intervention be driven by the client.

Understanding the Patient's Motivations

As alluded to previously, it is the patient's own reasons for change, rather than the clinicians, that will ultimately result in behavior change. When clients/patients are allowed to explore their own interests, concerns, and values with freedom and the clinician openly explores the patient's motivations for change, a better understanding of the patient's motivations and potential barriers to change will emerge.

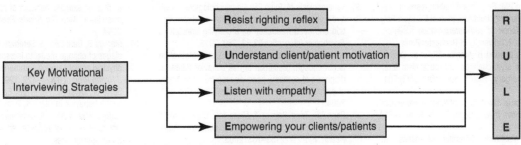

Figure 1-7 Motivational interviewing strategies.

Listening with Empathy

Effective listening skills are essential to understand what will motivate the patient, as well as the "pros" and "cons" of their situation. A general rule of thumb in MI is that equal amounts of time in a consultation should be spent listening and talking.

Empowering the Patient

Empowering one's client/patient involves the establishment of a collaborative therapeutic relationship that allows the patient to explore his or her own ideas about how one can make changes to improve his or her health. It permits patients to access personal knowledge about what has succeeded for them in the past.[131] Clients/patients will benefit from this relationship the most when the practitioner also embodies hope that change is possible.

SUMMARY

As is apparent from this chapter, the concepts of motivation, adherence, and compliance as they relate to physical activity, exercise, and rehabilitation are complex. There is no one factor that will help individuals want to engage in healthy habits. For behavior to change, a combination of factors needs to be incorporated to assist individuals in making decisions that will positively affect their quality of life. Health care practitioners and exercise professionals should make use of the many theories and models available in the literature, including the use of MI as an effective way to facilitate positive behavioral changes in their patients and clients. Listening and addressing the unique situations of each patient and client are needed to help empower and motivate patients and clients to be involved in their own care.

REFERENCES

1. U.S. Department of Health and Human Services, Physical Activity and Health: *A report of the surgeon general*, Atlanta, 1996, US Department of Health and Human Services, Center for Disease Control and Prevention, National Center for Chronic Disease Prevention and Promotion.
2. Robert Wood Johnson Foundation: National blueprint for increasing physical activity for adults 50 and older, *J Aging Phys Act* 9(suppl):S5–S12, 2001.
3. Physical Activity Guidelines Advisory Committee: *Physical activity guidelines advisory committee report 2008*, Washington, DC, 2008, US Department of Health and Human Services.
4. Centers for Disease Control and Prevention: *State indicator report on physical activity 2014*, Atlanta, 2014, US Department of Health and Human Services.
5. Blair SN: Physical inactivity: the biggest public health problem of the 21st century, *Br J Sports Med* 43:1–2, 2009.
6. The Latin Dictionary. Available at: http://latindictionary.wikidot.com/verb:movere. Accessed November 23, 2014.
7. Carver CS, Scheier MF: Dispositional optimism, *Trends Cogn Sci* 18(6):293–299, 2014.
8. Steptoe A, Wright C, Kunz-Ebrecht SR, et al: Dispositional optimism and health behaviour in community-dwelling older people: associations with healthy ageing, *Br J Health Psychol* 11:71–84, 2006.
9. Maslow A: *The farther reaches of human nature*, New York, 1971, Viking.
10. Freud S: *Beyond the pleasure principle*, New York, 1990, Norton.
11. Deci EL, Ryan RM: Self-determination research: reflections and future directions. In Deci EL, Ryan RM, editors: *Handbook of self-determination research*, Rochester, 2002, University of Rochester Press.
12. Ben-Zur H, Rappaport B, Ammar BR, et al: Coping strategies, life style changes, and pessimism after open-heart surgery, *Health Soc Work* 25(3):201, 2000.
13. Bandura A: *Social foundations of thought and action: a social-cognitive theory*, Upper Saddle River, 1986, Prentice Hall.
14. Huitt WG: Maslow's hierarchy of needs. In *Educational psychology interactive*, Valsdosta, 2007, Valdosta State University.
15. Ng J, Thogersen-Ntoumani EC, Ntoumanis N, et al: Self-determination theory applied to health contexts: a meta-analysis, *Perspect Psycholog Sci* 7:325–340, 2012.
16. Patrick H, Williams GC: Self-determination theory: its application to health behavior and complementarity with motivational interviewing, *Int J Beh Nutr Phys Act* 9:18, 2012.
17. Silva MN, Vieira PN, Coutinho SR, et al: Using self-determination theory to promote physical activity and weight control: a randomized controlled trial in women, *J Behav Med* 33:110–122, 2010.
18. Fortier MS, Sweet SN, O'Sullivan TL, et al: A self-determination process model of physical activity adoption in the context of a randomized controlled trial, *Psychol Sport Exerc* 8:741–757, 2007.
19. Gourlana M, Sarrazina P, Trouillouda D: Motivational interviewing as a way to promote physical activity in obese adolescents: a randomised-controlled trial using self-determination theory as an explanatory framework, *Psychol Health* 28(11):1265–1286, 2013.
20. Ajzen I, Fishbein M: *Understanding attitudes and predicting social behavior*, Englewood Cliffs, 1980, Prentice Hall.
21. Ajzen I: From intentions to actions: a theory of planned behavior. In Kuhl J, Beckmann J, editors: *Action-control: from cognition to behavior*, Heidelberg, 1985, Springer.
22. American College of Sports Medicine: In Nigg C, editor: *ACSM's behavioral aspects of physical activity and exercise*, Philadelphia, 2014, Lippincott Williams & Wilkins.
23. Vansteenkiste M, Ryan RM: On psychological growth and vulnerability: basic psychological need satisfaction and need frustration as a unifying principle, *J Psychother Integration* 23:63–280, 2013.
24. Johnston DW, Johnston M, Pollard B, et al: Motivation is not enough: prediction of risk behavior following diagnosis of coronary heart disease from the theory of planned behavior, *Health Psychol* 23(5):533–538, 2004.
25. Conn VS, Tripp-Reimer T, Maas ML: Older women and exercise: theory of planned behavior, *Public Health Nurs* 20(2):153–163, 2003.
26. Maslow AH: *Motivation and personality*, ed 2, New York, 1970, HarperCollins.
27. Prochaska JO, DiClemente CC: Stages and processes of self change of smoking: toward an integrative model of change, *J Consult Clin Psychol* 51:390–395, 1983.
28. Prochaska JO, Velicer WF: The transtheoretical model of health behavior change, *Am J Health Promot* 12:38–48, 1997.
29. Cancer Prevention Research Center: Summary overview of the transtheoretical model. Available at: http://www.uri.edu/research/cprc/transtheoretical.htm. Accessed November 24, 2014.
30. Adams J, White M: Are activity promotion interventions based on the transtheoretical model effective?: a critical review, *Br J Sports Med* 37:106–114, 2003.
31. Velicer WF, DiClemente CC, Prochaska JO, et al: A decisional balance measure for assessing and predicting smoking status, *J Pers Soc Psychol* 48:1279–1289, 1985.
32. Cancer Prevention Research Center: *Detailed overview of the transtheoretical model*. Available at: http://www.uri.edu/research/cprc/transtheoretical.htm. Accessed April 12, 2015.
33. Zimmerman GL, Olsen CG, Bosworth MF: A 'Stages of Change' approach to helping patients change behavior, *Am Fam Physician* 61(5):1409–1416, 2000.
34. Smith DE, Heckemeyer CM, Kratt PP, et al: Motivational interviewing to improve adherence to a behavioral weight-control program for older obese women with NIDDM. A pilot study, *Diabetes Care* 20:52–54, 1997.
35. Norcross JC, Krebs PM, Prochaska JO: Stages of change, *J Clin Psychol* 67(2):143–154, 2011.
36. Cardinal BJ, Kosma M, Mccubbin JA: Factors influencing the exercise behavior of adults with physical disabilities, *Med Sci Sports Exerc* 36(5):868–875, 2004.
37. Marcus B, Banspach S, Lefebvre R, et al: Using the stages of change model to increase the adoption of physical activity among community participants, *Am J Health Promot* 6:424–429, 1992.
38. Sallis JF, Owen N, Fisher EB: Ecological models of health behavior. In Glanz K, Rimer BK, Viswanath K, editors: *Health behavior and health education: theory research and practice*, ed 4, San Francisco, 2008, Jossey-Bass.
39. Schneider M, Stokols D: Multilevel theories of behavior change: a social ecological framework. In Shumaker SA,

Ockene JK, Riekert KA, editors: *The handbook of health behavior change*, ed 3, New York, 2008, Springer.

40. Stokols D: Establishing and maintaining healthy environments. Towards a social ecology of health promotion, *Am Psychol* 47:6–22, 1992.

41. Bouchonville M, Armamento-Villareal R, Shah K, et al: Weight loss, exercise or both and cardiometabolic risk factors in obese older adults: results of a randomized controlled trial, *Int J Obes* 38(3): 423–431, 2013.

42. Schutzer KA, Graves BS: Barriers and motivations to exercise in older adults, *Prev Med* 39:1056–1061, 2004.

43. Burton LC, Shapiro S, German PS: Determinants of physical activity initiation and maintenance among community-dwelling older persons, *Prev Med* 29(5):422–430, 1999.

44. McKenna J, Naylor PJ, McDowell N: Barriers to physical activity promotion by general practitioners and practice nurses, *Br J Sports Med* 32:242–247, 1998.

45. Cohen-Mansfield J, Marx MS, Biddison JR, editors: Socio-environmental exercise preferences among older adults, *Prev med* 38: 804–811, 2004.

46. Dorflinger L, Kerns RD, Auerback SM: Providers' roles in enhancing patients' adherence to pain self-management, *Traditional Behav Med* 3(1): 39–46, 2013.

47. Sluijs EM, Kok GJ, van der Zee J, et al: Correlates of exercise compliance in physical therapy, *Phys Ther* 73(11):771–786, 1993.

48. Klepps R: *Improving home exercise program adherence in physical therapy*, Published, June 20, 2013. Available at: http://blog.theravid.com/patient-care/improving-home-exercise-program-adherence-in-physical-therapy/, Accessed November 23, 2014.

49. World Health Organization: *Adherence to long-term therapies: evidence for action.* Available at: www.who.int/chp/knowledge/publications/adherence:report/en/. Accessed November 12, 2014.

50. Vanhees L, Lefevre JM, Philippaerts R, et al: How to assess physical activity? *Eur J Cardiovasc Prev Rehabil* 12:102–111, 2005.

51. Forkan R, Pumper B, Smyth N, et al: Exercise adherence following physical therapy intervention in older adults with impaired balance, *Phys Ther* 86:401–410, 2006.

52. Whaley DE, Schrider AF: The process of adult exercise adherence: self-perceptions and competence, *Sport Psychologist* 19:148–163, 2005.

53. Dishman RK, Ickes W: Self-motivation and adherence to therapeutic exercise, *J Behav Med* 4: 421–438, 1981.

54. Brewer BW, Van Raalte JL, Corneliuis AE, et al: Psychological factors, rehabilitation adherence, and rehabilitation outcome after anterior cruciate ligament reconstruction, *Rehabil Pysch* 45:20–37, 2000.

55. Brewer BW, Cornelius AE, Van Raalte JL, et al: Age-related differences in predictors of adherence to rehabilitation after anterior cruciate ligament reconstruction, *J Athl Train* 38(2):158–162, 2003.

56. Boyette LW, Lloyd A, Boyette JE, et al: Personal characteristics that influence exercise behavior of older adults, *J Rehab Res Dev* 39(1):95–103, 2002.

57. Izquierdo-Porrera AM, Powell CC, Reiner J, et al: Correlates of exercise adherence in an African American church community, *Cultur Divers Ethnic Minor Psychol* 8(4):389–394, 2002.

58. Lee JY, Jensen BE, Oberman A, et al: Adherence in the training levels comparison trial, *Med Sci Sports Exerc* 28(1):47–52, 1996.

59. Hawkins SA, Cockburn MG, Hamilton AS, et al: An estimate of physical activity prevalence in a large population-based cohort, *Med Sci Sports Exerc* 36(2):253–260, 2004.

60. McArthur D, Dumas A, Woodend K, et al: Factors influencing adherence to regular exercise in middle-aged women: a qualitative study to inform clinical practice, *BMC Womens Health* 14:49, 2014.

61. Keele-Smith R, Leon T: Evaluation of individually tailored interventions on exercise adherence, *West J Nurs Res* 25(6):623–640, 2003.

62. Epstein DE, Sherwood A, Smith PA, et al: Determinants and consequences of adherence to the dietary approaches to stop hypertension diet in African-American and White adults with high blood pressure: results from the ENCORE trial, *J Rehabil Res Dev* 112(11):1763–1773, 2012.

63. Anderson DR, Emery CF: Irrational health beliefs predict adherence to cardiac rehabilitation: a pilot study, *Health Psychol* 33(12):1614–1617, 2014.

64. Blanchard CM, Rodgers WM, Courneya KS, et al: Does barrier efficacy mediate the gender-exercise adherence relationship during phase II cardiac rehabilitation? *Rehabil Psychol* 47(1):106–120, 2002.

65. Cox KL, Flicker L, Almeida OP, et al: The FABS trial: a randomised control trial of the effects of a 6-month physical activity intervention on adherence and long-term physical activity and self-efficacy in older adults with memory complaints, *Prev Med* 7(6): 824–830, 2013.

66. Martin SB, Morrow JR, Jackson AW, et al: Variables related to meeting the CDC/ACSM physical activity guidelines, *Med Sci Sports Exerc* 32(12): 2087–2092, 2000.

67. Grubbs L, Carter C: The relationship of perceived benefits and barriers to reported exercise behaviors in college undergraduates, *Fam Community Health* 25(2):76–85, 2004.

68. DiMatteo MR: Social support and patient adherence to medical treatment: a meta-analysis, *Health Psychol* 23(2):207–218, 2004.

69. Seguin RA, Economos CD, Palombo R, et al: Strength training and older women: a cross-sectional study examining factors related to exercise adherence, *J Aging Phys Act* 18(2):201–218, 2010.

70. Conraads VM, Deaton C, Piotrowicz E, et al: Adherence of heart failure patients to exercise, *Eur J Heart Fail* 14(5):451–458, 2012.

71. Jack K, McLean SM, Moffett JK, et al: Barriers to treatment adherence in physiotherapy outpatient clinics: a systematic review, *Man Ther* 15:220–228, 2010.

72. Rimmer JH, Rubin SS, Braddock D: Barriers to exercise in African American women with physical disabilities, *Arch Phys Med Rehabil* 81:182–188, 2000.

73. Dunlap J, Barry HC: Overcoming exercise barriers in older adults, *Phys Sportsmed* 27(11):1–8, 1999.

74. Romero AJ: Low-income neighborhood barriers and resources for adolescents' physical activity, *J Adolesc Health* 36:253–259, 2005.

75. Christmas C, Andersen RA: Exercise and older patients: guidelines for the clinician, *J Am Geriatr Soc* 48(3):318–324, 2000.

76. Cohen-Mansfield J, Marx MS, Guralnik JM: Motivators and barriers to exercise in an older community dwelling population, *J Am Psychoanal Assoc* 11:242–253, 2003.

77. Lim K, Taylor L: Factors associated with physical activity among older people: a population-based study, *Prev Med* 40:33–40, 2005.

78. Cox KL, Burke V, Gorely TJ, et al: Controlled comparison of retention and adherence in home versus center initiated exercise interventions in women ages 40-65 years: the S.W.E.A.T. study (sedentary women exercise trial), *Prev Med* 36:17–29, 2003.

79. Morey MC, Dubbert PM, Doyle ME, et al: From supervised to unsupervised exercise: factors associated with exercise adherence, *J Aging Phys Act* 11:351–368, 2003.

80. Booth ML, Bauman A, Owen N, et al: Physical activity preferences, preferred sources of assistance, and perceived barriers to increased activity among physically inactive Australians, *Prev Med* 26:131–137, 1997.

81. Harada ND, Wilkins SS, Schneider B, et al: The influence of depression and PTSD on exercise adherence in older veterans, *Military Behav Health* 1(2):2, 2013.

82. McGrady A, McGinnis R, Badenhop D, et al: Effects of depression and anxiety on cardiac rehabilitation, *J Cardiopulm Rehabil Prev* 29(6):358–364, 2009.

83. Zen AL, Whooley MA, Zhao S, et al: Post-traumatic stress disorder is associated with poor health behaviors: findings from the heart and soul study, *Health Psychol* 31(2):194–201, 2012.

84. Shelbourne KD, Wilckens JH: Current concepts in anterior cruciate ligament rehabilitation, *Orthop Rev* 19:957–960, 1990.

85. Spetch LA, Kolt GS: Adherence to sport injury rehabilitation: implications for sports medicine providers and researchers, *Phys Ther Sport* 2:80–90, 2001.

86. Conraads VM, Deaton C, Piotrowicz E, et al: Adherence of heart failure patients to exercise: barriers and possible solutions. A position statement of the study group on exercise training in heart failure of the heart failure association of the european society of cardiology, *Eur J Heart Failure* 14:451–458, 2012.

87. Goodman ED, Ballou MB: Perceived barriers and motivators to exercise in hemodialysis patients, *Nephrol Nurs J* 3(1):23–30, 2004.

88. Alewijnse D, Mesters I, Metsemakers J, et al: Predictors of long-term adherence to pelvic floor muscle exercise therapy among women with urinary incontinence, *Health Educ Res* 18(5):511–524, 2003.

89. Blanchard CM, Courneya KS, Rodgers WM, et al: Determinants of exercise intention and behavior during and after phase 2 cardiac rehabilitation: an application of the theory of planned behavior, *Rehabil Psychol* 47(3):308–323, 2002.

90. Beswick AD, Rees K, West RR, et al: Improving uptake and adherence in cardiac rehabilitation: literature review, *J Adv Nurs* 49(5):538–555, 2005.

91. Sin MK, Sanderson B, Weaver M, et al: Personal characteristics, health status, physical activity, and quality of life in cardiac rehabilitation participants, *Int J Nurs Stud* 41:173–181, 2004.

92. Song R, Lee H: Effects of a 12-week cardiac rehabilitation exercise program on motivation and health-promoting lifestyle, *Heart Lung* 30:200–209, 2001.

93. Dorn J, Naughton J, Imamura D, et al: Correlates of compliance in a randomized exercise trial in myocardial infarction patients, *Med Sci Sports Exerc* 33(7):1081–1089, 2001.

94. Franklin BA, Swain DP, Shephard RJ: New insights in the prescription of exercise for coronary patients, *J Cardiovasc Nurs* 18(2):116–124, 2003.

95. Bray SR, Cowan H: Proxy efficacy: implications for self-efficacy and exercise intention in cardiac rehabilitation, *Rehabil Psychol* 49(1):71–75, 2004.

96. New Guidelines for a Growing Threat to Global Health: Chronic Obstructive Pulmonary Disease. Available at: http://www.prnewswire.com/news-releases/new-guidelines-for-a-growing-threat-to-global-health-chronic-obstructive-pulmonary-disease-82339587.html. Accessed November 24, 2014.

97. Mink BD: Exercise and chronic obstructive pulmonary disease: modest fitness gains pay big dividends, *Phys Sportsmed* 25(11):1–8, 1997.

98. Emery CF, Shermer RL, Hauck ER, et al: Cognitive and psychological outcomes of exercise in a 1 year follow-up study of patients with chronic obstructive pulmonary disease, *Health Psychol* 22(6):598–604, 2003.

99. Goldstein RS: Long-term compliance post-COPD rehabilitation—evidence-based interventions: science to the art of cardiopulmonary rehabilitation, *Am J Med Sports* 4:195–196, 2004 204.

100. McAuley E, Pena MM, Jerome GJ: Self-efficacy as a determinant and an outcome of exercise. In Roberts GC, editor: *Advances in motivation in sport and exercise*, Champaign, 2001, Human Kinetics.

101. Bandura A: *Social foundations of thought and action: a social-cognitive theory*, Upper Saddle River, 1986, Prentice Hall.

102. Uhl TL, Harrison A, English T, et al: Rehabilitation concerns of the middle age athlete, *Sports Med Arthrosc* 11:155–165, 2003.

103. Slovinec D'Angelo ME, Pelletier LG, Reid RD, et al: The roles of self-efficacy and motivation in the prediction of short- and long-term adherence to exercise among patients with coronary heart disease, *Health Psychol* 33(11):1344–1353, 2014.

104. Tierney S, Mamas M, Woods S, et al: What strategies are effective for exercise adherence in heart failure? A systematic review of controlled studies, *Heart Fail Rev* 17:107–115, 2012.

105. Dolansky MA, Stepanczuk B, Charvat JM, et al: Women's and men's exercise adherence after a cardiac event, *Res Gerontol Nurs* 3:30–38, 2010.

106. Bandura A: Self-efficacy. In Friedman H, editor: *Encyclopedia of mental health*, San Diego, 1998, Academic Press.

107. McAuley E, Lox C, Duncan TE: Long-term maintenance of exercise, self-efficacy, and physiological change in older adults, *J Gerontol* 48:218–224, 1993.

108. McAuley E, Courneya KS, Rudolph DL, et al: Enhancing exercise adherence in middle-aged males and females, *Prev Med* 23:498–506, 1994.

109. Wallace JP, Raglin JS, Jastremski CA: Twelve month adherence of adults who joined a fitness program with a spouse versus without a spouse, *J Sports Med Phys Fitness* 35:206–213, 1995.

110. Fraser SN, Spink KS: Examining the role of social support and group cohesion in exercise compliance, *J Behav Med* 25(3):233–249, 2002.

111. Nies MA, Reisenberg CE, Chruscial HL et al: Southern women's response to a walking intervention, *Public Health Nurs* 20(2):146–152, 2003.

112. McAuley E, Jerome GJ, Elavsky S, et al: Predicting long-term maintenance of physical activity in older adults, *Prev Med* 37:110–118, 2003.

113. Task Force on Community Preventive Services: Recommendations to increase physical activity in communities, *Am J Prev Med* 22(4S):67–72, 2002.

114. Coghill N, Cooper A: Motivators and de-motivators for adherence to a program of sustained walking, *Prev Med* 49:24–27, 2009.

115. Farley RL, Wade TD, Birchmore L: Factors influencing attendance at cardiac rehabilitation among coronary heart disease patients, *Eur J Cardiovasc Nurs* 2:205–212, 2003.

116. Löfvenmark C, Mattiasson AC, Billing E, et al: Perceived loneliness and social support in patients with chronic heart failure, *Eur J Cardiovasc Nurs* 8:251–258, 2009.

117. Weiss MR, Troxel RK: Psychology of the injured athlete, *Athl Train J* 21:104–109, 1986.

118. Piaazri T, McBurney H, Taylor NF, et al: Adherence to anterior cruciate ligament rehabilitation: a qualitative analysis, *J Sport Rehabil* 11:90–102, 2002.

119. Brewer BW: Fostering treatment adherence in athletic therapy, *Athl Ther Today* 3(1):30–32, 1998.

120. Culos-Reed SN, Rejeski WJ, McAuley E, et al: Predictors of adherence to behavior change interventions in the elderly, *Control Clin Trials* 21:200S–205S, 2000.

121. DiMatteo R: Evidence-based strategies to foster adherence and improve patient outcomes, *JAAPA* 17:18–21, 2004.

122. Cress M, Buchner DM, Prohaska T, et al: Physical activity programs and behavior counseling in older adult populations, *Med Sci Sports Exerc* 36(11):1997–2003, 2004.

123. Levensky ER, Forcehimes A, O'Donohue WT, et al: Motivational interviewing: an evidence-based approach to counseling helps patients follow treatment recommendations, *Am J Nurs* 107(10):50–58, 2007.

124. Miller WR, Rollnick S: Ten things that motivational interviewing is not, *Behav Cognitive Psychother* 37:129–140, 2009.

125. Miller WR, Rollnick S: *Motivational interviewing: preparing people to change addictive behavior*, New York, 1991, Guilford.

126. Rogers CR: Carl Rogers on the development of the person-centered approach, *Person-Centered Review* 1:257–259, 1986.

127. Carkhuff R: *The art of helping*, ed 7, Amherst, 1993, Human Resource Development Press.

128. Carkhuff RR, Anthony WA, Cannon JR, et al: *The skills of helping: an introduction to counseling skills*, Amherst, 1979, Human Resource Development Press.

129. Lundhal B, Moleni T, Burke B, et al: Motivational interviewing in medical care settings: a systematic review and meta-analysis of randomized controlled trials, *Patient Educ Couns* 93(2):157–168, 2013.

130. Lundhal B, Burke B: The effectiveness and applicability of motivational interviewing: a practice-friendly review of four meta-analyses, *J Clin Psychol* 65(11):1232–1245, 2009.

131. Rollnick S, Butler CC, Kinnersley P: Motivational interviewing, *BMJ* 27:340, 2010.

132. Miller WR, Rollnick S: *Motivational interviewing: preparing people for change*, ed 2, New York, 2002, Guilford.

133. Rollnick S, Miller WR, Butler C: *Motivational interviewing in health care: helping patients change behavior*, New York, 2008, Guilford.

134. Rubak S, Sandbaek A, Lauritzen T, et al: Motivational interviewing: a systematic review and meta-analysis, *Br J Gen Pract* 55:305–312, 2005.

135. Burke BL, Arkowitz H, Menchola M: The efficacy of motivational interviewing: a meta-analysis of controlled trials, *J Consult Clin Psychol* 71(5):843–861, 2003.

136. Hettema J, Steele J, Miller WR: Motivational interviewing, *Ann Rev Clin Psychol* 1:91–111, 2005.

137. Lundahl BW, Kunz C, Brownell C, et al: A meta-analysis of motivational interviewing: twenty-five years of empirical studies, *Res Soc Work Pract* 20:137–160, 2010.

138. West D, Dilillo V, Bursac Z, et al: Motivational interviewing improves weight loss in women with type 2 diabetes, *Diabetes Care* 30:1081–1087, 2007.

139. Kuyper L, de Wit J, Heijman T, et al: Influencing risk behavior of sexually transmitted infection clinic visitors: efficacy of a new methodology of motivational preventive counseling, *AIDS Patient Care STDS* 23:423, 2009.

140. Hardcastle S, Taylor AH, Bailey M, et al: A randomised controlled trial of the effectiveness of a primary health care based counselling intervention on physical activity, diet and coronary heart disease risk factors, *Patient Educ Couns* 70:31–39, 2008.

141. Armstrong MJ, Mottershead TA, Ronksley PE, et al: Motivational interviewing to improve weight loss in overweight and/or obese patients: a systematic review and meta-analysis of randomized controlled trials, *Obes Rev* 12:709–723, 2011.

142. Van Wormer K: Motivational interviewing: a theoretical framework for the study of human behavior and the social environment, *Adv Social Work* 8(1):19–29, 2007.

143. Rollnick S, Miller WR: What is motivational interviewing? *Behav Cognitive Psychother* 23:325–334, 1995.

CHAPTER 2

The Skin and Wound Healing

HOLLIE KIRWAN, ROSE PIGNATARO

ANATOMY AND FUNCTION OF SKIN

Skin is the largest organ in the body and performs a wide variety of different functions. It is composed of a predominantly cellular epidermis and an underlying dermis, which is composed of fibers of connective tissue relatively sparsely populated with cells (Figure 2-1). Both the epidermis and dermis play roles essential to the skin's function and response to injury.[1]

The **epidermis** contains mostly keratinocytes, among which are interspersed melanocytes, Merkel cells, Langerhans cells, and other resident immune cells. *Keratinocytes* represent 95% of the cellular content of the epidermis. They migrate from the dermo-epidermal junction between the dermis and epidermis toward the surface of the skin. During this migration, they undergo progressive flattening and loss of cellular "machinery," giving rise to four distinct layers: stratum basale, stratum spinosum, stratum granulosum, and stratum corneum.[1,2] Keratinocytes are responsible for the production of keratin, a fibrous structural protein that contributes to the strength and waterproofing of skin. *Melanocytes* protect against ultraviolet (UV) light, producing melanin, the dark pigment that gives the skin its color. *Langerhans cells* are professional antigen-presenting cells and play critical roles in both protective immune responses in the skin and maintenance of immune homeostasis.[3] *Merkel cells* are perhaps the least well characterized of the cutaneous cells but have been associated with discrimination of light touch.[4] The epidermis also contains dermal appendages, such as hair follicles, sebaceous glands, eccrine sweat glands, and apocrine glands. The **pilosebacious unit** is composed of hair follicle, hair shaft, and sebaceous gland. The pilosebacious unit contains epithelial stem cells, which are critical to the reepithelialization process because they have a high capacity for self-renewal.[2]

The **dermis** is the layer between the epidermis and the subcutaneous tissue. It is made up of collagen, elastic fibers, and an extrafibrillar matrix. The dermis can be subdivided into a papillary layer and recticular dermis. The *papillary layer* interweaves with the epidermis through papillae, which are fingerlike projections with capillaries that help to nourish the epidermis. The *reticular layer* of the dermis contains a network of collagen fibers, which provides skin turgor and elasticity.

The dermis is a highly vascularized structure containing major vascular networks or plexuses, the deepest of which is the fascial plexus, located at the level of the deep muscle fascia. Overlying this, at the level of the superficial fascia, is the subcutaneous plexus. The next level is the subdermal plexus, an extensive vascular network situated at the junction between the reticular dermis and the subcutaneous tissue directly below, which has an important role in the distribution of blood to other regions of the cutaneous system. Superficial to the subdermal plexus is the subpapillary plexus, situated between the papillary and reticular dermis with capillary loops extending into the papillae. Blood flow between the subdermal and subpapillary plexus is achieved through a series of arterioles and venules and has an important role in regulation of body temperature and the metabolic supply of the skin.

WOUNDS AND HEALING

Wounds can be separated into open or closed wounds. In a **closed wound** the surface of the skin is intact, but the underlying tissues may be damaged. Examples of closed wounds are contusions, hematomas, or stage 1 pressure ulcers. With **open wounds** the skin is split or cracked, and the underlying tissues are exposed to the outside environment. In terms of open wounds, the depth of tissue damage may be broadly divided into the following categories: superficial, partial thickness, or full thickness. Wound healing can occur by primary, secondary, or tertiary intention (Table 2-1). If the edges of the wound can be readily approximated, wound healing of superficial or partial-thickness wounds (i.e., epidermis and dermis) will usually occur by **primary intention**.

Depth of Wound Damage in Open Wounds

Superficial	Involving only the epidermis and upper dermis
Partial thickness	Skin loss up to the lower dermis
Full thickness	Skin and subcutaneous tissue loss

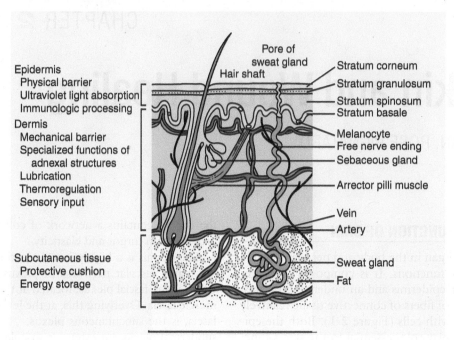

Figure 2-1 The anatomy of the human skin illustrating structures pertinent to wound repair. (From Cohen BA: *Pediatric dermatology*, ed 2, London, 1999, Mosby International Ltd.)

TABLE **2-1**

Types of Wound Healing

Primary Intention	Secondary Intention	Tertiary Intention
• Skin edges are approximated with sutures, staples, or adhesive • Enables quick closure with minimal scarring • Used when there is minimal epithelialization and new tissue	• Large, deep wounds in which edges cannot be approximated • Wound depth determines degree of new tissue matrix and epidermal surface needed for complete closure • Lengthier than healing by primary intention • Can be associated with substantial scarring	• Healing is promoted by leaving the wound open for a prescribed period before approximating the skin edges for primary closure • Used in infected or dehisced surgical wounds

Modified from Strodtbeck F: Physiology of wound healing, *Newborn Infant Nurs Rev* 1(1):43-52, 2001.

The wound will heal through the formation of granulation tissue and reepithelialization, and there should be little or no evidence of a scar. When the wound covers a larger surface area and the margins cannot be readily approximated and/or tissue damage extends deeper than the dermis and into the subcutaneous tissue, wound healing occurs by secondary intention. **Secondary intention** involves wound contraction, along with angiogenesis (i.e., formation of new blood vessels) and reepithelialization. Due to the presence of greater amounts of scar tissue for wounds that close by secondary intention, the regenerated tissues are not identical to the original tissues and only regain a portion of their original tensile strength, making them somewhat vulnerable to future injury. Wounds that heal by secondary intention should be monitored and protected until maturation of the scar tissue has occurred. In wounds that contain a large degree of tissue damage, necrosis, or foreign debris, treatment may include delayed closure to ensure removal of these materials before closure of the skin. This process is known as **delayed primary** or **tertiary healing**.

In adults, optimal wound healing should involve four continuous and overlapping phases: **hemostasis, inflammation, proliferation,** and **remodeling** (Table 2-2). The first-stage wound healing concentrates on achieving *hemostasis* (i.e., a relatively constant internal environment) and a provisional wound matrix. In open wounds, vascular constriction and fibrin clot formation will occur to prevent further blood loss. Damage to the tissues also stimulates vasodilation with an increase in capillary permeability due to the release of histamine by injured mast cells. This will influence the release of chemotactic factors leading to leukocyte infiltration and thus the release of cytokines and growth factors, which allow the tissues to progress to the inflammatory phase. When injury to the skin first occurs, keratinocytes release a store of interleukin-1 (IL-1). This proinflammatory cytokine is important in initiating the healing cascade.[5] Other cytokines released during the transition from hemostasis to

TABLE **2-2**

Physiology of Healing

Phases of Healing		Timeline
1	Homeostasis	Within hours of injury
2	Inflammation	1 to 5 days post injury
3	Proliferation	4 to 21 days post injury
4	Remodeling	21 days to 1 yr post injury

the inflammatory phase include epidermal growth factor (EGF) and platelet-derived growth factor (PDGF), another important substance in stimulating growth and function of fibroblasts and the formation of new tissue.

Neutrophil infiltration and migration of macrophages, shortly followed by lymphocyte infiltration into the wound, signal the start of the *inflammatory phase*. Macrophages play a central role in tissue healing through their production of growth factors, cytokines, and chemokines, which are important in the modulation of the inflammatory response. As the process of phagocytosis cleanses the wound of debris, such as denatured matrix and damaged cells, there is a shift toward the *proliferative* or *granulation phase* of healing. The focus of healing during the proliferative phase is to cover the surface of the wound and restore the vascular network through the generation of granulation tissue. This stage is characterized by epithelial proliferation and migration over the provisional matrix within the bed of the wound. As blood cells enter the site of tissue injury, monocytes are converted to macrophages with the assistance of transforming growth factor beta (TGF-β), a substance released by degranulating platelets. The macrophages release basic fibroblast growth factor (bFGF), a substance that increases the proliferation and function of fibroblasts. It is thought that macrophages also release vascular endothelial growth factor (VEGF), which contributes to angiogenesis. During the proliferative phase, reduction in the number of macrophages or impairment in function can contribute to impaired wound closure and delayed formation of granulation tissue.[6] Fibroblasts and endothelial cells are the predominant cell types in the wound during this phase, and they support capillary growth, collagen formation, and the formation of granulation tissue. Collagen is the major component of acute wound connective tissues. During the proliferative phase, its molecules are cross-linked and organized into bundles. In addition to producing collagen, fibroblasts also produce glycosaminoglycans and proteoglycans, all of which are major components of the extracellular substance of granulation tissue. Keratinocytes and endothelial cells produce autocrine growth factors, and, in synchrony with endothelial expansion, new blood vessels are formed by angiogenesis. As the fibrin clot and provisional matrix are degraded, there is simultaneous deposition of granulation tissue. Epithelial cells migrate inward until the wound is covered. Fibroblasts are transformed into myofibroblasts

through contact inhibition. Myofibroblasts are contractile cells, so wound contraction follows, leading to the final stage of wound healing, the remodeling or maturation phase.

The *maturation* or *remodeling phase* can last up to 1 year or longer post injury, particularly in full-thickness wounds and/or wounds involving larger surface areas of skin. During this time the formation of granulation tissue stops through the apoptosis (i.e., normal death of cells as part of the healing process) or exiting of macrophages, endothelial cells, and myofibroblasts. Therefore a mature wound can be classified as avascular and acellular. Collagen is remodeled into a more organized structure along lines of stress, thereby increasing the tensile strength of the healing tissues. Fibroblasts secrete matrix metalloproteinases. The enzymes facilitate remodeling of type III collagen to type I collagen, which is now organized in parallel bundles until the normal collagen ratio of 4 type III:1 type I is achieved.[7]

There are many factors that can affect tissue healing. These are listed in Table 2-3. Factors intrinsic to the patient can include age, nutrition, and hydration levels, location and depth of the wound, medications, and co-morbidities. Extrinsic factors include support surfaces, friction, and shear and effective repositioning schedules. Education of the patient and caregiver on factors that can affect wound healing is an integral part of the management strategy. More information on wound healing may be found in Chapter 1 - Injury, Inflammation, and Repair: Tissue Mechanics, the Healing Process and Their Impact on the Musculoskeletal System in *Scientific Foundations and Principles of Practice in Musculoskeletal Rehabilitation*, volume 2 of this Musculoskeletal Rehabilitation book series.

TABLE **2-3**

Systemic and Local Factors Affecting Wound Healing

Systemic Factors	Local Factors
• Nutrition and hydration	• Hypergranulation
• Diabetes mellitus	• Perfusion and oxygenation
• Peripheral vascular disease	• Infection
• Gastroesophageal reflux disease	• Edema
• Collagen disease	• Pressure, friction, shear, moisture
• End stage renal disease	• Sensation, neuropathy
• Immunosuppression	• Hyperkeratosis
• Aging	• Epibole
• Medications	• Cellulitis
• Social and health habits	• Nonviable tissue
• Functional status	• Lack of growth factors
• Infection	• Cytokines
• Paresthesia	• Matrix metalloproteinases
• Perfusion	
• Incontinence	
• Psychological function (i.e., stress, memory)	

WOUND ASSESSMENT

As will be evident from the extensive list of parameters that may affect wound healing, wound assessment must be performed in the context of a thorough patient evaluation. In severe cases, such as large burns, evaluation is most effectively performed by an interdisciplinary team, which can include physicians, nurses, occupational therapists, and physical therapists. A detailed patient history, systems review, and general physical examination (including cardiopulmonary and vascular testing, in addition to a musculoskeletal assessment and overall view of the integument) should precede local evaluation of the wound itself. There are a variety of tools available for local wound assessment, and these tools should contain the categories of examination reviewed in the following section. Any nonhealing wounds or suspicious lesions should be referred to a specialist physician to check for signs of malignancy.

Wound Dimensions: Surface Area and Depth Measurement Techniques

Keeping a record of wound dimensions is necessary to monitor changes in wound size to identify whether an exacerbation or progression of healing has occurred. There are various methods that can be used to measure and describe the size, shape, and location of a wound.

Clock Method

The clock method is one of the most common methods of wound measurement. The wound is considered as a face of a clock with the position of the wound based on the standard anatomical position of the patient (Figure 2-2). For wounds on the torso and extremities, the patient's head is considered as the landmark for 12 o'clock and the feet are considered 6 o'clock, whereas for wounds located on the foot, the heel is considered 12 o'clock and the toes are 6 o'clock. Key characteristics that can be measured and described using the clock method are length, width, depth, and the presence of dead space. **Dead space** represents tissue damage that is not immediately evident when inspecting visible aspects of the wound. All forms of dead space must be properly addressed during local treatment of the wound to prevent the accumulation of pathogens and exudate. This can be prevented by using wound fillers, such as calcium alginate or amorphous hydrogel, or in deeper wounds using gauze strips. In addition, the use of wound fillers to occupy dead space ensures that the wound will heal from the base to the surface without abscess formation or opportunities for deeper infection and sepsis.

Categories of dead space include sinus formation, tunneling, and undermining. **Tunneling** is generally located in the wound bed or along the wound margins and can connect one wound to another or a wound to a body cavity. Tunnels can descend deeper into the wound or to

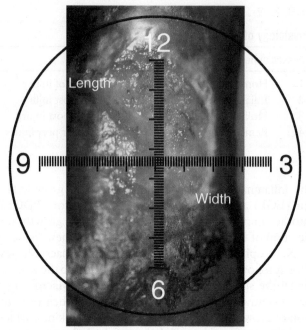

Figure 2-2 Demonstration of how the clock face method can be used to measure the size of a leg wound. (Modified from Morison M, Ovington LG, Wilkie K: *Chronic wound care*, St Louis, 2004, Mosby/Elsevier.)

the side of the wound bed. The deepest area of tunneling and its location on the clock should be recorded. **Sinus** formation may appear similar to tunneling but differs in that there is no exit point. Sinuses may extend beyond the visible margins of the wound and are often hidden beneath the surface of the skin. Both tunneling and sinus formation need to be carefully assessed due to possible infection, unrelieved pressure, or the presence of foreign bodies. **Undermining** is another category of dead space and can be described as a hidden shelf or ledge resting just beneath the wound margin but not visible from the surface of the skin. The presence of undermining can indicate shear or pulling at the wound bed and should be properly documented because the presence of preexisting damage to the subcutaneous tissues may later manifest as a visible increase in the length, width, or diameter of the wound. Undermining should be measured at each time of the clock, for example, 4 cm at 12 o'clock, 3 cm at 3 o'clock, 3 cm at 6 o'clock, and 2 cm at 9 o'clock.

Perpendicular Method

A quick method often used during brief patient encounters is a linear wound measurement. A perpendicular linear dimension is simple, reliable, costs little to implement, and is portable. However, it can have limited sensitivity to change in wound size, and limited information is gathered on wound shape. The perpendicular method assumes the wound is a simple shape, such as a circle or a rectangle. Using this method the size of the wound is estimated by measuring the maximum length and the maximum width perpendicular to the initial measurement, in centimeters or millimeters using a paper or plastic ruler.[8] Next the two measurements (length×width) are multiplied and recorded as total surface area. Although the perpendicular method can overestimate total size of the wound, particularly when tissue damage involves an irregularly shaped area, research has demonstrated a high degree of interrater reliability and the ability to document changes in wound area over time using serial measurements taken using the same standard procedures.[9]

Planimetry

Planimetry (i.e., wound tracing) is a technique that is more sensitive to changes in wound size than the perpendicular method. The outline of the wound is drawn onto a clear plastic sheet then transferred onto metric graph paper with a 4- or 8-cm grid. A second clear plastic sheet is placed between the tracing sheet and the wound to manage wound contamination. This sheet is discarded after use. The wound tracings are kept for sequential comparison. Wound tracings rely on the precise location of the wound edges and have good intrarater reliability.[8,10] A study comparing wound tracing to other techniques, including photographic area quantification, reported that wound tracing was highly correlated with the other techniques ($r \geq 0.93$, $p \leq 0.001$).[11]

Deepest Wound Base (Swab Measuring Technique)

Measurement of wound depth or volume is more reliable in deep wound cavities and less reliable for shallow and irregularly shaped wounds. Depth can be measured using a sterile cotton swab or curette inserted into the maximum depth in a particular dimension and documented on the wound tracing (Figure 2-3). Care must be taken with this method to avoid iatrogenic injury (i.e., injury caused by treatment or diagnostic procedures).

Photographs

The use of photographs in wound documentation allows a permanent record of wound size as well as appearance to be maintained in records for future comparison. High-resolution photographs are preferable to identify epithelial growth at wound margins.[12] Photo quality, lighting, and angle must all be considered. A variation in camera angle can lead to an underestimation of wound area by up to 10%.[13] Therefore it is recommended that photos contain a small ruler or tape measure within the vicinity of the wound to indicate scale. In addition, effort should be made to maintain consistent distance from the camera to the wound when taking serial photographs. In some facilities, digital film does not meet legal requirements for documentation due to its nature of being easily altered. In these cases special film integrating graph lines can facilitate wound measurement and comparison over time. Circumferential wounds or those on curved body surfaces may lead to apparent wound size discrepancy due to the two-dimensional (2D) nature of photography. It is

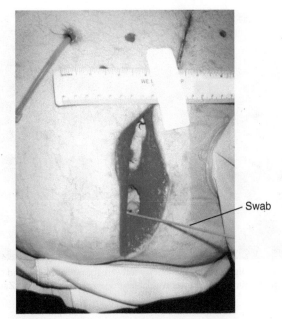

Figure 2-3 Demonstration of measuring wound depth using a swab. A sterile swab is inserted into the deepest portion of the wound and marked at surface level. The depth of the wound from the end of the swab to the mark is measured and recorded. (From Gallagher S, Gates JL: Obesity, panniculitis, panniculectomy, and wound care: understanding the challenges, *J Wound Ostomy Continence Nurs* 30(6):334-341, 2003.)

best to combine wound photography with other methods for assessing wound dimensions to obtain the most accurate results. Benefits of the photographic method include reduced risk of wound contamination, wound bed contact, and patient discomfort.

Photogrammetry

Computerized photogrammetry can give the practitioner precise objective information on wound size, shape, outline, area, color, and surrounding tissue changes.[8] The photogrammetry technique is based on color- and light-balanced computerized photographic image capture. A target plate is based in the same plane as the wound, and the software can extract dimensional and perspective information from the image (Figure 2-4). Marking a cotton swab showing the depth and placing the swab in the image allows calculation of wound depth.

Assessment of the Wound Bed

To determine the correct management and appropriate dressing selection, it is necessary to identify the shape and size of the wound and what types of tissue are present within the wound base.

Granulation tissue is the indication of healthy tissue—it can be yellow, red, or pink in color and will progress upward, filling in the base of the wound and providing a surface for the migration of new epithelial cells. It often has an appearance resembling cobblestones. **Unhealthy**

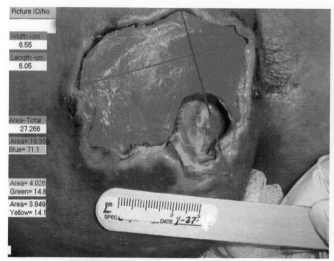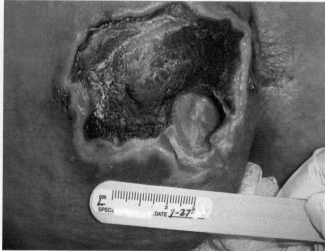

Figure 2-4 Digital photo-planimetry software for measuring wound size. This image displays output from PictZar software. (Images courtesy PictZar® Digital Planimetry Software. Available at: www.pictzar.com/PictZar%20Images.htm.)

granulation tissue is dark red in color, can bleed on contact, and may be indicative of wound infection. **Hypergranulation tissue** is red or pink in color and can rise above the wound bed. Evidence of hypergranulation can indicate that the cells contain excess fluid or have had contact with a caustic irritant causing chronic irritation and inflammation. It may also indicate the presence of an aerobic pathogen causing increased oxygen in the wound bed. **Slough** is nonviable, yellow or white, fibrous, necrotic tissue. It can vary from being loose and easily removed to being stringy and difficult to remove, as is often the case in chronic wounds. Slough is made up of fibrin, bacteria, dead cells, and wound fluid. It is necrotic tissue, and if left in the wound, healing cannot occur. Methods for debriding slough will depend on whether it is heavily adhered to underlying tissue. Slough that is loose and easily removed can be lifted from the wound bed using gentle mechanical debridement or through dressing choices that promote autolysis (i.e., enzymatic digestion of cells). Care must be taken because exposed tendons may be mistaken for slough. Tendons tend to be gleaming yellow or white and shinier than slough. In addition, upon close inspection, tendons contain a visible network of parallel fibers due to the presence of well-organized layers of collagen. **Eschar** is nonviable, hard, brown or black tissue. Sometimes the presence of eschar represents necrotic tissue that has remained in the wound and become desiccated, or dry. It may also represent necrotic tissue that has lost its blood supply. The presence of black eschar, slough, or any necrotic tissue will inhibit wound closure and may serve as a breeding ground for pathogens. Therefore removal of this tissue is usually required to promote full healing in most wounds. Black eschar and slough may be quantified as excessive (+++), moderate (++), minimal (+), or absent (−). The choice of an appropriate method of debridement, or removal of necrotic tissue from the wound bed, will depend on the type of necrotic tissue present, how firmly adhered the tissue is to the underlying layers of the wound, and the amount of necrotic tissue present relative to the presence of granulation tissue or new epithelium.

Epithelial tissue is the final visual sign of healing. Epithelial tissue is superficial, pink or pearly white tissue that migrates from the wound margins, hair follicle, or sweat glands.[14] As healing progresses, this new epithelial tissue will eventually cover the granulation tissue, resulting in full wound closure.

Assessment of Wound Edges

Examining the edges and margins of a wound may provide information on the wound etiology and assist in differential diagnosis. For example, venous leg ulcers often have sloping edges, irregular borders, and a shallow wound base. In contrast, arterial ulcers tend to be well demarcated with steep wound margins and greater depth. In some cases rolled or everted edges can indicate wound chronicity but may also raise suspicions of malignancy.[15]

Non-distinct wound edges occur when the wound bed is at the same level of the edges and can indicate that epithelialization is occurring. If the wound edges are calloused, it may indicate the presence of repetitive stresses, such as pressure or rubbing close to the wound. Calloused edges are a strong characteristic in neuropathic foot ulcers, often seen in diabetic patients. In these cases, the wound may fail to close because calloused tissue is not capable of epithelial regeneration. Rolled edges or epibole (i.e., wound edge rolls downward, and there is premature closure of wound) occur when the wound has been kept dry and the cells at the edges need moisture to continue healing. These rolled edges may also occur if there is a mechanical impediment to wound closure, such as the presence of necrotic tissue, foreign debris, or the use of an improper dressing or topical agent within the wound bed. When rolling occurs, application of silver nitrate or surgical reopening of the wound edges is required to allow migration of new epithelial cells from the margins of the wound. If the wound margin is macerated (i.e., showing damp white edges with a mushy consistency), then a review of the wound dressing is required. If wound drainage is not adequately controlled, the areas of maceration may lead to further tissue breakdown, extending the size of the wound.[16] In many cases the onset of maceration can be effectively prevented through use of an absorptive dressing and the application of a petroleum skin protectant on intact tissues surrounding the wound.

Wound Site

The position and location of the wound can also provide information on differential diagnosis. For example, pressure wounds occur at or near bony prominences. **Arterial wounds** typically occur at the most distal portion of the impaired vascular supply, and **venous wounds** also tend to occur in the distal lower extremity, at locations where the return of blood to the systemic circulation is challenged by gravity and dependent positioning of the affected body part. The location of a wound also influences dressing and treatment choices. A wound over a joint capsule may leak synovial fluid, which could be mistaken for wound exudate. Exposed bone should be treated with care to reduce the risk of developing osteomyelitis. In addition, if a wound is in close proximity to or in close communication with an organ, body cavity, large blood vessel, or peripheral nerve, care must be taken to protect the exposed tissues during wound cleansing and irrigation and through the appropriate choice and application of topical agents, if any, as well as selection of a dressing that will guard against injury and infection without adhering or applying tension or excessive compression to the site. It should also be noted that if the wound meets the criteria noted earlier, the use of negative pressure wound therapy (NPWT) may be contraindicated.[14]

Wound Exudate

Consistency, color, odor, and amount of exudate should be recorded. Exudate can range from frank pus to serous, viscous, or blood-stained fluid. **Serosanguineous fluid** is a combination of blood and serous drainage that is thin, watery, and pale red or pink in color. Serous exudate is clear in color, and sanguineous is blood red. **Purulent exudate** can be thick or thin and yellow or brown or green in color. Purulent exudate is present in the inflammatory stage of healing due to the breakdown of blood cells, necrotic tissue, and other vascular constituents but can sometimes be indicative of infection, especially when found in conjunction with wound odor or other signs,

such as warmth, redness, swelling, pain, or systemic symptoms, including fever, nausea, vomiting, and/or malaise. The amount of exudate may vary depending on the stage of wound healing. Wounds can produce exudate until the final stage of healing, epithelialization, is complete. The amount of moisture will determine the dressing choice. The quantity of exudate can be classified as heavy (+++ [dressing soaked]), medium (++ [dressing wet]), or minimal (+ [dressing dry]).[15] Wound infection or gross edema may cause excessive exudate, as may vascular congestion due to venous insufficiency. Each of these factors can lead to complications in wound healing if not properly addressed in the plan of care.

Tissue Classification Models

There are various models used in clinical practice to classify wound tissue or the extent of integumentary damage. These include, but are not limited to, pressure ulcer staging,[17] Wagner Wound Classification System for diabetic ulcers,[18] University of Texas classification for diabetic foot ulcers,[18,19] and Red-Yellow-Black (RYB) tissue color classification system.[20] In addition, there are objective tools and measures that can be used to document changes in wound status. These include the National Pressure Ulcer Association Pressure Ulcer Scale for Healing (PUSH) tool[21,22] and the Bates-Jensen Wound Assessment Tool (BWAT).[23]

Pressure Ulcer Staging

The National Pressure Ulcer Advisory Panel (NPUAP) redefined the definition of a pressure ulcer and the stages of pressure ulcers in 2007.[17] This definition is now considered the gold-standard system for staging or reporting pressure ulcers (Table 2-4). The original well-documented staging system was defined in 1975 by Shea[24] and was composed of four grades with each stage defined by the extent of soft tissue damage (I to IV and a closed pressure ulcer). When the NPUAP first developed its staging system, knowledge of pathology leading to pressure ulcers was very limited, and oftentimes, suspected deep tissue injuries were not considered and occasionally misclassified as stage I pressure ulcers. To help resolve this dilemma, the NPUAP has now defined deep tissue injury as the newest pressure ulcer stage in the current NPUAP staging system after examination of multiple clinical cases. Under the NPUAP system, the deep tissue stage has been defined as "purple or maroon localized area of discolored intact skin, or blood-filled blister resulting from damage of underlying soft tissue due to excessive pressure and/or shear."[17] The NPUAP acknowledged that deep tissue injuries could be more difficult to detect in individuals with dark skin tones. Therefore visual assessment should be augmented by additional observations, such as changes in skin temperature, texture, and turgor, as well as presence and degree of pain at the site of tissue damage.

TABLE **2-4**

National Pressure Ulcer Advisory Panel Staging System for Pressure Ulcers

Stage	Definition
(Suspected) Deep Tissue Injury	Purple or maroon localized area of discolored intact skin or blood-filled blister due to damage of underlying soft tissue from pressure and/or shear. The area may be preceded by tissue that is painful, firm, mushy, boggy, warmer, or cooler as compared with adjacent tissue.
Stage I	Intact skin with nonblanchable redness of a localized area usually over a bony prominence. Darkly pigmented skin may not have visible blanching; its color may differ from the surrounding area.
Stage II	Partial-thickness loss of dermis presenting as a shallow open ulcer with a red-pink wound bed, without slough. May also present as an intact or open/ruptured, serum-filled blister.
Stage III	Full-thickness tissue loss. Subcutaneous fat may be visible, but bone, tendon, or muscle is not exposed. Slough may be present but does not obscure the depth of tissue loss. May include undermining and tunneling.
Stage IV	Full-thickness tissue loss with exposed bone, tendon, or muscle. Slough or eschar may be present on some parts of the wound bed. Often include undermining and tunneling.
Unstageable	Full-thickness tissue loss in which the base of the ulcer is covered by slough (yellow, tan, gray, green, or brown) and/or eschar (tan, brown, or black) in the wound bed.

Note: This staging system should be used only to describe pressure ulcers.

Modified from the National Pressure Ulcer Advisory Panel (NPUAP): NPUAP Pressure Ulcer Stages/Categories. Available at: http://www.npuap.org/resources/educational-and-clinical-resources/npuap-pressure-ulcer-stagescategories/. Accessed April 28, 2015

Stage I pressure ulcers are areas where skin damage exists but has yet to manifest as a break in the epidermis and visible exposure of subcutaneous tissues. Stage I pressure ulcers are identified as areas of nonblanchable erythema–areas of redness that do not turn white in response to gentle external pressure. Stage I pressure ulcers may also be more difficult to detect in patients with higher levels of skin pigmentation and may instead be characterized by a darker, almost violet discoloration. In stage I pressure ulcers the site may also be painful, firm, soft, warmer, or cooler when compared with adjacent tissue. **Stage II** pressure ulcers may present as a shiny or dry shallow ulcer with partial-thickness damage that extends through the epidermis and into, but not through, the underlying dermis. It is inappropriate to use this stage to describe skin tears, tape burns, perineal dermatitis, maceration, or denudement. **Stage III** pressure ulcer depth may vary depending on anatomical location. The bridge of the nose, ear, occiput, and malleolus lack subcutaneous tissue meaning that, even at stage III, ulcers in these areas may still be shallow. However, in areas with significant amounts of adipose tissue, extremely deep stage III ulcers may occur. Stage III pressure ulcers involve full-thickness damage to the epidermis and dermis, extending to, but not through, the subcutaneous tissues. **Stage IV** pressure ulcer depth will also vary depending on anatomical location. If over areas with little or no subcutaneous tissue, the ulcer may be shallow, but in areas with significant adipose tissue, the ulcer may extend into muscle and supporting structures, such as fascia, tendon, or joint capsule. This can lead to increased risk of osteomyelitis. In stage IV ulcers, bone and tendon may be visible or directly palpable.

There are some limitations in use of the NPUAP staging system that should be noted. The depth of a pressure ulcer cannot be properly assessed until sufficient amounts of slough or eschar have been removed such that the base of the wound may be seen. Therefore wounds that are covered with overlying necrotic tissue should be categorized as "unstageable" until an accurate determination of depth may be obtained. Another limitation in use of the NPUAP staging system is that a wound stage cannot be reversed; for instance, a stage III cannot become a stage II as wound closure occurs.

Pressure Ulcer Scale for Healing (PUSH) Tool

As an alternative to reverse staging, the NPUAP developed the PUSH tool (Appendix 2-1).[21,22] The PUSH tool represents a biologically accurate, easy-to-use, and clinically practical instrument for tracking pressure ulcer status over time. The NPUAP recommends use of the PUSH tool at regular intervals or if the condition of the patient or of the wound deteriorates. The PUSH tool is designed to monitor three critical parameters that are most indicative of healing: surface area (length×width, in centimeters squared), exudate (none, light, moderate, or heavy), and type of tissue present at the wound bed (i.e., closed or resurfaced, epithelial tissue, granulation tissue, slough, or necrotic tissue [eschar]). In addition, the NPUAP recommends assessment of additional parameters, such as odor, color of exudate, and the presence of undermining, tunneling, or sinus formation, as well as the condition of the periwound skin, to develop the most appropriate treatment regime.

Bates-Jensen Wound Assessment Tool (BWAT)

As an alternative to the PUSH tool, which is specifically designed for use in assessing pressure ulcers only, the BWAT is used to assess and monitor healing of all types of wounds. The BWAT was developed by Bates-Jensen in the early 1990s and was initially called the Pressure Sore Status Tool (PSST). In 2001, the PSST was revised and renamed the BWAT—its new title reflecting its increasingly common use in wounds caused of various etiologies other than pressure (Appendix 2-2).[23] The BWAT is used to measure wound status at initial evaluation and then on at least a weekly basis or whenever a change in wound status occurs. It is more comprehensive than the PUSH tool and consists of 15 items (location and shape are not scored). The scored items are size, depth, edges, undermining, necrotic tissue type, necrotic tissue amount, exudate type, exudate amount, skin color, edema, induration, granulation, and epithelialization. Each item is scored from 1 to 5, with a lower score being preferable. The 13 subscores are totaled to get a total score. A BWAT score can be used to give an indication of the wound severity.

Bates-Jensen Wound Assessment Tool (BWAT) Score

13-20	Minimal severity
21-30	Mild severity
31-40	Moderate severity
41-65	Extreme severity

Wagner Wound Classification System for Diabetic Foot Ulcers

The well-established Wagner Wound Classification System for Diabetic Foot Ulcers (Table 2-5) has long been a popular tool for health care providers.[18] The Wagner system assesses ulcer depth and the presence of osteomyelitis or gangrene by using a grading system[25,26]; however, the disadvantage of this system is that it does not consider the presence of ischemia or infection of the ulcer.[27] Grading criteria for the Wagner system are as follows: Grade 0 signifies presence of bony foot deformities, callus formation, redness, or scar tissue indicative of a preulcerative or postulcerative state, but skin is intact. Grade 1 is used to describe a single, well-defined superficial ulcer. Grade 2 describes a deeper ulcer with exposure of the joint capsule or tendon. Grade 3 ulcers have involvement of deeper tissues, such as the muscle, fascia, or periosteum. Grades 4 and 5 involve more extensive tissue destruction with gangrene of the forefoot or more than two thirds of the foot, respectively.

The University of Texas San Antonio Diabetic Wound Classification System

The University of Texas classification system for diabetic foot ulcers is another commonly used tool. Similar to the Wagner Classification System, it uses four numeric stages focused on the depth of the wound, but within each stage, the University of Texas system also includes four letter grades based on the presence of infection and/or ischemia,[19] enabling better prediction of outcomes (Table 2-6).[18]

TABLE **2-5**

Wagner Wound Classification System for Diabetic Foot Ulcers

Grade	Description
0	Intact skin
1	Superficial diabetic ulcer
2	Ulcer extension involving ligament, tendon, joint capsule, or fascia. No abscess or osteomyelitis
3	Deep ulcer with abscess or osteomyelitis
4	Partial foot gangrene (i.e., forefoot)
5	Extensive or widespread gangrene (more than two thirds of foot)

Modified from Clayton W, Elasy TA: A review of the pathophysiology, classification, and treatment of foot ulcers in diabetic patients, *Clinical Diabetes* 27(2):54, 2009.

The Red-Yellow-Black (RYB) Color Classification System

The RYB tissue color classification system is a simple system for wound evaluation in chronic wounds or surgical sites. This system classifies wounds that are healing by secondary or delayed primary intention as red, yellow, black, or mixed. It can be applied to acute and chronic wounds. The classification is based on the continuum of the wound-healing process. Red wounds may be in the inflammatory phase, proliferation phase, or maturation phase of wound healing. Wounds that are not ready to heal are yellow wounds, which are infected or may contain fibrinous slough, and black wounds are those that contain necrotic tissue or eschar.[20]

Burns: Area and Depth Charts

There are three levels of burns: first, second, and third degree (Figure 2-5). In a first-degree burn, only the epidermis is affected, and pain, redness, and swelling may be present. With a second-degree burn (i.e., partial-thickness burn), the entire epidermis and upper layers of the dermis are affected, causing pain, redness, swelling, and blistering. Third-degree burns (i.e., full-thickness burns) destroy the entire epidermis and most of the dermis and will cause blackened and burned skin and may be accompanied by numbness or diminished sensation.[28] There are three methods that are commonly used to measure the size of a burn based on the amount total body surface area involved in the injury. These are the Rule of Nines, Palmar method, and Lund-Browder (LB) method.

Wallace Rule of Nines

The Rule of Nines was first developed in the 1940s but did not appear in the literature until the 1950s. It has now become a standard clinical method for determination of the percentage of the body affected by a burn (Table 2-7).[29] It is a quick way of estimating medium-to-large burns in adults, but it is not as accurate in children. Using a diagram, each region of the body is divided into regions

TABLE **2-6**

University of Texas Diabetic Wound Classification System

	Grade 0	Grade 1	Grade 2	Grade 3
Stage A	Areas of pressure which are sometimes called preulcerative lesion	Noninfected, nonischemic superficial ulceration not including tendon, capsule, or bone	Noninfected, nonischemic ulcer that penetrates to tendon or capsule	Noninfected, nonischemic ulcer that penetrates to bone or joint
Stage B	Infected, nonischemic epithelialized wound	Infected, nonischemic superficial ulceration	Infected, nonischemic ulcer that penetrates to tendon or capsule	Infected, nonischemic ulcer that penetrates to bone or joint
Stage C	Ischemic, noninfected epithelialized wound	Ischemic, noninfected superficial ulceration	Ischemic, noninfected ulcer that penetrates to tendon or capsule	Ischemic, noninfected ulcer that penetrates to bone or joint
Stage D	Infected and ischemic epithelialized wound	Infected and ischemic superficial ulceration	Infected and ischemic ulcer that penetrates to tendon or capsule	Infected and ischemic ulcer that penetrates to bone or joint

Modified from Armstrong DG, Lavery LA, Harkless LB: Validation of a diabetic wound classification system. The contribution of depth, infection, and ischemia to risk of amputation, *Diabetes Care* 21(5):855-859, 1998.

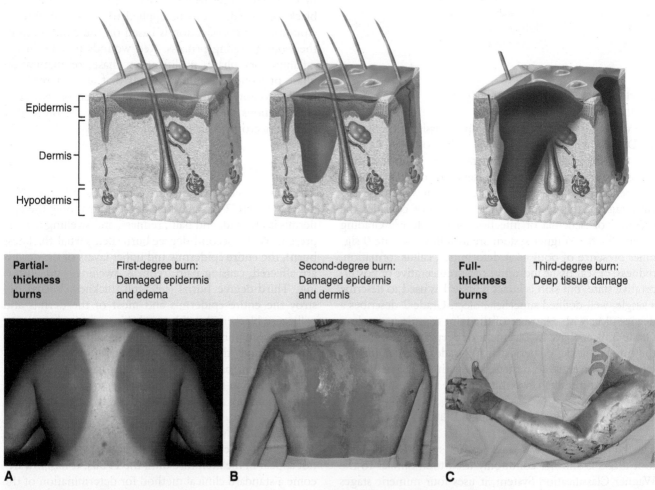

Figure 2-5 First-, second-, and third-degree burns and the layers of skin affected. **A,** In a first-degree burn, only the epidermis is affected and in pain. **B,** In a second-degree burn (partial-thickness burn), the entire epidermis and upper layers of the dermis are affected. **C,** Third-degree burns (full-thickness burns) destroy the entire epidermis and most of the dermis. (**A-C** [illustrations], From Patton KT, Thibodeau GA: *Anatomy and physiology*, ed 8, St. Louis, 2013, Mosby/Elsevier; **A** [photo], From Kliegman RM, Stanton B, St. Geme J et al: *Nelson textbook of pediatrics*, ed 19, Philadelphia, 2011, Saunders/Elsevier; **B** and **C** [photos], From Black JM, Hokanson Hawks J: *Medical-surgical nursing: clinical management for positive outcomes*, ed 8, St Louis, 2009, Saunders/Elsevier.)

TABLE **2-7**

Wallace Rule of Nines

BODY PARTS		PERCENTAGE OF BODY AREA	
		Adult (%)	Child (%)
Head and neck	Anterior	4.5	9
	Posterior	4.5	9
Trunk	Anterior–upper	9	18 (whole front)
	Anterior–lower	9	
	Posterior–upper	9	18 (whole back)
	Posterior–lower	9	
Upper extremities	Anterior	4.5 (each)	4.5 (each)
	Posterior	4.5 (each)	4.5 (each)
Lower extremities	Anterior	9 (each)	13.5 (each)
	Posterior	9 (each)	
Genitalia		1	1
TOTAL		**100**	**100**

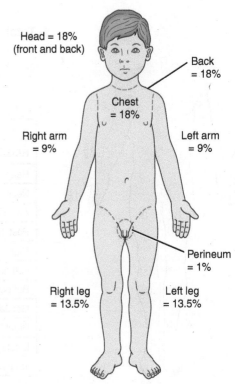

Head = 18%
(front and back)

Back = 18%

Chest = 18%

Right arm = 9%

Left arm = 9%

Perineum = 1%

Right leg = 13.5%

Left leg = 13.5%

Figure 2-7 Child Rule of Nines.

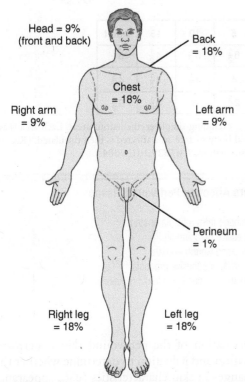

Head = 9%
(front and back)

Back = 18%

Chest = 18%

Right arm = 9%

Left arm = 9%

Perineum = 1%

Right leg = 18%

Left leg = 18%

Figure 2-6 Wallace Adult Rule of Nines. Using the diagram, each region of the body is divided into regions representing 9% of the total body surface area. Note: Rule of Nines tends to overestimate burn area by 1% to 3%.

representing 9% of the total body surface. Due to differences in anthropometric proportions, separate diagrams are available for use in the adult and pediatric populations (Figures 2-6 and 2-7). Location of the burn is documented and size of the burn calculated based on affected regions of the body diagram.

Lund-Browder (LB) Chart

The LB chart (Figure 2-8) is thought to be the most accurate assessment of a burn area when used correctly. It considers the body shape, size, and age of the patient when assigning total body surface area and therefore can be also used for children.[10] The LB chart consists of two drawings of the human body, one of the anterior body surface area and one of the posterior body surface area. The assessor draws the shape of the burn onto the chart, excluding simple erythematous areas. Each area is assigned a value of the body surface area percentage, which is entered into a table. The total body surface area affected by burn is then calculated.[30]

Palmar Surface Method

This method uses the surface area of the hand to estimate the surface area of a burn. The palmar surface area, including the fingers, represents roughly 1% of the total body surface area (Figure 2-9). Therefore the number of "palms" required to cover a burn injury can be used as an approximation of size. This method can be fairly accurate and reliable when evaluating smaller burns with irregular shapes or scattered distributions. However, accuracy and reliability steadily decline when measuring burns that involve more than 15% of total body surface area.[10]

Examination of Periwound Tissue

When caring for a patient with acute or chronic wounds, it is important to fully assess the area surrounding the wound. Skin surrounding a wound site is vulnerable, and

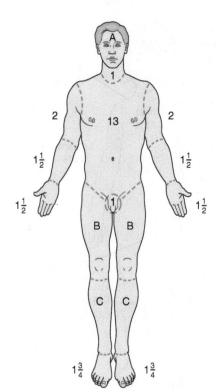

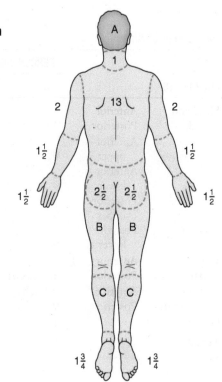

% Total Body Surface Area Burn

- Be clear and concise
- Do **not** include erythema

REGION	% Anterior	% Posterior
Head		
Neck		
Ant. trunk		
Post. trunk		
Right arm		
Left arm		
Buttocks		
Genitalia		
Right leg		
Left leg		
Total burn		

AREA	Age 0	1	5	10	15	Adult
A = $\frac{1}{2}$ OF HEAD	$9\frac{1}{2}$	$8\frac{1}{2}$	$6\frac{1}{2}$	$5\frac{1}{2}$	$4\frac{1}{2}$	$3\frac{1}{2}$
B = $\frac{1}{2}$ OF ONE THIGH	$2\frac{3}{4}$	$3\frac{1}{4}$	4	$4\frac{1}{2}$	$4\frac{1}{2}$	$4\frac{3}{4}$
C = $\frac{1}{2}$ OF ONE LOWER LEG	$2\frac{1}{2}$	$2\frac{1}{2}$	$2\frac{3}{4}$	3	$3\frac{1}{4}$	$3\frac{1}{2}$

Figure 2-8 Lund-Browder (LB) Chart. The shape of the burn is drawn onto the chart, excluding simple erythematous areas. Each area is assigned a value of the body surface area percentage, which is entered into the table and the total body surface area affected is then calculated. (Redrawn from Hettiaratchy S, Papini R: Initial management of a major burn: II—assessment and resuscitation, *BMJ* 329:101, 2004.)

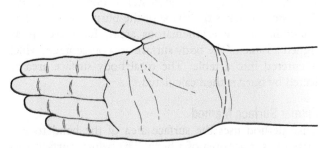

Figure 2-9 Palm and fingers represent 1% of total body surface area. (From Magee DJ: *Orthopedic physical assessment*, ed 6, St. Louis, 2014, Saunders.)

Factors Affecting Periwound Tissue

- Drainage from a fistula or stoma
- Excessive perspiration
- Increased wound exudate
- Removal of adhesive products
- Sensitivities, such as allergic reactions

periwound (i.e., skin surrounding the wound) problems are a frequent occurrence. Damage to periwound tissue may delay healing, increase the size of the original wound, and cause pain and discomfort that may adversely affect the patient's quality of life. Wounds such as venous leg ulcers, pressure ulcers, and diabetic foot ulcers may leave the periwound tissue more vulnerable due to the increased prevalence of maceration and exudate associated with these wound pathologies.[31] There are a number of wound-related factors that may also compromise the periwound skin, such as those listed in the following textbox.[32]

Examination of the periwound skin is performed by observation and palpation to determine whether there are any changes in skin characteristics (e.g., appearance, texture, temperature, or moisture content) with the skin being described in different ways (e.g., moist or dry, warm or cold, and rough or smooth).[33] If skin is devoid of hair, has a shiny appearance, and looks thin and fragile, it may indicate a chronic decrease in vascular supply. It is important to remember that skin lesions and inflammation may appear differently depending on the skin tone of the patient. Red or brown lesions on white skin may appear black or purple in people with darker skin pigment. It can also be difficult to identify areas of mild erythema (i.e., redness) in individuals with darker skin shades. The following items should be considered during the assessment of periwound tissue.

Callus (Hyperkeratosis)

Callus formation is most commonly observed on the soles of the feet or areas of increased pressure on the skin, uneven weight distribution, or friction on the skin.[33] The presence of excessive stresses on the upper layers of the epidermis may cause an increase in keratin production, leading to areas of skin that may be rough, thick, and yellow in color. Calluses tend to occur over bony prominences exposed to repeated pressure, friction, and shear. Although intended as a protective response to prevent damage to deeper tissue layers, when excessive callus formation occurs, the callus itself can lead to further problems in pressure distribution and may impair proper delivery of oxygen and nutrients to deeper tissue layers. In addition, the presence of callus may obscure underlying tissue damage, making it harder to identify areas of inflammation or infection. This is particularly true in patients with diabetic neuropathy in which damage to the autonomic nerve supply affects the function of sebaceous glands, leading to excessive dryness, cracking, and fissures at the sole of the foot. This increases the propensity toward callus formation and vulnerability toward tissue breakdown. Bony foot deformities resulting from the combined effects of motor and sensory neuropathy, as well as gait and balance impairments present in diabetic peripheral neuropathy, also contribute to excessive pressure and shear at the sole of the foot. These factors can also increase the likelihood of callus formation and subsequent tissue breakdown. Therefore, patients with a diabetic peripheral neuropathy should be advised to regularly apply emollient (a substance to soften tissue) to the heels and soles of the foot and have calluses regularly filed down or removed by a podiatrist.[31] Areas between the toes should be kept dry to decrease risk of fungal infection.

Color and Temperature

Warmth, increase in pain, and drainage at the wound site may indicate infection.[34] If capillaries in the periwound area around pressure ulcers have become damaged, the skin may become erythematous with the red color persisting despite removal of the pressure. This is more easily determined in white or lightly pigmented skin and is termed *unblanchable erythema*.[33] If the erythema persists after removing the pressure, it may signal a stage 1 pressure ulcer as defined by NPUAP.[17] Depending on the type of trauma, nonblanchable erythema may also indicate a superficial burn. If the skin tone of the patient makes it difficult to determine the presence of erythema, the clinician should compare the color on the opposite side of the body or ask the patient or family members, if appropriate, about color changes.

Induration (Hardening of the Tissue)

Presence of induration indicates excess fluid trapped within the tissue layers of the periwound skin and may signify a relapse to phase 1 of the inflammatory process. Induration may be described as an abnormal hardening of the tissue caused by consolidation of edema due to trauma or infection. Occasionally, induration will also be accompanied by visual changes including the appearance of small indentations or hollows in the skin resembling the peel or skin of an orange (i.e., *peau d'orange*).

Excoriation (Injury to Body Surface Caused by Trauma)

Excoriation is an abrasion of the superficial layers of the skin or linear erosion caused by itching, scratching, alteration of the natural moisture content, contact with topical irritants, presence of pathogenic microorganisms, or removal of adherent dressings. Repeated removal of adhesives in the same area can lead to a problem known as "skin stripping." Inflammatory skin damage, edematous changes, pain, and a negative effect on the skin barrier function may result.[35] Conditions that may predispose a patient to excoriation include urinary and/or fecal incontinence, excessive perspiration, use of harsh or caustic topical cleansers (which contribute to desiccation of the skin), and the presence of an artificial stoma, such as a tracheostomy or colostomy. In addition, older patients tend to be more vulnerable to both excoriation and stripping due to reductions in skin hydration, tissue turgor, and elasticity.

Fungal Infections

The alkaline nature of some wound fluid coupled with the increased humidity from the bandages can contribute to fungal growth.[36] Normally, the epidermis retains a slightly acidic pH. This *"acid mantle"* helps to protect against the excessive proliferation of surface bacteria and other pathogens. Alterations in the microenvironment of the skin due to illness or injury can lead to an increase in transient and resident flora, which are often the cause of mucocutaneous infections. Controlling the moisture content and temperature and maintaining normal pH balance will help to lower the risk of developing a fungal infection. It is prudent to have samples undergo laboratory analysis if fungal infection is suspected because incorrect treatment may lead to exacerbation of symptoms.[32]

Maceration (Skin Breakdown due to Prolonged Exposure to Moisture)

Prolonged exposure of the skin to moisture can lead to changes in the appearance of the skin, such as softening, swelling, and wrinkling of the epidermis. The moisture can be the result of wound exudate or body fluids, such as perspiration, urine, or fecal material. Macerated skin has been shown to be more sensitive to irritants[37] and may lead to breakdown of tissue in the periwound area leading to an enlarged wound. If the periwound tissue is white in color, it may mean there is maceration but little inflammation. However, red and inflamed periwound tissue may indicate erythematous maceration, which may be accompanied by contact dermatitis or weeping.[38] Maceration of periwound tissue may result in excoriation, pain, and discomfort. Maceration can be avoided by appropriate selection of skin protectants and dressings.

Scarring

Scar tissue that is immature will be thin, flexible, and more susceptible to skin breakdown than healthy tissue. A new scar will appear light pink in color regardless of skin pigmentation. Thick and rigid scarring may lead to susceptibility of future skin breakdowns in addition to impairing motion, specifically if the wound is at or near a joint surface. Formation of **hypertrophic scarring** (Figures 2-10 and 2-11) appears to have a genetic component and is excess scar tissue within the boundaries of the wound. Hypertrophic scarring can sometimes also result from repeated or excessive stresses on the wound site during the proliferative phase of healing. The body responds to the excessive stress with an increase in collagen formation, leading to scar tissue that extends above the original wound dimensions. In addition to cosmetic concerns, this type of scarring may adhere to underlying layers, causing problems in soft tissue mobility and range of motion. Hypertrophic scarring is a major concern in burn injuries, particularly ones that involve excessive tissue depth or cross the surface of the joint. **Keloid scars**, which "spill out" beyond the wound margins, tend to be more common in people with intensely pigmented skin, have a female to male ratio of 2:1, and most commonly occur on the upper trunk (Figure 2-12; see Figure 2-10). The exact etiology behind keloid scars is unknown, but it is thought that estrogen and growth factors are important influences, in addition to immunological influences and genetic predisposition.[39] Prevention and management may include the use of splinting to prevent contracture, as well as compression garments to encourage remodeling.

Edema

Edema is an accumulation of fluid in the intracellular tissues and may be characterized as acute, subacute, or chronic. Immediately following an injury, the presence of edema is an early sign of inflammation, resulting from a transient increase in capillary permeability to large plasma proteins and other constituents of the blood. When large

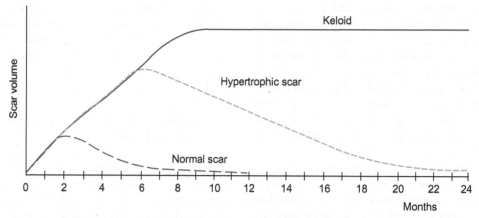

Figure 2-10 Growth of scar tissues. (From Nicoletis C, Bazin S, Le Lous M: Clinical and biochemical features of normal, defective, and pathologic scars, *Clin Plast Surg* 4:350, 1977.)

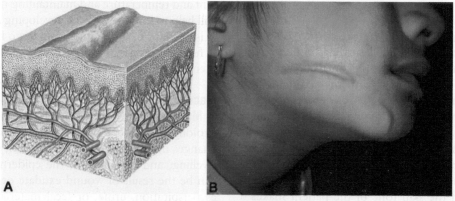

Figure 2-11 A, Diagrammatic hypertrophic scarring. Note how scar is larger than normal scar and stays within wound margin. **B,** Hypertrophic scar on cheek limited to original site of injury. Note normal scar on chin. (**A,** From Goldman MP, Fitzpatrick RE: Cutaneous laser surgery: the art and science of selective photothermolysis, ed 2, St. Louis, 1998, Mosby. **B,** From Zaoutis LB, Chiang VW, editors: *Comprehensive pediatric hospital medicine*, Philadelphia, 2007, Mosby/Elsevier.)

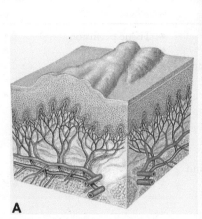
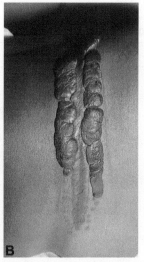

Figure 2-12 A, Diagrammatic keloid scarring. **B,** Keloid scars are thick scars that form in the lower area of the skin and expand beyond the original boundaries of the wound. This photo shows keloids that formed at suture holes after surgery. (**A,** From Weston WL, Lane AT: *Color textbook of pediatric dermatology,* ed 3, St. Louis, 2002, Mosby. **B,** From Thibodeau GA, Patton KT: *The human body in health and disease,* ed 4, St Louis, 2005, Mosby/Elsevier.)

plasma proteins leave the vascular bed, the oncotic pressure (a form of osmotic pressure) gradient is disrupted, causing excess fluids to follow. As the histamine reaction subsides, capillary permeability is restored to its usual level. These fluids are either reabsorbed into the local circulation or removed via the lymphatics. The presence of edema should be carefully evaluated before treatment. In patients with cardiovascular disease, localized edema (particularly within the extremities) may be indicative of cardiac pump failure. Care must be taken not to promote return of the fluid into the systemic circulation to avoid additional cardiac stresses. The same is true for patients with end-stage renal disease, in which the collection of excessive fluid within the abdomen (ascites) and extremities can indicate a protein imbalance and/or inability of the excretory system to remove fluids and toxins from the body. In certain cases the presence of excessive swelling can eventually lead to tissue breakdown because of increased pressures and secondary impairments in the delivery of adequate oxygen and nutrients to the affected area.[33] This is what often occurs in patients with venous insufficiency, in which chronic dependent edema in the lower extremities contributes to skin breakdowns in the gaiter area of the leg (i.e., the region that lies between the ankle and the knee, along the lower shin and calf area).

In closed traumas, such as fractures and crush injuries, excessive accumulation of fluid can cause compartment syndrome, resulting in the need for emergent surgery to alleviate pressures on the internal vasculature and nerve supply.

Hemosiderin Staining

Hemosiderin staining causes brownish discoloration of the legs and occurs when chronic venous stasis causes a change in skin elasticity and texture (Figure 2-13). The staining is caused by iron from hemoglobin leaking

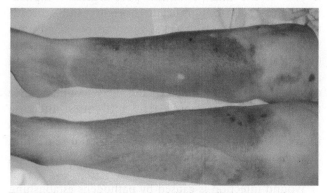

Figure 2-13 Hemosiderin staining of the lower limbs occurs when iron from hemoglobin leaks out of red blood cells that have broken due to venous pressure. This causes brownish discoloration of the legs.

out of red blood cells, which have broken down due to increased venous pressure. Eventually the build-up of swelling in the area causes the skin to fail and break open, and a venous stasis ulcer results.[34] The leakage of proteins and accumulation of fibrin around the capillaries can lead to impaired circulation and sluggish lymphatic turnover.

Infection

Infected wounds, such as pressure ulcers, can lead to delayed healing, temporary disability, and prolonged hospital stays, and in severe cases, the patient may develop septicemia (life-threatening infection), which causes thousands of deaths each year.[40] Infection is one of the greatest challenges in chronic wound closure. Many factors will influence healing in surgical, acute, and chronic wounds, and the most significant risk factor is the level of bacterial burden relative to the immune response of the patient or host. These risk factors are summarized in Table 2-8.[41,42]

TABLE **2-8**

Risk Factors for Wound Infection[41,42]

Patient Factors	Surgical Factors	Anesthetic Factors	Other
• Diabetes • Nutrition • Smoking • Alcohol intake • Chronic renal failure • Liver function • Body mass index • Age • Medications • Chemotherapy • Radiotherapy	• Surgical classification • Skin preparation • Site and duration of surgery • Complexity of surgery • Presence of suture or foreign body • Suturing quality • Preexisting infection • Hematoma • Mechanical stress on wound	• Tissue perfusion • Normovolemia • Hypovolemia • Body temperature • O_2 saturation • Blood transfusion	• Wounds with necrotic tissue • Wound near areas of contamination, such as the groin • Microbial virulence and pathogenicity

Early identification of wound infection is vital for timely implementation of the appropriate treatment and for improved patient outcomes. Wound infection is one of the most common postsurgical complications and leads to significant mortality and morbidity.[43] Reports indicate that as many as 5% of patients who undergo surgery develop a surgical site infection (SSI).[44] Infection rates for SSIs are typically grouped according to surgical classification: clean, clean-contaminated, contaminated, and dirty wounds. Since the introduction of prophylactic antibiotics, infection rates of SSIs have been greatly reduced. Infection rates in the U.S. National Nosocomial (Hospital) Infection Surveillance system are reported to be: 2.1% clean, 6.4% contaminated, and 7.1% dirty.[45]

Wound infection is caused by pathogens establishing themselves within the host tissue, multiplying and causing a host reaction. Direct contact and poor hand sanitization methods of health care professionals are thought to be significant factors for common entry of pathogens into a wound. Some of the risk factors for infection can be avoided by use of modern surgical techniques and prophylactic antibiotics. In acute and chronic wounds, prevention also relies on proper cleansing and debridement, as well as careful attention to clean and sterile technique.

Ways in Which Microorganisms Gain Access to a Wound[46]

• Direct contact: transfer from hands of care givers or from equipment
• Airborne dispersal: deposited from the surrounding air
• Self-contamination: physical migration from the patient's skin or gastrointestinal tract

Infection may be localized to the wound site or systemic. The classic signs of infection are purulent or excessive exudate, heat, edema, erythema, cellulitis, pyrexia (increased temperature), delayed healing, wound breakdown, fragile granulation tissue, and presence of pus.[47] However, not all of these features are present in some patients with chronic wounds, particularly with microvascular or macrovascular disease, immunocompromise, or patients on anti-inflammatory medications, such as corticosteroids.[48] In these patients the only sign of infection may be failure of the wound to heal.

Contamination of a wound in the absence of active bacterial proliferation in a wound is not considered to be relevant to clinical practice. Due to the presence of resident flora on the surface of healthy, intact skin, all open wounds have some level of bacterial contamination. Instead, the presence of bacteria in a wound should be thought of as a continuum that may progress from contamination, to colonization, to critical colonization, in which replication of bacteria begins to overwhelm the immune response of the patient or host. Colonization in a wound (i.e., healing by secondary intention) is considered to be a healthy stable state even though the bacteria may be growing and multiplying. If a patient's immune response is efficient, a balance will be maintained and presence of bacteria in the wound will not lead to an infection.[49] However, if the patient's defense mechanisms are suppressed, then critical colonization may occur. *Critical colonization* is the state between colonization and infection when multiplication of bacteria delays wound healing but without some of the common signs and symptoms of infection.[41] Wound management involves prevention of bacterial invasion, with early detection and intervention to prevent progression of contamination to infection.[49] In a colonized but not infected wound, there is the risk of obtaining a false positive result in wound culture tests, which can lead to unnecessary treatment. To avoid inappropriate testing and treatment, it is important to use clinical judgment to distinguish between contaminated and infected wounds. Testing should only be performed when the presence of infection is suspected due to patient symptoms and/or changes in the clinical presentation of the wound or the presence of delayed healing.

For patients with suspected infections, it is the current reference standard to perform a deep tissue biopsy. However, tissue biopsies are painful and invasive. Therefore most acute and chronic wounds are cultured using a wound surface swab. Use of wound cultures should be reserved for cases involving existing signs of infection or delayed healing due to the presence of surface bacteria in all open wounds and intact skin. The presence of bacteria alone does not indicate infection unless the number and virulence of the pathogen have overwhelmed or overburdened the immune response of the patient or host.

Three Techniques Commonly Used to Obtain a Wound Culture

- Tissue biopsy
- Needle aspiration
- Swab

Removal of a piece of tissue using a scalpel or punch biopsy is critical to achieve a quantitative culture of wound tissue, which is the gold standard for identification of wound infection.[50] Although tissue biopsies are considered the gold standard, they are time consuming, costly, and not within the scope of all wound care specialists. Swab culture is more cost effective and is noninvasive; therefore it is more commonly used in clinical settings. Quantitative swab culture technique is considered adequate by many to identify any bacterial species causing wound infection and can be used to guide antibiotic therapy.[51,52]

INTERVENTIONS

In the United States the Agency for Health Care and Policy Research (AHCPR, now known as the Agency for Healthcare Research and Quality [AHRQ]) recommends that initial pressure ulcer risk assessment be done on admission and reassessed at regular intervals.[53] The frequency of reevaluation will depend on the acuity of the individual and how rapidly a patient's condition changes over time.

Patients at higher risk of developing pressure-related wounds include older adults, patients with impaired mobility, under sedation, and having decreased motivation due to psychological overlay, and those with impaired cognition. Tools that can be used to assess the level of risk include the Norton[54] and Braden[55] Scales. The Norton Pressure Sore Risk Assessment Scale (Figure 2-14) was created in Britain in 1962 and examines five categories to calculate an overall score predicting likelihood of breakdown.[54] These categories include the patient's physical condition, activity level, mobility level, cognition, and presence of incontinence.

Lower scores indicate individuals at higher risk. The Braden Scale (Figure 2-15) is the most commonly used pressure ulcer assessment scale in the United States.[55] The Braden Scale has six subscales: sensory perception, moisture, activity, mobility, nutrition, and friction or shear. It addresses the main etiological factors behind pressure ulcer development, intensity and duration of pressure and tissue tolerance for pressure.[55] A lower score indicates a patient at higher risk. Positioning and pressure redistribution are key factors in the prevention and management of pressure ulcers.

Positioning and Pressure Redistribution

For patients at risk, as well as those who have already developed a pressure ulcer, there are a number of interventions commonly used for redistributing pressure (Figure 2-16).

Interventions Commonly Used for Pressure Redistribution

- Modified support surfaces
- Reducing duration of loading by increasing frequency of turning and positioning
- Positioning devices and posture
- Weight shifting

The use of support surfaces in the treatment of pressure ulcers includes reactive and active surfaces. A reactive surface responds to the load placed upon it, whereas an active surface dynamically changes the body–support surface interface.[56] The effectiveness of a support surface can be measured by monitoring physiological responses, such as blood flow and tissue oxygenation, or by directly measuring the interface pressure. Support surfaces can be foam, air, water, or elastomeric mattresses, cushions, and overlays.[57]

Reducing the duration of loading is pertinent for patients who may be unable to reposition themselves independently or for patients who do not have the sensory feedback that would prompt repositioning. Using turning schedules and teaching weight-shifting strategies are necessary interventions for these patients.

Turning frequency is dependent on the support surface. Recommendations derived from research studies investigating optimal turning frequency range from every 2 to 6 hours depending on the support surface, stage of the ulcer healing, and mobility level of the patient.[58-60] When it comes to positioning of the patient, alternating between side lying and supine is common practice. In side lying, the greater trochanter, the malleoli, and medial femoral epicondyles are at increased risk, but the use of positioning devices, such as pillows or wedges, can effectively unload these bony prominences. In addition, rather than lying directly on the lateral aspect of the hip, pressure on the greater trochanter can be alleviated by slightly rotating the body 5° to 10° laterally. When lying in a supine position, care must be taken to avoid friction or shear in

Norton Scale for Assessing Risk of Pressure Ulcers*

Instructions: Complete the form by scoring each item from 1 to 4. Put 1 for low level of functioning and 4 for highest level functioning,

Name: _____   Date: _____

Criterion	Score
Physical condition	4 = Good
	3 = Fair
	2 = Poor
	1 = Very bad
Mental condition	4 = Alert
	3 = Apathetic
	2 = Confused
	1 = Stupor
Activity	4 = Ambulant
	3 = Walk with help
	2 = Chair bound
	1 = Bed bound
Mobility	4 = Full
	3 = Slightly impaired
	2 = Very limited
	1 = Immobile
Incontinent	4 = Not
	3 = Occasionally
	2 = Usually/Urine (catheter)
	1 = Doubly (urine and feces)
TOTAL SCORE =	

Greater than 18 - Low risk
Between 18 and 14 - Medium risk
Between 14 and 10 - High risk
Less than 10 - Very high risk

Figure 2-14 Norton Scale for Assessing Risk of Pressure Ulcers. (Modified from Norton D, McLaren R, Exton-Smith AN: *An investigation of geriatric nursing problems in hospital,* London, 1962, National Corporation for the Care of Old People.)

the buttocks. The amount of pressure and shear on the buttock is increased if the head of the bed is elevated; so although this is a more functional position for eating or drinking, it should not be used for extended periods. Keeping the head of the bed below a 45° angle and raising the foot of the bed can counteract the sliding motion, but there is still increased pressure on the sacral area.

Weight-shifting maneuvers can be taught to wheelchair users and patients with limited mobility. In bed, repositioning may be facilitated by the use of rails and/or installation of an overhead frame or trapeze.

Weight-Shifting Maneuvers for Wheelchair Users and Patients with Limited Mobility

- Pushing on the arms of the chair with the arms to lift the buttocks off the cushion
- Leaning forward to rest the trunk on the lower limbs
- Leaning over to one side and then repeat leaning over to the opposite side
- Using the powered tilt and recline function on powered wheelchairs to redistribute the pressure

Patient's Name		Evaluator's Name		Date of Assessment			
SENSORY PERCEPTION Ability to respond meaningfully to pressure-related discomfort	**1. Completely limited:** Unresponsive (does not moan, flinch, or grasp) to painful stimuli, due to diminished level of consciousness or sedation. OR Limited ability to feel pain over most of body surface.	**2. Very Limited:** Responds only to painful stimuli. Cannot communicate discomfort except by moaning or restlessness. OR Has a sensory impairment that limits the ability to feel pain or discomfort over half of body.	**3. Slightly Limited:** Responds to verbal commands, but cannot always communicate discomfort or need to be turned. OR Has some sensory impairment that limits ability to feel pain or discomfort in one or two extremities.	**4. No Impairment:** Responds to verbal commands. Has no sensory deficit which would limit ability to feel or voice pain or discomfort.			
MOISTURE Degree to which skin is exposed to moisture	**1. Constantly Moist:** Skin is kept moist almost constantly by perspiration, urine, etc. Dampness is detected every time patient is moved or turned.	**2. Very Moist:** Skin is often, but now always moist. Linen must be changed at least once a shift.	**3. Occasionally Moist:** Skin is occasionally moist, requiring an extra linen change approximately once a day.	**4. Rarely Moist:** Skin is usually dry, linen only requires changing at routine intervals.			
ACTIVITY Degree of physical acitivity	**1. Bedfast:** Confined to bed	**2. Chairfast:** Ability to walk severely limited or non-existent. Cannot bear own weight and/or must be assisted into chair or wheelchair.	**3. Walks Occasionally:** Walks occasionally during day, but for very short distances, with or without assistance. Spends majority of each shift in bed or chair.	**4. Walks Frequently:** Walks outside the room at least twice a day and inside room at least once every 2 hours during waking hours.			
MOBILITY Ability to change and control body position	**1. Completely Immobile:** Does not make even slight changes in body or extremity position without assistance.	**2. Very Limited:** Makes occasional slight changes in body or extremity position but unable to make frequent or significant changes independently.	**3. Slightly Limited:** Makes frequent though slight changes in body or extremity position independently.	**4. No Limitations:** Makes major and frequent changes in position without assistance.			
NUTRITION Usual food intake pattern	**1. Very Poor:** Never eats a complete meal. Rarely eats more than a third of any food offered. Eats two servings or less of protein (meat or dairy products) per day. Takes fluids poorly. Does not take a liquid dietary supplement. OR Is NPO and/or maintained on clear liquids or IVs for more than 5 days.	**2. Probably Inadequate:** Rarely eats a complete meal and generally eats only about half of any food offered. Protein intake includes only three servings of meat or dairy products per day. Occasionally will take a dietary supplement. OR Receives less than optimum amount of liquid diet or tube feeding.	**3. Adequate:** Eats over half of most meals. Eats a total of four servings of protein (meat, dairy products) each day. Occasionally will refuse a meal, but will usually take a supplement if offered. OR Is on a tube feeding or TPN regimen that probably meets most of nutritional needs.	**4. Excellent:** Eats most of every meal. Never refuses a meal. Usually eats a total of four or more servings of meat and dairy products. Occasionally eats between meals. Does not require supplementation.			
FRICTION AND SHEAR	**1. Problem:** Requires moderate to maximum assistance in moving. Complete lifting without sliding against sheets is impossible. Frequently slides down in bed or chair, requiring frequent repositioning with maximum assistance. Spasticity, contractures, or agitation leads to almost constant friction.	**2. Potential Problem:** Moves feebly or requires minimum assistance. During a move, skin probably slides to some extent against sheets, chair, restraints, or other devices. Maintains relatively good position in chair or bed most of the time but occasionally slides down.	**3. No Apparent Problem:** Moves in bed and in chair independently and has sufficient muscle strength to lift up completely during move. Maintains good position in bed or chair at all times.				
				Total Score			

At risk = 15-18; Moderate risk = 13-14; High risk = 10-12; Severe Risk = 9.
Key: IV, intravenously; *NPO,* nothing by mouth; *TPN,* total parenteral nutrition.

Figure 2-15 Braden Scale for predicting pressure sore risk. (Copyright. Barbara Braden and Nancy Bergstrom, 1988. Reprinted with permission. All Rights Reserved.)

Splinting

Deciding on the appropriate splint for pressure relief, for protection, or to off-load a limb will depend on the mobility status of the patient. Factors to consider are whether the splint will be used while in bed only or if the patient will also be using the device for transfers and ambulation. The algorithm in Figure 2-17 displays some of the elements one needs to consider when providing a cast or splint.

Integumentary Repair and Protection Techniques

The presence of eschar or scab in dry wounds can delay epithelialization and wound contraction. Removal of impediments to healing can be done through cleansing or debridement. Cleansing typically uses fluid to remove debris and microorganisms on the wound surface.[61] Debridement (i.e., removal of damaged tissue or a foreign object from the wound[62]) involves the use of mechanical or chemical measures for the removal of adherent materials, such as necrotic tissue. There are numerous methods of cleansing, irrigating, and hydrating wound tissue. The size, location of the wound, and facilities available (e.g., inpatient versus outpatient clinic), as well as the knowledge, skill, and comfort level of the clinician, should all be considered when determining the appropriate method based on individual patient presentation.

Wound Cleansing

Prepackaged, single-dose, 8-psi, sterile irrigation can be used for simple cleansing. It is advisable to use splash guards during any irrigation procedures to avoid transfer of contaminated fluid to the treatment area. Sponges, cloths, or gauze may also be used for superficial cleansing when doused in saline or other cleansing detergents. The AHRQ has recommended avoiding use of antiseptic formulas or disinfectants on chronic wounds and limiting these agents to acute wound care.[63] The most commonly used irrigants are sterile water and sterile saline. Saline is preferred to maintain osmotic gradients within physiological tissues. The AHRQ guidelines[63]

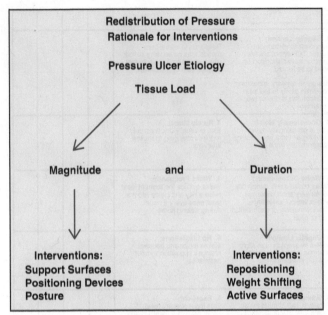

Figure 2-16 Redistribution of pressure: rationale for interventions. This model considers both magnitude and timing of loading to be important in pressure ulcer development. The magnitude of pressure can be controlled by strategies such as selection of support surfaces, and duration is addressed by turning and weight-shifting frequencies. (From Sprigle S, Sonenblum S: Assessing evidence supporting redistribution of pressure for pressure ulcer prevention: a review, *J Rehabil Res Dev* 48(3):203-213, 2011.)

also state that a pressure of less than 4 psi is unlikely to remove bacteria from the wound, and more than 15 psi might drive the bacteria or debris into the wound bed. Therefore, 4 to 15 psi is the recommended range for irrigation pressure.

Clinical Note

- When cleansing wounds, sterile irrigation should be between 4 and 15 psi

Debridement

Debridement is usually performed in conjunction with irrigation. Necrotic tissue may serve as a culture medium for bacteria, and often, wounds with necrotic tissue will not heal until the necrotic tissue is removed. The body may slough off the dead tissue on its own, but in cases in which this fails to happen, debridement may be necessary to facilitate wound healing. Debridement also allows removal of tissue samples for culture and sensitivity testing to confirm cases of suspected infection and to identify the best medication to facilitate recovery. For patients with intact neurological function, one of the negative side effects of debridement is pain. Use of topical anesthesia directly into the wound bed, regional anesthesia achieved

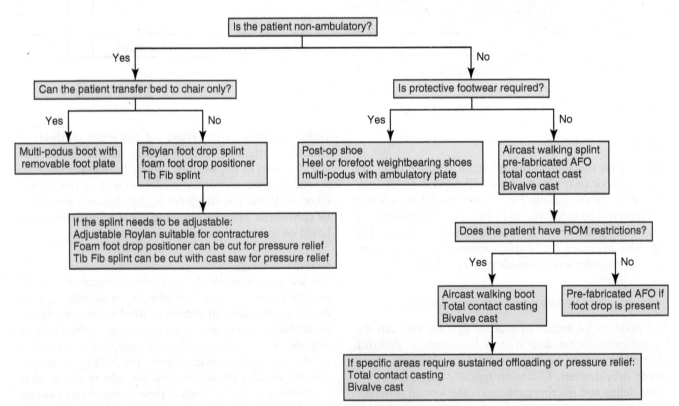

Figure 2-17 This algorithm for choice of splinting demonstrates the elements to consider when using a cast or splint for wound management. (Modified from Brigham and Women's Hospital: Standard of care: wound care/integumentary management. Physical Therapy management of the patient at risk for or with an integumentary disorder. Copyright © 2009 The Brigham and Women's Hospital, Inc., Department of Rehabilitation Services.)

by a nerve block, or in extreme cases, general, spinal, or epidural anesthesia may be required.[62]

As a rule, debridement methods (Table 2-9) may be divided into two distinct categories: selective and nonselective. Selective methods target only the necrotic tissue or debris and are preferred when a substantial proportion of the wound has already entered the proliferative phase, and care must be taken to protect the new granulation tissue and/or epithelial budding. Nonselective methods are used when the majority of the wound bed remains covered by necrotic tissue or debris or very little granulation tissue or new cell growth is present.

Surgical or Sharp Debridement. Surgical or sharp debridement is considered to be the gold standard for removal of necrotic tissue using selective methods. It is most commonly used when patients have increased risk of infection or gross contamination or for quick removal of large quantities of necrotic tissue. In surgical or sharp debridement, necrotic tissue and other foreign material can be removed using scalpels, scissors, and/or forceps. The clinician should use caution if sharp debridement is to be performed on patients on anticoagulant therapy or those with bleeding disorders. In addition, the clinician should be skilled in distinguishing necrotic tissue from underlying normal tissues because there is the risk of inadvertently removing viable tissue, such as a tendon, or other structures that may be mistaken as slough. Therefore clinicians should consider interprofessional consultation to identify the team member who is most skilled in performing this procedure. The choice of whether or not to use sharp debridement methods will also depend on the size and location of the wound, as well as the treatment setting and whether adequate support and resources are available in case of adverse events. Within the United States, physical therapists and other health professionals should consult their state practice acts to be sure this technique falls within their legal scope of practice.

Biological Debridement. The use of fly larvae (i.e., maggots) to debride nonviable tissue was first introduced following anecdotal observation that maggots will only ingest nonviable tissue, making this a form of selective debridement.[64,65] Although the method remained unpopular due to concerns for safety and potential psychological stresses for the patient, a series of research studies conducted in the early 1990s affirmed that this method is highly effective in promoting debridement and accelerated wound closure. The efficacy of this method relies on three modes of action: debridement of necrotic tissue, removal of microorganisms and pathogens that may contribute to infection, and release of growth factors or cytokines to enhance formation of new tissue. The therapeutic use of maggots for tissue debridement should be distinguished from maggot infestation that sometimes accompanies neglect, poor sanitation, and/or limited access to care. Biological debridement, or biotherapy, is a well-controlled intentional process. Evidence-based information suggests a therapeutic dose of five to eight larvae per square centimeter (0.5 square inch) of wound surface area. Larvae are placed onto a piece of gauze netting, which is inverted over the wound. The wound is surrounded by a halo of hydrocolloid, which prevents migration of the larvae from the wound bed, and covered by a layer of nylon or Dacron netting and adhesive tape to secure its position. A light gauze bandage is then used as a secondary bandage to absorb exudates and liquefied necrotic tissue produced during this process. The maggots remain in place for approximately 48 to 72 hours and can be removed through irrigation or pulsed lavage. Maggots and associated materials should be handled as biological waste. This process may be repeated over several cycles, as indicated, until a clean, granulating wound bed has been achieved.[65] Biological debridement has been successfully employed in several types of chronic wounds, particularly neuropathic (diabetic) foot ulcers and chronic leg ulcers of vascular etiology. Most patients report little, if any, associated physical discomfort, and detailed patient education regarding safety and treatment rationale is usually sufficient to allay psychological concerns.[66,67]

Autolytic Debridement. This selective method of debridement uses the individual's endogenous enzymes to remove the necrotic tissue. This is achieved by placing a moisture-retentive occlusive or semiocclusive dressing over the wound and allowing the proteases within the wound to liquefy the necrotic tissue. In well-perfused wounds, this method is painless and has the benefit of being easy to perform. The patient should be closely monitored for signs of infection, especially patients who are immunocompromised. This method is contraindicated in infected wounds because it may lead to more severe infection. In addition, this method can be somewhat slower than other means of selective debridement

TABLE 2-9

Types of Wound Debridement

Type	Description
Surgical or sharp	Necrotic tissue removed using scalpel, scissors, forceps, or curette
Biological	Maggot larvae: consume necrotic tissue and bacteria
Autolytic	Endogenous enzymes in wound fluid interact with moist dressings to soften and remove tissue
Enzymatic	Enzymes degrade and remove necrotic tissue
Mechanical	Wet-to-dry: moist dressings are allowed to dry on the wound and are then removed
Hydrotherapy: flowing water removes loose debris
Pulsed lavage: irrigation combined with suction

due to the time required for production and action of endogenous enzymes to occur. Therefore autolytic debridement is often used in combination with other methods, such as serial sharp debridement, whirlpool, or pulsed lavage.

Enzymatic Debridement. Use of topical enzymatic agents, such as papain or collagenase, is a popular treatment choice for nonviable or devitalized tissue.[62] Proteolytics, fibrinolytics, and collagenases act on necrotic tissue. However, papain urea debriding breaks down eschar and is the agent of choice in necrotic wounds. Cross-hatching or scoring the wound base allows for deeper penetration of the enzymatic agent. This method does not require a physician present and is relatively safe and effective without being cost prohibitive. Enzymatic debridement is often the selective debridement method of choice for patients who are not candidates for surgical debridement or for patients in long-term facilities and care homes where sharp debridement facilities are not available. Careful choice of dressings and cleaning substances is advised because metals, such as silver, may interfere with the enzymes, deactivating them. In addition, although this method is considered to be selective, repeated or prolonged exposure to enzymatic agents can damage viable tissue. Therefore specific application of topical ointments should be confined to areas of slough or eschar only. Topical antibiotic powder can be applied to the wound to prevent excessive bacterial growth on the liquefied material that can be produced during this method of debridement. In addition, a petroleum-based skin protectant can be used to reduce possible irritation of periwound tissues.

Mechanical Debridement. Mechanical debridement is nonselective because these methods target the entire wound bed as a whole. Mechanical methods can include wet-to-dry dressings, pulsed lavage, and whirlpool therapy.

Wet-to-dry dressings involve the placement of saline-soaked gauze on the wound surface. When the gauze is dry, it is removed, taking away devitalized tissue and debris on the gauze. However, because this method is notoriously painful and has a strong potential to damage viable tissue and underlying granulation tissue, it is rarely indicated and is no longer favored within clinical settings.[68]

Hydrotherapy or whirlpool therapy is one of the oldest therapies still in use in the modern era. Whirlpool therapy is jointly considered a method of wound cleansing as well as mechanical debridement. The agitation of water combined with injected air can remove necrotic tissue and foreign material and may dilute bacterial content. Care must be taken to control the pressure on the wound because excessive pressures or shearing forces may damage granulation tissue, extend the wound margins, or cause maceration.[69] Care must be taken to ensure the water and tank are clean before allowing the patient to receive treatment in the whirlpool tank. Cross-contamination is an issue if multiple patients are using the same tank, and although antibacterial agents in the water may help prevent this, these detergents may damage new tissues. In addition, even when care is taken to disinfect surfaces between patient use, it can be very challenging to properly cleanse and dry the internal mechanisms within the jets and turbines. However, the benefits of whirlpool therapy are numerous and beneficial in the following scenarios:

1. Patients for whom dressing changes are painful. The dressings can be soaked and removed gently by either the patient or the caregiver.
2. The warmth of the water promotes increased blood flow to the wound surface.
3. The resistance and buoyancy of the water can facilitate range-of-motion exercise, strengthening exercises, and functional exercises, such as aqua walking or jogging.

The frequency and duration of whirlpool sessions range from 20 to 30 minutes, 3 to 4 times per week.[69] Temperature of the water will vary and should be adjusted based on the stage of healing (e.g., avoid excessive warmth during the acute inflammatory stage or in the presence of excessive edema). The nature and presentation of the wound should also be considered because the affected limb will be in a dependent position throughout the treatment. For this reason, whirlpool therapy is generally deferred in patients with venous insufficiency, although when needed, parameters can be adjusted to include cooler temperatures and less exposure duration. Furthermore, to prevent infection or an increase in size of the wound, whirlpool therapy or soaking of the wound should be avoided in patients with stable, dry gangrene until restoration of necessary circulation has been achieved.

Pulsed lavage is the direct delivery into the wound of a cleansing solution or irrigant under pressure produced by a single-patient use, battery-powered device (Figure 2-18). This method has overtaken whirlpool treatment in popularity due to its portability, lower cross-contamination risks, and ease of use in patients with poor mobility or those being treated in isolation rooms. Like whirlpool, pulsed lavage is considered a wound cleansing method as well as a nonselective method of mechanical debridement. It is used to remove debris or infectious agents from the wound bed and surface. Pulsed lavage is particularly effective for neuropathic and venous ulcers, abscesses (pus in wound), or dehiscent (splitting open of wound)

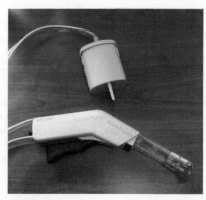

Figure 2-18 Pulsed lavage device.

wounds. It is also useful following sharp or surgical debridement to remove the necrotic tissue that remains or develops after surgical debridement. However, it is not effective at removing hard eschar. Patients with widespread wounds or burns may be more effectively treated using whirlpool therapy. Use of the appropriate pressure will be the key determinant in how effective pulsed lavage will be for wound cleansing. Low pressures may be used for cleansing, and higher pressures often used when more of a debriding effect is desired. Pressures of between 5 and 10 psi have been found to be effective at removing loose necrotic tissue, wound exudate, and loose surface debris.[61] Using pressure of greater than 10 psi is more effective at preventing gross wound infection. Use of a splash guard and personal protective equipment for all personnel and any family members or visitors in the immediate vicinity of the treatment areas is necessary to minimize risks associated with splashing of contaminated fluid and bacteria that may be aerosolized during treatment. For these reasons, patients must also be treated in closed quarters. All intravenous sites, ports, and other potential areas for access of bacteria should be covered to prevent cross-contamination during treatment. Sterile saline is the most commonly used irrigant for pulsed lavage, although sometimes sterile water is also used. Most pulsed lavage devices come equipped with suction to collect fluids and materials removed from the wound bed. Such materials should be treated as biohazardous waste and disposed of accordingly.

Low-Intensity Phototherapy

There is an array of terms used to describe the use of light for therapeutic effect, including phototherapy, low-level laser therapy, low-power laser therapy, low-intensity laser therapy, cold laser, therapeutic laser, light-emitting diode, low reactive-level laser, and diode laser.[70] Low-intensity phototherapy has been described as highly effective in the treatment of tissue repair but with stronger evidence coming from experimental animal research than from human studies.[71] There are a small number of studies that have shown that laser therapy can be beneficial in the treatment of diabetic foot ulcers that have been unresponsive to conventional treatment.[72,73] The variables to consider when using low-intensity phototherapy are wavelength, power, power density, energy, energy density, treatment duration, chronicity of the wound, and the mode of treatment. The clinician must also consider elements of patient presentation, including wound size, patient history, presence of co-morbidities, and any concomitant treatment of the wound.[71] Energy density has been found to have a predictable dose-dependent treatment effect.[74] The mechanisms of action of phototherapy include promoting fibroblast proliferation, collagen synthesis, cellular and subcellular processes needed to augment formation of type I and type III procollagen pools of mRNA, ATP synthesis, and lymphocytic action.[71,74] The range of variables that need to be accounted for can make it complicated to compare studies, and there is a need for more well-controlled, blinded studies in clinical populations. There are few contraindications and side effects associated with this intervention, so, despite the controversy surrounding its effectiveness in humans, it remains a popular treatment modality.

Wound Dressings

There are numerous factors to consider when selecting an appropriate dressing for wounds. These factors are summarized in Table 2-10 and include the nature of the wound, level of moisture or hydration of the wound and surrounding tissues, location of the wound, and types of materials available.[75] Determining the main aims of dressing application will also influence the choice of dressings.

Function of Wound Dressings

- Facilitate the healing process by retaining warmth, moisture, cells, enzymes, and growth factors in the wound bed
- Promote autolytic debridement
- Fill dead space to prevent formation of hematomas, abscesses, and sinus tracts
- Manage odor and exudate by drainage, evaporation, or occlusion
- Reduce pain
- Prevent or manage infection
- Improve patient quality of life, achieved by minimizing distress or disturbance, or by hiding or covering wounds

Primary dressings typically refer to the dressing in contact with the wound itself or materials placed directly in the wound bed. Secondary dressings are used to cover and secure the primary dressing. The Center for Medicare and Medicaid Services (CMS) recognizes the categories of dressings listed in the following textbox.[76]

Types of Wound Dressings

- Hydrogel (sheets)
- Biological and synthetic membranes
- Impregnated
- Silicone gel sheets
- Contact layers
- Silver technology
- Elastic gauzes
- Transparent films
- Wound fillers
- Gauzes and nonwoven dressings
- Liquid skin protectants
- Hydrocolloids
- Moisture barriers
- Hydrogels (amorphous)
- Therapeutic moisturizers
- Hydrogels (impregnated dressings)
- Skin substitutes
- Oxygen reconstituted cellulose

From Irion G: *Comprehensive wound management*, ed 2, Thorofare, 2010, SLACK.

TABLE **2-10**

Factors Influencing Wound Dressing Selection

Factor	Description
Wound type	• Superficial • Full thickness • Cavity
Wound description	• Necrotic • Sloughy • Granulating • Epithelializing
Wound characteristics	• Dry • Moist • Excessive exudate • Malodorous • Painful • Bleeds easily • Location
Bacterial profile	• Sterile • Colonized • Infected • Risk of serious cross-infection
Product-related factors	• Conformity and volume • Fluid-handling properties • Potential for sensitization • Ability to absorb odor • Antibacterial properties • Hemostatic properties • Permeability to fluid and microorganisms • Ease of use • Fiber-fast • Nontoxic
Patient-related factors	• Wound etiology • Continence • Sensitivity to medicated dressings • Fragile skin • Need to bathe or shower regularly • Compliance
Economic considerations	• Unit and treatment cost • Cost of alternative materials • Prescription required • Availability in stores or pharmacies • Availability in local formularies

Modified from Thomas S: *A structured approach to the selection of dressings*, World Wide Wounds, 1997. Available at: http://www.worldwide-wounds.com/1997/july/Thomas-Guide/Dress-Select.html. Accessed April 28, 2015.

Transparent Film Dressings

Transparent films can be used as primary or secondary dressings. They are clear polyurethane membranes with a semipermeable adhesive surface. These dressings will accumulate liquid and exudate underneath because they have no absorption properties and can therefore be used to enhance autolytic debridement in noninfected wounds. However, if used with wounds having excessive exudate, there is a risk of leakage and maceration of the periwound tissue. The impermeable nature of the film means they protect the wound from contamination, and the transparency allows the patient, clinician, and caregivers to monitor the wound without disturbing the dressing. Films may also be used as a secondary dressing to hold wound fillers or primary dressings in place and are often used in conjunction with gauze and alginates (a salt or ester of alginic acid).

Hydrogels

Hydrogels are hydrative dressings that add moisture to a wound and may be indicated when wounds are dry (i.e., desiccated) or may be used to provide a soothing effect on burns and superficial abrasions.[76] Hydrogels are manufactured as sheets or amorphous material. The sheet form of hydrogels can be used on partial-thickness and full-thickness wounds, and due to the high moisture content, they are easily removed without causing additional trauma to the wound. Hydrogel sheets usually require a secondary dressing to hold them in place. Amorphous (lacking definite form) hydrogels come in a tube and can be applied using a cotton swab to hydrate dry wounds, loosen slough, and protect structures, such as tendons, nerves, and ligaments, from desiccation. The use of sheet hydrogels is discouraged in infected wounds, but amorphous hydrogels may instead be used, usually in combination with a carrier material, such as gauze or another secondary dressing.

Hydrocolloid Dressings

These dressings are moisture-retentive dressings made of pectin, carboxymethylcellulose, and adhesives. When the wound side of the dressings interacts with exudate or wound fluid, a gel is formed, leading to a moist environment.[77] The dressing in contact with the periwound skin will remain adhesive until the exudate soaks through and migrates toward the edges of the dressing. Often a layer of skin protectant will be applied to periwound skin to prevent rolling of the edges of the sheet and minimize skin injury during removal of the dressing. These dressings are worn for several days and on application allow for limited wound visualization. Hydrocolloid dressings are semiocclusive in nature, so they are not suitable for use in contaminated or infected wounds. These dressings are also not advised in wounds with subcutaneous defects, such as tracts or tunnels, unless used as a secondary dressing in combination with wound fillers, such as gauze roping, alginate, or hydrofiber.

Alginates and Hydrofibers

Alginates are a very versatile and absorbent dressing. They are made of nonwoven fibers derived from seaweed, composed of calcium salts of alginic acid, and typically absorb at higher rates than hydrocolloids. When they are dry, alginates have a feltlike fibrous consistency, but when they absorb fluid, they turn into a gel. This gel conforms to the wound bed, maintaining a moist environment. Alginates can be combined with collagen, which promote wound healing as the combination is absorbed into the wound. Hydrofiber dressings are composed of sodium carboxymethylcellulose fibers, which have the ability to absorb large amounts of wound exudate. Alginates and hydrofiber dressings should not be used on dry dressings, hard eschar, or third-degree burns. They should also not be used in full-thickness wounds when tendon, nerve, or periosteum has been exposed. Removal of an alginate or hydrofiber dressing from a wound that has turned dry will have a similar effect to a wet-to-dry dressing, which can be painful to remove and cause trauma to the wound bed. Instead, the dressing should be moistened with saline before removal to prevent discomfort and associated tissue injury.

Foam Dressings

Foam dressings are typically made from a polyurethane base with a heat- and pressure-modified wound contact layer. They are highly absorbent, promote autolytic debridement, and are permeable to gases and water vapors. Foam dressings are used to provide a moist wound environment, most commonly in wounds with moderate-to-heavy exudate. They are very adaptable dressings and provide a cushioning effect, making them suitable for bony prominences or areas of increased friction. Not all foam dressings have adhesive edges, so they may need a secondary dressing to secure them in place. Foam dressings may be used in combination with enzymatic debriders and other agents, and newer-generation foams are available with ionic silver, a wide-spectrum antimicrobial. If changed daily, they can be used in the treatment of infected wounds, but the clinician should check the package insert before use.

Silver Technology

Silver has long been used in the management and treatment of wounds arising from burns, but the development of silver-containing dressings has led to a new interest in its use for wound management. It is the antimicrobial properties of silver that make it popular for use in nonhealing wounds. There are now ranges of proprietary silver dressings, which incorporate the metal into an alignate or hydrocolloid base, as well as fabric-based, silver-impregnated dressings.[78] It is thought that silver dressings provide immediate and sustained release of ionic silver and act as an effective barrier to bacterial penetration. In addition, silver ions are thought to interact with the cell membranes of bacteria, causing leakage, and apoptosis (i.e., cell death without release of harmful substances). Binding of the silver ions with proteins within the bacteria reduces the bacteria's ability to produce enzymes needed for replication.[79] For these reasons, silver dressings are often used in infected or highly colonized wounds and have proven effective in exerting antimicrobial effects in a variety of gram-positive and gram-negative pathogens, including methicillin-resistant staphylococcus aureus (MRSA), pseudomonas aeruginosa, and proteus.[80] Some reports have suggested that combining silver with suitable dressings may decrease some of the unwanted side effects, such as toxicity and staining, while increasing their antimicrobial efficacy.[81] Gradual, sustained release is thought to counteract some previous concerns associated with the use of silver, including studies that questioned whether silver might be cytotoxic to keratinocytes and fibroblasts.[82] In addition, due to concerns regarding the development of silver-resistant strains of bacteria, this intervention should be reserved for use in wounds showing overt signs of infection and should not be indiscriminately applied prophylactically unless there is evidence to suggest a high risk of contamination. In any case the use of silver should be reviewed at a 2-week minimum to ensure that effective progress is being made toward goals for appropriate wound management.

Honey Dressings

Honey has been used in the treatment of wounds for many years. Those typically used in the treatment of wounds are medical-grade honeys (MGHs) and are chosen for their bactericidal properties. *Leptospermum* honeys are the most widely studied, but local-regional honeys have also been reported in the literature. This presents a unique challenge in identifying which properties of honey are universal and those that are unique.[83] Honey has been used in the treatment of traumatic wounds, surgical incision sites, burns, sloughy wounds, and pressure ulcers.[84] It is also used for topical treatment of infected wounds or as a prophylactic treatment in patients susceptible to MRSA and other antibiotic-resistant bacteria.[85] Honey has been found to improve healing times in mild-to-moderate superficial and partial-thickness burns compared with conventional dressings; however, there is a conflicting report on its efficacy on other wound types.[86] The mechanisms of action of honey in promoting wound healing are summarized in Table 2-11.[87] The following practical considerations for the use of honey were described in a review by Molan.[85] The amount of fluid exudate will determine the amount of honey to be used. If the exudate is rapidly diluting the honey, then the frequency of application will need to be adjusted. It is preferable to apply the honey to an absorbent dressing rather than directly to the wound to prevent loss of honey from the wound before the dressing is applied. It may also be necessary to warm the honey to body temperature or to dilute it with 1 part water to 20 parts honey to facilitate soaking into the absorbent dressing. Depressions or cavities of wounds can be filled with honey to take advantage of the antibacterial components diffusing into the deeper

TABLE **2-11**

Beneficial Effects of Medical-Grade Honey on Wound Healing

Effects	Description
Antibacterial activity	• Broad spectrum of activity, including antifungal • Effective against antibiotic resistant species • Effective against bacteria in biofilms
Debriding action	• Activates plasminogen which lyses fibrin-attaching slough • Prevents formation of eschar and scabs
Anti-inflammatory activity	• Clinical observation of reduced symptoms of inflammation • Biochemical and histological studies show decreased inflammation • Inhibits phagocytosis, the start of the inflammatory response
Antioxidant activity	• Contains plant phenolics from the nectar source • Scavenges reactive oxygen species • Decreases oxidative activation of proteases which destroy the matrix and growth factors
Increasing healing rate	• Stimulates leukocytes to release cytokines and growth factors that activate tissue repair • Acidity of honey allows for increased oxygen availability from the circulation for tissue repair • Osmotic action leads to outflow of lymph fluid

Modified from Molan P: The evidence and the rationale for the use of honey as a wound dressing, *Wound Pract Res* 19(4):215, 2011.

wound tissues. For practical purposes, treatment is usually applied using commercially available dressings consisting of pads that are preimpregnated with MGH. It is important to remember that honey designed for medical use differs significantly from culinary honeys. Most culinary honeys are heat pasteurized, a process that destroys the natural enzymes that contribute to its antimicrobial properties, making them less effective when used in the treatment of wounds.

Scar Management

Scar tissue is the end product of wound healing. It serves to restore tissue continuity, along with some tensile strength, and tissue function. However, scar tissue lacks the strength and elasticity of normal skin. Scar tissue also lacks some functions of normal skin, including melanization, sweating, and oil secretion. Scar tissue does not have hair follicles and the pigmentation differs from that of normal skin. If there has been a period of immobilization during the healing phases, the presence of scar tissue can increase risk of adhesions to subcutaneous structures, which may cause pain, and loss of range of motion. During the healing phases, controlling unwanted stresses and increasing stresses that produce a better quality scar should be considered when selecting splints or positioning patients.

Topical interventions, such as pressure garments, are often used as part of scar management, notably in burn patients.

Considerations when Choosing Pressure Garments or Devices for Scar Management[88]

- Healing time
- Size of the scar area
- Fragility of the healed skin
- Location of the scar

Scar mobilization can be used to increase range of movement around a joint that has been limited due to scar tissue. There is a three-point scale that can be used to describe the extent to which mobility is limited due to scar tissue.[76] A score of 3/3 indicates normal mobility that is the same as normal skin, 2/3 indicates mild hypomobility, and 1/3 indicates moderate hypomobility. When using this scale, the clinician should assess range of motion in all planes of movement that would normally be available at that joint.

Many patients require some desensitization before scar mobilization. Desensitization can include gentle tapping, massage, or rubbing the scar with different textures, such as soft clothes and coarser textures. To gain a prolonged increase in range, scar mobilization should be performed regularly for a number of sessions before significant improvement is observed. The scar tissue should be pushed and pulled in all directions in a slow and sustained manner. Skin blanching indicates the beginning of relevant stretching of the scar tissue. Other techniques, such as plucking and rolling, can be used by the clinician to mobilize adherent scar tissue. It should be noted that patients are less likely to be as aggressive as a clinician in their own self-mobilization techniques due to the discomfort the techniques can cause. The patient should be educated on how to perform stretches correctly, and if appropriate, a home exercise program of stretching exercises should be given to the patient. Gravity and assistive devices, such as pulleys and traction devices, may also be of help.

ADJUNCTIVE INTERVENTIONS IN WOUND MANAGEMENT

Therapeutic Ultrasound

Ultrasound uses sound waves, which are transferred into a tissue through a hydrated medium, such as a gel or mist, through a treatment applicator. The depth of tissue reached by the ultrasound is dependent on the frequency. Typical therapeutic ultrasound frequencies used in wound management include frequencies of 1 and 3 MHz and noncontact low-frequency ultrasound (40 kHz). Because the frequency of the ultrasound device determines the depth of penetration, the approximate depth of penetration for a 3 to 3.3-MHz ultrasound is estimated at 0.5 to 1 cm beneath the surface of the skin, whereas a 1-MHz ultrasound is thought to penetrate 0.5 to 5 cm beneath the surface of the skin.[89] The benefits of therapeutic ultrasound can be classified into thermal or nonthermal effects. Thermal effects are achieved at intensities of 1.0 to 1.5 W/cm² and can improve scar or wound outcomes when used in the late stages of wound healing or during the remodeling phase. However, the frequencies at which therapeutic ultrasound is used by clinicians when treating open wounds tend to draw on the nonthermal effects. These effects are typically gained at intensities of 0.3 to 1.0 W/cm². The nonthermal effects include acoustic streaming, which is a unidirectional steady mechanical force, and cavitation. Cavitation is the production and vibration of small bubbles within the coupling medium and fluids within the tissues. The bubbles collect, condense, and are compressed. The movement and compression may lead to changes in cellular activities in the tissue. Both cavitation and acoustic streaming are thought to cause changes in cell membrane permeability and diffusion of cellular metabolites. Basic science and laboratory proof of the following effects of ultrasound have been reported in the literature.[69]

Beneficial Effects of Therapeutic Ultrasound on Wound Healing[69]

- Cellular recruitment
- Collagen synthesis
- Increased collagen tensile strength
- Angiogenesis
- Wound contraction
- Fibroblast stimulation
- Macrophage stimulation
- Fibrinolysis
- Reduction in inflammatory phase
- Promotion of proliferative phase

Research regarding the use of therapeutic, high-frequency ultrasound in wound management is sparse, and further studies using better methodology are required to reach a definitive decision on the effect of therapeutic ultrasound. When reviewing the use of therapeutic ultrasound for the treatment of venous leg ulcers, the Cochrane group reported that there was some available evidence suggesting accelerated wound closure with use of this modality.[90] A similar review of the use of therapeutic ultrasound for treatment of

pressure ulcers failed to find any substantial evidence of benefit.[91]

In terms of clinical evidence of the benefits of therapeutic ultrasound, there have been some studies that use noncontact ultrasound therapy, in which low-frequency ultrasound (40 kHz) is delivered through a fine, sterile saline mist, which transmitted the ultrasound energy (also known as "MIST therapy"). These studies were using ultrasound to achieve wound healing via wound cleansing and removal of the yellow slough, fibrin, tissue exudates, and bacteria.[92] It is suggested that therapeutic ultrasound used in this way is indicated until slough is removed and healthy granulation tissue covers the wound bed. Other effects of this modality may include an increase in the synthesis and release of growth factors, improved blood flow, accelerated angiogenesis, and better collagen content and alignment during the proliferative phases of healing. MIST therapy has been shown to be effective in promoting accelerated rates of wound closure for a variety of chronic wounds, including diabetic foot ulcers and vascular ulcers.[93,94]

Electrical Stimulation

Electrical stimulation is the application of electrical current through electrodes placed on the skin near the wound or directly within the wound. It allows clinicians to deliver exogenous electrical signals into wound tissue, which mimics the underlying natural bioelectrical response to injury. It has been found that within 1 mm of the wound edge, there is a natural steady electrical field that can be manipulated through therapeutic electrical stimulation to accelerate the wound-healing process.[95] The resulting electrical fields can cause the stimulation of biomolecular signaling pathways and cell migration.[69] Electrical stimulation has been found to promote cellular activity in nearly all phases of experimental wound healing.[96] The effects of electrical stimulation are summarized in Table 2-12.

Current research focuses in the area of electrical stimulation are to develop new technologies, including dressings with embedded batteries, which will make the electrical stimulation devices more tractable for clinical uses, and the design of devices for use in the community, which may be a more cost-effective therapy than current standard therapies.

Compression Therapy

Compression therapy has long been a mainstay of treatment for vascular management and treatment of wounds arising from venous insufficiency. Benefits of compression therapy include edema management and improved venous return. However, many patients cannot tolerate the stockings and compression bandages that are commonly used. External pneumatic pressure therapy or intermittent compression therapy (ICT) can yield similar effects to compression bandages and stockings. ICT

TABLE **2-12**

Effects of Electrical Stimulation on Wound Healing[69,96]

Negative Current	Positive Current	Both
• Decreases edema surrounding the electrode	• Promotes epithelial growth and organization	• Stimulate neovasculature
• Lyses necrotic tissue	• Acts as a vasoconstrictor	• Have a bacteriostatic effect
• Simulates growth of granulation tissue	• Denatures protein	• Stimulate receptor sites for specific growth factors
• Increases blood flow	• Aids in preventing postischemic lipid perioxidization	
• Causes fibroblasts to proliferate and produce collagen	• Decreases mast cells in healing wounds	
• Causes epidermal cell migration	• Attracts macrophages	
• Attracts neutrophils		
• Stimulates directional growth of neurites		

uses an air pump to inflate and deflate an airtight bag wrapped around the limb, causing intermittent compression of the limb. ICT can cause a collapse of the superficial venous system, forcing blood into the deep venous system with an increase in subcutaneous pressure. This can prevent blood, fibrins, and protein from leaking out of the skin capillaries. Some studies have proposed that enhancement of fibrinolysis is yielded through ICT.[97] A Cochrane review summarized that ICT might increase healing compared with no compression and when used in conjunction with compression bandages. However, more studies are required to determine if ICT can be a substitute for compression bandages. Rates of application of external pneumatic pressure can vary. The ICT bags can be rapidly inflated and deflated. One study compared a rapid inflation protocol with a slow inflation protocol (0.5 seconds to inflate, 6-second plateau, 12-second deflation versus 60-second inflation, 30-second plateau, 90-second deflation) and reported that rapid ICT healed more venous leg ulcers than slow ICT.[98] The use of ICT is contraindicated in patients with deep vein thrombosis and peripheral vascular disease. Patients with congestive heart failure should be very closely monitored if an ICT protocol is used in their treatment plan.

Negative Pressure Wound Therapy (NPWT)

NPWT is also known as topical NPWT, vacuum-sealing technique, sealed surface wound suction, vacuum-assisted closure, or vacuum pack technique. It involves the application of subatmospheric pressure to a healing wound. A porous dressing will allow for an even distribution of pressure throughout the wound. This dressing is placed in direct contact with the wound with a drain attached to the vacuum device. A polyurethane covering should extend approximately 2 cm beyond the wound edges to provide an airtight seal. There are ongoing discussions regarding the intensity, intermittent or constant pressure, and the filler material to cover the wound.[99] Negative pressures of -50 to -150 mm Hg have been reported in the literature.[99,100]

Treatment Goals for the Application of Negative Pressure Wound Therapy (NPWT)[101]

- Provide a temporary wound cover
- Manage wound fluid and edema
- Accelerate patient mobility
- Improve pain management
- Prevent wound progression
- Increase dermal and wound perfusion
- Stimulate formation of granulation tissue
- Enhance wound bed reepithelialization
- Improve matrix material availability
- Reduce bacterial load
- Provide a moist wound environment that is preferable for wound healing
- Influence expression of genes involved in the wound-healing process, such as growth factors, TGF-β expression, and genes that elicit angiogenesis and cellular proliferation

---

NPWT is often used in the treatment of acute wounds in which healing by primary intention is unlikely or not possible. This includes grossly contaminated wounds and complex soft tissue injuries. NPWT is also used to treat chronic wounds, such as pressure ulcers, trophic, and vascular ulcers. The absence of well-designed studies makes it challenging to draw reliable conclusions regarding the efficacy of NPWT in the treatment of chronic wounds.[100] However, single studies have suggested that NPWT can lead to accelerated closure of diabetic foot ulcers when compared with current standards of care using moist wound-healing principles.[102,103] NPWT is contraindicated in wounds with exposed viscera, intestinal fistulas, in the presence of invasive soft tissue infection, wound necrosis, or active bleeding. Clinicians should be aware that NPWT can cause pain, pressure necrosis around the wound edges, hemorrhage, and infection when the patient is not properly monitored and treatment is not properly adjusted in light of these adverse responses.[69,101]

Hyperbaric Oxygen Therapy

Hyperbaric oxygen treatment has been used in the treatment of a myriad of medical conditions since the 1960s. It involves the patient breathing 100% oxygen while being exposed to increased atmospheric pressure. The pressures in the chamber are typically 2 to 3 atmospheres absolute (ATA), and treatments can last 1 to 2 hours, 2 to 3 times daily depending on the reason for choosing this modality. A typical course may last 15 to 30 days.[104] Arterial oxygen tension can exceed 2000 mm Hg, and the pressure in tissues can reach 200 to 400 mm Hg during treatment.[105] It has been well established that breathing more than 1 ATA of oxygen will result in increased production of reactive oxygen species. This provides the molecular basis for the therapeutic benefits of this therapy through stimulation of pathways for growth factors, cytokines, and hormones. Wounds that should respond well to hyperbaric oxygen therapy include those with depletion of epithelial and stromal cells, chronic inflammation, fibrosis, and abnormalities in the components of the extracellular matrix and those with impaired keratinocyte function.[105] These characteristics are often seen in diabetic lower extremity wounds and delayed radiation injuries. However, it must be noted that reactive oxygen species can also cause detrimental effects on wound healing through damage to DNA and oxidation of lipids, amino acids, and enzymatic cofactors, leading to defective cellular functioning.[106] There is a lack of high-quality research reporting on the clinical benefits of hyperbaric oxygen therapy, with many of the studies demonstrating flaws in the study design and reporting. Therefore there is a need for further adequately powered research into the therapeutic and clinical benefits of hyperbaric oxygen therapy in acute and chronic wound healing.

Therapeutic Exercise

Therapeutic exercise can provide many benefits to patients with acute or chronic wounds. Exercise including gentle active or passive range of movement exercises can assist in edema management, increased perfusion, prevention of contractures, maintenance of mobility, and improved endurance (Table 2-13). It is thought that physical exercise may enhance cutaneous blood flow and accelerate angiogenesis due to its positive influence on production of vasoendothelial growth factor (VEGF).[108]

There are a very small number of studies that examine the effects of exercise on cutaneous wound healing. One such study[109] examined the effects of an exercise program on wound healing following a low-risk punch biopsy procedure in a group of older adults. This study found that the study participants assigned to the exercise group had a faster healing rate and increased cortisol secretion during stress testing following the intervention when compared with the participants assigned to the control group. The authors postulated that because exercise was associated with an enhanced neuroendocrine response, exercise might facilitate wound healing through neuroendocrine regulation and thus immune function changes. Another study,[110] which investigated the effects of exercise on subcutaneous wound healing in older mice,

found that moderate exercise elicited an improved healing response. This might be attributed to decreased levels of proinflammatory cytokines and chemokines found in the wound tissue. There is a need for further investigation on the effects of exercise on wound healing, but the research available to date would indicate that exercise can lead to improved wound healing due to the exercise-induced anti-inflammatory response.

SUMMARY

The objective of successful wound management is to achieve a clean wound bed, protect the wound bed, prevent and eliminate infection, and provide an optimal wound-healing environment. As the chapter shows, there are numerous tools available to assist in objectively monitoring a patient with an acute or chronic wound. These tools will assist in identifying signs of infection and documenting efficacy of treatment techniques and wound-healing progression. Using these tools will also allow the clinician to determine which treatment techniques are most suitable. Pressure management, dressing selection, and use of adjunctive therapies must be considered for patients at risk of integumentary disruption or for patients presenting with an acute or chronic wound.

TABLE 2-13

Types of Exercise Used in the Management of Patients with Wounds[107]

Type	Description
Therapeutic exercise	• Passive, active assisted, or active range of movement exercises in supine, sitting, or standing • Used for bilateral upper and lower extremities • Progression of intensity, duration, and frequency
Endurance training	• Increase out of bed tolerance • Progress time, distance, and frequency of ambulation • Develop an activity schedule with the patient, family, and caregivers
Gait training	• Preparation for gait • Education on weight-bearing restrictions and training of partial weight-bearing gait techniques • Gait retraining for patients with gait asymmetries • Assessment and prescription of assistive devices
Functional mobility	• Bed mobility • Transfers • Ambulation • Stair practice

APPENDIX 2-1

Pressure Ulcer Scale for Healing (PUSH) Tool 3.0
 (Copyright National Pressure Ulcer Advisory Panel (NPUAP), 2003 Reprinted with permission.)

Instructions for Using the Pressure Ulcer Scale for Healing (PUSH) Tool

To use the PUSH Tool, the pressure ulcer is assessed and scored on the three elements in the tool:
Length × Width –> scored from 0 to 10

Exudate Amount —> scored from 0 (none) to 3 (heavy)

Tissue Type —> scored from 0 (closed) to 4 (necrotic tissue)

In order to insure consistency in applying the tool to monitor wound healing, definitions for each element are supplied at the bottom of the tool.

Step 1: Using the definition for length × width, a centimeter ruler measurement is made of the greatest head to toe diameter. A second measurement is made of the greatest width (left to right). Multiple these two measurements to get square centimeters and then select the corresponding category for size on the scale and record the score.

Step 2: Estimate the amount of exudate after removal of the dressing and before applying any topical agents. Select the corresponding category for amount and record the score.

Step 3: Identify the type of tissue. Note: if there is ANY necrotic tissue, it is scored a 4. Or, if there is ANY slough, it is scored a 3, even though most of the wound is covered with granulation tissue.

Step 4: Sum the scores on the three element of the tool to derive a total PUSH Score.

Step 5: Transfer the total score to the Pressure Ulcer Healing Graph. Changes in the score over time provide an indication of the changing status of the ulcer. If the score goes down, the wond is healing. If it gets larger, the wound is deteriorating.

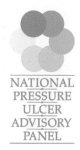

NATIONAL
PRESSURE
ULCER
ADVISORY
PANEL

Pressure Ulcer Scale for Healing (PUSH)
PUSH Tool 3.0

Patient Name_____ Patient ID# _____

Ulcer Location _____ Date _____

Directions:

Observe and measure the pressure ulcer. Categorize the ulcer with respect to surface area, exudate, and type of wound tissue. Record a sub-score for each of these ulcer characteristics. Add the sub-scores to obtain the total score. A comparison of total scores measured over time provides an indication of the improvement or deterioration in pressure ulcer healing.

LENGTH X WIDTH (in cm²)	**0** 0	**1** < 0.3	**2** 0.3 – 0.6	**3** 0.7 – 1.0	**4** 1.1 – 2.0	**5** 2.1 – 3.0	Sub-score
		6 3.1 – 4.0	**7** 4.1 – 8.0	**8** 8.1 – 12.0	**9** 12.1 – 24.0	**10** > 24.0	
EXUDATE AMOUNT	**0** None	**1** Light	**2** Moderate	**3** Heavy			Sub-score
TISSUE TYPE	**0** Closed	**1** Epithelial Tissue	**2** Granulation Tissue	**3** Slough	**4** Necrotic Tissue		Sub-score
							TOTAL SCORE

Length x Width: Measure the greatest length (head to toe) and the greatest width (side to side) using a centimeter ruler. Multiply these two measurements (length x width) to obtain an estimate of surface area in square centimeters (cm²). Caveat: Do not guess! Always use a centimeter ruler and always use the same method each time the ulcer is measured.

Exudate Amount: Estimate the amount of exudate (drainage) present after removal of the dressing and before applying any topical agent to the ulcer. Estimate the exudate (drainage) as none, light, moderate, or heavy.

Tissue Type: This refers to the types of tissue that are present in the wound (ulcer) bed. Score as a "4" if there is any necrotic tissue present. Score as a "3" if there is any amount of slough present and necrotic tissue is absent. Score as a "2" if the wound is clean and contains granulation tissue. A superficial wound that is reepithelializing is scored as a "1". When the wound is closed, score as a "0".

- 4 – **Necrotic Tissue (Eschar):** black, brown, or tan tissue that adheres firmly to the wound bed or ulcer edges and may be either firmer or softer than surrounding skin.
- 3 – **Slough:** yellow or white tissue that adheres to the ulcer bed in strings or thick clumps, or is mucinous.
- 2 – **Granulation Tissue:** pink or beefy red tissue with a shiny, moist, granular appearance.
- 1 – **Epithelial Tissue:** for superficial ulcers, new pink or shiny tissue (skin) that grows in from the edges or as islands on the ulcer surface.
- 0 – **Closed/Resurfaced:** the wound is completely covered with epithelium (new skin).

PUSH Tool Version 3.0: 9/15/98
©National Pressure Ulcer Advisory Panel

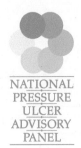

NATIONAL
PRESSURE
ULCER
ADVISORY
PANEL

Pressure Ulcer Healing Chart
To monitor trends in PUSH Scores over time
(Use a separate page for each pressure ulcer)

Patient Name_____ Patient ID# _____

Ulcer Location _____ Date _____

Directions:

Observe and measure pressure ulcers at regular intervals using the PUSH Tool.
Date and record PUSH Sub-scores and Total Scores on the Pressure Ulcer Healing Record below.

Pressure Ulcer Healing **Record**														
Date														
Length x Width														
Exudate Amount														
Tissue Type														
PUSH Total Score														

Graph the PUSH Total Scores on the Pressure Ulcer Healing Graph below.

PUSH Total Score	Pressure Ulcer Healing **Graph**													
17														
16														
15														
14														
13														
12														
11														
10														
9														
8														
7														
6														
5														
4														
3														
2														
1														
Healed = 0														
Date														

PUSH Tool Version 3.0: 9/15/98
©National Pressure Ulcer Advisory Panel

APPENDIX 2

Bates-Jensen Wound Assessment Tool.
  (Copyright 2001 Barbara Bates-Jensen.)

BATES-JENSEN WOUND ASSESSMENT TOOL
Instructions for use

<u>General Guidelines:</u>

Fill out the attached rating sheet to assess a wound's status after reading the definitions and methods of assessment described below. Evaluate once a week and whenever a change occurs in the wound. Rate according to each item by picking the response that best describes the wound and entering that score in the item score column for the appropriate date. When you have rated the wound on all items, determine the total score by adding together the 13-item scores. The HIGHER the total score, the more severe the wound status. Plot total score on the Wound Status Continuum to determine progress.

<u>Specific Instructions:</u>

1. **Size**: Use ruler to measure the longest and widest aspect of the wound surface in centimeters; multiply length x width.

2. **Depth**: Pick the depth, thickness, most appropriate to the wound using these additional descriptions:
   1 = tissues damaged but no break in skin surface.
   2 = superficial, abrasion, blister or shallow crater. Even with, &/or elevated above skin surface (e.g., hyperplasia).
   3 = deep crater with or without undermining of adjacent tissue.
   4 = visualization of tissue layers not possible due to necrosis.
   5 = supporting structures include tendon, joint capsule.

3. **Edges**: Use this guide:

Indistinct, diffuse	=	unable to clearly distinguish wound outline.
Attached	=	even or flush with wound base, <u>no</u> sides or walls present; flat.
Not attached	=	sides or walls <u>are</u> present; floor or base of wound is deeper than edge.
Rolled under, thickened	=	soft to firm and flexible to touch.
Hyperkeratosis	=	callous-like tissue formation around wound & at edges.
Fibrotic, scarred	=	hard, rigid to touch.

4. **Undermining**: Assess by inserting a cotton tipped applicator under the wound edge; advance it as far as it will go without using undue force; raise the tip of the applicator so it may be seen or felt on the surface of the skin; mark the surface with a pen; measure the distance from the mark on the skin to the edge of the wound. Continue process around the wound. Then use a transparent metric measuring guide with concentric circles divided into 4 (25%) pie-shaped quadrants to help determine percent of wound involved.

5. **Necrotic Tissue Type**: Pick the type of necrotic tissue that is <u>predominant</u> in the wound according to color, consistency and adherence using this guide:

White/gray non-viable tissue	=	may appear prior to wound opening; skin surface is white or gray.
Non-adherent, yellow slough	=	thin, mucinous substance; scattered throughout wound bed; easily separated from wound tissue.
Loosely adherent, yellow slough	=	thick, stringy, clumps of debris; attached to wound tissue.
Adherent, soft, black eschar	=	soggy tissue; strongly attached to tissue in center or base of wound.
Firmly adherent, hard/black eschar	=	firm, crusty tissue; strongly attached to wound base <u>and</u> edges (like a hard scab).

6.   **Necrotic Tissue Amount**: Use a transparent metric measuring guide with concentric circles divided into 4 (25%) pie-shaped quadrants to help determine percent of wound involved.

7.   **Exudate Type**: Some dressings interact with wound drainage to produce a gel or trap liquid. Before assessing exudate type, gently cleanse wound with normal saline or water. Pick the exudate type that is <u>predominant</u> in the wound according to color and consistency, using this guide:

Bloody	=	thin, bright red
Serosanguineous	=	thin, watery pale red to pink
Serous	=	thin, watery, clear
Purulent	=	thin or thick, opaque tan to yellow
Foul purulent	=	thick, opaque yellow to green with offensive odor

8.   **Exudate Amount**: Use a transparent metric measuring guide with concentric circles divided into 4 (25%) pie-shaped quadrants to determine percent of dressing involved with exudate. Use this guide:

None	=	wound tissues dry.
Scant	=	wound tissues moist; no measurable exudate.
Small	=	wound tissues wet; moisture evenly distributed in wound; drainage involves ≤ 25% dressing.
Moderate	=	wound tissues saturated; drainage may or may not be evenly distributed in wound; drainage involves > 25% to ≤ 75% dressing.
Large	=	wound tissues bathed in fluid; drainage freely expressed; may or may not be evenly distributed in wound; drainage involves > 75% of dressing.

9.   **Skin Color Surrounding Wound**: Assess tissues within 4cm of wound edge. Dark-skinned persons show the colors "bright red" and "dark red" as a deepening of normal ethnic skin color or a purple hue. As healing occurs in dark-skinned persons, the new skin is pink and may never darken.

10.   **Peripheral Tissue Edema & Induration**: Assess tissues within 4cm of wound edge. Non-pitting edema appears as skin that is shiny and taut. Identify pitting edema by firmly pressing a finger down into the tissues and waiting for 5 seconds, on release of pressure, tissues fail to resume previous position and an indentation appears. Induration is abnormal firmness of tissues with margins. Assess by gently pinching the tissues. Induration results in an inability to pinch the tissues. Use a transparent metric measuring guide to determine how far edema or induration extends beyond wound.

11.   **Granulation Tissue**: Granulation tissue is the growth of small blood vessels and connective tissue to fill in full thickness wounds. Tissue is healthy when bright, beefy red, shiny and granular with a velvety appearance. Poor vascular supply appears as pale pink or blanched to dull, dusky red color.

12.   **Epithelialization**: Epithelialization is the process of epidermal resurfacing and appears as pink or red skin. In partial thickness wounds it can occur throughout the wound bed as well as from the wound edges. In full thickness wounds it occurs from the edges only. Use a transparent metric measuring guide with concentric circles divided into 4 (25%) pie-shaped quadrants to help determine percent of wound involved and to measure the distance the epithelial tissue extends into the wound.

BATES-JENSEN WOUND ASSESSMENT TOOL   NAME

Complete the rating sheet to assess wound status. Evaluate each item by picking the response that best describes the wound and entering the score in the item score column for the appropriate date.

Location: Anatomic site. Circle, identify right **(R)** or left **(L)** and use **"X"** to mark site on body diagrams:

____ Sacrum & coccyx	____ Lateral ankle	
____ Trochanter	____ Medial ankle	
____ Ischial tuberosity	____ Heel	Other Site

Shape: Overall wound pattern; assess by observing perimeter and depth.

Circle and <u>date</u> appropriate description:

____ Irregular	____ Linear or elongated	
____ Round/oval	____ Bowl/boat	
____ Square/rectangle	____ Butterfly	Other Shape

Item	Assessment	Date Score	Date Score	Date Score
1. Size	1 = Length x width <4 sq cm 2 = Length x width 4--<16 sq cm 3 = Length x width 16.1--<36 sq cm 4 = Length x width 36.1--<80 sq cm 5 = Length x width >80 sq cm			
2. Depth	1 = Non-blanchable erythema on intact skin 2 = Partial thickness skin loss involving epidermis &/or dermis 3 = Full thickness skin loss involving damage or necrosis of subcutaneous tissue; may extend down to but not through underlying fascia; &/or mixed partial & full thickness &/or tissue layers obscured by granulation tissue 4 = Obscured by necrosis 5 = Full thickness skin loss with extensive destruction, tissue necrosis or damage to muscle, bone or supporting structures			
3. Edges	1 = Indistinct, diffuse, none clearly visible 2 = Distinct, outline clearly visible, attached, even with wound base 3 = Well-defined, not attached to wound base 4 = Well-defined, not attached to base, rolled under, thickened 5 = Well-defined, fibrotic, scarred or hyperkeratotic			
4. Undermining	1 = None present 2 = Undermining < 2 cm in any area 3 = Undermining 2-4 cm involving < 50% wound margins 4 = Undermining 2-4 cm involving > 50% wound margins 5 = Undermining > 4 cm or Tunneling in any area			
5. Necrotic Tissue Type	1 = None visible 2 = White/grey non-viable tissue &/or non-adherent yellow slough 3 = Loosely adherent yellow slough 4 = Adherent, soft, black eschar 5 = Firmly adherent, hard, black eschar			
6. Necrotic Tissue Amount	1 = None visible 2 = < 25% of wound bed covered 3 = 25% to 50% of wound covered 4 = > 50% and < 75% of wound covered 5 = 75% to 100% of wound covered			
7. Exudate Type	1 = None			

Item	Assessment	Date Score	Date Score	Date Score
	2 = Bloody 3 = Serosanguineous: thin, watery, pale red/pink 4 = Serous: thin, watery, clear 5 = Purulent: thin or thick, opaque, tan/yellow, with or without odor			
8. Exudate Amount	1 = None, dry wound 2 = Scant, wound moist but no observable exudate 3 = Small 4 = Moderate 5 = Large			
9. Skin Color Surrounding Wound	1 = Pink or normal for ethnic group 2 = Bright red &/or blanches to touch 3 = White or grey pallor or hypopigmented 4 = Dark red or purple &/or non-blanchable 5 = Black or hyperpigmented			
10. Peripheral Tissue Edema	1 = No swelling or edema 2 = Non-pitting edema extends <4 cm around wound 3 = Non-pitting edema extends ≥4 cm around wound 4 = Pitting edema extends < 4 cm around wound 5 = Crepitus and/or pitting edema extends ≥4 cm around wound			
11. Peripheral Tissue Induration	1 = None present 2 = Induration, < 2 cm around wound 3 = Induration 2-4 cm extending < 50% around wound 4 = Induration 2-4 cm extending ≥ 50% around wound 5 = Induration > 4 cm in any area around wound			
12. Granulation Tissue	1 = Skin intact or partial thickness wound 2 = Bright, beefy red; 75% to 100% of wound filled &/or tissue overgrowth 3 = Bright, beefy red; < 75% & > 25% of wound filled 4 = Pink, &/or dull, dusky red &/or fills ≤ 25% of wound 5 = No granulation tissue present			
13. Epithelialization	1 = 100% wound covered, surface intact 2 = 75% to <100% wound covered &/or epithelial tissue extends >0.5cm into wound bed 3 = 50% to <75% wound covered &/or epithelial tissue extends to <0.5cm into wound bed 4 = 25% to < 50% wound covered 5 = < 25% wound covered			
	TOTAL SCORE			
	SIGNATURE			

WOUND STATUS CONTINUUM

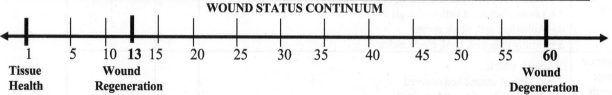

| 1 | 5 | 10 | **13** | 15 | 20 | 25 | 30 | 35 | 40 | 45 | 50 | 55 | **60** |

Tissue Health   **Wound Regeneration**   **Wound Degeneration**

Plot the total score on the Wound Status Continuum by putting an **"X"** on the line and the date beneath the line. Plot multiple scores with their dates to see-at-a-glance regeneration or degeneration of the wound.

REFERENCES

1. McGrath J, Eady R, Pope F: Anatomy and organization of human skin. In Burns T, Breathnach S, Cox N, et al, editors: *Rook's textbook of dermatology*, ed 8, Hoboken, 2010, Wiley-Blackwell.

2. Gantwerker EA, Hom DB: Skin: histology and physiology of wound healing, *Facial Plast Surg Clin North Am* 19(3):441–453, 2011.

3. Seneschal J, Clark RA, Gehad A, et al: Human epidermal Langerhans cells maintain immune homeostasis in skin by activating skin resident regulatory T cells, *Immunity* 36(5):873–884, 2012.

4. Maricich SM, Wellnitz SA, Nelson AM, et al: Merkel cells are essential for light-touch responses, *Science* 324:1580–1582, 2009.

5. Barrientos S, Stojadinovic O, Golinko MS, et al: Growth factors and cytokines in wound healing, *Wound Repair Regen* 16(5):585–601, 2008.

6. Koh TJ, DiPietro LA: Inflammation and wound healing: the role of the macrophage, *Expert Rev Mol Med* 13:e23, 2011.

7. Wild T, Rahbarnia A, Kellner M, et al: Basics in nutrition and wound healing, *Nutrition* 26(9):862–866, 2010.

8. Goldman RJ, Salcido R: More than one way to measure a wound: an overview of tools and techniques, *Adv Skin Wound Care* 15(5):236–243, 2002.

9. Bryant JL, Brooks TL, Schmidt B, et al: Reliability of wound measuring techniques in an outpatient wound center, *Ostomy Wound Manage* 47(4):44–51, 2001.

10. Hettiaratchy S, Papini R: Initial management of a major burn: II—assessment and resuscitation, *BMJ* 329:101–103, 2004.

11. Thomas AC, Wysocki AB: The healing wound: a comparison of three clinically useful methods of measurement, *Decubitus* 3(1):18–20, 1990.

12. Chang AC, Dearman B, Greenwood JE: A comparison of wound area measurement techniques: Visitrak versus photography, *Eplasty* 11:e18, 2011.

13. Palmer R, Ring E, Ledgard L: A digital video technique for radiographs and monitoring ulcers, *J Photographic Sci* 37(3-4):65–67, 1989.

14. Eagle M: Wound assessment: the patient and the wound, *Wound Essentials* 4:14–24, 2009.

15. Grey JE, Enoch S, Harding KG: Wound assessment, *BMJ* 332:285–288, 2006.

16. Meyer L: *Wound care: getting to the depth of the tissue*. Available at: https://www.nursece.com/courses/97. Updated 2014. Accessed May 11, 2014.

17. Black J, Baharestani MM, Cuddigan J, et al: National pressure ulcer advisory panel's updated pressure ulcer staging system, *Adv Skin Wound Care* 20(5):269–274, 2007.

18. Oyibo SO, Jude EB, Tarawneh I, et al: A comparison of two diabetic foot ulcer classification systems: the Wagner and the University of Texas wound classification systems, *Diabetes Care* 24(1):84–88, 2001.

19. Lavery LA, Armstrong DG, Harkless LB: Classification of diabetic foot wounds, *J Foot Ankle Surg* 35(6):528–531, 1996.

20. Krasner D: Wound care: how to use the red-yellow-black system, *Am J Nurs* 95(5):44–47, 1995.

21. The National Pressure Ulcer Advisory Panel: *PUSH tool*. Available at: http://www.npuap.org/resources/educational-and-clinical-resources/push-tool/. Accessed October 25, 2014.

22. Stotts NA, Rodeheaver GT, Thomas DR, et al: An instrument to measure healing in pressure ulcers: development and validation of the pressure ulcer scale for healing (PUSH), *J Gerontol A Biol Sci Med Sci* 56(12):M795–M799, 2001.

23. Harris C, Bates-Jensen B, Parslow N, et al: Bates-Jensen wound assessment tool: pictorial guide validation project, *J Wound Ostomy Continence Nurs* 37(3):253–259, 2010.

24. Shea JD: Pressure sores classification and management, *Clin Orthop* 112:89–100, 1975.

25. Wagner FW Jr: The dysvascular foot: a system for diagnosis and treatment, *Foot Ankle* 2(2):64–122, 1981.

26. Wagner FW Jr: The diabetic foot, *Orthopedics* 10(1):163–172, 1987.

27. Clayton W, Elasy TA: A review of the pathophysiology, classification, and treatment of foot ulcers in diabetic patients, *Clinical Diabetes* 27(2):52–58, 2009.

28. MedlinePlus Medical Encyclopedia: *Burns*. Available at: http://www.nlm.nih.gov/medlineplus/ency/article/000030.htm. Updated 2012. Accessed October 25, 2014.

29. Knaysi GA, Crikelair GF, Cosman B: The rule of nines: its history and accuracy, *Plast Reconstr Surg* 41(6):560–563, 1968.

30. Miminas DA: A critical evaluation of the Lund and Browder Chart, *Wounds UK* 3(3):58–66, 2007.

31. Langøen A, Lawton S: Dermatological problems and periwound skin, World Wide Wounds, 2009.

32. Lawton S, Langøen A: Assessing and managing vulnerable periwound skin, World Wide Wounds, 2009.

33. Sussman C: *Wound care—all modules*. Available at: https://www.atrainceu.com/course-all/wound-care-057. Accessed May 26, 2014.

34. Meyer L: *Wound care: getting to the depth of the tissue*. Available at: https://www.nursece.com/courses/97. Updated 2014. Accessed May 11, 2014.

35. Tokumura F, Umekage K, Sado M, et al: Skin irritation due to repetitive application of adhesive tape: the influence of adhesive strength and seasonal variability, *Skin Res Technol* 11(2):102–106, 2005.

36. Lawton S: Skin and fungal nail infections, *Independent Nurse*, 4–7, 2009, January(suppl).

37. Basketter D, Gilpin G, Kuhn M, et al: Patch tests versus use tests in skin irritation risk assessment, *Contact Dermatitis* 39(5):252–256, 1998.

38. Cameron J: Exudate and care of the peri-wound skin, *Nurs Stand* 19(7):62, 2004, 64, 66 passim.

39. Machens HG, Gunter CI, Bader A: Skin. In Steinhoff G, editor: *Regenerative medicine* Netherlands, 2011, Springer.

40. Redelings M, Lee N, Sorvillo F: Pressure ulcers: more lethal than we thought? *Adv Skin Wound Care* 18(7):367–372, 2005.

41. Swindon, Wiltshire, Bath and North East Somerset Wound Group: Identification, diagnosis and treatment of wound infection, *Nurs Stand* 26(11):44–48, 2011.

42. Gottrup F, Melling A, Hollander DA: An overview of surgical site infections: aetiology, incidence and risk factors, *EWMA J* 5(2):11–15, 2005.

43. Storm-Versloot MN, Vos CG, Ubbink DT, et al: Topical silver for preventing wound infection, *Cochrane Database Syst Rev* 3:CD006487, 2010.

44. Leaper DJ: Risk factors for and epidemiology of surgical site infections, *Surg Infect (Larchmt)* 11(3):283–287, 2010.

45. Culver DH, Horan TC, Gaynes RP, et al: Surgical wound infection rates by wound class, operative procedure, and patient risk index, *Am J Med* 91(3):S152–S157, 1991.

46. Collier M: Recognition and management of wound infections, *World Wide Wounds* 1–10:2004.

47. Benbow M, Stevens J: Exudate, infection and patient quality of life, *Br J Nurs* 19(20):S30, 2010, S32-S36.

48. Reddy M, Gill SS, Wu W, et al: Does this patient have an infection of a chronic wound? *JAMA* 307(6):605–611, 2012.

49. Santy J: Recognising infection in wounds, *Nurs Stand* 23(7):53–54, 2008, 56, 58 passim.

50. Bonham PA: Swab cultures for diagnosing wound infections: a literature review and clinical guideline, *J Wound Ostomy Continence Nurs* 36(4):389–395, 2009.

51. Gardner SE, Frantz RA, Saltzman CL, et al: Diagnostic validity of three swab techniques for identifying chronic wound infection, *Wound Repair Regen* 14(5):548–557, 2006.

52. Levine NS, Lindberg RB, Mason AD, et al: The quantitative swab culture and smear: a quick, simple method for determining the number of viable aerobic bacteria on open wounds, *J Trauma Acute Care Surg* 16(2):89–94, 1976.

53. US Department of Health and Human Services: Pressure ulcers in adults: prediction and prevention (AHCPR publication no. 92-0047), 1992, Rockville, MD.

54. Norton D, McLaren R, Exton-Smith AN: An investigation of geriatric nursing problems in hospital, London, 1962, National Corporation for the Care of Old People.

55. Ayello EA, Braden B: How and why to do pressure ulcer risk assessment, *Adv Skin Wound Care* 15(3):125–131, 2002.

56. Sprigle S, Sonenblum S: Assessing evidence supporting redistribution of pressure for pressure ulcer prevention: a review, *J Rehabil Res Dev* 48(3):203–213, 2011.

57. Cullum N, McInnes E, Bell-Syer S, et al: Support surfaces for pressure ulcer prevention, *Cochrane Database Syst Rev* 3:CD001735, 2004.

58. Clark M: Repositioning to prevent pressure sores—what is the evidence? *Nurs Stand* 13(3):58–60, 1998, 62, 64.

59. Defloor T, Bacquer DD, Grypdonck MH: The effect of various combinations of turning and pressure reducing devices on the incidence of pressure ulcers, *Int J Nurs Stud* 42(1):37–46, 2005.

60. Vanderwee K, Grypdonck M, De Bacquer D, et al: Effectiveness of turning with unequal time intervals on the incidence of pressure ulcer lesions, *J Adv Nurs* 57(1):59–68, 2007.

61. Luedtke-Hoffmann KA, Schafer DS: Pulsed lavage in wound cleansing, *Phys Ther* 80(3):292–300, 2000.

62. Steed DL: Debridement, *Am J Surg* 187(5):S71–S74, 2004.

63. Institute for Clinical Systems Improvement (ICSI): Pressure ulcer prevention and treatment protocol. Health care protocol, Bloomington, 2012, Institute for Clinical Systems Improvement, Agency for Healthcare Research and Quality, US Department of Health and Human Services.

64. Tanyuksel M, Araz E, Dundar K, et al: Maggot debridement therapy in the treatment of chronic wounds in a military hospital setup in turkey, *Dermatology* 210(2):115–118, 2005.

65. Fleischmann W, Grassberger M: *Maggot therapy: a handbook of maggot-assisted wound healing*, Stuttgart, 2004, Thieme.

66. Armstrong DG, Salas P, Short B, et al: Maggot therapy in "lower-extremity hospice" wound care: fewer amputations and more antibiotic-free days, *J Am Podiatr Med Assoc* 95(3):254–257, 2005.

67. Sherman RA: Maggot therapy for treating diabetic foot ulcers unresponsive to conventional therapy, *Diabetes Care* 26(2):446–451, 2003.

68. Cowan LJ, Stechmiller J: Prevalence of wet-to-dry dressings in wound care, *Adv Skin Wound Care* 22(12):567–573, 2009.

69. Hess CL, Howard MA, Attinger CE: A review of mechanical adjuncts in wound healing: hydrotherapy, ultrasound, negative pressure therapy, hyperbaric oxygen, and electrostimulation, *Ann Plast Surg* 51(2):210–218, 2003.

70. Whinfield A, Aitkenhead I: The light revival: does phototherapy promote wound healing? A review, *Foot* 19(2):117–124, 2009.

71. Fulop AM, Dhimmer S, Deluca JR, et al: A meta-analysis of the efficacy of phototherapy in tissue repair, *Photomed Laser Surg* 27(5):695–702, 2009.

72. Caetano KS, Frade MAC, Minatel DG, et al: Phototherapy improves healing of chronic venous ulcers, *Photomed Laser Surg* 27(1):111–118, 2009.

73. Minatel DG, Frade MAC, França SC, et al: Phototherapy promotes healing of chronic diabetic leg ulcers that failed to respond to other therapies, *Lasers Surg Med* 41(6):433–441, 2009.

74. Woodruff LD, Bounkeo JM, Brannon WM, et al: The efficacy of laser therapy in wound repair: a meta-analysis of the literature, *Photomed Laser Surg* 22(3):241–247, 2004.

75. Thomas S: A structured approach to the selection of dressings, *World Wide Wounds*, 1997.

76. Irion G: *Comprehensive wound management*, ed 2, Thorofare, 2010, SLACK.

77. Weir D: How to … Top tips for wound dressing selection, *Wounds Int* 3(4):2012.

78. Eardley WG, Watts SA, Clasper JC: Extremity trauma, dressings, and wound infection: should every acute limb wound have a silver lining? *Int J Low Extrem Wounds* 11(3):201–212, 2012.

79. Leaper D: Appropriate use of silver dressings in wounds: international consensus document, *Int Wound J* 9(5):461–464, 2012.

80. Ip M, Lui SL, Poon VK, et al: Antimicrobial activities of silver dressings: an in vitro comparison, *J Med Microbiol* 55(Pt 1):59–63, 2006.

81. Maillard J, Denyer SP: Focus on silver, *World Wide Wounds*, 2006.

82. Lansdown AB: A pharmacological and toxicological profile of silver as an antimicrobial agent in medical devices, *Adv Pharmacol Sci* 2010:910686, 2010.

83. Lee DS, Sinno S, Khachemoune A: Honey and wound healing, *Am J Clin Dermatol* 12(3):181–190, 2011.

84. Seckam A, Cooper R: Understanding how honey impacts on wounds: an update on recent research findings, *Wounds Int* 4(1):20–24, 2013.

85. Molan PC: Honey as a topical antibacterial agent for treatment of infected wounds, *World Wide Wounds* 1–13, 2001.

86. Jull AB, Rodgers A, Walker N: Honey as a topical treatment for wounds, *Cochrane Database Syst Rev* 4:CD005083, 2008.

87. Molan P: The evidence and the rationale for the use of honey as a wound dressing, *Wound Pract Res* 19(4):204–220, 2011.

88. Johnson CL: Physical therapists as scar modifiers, *Phys Ther* 64(9):1381–1387, 1984.

89. Robertson VJ, Ward AR, Jung P: The effect of heat on tissue extensibility: a comparison of deep and superficial heating, *Arch Phys Med Rehabil* 86(4):819–825, 2005.

90. Al-Kurdi D, Bell-Syer S, Flemming K: Therapeutic ultrasound for venous leg ulcers, *Cochrane Database Syst Rev* 1:CD001180, 2008.

91. Akbari Sari A, Flemming K, Cullum NA, et al: Therapeutic ultrasound for pressure ulcers, *Cochrane Database Syst Rev* 3:CD001275, 2006.

92. Bell AL, Cavorsi J: Noncontact ultrasound therapy for adjunctive treatment of nonhealing wounds: retrospective analysis, *Phys Ther* 88(12):1517–1524, 2008.

93. Kavros SJ, Liedl DA, Boon AJ, et al: Expedited wound healing with noncontact, low-frequency ultrasound therapy in chronic wounds: a retrospective analysis, *Adv Skin Wound Care* 21(9):416–423, 2008.

94. Ennis W, Foremann P, Mozen NM, et al: Ultrasound therapy for recalcitrant diabetic foot ulcers: results of a randomized, double-blind, controlled, multi-center study, *Ostomy Wound Manage* 51(8):24–39, 2005.

95. Pullar CE: The biological basis for electric stimulation as a therapy to heal chronic wounds, *J Wound Technol* 6:20–24, 2009.

96. Gentzkow GD: Electrical stimulation to heal dermal wounds, *J Dermatol Surg Oncol* 19(8):753–758, 1993.

97. Alpagut U, Dayioglu E: Importance and advantages of intermittent external pneumatic compression therapy in venous stasis ulceration, *Angiology* 56(1):19–23, 2005.

98. Nikolovska S, Arsovski A, Damevska K, et al: Evaluation of two different intermittent pneumatic compression cycle settings in the healing of venous ulcers: a randomized trial, *Med Sci Monit* 11(7):CR337–CR343, 2005.

99. Mouës C, Heule F, Hovius S: A review of topical negative pressure therapy in wound healing: sufficient evidence? *Am J Surg* 201(4):544–556, 2011.

100. Ubbink DT, Westerbos SJ, Evans D, et al: Topical negative pressure for treating chronic wounds, *Cochrane Database Syst Rev* 3:CD001898, 2008.

101. Barker JA, Carlson GL: Managing the open wound: Indications for topical negative pressure therapy, *Surgery (Oxford)* 29(10):507–512, 2011.

102. Page JC, Newswander B, Schwenke DC, et al: Retrospective analysis of negative pressure wound therapy in open foot wounds with significant soft tissue defects, *Adv Skin Wound Care* 17(7):354–364, 2004.

103. Blume PA, Walters J, Payne W, et al: Comparison of negative pressure wound therapy using vacuum-assisted closure with advanced moist wound therapy in the treatment of diabetic foot ulcers: a multicenter randomized controlled trial, *Diabetes Care* 31(4):631–636, 2008.

104. Kranke P, Bennett MH, Martyn-St James M, et al: Hyperbaric oxygen therapy for chronic wounds, *Cochrane Database Syst Rev* 4:CD004123, 2012.

105. Thom SR: Hyperbaric oxygen: its mechanisms and efficacy, *Plast Reconstr Surg* 127(suppl 1):131S–141S, 2011.

106. Dauwe PB, Pulikkottil BJ, Lavery L, et al: Does hyperbaric oxygen therapy work in facilitating acute wound healing: a systematic review, *Plast Reconstr Surg* 133(2):208e–215e, 2014.

107. Brigham and Women's Hospital: Standard of care: wound care/integumentary management. Physical Therapy management of the patient at risk for or with an integumentary disorder, 2009, The Brigham and Women's Hospital, Inc., Department of Rehabilitation Services.

108. Roy S, Khanna S, Sen CK: Redox regulation of the VEGF signaling path and tissue vascularization: hydrogen peroxide, the common link between physical exercise and cutaneous wound healing, *Free Radical Biol Med* 44(2):180–192, 2008.

109. Emery CF, Kiecolt-Glaser JK, Glaser R, et al: Exercise accelerates wound healing among healthy older adults: a preliminary investigation, *J Gerontol A Biol Sci Med Sci* 60(11):1432–1436, 2005.

110. Keylock KT, Vieira VJ, Wallig MA, et al: Exercise accelerates cutaneous wound healing and decreases wound inflammation in aged mice, *Am J Physiol Regul Integr Comp Physiol* 294(1):R179–R184, 2008.

CHAPTER 3

Cervical Spine

JIM MEADOWS, SUSAN L. ARMIJO-OLIVO, DAVID J. MAGEE

INTRODUCTION

The etiology of injury to the cervical spine and the causes of cervical spine pathology are numerous. They can be myogenic, mechanical, neurogenic, or psychosomatic in origin and can be further divided into acute and chronic states. Acute injuries may be due to trauma, unaccustomed activity, or a poor working or sleeping position. Chronic pathology usually is due to poor posture, poor muscle tone, or illness. In a young child, it may be the result of an idiopathic torticollis.

In young people, mechanical and myogenic types of cervical pathology are most commonly due to a ligament sprain or muscle strain, whereas in older adults, they are more commonly due to cervical spondylosis (disc degeneration). Spinal stenosis (narrowing of the spinal canal) also can lead to symptoms, as can facet syndrome (pathology in the zygapophyseal joints). Neurogenic neck pain is primarily due to facet impingement or disc degeneration or herniation, resulting in irritation of the cervical nerve roots and subsequent radicular pain into the shoulder and/or arm. Psychosomatic problems commonly are the result of depression, anxiety, hysteria, or, in some cases, malingering.

One reason the cervical spine is vulnerable to injury is its high degree of mobility with a heavy weight, the head, perched on top of it. The cervical spine is the most flexible and mobile part of the spine, with the intervertebral discs making up approximately 40% of its height.[1] However, neck pain tends to be less disabling than back pain.[2]

With regard to injuries, the cervical spine can be divided into two areas, the upper and lower cervical spine. Upper cervical injuries are associated with the vertebral segments CO (occiput) to C2; these injuries are referred to as cervicoencephalic injuries.[3,4] The term **cervicoencephalic** portrays the relationship between the cervical spine and the occiput. Cervicoencephalic injuries can be severe enough to involve the brain, brain stem, and spinal cord.[3,4] The symptoms of injury associated with these segments may arise from areas of the brain (cognitive dysfunction), autonomic nervous system (sympathetic dysfunction), cranial nerves (cranial nerve dysfunction), or vertebral and/or internal carotid artery (vascular dysfunction) and tend to be headache, fatigue, vertigo, poor concentration, and irritability to light.[3,4] This is important to understand because, once sympathetic system dysfunction, cognitive dysfunction, cranial nerve dysfunction, or vascular dysfunction is evident, the condition takes an inordinate amount of time to resolve, is more difficult to treat, and may have more severe consequences. Cognitive dysfunction includes altered mental functions of comprehension, judgment, memory, and reasoning. Sympathetic symptoms are a result of hypertonia of the sympathetic nervous system, affect emotions, and may include tinnitus, postural dizziness, blurred vision, photophobia, rhinorrhea, sweating, lacrimation, and weakness.[3,5] Cranial nerve dysfunction involves one or more of the cranial nerves, and vascular dysfunction involves either the vertebral, basilar, or internal carotid arteries. Patients with severe injuries often may also demonstrate numbness or pain, sharp reversal of the cervical lordosis, and restricted motion, especially at one particular vertebral level.

Sympathetic Symptoms Caused by Cervical Pathology

- Tinnitus (ringing in the ear)
- Postural dizziness
- Blurred vision
- Photophobia (intolerance to light)
- Rhinorrhea (runny nose)
- Abnormal sweating
- Lacrimation (tearing)
- Weakness

Symptoms of Cognitive Dysfunction

- From concussions, head injuries
- Memory dysfunction–retrograde amnesia, posttraumatic amnesia
- Concentration difficulties or difficulty remembering things
- Disorientation
- Balance problems or incoordination
- Dizziness
- Increased emotionality
- Feeling "in a fog"

Lower cervical spine injuries are associated with vertebral body segments C3 to C7; these injuries are referred to as **cervicobrachial** injuries. Pathology in this region commonly leads to pain in the upper extremity.[3,4] Neck pain or extremity pain may occur individually, or the two may occur together. One may be greater than the other, or they may be equal. In any case the clinician's main concern is whether the signs and symptoms are peripheralizing (i.e., moving more distally) or centralizing (i.e., moving more centrally). If they are peripheralizing, the condition usually is worsening. If they are centralizing, the condition is improving. Common signs of minor injury are neck stiffness and limited range of motion (ROM). Unfavorable signs of neck injury include the presence of paresthesia, muscle weakness into the upper extremity, radicular signs, and neurological deficit, all of which lead to longer recovery time.[5]

TORTICOLLIS

The term *torticollis* (wry neck) means scoliosis or "twisted neck" in the cervical spine. The condition may be acute or chronic. Congenital torticollis, seen in young children, involves the sternocleidomastoid (SCM) muscle. Congenital or infantile torticollis primarily affects females aged 6 months to 3 years. It results from unilateral contraction of the SCM muscle caused by ischemic changes in the muscle. The resulting deformity is side flexion to the same (affected) side and rotation to the opposite side (Figure 3-1). A lump, or pseudo-tumor, sometimes is felt over the muscle in the first month, but this disappears.[6] The contracture itself is not painful, but it can lead to developmental and cosmetic problems with altered head and neck posture and alignment.

The cause of congenital torticollis is unknown, but the condition may be related to abnormal blood supply to the SCM muscle, resulting in a structural abnormality in the muscle. Increased amounts of interstitial fibrous tissue are found in the muscle, and this fibrous tissue tends to contract over time, causing the deformity. If the condition is not corrected early, asymmetry of the face may develop, with the affected side not being as well developed. The asymmetry corrects itself if the condition is corrected early. However, the correction, which commonly involves repeated, painful stretching of the affected muscle, may take years. Torticollis often is associated with other cervical deformities, such as **Klippel-Feil syndrome**, which is characterized by shortness of the neck and fusion of two or three of the vertebral bodies.[6]

The treatment for congenital torticollis, from a rehabilitation standpoint, is stretching and overcorrection of the deformity at birth. Most cases of congenital torticollis can be corrected this way, provided the stretching is carried out diligently. The clinician must teach the parents how to do the stretching because it must be done 2 to 4 times a day for at least a year. Needless to say, the child will not like the stretching and will express herself

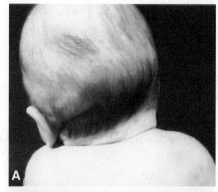
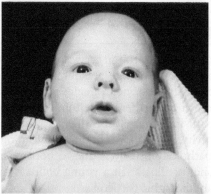
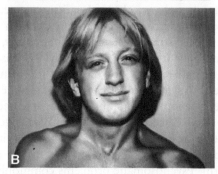

Figure 3-1 A, Congenital muscular torticollis on the left. The head is tilted to the left, and the chin is rotated to the right. **B,** Untreated right congenital muscular torticollis in a 19-year-old man. Note the asymmetry of the face. On the affected side, it is shortened from above downward and relatively wide from side to side. The level of the eyes and the ears is asymmetrical. (From Canale ST: *Campbell's operative orthopaedics*, St Louis, 2003, Mosby.)

or himself the only way she or he can— by crying. The clinician should prepare the parents for this so that they are not worried that the child is being injured.

Acute or acquired torticollis usually occurs in people 20 years of age or older. Spasm of one or more muscles (i.e., the SCM, splenius capitis, semispinalis capitus, or scalenus anterior) is commonly seen. The acute type of torticollis primarily is due to trauma or muscle strain; however, in some cases, it may be related to an upper respiratory tract infection, a viral infection, poor posture (with symptoms arising after the patient has been in an awkward posture for several hours), hearing problems, injury to the facet joints, dislocation, or even tumors.[6] Patients commonly awaken complaining of a "crick" or pain in the neck, and they may relate the condition to "sleeping in a draft" or a similar circumstance. More commonly the real cause is poor neck position for several hours. The pain is unilateral; ROM is decreased, especially to one side; and severe pain is noted at the end range on active and passive movement testing.[6] In the neutral position, resisted isometric strength is strong but may be uncomfortable; however, the discomfort is not as great as that seen at the end of ROM in active and passive movement.

Acute or acquired torticollis usually resolves on its own within 7 days to 2 weeks.[6] This type of torticollis is treated primarily with rest and heat and/or ice, if the patient is seen within the first 24 hours. Muscle and joint mobilization and manipulation techniques may also be helpful, and pain-relieving modalities may be effective. The patient also should be treated with nonsteroidal anti-inflammatory drugs (NSAIDs) or muscle relaxants.

WHIPLASH (ACCELERATION INJURY)

Whiplash has been recognized as a significant public health problem in industrialized countries because it is an important cause of chronic pain disability.[7] According to Carrol et al.,[8] the incidence of whiplash-associated disorders (WADs) in Western countries has increased since the 1980s, with an estimated yearly incidence of at least 300 per 100,000 inhabitants. The economic impact of whiplash disorders has been reported to be incredibly high. For example, Joslin et al.[9] reported that whiplash personal injury claims exceeded £3 billion per year in the United Kingdom. Similar economic impact has been reported in the United States, with costs reaching U.S. $230 billion per annum in 2000.[10]

The term *whiplash* is derived from the "whipping of a lash," indicating a quick change in direction or movement, often with a snap. The head goes through a ROM involving flexion often combined with rotation, followed very rapidly by extension, or vice versa. Whiplash is also called a *cervical sprain* or *cervical strain* or an *acceleration-deceleration injury* of the neck. The extent of injury depends on the force of impact. If the injury is caused by an automobile accident, the position of the head at the time of impact, whether the patient was aware of the impending collision, and the condition of the neck tissues (e.g., effects of aging) are all factors that affect the severity of the injury.[11-13] Seventy percent of patients with whiplash report an immediate occurrence of symptoms, but many also report delayed symptoms.[5,14-17] Common signs include neck pain and headaches originating from the occipital area. If the condition is serious enough, the patient may complain of more severe symptoms (Table 3-1).[5,18]

The Quebec Task Force (QTF) on WADs[18] defines whiplash as "an acceleration-deceleration mechanism of energy transfer to the neck. It may result from rear end

TABLE **3-1**

Grading System for Whiplash-associated Disorders

Grade 1	Grade 2	Grade 3	Grade 4
• Muscle strain • Neck stiffness • Neck pain/tenderness • No physical signs • Normal reflexes, dermatomes, and myotomes • X-ray film: Unnecessary • Accounts for approximately 43% of cases	• Muscle strain/ligament sprain • Neck and/or back stiffness • Neck and/or back pain • Paraspinal tenderness • Restricted ROM • Normal reflexes, dermatomes, and myotomes • X-ray film: No fracture/dislocation • Accounts for approximately 29% to 56% of cases	• Possible disc protrusion • Nerve root signs: Objective neurological signs (myotomes/dermatomes) • Neck or back pain • Restricted ROM • Abnormal reflexes (reduced), dermatomes (abnormal), and myotomes (weak) • Possible upper motor neuron signs • X-ray film: No fracture/dislocation • CT scan/MRI: May show area of nerve involvement • Accounts for approximately 3% to 2% of cases	• Cervical fracture/dislocation • Nerve root signs: Objective neurological signs (myotomes/dermatomes) • Neck pain • Restricted ROM • Abnormal reflexes (reduces), dermatomes (abnormal) and myotomes (weak) • Possible upper motor neuron signs (e.g., urinary incontinence, pathological reflexes) • X-ray film: Fracture/dislocation • CT scan/MRI: May show area of nerve/fracture/dislocation/spinal cord involvement • Accounts for approximately 6% of cases

Data from Spitzer WO, Skovron ML, Salmi LR et al: Scientific monograph of the Quebec Task Force on Whiplash-associated Disorders: redefining "whiplash" and its management, *Spine* 20:1S-73S, 1995.

TABLE **3-2**

Quebec Task Force Classification of the Severity of Whiplash-associated Disorders

Grade	Clinical Presentation
0	No neck symptoms, no physical signs
1	No physical signs except neck pain, stiffness, or tenderness only
2	Neck symptoms and musculoskeletal signs, such as decreased ROM and point tenderness
3	Neck symptoms and neurological signs, such as decreased or absent deep tendon reflexes, weakness, and sensory deficits
4	Neck symptoms and fracture or dislocation

From Spitzer WO, Skovron ML, Salmi LR et al: Scientific monograph of the Quebec Task Force on "Whiplash-Associated Disorders: redefining "whiplash" and its management, *Spine* 20:8S-58S, 1995.

or side impact motor vehicle collision, but can also occur during other mechanisms. The impact may result in bony or soft tissue injuries to the cervical spine (whiplash injury), which in turn may lead to a variety of clinical manifestations called **whiplash-associated disorders (WADs)**." Chronic WADs usually are defined as symptoms or disabilities that persist for longer than 6 months.[18,19] The QTF established a system of five grades for classifying the severity of these disorders (Table 3-2).[18] WADs include aching or stiffness in the neck. These symptoms usually appear within a few hours after the accident. In some cases, the patient may have difficulty swallowing because of injury to the esophagus and larynx. Headache is common and usually occurs in the occipital area, but it may also radiate to the vertex of the skull or the temples. In some cases, the pain may be retroocular. The pain may also be referred into the interscapular area, chest, and shoulders. The head commonly is held in flexion (with a loss of the lordotic curvature) as a result of muscle spasm, and ROM, especially side flexion or rotation, is limited. In some cases, the person may suffer a concussion during the accident, leading to loss of consciousness, amnesia, nausea, vomiting, and cognitive dysfunction. Older patients because of preexisting degenerative changes and those who have a psychosocial response to the injury tend to have a poor prognosis. Symptoms associated with any preexisting degenerative changes seem to come on faster after an accident.[20] Research has indicated that even minor trauma, such as low-velocity collisions, can lead to prolonged symptoms.[21]

Rear-end impact (i.e., acceleration type) injuries tend to cause the greatest disability from the whiplash mechanism primarily because the victim is unaware of the impending impact. Impact from behind causes the lower portion of the body to move forward abruptly while the head momentarily remains in place. The head then arches backward through a path of extension because it is heavy and suspended on a thin, flexible support (the cervical spine). This quick movement catches the protective muscle reflex unprepared; consequently the limiting influence of the ligaments is exceeded, resulting in hyperextension, especially if the head is not stopped by a headrest. Backward shearing may also occur in the cervical spine, possibly resulting in spinal cord damage from subluxation or fracture of the vertical body.[22] The hyperextension is followed by a protective flexor muscle contraction that causes a rebound, combined with compression that pulls the head forward from its hyperextended position; the result is a compressive hyperflexion, which may stress the intervertebral disc and posterior structures.

The position of the head at the time of impact affects ROM and the severity of injury. Normal extension is approximately 70°, but extension is decreased when the head is rotated 45°. Therefore head rotation can increase the probability and severity of cervical injury because of the decrease in available ROM.

In front-end impact (i.e., deceleration type) injuries, the body moves forward and then comes to a sudden stop. Actually, the body stops, but the head, because of its weight, continues to move forward as a result of inertia. The impact is abrupt, may be unexpected, or overpowers the extensor mechanism, resulting in hyperflexion. Movement of the head is stopped by the chin hitting the chest wall. A rebound then occurs, causing hyperextension as a result of reflexive contraction of the extensor muscles.

A third type of whiplash mechanism is a rotation injury. For example, people with long hair can cause a rotational sprain of the ligaments or strain of the muscles, or possibly damage the facet joint, by whipping the head around to get the hair out of their eyes.

The influence of crash-related factors on outcome is the subject of debate. Some studies have found a relationship between factors,[23] whereas others have reported that crash-related factors were not important predictors of poor outcome.[7] The evidence is not conclusive in this matter. Higher-intensity neck pain and headache, as well as radicular symptoms and signs, have been strongly associated with delayed recovery.[24,25] Cassidy et al.[7] reported that patients who consulted a medical physician and a physical therapist or a medical physician and a chiropractor took longer to recover than those who did not seek a health care provider. These findings were corroborated by Gun et al.[20] No explanation was given for the difference, except that people in greater pain and discomfort would be more likely to seek help.

In some cases the same mechanism of injury that occurs with whiplash, if assisted by contact with the nonyielding surface, can lead to more severe cervical injuries, such as dislocation or fracture of a cervical vertebra, or a combination of these two injuries. The result can be neurological damage and paralysis. This might occur in an individual who falls forward, striking the chin, face, or forehead against an object, causing forceful hyperextension or backward thrust of the neck or an individual who falls backward, striking the head, causing forceful hyperflexion or forward thrust of the neck. Another example is an individual who dives into shallow water, striking the head, causing forceful hyperflexion and compression of the cervical spine. Similar injury patterns can occur in football with spearing or in hockey when players are checked headfirst into the boards.

Although efforts have been made to classify and define WADs, the descriptive validity of the WAD classifications has been questioned because the two primary symptoms used to describe these conditions are nonspecific and prevalent in the general population.[26-29] Nederhand et al.[30] concluded that cervical muscle dysfunction was not specific to patients with grade 2 WAD and that it appeared to be a general sign of chronic pain. These findings do not support the validity of the WAD categories described by the QTF. Attempts have been made to modify this classification with no success due to the increase in complexity for classifying patients. Thus the QTF classification is still considered the criteria to classify WADs.[31]

According to Stovner[19] and Freeman et al.,[32] the estimated proportion of patients who report pain and disability 6 months after an accident ranges from 19% to 60%, and the percentage of patients who are absent from work after 6 months is 9% to 26%.[15,19] Styrke et al.[33] reported that 44% of subjects 5 years after suffering a whiplash presented with an inability to sustain previous workload and 43% fatigue at work. Only 39% of the sample were satisfied with their somatic health and 60% with their psychological health. Compared with healthy controls, the whiplash-injured individuals exhibited more symptoms and had lower life satisfaction, which could interfere with the recovery.

The natural course of whiplash disorders is unknown. Sterling et al.[34] have described three pathways to WAD recovery. The first is "good recovery," which involves people with initial mild-to-moderate disability after the accident. Generally 45% of patients follow this path. The second is characterized by initial moderate-to-severe pain-related disability, with "moderate recovery" at 12 months follow-up. Thirty-nine percent of people are predicted to follow this path of recovery. The last path is the "bad recovery." Subjects in this path start with moderate-to-severe disability and progress to some recovery with moderate-to-severe levels of disability at 1 year. Sixteen percent of the subjects follow this path.[34]

The area of prognostic factors for WAD has been of great interest because it is of paramount importance to recognize which patients will recover as well as the ones who will progress to high levels of disability, in order to target appropriate treatment strategies. Some prognostic factors have been described to distinguish between patients who are expected to experience either a normal or a delayed recovery. According to Stovner,[19] a causal link between trauma and chronic symptoms is not conclusive. Litigation issues have been related to the chronicity of symptoms. In countries where litigation appears to play a role in recovery, the disability of WADs is prolonged, and in countries where litigation is absent, the prevalence of chronic whiplash syndrome is low or nonexistent.[7]

It has been reported that long-term neck symptoms do not occur in any higher proportion in whiplash patients than in the general population.[27,35] However, 15% to 40% of whiplash patients may report persistent headaches and neck pain.[14] In a long-term longitudinal study of subjects with whiplash,[33] it was reported that the most common symptoms 5 years after whiplash injury were fatigue (41%), poor memory (39%), and headache (37%). These symptoms are typical of mild **traumatic brain injury (TBI)**; thus WAD patients can share some of the symptomatology of TBI, and as a result, assessment of these patients would be important to quantify TBI symptoms earlier in the rehabilitation process and target an appropriate treatment. Furthermore, it has been reported that subjects with WAD commonly present psychiatric disorders, such as posttraumatic stress disorder, major depressive episode, and generalized anxiety disorder, which can contribute to doubling the health care utilization and considerably greater time off work compared with those with physical injury alone.[31]

Clinicians can help patients understand the effect of the injury and reduce the impact of any disability by explaining the prognostic factors associated with these injuries. According to Scholten-Peeters et al.,[36] the physical prognostic factors associated with delayed recovery in WADs are decreased mobility of the cervical spine immediately after injury, preexisting neck trauma, older age, and female gender. Some psychological factors (e.g., inadequate cognition, fear-avoidance beliefs, catastrophizing, maladaptive copying strategies, depression, and anxiety) have been found to be related to delayed recovery in WADs, much as they have been in other pain conditions, such as low back pain.[20] More research is needed to develop a prognostic patient profile consisting of factors that predict outcome in whiplash patients.[35] Gun et al.[20] and others[37] found that patients who consulted a lawyer had a worse Neck Pain Outcome Score (NPOS); after 1 year, these patients had a sevenfold greater chance of still receiving treatment and a sevenfold lesser chance of claim settlement. For individuals with a history of a previous motor vehicle accident claim, improvement after 1 year in the NPOS was 10 points lower and improvement on the Visual Analogue Scale (VAS) was 1 point lower.

Factors Associated with Delayed Recovery in Whiplash-associated Disorders

- Decrease in cervical spine mobility immediately after injury
- Preexisting neck trauma
- Older age
- Female gender
- Psychological factors
- Pending litigation

According to a systematic review of prognostic factors in whiplash by Cote et al.,[24] reliable information on whiplash is still scarce, and the methodological quality of studies needs to be improved. Based on the reviewed studies, these researchers concluded that consistent evidence indicated that older age and female gender were associated with delayed recovery from whiplash. No consistent evidence was found for marital status, number of dependents, income, work activities, or education as predictors of recovery. No strong evidence was associated with a past history of headaches or neck pain with recovery. However, the studies that reported these associations lacked control of the confounders.

Cote et al.[24] also found that compensation or litigation issues could have an influence on claimants' behavior and recovery. The differences in the rating of prolonged symptoms between systems with and without compensation raises questions about the real incidence of chronic WADs.[19] In a meta-analysis by Walton et al.,[38] 12 prognostic factors were identified as related to persistent problems following WAD. The significant variables included high baseline pain intensity (greater than 5.5/10), report of headache at inception, less than postsecondary education, no seat belt in use during the accident, report of low back pain at inception, high Neck Disability Index (NDI) score (greater than 14.5/50), preinjury neck pain, report of neck pain at inception (regardless of intensity), high catastrophizing, female sex, WAD grade 2 or 3, and WAD grade 3 alone. In addition, they reported that catastrophizing but not depression was found to be an important risk factor for chronicity of WAD.[38] Psychological factors have been found to be more relevant than collision severity in predicting duration and severity of symptoms in WAD.[39] Helplessness, older age, and poor preinjury work status were found to predict poorer health and nonrecovery.[38,40] A study in a Swiss cohort[41] has partially corroborated these findings. They found that relief of depression and low baseline depression were highly associated with improved physical function in subjects with whiplash after a rehabilitation program (especially at the 6-month follow-up:

20.5% explained variance). In addition, low baseline catastrophizing and reduction of catastrophizing were associated with improvements in pain relief, physical function, and working capacity. For improved function at discharge, reduction of catastrophizing was the most important predictor (19.4% explained variance). Low baseline pain and relief of pain were associated with improvement of function and vice versa. Thus improved coping (i.e., decreasing catastrophizing and ability to decrease pain) and reduced depression may act as important predictors for pain relief and improved function in subjects with WAD. These findings shed light on the interrelation among psychological factors that could potentially affect recovery in subjects with WAD. These prognostic factors should be taken into consideration when planning therapy for subjects with chronic WAD. According to Sterling,[34] most of the studies investigating prognostic factors lacked validation, and thus more research is needed to develop a prognostic patient profile consisting of factors that predict outcome in whiplash patients.[24,29] Results from systematic reviews of prognostic factors' evidence were summarized by Sterling[34] and presented in Table 3-3.

A complete history of the whiplash patient should be taken. This should include details about specific symptoms (especially those related to cognitive, sympathetic, cranial nerve, and vascular dysfunction), preexisting symptoms, disabilities, participation problems, accident-specific information (e.g., velocity of the car, type of collision), recovery time, previous diagnostic tests and procedures, success of treatment (medical or other), attitude, cognition, present severity of symptoms, psychosocial issues, and medications used. This information can indicate the degree of compromise suffered by the patient and how the WAD affects his/her life. Some assessment tools are available for evaluating pain (VAS) and neck disability (NDI) (see *Orthopedic Physical Assessment*, volume 1 of this series). However, it should be pointed out that according to Stenneberg et al.,[42] these measurements do not cover important limitations for patients with WAD. For example, out of the

TABLE 3-3

Prognostic Indictors of Poor Functional Recovery Following Whiplash Injury Based on Findings of Systematic Reviews

Factors Showing Consistent Evidence for Being Prognostic Indicators for Poor Recovery	Factors Showing Consistent Evidence of Not Being Prognostic Indicators	Factors with Inconsistent Evidence
• Initial pain levels: > 5.5/1 • Initial disability levels: NDI>29% • Symptoms of posttraumatic stress • Negative expectations of recovery • High pain catastrophizing • Cold hyperalgesia	• Accident-related features (e.g., collision awareness, position in vehicle, speed of accident) • Findings on imaging • Motor dysfunction	• Older age • Female gender • Neck range of movement • Compensation related factors

From Sterling M: Physiotherapy management of whiplash-associated disorders (WAD), *J Physiother* 60(1):7, 2014.

40 limitations most important to patients with WAD, the NDI covers only six items.[43] In addition, Hoving et al.[44] concluded that the NDI and Northwick Park Neck Pain Questionnaire (NPQ) did not fully reflect the full spectrum of disabilities judged to be important by patients with WAD. Only three of the most important problems were included in the NDI, and only four were included in the NPQ.[44] Therefore, Stenneberg et al.[42] and Schmitt et al.[43] created a new scale to assess activity limitation and participation restriction in patients with WAD: the Whiplash Activity and Participation List (WAL). The WAL is a self-assessment instrument that is based on the International Classification of Functioning, Disability and Health (ICF) framework. The WAL is primarily developed for the Dutch language and consists of 35 activity and participation items, scored on a 5-point scale according to the ICF (World Health Organization [WHO], 2001). A sum score is calculated ranging from 0 (no limitations) to 140 (extremely limited). The development process involved a Delphi technique with experts as well as patients with subacute or chronic WAD. The validation study found excellent properties for this tool, which makes it a promising tool to be used specifically in subjects with WAD. Cronbach's alpha was high (0.95), and test-retest reliability was excellent (0.92, 95% confidence interval [CI] 0.87; 0.95). In addition, construct validity was supported by 14 out of 15 confirmed hypotheses, and the WAL showed statistically significant differences between known groups. The minimal detectable change (MDC) was 16 points, and the minimal clinically important change (MCIC) was 18 points (Table 3-4).

A study by Nederhand et al.[45] in 2000 demonstrated that patients with grade 2 WADs had higher activity of the upper trapezius than healthy controls and that they also were unable to relax these muscles after a dynamic task. These findings indicated that patients with grade 2 WADs exhibited abnormal muscle activation in situations in which no biomechanical demand for the activation existed. One of the symptoms described in the QTF WAD classification system[17,18] coincides with the description of "musculoskeletal signs." Nederhand et al.[45] considered the criteria used to determine musculoskeletal signs (e.g., the presence of "point tenderness" and "muscle spasm") to be inaccurate because assessment commonly is performed in the sitting or standing position, which results in only small differences in electromyography (EMG) levels between patients and controls. According to these authors, surface EMG may be a useful tool for differentiating patients with grade 2 WADs because it helps to determine the hyperactivity of the cervical muscles.

TABLE 3-4

Items Included in the Whiplash Activity and Participation List

Item	Rating*	Item	Rating*
Focusing attention	_____	Shopping	_____
Reading	_____	Preparing meals (such as slicing, cooking)	_____
Solving complex problems	_____	Doing housework (such as cleaning, washing clothes, window cleaning)	_____
Undertaking multiple tasks	_____		
Handling stress	_____	Using household appliances (such as vacuum cleaners)	_____
Conversing	_____	Gardening	_____
Using a desktop computer or laptop	_____	Interacting with people (such as friends, coworkers, partner, and children)	_____
Bending over	_____		
Maintaining a sitting position	_____	Maintaining relationships	_____
Looking over the shoulder	_____	Sexuality	_____
Lifting and carrying objects	_____	Following education or training	_____
Prolonged walking	_____	Work (maintaining a job, performing volunteer work)	_____
Running	_____	Engaging in recreational activity (such as sightseeing or visiting an amusement park)	_____
Overhead work	_____		
Using public transportation (bus, train, or subway)	_____	Engaging in social activities (such as organized religious ceremonies, political events, or activities in a social club)	_____
Cycling	_____		
Driving a motor vehicle (such as an automobile or motorcycle)	_____		
		Sports	_____
Wash or shower	_____	Going out (such as going to the theater, cinema, or museum)	_____
Caring for body parts (such as face, teeth) or washing hair	_____		
		Visiting friends or relatives	_____
To dress or undress	_____		

*Subjects are asked to rate from 0, no problem; 1, mild problem; 2, moderate problem; 3, severe problem; 4, complete problem.

Modified from Schmitt MA, Stenneberg MS, Schrama PPM et al: Measurement of clinically relevant functional health perceptions in patients with whiplash-associated disorders: The development of the whiplash specific activity and participation list (WAL), *Eur Spine J* 22(9):2103, 2013.

For treatment of WADs, the advice to stay active as well as follow a program of exercise has been advocated as a good choice to manage this condition. However, the evidence is not consistent as to which type of exercise might yield the best results (a general program of exercise to treat neck pain and associated disorders is described later in this chapter). It seems that no specific exercise is better than the advice to stay active for acute and chronic WAD. Nevertheless, what is clear from the synthesis of the best evidence is that activity and exercise are superior to restricting movement with a soft collar, which has shown to be ineffective for the management of acute WAD.[46] Furthermore, interdisciplinary approaches have been found to be beneficial for some patients. However, no clear conclusions can be established for all cases due to the limited evidence found in randomized controlled trials (RCTs). Thus future directions for the research process are to target factors associated with recovery after WAD because many of them are potentially modifiable with more specific interventions.[46]

CERVICAL SPONDYLOSIS

Cervical spondylosis is an age-related, degenerative condition sometimes referred to as *cervical arthritis, segmental instability, hypertrophic arthritis, degenerative spondylosis, cervical arthrosis,* or *degenerative disease.*[3] It is believed to be part of the normal aging process of the vertebral column and is commonly seen in people after the age of 40.[47] Radiological investigation of asymptomatic individuals has shown spondylotic changes of greater than 50% by age 50 and up to 90% by age 65.[48-50] Spondylosis has both an inflammatory component and a degenerative component, which eventually lead to arthritis of the cervical spine. The term *cervical spondylosis* implies a loss of mechanical integrity of a cervical intervertebral disc, leading to instability of the affected segment and, later on, nerve root or cord compression symptoms caused by stenosis in either the intervertebral foramen or the spinal canal (Table 3-5).[51] Although spondylosis appears most obviously in the cervical spine because of its mobility, it may occur in other areas of the spine, especially the lower lumbar spine. The condition begins with intervertebral disc degeneration, which can occur as a result of damage to the disc or poor nutrition. A state of poor nutrition

may result from changes at the cartilaginous end plate between the disc and the vertebral body, resulting in lack of nutritional interchange.

As the disc degenerates and loses bulk, a reduction of the mucopolysaccharides in the nucleus pulposus occurs, leading to an increase in collagen in the nucleus pulposus. These changes result in the loss of turgor in the disc[52,53] and a loss in the disc's ability to resist compressive forces. In time, the annulus, because it starts to act like an under-inflated tire, begins to protrude beyond the margins of the vertebral body. This results in a loss in the buffer qualities of the nucleus pulposus. Shock absorption is no longer spread or absorbed evenly by the annulus or the cartilaginous end plate. The increased mobility (because of the "underinflated tire" of the disc) leads to greater shearing, rotation, and traction stress on the disc and adjacent vertebra. The result of these actions is approximation of the vertebral bodies and loss of the normal lordotic curvature in the cervical spine. In addition, the pedicles begin to approximate, resulting in an overriding or subluxation of the facet joints, which leads to approximation of the lamina. This in turn can lead to possible infolding of the ligamentum flava, especially when the cervical spine is in the neutral position or extension, along with degeneration of the joints of von Luschka. These changes subsequently lead to decreased ROM, shortening of the cervical spine, and loss of spinal stiffness.[53,54]

As previously stated, as the disc degenerates, the nucleus pulposus begins to lose its turgor, and its gel-like tissue, which normally is under pressure, begins to fibrose and take on an appearance similar to the annulus. The disc also begins to lose height, causing slight overriding of the zygapophyseal joint articular surfaces; this in turn leads to translational instability (i.e., loss of arthrokinematic control). Over time this instability leads to the formation of protective osteophytes and limitation of movement.[51,53] Radiological evidence shows that these changes are found in 60% of patients over age 45 and 85% of those over age 65, even if symptoms are not present.[51,53-55] In the cervical spine, the areas most commonly and most severely affected are reported to be C5-6 and C6-7.[3] If symptoms are going to develop, they tend to appear between 35 and 55 years of age. A cadaveric study by Lee and Riew[56] found that the upper cervical specimens appeared to be affected by facet arthrosis more frequently than the lower levels. In the same study, it was found that in the older population, the prevalence of facet arthrosis was as high as 29.87% for the C4-C5 level, which was the segment affected most frequently, followed by the C3-C4 level, then C2-C3, C5-C6, and C6-C7.[3,55] If symptoms are going to develop, they tend to appear between 35 and 55 years of age.

Kirkaldy-Willis[55] divided spondylosis into three stages: dysfunctional, unstable, and stabilization. Although he developed these stages for the lumbar spine, they are equally applicable to any area of the spine. Based on Kirkaldy-Willis's description, these stages begin when the

---

Synonyms for Spondylosis

- (Cervical)* disc disease/degeneration
- Segmental instability
- Hypertrophic arthritis
- Degenerative spondylosis
- (Cervical)* arthrosis

*Also occurs in other areas of the spine

TABLE **3-5**

Assessment of Aging and Degeneration of the Human Intervertebral Disc

Disc Grade	Nucleus Pulposus	Annulus Fibrosus	End Plate	Vertebral Body
Assessment by Gross Morphology*				
I	Gel-like, bulging; blue-white	Discrete lamellae; white	Hyaline; uniform thickness	Margins rounded
II	Fibrous tissue band extending from the annulus fibrosus	Chondroid or mucinous material between lamellae	Irregular thickness of cartilage	Margins pointed
III	Consolidation of fibrous tissue	Extensive chondroid or mucinous material; loss of annulus-nucleus demarcation	Focal defects in cartilage	Early chondrophytes or osteophytes at margins
IV	Horizontal clefts parallel to end plate	Focal disruptions	Fibrocartilaginous tissue extending from subchondral bone; irregularity and focal sclerosis of subchondral bone	Osteophytes <2 mm
V	Clefts extending throughout	Clefts extending throughout	Diffuse sclerosis	Osteophytes <2 mm
Assessment of Magnetic Resonance Imaging Findings†				
I	Homogeneous; bright; demarcation distinct	Homogeneous; dark gray	Single dark line	Margins rounded
II	Horizontal dark bands extend across the annulus fibrosus centrally	Areas of increased signal intensity	Increase in central concavity	Tapering of margins
III	Signal intensity diminished; gray tone with dark and bright stippling	Indistinguishable from nucleus pulposus	Line less distinct	Small dark projections from margins
IV	Proportion of gray signal reduced; bright and dark regions larger	Indistinguishable from nucleus pulposus; some bright and dark signals contiguous with nucleus pulposus and annulus fibrosis	Focal defects in line	Projections <2 mm with same intensity as marrow
V	Gross loss of disc height; bright and dark signals dominant	Signals contiguous with nucleus pulposus	Defects and areas of thickening	Projections <2 mm with same intensity as marrow

*Based on data from Vernon-Roberts B: The pathology and interrelation of intervertebral disc lesions, osteoarthritis of the apophyseal joints, lumbar spondylosis and low back pain. In Jayson MIV, editor: *The lumbar spine and backpain,* ed 2, pp 83-114, London, 1980, Pitman Medical.

†Using T2-weighted spin-echo images. TR 2000 msec and TE 90 msec.

Based on data information from Frymoyer JW, Gordon SL: *New perspectives on low back pain,* p 193, Park Ridge, 1989, American Academy of Orthopedic Surgeons.

patient complains of symptoms. However, the condition begins long before symptoms are evident. Initially spondylosis develops insidiously (silently) and is asymptomatic.[6]

In the **dysfunctional stage**,[55] the patient complains of nonspecific neck pain with localized tenderness (Table 3-6). On radiographic examination, the disc degeneration is obvious, as seen in the loss of height and the bulging of the annulus beyond the vertebral margins. Abnormal function of the facet joints (i.e., subluxation caused by disc degeneration) and synovitis may occur, along with protective muscle spasm, although this subluxation is seldom seen on x-ray films. Side flexion or rotation commonly is limited or stiff and painful, especially to one side. The same is true for cervical extension. A neurological examination at this stage frequently is negative. In some cases symptoms may be attributed to a recent injury, such as a car accident, when in fact they already were present, even though the patient did not complain of symptoms.

TABLE **3-6**

Signs, Symptoms, and Radiological Changes in the Dysfunctional Stage of Spondylosis

Signs	Symptoms	Radiological Changes

• Local tenderness
• Muscle contraction
• Hypomobility
• Pain on extension
• Neurological exam usually normal
	• Low back pain:
	  ○ Often localized
	  ○ Sometimes referred
	• Pain with movement
		• Abnormal decreased movement
		• Malalignment of spinous processes
		• Irregular facets
		• Early disc changes

From Kirkaldy-Willis WH: *Managing low back pain*, p 79, New York, 1983, Churchill Livingstone.

The **unstable stage**[55] is marked by increased zygapophyseal or facet capsular laxity (Table 3-7). An abnormal "spinal rhythm" or "instability jog" (i.e., a flickering of the skin over the spine during movements) may become evident. This instability jog is an indication of lack of arthrokinematic motion control (i.e., a motor control deficit exists) as the patient moves the neck and head. The disc continues to degenerate and in some cases may herniate, and more bulging can occur in unstable stages and lead to hypermobility. This leads to segmental hypermobility (i.e., translational instability). Progressive degeneration of the facet joints is seen, which may lead to facet joint syndrome.[56] Radicular pain also may be seen because the lateral nerve roots can become trapped in the intervertebral foramen.[57] Traction spurs (usually found anteriorly) are sometimes seen on radiological examination.[58] Traction spurs are caused by abnormal stresses on the outermost attachments of the annulus and are thought to be related to the excessive mobility caused by the degenerative disc.[51,59] Traction spurs generally are seen 2 to 3 mm from the discal edge of the vertical body and project horizontally.

Traction spurs are not true claw, or marginal, osteophytes, which occur at the edge of the vertebral body (Figure 3-2). A claw osteophyte is commonly related to loss of disc height and annular bulging, which lifts the

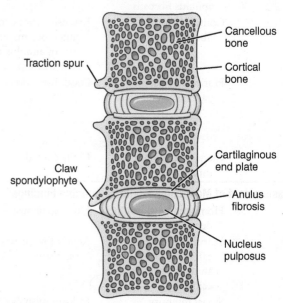

Figure 3-2 A traction spur projects horizontally from the vertebral body approximately 1 mm from the discal border. Traction spurs are indicators of segmental instability. In contrast, the common claw spondylophyte extends from the rim of the vertebral body and curves as it grows around the bulging intervertebral disc. Claw spondylophytes are associated with disc degeneration; they are *not* radiological manifestations of osteoarthritis. (Redrawn from Wong DA, Transfeldt E: *MacNab's backache*, ed 4, Philadelphia, 2007, Lippincott, Williams & Wilkins.)

TABLE **3-7**

Signs, Symptoms, and Radiological Changes in the Unstable Stage of Spondylosis

Signs	Symptoms	Radiological Changes
• Detection of abnormal movement (inspection, palpation) • Observation of "catch" in the back (on movement) • Pain on coming to standing position after flexion	• Symptoms of dysfunction • Giving way of back (i.e., "catch" in back on movement) • Pain on coming to standing position after flexion	Anteroposterior view: • Lateral shift • Rotation • Abnormal tilt • Malaligned spinous processes Oblique view: • Opening of the facets Lateral view: • Spondylolisthesis (in flexion) • Retrospondylolisthesis (in extension) • Narrowing of the foramen (in extension) • Abnormal opening of the disc • Abrupt change in pedicle height CT changes

From Kirkaldy-Willis WH: *Managing low back pain*, p 81, New York, 1983, Churchill-Livingstone.

periosteum from the vertebral edge, causing new bone to be laid down. A claw osteophyte or spur may also hook over the disc at the discal margin. Osteophytes are a physiological response to a compression load that reflects the body's attempts to stabilize the spine.[59,60]

With disc degeneration in the cervical spine, the joints of von Luschka, also called uncovertebral joints, are approximated, leading to a third location of osteophyte formation. Intraforaminal osteophytes encroach on the intervertebral foramen and possibly the vertebral artery, resulting in neurological symptoms and an increased possibility of vertebral artery syndrome.[61] The anterior spinal artery may thicken, leading to vascular insufficiency, or compression of the nutrient vessels may occur. Silberstein[61] contends that the joints of von Luschka are actually formed by this degeneration and rubbing and that they are not true synovial joints. Intraforaminal osteophytes limit movement and eventually stabilize the joint containing the fragmented disc.

In the unstable stage, patients complain primarily of neck dysfunction (see Table 3-7). They also commonly complain of a "catch" or sudden pain in the neck in part of the ROM during movement.[54] Greater restriction of movement is seen in this stage than in the dysfunctional stage, as well as uncoordinated movement (i.e., abnormal movement patterns) caused by dysfunction of the functional spinal unit (i.e., the disc and two apophyseal joints). Circumferential tears of the annulus fibrosus and radial tears extending from the annulus fibrosus to the nucleus pulposus may also be seen in this stage.

In the final stage, or **stabilization stage**,[55] fibrosis of the facet joints occurs, along with even greater disc degeneration and osteophyte formation (Table 3-8). Osteophytes form along the edges of the facet joints, leading to enlarged facets. Lateral nerve root entrapment becomes more common in this stage, leading to radicular signs and lateral stenosis in the intervertebral foramen. At the same time, osteoarthritis (OA) of the facet joints becomes more obvious.

Narrowing of the degenerating disc through the different stages of spondylosis can lead to anterior impingement

by the uncovertebral spurs, anterior impingement by the annular bulging, and posterior impingement by the osteophytes of the facet joints and fibrosis of the epidural nerve sleeves.[51,57] Facet joint degeneration leads to erosion of the joint cartilage and lipping around the joint edge, with formation of facet osteophytes. The synovial membrane thickens, and this, combined with the formation of facet osteophytes, leads to a decrease in the size of the intervertebral foramen and a greater possibility of radicular signs and symptoms. Nerve root fibrosis may also result from disc degeneration, leading to inflammatory changes, rubbing of the nerve root and sheath against the rough pedicles during movement, or injury to the nerve root. The cartilaginous end plate of the vertebral body degenerates throughout the development of spondylosis, showing thinning, fibrillation, and fissuring. The fissuring may extend the whole thickness of the end plate, and granulation tissue may grow through into the disc, adding to the fibrosis of the disc.[54]

The signs and symptoms of cervical spondylosis are mainly pain, restriction of motion, and in later stages, radicular signs. Cervical radiculopathy is the most common symptom of cervical degenerative disease that leads patients to seek treatment.[62] This occurs due to a combination of degenerative changes in the cervical spine, such as disc herniation, OA of uncovertebral and facet joints, decreased intervertebral height, and spondylolisthesis of cervical vertebrae. In some cases, the spinal cord or anterior spinal vessels may be compressed, leading to myelopathic symptoms.[63,64] It has been reported that cervical spondylotic myelopathy is the most serious and disabling progression of this disease.[48] The pain may be vague or ill defined, or it may be a dull, aching pain that increases over time and then tends to be referred to the shoulder or arm rather than the neck. Pain tends to be accentuated by movement and more often is evident toward end range. Radicular pain is referred into the appropriate dermatome initially, and the myotomes are affected later. Radiographic examination shows narrowing of one or more of the intervertebral discs and osteophyte spurring and irregularity, along with sclerosis of the vertebral body.[54,64,65]

Kellgren and Lawrence[66] developed a set of criteria to classify degenerative spondylosis based upon lateral cervical spine radiographs in a normal population sample. The classification is qualitative and has been extensively used to describe radiological changes in the cervical spine. This classification is a five-grade scale, ranging from "0" (absence of degeneration) up to "4" (severe narrowing of the disc space with sclerosis and large osteophytes). Gore et al.[67] added some criteria regarding the disc space narrowing, end plate sclerosis, and anterior and posterior osteophytes. According to a study by Ofiram et al.,[68] although the classification postulated by Kellgren and Lawrence has been shown to be reliable, it provides only a qualitative and general description of the degenerative changes. Therefore they created a quantitative radiographic index: the Cervical Degenerative Index (CDI) to measure cervical

TABLE 3-8

Signs, Symptoms, and Radiological Changes in the Stabilization Stage of Spondylosis

Signs	Symptoms	Radiological Changes
• Muscle tenderness • Stiffness • Reduced movement • Scoliosis	• Low back pain of decreasing severity	• Enlarged facets • Loss of disc height • Osteophytes • Small foramina • Reduced movement • Scoliosis

From Kirkaldy-Willis WH: *Managing low back pain*, p 86, New York, 1983, Churchill Livingstone.

TABLE **3-9**

Cervical Degenerative Index (CDI) and Scoring System

FACTOR	CDI SCORE			
	0	1	2	3
Disc space narrowing (%)	None-25	25-50	50-75	75-100
Sclerosis	None	Minimal	Moderate	Severe
Osteophytes	None	Small, less than 2 mm	Moderate, 2-4 mm	Large, more than 4 mm
Olisthesis	None	Less than 3 mm	3-5 mm	More than 5 mm

From Ofiram E, Garvey TA, Schwender JD et al: Cervical degenerative index: a new quantitative radiographic scoring system for cervical spondylosis with interobserver and intraobserver reliability testing, *J Orthop Traumatol* 10(1):22, 2009.

spondylosis.[68] The CDI includes four factors: disc space narrowing, end plate sclerosis, osteophyte formation, and olisthesis (either anterior or posterior), which makes the index more specific. The index is calculated based on a standard four-view cervical radiograph series (antero-posterior, lateral, flexion, and extension views), summing the four factors to achieve the final score for the CDI. A low score represents normal or very few signs of degenerative changes, and a high value represents more degenerative spondylytic changes of the cervical spine on the radiograph. Details of the scoring system can be found in Table 3-9. The overall CDI is thus calculated as the sum of the factor scores at all levels (equivalent to the sum of the level scores across all factors), resulting in a possible CDI score ranging from 0 (normal appearance) to 60 (most severe degeneration at each level). This index is innovative and can provide a score per cervical spine level, per independent factor, and a total for the entire cervical spine. It has been reported to have good intra-rater (0.87-0.89) and inter-rater (0.86) reliability, especially for senior raters. Thus, this index is useful and clinically relevant for the assessment of cervical spondylosis and can have a direct applicability for longitudinal studies of cervical spondylosis.

CERVICAL OSTEOARTHRITIS (OA)

OA in the cervical spine is in effect the later stage of spondylosis, marked by progressive degeneration of the intervertebral disc and especially the zygapophyseal joints (trijoint complex). Although the condition commonly is silent and asymptomatic, osteoarthritic changes can include osteophyte formation, hypertrophy of the synovial membrane, and in some cases a chronic inflammatory response (Figure 3-3). OA involves the zygapophyseal (facet) joints, which show degeneration of the articular surfaces and increased stiffness of the subchondral bone.[6] These changes lead to a decrease in the intervertebral disc space, osteophyte encroachment into the intervertebral foramen, hypertrophy of soft tissue (e.g., the ligamentum flava), and in some cases, encroachment on the spinal cord or vertebral artery.

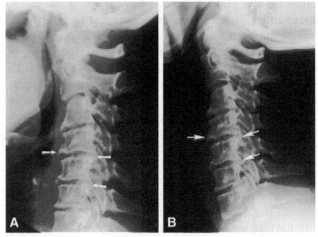

Figure 3-3 X-ray films of a 68-year-old man with multiple radiological signs of cervical osteoarthritis (*arrows*). **A,** The cervical spine in flexion, which is very limited. Note that the atlas tips up, compared with the one shown in **B.** All intervertebral disc spaces below C2-3 are very narrow, and anterior and posterior osteophytes are apparent (*arrows*). The spine extends very little in **B** and is quite straight in **A** (i.e., no significant flexion). (From Bland JH: *Disorders of the cervical spine,* p 213, Philadelphia, 1994, WB Saunders.)

Because of the structures involved and their proximity to the spinal cord, nerve roots, peripheral nerves (especially the sinuvertebral nerve), and in some cases, components of the autonomic system, symptoms can vary widely. They can range from relatively benign effects (e.g., limited ROM with minimal pain) to more severe symptoms involving the spinal cord (myelopathy), nerve roots (painful radiculopathy, sometimes without a predictable pattern), severe pain and muscle spasms, and in some cases, autonomic and brain stem responses.[6] Symptoms commonly are aggravated by movement.

CERVICAL SPINE INSTABILITY

According to Cook et al.,[69] "instability associated with active and neural cervical subsystem failure is identified as clinical cervical spine instability (CCSI)" (p. 896). It also has been called minor cervical instability.[70] Loss of cervical spine stability may be a significant factor in neck pain in many cases.[71-74] Cervical instability has not been fully defined, and many of the concepts used to describe it are extrapolated from work done on the lumbar region.[75] Panjabi et al.[76] defined clinical stability as "the ability of the spine, under physiological loads, to limit patterns of displacement so as not to damage or irritate the spinal cord or nerve roots, and, in addition, to prevent incapacitating deformity or pain due to structural changes" (p. 313). When the cervical spine demonstrates instability, failure to maintain correct vertebral alignment has occurred,[77] a result either of bony changes or of neuromuscular pathology. The essential feature of stability is therefore the ability of the body to control the full range of joint motion.[78] Thus normally the limits of the stability should provide sufficient support yet allow for the flexibility of normal activities.[54,79-82]

Clinical instability of the spine occurs when the neutral zone increases relative to the total ROM (Figure 3-4). The neutral zone has been shown to increase with intersegmental injury and intervertebral disc degeneration (see the Cervical Spondylosis section)[80,83-85] and to be decreased by the activation of the stabilizing muscle forces across the motion segment. Degeneration and mechanical injury of the cervical stabilization components (e.g.,

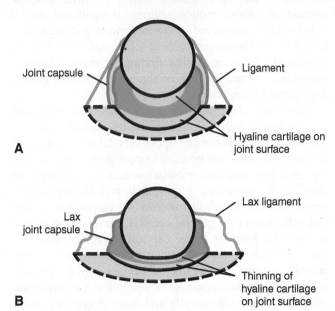

Figure 3-4 Articular instability. **A,** Normal joint with normal stability. Glides and nonphysiological mobility are limited by the joint surfaces and tension in the ligaments and joint capsules. **B,** Degenerative joint with articular instability. Note that the degeneration permits the bone ends to move closer to each other and thereby slacken off the capsule and ligaments. This allows increased nonphysiological motion on stability testing with a normal end feel. Glides and nonphysiological mobility are less limited by the flattened joint surfaces and slackened ligaments and joint capsules. (Modified from Panjabi M: The stabilizing system of the spine. Part II. Neutral zone and instability hypothesis, *J Spinal Disord* 5:390–396, 1992. In Magee DJ, Zachazewski JE, Quillen WS: *Scientific foundations and principles of practice in musculoskeletal rehabilitation*, p 516, St Louis, 2007, Mosby.)

discs, ligaments, and muscles) are the primary causes of increases in the neutral zone.[86]

Cervical instability can be secondary to several cervical spine conditions, such as chronic whiplash dysfunction, rheumatoid arthritis, OA, and segmental degeneration, situations involving trauma, genetic predisposition, disk degeneration, cervicogenic headache, systemic disease, or tumors. However, most patients diagnosed with cervical instability suffer from degenerative changes to the motion segment. Niere and Torney[70] defined minor cervical instability as "an increase in the neutral zone associated with one or more segments within the cervical spine. This condition may be associated with a number of signs and symptoms but does not include severe incapacitating pain nor symptoms indicative of spinal cord compression or vertebral artery disruption" (p. 145). It has been proposed that cervical instability may exist where pain and disability occur as a result of lack of control of the neutral zone motion, without compromise of the vascular or neural structures.[70] Minor cervical instability can be demonstrated only through clinical features that make the diagnosis more difficult (Table 3-10).[70]

Unfortunately, there is no gold standard for diagnosing minor cervical instability, nor even an accepted set of associated clinical signs and symptoms.[70] Clinical reasoning plus certain clinical characteristics could help with an approximated diagnosis. Clinical tests have been described to determine cervical instability. However, they have been considered unreliable,[87] or they have been reported to be uncommonly used by practitioners for diagnosing cervical instability.[88] According to Niere and Torney,[70] clinicians have described traction spurs, hypermobility, and anterolithesis on x-rays and clinical signs similar to those seen in Kirkaldy-Willis' unstable phase of cervical spondylosis as a sign of minor cervical instability. Poor motor control has been recognized as a major component of clinical instability.[70] Studies on the lumbar spine have demonstrated that this alteration in motor control can be a factor in the development of lumbar instability.[89-93] It has been hypothesized that aberrant motion (i.e., an instability jog), which is seen with sudden acceleration or deceleration that occurs outside the intended plane of movement in the midranges of active cervical movement, is a cardinal sign of instability.[94]

Other signs of clinical instability are reported to be general tenderness in the cervical region, referred pain to the shoulder and parascapular area, cervical radiculopathy, cervical myelopathy, occipital and frontal or retroorbital headaches, paraspinal muscle spasm, decreased cervical lordosis, and pain with sustained postures.[70,95] According to Niere and Torney[70] and Swinkels et al.,[96] clinical findings associated with cervical instability include neck pain, complaints of catching or locking in the neck, weakness, altered ROM, a history of major trauma or repetitive microtrauma, neck pain and headaches that are provoked by a sustained weight-bearing posture (e.g., sitting) and

TABLE **3-10**

Signs and Symptoms of Minor Clinical Cervical Instability

Main Signs and Symptoms	Secondary Signs and Symptoms	Other Signs and Symptoms
• History of major trauma • Catching/locking/giving way • Poor muscular control • Excessively free end feel on palpation • Signs of hypomobility on x-ray film • Unpredictability of symptoms • Spondylolisthesis	• History of repeated microtrauma • Neck weakness (subjective) • Traction spurs • Altered ROM • Neck pain • Muscle spasms • Muscular atrophy • Headaches	• Apprehension when moving into neck extension • Feeling of "heavy head" • Feeling as if the head is dropping off • Episodes with no precipitating cause • Crepitus • Feeling of a lump in the throat • Difficulty returning from extension • Poor response to previous treatment and good response to stabilizing treatment • Shoulder girdle weakness and atrophy

Modified from Niere KR, Torney SK: Clinicians' perceptions of minor cervical instability, *Man Ther* 9:144-150, 2004; and Cook C, Brismée JM, Fleming R et al: Identifiers suggestive of clinical cervical spine instability: a Delphi study of physical therapists, *Phys Ther* 85(9):895-906, 2005.

relieved by non–weight-bearing postures (e.g., lying supine), hypermobility with a soft end feel during passive intervertebral motion testing, and poor cervical muscle strength (e.g., the multifidus, longus colli, and longus capitis).[69] Shaking and poorly controlled (aberrant) motion during active cervical ROM also have been mentioned.[71] Cook et al.[69] used similar signs and symptoms when describing cervical spinal instability when questioning practitioners about key features of cervical instability. For example, they found that "intolerance to prolonged static postures" was the symptom identifier that was most related to cervical instability. "Fatigue and inability to hold head up" ranked second, followed by "better with external support, including hands or collar." Regarding physical examination findings, clinicians thought that "poor coordination and neuromuscular control, including poor recruitment and disassociation of cervical segments with movement" were the most related physical examination findings to cervical instability followed by "abnormal joint play."[69] In a survey conducted in Australia on upper cervical instability, practitioners felt that increased mobility on passive testing, dizziness, headaches, upper cervical pain, nausea and/or vomiting, suboccipital pain, and bilateral or quadrilateral paresthesia were signs and symptoms that characterized this condition.[9] According to Paris,[97] instability exists only when an aberrant motion, such as a visible slip, catch, or shaking, occurs (i.e., an instability jog) or when a palpable difference in bony position can be noted between standing and lying supine. Poor motor control and an inability to initiate cocontraction of the local muscle system in the neutral zone have been observed in many patients.[93]

Generally patients with cervical instability develop compensatory movements to stabilize the motion segment. Because the patient does not have good control of deep spinal muscles (e.g., the multifidus, intertransversarii, and longissimus), the body tries to recruit global muscles to maintain segmental stability. This action also has been seen

in patients with neck pain and whiplash.[98–100] Tables 3-11 and 3-12 present summaries of the variables and factors related to minor cervical instability as described by Niere and Torney.[70]

The lack of specific or sensitive diagnostic tools complicates the diagnosis of cervical instability. O'Sullivan[92] maintains that radiological evidence of intersegmental motion of a single motion segment is significant only if this finding is supported by clinical evidence of segmental instability at the corresponding segmental level. The diagnosis still relies on clinical findings: history, subjective complaints, visual analysis of the active motion quality, and manual examination.[71]

Upper cervical instability is a controversial topic, and the literature lacks consensus on its clinical aspects.[96] However, instability in the upper cervical spine is a major concern for clinicians because inappropriate treatment in this area can have severe consequences (i.e., paralysis or death).[71,101] According to Swinkels and Oostendorp,[102] upper cervical instability should be considered a special subcategory of general cervical instability because it is doubtful whether upper cervical instability occurs in patients without an inflammatory process (e.g., rheumatoid arthritis) or congenital problems (e.g., Down's syndrome). In fact atlantoaxial instability and hypermobility occur more frequently and most clearly in patients with rheumatoid arthritis, and in most cases without neurological signs.[102] Muscle action compensation could be argued to be a response of upper cervical instability without symptoms. A case study of upper cervical instability secondary to rheumatoid arthritis was published showing typical signs and symptoms of this condition.[103] This highlighted the importance of a good physical assessment performed by first contact practitioners to be able to recognize upper cervical instability, a condition which contraindicates manual treatment and requires immediate referral and further investigation of symptomatology. Practitioners working with manual techniques must be

TABLE **3-11**

Frequency of Response of Clinicians in Each Category for Cervical Clinical Stability

FINDING	NO IMPORTANCE		MINOR IMPORTANCE		SOMEWHAT IMPORTANT		VERY IMPORTANT		VITALLY IMPORTANT		% RESPONSES OF VERY OR VITALLY IMPORTANT
	N	%	N	%	N	%	N	%	N	%	%
History of major trauma	0	0	5	4	36	25	70	48	33	23	71
Catching/locking/giving way	1	1	13	9	29	20	66	46	34	24	70
Poor motor control	0	0	16	11	34	24	69	48	24	17	65
Excessively free end feel on palpation	4	3	8	6	40	28	63	44	27	19	63
Signs of hypomobility on x-ray film	3	2	16	11	34	24	56	39	34	24	63
Unpredictability of symptoms	1	1	16	11	46	32	63	44	16	11	56
Spondylolisthesis	7	5	21	15	43	30	50	35	21	15	50
History of repeated trauma	4	3	22	15	46	32	58	40	13	9	49
Neck weakness (subjective)	3	2	20	14	63	44	46	32	11	8	40
Traction spurs	11	8	26	18	59	41	36	25	11	8	33
Altered ROM	8	6	48	33	45	31	36	25	7	5	30
Neck pain	10	7	36	25	56	39	34	24	7	5	29
Muscle spasm	4	3	46	32	61	42	27	19	5	4	23
Muscular atrophy	14	10	56	39	50	35	17	12	7	5	17
Headaches	16	11	62	43	45	31	19	13	1	1	14

From Niere KR, Torney SK: Clinicians' perceptions of minor cervical instability, *Man Ther* 9(3):144-150, 2004.

TABLE **3-12**

Factors Related to Cervical Instability

Passive Dysfunction	Active Dysfunction	Cervical Pattern	Movement Abnormality
• Traction spurs • Signs of hypomobility on x-ray films • Spondylolisthesis • History of repeated microtrauma • History of major trauma	• Poor motor control • Neck weakness (subjective) • Unpredictability of symptoms • Catching/locking/giving way, as well as muscular atrophy	• Headaches • Neck pain • Muscle spasm • Muscular atrophy	• Excessively free end feel on palpation • Altered ROM • History of major trauma

From Niere KR, Torney SK: Clinicians' perceptions of minor cervical instability, *Man Ther* 9(3):144-150, 2004.

aware of this condition and have the skills to detect it to avoid negative outcomes.

Atlantoaxial subluxation is the most common type of cervical spine instability in patients with rheumatoid arthritis, with a quoted incidence of 50% to 70%.[104] Inflammation and pannus formation in and around the transverse and alar ligaments cause the instability seen in rheumatoid arthritis. Other conditions associated with upper cervical instability are ankylosing spondylitis, psoriatic arthritis, and Reiter's syndrome.[104]

Suspicion of upper cervical instability is based on clinical signs, such as neck pain, the most common symptom (Table 3-13). Seventy percent of patients have pain in the upper cervical or suboccipital area, with variable radiation to the mastoid, occipital, temporal, or frontal region. Other signs that may be present include limitation of neck movements, torticollis (a cardinal sign in the early phase), and neurological signs (e.g., hyperreflexia, paresthesia, coordination problems when walking, and spasticity or pareses). Hypoesthesia is seen less frequently.

Upper cervical instability is commonly diagnosed using a radiological criterion known as the **Atlas-Dens Interval (ADI)**.[105] A consensus meeting of the American Roentgen Ray Society[106,107] set the upper limit for the ADI at 2.5 to 3 mm for adults and 4.5 to 5 mm for children. X-ray examinations have some restrictions, and other concerns include standardization of techniques, faults in measurements, and problems with standards of normalization. Thus a conventional x-ray study can fail to provide adequate information about atlantoaxial stability. According to some radiographic studies, no correlation has been found

TABLE 3-13

Signs and Symptoms of Upper Cervical Instability

Neurological Signs	Clinical Symptoms	Radiological Signs

• Hyperreflexia
• Paraesthesia
• Coordination problems in walking
• Spasticity or pareses
• Hypoesthesia in the area of the occipitalis major nerve (less frequent)
	• Pain in the upper cervical or suboccipital areas (70%)
	• Variable radiation to mastoid, occipital, temporal, or frontal regions
	• Limitation of neck movement
	• Torticollis
		• Atlas-Dens Interval (ADI):
		  • Adult limit: 2.5-3 mm
		  • Child limit: 4.5-5 mm

Modified from Swinkles R, Beeton K, Alltree J: Pathogenesis of upper cervical instability, *Man Ther* 1:127-132, 1996; and Swinkles RA, Oostendorp RA: Upper cervical instability: fact or fiction? *J Manip Physiol Ther* 19:185-194, 1996.

between the amount of atlantoaxial dislocation and the presence of neurological symptoms.[105,106] Most patients with rheumatoid arthritis tolerate atlantoaxial instability without neurological symptoms because the spinal cord tolerates gradually applied pressure surprisingly well.[98]

Clinical tests to detect upper cervical instability, such as the lateral shift test of C1, upper cervical flexion test, Sharp-Purser test, rotation test of C2 coupled with side flexion of the head, and anterior shift of the atlas compared with the dens axis,[107] are disputable, and according to Swinkels and Oostendorp,[102] no information is available about the reliability and validity of these tests. Surgical treatment for cervical instability is reserved for patients with severe neurological involvement. The objective of conservative treatment of clinical cervical instability is to increase the function of the muscular and neural systems so as to decrease the stress on the spinal segments.[77,81] Slater et al.[103] recommended cervical isometric stabilization exercises, controlled soft tissue stretches within the pain-free range, advice on the use of active ROM rotational and side flexion exercises, and information about symptoms that could prompt a patient to seek further assessment to treat cervical instability.

The objective of the stabilization exercises commonly incorporated into rehabilitation programs is to restore (i.e., reduce) the size of the neutral zone in order to restore the normal arthrokinematic motion that occurs when minimal forces are imposed on the spine.[104] The methods of restoring the neutral zone in rehabilitation are evident, and they include reeducation of the neurofeedback loop system, which includes muscles, tendons, and receptors.[104]

FACET (APOPHYSEAL OR ZYGAPOPHYSEAL) JOINT SYNDROME

The posterior joints of the vertebrae have a surface area that is approximately two thirds the size of the surface area of the intervertebral disc; they also have relatively lax and richly innervated capsules, and they are covered with hyaline cartilage.[6] The joints aid stability but are not primarily weight bearing.[6] As a result of disc degeneration or trauma, the mechanical load on the facet joints can be increased. This increased load may cause a synovial reaction, cartilage fibrillation, erosion of the joint surface, and in rare cases loose bodies. In most cases facet joint syndrome is believed to be the result of a synovial reaction that manifests itself symptomatically as muscle spasm and pain. These symptoms (i.e., pain and spasm) may be referred into specific areas, depending on the facet joint involved (Figure 3-5). This pattern of symptom referral is different from normal dermatome patterns.[108,109] Similarly ROM may be decreased. In some patients the condition is thought to be an early case of OA of the facet joints.

DISC HERNIATION

Disc herniation can occur in the cervical spine, although it is much less common than in the lumbar spine. The condition seems particularly to affect males in their 30s, and the discs most commonly affected are those between

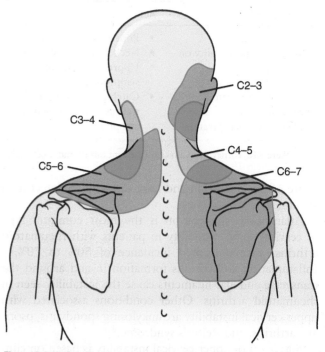

Figure 3-5 Referred pain patterns that can occur with pathology of the zygapophyseal joints. (Redrawn from Porterfield JA, DeRosa C: *Mechanical neck pain: perspective in functional anatomy,* p 104, Philadelphia, 1995, Saunders; modified from Dwyer A, Aprill C, Bogduk N: Cervical zygapophyseal joint pain patterns, *Spine* 15:453-457, 1990.)

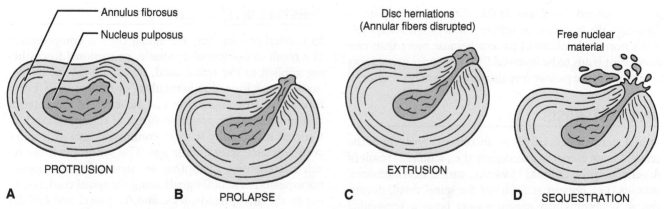

Figure 3-6 Types of disc herniations. **A,** Protrusion. **B,** Prolapse. **C,** Extrusion. **D,** Sequestration. (From Magee DJ: *Orthopedic physical assessment,* ed 6, p 553, St Louis, 2014, Elsevier/Saunders.)

C5-6 and C6-7.[110] Disc herniations can range from protrusion and bulging of the disc without rupture of the annulus fibrosus to sequestration of the disc, which results in discal fragments from the annulus fibrosus and nucleus pulposus outside the disc proper (Figure 3-6).[107–111] Between these two extremes are disc prolapse, in which the outermost fibers of the annulus fibrosus contain the nucleus, and disc extrusion, in which the annulus fibrosus is perforated and discal material moves into the epidural space.[107,111]

Disc herniations may occur in any direction, but posterior and posterolateral herniations produce the greatest number of clinical signs and symptoms. Central posterior herniations lead to pain that radiates into the limbs bilaterally and to myelopathic symptoms (Table 3-14).[3] However, because of the strength of the posterior longitudinal ligament, patients more commonly present with posterolateral protrusions that cause unilateral symptoms (radicular pain) in the upper extremity.[3] In most cases cervical disc herniations are acute, and the patient complains of pain or aching

TABLE 3-14

Signs and Symptoms of Motor and Sensory Changes in Cervical Myelopathy

Initial Symptoms (Predominantly Lower Limbs)	Later Symptoms (In Order of Occurrence)
• Spastic paraparesis • Stiffness and heaviness, scuffing of the toe, difficulty climbing stairs • Weakness, spasms, cramps, easy fatigability • Decreased power, especially of flexors (dorsiflexors of ankles and toes; flexors of hips) • Hyperreflexia of knee and ankle jerks, with clonus • Positive Babinski's sign, extensor hypertonia • Decreased or absent superficial abdominal and cremasteric reflexes • Drop foot crural monoplegia	• Various combinations of upper and lower limb involvement • Mixed picture of upper and lower motor neuron dysfunction • Atrophy, weakness, hypotonia, hyperreflexia to hyporeflexia, and absent deep tendon reflexes • Headache and head pain • Neck, eye, ear, throat, or sinus pain • Sensory symptoms in the pharynx and larynx • Paroxysmal hoarseness and aphonia • Rotary vertigo • Tinnitus synchronous with pulse or continuous whistling noises • Deafness • Oculovisual changes: Blurring, photophobia, scintillating scotomata, diplopia, homonymous hemianopsia, and nystagmus • Autonomic disturbance: Sweating, flushing, rhinorrhea, salivation, lacrimation, nausea, and vomiting • Weakness in one or both legs, drop attacks with or without loss of consciousness • Numbness on one or both sides of the body • Dysphagia or dysarthria • Myoclonic jerks • Hiccups • Respiratory changes: Cheyne-Stokes respiration, Biot's respiration, or ataxic respiration

Data from Bland J: *Disorders of the cervical spine: diagnosis and medical management,* Philadelphia, 1994, Saunders.

and has limited functional ROM of the cervical spine.[112] Although the pain may be referred, it does not always follow a normal dermatomal pattern because more than one nerve root tends to be involved.[112] If the upper nerve roots are involved, the patient may also complain of headaches.[112]

SPINAL STENOSIS

Spinal stenosis generally is an uncommon problem in the cervical spine except as a secondary (i.e., acquired) result of degeneration or trauma. However, with a developmental stenosis (i.e., present at birth) of the spinal canal, degenerative symptoms may appear sooner because congenital spinal stenosis has been combined with the acquired spinal stenosis from spondylosis or trauma (Table 3-15).[113,114] With activities that put stress on the head, resulting in spinal compression, unilateral or bilateral neurological signs may result.[115] Spinal stenosis is diagnosed if the sagittal diameter of the spinal canal is less than 13 mm.[6] Acquired spinal stenosis may be due to disc herniation (all four types), hypertrophy of the ligamentum flava, osteophytes, an inflammatory response, or hypertrophy of the lamina or facet joints. Differential diagnosis of spinal stenosis must include elimination of other conditions (see the following sections). If the problem is due to an inflammatory response, physical therapy may be useful. If the problem is due to structural change, surgery may be indicated.

Differential Diagnosis of Central Spinal Stenosis

- Vascular claudication
- Diabetic neuropathy
- Other peripheral neuropathies
- Motor neuron disease
- Multiple sclerosis
- Other central nervous system lesions
- Spinal infections (acute, subacute, and chronic)
- Neoplasms (involving the cauda equina, spinal nerves, or vertebrae)

From Kirkaldy-Willis WH: *Managing low back pain*, p. 103, New York, 1983, Churchill-Livingstone.

TABLE 3-15

Classification of Spinal Stenosis

Congenital/Developmental

Acquired
- Degenerative (central, lateral, or both)
- Combined (with disc herniation, with developmental stenosis, or with both)
- After laminectomy (scarring)
- After fusion (above the fusion, beneath the fusion)
- Trauma (early and late changes)
- Paget's disease
- Fluorosis

From Kirkaldy-Willis WH: *Managing low back pain*, p 103, New York, 1983, Churchill Livingstone.

CERVICAL MYELOPATHY

In cervical myelopathy, the spinal cord is compromised as a result of compressive, tensile, or torsional forces being applied to the spinal cord, which are caused by stenosis, spondylosis, disc herniation, or trauma.[116,117] These forces lead to compression and ischemia of the anterior and sometimes the posterior aspect of the spinal cord.[6,51] Cervical myelopathy is most commonly seen as a spinal cord "disease" after middle age. This syndrome is the result of something disrupting or interrupting the normal transmission of neural signals along the spinal cord, resulting in the arms, hands, legs, and/or bowel and bladder being affected. This "something" may include trauma, inflammatory and autoimmune disorders, tumors, viral infections, or degenerative processes. The condition usually has an insidious onset, and the signs and symptoms can be quite variable depending on the spinal level involved and the pattern of involvement. These signs and symptoms are highly variable (see Table 3-14) and may be progressive and unrelenting or intermittent and steplike. They may also be associated with multiple remissions.[116] Cervical pain and signs related to cervical movement are not common.[116] This variability of symptoms often results in confusing diagnoses; consequently, the interval between the development of initial symptoms and final diagnosis can be as long as 1.5 to 4 years.[6] Decompression surgery is commonly performed to prevent progression of symptoms by removing the structures causing the pressure, although it should be noted that the surgery may not result in a clinical improvement.

VERTEBROBASILAR ARTERY INSUFFICIENCY

Vertebrobasilar artery insufficiency is not a common condition. However, both vertebrobasilar artery insufficiency and internal carotid artery insufficiency can lead to significant problems.[6] Injury to the lining of the vessels can lead to thrombotic occlusion, artery dissection, pseudoaneurysm, or subintimal hematoma from manipulation of the spine, overhead work, or traction.[118] Normally the vertebral artery, which supplies approximately 20% of the blood to the brain (the internal carotid supplies approximately 80%), runs cephalically through openings in the transverse processes of the cervical spine. Once past the transverse processes of C2, the course that the arteries must take to enter the skull en route to the brain causes them to "kink." As a consequence of this route and because the artery is tethered at the atlantooccipital membrane, at the C1 transverse foramen and at the C2 transverse process along with the kinking, these arteries are at risk from forces that cause excessive traction or compressive stress on the vessels. Excessive force or motion in rotation and extension can reduce the circulation and potentially injure the vessel lining of these arteries.[6,118,119] If this reduction in circulation with movement, which is normal, especially in rotation or extension, is combined with degenerative or other changes in the area, the circulation to the brain stem may be further compromised; this can lead to signs and symptoms of vertebrobasilar artery insufficiency (Tables 3-16 and 3-17) or internal carotid artery insufficiency (Table 3-18), resulting from ischemia of the brain stem, cerebellum, cerebrum visual cortex, and vestibular apparatus.[6,119] Injury to the vessels can lead to quadriplegia or death.[119] Although injury to the vertebral artery and internal carotid artery is rare, clinicians treating the cervical spine should always have an understanding of possible accompanying risk factors as well as what factors should be assessed when looking for vascular problems.

Vascular Risk Factors

- Hypertension
- Hypercholesterolemia (high cholesterol)
- Hyperlipidemia (high fat)
- Hyperhomocysteinemia (hardening of the arteries)
- Diabetes mellitus
- General clotting disorders
- Infection
- Smoking
- Direct vessel trauma
- Iatrogenic causes (surgery, medical interventions)

Data from Kerry R, Taylor AJ: Cervical arterial dysfunction assessment and manual therapy, *Man Ther* 11:243-253, 2006.

TABLE 3-16

Classic Signs and Symptoms of Vertebrobasilar Insufficiency with Associated Neuroanatomy

Sign or Symptom	Associated Neuroanatomy
Dizziness (vertigo, giddiness, lightheadedness)	Lower vestibular nuclei (vestibular ganglion = nuclei of CN VIII vestibular branch)
Drop attacks (loss of consciousness)	Reticular formation of midbrain Rostral pons
Diplopia (amaurosis fugax; corneal reflux)	Descending spinal tract, descending sympathetic tracts (Horner's syndrome); CN V nucleus (trigeminal ganglion)
Dysarthria (speech difficulties)	CN XII nucleus (medulla, trigeminal ganglion)
Dysphagia (+ hoarseness/hiccups)	Nucleus ambiguous of CN IX and X, medulla
Ataxia	Inferior cerebellar peduncle
Nausea	Lower vestibular nuclei
Numbness (unilateral)	Ipsilateral face: descending spinal tract and CN V Contralateral body: ascending spinothalamic tract
Nystagmus	Lower vestibular nuclei + various other sites depending on type of nystagmus (at least 20 types)

From Kerry R, Taylor AJ: Cervical arterial dysfunction assessment and manual therapy, *Man Ther* 11:245 2006.

TABLE 3-17

Presentations of Vertebral Artery Dissection

Nonischemic (Local) Signs and Symptoms	Ischemic Signs and Symptoms
- Ipsilateral posterior neck pain/occipital headache - C5-6 cervical root impairment (rare)	- Hindbrain transient ischemic attack (dizziness, diplopia, dysarthria, dysphagia, drop attacks, nausea, nystagmus, facial numbness, ataxia, vomiting, hoarseness, loss of short-term memory, vagueness, hypotonia/limb weakness [arm or leg], anhidrosis [lack of facial sweating], hearing disturbances, malaise, perioral dysthesia, photophobia, papillary changes, clumsiness and agitation) - Hindbrain stroke (e.g., Wallenberg's syndrome, locked-in syndrome) - Cranial nerve palsies

Nonischemic symptoms may precede ischemic events by a few days to several weeks.

From Kerry R, Taylor AJ: Cervical arterial dysfunction assessment and manual therapy, *Man Ther* 11:245, 2006.

TABLE 3-18

Clinical Features of Internal Carotid Artery Dissection

Nonischemic (Local) Signs and Symptoms	Ischemic (Cerebral or Retinal) Signs and Symptoms

- Head/neck pain
- Horner's syndrome
- Pulsatile tinnitus
- Cranial nerve palsies (most commonly CN IX to XII)
- Less common local signs and symptoms include:
  - Ipsilateral carotid bruit
  - Scalp tenderness
  - Neck swelling
  - CN VI palsy
  - Orbital pain
  - Anhidrosis (facial dryness)
	- Transient ischemic attack (TIA)
	- Ischemic stroke (usually middle cerebral artery territory)
	- Retinal infarction
	- Amaurosis fugax

Nonischemic signs and symptoms may precede cerebral/retinal ischemia by anything from a few days to over a month.

From Kerry R, Taylor AJ: Cervical arterial dysfunction assessment and manual therapy, *Man Ther* 11:248, 2006.

Assessing for Vascular Problems

- Risk factors
- Position testing (especially rotation and extension) for symptoms
- Cranial nerve examination
- Eye examination
- Blood pressure examination
- "Headache like no other"
- Autonomic nervous system examination

Data from Kerry R, Taylor AJ: Cervical arterial dysfunction assessment and manual therapy, *Man Ther* 11:243-253, 2006.

Barré-Léou syndrome, also known as *posterior cervical sympathetic syndrome*, involves both the sympathetic nervous system and the vertebral artery. It causes a widespread and diverse combination of signs and symptoms.[6] Basically, the symptoms are the result of compression on the posterior cervical sympathetic system and its innervation of the vertebral artery, which lies close by.

CERVICAL ANOMALIES

Although relatively rare, congenital anomalies can be found in the cervical spine. They are not usually found in isolation but are associated with other developmental skeletal defects, such as dysplasia.[6,120] Many anomalies cause no signs or symptoms and are discovered on a cervical x-ray film taken for other reasons. Some patients present with signs and symptoms later in life as degeneration contributes to the effect of the anomaly; other anomalies, although rare, may be incompatible with life.[6]

Cervical anomalies may combine bone and nerve defects.[121-124] Bony anomalies are of concern primarily in terms of their effect on cervical stability, especially in the upper cervical spine, as well as the narrowing (stenosis) of the spinal canal and the effect this narrowing may have on the neural structures.[120,122,123]

As mentioned previously, Klippel-Feil syndrome (Figure 3-7) is a condition in which two or more vertebral bodies are fused, which occurs during embryological development.[124] Approximately 50% of patients with Klippel-Feil syndrome have a low posterior hairline, limited ROM, and an apparent short neck,[124] although some may appear normal.

Cervical ribs (Figure 3-8) are another anomaly that may be related to the cervical spine, and this condition is often grouped with a number of conditions under thoracic outlet syndrome. These anomalous ribs, which may be bony or cartilaginous, arise from the costal processes of the vertebral bodies. They usually are asymptomatic but may cause brachial plexus symptoms, especially of the lower nerve roots (C7, C8, and T1), as well as evidence of nervous or arterial compression.[6]

CERVICOGENIC HEADACHE

Cervicogenic headache is pain referred to the head from a source in the cervical spine.[125] Although the International Headache Society recognizes cervicogenic headache as a distinct disorder,[126] the concept of cervicogenic headache has not been fully accepted. The prevalence of cervicogenic headache is variable depending on the population and diagnosis criteria used to make the diagnosis. It has been reported to be 1%, 2.5%,[127] or 4.1%[128] in the general population when the clinical criteria has been used and as high as 17.5% among patients with severe headaches.[128] Patients after WAD present a prevalence of cervicogenic headache as high as 53%.[129] In fact the presence of trauma has been considered one of the distinct criteria for cervicogenic headache because all studies that have implicated the C2-3 zygapophyseal joint as a source of cervicogenic headache have been conducted in patients with a history of trauma.[125] As occurs in most headache forms, the incidence of cervicogenic headache is more prevalent in females.[130] The onset of cervicogenic headache is not age specific and can be associated with degenerative joint disease or a sedentary lifestyle. The history is often prolonged.[130] According to Andersen et al.,[131] cervicogenic headache is a complex syndrome, and its pathophysiology is far from simple. The involvement of musculoskeletal structures (i.e., nociceptive pain), sensory nerves and nerve roots (i.e., neuropathic pain), and referred pain can be implicated. Even if no definitive damage can be found in patients with cervicogenic headache, the presence of some axonal dysfunction cannot be excluded. Also, central sensitization of the central nervous system (CNS) may explain the chronicity of this syndrome.

The pathophysiological mechanisms underlying cervicogenic headache have not been clearly demonstrated; however, there is some evidence that the fundamental mechanism must be convergence.[64,132,133] The neuroanatomic relationship between the cervical spine and craniofacial pain is provided by the interconnection between the trigeminal nerve and first cervical nerve roots. Studies in animals have supported this connection.[134-137] The communication between the trigeminal nerve and first three levels of the cervical spine is so close that they merge into a single column of gray matter, and, as a result, they are not differentiated anatomically, functionally, or pathologically.[127] This convergence is the foundation of referred pain in the head and upper neck. Nevertheless, the reference pattern is more common in the region innervated by the ophthalmic branch of the trigeminal nerve than in the maxillary or mandibular branches because the maxillary and mandibular afferents in the spinal tract of the trigeminal nerve do not extend as far caudally into the cervical segments as do the ophthalmic afferents.[138,139]

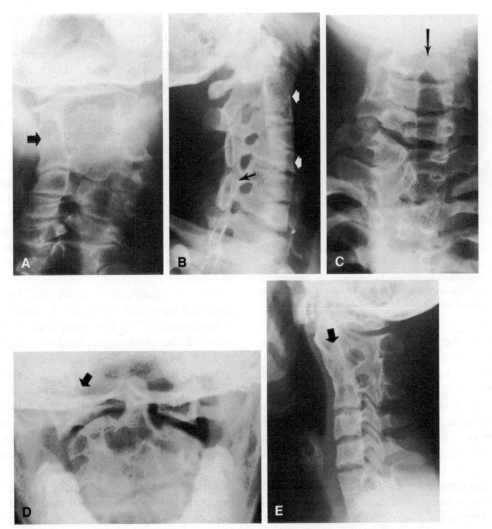

Figure 3-7 A, Anteroposterior view of the cervical spine of a 31-year-old man with Klippel-Feil syndrome shows fused C2 and C3 vertebrae (*arrow*), a hemivertebra at C5, spina bifida, and scoliosis of the cervical spine. The patient was asymptomatic and had an incidental radiological study for an injury. **B,** Lateral view of the cervical spine of a 12-year-old boy with Klippel-Feil syndrome shows fusion of the C2 and C3 vertebrae (*upper white arrow*) and only partial fusion with poorly developed disc spaces at C3-4, C4 to C6, and C6-7. A hemivertebra is seen at C5 (*lower white arrow*). The zygapophyseal joint is fused at C3-4 and C5-6 (*black arrow*). **C,** Anteroposterior view of **B** shows a butterfly vertebra (C3 and C4, *arrow*) and hemivertebrae (C7 to T1). T2 and spina bifida are seen just above the level of the first rib. In other views, a surprising amount of remodeling and osteophytosis is seen. **D,** Open-mouth view of **B** shows deviation of the odontoid process to the right, the result of having two sets of posterior elements on the left (*arrow*) and only one on the right. **E,** Lateral view of the cervical spine of a 15-year-old girl with Klippel-Feil syndrome shows fusion of the C2-3-4 vertebrae (*arrow*) and a kyphotic deformity of the cervical spine. Fusion also occurred at C7 through T3, and a hemivertebra is seen at C7. The neck was not short, and no evidence of basilar impression or occipitalization of the atlas was noted. The patient was asymptomatic. (From Bland JH: *Disorders of the cervical spine,* p 425, Philadelphia, 1994, Saunders.)

Another source of referred pain from the cervical spine to the head is provided by the innervation coming from the upper cervical nerve roots (Table 3-19).[138,140–142] The atlantooccipital joint is innervated by the C1 ventral ramus and the lateral atlantoaxial joint by the C2 ventral ramus; the C2-3 zygapophyseal joints are innervated by the C3 dorsal ramus. All three nerves of the upper cervical spine intermingle at multiple segments and converge with the trigeminal afferents on cells in the dorsal gray column of the C1 to C3 segments. Because of this convergence, pain from any of the upper three cervical synovial joints could be perceived in the same region and referred to the occiput and to regions innervated by the trigeminal nerve.[142–149]

The Quebec Headache Study group has stated that cervical facet dysfunction is probably the most important clinical source of cervicogenic headache.[150] In addition, the best available evidence indicates that the C2-3 zygapophyseal joints are the most common source of cervicogenic headache[129,145,151,152] accounting for approximately 70% of cases.[147] Some investigators have proposed the idea that cervicogenic headache can be caused by dysfunction of the lower cervical segments based on the evidence that some patients with lower cervical radiculopathy also have headache and were relieved of their headache pain after the radiculopathy had been treated surgically.[153] Although these data show an association between headache and lower cervical segments,

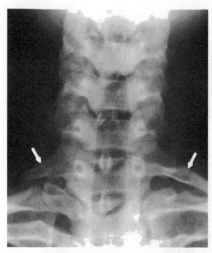

Figure 3-8 Anteroposterior view of the cervical spine of a 21-year-old man whose incidentally discovered cervical ribs became typically symptomatic after an automobile accident resulted in a neck injury (*arrows*). (From Bland JH: *Disorders of the cervical spine,* p 427, Philadelphia, Saunders, 1994.)

cervical structures, such as the skin, the cervical muscles and their attachments, the capsules of the cervical joints, and discs, ligaments, nerves, and nerve roots, are thought to be possible origins of cervicogenic headache.[142]

According to Pereira Monteiro,[155] the clinical limits of cervicogenic headache have not yet been well defined. Cervicogenic headache is estimated to account for 15% to 20% of all chronic and recurrent headaches,[156,157] and cervicogenic headache is the most common persistent symptom following neck trauma.[144,145] According to Sjaastad et al.,[158] cervicogenic headache is characterized by predominantly unilateral symptoms, always on the same side, that are precipitated by neck movement or sustained neck postures or by pressure on certain tender spots in the neck. There is a variable presence of pain, stiffness, and decreased ROM of the neck and ipsilateral shoulder or arm pain.

From a classification standpoint, the implication of unilateral signs and symptoms in cervicogenic headache is fundamental.[159-161] However, Watson and Trott[162] have reported that cervicogenic headache can be bilateral with one side predominant. Side consistency is evident with cervicogenic headache; this means that the side on which the signs and symptoms appear should not change with different attacks, as occurs with migraine headaches. Although unilaterality has been used as diagnostic criteria, Sjaastad and Bakketeig,[163] the authors of the diagnosis criteria, have recognized that unilaterality is rare and generally is seen only in mild cases of cervicogenic headache. When the headache is severe, bilateral pain is present. Cervicogenic headache headache is typically associated with pain in the neck or suboccipital region.[164] By definition, the pain can be mechanically provoked or intensified, and it radiates in

neuroanatomically, there is no direct link between lower cervical afferents and the trigeminocervical nucleus, and thus it does not seem plausible that cervicogenic headache can be caused by the lower cervical segments.

Another origin of cervicogenic headache may be the dura mater; headache can occur as a result of tension and/or pressure on the dura mater. The cranial dura mater is innervated by the trigeminal, vagus, and hypoglossal nerves and the upper cervical nerves. Hack et al.[154] found that an anatomical connection existed between the rectus posterior minor muscle and the dura mater, and as a result contraction of the rectus posterior muscle might cause tension on the dura mater, leading to a headache. Several

TABLE **3-19**

Innervation Provided by Upper Cervical Nerves (C1, C2, and C3) to Different Structures

Structures	C1	C2	C3
Tissues	Sensory information to deep suboccipital tissues Vertebral internal carotid Paramedian dura of the posterior cranial fossa	Skin of the occiput, transverse ligament of Atlas, and membrane tectoria Vertebral internal carotid Paramedium dura (through its sinuvertebral nerve itinerates)	Atlantoaxial ligaments and the dura matter of the spinal cord and clivus Vertebral internal carotid
Muscles	Sensory of cervical prevertebral muscles (longus capitis, longus cervicis, rectus capitis anterior, lateralis, ECM, and trapezius)	Major part of the upper neck muscles, splenius capitis, semispinalis capitis, and longissimus capitis	Splenius capitis, splenius cervicis, and longissimus capitis Deeper branch supplies semispinalis cervicis and multifidus Superficial branch innervates semispinalis capitis
Joints	Atlantooccipital joint Median atlantoaxial joint	Atlantoaxial joint; through its sinuvertebral nerve innervates the median atlantoaxial joint	C2-C3 zygapophyseal joint C2-C3 disc

From Bogduk N: Cervicogenic headache: anatomic basis and pathophysiologic mechanisms, *Curr Pain Headache Rep* 5:382-386, 2001.

an atypical distribution from the occipital to the fronto-temporal and orbital regions. In some cases, the face and ipsilateral shoulder and arm, without any definitive radicular pattern, are also affected. Nausea, vomiting, phonophobia and photophobia, and ipsilateral visual blurring may occur, as well as dizziness and difficulty swallowing.[165]

The intensity of cervicogenic headache can be mild, moderate, or severe, but it most commonly is moderate. It can fluctuate in intensity between headache periods and even within a single headache period. Lying down and resting may help, as does simple analgesia for some patients. Table 3-20 presents Sjaastad's diagnostic criteria[160,161] for cervicogenic headache. Alteration of the neck ROM generally is seen with cervicogenic headache, and it has been defined as a distinctive feature in the diagnosis of these patients.[151,155] Impaired neck mobility in the cardinal plane is a diagnostic criterion of cervicogenic headache.[161-166]

A systematic review[167] and meta-analysis about cervical impairments in cervicogenic headache supported the statement that patients with cervicogenic headache presented with altered ROM in all planes when compared with normal subjects. Moreover, it was found that cervical rotation movement with cervical flexion (i.e., the cervical flexion-rotation test) was very limited in patients with cervicogenic headache, supporting the finding that patients with cervicogenic headache have limited function in the upper cervical segments.[142] When all studies were added together for the meta-analysis,[168-171] it was found that patients with cervicogenic headache had a reduced ROM in all directions (i.e., flexion-extension, lateral bending, and rotation) when compared with a control group. Complete cervical rotation and flexion-extension movements were the most affected in patients with cervicogenic headache when compared with control subjects. When pooling the results of two studies[169,172] investigating the cervical ROM of rotation with cervical flexion, it was found that patients with cervicogenic headache presented with reduced ROM when compared with control groups. This information has been confirmed by a systematic review performed by Snodgrass et al.[173] Restricted cervical extension and altered cervical rotation test appeared to

TABLE 3-20

Major and Minor Criteria for Cervicogenic Headache

Major Criteria	Symptoms and signs of neck involvement. One or more of the following three phenomena must be present:
	• Precipitation of head pain similar to that which usually occurs by:
	  ○ Neck movement and/or a sustained, awkward head position, and/or
	  ○ External pressure over the upper cervical or occipital region on the symptomatic side
	• Restriction of ROM in the neck
	• Ipsilateral neck, shoulder, or arm pain of a rather vague, nonradicular nature or occasionally arm pain of a radicular nature
	
	Confirmatory evidence by diagnostic anesthetic blockages
	
	Unilateral head pain without side shift
	
	Head pain characteristics:
	• Moderate-to-severe, nonthrobbing pain that usually starts in the neck
	• Episodes of varying duration or fluctuating, continuous pain

Minor Criteria	Other characteristics of some importance:
	• Only marginal effect or lack of effect of indomethacin
	• Only marginal effect or lack of effect of ergotamine and sumatriptan
	• Female gender
	• Not infrequent head or indirect neck trauma by history, usually of more than moderate severity
	
	Other features of lesser importance:
	• Various attack-related phenomena that are only occasionally present and/or moderately expressed when present:
	  ○ Nausea
	  ○ Phonophobia
	  ○ Photophobia
	  ○ Dizziness
	  ○ Ipsilateral blurred vision
	  ○ Difficulty swallowing
	  ○ Ipsilateral edema, mostly in the periocular area

Modified from Sjaastad O, Fredriksen T, Bono G et al: *Cervicogenic headache: basic concepts*, European Headache Federation, p 43, London, 2003, Smith-Gordon; and Pikus H, Philips J: Characteristics of patients successfully treated for cervicogenic headache by surgical decompression of the second cervical root, *Headache* 35:621-629, 1995.

be useful when classifying individuals with cervicogenic headache if the patient also exhibited pain during manual examination of the upper cervical spine.[174] Thus ROM evaluation may be a useful tool in clinical practice to identify individuals with this disorder. In addition, this information could be used to determine appropriate treatment options and subjects who could benefit from therapies targeted to increase ROM because it has been shown to be effective in this population. However, several earlier studies have found that active cervical mobility is unreliable in differential diagnosis.[169,174-176]

In addition, the onset of cervicogenic headache may be related to a traumatic incident. Whiplash is among the first diagnostic criteria for cervicogenic headache,[157,162,168,169] but cervicogenic headache can be present in individuals without a history of trauma.[157,162,169,177-179] As with most forms of headache, the incidence of cervicogenic headache is higher in females.[180] The onset of cervicogenic headache is not age specific, and the condition can be associated with degenerative joint disease or a sedentary lifestyle. The history often is prolonged.[180]

Despite efforts to clarify the clinical diagnosis of cervicogenic headache, diagnosis is still a problem because of the overlap of symptoms with other types of headaches, such as migraine and tension-type headaches (Table 3-21). Furthermore, the validity of the clinical diagnosis of cervicogenic headache has been questioned. According to several experts in cervicogenic headache, making the diagnosis of cervicogenic headache remains problematic and cervicogenic headache remains a controversial topic.[125,181] Because the clinical diagnosis of cervicogenic headache has not been completely validated, diagnostic blocks of cervical joints or nerves have been the most accepted method used to diagnose cervicogenic headache by practitioners of interventional pain medicine.[125] Without other evidence, controlled diagnostic blocks become the only means of establishing the diagnosis. However, this way to diagnose cervicogenic headache is impractical for clinicians working with these patients, and still the clinical criteria are commonly used to diagnose it in general practice.

Although Jull and Stanton[182] did not find any consistent pattern of predictors for improving cervicogenic headache, Fleming et al.[183] found that increased patient age, provocation or relief of headache with movement, and being gainfully employed were all patient factors that were found to be significantly related to improved outcomes.

TABLE **3-21**

Diagnosing Different Headaches

Cervicogenic Headache	Migraine	Tension-type Headache
Unilateral pain; never changes sides	Unilateral pain but may be bilateral and can change sides with different attacks	Usually bilateral pain
Throbbing pain	Throbbing pain	Pressing, tightening pain
Moderate-to-severe intensity	Moderate-to-severe intensity	Mild-to-moderate intensity
Autonomic symptoms	Autonomic symptoms	Not accompanied by autonomic symptoms
Pain starting in the neck and pain triggered by neck movement and/or sustained awkward position	Pain is not triggered by neck movement	Pain usually is not triggered by neck movement
Affecting mainly females	Affecting mainly females	Affecting mainly females
Requires individual to lie down to feel better	Aggravation by routine physical activity	Does not worsen with routine physical activity
Reduced ROM in the cervical spine	No reduced ROM in the cervical spine	No remarkable unilateral restriction of neck motion
No precipitant mechanism	Precipitant mechanism (i.e., food, light, stress)	Not attributed to some other disorder
No response to medications	Response to ergot/sumatriptan treatment	Presence of trigger points; tenderness extending to shoulders and cervical muscles and also present in pericranial muscles
Good response to blockage of cervical joints or nerves	No response to blockage of cervical joints or nerves	Blockage of greater occipital nerve reduces pain only in area of blockage; does not abolish headache

Modified from Bono G, Antonaci F, Ghirmai S et al: Unilateral headaches and their relationship with cervicogenic headache, *Clin Exp Rheumatol* 18(suppl 19): S11-S15, 2000; and Vincent MB, Luna RA: Cervicogenic headache: a comparison with migraine and tension-type headache, *Cephalalgia* 19:11-16, 1999.

In addition, in a recent survey conducted in Australia regarding factors associated to nonresponsiveness to treatment in subjects with cervicogenic headache, clinicians considered a history of trauma, minimal mechanical signs, family history of headache, genetic predisposition, neural sensitivity, and the presence of co-morbidities to be features associated with nonresponsiveness to cervicogenic headache management.[184] Thus it is important that clinicians consider these factors when evaluating and treating patients with cervicogenic headache, especially those which are modifiable. Therefore relying on the patient's history and symptoms may not be the best way to reach an accurate diagnosis. Also, patients can suffer a "mixed" headache form or two types of headaches concurrently.[180] The differences between the available classifications for headaches of cervical origin make the study of cervicogenic headache confusing and the diagnosis of this condition more difficult.[158]

According to Jull,[130] evaluation of physical impairments of the cervical spine can help in the diagnosis of cervicogenic headache. Also, treatment of the musculoskeletal impairments associated with cervicogenic headache has been proposed as an essential part of the condition's overall treatment.[130,185] This means that the physical examination is crucial. Deep flexor muscles, including the longus capitis and longus colli, are important for cervical segmental and postural control. Alteration of the strength and endurance of the deep flexor muscles has been found in patients with neck pain and those with cervical dysfunction.[130] Dumas et al.[168] and Watson and Trott[162] investigated the relationship between strength of the upper neck flexor muscles and endurance of the same group of muscles in patients with cervicogenic headache. Both studies concluded that strength of the upper neck flexors was significantly different between patients with nontraumatic cervicogenic headache compared with controls. In both studies, patients with nontraumatic cervicogenic headache had smaller values of endurance compared with normal subjects.

The treatment of cervicogenic headache involves many specialists, including physicians, neurologists, orthopedic surgeons, rheumatologists, neurosurgeons, physical therapists, chiropractors, and osteopaths. Conservative therapies are recommended as the first choice. According to Jull,[130] the physical therapy approach to cervicogenic headache should include treating the patient's physical impairments not only to reduce symptoms but also to provide preventive maintenance. In addition, education of the patient in the predisposing and precipitating factors that aggravate the condition is essential for the overall management of these patients. There is some evidence from randomized controlled trials (RCTs) that supports the use of both manipulative therapy and specific exercise to reduce the frequency and intensity of the headaches and neck pain in a 1-year follow-up period. However, the combined therapy was not superior to either therapy alone.[186] Exercise therapy consisted of exercises directed toward improving motor control of the deep and superficial cervical muscles and training of the scapular muscles. Stretching and postural exercises were also recommended to improve body mechanics.[187] A study by Sharma et al.[188] also provided evidence in favor of stabilization exercises for the cervical spine to reduce headache dysfunction and improve proprioception of the neck.[188]

Five systematic reviews regarding the effectiveness of manipulative therapy in cervicogenic headache have shown some evidence supporting its effectiveness.[189-193] Bronfort et al.[190] reported that spinal manipulation appeared to have a better effect than massage for cervicogenic headache. It also appeared that spinal manipulation has an effect that is comparable to commonly used, first-line, prophylactic prescription medications for tension-type headache and migraine headache. Although Posadzki and Ernst[192] found that the majority of the RCTs showed that spinal manipulation was more effective than physical therapy, gentle massage, drug therapy, or no intervention, three out of nine RCTs showed no difference in pain, duration, or frequency of headaches compared with placebo, manipulation, physical therapy, massage, or wait-list controls. From all of these trials, only one was able to adequately control for a placebo effect, and this trial showed no benefit of spinal manipulations beyond a placebo effect. Thus the authors concluded that, based on these studies' methodological quality, the evidence cannot be conclusive regarding the use of spinal manipulation to treat cervicogenic headache. However, another systematic review[191] investigating the effect of physical therapy and manual therapies for cervicogenic headache found positive results. They concluded that physical therapy and spinal manipulation might be an effective treatment in the management of cervicogenic headache, although the patients included had infrequent cervicogenic headache and there was a lack of a true control group. These results were supported by the systematic review by Raciki et al.[193] They found that a combination of therapist-applied cervical manipulation and mobilization with cervicoscapular strengthening was most effective for decreasing pain outcomes in those with cervicogenic headache. However, due to the limited number of included studies in these reviews, more research is necessary investigating the effect of physical therapy and manipulative therapy treatment in patients with cervicogenic headache to be supported clinically.

In the early stages, conservative treatment through medication, change of lifestyle, physical therapy modalities, and acupuncture can be used. If the symptoms persist, blocks or radiofrequency treatment of the facet joints may be useful. More aggressive procedures, such as surgical cervical stabilization (e.g., foraminectomy, laminectomy, and unectomy), are reserved for patients with severe symptoms.

ASSESSMENT OF THE CERVICAL SPINE

The assessment of the cervical spine follows the method presented in *Orthopedic Physical Assessment* (volume 1 of this series). However, if the examiner is assessing primarily for hypomobility, then an understanding of the biomechanics in the cervical spine becomes important. In this context, *coupling* becomes an important factor in the assessment of the cervical spine. In effect, coupling is the conjunct rotation of a spinal segment. Side flexion and rotation have very small amounts of pure movement, and for all practical purposes, the two movements are combined. If side flexion initiates coupled movement, a small amount of rotation is combined with it. Similarly, if rotation initiates a movement, a small amount of side flexion accompanies it. In this context, rotation implies rotation and side flexion occurring together, not separately. Experts have many opinions about how a spinal segment couples, whether ipsilaterally (right rotation with left side flexion) or contralaterally (right rotation with right side flexion). For the most part, no one really knows the exact coupling action. Fortunately, with regard to the cervical spine (unlike with the lumbar spine), most of the opinions about coupling are convergent, which strengthens their validity. That being said, the reliability and validity of these tests have not been confirmed. The following section is based on the clinical experience of the chapter's first author, Jim Meadows.

Atlanto-occipital Segment

Considerable motion occurs at the atlanto-occipital joint, certainly enough for the movement to be appreciated and not just the end feel. Table 3-22 outlines the movement and ROM that occur at the left occipital joint.

As with most of the cervical spine, the key to understanding the function of the atlanto-occipital joint is to remember that it is primarily capable of flexion and extension. A considerable degree of rotation and side flexion is also available. The second point to keep in mind is that the arthrokinematics are the reverse of

TABLE **3-22**

Movement and Range of Motion of the Left Atlanto-occipital Joint

Movement	Range (Degrees)
Flexion	3.5
Extension	21.0
Right side flexion	5.4
Left side flexion	5.6
Right rotation	6.6
Left rotation	7.9
Combined flexion-extension	24.5
Combined side flexions	11.0
Combined rotations	14.5

those in the other zygapophyseal joints, and they occur in a different plane (i.e., horizontal). Although clinicians may know this intellectually, intuitively it "goes against the grain," and practitioners have a tendency to forget this point.

Mobility Tests

With the patient supine, the patient's head is extended around the axis for the atlanto-occipital joint (an axis approximately common with that of the atlantoaxial joint and running through the external auditory meatus). The head then is side-flexed left and right around a common craniovertebral axis running roughly through the nose. As the side flexion is performed, a gradual translation force is applied in the opposite direction to the side flexion. The translation is economical in that it maintains the axes of motion, reduces the degree of angular displacement necessary to obtain full ROM, and allows the clinician to detect an end feel. The ROM of side flexion is assessed from side to side, as is (more important) the end feel of the translation. The end feel allows the barrier to be assessed and can be muscular, capsular or tissue stretch (pericapsular tissue), or pathomechanical (subluxation or "jamming" of the joint). The side flexion procedure is then repeated for flexion.

During extension, the occipital condyles glide anteriorly to the limit of their symmetrical extension range. During side flexion and right translation, the coupled right rotation is produced. As rotation causes the right occipital condyles to retreat toward a neutral position, the left condyle must advance into the extension barrier. If side flexion is limited, the limiting factor must be on the left side of the segment (i.e., ipsilateral to the side flexion), preventing the advance of the condyle into its normal position (or with hypermobility, allowing it to advance too far).

An alternate method is to extend the segment and then rotate it rather than side-flex it. This method may be preferable because it eliminates the need to consider the coupling motion. Right rotation must flex the right joint and extend the left, but in practical terms this is problematic. Limiting the rotation to the atlantoaxial segment is quite difficult, and the examiner cannot be confident that any range restriction is a result of hypomobility at the atlanto-occipital joint rather than the segment below.

During flexion, the occipital condyles move posteriorly. The right rotation that occurs as a consequence of the left side flexion causes the left condyle to move away from the flexion barrier toward the neutral position while the right condyle is moved posteriorly into the flexion barrier. Therefore the limiting factor must lie on the right side of the segment that is contralateral to the side flexion. Again, rotation of the segment can be used instead of side flexion, but the practical difficulties remain.

It is apparent that the arthrokinematic and osteokinematic movements occur simultaneously. In fact the arthrokinematic movement in itself does not afford as much information about the type of hypomobility in these craniovertebral segments as it does elsewhere. This is due to the orientation of some of the suboccipital muscles that are oriented parallel to the plane of the joint so that they can restrict the glide of the joint and the bone movement. Consequently whether the hypomobility is myofascial, pericapsular, or pathomechanical in nature must be determined by other means. End feel would be the obvious answer to this question, but hypertonic muscles sometimes alter the axis of rotation in such a manner as to cause a false pathomechanical end feel. The more useful approach is to try a hold-relax technique and determine how much improvement occurs. If substantial improvement is seen, an extraarticular restriction is playing a major role; if little improvement is noted, an articular restriction is present.

It is important for the clinician to determine the side that is affected. If manipulation is used, the force must be as local as possible. The side of hypomobility is less important if mobilization is used because the direction of the mobilization is into the hypomobility.

Atlantoaxial Segment

Although rotation is the main movement at the atlantoaxial joints, a surprisingly large amount of flexion, extension, and side flexion also occurs at the segment (Table 3-23).

Mobility Tests

The atlantoaxial joints can be tested using the coupled movements of rotation and side flexion. According to cadaveric and in vivo studies, this segment has considerable ROM (see Table 3-23).

Rotation. The advantage of using rotation to assess ROM is that coupling is not an issue. The disadvantage is that many clinicians find this a less sensitive means of testing. (*Sensitive* here means being able to feel the movement.)

The patient sits with the clinician standing to one side. C2 is stabilized with a wide pinch grip, and the clinician's other hand reaches around the head to hold the occiput and C1. The patient's head is held against the clinician's chest, and a very light compressive force is applied as the head is rotated toward the clinician. The compressive force allows the descent of the head that normally occurs as the C1 facets descend on those of C2. The ROM is assessed and the end feel evaluated (Figure 3-9).

Side Flexion. With the patient lying supine, the clinician reaches under the neck such that a finger wraps around the spinous process of C2, compressing the soft tissue against the process. The clinician side-flexes the occiput around the craniovertebral axis while palpating the movement of the C2 vertebra via the motion of its spinous process (Figure 3-10). The movement is in the opposite direction to the side flexion, indicating rotation of the C2 vertebra to the same side with consequential rotation of the segment to the opposite side. For example, if the head is side-flexed to the right, the spinous process of C2 moves to the left as the vertebral body rotates to the right. Because by convention segmental movement is named by the movement

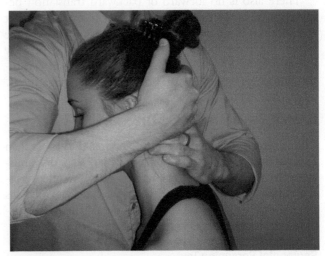

Figure 3-9 Atlantoaxial mobility test in rotation.

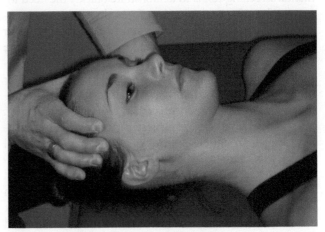

Figure 3-10 Atlantoaxial mobility test in side flexion.

TABLE 3-23

Movement and Range of Motion of the Left Atlantoaxial Joints

Movement	Range (Degrees)
Flexion	11.5
Extension	10.9
Right side flexion	9.4
Left side flexion	4.0
Right rotation	39.5
Left rotation	38.3
Combined flexion-extension	22.4
Combined side flexions	13.4
Combined rotations	77.8

of the superior vertebra, the C1-2 segment is rotated to the left. As the head is side-flexed, the clinician assesses the amount of spinous process displacement to gain an idea of the range of C2 rotation. The clinician stabilizes the head when all movement has ended and then pulls the C2 spinous process further into its passive range to gain the end feel of rotation. When right side flexion is produced, the clinician assesses left rotation and vice versa.

Flexion and Extension. These movements are most easily assessed in the sitting position when a rocking motion is produced and no glide is available. However, given that combined rotation has approximately 4 times the range of combined flexion-extension (see Table 3-23), if rotation is restored at the zygapophyseal joint, flexion and extension must also be restored, and this precludes the need to test the motion except in the extremely unlikely event that scarring has occurred in the flexor or extensor muscles. In trauma patients, who may have such scarring, flexion or extension is likely to be much more limited than rotation and side flexion. In addition, isometric testing reasonably can be expected to be either weak or painful (in the acute case, painfully weak) and the muscle to be tender to palpation. In such cases, stretching techniques must be undertaken for these muscles.

There also is no forward or backward translation because the dens and the transverse ligament severely restrict this motion; therefore no deductive determination of the side of the hypomobility can be made. Complex and very careful testing by a skilled practitioner may elicit this information, but in reality it is not necessary for treatment.

Cervical Segments (C2 to C7)

The cervical spine proper is more complicated to assess than the craniovertebral articulations because it has not only muscles and zygapophyseal joints but also discs and uncovertebral joints (i.e., joints of von Luschka). Consequently this examination needs to be somewhat more detailed and complex to obtain information on these additional structures.

Segmental Screening Test

As with any other screening tests, the purpose of the segmental screening test is to demonstrate quickly the need for more exhaustive testing and to focus the clinician's attention on a specific level or levels and specific movement or movements. However, it also can be used to determine the direction of treatment without concern about which structure is limiting the movement. This is particularly true for mobilization, but the information gained from the screening test may also be used with certain types of manipulation.

The segmental screening test is performed in a fashion similar to mobility testing of the atlantooccipital joint. The segment is extended, which lifts the superior vertebra forward (eliminating the need to extend the entire cervical spine). While the extended position is maintained, the segment is side-flexed left and right around its axis of motion and simultaneously translated

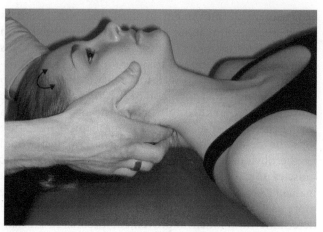

Figure 3-11 Segmental screening test for cervical segments C5 to C7.

contralaterally (Figure 3-11). During left side flexion, the left side of the segment is maximally extended while the right side is moving toward its neutral position. The ROM of the side flexion and the end feel of the translation are evaluated for normal, excessive, or reduced motion. If left side flexion is restricted, extension of the flexor muscles or one of the joints on the left likely is the problem. If the end feel of the translation is normal but side flexion is restricted, the hypomobility is extraarticular (i.e., myofascial). If left side flexion is restricted in flexion, then the right side of the segment is not flexing normally.

Occasionally side flexion appears to be normal but translation is restricted in all three positions. The likeliest cause of this restriction is uncovertebral joint dysfunction because these "joints" are involved in (or are the result of) side flexion and rotation and are largely unaffected by flexion or extension.

Deduction within the limits of theoretical knowledge can be used to determine the dysfunction, but direct testing, of course, is better. To this end, the arthrokinematics of the zygapophyseal and uncovertebral joints are evaluated.

Zygapophyseal Arthrokinematic Tests: Posteroanterior Intervertebral Movements (PAIVMs)

The orientation of the zygapophyseal joints is craniocaudal, mainly in the coronal plane. The patient lies supine. If extension is to be tested, the clinician lifts the superior vertebra of the segment by using the hand to gain extension, and the fingers are placed over the inferior processes of the superior vertebra (the superior facet). The two facets of the hypomobile side are compressed against each other by lifting upward while the superior facet is pushed caudally (Figure 3-12). The end feel is assessed by comparing it with the other side and/or the joints above and below.

For flexion, the segment is flexed and the superior facet of the suspected hypomobile joint is pulled cranially, again to assess the end feel. To do this the clinician must move the bone and not the overlying soft tissue; therefore it is useful for the clinician to attempt to put the fingertips between the two facets (Figure 3-13).

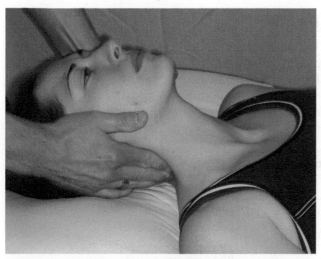

Figure 3-12 Posteroanterior intervertebral movement in extension.

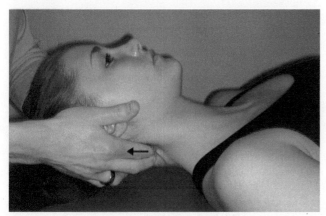

Figure 3-13 Posterior intervertebral movement in flexion.

Uncovertebral Arthrokinematic Tests: Posteroanterior Intervertebral Movements (PAIVMs)

The uncovertebral joints are oriented inferomedially and superolaterally in a mainly sagittal plane. Hypomobility of the joint restricts translation with or without perceptible limitation of side flexion itself. The restriction is felt in flexion, extension, and neutral; flexion generally is the least affected. The patient lies supine. If left translation is restricted, the right joint's inferomedial glide is tested by pushing inferomedially on the right superior transverse process while the inferior bone is stabilized by holding the left inferior transverse process (Figure 3-14). Superolateral glide of the left joint is tested by pushing the left inferior transverse process inferomedially while the superior bone is stabilized via the right superior transverse process.

Analysis of the Assessment Results

The assessment can yield information about the severity of the pain, the onset of the pain relative to the onset of tissue resistance (i.e., simultaneously, before,

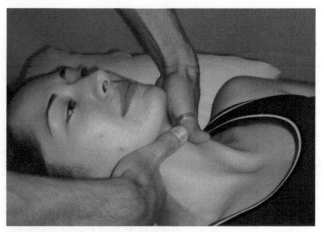

Figure 3-14 Uncovertebral arthrokinematic testing.

or after), and the type of tissue resistance (e.g., normal or abnormal, muscle spasm, capsular, or pathomechanical). Knowing these results and correlating them with the history findings enable the clinician to determine the degree of inflammation, if any, and the direction and type of hypomobility (i.e., flexion or extension, pathomechanical, pericapsular, extraarticular, or subacute inflammatory) and thus establish a viable treatment plan. Table 3-24 outlines the vertebral segments and the hypomobility diagnoses based on hypomobility findings.

Cervical Spine Hypomobility Considerations

- Limited motion with a spasm end feel plus a history of relatively severe pain and a proportional amount of irritability is strongly indicative of arthritis (systemic or traumatic), the treatment of which must be rest from adverse stress. This may mean mobilizing a nearby hypomobile segment that is putting undue stress on the painful joint.
- Limited motion with a hard capsular end feel requires rhythmical oscillations that stretch the capsular tissues. The joint may or may not be painful but is almost certainly contributing to the patient's neck pain by stressing a painful joint.
- Limited motion with a pathomechanical end feel (i.e., abrupt and lightly springy) requires nonrhythmical techniques, such as high-velocity, low-amplitude thrusts (manipulation) or minithrusts (oscillations).
- Minor pain or discomfort, which usually occurs when the barrier is stretched (i.e., pain after resistance), requires true grade 3 or grade 4 techniques; that is, near–end range oscillatory mobilizations that do not reproduce the pain but also do not retreat to the beginning of the range.
- Acute and subacute pain states (i.e., pain before or with the onset of resistance) require grade 1 or grade 2 oscillations for neurophysiological pain modulation.
- Any technique that provokes spasms should be avoided. If an alternative cannot be found, manual treatment should be abandoned until the pathology subsides.

Inflammation of the joint is characterized by relatively intense, continuous pain with high levels of irritability. In deeper joints, such as the vertebral articulations, other characteristics of inflammation, such as heat and swelling, cannot be observed. However, in the neck swelling may be palpated, and any redness is an indication of a systemic arthritis or infection (Table 3-25).

TREATMENT

Treatment of the cervical spine revolves primarily around patient complaints of pain, weakness, and restricted ROM. Several systematic reviews have been conducted to determine the best-quality evidence to treat neck pain and related disorders. Most of these reviews have found

TABLE **3-24**

Cervical Segment, Hypomobility Findings, and Subsequent Hypomobility Diagnosis

Segment	Hypomobile Findings	Hypomobility Diagnosis
Atlanto-occipital	Flexion/right side-flexion/left translation Hold/relax substantially improves Hold/relax no improvement	Left extensor hypertonicity Left joint hypomobility
	Flexion/left side-flexion/left translation Hold/relax substantially improves Hold/relax no improvement	Right extensor hypertonicity Right joint hypomobility
	Extension/left extensor hypertonicity Hold/relax substantially improves Hold/relax no improvement	Left flexor hypertonicity Right joint hypomobility
	Extension/left extensor hypertonicity Hold/relax substantially improves Hold/relax no improvement	Right flexor hypertonicity Left joint hypomobility
Atlantoaxial	Right rotation Hold/relax substantially improves Hold/relax no improvement	Left rotator hypertonicity Right rotation articular
	Left rotation Hold/relax substantially improves Hold/relax no improvement	Left rotator hypertonicity Right rotation articular hypomobility
	Flexion loss leading to rotation loss Hold/relax substantially improves Hold/relax no improvement	Extensor hypertonicity Bilateral articular
	Extension loss leading to rotation loss Hold/relax substantially improves Hold/relax no improvement	Extensor hypertonicity Bilateral articular
C2 to C7	Flexion/right side flexion/left translation Z- and U-joint PAIVM: − Left Z-joint PAIVM: + Right U-joint PAIVM: + Left U-joint PAIVM: +	Left side-flexion hypomobility Left extensor hypertonicity Left Z-joint superior glide (flexion) Right U-joint inferomedial glide Left U-joint superolateral glide
	Flexion/left side flexion/right translation Z- and U-joint PAIVM: − Left Z-joint PAIVM: + Right U-joint PAIVM: + Left U-joint PAIVM: +	Left side-flexion hypomobility Right extensor hypertonicity Left Z-joint superior glide (flexion) Right U-joint inferomedial glide Left U-joint superolateral glide
	Extension/right side flexion/left translation Z- and U-joint PAIVM: − Left Z-joint PAIVM: + Right U-joint PAIVM: + Left U-joint PAIVM: +	Right side extension hypomobility Left extensor hypertonicity Right Z-joint inferior glide (extension) Right U-joint inferomedial glide Left U-joint superolateral glide
	Extension/left side flexion/left translation Z- and U-joint PAIVM: − Left Z-joint PAIVM: + Right U-joint PAIVM: + Left U-joint PAIVM: +	Left side-flexion hypertonicity Right flexor hypertonicity Left Z-joint inferior glide (extension) Right U-joint superolateral glide Left U-joint inferomedial glide

PAIVM, Posteroanterior intervertebral movement; *U-joint,* uncovertebral joint; *Z-joint,* zygapophyseal joint.

TABLE 3-25

Pain-Resistance Relationship, Acuteness, and Possible Treatment in the Cervical Spine

Pain-Resistance Relationship	Acuteness	Treatment
Severe pain with no resistance	Empty feel (severe pathology)*	None
True constant pain†	Visceral	None
Severe continuous pain‡	Hyperacute	Rest, ice, compression, and elevation (RICE)
Pain before resistance	Acute	Grade 1 mobilization
Pain with resistance	Subacute	Grade 2 mobilization
Pain after resistance	Nonacute	Grade 3 or 4 mobilization
Resistance without pain	Stiff or pathomechanical	Grade 4++ mobilization
		Minithrusts or manipulation

*This is true empty end feel, not the feeling caused by torn ligaments, which usually is a soft capsular end feel.

†No physical stress or rest changes the intensity of the pain.

‡High-intensity rest pain that worsens with mechanical stress.

limited-to-moderate evidence regarding the effectiveness of manual therapy alone or in combination with physical modalities or exercises to decrease pain.[194-196] For example, Gross et al.[194] found moderate-quality evidence that cervical manipulation and mobilization had similar beneficial effects on pain, function, and patient satisfaction. In addition, they found low-quality evidence suggesting that cervical manipulation might provide greater short-term pain relief than a control group (standardized mean difference [SMD]: -0.90; 95% confidence interval [CI]: -1.78 to -0.0]). Miller et al.[196] concluded that the combination of manual therapy and exercise for treating neck pain was better than no treatment or exercise alone. When compared with no treatment, manual therapy plus exercises showed a clinically important long-term improvement in pain (SMD: -0.87 [95% CI: -0.69 to 0.06]), function and disability, and a global perceived effect. In addition, the combination of these two treatment modalities was superior to exercises alone or manual therapy alone for improving pain and quality of life for chronic neck pain sufferers. Yamato et al.[197] also investigated the use of therapeutic exercise in managing neck pain. They found that exercises in the form of strength training, stretching, deep muscle activation and coordination, endurance, and dynamic and postural exercises help to reduce pain in short (i.e., up to 1 month) and intermediate (i.e., 1 to 6 months) time periods. The effect sizes obtained ranged from 0.45 to 0.53, which are considered moderate effect sizes according to Cohen guidelines.[198] Another systematic review[199] that looked at exercises for neck pain found similar results. However, these authors' recommendations were more precise for different disorders. For example, they found that exercises, such as supervised qigong (a traditional Chinese practice of aligning body, mind, and breathing for health, meditation, and martial arts) and combined strengthening, ROM, and flexibility exercises, were more beneficial than a waiting list for subjects with persistent neck pain and a WAD grade 1/2. However, unsupervised exercise had no more superior effect than nonsteroidal anti-inflammatory drugs (NSAIDs) and acetaminophen, nor was manual therapy for acute neck pain or WAD, or a supervised high-dose strengthening superior to home exercises or advice. For acute neck pain grade 3, supervised graded strengthening was more effective than advice but was equally effective as a cervical collar in the short term.

Patient education for neck pain has also being investigated. Two systematic reviews[200,201] found that trials looking at different types of education, such as advice on how to activate certain muscles, advice on stress coping skills, and neck school, were not superior to other treatments, such as therapeutic exercise, manual therapy, or cognitive behavioral therapy. These results contrast to the results of Sutton et al.,[202] who found that multimodal care involving manual therapy, education, and exercise might benefit patients with grades 1 and 2 WAD, neck pain, and associated disorders. The systematic review by Yu et al.[201] found that structured patient education might provide small benefits when combined with physical therapy regardless of the mode of delivery (i.e., oral or written education). The differences between these reviews was that the Haines et al.[200] and Yu et al.[201] reviews looked at education as a single modality; however, Sutton et al.[202] looked at education as part of a multimodal treatment. Based on these findings, it is recommended that clinicians reassure patients to stay active and carry on regular activities for the early management of WAD grades 1 and 2 as part of a multimodal management program. In addition, clinicians should not provide high levels of treatment for patients with WAD, neck pain, and associated disorders because these patients had demonstrated poorer outcomes than those who receive fewer treatments. According to Jull and Richardson,[203] it is not wise to think that the "one-size-fits-all" approach is the solution for treating neck disorders. Rather, a tailored program of exercise should be planned because of the great variability of motor control impairment found in subjects with spinal pain.

The remainder of the chapter discusses treatment methods used in the cervical spine to increase ROM, improve strength, and provide relief of pain. However, before beginning the treatment, the clinician must clear any cautions or contraindications to such treatment (Table 3-26).

TABLE **3-26**

Cautions and Contraindications to Joint Play Mobilization of the Cervical Spine

Cautions	Contraindications
• Osteoporosis	• Vertebral artery symptoms
• Bone disease	• Spinal cord lesions
• Congenital anomalies	• Multiple nerve root involvement
• Coagulation problems	• Active collagen disease
• Dizziness/vertigo	• Active rheumatic disease
• Nonmechanical reason for hypomobility	• Joint instability
• Atypical patterns of restriction	• Ankylosed joint
• Neurotic patient	• Hyperacute pain
• Acute inflammation	
• Pending litigation	
• History of cancer in the area	
• History of poor response to manual techniques	

Exercise Therapy

Exercise therapy is one of the most commonly used approaches to treat neck pain and associated disorders. Therapeutic exercise has grown enormously in physical therapy due to its benefits in chronic conditions.[204-207] Physical exercise represents a relevant component of rehabilitation for subjects suffering from musculoskeletal pain. Therapeutic exercise has been widely used in a variety of painful musculoskeletal conditions, such as low back pain, shoulder pain, neck pain, patellofemoral pain syndrome, and OA, to reduce pain and improve function of the musculoskeletal system.[204-207] Besides its effects on function and health, therapeutic exercise is known to have some pain-relieving effects,[208,209] and specific exercises targeted at the neck can enhance the neural control of the cervical spine in patients with neck pain.[210] According to Jordan and Ostergaard,[211,212] the goal of any rehabilitation protocol using exercises is to restore lost functional capabilities, such as ROM and muscular strength and endurance, as well as the ability to manage daily tasks at home and in the workplace. O'Leary et al.[213] have highlighted that regardless of the approach, "the focus underlying all exercise strategies is towards the restoration of the patient's key functional deficits, and this should be reflected in all exercise prescription. This function-oriented approach is meaningful to the patient and encourages patient compliance" (p. 329). Exercise should be implemented early in the rehabilitation process and has to be free of pain to avoid exacerbation of symptoms and fear avoidance behavior.[213] Although evidence supports the use of exercise to treat neck pain conditions, successful treatment relies on clinician skills and abilities to optimally assess and treat cervical muscle function and respond to requirements of each patient.[213]

Exercise therapy trials have shown that certain parameters are important for a successful outcome. Richardson and Jull[214] and Bird et al.[215] have reported that appropriate exercises must ensure proper motor control, performance, and endurance of a certain part of the body. Furthermore, it has been found that specific types of training, such as resistance, coordination, or mobility, improve motor performance domains specifically, without improving other domains.[216] Therefore the clinician must decide on the type of muscle contraction (i.e., concentric, eccentric, or isometric), patient's body position (i.e., supine, prone, or standing), level of resistance or load (i.e., high or low intensity), number of repetitions, and method of progression.[217]

Type of Muscle Contraction

Based on the biomechanical and physiological characteristics of local cervical muscles, isometric exercises are more beneficial for reeducating the stabilization role of the deep muscles in the spine because these muscles support low loads for longer periods and work to control fine movement. However, in later stages, isometric exercises can be combined with dynamic and global exercises.

Exercises involving a coordinated contraction between deep anterior and posterior muscles (the multifidus posteriorly and the longus colli and longus capitis anteriorly) are also part of the protocol requirements. In the cervical spine, stability is obtained by the coordinated activity of deep muscles.

Tonic motor units and tonic fibers work best in a stabilization function. Disuse and reflex inhibition are shown to affect the slow twitch and tonic fiber function. A good training program focuses on improving the holding capacity (i.e., endurance) of these muscles; therefore prolonged tonic isometric contractions using a percentage of the maximum voluntary contraction (MVC) (approximately 30%) are most effective in retraining the stability in the affected muscles.[218] In addition, specific exercises that isolate the local muscles from the global muscles are preferred because they have been shown to obtain a better result in posture control and symptomatology.[186,203] These suggestions are in agreement with those postulated by Bird et al.[215] and Falla et al.[217] According to Bird et al.,[215] low loads are used for muscular endurance in the range of 20 or more repetition maximum (RM) (i.e., the greatest amount of weight lifted with a correct technique for a specific number of repetitions).

Body Position and Level of Resistance

In general, the body positions used depend on the objectives of treatment. Because the required level of resistance is low, to obtain a focused reeducation of the muscles, positions such as supine, prone, or kneeling have been suggested to help better obtain motor control in the spinal segments.[214] Therefore reduced loads to the local muscles should be used as much as possible, along with positions and exercises involving minimal external loading to reduce the possibility of pain and reflex inhibition. Thus high-intensity exercises are not appropriate in the early stages of rehabilitation or when the objective is reeducation of specific muscles.

Low loads also help to restore tonic function in the spinal muscles. Muscle contractions below 30% to 40% of MVC can be used to restore this function.[218] Loads as low as approximately 25% of the MVC have been shown to develop increased muscle stiffness to stabilize the spine. It has been shown that exercise at low load (20% MVC) facilitated a more selective activation of the deeper cervical muscles compared with exercise at moderate (50% MVC) and maximal (100% MVC) intensities.[219] At higher intensities, superficial muscles that are not stabilizers of the cervical spine increase their activity. However, if the patient requires a higher level of training due to his or her activity demands, high-load training should be implemented mainly in later stages of training. However, the load has to be tailored to each patient and based on symptom control. In this way, improved function without increasing symptoms can be attained.

In summary, low loads used with positions and exercises that involve minimal external loading are the ideal combination for rehabilitating local muscles in any spinal stabilization program.[203,213,213]

Number of Repetitions

To rehabilitate motor control and coordination among muscles in the cervical spine, the local (deep) muscles must be isolated. Therefore, to gain maximum benefit, the exercise must be repeated as many times as possible during the day until the patient acquires the desired control of the muscle. In addition, the patient must be able to hold the determined position before progressing to advanced stages. According to Bird et al.,[215] to improve endurance, a repetition of four to six sets per exercise, with rest periods of 30 to 60 seconds between sets, is appropriate.

Methods of Progression

According to Richardson and Jull[214] and corroborated by others,[213,220] progression proceeds in the following stages: first, the hold time of a determined action (isometric co-contraction) is increased. This is followed by increasing the number of repetitions of this holding activity (i.e., static stabilization). Ideally patients should be able to stabilize and isolate the correct muscle action in all exercise positions and develop this holding activity. As patients progress, they should be able to reproduce and maintain the contraction during dynamic functional movements. The time taken to achieve this varies from patient to patient and with the severity of the dysfunction. The first treatment sessions commonly focus on teaching the patient the correct contraction procedure, which can take several weeks.

Duration

According to Jordan and Ostergaard,[211,212] supervised instruction should be provided for a minimum of 2 months, with two or three sessions per week. To ensure compliance with the treatment, sessions should last no longer than 1 hour. Home exercises must be performed in addition to these supervised exercises.[213,220–224]

Cervical Muscle Retraining

It has been shown that motor dysfunction appears early after injury and does not automatically resolve with pain reduction.[225] Therefore therapeutic exercises have an important role to play in improving motor function because pain reduction alone does not seem to restore motor function fully. In addition, early intervention is preferred in patients suffering from pain and cervical dysfunction to prevent chronicity and perpetuation of symptoms and dysfunctional patterns.[213,217]

According to O'Leary et al.[213] and Falla et al.,[217] two basic approaches can be used to treat neck pain conditions with exercises. One exercise regimen consists of general strengthening and endurance exercises for the neck flexor muscles.[211,226,227] This exercise program involves high-load training and recruiting of all synergist muscles (i.e., deep and superficial muscles).

The other exercise approach focuses on the muscle control aspects, and its objective is to improve coordination and control of the muscles (e.g., during a controlled flexion movement).[213,218] With this approach, low-intensity contractions of the deep cervical flexors are used during the craniocervical flexion (CCF) movement. After the patient acquires control between the deep and superficial muscles, through training of the CCF movement holding capacity and progression, general strengthening exercises can be added.

O'Leary et al.[213] highlighted that both regimens could be used, but they must be applied at different times. Low-intensity exercises and control pattern movements must be applied in the initial stages when the subjects' pain and disability might impede high-load exercises, whereas global exercises involving a greater number of muscles must be used after reeducation of and coordination between the deep and postural neck muscles have been established.[217,221] Both approaches have been found to have successful outcomes.[213]

Evidence supports the use of exercises that address neck muscular impairments to reduce symptoms and to improve functionality in the cervical spine in conditions such as chronic neck pain, WAD, and cervicogenic headache.[186,228–230] Several clinical trials have been conducted to address muscular impairments in patients with cervical involvement. Training the endurance capacity of these muscles as well as exercises focused on fine motor control through the reeducation of normal patterns of contraction have obtained good results in reducing pain and improving function in these subjects.[186,228,230–232] Deep flexor training in patients with cervicogenic headache has been shown to decrease pain and the frequency of headaches.[186] The same findings were corroborated by van Ettekoven and Lucas[233] in a sample of subjects with tension-type headache using craniocervical (i.e., deep flexor) training, by Dusunceli et al.,[234] who found positive results at long-term follow-up (i.e., 12 months) in a group of subjects with neck pain, and by Deep Gupta et al.[230] in a group of dentists with neck pain. In addition, subjects participating in a training program involving CCF and cervical flexion exercises improved endurance as well as strength in the cervical flexor muscles after training.[219] Furthermore, an endurance program targeting the cervical flexor muscles found that subjects who underwent this type of training improved cervical flexor strength and showed reduced myoelectric manifestations of fatigue of the cervical flexor muscles, along with a decrease in pain and disability of the neck.[228] The same effects were found when training the endurance of the cervical extensor muscles in a group of patients with neck pain and cervical disk disease after anterior cervical decompression and fusion.[235] According to Falla et al.,[228] the improvements in strength and endurance capacities after treatment could have been responsible for the reported efficacy of this type of exercise program in musculoskeletal pain conditions. They reported that this type of exercise program decreased pain intensity and improved function of the neck.[228] The effects of this program were attributed to an increase in stabilization, improvement in motor control of the cervical spine, and an afferent input produced by joint mobilization during the exercises, which, in turn, modulated pain perception at different levels of spinal cord.[236] Although the majority of studies looking at these exercises found positive results, Griffiths et al.[237] in an RCT did not find any statistical difference between a specific neck stabilization exercise program when compared with general neck advice and an exercise program for subjects with chronic neck pain. Nevertheless, subjects receiving a specific exercise program showed clinically significant improvement at 6 months and also reduced the use of pain medications at 6 weeks.

It has also been shown that exercises addressing the neck extensor muscles increased the total neck cross-sectional area (CSA) by approximately 13%. The hypertrophy obtained after 12 weeks of training was mainly due to increases in CSA for the splenius capitis (24%), semispinalis capitis (24%), and semispinalis cervicis and multifidus muscles (24.9%).[238] A positive training effect for the cervical muscles was demonstrated by an increased CSA of the SCM and trapezius muscles as well as decreased fatigability of the cervical muscles after 8 weeks of training.[239] It is known that an increase in neck muscle size is expected to stabilize the cervical spine and prevent or reduce the severity of cervical impairments and cervical pain.

Jull et al.[221] proposed a treatment protocol for training dysfunctional cervical muscles, which has been used successfully in several trials to treat both patients with cervicogenic headache and those with painful neck conditions.[186,234,239,240] The protocol emphasizes motor control rather than muscle strength. The same principles have been stated by O'Grady and Tollan.[241] Both groups of researchers divided the treatment into two phases: retraining the cervical muscles and retraining the scapular muscles. The following sections describe retraining of the cervical muscles.

Reeducation of the Craniocervical Flexion Movement. According to Jull et al.,[221] the reeducation of the correct CCF movement is the first indispensable component of the exercise program. The clinician must teach the patient to perform the movement correctly and to control and to eliminate any compensation strategy, such as neck retraction, excessive cervical flexion, and/or jaw clenching. For the treatment to progress, the CCF movement must be performed correctly. Emphasis on the precision of the movement, rather than the number of repetitions, is essential.[213,217,221,240]

Training of the Holding Capacity of the Deep Neck Flexors. Once the patient can correctly perform the CCF movement, training to improve the holding capacity of the deep flexors is begun. A preinflated, air-filled pressure sensor is used to guide and control the training of deep neck flexor muscles (Figure 3-15). This sensor, which has a visual feedback device (a pressure gauge), is essential to guide the patient in controlling the level of pressure and the desired level of muscle contraction. In addition, the feedback device helps motivate the patient and provides quantification of the degree of improvement.[217,221,240]

The starting point for holding capacity training (HCT) usually is the pressure level the patient has reached and

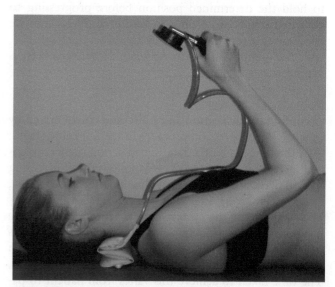

Figure 3-15 Craniocervical flexion test and craniocervical flexion training. Patients are instructed to perform a gentle nodding movement (craniocervical flexion) and practice progressive targeting using the air-filled pressure sensor at five incremental levels with the aid of a visual feedback device.

can hold without compensation for at least 10 seconds.[214,221,241] Patients commonly start at 22 or 24 mm Hg. The training consists of teaching the patient to achieve the determined pressure level and then to hold it for a time without evidence of compensation or poor motor patterns. Ideally the patient is asked to practice the exercise at least twice a day, as long as it does not interfere with daily activities. For each pressure level, the patient holds the position for 10 seconds and repeats this 10 times. Reaching an ideal pressure level between 28 and 30 mm Hg may be somewhat difficult for patients.[221] The duration of training needed to acquire holding capacity for the deep flexors varies from patient to patient; however, according to Jull et al.,[221] an average of 4 to 6 weeks is necessary to obtain a good performance (i.e., holding 28 to 30 mm Hg for 10 seconds, 10 times), but some patients with major muscle dysfunctions could take up to 12 weeks. The patient can use the feedback device at home to practice the training, and once the correct performance is achieved, the individual can be weaned from the visual feedback. Beer et al.[242] have tested the training of the CCF movement in the sitting position. They asked subjects to gently lift the base of the skull from the top of the neck as if lengthening the cervical spine. This type of exercise has been demonstrated to activate the longus colli muscle. Subjects were asked to perform the exercise holding the position for 10 seconds, ideally every 15 to 20 minutes throughout the day, as a daily routine. They found that this simple exercise improved performance in the CCF and decreased the EMG activity of the SCM. Thus these authors recommended the inclusion of this type of exercise in training programs because it is an easy and convenient exercise that can be performed during the day and does not interfere with daily routine.

Retraining of Cervical Spine Extension in the Upright Position. Once the patient is able to perform the CCF movement in the supine position without compensations, the movement is progressed to the sitting and standing positions. The first part of this next stage consists of moving the head and cervical spine into an extension movement in the sitting or standing position. The patient is instructed to first lift the chin and then look up to the ceiling and to continue this movement, trying to look farther along the ceiling, until the end of the comfortable range of extension is reached. The patient then returns to the neutral position (i.e., natural head position). The first part of this exercise trains the cervical flexor muscles to contract eccentrically. Any compensation, such as chin retraction or cervical retraction, should be discouraged.

The second part of the exercise is the return to the upright position by concentric contraction of the cervical flexors muscles. The movement must be started with CCF. It is important that the movement be performed mainly at the level of the craniocervical region rather than having dominant action of the SCM (Figure 3-16).

These exercises can be progressed in two ways: first, by increasing the range of the head extension movement as control improves and second, by adding isometric hold exercises in different parts of the range of cervical returning movement (i.e., concentric flexion) to improve the cervical flexion synergy through functional ranges of extension. The exercises consist of performing neck extension in a comfortable (i.e., pain-free) range and then initiating the CCF movement toward the standing position, without reaching the full upright position, and holding it for 5 seconds. These exercises should be repeated and progressed according to the patient's tolerance because they are potentially high-load exercises.

Retraining of the Extensors of the Craniocervical Spine. To retrain the extensors of the cervical spine along with the training of the deep flexor muscles, exercises are started

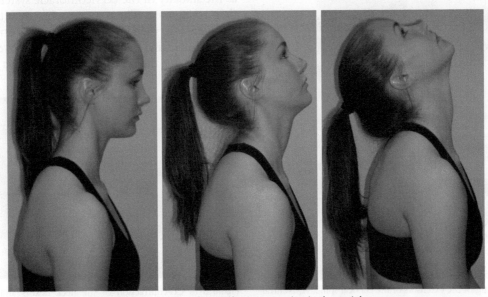

Figure 3-16 Retraining of cervical spine extension in the upright posture.

with the patient in the sitting or standing positions, with progression to the prone and four-point kneeling positions. In the sitting position, for example, the patient is instructed to perform slow head flexion, controlling the speed against gravity and working the extensors eccentrically, and then to return to the neutral position without any compensation. Chin poking, for example, is one of the most common compensations seen with this movement, and it indicates excessive craniocervical extension, which usually is caused by dominance of the superficial muscles (e.g., semispinalis capitis). This exercise can be progressed by asking the patient to alternate small ranges of craniocervical extension and flexion while maintaining the cervical spine in the neutral position in the prone on elbows position or the four-point kneeling position (Figure 3-17). In addition, isometric holds during this movement in the intermediate ranges can be encouraged. The objective of these exercises is to train the coordinated movement among the deep cervical extensor muscles (e.g., the semispinalis cervicis and multifidus), deep craniocervical extensors (e.g., rectus capitis and the suboccipital muscles in the upper cervical levels), and deep flexor muscles (e.g., longus colli and longus capitis). In this exercise, semispinalis and multifidus help

to control the cervical spine in the neutral position and the deep flexor muscles (especially longus colli) stabilize the neck,[243] while the deep small craniocervical extensor muscles perform controlled eccentric, concentric, or isometric contractions.[217,221,240]

Co-contraction of the Neck Flexors and Extensors. This exercise is started once the patient has achieved control of the correct pattern of contraction for the cervical flexor and extensor muscles. The exercise consists of a self-resisted isometric rotation in the supine, correct sitting, or standing position. The resistance must be gentle (approximately 10% to 30% of the MVC) (Figure 3-18). The patient alternates the resistance as an alternating rhythmic stabilization exercise. The exercise must be done smoothly and slowly, with the focus on control rather than speed. This exercise is easy to perform and can be done throughout the day.[213,217,221,240]

Murphy[222,223] has proposed a progression for retraining of the cervical muscles through retraining of the cervical flexors and extensors in the four-point ("all fours" or "bird dog") kneeling position. This method is designed to help the dynamic stability system of the cervical spine work functionally and optimally. The first step is a maneuver called **cervical bracing**, which consists of training the cocontraction of the deep cervical flexors and lower cervical and upper thoracic extensors. While in the four-point kneeling position (Figure 3-19, *A*), the patient first protracts the head and then performs upper cervical flexion, while keeping the lower cervical spine in a neutral position. This configuration is maintained by the patient, who is encouraged to keep the spine and the rest of the body stabilized.[223] When this movement can be performed correctly and held for at least 10 seconds, the patient progresses to the next stage in which the patient combines head and neck control movement with arm and leg movements (Figure 3-19, *B* and *C*). The patient raises an arm and maintains the stability of the body, as well as the stability of the cervicothoracic system. The patient then raises a leg. These movements are alternated (right arm, left leg; then right leg, left arm) until the patient can maintain and perform the correct movement pattern. In addition, the patient can balance a light weight

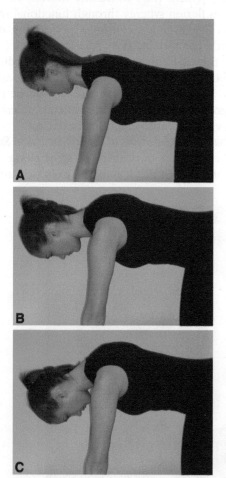

Figure 3-17 Retraining of the extensors of the cervical spine. **A,** Neutral position. **B,** Nod. **C,** Flexion.

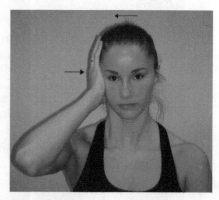

Figure 3-18 Co-contraction of the neck flexors and extensors using self-resisted isometric rotation contraction in a correct upright position.

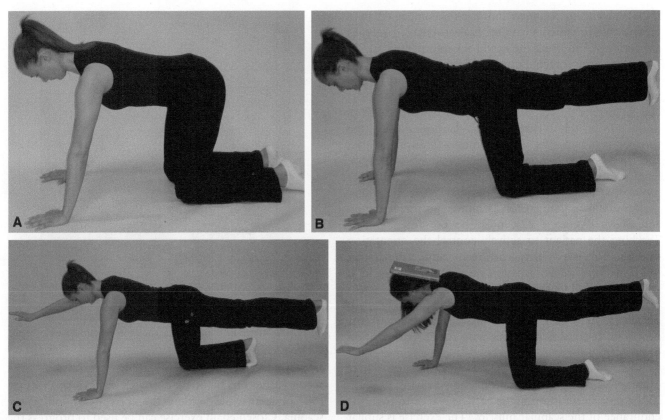

Figure 3-19 Sensorimotor training and cervical stabilization. **A,** Four-point kneeling position. **B,** Patient lifts one leg. **C,** Patient lifts one leg and the opposite arm. **D,** Patient lifts a leg and the opposite arm while maintaining head posture holding a book.

(e.g., a book) on the head to increase the difficulty of the exercise and to retrain stability in the same sequence (Figure 3-19, *D*).[222-224]

O'Grady and Tollan[241] have proposed a further progression of these exercises using foam rolls or a gym ball. The exercises performed with these tools are advanced-stage exercises of increased difficulty, as they are two- and three-dimensional, unstable exercises, so they must be performed with care. The patient co-contracts the deep cervical flexors and extensors while balancing on the foam rolls or gym ball (Figure 3-20). These exercises can be made more challenging by having the patient contract the neck (i.e., cocontraction) in different positions.

Retraining of Scapular Orientation and Position. The position of the scapula commonly is altered in patients with cervical pain resulting in tight and weak muscles. The altered muscular patterns contribute to increased vertical compressive loads on the joints of the cervical spine.[184] Retraining of the scapular position is a very complex and difficult task because patients have difficulty understanding the position of the scapula and cannot correct it through visual cues; they must be taught to feel the correct position and movement.[207,221,240]

The scapula generally is seen to be protracted and downwardly rotated (inferior angle moves toward the

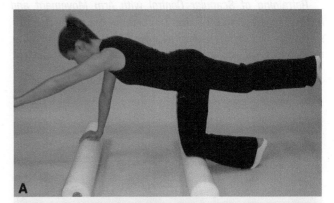

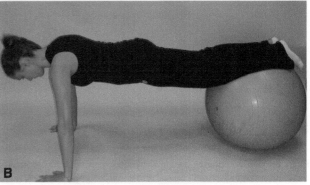

Figure 3-20 Advanced cervical stabilization exercises. **A,** Two-dimensional exercises. **B,** Three-dimensional exercises.

spine) leading to rounded shoulders accompanied by a poking chin in patients with cervical problems. Exercises are performed to bring the head back into neutral and to try to bring the coracoid upward and the acromion backward to retract and put the scapula in the normal resting position. This action results in a slight retraction and lateral rotation of the scapula. The objective is to activate all of the muscles that control the scapular position (i.e., the three parts of trapezius, serratus anterior, levator scapulae, and rhomboids). However, before retraining can begin, lengthening and relaxation of the hyperactive and tight muscles, such as the upper trapezius (Figure 3-21) and the levator scapulae, pectoralis minor, pectoralis major, and SCM (Figure 3-22), must be promoted.[217,221,240] Teaching the patient to actively control the orientation of the scapula is a priority when reeducating axioscapular muscles.[213] (More information on scapular stabilization may be found in Chapter 6.)

Training of the Endurance Capacity of the Scapular Stabilizers. Increasing scapular muscle endurance is the next step. It consists of maintaining the correct position of the scapula for at least 10 seconds and then progressing to holding longer based on the patient's tolerance. These exercises can be progressed from the side-lying position to the prone position using gravity resistance to train the endurance of the scapular muscles. The exercise is similar to the retraction and depression test. The clinician usually needs to facilitate this training until the patient is able to perform the movement and hold it for the required time.[217,221,240]

Retraining of Scapular Control with Arm Movement and Load. The objective of this stage is to maintain the position of the scapula (i.e., "locking" it) while performing movements of the arm (i.e., "loading" it). The patient

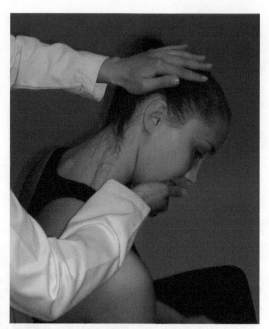

Figure 3-22 Stretching of the cervical and shoulder girdle muscles (here, the sternocleidomastoid).

accomplishes this by doing exercises within a small ROM (60° or less) while holding the correct position of the scapula. Closed chain exercise can be used to progress the difficulty of these exercises. For example, in the four-point kneeling, "prone on elbows" position, the patient can perform concentric and eccentric scapular control exercises of the scapula while maintaining the cervical spine in the neutral position. The objective is to improve the holding capacity of serratus anterior by holding set positions in the intermediate ranges for 10 seconds; this is repeated 10 times (Figure 3-23).

Postural Re-education. Postural retraining is one of the main objectives of treatment of patients with neck pain. Correcting the patient's posture and alignment ensures a regular reduction in harmful loads applied to the cervical joints by the poor postural pattern of the head, cervical spine, and scapula and is especially useful in patients having postural alterations as an aggravating factor.[213] In addition, postural correction helps retrain the deep and postural stabilizing muscles during functional postures. Postural training should be performed repeatedly during the day so that it becomes a habit for the patient and also to give constant positive feedback to the muscles needing to be activated. Postural training is performed first in the sitting position and then in the standing and functional positions (Figures 3-24 and 3-25). This retraining cannot just concentrate on the cervical spine and head and their relation to the trunk and pelvis. It must involve training of the thoracic spine, scapula, and especially the pelvic core. The complete kinetic chain must be trained. An interesting postural exercise, the action of lifting the occiput from the atlas, has been shown to activate the longus colli, an important postural muscle.[244]

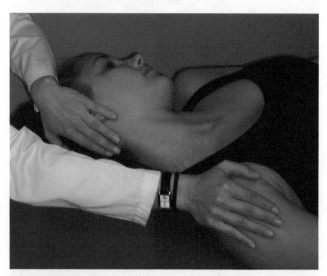

Figure 3-21 In addition to having the patient perform active exercises, the clinician stretches the cervical and shoulder girdle muscles (here, the upper trapezius) to maintain the biomechanical environment and to allow reeducation of muscular function.

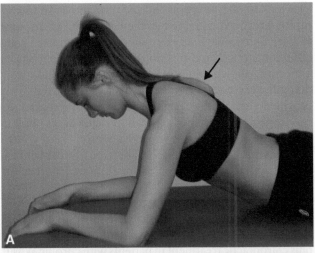

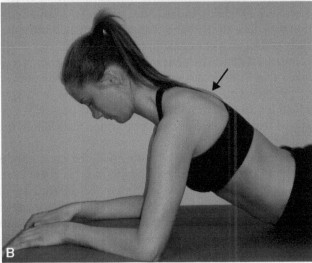

Figure 3-23 Training of the scapular stabilizing muscles. The patient is positioned with the elbows supported in the bed. She then trains the scapulae in both eccentric and concentric control and in holding capacity. The head and neck must maintain a neutral position to retrain the capacity of the cervical extensors. **A,** Scapular winging. **B,** Scapula engaged.

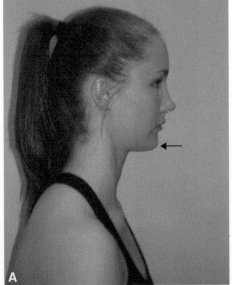

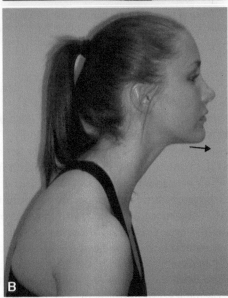

Figure 3-24 Postural control is essential to maintain the functionality of the muscles and the stability of the craniocervical system. **A,** Retraction. **B,** Protraction.

Treatment of Postural Control Disturbances

In some patients, especially those with chronic WADs, dizziness and unsteadiness are common symptoms.[220] Patients with idiopathic chronic neck pain and those with acute and persistent WADs also have been found to have greater cervical joint position errors.[245-248] In addition, patients with whiplash who complain of dizziness have a greater joint position deficit than those who do not have these symptoms.[221] Deficits in standing balance have been demonstrated in people with persistent neck pain of both idiopathic and traumatic origin.[221] According to Humphreys and Irgens,[247] *"There is a dissociation or dysfunction in the integrated visual, vestibular and proprioceptive systems of the neck due to trauma and/or continuing mechanical problems in chronic neck patients (p. 100)."* Most of the time these symptoms (i.e., dizziness and unsteadiness) are related to altered

joint position error or disruptions of balance or eye movement control.[247-249] The treatment should include exercises to address these conditions (although research into the effectiveness of these exercises is needed). According to Kristjansson and Treleaven,[220] specific programs targeting cervical joint position sense, eye-neck coordination, and gaze stability have demonstrated a better success at improving pain, neck disability, and ROM in subjects with neck pain than other nonspecific programs. For example, Hansson et al.[250] showed that a specific vestibular rehabilitation program improved balance and dizziness in patients suffering from whiplash injury. Thus, subjects with neck pain need to be evaluated for these disturbances to provide a more focused management to obtain better results.

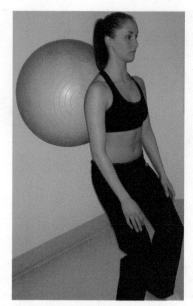

Figure 3-25 Postural training in the upright position using a gym ball. The patient is encouraged to lift the occiput from the atlas and to maintain the shoulder girdle in neutral position. Scapula position also is encouraged.

The following section focuses on the retraining of these impairments.

Retraining Exercises for Repositioning the Head in Natural Head Posture. These exercises are applied only if the patient has an impairment of the joint position sense of the head and the patient is able to hold the neutral head position.[251,252] The patient practices relocating the head to the natural head posture and to specific positions through the ROM. The patient trains first with the eyes open and then with the eyes closed. All movements (i.e., flexion, extension, rotation, and side flexion) are used to retrain the head position.[221,247]

Retraining Balance. Training of balance is important and depends on the level of impairment. The positions and exercises commonly use unstable positions or surfaces to train body balance first in "low" positions (e.g., lying down) and then progress to the sitting and standing positions.

Oculomotor Exercises. Ocular exercises progress through several stages. They start with the head stationary and progress to head movements but with the eyes fixed on a target.[221,247,248] These exercises cannot be performed if the patient is in pain, and they should be stopped if symptoms, such as dizziness and unsteadiness, appear. According to Fitz-Ritson,[249] the exercises must begin slowly, and the patient must focus on different components of each exercise. Some exercises for eye and head coordination are also used. For these, the patient must combine eye movements and head movement in a synchronized fashion. For example, the patient first rotates the head and the eyes at the same time in the same direction; then, progressively, the patient moves the eyes first to the target and then rotates or moves the head toward the target. Movement in opposite directions (i.e., the eyes look in one direction and the head moves in the opposite direction) is trained at the end of the progression (Figure 3-26). All these exercises can be progressed using different surfaces and positions (e.g., the patient sits on a therapy ball, wobble board, or foam roll or walks while doing the exercises).[247] Kristjansson and Treleaven[220] have provided a detailed example for an exercise program for cervicogenic dizziness or unsteadiness and an example of progression of exercises to improve sensorimotor control in neck disorders (Table 3-27). This type of treatment can be embedded with the general multimodal approach to treat neck disorders.

Fitz-Ritson[249] used these types of exercises in an RCT to evaluate the effect of "phasic exercises" plus chiropractic treatment compared with standard exercise treatment plus chiropractic treatment in patients with chronic WADs. The Neck Disability Index (NDI) was used as an evaluation tool. The study found that patients treated with phasic exercises plus chiropractic treatment improved 48.3% compared with the baseline evaluation. The author recognized that in the past these phasic exercises were applied to patients with acute and chronic neck pain or WADs, which led to poor results. Therefore Fritz-Ritson[249] suggested that tonic exercises be performed first, before the patient is progressed to phasic exercises.

Humphreys and Irgens[247] obtained the same results using oculomotor exercises. They found that these exercises reduced pain intensity and improved the accuracy of repositioning of the head after 4 weeks of treatment in patients with chronic neck pain compared with patients who did not receive treatment. However, even with these good results, the authors recognized that a link still had to be established connecting cervicocephalic kinesthesia, head reposition accuracy (HRA), and neck pain.

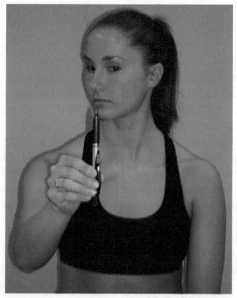

Figure 3-26 Oculomotor training. The patient trains the coordination between head and eye movements.

TABLE **3-27**

Example of Task and Progression to Improve Sensorimotor Control in Subjects with Neck Disorders and Postural Disturbances

Aim	Task	Progression
Cervical position sense	With laser on headband for feedback, relocate back to neutral head position from all head movements with eyes open	• Eyes closed, check eyes open • Relocate to points in range place on a wall, eyes closed, check eyes open • Increase in speed • Perform in standing • Perform on unstable surfaces
Cervical movement sense	With laser mounted on headband practice trace over a pattern placed on the wall, eyes open	• Increase in speed • More difficult and intricate pattern • Small finer movements
Eye follow	Sit in a neutral neck position, keeping the head still and the hands in the laps. Move the laser light back and forth across the wall, while following the laser with the eyes	• Sit with neck in a relative neck torsion position • Eyes up and down, H pattern • Increase in speed • Increase range of movements • Perform in standing • Perform on unstable surfaces
Saccades	Quick simultaneous movement of both eyes to focus on selected dots on a wall	• Increase distance • Add busy background, such as stripes
Gaze stability	Maintain gaze on a dot on the wall as therapist passively moves the patient's trunk and/or the head/neck Maintain gaze on a dot placed on the wall or ceiling as patient actively moves the head/neck in all directions	• Fix gaze, close eyes, move head and open eyes to check if gaze was maintained • Check the background of the target, plain, stripes, checks • Change focus point to words or a business card • Increase in speed • Increase range of movements • Perform in standing • Perform on unstable surfaces
Eye-head coordination	Move eyes to a new focus point and then move head in the same direction and return to neutral	• Actively move head and eyes together same direction • Move eyes one direction and head opposite direction • Move eyes and head together when peripheral vision restricted • Move eyes, head, neck, and arm with or without vision restricted • Rotate eyes, head, and trunk looking as far behind as possible with or without vision restricted • Hold a target, keep eyes fixed and move target, head and eyes move together
Balance	Maintain standing position for 30 seconds	• Eyes open then closed • Firm then soft surface • Different stances: comfortable, narrow, tandem, single limb • Walking with head movements-rotation, flexion, and extension-maintaining direction and velocity of gait • Performing oculomotor or movement or position sense exercises while balance training

Adapted from Treleaven J: Sensorimotor disturbances in neck disorders affecting postural stability, head and eye movement control - Part 2: case studies, *Man Ther* 13:266-275, 2008. In Kristjansson E, Treleaven J: Sensorimotor function and dizziness in neck pain: Implications for assessment and management, *J Orthop Sports Phys Ther* 39(5):372, 2009.

Traction

Traction is used in the cervical spine to distract the zygapophyseal joints, increase the space between the vertebrae, and enlarge the intervertebral foramina. Traction may also be used to stretch joint capsules and ligaments that are hypomobile, reduce muscle spasm and pain by reducing α-neuron excitability and improve blood supply through use of intermittent traction.[253,254] Although traction is commonly used in the treatment of the cervical spine and has been found clinically effective in some cases (e.g., nerve root irritation), there are some who have questioned its effectiveness.[255-258]

Manual traction usually is the first form applied. It is used to relax the patient, test the tissues' reaction to traction, and test the reaction of the patient's signs and symptoms to traction.

Specific manual traction involves applying longitudinal traction to a segment while stabilizing the segments above and below to safeguard them from the effects of the treatment. This technique generally is used to reduce pain and muscle spasm and thereby indirectly increase the ROM. The technique also is used to reduce the mechanical effects of traction when pain relief is not the primary response required. For example, in certain patients with multiple levels that are unstable or painful or in a patient who is unable to tolerate lying down, mechanical traction may be difficult or even contraindicated.

Manual traction may be used with the patient in either the sitting or the supine lying position (the sitting position is described). The patient is seated comfortably at a height suitable for the clinician (the top of the patient's head should be approximately level with the clinician's humerus when the arm is held at 90° of elevation). To achieve this, the patient may have to slump in the seat if the chair is not adjustable. The clinician stands just behind the patient's shoulder on either side, depending on which is more comfortable for the clinician. The clinician cradles the patient's forehead with the arm that is anterior with respect to the patient, reaching around the patient's head to hold the occiput. The clinician's other hand holds across a posterior aspect of the inferior bone of the segment to be treated in a lumbrical grip. The segments above are now locked by a sequence of movements that, all else being equal, are at the discretion of the clinician (Figure 3-27). This sequence includes flexion, rotation, and side flexion or extension, and rotation and side flexion to the left or right, depending on whether instability is present above the target segment.

Mechanical traction usually is applied to the cervical spine with the patient in the supine position on a traction table (Figure 3-28), although seated traction may be used in some cases, especially if the patient has respiratory difficulties.[259] This is often an effective technique for patients with cervical spondylosis or those showing radicular signs. The patient is placed in a relaxed position with pillows under the head, shoulders, and knees.

The amount of traction applied to the cervical spine will vary; the minimum is 1.8 to 4.5 kg (4 to 10 lb). Gentle, sustained traction of 4.5 to 7 kg (10 to 15 lb) for 3 to 5 minutes is appropriate for relieving muscle spasm; intermittent traction of 7 to 14 kg (15 to 30 lb) is appropriate for causing a "pumping action" to aid circulation and to relieve pressure on the nerve and nerve roots by separating the joint structures. Traction increases the pressure in a normal disc, and machine traction has a greater effect than manual traction.[260]

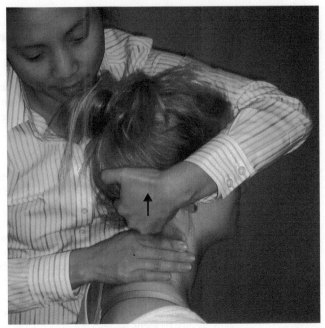

Figure 3-27 Specific manual traction.

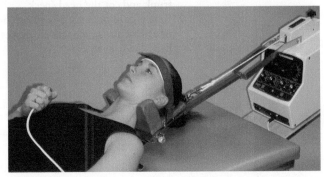

Figure 3-28 Mechanical traction using the Saunders device with the patient in the supine position.

Sustained, or **static,** mechanical traction is traction that is applied continuously for a number of minutes. Sustained traction is indicated for patients with high joint and/or nerve root irritability, those with recent or developing neurological signs that have been associated with irritability, and patients with severe arm pain combined with reduced neck movement toward the painful site.

Intermittent, or **rhythmic,** mechanical traction is probably the most common form of cervical traction used by clinicians because it enables patients to tolerate greater traction forces.[261] This type of traction is applied for short periods (i.e., seconds or minutes) with equal or longer rest periods (i.e., seconds or minutes) in between. Intermittent traction is indicated for patients with an acute joint derangement (less than 6 weeks), unless joint or root irritability is high, and for those needing generalized joint mobilization (facet OA), or suffering from spondylosis, cervical problems that do respond to mobilization, nonirritable neurological (radicular) signs, headaches coming from the neck, muscle spasm, or pain. Intermittent traction is reported to produce twice as much separation as sustained traction.[261]

Studies have shown that 24° to 35° of cervical flexion allows maximum separation of the zygapophyseal joints, providing maximum enlargement of the intervertebral foramina.[261-265] In the supine lying position, the most effective angle of pull for treating the cervical spine is approximately 60° from the horizontal. Researchers also have found that approximately 11.3 kg (25 lb) is necessary to separate the cervical vertebrae, with maximum separation occurring with 20.4 kg (45 lb); at these weights, separation occurred within 7 seconds.[266] Ten to 4.5 to 6.8 kg (15 lb) may be necessary to overcome the weight of the head and the force of gravity if the head is upright. In the lying position, the force is reduced. However, the clinician must keep in mind that the head accounts for approximately 7% of the total body weight.

It has been shown that 9.1 to 11.3 kg (20 to 25 lb) is necessary to straighten the lordotic curvature of the cervical spine.[267,268] Table 3-28 provides a traction guide that is based on signs and symptoms as an indication of when the duration (time) or weight should be altered. Normally, the clinician starts with a weight approximately equivalent to the weight of the head (i.e., 3.6 to 4.5 kg [8 to 10 lb] or less) and increases or decreases either the duration or the load, depending on the reaction of the signs and symptoms.[261] Treatment usually is given for 20 to 30 minutes daily or every second day for 2 to 3 weeks.[262]

Cervical traction must be applied with caution in patients whose history indicates osteoporosis, hypertension, cardiovascular disease, congenital anomalies, evidence of instability, vertigo, "drop attacks," possible arteriosclerosis of the vertebral or carotid arteries, or claustrophobia, as well as in patients with respiratory problems or coughing. The immediate disappearance of nerve root pain on the first application of traction may indicate a high probability of severe pain occurring when the traction is removed. It has been reported that intermittent cervical traction may lead to lumbar radicular discomfort in some cases.[180]

Manual Traction with a Locking Technique

To apply manual traction with locking, the clinician flexes or extends (depending on the clinician's preference or the patient's requirement) the segments from the occiput down to the superior bone of the segment of interest while palpating a superior vertebra for movement. As soon as any movement is felt, the flexion or extension is backed off slightly to ensure that the target segment remains in neutral. The superior segments then are side-flexed away from the clinician, who ensures by palpation of the superior vertebra that the side flexion is not carried into the target segment. At this point, the levels above the target segment are locked into flexion, side flexion, and rotation, whereas the levels below it are stabilized by the clinician's lumbrical grip (see Figure 3-27). Traction is produced by slight straightening of the clinician's legs at the knees, to the degree required. When only neurophysiological effects are required, very little lifting is necessary. If a mechanical effect is required, the clinician provides more knee extension.

Cervical Orthosis

Cervical collars are used primarily to treat muscle spasm, provide stabilization, and limit ROM. The physiological effectiveness of these devices has been questioned, but they can limit movement, depending on the collar chosen.[6,269-272] No studies have been performed to determine the clinical effectiveness of these devices or the outcomes when they are used. The clinician must also be aware that the patient may become dependent on the device, which is visible and may contribute to a sympathy factor. In most

TABLE **3-28**

Traction Guide

	Symptoms	Signs	Duration	Weight	Comment
Case 1	↓	↓	↗	↗	Work slowly if joint is irritable
Case 2	No change	No change	↑	= or ↑	
Case 3	↓	No change	↑	=	
Case 4	↓	↑	=	=	
Case 5	↑	↓	=	=	
Case 6	↑	No change	=	0.5 ↓	
Case 7	↑	↑	0.5 ↓	0.5 ↓	

Note: 1. Do *not* increase weight and duration at the same time; 2. Increase in units of 3-5 each time.

Modified from Grieve GP, editor: *Modern manual therapy of the vertebral column*, New York, 1986, Churchill Livingstone. ↑, Increase; ↓, decrease; ↗, slight increase; =, leave the same.

cases, except when bony or ligamentous instability has been diagnosed, the patient should be weaned off the collar as soon as possible.

Mobilization of the Cervical Spine

The results of the segmental examination, leading to treatment and the assessment described previously, can be used as the basis for treatment of both acute pain states in which a neurophysiological but nonmechanical effect is desired and for nonacute conditions in which primarily a mechanical effect is needed. The advantage of using the assessment technique for mobilization is that it requires no "levering" through a proximal segment, and therefore there is no need to lock the cervical spine segments above and below the segment of interest. This means that minimal risk of stressing either the other segments or the vertebral arteries at levels different from that being treated is incurred. The assessment approach is also a simpler technique and consequently easier to master. The following section is based on the clinical experience of the chapter's first author, Jim Meadows.

Treatment of the Non-acutely Painful Segment

When the cervical spine is treated with manual techniques for nonacute or nonpainful hypermobilities for which a mechanical effect on the barriers is required, multiple barriers are likely to be encountered during the treatment, and each barrier must be dealt with as it becomes evident. Muscle resistance usually is the first barrier the clinician meets, and this resistance can be reduced or eliminated by using very light hold-relax (10% to 30% MVC contraction) techniques or muscle energy techniques.[273–275] The patient is asked to produce resistance that matches the clinician's light push into the direction to be mobilized, holds the contraction for approximately 10 seconds to allow inhibition of the muscle spindle, and then relaxes. The clinician then takes up the slack, and the sequence is repeated until a new barrier is met or until no new range is achieved with each contraction. If full range and normal end feels are found after this, the barrier was entirely increased muscle tone (e.g., muscle spasm). If motion is still restricted and the end feel changes from a muscular end feel, different techniques may be required. For example, the next barrier may be mild pain or discomfort, for which grade 4 Maitland oscillatory techniques may be used until the discomfort is abolished.[276] If the grade 4 techniques provoke pain, the clinician should perform grade 3 techniques. If an early collagen end feel is detected, a technique specific to that barrier is used, such as grade 4+ oscillatory techniques for pericapsular extensibility or minithrust or manipulation for pathomechanical problems. Treating each barrier as it appears, with the appropriate technique, makes the entire treatment more effective and economical.

The duration of mobilization treatment varies and depends on the effect required, irritability of the patient's

Mobilization Sequence of Progression

1. Hold-relax or muscle energy techniques for muscle spasm
2. Maitland grades 2-4 mobilization techniques for pain modulation (depending on acuteness); grades 3-4 techniques for mobilization
3. Maitland grade 4+ mobilizations or minithrusts for end-range mobilization
4. Isometric contractions for reeducation

tissues, and patient's response during treatment. If the patient's tissues or joints are all irritable, the additional treatment should be relatively short, especially if it is performed at the same session as the extensive assessment. Once the clinician knows that the treatment responses are good or at least neutral, the dose (i.e., the duration) can be increased. If the clinician hears a click or other noise or feels the vertebra shift, the treatment should be stopped and the segment and regional movements should be reassessed. Before the segment is taken out of its end-range position, four or five isometric contractions should be performed by the agonist muscles. This tends to reduce the amount of relapse between treatment sessions.

Neurophysiological Techniques for Pain

Midrange Techniques. For the purposes of this chapter, midrange is the biomechanical neutral or resting position of the joint. It is the point where the joint capsule has maximum laxity, the volume of the joint is at its greatest, and as a result the joint is in its least irritable position.[109] Therefore as a starting point, this position is ideal for techniques that are not intended to stress the barrier and that are intended to avoid causing pain and increasing inflammation.

Using the starting point, a **grade 1** Maitland technique can be defined as a small-amplitude technique (approximately 25%) at the beginning of the available range; a **grade 2** Maitland technique is a large-amplitude movement in the middle of the ROM (i.e., the middle 50%); a **grade 3** Maitland technique is a large-amplitude movement at the end of the ROM (i.e., the last 50%); and a **grade 4** Maitland mobilization is a small-amplitude movement at the end of the ROM (the last 25%).[276] Although grades 3 and 4 are not primarily intended to stress the barrier, but just to reach it, in practice most clinicians do stress the barrier with these techniques; therefore properly speaking, they should be described as grade 3+ and grade 4+ mobilizations. A **grade 5** mobilization generally is referred to as exceeding the barrier and is in fact a manipulation; however, for most models of biomechanical dysfunction, this definition is lacking in accuracy; therefore in this chapter, it is defined as a grade 4+ mobilization.

With the exception of traction or distraction, techniques that work at the beginning of joint play are intended to reduce pain by achieving a neurophysiological modulation of the pain rather than by exerting a mechanical effect on the abnormal movement barrier.

Neutral Side Glide Techniques. Neutral side glide techniques may be general or specific. For the general techniques, the patient lies supine, and the clinician stands at the head of the bed. The clinician lifts the patient's head slightly off the pillow using both hands and then side glides the head, keeping it parallel with the shoulders (Figure 3-29). This causes a side translation in the whole cervical spine.

With regard to specific techniques, those described in the following sections can be used for pain modulation. When they are used for this purpose, no flexion or extension is added to the technique for the atlantooccipital joint and the C2 to C7 segments, and very low amplitude translation oscillations are used. For the atlantoaxial segments, the supine techniques work well when grade 1 or grade 2 techniques are required.

Common Requirements for a Safe, Effective, and Economical Mobilization Treatment

- Most importantly, all cautions and contraindications must be recognized and respected
- A precise and accurate diagnosis is essential
- The mobilizing force must be focused at the affected segment
- Each barrier must be recognized as it is encountered and treated appropriately
- The mobilization technique must be appropriate for the direction, grade, and type of mobilization; this will depend on the barrier met.
- All other segments must be safeguarded from the force of the mobilization as much as possible
- Definitive therapeutic exercise and patient instruction must follow up manual therapy for both hypomobility and instability (hypermobility) if long-term results are to be accomplished

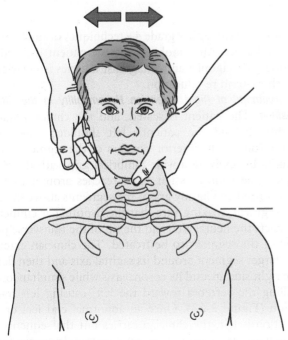

Figure 3-29 Side glide of the cervical spine: Glide to the right. (From Magee DJ: *Orthopedic physical assessment,* ed 6, p 204, St Louis, 2014, Elsevier/Saunders.)

Treatment of the Atlanto-occipital Joint

The first technique to treat the atlanto-occipital joint simply takes the assessment and, using grades, converts it into a treatment method. The techniques described are for the right side of the segments; therefore when the joints on the left are treated, the patient's and clinician's positions, the hand positions, and the directions of forces must be reversed.

Treatment of Right Flexion Hypomobility in the Supine Position. The patient lies supine, and the clinician sits or stands at the head of the bed. Both of the clinician's hands are placed on top of the patient's head, slightly forward of midline (Figure 3-30, *A*). The clinician flexes the patient's head by pushing down on the head so that the chin tucks in. Hold-relax or muscle energy techniques then are used to relax the muscles, and any discomfort that may be present is dealt with using grade 4 oscillations. Then mobilization is performed using either grade 4+ techniques or minithrusts to the barrier. The clinician then side-flexes the head to the left, trying to take the left ear onto the

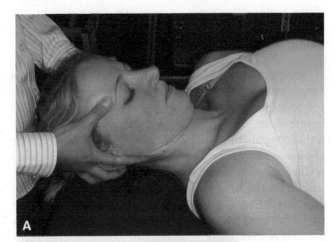

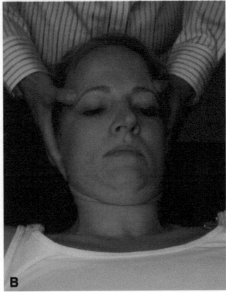

Figure 3-30 A, Axially specific mobilization of extension of right flexion atlantooccipital joint. **B,** Supine side flex of the right atlantooccipital joint.

neck and simultaneously translating the head to the right until the barrier is felt (Figure 3-30, *B*). Mobilization is performed using either grade 4+ techniques or minithrusts to the barrier. After mobilization the patient is asked to contract the agonist and antagonist muscles isometrically for short-term re-education.

Treatment of Right Flexion Hypomobility in the Sitting Position. The patient is seated, and the clinician stands slightly behind the patient's right shoulder. The clinician stabilizes the atlas by applying a wide lumbrical grip with the left hand. The clinician's other hand reaches around the patient and lightly grasps the occiput. The clinician flexes the occiput around its own sagittal axis (i.e., through the ear) and then side flexes it to the left around its coronal axis (i.e., through the nose) and simultaneously translates it to the right, being careful to minimize movement in the adjacent segment (Figure 3-31). When the abnormal end feel is felt, the clinician performs the sequence for muscle relaxation (i.e., hold-relax or muscle energy techniques) or pain modulation (i.e., grades 2 to 4 mobilizations); when the definitive barrier of translation is encountered, the clinician applies either grade 4+ mobilizations or minithrusts. Afterward, the patient performs isometric contractions using the antagonist and agonist muscles to move the joint actively through the available ROM.

Treatment of Right Extension Hypomobility in the Supine Lying Position. The patient lies supine, and the clinician sits or stands at the head of the bed. The patient's head is extended. Both of the clinician's hands are placed on top of the patient's head, slightly behind the midline. The clinician extends the patient's head by pushing it down so that the chin is lifted up and back. The clinician then side-flexes the head to the right, trying to tuck the right ear onto the neck and simultaneously translating the head to the left until a barrier is felt (Figure 3-32). The muscles are first relaxed using hold-relax or muscle energy techniques, and any discomfort that may be present is dealt with using grades 2 to 4 oscillations. Mobilization is then

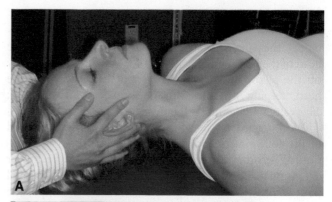

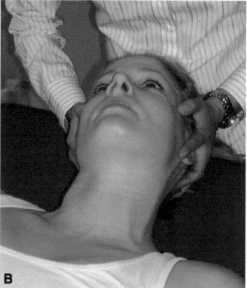

Figure 3-32 A, Axially specific mobilization of extension of right flexion atlantooccipital joint. **B,** Extension of the right atlantooccipital joint.

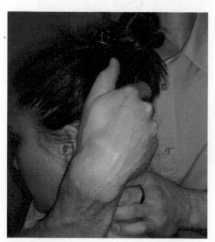

Figure 3-31 Treatment of right flexion hypomobility in the sitting position.

performed with either grade 4+ techniques or minithrusts to the barrier. After mobilization the patient is asked to contract the agonist and antagonist muscles isometrically for short-term re-education.

Treatment of Right Extension Hypomobility in the Sitting Position. The patient is seated, and the clinician stands slightly behind the patient's left shoulder. The clinician stabilizes the inferior vertebra of the segment to be treated by applying a wide lumbrical grip with the right hand. The clinician's left hand reaches around the patient's head and lightly grasps the segments above the target segment, making sure that the hypothenar eminence contacts the neural arch and the tip of the transverse process of the segment to be treated. The clinician extends the target segment around its sagittal axis and then flexes the right side around its coronal axis while simultaneously pulling the vertebra toward the left, causing left translation (Figure 3-33). Once an abnormal end feel or restriction is felt, the clinician carries out the sequence of muscle relaxation (i.e., hold-relax or muscle energy techniques) until no further relaxation is produced (usually 4 to 5 contractions). If necessary, pain modulation can be

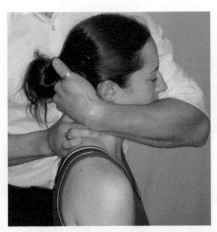

Figure 3-33 Treatment of right extension hypomobility in the sitting position.

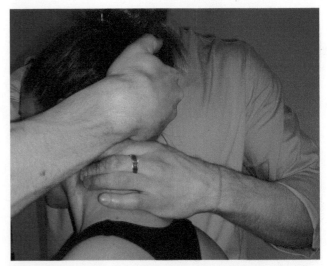

Figure 3-34 Treatment of bilateral flexion hypomobility in the sitting position.

achieved using oscillatory mobilization graded according to the degree of pain (i.e., grades 1 to 4) until the pain is relieved, at which point the definitive restricted end feel (i.e., capsular or pathomechanical) is encountered. This definitive barrier or abnormal end feel can then be treated with grade 4+ mobilizations, minithrusts, or a manipulation technique. The mobilizations are continued as long as the clinician feels necessary or prudent. Afterward the patient performs agonist and antagonist isometric contractions at the end of the newly gained range.

Note: In the preceding descriptions, side flexion is always away from the clinician, and translation is always toward the clinician. The clinician can stand on the other side of the patient and side-flex toward and translate away, but the method described is the easiest one.

Treatment of Bilateral or Symmetrical Hypermobilities. Bilateral hypermobilities can be treated with unilateral techniques performed to each side, and this approach is preferable when only the last part of the range of movement is absent. However, a bilateral technique for symmetrical dysfunction can also be used and may save time and effort. Such symmetrical restrictions can be due to scarring or adhesions resulting from trauma or to adaptive shortening; that is, structural shortening that results when the tissue does not go through its full ROM frequently enough.

Treatment of Bilateral Flexion Hypomobility. The treatment for bilateral flexion hypomobility can be performed with the patient either seated or lying down. If the patient is seated, the clinician stands to one side of the patient (in this case description, the clinician stands on the right). The clinician's left hand stabilizes the atlas with a wide lumbrical pinch grip around the neural arch; the right hand reaches around the patient's head and the fingers wrap around the lower occiput, so that the fingers of both hands touch each other. The occiput is flexed around the craniovertebral sagittal axis and simultaneously glided posteriorly (Figure 3-34). Hold-relax or muscle energy techniques are used to reduce muscle tone or spasm, and grades 2 to 4 oscillations are performed to reduce any discomfort that may

be present. Then grade 4+ techniques are used to stretch the abnormal barrier to posterior gliding.

If the lying position is preferred, the patient is placed in the supine lying position with the head on a pillow, and the clinician stands at the head of the bed. The clinician uses both hands to hold the patient's head slightly forward of midline. The chin is tucked into the throat until the clinician detects the end feel. Muscle spasm and pain are dealt with first as noted previously (Figure 3-35). Using 4+ mobilizations, the glide is increased by applying further pressure into the end feel.

If a locking technique is desired (some clinicians feel that it is more specific), only one hand is placed on the head, and the other hand stabilizes the atlas in the same wide lumbrical grip described for the sitting technique.

Treatment of Bilateral Extension Hypomobility. The treatment for bilateral extension hypomobility can be performed with the patient either seated or lying down. If the patient is seated, the clinician stands to one side of the patient (in this case description, the clinician stands on the right). The clinician's left hand stabilizes the atlas with a wide lumbrical pinch grip around the neural arch,

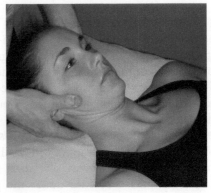

Figure 3-35 Treatment of bilateral flexion hypomobility in the supine lying position.

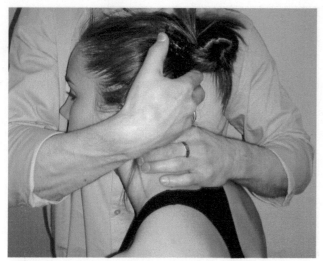

Figure 3-36 Treatment of bilateral extension hypomobility in the sitting position.

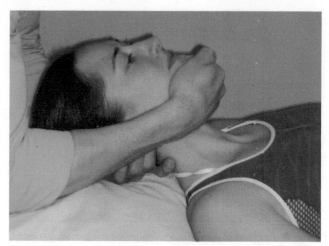

Figure 3-37 Treatment of bilateral extension hypomobility in the supine lying position.

if possible coming a little anterior around the transverse process; the right hand reaches around the patient's head and the fingers wrap around the lower occiput, such that the fingers of both hands touch each other. The occiput is extended around the craniovertebral sagittal axis and simultaneously glided anteriorly (Figure 3-36). The clinician then applies the appropriate mobilization technique, which depends on the barrier encountered. The technique using grade 4+ mobilizations to stretch the abnormal barrier to posterior gliding is a little more difficult because the atlas must be prevented from moving forward during the mobilization.

If the lying position is preferred, the patient is placed in the supine lying position with the head on a pillow, and the clinician stands at the head of the bed. The clinician uses one hand to reach under the patient's head to stabilize the atlas, using the usual wide lumbrical grip, by holding the head back; the other hand reaches around the chin so that the head rests in the crook of the clinician's arm. The head is extended and glided anteriorly on the stabilized atlas until an end feel is appreciated (Figure 3-37). Grade 4+ mobilizations are applied in the manner described previously.

Treatment of the Atlantoaxial Segment

As with the treatment techniques for the atlanto-occipital segment, the techniques for the atlantoaxial segment are simply modifications of the assessment techniques. Right hypomobility restriction is described. Similar techniques can be used for left hypomobility restriction but in the opposite direction.

Treatment of Right Rotation Hypomobility Using Side Flexion. With the patient lying supine with a pillow supporting the head, the clinician stands or sits at the head of the bed. The clinician reaches under the patient's neck with the right hand such that his or her finger wraps around the spinous process of C2, compressing

the soft tissue against the spinous process; the other hand holds the top of the patient's head. The clinician left side-flexes the occiput around the craniovertebral coronal axis (i.e., through the nose) while pulling on the spinous process of the C2 vertebra until an end feel is appreciated. At this point, C2 is rotated to the left, but the segment is rotated to the right as C1 is relatively right rotated (Figure 3-38, *A*). As mentioned previously, convention dictates that the segmental movement be named by the relative or absolute movement of the superior vertebra.

The clinician stabilizes the head when all movement has occurred and the end feel has been reached, and then starts to mobilize into right rotation (Figure 3-38, *B*). Muscle relaxation consists of hold/relax or muscle energy techniques to the right side flexors; left side-flexion slack is taken up in the relaxation phase. If soreness intervenes, grades 2 to 4 mobilizations are performed by oscillations to the spinous processes, and the barrier then is mobilized by grade 4+ mobilizations or minithrusts. Isometric exercises of the right and left side flexors are performed to produce some short-term re-education.

Treatment of Right Rotation Hypomobility Using Rotation. The patient is seated, and the clinician stands on the right side, slightly behind the patient. The clinician's left hand holds C2 in a wide lumbrical grip around its neural arches so that the thumb stabilizes the posterior aspect of the right transverse process. The clinician's right hand wraps around the occiput, with the little finger lying over the left neural arch of C1. Care must be taken that the clinician's arm does not compress the patient's nose or face. One of two things now must be done to take the slack off the alar ligament and allow rotation to occur; either the occiput must be side-flexed to the left or a light compressive force must be imparted so that when rotation starts, C1 can descend onto C2. The clinician achieves compression by allowing a small amount of his or her weight to fall onto the patient's head, so that the head is not being

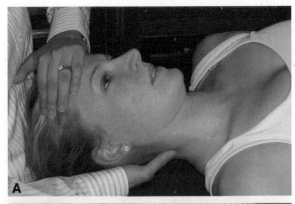

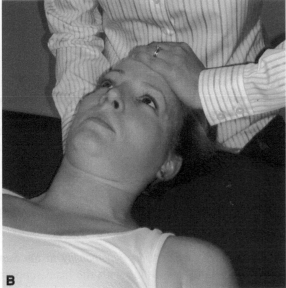

Figure 3-38 Right rotation assessment and mobilization of the atlantoaxial joints. **A,** Side view. **B,** Overhead view.

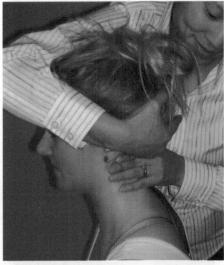

Figure 3-39 Assessment and mobilization for right rotation of the atlantoaxial joint in the sitting position.

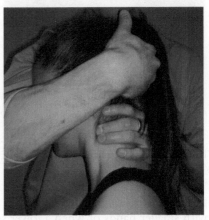

Figure 3-40 Treatment of flexion hypomobility of the atlantoaxial joint.

inadvertently held up by the clinician (Figure 3-39). The appropriate mobilization technique is used for the type of barrier encountered, followed by the appropriate isometric contractions.

Treatment of Flexion Hypomobility. On the rare occasion that the posterior muscles are structurally shortened and require stretching, the following technique may be useful. The patient is seated, and the clinician stands on either side of the patient (for the purpose of this description, the clinician is on the right side). The clinician's left hand stabilizes the axis (i.e., C2); the right hand reaches around the occiput and atlas (i.e., C1), as low as possible, such that both hands are touching. Care must be taken that the clinician's forearm does not compress the patient's face. The clinician flexes the occiput and atlas around the craniovertebral sagittal axis until the end feel is appreciated (Figure 3-40). The appropriate mobilization technique is then performed. These mobilizations are *osteokinematic* (i.e., they follow a normal ROM), rather than arthrokinematic, and they consist of a rollover movement because the dens-transverse ligament complex, when intact, prevents anterior and posterior gliding at this segment.

Treatment of Extension Hypomobility. The patient and clinician positions, as well as the positions of the clinician's hands, as described in the previous section, are adapted for the flexion technique, except that the occiput and atlas are extended around the craniovertebral sagittal axis, and extension osteokinematic mobilizations are applied at the appropriate barrier (Figure 3-41).

Minithrusts are not indicated for either flexion or extension hypomobility because neither type of hypomobility is a pathomechanical dysfunction.

Treatment of C2 to C7

Treatment of Right Side Flexion/Flexion Hypomobility in the Supine Lying Position. The patient lies supine, and the clinician sits or stands at the head of the bed. The patient's head and neck are fully flexed and resting on a pillow or the clinician's abdomen. The clinician uses the middle fingers of both hands to hold the superior vertebra of the target segment under the neural arches; the pads of the index fingers are pressed gently against the transverse

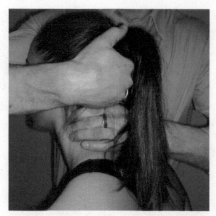

Figure 3-41 Treatment of extension hypomobility of the atlantoaxial joint.

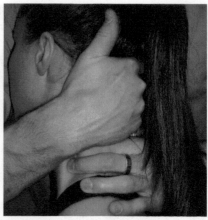

Figure 3-43 Treatment of right side-flexion hypomobility of C2 to C7 in the sitting position.

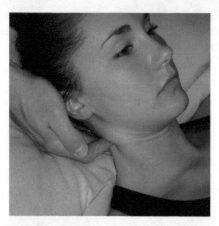

Figure 3-42 Treatment of right side-flexion hypomobility of C2 to C7 in the supine lying position.

process tips (Figure 3-42). As an alternative, especially for those with smaller hands or when a lower segment is treated, the index fingers reach around the neural arches and the first metacarpal head is pressed against the transverse process tip. The first technique is likely to be more sensitive for most clinicians.

With either grip, a small amount of left side flexion is applied to fix the axis and then combined with rotation to the right until an end feel is appreciated. The barrier to the translation is then addressed with the appropriate mobilization technique, as determined by the end feel. As more range becomes available as a result of the treatment, the slack is taken up. The maximum duration of the treatment has been reached when no further improvement in movement is noted or when the technique can no longer be controlled because of clinician limitations (e.g., fatigue).

Treatment of Right Side-Flexion/Flexion Hypomobility in the Sitting Position. The patient is seated, and the clinician stands slightly behind the patient's right shoulder. The clinician uses the left hand to stabilize the lower vertebra of the target segment, using a wide lumbrical grip around its neural arches. The clinician's right hand reaches around the patient to lightly grasp the segment above the level to

be treated, making sure that the little finger wraps around the right neural arch of the superior vertebra of the target segment and that the hypothenar eminences are over the left transverse process tip. The clinician flexes the segment around its own sagittal axis and then side-flexes it to the left around its coronal axis while simultaneously translating it to the right, taking care to minimize movement in the adjacent segments (Figure 3-43). When the abnormal end feel is appreciated, the clinician applies the appropriate mobilization technique, followed by the appropriate isometric contractions.

Treatment of Right Extension Hypomobility in the Supine Position. The patient lies supine with the head supported on a low pillow, and the clinician sits or stands at the head of the bed. The clinician uses the middle fingers to hold the superior vertebra of the target segment under the neural arches; the pads of the index fingers are pressed gently against the transverse process tips (Figure 3-44). As an alternative, especially for those with smaller hands or when a lower segment is treated, the index fingers reach around the neural arches and the metacarpal head

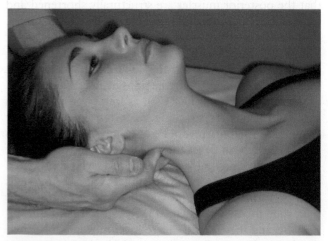

Figure 3-44 Treatment of right side-extension hypomobility of C2 to C7 in the supine position.

of the second finger is pressed against the transverse process tip. Using either grip, the clinician lifts the vertebra so that the segment extends. A small amount of right side-flexion is applied to fix the axis and then combined with left translation until an end feel is felt. The barrier to the translation is then addressed with the appropriate mobilization technique, as determined by the end feel. As more range becomes available as a result of the technique, the slack is taken up.

Treatment of Right Extension Hypomobility in the Sitting Position. The patient is seated, and the clinician stands slightly behind the patient's left shoulder. The clinician stabilizes the lower vertebra of the target segment with the right hand, using a wide lumbrical grip around the neural arches. The clinician's left hand reaches around the patient to lightly grasp the segments above the level to be treated, making sure that the little finger wraps around the right neural arch of the superior vertebra of the target segment and that the hypothenar eminence is over the right transverse process tip (Figure 3-45). The clinician extends the segment around its own sagittal axis and then side-flexes it to the right around its coronal axis while simultaneously translating it to the left, taking care to minimize movement in the adjacent segment. The barrier to the translation is then addressed with the appropriate mobilization technique, as determined by the end feel. This is followed by the appropriate isometric muscle techniques.

Note: In the preceding descriptions, side flexion is always away from the clinician, and translation is always toward the clinician. To treat hypomobility to the left, the same techniques are used, but in the opposite direction.

Treatment with a Flexion, Extension, or Rotation Locking Technique. The segments from the occiput down to the superior bone of the segment of interest are flexed or extended (depending on the clinician's preference or the patient's requirement) while the superior vertebra is palpated for movement. As soon as any movement is felt, the clinician backs off the flexion or extension to ensure that the target segment remains in neutral. The superior segments then are side-flexed (the clinician palpates the superior vertebra to ensure that the side flexion is not carried into the target segment) (Figure 3-46). At this point, the levels above the target segment are locked into flexion, side flexion, and rotation while the levels below are stabilized by the clinician's lumbrical grip. If flexion is mobilized, the spine must be locked into extension, and if extension is mobilized, the spine must be locked into flexion; otherwise, the mobilizing force will extend to unlock the superior segments. The clinician provides flexion by flexing the head and spine while holding the locked position. Extension is performed in a similar fashion. The clinician provides rotation by rotating the head and spine while holding the locked position.

Summary of Mobilization Techniques

Specific manual mobilization techniques are many and varied. They may include complex locking techniques that allow the clinician to lever through unaffected segments, or they may be simple techniques with no preparatory locking if direct force to the affected vertebra is intended. Passive mobilization is an effective and satisfying method of treating mechanical segment dysfunction, but it is only part of the treatment, and it opens a window of opportunity for rehabilitation. Passive mobilization is not a definitive treatment in and of itself. Nonetheless, it is perhaps the most effective way to control the sequencing of other interventions because it results in rapid improvement in pain intensity, ROM, willingness to move, and patient compliance, and it allows the clinician to dictate when rehabilitation of movement begins.

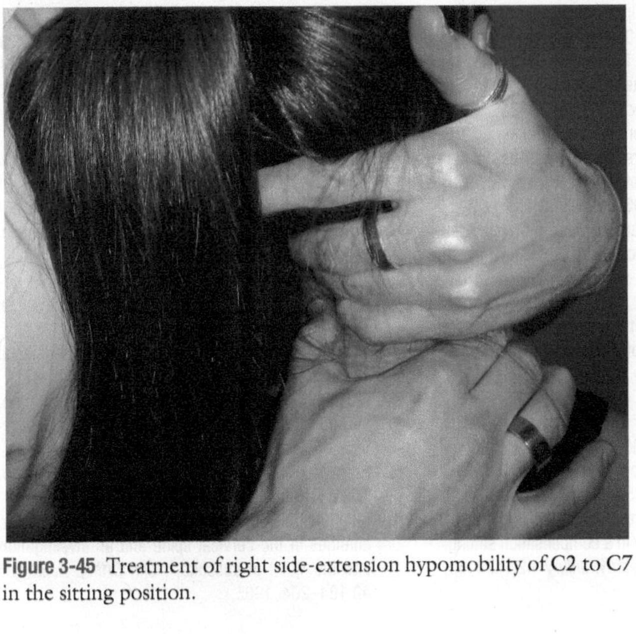

Figure 3-45 Treatment of right side-extension hypomobility of C2 to C7 in the sitting position.

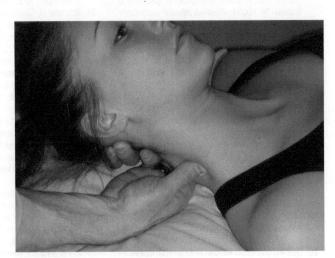

Figure 3-46 Locking techniques for C2 to C7 in supine lying flexion, side flexion, and rotation.

REFERENCES

1. Adams M: Biomechanics of the cervical spine. In Gunzburg R, Szpalski M, editors: *Whiplash injuries: current concepts with prevention, diagnosis, and treatment of cervical whiplash syndrome*, Philadelphia, 1998, Lippincott-Raven.
2. Makela M, Heliovaara M, Sievers K, et al: Prevalence, determinants, and consequences of chronic neck pain in Finland, *Am J Epidemiol* 134:1356–1367, 1991.
3. Porterfield J, DeRosa C: *Mechanical neck pain: perspectives in functional anatomy*, Philadelphia, 1995, Saunders.
4. Radanov BP, Dvorak J, Valach L: Cognitive deficits in patients after soft tissue injury of the cervical spine, *Spine* 17:127–131, 1992.
5. Dvorak J: Soft-tissue injuries of the cervical spine (whiplash injuries): classification and diagnosis. In Gunzburg R, Szpalski M, editors: *Whiplash injuries: current concepts with prevention, diagnosis, and treatment of cervical whiplash syndrome*, Philadelphia, 1998, Lippincott-Raven.
6. Bland J: *Disorders of the cervical spine: diagnosis and medical management*, Philadelphia, 1994, Saunders.
7. Cassidy JD, Carroll LJ, Cote P, et al: Effect of eliminating compensation for pain and suffering on the outcome of insurance claims for whiplash injury, *N Engl J Med* 342:1179–1186, 2000.
8. Carroll L, Cassidy J, Côté P: Frequency, timing, and course of depressive symptomatology after whiplash, *Spine* 31(16):551–556, 2006.
9. Joslin CC, Khan SN, Bannister GC: Long-term disability after neck injury, *J Bone Joint Surg Br* 86(7):1032–1034, 2004.
10. Blincoe L, Seay A, Zaloshnja E, et al: *The economic impact of motor vehicle crashes*, 2000, Washington, DC, 2002, US Department of Transportation.
11. Burke JP, Orton HP, West J, et al: Whiplash and its effect on the visual system, *Graefes Arch Clin Exp Ophthalmol* 230:335–339, 1992.
12. Kumar S, Ferrari R, Narayan Y: The effect of trunk flexion in healthy volunteers in rear whiplash-type impacts, *Spine* 30:1742–1749, 2005.
13. Norris S, Watt I: The prognosis of neck injuries resulting from rear-end vehicle collisions. In *Tenth international technical conference on experimental safety vehicles*, Washington, DC, 1985, Oxford Press.
14. Benoist M: Natural evolution and resolution of the cervical whiplash syndrome. In Gunzburg R, Szpalski M, editors: *Whiplash injuries: current concepts with prevention, diagnosis, and treatment of cervical whiplash syndrome*, Philadelphia, 1998, Lippincott-Raven.
15. Deans GT, Magalliard JN, Kerr M, et al: Neck sprain: a major cause of disability following car accidents, *Injury* 18:10–12, 1987.
16. Evans RW: Some observations on whiplash injuries, *Neurol Clin* 10:975–997, 1992.
17. Suissa S, Veilleux M: The Quebec whiplash-associated disorders cohort study, *Spine* 20: 12S–20S, 1995.
18. Spitzer WO, Skovron ML, Salmi LR, et al: Scientific monograph of the Quebec task force on whiplash-associated disorders: redefining "whiplash" and its management, *Spine* 20:1S–73S, 1995.
19. Stovner LJ: The nosologic status of the whiplash syndrome: a critical review based on a methodological approach, *Spine* 21:2735–2746, 1996.
20. Gun RT, Osti OL, O'Riordan A, et al: Risk factors for prolonged disability after whiplash injury: a prospective study, *Spine* 30:386–391, 2005.
21. Duffy MF, Stuberg W, DeJong S, et al: Case report: whiplash-associated disorder from a low-velocity bumper car collision—history, evaluation, and surgery, *Spine* 29:1881–1884, 2004.
22. Kumar S, Ferrari R, Narayan Y: Looking away from whiplash: effect of head rotation in rear impacts, *Spine* 30:760–768, 2005.
23. Provinciali L, Baroni M, Illuminati L, et al: Multimodal treatment to prevent the late whiplash syndrome, *Scand J Rehabil Med* 28:105–111, 1996.
24. Cote P, Cassidy JD, Carroll L, et al: A systematic review of the prognosis of acute whiplash and a new conceptual framework to synthesize the literature, *Spine* 26:1, 2001.
25. Schellhas KP, Smith MD, Gundry CR, et al: Cervical discogenic pain: prospective correlation of magnetic resonance imaging and discography in asymptomatic subjects and pain sufferers, *Spine* 21:300–311, 1996, discussion, 311-312.
26. Andersson HI, Ejlertsson G, Leden I, et al: Chronic pain in a geographically defined general population: studies of differences in age, gender, social class, and pain localization, *Clin J Pain* 9:174–182, 1993.
27. Bovim G, Schrader H, Sand T: Neck pain in the general population, *Spine* 19(12):1307–1309, 1994.
28. Brattberg G, Parker MG, Thorslund M: A longitudinal study of pain: reported pain from middle age to old age, *Clin J Pain* 13(2):144–149, 1997.
29. Makela M, Heliovaara M, Sievers K, et al: Prevalence, determinants, and consequences of chronic neck pain in Finland, *Am J Epidemiol* 134(11):1356–1367, 1991.
30. Nederhand MJ, Hermens HJ, IJzerman MJ, et al: Cervical muscle dysfunction in chronic whiplash-associated disorder grade 2: the relevance of the trauma, *Spine* 27:1056–1061, 2002.
31. Sterling M: Physiotherapy management of whiplash-associated disorders (WAD), *J Physiother* 60(1):5–12, 2014.
32. Freeman MD, Croft AC, Rossignol AM: Whiplash associated disorders: redefining whiplash and its management, by the Quebec task force [see comment], *Spine* 23:1043–1049, 1998.
33. Styrke J, Sojka P, Björnstig U, et al: Symptoms, disabilities, and life satisfaction five years after whiplash injuries, *Scand J Pain* 5:229–236, 2014.
34. Sterling M, Hendrikz J, Kenardy J: Compensation claim lodgement and health outcome developmental trajectories following whiplash injury: a prospective study, *Pain* 150:22–28, 2010.
35. Schrader H, Obelieniene D, Bovim G, et al: Natural evolution of late whiplash syndrome outside the medicolegal context, *Lancet* 347:1207–1211, 1996.
36. Scholten-Peeters GG, Verhagen AP, Bekkering GE, et al: Prognostic factors of whiplash-associated disorders: a systematic review of prospective cohort studies, *Pain* 104(1-2):303–322, 2003.
37. Osti OL, Gun RT, Abraham G, et al: Potential risk factors for prolonged recovery following whiplash injury, *Eur Spine J* 14:90–94, 2005.
38. Walton DM, Macdermid JC, Giorgianni AA, et al: Risk factors for persistent problems following acute whiplash injury: update of a systematic review and meta-analysis, *J Orthop Sports Phys Ther* 43(2): 31–43, 2013.
39. Richter M: Correlation of clinical findings, collision parameters, and psychological factors in the outcome of whiplash associated disorders, *J Neurol Neurosurg Psychiatry* 74(5):758–764, 2004.
40. Casey PP, Feyer AM, Cameron ID: Identifying predictors of early non-recovery in a compensation setting: the whiplash outcome study, *Injury* 42(1):25–32, 2011.
41. Angst F, Gantenbein AR, Lehmann SG-K, et al: Multidimensional associative factors for improvement in pain, function, and working capacity after rehabilitation of whiplash associated disorder: a prognostic, prospective outcome study, *BMC Musculoskelet Disord* 15(1):130, 2014.
42. Stenneberg MS, Schmitt MA, van Trijffel E, et al: Validation of a new questionnaire to assess the impact of whiplash associated disorders: the whiplash activity and participation list (WAL), *Man Ther*, July 16, 2014 (Epub ahead of print).
43. Schmitt MA, Stenneberg MS, Schrama PPM, et al: Measurement of clinically relevant functional health perceptions in patients with whiplash-associated disorders: The development of the whiplash specific activity and participation list (WAL), *Eur Spine J* 22(9):2097–2104, 2013.
44. Hoving JL, O'Leary E, Niere KR, et al: Validity of the neck disability index, Northwick Park neck pain questionnaire, and problem elicitation technique for measuring disability associated with whiplash-associated disorders, *Pain* 102:273–281, 2003.
45. Nederhand MJ, IJzerman MJ, Hermens HJ, et al: Cervical muscle dysfunction in the chronic whiplash associated disorder grade II (WAD-II), *Spine* 25:1938–1943, 2000.
46. Teasell RW, McClure JA, Walton D, et al: A research synthesis of therapeutic interventions for whiplash-associated disorder (WAD): part 2—interventions for acute WAD, *Pain Res Manage* 15(5):295–304, 2010.
47. Croft PR, Lewis M, Papageorgiou AC, et al: Risk factors for neck pain: a longitudinal study in the general population, *Pain* 93:317–325, 2001.
48. McCormack BM, Weinstein PR: Cervical spondylosis—an update, *West J Med* 165:43–51, 1996.
49. Mahbub M, Laskar MS, Seikh FA, et al: Prevalence of cervical spondylosis and musculoskeletal symptoms among coolies in a city of Bangladesh, *J Occup Health* 48(1):69–73, 2006.
50. Oguntona S: Cervical spondylosis in South West Nigerian farmers and female traders, *Ann Afr Med* 13(2):61–64, 2014.
51. Macnab IL: Cervical spondylosis, *Clin Orthop Relat Res* 109:69–77, 1975.
52. Frymoyer JW, Gordon SL: *New perspectives on low back pain*, Park Ridge, 1989, American Academy of Orthopedic Surgeons.
53. Lestini WF, Wiesel SW: The pathogenesis of cervical spondylosis, *Clin Orthop Relat Res* 239:69–93, 1989.
54. Dupuis PR, Yong-Hing K, Cassidy JD, et al: Radiologic diagnosis of degenerative lumbar spinal instability, *Spine* 10:262–276, 1985.
55. Kirkaldy-Willis WH: *Managing low back pain*, New York, 1983, Churchill Livingstone.
56. Lee MJ, Riew KD: The prevalence cervical facet arthrosis: an osseous study in a cadveric population, *Spine J* 9(9):711–714, 2009.
57. Murphy RW: Nerve roots and spinal nerves in degenerative disk disease, *Clin Orthop Relat Res* 129: 46–60, 1977.
58. Macnab I: The traction spur: an indicator of segmental instability, *J Bone Joint Surg Am* 53:663–670, 1971.
59. Macnab I: Symptoms in cervical disc degeneration. In Cervical Spine Research Society, editors: *The cervical spine*, 2 ed., Philadelphia, 1989, JB Lippincott.
60. Kramer J: *Intervertebral disk disease*, Chicago, 1981, Year Book Medical.
61. Silberstein CE: The evolution of degenerative changes in the cervical spine and an investigation into the "joint of Luschka,", *Clin Orthop Relat Res* 40:184–204, 1965.

62. Kirkaldy-Willis W: The three phases and three joints. In Kirkaldy-Willis W, Bernard TN, editors: *Managing low back pain*, 4 ed., New York, 1999, Churchill Livingstone.

63. Yu YL, Woo E, Huang CY: Cervical spondylotic myelopathy and radiculopathy, *Acta Neurol Scand* 75:367–373, 1987.

64. Fukui S, Ohseto K, Shiotani M, et al: Referred pain distribution of the cervical zygapophyseal joints and cervical dorsal rami, *Pain* 68:79–83, 1996.

65. Friedenberg ZB, Broder HA, Edeiken JE, et al: Degenerative disk disease of the cervical spine: clinical and roentgenographic study, *JAMA* 174:375–380, 1960.

66. Kellgren JH, Lawrence JS: Osteo-arthrosis and disk degeneration in an urban population, *Ann Rheum Dis* 17(4):388–397, 1958.

67. Gore DR, Sepic SB, Gardner GM: Roentgenographic findings of the cervical spine in asymptomatic people, *Spine* 11:521–524, 1986.

68. Ofiram E, Garvey TA, Schwender JD, et al: Cervical degenerative index: a new quantitative radiographic scoring system for cervical spondylosis with interobserver and intraobserver reliability testing, *J Orthop Traumatol* 10(1):21–26, 2009.

69. Cook C, Brismée JM, Fleming R, et al: Identifiers suggestive of clinical cervical spine instability: a Delphi study of physical therapists, *Phys Ther* 85(9):895–906, 2005.

70. Niere KR, Torney SK: Clinicians' perceptions of minor cervical instability, *Man Ther* 9(3):144–150, 2004.

71. Olson KA, Joder D: Diagnosis and treatment of cervical spine clinical instability, *J Orthop Sports Phys Ther* 31:194–206, 2001.

72. Hensinger RN: Osseous anomalies of the craniovertebral junction, *Spine* 11:323–333, 1986.

73. Aspinall W: Clinical testing for the craniovertebral hypermobility syndrome, *J Orthop Sports Phys Ther* 12:47–54, 1990.

74. Derrick LJ, Chesworth BM: Post–motor vehicle accident alar ligament laxity, *J Orthop Sports Phys Ther* 16:6–11, 1992.

75. Ng H-W, Teo E-C, Lee K-K, et al: Finite element analysis of cervical spinal instability under physiologic loading, *J Spinal Disord Tech* 16:55–65, 2003.

76. Panjabi M, Thibodeau L, Crisco JJ, et al: What constitutes spinal stability, *Clin Neurosurg* 34:313–319, 1988.

77. Norris C: Spinal stabilisation: active lumbar stabilisation concepts, *Physiotherapy* 81:61–64, 1995.

78. Norris C: What is back stability? In Norris C, editor: *Back stability*, Champaign, 2000, Human Kinetics.

79. Handal J, Selby D: Spine instability. In Hochschuler S, Cotler H, Guyer R, editors: *Rehabilitation of the spine*, St Louis, 1993, Mosby.

80. Panjabi M, Abumi K, Duranceau J, et al: Spinal stability and intersegmental muscle forces: a biomechanical model, *Spine* 14:194–200, 1989.

81. Panjabi MM: The stabilizing system of the spine. Part I. Function, dysfunction, adaptation, and enhancement, *J Spinal Disord* 5:383–389, 1992.

82. Panjabi MM: The stabilizing system of the spine. Part II. Neutral zone and instability hypothesis, *J Spinal Disord* 5:390–396, 1992.

83. Kaigle AM, Holm SH, Hansson TH: Experimental instability in the lumbar spine, *Spine* 20:421–430, 1995.

84. Mimura M, Panjabi MM, Oxland TR, et al: Disc degeneration affects the multidirectional flexibility of the lumbar spine, *Spine* 19:1371–1380, 1994.

85. Panjabi M: Dysfunction of the spinal stability system and its restabilization. In Singer K, editor: *Clinical anatomy and management of cervical spine pain*, Oxford, 1990, Butterworth Heinemann.

86. Farfan HF, Gracovetsky S: The nature of instability, *Spine* 9:714–719, 1984.

87. Olson KA, Paris SV, Spohr C, et al: Radiographic assessment and reliability study of the craniovertebral sidebending test, *J Man Manip Ther* 6(2):87–96, 1998.

88. Osmotherly PG, Rivett DA: Knowledge and use of craniovertebral instability testing by Australian physiotherapists, *Man Ther* 16(4):357–363, 2011.

89. Cholewicki J, Polzhofer GK, Radebold A: Postural control of trunk during unstable sitting, *J Biomech* 33:1733–1737, 2000.

90. Hodges PW, Richardson CA: Inefficient muscular stabilization of the lumbar spine associated with low back pain: a motor control evaluation of transversus abdominis, *Spine* 21:2640–2650, 1996.

91. Hungerford B, Gilleard W, Hodges P: Evidence of altered lumbopelvic muscle recruitment in the presence of sacroiliac joint pain, *Spine* 28:1593–1600, 2003.

92. O'Sullivan PB: Manual therapy master classes: lumbar segmental and instability—clinical presentation and specific stabilizing exercise management, *Man Ther* 5:2–12, 2000.

93. Silfies SP, Squillante D, Maurer P, et al: Trunk muscle recruitment patterns in specific chronic low back pain populations, *Clin Biomech (Bristol, Avon)* 20:465–473, 2005.

94. Fritz JM, Erhard RE, Hagen BF: Segmental instability of the lumbar spine, *Phys Ther* 78:889–896, 1998.

95. Falla D, Jull G, Dall'Alba P, et al: An electromyographic analysis of the deep cervical flexor muscles in performance of craniocervical flexion, *Phys Ther* 83:899–906, 2003.

96. Swinkels R, Beeton K, Alltree J: Pathogenesis of upper cervical instability, *Man Ther* 1:127–132, 1996.

97. Paris SV: Physical signs of instability, *Spine* 10:277–279, 1985.

98. Falla D, Jull G, Rainoldi A, et al: Neck flexor muscle fatigue is side specific in patients with unilateral neck pain, *Eur J Pain* 8:71–77, 2004.

99. Falla D, Rainoldi A, Merletti R, et al: Myoelectric manifestations of sternocleidomastoid and anterior scalene muscle fatigue in chronic neck pain patients, *Clin Neurophysiol* 114:488–495, 2003.

100. Falla DL, Jull GA, Hodges PW: Patients with neck pain demonstrate reduced electromyographic activity of the deep cervical flexor muscles during performance of the craniocervical flexion test, *Spine* 29:2108–2114, 2004.

101. Beck RW, Holt KR, Fox MA, et al: Radiographic anomalies that may alter chiropractic intervention strategies found in a New Zealand population, *J Manipulative Physiol Ther* 27:554–559, 2004.

102. Swinkels RA, Oostendorp RA: Upper cervical instability: fact or fiction? *J Manipulative Physiol Ther* 19(3):185–194, 1996.

103. Slater H, Briggs AM, Fary RE, et al: Upper cervical instability associated with rheumatoid arthritis: what to "know" and what to "do," *Man Ther* 18(6):615–619, 2013.

104. Allen SC: Pathoanatomic and etiological aspects of cervical spine instability, *Orthop Phys Ther Clin North Am* 10:409–415, 2001.

105. Hildebrandt G, Agnoli AL, Zierski J: Atlanto-axial dislocation in rheumatoid arthritis: diagnostic and therapeutic aspects, *Acta Neurochir* 84:110–117, 1987.

106. Mathews JA: Atlantoaxial subluxation in rheumatoid arthritis, *Ann Rheum Dis* 28:260–266, 1969.

107. Dobbs AG: Manual therapy assessment of cervical instability, *Orthop Phys Ther Clin North Am* 10:431–454, 2001.

108. Aprill C, Dwyer A, Bogduk N: Cervical zygapophyseal joint pain patterns. II. A clinical evaluation, *Spine* 15:458–461, 1990.

109. Dwyer A, Aprill C, Bogduk N: Cervical zygapophyseal joint pain patterns. I. A study in normal volunteers, *Spine* 15:453–457, 1990.

110. Kelsey JL, Githens PB, Walter SD: An epidemiological study of acute prolapsed cervical intervertebral disc, *J Bone Joint Surg Am* 66:907–914, 1984.

111. Macnab I: *Backache*, Baltimore, 1977, Williams & Wilkins.

112. Rothman RH, Marvel JP: The acute cervical disk, *Clin Orthop Relat Res* 109:59–68, 1975.

113. Arnoldi CC, Brodsky AE, Cauchoix J: Lumbar spinal stenosis and nerve root entrapment syndromes: definition and classification, *Clin Orthop Relat Res* 115:4–5, 1976.

114. McIvor GWD, Kirkaldy-Willis WH: Pathological and myelographic changes in the major types of lumbar spinal stenosis, *Clin Orthop Relat Res* 115:72–76, 1976.

115. Grant TT, Puffer J: Cervical stenosis: a developmental anomaly with quadriparesis during football, *Am J Sports Med* 4:219–221, 1976.

116. Lunsford LD, Bissonette DJ, Zorub DS: Anterior surgery for cervical disc disease. Part 2. Treatment of cervical spondylotic myelopathy in 32 cases, *J Neurosurg* 53:12–19, 1980.

117. Wilberger JE Jr., Chedid MK: Acute cervical spondylytic myelopathy, *Neurosurgery* 22:145–146, 1988.

118. Pierce DS: Fracture and dislocations at the base of the skull and upper cervical spine. In Cervical Spine Research Society, editors: *The cervical spine*, 2 ed., Philadelphia, 1989, JB Lippincott.

119. Kerry R, Taylor AJ: Cervical arterial dysfunction assessment and manual therapy, *Man Ther* 11:243–253, 2006.

120. Hensinger RN: Congential anomalies of the atlantoaxial joint. In Cervical Spine Research Society, editors: *The cervical spine*, 2 ed., Philadelphia, 1989, JB Lippincott.

121. Raynor RB: Congenital malformations of the base of the skull: the Arnold-Chiari malformation. In Cervical Spine Research Society, editors: *The cervical spine*, 2 ed., Philadelphia, 1989, JB Lippincott.

122. Torg J: Risk factors in congenital stenosis of the cervical spine canal. In Cervical Spine Research Society, editors: *The cervical spine*, 2 ed., Philadelphia, 1989, JB Lippincott.

123. Hensinger RN: Congenital anomalies of the odontoid. In Cervical Spine Research Society, editors: *The cervical spine*, ed 2 Philadelphia, 1989, JB Lippincott.

124. Pizzutillo PD: Klippel-Feil syndrome. In Cervical Spine Research Society, editors: *The cervical spine*, ed 2 Philadelphia, 1989, JB Lippincott.

125. Bogduk N, Govind J: Cervicogenic headache: an assessment of the evidence on clinical diagnosis, invasive tests, and treatment, *Lancet Neurol* 8(10):959–968, 2009.

126. Headache Classification Subcommittee of the International Headache Society: The International Classification of Headache Disorders: 2nd edition, *Cephalalgia* 24(suppl 1):9–160, 2004.

127. Evers S: Comparison of cervicogenic headache with migraine, *Cephalalgia* 28:16–17, 2008.

128. Sjaastad O: Cervicogenic headache: comparison with migraine without aura; Vågå study, *Cephalalgia* 28:18–20, 2008.

129. Lord S, Barnsley L, Wallis BJ, et al: Third occipital nerve headache: a prevalence study, *J Neurol Neurosurg Psychiatry* 57(10):1187–1190, 1994.

130. Jull G: Management of cervical headache, *Man Ther* 2(4):182–190, 1997.

131. Andersen N, Vingen J, Westgard R, et al: Pathophysiology of cervicogenic headache: a review. In Sjaastad O, Fredriksen TA, Bono G, Nappi G, editors: *Cervicogenic headache: basic concepts*, London, 2003, Smith-Gordon.

132. Hu JW, Yu XM, Vernon H, et al: Excitatory effects on neck and jaw muscle activity of inflammatory irritant applied to cervical paraspinal tissues, *Pain* 55:243–250, 1993.

133. Svensson P, Wang K, Sessle BJ, et al: Associations between pain and neuromuscular activity in the human jaw and neck muscles, *Pain* 109:225–232, 2004.

134. Hu JW, Sessle BJ, Amano N, et al: Convergent afferent input patterns in medullary dorsal horn (trigeminal subnucleus caudalis): A basis for referred orofacial pain? *Pain* 18(suppl 1):S281, 1984.

135. Kerr FW: The fine structure of the subnucleus caudalis of the trigeminal nerve, *Brain Res* 23(2):129–145, 1970.

136. Kerr FW: Central relationships of trigeminal and cervical primary afferents in the spinal cord and medulla, *Brain Res* 43:561–572, 1972.

137. Kerr FW: The potential of cervical primary afferents to sprout in the spinal nucleus of V following long term trigeminal denervation, *Brain Res* 43:547–560, 1972.

138. Bogduk N: Anatomy and physiology of headache, *Biomed Pharmacother* 49:435–445, 1995.

139. Berry M, Standring SM, Bannister LH: Nervous system. In Williams PL, Bannister LH, Berry MH, et al, editors: *Gray's anatomy*, New York, 1995, Churchill Livingstone.

140. Bogduk N: Cervical causes of headache. In Grieves BJ, Palastanga N, editors: *Grieve's modern manual therapy: the vertebral column*, Edinburgh, 1994, Churchill Livingstone.

141. Bogduk N: The clinical anatomy of the cervical dorsal rami, *Spine* 7:319–330, 1982.

142. Bogduk N: Cervicogenic headache: anatomic basis and pathophysiologic mechanisms, *Curr Pain Headache Rep* 5:382–386, 2001.

143. Bogduk N: Biomechanics of the cervical spine. In Grant R, editor: *Physical therapy of the cervical and thoracic spine*, New York, 2002, Churchill Livingstone.

144. Bogduk N, Crosbie J, McConnell J: *The anatomy and physiology of nociception*, Toronto, 1993, Butterworth Heinemann.

145. Bogduk N, Marsland A: The cervical zygapophysial joints as a source of neck pain, *Spine* 13:610–617, 1988.

146. Amevo B, Aprill C, Bogduk N: Abnormal instantaneous axes of rotation in patients with neck pain, *Spine* 17(7):748–756, 1992.

147. Dwyer A, Aprill C, Bogduk N: Cervical zygapophyseal joint pain patterns. I. A study in normal volunteers, *Spine* 15:453–457, 1990.

148. Edmeads J: Headache of cervical origin, *Rev Prat* 40:399–402, 1990.

149. Ehni G, Benner B: Occipital neuralgia and the C1-2 arthrosis syndrome, *J Neurosurg* 61:961–965, 1984.

150. Meloche J, Bergeron Y, Bellavance A, et al: Painful intervertebral dysfunction: Robert Maigne's original contribution to headache of cervical origin. The Quebec headache study group, *Headache* 33(6):328–334, 1993.

151. Cooper G, Bailey B, Bogduk N: Cervical zygapophysial joint pain maps, *Pain Med* 8(4):344–353, 2007.

152. Bogduk N, Marsland A: On the concept of third occipital headache, *J Neurol Neurosurg Psychiatry* 49(7):775–780, 1986.

153. Diener HC, Kaminski M, Stappert G, et al: Lower cervical disc prolapse may cause cervicogenic headache: Prospective study in patients undergoing surgery, *Cephalalgia* 27(9):1050–1054, 2007.

154. Hack GD, Koritzer RT, Robinson WL, et al: Anatomic relation between the rectus capitis posterior minor muscle and the dura mater, *Spine* 20:2484–2486, 1995.

155. Pereira Monteiro J: Epidemiology of cervicogenic headache. In Sjaastad O, Fredriksen TA, Bono G, et al, editors: *Cervicogenic headache: basic concepts*, London, 2003, Smith-Gordon.

156. Drottning M: Cervicogenic headache after whiplash injury, *Curr Pain Headache Rep* 7:384–386, 2003.

157. Sjaastad O: The headache of challenge in our time: cervicogenic headache, *Funct Neurol* 5:155–158, 1990.

158. Sjaastad O, Sauntec C, Hovdal H, et al: "Cervicogenic" headache. An hypothesis, *Cephalalgia* 3:249–256, 1983.

159. Antonaci F, Ghirmai S, Bono G, et al: Cervicogenic headache: evaluation of the original diagnostic criteria, *Cephalalgia* 21:573–583, 2001.

160. Sjaastad O, Fredriksen TA: Cervicogenic headache: criteria, classification and epidemiology, *Clin Exp Rheumatol* 18:S3–S6, 2000.

161. Sjaastad O, Fredriksen TA, Pfaffenrath V: Cervicogenic headache: diagnostic criteria, *Headache* 38(6):442–445, 1998.

162. Watson DH, Trott PH: Cervical headache: an investigation of natural head posture and upper cervical flexor muscle performance, *Cephalalgia* 13:272–284, 1993.

163. Sjaastad O, Bakketeig LS: Prevalence of cervicogenic headache: Vågå study of headache epidemiology, *Acta Neurol Scand* 117(3):173–180, 2008.

164. Bogoluk N: The neck and headaches, *Neurol Clin* 22:151–171, 2004.

165. Pfaffenrath V, Dandekar R, Pollmann W: Cervicogenic headache: the clinical picture, radiological findings and hypotheses on its pathophysiology, *Headache* 27:495–499, 1987.

166. Mersky HB, Bogduk N: *Classification of chronic pain*, ed 2, Seattle, 1994, IASP Press.

167. Gadotti IC, Armijo-Olivo S, Magee DJ: Cervical musculoskeletal impairments in cervicogenic headache: a systematic review and a meta-analysis, *Phys Ther Rev* 13(3):149–166, 2008.

168. Dumas JP, Arsenault AB, Boudreau G, et al: Physical impairments in cervicogenic headache: traumatic versus nontraumatic onset, *Cephalalgia* 21:884–893, 2001.

169. Hall T, Robinson K: The flexion-rotation test and active cervical mobility: a comparative measurement study in cervicogenic headache, *Man Ther* 9:197–202, 2004.

170. Zito G, Jull G, Story I: Clinical tests of musculoskeletal dysfunction in the diagnosis of cervicogenic headache, *Man Ther* 11(2):118–129, 2006.

171. Zwart JA: Neck mobility in different headache disorders, *Headache* 37(1):6–11, 1997.

172. Ogince M, Hall T, Robinson K, Blackmore A: The diagnostic Validity of the cervical flexion-rotation test in C1/C2 related cervicogenci headache, *Man Ther* 12(3):256–262, 2007.

173. Snodgrass SJ, Cleland JA, Haskins R, Rivett DA: The clinical utility of cervical range of motion in diagnosis, prognosis, and evaluating the effects of manipulation: a systematic review, *Physiotherapy* May 2, 2014 [Epub ahead of print].

174. Jensen OK, Nielsen FF, Vosmar L: An open study comparing manual therapy with the use of cold packs in the treatment of post-traumatic headache, *Cephalalgia* 10:241–250, 1990.

175. Jull G: Headache of cervical origin. In Grant R, editor: *Physical therapy of the cervical and thoraxic spine*, New York, 1988, Churchill Livingstone.

176. Placzek JD, Pagett BT, Roubal PJ, et al: The influence of the cervical spine on chronic headache in women: a pilot study, *J Man Manip Ther* 7:33–39, 1999.

177. Sandmark H, Nisell R: Validity of five common manual neck pain provoking tests, *Scand J Rehabil Med* 27:131–136, 1995.

178. Treleaven J, Jull G, Atkinson L: Cervical musculoskeletal dysfunction in post-concussional headache [see comment], *Cephalalgia* 14:273–279, 1994.

179. Wight S, Osborne N, Breen AC: Incidence of ponticulus posterior of the atlas in migraine and cervicogenic headache, *J Manipulative Physiol Ther* 22:15–20, 1999.

180. Lance J: *Mechanisms and management of headache*, ed 5, Oxford, 1993, Buttherworth-Heinemann.

181. Becker WJ: Cervicogenic headache: evidence that the neck is a pain generator, *Headache* 50(4):699–705, 2010.

182. Jull GA, Stanton WR: Predictors of responsiveness to physiotherapy management of cervicogenic headache, *Cephalalgia* 25(2):101–108, 2005.

183. Fleming R, Forsythe S, Cook C: Influential variables associated with outcomes in patients with cervicogenic headache, *J Man Manip Ther* 15(3):155–164, 2007.

184. Liebert A, Rebbeck T, Elias S, et al: Musculoskeletal physiotherapists' perceptions of non-responsiveness to treatment for cervicogenic headache, *Physiother Theory Pract* 29(8):616–629, 2013.

185. Janda V: Muscles and cervicogenic pain syndromes. In Grant EE, editor: *Physical therapy of the cervical and thoracic spine*, New York, 1988, Churchill Livingstone.

186. Jull G, Trott P, Potter H, et al: A randomized controlled trial of exercise and manipulative therapy for cervicogenic headache, *Spine* 27:1835–1843, 2002.

187. Mark BM: Cervicogenic headache differential diagnosis and clinical management: literature review, *Cranio* 8(4):332–338, 1990.

188. Sharma D, Sen S, Dhawan A: Effects of cervical stabilization exercises on neck proprioception in patients with cervicogenic headache, *Int J Pharma Bio Sci* 5(1):B405–B420, 2014.

189. Astin JA, Ernst E: The effectiveness of spinal manipulation for the treatment of headache disorders: a systematic review of randomized clinical trials, *Cephalalgia* 22:617–623, 2002.

190. Bronfort G, Assendelft WJJ, Evans R, et al: Efficacy of spinal manipulation for chronic headache: a systematic review, *J Manipulative Physiol Ther* 24:457–466, 2001.

191. Chaibi A, Russell MB: Manual therapies for cervicogenic headache: a systematic review, *J Headache Pain* 13(5):351–359, 2012.

192. Posadzki P, Ernst E: Spinal manipulations for cervicogenic headaches: a systematic review of randomized clinical trials, *Headache* 51(7):1132–1139, 2011.

193. Racicki S, Gerwin S, DiClaudio S, et al: Conservative physical therapy management for the treatment of cervicogenic headache: a systematic review, *J Man Manip Ther* 21(2):113–124, 2013.

194. Gross A, Miller J, D'Sylva J, et al: Manipulation or mobilisation for neck pain: a Cochrane review, *Man Ther* 15(4):315–333, 2010.

195. D'Sylva J, Miller J, Gross A, et al: Manual therapy with or without physical medicine modalities for neck pain: a systematic review, *Man Ther* 15(5):415–433, 2010.

196. Miller J, Gross A, D'Sylva J, et al: Manual therapy and exercise for neck pain: a systematic review, *Man Ther* 15(4):334–354, 2010.

197. Yamato TP, Saragiotto BT, Maher C: Therapeutic exercise for chronic non-specific neck pain, *Br J Sports Med* Aug 18, 2014 [Epub ahead of print].

198. Cohen J: The concepts of power analysis. In Cohen J, editor: *Statistical power analysis for the behavioral sciences*, ed 2 Hillsdale, 1988, Academic Press.

199. Southerst D, Nordin MC, Côté P, et al: Is exercise effective for the management of neck pain and associated disorders or whiplash-associated disorders? A systematic review by the Ontario Protocol for Traffic Injury Management (OPTIMa) collaboration, *Spine* J Feb 15, 2014 [Epub ahead of print].

200. Haines T, Gross AR, Burnie S, et al: A Cochrane review of patient education for neck pain, *Spine* J 9(10):859–871, 2009.

201. Yu H, Côté P, Southerst D, et al: Does structured patient education improve the recovery and clinical outcomes of patients with neck pain? A systematic review from the Ontario Protocol for Traffic Injury Management (OPTIMa) collaboration, *Spine J* Apr 7, 2014 [Epub ahead of print].

202. Sutton DA, Côté P, Wong JJ, et al: Is multimodal care effective for the management of patients with whiplash-associated disorders or neck pain and associated disorders? A systematic review by the Ontario Protocol for Traffic Injury Management (OPTIMa) collaboration, *Spine J* Jul 8, 2014 (Epub ahead of print].

203. Jull GA, Richardson CA: Motor control problems in patients with spinal pain: a new direction for therapeutic exercise, *J Manipulative Physiol Ther* 23(2):115–117, 2000.

204. Gross AR, Goldsmith C, Hoving JL, et al: Conservative management of mechanical neck disorders: a systematic review, *J Rheumatol* 34(5):1083–1102, 2007.

205. Macedo LG, Maher CG, Latimer J, et al: Motor control exercise for persistent, nonspecific low back pain: a systematic review, *Phys Ther* 89(1):9–25, 2009.

206. McNeely M, Armijo Olivo S, Magee D: A systematic review of physical therapy intervention for temporomandibular disorders, *Phys Ther* 86(5):710–720, 2006.

207. Fransen M, McConnell S: Exercise for osteoarthritis of the knee, *Cochrane Database Syst Rev* 4:CD004376, 2008 Oct 8.

208. Sokunbi O, Moore A, Watt P: Plasma levels of beta-endorphin and serotonin in response to specific spinal base exercises, *South Afr J Physiother* 64(1):31–37, 2008.

209. Sokunbi O, Watt P, Moore A: Changes in plasma concentration of serotonin in response to spinal stabilization exercises in chronic low back pain patient, *Nig Qt J Hosp Med* 17:108–111, 2007.

210. Falla D, Lindstrøm R, Rechter L, et al: Effectiveness of an 8-week exercise programme on pain and specificity of neck muscle activity in patients with chronic neck pain: a randomized controlled study, *Eur J Pain* 17(10):1517–1528, 2013.

211. Jordan A, Ostergaard K: Rehabilitation of neck/shoulder patients in primary health care clinics, *J Manipulative Physiol Ther* 19(1):32–35, 1996.

212. Jordan A, Ostergaard K: Implementation of neck/shoulder rehabilitation in primary health care clinics, *J Manipulative Physiol Ther* 19(1):36–40, 1996.

213. O'Leary S, Falla D, Elliott JM, et al: Muscle dysfunction in cervical spine pain: Implications for assessment and management, *J Orthop Sports Phys Ther* 39(5):324–333, 2009.

214. Richardson CA, Jull GA: Muscle control–pain control: what exercises would you prescribe? *Man Ther* 1:2–10, 1995.

215. Bird SP, Tarpenning KM, Marino FE: Designing resistance training programmes to enhance muscular fitness: a review of the acute programme variables, *Sports Med* 35:841–851, 2005.

216. O'Leary S, Jull G, Kim M, et al: Training mode-dependent changes in motor performance in neck pain, *Arch Phys Med Rehabil* 93(7):1225–1233, 2012.

217. Falla D, Bilenkij G, Jull G: Patients with chronic neck pain demonstrate altered patterns of muscle activation during performance of a functional upper limb task, *Spine* 29(13):1436–1440, 2004.

218. McArdle W, Katch F, Katch V: *Exercise physiology, energy, nutrition, and human performance*, ed 6, Philadelphia, 1991, Lea & Febiger.

219. O'Leary S, Jull G, Kim M, et al: Specificity in re-training craniocervical flexor muscle performance, *J Orthop Sports Phys Ther* 37(1):3–9, 2007.

220. Kristjansson E, Treleaven J: Sensorimotor function and dizziness in neck pain: implications for assess-ment and management, *J Orthop Sports Phys Ther* 39(5):364–377, 2009.

221. Jull G, Falla D, Treleaven M, et al: A therapeutic exercise approach for cervical disorders. In Boyling J, Jull G, editors: *Grieve's modern manual therapy*, London, 2004, Churchill Livingstone.

222. Murphy D: Sensorimotor training and cervical stabilization. In Murphy D, editor: *Conservative management of cervical spine syndromes*, New York, 2000, McGraw-Hill.

223. Murphy D: A clinical model for the diagnosis and management of patients with cervical spine disorders, *Aust J Chiropr Osteop* 12(2):57–71, 2004.

224. Murphy DR: Chiropractic rehabilitation of the cervical spine, *J Manipulative Physiol Ther* 23(6):404–408, 2000.

225. Sterling M, Jull G, Vicenzino B, et al: Development of motor system dysfunction following whiplash injury, *Pain* 103:65–73, 2003.

226. Berg HE, Berggren G, Tesch PA: Dynamic neck strength training effect on pain and function, *Arch Phys Med Rehabil* 75(6):661–665, 1994.

227. Jordan A, Manniche C: Rehabilitation and spinal pain, *J Neuromusc Sys* 4(3):89–93, 1996.

228. Falla D, Jull G, Hodges P, et al: An endurance-strength training regime is effective in reducing myoelectric manifestations of cervical flexor muscle fatigue in females with chronic neck pain, *Clin Neurophysiol* 117(4):828–837, 2006.

229. Falla D, Jull G, Russell T, et al: Effect of neck exercise on sitting posture in patients with chronic neck pain, *Phys Ther* 87(4):408–417, 2007.

230. Deep Gupta B, Aggarwal S, Gupta B, et al: Effect of deep cervical flexor training vs. conventional isometric training on forward head posture, pain, neck disability index in dentists suffering from chronic neck pain, *J Clin Diagn Res* 7(10):2261–2264, 2013.

231. Ylinen J, Takala EP, Nykanen M, et al: Active neck muscle training in the treatment of chronic neck pain in women: a randomized controlled trial, *JAMA* 289(19):2509–2516, 2003.

232. Ylinen J, Yelland M, Takala EP, et al: Both endurance training and strenght training reduced disability and pain in chronic non-specific neck pain in women, *Evid Based Med* 8(6):184, 2003.

233. van Ettekoven H, Lucas C: Efficacy of physiotherapy including a craniocervical training programme for tension-type headache: a randomized clinical trial, *Cephalalgia* 26(8):983–991, 2006.

234. Dusunceli Y, Ozturk C, Atamaz F, et al: Efficacy of neck stabilization exercises for neck pain: A randomized controlled study, *J Rehabil Med* 41(8):626–631, 2009.

235. Peolsson A, Kjellman G: Neck muscle endurance in nonspecific patients with neck pain and in patients after anterior cervical decompression and fusion, *J Manipulative Physiol Ther* 30(5):343–350, 2007.

236. Armstrong BS, McNair PJ, Williams M: Head and neck position sense in whiplash patients and healthy individuals and the effect of the cranio-cervical flexion action, *Clin Biomech* 20(7):675–684, 2005.

237. Griffiths C, Dziedzic K, Waterfield J, et al: Effectiveness of specific neck stabilization exercises or a general neck exercise program for chronic neck disorders: a randomized controlled trial, *J Rheumatol* 36(2):390–397, 2009.

238. Conley MS, Stone MH, Nimmons M, et al: Specificity of resistance training responses in neck muscle size and strength, *Eur J Appl Physiol Occup Physiol* 75(5):443–448, 1997.

239. Portero P, Bigard AX, Gamet D, et al: Effects of resistance training in humans on neck muscle performance, and electromyogram power spectrum changes, *Eur J Appl Physiol* 84(6):540–546, 2001.

240. O'Leary S, Falla D, Jull G: Recent advances in therapeutic exercise for the neck: implications for patients with head and neck pain, *Aust Endodont J* 29:138–142, 2003.

241. O'Grady WH, Tollan MF: The role of exercise in treating cervical hypermobility or instability, *Orthop Phys Ther Clin North Am* 10:475–501, 2001.

242. Beer A, Treleaven J, Jull G: Can a functional postural exercise improve performance in the cranio-cervical flexion test?—a preliminary study, *Man Ther* 17(3):219–224, 2012.

243. Mayoux-Benhamou MA, Revel M, Vallee C, et al: Longus colli has a postural function on cervical curvature, *Surg Radiol Anat* 16(4):367–371, 1994.

244. Fountain FP, Minear WL, Allison RD: Function of longus colli and longissimus cervicis muscles in man, *Arch Phys Med Rehabil* 47:665–669, 1966.

245. Heikkilä H, Astrom PG: Cervicocephalic kinesthetic sensibility in patients with whiplash injury, *Scand J Rehabil Med* 28(3):133–138, 1996.

246. Heikkilä HV, Wenngren BI: Cervicocephalic kinesthetic sensibility, active range of cervical motion, and oculomotor function in patients with whiplash injury, *Arch Phys Med Rehabil* 79(9):1089–1094, 1998.

247. Humphreys BK, Irgens PM: The effect of a rehabilitation exercise program on head repositioning accuracy and reported levels of pain in chronic neck pain subjects, *J Whiplash Relat Disord* 1(1):99–112, 2002.

248. Revel M, Minguet M, Gregoy P, et al: Changes in cervicocephalic kinesthesia after a proprioceptive rehabilitation program in patients with neck pain: a randomized controlled study, *Arch Phys Med Rehabil* 75(8):895–899, 1994.

249. Fitz-Ritson D: Phasic exercises for cervical rehabilitation after "whiplash" trauma, *J Manipulative Physiol Ther* 18:21–24, 1995.

250. Hansson EE, Månsson NO, Ringsberg KAM, Håkansson A: Dizziness among patients with whiplash-associated disorder: a randomized controlled trial, *J Rehabil Med* 38(6):387–390, 2006.

251. Petersen CM, Zimmermann CL, Tang R: Proprioception interventions to improve cervical position sense in cervical pathology, *Int J Ther Rehabil* 20(3):154–163, 2013.

252. Morimoto H, Asai Y, Johnson EG, et al: Effect of oculo-motor and gaze stability exercises on postural stability and dynamic visual acuity in healthy young adults, *Gait Posture* 33(4):600–603, 2011.

253. Bradnan L, Roohester L, Vujnovich A: Manual cervical traction reduces alpha-motoneuron excitability in normal subjects, *Electromyogr Clin Neurophysiol* 40:259–266, 2000.

254. Harris PR: Cervical traction: review of literature and treatment guidelines, *Phys Ther* 54:910–914, 1977.

255. *The Cochrane database of systematic reviews*, 2006.

256. Jette D, Falkel JE, Trombly C: Effect of intermittent, supine cervical traction on the myoelectric activity of the upper trapezius muscle in subjects with neck pain, *Phys Ther* 65:1173–1176, 1985.

257. Onel D, Tuzlaci M, Sari H, et al: Computed tomographic investigation of the effect of traction on lumbar disc herniations, *Spine* 14:82–90, 1989.

258. Rattanatharn R, Sanjaroensuttikul N, Anadirekkul P, et al: Effectiveness of lumbar traction with routine conservative treatment in acute herniated disc syndrome, *J Med Assoc Thailand* 87(2):S272–S277, 2004.

259. Deets D, Hands KL, Hopp SS: Cervical traction: a comparison of sitting and supine positions, *Phys Ther* 57:255–261, 1977.

260. Andersson GBJ, Schultz AB, Nachemson AL: Intervertebral disc pressures during traction, *Scand J Rehabil Med* 15:88–91, 1983.

261. Kekosz VN, Hilbert L, Tepperman PS: Cervical and lumbopelvic traction: to stretch or not to stretch, *Postgrad Med* 80:187–194, 1986.

262. Harris PR: Cervical traction: review of literature and treatment guidelines, *Phys Ther* 57:910–914, 1977.

263. Humphreys SC, Chase J, Patwardhan A, et al: Flexion and traction effect on C5-C6 foraminal space, *Arch Phys Med Rehabil* 79:1105–1109, 1998.

264. Pio A, Rendina M, Benazzo F, et al: The statics of cervical traction, *J Spinal Disord* 7(4):337–342, 1994.

265. Wong AMK, Chau Peng L, Chen CM: The traction angle and cervical intervertebral separation, *Spine* 17:136–138, 1992.

266. Colachis SC, Strohm BR: Radiographic studies of cervical spine motion in normal subjects: flexion and hyperextension, *Arch Phys Med Rehabil* 46:753–760, 1965.

267. Grieve GP: Neck traction, *Physiotherapy* 68:260–265, 1982.

268. LaBan MM, Macy JA, Meerschaert JR: Intermittent cervical traction: a progenitor of lumbar radicular pain, *Arch Phys Med Rehabil* 73:295–296, 1992.

269. Hart DL, Johnson RM, Simmons EF, et al: Review of cervical orthoses, *Phys Ther* 58(7):857–860, 1978.

270. Johnson RM, Hart DL, Simmons EF, et al: Cervical orthoses: a study comparing their effectiveness in restricting cervical motion in normal subjects, *J Bone Joint Surg Am* 59(3):332–339, 1977.

271. Johnson RM, Owen JR, Hart DL, et al: Cervical orthoses: a guide to their selection and use, *Clin Orthop Relat Res* 154:34–45, 1981.

272. Colachis SC, Strohm BR, Ganter EL: Cervical spine motion in normal women: radiographic study of effect of cervical collars, *Arch Phys Med Rehabil* 54(4):161–169, 1973.

273. Chaitow L: *Muscle energy techniques*, Edinburgh, 2001, Churchill Livingstone.

274. Mitchell FL, Moran PS, Pruzzo NA: *An evaluation and treatment manual of osteopathic muscle energy procedures*, Valley Park, 1979, Mitchell, Moran & Pruzzo.

275. Mitchell FL: Elements of muscle energy. In Basmajian JV, Nyberg R, editors: *Rational manual therapies*, Baltimore, 1993, Williams & Williams.

276. Maitland GD: *Vertebral manipulation*, London, 1986, Butterworth.

CHAPTER 4

Temporomandibular Disorders

SUSAN L. ARMIJO-OLIVO, INAE C. GADOTTI*

INTRODUCTION

Temporomandibular disorders (TMDs) consist of a group of pathologies that affect the masticatory muscles and the temporomandibular joint (TMJ) and related structures. TMDs interfere greatly with daily activities and can significantly affect the patient's lifestyle, diminishing the individual's ability to work and interact in a social environment. In the United States alone approximately $2 billion is spent each year on direct care for TMDs.[1]

Chronic pain caused by TMDs has been shown to produce the same individual impact and burden as back pain and severe headache. TMDs are commonly associated with other conditions of the head and neck region, such as headache, neck pain, and neck muscular dysfunction. To date, studies have shown a clinical association between cervical spine dysfunction and TMD.[2-8]

Research supports the use of conservative and reversible treatments to treat most patients with TMDs.[9,10] A TMD is recognized as a complex disorder, and the treatment of these patients involves many health care professionals, such as dentists, speech pathologists, physicians, psychologists, and physical therapists. Occlusal splint therapy, medications, psychotherapy, behavioral therapy, acupuncture, and physical therapy have been used to improve patients' symptomatology. The effectiveness of the treatment also depends on the patient. Most treatments have not been researched, and their use depends on the experience of the clinicians.

Physical therapy does not escape the rigor of scientific evaluation. The procedures of physical therapy intervention are not well described in the literature in this area. Basically, physical therapy treatment is used to relieve pain, improve range of motion (ROM), and improve the function of the masticatory system through physical modalities, exercises, and manual techniques. Physical therapy also addresses the craniocervical system as a whole, improving the balance between various muscles to maintain the equilibrium of the craniomandibular system (CMS) (i.e., postural equilibrium) and to prevent additional problems sometimes seen in patients with TMDs, such as spasm of the cervical muscles, cervical pain, and referred pain from the cervical spine to the masticatory system.

From a physical therapy perspective, clinicians work with patients who require treatment of the TMJ and its surrounding structures. Treatment goals are the same as for any other musculoskeletal structure. However, the clinician must always keep in mind that this is a special joint: bilateral in nature and having structural and anatomical features that are different from the other joints in the body.[11] Pain is the most common symptom and the one that usually causes the patient to seek help in the first place. For this reason any clinician treating patients with TMDs must address pain management in addition to possible causes or factors associated with pain.

If the TMJ is hypomobile, normal mobility should be restored through mobilization and exercise and then should be maintained through exercise and function. If the TMJ is hypermobile, the hypermobility must be restricted through patient education, modification of use, and exercises to restore normal function. If muscle spasm is present, the spasm has to be reduced through mobilization, exercise, or perhaps with the assistance of physical agents. If inflammation is a factor, the effects of the inflammation must be controlled with rest, change of function, an increase in the blood supply to the area, and adjunctive pharmaceutical therapy.

This chapter provides a general overview of the etiology, epidemiology, classification, and treatment of TMDs. It deals only with disorders that are commonly presented or referred for rehabilitation (usually to a physical therapy department). The reader interested in more in-depth knowledge about TMDs is encouraged to refer to more specific references.[12,13]

TEMPOROMANDIBULAR DISORDERS (TMDS)

Definition

TMDs is a broad, nonspecific term that encompasses several clinical problems involving the stomatognathic

*The authors, editors, and publisher wish to acknowledge Martin Parfitt for his contributions on this topic in the previous edition.

system (which is responsible for speech, swallowing, breathing, and mastication functions), TMJ, masticatory muscles, and craniocervical system.[14] Use of the term **temporomandibular joint (TMJ) dysfunction** as an overall descriptor of TMDs has been discontinued because it is considered misleading and inaccurate, implying structural conditions when in fact most of the time these conditions are not the cause of the dysfunction.[15] TMDs usually are manifested by one or more of the following signs or symptoms: pain, joint sounds, limitation of jaw movement, muscle tenderness, and joint tenderness.[16] In addition, TMDs are commonly associated with other symptoms affecting the head and neck region, such as headache, ear-related symptoms (e.g., tinnitus [ringing in the ear] and otalgia [pain in the ear]), and cervical spine disorders (e.g., fatigue of the masticatory, cervical, and scapular muscles).[17-20] TMDs are considered musculoskeletal disorders of the masticatory system, and they affect more than 25% of the general population.[17] According to Goldstein "chronic TMD is considered as a psychophysiologic disorder of the central nervous system that modulates emotional, physiologic, and neuroendocrine responses to emotional and physical stressors" (p. 380).[15]

Epidemiology

According to a study by Drangsholt and LeResche,[1] TMDs affected approximately 20 million adults in the United States and 450 million adults worldwide in 1998. One in three adults will develop TMD pain.[21] Therefore TMDs are very common conditions. However, only 1% to 3% of the population seeks care for their TMDs, and 3.6% to 7% of the general population is in need of treatment.[21] Various studies demonstrate that 50% to 75% of adults have at least one sign and/or symptom related to TMD.[22] According to Auvenshine,[23] approximately 10% of the adult population has pain in the temporomandibular region. Some signs seem to be more common in the healthy population than others; for example, joint sounds or mandibular deviation occurs in 50% of the population.[17,24,25] Limitation of mouth opening is thought to be rare (seen only in 5%).[23]

In a representative urban sample of 1230 subjects from the Brazilian population, at least one TMD symptom was reported by 39.2% of the individuals and pain related to TMD was noted by 25.6% of the population. The most common symptom was TMJ sound, followed by TMJ pain and masticatory muscle pain.[26] All symptoms were more prevalent in women than in men. In a prospective study a cohort of 2737 TMD-free subjects were followed for up to 5.2 years.[27] According to the study, 260 people developed first onset of TMD, which indicates an annual incidence rate of 4%. Although the literature about the natural course of TMD is limited, evidence shows that progression to chronic condition is uncommon.[28]

Some studies have found that signs and symptoms of TMD in the general population occur twice as often in females as in males (2:1).[29-32] However, other studies have found the ratio of females to males to be approximately the same[33] or 3:1.[34] For example, one study found that more than 70% of patients with TMD were women, and the ratio of affected females to males was 2.4:1 for arthralgia, 2.5:1 for osteoarthritis, 3.4:1 for myofascial pain, and 5.1:1 for disc displacement (DD).[35] The literature supports the fact that women are more sensitive to pain conditions and that they report pain that is more severe, more frequent, and of longer duration than that reported by men.[36-43] In addition, women are more likely to seek help than men.[1]

Women have also been found to have more TMJ clicking and tenderness, headaches, and muscle tenderness than men.[44] According to data presented by LeResche,[45] only 25% of the community cases met the criteria for a diagnosis of myalgia or myofascial pain; 3.3% met the criteria for a diagnosis of internal derangement; and 4.2% met the criteria for a diagnosis of an arthrogenic condition. Most subjects presented with a mixed diagnosis and were classified into more than one group. Muscle and disc diagnoses were made in 8.3%; myogenic and arthrogenic diagnoses were made in 21.7%; and myogenic, arthrogenic, and DD diagnoses were made in 7.5%.

Etiology

The etiology of TMDs has been hypothesized to be multifactorial. As stated by Goldstein,[15] the medical cause of most TMDs has not yet been established or is unknown (idiopathic). Some factors, such as bad posture, bruxism, anatomical factors (related to dental occlusion alterations that can cause internal derangement of the TMJ), occlusal disharmony, malposition or malformation of the condyle or fossa, trauma, orthodontic treatment, and psychological factors (e.g., stress),[46] have been hypothesized to initiate or precipitate TMD or to increase a person's predisposition to develop these disorders.[47] However, most of these factors are not based on solid scientific grounds. According to Drangsholt and LeResche,[1] factors associated with female gender, the number of preexisting pain conditions, and depression appear to be strongly associated with TMDs. The remaining factors mentioned previously have failed to demonstrate a strong relationship with TMDs, and more research is needed to clarify their role in causing or perpetuating TMD pain.

It is unknown why people develop TMDs and why they progress to chronicity. A variety of physical and psychological factors could be implicated in chronic TMDs, such as oral habits, secondary gain, and higher levels of pain and disability. Such factors are also seen in other chronic pain conditions, including low back pain, headache, and neck pain. Thus, the most accepted theory related to the etiology, assessment, and management of TMD is supported by the biopsychosocial model.[48] Therefore TMD is recognized as a multidimensional disorder that is a result of biological, psychological, and social alterations.

CLASSIFICATION OF TEMPOROMANDIBULAR DISORDERS

Various professional organizations have classified TMDs in various ways. The American Academy of Orofacial Pain has established a set of diagnostic criteria that has been presented as an addendum to the classification of and diagnostic criteria for headache disorders, cranial neuralgias, and facial pain.[49] A number of classification schemes used in epidemiological studies of TMDs include clinical signs. The differential diagnosis of TMD is based on the patient's chief complaint, clinical evaluation of the patient's signs and symptoms, and TMJ imaging, when necessary. Most of the tools have been based on clinical experience and patients' reports.

Several classification systems have been used in epidemiological studies to define TMDs. However, not all of them have been validated or tested for reliability and responsiveness. The *Research Diagnostic Criteria for Temporomandibular Disorders* (RDC/TMD)[1] for diagnosing TMDs developed by the Department of Oral Surgery, University of Washington has been the accepted criteria to diagnose TMDs. The RDC/TMD is a guide that provides clinical researchers with a standardized system for examining, diagnosing, and classifying the most common subtypes of TMDs with clear face and criterion validity.[1] It was introduced in 1992 and has been widely used in clinical research settings around the world where TMD and facial pain are managed. Some studies have demonstrated good reliability of the RDC/TMD in different settings, not only for determining signs and symptoms[50] but also for making reliable diagnoses.[51] Wahlund et al.[52] found good to excellent reliability ($\kappa > 0.78$) for each of the RDC/TMD major groups. This guide has been recommended as a model system for standardizing the investigation into the diagnosis and classification of any chronic pain condition. The guide is divided into two sections—axis I: clinical TMD conditions and axis II: pain-related disability and psychological status.[53] The axis I diagnosis classification will be described in this section of the chapter. The axis II classification will be discussed later.

Although the RDC/TMD has been used extensively in the TMD area since its inception in 1992, several researchers have revised it, and several studies have been performed to improve its psychometric properties as well as its usability for clinical practice and research.[54-59] Steenks and de Wijer,[60] for example, felt that the RDC/TMD criteria were unbalanced in the number of muscular and articular palpation sites which could lead to an overrepresentation of muscular conditions at the expense of articular pain conditions when determining TMD diagnoses. In addition, the use of some unreliable muscle palpation sites, such as intraoral muscles and submandibular muscles, and

the arbitrary cutoff of three painful palpation sites could increase the probability of false positive results for myogenous muscular pain as well. Furthermore, the algorithm to determine articular compromise from the RDC/TMD was only based on ongoing pain. Compression, retrusion, and joint play (i.e., a traction test) were not included in the examination protocol used by the RDC/TMD. Thus these suggestions were compiled as well as other suggestions from several experts, and a new version of the RDC/TMD has been launched.[61]

Now it is called *Diagnostic Criteria for Temporomandibular Disorders* (DC/TMD). This new diagnostic classification is intended to be used in clinical as well as research settings. It includes 12 common diagnoses of TMD: arthralgia, myalgia, local myalgia, myofascial pain, myofascial pain with referral, four disc displacement (DD) disorders (i.e., DD with reduction [DDwithR], DDwithR with intermittent locking, DD without reduction [DDwithoutR] with limited opening, and DDwithoutR without limited opening), degenerative joint disease (DJD), subluxation, and headache attributed to TMD. A complete outline of the main diagnoses proposed by the DC/TMD can be found in Table 4-1. Several new diagnoses were created and some of the old diagnoses were deleted because their clinical applicability was minimal.[53,62] For instance, because the terms osteoarthrosis and arthritis are not used consistently in medicine, there is a change in nomenclature and these terms are considered to denote subclasses of DJD according to the new DC/TMD. If pain co-occurs with DJD, the diagnosis of arthralgia can be used as well. Thus, the previous diagnosis of osteoarthritis is now called DJD and arthralgia. This new classification has been found to be valid for differentiating the most common pain-related TMDs, such as myalgia with a sensitivity of ≥ 0.90 and a specificity of 0.99. Myofascial pain with referral showed a sensitivity of ≥ 0.86 and a specificity of ≥ 0.98. Arthralgia had a sensitivity of 0.89 and specificity of 0.98. In addition, DDwithoutR with limited opening had a sensitivity of 0.80 and specificity of 0.97. The diagnostic accuracy of the rest of the classifications was poor. Interexaminer reliability for myalgia was found to be excellent ($\kappa = 0.94$) as well as for myofascial pain with referral ($\kappa \geq 0.85$) and arthralgia ($\kappa = 0.86$), which is considered excellent. Nevertheless, other intracapsular diagnoses had poor reliability.

Some authors classify TMDs as **arthrogenic TMDs**, which involve an alteration in the TMJ (e.g., congenital disorders, DD, fracture, dislocation, inflammation, hypermobility, ankylosis, and osteoarthritis) and **myogenic TMDs**, which involve the masticatory muscles (e.g., myalgia [local muscle soreness], myofascial pain, myositis, myospasm [protective co-contraction], myofibrotic contracture, and centrally mediated myalgia).[9,23,63]

Because the classification proposed by the new DC/TMD is the most up to date and accepted, it will be described in more detail in this chapter. In addition, only

TABLE 4-1

Expanded Taxonomy for Temporomandibular Disorders Proposed by the New Diagnostic Criteria for Temporomandibular Disorders (DC/TMD)

I. TEMPOROMANDIBULAR JOINT DISORDERS
1. Joint pain
   A. Arthralgia
   B. Arthritis
2. Joint disorders
   A. Disc disorders
      1. Disc displacement with reduction
      2. Disc displacement with reduction with intermittent locking
      3. Disc displacement without reduction with limited opening
      4. Disc displacement without reduction without limited opening
   B. Hypomobility disorders other than disc disorders
      1. Adhesions/Adherence
      2. Ankylosis
         a. Fibrous
         b. Osseous
   C. Hypermobility disorders
      1. Dislocations
         a. Subluxation
         b. Luxation
3. Joint diseases
   A. Degenerative joint disease
      1. Osteoarthrosis
      2. Osteoarthritis
   B. Systemic arthritides
   C. Condylysis/idiopathic condylar resorption
   D. Osteochondritis dissecans
   E. Osteonecrosis
   F. Neoplasm
   G. Synovial Chondromatosis
4. Fractures
5. Congenital/developmental disorders
   A. Aplasia
   B. Hypoplasia
   C. Hyperplasia

II. MASTICATORY MUSCLE DISORDERS
1. Muscle pain
   A. Myalgia
      1. Local myalgia
      2. Myofascial pain
      3. Myofascial pain with referral
   B. Tendonitis
   C. Myositis
   D. Spasm
2. Contracture
3. Hypertrophy
4. Neoplasm
5. Movement Disorders
   A. Orofacial dyskinesia
   B. Oromandibular dystonia
6. Masticatory muscle pain attributed to systemic/central pain disorders
   A. Fibromyalgia/widespread pain

III. HEADACHE
1. Headache attributed to temporomandibular disorders

IV. ASSOCIATED STRUCTURES
1. Coronoid hyperplasia

From Peck CC, Goulet JP, Lobbezoo F et al: Expanding the taxonomy of the diagnostic criteria for temporomandibular disorders, *J Oral Rehabil* 41(1):6, 2014. In consultation with Schiffman E, Ohrbach R, Truelove E et al: Diagnostic criteria for temporomandibular disorders (DC/TMD) for clinical and research applications: recommendations of the International RDC/TMD Consortium Network and Orofacial Pain Special Interest Group, *J Oral Facial Pain Headache* 28(1):6-27, 2014.

common TMD alterations are described. For a more detailed description of other less common disorders, the reader is encouraged to review the expanded taxonomy of DC/TMD elaborated by Peck et al.[64]

Joint Pain

Temporomandibular Joint (TMJ) Arthralgia

TMJ arthralgia is pain of joint origin. It is characterized by pain and tenderness in the TMJ capsule and/or the synovial lining. Pain is present in one or both joints during palpation, and the patient has at least one of the following symptoms: pain in the joint region, pain during maximum unassisted opening, pain during assisted opening, or pain during lateral movements. Crepitus should not be present with a diagnosis of simple arthralgia.[53] Capsulitis commonly is present in patients with TMJ arthralgia. Pain

occurs with provocation testing of the TMJ. Patients report familiar pain (i.e., reproduction of the patient's pain) in the TMJ on palpation at the lateral pole or around the lateral pole or with jaw movements.[64]

Arthritis (Synovitis, Capsulitis)

Patients will complain of pain of joint origin with clinical characteristics of inflammation or infection over the affected joint (i.e., edema, erythema, and/or increased temperature). Arthritis is also called synovitis or capsulitis, but these terms limit the sites of pain perception; thus the term *arthralgia* is more global and involves them both. Pain on palpation over the superior pole and/or posterior part of the TMJ is thought to indicate a capsulitis of the joint. This can be present in an acute stage (e.g., after trauma, such as a blow to the jaw) or in a chronic stage, after repeated minor trauma or insults to the joint itself (e.g., with bruxism in the presence of a class II malocclusion).* The clinician should keep in mind that capsulitis also may be present in the first stages of some general systemic diseases (e.g., rheumatoid arthritis, ankylosing spondylitis) and with local or systemic infection, although cases involving infection are rarely seen in the private practice setting.

Along with pain on palpation, the patient may have some swelling within the joint (although this is rarely seen except in cases of direct acute trauma). Patients often complain of swelling or a sense of fullness over the temporomandibular region. However, this is not often seen clinically unless the area has suffered a severe degree of trauma. Patients are likely to have pain on occlusion and to complain of discomfort with mastication (which of course causes compression within the joint and distention of the joint capsule). The capsular pattern of the TMJ is thought to be reduction of mandibular opening. Sometimes the patient also reports having pain with activities such as yawning or opening wide to bite, which involve stretching of the joint capsule. Capsulitis can be accompanied by spasm of the muscles of mastication, particularly the masseter and the medial and lateral pterygoid muscles. Muscle spasm is present on the ipsilateral side, and during the assessment the examiner will note deviation of the mandible to that side on opening. Condylar translation (i.e., the movement of the condyle forward within the joint) is likely to be present, and this clinical finding is one of the differential diagnostic indicators that distinguish an isolated capsulitis from other internal derangements of the TMJ.

In the acute stage, treatment is aimed at reducing the inflammation and resultant swelling, resting the involved structures, and reducing any muscle spasm. Pain reduction should follow as a result of these measures.

Three of the four basic principles represented by the acronym RICE (rest, ice, and compression; elevation is not really possible with the TMJ) can be used in the treatment of acute capsulitis. The patient should be instructed to eat only soft foods to avoid compressing the joint and aggravating the muscle spasm. The use of an occlusal splint to rest the joint sometimes is effective; however, if the surrounding muscle spasm is severe, a splint can actually increase the spasm because it increases the vertical dimension, thus stretching the contracted muscles. Ice can be applied to the side of the face over the TMJ region to reduce any heat caused by an acute inflammation, as well as the effects of the inflammation and swelling. The authors' experience has been that, apart from cases involving an acute traumatic inflammatory problem,

patients usually find moist heat more comfortable and efficacious. As mentioned, elevation is not possible for cases involving the TMJ; however, symptoms can be controlled through use of the usual principles for treating an acutely traumatized musculoskeletal joint. Nonsteroidal anti-inflammatory drugs (NSAIDs) may be prescribed to reduce pain and/or inflammation.

Joint Disorders

Temporomandibular Joint Disc Displacements

Internal derangement of the TMJ is defined as an abnormal relationship between the mandibular condyle and the disc. This abnormal relationship may involve DDwithR or DDwithoutR. Patients with DD can present with a clinical sign, such as clicking, that is characteristic but not necessarily confirmation of a reducing DD.[65]

Disc Displacement with Reduction (DDwithR)

DDwithR is an intracapsular biomechanical disorder involving the condyle-disc complex. DD can occur anteriorly, medially, anteromedially, or (the most rarely seen) posteriorly. The etiology of DD can be either direct trauma to the mandible (e.g., a blow during a motor vehicle accident [MVA] or contact sports) or indirect trauma. Some researchers postulate that small, repeated episodes of trauma to the joint eventually can cause enough internal tissue damage to produce displacement.[66] It is thought that microtrauma occurs to the structure of the disc itself and/or in some cases to the posterior ligament attached to the disc. This damage causes histological changes within the cell structures of the disc and reduces the disc's load-bearing or compression capacity.

Repeated microtrauma eventually leads to macrotrauma and a further breakdown in tissue and in the disc's ability to function properly. Eventually the disc begins to sublux off the head of the condyle; clinically this produces a click, which can be heard by the patient (and sometimes by others) or can be felt by the clinician during palpation over the poles of the joint during mandibular movement. The patient may present with a reducing disc (i.e., a disc that is displaced and reduces back to its proper position on the condyle), which the patient and clinician may or may not be able to feel. According to the new DC/TMD, to diagnose a DDwithR, clicking or popping and/or snapping noise is detected during both opening and closing with palpation during at least one of three repetitions of jaw opening and closing or clicking or popping and/or snapping noise with palpation during at least one of three repetitions of jaw opening or closing or lateral or protrusive movements. A confirmatory diagnosis of subluxed or dislocated disc can be made only with the backup of an appropriate radiological examination (i.e., MRI). In this case, in the maximum intercuspal position, the posterior band of the disc is located anterior to the 11:30 position

---

*Details on malocclusion, internal derangement, clinician observation, and the patient history can be found in volume 1 of this series, *Orthopedic Physical Assessment*, Chapter 4.

and the intermediate zone of the disc is anterior to the condylar head, or on full opening the intermediate zone of the disc is located between the condylar head and the articular eminence.

In the initial stage of DD, the click during displacement is present early in the opening phase. As the disc and posterior ligament become further traumatized and further displaced, the click is noted later in the opening phase. Therefore a patient who has a click after opening the mandible at least 5 mm of intraincisal distance is likely to have a fairly recent dysfunction, whereas a patient who does not have a click until 45 mm of opening is likely to have had a dysfunction for a longer time (Figures 4-1 and 4-2). In the dental profession a click that is felt during both the opening and closing phases is called a **reciprocal click**; in other cases a click at the joint may be felt either during opening or during closing. When the DD with reduction is unilateral, the mandible can deviate to the affected side during mouth opening.[67]

Patients with DDwithR can have symptoms of joint tenderness on palpation, joint pain that is increased with function, and aberrant mandibular movement with opening.[67]

From a clinical standpoint, it is important to make the patient aware of the likely biomechanical dysfunction occurring in the joint and to emphasize the fact that no form of treatment is likely to reduce the displaced disc. Patients tend to focus on the click, and it is vital to explain as an educational part of the treatment that it is possible to have a clicking joint that is pain free and functional. Indeed, because the disc is crucial to lubrication and nutrition of the structures within the joint,[11] a joint with a clicking disc is preferable to one that is silent and displaced.

Treatment should focus on attempting to produce a symmetrical opening so that the heads of the mandibular condyles translate equally during opening. Making sure that muscle activity is symmetrical also is necessary. As part of the education process, the clinician must teach the patient to avoid any activities that might cause additional trauma to the involved joint or even to the opposite joint. As a result of the dysfunction or the pain caused by the dysfunction, patients not uncommonly isolate any mastication to the side away from the dysfunction. Patients must be coached to chew equally on both sides. They also must be taught to avoid any habit that might increase trauma to the joint, such as nail biting, chewing on toothpicks, bruxing, or chewing gum; these activities can adversely affect the TMJ.

Disc Displacement Without Reduction (DDwithoutR)

DDwithoutR (also called a **clinical closed lock**) (Figures 4-3) is an intracapsular biomechanical disorder involving the condyle-disc complex. In some cases DDwithR causes enough trauma to the disc and its attached

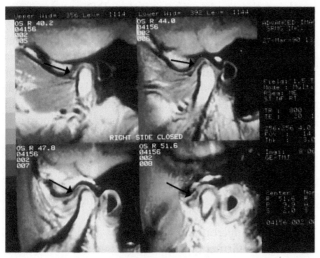

Figure 4-1 MRI of disc displacement with reduction. *Arrows* indicate disc. (Courtesy Dr. L. Kamelchuk, Calgary, Alberta.)

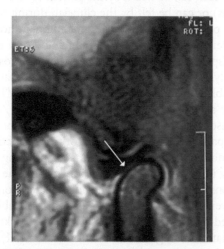

Figure 4-2 MRI of disc displacement with reduction showing reduced disc opening. (Courtesy Dr. D. Hatcher, Sacramento, California.)

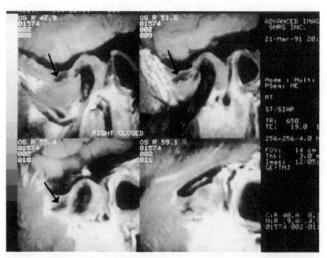

Figure 4-3 MRI of disc displacement without reduction. *Arrows* indicate disc. (Courtesy Dr. L. Kamelchuk, Calgary, Alberta.)

ligaments that the disc does not slide back into its normal position over the pole of the condyle. This can happen asymptomatically, although classically patients present with a history of a clicking functional joint that suddenly changes to a nonclicking, reduced opening joint (e.g., "My jaw clicked for 5 years, and then all of a sudden I woke up [or bit down on some popcorn or yawned], there was a big crack, and my jaw did not click any more, but I couldn't open my mouth as far."). In a study by Stegenga and De Bont,[65] 9% of patients with reducing DD progressed to nonreducing DD within 3 years. The main complaint of these patients is inability to open the mouth wide, and it does not resolve with the clinician or patient performing a specific manipulative maneuver. In the case of a unilateral problem, the mandible is deviated to the affected side during attempted opening without returning to the midline.[67] In the closed-mouth position, the disc is in an anterior position relative to the condylar head, and the disc does not reduce with opening of the mouth. Medial and lateral displacement of the disc may also be present. Presence of TMJ noise (e.g., click with full opening) does not exclude this diagnosis.[64]

As previously noted, the closed lock can be present with or without symptoms; however, a person with a clinical closed lock is more likely to have accompanying symptoms, such as pain, muscle spasm, and reduced function. If the pain is from the TMJ itself, the patient probably will point to the joint and indicate that it hurts there. Sometimes pain can be referred from the TMJ to other areas. It often manifests as a parietal headache on the same side or as pain under the angle of the jaw, or both. Pain also can be referred to the temporomandibular area from other structures; for example, a trigger point in the midbelly of the sternocleidomastoid muscle refers pain directly over the TMJ. Therefore, it is very important that the clinician perform a complete musculoskeletal assessment, which includes not only the masticatory system but also other structures that could be involved, especially the cervical spine.

Treatment of a clinical closed lock is aimed at restoring more normal function. Because of the kinematics of the joint, a degree of opening can be achieved with the disc in a displaced position. Opening produces condylar translation and rotation. In the first movement, which takes place in the superior part of the joint, the mandibular condyle articulates with the disc; in the second movement, which takes place in the inferior part of the joint, the disc and condyle articulate with the temporal fossa. With the disc displaced, translation is reduced; this can be seen during the examination, and it differentiates the clinical closed lock from a straightforward capsulitis. Unless a large amount of muscle spasm disrupts the normal condylar movement, when capsulitis is present without DD, the head of the condyle is still able to translate forward during mandibular opening. In both disorders the condyle can still rotate, and an opening of up to 30 mm of intraincisal distance can be achieved using only condylar rotation.

In most cases if the joint is left untreated, the structures in the joint gradually are stretched so that eventually a more functional opening is achieved. However, secondary adaptive changes can occur in the masticatory structures and can cause other dysfunctions. For example, a joint with a clinical closed lock (a hypomobile joint) stresses the contralateral mandibular joint and causes hypermobility of that joint, which may become symptomatic. For this reason, one of the aims of treatment should be to speed up the stretching that normally occurs in the dysfunctional joint to alleviate the stress on the opposite joint. Thus mobilization of the hypomobile joint becomes vital to restoration of a more symmetrical opening. The patient should be informed that the clinician is not actually trying to relocate the disc but rather to speed up what the body eventually would achieve anyway; that is, a stretching out of tight structures to obtain a more normal function.

Estimates are that 9% to 13% of asymptomatic joints have some type of TMD-related problem. However, not all patients with pain over the TMJ region have an internal derangement; likewise the absence of pain in the TMJ region does not necessarily mean that no internal derangement is present. It has been shown that in so-called normal, symptom-free populations, a certain percentage of joints actually have internal derangements. This fact emphasizes the importance of the history, musculoskeletal assessment, and radiological survey in determining the condition present.

The clinician cannot determine the type of pathology taking place in the joint by using just one type of diagnostic imaging. In the past some practitioners thought that a lateral x-ray film of the TMJ was enough to allow determination of the pathological condition at the TMJ and even the position of the condylar head in the temporal fossa. However, it has since been shown that a full set of diagnostic images is needed to ascertain properly what is going on in the joint. Many practitioners now require a Panorex (a radiograph that gives an overall impression of the maxilla-mandible structure) (Figure 4-4), tomograms that show both the opening and resting positions of the condyle, and cephalograms, which orthodontists use to define growth patterns, particularly the skull structure (Figure 4-5). Magnetic resonance imaging (MRI) of the joint demonstrates the state and position of the disc and surrounding soft tissues in much greater detail (Figure 4-6) than an x-ray film.

Disc Displacement Without Reduction Without Limited Opening

Similar to DDwithoutR, this condition is an intracapsular biomechanical disorder involving the condyle-disc complex. The only difference with the DDwithoutR is that this kind is *not* associated with limited mandibular opening.[64]

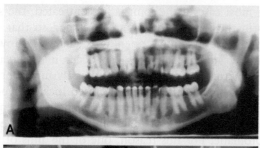

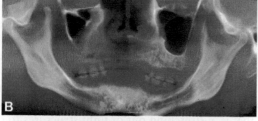

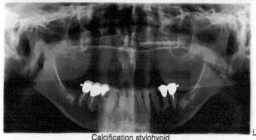

Calcification stylohyoid

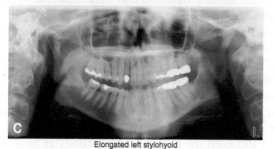

Elongated left stylohyoid

Figure 4-4 A, Panorex image of the maxilla and mandible. **B,** Panorex image of an edentulous patient. **C,** Panorex image of a patient with Eagle syndrome. (**A,** Courtesy Dr. L. Kamelchuk, Calgary, Alberta. **B** and **C,** Courtesy Dr. D. Hatcher, Sacramento, California.)

Joint Diseases

Degenerative Joint Disease (DJD)

DJD is a degenerative disorder characterized by deterioration of articular tissue of the joint with concomitant osseous changes in the condyle and/or articular eminence. DJD can be subclassified: DJD without arthralgia is defined as osteoarthrosis and DJD with arthralgia is defined as osteoarthritis.

As mentioned previously, the disc is an important structure in the lubrication and nutrition of the joint. When the disc stops functioning properly (e.g., immobile, disc in the anterior position), changes occur in the joint structures that can be seen with diagnostic imaging. The hypomobility affects the pumping action that delivers nutrients from the synovial fluid to the articular cartilage.

The deficiency in lubrication and nutrients may induce or aggravate degeneration.[65] Changes that occur in the joint structures include erosion, cavitation, osteophyte formation, and a reduction in the normal joint line (Figure 4-7).

TMDs that arise from degenerative joint changes most often are seen after age 40.[68] Some small x-ray changes usually can be seen in a joint that has DDwithR, such as flattening of the condylar head, subchondral sclerosis, and slight remodeling; however, the major degenerative changes do not occur until the disc is displaced and is not reducing. According to the new DC/TMD classification, flattening and/or cortical sclerosis are considered indeterminant findings for DJD and may represent normal variation, aging, remodeling, or a precursor to frank DJD. All these changes can occur without symptoms. When symptoms do occur, they usually include pain, muscle spasm, headaches, and a change in function of the masticatory system. For example, the patient is unable to chew hard foods, or crepitus is experienced at the TMJ with function. The main aim of treatment for DJD of the TMJ is to restore the area to normal function. In addition, it bears repeating: "*as part of the educational process, the clinician must emphasize to the patient that the treatment is not about restoring the disc or disc function, but more about speeding along what the body would normally do.*"

Based on the new DC/TMD, DJDs include TMJ osteoarthritis and osteoarthrosis.

TMJ Osteoarthritis and Osteoarthrosis. Osteoarthritis is an inflammatory condition in the joint, and it can manifest in different forms, such as osteoarthritis and rheumatoid arthritis (RA). Osteoarthritis results in erosion and fibrillation of the cartilage and degeneration of subchondral bone. Symptoms of osteoarthritis include pain, restricted jaw movement, and joint sounds (crepitus). RA is a chronic systemic inflammatory disease that involves the synovial joints, including the TMJ. RA produces symptoms such as fatigue, fever, anemia, and neuropathy.[69]

According to the new DC/TMD, a diagnosis of osteoarthritis requires the presence of arthralgia plus either crepitus in the joint or imaging evidence of at least one degenerative characteristic, specifically subchondral cyst, erosion of normal cortical delineation, generalized sclerosis of the condyle and articular eminence, or osteophyte formation.[64] TMJ osteoarthrosis is a degenerative disorder in a joint with an abnormal joint structure. For this diagnosis, the same characteristics must be present as for the osteoarthritis diagnosis, but the arthralgia symptoms must be absent.[53,64]

Osteoarthrosis presents degenerative changes similar to those seen with osteoarthritis, but it is a noninflammatory condition.

Masticatory Muscle Disorders

Myalgia

Myalgia is an acute, local, noninflammatory pain in the masticatory muscles that is the result of protective

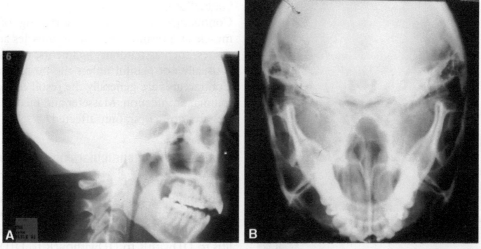

Figure 4-5 Cephalograms of the skull. **A,** Lateral view. **B,** Basilar view. (Courtesy Dr. L. Kamelchuk, Calgary, Alberta.)

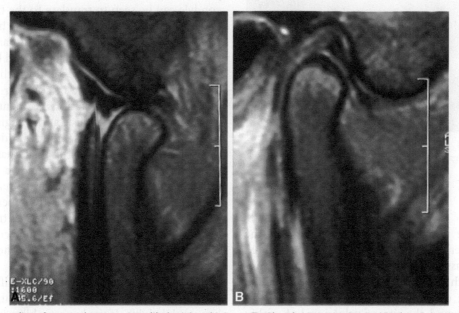

Figure 4-6 MRI studies of a normal temporomandibular joint. **A,** Open. **B,** Closed. (Courtesy Dr. D. Hatcher, Sacramento, California.)

muscle splinting, postexercise muscle soreness, muscle fatigue, trauma, and/or pain from ischemia. It is a pain of muscle origin affected by jaw movement, function, or parafunction, and replication of this pain with provocation testing of the masticatory muscles. Limitation of the mandibular movement(s) secondary to pain may be present.[61] Its causes and pathology are not clearly defined.[62] It is called "local myalgia" when the localization of pain is only at the site of palpation (i.e., localized to the area of the palpating finger) when using the examination protocol stated by the DC/TMD.[61,64] According to Okeson,[70] it is characterized by changes in the local environment of the muscle tissues, mainly through release of algogenic substances that produce pain.

The diagnosis of myalgia is made based on examination of the masseter and temporalis muscles. However, a positive finding with the specified provocation tests when examining the other masticatory muscles can help to corroborate this diagnosis. Based on the new DC/TMD classification scheme, there are three subclasses of myalgia: local myalgia, myofascial pain, and myofascial pain with referral, which are described later. When myalgia is further subclassified as local myalgia, myofascial pain, or myofascial pain with referral, the latter diagnoses are based on using only the examination findings from palpation protocol stated by the DC/TMD. The palpation pressure being held over the site being palpated for myofascial pain with referral is 5 seconds compared with 2 seconds for myalgia.

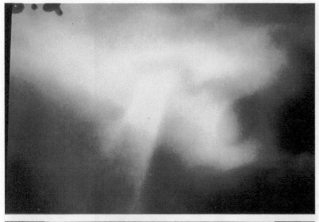

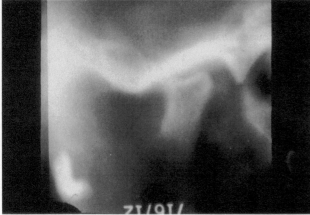

Figure 4-7 CT scans of degenerative joint disease. (Courtesy Dr. L. Kamelchuk, Calgary, Alberta.)

Myofascial Pain

According to the new classification scheme from the DC/TMD, the term "myofascial pain" can be divided in two new subclassifications: **myofascial pain** and **myofascial pain with referral**. Myofascial pain is defined as pain of muscle origin as described for myalgia with pain spreading beyond the site of palpation but within the boundary of the muscle at palpation. Myofascial pain with referral describes the pain that is characterized by referral of pain beyond the muscle being palpated when using the examination protocol described by the DC/TMD.[61,64] It can be characterized by stiffness, muscle pain that increases with function, and the possible presence of trigger points.[53,62] The recommended treatments include manual therapy (e.g., therapeutic massage, acupressure, and acupuncture) and osteopathic manipulation. Some of these treatments are discussed in detail later in the chapter.

Myospasm

Myospasm is a rare, acute condition of the masticatory muscles. It is a sudden, involuntary, and reversible muscle contraction characterized by localized pain and limited ROM of the jaw.[62] It usually is of short duration.[70] It may affect any of the masticatory muscles.[64]

Contracture

Contracture is a painless shortening of a masticatory muscle as a result of fibrosis in muscles and surrounding tissues, such as tendons, ligaments, or muscle fibers.[62] It is usually not painful unless the muscle is overstretched. Contractures are generally the result of radiation therapy, trauma, or infection. Masseter and medial pterygoid muscles are most commonly affected.[64]

Other Temporomandibular Joint Problems

Hypermobility

Hypermobility can be viewed in two ways: as a joint dysfunction entity in itself or as an end process in the natural history of joint dysfunction, which progresses from capsulitis to DDwithR to DDwithoutR to DJD and eventually to hypermobility.

For a joint to be labeled hypermobile, radiological hypermobility must be present. Normally the head of the condyle can be seen to translate to the tip of the articular eminence; however, with radiographic hypermobility, the condylar head translates beyond the articular eminence (Figure 4-8). This often is accompanied by a change in the normal biomechanics of the joint, which means the examiner would see an increase in condylar translation and a reduction in condylar rotation. As mentioned previously, rotation normally takes place at the beginning of mandibular opening; midopening requires a degree of rotation and some translation; and the final phase of opening involves mainly translation of the condyle. In a hypermobile joint, posterior disc structures usually are stretched and the posterior ligament frequently is perforated. Because of the soft tissue laxity, a great deal of translation can occur at the beginning of opening, and very little rotation is felt at all. This is almost a reversal of the normal articular mechanics of the joint.

If the hypermobility is the result of stiffness in the opposite joint, treatment obviously includes mobilization of the hypomobile joint. If the hypermobility is the end result of degenerative changes within the joint, treatment focuses more on restricting the extra mobility within the joint. If the biomechanics of the joint have been changed, part of the treatment should include exercise to try to return joint movement to a more normal form. For example, some hypermobility can cause increased translation and reduced rotation. One way to restrict translation is to coach the patient in using the tongue to control movement. The tip of the tongue is placed behind the top teeth, the lips are placed together, and the teeth are left in their resting position in slight dysocclusion (the upper and lower teeth have a slight distance between them [1 to 3 mm at rest]; this is called the *free way space*). Then the patient is instructed to keep the lips together and drop the jaw. By placing an index finger over the head of the condyle, the examiner can feel a reduction in the condylar translation and a return to some rotation. The patient is instructed to repeat this exercise once an hour so that the different movement

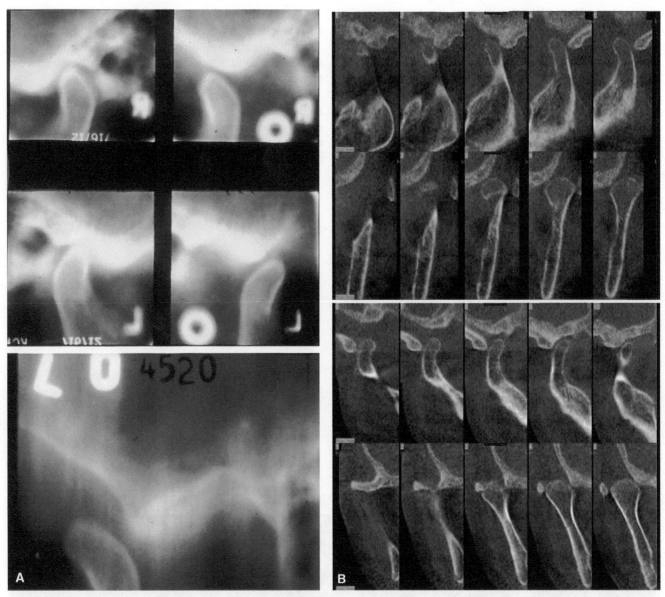

Figure 4-8 A, Tomograms showing hypermobility of the temporomandibular joint (TMJ). **B,** Tomograms of a hypermobile TMJ showing dislocation of the condyle. (**A,** Courtesy Dr. L. Kamelchuk, Calgary, Alberta. **B,** Courtesy Dr. D. Hatcher, Sacramento, California.)

patterns produced by the motor units are reprogrammed as a new engram into the motor cortex.

The tongue can also be used to restrict hypermobility. If the patient is instructed to keep the tip of the tongue behind the top teeth and to open the mouth as far as possible with the tongue in place, in most cases the joint will not be stretched into its hypermobile range. In some cases a patient with a long tongue will not be able to restrict the opening sufficiently; the individual should then be instructed to place the tip of the tongue in the roof of the palate. If this still does not restrict the opening movement sufficiently, the patient can be coached to fold the upper one third of the tongue into the roof of the mouth. Normal opening should be assessed as 40 to 50 mm interincisal distance. Opening past 50 mm frequently can be present with normal joint biomechanics, indicating laxity. Increased translation also can occur at the cost of lost condylar rotation (less than 50 mm), which often is seen in individuals with Asian features.

Patient Education to Limit Hypermobility

- Control opening wide (hypermobility)
- Put the tip of your tongue against the back of your upper teeth. Keeping your tongue in this position, open your mouth as far as the tongue will allow. This is as far as you should allow yourself to open, so that the soft tissue around the jaw is not overstretched and is allowed to rest
- Cut your food into bite-sized (i.e., small) pieces. Do not take big bites out of hamburgers or other foods
- When you feel a yawn coming on, make sure to control the amount of mouth opening, using the tongue positioning technique described in the second point

Temporomandibular Joint Ankylosis

Ankylosis of the TMJ is a complete fusion of the condyle to the temporal fossa (true ankylosis). Ankylosis is classified as congenital, traumatic, inflammatory (i.e., RA), systemic (e.g., ankylosing spondylitis), or neoplastic (e.g., osteochondroma).[67]

TMJ ankylosis causes restriction of opening and stress on the opposite joint; in fact patients often present with symptoms arising from the joint opposite the ankylosed joint. In children, TMJ ankylosis impairs mandibular growth and can result in mandibular micrognathia (underdevelopment).

This condition has functional and aesthetic implications. It also causes difficulties related to nutrition and oral hygiene. Treatment (i.e., surgical correction) should be initiated as soon as the condition is recognized. The main objective is to reestablish joint and jaw functions.[71]

During mobilization as part of the physical therapy treatment, no distraction of the condyle on the ankylosed side occurs, and radiographic restriction also is noted. Apart from treating the opposite joint symptomatically, therapy is not effective in improving movement (Figure 4-9).

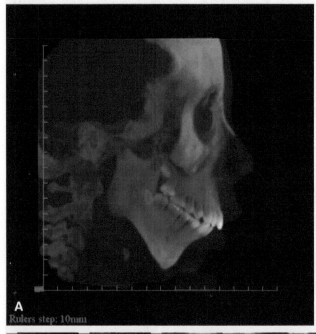

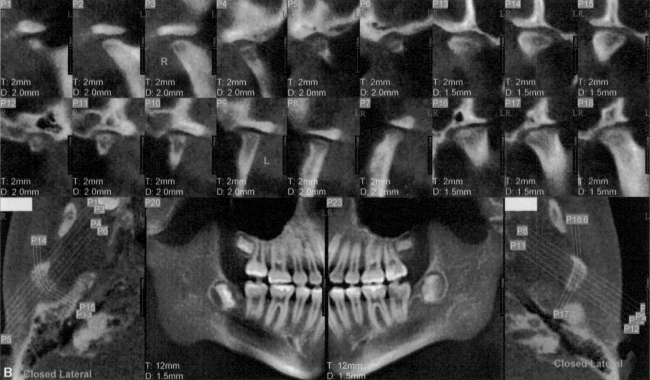

Figure 4-9 Tomogram of (**A**) ankylosis of the temporomandibular joint and (**B**) juvenile rheumatoid arthritis (right closed). (Courtesy Dr. D. Hatcher, Sacramento, California.)

TEMPOROMANDIBULAR DISORDER-RELATED FACTORS

Any discussion of TMDs must include factors and dysfunctions associated with TMDs. As mentioned previously, bruxism, forward head posture, whiplash injury, cervical spinal dysfunction, alterations in occlusion, and psychosocial stress have been hypothesized to initiate or precipitate a TMD or to increase a person's predisposition to developing a TMD. These factors will be described briefly in this chapter.

Bruxism

Parafunctional (abnormal) habits, such as bruxism, teeth clenching, jaw thrusting, gum chewing, and jaw testing (repeatedly moving the jaw to cause a click or moving the jaw into a painful position to see if the click or pain is still present), can add repetitive strain to the masticatory muscles and cause tenderness and pain.

According to Lobbezoo and Naeije,[72] the etiology of bruxism is related to morphological, pathophysiological, and psychological factors. Pathophysiological factors in the etiology of bruxism are increasingly related to sleep disturbances, chemical alterations in the brain, use of medication, and use of cigarettes and alcohol. Bruxism can cause muscle pain, TMJ noise, limited jaw movements, and headache.

One of the most common characteristics seen in patients with myogenic TMDs is the hyperactivity of the masticatory muscles that can be caused by bruxism. This hyperactivity is caused by the dynamic imbalance of the masticatory system,[74] and it can contribute to internal derangement.[68]

In 1997, Kampe et al.[74] investigated subjects between 23 and 68 years of age with more than 5 years of bruxism. The authors suggested a causal relationship between the bruxism and TMD signs and symptoms, including headache and pain in the neck and shoulder. People with TMDs commonly have parafunctional habits (e.g., bruxism, clenching the teeth, and nail biting [neuromuscular factors]). However, the relationship between bruxism, stress, and TMDs is unclear. Some studies have found that bruxism is not always present in people with a TMD; therefore a causal relationship cannot be claimed.[48]

Bruxism (clenching the teeth) often can be done unconsciously and may be the body's response to an aggravating stimulus (e.g., a high restoration on a tooth, malocclusion, stress, habit, or a combination of factors). Some authors believe that bruxing can trigger problems within the TMJ apparatus, whereas others deny such a claim.[15,75] Either way, bruxing definitely can aggravate TMDs and hinder treatment and recovery.

Because bruxism often is an unconscious habit, it can be very difficult to control. Sometimes just pointing out the habit to patients can be enough to make them aware of the problem and prompt them to take steps to control it themselves. In other cases some form of relaxation technique, biofeedback, or stress management might be necessary to help control the problem. Exercise that promotes the contraction of muscles antagonistic to the masseters and temporalis can help (e.g., a resisted mandibular opening). If the bruxing is aggravated by gum chewing or holding a toothpick between the teeth, removal of the offending object often is enough to control the symptoms.

Signs and Symptoms of a "Bruxer"

- The patient regularly and consistently clenches and relaxes the masseters
- A masseter "bump" is present. (The clinician lightly palpates the masseters as the patient opens and closes the mouth. Normally, on closing, the teeth lightly come together before resting. A "bruxer" shows a definite and obvious overcontraction as the teeth occlude)
- Hypertrophy of the masseters is obvious (this may give the patient a heavyset jaw)
- The patient regularly and consistently purses the lips or squeezes them together
- The teeth show facet wearing
- The tongue shows scalloping (this occurs as a result of the teeth constantly biting on the edges of the tongue)

Patient Management Program: Controlling Bruxism

- One of the most important steps in breaking the habit of clenching and grinding the teeth (bruxism) is to become conscious of when it occurs and then to stop doing it. Many people are unaware they have the habit until it is pointed out to them. This awareness must occur before you can control the habit. An excellent way to avoid clenching the teeth is to learn to keep your lips together and your teeth apart. This simple step makes clenching the teeth impossible; even more important, it relaxes the muscles that become tense and taut. As an extra dividend, this relaxation technique improves your facial expression and appearance. It also promotes a more normal resting position of the TMJs.
- The more conscious you become about this basic procedure of relaxing the jaw muscle, the greater control you will have in overcoming this harmful habit. First, you need to identify when you are most likely to clench or grind your teeth during waking hours, such as while driving on the freeway, during physical exertion or sports, or when you are under emotional tension or stress. At these times you should repeat to yourself, "lips together, teeth apart."
- By sealing your lips and gently blowing or puffing air, you will automatically separate your teeth and simultaneously relax your jaw and facial muscles.
- Remember, you probably have had this habit for a long time, and it will not vanish overnight. You must persevere and practice this exercise each time you find your teeth clenched.

Forward Head Posture

According to some researchers, forward head posture can cause TMDs.[76-78] Head posture and its relation to occlusion, to the development and function of the dentofacial structures, and to TMDs have been studied. Head posture alterations have been associated with changes in the stomatognathic system, influencing the biomechanical behavior of the TMJ and associated structures. Some have suggested that the position of the head affects the resting position of the mandible,[78,79] produces greater muscular activity in the temporal and masseter muscles,[76,78–85] and alters the TMJ internal relationships.[86] This can be explained by the relationship between the masticatory system and the cervical spine, as a result of neurophysiological, anatomical, and biomechanical interactions.[73]

The association between cervical and head posture in the presence of TMDs has been a matter of debate for many years. Physical therapists have commonly used cervical-head posture reeducation techniques to address postural abnormalities in patients with neck involvement.[87] Postural alterations have been associated with changes in the distribution of loads between the anterior and posterior cervical segments as well as with changes in cervical muscular length.[78]

A systematic review done in 2006 studied the association between the head and the cervical posture and TMD.[88] Of the 12 papers included in the study, nine concluded that postural alteration could be associated with TMD. However, the studies included in the review were of poor methodological quality. According to the authors, it was not clear that head and cervical posture were associated with TMD because of the level of evidence in the studies.

A study investigating head and neck posture in subjects with TMD[89] found that subjects with TMD had neither statistically nor clinically significant differences in most of the head and cervical posture variables when compared with pain-free subjects. According to the results of this study along with a systematic review,[90] there is a lack of a scientific validation of a correlation between postural alteration and TMD. The study results indicated that static posture of the craniocervical system in patients with TMD (evaluated through the tragus-C7-horizontal, pogonion-tragus-C7, eye-tragus-horizontal, and tragus-C7-shoulder angles) was not significantly altered and thus static posture evaluation of the craniocervical system was not recommended for these patients. However, it is still unknown whether dynamic posture (i.e., posture that subjects adopt when performing functional activities) is significantly different in subjects with TMD when compared with healthy subjects. Falla et al.[91] evaluated posture when subjects were performing a functional activity. They found that subtle changes in head and cervical posture over time (approximately 4°) could reflect poor muscle control of the deep cervical flexor muscles when evaluating sustained postures in patients with pain in the upper quarter. Thus, a more functional evaluation of posture between patients with TMD and healthy controls could provide a better understanding of the muscular impairments of these patients and also explain more accurately the symptomatology in these patients.

Although there is a lack of a scientific validation of an association between postural alteration and TMD, a systematic review that focused on the effectiveness of physical therapy interventions for TMD found that postural training was one of the interventions recommended to restore or optimize the alignment of the CMS and to reduce pain in patients who have TMDs with muscular involvement (i.e., myogenic TMD).[92] According to O'Leary et al.,[87] postural evaluation and treatment could be considered based on individual needs. For example, patients who reported posture as an aggravating factor and who reported an improvement of symptoms when performing postural corrections could use postural correction to improve their symptoms. Thus clinicians who work with patients with TMD having postural abnormalities as an aggravating factor could consider these recommendations for treating these subjects in clinical practice.

Occlusal Alterations

Dental occlusion is very important for masticatory function. It has been suggested that a significant relationship exists between alterations in the masticatory system and dental occlusion. Occlusion relationships should be routinely considered as part of the examination in patients with TMD.[93]

Occlusion alterations influence the TMJ and the functions of the masticatory muscles. According to Okeson,[63] occlusion alterations can be associated with parafunctional habits, such as squeezing, bruxism, and clenching the teeth, which lead to muscle spasm and hyperactivity. Celic et al.[94] investigated the prevalence of TMD and relationship between dental occlusion and parafunctional habits using clinical assessment and patient histories. They found a significant correlation between occlusion alterations, parafunctional habits, and TMD. Another study[95] found that the electromyographic (EMG) responses of the temporal and masseter muscles were modified in subjects with a class II occlusion alteration (Angle classification). Subjects with a class II occlusion showed hyperactivity of the temporal muscles, which altered the normal EMG pattern between the temporal and masseter muscles and also led to a higher occurrence of forward head posture. Conversely, many clinical studies have failed to demonstrate any significant differences between patients with TMD and controls in terms of occlusal variables.[96–98] For example, a study that evaluated 4310 subjects did not find any association between any occlusal variable and subjective TMD symptoms.[97] Neither convincing nor powerful evidence supports the theory of occlusal alterations as an important factor in TMD.[15]

Stress, Anxiety, and Depression

Psychological factors, such as stress and anxiety, can play a significant role in TMDs—they can either initiate problems or aggravate an existing dysfunction. The clinician should include an explanation of the effects of stress in the initial history and interview process because if stress appears to be a major concern, it may be necessary to involve a health professional (e.g., a clinical psychologist) who is experienced in stress management techniques, relaxation techniques, biofeedback, and counseling. The authors have found that a patient is much more willing to accept a referral to a clinical psychologist if this is brought up as a possibility before any therapy is initiated. If the whole concept of stress as a factor in the pathology and treatment of the condition is left until after therapy has been initiated, the patient is more inclined to believe that the clinician thinks the problem is all in the patient's head; patients can be very averse to referral to a clinical psychologist after therapy has been unsuccessful or only partially successful.

Discussions with clinical psychologists have revealed that people commonly are able to cope with a severe life stress at the time of the event and that symptoms become apparent approximately 6 months after the stressful period. Therefore when taking the history, the clinician should ask about previous life stressors to determine whether they are coincident with the latest exacerbation of symptoms. Clinically, some patients have been found not to be *psychologically aware;* that is, they are unable (or unwilling) to comprehend the effects of the psyche on the body and on an individual's well-being. Involvement in the psychological side of therapy might not be practical. Similarly the clinician may have encountered people who are not *body aware;* that is, they seem to have no awareness of the physical functioning of the body or its specific control. This can make treatment for certain individuals challenging.

To help a patient understand the problem and identify some of the initiating factors, the clinician may find it worthwhile to get the patient to keep a daily diary of the symptoms or pain. The myofascial pain caused by stress and fatigue can occur not only in the region of the masticatory muscles but also in the neck and shoulder region. This symptom is commonly present in patients with TMD. The sternocleidomastoid and trapezius muscles often are affected. Stress also can cause the patient to develop parafunctional habits, such as bruxism and clenching the teeth, which contribute to the hyperactivity of the masticatory muscles and consequently cause pain in this region.

A group of patients with TMD have been differentiated from a control group by levels of pain, anxiety, depression, and sleep disturbances.[99] Patients with TMD frequently have symptoms of fibromyalgia, chronic fatigue syndrome, headaches, panic disorder, irritable bowel syndrome, and posttraumatic stress disorders.[100]

In a multicenter study[101] including 1149 patients seeking for TMD treatment, a strong relationship of depression and somatization levels with pain-related disability was found ($p < 0.001$). In addition, pain lasting more than 6 months (i.e., chronic conditions) was found to be significantly correlated with high scores of pain-related disability in subjects with TMD ($p < 0.001$). In another study,[102] chronic female patients presented significantly higher depression and somatization scores in comparison with acute patients. In addition, acute patients self-perceive higher levels of anxiety in relation to the control group (healthy females). Patients reporting higher levels of depression were more inclined to somatization and had experienced a greater number of stress events in the past 6 months.

The presence of mood and panic-agoraphobic symptoms in different groups of TMD patients has been investigated.[103] Patients classified as having myofascial pain differed from those with DD, joint disorders, and no TMD in relation to some psychopathological symptoms. A higher prevalence of both mood ($p < 0.001$) and panic-agoraphobic ($p < 0.01$) symptoms was found in this group classification.

In a large prospective cohort study (Orofacial Pain: Prospective Evaluation and Risk Assessment, OPPERA) designed to discover causal determinants of TMD pain,[104] 3263 TMD-free subjects completed several psychological tests assessing general psychological adjustment and personality, affective distress, psychosocial stress, somatic symptoms, and pain coping and catastrophizing. The follow-up data (after 2.8 years) from 2737 subjects revealed that several psychological variables predicted increased risk of first-onset TMD, including reported somatic symptoms, psychosocial stress, and affective distress.

In summary, physiological factors, such as stress, depression, and anxiety, may play a predisposing role in the etiology of TMD. Therefore these factors should be taken into account in the management of these patients. Because patients with TMD present with cognitive, emotional, and behavioral responses to pain, the new DC/TMD recommended assessing the psychosocial functioning of these subjects by applying the questionnaires described in Table 4-2. These tools can be used when indicated by clinicians or researchers. These tools follow the Initiative on Methods, Measurements, and Pain Assessment in Clinical Trials (IMMPACT) recommendations. The axis II screening instruments consist of 41 questions from the Patient Health Questionnaire 4 (PHQ-4), Graded Chronic Pain Scale (GCPS), Oral Behaviors Check List (OBC), and Jaw Functional Limitation Scale (JFLS, short form), as well as pain drawing. It was strongly recommended that these instruments be used in patients with a history of pain longer than 6 months and presence of previous unsuccessful treatments.[61] The JFLS (short and long versions) is described here because this tool is generally used to determine dysfunction associated with TMDs and can be used to test effectiveness of treatments in clinical practice as well as research. The remaining tools are described in detail elsewhere.[105]

The JFLS is a valid and reliable tool comprising 8 and 20 items (short and long forms, respectively) clustered in three domains. These three constructs (mastication, vertical jaw mobility, and emotional and verbal expression) were obtained through a complete validation process

TABLE **4-2**

Diagnostic Criteria for Temporomandibular Disorders (DC/TMD) Axis II Recommended Tools to Assess the Psychosocial Functioning of Subjects with TMD

Domain	Instrument	Number of Items
Pain intensity	Graded Chronic Pain Scale (GCPS)	3
Pain locations	Pain Drawing	1
Physical function	Graded Chronic Pain Scale (GCPS)	4
Limitation	Jaw Functional Limitation Scale (JFLS)—short and long form	8 and 20 items, respectively
Distress	Patient Health Questionnaire 4 (PHQ-4)	4
Depression	Patient Health Questionnaire 9 (PHQ-9)	9
Anxiety	General Anxiety Disorder-7 (GAD-7)	7
Physical symptoms	Patient Health Questionnaire-15 (PHQ-15)	15
Parafunction	Oral behaviors Checklist (OBC)	21

Modified from Schiffman E, Ohrbach R, Truelove E et al: Diagnostic criteria for temporomandibular disorders (DC/TMD) for clinical and research applications: Recommendations of the International RDC/TMD Consortium Network and Orofacial Pain Special Interest Group, *J Oral Facial Pain Headache* 28(1):6-27, 2014.

using expert consensus as well as psychometric testing by a Rash analysis. A global functional limitation score is obtained from both versions (short and long). In addition, both scales can be administered independently, which allows the clinician or researcher to tailor the administration of this scale. The tool has exhibited excellent psychometric properties with respect to modeled variance, item fit, reliability, and internal consistency.[106] The items for short and long versions can be found in Table 4-3.

Whiplash Injury

Whiplash injury may cause symptoms associated with TMDs in addition to other symptoms, such as neck pain,

TABLE **4-3**

Jaw Functional Limitation Scale (JFLS)

Items 1 to 6 represent mastication, items 7 to 10 represent mobility, and items 11 to 20 represent verbal and emotional communication. Items with an asterisk (*) are those used for the JFLS-8 (short form). Responses used a 0 to 10 NRS, with 0 anchored as "no limitation" and 10 anchored as "severe limitation."

For each of the items below, indicate the level of limitation during the past month. If the activity was completely avoided because it is too difficult, indicate "10." If you avoid an activity for reasons other than pain or difficulty, then leave the item blank.

1* Chew tough food
2　Chew hard bread
3* Chew chicken (e.g., prepared in oven)
4　Chew crackers
5　Chew soft food (e.g., macaroni, canned or soft fruits, cooked vegetables, fish)
6* Eat soft food requiring no chewing (e.g., mashed potatoes, apple sauce, pudding, pureed food)
7　Open wide enough to bite from a whole apple
8　Open wide enough to bite into a sandwich
9　Open wide enough to talk
10* Open wide enough to drink from a cup
11* Swallow
12* Yawn
13* Talk
14　Sing
15　Putting on a happy face
16　Putting on an angry face
17　Frown
18　Kiss
19* Smile
20　Laugh

From Ohrbach R, Larsson P, List T: The jaw functional limitation scale: Development, reliability, and validity of 8-item and 20-item versions, *J Orofacial Pain* 22(3):219-230, 2008.

headache, and cognitive disturbances. TMDs following a motor vehicle accident (MVA)-related whiplash may result from direct trauma to the orofacial region, or symptoms could also occur later following the accident.[107]

Salé and Isberg[108] found the incidence of new symptoms of TMD among patients who suffered whiplash due to MVA was 5 times that found in a control group. TMD was reported as the primary complaint by 5% of the patients at the first visit and by 19% at 1-year follow-up. Delayed onset of new symptoms of TMDs was seen in a third of patients with whiplash-associated disorder (WAD) versus 7% of the control group.[108] Therefore approximately 33% of people with whiplash history are at risk of developing TMD.[107]

According to a systematic review, the prevalence of whiplash trauma is higher in patients with TMD compared with non-TMD controls.[109,110] TMD patients with history of whiplash present with more jaw pain and more severe jaw dysfunction compared with TMD patients without a history of head-neck trauma. Symptoms such as limited jaw opening, TMD pain, headaches, and stress were reported more by TMD patients with history of whiplash. According to the authors of the papers, whiplash trauma may be an initiating and/or aggravating factor as well as a co-morbid condition for TMD.

According to Epstein et al.,[107] TMDs may represent a component of the whiplash symptom cluster, and therefore the masticatory region should be evaluated not only at the beginning but also later during the treatment for neck pain due to whiplash injury.

Cervical Spine Dysfunction

Some clinical evidence of the interconnection between the cervical spine and TMDs has been demonstrated, and thus cervical spine dysfunction (CSD) has been associated with TMD.[18,20,111,112] De Wijer et al.[18-20,113] concluded that symptoms of the stomatognathic system overlap in patients with TMD and CSD, and symptoms from the cervical spine overlap in the same group of patients (TMD and CSD). It has also been found that patients with chronic TMD more often suffered from cervical spine pain than those without this disorder[111] and asymptomatical functional disorders of the cervical spine occurred more frequently in patients with internal derangement of the TMJ than in a control group.[114] Sipila et al.[115] found that facial pain was associated with reported neck pain and clinical pain resulting from palpation in the muscles of the neck-occiput area. Ciancaglini et al.[116] demonstrated that patients suffering from TMD had more than double the risk (odds ratio [OR]=2.33) of suffering neck pain than patients without TMD (OR=1). Plesh et al.[117] in a population study from the United States found that TMD-type pain was most often associated with other common pains and seldom existed alone (only 0.77% overall reported TMJ and muscle disorders [TMJ/MDs] without co-morbid headache and migraine, neck, or low back pain). In addition, almost 55% of those who reported TMJ/MD-type pain also reported neck pain versus 13% of those who did not report TMJ/MD-type pain (OR=7.9, $p<0.001$). Thus neck pain was most strongly associated with TMJ/MD-type pain, followed by headache and migraine pain, low back pain, and then joint pain. Armijo-Olivo and coworkers investigated the relationship between cervical impairments and TMD.[3,4,118] They found a strong relationship between neck disability and jaw disability ($r=0.82$). No statistically significant differences were found in EMG activity of the sternocleidomastoid or the anterior scalene muscles in patients with TMDs when compared with healthy subjects while executing the craniocervical flexion test ($p=0.07$). However, clinically important effect sizes (0.42 to 0.82) were found.[3] Subjects with TMDs presented with reduced cervical flexor as well as extensor muscle endurance while performing the flexor and extensor muscle endurance tests when compared with healthy individuals.[3] Therefore subjects with TMD presented with impairments of the cervical flexors and extensors muscles. Based on these results, they suggested that an association between neck pain and TMD may be possible and a systematic clinical examination of cervical spine areas could be important in identifying possible causes of craniofacial pain and guide possible treatments. These results could help guide clinicians in the assessment and prescription of more effective interventions for individuals with TMD.

PHYSICAL THERAPY TREATMENT

The American Academy of Craniomandibular Disorders (AACD) and the Minnesota Dental Association (MDA) have cited physical therapy as an important treatment for TMD.[119] The role of physical therapy has been shown to be one of the most effective conservative treatments for TMDs.[120] The most important contribution by physical therapists is the identification of the musculoskeletal components that contribute to the symptoms of the patient.[9] Because the TMJs are synovial joints, physical therapists can treat the joints with similar interventions as they would most other joints in the body. Physical therapy includes a large number of modalities to treat TMDs secondary to inflammation, hypermobility, DD, masticatory muscle pain, bruxism, and fibrous adhesion, among other conditions.[9] Physical therapy is prescribed with the intent to relieve musculoskeletal pain, reduce inflammation, and restore oral and neck motor function.

Numerous therapeutic interventions may prove effective in the treatment of TMDs, including electrophysical modalities, acupuncture, exercises, and manual therapy techniques. Electrophysical modalities include ultrasound (US), microwave, laser, and electroanalgesic techniques (e.g., transcutaneous electrical nerve stimulation [TENS]), interferential current, and biofeedback. Interventions often include therapeutic exercises for the masticatory and/or cervical spine muscles to improve strength, coordination, resistance, and mobility in the region.[121] Manual therapy techniques are commonly used to reduce pain, restore mobility, or both. Interventions may also include or focus on associated impairments of the craniocervical system, such as poor posture, cervical muscle spasm, cervical pain, and referred pain from the cervical spine,[121] because a connection between cervical spine dysfunction and TMDs has been seen clinically.[2,3,5,7,122]

Several systematic reviews have been conducted regarding the effectiveness of physical therapy interventions in subjects with TMDs.[92,123-125] The information has expanded in the past 10 years, and new randomized clinical trials have been performed. However, the quality of the current evidence supporting the effectiveness of physical therapy in TMDs is still limited.[126] Because of the lack of published research on the efficacy of physical therapy in the treatment of TMDs, only limited evidence is available upon which to base practice guidelines. Consequently, clinical decision making must still be based on empirical evidence. For this reason the information about treatment interventions that follows is based on evidence and on the authors' clinical experience. For practical reasons, the information is divided into three general categories:

1. *Exercise,* including isotonic and isometric exercises to reestablish the correct working postures of the masticatory, cranial, and cervical systems, along with exercises to improve strength, resistance, and motor control of the masticatory and cervical muscles
2. *Manual therapy,* including various mobilization techniques to improve ROM, reduce muscle spasm, and diminish pain
3. *Electrophysical modalities,* including heat sources (e.g., hot packs), US, TENS, and acupuncture

Clinicians practicing in this area can use any combination of these treatments that they feel suits their needs. However, after a stringent search of the literature, the authors must emphasize that the methods and combinations chosen are purely a matter of preference; there is no "gold standard" physical therapy treatment for any particular TMJ condition.

Exercise

Therapeutic exercises are prescribed to address specific TMJ impairments and to improve the function of the TMJ.[127] The most useful techniques for reeducation and rehabilitation of the masticatory muscles have been reported to be muscle stretching and strengthening exercises.[128] Passive and active stretching of muscles and/or ROM are performed to increase oral opening and reduce pain.[128] Postural exercises also are recommended to restore or optimize the alignment of the CMS.[121]

All of the systematic reviews published[92,123,125] provided evidence in support of postural exercises and active and passive oral exercises to reduce pain and improve mouth opening in people with TMD due to DD, acute arthritis, and chronic myofascial pain. Effectiveness of different types of exercise therapy by specific TMD conditions bringing together the results of these systematic reviews plus up-to-date information of physical therapy interventions used to manage TMDs will be discussed later. A summary of the results found in the latest systematic reviews are described in the following section.[125]

Posture Correction Exercises in Myogenous Temporomandibular Disorders

Two studies[129,130] evaluated the effectiveness of posture correction exercises for patients with myofascial pain. One of them[130] compared posture correction exercises with self-management instructions, and the other[129] assessed the postural exercises plus behavioral therapy versus behavioral therapy alone and versus a control group. Both studies found positive results of postural exercises for improving symptoms of muscular TMDs. Based on the results of Armijo-Olivo et al.[125] when pooling the data from both studies, it was found that maximum pain-free opening significantly increased in patients receiving postural training when compared with a control group. The mean difference in maximum pain-free opening was 5.54 mm (95% confidence interval [CI] = 2.93, 8.15) (Table 4-4). This difference has been found to be clinically significant.[131] Furthermore, patients treated with postural training had significantly fewer symptoms and disturbance with daily living when compared with a control group. The standardized mean difference (SMD) in symptoms and disturbance of symptoms with daily life was 1.13 (95% CI = 0.48, 1.78) which indicated a big effect size for this pooled outcome.

These results are encouraging and support the use of physical therapy interventions including exercises to correct head and neck posture to relieve musculoskeletal pain and to improve oral motor function[129,130] in subjects with myogenous TMDs. More information is required, however, on the optimal exercise prescription. In particular, details on frequency, intensity, time, and type of the specific exercise used in treatment protocols are essential to allow for replication in the clinical setting.

General Exercise Program in Myogenous Temporomandibular Disorders

Seven studies[132-138] looked at the effect of exercises alone or combined with other therapies for myogenous TMDs. When pooling the data from all of these studies, there was a trend to favor exercise therapy for pain-free maximum opening and pain intensity when compared with a control group. The mean difference for pain-free maximum opening was 5.94 mm (95% CI = -1.0, 12.87), which is clinically significant (Table 4-5).[131] The SMD for pain

TABLE 4-4

Maximum Pain-Free Opening: Postural Training versus Control Group in Myogenous TMD Patients

	POSTURAL CORRECTION			CONTROL				
STUDY OF SUBGROUP	Mean	SD	Total	Mean	SD	Total	WEIGHT	MEAN DIFFERENCE IV, RANDOM, 95% CL
Komiyama et al.[129]	16.35	5.06	20	9.58	6	20	53.8%	6.77 [3.33, 10.21]
Wright et al., 2000 [130]	5.3	8.8	30	1.2	5.6	30	46.2%	4.10 [0.37, 7.83]
Total (95% Cl)			**50**			**50**	**100.0%**	**5.54 [2.93, 8.15]**

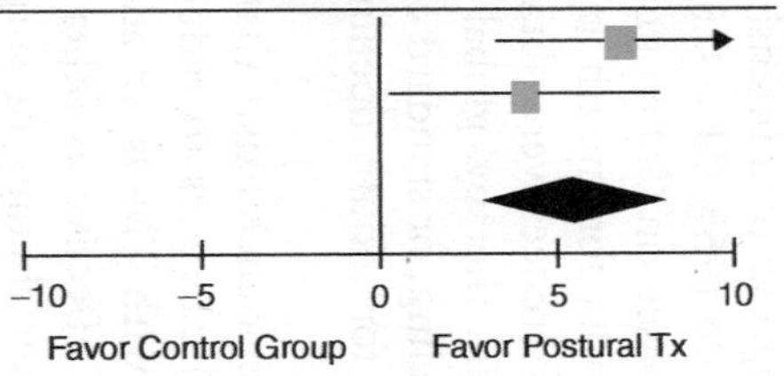

MEAN DIFFERENCE IV, RANDOM, 95% CL

Heterogeneity: $\tau^2 = 0.21$; $X^2 = 1.06$, $df = 1$ ($p = 0.30$); $I^2 = 6\%$
Test for overall effect: $Z = 4.16$ ($p < 0.0001$)

TABLE 4-5

Mean Difference (MD) for Pain Free Maximum Opening: General Exercise Physical Therapy Program versus Control Group in Myogenous TMD Patients

	GENERAL EXERCISES			CONTROL				
STUDY OF SUBGROUP	Mean	SD	Total	Mean	SD	Total	WEIGHT	MEAN DIFFERENCE IV, RANDOM, 95% CL
Craane et al., 2012 [132]	-0.4	6.54	22	0.9	5.59	25	27.3%	-1.30 [-4.80, 2.20]
Magnusson et al., 1999 [134]	7	10.37	9	2	7.4	9	20.6%	5.00 [-3.32, 13.32]
Maloney et al., 2002 [135]	16.29	5.93	7	0.8	5.31	10	24.8%	15.49 [10.00, 20.98]
Michelotti et al., 2004 [136]	9.4	6.3	26	4.2	6.3	23	27.3%	5.20 [1.67, 8.73]
Total (95% Cl)			**64**			**67**	**100.0%**	**5.94 [-1.00, 12.87]**

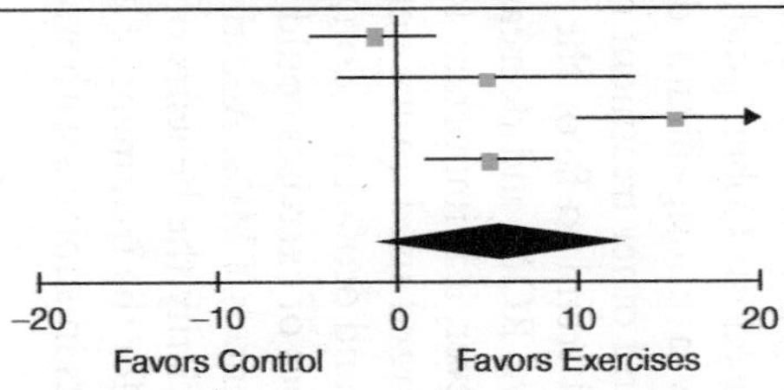

MEAN DIFFERENCE IV, RANDOM, 95% CL

Heterogeneity: $\tau^2 = 42.72$; $X^2 = 26.06$, $df = 3$ ($p < 0.00001$); $I^2 = 88\%$
Test for overall effect: $Z = 1.68$ ($p = 0.09$)

intensity was 0.43 (95% CI = −0.02, 0.87) with a moderate effect size based on Cohen guidelines.[139] Although these results show a nonsignificant difference between general exercises and other treatment modalities, they do highlight a clinical trend to favor the use of therapeutic exercise to improve ROM and decrease pain in this patient group. However, it is important to highlight that all of the studies analyzed used a very general exercise program for the TMJ and orofacial region, and it is uncertain if more specific types of exercises could be more beneficial for treating myogenous TMDs. Additional research studies are needed to clarify the benefits of a specific physical therapy treatment for the treatment of jaw pain over other forms of treatments in subjects with myogenous TMDs.

Exercises Alone or as Part of a Conservative Regime in Arthrogenous Temporomandibular Disorders

Nine studies[135,140-147] looking at subjects with arthrogenous TMDs focused on exercises alone or combined with other therapies, such as medications, surgery, or self-care recommendations. Most of the studies tended to favor exercises to improve ROM and decrease pain intensity in patients with arthrogenous TMDs. When the results of the studies investigating the effectiveness of exercise alone or in combination with other conservative therapies on pain intensity at 4 to 6 weeks of treatment were pooled, it was found that there was no statistically significant difference in pain between the exercise and control groups. Nevertheless, there was a trend to favor the exercise group when compared with the control group. The SMD for pain intensity was 0.68 (95% CI = −0.04, 1.40) with a moderate effect size favoring exercise therapy based on Cohen guidelines.[139] Regarding active mouth opening, a nonsignificant effect was found between general exercise and the control group. The mean difference for active mouth opening was 3.13 mm (95% CI = −1.96, 8.23), although a trend to favor exercises was observed.

When pooling the studies that looked at exercises plus arthrocentesis or arthroscopy versus conservative therapy including exercises alone on active mouth opening at 6 months, it was found that no differences between these approaches existed. The mean difference was −1.01 mm (95% CI = −5.43, 3.42), implying that conservative treatment plus exercises is appropriate to treat DDwithoutR or restricted mandibular movement. In addition, these results highlight that arthrocentesis or arthroscopy, procedures that are more invasive than conservative treatment, should not be conducted as a routine treatment for these patients.

Exercise in Mixed Temporomandibular Disorders

Several studies[148-160] looked at exercises alone or as part of a general conservative therapeutic regime to treat subjects with mixed TMDs. When the results of studies with available data were pooled, it was found that exercises in the form of general jaw exercises plus conventional treatment or with the addition of an oral device[156] were equally

effective when compared with other treatment modalities, such as splint therapy, global reeducation posture, splint plus counseling, acupuncture, or standard conservative care, to improve pain intensity. The SMD for pain intensity was −0.06 (95% CI = −0.50, 0.38) with a very small effect size based on Cohen guidelines.[139]

When the results for mouth opening were pooled, nonsignificant differences were obtained between general exercises and splint therapy, global reeducation posture, splint plus counseling, or standard conservative care. The mean difference for mouth opening was 0.4 mm (95% CI = 1.64, 2.51).

In summary, evidence exists that supports the use of oral and postural exercises to reduce pain and improve ROM in people with TMDs. In addition, exercise therapy is equally as effective as other more costly modalities, such as splint therapy or surgery. This can guide clinicians in making the best choice for treating TMD patients. Exercises can help reduce muscle spasm, restore muscle function, improve muscle strength and resistance, diminish pain, and aid muscle motor control. Different types of exercises can be performed to the jaw and cervical region. (Information on cervical spine exercises can be found in Chapter 3.) Evidence supports the use of cervical and postural exercises to improve TMD symptoms. The following exercises focus on the TMJ and masticatory muscles.

Isotonic, isometric, and resistive exercises can be used, depending on the patient's condition. For example, the patient can actively perform exercises to improve ROM by moving the jaw in all directions (open-close and lateral movements) to the end of ROM. These types of exercises stimulate lubrication of the TMJ, improve the proprioceptive information to the joint receptors, and help control pain.[161-163] In addition, these active exercises can be assisted by the clinician or self-assisted by the patient at the end of opening ROM. Mandibular opening can be achieved by placing the thumbs and forefingers between the teeth and causing a passive stretch against the mandible and maxilla (Figure 4-10). The stretch should be held for at least 30 seconds to cause changes in the soft tissues.[164]

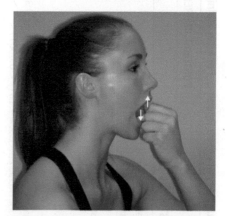

Figure 4-10 Passive stretch of the mouth opening.

Active exercises also have been used to improve coordination and retraining of the jaw muscles. As mentioned previously, patients with TMD usually present with impaired masticatory muscle contraction patterns. These impaired patterns can cause abnormal distribution of loads to the TMJ and reinforce abnormal equilibrium between muscular groups. The objective of active coordination exercises is to train the patient to open and close the mouth and to perform lateral movements smoothly, trying to avoid abnormal patterns of contraction. This often can best be done if the patient works in front of a mirror. The patient opens and closes the mouth and performs lateral movements using the visual feedback on the position of the jaw (Figure 4-11).

A mastication device can be used to improve coordination of jaw movements and muscle strength during the movements. The hyperboloid is a mastication device invented by a Brazilian dentist (patent no. 8901216-0) that has a hyperbolic shape and is made of soft, nontoxic, odorless, tasteless silicone (Figure 4-12).[165] Its hardness and texture are compatible with the ideal force applied during mastication.[166] This device is used to assist with the treatment of patients with TMD.[167] The proprioceptive mechanism of excitation is the explanation for the ef-

fectiveness of the hyperboloid device.[165,167] This device has also been used to treat abnormal orodental development, abnormal occlusion, and bruxism.[165]

Few studies have investigated the effect of the hyperboloid. Its effect on EMG activity in the jaw-closing muscles and on the reduction of sleep bruxism in a child with cerebral palsy was investigated by Giannasi et al.[166] They found that 9 months of treatment using specific exercises with the hyperboloid (6 times a day for 5 minutes) resulted in an improvement of EMG activity of the jaw-closing muscles and a reduction of sleep bruxism. The authors concluded that the mastication device positively affected the processes of chewing and swallowing, improving oral function associated with improvement of muscle tone. The hyperboloid was also included in a physical therapy program of a patient with TMD.[168] Treatment also included exercises, manual therapy, massotherapy, laser, and US. Results indicated a reduction of pain in the masticatory muscles and cervical region, parafunctional habits (i.e., habitual use of the mouth, tongue, or jaw for activities unrelated to eating, drinking, or speaking—e.g., bruxism [tooth clenching or grinding], tongue thrusting, fingernail biting, pencil or pen chewing, mouth breathing), improvement of posture, and better coordination of jaw movements. The effectiveness of physical therapy, including the use of the hyperboloid, was also evaluated in 11 patients suffering from oral cancer and TMDs.[169] Exercises for proprioception using the hyperboloid are performed at the end of treatment after a series of treatment techniques, including muscle relaxation, cervical spine, and TMJ mobilization. The results showed an increase of mouth opening and relief of symptoms, such as pain and difficulty to chew and talk. Figures 4-13 and 4-14 show some exercises of coordination and proprioception with the hyperboloid. The patient is asked to place the device between central incisors and perform deviation of the mandible to the side (see Figure 4-13, *A*). The same can be done by asking the patient to perform

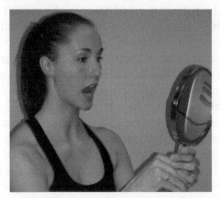

Figure 4-11 Visual feedback on jaw movement using a mirror.

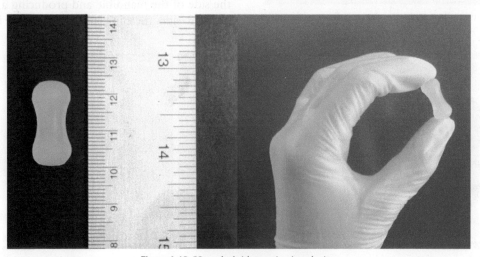

Figure 4-12 Hyperboloid: mastication device.

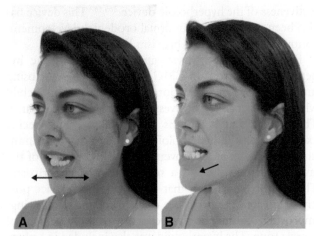

Figure 4-13 Exercises using the mastication device. **A,** With mandible side movement. **B,** With mandible protrusion.

protrusion (see Figure 4-13, *B*). The exercises can be performed with the patient positioned in front of a mirror for visual feedback (see Figure 4-14).

The other exercise used for coordination of jaw movements is to ask the patient to open and close the mouth in front of a mirror using a paper covering half of the patient's face (Figure 4-15). The edge of the paper will guide the jaw to a more straight down movement during

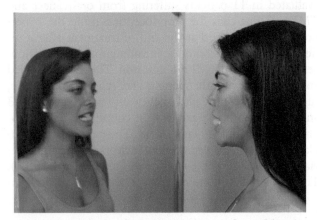

Figure 4-14 Exercise using the mastication device in front of the mirror for visual feedback.

opening.[63] The tongue positioned on the palate during this exercise can also be added to help the jaw to achieve a straight movement and to limit excessive opening in patients with TMJ hypermobility.

As mentioned earlier, in patients with hypermobility, the active exercises can be controlled with the tongue positioned in the roof of the palate (Figure 4-16). If strengthening is the aim, gentle resistance can be provided in all directions (Figures 4-17 and 4-18). Sensory input can be achieved by the clinician placing the fingers lightly beneath or on the side of the mandible and having the patient push into the slight resistance to get the muscles to contract and achieve the required movement. As an alternative, the clinician can have the patient use his or her own fingers to supply the necessary light resistance. Jaw strengthening is performed with low loads (i.e., low resistance). The clinician must always keep in mind the patient's symptoms. If the patient is in an acute phase or if pain is intense, strengthening exercises should be delayed and treatment should begin with only gentle active or passive exercises.

Proprioceptive neuromuscular facilitation (PNF) techniques are another type of active-assisted exercises that physical therapists commonly use to reduce muscular activity in the jaw (e.g., the masseter and pterygoid muscles).[170] The patient is asked to open the mouth within a comfortable range; this takes pressure off the inflamed or painful posterior structures and prevents condylar loading when resistance is applied. The clinician then places the hands under the mandible and, using light, gradually increasing pressure, attempts to close the mandible while the patient resists the closure (Figure 4-19). This causes contraction of the hyoid muscles and produces a reciprocal inhibition of the masseter, temporalis, and pterygoid muscles. Resistance is applied for a number of seconds and then slowly withdrawn, and the sequence is repeated a number of times, as required. Pain and fatigue are limiting factors and should guide the clinician in the number of repetitions to be performed. By placing one hand on the side of the mandible and producing a pressure to the opposite side, the clinician can encourage lateral glide and

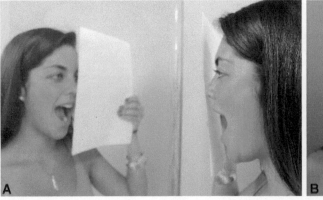
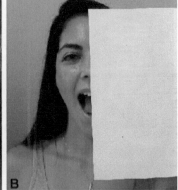

Figure 4-15 Using a piece of paper as a guide to opening and closing jaw in a straight line. **A,** Oblique view showing mirror. **B,** Front view.

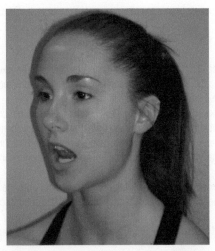

Figure 4-16 Tongue positioned in the roof of the palate.

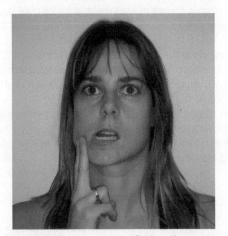

Figure 4-17 Resistive exercise for lateral excursion.

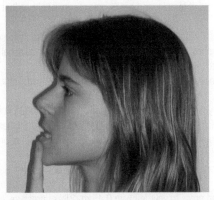

Figure 4-18 Resistive exercise for protrusion.

exercise of the muscles. Again using the PNF technique of reciprocal inhibition, the muscles on the side of the resistance contract and the muscles on the opposite side relax. Even though these exercises are effective at improving ROM of the jaw and probably improve the flexibility of the relaxed muscles, the mechanisms of that improvement are still under study.[170,171]

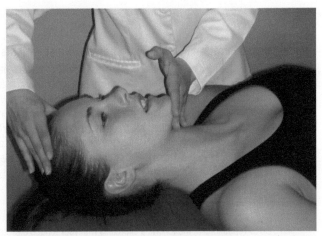

Figure 4-19 PNF technique for inhibition of closing of the masticatory muscles.

Clinicians must keep in mind that exercise and/or mobilization can easily be overdone in the treatment of the temporomandibular region. This is a sensitive area, which is made more sensitive by any dysfunction within it. Instead of exercising once or twice a day for 5 minutes at a time, a far more effective approach is to exercise a little bit and often. Some clinicians, such as Rocabado,[172] have instituted a 6×6×6 exercise routine: six exercises performed six times a day, with six repetitions of each exercise. This is easy for the patient to remember and to follow. Other clinicians prefer to have the patient perform one or two exercises each hour, using a few repetitions of each exercise. Either way, the patient must be continually reminded to perform the exercises, not only to maintain any restored function but also as a reminder to avoid performing any movements or habituations that might aggravate the condition. A home exercise program is described in Box 4-1.

Manual Therapy

Kalamir et al.[173] stated that, "the biopsychosocial health paradigm emphasizes a reversible and conservative approach to chronic pain management. Manual therapy for TMD claims to fulfill these criteria." Mobilization of the mandible aims to restore the normal ROM, reduce local ischemia, stimulate proprioception, break fibrous adhesions, stimulate synovial fluid production, and reduce pain.[173] Manual therapy has been used for many years as an adjunct treatment, along with exercises, physical modalities, and splint therapy. Evidence suggests that manual therapy is a legitimate treatment for TMDs, superior to splint therapy and even more effective when combined with exercises.[174]

Before the TMJ can be mobilized (Figure 4-20), any inflammation and local muscle spasm in the area must be reduced because both of these conditions can be aggravated by attempts to stretch the affected joint. Unless the dysfunction is fairly recent (fewer than 6 weeks), the

BOX 4-1

Home Exercise Program for the Temporomandibular Patients

Do all of the exercises (or those assigned) hourly or as instructed, with a repetition of 5 times each. The five repetitions of each exercise should take 1 minute or less. Doing these exercises throughout the day will take only a few minutes of your time. Do the exercises for 1 month or longer if so instructed. Do them at home, at work, in the car, and so on. However, if any exercise causes you pain, discontinue it immediately and consult your therapist.

Exercise 1: Place the top of your tongue against the roof of your mouth, and make a clucklike sound. Your lower jaw will drop downward to a comfortable position, and your upper and lower teeth will be apart. Return the top of your tongue to the position it was in immediately before you made the sound, exerting slight upward pressure with the tongue; your teeth are still apart. Place the palm of your left hand just below your navel, and breathe in and out through your nose 5 times using only your stomach muscles to breathe. Feel your stomach rise and fall the 5 times. Do not use the muscles of your chest or shoulders to breathe.

Exercise 2: Return the top of your tongue to the position against the roof of your mouth as in exercise 1, exerting slight upward pressure. Continue to breathe through your nose using your stomach muscles. Now, open and close your mouth farther 5 times without moving your tongue. At the end of the second week, chew all your food this way.

NOTE: Do all repetitions of the following exercises with your tongue elevated against the roof of your mouth; breathe through your nose using your stomach muscles.

Exercise 3: Grasp the back of your neck with both hands with your elbows pointing forward. Holding your neck rigid, nod your head, trying to touch your chin to your Adam's apple. If you do this correctly, your head will be able to move only about 2.5 to 3.8 cm (1 to 1.5 inches). Do not flex your neck forward. Your head should just rotate forward at the very top of your neck. Hold this position for a few seconds. Feel the muscles stretch at the top of the back of your neck, just beneath your skull. Repeat 5 times. Continue breathing through your nose using your stomach muscles and with your tongue against the roof of your mouth.

Exercise 4: Move your face straight backward keeping your chin down and your face perpendicular to the floor (i.e., as if you were bracing at attention). Do not raise your head while doing this exercise. Continue to breathe through your nose. Pause for a few seconds when your head is in the backward position, as far back as you can get it, and then relax. To help maintain the head in the correct position, you can focus your eyes on a point directly in front of you while performing the exercise. Repeat 5 times. Continue correct breathing.

Exercise 5: Repeat the position in exercise 4. With your head braced back, rotate your head forward, and try to touch your chin to your Adam's apple. You do not need to immobilize your neck with your hands, but do not bend your neck forward. Hold for a few seconds. Repeat 5 times.

Exercise 6: Grasp your hands behind your waist. Roll your shoulders backward as far as they will go. Mentally picture your left and right shoulder blades touching each other. Hold for a few seconds and then relax. Repeat 5 times. Continue correct breathing.

Exercise 7: Simultaneously elevate your left and right shoulders upward, attempting to touch your ears. Hold for a few seconds and then relax. Repeat 5 times.

Exercise 8: Without elevating your left shoulder, bend your head to the left and attempt to touch your left ear to your left shoulder. Hold for a few seconds and then relax. Repeat 5 times.

Exercise 9: Without elevating your right shoulder, bend your head to the right, and attempt to touch your right ear to your right shoulder. Hold for a few seconds, and then relax. Repeat 5 times.

Exercise 10: With your head in a neutral position, place the heel of your right hand against your right temple, and gently press to your left so that your head bends an additional 1.3 cm (0.5 inch) toward your shoulder. Repeat 5 times.

Exercise 11: With your head in a neutral position, place the heel of your left hand against your left temple, and gently press to your right so that your head bends an additional 1.3 cm (0.5 inch) toward your shoulder. Repeat 5 times.

Exercise 12: With your head braced back and your chin rotated toward your Adam's apple, intertwine the fingers of your hands, and place them so that they cup the back of your head. Gently press forward to rotate your chin an additional 1.3 cm (0.5 inches) toward your Adam's apple. Feel this additional stretching pressure at the top of your neck just beneath your skull. Hold for a few seconds, and then relax. Repeat 5 times.

Exercise 13: This is an *isometric* exercise; that is, the muscles contract, but you will not see or feel any appreciable movement of the head. Throughout this exercise, *do not* let the position of your head change.
  a. With your head bent forward 30°, place the heel of either your left or right hand against your forehead and press upward with 0.45 kg (2 lb) of pressure. Resist this upward pressure with your neck muscles so that your head does not move. Hold for a few seconds, and then relax. Repeat 5 times.
  b. With your head upright, place the palm of your left or right hand against the back of your head, and press forward with 0.45 kg (2 lb) of pressure. Resist this pressure for a few seconds, and then relax. Repeat 5 times.
  c. With your head upright, place the heel of your left hand against your left temple, and press to your right with 0.45 kg (2 lb) of pressure. Resist this pressure for a few seconds, and then relax. Repeat 5 times.
  d. With your head upright, place the heel of your right hand against your right temple, and press to your left with 0.45 kg (2 lb) of pressure. Resist this pressure for a few seconds, and then relax. Repeat 5 times.

Exercise 14: Place the top of your tongue in the same position against the roof of your mouth as in exercise 1, exerting slight upward pressure. Continue to breathe through your nose using your stomach muscles. The upper and lower teeth are still apart. Throughout this exercise, *do not* let the position of your jaw move.
  a. This is an isometric exercise. Place your thumbs beneath your chin and push upward with 170 g (6 oz) of pressure to close your mouth. Resist this closing force with an equal opening force so that your jaw does not move from its original position. Hold for a few seconds. Repeat 5 times.
  b. Resume the tongue and jaw positions described in exercise 1. Place the ends of the index and middle fingers of your right hand against the right side of your lower jaw and push to your left with 170 g (6 oz) of pressure. Resist this by holding your jaw steady with an equal force so that your jaw does not move. Hold for a few seconds. Repeat 5 times.
  c. Repeat exercise 14b using the index and middle fingers of the *left* hand against the *left* side of your lower jaw and pushing to the *right* with 170 g (6 oz) of pressure. Do not let your jaw move. Hold for a few seconds. Repeat 5 times.

Box 4-1—Cont'd

Exercise 15: Throughout this exercise, *do not* let the position of your tongue change.
   a. Place the index finger of your right or left hand on top of your tongue with your finger pointing toward your throat. Press downward with approximately 170 g (6 oz) of pressure and simultaneously lift your tongue with an equal force so that the index finger does not press the tongue down. Hold for a few seconds, and then relax. Repeat 5 times.
   b. Place your index finger under your tongue with your fingernail upward. Press upward against the undersurface of your tongue with 170 g (6 oz) of pressure and simultaneously press down with your tongue with an equal force so that the index finger does not push the tongue up. Hold for a few seconds, and then relax. Repeat 5 times.
   c. Place your left index finger against the left side of your tongue. Press to your right with 170 g (6 oz) of pressure and simultaneously resist this pressure with an equal force so that your tongue does not move. Hold for a few seconds, and then relax. Repeat 5 times.
   d. Place your right index finger against the right side of your tongue. Press to your left with 170 g (6 oz) of pressure and simultaneously resist this pressure with an equal force so that your tongue does not move. Hold for a few seconds, and then relax. Repeat 5 times.

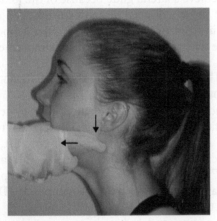

Figure 4-20 Mobilization to reduce acute disc displacement without reduction.

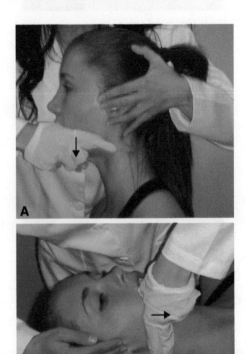

Figure 4-21 A, Axial intraoral mobilization in the sitting position. **B,** Axial intraoral mobilization in the supine position.

clinician should not look to mobilization to restore the disc-condyle relationship to normal. Rather, mobilization should be used to achieve what the body would do on its own over an extended period; that is, stretch out the tight structures to restore a more functional movement. The clinician must be sure to explain this so that the patient does not get the idea that mobilization will cure the clicking or tight joint by "getting everything back to normal." In addition to restoring function, mobilization attempts to prevent the development of adaptive problems elsewhere. For example, stiffness in the affected joint causes torsion of the unaffected joint on the opposite side, which eventually could cause hypermobility of that joint.

To mobilize the joint, the clinician asks the patient to open the mouth and then places the thumb along the superior surface of the lower teeth on the side of the joint to be mobilized (Figure 4-21). The index finger is curled under the angle of the mandible so that the bone is cupped by the finger. The index finger of the opposite hand can be used to palpate the joint. Mobilization is brought about by exerting pressure on the teeth with the thumb; this causes a distraction of the head of the condyle meeting the head of the mandibular joint. If some condylar translation is lost, this can be restored by performing an anterior glide of the condyle after some distraction of the joint.

Jaw mobilization can also be performed in the lateral and medial directions to provide joint stretching in all structures. For lateral mobilization the clinician positions the thumb in the lateral aspect of the last molar and pushes the condyle in a lateral direction. For medial mobilization (i.e., internal mobilization of the condyle), the clinician positions the second and third fingers outside the mouth and pushes the condyle in a medial direction. Sometimes the clinician can guide the lateral or medial movements using intraoral mobilization (Figure 4-22).

Patients can be taught to perform self-mobilization of the joint according to the techniques just described (Figure 4-23). It is important to teach the patient to perform these mobilizations appropriately and to hold the

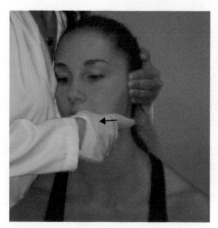

Figure 4-22 Guided jaw mobilization.

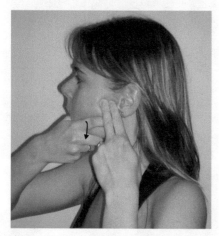

Figure 4-23 Patient self-mobilization of the TMJ.

positions for the amount of time required to achieve a positive effect on the TMJ.

Patients with a hypomobile joint on one side and a symptomatic hypermobile joint on the other side frequently complain that mobilization on the hypomobile side causes pain on the hypermobile side because of stretching of symptomatic tissue. This is a problem that requires graduated mobilization to lessen the effects of any torsion of the opposite mandible. In these cases Maitland-type graduated mobilization can be used. The regimen starts with mobilization grade 1 techniques and progresses through grades 2 and 3 to a strong grade 4 (4+). Oscillation at the end of the available range can be added to reduce spasm and to add more proprioceptive input, thereby reducing pain.[175] Although mobilization is used primarily to restore movement, the clinician should keep in mind that the lighter grades (1,2) can be used on a hypermobile joint to reduce muscle spasm and for proprioceptive effect. The stronger grades of mobilization should not be used on a hypermobile joint because they would stretch tissue that already is in a lax state.

Once a joint has been mobilized, the patient should be instructed to perform some regular exercises to maintain the regained mobility. Opening the mouth to the end of the newly acquired range, repeated a few times every hour, is one such exercise. The patient might need the visual feedback afforded by performing the exercise in front of a mirror to ensure that the mandibular motion can be produced symmetrically in the midline. Unless the patient is coached properly, maintenance exercises will not return the mandible to its normal function. For example, an anteromedially displaced disc on one side will stop condylar movement during opening and also during lateral glide. If mobilization has succeeded in stretching out the tight tissue, more opening should be available, together with more lateral glide. However, if the patient has not been able to achieve a lateral glide because of the joint dysfunction, she or he will need visual feedback (i.e., doing the exercise in front of a mirror) to see what happens to the mandible when she or he performs the movement.

Manual Therapy Targeted to the Orofacial Region in Myogenous Temporomandibular Disorders

Four studies[176-179] looked at manual therapy techniques, such as facial manipulation versus botulinum toxin[176] or intraoral myofascial therapy versus waiting list, and self-care education and exercises for subjects with myogenous TMDs.[177-179] The results of these studies supported the use of manual therapy to treat myogenous TMDs because subjects treated with all of these approaches improved mouth opening and reduced jaw pain related to their baseline. Although intraoral myofascial therapy and exercise groups were superior to a waiting list control group, they did not have any statistically significant difference between them. In addition, facial manipulation had the equivalent effect as botulinum toxin. However, fascial manipulation was slightly superior in reducing subjective pain perception, and botulinum toxin injections were slightly superior in increasing jaw ROM at 3 months following treatment. When pooling the results from three of these studies,[176,178,179] it was found that there was a trend in favor of manual therapy to improve pain at 4 to 6 weeks of treatment when compared with an exercise waiting list group. However, the difference was not clinically relevant. The mean difference for pain intensity was 0.95 cm (95% CI = −0.07, 1.83).

Manual Therapy Targeted to the Cervical Spine and Cervical Exercises in Myogenous Temporomandibular Disorders

A randomized controlled trial (RCT) conducted by La Touche et al.[180] testing a more specific approach directed to the cervical spine to treat patients with cervicocraniofacial pain of myofascial origin was performed. They investigated the effects of anterior-posterior upper cervical mobilization (APUCM) when compared with placebo on pressure pain thresholds (PPTs) in the craniofacial and cervical regions and pain intensity after three sessions of treatment. This preliminary study found that mobilizations targeted at the cervical spine drastically decreased pain intensity and pain sensitivity (through the PPT evaluation) in patients with cervicocraniofacial pain of myofascial origin immediately after the application of the technique when compared with placebo treatment. The effect sizes found by this study for pain intensity were 28.75 points (95% CI = 21.65, 35.85) and 1.12 kg/cm² (95% CI = 0.96, 1.29) for pain and PTT, respectively, which is encouraging. These results exceeded suggested values for the minimum clinically important differences for pain[181–184] and for PPT outcomes.[185,186] The minimal important difference (MID) for Pain and PPT outcomes have been reported to be from 15 to 32 points[181–184,187] and ≥1.10 kg/cm² per second,[185,186] respectively, which suggest a potentially beneficial effect for this specific treatment to improve symptoms in patients with myogenous TMDs.

This early evidence provides support for more specific treatment directed at the cervical spine to treat pain and impairments found in TMD patients. Furthermore, preliminary evidence has found that exercises addressing the cervical impairments through the training of neck flexor muscles as part of cervical spine treatment in people with TMDs reduced pain and improved function (i.e., increasing pain-free mouth opening), which potentially supports the fact that patients with TMDs could benefit from treatment to impaired cervical flexor muscles.[188] Thus these results testing the effectiveness of exercise protocols to improve cervical muscular impairments and consequently decrease pain intensity and improve function are promising and might be translated to the area of TMD because, up to now, this type of training has not been proven in a large clinical trial. Therefore future research should be conducted with larger RCTs in this area to confirm these results as well as using a longer follow-up period to evaluate the long-term effects of these types of interventions.

Manual Therapy plus Exercises in Arthrogenous Temporomandibular Disorders

Seven studies[174,189–195] looked at the combined effect of manual therapy plus exercises for subjects with arthrogenous TMDs. Three studies[174,189,190] compared manual therapy and exercises versus splint therapy. One study[191,192] compared them with self-care and advice regarding prognosis, and two studies used medications as a comparison.[143,193] In addition, one study[194] compared anesthetic blockage of the auriculotemporal nerve versus manual therapy and exercises.

In general, it was found that manual therapy plus exercises was successful in reducing symptoms and increasing the ROM for patients with arthrogenous TMDs, especially in subjects with a closed lock.[195] When studies with homogeneous interventions and available data were pooled, it was found that pain was significantly reduced in subjects receiving manual therapy combined with exercises when compared with splint therapy, self-care, or medications. The SMD for pain intensity at 4 weeks to

3 months was 0.40 (95% CI = 0.13, 0.68) with a moderate effect size, based on Cohen guidelines.[139] When looking at active mouth opening, it was found that manual therapy plus exercises significantly increase active mouth opening when compared with splint therapy, self-care, or medications. The mean difference for active mouth opening at 4 weeks to 3 months was 3.58 mm (95% CI = 1.46, 5.70).

Manual Therapy and Mixed Temporomandibular Disorders

Four studies[196–199] looked at manual therapy to mobilize the atlantoaxial joints,[197,199] at another level of cervical spine,[198] or mobilizations to the TMJ joint[196] for subjects with mixed TMDs. When the data from Mansilla-Ferragud et al. and Otano et al. were pooled, it was found that there was no statistically significant difference in mouth opening between mobilization of the atlantoaxial joint[197,199] when compared with a control group receiving no mobilization. The mean difference in mouth opening between control and manual therapy groups was 17.33 mm (95% CI = −10.39, 45.06), which is considered to be a clinically important difference between groups in favor of the manual therapy treatment.[131]

Manual Therapy plus Exercises for Mixed Temporomandibular Disorders

Two studies[200–202] investigated the effect of manual therapy combined with exercises in subjects with mixed TMDs (i.e., both muscular and joint involvement). Tuncer et al.[200] looked at the specific effect of orofacial and cervical manual therapy involving soft tissue mobilization (i.e., intraoral and extraoral deep friction massage to painful muscles), TMJ mobilization (i.e., caudal and ventrocaudal traction, ventral and mediolateral translation), TMJ stabilization (i.e., gentle isometric tension exercises against resistance), coordination exercises (i.e., guided opening and closing jaw movements), cervical spine mobilization (i.e., traction and translation), and postisometric relaxation and stretching techniques for the masticatory and neck muscles. Von Piekartz et al.[202] compared the effect of orofacial physical therapy involving (translatory) movements of the temporomandibular region and/or masticatory muscle techniques, such as tender trigger point treatment and muscle stretching, active and passive movements facilitating optimal function of cranial nerve tissue, coordination exercises, and home exercises with treatment targeted at the cervical spine in subjects with signs and symptoms of TMDs. When the results of these two studies regarding mouth opening were pooled, it was found that manual therapy targeted to the orofacial region or in combination with cervical treatment was better than home exercises or treatment to the cervical spine alone. The mean difference in mouth opening between control and manual therapy groups was 6.10 mm (95% CI = 1.11, 11.09), favoring the manual therapy groups. This difference is considered to be clinically relevant.[131]

Electrophysical Modalities

Electrophysical modalities, such as shortwave diathermy, US techniques, laser treatments, and TENS, are commonly used in the clinical setting.[203] The purpose of these modalities is to reduce inflammation and increase blood flow by altering capillary permeability.[203] The literature suggests that treatments with electrophysical modalities performed early in the course of TMDs are beneficial in reducing symptoms.[203] A discussion of some of the common physical modalities used for treating the TMJ and associated structures and the evidence from a meta-analysis[125] of their effectiveness follows.

Laser

The use of low-level laser therapy (LLLT) has increased in the treatment of TMD due to its pain-relieving effects as well as its simplicity. "The LLLT can be defined as a non-thermal type of light, which causes internal changes in cells and tissues, leading to different types of metabolic activation."[204] It has been reported that LLLT could cause analgesia as well as anti-inflammatory effects[204] by causing a reduction of prostaglandin E_2 (PGE_2), which is involved in inflammation. The dosage associated with PGE_2 reduction has been reported to be between 0.4 and 19 J and within a range of power density between 5 and 21.2 mW/cm².

At least two recent systematic reviews[204,205] have been conducted regarding the effectiveness of laser therapy for TMDs. Although both systematic reviews had different studies, both agree that the evidence of LLLT is not conclusive regarding the usefulness of LLLT for treating TMDs. The systematic review of Petrucci et al.[204] involved six[206-211] RCTs, and the systematic review of Melis et al. included 14 RCTs.[206-219] Petrucci et al.[204] performed a meta-analysis of the six analyzed trials. They evaluated the effect of LLLT on pain intensity as well as on mouth opening and mouth lateral movements. They concluded that LLLT was no more effective than a placebo in reducing pain intensity. The mean difference was 7.77 mm (95% CI = −2.49, 18.02), which was not statistically significant. Although this result cannot be considered statistically significant, the 95% CI of the difference between a placebo and LLLT shows a trend indicating that LLLT could be clinically meaningful at reducing pain in patients with TMD.[220] LLLT was significantly more effective than a placebo in improving vertical mouth opening (4.04 mm [95% CI = 3.06, 5.02]) and right lateral movement (1.64 mm [95% CI = 0.10, 3.17]). Interestingly, LLLT was not significantly different from a placebo in increasing left lateral mouth movement (1.90 [95% CI = −4.08, 7.88]). The similarities between LLLT and placebo effect could indicate that LLLT could have a strong placebo effect.

There was great heterogeneity between studies regarding the site of application of the beam, the number of applications performed (between 3 and 20 sessions), their duration (between 10 and 180 seconds), and the dosage used by each study in terms of wavelength, frequency, and output. According to Melis et al.,[205] output varied from 17 mW and 27 W. Frequency varied between 0 and 1.500 Hz; wavelength between 632.8 and 910 nm, and density dosage between 1 and 105 J/cm². In addition, different outcome measures were used. According to Petrucci et al.,[204] only one study[208] used doses inside the dose range recommended as effective by Bjordal et al.[221] Power density could not be calculated for most of the studies. This is a serious methodological flaw because it highlights that LLLT could have been ineffective due to the inadequacy of dosages used by the analyzed studies. Thus, it is uncertain if LLLT is effective when applied using the right dosages. More studies using an acceptable level of intensity are needed.

Biofeedback

EMG biofeedback therapy is a muscular relaxation technique in which a signal constantly provides patients with feedback about their masticatory muscles activity level. Biofeedback is based on the idea that stress-induced hyperactivity may be an important component of muscular TMDs. The feedback information assists patients in the self-control and management of their own levels of muscular tension, which may be a contributing factor for the onset, maintenance, or exacerbation of pain.[222]

The mechanisms underlying the apparent efficacy of EMG biofeedback for TMDs are not well understood. Several theories support its use in TMDs. For example, it has been suggested that the clinical improvement obtained with biofeedback is the consequence of reduced EMG activity in facial and/or masticatory muscles, or that biofeedback could enhance awareness of activity in facial and masticatory muscles, thereby improving patients' ability to detect, label, and voluntarily reduce muscle tension before it reaches uncomfortably high levels. In addition, it has been hypothesized that EMG biofeedback could induce patients to believe in their ability to manage and to cope with the environmental stressors and their own psychophysiological states, which in turn may help decrease symptoms associated with TMDs.[223]

A meta-analysis published in 1999 examined the efficacy of EMG biofeedback for TMDs.[224] Based on a meta-analysis of 13 studies (both controlled and uncontrolled trials), the authors concluded that there was evidence to support the use of EMG biofeedback in the treatment of TMD. The results of a recent meta-analysis of these studies,[125] pooling data from all studies regardless of diagnosis (i.e., controlled and RCT studies) investigating the effectiveness of biofeedback versus control or other treatments, such as splint and physical therapy exercises[138,225-229] on pain intensity, found a beneficial effect favoring biofeedback therapy. The SMD for pain intensity outcome was 1.37 (95% CI = 0.24, 2.50), which is statistically significant. The magnitude of effect size is considered high, based on Cohen guidelines.[139] However, the heterogeneity of studies was high as well (90%). Thus, these results should be interpreted with caution. When eliminating an outlier[226] with a very high positive effect for biofeedback, a positive effect of biofeedback against other treatment on pain intensity was still found (0.87 [95% CI = 0.24, 2.50]). When analyzing only RCTs without the outlier previously mentioned, a small-to-moderate effect favoring biofeedback still remained. The SMD difference for pain intensity outcome was 0.37 (95% CI = 0.00, 0.74), reducing greatly the heterogeneity to 21%.

Transcutaneous Electrical Nerve Stimulation (TENS)

TENS has been a common modality used for physical therapists. It deserves special attention because it presents no side effects and enables both pain reduction and reestablishing the function of the masticatory muscles by modifying the perception of pain and, according to some, it changes the level of activity of masticatory muscles.[230,231] Studies looking at TENS and its effectiveness on masticatory muscles have shown that it is effective in relieving pain, in decreasing the EMG activity of the masticatory muscles at rest, in reducing the myoelectric activity of the jaw-closing muscles during the opening phase of the jaw, and in increasing the muscular electrical activity recorded during clenching in TMD patients.[230,231]

TENS applies a low-voltage, low-amperage, biphasic current at varying frequencies to provide counterstimulation, with the main purpose of pain relief.[232] TENS therapy is supposed to stimulate large, fast, myelinated, nonnociceptive neurons in the painful area, "closing the central gate" for those stimuli generated by pain-specific fibers. This system, associated to the activation of an endogenous opioid system, is supposed to be responsible for the analgesic effect of the TENS.

TENS is regularly employed in patients with TMDs, in view of its analgesic and muscle-relaxing effect, with positive results. Hence TENS therapy is recommended in patients presenting with signs of myofascial dysfunction, limited mouth opening, and pain or tenderness in the masticatory muscles.[233] It should be pointed out that the efficacy of TENS procedures has been challenged. Several controlled trials have indicated that TENS had no greater benefit than a placebo therapy program.[234,235] Furthermore, the antalgic effect of TENS application is still a debated question because contrasting results have been reported in the literature and the possibility of a placebo effect has been suggested.[231]

According to a recent meta-analysis,[125] eight studies have examined the efficacy of TENS for treating TMDs. Five of them[230,236-239] focused on myogenous TMDs, and the remaining focused on arthrogenous TMD.[231,240,241] Because these studies were very heterogeneous in terms of outcomes, pooling of the data was not possible. In general, the studies included in this meta-analysis provided conflicting evidence regarding the effectiveness of TENS therapy. TENS was not found to be significantly better than muscular awareness relaxation, biofeedback, sham TENS, splint, laser therapy, or a control group for

patients with myogenous TMDs.[230,236-239] In addition, when analyzing the results for the studies investigating patients with arthrogenous TMDs, conflicting results were also obtained. Myostad et al.[240] and Monaco et al.[231] found that TENS helped at reducing functional pain and decreasing EMG activity of the masticatory muscles when compared with placebo TENS therapy; however, Linde et al.[241] found no significant differences between TENS and splint therapy.

Electromagnetic Fields and Shortwave Diathermy

Only four studies have looked at the effectiveness of electromagnetic fields or shortwave diathermy for treating TMDs versus placebo, muscle relaxants, or other physical agents.[242-245] Some studies[244,245] have favored the use of pulsed electromagnetic fields, whereas others[242,243] have not. Statistical analysis did indicate a borderline positive effect in its use.[243-245]

Iontophoresis

Two trials have been reported in a meta-analysis by Armijo-Olivo et al.[125] investigating the effectiveness of iontophoresis delivering dexamethasone therapy to manage arthrogenous TMDs when compared with placebo therapy.[246,247] The two studies had opposite results. Schiffman et al.[246] found that iontophoresis was helpful in improving pain in a short term, whereas Reid et al.[247] found that the placebo group presented with greater pain reduction than the subjects receiving iontophoresis. The SMD for the pool estimate reported by this meta-analysis[125] was −0.68 [95% CI = −2.83, 1.48], which is not statistically significant.

Ultrasound (US) Therapy

Therapeutic US refers to mechanical vibrations (i.e., sound waves) that are beyond the range of human hearing, commonly at either 1 or 3 MHz (million cycles per second).[248] These waves travel through tissue and are preferentially absorbed in dense collagen structures with lower water content and high protein content (i.e., tendon, ligament, joint capsule).[249] Therapeutic US has a long history of use in physical therapy practice, and its clinical application has evolved during the last decades from being used as a thermal modality to being employed for its nonthermal effects particularly in tissue repair and wound healing.[249] Clinically US has commonly been used for treating inflammation in the TMJ as well as masticatory muscles.

According to a meta-analysis,[125] three studies have looked at the effectiveness of US therapy for treating TMD. Two focused on myogenous TMD[244,250] and one[242] on mixed TMD (i.e., myogenous and arthrogenous TMD). The results of this meta-analysis showed that when the results from Gray et al.[242] and Taube et al.[250] were pooled, the proportion of improvement at the end of the treatment with US in patients with TMD, a nonsignificant risk ratio (RR) was found to exist with the use of US compared with a placebo (RR: 1.90 [95% CI = 0.35, 10.26]), although a high tendency to favor US therapy was observed when analyzed at the 95% CI. However, these results should be taken with caution due to the high heterogeneity between the studies (93%).

OTHER TEMPOROMANDIBULAR JOINT TREATMENTS

Orthodontics and Other Dental Treatments

Some authors, including Mew,[24] have postulated that orthodontic treatment can cause TMDs. Some studies refute this.[15,97,98] Even more, the orthodontic treatment used in patients with TMDs to improve symptomatology has been debated in the literature.[15] Because no clear link has been shown between malocclusion and the development of TMDs, orthodontics and other dental treatments that alter the bite or teeth (e.g., occlusal adjustment,[251] dental restorations, and TMJ surgery) are inappropriate as initial management methods for TMDs. This is supported by evidence from an overview published by List and Axelsson.[126] They found that no systematic review found evidence that occlusal adjustments are more or less effective than placebo in the treatment of TMD pain. All systematic reviews were restrictive in recommending the use of occlusal adjustments for treatment for TMD pain, especially because this therapy is nonreversible. Sometimes a patient starts to show signs and symptoms of TMDs during orthodontic treatment. These patients may need to be taught ways to reduce any stress through the joints during the period of orthodontic care. During orthodontic treatment a patient who is banded and fitted with elastics to control mandibular motion may develop muscle spasm and reduced mobility. In these cases treatment of the condition and mobilization must be coordinated with the orthodontist so that the elastics can be removed and joint mobilization provided.

Cognitive Behavioral Therapy

It is important that clinicians understand TMD as a complex disorder and that they keep in mind the biopsychosocial model as a basis for the etiology, assessment, and management of TMDs. In this context, cognitive behavioral therapy has emerged as an important option for treating patients with TMDs because it addresses the mind and body as a whole. Counseling, stress management, biofeedback, relaxation therapy, cognition, psychoeducation, and even primary therapeutic exercises are recognized components of a cognitive behavioral program.[48,252] List and Axelsson[126] concluded that this type of treatment was effective in treating TMD pain. Thus the authors recommended that patients with TMD pain and major psychological disturbances were in need of a combined therapeutic approach. Thus clinical examination

with a behavioral assessment needs to be combined to direct the patient to the proper mode of treatment.

Acupuncture

Acupuncture increasingly is being used in the treatment of musculoskeletal conditions in North America.[253] Currently the mechanisms underlying the action of acupuncture are unclear.[254] Acupuncture may relieve pain according to the principles of the gate control theory or by acting as a noxious stimulus. Some evidence indicates that acupuncture may stimulate the production of endorphins, serotonin, and acetylcholine within the central nervous system.[254]

In 1999 a systematic review examined the data of preliminary studies and reported that acupuncture was a potentially effective therapy for TMDs, although more rigorous studies were needed to confirm their conclusions.[255] Based on a systematic review and meta-analysis of acupuncture for TMDs[256] including nine trials,[257-265] acupuncture was effective in reducing pain when analyzing the differences before and after treatment and also when comparing with a control group (no numerical data provided). In addition, acupuncture was more effective at reducing pain when compared with a placebo or sham acupuncture treatment.[256] According to a meta-analysis of four trials[257,262,263,265] that provided numerical data performed within the systematic review, it was found that the SMD between acupuncture and placebo acupuncture was 0.83 (95% CI = 0.41, 1.25) for pain intensity, which is considered a high effect size.[139] These results indicated that acupuncture was more effective than a placebo or sham treatment at reducing pain intensity. Acupuncture demonstrated more effectiveness than other interventions, such as occlusal splint therapy. Results suggest that acupuncture is a reasonable adjunctive treatment for producing an analgesic effect in TMD patients; however, methodological issues, such as being the type of technique that can create placebo effects, are unknown, and placebo acupuncture response may rely on patient psychological and physiological expectations.[266]

Surgery

Surgery on the TMJ itself has become rare; only approximately 5% of patients who undergo treatment for TMDs require surgery.[267] There are no generally recognized surgical protocols for TMD, although some guidelines have been proposed as requirements for TMJ surgery.[15] Surgery should be reserved for cases in which surgical treatment can warrant success. According to a systematic review overview, List and Axelsson[126] found that for patients with DDwithR, one systematic review reported similar treatment effects for arthrocentesis, arthroscopy, and discectomy.[268] In patients with DDwithoutR, another review reported similar effects for arthrocentesis, arthroscopy, and physical therapy.[269] A third review reported an overall high success rate for arthrocentesis but made no comparison of arthrocentesis with other interventions.[270] In patients with TMD pain, a systematic review reported contradictory results following orthognathic surgery.[271] According to List and Axelsson,[126] all of these published systematic reviews dealing with surgery for TMDs showed low levels of evidence, and thus firm conclusions could not be made. Based on a general rule of thumb, conservative treatments are the choice for treating TMD. Surgical or other more invasive treatments should be reserved only for cases unresponsive to conservative approaches.

When surgery is performed, the procedure most often is an arthroscopic technique and includes lavage to free up any joint restrictions and to flush the joint to allow for better function. An ankylosed joint or a joint with a clinical closed lock that has not responded to conservative treatment fits the category of conditions requiring surgery. After surgery, therapy focuses on improving joint function as quickly as possible. The initial treatment is based on the same criteria used for acute capsulitis.

Guidelines for Temporomandibular Joint Surgery

- The TMJ is the source of pain and/or dysfunction that results in significant impairment
- Appropriate nonsurgical management was unsuccessful
- The pain is localized in the TMJ (when loading and with movement)
- Interferences with proper TMJ function are the mechanical type
- The patient requests the surgical approach
- The patient has no medical or psychological contraindications to surgery

---

Post-Radiation Therapy for Hypomobility of the Temporomandibular Joint

Patients who have had surgery and radiation therapy for treatment of cancer of the neck and oropharyngeal structures can present with severe restriction of ROM of the mandible. Extensive therapy, including mobilization, in an attempt to improve function has not been successful. Radiation therapy appears to cause severe fibrosis of the masticatory and neck musculature that does not respond to therapy. Surgical intervention can cause postoperative muscle spasm that makes swift mobilization difficult. The authors believe that if these unfortunate individuals are to be helped effectively, therapy must be instituted almost immediately after treatment, which entails the use of resources at the hospital where the treatment is given. If physical therapy is not introduced until after the patient has been discharged from hospital, it often is too late to effect any improvement.

PATIENT EDUCATION

As mentioned previously, it is vital that patients know the intent of the treatment so that they do not harbor any incorrect expectations for the treatment outcome. Patients also must be made aware of the likely biomechanical changes caused by the dysfunction, so that they become fully involved in the rehabilitation process and understand why certain activities must be avoided. A useful educational tool is a simple diagram of the anatomy of the TMJ; it need not be anatomically specific nor drawn with an excruciating degree of detail. The objectives of education are to reassure the patient, to explain the nature, etiology, and prognosis of the problem, to reduce repetitive strain of the masticatory system (e.g., daytime bruxism), to encourage relaxation, and to control the amount of the masticatory activity.[136,270,272,273]

The education process can be split into several parts. The first part should provide an explanation of the basic anatomy, joint position, and normal disc-condyle relationship. The second part should include some description of the patient's probable pathological condition. The third part should be a description of possible aggravating factors and various activities to be avoided. The fourth part should include a description of some things patients can do for themselves at home, including a list of required exercises. The fifth part should provide some indication of the extent of recovery expected, the likelihood of recurrence of problems, and the need to bring other health care professionals into the rehabilitation process.

Increased self-management is closely linked to successful rehabilitation, which includes three separate domains: physical, functional, and social.[270] The patient has to be reassured by explaining the problem, supposed etiology, and good prognosis of this benign disorder. Patients require good information to assist them in making choices, overcoming unhelpful beliefs, and modifying behavior. The relationship between chronic pain and psychosocial distress must also be considered. Normal jaw muscle function has to be explained, stressing how to avoid overloading the masticatory system, which could be the major cause of the complaints. The patients have to pay close attention to the jaw muscle activity, they should be informed about normal jaw function and that parafunctions could be a cause of their complaints. They should be instructed to avoid bad oral habits and excessive mandibular movements and to keep the jaw muscles relaxed and the teeth apart except for swallowing or eating. In acute conditions they have to avoid hard food, cut hard and tough food into small pieces, chew with the back teeth on both sides, and avoid chewing gum and nail biting. Later in the rehabilitation program, training of restrictive activities of daily living as mentioned previously (i.e., avoid bad oral habits and excessive mandibular movements) is part of the procedure to return to normal or desired levels of activity and participation and to prevent the development of chronic complaints. Patients must learn to keep the muscles relaxed by holding the mandible in the resting position (i.e., teeth apart) rather than in occlusion because occlusion requires "unintentional" muscle contraction.[271] The mandibular resting position can be determined by asking the patients to pronounce the letter "N" several times and to maintain the tongue behind the upper incisor teeth, with the lips in slight contact or as an alternative, to exhale through the mouth. Approaches aiming at changing maladaptive habits and behaviors, such as jaw clenching and grinding of the teeth, are important in treating painful tissues. Behavior-modification strategies, such as habit reversal, are commonly used. Although many habits are abandoned when the patients become aware of them, changing persistent habits requires a structured program. Patients should be aware that habits do not change spontaneously and that they are responsible for the change. For this reason, it is important to stress the need for the patients to practice what they have learned at home and during their common activities, often with the help of visual feedback.

Patient Management Program: Everyday Activities

Successful treatment and management of temporomandibular joint/muscle dysfunction depends in large part on the way these injured areas are treated. The following instructions can greatly enhance the correction and healing of this area.

- For the next few months, be sure to cut all your food into bite-sized (i.e., small) pieces. Try not to open your mouth any wider than the thickness of your thumb.
- Do not eat hard crusts of bread, tough meat, raw vegetables, or any other food that requires prolonged chewing.
- Do not chew gum during this period of treatment.
- Be sure not to protrude your jaw, as you must do in biting off a piece of meat.
- Do not bite any food with your front teeth.
- When you chew, make sure you chew equally on each side of your mouth. Do not get in the habit of doing all your chewing on one side only.
- If you wear lipstick, do not bring your jaw forward when applying it.
- Avoid protruding your jaw during any other activities (e.g., smoking, conversation).
- Make every effort not to strain your joint ligaments unnecessarily. For example, do not stretch your mouth open when yawning.
- If you find yourself clenching your teeth, try to remember, "lips together, teeth apart."
- Try to sleep on your back or side. Avoid sleeping on your jaw or in the prone position.

Patient Management Program: Diaphragmatic Breathing

- If you breathe through your mouth, you are breathing abnormally. Consequently, your jaw will be dropped and can never be in a normal resting position unless you change your breathing habits. Your symptoms will never entirely go away, and you will not receive maximum benefit from your treatment.
- When breathing and at rest, hold the tip of your tongue against the back of your top teeth. Keep your lips lightly together; the upper and lower teeth should be slightly separated. This technique will prevent mouth breathing. All breathing should be done through your nose, with your tongue elevated, for the rest of your life. Your teeth should be slightly apart (0.32 to 0.63 cm [0.125 to 0.25 inches]).
- Do not suck in air through your mouth.
- Concentrate your breathing on your stomach. Your stomach should expand and contract, *not* your chest. Put your hand on your stomach and feel it go in and out; this is called *abdominal*, or *diaphragmatic, breathing.* This is the way you should breathe from now on. Simultaneously, keep your tongue against the roof of your mouth.
- Do five breaths every hour (i.e., at 1-hour intervals, consciously inhale and exhale from your stomach five times; hopefully you will also be breathing this way subconsciously in between).
- Never use nasal inhalants or sprays.
- Never put your tongue between the biting surfaces of your teeth.

In summary, patient education involves explaining the nature of the pain and ways to avoid painful conditions. Information about the biopsychosocial model of TMDs, chronic pain, and self-management needs to be included in the education program.[272] In addition, the patient needs to be advised about posture and ergonomic conditions (e.g., work-related postures or loads) and the adverse effects of certain positions and oral behaviors, such as biting, chewing, and grinding, that create constant microtrauma in the tissues. Patient education has been found to be crucial to the success of treatment.[252]

Temporomandibular Joint Education Process

The following points are covered at the first visit:

- Explanation of anatomy, joint position, and the normal disc-condyle relationship
- Description of the probable pathology
- Description of the aggravating factors and activities to avoid
- Guidelines the patient can follow at home, including exercises
- Likely extent of recovery
- Likelihood of problem recurrence
- Inclusion of other health care professionals in the treatment process (if needed)

SUMMARY

Treatment of TMDs and related dysfunctions follows the same principles as treatment of any other musculoskeletal problem. After a comprehensive history has been taken and an assessment performed, a hierarchy of signs and symptoms is formulated, together with a hierarchy of treatments aimed at helping to alleviate the signs and symptoms and restore normal functioning of the CMS. The objective is to return the patient to maximum possible function. To do this, the clinician must have the patient's cooperation and participation; to give these, the patient must understand the condition, what will be required for recovery, and the goals set by the clinician.

Frequently treatment is not only multifaceted but also requires the participation and skills of practitioners from different specialties, such as physical therapists, dentists, clinical psychologists, speech pathologists, and physicians. Concentrating on one area alone does not provide successful outcomes or ensure a happy patient. TMD is recognized as a multidimensional disorder, the result of biological, psychological, and social alterations. Therefore assessment and management of TMD must address the biological, psychological, and sociological aspects of the individual as a whole.[48]

REFERENCES

1. Drangsholt M, LeResche L: Temporomandibular disorder pain. In Crombie I, Croft P, Linton S, et al, editors: *Epidemiology of pain*, Seattle, 1999, IASP.
2. Armijo-Olivo S, Magee D, Parfitt M, et al: The association between the cervical spine, the stomatognathic system, and craniofacial pain: a critical review, *J Orofac Pain* 20:271–287, 2006.
3. Armijo-Olivo S, Magee D: Cervical musculoskeletal impairments and temporomandibular disorders, *J Oral Maxillofac Res* 3(4):1–18, 2012.
4. Armijo-Olivo S: Relation entre les désordres de la colonne cervicale et les dysfonctions temporomandibulaires: mise au point et implications cliniques, *KINE Kinésithérapie, la revue* 13(134):12, 2013.
5. Armijo-Olivo S, Fuentes JP, da Costa BR, et al: Reduced endurance of the cervical flexor muscles in patients with concurrent temporomandibular disorders and neck disability, *Man Ther* 15(6):586–592, 2010.
6. Armijo-Olivo S, Silvestre R, Fuentes J, et al: Electromyographic activity of the cervical flexor muscles in patients with temporomandibular disorders while executing the craniocervical flexion test (CCFT): a cross sectional study, *Phys Ther* 91(8):1184–1197, 2011.
7. Armijo-Olivo S, Silvestre RA, Fuentes JP, et al: Patients with temporomandibular disorders have increased fatigability of the cervical extensor muscles, *Clin J Pain* 28(1):55–64, 2012.
8. Armijo-Olivo SL, Fuentes JP, Major PW, et al: Is maximal strength of the cervical flexor muscles reduced in patients with temporomandibular disorders? *Arch Phys Med Rehabil* 91(8):1236–1242, 2010.
9. Kraus S: Temporomandibular disorders, head and orofacial pain: cervical spine considerations, *Dental Clin North Am* 51(1):161–193, 2007.
10. Greene C: Concepts of TMD etiology: effects on diagnosis and treatment. In Laskin D, Green C, Hylander W, editors: *TMDs: an evidence-based approach to diagnosis and treatment*, Chicago, 2006, Quintessence.
11. Hylander W: Functional anatomy and biomechanics of the masticatory apparatus. In Laskin D, Green C, Hylander W, editors: *TMDs: an evidence-based approach to diagnosis and treatment*, Chicago, 2006, Quintessence.
12. Okeson JP: *Bell's orofacial pains. The clinical management of orofacial pain*, ed 6, Chicago, 2005, Quintessence.
13. Laskin D, Green C, Hylander W: *TMDs: an evidence-based approach to diagnosis and treatment*, Chicago, 2006, Quintessence.
14. Di Fabio RP: Physical therapy for patients with TMD: a descriptive study of treatment, disability, and health status, *J Orofac Pain* 12(2):124–135, 1998.
15. Goldstein BH: Temporomandibular disorders: a review of current understanding, *Oral Surg Oral Med Oral Pathol Oral Radiol Endod* 88(4):379–385, 1999.
16. Benoit P: History and physical examination for TMD. In Kraus S, editor: *Clinics in physical therapy: temporomandibular disorders*, ed 2 New York, 1994, Churchill Livingstone.
17. Gremillion HA, Mahan PE: The prevalence and etiology of temporomandibular disorders and orofacial pain, *Tex Dent J* 117:30–39, 2000.
18. De Wijer A, De Leeuw JRJ, Steenks MH, et al: Temporomandibular and cervical spine disorders: self-reported signs and symptoms, *Spine* 21(14):1638–1646, 1996.
19. De Wijer A, Steenks MH, Bosman F, et al: Symptoms of the stomatognathic system in temporomandibular and cervical spine disorders, *J Oral Rehabil* 23(11):733–741, 1996.
20. De Wijer A, Steenks MH, de Leeuw JR, et al: Symptoms of the cervical spine in temporomandibular and cervical spine disorders, *J Oral Rehabil* 23(11):742–750, 1996.
21. Dworkin SF, Huggins KH, LeResche L, et al: Epidemiology of signs and symptoms in temporomandibular disorders: clinical signs in cases and controls, *J Am Dental Assoc* 120(3):273–281, 1990.
22. McNeill C: Epidemiology. In McNeill C, editor: *Temporomandibular disorders: guidelines for classification, assessment, and management*, Carol Stream, 1993, Quintessence.
23. Auvenshine RC: Temporomandibular disorders: associated features, *Dent Clin North Am* 51(1):105–127, 2007.
24. Mew J: The aetiology of malocclusion. Can the tropic premise assist our understanding? *Brit Dent J* 151(9):296–302, 1981.
25. Ribeiro RF, Tallents RH, Katzberg RW, et al: The prevalence of disc displacement in symptomatic and asymptomatic volunteers aged 6 to 25 years, *J Orofac Pain* 11(1):37–47, 1997.
26. Gonçalves DA, Dal Fabbro AL, Campos JA, et al: Symptoms of temporomandibular disorders in the population: an epidemiological study, *J Orofac Pain* 24(3):270–278, 2010.
27. Greenspan JD, Slade GD, Bair E, et al: Pain sensitivity and autonomic factors associated with development of TMD: the OPPERA prospective cohort study, *J Pain* 14(12 suppl):T63–T74, 2013.
28. Egermark I, Carlsson GE, Magnusson T: A 20-year longitudinal study of subjective symptoms of temporomandibular disorders from childhood to adulthood, *Acta Odontol Scand* 59(1):40–48, 2001.
29. Agerberg G, Carlsson GE: Functional disorders of the masticatory system. I. Distribution of symptoms according to age and sex as judged from investigation by questionnaire, *Acta Odontol Scand* 30(6):597–613, 1972.
30. Glass EG, McGlynn FD, Glaros AG, et al: Prevalence of temporomandibular disorder symptoms in a major metropolitan area, *Cranio* 11(3):217–220, 1993.
31. Hirata RH, Heft MW, Hernandez B, et al: Longitudinal study of signs of temporomandibular disorders (TMD) in orthodontically treated and nontreated groups, *Am J Orthod Dentofacial Orthop* 101(1):35–40, 1992.
32. Schiffmann E, Fricton J: *Epidemiology of TMJ and craniofacial pain: diagnosis and management*, St Louis, 1988, IEA.
33. Armijo-Olivo S, Frugone R, Armijo-Olivo L, et al: Prevalence of signs and symptoms of temporomandibular disorders in patients who attended dental practice in public health centers of Talca-Chile, *Kinesiologia* 60:10–15, 2000.
34. Carlsson G: Epidemiology and treatment need for temporomandibular disorders, *J Orofac Pain* 13(4):232–237, 1999.
35. Kino K, Haketa T, Amemori Y, et al: The comparison between pains, difficulties in function, and associating factors of patients in subtypes of temporomandibular disorders, *J Oral Rehabil* 32(5):315–325, 2005.
36. Robinson ME, Dannecker EA, George SZ, et al: Sex differences in the associations among psychological factors and pain report: a novel psychophysical study of patients with chronic low back pain, *J Pain* 6(7):463–470, 2005.
37. Dannecker EA, Hausenblas HA, Kaminski TW, et al: Sex differences in delayed onset muscle pain, *Clin J Pain* 21(2):120–126, 2005.
38. Robinson ME, George SZ, Dannecker EA, et al: Sex differences in pain anchors revisited: further investigation of "most intense" and common pain events, *Eur J Pain* 8(4):299–305, 2004.
39. Robinson ME, Wise EA: Prior pain experience: influence on the observation of experimental pain in men and women, *J Pain* 5(5):264–269, 2004.
40. Robinson ME, Wise EA, Gagnon C, et al: Influences of gender role and anxiety on sex differences in temporal summation of pain, *J Pain* 5(2):77–82, 2004.

41. Robinson ME, Wise EA: Gender bias in the observation of experimental pain, *Pain* 104(1-2):259–264, 2003.

42. Myers CD, Riley III JL, Robinson ME: Psychosocial contributions to sex-correlated differences in pain, *Clin J Pain* 19(4):225–232, 2003.

43. Robinson ME, Gagnon CM, Price DD, et al: Altering gender role expectations: Effects on pain tolerance, pain threshold, and pain ratings, *J Pain* 4(5):284–288, 2003.

44. De Leeuw R: American Academy of Orofacial Pain: introduction to orofacial pain. In De Leeuw R, American Academy of Orofacial Pain, editors: *Orofacial pain: guidelines for assessment, diagnosis, and management*, Chicago, 2008, Quintessence.

45. LeResche L: Research diagnostic criteria for temporomandibular disorders. In Fricton J, Dubner R, editors: *Orofacial pain and temporomandibular disorders*, New York, 1995, Raven.

46. Steenks M, De Wijer A: Epidemiology, symptomatology, and etiology of craniomandibular dysfunctions [in portuguesse]. In Steenks M, De Wijer A, editors: *Temporomandibular joint dysfunction from a physical therapy and a dentistry perspective: diagnosis and treatment [in Portuguese]*, São Paulo, 1996, Santos.

47. Mew JR: The aetiology of temporomandibular disorders: a philosophical overview, *Eur J Orthodont* 19(3):249–258, 1997.

48. Suvinen TI, Reade PC, Kemppainen P, et al: Review of aetiological concepts of temporomandibular pain disorders: towards a biopsychosocial model for integration of physical disorder factors with psychological and psychosocial illness impact factors, *Eur J Pain* 9(6):613–633, 2005.

49. Clark GT, Delcanho RE, Goulet JP: The utility and validity of current diagnostic procedures for defining temporomandibular disorder patients, *Adv Dent Res* 7(2):97–112, 1993.

50. John MT, Zwijnenburg AJ: Interobserver variability in assessment of signs of TMD, *Int J Prosthodont* 14(3):265–270, 2001.

51. John MT, Dworkin SF, Mancl LA: Reliability of clinical temporomandibular disorder diagnoses, *Pain* 118(1-2):61–69, 2005.

52. Wahlund K, List T, Dworkin SF: Temporomandibular disorders in children and adolescents: reliability of a questionnaire, clinical examination, and diagnosis, *J Orofac Pain* 12(1):42–51, 1998.

53. Dworkin SF, LeResche L: Research diagnostic criteria for temporomandibular disorders: review, criteria, examinations and specifications, critique, *J Craniomandib Disord* 6(4):301–355, 1992.

54. Anderson GC, Gonzalez YM, Ohrbach R, et al: The research diagnostic criteria for temporomandibular disorders. VI: future directions, *J Orofac Pain* 24(1):79–88, 2010.

55. Look JO, John MT, Tai F, et al: The research diagnostic criteria for temporomandibular disorders. II: reliability of Axis I diagnoses and selected clinical measures, *J Orofac Pain* 24(1):25–34, 2010.

56. Ohrbach R, Turner JA, Sherman JJ, et al: The research diagnostic criteria for temporomandibular disorders. IV: evaluation of psychometric properties of the Axis II measures, *J Orofac Pain* 24(1):48–62, 2010.

57. Schiffman EL, Ohrbach R, Truelove EL, et al: The research diagnostic criteria for temporomandibular disorders. V: methods used to establish and validate revised Axis I diagnostic algorithms, *J Orofac Pain* 24(1):63–78, 2010.

58. Schiffman EL, Truelove EL, Ohrbach R, et al: The research diagnostic criteria for temporomandibular disorders. I: overview and methodology for assessment of validity, *J Orofac Pain* 24(1):7–24, 2010.

59. Truelove E, Pan W, Look JO, et al: The research diagnostic criteria for temporomandibular disorders. III: validity of Axis I diagnoses, *J Orofacial Pain* 24(1):35–47, 2010.

60. Steenks MH, de Wijer A: Validity of the research diagnostic criteria for temporomandibular disorders axis. I: in clinical and research settings, *J Orofac Pain* 23(1):9–16, 2009.

61. Schiffman E, Ohrbach R, Truelove E, et al: Diagnostic criteria for temporomandibular disorders (DC/TMD) for clinical and research applications: recommendations of the International RDC/TMD Consortium Network and Orofacial Pain Special Interest Group, *J Oral Facial Pain Headache* 28(1):6–27, 2014.

62. Gonzalez Y, Mohl N: Masticatory muscle pain and dysfunction. In Laskin D, Green C, Hylander W, editors: *TMDs: an evidence-based approach to diagnosis and treatment*, Chicago, 2006, Quintessence.

63. Okeson JP: *American Academy of Orofacial Pain. Orofacial pain: guidelines for assessment, diagnosis and management*, Chicago, 1996, Quintessence.

64. Peck CC, Goulet JP, Lobbezoo F, et al: Expanding the taxonomy of the diagnostic criteria for temporomandibular disorders, *J Oral Rehabil* 41(1):2–23, 2014.

65. Stegenga B, De Bont L: TMJ disc derangements. In Laskin D, Green C, Hylander W, editors: *TMDs: an evidence-based approach to diagnosis and treatment*, Chicago, 2006, Quintessence.

66. Tropkova B: *Posterior anterior cephalometric assessment of adolescent with TMJ internal derangement*, Edmonton, 1998, Department of Dentistry, University of Alberta.

67. Laskin D: Internal derangements. In Laskin D, Green C, Hylander W, editors: *TMDs: an evidence-based approach to diagnosis and treatment*, Chicago, 2006, Quintessence.

68. Biazotto-Gonzalez D: Temporomandibular dysfunction. In Biazotto-Gozalez D, editor: *Interdisciplinary approach in temporomandibular dysfunctions [Portuguese]*, Sao Paulo, 2005, Manole.

69. Landesberg R, Huang L: Analysis of TMJ synovial fluid. In Laskin D, Green C, Hylander W, editors: *TMDs: an evidence-based approach to diagnosis and treatment*, Chicago, 2006, Quintessence.

70. Okeson JP: Pain of muscular origin. In Okeson JP, editor: *Bell's orofacial pains. The clinical management of orofacial pain*, ed 6 Chicago, 2005, Quintessence.

71. McFadden LR, Rishiraj B: Treatment of temporomandibular joint ankylosis: a case report, *J Can Dent Assoc* 67(11):559–563, 2001.

72. Lobbezoo F, Naeije M: Bruxism is mainly regulated centrally, not peripherally, *J Oral Rehabil* 28(12):1085–1091, 2001.

73. Okeson J: *Bell's orofacial pain*, ed 5, Chicago, 1995, Quintessence.

74. Kampe T, Tagdae T, Bader G, et al: Reported symptoms and clinical findings in a group of subjects with longstanding bruxing behaviour, *J Oral Rehabil* 24(8):581–587, 1997.

75. Greene CS: The etiology of temporomandibular disorders: implications for treatment, *J Orofac Pain* 15(2):93–105, 2001 discussion 106–116.

76. Boyd CH, Slagle WF, Boyd CM, et al: The effect of head position on electromyographic evaluations of representative mandibular positioning muscle groups, *Cranio* 5(1):50–54, 1987.

77. Darnell MW: A proposed chronology of events for forward head posture, *J Cranio-Mandib Pract* 1(4):49–54, 1983.

78. Gonzalez HE, Manns A: Forward head posture: its structural and functional influence on the stomatognathic system, a conceptual study, *Cranio* 14(1):71–80, 1996.

79. Goldstein DF, Kraus SL, Williams WB, et al: Influence of cervical posture on mandibular movement, *J Prosthetic Dent* 52(3):421–426, 1984.

80. Yamabe Y, Yamashita R, Fujii H: Head, neck and trunk movements accompanying jaw tapping, *J Oral Rehabil* 26(11):900–905, 1999.

81. Schwarz A: Positions of the head and malrelations of the jaws, *Int J Orthod Oral Surg Radiography* 14:56–68, 1928.

82. Preiskel H: Some observations on the postural position of the mandible, *J Prosthet Dent* 15:625–633, 1965.

83. Posselt U: Studies in the mobility of the human mandible, *Acta Odontol Scand* 10(suppl 10):1–153, 1952.

84. McLean LF, Brenman HS, Friedman MG: Effects of changing body position on dental occlusion, *J Dent Res* 52(5):1041–1045, 1970.

85. Solow B, Tallgren A: Head posture and craniofacial morphology, *Am J Phys Anthropol* 44(3):417–435, 1976.

86. Visscher CM, Slater J, Lobbezoo F, et al: Kinematics of the human mandible for different head posture, *J Oral Rehabil* 27(4):299–305, 2000.

87. O'Leary S, Falla D, Elliott JM, et al: Muscle dysfunction in cervical spine pain: Implications for assessment and management, *J Orthop Sports Phys Ther* 39(5):324–333, 2009.

88. Armijo-Olivo S, Bravo J, Magee DJ, et al: The association between head and cervical posture and temporomandibular disorders: A systematic review, *J Orofac Pain* 20(1):9–23, 2006.

89. Armijo-Olivo S, Rappoport K, Fuentes J, et al: Head and cervical posture in patients with temporomandibular disorders (TMD), *J Orofac Pain* 25(3):199–209, 2011.

90. Armijo-Olivo S, Bravo J, Magee DJ, et al: The association between head and cervical posture and temporomandibular disorders: A systematic review, *J Orofac Pain* 20(1):9–23, 2006.

91. Falla D, Jull G, Russell T, et al: Effect of neck exercise on sitting posture in patients with chronic neck pain, *Phys Ther* 87(4):408–417, 2007.

92. McNeely M, Armijo-Olivo S, Magee D: A systematic review of physical therapy intervention for temporomandibular disorders, *Phys Ther* 86(5):710–720, 2006.

93. Stohler D: Management of dental occlusion. In Laskin D, Green C, Hylander W, editors: *TMDs: an evidence-based approach to diagnosis and treatment*, Chicago, 2006, Quintessence.

94. Celic R, Jerolimov V, Panduric J: A study of the influence of occlusal factors and parafunctional habits on the prevalence of signs and symptoms of TMD, *Int J Prosthodont* 15(1):43–48, 2002.

95. Gadotti IC, Bérzin F, Biasotto-Gonzalez D: Preliminary rapport on head posture and muscle activity in subjects with class I and II, *J Oral Rehabil* 32(11):794–799, 2005.

96. Carlsson GE, Egermark I, Magnusson T: Predictors of signs and symptoms of temporomandibular disorders: a 20-year follow-up study from childhood to adulthood, *Acta Odontolog Scand* 60(3):180–185, 2002.

97. Gesch D, Bernhardt O, Mack F, et al: Association of malocclusion and functional occlusion with subjective symptoms of TMD in adults: results of the Study of Health in Pomerania (SHIP), *Angle Orthod* 75(2):183–190, 2005.

98. Gesch D, Bernhardt O, Kocher T, et al: Association of malocclusion and functional occlusion with signs of temporomandibular disorders in adults: Results of the population-based study of health in Pomerania, *Angle Orthod* 74(4):512–520, 2004.

99. Carlson CR, Reid KI, Curran SL, et al: Psychological and physiological parameters of masticatory muscle pain, *Pain* 76(3):297–307, 1998.

100. Aaron LA, Burke MM, Buchwald D: Overlapping conditions among patients with chronic fatigue syndrome, fibromyalgia, and temporomandibular disorder, *Arch Int Med* 160(2):221–227, 2000.

101. Manfredini D, Winocur E, Ahlberg J, et al: Psychosocial impairment in temporomandibular disorders patients. RDC/TMD axis II findings from a multicentre study, *J Dent* 38(10):765–772, 2010.

102. Lajnert V, Franciskovic T, Grzic R, et al: Depression, somatization and anxiety in female patients with temporomandibular disorders (TMD), *Coll Antropol* 34(4):1415–1419, 2010.

103. Manfredini D: Bandettini di Poggio A, Cantini E et al: Mood and anxiety psychopathology and temporomandibular disorder: a spectrum approach, *J Oral Rehabil* 31(10):933–940, 2004.

104. Fillingim RB, Ohrbach R, Greenspan JD, et al: Psychological factors associated with development of TMD: the OPPERA prospective cohort study, *J Pain* 14(12 suppl):T75–T90, 2013.

105. Diagnostic criteria for temporomandibular disorders: clinical protocol and assessment instruments. http://www.rdc-tmdinternational.org/Portals/18/protocol_DC-TMD/DC-TMD%20Axis%20I%20&%20Axis%20II%20Protocol%20-%202013_06_08.pdf. Accessed September 10, 2014.

106. Ohrbach R, Larsson P, List T: The jaw functional limitation scale: development, reliability, and validity of 8-item and 20-item versions, *J Orofac Pain* 22(3):219–230, 2008.

107. Epstein JB, Klasser GD, Kolbinson DA, et al: Orofacial injuries due to trauma following motor vehicle collisions: part 2. Temporomandibular disorders, *J Can Dent Assoc* 76(1):a172, 2010.

108. Salé H, Isberg A: Delayed temporomandibular joint pain and dysfunction induced by whiplash trauma a controlled prospective study, *J Am Dent Assoc* 138(8):1084–1091, 2007.

109. Häggman-Henrikson B, List T, Westergren HT, et al: Temporomandibular disorder pain after whiplash trauma: a systematic review, *J Orofac Pain* 27(3):217–226, 2013.

110. Häggman-Henrikson B, Rezvani M, List T: Prevalence of whiplash trauma in TMD patients: a systematic review, *J Oral Rehabil* 41(1):59–68, 2014.

111. Visscher CM, Lobbezoo F, de Boer W, et al: Prevalence of cervical spinal pain in craniomandibular pain patients, *Eur J Oral Sci* 109(2):76–80, 2001.

112. Fink M, Tschernitschek H, Stiesch-Scholz M: Asymptomatic cervical spine dysfunction (CSD) in patients with internal derangement of the temporomandibular joint, *Cranio* 20(3):192–197, 2002.

113. De Wijer A, Steenks MH: Cervical spine evaluation for the temporomandibular disorders patient—a review. In Fricton J, Dubner R, editors: *Orofacial pain and temporomandibular disorders*, New York, 1995, Raven.

114. Stiesch-Scholz M, Fink M, Tschernitschek H: Comorbidity of internal derangement of the temporomandibular joint and silent dysfunction of the cervical spine, *J Oral Rehabil* 30(4):386–391, 2003.

115. Sipila K, Zitting P, Siira P, et al: Temporomandibular disorders, occlusion, and neck pain in subjects with facial pain: a case-control study, *Cranio* 20(3):158–164, 2002.

116. Ciancaglini R, Testa M, Radaelli G: Association of neck pain with symptoms of temporomandibular dysfunction in the general adult population, *Scand J Rehabil Med* 31(1):17–22, 1999.

117. Plesh O, Adams SH, Gansky SA: Temporomandibular joint and muscle disorder-type pain and comorbid pains in a national US sample, *J Orofac Pain* 25(3):190–198, 2011.

118. Armijo-Olivo S: *Relationship between cervical musculoskletal impairments and temporomandibular disorders: clinical and electromyographic variables*, Edmonton, 2010, Faculty of Rehabilitation Medicine, University of Alberta.

119. Sturdivant J, Fricton JR: Physical therapy for temporomandibular disorders and orofacial pain, *Curr Opin Dent* 1(4):485–496, 1991.

120. Melis M: The role of physical therapy for the treatment of temporomandibular disorders, *J Orthodont Sci* 2(4):113–114, 2013.

121. Rocabado M: The importance of soft tissue mechanics in stability and instability of the cervical spine: a functional diagnosis for treatment planning, *Cranio* 5(2):130–138, 1987.

122. Armijo-Olivo SA, Fuentes J, Major PW, et al: The association between neck disability and jaw disability, *J Oral Rehabil* 37(9):670–679, 2010.

123. Medlicott MS, Harris SR: A systematic review of the effectiveness of exercise, manual therapy, electrotherapy, relaxation training, and biofeedback in the management of temporomandibular disorder, *Phys Ther* 86(7):955–973, 2006.

124. Brantingham JW, Cassa TK, Bonnefin D, et al: Manipulative and multimodal therapy for upper extremity and temporomandibular disorders: a systematic review, *J Manip Physiol Ther* 36(3):143–201, 2013.

125. Armijo-Olivo S, Michelotti A, Thie N: Advances in physical therapy interventions for managing orofacial pain. In Sessle BJ, editor: *Orofacial pain: recent advances in assessment, management, and understanding of mechanisms*, Washington, DC, 2014, IASP.

126. List T, Axelsson S: Management of TMD: evidence from systematic reviews and meta-analyses, *J Oral Rehabil* 37(6):430–451, 2010.

127. Blackney M, Hertling D: The cervical spine. In Hertling D, Kessler R, editors: *Management of common musculoskeletal disorders: physical therapy principles and methods*, ed 3 Philadelphia, 1996, Lippincott Williams & Wilkins.

128. Fricton JR: Management of masticatory myofascial pain, *Sem Orthodont* 1(4):229–243, 1995.

129. Komiyama O, Kawara M, Arai M, et al: Posture correction as part of behavioural therapy in treatment of myofascial pain with limited opening, *J Oral Rehabil* 26(5):428–435, 1999.

130. Wright E, Domenec M, Fischer JJ: Usefulness of posture training for patients with temporomandibular disorders[see comment], *J Am Dent Assoc* 131(2):202–210, 2000.

131. Kropmans TJB, Dijkstra RU, Stegenga B, et al: Smallest detectable difference in outcome variables related to painful restriction of the temporomandibular joint, *J Dent Res* 78(3):784–789, 1999.

132. Craane B, Dijkstra PU, Stappaerts K, et al: One-year evaluation of the effect of physical therapy for masticatory muscle pain: a randomized controlled trial, *Eur J Pain* 16(5):737–747, 2012.

133. Gavish A, Winocur E, Astandzelov-Nachmias T, et al: Effect of controlled masticatory exercise on pain and muscle performance in myofascial pain patients: a pilot study, *Cranio* 24(3):184–190, 2006.

134. Magnusson T, Syren M: Therapeutic jaw exercises and interocclusal appliance therapy. A comparison between two common treatments of temporomandibular disorders, *Swedish Dent J* 23(1):27–37, 1999.

135. Maloney GE, Mehta N, Forgione AG, et al: Effect of a passive jaw motion device on pain and range of motion in tmd patients not responding to flat plane intraoral appliances, *Cranio* 20(1):55–65, 2002.

136. Michelotti A, Steenks MH, Farella M, et al: The additional value of a home physical therapy regimen versus patient education only for the treatment of myofascial pain of the jaw muscles: short-term results of a randomized clinical trial, *J Orofac Pain* 18(2):114–125, 2004.

137. Mulet M, Decker KL, Look JO, et al: A randomized clinical trial assessing the efficacy of adding 6×6 exercises to self-care for the treatment of masticatory myofascial pain, *J Orofac Pain* 21(4):318–328, 2007.

138. Crockett DJ, Foreman ME, Alden L, et al: A comparison of treatment modes in the management of myofascial pain dysfunction syndrome, *Biofeedback Self Regul* 11(4):279–291, 1986.

139. Cohen J: The concepts of power analysis. In Cohen J, editor: *Statistical power analysis for the behavioral sciences*, ed 2 Hillsdale, 1988, Academic Press.

140. Craane B, Dijkstra PU, Stappaerts K, et al: Randomized controlled trial on physical therapy for TMJ closed lock, *J Dent Res* 91(4):364–369, 2012.

141. de Felicio CM, Melchior Mde O, Ferreira CL, et al: Otologic symptoms of temporomandibular disorder and effect of orofacial myofunctional therapy, *Cranio* 26(2):118–125, 2008.

142. Diracoglu D, Bayraktar Saral I, Keklik B, et al: Arthrocentesis vs conventional methods in the pain and functional status of the patients with temporomandibular disc displacement without reduction, *Pain Pract* 9:47, 2009.

143. Stegenga B, De Bont LGM, Dijkstra PU, et al: Short-term outcome of arthroscopic surgery of temporomandibular joint osteoarthrosis and internal derangement: A randomized controlled clinical trial, *Br J Oral Maxillofac Surg* 31(1):3–14, 1993.

144. Tavera AT, Montoya MC, Calderon EF, et al: Approaching temporomandibular disorders from a new direction: a randomized controlled clinical trial of the TMDs ear system, *Cranio* 30(3):172–182, 2012.

145. Yoda T, Sakamoto I, Imai H, et al: A randomized controlled trial of therapeutic exercise for clicking due to disk anterior displacement with reduction in the temporomandibular joint, *Cranio* 21(1):10–16, 2003.

146. Yoshida H, Sakata T, Hayashi T, et al: Evaluation of mandibular condylar movement exercise for patients with internal derangement of the temporomandibular joint on initial presentation, *Br J Oral Maxillofac Surg* 49(4):310–313, 2011.

147. Yuasa H, Kurita K, Ogi N, et al: Randomized clinical trial of primary treatment for temporomandibular joint disk displacement without reduction and without osseous changes: A combination of NSAIDs and mouth-opening exercise versus no treatment, *Oral Surg Oral Med Oral Pathol Oral Radiol Endod* 91(6):671–675, 2001.

148. de Felicio CM, de Oliveira MM, da Silva MA: Effects of orofacial myofunctional therapy on temporomandibular disorders, *Cranio* 28(4):249–259, 2010.

149. Ficnar T, Middelberg C, Rademacher B, et al: Evaluation of the effectiveness of a semi-finished occlusal appliance—a randomized, controlled clinical trial, *Head Face Med* 9:5, 2013.

150. Niemela K, Korpela M, Raustia A, et al: Efficacy of stabilisation splint treatment on temporomandibular disorders, *J Oral Rehabil* 39(11):799–804, 2012.

151. Raustia AM: Diagnosis and treatment of temporomandibular joint dysfunction. Advantages of computed tomography diagnosis. Stomatognathic treatment and acupuncture—a randomized trial, *Proceedings of the Finnish Dental Society, Suom Hammaslaak Toim* 82:9–10, 1986.

152. Raustia AM, Pohjola RT: Acupuncture compared with stomatognathic treatment for TMJ dysfunction. Part III: effect of treatment on mobility, *J Prosthet Dent* 56(5):616–623, 1986.

153. Raustia AM, Pohjola RT, Virtanen KK: Acupuncture compared with stomatognathic treatment for TMJ dysfunction. Part I: a randomized study, *J Prosthet Dent* 54(4):581–585, 1985.

154. Maluf S, Moreno BGD, Osvaldo C, et al: A comparison of two muscular stretching modalities on pain in women with myogenous temporomandibular disorders, *Pain Pract* 9:49, 2009.

155. Truelove E, Huggins KH, Mancl L, et al: The efficacy of traditional, low-cost and nonsplint therapies for temporomandibular disorder: a randomized controlled trial, *J Am Dent Assoc* 137(8):1099–1107, 2006.

156. Grace EG, Sarlani E, Reid B: The use of an oral exercise device in the treatment of muscular TMD, *Cranio* 20(3):204–208, 2002.

157. Klobas L, Axelsson S, Tegelberg A: Effect of therapeutic jaw exercise on temporomandibular disorders in individuals with chronic whiplash-associated disorders, *Acta Odontol Scand* 64(6):341–347, 2006.

158. Burgess JA, Sommers EE, Truelove EL, et al: Short-term effect of two therapeutic methods on myofascial pain and dysfunction of the masticatory system, *J Prosthet Dent* 60(5):606–610, 1988.

159. Tegelberg A, Kopp S: Short-term effect of physical training on temporomandibular joint disorder in individuals with rheumatoid arthritis and ankylosing spondylitis, *Acta Odontol Scand* 46(1):49–56, 1988.

160. Tegelberg A, Kopp S: A 3-year follow-up of temporomandibular disorders in rheumatoid arthritis and ankylosing spondylitis, *Acta Odontol Scand* 54(1):14–18, 1996.

161. Koltyn KF: Analgesia following exercise: a review, *Sports Med* 29(2):85–98, 2000.

162. Kadetoff D, Kosek E: The effects of static muscular contraction on blood pressure, heart rate, pain ratings and pressure pain thresholds in healthy individuals and patients with fibromyalgia, *Eur J Pain* 11(1):39–47, 2007.

163. Kosek E, Lundberg L: Segmental and plurisegmental modulation of pressure pain thresholds during static muscle contractions in healthy individuals, *Eur J Pain* 7(3):251–258, 2003.

164. Feland JB, Myrer JW, Schulthies SS, et al: The effect of duration of stretching of the hamstring muscle group for increasing range of motion in people aged 65 years or older, *Phys Ther* 81(5):1110–1117, 2001.

165. Cheida A: Hiperboloid—mastication tool, *Brazilian J Ortodont Maxillo Orthop* 2(11):49–53, 1997.

166. Giannasi L, Batista S, Matsui M, et al: Effect of a hyperboloid mastication apparatus for the treatment of severe sleep bruxism in a child with cerebral palsy: long-term follow-up, *J Bodyw Mov Ther* 18:62–67, 2014.

167. Biazotto-Gonzalez D: Evaluation and physical therapy treatment. In Biazotto-Gozalez D, editor: *Interdisciplinary approach in temporomandibular dysfunctions [Portuguese]*, Sao Paulo, 2005, Manole.

168. Garcia J, Oliveira A: Physical therapy for signs and symptoms of temporomandibular joint dysfunction, *Revista Hórus* 5(1):113–124, 2001.

169. De Abreu K, Tenorio F, Nepomuceno R: Physical therapy intervention insubjects with oral cancer sequelae associated with temporomandibular dysfunction, *Revista Semente* 6(6):164–172, 2011.

170. Armijo-Olivo S, Magee DJ: Electromyographic activity of the masticatory and cervical muscles during resisted jaw opening movement, *J Oral Rehabil* 34(3):184–194, 2007.

171. Armijo-Olivo SA, Magee DJ: Electromyographic assessment of the activity of the masticatory using the agonist contract-antagonist relax technique (AC) and contract-relax technique (CR), *Man Ther* 11(2):136–145, 2006.

172. Rocabado M: *Head and neck: joint treatment*, Buenos Aires, 1979, Intermedica.

173. Kalamir A, Pollard H, Vitiello AL, et al: Manual therapy for temporomandibular disorders: a review of the literature, *J Bodyw Mov Ther* 11(1):84–90, 2007.

174. Carmeli E, Sheklow SL, Bloomenfeld I: Comparative study of repositioning splint therapy and passive manual range of motion techniques for anterior displaced temporomandibular discs with unstable excursive reduction, *Physiother* 87(1):26–36, 2001.

175. Maitland G: *Maitland's vertebral manipulation*, ed 6, Oxford, Boston, 2001, Butterworth Heineman Publisher.

176. Guarda-Nardini L, Stecco A, Stecco C, et al: Myofascial pain of the jaw muscles: comparison of short-term effectiveness of botulinum toxin injections and fascial manipulation technique, *Cranio* 30(2):95–102, 2012.

177. Kalamir A, Bonello R, Graham P, et al: Intraoral myofascial therapy for chronic myogenous temporomandibular disorder: a randomized controlled trial, *J Manip Physiol Ther* 35(1):26–37, 2012.

178. Kalamir A, Pollard H, Vitiello A, et al: Intra-oral myofascial therapy for chronic myogenous temporomandibular disorders: a randomized, controlled pilot study, *J Man Manipul Ther* 18(3):139–146, 2010.

179. Kalamir A, Graham PL, Vitiello AL, et al: Intra-oral myofascial therapy versus education and self-care in the treatment of chronic, myogenous temporomandibular disorder: a randomised, clinical trial, *Chiropract Man Ther* 21(1):17, 2013.

180. LaTouche R, Paris-Alemany A, Mannheimer JS, et al: Does mobilization of the upper cervical spine affect pain sensitivity and autonomic nervous system function in patients with cervico-craniofacial pain?: a randomized-controlled trial, *Clin J Pain* 29(3):205–215, 2013.

181. Farrar JT, Young JJP, LaMoreaux L, et al: Clinical importance of changes in chronic pain intensity measured on an 11-point numerical pain rating scale, *Pain* 94(2):149, 2001.

182. Van Der Roer N, Ostelo RWJG, Bekkering GE, et al: Minimal clinically important change for pain intensity, functional status, and general health status in patients with nonspecific low back pain, *Spine* 31(5):578–582, 2006.

183. Maughan EF, Lewis JS: Outcome measures in chronic low back pain, *Eur Spine J* 19(9):1484–1494, 2010.

184. Dworkin RH, Turk DC, Wyrwich KW, et al: Interpreting the clinical importance of treatment outcomes in chronic pain clinical trials: IMMPACT recommendations, *J Pain* 9(2):105–121, 2008.

185. Chesterton LS, Foster NE, Wright CC, et al: Effects of TENS frequency, intensity and stimulation site parameter manipulation on pressure pain thresholds in healthy human subjects, *Pain* 106(1-2):73–80, 2003.

186. Fuentes CJ, Armijo-Olivo S, Magee DJ, et al: A preliminary investigation into the effects of active interferential current therapy and placebo on pressure pain sensitivity: A random crossover placebo controlled study, *Physiother* 97(4):291–301, 2011.

187. Kovacs FM, Abraira V, Royuela A, et al: Minimal clinically important change for pain intensity and disability in patients with nonspecific low back pain, *Spine* 32(25):2915–2920, 2007.

188. La Touche R, Fernandez-De-Las-Penas C, Fernandez-Carnero J, et al: The effects of manual therapy and exercise directed at the cervical spine on pain and pressure pain sensitivity in patients with myofascial temporomandibular disorders, *J Oral Rehabil* 36(9):644–652, 2009.

189. Haketa T, Kino K, Sugisaki M, et al: Randomized clinical trial of treatment for TMJ disc displacement, *J Dent Res* 89(11):1259–1263, 2010.

190. Ismail F, Demling A, Hessling K, et al: Short-term efficacy of physical therapy compared to splint therapy in treatment of arthrogenous TMD, *J Oral Rehabil* 34(11):807–813, 2007.

191. Minakuchi H, Kuboki T, Maekawa K, et al: Self-reported remission, difficulty, and satisfaction with nonsurgical therapy used to treat anterior disc displacement without reduction, *Oral Surg Oral Med Oral Path Oral Radiol Endod* 98(4):435–440, 2004.

192. Minakuchi H, Kuboki T, Matsuka Y, et al: Randomized controlled evaluation of non-surgical treatments for temporomandibular joint anterior disk displacement without reduction, *J Dent Res* 80(3):924–928, 2001.

193. Yoshida H, Fukumura Y, Suzuki S, et al: Simple manipulation therapy for temporomandibular joint internal derangement with closed lock, *Asian J Oral Maxillofac Surg* 17(4):256–260, 2005.

194. Nascimento MM, Vasconcelos BC, Porto GG, et al: Physical therapy and anesthetic blockage for treating temporomandibular disorders: a clinical trial, *Med Oral Patol Oral Cir Bucal* 18(1):e81–e85, 2013.

195. Schiffman EL, Look JO, Hodges JS, et al: Randomized effectiveness study of four therapeutic strategies for TMJ closed lock, *J Dent Res* 86(1):58–63, 2007.

196. Cuccia AM, Caradonna C, Annunziata V, et al: Osteopathic manual therapy versus conventional conservative therapy in the treatment of temporomandibular disorders: A randomized controlled trial, *J Bodywork Movement Ther* 14(2):179–184, 2010.

197. Mansilla Ferragud P, Bosca Gandia JJ: Effect of upper cervical spine manipulation on mouth opening, *Osteopatia Cientifica* 3(2):45–51, 2008.

198. O'Reilly A, Pollard H: TMJ pain and chiropractic adjustment—a pilot study, *Chiropract J Australia* 26(4):125–129, 1996.

199. Otano L, Legal L: Radiological changes in the atlanto-occipital space after Fryette global manipulation (OAA), *Osteopatia Cientifica* 5(2):38–46, 2010.

200. Tuncer AB, Ergun N, Tuncer AH, et al: Effectiveness of manual therapy and home physical therapy in patients with temporomandibular disorders: a randomized controlled trial, *J Bodyw Mov Ther* 17(3):302–308, 2013.

201. von Piekartz H, Hall T: Orofacial manual therapy improves cervical movement impairment associated with headache and features of temporomandibular dysfunction: a randomized controlled trial, *Man Ther* 18(4):345–350, 2013.

202. von Piekartz H, Ludtke K: Effect of treatment of temporomandibular disorders (TMD) in patients with cervicogenic headache: a single-blind, randomized controlled study, *Cranio* 29(1):43–56, 2011.

203. Gray RJ, Quayle AA, Hall CA, et al: Physiotherapy in the treatment of temporomandibular joint disorders: a comparative study of four treatment methods, *Br Dent J* 176(7):257–261, 1994.

204. Petrucci A, Sgolastra F, Gatto R, et al: Effectiveness of low-level laser therapy in temporomandibular disorders: a systematic review and meta-analysis, *J Orofac Pain* 25(4):298–307, 2011.

205. Melis M, Di Giosia M, Zawawi KH: Low level laser therapy for the treatment of temporomandibular disorders: a systematic review of the literature, *Cranio* 30(4):304–312, 2012.

206. Carrasco TG, Mazzetto MO, Mazzetto RG, et al: Low intensity laser therapy in temporomandibular disorder: A phase II double-blind study, *Cranio* 26(4):274–281, 2008.

207. Conti PCR: Low level laser therapy in the treatment of temporomandibular disorders (TMD): a double-blind pilot study, *Cranio* 15(2):144–149, 1997.

208. Da Cunha LA, Firoozmand LM, Da Silva AP, et al: Efficacy of low-level laser therapy in the treatment of temporomandibular disorder, *Int Dent J* 58(4):213–217, 2008.

209. De Abreu Venancio R, Camparis CM: De Fátima Zanirato Lizarelli R: Low intensity laser therapy in the treatment of temporomandibular disorders: a double-blind study, *J Oral Rehabil* 32(11):800–807, 2005.

210. Emshoff R, Bösch R, Pümpel E, et al: Low-level laser therapy for treatment of temporomandibular joint pain: a double-blind and placebo-controlled trial, *Oral Surg Oral Med Oral Pathol Oral Radiol Endod* 105(4):452–456, 2008.

211. Kulekcioglu S, Sivrioglu K, Ozcan O, Parlak M: Effectiveness of low-level laser therapy in temporomandibular disorder, *Scand J Rheumatol* 32(2):114–118, 2003.

212. Bertolucci LE, Grey T: Clinical analysis of mid-laser versus placebo treatment of arthralgic TMJ degenerative joints, *Cranio* 13(1):26–29, 1995.

213. Bertolucci LE, Grey T: Clinical comparative study of microcurrent electrical stimulation to mid-laser and placebo treatment in degenerative joint disease of the temporomandibular joint, *Cranio* 13(2):116–120, 1995.

214. Carrasco TG, Guerisoli LDC, Guerisoli DMZ, et al: Evaluation of low intensity laser therapy in myofascial pain syndrome, *Cranio* 27(4):243–247, 2009.

215. Marini I, Gatto MR, Bonetti GA: Effects of superpulsed low-level laser therapy on temporomandibular joint pain, *Clin J Pain* 26(7):611–616, 2010.

216. Mazzetto MO, Carrasco TG, Bidinelo EF, et al: Low intensity laser application in temporomandibular disorders: A phase I double-blind study, *Cranio* 25(3):186–192, 2007.

217. Mazzetto MO, Hotta TH, Pizzo RCA: Measurements of jaw movements and TMJ pain intensity in patients treated with GaAlAs laser, *Brazilian Dent J* 21(4):356–360, 2010.

218. Shirani AM, Gutknecht N, Taghizadeh M, et al: Low-level laser therapy and myofacial pain dysfunction syndrome: A randomized controlled clinical trial, *Lasers Med Sci* 24(5):715–720, 2009.

219. Venezian GC, da Silva MA, Mazzetto RG, et al: Low level laser effects on pain to palpation and electromyographic activity in TMD patients: a double-blind, randomized, placebo-controlled study, *Cranio* 28(2):84–91, 2010.

220. McNeely M, Warren S: Value of confidence intervals in determining clinical significance, *Physiother Can* 58:205–211, 2006.

221. Bjordal JM, Couppe C, Chow RT, et al: A systematic review of low level laser therapy with location-specific doses for pain from chronic joint disorders, *Austr J Physiother* 49(2):107–116, 2003.

222. Sherman JJ, Turk DC: Nonpharmacologic approaches to the management of myofascial temporomandibular disorders, *Curr Pain Headache Rep* 5(5):421–431, 2001.

223. Shedden Mora MC, Weber D, Neff A, et al: Biofeedback-based cognitive-behavioral treatment compared with occlusal splint for temporomandibular disorder, *Clin J Pain* 29(12):1057–1065, 2013.

224. Crider AB, Glaros AG: A meta-analysis of EMG biofeedback treatment of temporomandibular disorders, *J Orofac Pain* 13(1):29–37, 1999.

225. Dalen K, Ellertsen B, Espelid I, et al: EMG feedback in the treatment of myofascial pain dysfunction syndrome, *Acta Odontol Scand* 44(5):279–284, 1986.

226. Dohrmann RJ, Laskin DM: An evaluation of electromyographic biofeedback in the treatment of myofascial pain-dysfunction syndrome, *J Am Dent Assoc* 96(4):656–662, 1978.

227. Hijzen TH, Slangen JL, van Houweligen HC: Subjective, clinical and EMG effects of biofeedback and splint treatment, *J Oral Rehabil* 13(6):529–539, 1986.

228. Stenn PG, Mothersill KJ, Brooke RI: Biofeedback and a cognitive behavioral approach to treatment of myofascial pain dysfunction syndrome, *Behavior Ther* 10(1):29–36, 1979.

229. Turk DC, Zaki HS, Rudy TE: Effects of intraoral appliance and biofeedback/stress management alone and in combination in treating pain and depression in patients with temporomandibular disorders, *J Prosthet Dent* 70(2):158–164, 1993.

230. Kato MT, Kogawa EM, Santos CN, et al: TENS and low-level laser therapy in the management of temporomandibular disorders, *J Appl Oral Sci* 14(2):130–135, 2006.

231. Monaco A, Sgolastra F, Ciarrocchi I, et al: Effects of transcutaneous electrical nervous stimulation on electromyographic and kinesiographic activity of patients with temporomandibular disorders: a placebo-controlled study, *J Electromyogr Kinesiol* 22(3):463–468, 2012.

232. Fricton JR: Management of masticatory myofascial pain, *Sem Orthodont* 1(4):229–243, 1995.

233. Nunez SC, Garcez AS, Suzuki SS, et al: Management of mouth opening in patients with temporomandibular disorders through low-level laser therapy and transcutaneous electrical neural stimulation, *Photomed Laser Surg* 24(1):45–49, 2006.

234. Deyo RA, Walsh NE, Martin DC, et al: A controlled trial of transcutaneous electrical nerve stimulation (TENS) and exercise for chronic low back pain, *New Engl J Med* 322(23):1627–1634, 1990.

235. Rodrigues D, Siriani AO, Berzin F: Effect of conventional TENS on pain and electromyographic activity of masticatory muscles in TMD patients, *Braz Oral Res* 18(4):290–295, 2004.

236. Alvarez-Arenal A, Junquera LM, Fernandez JP, et al: Effect of occlusal splint and transcutaneous electric nerve stimulation on the signs and symptoms of temporomandibular disorders in patients with bruxism, *J Oral Rehabil* 29(9):858–863, 2002.

237. Kruger LR, Van Der Linden WJ, Cleaton-Jones PE: Transcutaneous electrical nerve stimulation in the treatment of myofascial pain dysfunction, *S Afr J Surg* 36(1):35–38, 1998.

238. Treacy K: Awareness/relaxation training and transcutaneous electrical neural stimulation in the treatment of bruxism, *J Oral Rehabil* 26(4):280–287, 1999.

239. Wieselmann-Penkner K, Janda M, Lorenzoni M, et al: A comparison of the muscular relaxation effect of TENS and EMG-biofeedback in patients with bruxism, *J Oral Rehabil* 28(9):849–853, 2001.

240. Moystad A, Krogstad BS, Larheim TA: Transcutaneous nerve stimulation in a group of patients with rheumatic disease involving the temporomandibular joint, *J Prosthet Dent* 64(5):596–600, 1990.

241. Linde C, Isacsson G, Jonsson BG: Outcome of 6-week treatment with transcutaneous electric nerve stimulation compared with splint on symptomatic temporomandibular joint disk displacement without reduction, *Acta Odontol Scand* 53(2):92–98, 1995.

242. Gray RJ, Quayle AA, Hall CA, et al: Physiotherapy in the treatment of temporomandibular joint disorders: a comparative study of four treatment methods, *Br Dent J* 176(7):257–261, 1994.

243. Peroz I, Chun YH, Karageorgi G, et al: A multicenter clinical trial on the use of pulsed electromagnetic fields in the treatment of temporomandibular disorders, *J Prosthet Dent* 91(2):180–187, 2004.

244. Talaat AM, El-Dibany MM, El-Garf A: Physical therapy in the management of myofacial pain dysfunction syndrome, *Ann Otol Rhinol Laryngol* 95(3I):225–228, 1986.

245. Al-Badawi EA, Mehta N, Forgione AG, et al: Efficacy of pulsed radio frequency energy therapy in tem-poromandibular joint pain and dysfunction, *Cranio* 22(1):10–20, 2004.

246. Schiffman EL, Braun BL, Lindgren BR: Temporomandibular joint iontophoresis: a double-blind randomized clinical trial, *J Orofac Pain* 10(2):157–164, 1996.

247. Reid KI, Dionne RA, Sicard-Rosenbaum L, et al: Evaluation of iontophoretically applied dexamethasone for painful pathologic temporomandibular joints, *Oral Surg Oral Med Oral Pathol* 77(6):605–609, 1994.

248. Robertson VJ, Baker KG: A review of therapeutic ultrasound: effectiveness studies, *Phys Ther* 81(7):1339–1350, 2001.

249. Watson T: Ultrasound in contemporary physiotherapy practice, *Ultrasonics* 48(4):321–329, 2008.

250. Taube S, Ylipaavalniemi P, Könönen M, et al: The effect of pulsed ultrasound on myofacial pain, *A placebo controlled study*, *Proc Finn Dent Soc* 84(4):241–246, 1988.

251. Tsukiyama Y, Baba K, Clark GT: An evidence-based assessment of occlusal adjustment as a treatment for temporomandibular disorders, *J Prosthet Dent* 86(1):57–66, 2001.

252. Ohrbach R: Biobehavioral therapy. In Laskin D, Green C, Hylander W, editors: *TMDs: an evidence-based approach to diagnosis and treatment*, Chicago, 2006, Quintessence.

253. Sarlani E, Greenspan JD: Evidence for generalized hyperalgesia in temporomandibular disorders patients, *Pain* 102(3):221–226, 2003.

254. van Tulder MW, Touray T, Furlan AD, et al: Muscle relaxants for non-specific low back pain, *Cochrane Database Syst Rev* (2):2003 CD004252.

255. Ernst E, White AR: Acupuncture as a treatment for temporomandibular joint dysfunction: a systematic review of randomized trials, *Arch Otolaryngol Head Neck Surg* 125(3):269–272, 1999.

256. La Touche R, Goddard G, De-La-Hoz JL, et al: Acupuncture in the treatment of pain in temporomandibular disorders: A systematic review and meta-analysis of randomized controlled trials, *Clin J Pain* 26(6):541–550, 2010.

257. Goddard G, Karibe H, McNeill C, Villafuerte E: Acupuncture and sham acupuncture reduce muscle pain in myofascial pain patients, *J Orofac Pain* 16(1):71–76, 2002.

258. Johansson A, Wenneberg B, Wagersten C, et al: Acupuncture in treatment of facial muscular pain, *Acta Odontol Scand* 49(3):153–158, 1991.

259. List T, Helkimo M: Acupuncture and occlusal splint therapy in the treatment of craniomandibular disorders. II. A 1-year follow-up study, *Acta Odontol Scand* 50(6):375–385, 1992.

260. List T, Helkimo M, Andersson S, et al: Acupuncture and occlusal splint therapy in the treatment of craniomandibular disorders. Part I. A comparative study, *Swedish Dent J* 16(4):125–141, 1992.

261. List T, Helkimo M, Karlsson R: Pressure pain thresholds in patients with craniomandibular disorders before and after treatment with acupuncture and occlusal splint therapy: a controlled clinical study, *J Orofac Pain* 7(3):275–282, 1993.

262. Schmid-Schwap M, Simma-Kletschka I, Stockner A, et al: Oral acupuncture in the therapy of craniomandibular dysfunction syndrome—a randomized controlled trial (RCT), *Wien Klin Wochenschr* 118(1-2):36–42, 2006.

263. Shen YF, Goddard G: The short-term effects of acupuncture on myofascial pain patients after clenching, *Pain Pract* 7(3):256–264, 2007.

264. Shen YF, Younger J, Goddard G, Mackey S: Randomized clinical trial of acupuncture for myofascial pain of the jaw muscles, *J Orofac Pain* 23(4):353–359, 2009.

265. Smith P, Mosscrop D, Davies S, et al: The efficacy of acupuncture in the treatment of temporomandibular joint myofascial pain: a randomised controlled trial, *J Dent* 35(3):259–267, 2007.

266. Greene CS, Goddard G, Macaluso GM, et al: Topical review: placebo responses and therapeutic responses. How are they related? *J Orofac Pain* 23(2):93–107, 2009.

267. McNeill C: Orofacial pain and temporomandibular disorders. In McNeill C, editor: *Temporomandibular disorders: guidelines for classification, assessment, and management*, Carol Stream, 1993, Quintessence.

268. Glaros A, Kim-Weroha N, Lausten L, et al: Comparison of habit reversal and a behaviorally-modified dental treatment for temporomandibular disorders: a pilot investigation, *Appl Psychophysiol Biofeedback* 32(3-4):3–4, 2007.

269. Michelotti A, Cioffi I, Landino D, et al: Effects of experimental occlusal interferences in individuals reporting different levels of wake-time parafunctions, *J Orofac Pain* 26(3):168–175, 2012.

270. Michelotti A, Farella M, De Wijer A, et al: Home-exercise regimes for the management of non-specific temporomandibular disorders, *J Oral Rehabil* 32(11):779–785, 2005.

271. Michelotti A, Farella M, Vollaro S, et al: Mandibular rest position and electrical activity of the masticatory muscles, *J Prosthetic Dent* 78(1):48–53, 1997.

272. Dworkin S: Psychological and psychosocial psessment. In Laskin D, Green C, Hylander W, editors: *TMDs: an evidence-based approach to diagnosis and treatment*, Chicago, 2006, Quintessence.

273. Michelotti A, Cioffi I, Landino D, et al: Effects of experimental occlusal interferences in individuals reporting different levels of wake-time parafunctions, *J Orofac Pain* 26(3):168–175, 2012.

CHAPTER 5

Shoulder Trauma and Hypomobility

JUDY C. CHEPEHA

INTRODUCTION

Optimal functioning of the shoulder and arm can take place only if the delicate balance of healthy anatomy, proper biomechanics, and normal physiology is maintained. Disruption of any one of these three factors may lead to overload and injury, resulting in pain and dysfunction. A vast amount of information regarding the pathoanatomy and biomechanics of the shoulder has contributed to the clinician's ability to understand and manage patients with shoulder complaints more accurately and effectively.[1-11] Surgical techniques grounded in basic scientific principles related to the restoration of normal anatomy, biomechanics, and the physiology of injured or compromised structures have changed to allow for earlier introduction of rehabilitation. Keeping pace with changes in surgical intervention, rehabilitation programs are now based upon principles derived from pathophysiology, functional anatomy, and restoration of the entire kinetic chain from the lower extremity through the trunk, shoulder girdle, and arm.

Proper rehabilitation of the injured shoulder should be based on knowledge of the normal anatomy and function of the entire shoulder girdle complex and the inherent demands and potential mechanisms that may contribute to or cause injury to this region. Goals of simply increasing range of motion (ROM) and/or improving strength at the glenohumeral joint are no longer acceptable; rather, clinicians must be mindful of how the glenohumeral and scapulothoracic complex functions as part of the entire kinetic chain and understand the subtle relationships among all these interrelated components. Rehabilitation programs prescribed for the treatment of shoulder conditions should be centered on **principles of treatment** as well as specific condition exercise protocols, and these principles should be coupled with the clinician's knowledge of the shoulder, particularly how it functions under both normal and abnormal circumstances. Hopefully, advances in management of the injured shoulder are reflected in improved and earlier return to functional status for patients.

An advantage of managing the injured shoulder according to general treatment principles, rather than specific protocols, is the adaptability of these principles to many different situations. In other words, patients with different shoulder pathologies can benefit from the application of some or all of these treatment principles as they share the same goals of "normalizing" shoulder anatomy, biomechanics, and physiology.

Principles of Shoulder Treatment

- Proper and thorough assessment
- Early protected motion after a period of immobilization
- Proper evaluation and treatment of local and distant deficits
- Scapular control
- Pain management
- Sensorimotor control
- Progressions
- Closed chain axial loading exercise
- Functional exercises

Common Principles of Treatment

1. *Proper and Thorough Assessment:* As with any musculoskeletal pathology, treatment of the patient with a shoulder injury must begin with a thorough history and physical assessment. Assessment should include an evaluation of all shoulder girdle tissue as well as the cervical and thoracic spine regions. Depending on the patient and his or her shoulder condition, the lumbar spine and lower extremity may be important to also include in the assessment. Patients should be examined statically and dynamically and while they are performing functional activities.

2. *Protected Motion After a Period of Immobilization:* The shoulder complex, particularly the glenohumeral joint, is prone to stiffness after trauma or immobilization.[12,13] Early intervention through gentle ROM exercises and joint mobilization techniques may prevent this restriction of ROM, reduce the associated pain, and allow the shoulder to move into positions that can best address normalization of muscle activity and function. Special consideration must always be

given to surgically repaired tissue as well as the adaptive tightening of the glenohumeral posterior capsule, which presents clinically as a medial rotation deficit (i.e., glenohumeral internal rotation deficit [GIRD]), and finally the anterior shoulder muscles (e.g., pectoralis minor), which also tend to shorten.

3. *Evaluation and Treatment of Local and Distal Deficits:* Many shoulder injuries are associated with local and/or distal deficits in flexibility, strength, muscle balance, and proper mechanics that affect the whole kinetic chain. For example, hip and lumbar spine inflexibility, altered scapulohumeral rhythm, and reduced medial rotation motion may be part of the cause of the shoulder injury or may occur as a result of the injury. Regardless of the onset, all deficits of the kinetic chain must be noted on assessment and incorporated into a proper treatment plan.

4. *Scapular Control:* Scapular dyskinesis, an alteration in the position or motion of the scapula, is caused by weakness or inhibition of the periscapular muscles, especially the lower trapezius and serratus anterior.[14] The resultant loss of scapular control, coupled with an often overactive upper trapezius, can contribute to shoulder impingement and instability syndromes, acromioclavicular (AC) dysfunction, and rotator cuff weakness.[14-17] Proper shoulder rehabilitation must always include a thorough examination of the scapula and correction of any deficits.

5. *Pain Management:* Pain is a powerful inhibitor of muscle activation throughout the body. This is especially true at the shoulder because of the degree of muscle activity required to coordinate joint motion, stability, and function. Clinicians must closely monitor and manage pain, making certain that it is not causing inhibition of the weaker, targeted muscles and encouraging perpetuation of an improper muscle recruitment pattern.

6. *Sensorimotor Control:* Sensorimotor control is the neuromuscular control basis of sensory input, often known as proprioception. With the increased knowledge about the effect of changes in proprioception and neuromuscular control of joint stabilization in the shoulder, exercises that address retraining of this important factor have been integrated into treatment approaches.[16,18]

7. *Progressions:* Indications for progressing a patient to more challenging exercises are based in part on physiological principles of tissue healing and tissue response to injury. Decisions should also be made through the evaluation of the patient's ability to perform key functions at the shoulder girdle (i.e., scapular stabilization) and the entire kinetic chain; these include adequate hip and trunk extension, normal pelvic control, proper scapular control (especially into retraction and depression), normal scapulohumeral rhythm, and glenohumeral joint ROM.

8. *Closed Chain Axial Loading Exercises:* Closed chain rehabilitation exercises link the trunk to the scapula and the scapula to the arm; this allows strengthening of the scapular and arm musculature as a functional unit. These exercises should be performed along with early postoperative ROM techniques because they minimize the shear effect and reduce the open kinetic chain loading applied to the glenohumeral joint.[19-22]

9. *Functional Exercises:* Rehabilitation of the injured shoulder should always include exercises that are considered functional. However, clinicians must keep in mind that, for an exercise to be considered functional, it must reflect the individual patient's functional activities and goals for work, daily life, and recreation.

These nine shoulder rehabilitation principles form the foundation of treatment for most shoulder pathologies managed conservatively. Greater detail on specific treatments and exercise guidelines are presented throughout the remainder of this chapter and in Chapters 6 and 7.

SHOULDER ANATOMY

When considering the shoulder, the clinician must include the entire shoulder girdle, consisting of three bones (scapula, clavicle, and humerus) linked to each other and to the body by four joints (glenohumeral, AC, sternoclavicular, and scapulothoracic articulation). The combined effect of these four articulations is a high degree of mobility, which not only allows the arm and hand great functional capacity but also makes the shoulder particularly vulnerable to injury because stability is sacrificed for mobility. The glenohumeral joint has an almost global ROM due to the shallow glenoid socket, which is approximately one third to one fourth the size of the humeral head. The glenoid labrum, attached tightly to the bottom half of the glenoid and loosely to the top half, increases the glenoid depth approximately 2 times, adding to glenohumeral stability.[3,4] Normally when the humeral head is moved through its large ranges of motion, only a small amount of translation or excursion occurs between the humeral head and the glenoid. If the dynamic structures controlling this translation (primarily the rotator cuff) are injured, translation may increase, leading to increased wear on the glenoid labrum, failure of the static restraints, and eccentric overload of the dynamic restraints, resulting in instability, impingement, or both.[2,4,6,7,23-25]

The restraints of the glenohumeral joint typically are classified as either active (dynamic) or passive (static). Table 5-1 presents a list of the two groups. It is worth noting that even though the stabilizing components are divided into two groups, the actual mechanism of stability is not achieved through distinctive, separate processes but rather by one that is highly interconnected.

TABLE **5-1**

Restraints about the Glenohumeral Joint

Passive (Static)	Active (Dynamic)	
Capsule Labrum Coracohumeral ligament Superior glenohumeral ligament	Suprapinatus Infraspinatus Subscapularis Teres minor	Humeral stabilizers
Middle glenohumeral ligament Inferior glenohumeral ligament Geometry of humeral articular surface Geometry of glenoid articular surface Coracoacromial ligament Articular cartilage compliance Joint cohesion	Pectoralis major Latissimus dorsi Long head of the biceps Triceps Deltoid Teres major	Movers of glenohumeral joint
	Serratus anterior Latissimus dorsi Trapezius Rhomboids Levator scapulae Pectoralis minor	Scapular stabilizers

Modified from Zachazewski JE, Magee DJ, Quillen WS, editors: *Athletic injuries and rehabilitation*, p 510, Philadelphia, 1996, WB Saunders.

SHOULDER FUNCTION

The shoulder is the most proximal link of the upper extremity kinetic chain. It has evolved to allow humans great mobility so that they can position the most distal segment, the hand, for function. This seemingly simple task is achieved through a highly coordinated pattern of movement that begins in the lower extremities and moves sequentially to the trunk, scapulothoracic joint, glenohumeral joint, and elbow and eventually to the wrist and hand, where the function is performed.

Specific shoulder girdle function relies on the combined motion of the sternoclavicular, AC, glenohumeral, and scapulothoracic joints. This collective motion is achieved through the interaction of the muscles that influence the movement of the scapula, clavicle, and humerus relative to the axial skeleton. Research (in vivo and in vitro) has been done to try to elucidate the complex mechanism by which the shoulder moves and muscles act to facilitate these movements.[26,27] Early radiographic studies of arm elevation identified a 2:1 ratio of glenohumeral to scapulothoracic motion when the humerus is elevated in the coronal plane (Figure 5-1).[28] A similar analysis of elevation in the scapular plane found a ratio of 5:4 after the first 30° of elevation.[29,30] Similar studies carried out by other researchers found slight variations of these earlier observations.[31]

Elevation in a 30° to 40° anterior to the coronal plane customarily is referred to as *scapular plane elevation* or *scaption*. However, the scapula is a highly mobile reference point that not only moves with arm elevation but also inclines forward early in motion, obviously in a different direction from that of the intended elevation. Relative motion between the scapulothoracic joint and the glenohumeral joint has been referred to as the *scapulohumeral* or *glenohumeral rhythm*. The ratios of 2:1 and 5:4 are commonly accepted as representing the ratio of glenohumeral to scapulothoracic motion, but these values are only a limited reflection of the scapulothoracic and scapulohumeral combinations possible to achieve a given arm position. These ratios are based on two-dimensional radiographic projections of angular rotations taken at discrete positions of elevation; however, the arm moves in three dimensions, and for positions other than elevation, much of this motion is under voluntary control. These findings and others are not intended to dismiss completely all of our earlier understanding of scapulohumeral motion but rather to broaden awareness of the dynamic, multiplane model of the shoulder.

Muscle function at the shoulder is considered one of the highly intricate systems in the body. The function of a muscle with respect to any joint depends on the position of the skeletal components, distance of the muscle from the joint's center of rotation, and external and

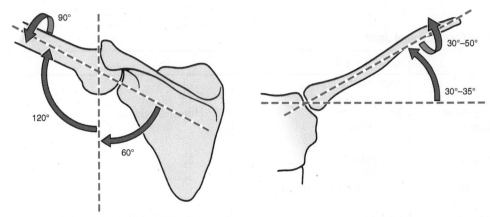

Figure 5-1 Movements of the scapula, humerus, and clavicle during scapulohumeral rhythm. (From Magee DJ: *Orthopedic physical assessment,* ed 6, p 274, St Louis, 2014, Saunders/Elsevier.)

internal forces acting at the time of muscle contraction. Given the three-dimensional, highly mobile nature of the shoulder joint, it is easy to understand why proper functioning of its muscles is essential for a normal, healthy shoulder.

The prime movers of the shoulder are the deltoid, pectoralis major, latissimus dorsi, and teres major muscles. Electromyographic studies[26,32-34] have shown that these muscles function predictably along their line of pull and that they form a drapelike effect over the shoulder, creating the potential for infinite lines of pull that may allow an almost 360° arc of motion.

The rotator cuff contributes to shoulder motion through a variety of means. The muscles of the rotator cuff can function as important movers of the upper extremity if the muscles' line of action is consistent with the intended direction of motion. This group of muscles also serves as a key set of stabilizing muscles for the glenohumeral joint by creating a compressive force that maintains the humeral head on the glenoid surface, and it can function to produce axial rotation of the humerus.

Finally, muscles that attach to the scapula and therefore control scapulothoracic joint motion have been decisively reported as playing a fundamental role in how the shoulder functions or, more appropriately, how *well* the shoulder functions. The work of researchers, such as Kibler[15] and Kibler and Livingstone,[21] has taught clinicians to be mindful of the trapezius, rhomboids, levator scapulae, teres minor, serratus anterior, and latissimus dorsi muscles because their attachments to the scapula allow for control of motion at the scapulothoracic articulation. Dysfunction or inhibition of any of these muscles has been shown to alter the position of the glenoid significantly, which in turn may result in abnormal centering of the humeral head within the glenohumeral joint.[6,15,35] The importance of proper scapulothoracic positioning at rest and during movement cannot be overemphasized, and clinicians must be cognizant of dysfunction at this region of the shoulder girdle.

STERNOCLAVICULAR AND ACROMIOCLAVICULAR JOINT INJURIES

Sternoclavicular (SC) Joint

The sternoclavicular joint is unique because it is the only true articulation between the clavicle of the upper extremity and axial skeleton. It is a diarthrodial type of joint, with the enlarged medial end of the clavicle creating a saddle-type articulation with the clavicular notch of the sternum. The clavicle is the first long bone in the body to ossify. The epiphysis at the medial end of the clavicle, however, is the last long bone to appear and is the last epiphysis to close at approximately 18 to 20 years of age. The epiphysis does not fuse with the shaft of the clavicle until 23 to 25 years of age; therefore the growth plate is the weakest point and more likely to sustain a displaced physeal fracture than a true dislocation.[36] This joint has the distinction of having the least amount of bony stability; therefore it relies heavily on support from the surrounding capsule and ligaments. These ligaments include the intra-articular disc ligament, extraarticular costoclavicular (rhomboid) ligament, interclavicular ligament, and capsular ligament.

The intra-articular disc ligament is a very dense, fibrous tissue that originates from the synchondral junction of the first rib to the sternum and travels through the sternoclavicular joint, dividing it into two distinct joint spaces (Figure 5-2). Anteriorly and posteriorly, the disc blends with the fibers of the capsular ligament. The intra-articular disc ligament functions as a checkrein for medial displacement of the proximal clavicle.

The costoclavicular, or rhomboid, ligament is short and strong and is made up of an anterior fasciculus and a posterior fasciculus. These two different parts give the ligament a slightly twisted appearance. Below, the costoclavicular ligament attaches to the upper surface of the first rib and at the adjacent part of the synchondral junction

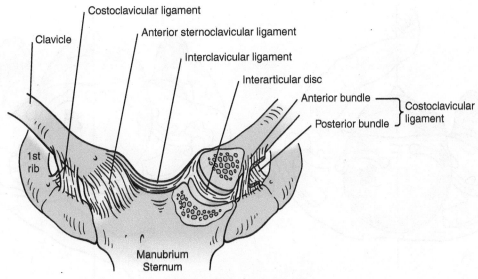

Figure 5-2 Sternoclavicular joint.

with the sternum; above, it attaches to the margins of the impression on the inferior surface of the medial end of the clavicle, sometimes called the *rhomboid fossa*.[37,38] Bearn[39] has shown that the anterior fibers resist excessive upward rotation of the clavicle and the posterior fibers resist excessive downward rotation. Specifically the anterior fibers resist lateral displacement, and the posterior fibers resist medial displacement.

The interclavicular ligament connects the superomedial aspects of each clavicle with the capsular ligaments and the upper aspect of the sternum (see Figure 5-2). Along with the capsular ligaments, the interclavicular ligament helps to hold up the shoulder. To demonstrate this, the clinician can place a finger in the superior sternal notch; the ligament is lax with elevation of the arm but becomes taut when both arms are left to hang at the sides.

The capsular ligament of the sternoclavicular joint, which extends over the anterosuperior and posterior aspects of the joint, represents thickenings of the joint capsule. The posterior capsule is the most important restraint for anterior and posterior translation of the sternoclavicular joint, whereas the anterior capsule acts mostly to prevent anterior translation. These capsular ligaments are considered the most important and strongest ligaments of the sternoclavicular joint and the structures most responsible for preventing upward displacement of the medial clavicle in the presence of a downward force on the distal end of the shoulder.[39]

Function of the Sternoclavicular Joint

The sternoclavicular joint is the most frequently moved, nonaxial joint in the body.[40] It acts similar to a ball and socket joint, allowing for motion in almost all planes, including rotation. In normal shoulder motion, the joint accounts for 30° to 35° of upward elevation, 35° of combined forward and backward movement, and 45° to 50° of rotation about the long axis of the clavicle and sternoclavicular joint.[28,41,42] It is important that clinicians appreciate that almost all motions of the upper extremity impact the sternoclavicular joint and conversely that motion at the sternoclavicular joint influences movement distally, along the upper extremity kinetic chain.

Sternoclavicular Joint Dislocations

Dislocations of the sternoclavicular joint are quite rare, accounting for approximately 3% of all fractures and dislocations affecting the shoulder girdle.[43,44] This is mostly due to the strength and integrity provided by the joint's surrounding capsuloligamentous tissue. Anterior dislocations are 2 to 3 times more common than posterior dislocations, fortunately, because posterior dislocations have a high complication rate with potentially life-threatening consequences (Figure 5-3).[36,38,45] The amount of force required to dislocate the sternoclavicular joint posteriorly is more than 1.5 times the force required for anterior dislocation. In addition, a posterior dislocation may put pressure on the underlying mediastinal structures, including the brachial plexus, vascular structures, trachea, and esophagus (Figure 5-4).[46,47] Complications include brachial plexus lesions, pneumothorax and respiratory distress, vascular injury, dysphagia, and hoarseness.[48,49] Motor vehicle accidents are reported as the most common cause of dislocation of the sternoclavicular joint, followed by direct or indirect trauma during a sporting activity. An example of a direct trauma in a sporting activity might be a hockey player hitting the medial side of the clavicle on the goalpost or on another player's knee. With an indirect injury, the athlete may be lying on his side, and the uppermost shoulder is compressed and rolled backward, resulting in an anterior sternoclavicular dislocation on that side. If the shoulder rolls forward and is compressed, a posterior dislocation is more likely.[45,50]

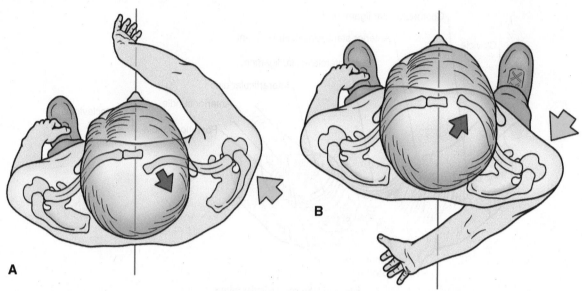

Figure 5-3 Mechanism of injury to the sternoclavicular joint. **A,** Posterior applied force (*green arrow*) directed anteriorly causes proximal end of clavicle to move posteriorly (*red arrow*). **B,** Anterior applied force (*green arrow*) directed posteriorly causes proximal end of clavicle to move anteriorly (*red arrow*). (Redrawn from Emery R: Acromioclavicular and sternoclavicular joints. In Copland SA, editor: *Shoulder surgery*, Philadelphia, 1997, WB Saunders; and Rockwood CA, Green DP, editors: *Fractures*, vol 1, ed 2, Philadelphia, 1984, JB Lippincott.)

Sternoclavicular dislocations are classified according to patient age, severity, and direction of dislocation. Mild sternoclavicular joint injuries are those in which the joint is stable and the ligamentous integrity has been maintained. Moderate injuries have had part of the ligamentous tissue disrupted, and the sternoclavicular joint has partially separated or subluxed. Complete ligamentous disruption, resulting in an unstable sternoclavicular joint, is considered a severe injury. The degree of separation can also be classified as first, second, or third, but this classification is based more on injury to the ligaments supporting the joint rather than injury to the joint itself. A first-degree sternoclavicular dislocation results in minor tearing (first- or second-degree sprain) of the sternoclavicular and costoclavicular ligaments, with no true displacement of the joint. A complete tear (third-degree sprain) in the sternoclavicular ligaments and a second-degree sprain of the costoclavicular ligament constitute a second-degree sternoclavicular dislocation and actually result in subluxation of the joint. A third-degree sternoclavicular dislocation is a true dislocation of the joint, caused by third-degree sprains in the sternoclavicular and costoclavicular ligaments.[51]

Clinical Presentation of Sternoclavicular Joint Dislocations

Sternoclavicular dislocations are characterized by deformity, ecchymosis, crepitus, and local pain or tenderness, especially with arm movements that roll the shoulders forward and/or lying supine. In the acute situation, clinicians should note any tenting of the skin, which could be indicative of an underlying fracture or dislocation of the sternoclavicular joint. A careful neurological and vascular examination should always be performed because of the joint's proximity to these key structures. Observation of an anterior sternoclavicular dislocation will show a prominent medial clavicle that is more anterior compared with the sternum, whereas a posterior dislocation will reveal a medial clavicle that is less visible and often not palpable. With a posterior dislocation or subluxation, some shortness of breath or even venous congestion in the neck may be seen, with decreased circulation sometimes evident in the arm. Reduction of a posterior sternoclavicular dislocation usually is accomplished by extending the shoulders while using some form of roll or sandbag as a fulcrum along the spine. Reduction most often occurs easily, although in some cases supplemental anesthesia may be required. The practitioner also may need to grasp the clavicle with the fingers or, if the anatomy is less defined, with some type of surgical instrument, such as a towel clip.

Treatment of Sternoclavicular Joint Dislocations

Goals of treatment following a sternoclavicular injury include pain control, reduction and/or immobilization as indicated, identification and management of associated injuries, and education regarding protection and prevention of subsequent injury. If the sternoclavicular joint has incurred only a first- or second-degree sprain and the joint is deemed stable, treatment follows a course similar to that for any other injured joint. The patient's shoulder should be immobilized for 3 to 4 days, as pain dictates, and then should make a gradual return to normal use of the shoulder and arm. Local electrical modalities and the use of ice and heat may be helpful for reducing pain and inflammation at the sternoclavicular joint. The clinician should be aware of the impact of a sternoclavicular injury on the entire shoulder complex because the effects of the initial injury may be far-reaching and can lead to compensatory patterns of movement.

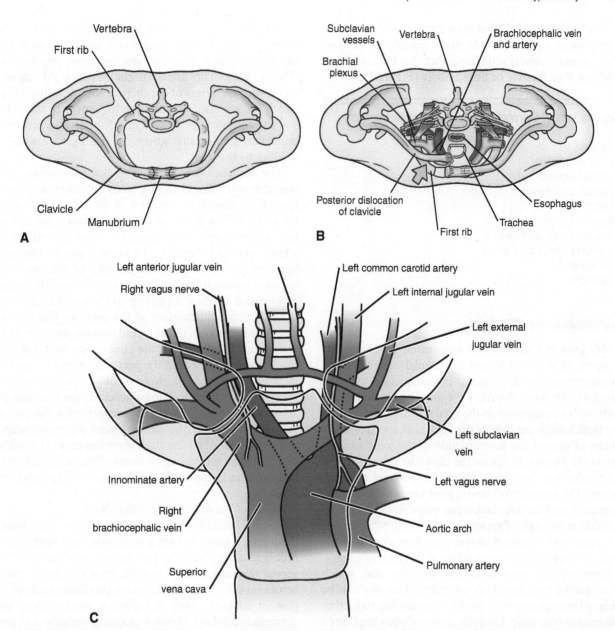

Figure 5-4 Sternoclavicular joint posterior dislocation. **A,** Overhead view of normal anatomical relationships. **B,** Posterior dislocation of the sternoclavicular joint. Note proximity of vessels which could be compressed with dislocation. *Arrow* indicates direction of force. **C,** Anterior view of retrosternal anatomy. Note the proximity of the sternoclavicular joint to the trachea, aortic arch, and brachiocephalic vein. (**C,** From Magee DJ: *Orthopedic physical assessment,* ed 6, p 257, St Louis, 2014, Saunders/Elsevier; redrawn from Higginbotham TO, Kuhn JE: Atraumatic disorders of the sternoclavicular joint, *J Am Acad Orthop Surg* 13:139, 2005.)

In second- or third-degree sprains of the sternoclavicular joint, if the main complaint after reduction is instability, treatment frequently requires sling support for an anterior dislocation or a figure-of-eight bandage for the posterior dislocation. The sling is worn for at least 2 to 3 weeks. Chronic instability may require surgical stabilization of the sternoclavicular joint, which is by no means uniformly successful. Chronic subluxation or damage to the intra-articular disc can produce long-term discomfort with repetitive strong movements of the upper limb.

Complications of anterior sternoclavicular dislocation include cosmetic deformity, recurrent instability, and late osteoarthrosis; complications of posterior dislocation include all of these plus pressure on or rupture of the trachea,

pneumothorax, rupture of the esophagus, pressure on the subclavian artery or brachial plexus, voice change, and dysphagia. Although the incidence of one of these complications can be as high as 25%, only about three deaths have been reported in the literature from the more serious complications associated with this injury.[45,51]

Atraumatic anterior subluxation of the sternoclavicular joint during arm elevation is occasionally reported in patients younger than 30 years of age. Many individuals affected by this condition demonstrate signs of generalized ligamentous laxity. Patients report a nontraumatic, spontaneous subluxation of the medial end of the clavicle, occasionally with a pop, that reduces when the arm lowers back down. Most cases are not painful and do not interfere with functional activities; therefore management is conservative with the focus on patient education regarding the anatomical events involved and reassurance that the condition should not alter lifestyle or limit activity (Figure 5-5).[52,53]

Complications of Sternoclavicular Posterior Dislocation

- Cosmetic deformity
- Recurrent instability
- Late osteoarthritis
- Pressure on or rupture of the trachea
- Pneumothorax
- Rupture of the esophagus
- Pressure on the subclavian artery
- Pressure on the brachial plexus
- Voice change
- Dysphagia

Acromioclavicular (AC) Joint

The AC joint is a diarthrodial joint made up of the lateral aspect of the clavicle and the medial margin of the acromion process of the scapula. In conjunction with the sternoclavicular joint, the AC joint provides the upper extremity with a connection to the axial skeleton. The articular surfaces initially are hyaline cartilage until approximately 17 years of age on the acromial side of the joint and approximately 24 years of age on the clavicular side. After this time, the hyaline cartilage acquires the structure of fibrocartilage. The anatomy of the AC joint varies considerably; the articular surface orientation can range from vertical to overriding at an angle of approximately 50°.[45,54-56] The dramatic variation in anatomy may explain why some individuals seem more susceptible to injury at this joint.

Within the AC joint is an intra-articular disc, which may be partial (meniscoid) or complete. This disc can be damaged through injury to the AC joint leading to further degeneration over time. Unstable discs are often implicated as the cause of clicking and recurrent pain at the AC joint.

The AC joint is surrounded by a thin capsule that is reinforced above, below, anteriorly, and posteriorly by the superior, inferior, anterior, and posterior AC ligaments (Figure 5-6). The fibers of the superior AC ligament blend with the fibers of the deltoid and trapezius muscles, which are attached to the superior aspect of the clavicle and the acromion process. These muscle attachments are important as they strengthen the AC ligaments and add stability to the joint.

The coracoclavicular ligament is a very strong, heavy ligament with fibers running from the outer, inferior surface of the clavicle to the base of the coracoid process of the scapula. The ligament consists of two individual ligaments, the conoid and trapezoid, which sometimes have a bursa between them. As the name suggests, the conoid ligament is cone shaped, with the apex of the cone attaching on the posteromedial aspect of the base of the coracoid process and the base attaching to the conoid tubercle on the posterior undersurface of the clavicle. The trapezoid ligament arises from the coracoid process, anterior and lateral to the attachment of the conoid ligament just posterior to the attachment of the pectoralis minor tendon. The ligament travels superiorly to a rough line on the undersurface of the clavicle. The coracoclavicular ligament plays an important role not only in strengthening the AC joint but also in assisting the glenohumeral joint with scapulohumeral motion. As the clavicle rotates upward, it dictates scapulothoracic rotation by virtue of its attachment to the scapula, that is, the conoid and trapezoid ligaments.[55,57]

Function of the Acromioclavicular Joint

Codman[58] described the motion at the AC joint as "swinging a little, rocking a little, twisting a little, sliding a little and acting like a hinge." Subsequent authors[59,60] observed relatively little motion between the clavicle and the acromion during studies involving percutaneous implanted pins in subjects. They described a synchronous, three-dimensional linkage between clavicular rotation and scapular rotation, such that when the clavicle rotates, the scapula

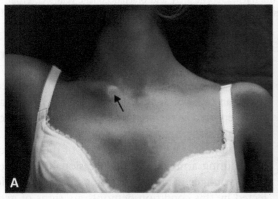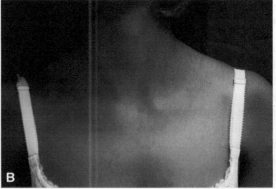

Figure 5-5 Spontaneous subluxation of the sternoclavicular joint. **A,** With the arms in the overhead position, the medial end of the right clavicle spontaneously subluxes out anteriorly (*arrow*) without any trauma. **B,** When the arm is brought back down to the side, the medial end of the clavicle spontaneously reduces. This usually is associated with no significant discomfort. (From Rockwood CA, Matsen FA, Wirth MA, et al, editors: *The shoulder,* ed 4, p 535, Philadelphia, 2009, Saunders.)

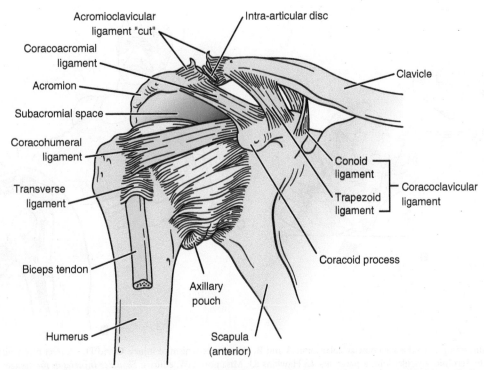

Figure 5-6 Anterior view of the right glenohumeral and acromioclavicular joints. Note the subacromial space or supraspinatus outlet located between the top of the humeral head and the underside of the acromion. The **coracoacromial arch** forming the ceiling of the subacromial space is made up of the undersurfaces of the acromion process, the coracoacromial ligament, and the coracoid process. (From Magee DJ: *Orthopedic physical assessment,* ed 6, p 256, St Louis, 2014, Saunders/Elsevier; modified from Neumann DA: *Kinesiology of the musculoskeletal system: foundations for rehabilitation,* ed 2, St Louis, 2010, Mosby.)

also rotates, concluding that most scapulothoracic motion occurs through the sternoclavicular joint, not the AC joint.

In a classic article published in 1944, Inman[41] suggested that the total ROM of the AC joint was 20° and that clavicular rotation was a fundamental feature of shoulder motion. He noted that motion occurred in the first 30° of abduction and then again after 135° of arm elevation. He also showed that with full elevation, the clavicle rotates upward 40° to 50°. Since these original observations, researchers have disputed the amount of motion that occurs at the AC joint relative to the glenohumeral joint.[54,61,62] Despite the controversy, researchers agree on the important relationship between the two joints and recognize that scapulohumeral rhythm is a delicate balance achieved through a combination of elevation and rotation of the clavicle and proper scapulothoracic and glenohumeral joint motion.

Acromioclavicular Joint Injuries

The AC joint is one of the most frequently injured joints in the body, particularly in sports and activities that require overhead involvement of the shoulder and arm and/or that have a high risk of collision and impact. Injuries to the AC joint result in what is often called a "separated" shoulder, and they account for 9% to 10% or acute injuries to the shoulder girdle in the general population, whereas separations of the AC joint account for 40% of shoulder girdle injuries in athletes.[40,61–64] Common mechanisms of injury include falls on an outstretched hand or elbow

(i.e., FOOSH injury), direct blows to the shoulder, or falling onto the point of the shoulder (Figure 5-7).

As with the sternoclavicular joint, AC joint injuries are classified according to ligamentous injury rather than injury to the joint itself. Table 5-2 describes the features and management of the six classifications of AC joint injury (Figures 5-8 and 5-9). Some have suggested that third-degree (type III) disruptions can be further divided according to the magnitude of displacement and the potential accompanying muscle and soft tissue stripping and tearing as well as the direction of displacement of the distal clavicle.[45,59] For instance, displacement of the clavicle of more than 100% is often classified as a fourth-degree (type IV) injury. Type V injuries involve very severe deformity because the distal end of the clavicle is displaced upward a significant degree toward the base of the neck (Figure 5-10). In addition, displacements may occur posteriorly through the trapezius or, in rare cases, inferiorly below the coracoid (type VI). Fourth-degree injuries are associated with considerable disruption of the deltoid and trapezius muscles. A third-degree separation may be treated without surgery, but surgery does have a role in the treatment of fourth-, fifth-, and sixth-degree injuries because of the associated ligamentous disruption and because of cosmetic considerations in leaner individuals (see Figure 5-8).[65–68]

Clinical Presentation of Acromioclavicular Joint Injuries

Patients who have suffered an injury to the AC joint typically present with a history of either a distinctive, traumatic

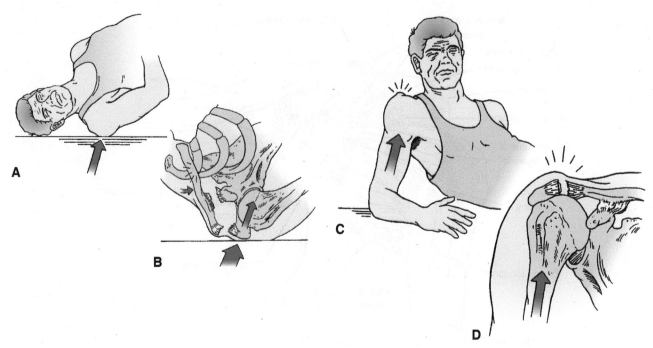

Figure 5-7 Mechanisms of injury to the acromioclavicular joint. **A** and **B**, Direct mechanism of injury. **C** and **D**, Indirect mechanism of injury. (From Field LD, Warren RF: Acromioclavicular joint separations. In Hawkins RJ, Misamore GW, editors: *Shoulder injuries in the athlete: surgical repair and rehabilitation*, p 206, New York, 1996, Churchill Livingstone.)

mechanism of injury or a more insidious type of onset that began with pain and dysfunction. The diagnosis is made in part by assessing the site of local tenderness, the degree of deformity, and whether instability is present. As with the sternoclavicular joint, injury to the AC joint tends to cause localized pain with minimal referral. Stressing the joint with horizontal adduction elicits pain in the injured AC joint, as does loading the joint by applying leverage at the distal arm. A palpable gap (i.e., a step deformity) may be present with the higher degrees of separation (Figure 5-11). With trauma to the AC joint, the clinician must take care to assess for secondary injury to the surrounding soft tissues (e.g., the rotator cuff) and to the other three articulations of the shoulder complex. Long term, most people function well

TABLE 5-2

Classification of Acromioclavicular Joint Trauma

Classification	Salient Features	Management
First degree (type I)	• Minimal structural damage • First-degree sprain of the acromioclavicular ligament • Local tenderness on palpation • Full range of motion (may have pain at extreme) • No loss of structural strength • Normal stress x-ray film	• Re-establish full range of motion and strength
Second degree (type II)	• Subluxation of the acromioclavicular joint • Tearing of the acromioclavicular capsule • Second- or third-degree sprain of the acromioclavicular ligament • First- or second-degree sprain of the coracoclavicular ligament • May affect the deltoid and trapezius muscles • No significant increase in the costoclavicular space on stress x-ray film • Slight widening of the acromioclavicular joint on stress x-ray film • Definite structural weakness • Detectable instability on stress • Palpable gap or step deformity possible • Obvious swelling initially with later ecchymosis	• Requires 6 weeks to heal, although ligaments have good structural strength after approximately 3 weeks • Limb support (sling) • Treatments for pain relief (e.g., ice, transcutaneous electrical nerve stimulation [TENS], interferential therapy) • Therapeutic ultrasound therapy for collagen enhancement • Functional exercises (activities at functional speed control)

TABLE **5-2**

Classification of Acromioclavicular Joint Trauma—Cont'd

Classification	Salient Features	Management
Third degree (type III)	• Dislocation of the acromioclavicular joint • Complete disruption of the acromioclavicular joint • Third-degree sprain of the acromioclavicular ligament • Third-degree sprain of the coracoclavicular ligament • Tearing of the deltoid and trapezius muscles from the distal end of the clavicle • Obvious step deformity, often without stress • Increased costoclavicular space on stress x-ray film • Widening of the acromioclavicular joint on stress x-ray film	• May be treated surgically or conservatively • If treated conservatively, deformity remains but athlete will function remarkably well with only slight discomfort or instability at high loads • Conservative treatment as above
Fourth degree (type IV)	• Modifications of type III trauma (rare injuries)	• Require surgical repair
Fifth degree (type V)	• Modifications of type III trauma (rare injuries)	• Require surgical repair
Sixth degree (type VI)	• Modifications of type III trauma (rare injuries)	• Require surgical repair

Modified from Zachazewski JE, Magee DJ, Quillen WS, editors: *Athletic injuries and rehabilitation*, p 519, Philadelphia, 1996, WB Saunders.

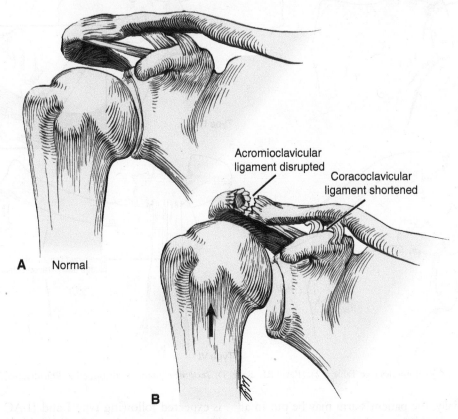

Figure 5-8 Disruption of the acromioclavicular ligament with preservation of the coracoclavicular ligaments. (Redrawn from Rockwood CA, Green DP, editors: *Fractures*, vol 1, ed 2, Philadelphia, 1984, JB Lippincott.)

without surgery, although degenerative changes, including clavicular osteolysis, may be seen in some individuals.

Treatment of Acromioclavicular Joint Injuries

Management of an AC joint injury depends on the type of separation. It is generally agreed upon that higher-grade lesions (i.e., type IV to VI) should be treated surgically, whereas lower-grade lesions (i.e., type I and II) are best

managed conservatively. How to best treat type III injuries remains controversial; however, current literature suggests the decision should be made on a case-by-case basis with an emphasis on initial nonoperative treatment.[69,70] The ultimate function of the AC joint depends not so much on the amount of separation as on the amount of pain that persists in the joint. Therefore early conservative treatment for first- and second-degree separations focuses

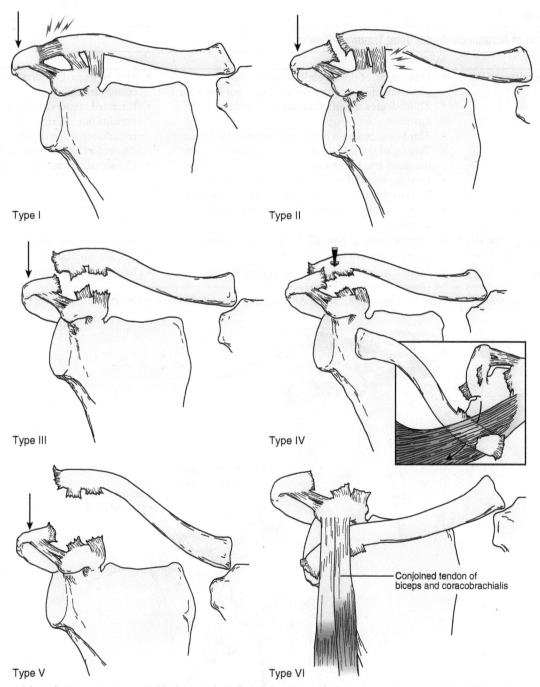

Figure 5-9 Acromiclavicular joint injuries (see Table 5-2). (Rakel RE, Rakel D: *Textbook of family medicine*, ed 9, Philadelphia, 2016, Saunders.)

on pain relief. Initially, the patient's arm may be put in a sling, often accompanied by a swath, to remove the stress of the weight of the limb on the joint and to protect the joint from further damage. This period of immobilization is accompanied by ice and oral analgesic medication, if tolerated. As the pain decreases (within 3 to 7 days), ROM and strengthening exercises, especially for the scapular stabilizers, deltoid, and upper trapezius muscles, are initiated. During this time, heavy lifting and contact sports are avoided to encourage optimal ligament healing. Patients generally return to light-moderate activities 2 to 6 weeks after injury. Return to sport and/or heavy labor

is expected following type I and II AC joint separations; however, the timeframe for this is highly dependent upon the individual and his or her specific activity. Associated soft tissue trauma in type II and III injuries typically is more extensive; therefore the time frame is likely to be prolonged for all the suggested treatments.

With third-degree (type III) AC joint injuries, complete reduction is not necessary for satisfactory function; in fact, in terms of strength, endurance, and function, nonsurgical and surgical treatments have been reported to be equally effective.[67-74] Depending on the preference of the surgeon, type III injuries may be treated surgically,

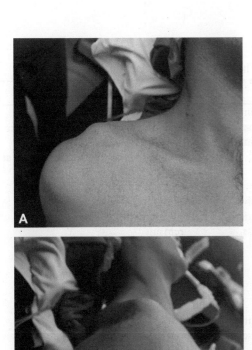

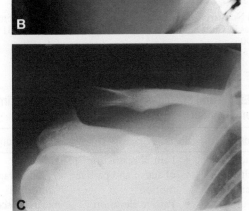

Figure 5-10 Typical findings after a type V AC joint injury, anterior view (**A**) and lateral view (**B**). There is a twofold to threefold increase in the coracoclavicular distance as well as a stripping of the deltoid and trapezial fascia from the clavicle. This patient was unable to reduce the AC joint with an active shoulder shrug, indicating a true type V injury instead of a type III injury. **C,** Anteroposterior radiographic view demonstrates widening, evidence of a type V injury. (From Miller MD, Thompson SR: *DeLee & Drez's orthopaedic sports medicine: Principles and practices,* ed 3, Philadelphia, 2010, Saunders.)

but the results are seldom better than with conservative treatment, recovery period is longer, and complications of surgery must be considered. For these reasons, most surgeons opt for initial nonoperative treatment, focused on attaining full ROM and scapular stabilization. Surgical consideration is given only to those patients who fail conservative management and present with persistent symptoms and functional limitations.

Types IV, V, and VI require surgical repair to stabilize the joint.

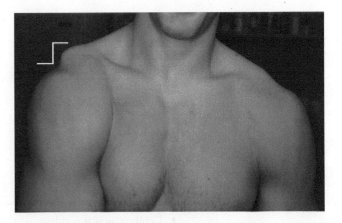

Figure 5-11 Step deformity resulting from acromioclavicular joint trauma (note "step"). (From Magee DJ: *Orthopedic physical assessment,* ed 6, p 265, Philadelphia, 2014, WB Saunders.)

Complications of an AC joint injury include a step deformity produced by the elevated distal end of the clavicle, early skin necrosis if the clavicle is widely displaced in a thin individual, osteoarthrosis, osteolysis, and continuing pain in the long term. For surgical procedures, complications include infection, wound dehiscence, pin migration, and recurrence of the instability, as well as the normal risks of general anesthesia.

FROZEN SHOULDER

The first reported description of frozen shoulder was made by Duplay in the late 1800s.[75] They used the label *scapulohumeral periarthritis* to describe a broad spectrum of pathologies of the shoulder that resulted in pain, stiffness, and dysfunction. This label served as an umbrella term that encompassed disorders such as rotator cuff tendonitis and tears, biceps tendonitis and tears, calcific deposits, AC arthritis, and other painful shoulder syndromes. The term *frozen shoulder* was later coined in 1934 by Codman,[76] who characterized the condition as involving a slow onset, pain near the deltoid insertion, inability to sleep on the affected side, painful and restricted elevation and lateral (external) rotation, and a normal radiological appearance. Even then, Codman described the condition as "difficult to define, difficult to treat and difficult to explain from the point of view of pathology." Subsequent to Codman's observations, Neviaser[77] in 1945 recorded his operative and histological observations from 10 patients with frozen shoulder, noting it was the capsule not the bursa that was thickened and adhered to the humeral head. As a result, he suggested *adhesive capsulitis* as a more descriptive term for shoulders that appeared frozen. More recent investigations have shown that frozen shoulders do not always possess capsular adhesions or, if they do, the adhesions are not always on to the humerus, as first described. Therefore the term *adhesive capsulitis* has been suggested as not appropriate to describe frozen shoulders and should not be used.[78–80]

TABLE 5-3

Types of Secondary Frozen Shoulder

Type	Contributing Causes
Intrinsic	• Calcific tendinosis • Rotator cuff tendinopathy • Biceps tendinopathy • Shoulder surgery
Extrinsic	• Humeral fractures • Clavicular fractures • Cervical radiculopathy • Ipsilateral breast surgery • Chest wall tumor • Cerebrovascular accident
Systemic	• Diabetes • Thyroid abnormalities • Heart disease

TABLE 5-4

Three Phases of Primary (Idiopathic) Frozen Shoulder

Phase	Clinical Presentation
Freezing phase (painful)	Duration: 10 to 36 weeks Pain and stiffness around the shoulder No history of injury Nagging, constant pain that is worse at night Little or no response to NSAIDs
Adhesive/ restrictive phase	Duration: 4 to 12 weeks Pain gradually subsides but stiffness remains Pain apparent only at extremes of movement Gross reduction of glenohumeral movements with near total loss of lateral (external) rotation
Resolution phase	Duration: 12 to 42 weeks Spontaneous improvement in ROM Mean duration from onset of frozen shoulder to greatest resolution exceeds 30 weeks

NSAIDs, Nonsteroidal anti-inflammatory drugs; *ROM,* range of motion. From Dias R, Cutts S, Massoud S: Frozen shoulder, *Br Med J* 331:1453-1456, 2005.

Lundberg[81] introduced the terms *primary* and *secondary* to further describe frozen shoulders in 1969. Primary frozen shoulders are those with an idiopathic onset (i.e., no detectable underlying cause), whereas secondary frozen shoulders occur following trauma and/or immobilization. Secondary frozen shoulders have been further classified into intrinsic, extrinsic, and systemic categories by Zuckerman and Rokito[82] and are presented along with contributing causes in Table 5-3.

Despite frozen shoulder being recognized for more than 100 years, there still remains a lack of evidence regarding its etiology, natural history, and best method of management. Clinicians must work closely with their patients with frozen shoulders to tailor treatment plans that best meet the needs of each individual patient, depending on factors such as stage of disease, symptom severity, age, occupation, and expected goals.

Clinical Presentation of Frozen Shoulder

Patients with an idiopathic frozen shoulder tend to progress through three overlapping clinical phases (Table 5-4).[83,84] Phase 1 lasts anywhere from 2 to 9 months and is referred to as the *painful* or *freezing* phase because it is characterized mostly by pain and a progressive loss of glenohumeral joint ROM. Phase 2 is the *stiff* or *frozen* phase and it typically lasts between 4 to 12 months. During this phase considerable stiffness predominates, with a gradual reduction of pain. The final phase (phase 3) is the *resolution* or *thawing* phase, in which there is improvement in ROM and resolution of stiffness. This last phase can range anywhere between 12 and 42 months.[84,85]

Because of the past challenges associated with defining frozen shoulder, authors have begun to adopt definitions of this condition that encompass signs, symptoms, and investigations.[82,86] Table 5-5 presents the symptoms, signs, and investigations that constitute the British Elbow and Shoulder Society's definition of idiopathic frozen shoulder.

TABLE 5-5

British Elbow and Shoulder Society (BESS) Survey Definition of Frozen Shoulder

Symptoms	Signs	Investigations
• True (deltoid insertion) shoulder pain • Night pain of insidious onset	• Painful restriction of active and passive motion • Passive elevation less than 100° • Passive lateral (external) rotation less than 30° • Passive medial (internal) rotation less than reaching the level of L5 • All other shoulder conditions excluded	• Plain radiographs normal • Arthroscopy shows vascular granulation tissue in the rotator interval

Modified from Guyver PM, Bruce DJ, Rees JL: Frozen shoulder—a stiff problem that requires a flexible approach, *Maturitas* 78:12, 2014.

The two defining symptoms in patients with frozen shoulders are pain and restricted ROM of the glenohumeral joint (Figure 5-12). The pain is characteristically felt around the deltoid insertion but can also be described as diffuse around the entire shoulder. Patients usually describe the pain as severe, affecting sleep and most activities of daily life. As mentioned earlier, pain is often noted first, followed by a decrease in glenohumeral motion.

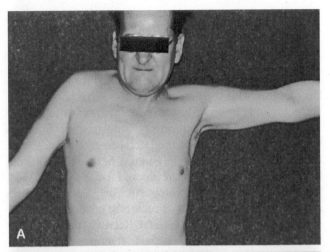

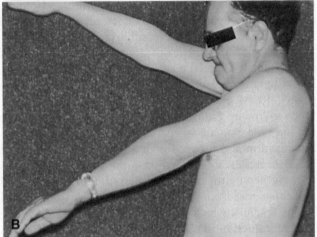

Figure 5-12 A and **B,** A 45-year-old man whose right shoulder is in the painful freezing phase of primary frozen shoulder. Note the distress and discouragement in the patient's face. (From Rowe CR, Leffet RD: Frozen shoulder. In Rowe CR, editor: *The shoulder,* p 158, New York, 1988, Churchill Livingstone.)

Patients describe either a slow, progressive loss of movement or occasionally a sudden loss. The reduced ROM follows a *capsular pattern of restriction,* a characteristic pattern of motion loss, secondary to capsular involvement in synovial joints. In the glenohumeral joint, the capsular pattern of restriction is lateral rotation most affected, followed by abduction, and medial rotation. Many clinicians believe that lateral rotation should be reduced more than 50% compared with the unaffected side to consider a diagnosis of frozen shoulder. Plain radiographs are used to rule out bony causes of pain and restricted ROM. To date, there is no evidence to support the use of ultrasound and/or magnetic resonance imaging in diagnosing frozen shoulder.[87]

Clinicians should be mindful of the secondary signs and symptoms that may develop in the patient with a frozen shoulder. Weakness of the glenohumeral and scapular stabilizer muscles is very common as a result of disuse or improper use. This usually occurs in the deep stabilizers of the glenohumeral joint (i.e., the rotator cuff) and

in the more superficial movers, such as the three parts of the deltoid muscle. The upper trapezius is often overused in its attempt to compensate for weak and painful shoulder elevation, leading to a reversal of normal scapulohumeral rhythm and further muscle imbalance about the scapula.

Treatment of Frozen Shoulder

Given the uncertainty about the etiology of frozen shoulder syndrome, it is not surprising that the theories of treatment for this condition are equally inconsistent. Systematic reviews regarding the effectiveness of physical therapy[88-91] have concluded limited overall clinical evidence, based upon low-moderate quality evidence, for exercise and manual therapy and low-level laser therapy. The effects of treatment were reported to be greatest during phases 2 and 3 of the condition.

Most patients with a frozen shoulder can be managed successfully with nonoperative treatment, using a multidisciplinary approach of patient education, physical therapy, analgesic medication, and injection therapy.[85,87,88,92] Secondary frozen shoulder requires management of the preceding factor (e.g., shoulder surgery) or contributory factor (e.g., diabetes) as well. Although there is a lack of evidence to support these common treatment interventions, they are noninvasive, inexpensive, and have minimal risk.

Traditional rehabilitation programs focus on exercises and manual therapy techniques that improve glenohumeral ROM and pain-relieving modalities.[87,88,93,94] Joint mobilization techniques, stretching, and passive ROM exercises are done initially because pain usually prevents patients from doing these exercises independently. Some patients may not tolerate any mobility within the first phase of this condition, due to severe pain. In these cases, physical therapy management should focus on patient education and reassurance, pain-relieving strategies and gentle posture, and scapular setting exercises. Patients should also be encouraged to participate in some form of activity that promotes general health and wellness during the time they are dealing with their frozen shoulder. All exercises and techniques should be performed within the limitations of pain to avoid aggravating the affected tissue, especially during the painful, freezing phase.

Clearly no preponderance of evidence points to the best treatment for patients with frozen shoulder syndromes. However, it seems plausible that some, if not all, of the basic principles of shoulder rehabilitation could be applied in dealing with this condition. Patient education about the condition and its expected phases and outcome, postural awareness and treatment (especially of the adjacent cervical and thoracic spine levels), and exercises for the remaining shoulder girdle musculature are all important considerations. In addition, significant care should always be given to reeducate these patients to control movements of the glenohumeral and scapulothoracic joints because these muscles tend to become "detrained" as a result of the disease and the consequent loss of movement.

SHOULDER FRACTURES

Fractures of the shoulder girdle are relatively uncommon, ranging from minor, nondisplaced, hairline fractures to major, comminuted, displaced fractures with life-threatening consequences.[45] Most fractures in this region require some type of immobilization and/or period of protected motion. This immobilization, although essential for bone healing, often results in secondary stiffness of the glenohumeral joint, generalized muscle weakness, and altered scapulothoracic mechanics. Therefore it is important that the objectives of rehabilitation following a shoulder fracture include normalization of the entire shoulder girdle and trunk, not just the joint adjacent to the local fracture site.

Scapular Fractures

Fractures of the scapula account for only 1% of all fractures, 3% of all shoulder injuries, and 5% of fractures involving the entire shoulder.[95-97] They typically occur as a result of a high-energy situation involving a fall or direct blow and often occur in conjunction with other traumatic injuries. With less severe fractures, the muscles effectively stabilize the fracture, and the patient typically can expect a good functional outcome. However, patients may present with associated injuries to the involved arm, shoulder girdle, and thoracic cage; ipsilateral rib fractures are the most common associated injury, occurring in approximately 27% to 50% of patients.[95] Pulmonary trauma (e.g., pneumothorax, hemothorax, or both) is reported in 16% to 40% of patients, and clavicular fractures and injuries to the brachial plexus and subclavian artery reportedly occur in 26% and 12% of patients, respectively.[95-98]

Scapular fractures are classified according to the location of the fracture, specifically the body, neck, glenoid fossa, acromion, spine, or coracoid. The distribution of the different fracture sites has been reported as 35% to 43% at the scapular body, 26% at the neck, 10% at the glenoid fossa, 8% to 12% at the acromion, 6% to 11% at the spine, and 5% to 7% at the coracoid.[95,98-100]

Clinical Evaluation of Scapular Fractures

Most patients with a scapular fracture have experienced a traumatic, well-defined mechanism of injury; therefore clinical evaluation usually is precluded by a thorough radiographic and neurological examination. Local physical findings, such as swelling, ecchymosis, and crepitus with ROM, are common, as are subjective complaints of pain in the scapular region. In most cases, a detailed assessment of the entire shoulder girdle and the cervical and thoracic spine should be performed (see Volume 1 of this series, *Orthopedic Physical Assessment*).

Treatment of Scapular Fractures

Nonoperative treatment is recommended for most scapular fractures, with the exception of those that occur at specific sites and/or according to certain classifications.[101,102] These include (1) acromion or scapular spine fractures with downward tilting of the lateral fragment and resultant subacromial narrowing (Figure 5-13), (2) coracoid fractures that extend into the glenoid fossa (Figure 5-14), and (3) glenoid rim and intra-articular glenoid fractures associated with persistent or recurrent glenohumeral instability (Figures 5-15 and 5-16). Relative indications for the surgical treatment of scapular fractures include displaced acromion or coracoid process fractures (>10 mm), displaced intra-articular glenoid fractures (>5 mm), and those associated with humeral subluxation.[101,103]

Nonsurgical treatment of scapular fractures consists of approximately 7 to 10 days of sling immobilization, followed by a progressing regimen of pendular and gentle passive ROM exercises as comfort and control allow. Once follow-up radiographic findings indicate sufficient healing, the patient is encouraged to discontinue immobilization and proceed with active-assisted and active ROM exercises. Consideration must always be given to restrengthening the muscles that attach to the scapula and those that arise from the scapula (i.e., the rotator cuff and biceps brachii), which may have been affected by disuse and painful inhibition. In a number of cases, patients with a scapular fracture develop stiffness in the adjacent spine, specifically the lower cervical spine to the midthoracic spine. Clinicians must take care to assess these regions and treat accordingly. Failure to address this important

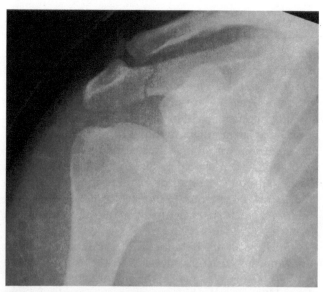

Figure 5-13 Radiograph demonstrating a fracture at the base of the acromion. (From Sanders R: *Core knowledge in orthopaedics: trauma,* Philadelphia, 2008, Saunders.)

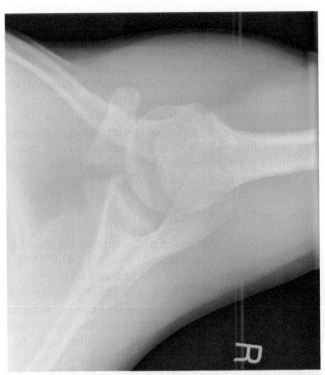

Figure 5-14 Axial radiograph of shoulder, demonstrating the coracoid base fracture. (From Alsey KJ, Mahapatra AN, Jessop JH: Coracoid fracture in an adolescent rugby player – case report and review of the literature, *Radiography* 18(4):301-302, 2012.)

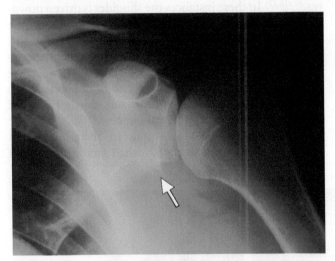

Figure 5-15 True anteroposterior plain radiograph demonstrating an anteroinferior glenoid fracture (*arrow*). (From Browner BD, Levine AM, Jupiter JB, et al: *Skeletal trauma*, ed 4, Philadelphia, 2009, Saunders.)

part of the kinetic chain may lead to further problems in the shoulder region and most certainly will result in a less than optimal outcome. Most minor scapular fractures are sufficiently healed by 6 to 12 weeks and able to withstand the progressive load delivered through ROM and strengthening exercises at this time. Clinicians and patients must keep in mind that maximum functional recovery, which encompasses more than just bone healing, may take as long as 6 to 12 months.[104,105]

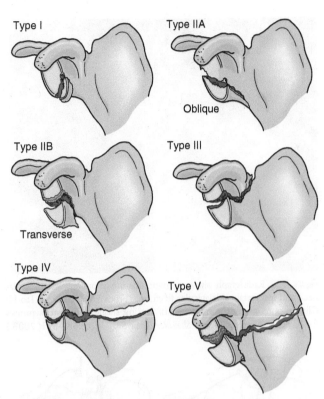

Figure 5-16 Ideberg's classification of glenoid fractures. (From Sanders R: *Core knowledge in orthopaedics: trauma*, Philadelphia, 2008, Saunders.)

"Floating Shoulder"

The term *floating shoulder* was introduced by Herscovici[106] in 1992 to describe an ipsilateral fracture of the clavicular shaft and the scapular neck (Figure 5-17). The combination of these two types of fractures has a significant effect on the stabilizing role of the clavicle. Goss[107] defined *floating shoulder* as "a double disruption of the superior suspensory shoulder complex (SSSC)." He described three struts of this complex: (1) the AC joint–acromial strut, (2) the clavicular–coracoclavicular ligament–coracoid linkage, and (3) the three process–scapular body junction. A potentially unstable anatomical condition exists when the complex is disrupted in at least two places with significant displacement at either or both sites (Figure 5-18). This condition has a high risk of poor bone healing from delayed union or malunion of the clavicle, the scapular neck, or both.

Combined clavicular and ipsilateral scapular neck fractures are usually caused by a high-energy mechanism of injury, most commonly motor vehicle accidents (80% to 100%).[108] Other causes have been cited, such as a direct blow, fall onto the tip of the shoulder, or a FOOSH injury.[106,107] As with most scapular fractures, combined clavicular and ipsilateral scapular neck fractures have a high incidence of associated traumatic lesions, and when severe accompanying injuries are present, the clinical signs and symptoms of this specific fracture type often are overlooked. The definitive diagnosis therefore is made on the basis of radiographic findings.

Very little research to date has addressed the most effective way to treat a floating shoulder. Literature related

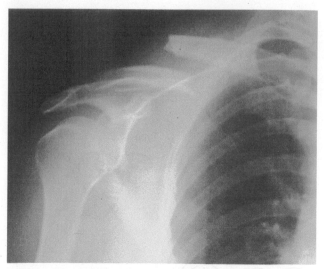

Figure 5-17 Radiograph showing right floating shoulder with scapular neck and ipsilateral midclavicular fractures. (From Hashiguchi H, Ito H: Clinical outcome of the treatment of floating shoulder by osteosynthesis for clavicular fracture alone, *J Shoulder Elbow Surg* 12(6):589-591, 2003.)

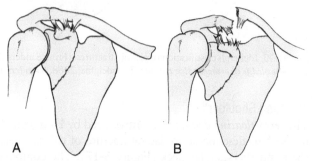

Figure 5-18 Fracture of the scapular neck. **A,** If the coracoclavicular and acromioclavicular ligaments are intact, there is little displacement of the glenoid (stable scapular neck fracture). **B,** Fracture of the scapular neck with disruption of the coracoclavicular and acromioclavicular ligaments creates a floating shoulder (unstable neck fracture). (From Herring JA: *Tachdjian's pediatric orthopaedics: from the Texas Scottish Rite Hospital for Children,* ed 5, Philadelphia, 2014, Saunders.)

to this fracture type is limited to case reports and retrospective studies of small patient series.[106-108] Treatment options mentioned range from conservative management with or without early mobilization to operative treatment through open reduction and internal fixation of the clavicle only or of the clavicle and the scapular neck fracture sites together. Clearly, further research and clinical study are necessary to elucidate this interesting pathology. Any rehabilitation plan should be derived from a careful analysis of the anatomy involved and a thorough examination of the entire shoulder girdle and adjacent spine.

Clavicular Fractures

The most commonly reported fracture of the shoulder girdle is the clavicular fracture (Figure 5-19).[109,110] The incidence is highest among children and adolescents, in whom the mechanism of injury is either a direct blow from a fall onto the affected shoulder or an impact such as a tackle in football. In a direct blow, the compressive force causes buckling of the clavicle, which leads to a fracture once the compressive force exceeds the tensile strength of the clavicle. The clavicle can also sustain a direct impact that results in a fracture. Eighty-seven percent of clavicular fractures occur from falls onto the shoulder, whereas direct impact to the shoulder accounts for 7%. FOOSH injuries account for 6% of clavicle fractures.[40,110,111] In these instances the shoulder is driven downward, causing the clavicle to forcefully impinge on the underlying first rib, resulting in a fracture (Figure 5-20).

Although a fracture can occur anywhere along the clavicle, the most common site is reported to be between the medial two thirds and lateral one third of the bone (80%) followed by fractures in the distal one third (17%) and those that occur in the proximal one third (2%).[45,109,110,112] Fractures are classified according to their anatomical location: group I are in the midshaft (middle third) of

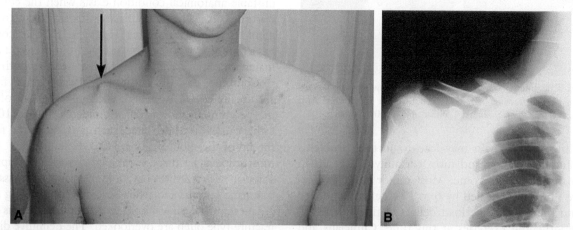

Figure 5-19 A, Clinical photograph of patient with a right clavicle fracture (*arrow*). Note "tenting" of skin. (From Ristevski B, Hall JA, Pearce D, et al: The radiographic quantification of scapular malalignment after malunion of displaced clavicular shaft fractures. *J Shoulder Elbow Surg* 22(2): 240-246, 2013.) **B,** Anteroposterior view of a fractured clavicle showing a comminuted fracture of the midshaft with upward displacement of the proximal fragment. (From Eiff MP, Hatch RL: *Fracture management for primary care,* ed 3, Philadelphia, 2012, Saunders.)

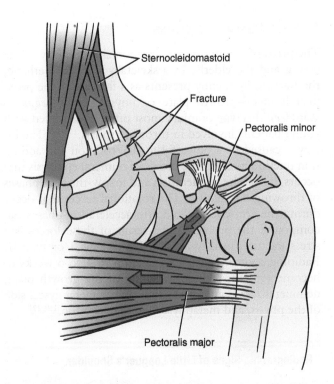

Figure 5-20 Clavicular fracture. With displacement, the proximal fragment is pulled superiorly by the sternocleidomastoid and the distal segment drops forward pulled down by pectoralis minor on coracoid process and pectoralis major on humerus.

TABLE 5-6

Subclassification of Group II Clavicular Fractures

Type	Description
Type I	Fractures lateral to the coracoclavicular ligaments
Type II	Fractures medial to the coracoclavicular ligaments
Type III	Fractures extending into the acromioclavicular joint
Type IV	Fractures in which the proximal fragment is displaced out of its periosteal tube
Type V	Comminuted fractures in which coracoclavicular ligaments remain attached to an inferior bone fragment but are not attached to the proximal or distal fragment

From Craig EV: Fractures of the clavicle. In Rockwood CA, Matsen FA, editors: *The shoulder*, Philadelphia, 1998, WB Saunders.

the clavicle, group II are in the distal (lateral) third of the clavicle, and group III are in the medial (proximal) third of the clavicle. Craig[112] devised a five-part subclassification system of the group II clavicular fractures (Table 5-6).

Clinical Evaluation of Clavicular Fractures

Because of their superficial location, clavicular fractures are easily recognizable through inspection and direct palpation. Patients are able to recall a specific mechanism of injury, describing localized pain and possibly a cracking or popping sound or sensation. If the patient is seen directly

following the injury, they may be holding the ipsilateral arm with the contralateral arm or it may be held in adduction at the side. Swelling, ecchymosis, and gross deformity may be visible with possible tenting of the skin. Tenderness to palpation and crepitus may be palpated over the fracture site. If the patient is able to move his or her arm, a grinding sensation may be felt or described.

The degree of deformity depends on the location of the fracture and the amount of displacement (see Figure 5-19, *A*). Associated injuries, although not common, may occur, including scapular fractures, scapulothoracic dissociation, rib fractures, pneumothorax, and neurovascular compromise (Figures 5-21 and 5-22). The brachial plexus is of particular concern because of its proximity to the clavicle, which makes it susceptible to injury.[111,112]

Treatment of Clavicular Fractures

The goal of treatment, relative to clavicular fractures, is to minimize the risk of nonunion and malunion. **Nonunion** is defined as the absence of clinical radiographic healing after 4 to 6 months, whereas **malunion** is associated with angulation, shortening, and poor cosmetic appearance. Generally it was believed that malunion did not affect functional capacity; however, studies have discovered that malunion may lead to weakness and fatigability.[113–116] Most

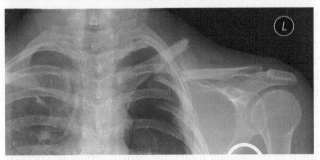

Figure 5-21 Fracture of the left clavicle and ribs with associated pneumothorax. Note the displaced midshaft clavicle fracture. (From Kim W, McKee MD: Management of acute clavicle fractures, *Orthop Clin North Am* 39(4): 491-505, 2008.)

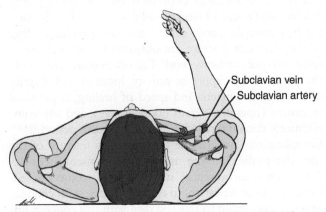

Figure 5-22 Potential injury to the subclavian vessels resulting from a fractured clavicle. (From Rockwood CA, Matsen FA, Wirth MA, et al, editors: *The shoulder*, ed 4, p 400, Philadelphia, 2009, Saunders.)

minimally displaced clavicular fractures do not require surgical intervention and can be treated conservatively with immobilization using either a sling or a figure-of-eight brace for approximately 4 to 6 weeks.[112,114–116] Both immobilizers appear to be effective; however, the sling is reported to provide more comfort with fewer complications, such as skin breakdown because the figure-of-eight brace must be kept in some degree of tension. In addition, the sling allows the patient to more easily perform light ROM exercises.

Clavicular fractures that require surgical consideration include open fractures, concomitant displaced scapular neck fractures that disrupt the superior shoulder suspensory complex, the presence of neurovascular or skin compromise, and a patient with multiple trauma who needs assistance with early mobilization.[116,117] Surgical treatment may be considered in some cases, for certain high-demand patients (such as heavy laborers or athletes), who are exposed to large, repetitive, potentially deforming forces, and individuals who have had a previous nonunion at the same site. However, careful patient selection and preoperative counseling are recommended because of the potential risks (e.g., implant infection, migration of intramedullary wires, neurovascular injuries) and sometimes less than optimal outcomes of the procedure.

Once bone healing is well established (**clinical union** occurs in 2 to 3 weeks), the patient can be guided through active-assisted and then active ROM exercises. Because most clavicular fractures do not involve the adjacent articulations, ROM is quite easily regained. Care must always be taken not to overload the healing fracture site with activities that produce too great a leverage point on this important fulcrum. Restrengthening exercises are prescribed for any muscles that were weakened as a result of painful inhibition and/or the immobilization period. As with any type of shoulder injury, the patient should be checked to ensure that the scapulohumeral rhythm is normal and symmetrical and that the essential stabilizing musculature of the glenohumeral joint is intact. Normal healing times vary slightly depending upon the site of the clavicular fracture but generally range between 6 and 9 weeks in young children and 8 and 12 weeks in adults.[109,111,112] It is important to ensure that both clinical and radiographic healing of the clavicular fracture are obtained before a patient's return to sport or heavy work. Factors to consider include the patient's age, sport or activity, location and severity of the fracture, extent and speed of healing, method of treatment (operative versus nonoperative), and any complications encountered during the recovery period.[114,116] Complications are possible following any fracture of the shoulder girdle, but the most serious consequences occur when neurovascular structures are compromised. Clinicians must be careful to continually assess for changes in sensation related to this and deal with this concern immediately. Less severe clavicular fracture complications include malunion (which results in a bony prominence but rarely a functional deficit), nonunion, and poor cosmesis.

Proximal Humeral Fractures

The proximal humerus is a common site of injury in the young and the elderly. In a skeletally immature athlete, the fracture frequently presents as a fracture at the proximal humeral growth plate or physis (*Little Leaguer's shoulder*); this type of injury most often is associated with young patients involved in throwing sports.[118–121] The injury is caused by a powerful medial rotation and adduction traction force on the proximal humeral epiphysis that occurs during the deceleration and follow-through phases of throwing or pitching. The rotational forces that occur during the arm-cocking and arm-acceleration phases can compound the problem. The result of these forces is a stress fracture, usually a Salter-Harris type I or type II. Radiologic signs, which may take up to 4 to 6 weeks to become evident, include widening of the growth plate, demineralization and rarefaction on the metaphyseal side of the physis, and metaphyseal bone separation.[119–121]

Radiographic Signs of Little Leaguer's Shoulder

- Widening of the epiphyseal plate
- Demineralization and rarefaction of the metaphyseal side of the physis
- Metaphyseal bone separation

The athlete typically complains of acute shoulder pain when attempting to throw hard. If these complaints are ignored, it can result in acute displacement of the weakened physis. Rest is the primary treatment, along with patient education regarding why absolute cessation from activity, at least initially, is essential. The bone may require up to 8 to 12 months to reossify and remodel.

Following a period of rest, rehabilitation should include activities to improve strength, coordination, proprioception, endurance, and ROM. The exact timing for beginning active exercises, as well as when and how much to progress these exercises, varies, depending on the stage of bone healing evident, the patient's tolerance of pain, and the condition of the surrounding soft tissue and adjacent joints. The most prudent decisions related to exercise prescription for these young patients is guided by the radiologic evidence and a thorough assessment and monitoring of the patient's clinical signs and symptoms. Clinicians must proceed cautiously, applying gentle stress to the area to encourage healing but never exceeding what the tissue can sustain.

In the elderly, proximal humeral fractures usually occur in patients with osteoporosis, and women are affected twice as often as men are. Predictions of incidence are estimated to triple during the next three decades as the population ages.[122] Most fractures are caused by minimal trauma, such as a FOOSH injury from a standing height or lower, or a direct blow to the lateral aspect of the shoulder (Figure 5-23).[123,124] Occasionally, they occur in association with a dislocation

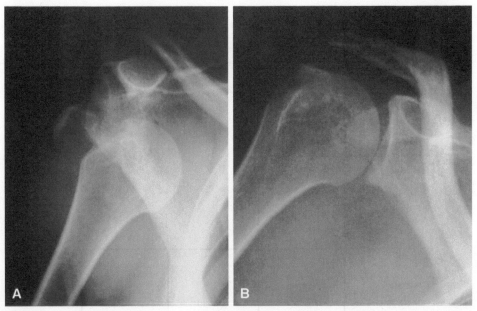

Figure 5-23 A, Anteroposterior x-ray film of a two-part anterior fracture-dislocation with a displaced greater tuberosity fracture. **B,** After a closed reduction, the greater tuberosity fracture reduced and healed without further displacement. (From Rockwood CA, Green DP, Bucholz RW, Heckman JD: *Fractures in adults,* ed 4, p 1069, Philadelphia, 1996, Lippincott-Raven.)

or with excessive rotation of the arm, especially while in the abducted position.[58] In this situation, the humerus locks against the acromion in a pivotal position, resulting in a fracture.

Most proximal humeral fractures are nondisplaced or minimally displaced; these should be differentiated from the more serious displaced fractures, which are managed quite differently. The most commonly used classification system is the four-part fracture classification developed by Neer in 1970, in which he divided fractures into displaced and nondisplaced (Figure 5-24).[125,126] Displaced fractures, according to this classification, have more than 1 cm of displacement or more than 45° of angulation. Nondisplaced fractures may be called *one-part fractures,* regardless of how many fracture lines are seen. A *two-part fracture* involves displacement of the anatomical neck, surgical neck, lesser tuberosity, or greater tuberosity in relation to the remaining intact proximal humerus. Similarly *three-* and *four-part fractures* involve displacement of two or three fragments in relation to the main humeral fragment.

According to Neer's classification, the most commonly reported fracture of the proximal humerus is a displaced or nondisplaced (one-part or two-part) fracture involving the surgical neck (Figure 5-25). Researchers have investigated the clinical impact of greater tuberosity displacements less than 1 cm and found that the shoulder has very little tolerance for greater tuberosity displacement. Displacements of 5 mm to 1 cm were found to result in substantial dysfunction from either impingement or rotator cuff tearing.[122,126,127]

Clinical Presentation of Proximal Humeral Fractures

Because most proximal humeral fractures present acutely, common symptoms are pain, swelling, and tenderness about the shoulder, particularly in the region of the greater tuberosity. Crepitus may be evident with movement of the shoulder, but in most cases the patient is reluctant to initiate any active movement and holds the arm closely against the chest wall. The definitive diagnosis is made through radiographic evaluation.

A thorough assessment should be performed, including evaluation of the integrity of the bony tissue and careful examination of the neurovascular and musculotendinous structures intimately situated in this region. A fracture-dislocation or a fracture resulting from a high-energy trauma is much more likely to be associated with neurovascular injuries. The axillary nerve can be injured during a shoulder fracture–dislocation; in most patients the injury results in axonotmesis and a full recovery is expected. Of particular concern is the rotator cuff, which attaches to the different tuberosities of the humerus and consequently may have a deforming effect, depending on where the proximal humerus has been injured. For example, with a fracture of the greater tuberosity, the fracture fragment is pulled superiorly and posteriorly due to the muscle action of the supraspinatus, infraspinatus, and teres minor muscles. Conversely, in a fracture of the lesser tuberosity, the fragment is pulled anteriorly and medially by the subscapularis muscle (Figure 5-26).[127,128]

The deltoid and pectoralis major muscles must also be evaluated in patients with a proximal humeral fracture. Because the deltoid muscle attaches to the lateral shaft of the humerus, it can cause displacement of fractures of the proximal humeral shaft. Similarly, the pectoralis major muscle's insertion onto the lower portion of the bicipital groove can displace the proximal shaft of the humerus medially, as is typically seen in surgical neck fractures.

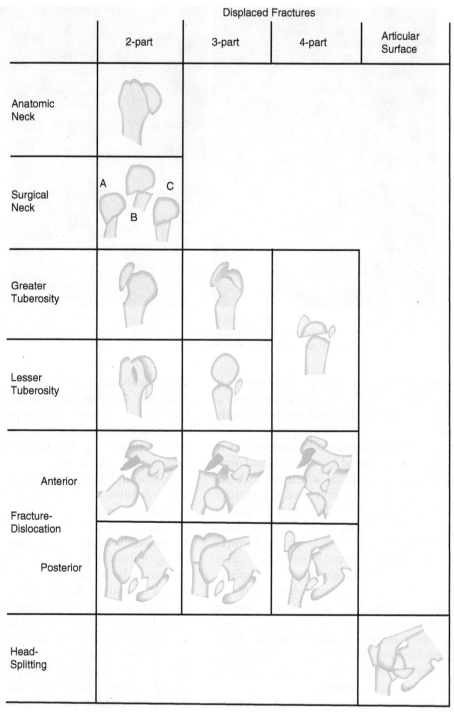

Figure 5-24 Neer four-segment classification of displaced proximal humeral fractures. A fragment is considered displaced when greater than 1 cm of displacement or 45 degrees of angulation is present. A fracture-dislocation is present if the articular segment is no longer in contact with the glenoid. (Redrawn from Neer CS: Displaced proximal humeral fractures. Part I. Classification and evaluation, *J Bone Joint Surg Am* 52:1077-1089, 1970.)

Treatment of Proximal Humeral Fractures

Most proximal humeral fractures are minimally displaced and are successfully treated without surgery.[121,127,129] If the fracture is classified as nondisplaced and is impacted or stable, an initial period of immobilization is indicated, using either a conventional sling or a collar and cuff sling that allows the weight of the arm to apply slight traction to the fracture. Early ROM exercises follow, at approximately 2 weeks after injury. If the fracture is classified as nondisplaced but is considered unstable, the immobilization period is more strictly adhered to with ROM exercises beginning after approximately 4 weeks when clinical union has occurred.

Diminished pain and an easing of the patient's apprehension are reasonable indicators for beginning gentle exercises. Obtaining intermittent radiographs before

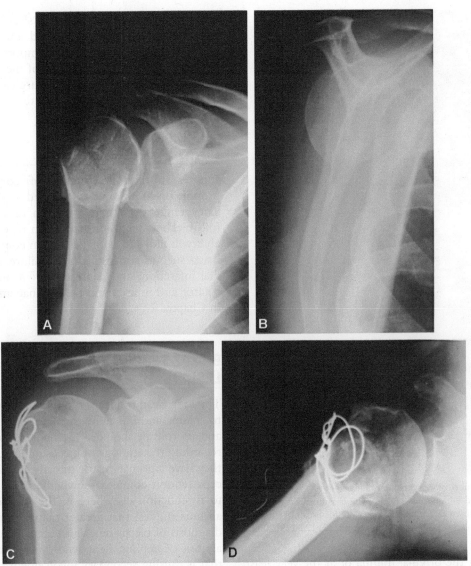

Figure 5-25 Displaced fracture of the surgical neck. **A** and **B,** Anteroposterior and lateral x-ray films of a displaced surgical neck fracture. The fracture was treated for 3 weeks as an undisplaced fracture on the basis of an anteroposterior x-ray film only (**A**). The follow-up lateral x-ray film (**B**) in the scapular plane revealed a significant anterior shaft displacement. **C** and **D,** Anteroposterior and lateral x-ray films after open reduction and internal fixation with two figure-of-eight wires. (From Rockwood CA, Matsen FA, editors: *The shoulder,* p 353, Philadelphia, 1998, WB Saunders.)

beginning rehabilitation is important to establish the fracture is clinically stable and the bone moves as a unit. Rehabilitation programs should follow general shoulder treatment principles of patient education, mobility of the entire shoulder girdle and relevant kinetic chain segments, optimal neuromuscular strength, and return to functional activities. Bertoft et al.[129] reported that the greatest amount of improvement in ROM occurs between 3 and 8 weeks after injury.

Management of the young athlete with an epiphyseal fracture of his or her proximal humeral growth plate is nonoperative with a 3-month period of rest followed by a program of shoulder ROM exercises, scapular and rotator cuff strength, and endurance exercise and functional exercises incorporating the entire kinetic chain. A progressive throwing program and subsequent return to play are

considered when the athlete demonstrates resolution of symptoms as well as optimal shoulder ROM and neuromuscular control.

Complications following nonoperative management of a proximal humeral fracture are primarily related to shoulder stiffness and limited motion or to the consequences of displacement of the greater tuberosity. Early initiation of passive and active-assisted ROM exercises compared with delaying exercises until 3 weeks post injury results in less pain and faster recovery in people with stable fractures.[130] Additional complications that may affect outcomes in patients with proximal humeral fractures are those related to associated soft tissue damage (e.g., rotator cuff) and neurovascular injury. Clinicians must be diligent in evaluating for and treating any associated injuries that may have been injured, along with

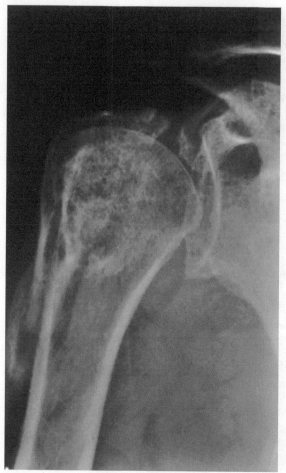

Figure 5-26 Greater tuberosity malunion resulting from unopposed pull of the supraspinatus and infraspinatus muscles. (From Antuña SA, Sperling JW, Sánchez-Sotelo J, et al: Shoulder arthroplasty for proximal humeral malunions: long-term results, *J Shoulder Elbow Surg* 11(2):122-129, 2002.)

the humerus, in the original trauma or at the very least may have been strained or traumatized as a result of the fracture.

Surgical indications for a fracture of the proximal humerus are not straightforward. Humeral head vascularity, fracture pattern, bone quality, and overall geometry are important considerations in determining appropriate treatment. Osteoporosis influences the degree of comminution, magnitude of cancellous defects secondary to impaction, and likelihood of fixation failure or loss of reduction.[131] Surgery is reserved primarily for fractures that are significantly displaced; it involves mainly closed reduction with or without percutaneous pinning or open reduction and internal fixation.[131,132] An osteoporotic fracture is often more appropriately treated with arthroplasty than with reduction and internal fixation. Treatment of proximal humeral fractures with surgery is considered difficult, not only because of the complex anatomy of the shoulder girdle but also because of the difficulty achieving and maintaining anatomical reduction and stable fixation. Rehabilitation following these types of surgical procedures is rigorous

and involved, and practitioners should ensure patients are well informed and educated about the procedure and are suited to handle the important postoperative period. In some cases, because of the co-morbidity status and the patient's age, nonsurgical treatment is the most appropriate choice despite substantial fracture displacement.

ROTATOR CUFF INJURIES

Injuries affecting the rotator cuff comprise the largest proportion of all injuries reported at the shoulder.[133–136] They range from minor tendon or muscle injuries to full-thickness tears and have been reported to cause disability in individuals that has been compared with health issues such as congestive heart failure, diabetes, myocardial infarction, and depression.[137] More information on rotator cuff injuries and their management can be found in Chapter 7.

BICEPS TENDON AND SUPERIOR LABRAL LESIONS

The long head of biceps is a tendinous tissue, susceptible to trauma and injury by the nature of its anatomical site and its role in shoulder mechanics. Some debate exists regarding the etiology of biceps injuries, namely, whether they have a primary cause directly associated with the biceps tendon complex or whether they occur secondary to dysfunction elsewhere in the shoulder girdle. Some authors suggest that greater than 90% of patients with a diagnosis of biceps tendonitis actually have a primary diagnosis of impingement syndrome or scapular instability that is causing secondary involvement of the biceps tendon.[138,139] Studies based on the results of magnetic resonance imaging and arthroscopic procedures have shed new light on the pathophysiology of the long head of the biceps tendon.[138–142]

One of the most significant contributions to understanding biceps injuries has come as a result of studies that have investigated the superior glenoid labrum. Andrews et al.[143] in 1985 described tears in the superior labrum of the glenohumeral joint noting the placement of these tears at the attachment of the biceps tendon (Figure 5-27). In 1990, Snyder et al.[144] first described the superolabral anterior to posterior (SLAP) lesion, a lesion of the superior labrum and adjoining biceps anchor. They categorized SLAP lesions into four types. Type I lesions show degenerative fraying with no detachment of the biceps insertion; type II lesions show detachment of the biceps insertion; type III lesions show a bucket handle tear of the superior aspect of the labrum with an intact biceps tendon insertion to bone; and type IV lesions show an intrasubstance tear of the biceps tendon with a bucket handle tear of the superior aspect of the labrum.

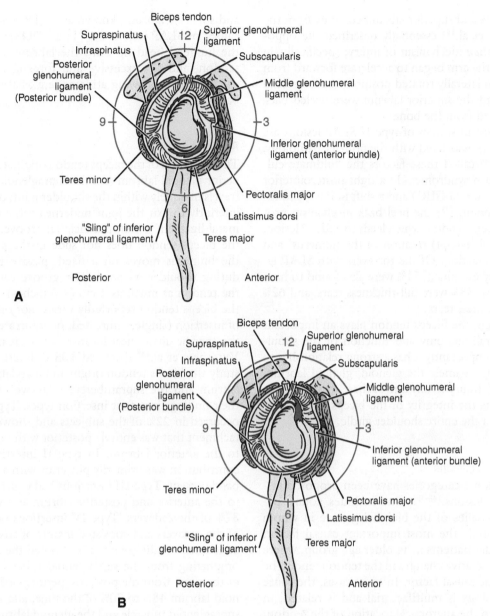

Figure 5-27 Labral lesions of the right shoulder. **A**, Bankart lesion. **B**, SLAP lesion. (From Magee DJ: *Orthopedic physical assessment*, ed 6, p 320, Philadelphia, 2014, WB Saunders.)

Morgan[145] further divided type II SLAP lesions into three subtypes, depending on whether the detachment of the labrum involved the anterior aspect of the labrum alone, the posterior aspect, or both.

In their three-part series, *"The Disabled Throwing Shoulder,"* Burkhart et al.[5,14,146] described the type II SLAP lesion (i.e., involving detachment of the biceps tendon) as the most common pathological entity associated with a "dead arm" syndrome, which they defined as any pathological shoulder condition that deems an athlete unable to throw due to pain and subjective unease in the shoulder. In an arthroscopic study done earlier, these same authors observed what they called a dynamic "peel-back phenomenon" in throwers with posterior and combined anteroposterior SLAP lesions.[147] They found

that with the arm in the cocked position of abduction and lateral rotation the peel-back occurred as a result of the effect of the biceps tendon as its vector shifted to a more posterior position in late cocking. The change in angle and the twist of the biceps tendon produced a torsional force to the posterosuperior labrum, causing detachment if the superior labrum was not well anchored to the glenoid. These findings suggested a mechanism of injury for SLAP lesions in throwers that was different from the mechanism postulated earlier by Andrews et al.[143] These researchers had described a *deceleration* mechanism of labral injuries in throwers, which occurred as the biceps contracted to slow the rapidly extending elbow in the follow-through phase. They believed that this created a high tensile load in the biceps that acted to pull the biceps and superior labrum complex from the bone. Burkhart et al.[146] essentially described the opposite, an *acceleration* mechanism of injury; specifically, in late cocking, as the arm began to accelerate forward from an abducted and laterally rotated position, the long head of the biceps and the superior labrum were peeled back rather than pulled from the bone.

Also of interest in studies of type II SLAP lesions are the clinical factors associated with the primary pathology. Burkhart et al.[146] called these factors the "ultimate culprits" in dead arm syndrome: (1) a tight posteroinferior capsule, which causes a GIRD and a shift in the glenohumeral rotation point, (2) the peel-back mechanism produced by the biceps tendon, which leads to a SLAP lesion, (3) hyperexternal (lateral) rotation of the humerus, and (4) scapular protraction. Of the throwers with SLAP lesions whom they examined, 31% were also found to have rotator cuff tears (38% were full-thickness tears, and 62% were partial-thickness tears).

As can be seen, the biceps tendon plays an important role in the overall anatomy and function of the shoulder joint. Most importantly it has a strong relationship to its adjacent tissue, namely the glenoid, glenoid labrum, and rotator cuff. Injury to any one of these structures undoubtedly affects the integrity of the biceps tendon and the well-being of the entire shoulder girdle.

Etiology of Biceps Lesions

Two main etiologic categories have been proposed relative to biceps lesions.[148–151] One includes young patients with anomalies of the bicipital groove in whom repetitive trauma is the most important causal factor; the other includes patients in an older age group, where associated degenerative changes in the tendon tend to be the predominant causal factor. In most cases, the cause of biceps pathology is multifactorial and is related, in some manner, to the anatomical location of the tendon. As mentioned, the potential for impingement of the biceps tendon under the coracoacromial arch is great, especially if dysfunction of the rotator cuff and/or scapular misalignment are present. The blood supply of the biceps has been shown to be diminished in the long tendon region, with a "critical zone" similar to that seen in the supraspinatus tendon.[152] In abduction, a zone of avascularity exists in the intracapsular portion of the biceps tendon, which is felt to be caused by pressure from the head of the humerus, a phenomenon referred to as *wringing-out*. Considering these positions, it is easy to see why patients involved in overhead lifting and throwing are more susceptible to ruptures, elongations, and dislocations of the biceps tendon. The past several years have produced a proliferation of information about the superior labrum and its relationship to the biceps tendon.[138,140,142–146] As noted earlier, Andrews et al.[143] and Snyder et al.[144] originally described lesions of the biceps

and superior labrum, known as *SLAP lesions*. Two cited causes of SLAP lesions are (1) a FOOSH, which drives the humeral head up onto the labrum and the biceps tendon, and (2) excessive and forceful contraction of the biceps in throwing athletes (e.g., baseball and football players).

Relevant Anatomy

The long head of the biceps tendon originates from the superior glenoid labrum and the supraglenoid tubercle and travels obliquely within the shoulder joint, turning sharply inferiorly to exit the joint underneath the transverse humeral ligament within the bicipital groove. Interestingly, the biceps tendon does not slide in the groove; rather, the humerus moves on a fixed, passive biceps tendon during shoulder motions. The groove can move along the tendon as much as 4 cm (1.5 inches). The origin of the biceps tendon reportedly varies, not only in the type of insertion (single, bifurcated, or trifurcated) but also in the specific anatomical location where it inserts.[148,153,154] Vangsness et al.[148] dissected 105 cadaveric shoulders to study the biceps tendon origin and its relationship to the labrum and the supratubercular groove. They classified their findings into four insertion types. Type I insertions occurred in 22% of the subjects and showed a labral attachment that was entirely posterior with no contribution to the anterior labrum. In type II insertions the labral contribution was primarily posterior with a small anterior band present. Type III insertions had equal contributions to the anterior and posterior labrum and were found in 37% of the cadavers. Type IV insertions occurred in 8% of the cadavers and consisted mainly of an anterior labral attachment. A different study[138] noted the biceps tendon originating from the supraglenoid tubercle 20% to 30% of the time, from the posterosuperior portion of the glenoid labrum 48% to 70% of the time, and from both the supraglenoid tubercle and the glenoid labrum 25% to 28% of the time. It is clear to see from these studies why the biceps tendon and superior labrum are commonly injured together.

The biceps tendon is surrounded by a synovial sheath, which ends at the distal end of the bicipital groove, making the tendon an intra-articular but extrasynovial structure. As the long head of the biceps tendon moves from its origin on the superior glenoid labrum and supraglenoid tubercle to its muscle insertion, it is stabilized in position by the supraspinatus and subscapularis tendons and the capsuloligamentous tissues. The triangular-shaped area between the supraspinatus and the subscapularis tendons is referred to as the *rotator interval*. It contains the coracohumeral and the superior glenohumeral ligaments and has on its medial side the coracoid process. Histoanatomical studies have found that both the superior glenohumeral ligament and the coracohumeral ligament are important structures in the stabilization of the biceps tendon in its groove, and lesions associated with any of the components of the rotator interval leave the biceps tendon and the rotator cuff vulnerable to injury.[141,152,155]

Function of the Biceps

The biceps extends from the scapula to the forearm and as a result plays an important role in function of the shoulder and elbow. Basmajian and Latif[150] characterized the action of biceps as flexion of the elbow when the forearm is in the neutral or supinated position. The muscle is also described as having an important role in decelerating the rapidly moving arm during activities such as forceful overhand throwing. The exact function of the biceps at the shoulder is not well understood. Most references regard it as a weak flexor,[140,153,155] but its proposed role as a humeral head depressor remains controversial.[152,154,155] One study, which used simulated muscle forces on a biomechanical cadaver model, showed that the biceps tendon force restrained superior humeral translation. A key factor in this study was that this occurred in the presence of a large rotator cuff tear.[141] A similar study demonstrated that the biceps assisted glenohumeral anterior stability through increased resistance to torsional forces. Other studies have disputed biceps role as a shoulder stabilizer, finding only a small amount of muscle activity during shoulder motion.[140,155-157] Despite the debate, the relationship between the long head of biceps and the function and stability of the glenohumeral joint is an important clinical feature, which must always be considered in the management of patients with a shoulder dysfunction.

Classification of Biceps Lesions

Historically, lesions involving the biceps tendon have been categorized as being either a *tendonitis* or *instability.* Tendonitis can be further divided into *primary tendonitis,* which occurs as a result of pathology of the tendon sheath, or *secondary tendonitis,* which occurs secondary to an underlying injury that causes subsequent biceps irritation and injury. Many believe that the pathology seen in the biceps is directly related to its intimate relationship with the rotator cuff because they both pass under the coracoacromial arch and are therefore susceptible to impingement. "Isolated" ruptures of the long head of the biceps tendon are reportedly uncommon. Neer believed that most ruptures of the long head of the biceps tendon were associated with supraspinatus tears.[158,159] One study documented isolated biceps tendon ruptures in as many as 25% of patients,[145] but this incidence has not been reproduced in subsequent studies.

Slatis and Aalto[160] developed a three-part classification for biceps lesions. A type A lesion is referred to as *impingement tendonitis* because it occurs secondary to an impingement syndrome and rotator cuff disease. The defective cuff exposes the biceps to a rigid coracoacromial arch, resulting in tendonitis. This is the most common cause of biceps tendonitis. Type B lesions describe a *subluxation of the biceps tendon*. All subluxations and dislocations of the biceps tendon are included in this category. Lesions of the coracohumeral ligament allow the biceps tendon gradually to displace medially; the slipping of the tendon into and out of its groove leads to inflammation and fraying. A type C lesion is called *attrition tendonitis.* These are primary lesions of the biceps tendon that occur inside the canal, resulting in inflammation and eventual degeneration of the biceps tendon. Often spurring and fraying are evident with this type of tendonitis.

Biceps lesions have also been classified according to their anatomical location, specifically, at their origin, in the rotator interval, or in association with rotator cuff tears.[138] As noted earlier, the third category has spurred considerable study regarding the intimate relationship between the rotator cuff and the biceps tendon complex.

Clinical Presentation of Biceps Lesions

Patients with biceps tendon injuries typically present with pain in the proximal anterior area of the shoulder directly over the biceps tendon, with occasional radiation of pain down into the muscle belly. Similar to rotator cuff impingement syndromes, the pain can also be described at the deltoid insertion. It is unusual for biceps-related pain to radiate into the neck or distally beyond the elbow joint. Night pain is sometimes reported with biceps lesions. However, this likely can be explained by overall problems associated with trying to sleep with a painful shoulder. Most shoulder conditions are worse at night for a number of reasons. A compressive load may be present (e.g., lying on the affected shoulder) or in some instances traction may be applied to the shoulder (e.g., arm hanging over the bed); either of these results in pain. Positioning to avoid pain is difficult; however, most patients find that, with the use of many pillows, lying on the contralateral side with the affected arm in neutral, resting on the pillows, is among the most comfortable positions. Many patients with a painful shoulder report that their best rest is achieved in a semireclined position, such as in a recliner, with the arm resting on a pillow in the shoulder resting position.

Patients with a biceps injury usually describe an insidious onset of their symptoms; however, the pattern of pain can be linked to repetitive types of activities. Acute trauma may be part of the original injury that predisposed the biceps tendon to subsequent rupture or dislocation. Patients with bicipital tendonitis tend to be young or middle aged, with a pain pattern that is less at rest and more intense with activity. This is especially true with overhead activities in daily living, work, and/or sports. Rotation of the humerus at or above the horizontal level brings the tuberosities, bicipital groove, biceps tendon, and rotator cuff in direct contact with the anterior acromion and the coracoacromial ligament. Biceps instability is most commonly associated with the throwing athlete, where in certain positions of overhead rotation, the motion is accompanied by a palpable snap and pain. Pain is felt locally at the anterior aspect of the shoulder and is aggravated by elevating the arm to around 90°. If the biceps tendon ruptures, there is associated acute pain and sometimes an audible pop in the shoulder, followed in a few days by a notable change in the contour of the arm, with ecchymosis that often tracks downward to the distal muscle belly.

Numerous special tests have been described that can assist in the diagnosis of biceps conditions; however, their findings should be interpreted in combination with other clinical tests because the sensitivity and specificity of these tests have been reported to be only moderate (see Volume 1 of this series, *Orthopedic Physical Assessment,* Chapter 5). Most biceps lesions present with tenderness on palpation in the bicipital groove, which often disappears as the lesser tuberosity and groove rotate medially under the short head of the biceps and coracoid process. This is different from the tenderness noted with subdeltoid bursitis and impingement syndromes, which has a more diffuse pattern that does not change with arm rotation. According to Burkhead et al.,[153] this "tenderness in motion" sign is among the most specific for differentiating biceps lesions. ROM may be slightly restricted and painful into full abduction and medial and lateral rotation, usually as a result of pain rather than capsular constriction. Resisted isometric testing reveals a painful weakness with forward flexion of the shoulder.

Treatment of Biceps Injuries

As is almost universally true of all injuries, the most effective form of treatment of a biceps injury is prevention. As noted, the biceps is often part of the domino effect that occurs as a result of other primary shoulder pathologies. Therefore prevention of injury and overuse in these regions of the shoulder (e.g., rotator cuff) conceivably could prevent injuries to the biceps tendon. Individuals involved in manual labor with either repetitive overhead work or heavy lifting, as well as individuals participating in sports that demand overhand motions, are particularly at risk for biceps injury and should be educated on how to monitor and prevent injuries in this region. Developing a balanced shoulder musculature that includes a strong, healthy rotator cuff and scapular muscle region can help prevent the vicious cycle of impingement tendonitis, irritation, and muscle weakness that leads to altered kinematics, instability, and further impingement of tissue, such as the long head of the biceps.

Once the biceps tendon has been injured, the first step in proper management is a thorough examination of the anterior shoulder, structures of the shoulder girdle, and, if appropriate, kinetic chain. Failure either to identify associated lesions (e.g., those affecting the glenoid labrum and rotator cuff) or to note contributing factors (e.g., poorly stabilized scapula, hypomobile cervical and/or

thoracic spine, or altered muscle recruitment patterning) may lead the clinician to direct the sole treatment to the affected biceps tendon rather than addressing the true cause of the shoulder injury. Depending on the specific nature and severity of the biceps injury, treatment can range from managing an early, acute inflammatory situation locally at the tendon to treating the biceps tendon by retraining the scapular stabilizing muscles and rotator cuff to properly position the glenohumeral joint and therefore reduce impingement on the long head of the biceps anteriorly. Whichever is the case, the message is always the same: the clinician must make sure that treatment encompasses not only the affected tissue but also the causal tissue.

NERVE INJURIES OF THE SHOULDER

Nerve injuries of the shoulder represent a relatively small percentage of overall problems reported.[43,161-165] They are most commonly caused by direct trauma but also may occur as a result of repetitive microtrauma. In some instances, nerve injuries affecting the shoulder occur secondary to the predominant injury (e.g., axillary nerve damage from an anterior glenohumeral dislocation) or they may be the consequence of an underlying shoulder condition (e.g., poor posture and/or scapular instability that leads to thoracic outlet syndrome). Nerve injuries affecting the shoulder are being recognized with increasing frequency in sports, such as football and rugby, that comprise higher risk of injury from direct contact.[162-164,166] Nerve injuries as a result of compression and/or stretching from muscle hypertrophy have been reported in weight lifters, body builders, and/or volleyball players as well as individuals who perform repetitive motions in their occupations, such as computer analysts and assembly line workers.[161,163]

It is important to note that a fair number of neurological-like symptoms that patients experience may originate from sites well beyond the actual shoulder. These could include the spinal cord, cervical disc, cervical or thoracic nerve roots, nerve branches, and peripheral nerves, as well as unsuspected sites (e.g., the pleural or abdominal cavity) that can refer pain to the shoulder. Patients with nerve injuries often describe inconsistent, vague symptoms that may involve some combination of pain, paresthesia, or motor weakness in the limb; however, this is highly variable and depends on the patient's particular injury and the component of the nerve affected.[161,163,165] To make a diagnosis, the clinician must recognize the muscles innervated, sensory distribution, muscle stretch reflex, and compressive sites associated with a particular nerve. Commonly affected nerves in the shoulder region include the dorsal scapular, long thoracic, suprascapular, axillary, and musculocutaneous nerves. Table 5-7 presents the clinical features associated with injury to these nerves. Conservative management of most nerve injuries includes avoidance of precipitating factors to allow

TABLE **5-7**

Clinical Findings of Nerve Injuries About the Shoulder

Nerve	Injury Site	Motor Findings	Sensory Findings	Other Findings
Dorsal scapular nerve	Within scalenus medius muscle	Weakness in pressing the elbow backwards against resistance while hand is on hip or in pushing the palm backward against resistance with arm folded behind the back	None	Scapular winging with lateral displacement; shoulder pain
Long thoracic nerve	Supraclavicular region	Weakness in raising arm above the head	None	Scapular winging when patient pushes arm against the wall while elbow is extended
Suprascapular nerve	Suprascapular notch Spinoglenoid notch	Weakness in both abduction and lateral (external) rotation of arm Weakness of only lateral (external) rotation of arm	None	Deep scapular pain
Axillary nerve	Lateral aspect of the humerus and quadrilateral space	Weakness of abduction of shoulder between 15° and 90°	Lateral shoulder	Deltoid atrophy
Musculocutaneous nerve	At the level of the coracobrachialis	Elbow flexor and forearm supination weakness	Lateral forearm	Proximal forearm pain aggravated by elbow extension; reduced biceps reflex

recovery, physical therapy, and anti-inflammatory medications. Most injuries resolve spontaneously within 6 to 24 months.[161-165] For nerve injuries that have failed conservative treatment, surgical techniques involving various combinations of fascial graft or transfer of adjacent muscles may be effective.[167] A more detailed description of nervous tissue and the pathology of nerve injuries about the shoulder can be found in Chapter 25 and in Volume 2 of this series, *Scientific Foundations and Principles of Practice in Musculoskeletal Rehabilitation*, Chapter 8.

REFERENCES

1. Warner JJ: The gross anatomy of the joint surfaces, ligaments, labrum and capsule. In Matsen FA, Fu FH, Hawkins RJ, editors: *The shoulder: a balance of mobility and stability*, Rosemont, 1993, American Academy of Orthopedic Surgeons.
2. Bowen MK, Warren RF: Ligamentous control of shoulder stability based on selective cutting and static translation experiments, *Clin Sports Med* 10:757–782, 1991.
3. Soslowsky L, Flatlow E, Bigliani L, et al: Articular geometry of the glenohumeral joint, *Clin Orthop Relat Res* 285:181–190, 1992.
4. Harryman D, Sidles J, Clark J, et al: Translation of the humeral head on the glenoid with passive glenohumeral motion, *J Bone Joint Surg Am* 72:1334–1343, 1990.
5. Burkhart SS, Morgan CD, Kibler WB: The disabled throwing shoulder: spectrum of pathology. I. Pathoanatomy and biomechanics, *Arthroscopy* 19(4):404–420, 2003.
6. Abboud JA, Soslowsky LJ: Interplay of the static and dynamic restraints in glenohumeral instability, *Clin Orthop Relat Res* 400:48–57, 2002.
7. Wuelker N, Wirth CJ, Plitz W, et al: A dynamic shoulder model: reliability testing and muscle force study, *J Biomech* 28:489–499, 1995.

8. Clark JM, Harryman DT: Tendons, ligaments and capsule of the rotator cuff: gross and microscopic anatomy, *J Bone Joint Surg Am* 74:713–725, 1992.
9. De Franco MJ, Cole BJ: Current perspectives on rotator cuff anatomy, *J Arthrosc Relat Surg* 25(3):305–320, 2009.
10. Ludewig PM, Braman JP: Shoulder impingement: Biomechanical considerations in rehabilitation, *Man Ther* 16:33–39, 2011.
11. Labriola JE, Lee TQ, Debski RE, et al: Stability and instability of the glenohumeral joint: The role of shoulder muscles, *J Shoulder Elbow Surg* 14:32S–38S, 2005.
12. Vermeulen HM, Rozing PM, Obermann WR, et al: Adhesive capsulitis, *Phys Ther* 86(3):355–368, 2006.
13. Tauro JC: Stiffness and rotator cuff tears: incidence, arthroscopic findings, and treatment results, *Arthroscopy* 22(6):581–586, 2006.
14. Burkhart SS, Morgan CD, Kibler WB: The disabled throwing shoulder: spectrum of pathology. III. The SICK scapula, scapular dyskinesis, the kinetic chain and rehabilitation, *Arthroscopy* 19(6):641–661, 2003.
15. Kibler WB: The role of the scapula in athletic shoulder function, *Am J Sports Med* 26:325–337, 1998.

16. Barden JM, Balyk R, Raso VJ, et al: Atypical shoulder muscle activation in multidirectional instability, *Clin Neurophysiol* 116(8):1846–1857, 2005.
17. Smith J, Dahm DL: Electromyographic activity in the immobilized shoulder girdle musculature during scapulothoracic exercise, *Arch Phys Med Rehabil* 87:923–927, 2006.
18. Barden JM, Balyk R, Raso VJ, et al: Dynamic upper limb proprioception in multidirectional shoulder instability, *Clin Orthop Relat Res* 420:181–189, 2004.
19. Burkhead W, Rockwood C: Treatment of instability of the shoulder with an exercise program, *J Bone Joint Surg Am* 70:890–896, 1992.
20. Wilk KE, Meister K, Andrews JR: Current concepts in the rehabilitation of the overhead throwing athlete, *Am J Sports Med* 30(1):136–151, 2002.
21. Kibler WB, Livingstone BP: Closed chain rehabilitation for the upper and lower extremities, *J Am Acad Orthop Surg* 9:412–421, 2001.
22. Lephart SM, Henry TJ: The physiologic basis for open and closed chain rehabilitation for the upper extremity, *J Sport Rehabil* 5:71–87, 1996.
23. O'Brien SJ, Arnoczky SP, Warren REF, et al: Developmental anatomy of the shoulder and anatomy of the glenohumeral joint. In Rockwood CA, Matsen FA, editors: The shoulder, vol 1, Philadelphia, 1990, WB Saunders.

24. Ardic F, Kahraman Y, Kacar M, et al: Shoulder impingement syndrome: Relationships between clinical, functional, and radiological findings, *Am J Phys Med Rehabil* 85(1):53–60, 2006.

25. Mehta S, Gimbel JA, Soslowsky LJ: Etiologic and pathogenetic factors for rotator cuff tendinopathy, *Clin Sports Med* 22:791–812, 2003.

26. Bradley JP, Tibone JE: Electromyographic analysis of muscle action about the shoulder, *Clin Sports Med* 10:789–805, 1991.

27. Morrey BF, Itoi E, An K: Biomechanics of the shoulder. In Rockwood CA, Matsen FA, editors: *The shoulder*, Philadelphia, 1998, WB Saunders.

28. Inman VT, Saunders JB, Abbott LC: Observations on the function of the shoulder joint, *J Bone Joint Surg* 26:1–30, 1944.

29. Doody SG, Waterland JC, Freedman L: Scapulohumeral goniometer, *Arch Phys Med Rehabil* 51:711–713, 1970.

30. Doody SG, Freedman L, Waterland JC: Shoulder movements during abduction in the scapular plane, *Arch Phys Med Rehabil* 51:595–604, 1970.

31. Poppen NK, Walker PS: Normal and abnormal motion of the shoulder, *J Bone Joint Surg Am* 58:195–199, 1976.

32. Freedman L, Munro RH: Abduction of the arm in the scapular plane: scapular and glenohumeral movements, *J Bone Joint Surg Am* 18:1503–1507, 1966.

33. Basmajian JV, Bazant FJ: Factors preventing downward dislocation of the adducted shoulder joint: an electromyographic and morphological study, *J Bone Joint Surg Am* 41:1182–1186, 1959.

34. Flanders M: Shoulder muscle activity during natural arm movements: what is optimized? In Matsen FA, Fu FH, Hawkins RJ, editors: *The shoulder: a balance of mobility and stability*, Rosemont, 1993, American Academy of Orthopaedic Surgeons.

35. Mell AG, LaScalza S, Guffey P, et al: Effect of rotator cuff pathology on shoulder rhythm, *J Shoulder Elbow Surg* 14(1 suppl S):58S–64S, 2005.

36. Van Tongel A, De Wilde L: Sternoclavicular joint injuries: a literature review, *Muscles, Ligaments Tendons J* 1(3):100–105, 2011.

37. Goss CM, editor: *Anatomy of the human body*, ed 28, Philadelphia, 1966, Lea & Febiger.

38. Rowe CR, editor: *The shoulder*, New York, 1988, Churchill Livingstone.

39. Bearn JG: Direct observations on the function of the capsule of the sternoclavicular joint in clavicular support, *J Anat* 101:159–170, 1967.

40. Rudzinski JP, Pittman LM, Uehara DT: Shoulder and humerus injuries. In Tintinalli JE, et al, editors: *Tintinalli's emergency medicine: a comprehensive study guide*, ed 7, New York, 2011, McGraw-Hill.

41. Inman VT: Observations on the function of the clavicle, *California Med* 63:158–166, 1946.

42. Lucas DB: Biomechanics of the shoulder joint, *Arch Surg* 107:425–432, 1973.

43. Kaplan LD, Flanigan DC, Norwig J, et al: Prevalence and variance of shoulder injuries in elite collegiate football players, *Am J Sports Med* 33(8):1142–1146, 2005.

44. Cave EM: *Fractures and other injuries*, Chicago, 1961, Year Book.

45. Rockwood CA, Green DP: *Fractures in adults*, Philadelphia, 1984, JB Lippincott.

46. Ferrera PC, Wheeling HM: Sternoclavicular joint injuries, *Am J Emerg Med* 18(1):58–61, 2000.

47. Phillipson MR, Wallwork N: Traumatic dislocation of the sternoclavicular joint, *Orthop Trauma* 26(2):128–135, 2012.

48. Jain S, Monbaliu D, Thompson JF: Thoracic outlet syndrome caused by chronic retrosternal dislocation of the clavicle. Successful treatment by transaxillary resection of the first rib, *J Bone Joint Surg Br* 84(1):116–118, 2002.

49. Nakayama E, Tanaka T, Noguchi T, et al: Tracheal stenosis caused by retrosternal dislocation of the right clavicle, *Ann Thorac Surg* 83(2):685–687, 2007.

50. Gleason BA: Bilateral, spontaneous, anterior subluxation of the sternoclavicular joint: a case report and literature review, *Mil Med* 171(8):790–792, 2006.

51. Rockwood CA, Wirth MA: Disorders of the sternoclavicular joint. In Rockwood CA, Matsen FA, editors: *The shoulder*, Philadelphia, 1998, WB Saunders.

52. Wirth MA, Rockwood CA: Complications following repair of the sternoclavicular joint. In Bigliani LU, editor: *Complications of the shoulder*, Baltimore, 1993, Williams & Wilkins.

53. Higginbotham TO, Kuhn JE: Atraumatic disorders of the sternoclavicular joint, *J Am Acad Orthop Surg* 13(2):138–145, 2005.

54. Beim GM: Acromioclavicular joint injuries, *J Athl Train* 35(3):261–267, 2000.

55. Rockwood CA, Williams GR, Young DC: Disorders of the acromioclavicular joint. In Rockwood CA, Matsen FA, editors: *The shoulder*, Philadelphia, 1998, WB Saunders.

56. Bosworth BM: Complete acromioclavicular dislocation, *N Engl J Med* 241:221–225, 1949.

57. Magee DJ, Reid DC: Shoulder injuries. In Zachazewski JE, Magee DJ, Quillen WS, editors: *Athletic injuries and rehabilitation*, Philadelphia, 1996, WB Saunders.

58. Codman EA: *The shoulder*, Boston, 1934, Thomas Todd.

59. Rockwood CA: Injuries to the acromioclavicular joint. In Rockwood CA, Green DP, editors: *Fractures in adults*, vol 1, ed 2, Philadelphia, 1984, JB Lippincott.

60. Rockwood CA, Guy DK, Griffin JL: Treatment of chronic, complete acromioclavicular joint dislocation, *Orthop Trans* 12:735–739, 1988.

61. Dias JJ, Gregg PJ: Acromioclavicular joint injuries in sport, *Sports Med* 11:125–132, 1991.

62. Beitzel MA, Cote MP, Apostolakos J: Current concepts in the treatment of acromioclavicular joint dislocations, *Arthroscopy* 29(2):387–397, 2013.

63. Johansen JA, Grutter PW, McFarland EG, et al: Acromioclavicular joint injuries: indications for treatment and treatment options, *J Shoulder Elbow Surg* 20(2):S70–S82, 2011.

64. Petron DJ, Hanson RW: Acromioclavicular joint disorders, *Curr Sports Med Rep* 6(5):300–306, 2007.

65. Wojtys EM, Nelson G: Conservative treatment of grade III acromioclavicular dislocations, *Clin Orthop Relat Res* 268:112–119, 1991.

66. Bannister GC, Wallace WA, Stableforth PG, et al: The management of acute acromioclavicular dislocation: a randomized prospective controlled trial, *J Bone Joint Surg Br* 71:848–850, 1989.

67. Bach BR, Van Fleet TA, Novak PJ: Acromioclavicular injuries: controversies in treatment, *Phys Sportsmed* 20(12):87–101, 1992.

68. Tibone J, Sellers R, Tonino P: Strength testing after third degree acromioclavicular dislocation, *Am J Sports Med* 20:328–331, 1992.

69. Trainer G, Arciero RA, Mazzocca AD: Practical management of grade III acromioclavicular separations, *Clin J Sports Med* 18:162–166, 2008.

70. Murena L, Canton G, Vulcano E, et al: Scapular dyskinesis and SICK scapula syndrome following surgical treatment of type III acute acromioclavicular dislocations, *Knee Surg Sports Traumatol Arthrosc* 21(5):1146–1150, 2013.

71. Walsh WM, Peterson DA, Shelton G, et al: Shoulder strength following acromioclavicular injury, *Am J Sports Med* 13:153–158, 1985.

72. Larsen E, Bjerg-Nielsen A: Conservative or surgical treatment of acromioclavicular dislocation, *J Bone Joint Surg Am* 68(4):552–555, 1986.

73. Schlegel TF, Burks RT: A prospective evaluation of untreated acute grade three acromioclavicular separations, *Am J Sports Med* 29(6):699–703, 2001.

74. Kim S, Blank A, Strauss E: Management of type 3 acromioclavicular joint dislocations: Current controversies, *Bull Hosp Joint Dis* 72(1):53–60, 2014.

75. Duplay ES: De la periarthrote scapulohumerale, *Arch Gen Med* 20:513–542, 1872.

76. Codman EA: Tendinitis of the short rotators. In Codman EA, editor: *The shoulder: rupture of the supraspinatus tendon and other lesions in or about the subacromial bursa*, Boston, 1934, Thomas Todd.

77. Neviaser JS: Adhesive capsulitis of the shoulder, *J Bone Joint Surg* 27:211–222, 1945.

78. Wiley AM: Arthroscopic appearance of frozen shoulder, *Arthroscopy* 7:138–143, 1991.

79. Bunker TD, Anthony PP: The pathology of frozen shoulder. A Dupuytren-like disease, *J Bone Joint Surg Br* 77:677–683, 1995.

80. Bunker TD: Time for a new name for frozen shoulder-contracture of the shoulder, *Shoulder Elbow* 1:4–9, 2009.

81. Lundberg BJ: The frozen shoulder, *Acta Orthop Scand* 119:1–59, 1969.

82. Zuckerman JD, Rokito A: Frozen shoulder: a consensus definition, *J Shoulder Elbow Surg* 20:322–325, 2011.

83. Zuckerman JD, Cuomo F: Frozen shoulder. In Matsen FA, Fu FH, Hawkins RJ, editors: *The shoulder: a balance of mobility and stability*, Rosemont, 1993, American Academy of Orthopedic Surgeons.

84. Reeves B: The natural history of the frozen shoulder syndrome, *Scand J Rheumatol* 4:193–196, 1975.

85. Dias R, Cutts S, Massoud S: Frozen shoulder, *Br Med J* 331:1453–1456, 2005.

86. Bunker TD, Schranz PJ: Clinical challenges in orthopaedics: the shoulder, Oxford, 1998, ISIS Medical Media.

87. Guyver PM, Bruce DJ, Rees JL: Frozen shoulder—a stiff problem that requires a flexible approach, *Maturitas* 78:11–16, 2014.

88. Jain TK, Sharma NK: The effectiveness of physiotherapeutic interventions in treatment of frozen shoulder/adhesive capsulitis: a systematic review, *J Back Musculoskelet Rehabil* 27(3):247–273, 2014.

89. Maund E, Craig D, Suekarran S: Management of frozen shoulder: a systematic review and cost-effectiveness analysis, *Health Technol Assess* 16(11):1–264, 2012.

90. Page MJ, Green S, Kramer S, et al: Manual therapy and exercise for adhesive capsulitis (frozen shoulder): Systematic review, *Cochrane Database Syst Rev* 8,2014, CD011275.

91. Page MJ, Green S, Kramer S, et al: Electrotherapy modalities for adhesive capsulitis (frozen shoulder), *Cochrane Database Syst Rev* 10, 2014, CD011324.

92. Griggs SM, Ahn A, Green A: Idiopathic adhesive capsulitis: A prospective functional outcome study of nonoperative treatment, *J Bone Joint Surg Am* 82(10):1398–1407, 2000.

93. Farrell CM, Sperling JW, Cofield RH: Manipulation for frozen shoulder: long-term results, *J Shoulder Elbow Surg* 14(5):480–484, 2005.

94. Lewis J: Frozen shoulder contracture syndrome—aetiology, diagnosis and management, *Man Ther*, 2014 Jul 18 [Epub ahead of print].

95. Ada JR, Miller ME: Scapular fractures: analysis of 113 cases, *Clin Orthop* 269:174–180, 1991.

96. Ideberg R, Grevsten S, Larsson S: Epidemiology of scapular fractures: incidence and classification of 338 fractures, *Acta Orthop Scand* 66:395–397, 1995.

97. Sudkamp NP, Jaeger N, Bornebusch L: Fractures of the scapula, *Acta Chir Orthop Traumatol Cech* 78(4):297–304, 2011.

98. Imatani RJ: Fractures of the scapula: a review of 53 fractures, *J Trauma* 15:473–478, 1975.

99. Bartonicek J, Tucek M, Fric V, et al: Fractures of the scapular neck: diagnosis, classifications and treatment, *Int Orthop* 38:2163–2173, 2014.

100. Goss TP: The scapula: coracoid, acromial and avulsion fractures, *Am J Orthop* 25:106–115, 1996.

101. Bauer G, Fleischmann W, Dussler E: Displaced scapular fractures: Indications and long term results of open reduction and internal fixation, *Arch Orthop Trauma Surg* 114:215–219, 1995.

102. Hardegger FH, Simpson LA, Weber BG: The operative treatment of scapular fractures, *J Bone Joint Surg Br* 66:725–731, 1984.

103. Jeray KJ, Cole PA: Clavicle and scapula fracture problems: functional assessment and current treatment strategies, *Instr Course Lect* 60:51–71, 2011.

104. McGahan JP, Rab GT, Dublin A: Fractures of the scapula, *J Trauma* 20:880–883, 1980.

105. Nordqvist A, Petersson C: Fracture of the body, neck or spine of the scapula: a long term follow up study, *Clin Orthop Relat Res* 283:139–144, 1992.

106. Herscovici D, Fiennes AG, Allgower M, et al: The floating shoulder: ipsilateral clavicle and scapular neck fractures, *J Bone Joint Surg Br* 74:362–364, 1992.

107. Goss TP: Double disruptions of the superior shoulder suspensory complex, *J Orthop Trauma* 7:99–106, 1993.

108. Noort A, Werken C: The floating shoulder, *Int J Care Injured* 10:1–10, 2005.

109. Sanders JO, Song KM: Fractures, dislocations and acquired problems of the shoulder in children. In Rockwood CA, Matsen FA, editors: *The shoulder*, Philadelphia, 1998, WB Saunders.

110. Robinson CM: Fractures of the clavicle: epidemiology and classification, *J Bone Joint Surg Br* 80:476–484, 1998.

111. Egol KA, Koval KJ, Zuckerman JD: *Handbook of fractures*, ed 4, Philadelphia, 2010, Lippincott Williams.

112. Craig EV: Fractures of the clavicle. In Rockwood CA, Matsen FA, editors: *The shoulder*, Philadelphia, 1998, WB Saunders.

113. Balcik BJ, Monseau AJ, Krantz W: Evaluation and treatment of sternoclavicular, clavicular and acromioclavicular injuries, *Prim Care Clin Office Pract* 40:911–923, 2013.

114. Pujalte GG, Housner JA: Management of clavicle fracture, *Curr Sports Med Rep* 7(5):275–280, 2008.

115. Nordqvist A, Petersson CJ, Redlund-Johnell I: Mid-clavicle fractures in adults: end result study after conservative treatment, *J Orthop Trauma* 12:572–576, 1998.

116. Van der Meijden OA, Gaskill TR: Treatment of clavicle fractures: current concepts review, *J Shoulder Elbow Surg* 21(3):423–429, 2012.

117. Kong L, Zhang Y, Shen Y: Operative versus nonoperative treatment for displaced midshaft clavicular fractures: a meta-analysis of randomized clinical trials, *Arch Orthop Trauma Surg* 134:1493–1500, 2014.

118. Barnett LS: Little league shoulder syndrome: proximal humeral epiphysiolysis in adolescent baseball pitchers—a case report, *J Bone Joint Surg Am* 67:495–496, 1985.

119. Zairns B, Andrews JR, Carson WG: *Injuries to the throwing arm*, Philadelphia, 1985, WB Saunders.

120. Osbahr DC, Kim HJ, Dugas JR: Little league shoulder, *Curr Opin Pediatr* 22(1):35–40, 2010.

121. Shanley E, Thigpen C: Throwing injuries in the adolescent athlete, *Int J Sports Phys Ther* 8(5):630–640, 2013.

122. Lauritzen JB, Schwarz P, Lund B: Changing incidence and residual lifetime risk of common osteoporosis-related fractures, *Osteoporos Int* 3:127–132, 1993.

123. Court-Brown CM, Garg A, McQueen MM: The epidemiology of proximal humeral fractures, *Acta Orthop Scand* 72:365–371, 2001.

124. Palvanen M, Kannus P, Parkkari J: Injury mechanisms of osteoporotic upper limb fractures, *J Bone Miner Res* 15:S539, 2000.

125. Neer CS: Displaced proximal humeral fractures: classification and evaluation, *J Bone Joint Surg Am* 52:1077–1089, 1970.

126. Neer CS: Displaced proximal humeral fractures. II Treatment of three-part and four-part displacement, *J Bone Joint Surg Am* 52:1090–1103, 1970.

127. Koval KJ, Gallagher MA, Marsicano JG, et al: Functional outcome after minimally displaced fractures of the proximal part of the humerus, *J Bone Joint Surg Am* 79:203–207, 1997.

128. Green A, Norris T: Proximal humerus fractures and fracture dislocations. In Jupiter J, editor: *Skeletal trauma*, ed 3 Philadelphia, 2003, Saunders.

129. Bertoft ES, Lundh I, Ringqvist I: Physical therapy after fracture of the proximal end of the humerus, *Scand J Rehabil Med* 16:11–16, 1984.

130. Handoll HHG, Ollivere BJ, Rollins KE: Interventions for treating proximal humeral fractures in adults, *Cochrane Database Syst Rev* 12,2012, CD000434.

131. Zuckerman JD: Fractures of the proximal humerus: diagnosis and management. In Iannotti JP, editor: *Disorders of the shoulder: diagnosis and management*, Philadelphia, 1999, Lippincott Williams & Wilkins.

132. Herscovici Jr. D, Saunders DT, Johnson MP, et al: Percutaneous fixation of proximal humeral fracture, *Clin Orthop* 375:97–104, 2000.

133. Kooijman M, Swinkels I, Dijk CV, et al: Patients with shoulder syndromes in general and physiotherapy practice: an observational study, *BMC Musculoskel Dis* 14:128–137, 2013.

134. Arce G, Bak K, Bain G, et al: Management of disorders of the rotator cuff: proceedings of the ISAKOS Upper Extremity Committee Consensus Meeting, *J Arthrosc Relat Surg* 29(11):1840–1850, 2013.

135. Luime JJ, Koes BW, Heridriksen IJ, et al: The prevalence and incidence of shoulder pain in the general population; a systematic review, *Scand J Rheumatol* 33(2):73–81, 2004.

136. Jain NB, Higgins LD, Losina E, et al: Epidemiology of musculoskeletal upper extremity ambulatory surgery in the United States, *BMC Musculoskel Dis* 15:4–7, 2014.

137. Mighell M: Massive irreparable rotator cuff tears. In Frankle MA, editor: *Rotator cuff deficiency of the shoulder*, New York, 2008, Thieme Medical.

138. Burkhart SS, Parten PM: Dead arm syndrome: torsional SLAP lesions versus internal impingement, *Tech Shoulder Elbow Surg* 2(2):74–84, 2001.

139. Habermeyer P, Walch G: The biceps tendon and rotator cuff disease. In Burkhead WZ Jr., editors: *Rotator cuff disorders*, Media, 1996, Williams & Wilkins.

140. Rodowsky MW, Harner CD, Fu FH: FH: The role of the long head of the biceps muscle and superior glenoid labrum in anterior stability of the shoulder, *Am J Sports Med* 22:121–130, 1994.

141. Itoi E, Kuechle DK, Newman SR, et al: Stabilizing function of the biceps in stable and unstable shoulders, *J Bone Joint Surg Br* 75:546–550, 1993.

142. Pal GP, Bhatt RH, Patel VS: Relationship between the tendon of the long head of biceps brachii and the glenoid labrum in humans, *Anat Rec* 229:278–280, 1991.

143. Andrews J, Carson W, McLeod W: Glenoid labrum tears related to the long head of the biceps, *Am J Sports Med* 13:337–341, 1985.

144. Snyder SJ, Karzel RP, Del Pizzo W: SLAP lesions of the shoulder, *Arthroscopy* 6:274–279, 1990.

145. Morgan CD: The thrower's shoulder. In McGinty JB, editor: *Operative arthroscopy*, ed 3, Philadelphia, 2003, Lippincott.

146. Burkhart SS, Morgan CD, Kibler WB: The disabled throwing shoulder: spectrum of pathology. Part II: evaluation and treatment of SLAP lesions in throwers, *Arthroscopy* 19(5):531–539, 2003.

147. Burkhart SS, Morgan CD: The peel-back mechanism—its role in producing and extending posterior type II SLAP lesions and its effect on SLAP repair rehabilitation, *Arthroscopy* 14:637–640, 1998.

148. Vangsness CT, Jorgenson SS, Watson T, et al: The origin of the long head of the biceps from the scapula and glenoid labrum, *J Bone Joint Surg Br* 76:951–954, 1994.

149. Meyer AW: Spontaneous dislocation of the tendon of the long head of the biceps brachii, *Arch Surg* 13:109–119, 1926.

150. Basmajian JV, Latif MA: Integrated actions and function of the chief flexors of the elbow, *J Bone Joint Surg Am* 39:1106–1118, 1957.

151. Glousman R, Jobe FW, Tibone JP: Dynamic electromyographic analysis of the throwing shoulder and glenohumeral instability, *J Bone Joint Surg Am* 70(2):220–226, 1988.

152. Ting A, Jobe FW, Barto P: An EMG analysis of the lateral biceps in shoulders with rotator cuff tears, San Francisco, 1987, Third Open Meeting of the Society of American Shoulder and Elbow Surgeons.

153. Burkhead WZ, Arcand MA, Zeman C, et al: The biceps tendon. In Rockwood CA, Matsen FA, editors: *The shoulder*, Philadelphia, 1998, WB Saunders.

154. Enad JG: Bifurcate origin of the long head of the biceps tendon, *Arthroscopy* 20:1081–1083, 2004.

155. Yamaguchi K, Riew KD, Galatz CM: Biceps function in normal and rotator cuff deficient shoulders: an EMG analysis, *Orthop Trans* 18:191, 1994.

156. Kumar VP, Satku K, Balasubramaniam P: The role of the long head of biceps brachii in the stabilization of the head of the humerus, *Clin Orthop Relat Res* 244:172–175, 1989.

157. Yamaguchi K, Riew KD, Galatz LM, et al: Biceps activity during shoulder motion: An electromyographic analysis, *Clin Orthop Relat Res* 336:122–129, 1997.

158. Neer CS: Impingement lesions, *Clin Orthop* 173:70–77, 1983.

159. Neer CS, Poppen NK: Supraspinatus outlet, *Orthop Trans* 11:234, 1987.

160. Slatis P, Aalto K: Medical dislocation of the tendon of the long head of the biceps brachii, *Acta Orthop Scand* 50:73–77, 1979.

161. Neal S, Fields K: Peripheral nerve entrapment and injury in the upper extremity, *Am Fam Physician* 81(2):147–155, 2010.

162. Safran MR: Nerve injury about the shoulder in athletes. Part 2. Long thoracic nerve, spinal accessory nerve, burners/stingers, and thoracic outlet syndrome, *Am J Sports Med* 32(4):1063–1076, 2004.

163. Schoen DC: Upper extremity nerve entrapments, *Orthop Nurs* 21(2):15–32, 2002.

164. Toth C, McNeil S, Feasby T: Peripheral nervous system injuries in sport and recreation: a systematic review, *Sports Med* 35(8):717–738, 2005.

165. McKenzie K, Kin G, Tamir S: Thoracic outlet syndrome part I: a clinical review, *J Am Chiropractic Assoc* January:17-24, 2004.

166. Robinson L: Traumatic injury to peripheral nerves, *Muscle Nerve* 23:863–873, 2000.

167. Galano G, Bigliani L, Ahmad C, et al: Surgical treatment of winged scapula, *Clin Orthop Relat Res* 466(3):652–660, 2008.

CHAPTER 6

Shoulder Instability

RONALD R. MATTISON, MARTIN J. BOULIANE, DAVID J. MAGEE*

INTRODUCTION

The impression gained from a cursory glance at the shoulder belies its complexity. This proximal part of the upper kinetic chain starts at the trunk and includes the scapula, glenohumeral joint, acromioclavicular joint, and sternoclavicular joint.[1] As part of the kinetic chain, the shoulder acts as a funnel, transferring the forces generated by the lower extremity and trunk to the arm.[2-5] The human shoulder has evolved to allow an incredible range of motion (ROM) for reaching and placing the human hand through a large functional arc, largely at the expense of bony stability. Elevation, depression, protraction, retraction, and rotation of the scapula, along with elevation and rotation of the clavicle, enhance or facilitate the motions of forward flexion, extension, abduction, adduction, medial and lateral rotation, and circumduction of the glenohumeral joint, which allow the arm and hand to be placed in many positions. Unfortunately, every anatomical adaptation toward mobility creates the potential for problems, which can be compounded by the large ROMs needed, frequent repetitions, and high stress loads seen in sports and occupations involving the upper limbs.

It is imperative that clinicians consider the whole kinetic chain as well as the shoulder girdle, rather than any one articulation when assessing the shoulder. With less bony support than other articulations, the shoulder girdle must be supplemented by strong ligaments and careful arrangement of all muscle groups to ensure stability.[7,8] With such a large ROM available at the shoulder, glenohumeral stabilization comes from the osseous anatomy, specifically the "pear-shaped" glenoid (Figure 6-1), as well as joint compression. This "concavity" compression is the result of precise sequencing of all the shoulder muscle groups involved along with the labrum, glenohumeral ligaments, and joint capsule.[9-12]

FUNCTIONAL ANATOMY

Although bony containment is lacking in the scapulohumeral articulation, the articular surfaces are positioned to contribute to stability, especially with the arm in elevated positions. For example, the scapula faces 30° anteriorly to the chest wall and is tilted upward 3° to augment functional reaching motions above shoulder height.[3,13,14] The "pear-shaped" glenoid is almost a perfect circle, being much wider in the lower half than in the superior half. It is also tilted upward 5° to help to control inferior instability and to further augment movements above shoulder height (see Figure 6-1).[15]

At the glenohumeral joint, a large humeral head articulates with the shallow glenoid cavity, which is deepened by the glenoid labrum. The surface area of the humeral head is significantly larger than the glenoid.[13,16,17] However, the articular surfaces of the humeral head and glenoid are functionally congruent, having radii within 3 mm. During movement, the area in contact between the two surfaces constantly changes, with the greatest contact in mid-elevation rather than at the extremes of glenohumeral motion, where the potential for instability is greatest.[18] Only approximately 25% to 30% of the large, spherical humeral head is in contact with the glenoid surface at any one time.[13,19] Stability in the glenohumeral joint is achieved through several factors: the bony glenoid, labrum, glenohumeral ligaments, rotator cuff, negative pressure within the joint capsule, and coefficient of friction of the synovial fluid.

During 180° of elevation of the arm, there is 120° of glenohumeral motion, along with 60° of scapulothoracic motion. This large ROM (i.e., scapulohumeral rhythm) is brought about by precise muscle sequencing, and the resultant force couples generate rotary torques on the scapula and humerus, creating complex arm movement patterns. The term *force couple* refers to muscles working together by applying different forces to create a common motion—some act concentrically to initiate and provide movement or control movement and others act isometrically, concentrically, or eccentrically to control or decelerate movement (Figure 6-2).[20] For example, abduction by the deltoid, which is part of a force couple, is counterbalanced by the supraspinatus, infraspinatus, and subscapularis, the other part of the force couple, to allow abduction by compressing the humeral head in the glenoid and preventing its

*The authors, editors, and publisher wish to acknowledge David C. Reid for his contributions on this topic in the previous edition.

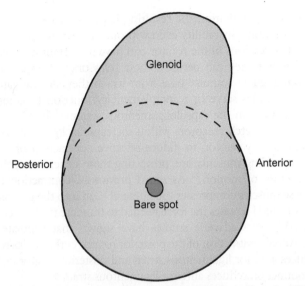

Figure 6-1 "Pear shape" of the right glenoid. (Redrawn from Lo IKY, Parten PM, Burkhart SS: The inverted pear glenoid: an indicator of significant glenoid bone loss, *Arthroscopy* 20(2):171, 2004.)

elevation under the acromion (see Figure 6-2, *A*). Similarly the serratus anterior is counterbalanced by the three parts of trapezius, levator scapulae, and rhomboids to control the scapula (see Figure 6-2, *B*).

Any structural injury, scapular dyskinesia (i.e., abnormal positions or patterns of movement of the scapula),

or dysplasia (i.e., abnormal development) of the humerus or the glenoid or its labrum can affect the stability of the glenohumeral joint.[21] Normally, translation of the humeral head on the glenoid is limited to a few millimeters in every direction during movement.[20,22-24] If the dynamic structures controlling this translation (i.e., primarily the rotator cuff) or the passive structures (e.g., the labrum or ligaments) are injured, this translation increases. The increased translation leads to increased stress on the glenoid labrum, failure of the static restraints (i.e., ligaments) (see Table 5-1), and eccentric overload of the dynamic restraints (i.e., rotator cuff and biceps), which work individually and in unison to provide stability in the joints of the shoulder, where mobility is paramount. The result is instability, impingement because of the translation and/or abnormal movement, or both.[25,26]

Any alteration in biomechanics or trauma may lead to a tear in the glenoid labrum. The glenoid labrum increases the glenoid depth approximately twofold, which contributes to glenohumeral stability.[13,16,17,19] However, labral anatomy can be quite variable, even being deficient in certain locations. Such variations often occur in the anterosuperior location and are referred to as a sublabral foramen or **Buford complex**.[27-29] A **Bankart lesion** is a traumatic labral tear that usually occurs with an anterior dislocation. However, the labrum can tear anywhere along its attachment on the glenoid. A Bankart lesion can also be a bony lesion. This typically occurs in the anteroinferior quadrant of the glenoid

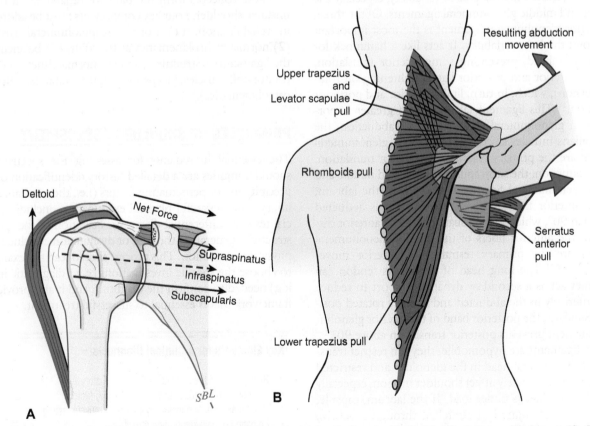

Figure 6-2 Force-couple examples about the shoulder. **A,** Glenohumeral joint. **B,** Scapula. (**A** Modified from Matsen FA, Lippett SB, Sidles JA, Harryman DT, editors: *Practical evaluation and management of the shoulder,* p 98, Philadelphia, 1994, WB Saunders.)

after traumatic anterior glenohumeral dislocation. As the size of the bone fragment increases, so does the risk of recurrent dislocation, especially in young, contact athletes. A **Hill-Sachs lesion** is the corresponding lesion or impaction fracture that usually occurs in the posterolateral aspect of the humeral head as the soft cancellous bone of the humeral head rests on the hard cortical glenoid bone during a traumatic glenohumeral dislocation. A condition that occurs in the superior labrum anterior and posterior (SLAP) to the biceps, **SLAP lesion**, is a lesion around the long head of the biceps where it crosses over the glenohumeral joint. Single or repetitive trauma can cause the labrum to fray, tear, or peel back from the bone, resulting in a SLAP lesion.[2-4]

The surrounding soft tissue envelope (i.e., the capsule) is the primary contributor to stability in the normal glenohumeral joint, with a normal lax inferior capsule allowing movement into full elevation. The capsule is reinforced by the coracohumeral and glenohumeral ligaments, which act as checkreins at the extreme ROM, assisting the compression caused by the dynamic rotator cuff.[21,29] These two components augment normal scapulohumeral rhythm to create functional stability. The concavity formed by the glenoid labrum, along with the muscles that provide compression and the unique tightening mechanism of the inferior glenohumeral ligament, provides a "concavity-compression" mechanism that stabilizes the glenohumeral joint.[13,21]

The glenohumeral ligaments, which are thickenings in the capsule, show a high degree of variability, especially the superior and middle glenohumeral ligaments. Of the three, the inferior glenohumeral ligament is the most important and shows the least variability. It acts like a hammock for the humeral head, preventing some inferior translation, with the anterior and posterior bands tightening on rotation (torsion), which, in turn, limits anterior and posterior translation.[24] This ligament takes on even greater importance with glenohumeral elevation. At 0° abduction, the subscapularis muscle, labrum, and superior glenohumeral ligament are the primary restraints to anterior translation. At 45° abduction, the subscapularis muscle and middle and inferior glenohumeral ligaments, along with the labrum, prevent anterior translation. When the arm is abducted more than 90°, which is the usual position of anterior dislocation, the anterior fibers of the inferior glenohumeral ligament are the primary restraints to anterior movement.[13,16,17,19,30] The long head of the biceps tendon can sometimes act as a secondary dynamic support to reduce stress anteriorly in the abducted and laterally rotated position.[31] Similarly, the posterior band of the inferior glenohumeral ligament prevents posterior translation above 90°.[16]

If the ligaments are hypomobile, they can restrict translation of the humeral head in the glenoid,[32] and restricted translation can adversely affect shoulder motion, especially when the shoulder is under load. If the labrum, capsule, or ligaments are injured or stretched through repetitive microtrauma, such as occurs with repetitive throwing or swimming activities, the resulting hypermobility can lead to functional instability even without major trauma.

The tendons of the rotator cuff have important dynamic roles, but they can perform these roles only when acting from a stable scapular base from which they all originate. The muscles serve in a complementary function to adjust the tension in the capsuloligamentous system.[33] It is possible that stretch receptors within the capsular ligaments are activated by tension to induce selective contraction of the surrounding musculature, protecting these structures at the extremes of motion.[34] As stated previously, contraction of these muscles compresses the humeral head into the glenoid cavity and increases the force needed to translate the humeral head.[16,35,36] Cadaveric studies have shown that simulated maximal contraction of the posterior rotator cuff muscles reduces anterior ligamentous strain and posterior rotator cuff contraction reduces anterior ligamentous strain.[37]

A second and equally important group of muscles that affects glenohumeral stability is the scapular control muscles (see Table 5-1). These muscles control (stabilize) the scapula, which is the dynamic base (i.e., the origin) for the rotator cuff, biceps, and triceps (long head) muscles. Through their action on the scapula, these muscles position the glenoid beneath the humeral head, adjusting for the changing position of the arm. With scapular dyskinesia, failure to maintain the stable glenoid platform (i.e., the scapula) may occur, causing an alteration in scapulohumeral rhythm and mild-to-severe winging of the scapula.

These concepts form the basis for rehabilitation of the unstable shoulder. Four key components must be addressed in rehabilitation: (1) normal scapulohumeral rhythm, (2) normal arthrokinematics at the joint, (3) balancing of the ligamentous structures, and (4) normal function of the rotator cuff muscles, biceps and scapular stabilizers (normal osteokinematics).[1]

PRINCIPLES OF SHOULDER ASSESSMENT

The essential ingredients for assessing the spectrum of shoulder injuries are a detailed history, identification of the precipitating or perpetuating factors (i.e., the mechanism of injury), and a careful physical examination, including special tests for differential diagnosis. Palpation of the specific structures generating the pain or dysfunction concludes the physical examination. This process should lead the examiner to choose the specific investigations (e.g., diagnostic imaging) needed to confirm the diagnosis, and it also provides a framework that is essential to successful treatment.

Key Elements for a Clinical Diagnosis

- Recognition of the salient points in the history
- Identification of precipitating or perplexing factors
- Careful examination including individual muscle testing
- Palpation of pain-generating structures

In the shoulder, dysfunction and pain may arise from a variety of sources, including the scapulohumeral complex, acromioclavicular or sternoclavicular articulations, rotator cuff and other shoulder muscles, associated subacromial (subdeltoid) bursa, biceps tendon, or labrum. Pain may even be referred from the cervical and thoracic spine and ribs. Shoulder pathology shows a common pattern of pain along the anterior glenohumeral joint line and biceps tendons, at the origin of the levator scapulae, and at the teres minor on the posterior joint line. Pain also may be present at the deltoid insertion and upper trapezius, along the medial border of the scapula and, in some cases, over the whole scapula.

When evaluating pain, clinicians should keep in mind the patient's age, occupation, recreational goals, and side dominance. The examiner must make sure that the patient is not confusing pain with weakness, instability, or apprehension. The mode of onset is important and may present as a spectrum of injury mechanisms, from a single traumatic episode to repetitive microtrauma.

Detailed examination of the shoulder can be found elsewhere (see Volume 1 of this series, *Orthopedic Physical Assessment,* Chapter 5). When assessing the shoulder, the examiner must keep in mind several important concepts:

1. *Shoulder pain must always be distinguished from referred pain arising from the cervical spine* (Table 6-1). The embryological derivation of the shoulder girdle from the cervical myotomes results in a close relationship for specific innervation, as well as for referred pain. With any complaint of shoulder girdle discomfort, cervical pathology must be ruled out. Neck pain and dysesthesia (i.e., numbness, tingling, burning) that radiate past the elbow in a dermatomal distribution normally implicate cervical disc disease, although nerve entrapment at the elbow or wrist or a local pathological lesion in the hand must be considered.[1] True shoulder pain rarely extends below the elbow. In any patient over age 50, a coexisting cervical degenerative abnormality must also be considered.[38]

2. *Generally shoulder pathology is characterized by pain on use, weakness, stiffness, and guarded apprehension.* (In many cases, the patient reports that the shoulder "just doesn't feel right.") These findings help distinguish shoulder pathology from cervical pain, which often is present even at rest and generally is aggravated by chronic compensatory postures, such as sitting, reading, or studying at a desk. Neck and shoulder pain cannot be totally isolated. The clinical points that are most suggestive of pain of spinal origin include absence of shoulder tenderness, guarded cervical spine motion, decreased biceps strength and reflex, and a positive cervical compression test (see volume I of this series, *Orthopedic Physical Assessment,* Chapter 3).[1] The most common pattern of cervical disc disease (i.e., spondylosis) refers into the C5-C6 dermatome with pain and/or paresthesia over the shoulder, the lateral arm, and even into the forearm and the thumb side of the hand.

3. *The patient's ability to maintain a static and dynamic stable core is important in shoulder rehabilitation.* A stable core (i.e., the ability to maintain control of the pelvis and spine) is the transfer zone between the lower extremity and the upper extremity, and as such, it plays a significant role in shoulder rehabilitation. If the practitioner tries to correct shoulder and/or cervical posture without addressing the unstable or incorrectly positioned core, treatment will be unsuccessful.

4. Neer[39] thought that mechanical *"impingement" could sometimes occur against the anterior edge of the acromion, coracoacromial ligament, or inferior acromioclavicular joint.* Others think that the anterior pain is due more to a complex interplay of rotator cuff dysfunction and degeneration ("rotator cuff disease") rather than impingement.[40] Structural narrowing of the subacromial space may occur secondary to inferior acromial tilting (i.e., anti-tilt), the so-called hooked acromion (i.e., type III), an unfused acromial ossification center called an **os acromiale**, or subacromial spurring. In addition, acromioclavicular joint hypertrophy and marginal osteophytes may irritate the rotator cuff.[9] Postural changes, particularly slouching with rounded shoulders and a protruding, chin-forward head posture, contribute to impingement. Magnetic resonance imaging (MRI) has demonstrated narrowing of the subacromial space as the shoulder girdle moves from a retracted to a protracted position.[41]

5. *Stability of the shoulder complex depends on an intimate relationship between the muscles controlling the scapula and those controlling the humerus.* The examiner must ensure correct functioning of the periscapular

TABLE 6-1

Factors Suggesting the Site of Origin of Shoulder Pain

Neck Pathology	Shoulder Pathology
• Pain at rest	• Pain with use
• Pain with neck motion	• Pain when working overhead
• Pain with overpressure on the neck	• Feeling of instability
• Pain aggravated by postural positions	• Local palpable tenderness
• Pain past the shoulder	• Painful arc of motion
• Reflex changes	• Pain into the deltoid area
• Altered peripheral sensation	• Pain mainly on the dominant side
• Guarded cervical spine motion	• Pain relief with local injections

From Zachazewski JE, Magee DJ, Quillen WS, editors: *Athletic injuries and rehabilitation,* p 511, Philadelphia, 1996, WB Saunders.

stabilizers and the rotator cuff (i.e., inner cone muscles). Commonly, the power (i.e., outer cone) muscles (i.e., the pectoralis major, deltoid, and latissimus dorsi) are not the problem, although they may contribute to the problem by being tight or substituting for the inner core muscles. Weakness or injury in any of the inner cone muscles leads to an imbalance of the synergistic inner cone (i.e., stabilizer) and outer cone (i.e., mobilizer) muscles and the prime mover muscles, resulting in abnormal shear forces which, in turn, can lead to instability (i.e., functional subluxation), labral injury, impingement, muscle imbalance, abnormal joint mechanics, and/or rotator cuff tears.[6,7,42] A thorough, detailed assessment of the strength and flexibility of each individual muscle of the shoulder complex is essential to identify weak and tight links in the kinetic chain and to ensure proper return to correct function. (For muscle testing, the reader is referred to the appropriate muscle testing books.[43–45])

6. *The examiner should watch for scapular dyskinesia, especially if the patient is under 35 and has anterior shoulder pain.*[2–4,46–48] If the scapula cannot be controlled by its stabilizer muscles, extra load is transferred to the humeral control muscles and they become overused, which leads to tendon and labral problems. Scapular instability is a common cause of rotator cuff and bicipital tendonitis or tendinosis and secondary impingement. A functional scapular base is essential for correct shoulder movement, especially in sports.[49]

7. *Hypomobility can be a major issue in shoulder instability and impingement.* The clinician must determine the mobility of the glenohumeral joint capsule (especially posteroinferiorly), ribs, scapula, and acromioclavicular and sternoclavicular joints, as well as assessing for tight muscles (e.g., pectoralis major and minor). Addressing tight structures helps to ensure normal shoulder arthrokinematics and function.[2–4] For example, glenohumeral arthrokinematics are markedly altered by a **glenohumeral internal (medial) rotation deficit (GIRD)** or by a tight posterior capsule when medial (internal) rotation is limited and lateral (external) rotation is excessive (also called **glenohumeral external (lateral) rotation gain [GERG]**). One theory proposed by Burkhart and coworkers[2–4,29] states that GIRD of 10° to 20° has a beneficial effect of offsetting the center of rotation of the glenohumeral joint posterosuperiorly. The advantage is that the greater tuberosity can "clear" the posterosuperior glenoid and labrum. Unfortunately, this process can get worse; with medial (internal) rotation deficits greater than 20° of the contralateral shoulder, combined with loss of the total motion arc, there continues to be stress on the

superior labrum, and a SLAP lesion eventually results. Thus, a tight posterior capsule results in a pathological "decentering" of the humeral head.

8. *Immobility of the thoracic spine and ribs can significantly influence the movement patterns of the shoulder complex and can affect the dimensions of the subacromial space.* A careful assessment of the cervical and thoracic spine and ribs is an important part of any shoulder assessment.[50]

9. *Any shoulder rehabilitation program must involve assessment of the whole kinetic chain.*[3] The clinician cannot assess the upper quadrant in isolation. Power movements and accelerating motions begin in the lower limb and trunk musculature. In patients with shoulder problems, the clinician should look for inflexibility in the hips (especially on the nondominant side) and in trunk rotation and the anterior shoulder muscles, along with weakness of the hip abductors and the pelvic core.[2]

10. *Exertional left shoulder pain in individuals over age 45 with coronary risk factors should be considered as cardiac pain until proven otherwise.* Coronary risk factors include smoking, obesity, hypertension, and a family history of cardiac disease.

11. *Pain from the lungs and abdominal organs can be referred to the shoulder, and injury to these structures should be considered in conditions involving trauma.*

12. *The initial observation should include the thoracic spine, ribs, and shoulder girdle and requires adequate exposure of the patient.* Viewing the disrobed patient from behind allows the clinician to note any wasting of the shoulder girdle muscles, especially the supraspinatus, infraspinatus, serratus anterior, and posterior deltoid. Such wasting may indicate a nerve injury (e.g., suprascapular, long thoracic, or axillary nerve)[51] or apparent hypertrophy of the upper trapezius as a result of superior migration of the scapula (i.e., type III dyskinesia).[2–4,46–48] The presence and size of stretch marks or scars often reflect poor quality collagen and may be a clue to the possibility of generalized ligamentous laxity or steroid abuse in athletes. Excessive lordotic curvature, a kyphotic thoracic spine, and/or associated poking chin with rounded shoulders should be noted. The clinician must assess for lack of pelvic or core control with these postural problems, which often contributes to shoulder problems. In addition, these anterior and posterior postural imbalances can lead to a tight pectoralis major and minor, resulting in increased stress on the anterior capsule, tightness of the posterior capsule, and overuse of scapular control muscles.[51]

13. *The examiner must always be aware of the possibility of referred pain.* The response to palpation must be put in the context of the patient's presentation and the implications of this presentation (e.g., secondary gain, pain threshold) must be judged correctly.

14. *Clinicians must know their patients.* The patient may have other issues and agendas that affect the clinical presentation.

ROTATOR CUFF DEGENERATION AND DYSFUNCTION (SHOULDER "IMPINGEMENT")

Shoulder impingement or "pinching" is associated with various degrees of inflammation or rotator cuff degeneration. It frequently occurs as a result of microtrauma, macrotrauma, or functional instability. The suspicion of impingement is raised by the presence of a painful arc during attempted active abduction or forward flexion or in patients with a complaint of anterosuperior or posterior shoulder pain with no history of trauma. There has been a tendency to move away from calling pain in the anterior region "impingement" because this implies that this is largely a mechanical phenomenon alone, when, in fact, it may be a more complex interplay of rotator cuff dysfunction and degeneration and less to do with attritional irritation from rotator cuff impingement.[40]

The subacromial space can be identified as a source of impingement by taking the arm passively into full forward elevation with gentle overpressure (i.e., Neer impingement test).[51] This test can be supplemented with the Hawkins-Kennedy impingement test, which involves taking the patient's arm to 90° of abduction and then moving it into horizontal adduction, followed by forced medial rotation.[51] The Hawkins-Kennedy impingement test can be enhanced by having the patient resist a force applied downward to the dorsum of the hand. A positive Hawkins-Kennedy test result implies impingement of the rotator cuff under the acromion. Historically a positive Neer impingement test result is thought to represent impingement of the rotator cuff on the anterosuperior glenoid rim or coracoacromial ligament.[52] Unfortunately, the sensitivity and specificity of these tests are quite poor and localizing the pain to one area is quite difficult.[53] Many sources of pain exist in this anterior region, including the bursa, rotator cuff, long head of biceps, anterosuperior labrum, and even the acromioclavicular joint.

Shoulder pain caused by impingement would seem to be easily distinguishable from that caused by post-traumatic instability. However, over time, clinicians have come to recognize that these conditions comprise a spectrum of both injury and pathology (Figure 6-3). At one end of the spectrum is an unstable painful shoulder along with rotator cuff degeneration and dysfunction, and at the other end is frank dislocation.[54,55] Rotator cuff degeneration is most often the result of a gradual attrition and irritation of the tendons that is associated with pain and dysfunction and that often is the result of repetitive overuse. Frank dislocation frequently goes on to become a recurrent dislocating joint. Similarly the spectrum of natural collagenous laxity ranges from extreme tightness to abnormal looseness; therefore the degree of

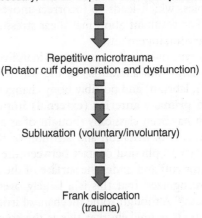

Vague sense of shoulder dysfunction
Unstable, painful shoulder

(**A**ltraumatic **M**ultidirectional Instability in **B**oth shoulders that responds to Intensive **R**ehabilitation. If surgery necessary, **I**nferior Capsular Shift used [**AMBRI**])

Repetitive microtrauma
(Rotator cuff degeneration and dysfunction)

Subluxation (voluntary/involuntary)

Frank dislocation
(trauma)

(**T**raumatic **U**nidirectional Instability with **B**ankart Lesion requiring **S**urgery [**TUBS**])

Figure 6-3 Shoulder instability spectrum. (Modified From Zachazewski JE, Magee DJ, Quillen WS, editors: *Athletic injuries and rehabilitation,* p 520, Philadelphia, 1996, WB Saunders.)

trauma or overuse required to generate a dislocation or subluxation varies.

Between these extremes lies the mildly unstable shoulder that predisposes the patient to impingement and pain; this condition is often seen in athletes, such as swimmers, and assembly line workers. The throwing shoulder in which the pitcher alters the mechanics to increase range of lateral rotation to get into the "slot" is another example.[2]

The aging process also fits into this spectrum, and its effects are manifested more in the soft tissue rotator cuff and in the joint surface itself.[52] Furthermore, internal derangements in the form of labral tears, attrition of the rotator cuff muscles, and degeneration of or partial tears in the biceps tendon have begun to be diagnosed with more prevalent use of the arthroscope and the increasing availability of MRI and computed tomography (CT) scanning. As a result, the previously simple, distinct diagnostic categories have become blurred into a spectrum of injuries.

Rotator cuff degeneration and dysfunction is often the result of cyclical repetitive abduction, forward flexion, and medial rotation motion at the glenohumeral joint.[56,57] Such movement is seen in swimmers who commonly swim approximately 10,000 to 14,000 m (6.2 to 8.7 miles) or more per day.[52] Impingement may also occur when the arm is forward flexed, medially rotated, and abducted within the coracohumeral space. This **coracoid impingement syndrome** occurs when the lesser tuberosity of the humerus encroaches on the coracoid process and has been associated with subscapularis tears.[58,59] The condition has been reported in swimmers, tennis players, weight lifters, and brick layers. With force overload, the humeral and scapular control muscles (see Figure 6-2) become fatigued, resulting in muscle weakness and muscle imbalance in the scapulohumeral force couples, which leads to incorrect movement patterns.[56,57] The resultant abnormal shear stresses can lead to secondary impingement.

Another type of impingement occurs in individuals over age 40, arising from alterations in the soft tissues (e.g., rotator cuff, labrum) and possibly bony changes. This has been called **primary anterior (external) impingement**. Although it has been classically thought of as a pure mechanical process of irritation and attrition of the rotator cuff secondary to physical contact between the anterosuperior rotator cuff and under the surface of the acromion, it is now recognized that this is a largely oversimplified point of view.[40] Although some mechanical irritation certainly occurs, it is unlikely that this is the source of the problem and is more likely the result of an aging, fatigued, and degenerating rotator cuff. This patient seldom has instability.[5,60,61]

In younger patients (ages 15 to 35), muscle dynamics is the primary problem (i.e., weakness of the scapular and humeral stabilizers). This has been called **secondary anterior (external) impingement**, which primarily is due to scapular dyskinesia and posterior rotator cuff fatigue.[5,60,61]

The fourth type of impingement is **posterior internal impingement** (Figure 6-4), which involves contact of the undersurface of the rotator cuff with the posterior superior glenoid labrum.[62-64] Burkhart et al.[3] reported that posterior internal impingement is a normal phenomenon that sometimes can result in pathology of the rotator cuff and labrum.

If significant inflammation is present, impingement tests are less specific because all testing positions tend to be uncomfortable. Very inflamed tissues are uncomfortable even on passive stretching or when put under tension by contraction of the associated muscle. By testing for pain in the nonimpingement position for each specific structure, the clinician can distinguish and isolate the inflammatory response of the tendon from a simple impingement area. For example, a partial rupture of the biceps tendon within the joint may give positive impingement signs and may also be maximally painful with resisted forward flexion. The clinician can further confirm the diagnosis by injecting approximately 3 mL of 0.25% to 1% lidocaine (Xylocaine) directly around the most painful areas (or 5 mL into the subacromial space) and then waiting a suitable interval (usually a few minutes) before repeating the impingement test.[62] Relief of at least 50% of the patient's pain through the painful arc or the impingement positions helps to confirm the source of the pain. However, it is important to keep in mind that although the source of the pain has been found, the source of the real problem may be more elusive. Most nontraumatic shoulder pain is the result of poste-

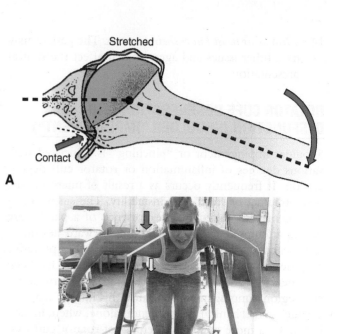

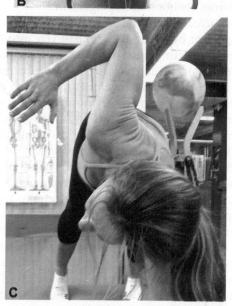

Figure 6-4 Posterior internal impingement. **A,** Posterior contact between the glenoid lip and the insertion of the cuff to the tuberosity occurs in the apprehension, or fulcrum, position, especially if the anteroinferior capsule has been stretched, allowing the humerus to extend to an unusually posterior scapular plane. This contact can challenge the integrity of the posterior cuff insertion and the tuberosity. **B** and **C,** Activity positions causing potential posterior impingement. (**A,** From Matsen FA: Stability. In Matsen FA, Lippett SB, Sidles JA, Harryman DT, editors: *Practical evaluation and management of the shoulder,* p 98, Philadelphia, 1994, WB Saunders.)

rior muscle problems involving the muscles stabilizing the scapula resulting in loss of scapular stabilization or control, overuse of the rotator cuff, loss of dynamic thoracic and pelvic control, and muscle imbalance in all four areas. In addition, when a rotator cuff tear is suspected, elimination of most of the pain allows a more specific examination of strength. The classic findings with a rotator cuff tear are pain even at rest (and especially at night), wasting of the supraspinatus and infraspinatus muscles, weakness of scaption (i.e., abduction in the scapular plane), and loss of lateral rotation strength. Small tears or partial-thickness tears may generate impingement signs without significant loss of rotator cuff strength. Diagnostic tests, such as ultrasound, MRI, or CT arthrograms can help to identify the true problem.

Functional Assessment of the Unstable or Dysfunctional Rotator Cuff and "Impinging" Shoulder

As the clinician goes through the assessment of the shoulder, he or she should carefully watch how patients position themselves and their shoulders to do the tasks they are asked to do. Proper alignment and a "streamlined" posture (i.e., major joints in line, ears squeezed by the arms, pelvis in neutral, feet and hands together, head in neutral) both in standing and sitting are key both during assessment and when doing exercises (Figure 6-5). Patients must be able to place the pelvis "in neutral" (anterior superior iliac spine [ASIS] one to two finger widths lower than posterior superior iliac spine [PSIS]) with the lower spine in proper postural alignment. Any alteration resulting in poor posture or altered scapular stabilization can lead to alterations in the position of the glenoid fossa, which can, in turn, lead to several different sequelae. For

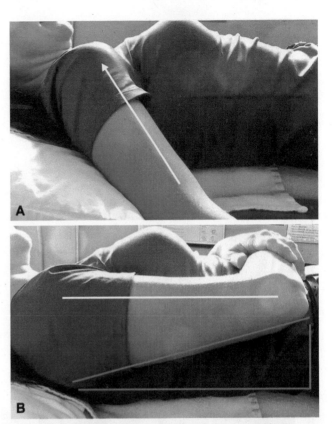

Figure 6-6 Compensatory "shoulder poke" position. **A**, Note how humeral head is translated anteriorly ("pokes" forward) in glenoid as arm extends. **B**, Correct resting position with head of humerus placed "neutrally" in glenoid.

example, when the patient is lying, supine or prone, the humeral head should align with the cervical spine and not project anteriorly (Figure 6-6). Similarly there should be no "shoulder bump" (i.e., shoulder hiking) (Figure 6-7). If the patient is slouching, the head of the humerus shifts anteriorly against the anterior capsule and labrum, resulting in undue pressure on these anterior structures. Shoulder ROM and rib motion both must be observed with motion on both sides of the body compared during the assessment.

Scapular posture should show the medial border of the scapula parallel to the normally straight thoracic spine and approximately 5 to 8 cm (2 to 3 inches) apart (Figure 6-8). There should be no scapular tilt (i.e., the inferior angle tilted away from the ribs), and the inferior angles of both scapula should be horizontally level and equidistant from the thoracic spine. The upper trapezius and levator scapulae should not be tight on palpation. To observe scapular functional movement, the examiner can have the patient hold the core and do a squat posture (Figure 6-9, *A*), with the shoulders in the power square position (Figure 6-9, *B*), open or closed shutters (Figure 6-9, *C*), and fly shutters. Lateral plank exercises may be performed from the knees or ankles as long as the patient can hold proper alignment (Figure 6-10).

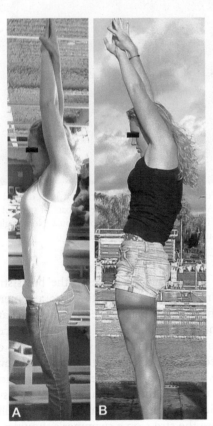

Figure 6-5 Postural alignment. **A**, Correct postural alignment. **B**, Compensatory postures due to hypomobility and weakness.

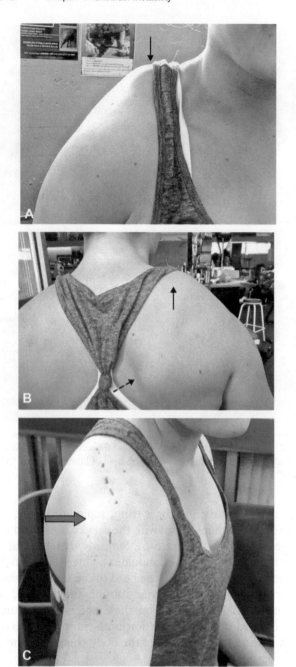

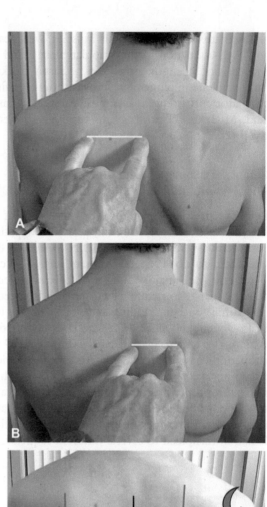

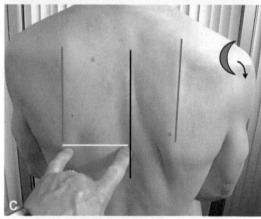

Figure 6-7 Compensatory "shoulder bump." **A,** Tight upper trapezius (*solid arrow*) causing bump. **B,** Tilting of inferior angle of scapula (*dotted arrow*) and tight trapezius (*solid arrow*). **C,** Forward position of humeral head in glenoid (*red arrow*).

Figure 6-8 Position of scapula. **A,** Normal at level of base of spine of scapula. **B,** Abnormal retraction at level of base of spine of scapula. **C,** Normal position of left inferior angle of scapula. Note angle of scapula on right, resulting in anti-tilt of glenoid.

Treatment of the Unstable Shoulder and Impingement

In the early clinical stages, the patient may complain of aching only after activity, and ROM is preserved. The clinician seldom sees the patient at this point, which is unfortunate, because postural correction involving the scapula, spinal postural line, and pelvis (see Figure 6-5, *A*) along with patient education could play a significant role. If the patient detects the early onset of symptoms, preventive measures can be instituted, such as modification of an activity. For example, during their workouts, swimmers could use a different stroke (e.g., the breaststroke), do only kicking drills, use speed fins, use a center snorkel, or alter their stroke pattern (e.g., different hand entry, altered body roll). The use of resistance devices should be kept to a minimum or, if used, monitored closely to ensure incorrect movement patterns do not develop and the arm is not being positioned in compromising positions. For example, the use of hand paddles or swimming with elastic cords, use of water barrels, or pulling foam can increase the stress on a swimmer's shoulder. In addition, using a flutter board held in front of the head while

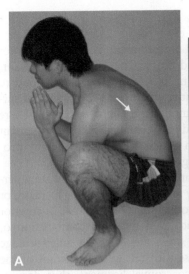
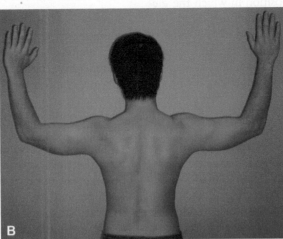
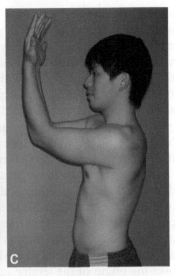

Figure 6-9 Scapular functional movement exercises. **A,** Core-hold squat posture (push against knees, scapula pulled down and back). **B,** Power square position. Also "open" start position for open or closed shutter. **C,** Closed shutters end position.

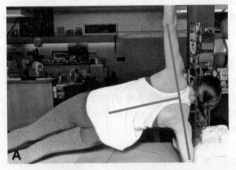
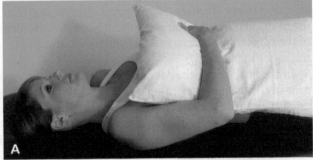
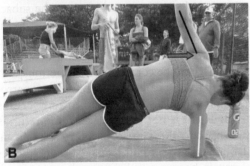
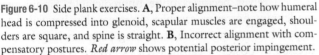
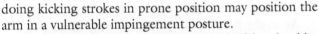
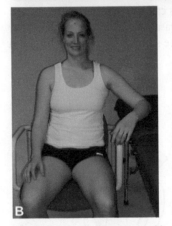
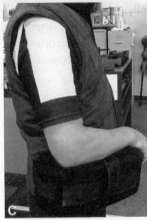

Figure 6-10 Side plank exercises. **A,** Proper alignment–note how humeral head is compressed into glenoid, scapular muscles are engaged, shoulders are square, and spine is straight. **B,** Incorrect alignment with compensatory postures. *Red arrow* shows potential posterior impingement.

Figure 6-11 Protecting the shoulder. The shoulder should NOT be allowed to poke forward. **A,** In supine. Pillow used to put shoulder in its resting position (40°-55° abduction, 30° horizontal adduction [scapular plane]). **B,** Sitting support (note shoulder is not elevated). **C,** Standing support with bolster.

doing kicking strokes in prone position may position the arm in a vulnerable impingement posture.

The patient should be instructed in healthy shoulder care (e.g., positioning or supporting the shoulder in resting positions) (Figure 6-11), the application of ice, especially after a workout, and how to take the shoulders slowly through a full ROM in a controlled fashion while ensuring a dynamically stabilized scapula and normal shoulder activation patterns. The patient should avoid compensatory shoulder impingement positions in activities of daily living and dry land training programs. Ideally, muscle strength

should be monitored regularly for weakness of the scapular stabilizers, compensatory movement patterns, loss of ROM (which is demonstrated by unequal movement or range when comparing both sides), pain, and compensatory postures. *Correct posture is an important concept that clinicians must keep in mind and continuously monitor when asking patients to do shoulder exercises.* The practitioner should not allow poor posture with protracted scapulae, which leads to **anti-tilt,** or the position in which the glenoid fossa is no longer superiorly and anteriorly tilted. This anti-tilt position allows the humeral head to "fall" out of the glenoid (Figure 6-12). With instability and impingement, any combination of poor posture or altered scapular stabilization and control can lead to compensation with the glenoid fossa facing inferiorly (anti-tilt). Matsen's "scapular dumping" seen in dislocations[32] is another, more traumatic, example of this glenoid anti-tilt.

As the pathology progresses, the patient experiences discomfort and pain during and after the activity. A positive impingement sign is elicited on examination (i.e., positive Hawkins and Neer tests, restriction in abduction and scaption). Palpation may demonstrate tenderness along the upper corner and medial border of the scapula, over the origin of the levator scapulae, around the insertion of deltoid, and long head of biceps, anterior capsule, and off the lateral edge of the acromion. These patients may also present with tenderness over the infraspinatus and teres minor muscles. Pathological changes may consist of thickening and fibrosis of the tendon, involvement of the subacromial bursa, residual adhesions, and possibly fraying of the labrum.

In the final stages, the patient complains of continuous pain over the supraspinatus and biceps tendons and tenderness over the coracoacromial ligament. A painful arc, especially in the empty can (Jobe's) position, is commonly demonstrated, and ROM can be restricted into medial and lateral rotation motions, which are not equal bilaterally, and impingement signs can be grossly positive. X-ray films may demonstrate infra-acromial and infraclavicular spurs, bony sclerosis near the supraspinatus insertion, and subacromial erosion.

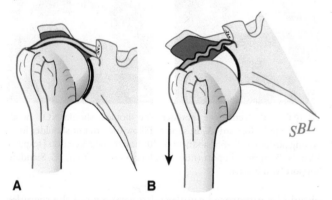

Figure 6-12 Scapular anti-tilt or dumping. With the scapula in a normal position (**A**), the superior capsular mechanism is tight, supporting the head in the glenoid concavity. Drooping of the lateral scapula (**B**) relaxes the superior capsular structures and rotates (anti-tilts) the glenoid concavity so that it does not support the head of the humerus. Conversely, stability is enhanced by elevating the lateral aspect of the scapula. (From Matsen FA, Lippett SB, Sidles JA et al: *Practical evaluation and management of the shoulder*, p 81, Philadelphia, 1994, WB Saunders.)

Surgical Treatment of Rotator Cuff Dysfunction

Surgery is considered a treatment of last resort for impingement-type syndromes. The indications for surgery include unremitting pain and failure to respond to nonoperative, conservative treatment. The timing of surgery depends on the functional disability and pain. There has been a strong trend away from surgical management of this condition, with aggressive physical therapy programs having equal or greater success to surgery.[65-67]

The surgical procedures used historically have been performed arthroscopically and were designed to increase, or decompress, the subacromial space. In the case of anterior impingement, this is achieved by some combination of shaving or excising the undersurface of the anterior edge of the acromion process with release or resection of the distal part of the coracoacromial ligament, thus decompressing the acromioclavicular space. The decision to remove inferior osteophytes or resect the acromioclavicular joint, combining the procedure with diagnostic arthroscopy of the glenohumeral joint and varying degrees of correction of labral lesions, and bicipital tendon pathology usually is a preoperative determination refined by intraoperative findings. It should be noted that several randomized controlled trials all have failed to show the benefit of subacromial decompression in the setting of anterosuperior shoulder pain.[65,66,68-70] Even in the setting of rotator cuff repair, routine use of subacromial decompression appears to not be warranted.[65,66,69,70] Select cases do still exist in which the degree of bony pathology is severe, such as those with huge subacromial spurs encroaching into the subacromial space, and may still warrant a subacromial decompression.[71] Surgical management of coracoid impingement is directed toward subscapularis repair and debridement of the undersurface of the coracoid if it is determined that the space between the coracoid and the humerus is narrowed.[72] Internal impingement is best identified early because surgical management is not often successful in returning the individual back to the same level of activity.[2-4] Once superior labral and rotator cuff damage occurs, the result of surgical repair becomes quite unpredictable. Significant, recalcitrant posterior capsular tightness that has failed to respond to an aggressive stretching program may be addressed by posterior capsular release, which is aimed at reducing GIRD. Associated labral and rotator cuff tearing may warrant debridement and/or repair.[3,73]

As might be expected with the array of surgical decisions to be made, the progress of postoperative rehabilitation varies. The clinician should have accurate and detailed information before starting the planning of the treatment regimen. In the simplest scenarios of surgical debridements and arthroscopic subacromial decompression, gentle ROM can be commenced within the tolerance of discomfort. The initial emphasis is on isometric muscle contractions, with progression to ROM exercises and strengthening. This progression is dictated by the ability to restore appropriate scapulohumeral rhythm and functional scapular control. Impingement positions must be avoided, and the exercises should focus on medial and lateral rotation in neutral, along with forward flexion motions, before abduction motions are initiated. It is better to go slow early, until most of the discomfort has subsided. The clinician should follow the principles of rehabilitation outlined later in this chapter, including those for nonoperative treatment of impingement.

SHOULDER INSTABILITY, SUBLUXATION, AND DISLOCATIONS

Shoulder instability, due either to significant trauma or to inherent ligamentous laxity and overuse with associated functional instability, is a common problem, especially in those under 35 years of age and in individuals who engage in a lot of overhead activity. The condition may be compounded by pseudo-laxity, which is an apparent increase in anterior laxity that results from a decreased cam effect, along with a tear of the superior labrum (i.e., SLAP lesion), congenital joint laxity (i.e., hypermobility), congenital muscle weakness, congenital anomalies, and/or muscle weakness or atrophy after injury.[2]

The glenohumeral joint is the most frequently dislocated major joint in the body. In one case series, glenohumeral dislocations are more common than all other joint dislocations combined.[63] Anterior dislocations of the shoulder account for 80% to 95% of all initial shoulder girdle dislocations, and recurrence is common.[64,74,75]

Classification of these injuries is necessary to develop a logical treatment plan. As previously mentioned, instabilities can range from subtle subluxation to a frank dislocation in which the articular surfaces are no longer in contact (i.e., true dislocation). Recurrent transient subluxation results in a feeling of instability or loss of control due to positioning of the arm. An example of this is forced hyperextension of the arm in elevation and/or lateral rotation, which may result in the "dead arm" syndrome seen in throwing athletes or in tennis players during a serve. In these cases, altered mechanics or traction, or pressure on the nerves generates the symptoms.[2,76,77]

Instabilities are basically classified as traumatic or atraumatic instabilities; Neer added a third type, acquired instabilities.[78] A traumatic dislocation is caused by a single force that applies excessive overload to the joint. This often damages the bony glenoid and/or the labrum and may even disrupt the capsule. This type of dislocation is seen in patients who present with a condition known as a **TUBS lesion** (i.e., *T*raumatic *U*nidirectional instability with a *B*ankart lesion that responds well to *S*urgery), as described by Matsen et al.[32] An atraumatic dislocation usually occurs in patients with multiple joint laxities who frequently have experienced episodes of subluxation before a relatively minor injury results in a dislocation. These individuals often show functional instability (i.e., lack of muscular

control) as a result of congenital hypermobility or congenital muscle weakness. This classification includes patients who present with an **AMBRI lesion** (i.e., *A*traumatic *M*ultidirectional instability that is *B*ilateral and the primary treatment is *R*ehabilitation, not surgery;[32] if surgery is required, an *I*nferior capsular shift is often recommended). Capsular laxity is common in these patients, and Bankart lesions are not seen, although the labrum may be frayed.[48]

However, the clinician must keep in mind that overlapping gradations of instability cover the entire spectrum, from TUBS to AMBRI lesions (see Figure 6-3).[25] Individuals with acquired instability who become symptomatic usually are engaged in overhead occupational or recreational activities, such as plastering ceilings, installing ceiling lighting, swimming, gymnastics, and baseball (i.e., pitching), in which the repetitive microtrauma of ill-conceived stretching or rapid, large range motion gradually contributes to capsular stretching. Although the shoulder becomes hypermobile, other joints may test within the normal range. A traumatic episode may push the joint over the edge and produce the first dislocation, but this major episode is only a small component of the problem.[63]

Many clinicians recognize functional instability as a pathological entity, particularly when the joint is put under high stress loads. Scapular control is lacking in these patients, which is one of the clinician's primary concerns.[3] This instability manifests itself from muscle fatigue or scapular dyskinesia after excessive load or repetitions. The mechanical etiology of **functional instability** is uncontrolled translation (i.e., loss of the arthrokinematic control) of the humeral head within the glenoid cavity.[19,56,79–83] Strong, coordinated muscle activity and proper neuromuscular balance contribute significantly to a reduction in functional instability and the often accompanying impingement, and these elements form the basis of treatment.

The glenohumeral instability, which is commonly due to asynchronous firing and fatigue of the scapular and humeral control muscles, can lead to subluxation, rotator cuff strains, and tendonitis or tendinosis injuries. Therefore movement control becomes the primary focus of the clinician.[3,21,84–87] Movement control focuses on maximizing coordinated and correct contraction of muscles through strength, endurance, proprioception, and coordination. Burkhead and Rockwood[8] reported that 80% of patients with atraumatic subluxations had good or excellent results with conservative treatment when appropriate rehabilitation was used. Other researchers are more conservative regarding the efficacy of the outcomes.[88–90] An accurate diagnosis and an appropriate, conservative treatment program can lead to a successful outcome in most patients and are essential for successful rehabilitation.[88] Functional instabilities occur primarily in one direction. However, they can present with global laxity, commonly referred to as *multidirectional instability*.[91]

Voluntary instability, another classification of instability, is usually due to congenital hypermobility or laxity combined with the patient using the shoulder muscles to purposely and spontaneously subluxate the joint.[63,92] For example, these patients commonly say, "Look what happens when I do this," as they voluntarily sublux the shoulder. This condition may provide an element of secondary gain for these individuals, and treatment is difficult. *Involuntary instability* is a recurrent dislocation in a person whose shoulder is so unstable that it dislocates spontaneously.[9]

A dislocation may be acute or chronic. An *acute, frank dislocation* is commonly traumatic and is usually reducible with a variety of manipulation techniques described elsewhere.[93,94] Reduction of a traumatic dislocation by manipulation should be attempted only by an experienced clinician. Occasionally the dislocation is irreducible, and open reduction may be required to extricate the structures preventing reduction. This condition is called a *complex dislocation,* in which interpositioning soft tissue blocks reduction.

With a *chronic dislocation,* the humeral head has been out of contact with the glenoid cavity for a protracted period (i.e., days to years). Unreduced posterior dislocations are the most common chronic dislocations because of the incidence of missed diagnosis. If the chronic nature of the dislocation is not recognized, attempts at closed reduction will be unsuccessful or may even result in a fracture.[75] Chronic dislocations invariably require open reduction. In studies of posterior instability, damage occurs to both the anterior and posterior aspects of the capsule.[94,95]

The principles of diagnosis of a dislocated or unstable shoulder were outlined earlier in the chapter. Usually the diagnosis is self-evident from the history, signs, and symptoms. The two most common mechanisms of traumatic injury are the arm being forced into 90° or more abduction and 90° lateral rotation and falling backward with the arm in extension.

The signs and symptoms of any dislocation or instability vary, depending on the severity. Patient complaints range from a vague sense of shoulder dysfunction to marked apprehension and pain, especially if the injury has been traumatic and the dislocation is unreduced. Reduction of the dislocation or subluxation usually provides immediate relief of pain, which is followed by a residual dull ache. Muscle spasm may make reduction difficult without the use of muscle relaxants, especially for the glenohumeral joint. A step deformity and loss of ROM are evident with a dislocation. Several days later, bruising and ecchymosis may be seen. If the patient complains of paresthesia, numbness, or muscle weakness, the clinician must be alert to the possibility of nerve injury, especially to the axillary nerve.

For dislocations, at least two radiographic views of the shoulder from two different angles are desirable to prevent a missed diagnosis, particularly with a posterior dislocation. X-ray films for an anterior dislocation should include a true anteroposterior (AP) view of the shoulder and a true lateral view of the scapula (Table 6-2).[51] An axillary view is difficult to obtain in an acutely injured shoulder but is extremely useful in ruling out a dislocation and thus

TABLE 6-2

Radiographic Imaging for Different Shoulder Pathologies

Pathology	Radiographic Imaging
Impingement	Anteroposterior (AP) x-ray film in the plane of the scapula Supraspinatus outlet view Axillary AP x-ray film, 30° caudal view (anterior acromial view)
Instability	AP x-ray film in the plane of the scapula Stryker Notch view West Point axillary view Axillary
Arthritis	AP x-ray film in the plane of the scapula Full humerus AP x-ray film in the plane of the scapula with laterally rotated 30° Axillary
Trauma	AP x-ray film in the plane of the scapula Axillary True scapular lateral view (Y view)

should be obtained whenever possible. Specialized x-ray views, including Stryker Notch and a West Point Axillary, are required to further elucidate the size of Hill-Sachs lesion and Bankart fractures, respectively, but are not typically obtained in the acute setting.

Anterior Dislocations

Anterior dislocations account for approximately 95% of acute traumatic glenohumeral injuries.[95] They occur most frequently in young adults. With an anterior glenohumeral dislocation, the head of the humerus is driven or levered anteroinferiorly. Typically, the glenoid labrum is stripped from the anteroinferior aspect of the glenoid (i.e., Bankart lesion). As previously noted, it frequently involves the anteroinferior glenoid bone (Bankart fracture) (Figure 6-13) and an impaction fracture in the posterolateral aspect of the humeral head (Hill-Sachs lesion) (Figure 6-14). The bony Bankart lesion can be an acute fracture or an erosive process in which the glenoid slowly becomes deficient anteroinferiorly with multiple recurrent dislocations[96] (see Figure 6-13). If no Bankart lesion is found, the anterior or lateral capsule may be disrupted at the humeral insertion site. This is called **humeral avulsion of the glenohumeral ligament**, or **HAGL lesion** (Figure 6-15).[94,96] With significant labrum damage, especially with increasing bone loss, the chances for recurrent dislocation are greater because the potential for healing and spontaneous reattachment of the fibrocartilaginous labrum and/or Bankart fracture fragment back to its anatomical location is poor. The disrupted osseous or soft tissue Bankart lesions do heal back to the glenoid but often in a more medial position along the glenoid neck,

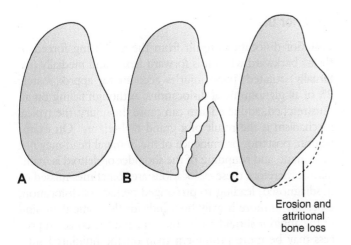

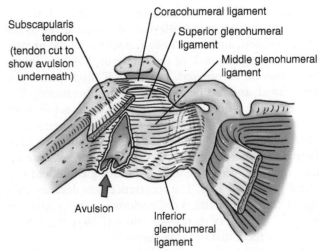

Figure 6-13 Bankart lesion. **A,** Pear-shaped normal glenoid. **B,** Bankart fracture. **C,** Erosive or attritional bone loss. (Redrawn from Burkhart SS, De Beer JF: Traumatic glenohumeral bone defects and their relationship to failure of arthroscopic Bankart repairs: significance of the inverted-pear glenoid and the humeral engaging Hill-Sachs lesion, *Arthroscopy* 16(7):684, 2000.)

Figure 6-15 Schematic of humeral avulsion (*arrow*) of the glenohumeral ligament (HSGL Lesion) showing avulsion of middle and inferior glenohumeral ligaments from the humerus (subscapularis tendon cut for clarity). (Redrawn from Wolf EM, Cheng JC, Dickson K: Humeral avulsion of the glenohumeral ligaments as a cause of anterior shoulder instability, *Arthroscopy* 11(5):602, 1995.)

resulting in an inadequate anterior buttress to humeral head translation. This is further exacerbated if there is a large Hill-Sachs lesion.

The intact labrum is important for maintaining a suction-like vacuum effect to hold the humeral head in the glenoid cavity and for its buttress effect. Although it is most important as a static stabilizer, it also enhances dynamic support of the joint.[16,17] The glenohumeral joint usually is bathed in less than 1 mL of synovial fluid,[97] which helps hold the articular surfaces together and enhances the normal negative intra-articular pressure.[18,33] However, excessive fluid (usually blood) in the joint can negate this effect.

On examination, an acutely dislocated shoulder demonstrates a deformity (i.e., step deformity), or a space usually is detected under the tip of the acromion, resulting in prominence of the acromion, flattening of the deltoid muscle, pain, and loss of motion. The patient tends to support the arm in 30° of abduction with the other arm while listing or leaning to the affected side. Attempts

at movement in any direction are painful, and the humeral head may be palpable in the axilla.

Anterior glenohumeral dislocations have several associated complications (of which recurrence is the most common). These may include injury to the axillary, musculocutaneous, or median nerves or more rarely the brachial plexus.[20] Only approximately 20% of these dislocations show minimal clinical signs, and 5% show significant evidence of neurological involvement; however, Rockwood demonstrated that up to 80% of individuals show electromyographic evidence of nerve injury.[63] This damage initially may be subclinical, with the patient showing no detectable weakness. Consequently *it is essential that the clinician repeatedly check and monitor for paresthesia and changes in the strength of the deltoid muscle.* Other complications include rotator cuff tears

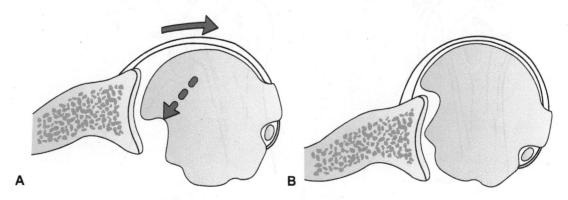

Figure 6-14 **A,** Hill-Sachs lesion (*dashed arrow*). **B,** Hill-Sachs lesion causes engagement of the humeral head in the anterior glenoid with lateral rotation. (Redrawn from Burkhart SS, De Beer JF: Traumatic glenohumeral bone defects and their relationship to failure of arthroscopic Bankart repairs: significance of the inverted-pear glenoid and the humeral engaging Hill-Sachs lesion, *Arthroscopy* 16(7):681, 2000.)

(the likelihood of these tears increases with advancing age, typically greater than 40 years of age), damage to the biceps tendon, and, on occasion, fractures of the greater tuberosity or the neck of the humerus. Vascular injury must also be considered, especially if distal pulses are diminished, and can be potentially limb threatening.[98]

Recurrent dislocations typically occur in active male patients under age 20, with recurrence rates being possibly as high as 90% after a traumatic dislocation.[95] Other factors that increase the risk of occurrence include contact, overhead activities, and significant glenoid and humeral head bone loss. The recurrence rate declines with age, with fewer recurrent dislocations occurring after age 40.[22,24,99,100] Most of these dislocations (75%) occur within 2 years of the initial traumatic event.[99]

Examination of a patient with recurrent instability is confirmed by a positive apprehension and relocation test. Signs of hyperlaxity, including lateral (external) rotation beyond 85° or hyperabduction of greater than 105°, should be watched for because these patients have a higher incidence of failure of a surgical repair.[101,102] Intact rotator cuff function should be confirmed. If there is concern for rotator cuff integrity, ancillary imaging, such as an ultrasound or an MRI, should be performed.

Nonoperative treatment may be successful in some patients with recurrent dislocations because restoration of kinetic chain function, shoulder strength, and proprioception may suffice in rendering the joint stable. Unfortunately, it is ineffective for most individuals with recurrent episodes; therefore, surgical stabilization is appropriate for those with significant functional instability, and excellent success rates usually are achieved.[24] The choice of surgical technique and the timing and extent of surgery depend on the degree and direction of instability, the requirements for ROM, the associated soft tissue and bone damage, and the surgeon's preference and skills.

Posterior Dislocations

Posterior dislocations result from the arm being forced or thrust backward when it is forward flexed and medially (internally) rotated; these injuries account for approximately 2% of all glenohumeral dislocations. Although falling on an outstretched, adducted arm can cause the injury, the typical mechanism is the result of a grand mal seizure. On examination, posterior prominence of the humeral head may not be evident, and rounding of the shoulder or deltoid is maintained; therefore these dislocations are sometimes missed or misdiagnosed, leading to prolonged periods of dislocation, especially in more heavily built individuals. Some flattening of the anterior shoulder may be seen, and the coracoid process may be more prominent than on the uninjured side. The patient will have limited lateral (external) rotation (less than 0°) and limited elevation (less than 90°), which are signs that further investigation is needed. In addition, medial rotation and cross-flexion (horizontal adduction) cause pain and apprehension. Posterior dislocations are recognized by the "empty glenoid" sign on the x-ray film (Figure 6-16). The true glenohumeral AP view of the posteriorly dislocated shoulder shows abnormal overlapping of the humeral head and glenoid shadows, which are normally on this view. Again, an axillary view will clearly show this dislocation but is often difficult to obtain in cases of an acutely posterior shoulder dislocation. If this injury is missed, it results in considerable morbidity because the relatively soft humeral head becomes severely damaged as it rests on the edge of the hard glenoid. Reduction becomes very difficult and it can often only be achieved through operative intervention.

In recurrent posterior dislocations, the patients complain of apprehension with shoulder elevation, especially with the arm adducted. Physical examination confirms excessive posterior translation of the humerus and subluxation, or even frank dislocation, with a posteriorly directed force on the humerus. The complex pathophysiology

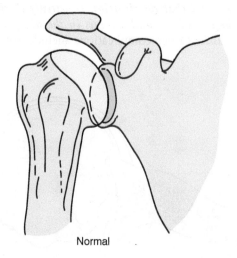
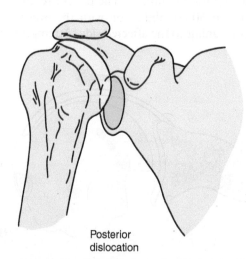

Normal

Posterior dislocation

Figure 6-16 "Empty glenoid" sign of posterior dislocation on an anteroposterior x-ray film. Note that the head of the humerus fills the glenoid in the normal x-ray film (*left*). With a posterior dislocation, the glenoid is "empty," especially in its anterior portion (*right*). (From Zachazewski JE, Magee DJ, Quillen WS: *Athletic injuries and rehabilitation*, p 523, Philadelphia, 1996, WB Saunders.)

involved in posterior shoulder dislocations has led to the development of numerous surgical techniques to address this problem.[100] Soft tissue techniques range from a simple arthroscopic posterior labral and capsular plication to a posteroinferior capsular shift.[103] Additional bony techniques include wedge osteotomies with or without a bone block, and humeral rotation osteotomies can be performed in only the most severe and rare cases.[104] With advanced arthroscopic techniques, surgeons have been able to perform arthroscopic stabilization with fairly good functional outcomes.[105] Postoperative care varies widely, but if the practitioner has an appreciation of the techniques used and follows the treatment principles outlined in this chapter, a customized treatment program can be developed to suit each specific situation. However, in all cases of posterior stabilization, the patient is immobilized in neutral to slight lateral rotation to protect the repaired posterior structures.

TREATMENT PRINCIPLES FOR A DISLOCATED SHOULDER

In the management of acute dislocations of the shoulder, an attempt must be made to characterize the injury. A major difficulty in developing a treatment plan from the older literature is the failure of the literature to separate groups adequately according to the underlying degree of injury and the direction of laxity.[106] A glenohumeral dislocation usually is reduced using closed techniques and adequate anesthesia. Post reduction, it is important to recheck the patient's neurovascular status both before and after reduction and to obtain second AP and lateral x-ray films to ensure proper positioning.

With dislocations, subluxations, or instability, a concerted, focused effort at nonoperative treatment with a well-planned, well-coordinated therapy program must be attempted. This principle is more important in cases in which the shoulder is more lax, the collagen hyperelasticity is greater, and/or less trauma is involved in the initial dislocation. If a larger Bankart fracture (i.e., greater than 25% of glenoid area) or other structural deficiencies, such as an acute rotator cuff tear, are found, they usually are dealt with surgically as soon as possible.

For acute anterior dislocations, treatment begins with early controlled immobilization. After closed reduction, the shoulder may be immobilized with a swath and sling or just a sling for up to 6 weeks (in young adults) to prevent extension, abduction, and lateral rotation, which helps to promote capsular healing. Commonly, after 3 weeks, the sling is used primarily to protect the glenohumeral joint from potential injurious outside forces (e.g., a fall, bumping into people) Some researchers have reported that the period or position of immobilization bears little relation to the recurrence of the dislocation,[100] and some authors advocate a shorter period of immobilization (1 to 3 weeks).[36,99] The duration of immobilization depends on the philosophy of the physician or surgeon and the type of reconstruction, if surgical repair is performed.

In the first 2 weeks following reduction, a program of strong isometric deltoid, shoulder abductor, adductor, and biceps work is instituted within the limits of pain tolerance. Scapular control exercises should be initiated right away within a pain-free ROM in standing or prone positions (Figure 6-17). This minimizes muscle wasting, keeping the muscles active following injury and decreases pain as the edema and hemorrhage resolve and the shoulder becomes more comfortable. The sling can be removed for exercises, controlled ROM, and unresisted eccentric exercises (to biceps and triceps) "in the cone" several times a day. When doing biceps exercises, the clinician should use a "block brace" or towel (Figure 6-18) to ensure the

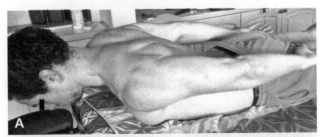
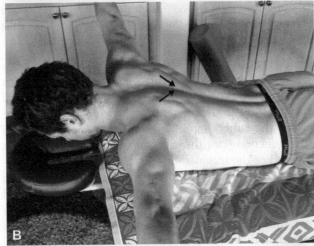
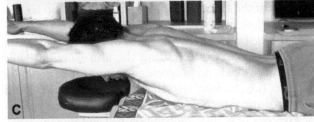

Figure 6-17 "Prone series of 3" scapular exercises used to engage scapula in streamlined position. **A,** Patient lies in prone with hands on gluteals, palms up. Patient then reaches for feet, lifting head and chest off bed, maintaining a straight spine with scapula engaged, core set, and neck in neutral (i.e., not looking up). **B,** Shoulders brought to 90° ("T" position) with thumbs facing forward. Patient then squeezes scapulae together and down (*arrows*) while maintaining a straight spine, core set, and neck in neutral. **C,** Patient brings arms over head and then pulls scapulae down and toward opposite hips while maintaining a straight spine, core set, and neck in neutral.

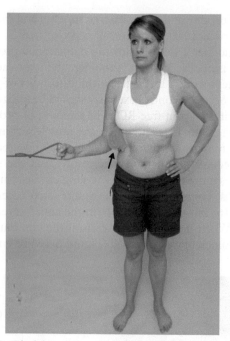

Figure 6-18 "Block brace" (towel or wedge) to prevent arm adduction in early rehabilitation. Note: The "block" (*arrow*) should be used with caution for glenohumeral rotator cuff exercises especially if the patient does not have good control of scapula. When using a towel at the elbow, the clinician must ensure that the scapula is able to stabilize. If the patient does not have good control of the scapula, stabilization of the shoulder occurs through the elbow with the rotator cuff working through reverse origin insertion to stabilize the scapula.

arm does not adduct or stays in alignment with the body line during elbow movement. Adduction may result in the humeral head being laterally levered against the lateral structures of the glenohumeral joint.

"**In the cone**" implies movement at the shoulder of 30° abduction (i.e., the range in which scapula becomes engaged or the scapular muscles begin to contract to stabilize the scapula and allow it to move in coordination with the moving arm), 30° to 60° forward flexion, and lateral (external) rotation to neutral (the hand does not move outside the plane of the body), with the elbow never extending through the frontal plane (behind) of the body (to prevent the humeral head from translating too far forward) (Figure 6-19). Pendular exercises may also be initiated at this stage (Figure 6-20), starting with momentum pendular exercises (i.e., leaving the arm hanging while rotating the hips) and progressing to controlled pendular exercises (i.e., moving relaxed arm in circles, forward and backward and side to side), and finally to modified pendular exercises (e.g., placing hand on ball and moving ball). Small range, gentle, closed kinetic chain exercises can be initiated, provided the movement is pain free.

The emphasis in the early stages is still on isometric activities, with neutral (i.e., not outside the body plane) shoulder medial and lateral rotator isometric exercises taking precedence using "closed stick" and "power square" drills in the supine position (Figure 6-21). The clinician must ensure that the patient is able to maintain and hold

starting postures when doing the exercises. The patient should always start in supine position (to help to stabilize the scapula), performing the exercises in three positions—at the level of the diaphragm, shoulder, and forehead. Exercises should be colinear and coupled so the Hawkins position (which stabilizes the glenoid under the humerus) (Figure 6-22), and the "power square" position (which is the basis of many shoulder movements) may be used as foundations for a number of different exercises.

In addition, concentric exercises through a limited range ("in the cone") are permitted, with the clinician bearing in mind that capsular healing is well under way at 3 weeks. The limits of range are determined by pain and whether the patient can comfortably control the movement. When stability is obtained "within the cone," the patient can carefully begin to increase the ROM outside the cone.

Controlled movements are essential during proper rehabilitation. The controlled active movement applies small amounts of stress to the joint structures to reduce the adverse effects of immobilization on the glenohumeral joint.[36,42,107,108] During this time, active abduction beyond 20° to 30°, forward flexion beyond 90°, or lateral rotation past neutral (outside the cone) should be performed carefully. In older individuals, in whom the danger of stiffness leading to adhesive capsulitis and frozen shoulder is greater than the risks of redislocation, the movement program is initiated at the beginning. Once immobilization has ended and dynamic control achieved, the treatment protocol follows the same principles as for treatment of patients with instability (see later discussion).

SURGICAL TREATMENT OF SHOULDER INSTABILITY

Indications for surgery and open reduction include the inability to reduce by closed reduction, presence of a large flake of avulsed bone on the inferior glenoid margin (which may contribute to future instability), a fracture through a significant portion of the articular surface, vascular impairment, and an associated displaced tuberosity fracture or a fracture of the neck of the humerus. On occasion, very athletic individuals may want a guarantee of stability in the shoulder by having early surgery. Postoperative care depends on the type and degree of associated problems that led to open reduction and repair.

Surgical procedures may be arthroscopic or open and involve either a soft tissue or bony reconstruction. The spectrum of surgical approaches depends largely on the pathology involved. Patients with largely soft tissue lesions, such as simple labral tears, are ideal candidates for a simple arthroscopic Bankart repair. If the inferior capsule is avulsed from the humeral side (i.e., an HAGL lesion), an open or arthroscopic capsular repair is indicated. A capsular plication is indicated for the rare occasion when surgery is indicated for the patient with multidirectional instability. Bony procedures also may be performed,

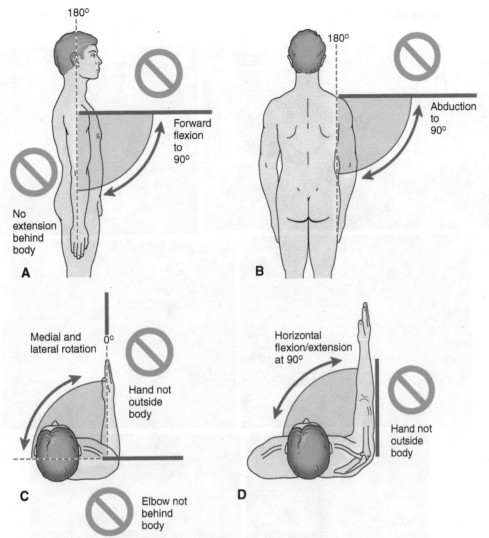

Figure 6-19 Low-risk postsurgical movement allowed "in the cone." **A,** Forward flexion to 90°. **B,** Abduction to 90°. **C,** Lateral rotation—hand not outside the body, elbow not behind body. **D,** Horizontal flexion—hand not outside body. Note: Horizontal flexion/extension is also called horizontal adduction/abduction. (Modified from Magee DJ: *Orthopedic physical assessment*, ed 6, p 273, Philadelphia, 2014, WB Saunders.)

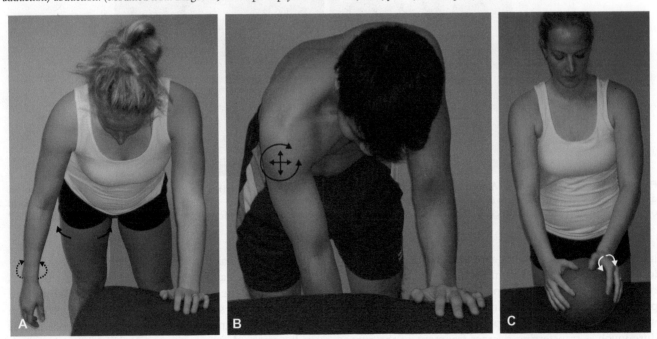

Figure 6-20 Pendular exercises. **A,** Injured arm hangs down free. "Momentum" pendular movement achieved by swinging hips to initiate movement in different directions. **B,** Active controlled pendular movement—muscles control movement in different directions. **C,** Ball pendular movement. Both hands press down on a ball to compress humeral head into glenoid. The unaffected left arm moves the ball in circles, back and forth, or side to side while injured right arm "goes along for a ride."

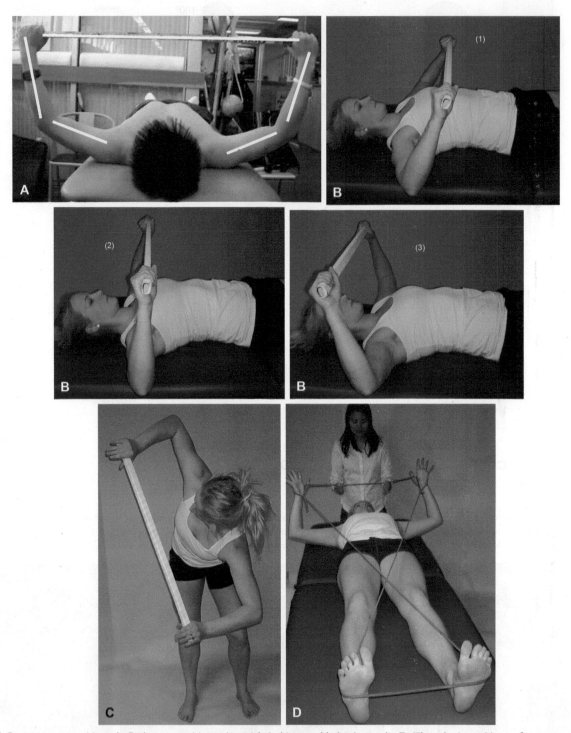

Figure 6-21 Power square position. **A,** Basic start position using stick (tubing could also be used). **B,** Three basic positions of power square—at diaphragm-nipple-xiphysternum line (*1*), at shoulder height (*2*), and at forehead/nose height (*3*)—to do co-contractions. **C,** Functional movement out of power square position with stick. **D,** "Spiderman" exercise out of power square position. Clinician is providing perturbations on "thumb-tube."

mainly focusing on restoring anteroinferior glenoid bone loss with local bone graft from a transferred coracoid and the attached conjoined tendon. Historically the Bristow procedure involves transferring the tip of the coracoid, whereas the more recently popularized Latarjet procedure involves transferring a larger fragment of the coracoid, allowing for a more robust bony reconstruction of the anteroinferior glenoid bone stock (Figure 6-23).[29]

This procedure has the added stabilizing effect of lowering the inferior half of the subscapularis muscle belly, as well as adding the dynamic sling effect of the conjoined tendon with the shoulder in positions of apprehension (i.e., abduction and lateral rotation). This procedure is usually reserved for severe cases of instability in which there is substantial glenohumeral bone loss and patients who require a robust repair, such as athletes involved

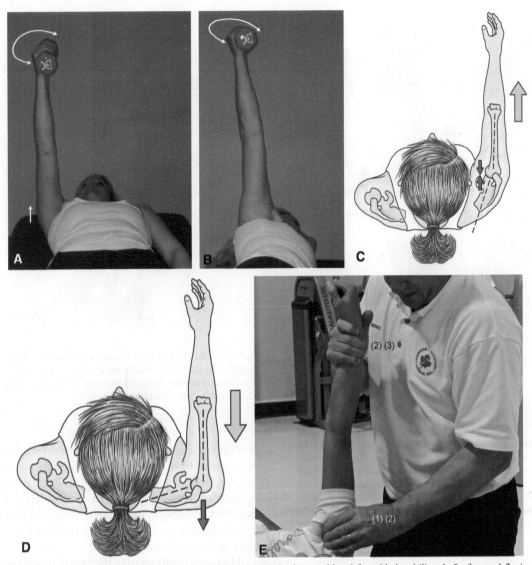

Figure 6-22 Hawkins ("punch out") position ensuring glenoid is sitting under humeral head for added stability. **A,** In forward flexion doing circles, horizontal, or up and down movement. **B,** In abduction. **C,** Line drawing shows how the glenohumeral joint is more stable with the glenoid lying under the head of the humerus in the Hawkins position than in **D. E,** To gain arthrokinematic control, the clinician applies resistance in all directions at the glenohumeral joint (*1*). To ensure arthrokinematic control at the glenohumeral joint while doing osteokinematic movement, the examiner applies resistance at the glenohumeral joint (arthrokinematic stabilization) and the wrist (osteokinematic movement) (*2*). To strengthen osteokinematic movement, the clinician applies resistance at the wrist (*3*) while palpating the glenohumeral joint to ensure there is minimal translation and to ensure arthrokinematic control during the perturbations. (**C** and **D,** modified from Matsen FA: Stability. In Matsen FA, Lippett SB, Sidles JA et al: *Practical evaluation and management of the shoulder,* p 64, Philadelphia, 1994, WB Saunders.)

in contact sports. The inferior glenoid can also be augmented by other bone graft options, including iliac crest and other cadaveric sources.[109] Large Hill-Sachs lesions have been addressed using allograft bone implantation to the humeral head defect or suturing the posterior cuff into the Hill-Sachs lesion. The latter procedure is called a *Remplissage*, which is the French word meaning "to fill" (Figure 6-24).[110,111] Other procedures have been described and may now be only of historical interest. Such procedures as the Putti-Platt and Magnuson-Stack involved excessive tightening of the anterior structures of the shoulder, specifically the subscapularis and anterior capsule, thus restricting lateral rotation and thereby preventing pathological translation and engagement of the Hill-Sachs lesion. Unfortunately, there is a report of

these procedures directly resulting in early osteoarthritis of the glenohumeral joint.[112] Excessive anterior capsular tightness results in posterior subluxation of the humeral head on the glenoid, and this eccentric loading of the glenohumeral joint can lead to the rapid development of arthritis. In addition, any procedure that involves restriction of lateral rotation is very undesirable to an athlete who requires full shoulder motion.[36,113–128]

Complication rates of instability surgery vary depending on the procedure performed. Arthroscopic procedures carry a higher risk of recurrent dislocation, especially in young athletes involved in contact sports with significant bone loss.[29,129] In the past, these arthroscopic approaches have been associated with worrisome redislocation rates.[130,131] With strict technical criteria,

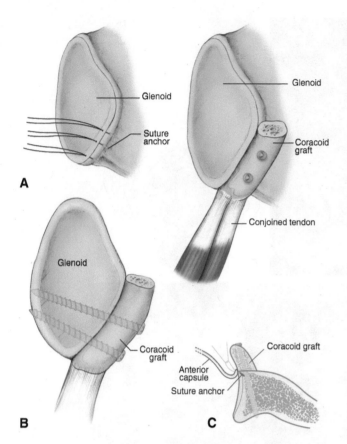

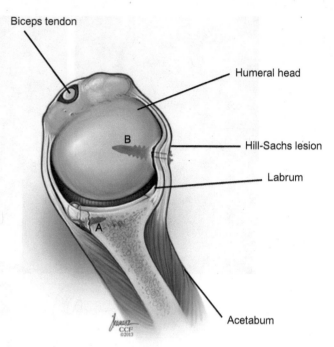

Figure 6-24 **A**, Bankart repair–reattachment of the anterior labrum. **B**, Remplissage (to fill in): Hill-Sachs lesion with the posterior capsule and infraspinatus muscle anchored into the lesion. (Courtesy of Cleveland Clinic Foundation, Cleveland, OH.)

Figure 6-23 Latarjet procedure. **A**, Conjoined tendon of biceps sutured to glenoid. **B**, Screws hold conjoint tendon. Note how graft restores pear shape of glenoid. **C**, Graft is placed so that it acts as an extension of the articular arc of the glenoid. (Redrawn from Burkhart SS, De Beer JF: Traumatic glenohumeral bone defects and their relationship to failure of arthroscopic Bankart repairs: significance of the inverted-pear glenoid and the humeral engaging Hill-Sachs lesion, *Arthroscopy* 16(7):677-694, 2000.)

including restoration of the proper resting length of the anterior-inferior glenohumeral ligament and recreation of the labral "bumper" or "chalk-block" effect, current arthroscopic techniques offer success rates comparable to open techniques. Strict clinical guidelines for suitable patient selection also are important. Open bone grafting procedures, such as the Latarjet procedure, have lower recurrence rates documented in the literature but unfortunately have higher rates of infection, hematoma formation, iatrogenic nerve injury, and degenerative changes related to poor bone graft positioning.[132,133]

With soft tissue surgical techniques, it is important to allow sufficient time for capsular healing with minimal stress to these tissues. With bony techniques, such as the Latarjet procedure, a period of approximately 4 to 6 weeks is required to allow for union of the bone block before stress is applied. After operative treatment, the traditional Putti-Platt procedure has a 1% to 5% incidence of recurrent dislocation; the Magnuson-Stack operation, 1% to 9%; and the Bristow repair, 1% to 6%.[125] These results should be compared with the increasingly successful

outcomes of arthroscopically assisted techniques, which, as surgeons have become more experienced, have reached and surpassed the open techniques. Return to a high level of function is the rule with an appropriately selected and executed technique performed with due regard for the pathological lesion, follow-up rehabilitation, and the activity goals of the patient.

Although postoperative therapy is based on tissue healing principles and proper stress to the tissues, each surgeon has certain criteria that he or she wants to be followed in a rehabilitation program. The clinician must be aware of these criteria, including the reasons for them, along with any restrictions or modifications to treatment, to prevent any misunderstanding with the surgeon and patient's desired outcome.

POSTSURGICAL TREATMENT OF THE SHOULDER

The basic rehabilitation plan may be modified, depending on the type of surgical procedure performed, precautions to treatment noted by the surgeon, the individual surgeon's preferences, and whether pain, restriction, or both are factors. For the most part, the treatment of patients who have undergone arthroscopic procedures parallels that for patients who have had open techniques, although the former have less tissue disruption and muscle wasting. The patient's willingness to move and the quality of the patient's movements also are of concern to the clinician. Only broad guidelines are given here for progression. The treatment principles remain constant: to relieve pain, observe for complications, regain muscle control, strengthen, regain ROM safely, improve endurance, and retrain proprioceptive control. These guidelines form the foundation of an activity-based protocol. Specificity plays a major role with each program being individualized to the patient and his or her activities.

Principles of Specificity Related to Sports and Rehabilitation

Every activity makes specific demands in terms of load (stress), rate, repetitions, duration, and neurophysiological adjustment. When a new or modified task with a different demand in intensity, load, rate, repetitions, duration, or neurophysiological adjustment is instituted, an entirely new pattern of adjustment must be acquired. Therefore training and rehabilitation must be specific to the sport or activity in which the patient hopes to take part or return to. This principle applies to all of the following:
1. Cardiovascular fitness (aerobic and anaerobic activities)
2. Strength training (isometric, isotonic [concentric and eccentric], econcentric, isokinetic)
3. Open-chain and closed-chain activities
4. Motor skills and motor learning
5. Flexibility (static, dynamic)
6. Coordination
7. Proprioceptive or kinesthetic control (stimulation of different mechanoreceptors)
8. Timing, reaction time, and movement time
9. Progressions
10. Biomechanical demands
11. Tissue healing and stress on tissues

To achieve progression in these areas, the clinician proceeds from:
1. General to specific
2. Simple to complex
3. Easy to difficult
4. Lesser to greater volume
5. Lesser to greater intensity
6. Lesser to greater frequency
7. Smaller to greater ROM

Modified from Zachazewski JE, Magee DJ, Quillen WS, editors: *Athletic injuries and rehabilitation*, p 527, Philadelphia, 1996, WB Saunders.

Postsurgical treatment initially concentrates primarily on the scapula. Scapular control exercises focus primarily on the lower and middle trapezius and serratus anterior. These exercises include scapular retraction, depression, protraction, and elevation with the arm at the side. Careful observation should detect compensatory trunk, pelvic, and especially shoulder postures that indicate incorrect firing (i.e., contraction) sequences and lack of proper stabilization. As the patient improves, the glenohumeral joint can be taken out of "the cone" into abduction, scaption (i.e., plane of the scapula), forward flexion, and other elevation movements, provided the patient can maintain control of the scapula and can stabilize the humerus in the glenoid. Lateral rotation should be performed only with extreme care and never beyond neutral in the early stages of rehabilitation (i.e., the hand should never go outside the sagittal plane of the body, and the elbow should never go behind

the frontal plane of the body). These are important early rules, regardless of the surgical procedure used. Keeping inside "the cone" reduces the stress on the anterior labrum and the repaired soft tissues to a minimum. During rotation exercises, the clinician should watch for excessive scapular winging or motion because the scapula may be compensating for tight medial or lateral rotators. If present, this can be treated with joint play techniques or muscle energy or proprioceptive neuromuscular facilitation (PNF) techniques, depending on whether the restriction is caused by inert (i.e., collagen) or contractile (i.e., muscle) tissues.

As control of the scapula is being achieved, isometric exercises to the muscles that control the humeral head can be initiated, starting with light contractions (importantly, not maximum voluntary contraction [MVC]) and progressing to stronger isometric contractions for the deltoid and rotator cuff muscles. Initially the clinician should start with exercises that cause the muscles controlling movement at the glenohumeral joint to compress the humeral head into the glenoid for stability (see Figure 6-22). If the patient has good pelvic and scapular control, plank exercises may be performed as long as correct posture can be maintained while doing the exercise (see Figure 6-10).

Postoperative exercises for the shoulder should not cause sharp or severe pain. It is acceptable for the patient to be slightly uncomfortable when doing exercises, but the exercises must be performed with confidence and a sense of control. The discomfort should disappear when the exercise stops. The clinician must ensure that the exercises are performed correctly. Correct movement patterns are more important than load or speed. Once proper scapular control is achieved up to 30° of abduction, the clinician can move to 30° to 90°, and when proper dynamic control has been gained in that range, the patient can be progressed to 180°.[134]

Once control of the scapula is achieved, isometrics to the muscles of the glenohumeral joint are instituted at several positions in the ROM below shoulder level, with no lateral rotation beyond 0°. The positioning and resistance depend on the patient's response to pain and discomfort. The clinician must ensure that compensatory pelvic, trunk, and cervical postures are addressed and that the scapular and humeral control (i.e., stabilization) muscles receive attention.[35] The patient is instructed to perform proper functional isometric position exercises in abduction, medial rotation, lateral rotation (to 0°), extension, and a "full can" (neutral with thumb up) scaption (below horizontal) for the supraspinatus.

Rhythmic stabilization exercises and co-contraction at the joint (e.g., supine or lateral Hawkins positions [see Figure 6-22, *C*]) can be performed to the affected shoulder. The progression of stabilization-co-contraction sequence follows three steps in each selected isometric position. Ensuring the patient has assumed a correct posture and has the appropriate scapular muscles engaged and, if possible, the glenoid under the head of the humerus for greater stability (e.g., supine Hawkins with punch out [see Figure 6-22, *C*], the clinician places one hand around the glenohumeral joint and one hand distally near the wrist. For the first step, the clinician applies perturbations to the humeral head while asking the patient to hold the head of the humerus stabilized (i.e., not moving or translating) in the glenoid. This is called **establishing arthrokinematic control** at the joint. The hand around the wrist offers no resistance but is there to keep the patient's arm extended. Once arthrokinematic control at the glenohumeral joint is gained, the clinician can progress to the second step, in which the clinician applies perturbations not only to the humeral head but also at the wrist. It is important that the clinician ensures that minimal translation occurs at the glenohumeral joint during the double perturbations and the hand applying the perturbations to the humeral head applies only enough counterforce that translation does not occur. Thus this hand is applying perturbations while palpating to ensure no unwanted translation occurs at the glenohumeral joint. If translation does occur, the wrist perturbations being applied at the wrist are too strong. The hand at the wrist can also apply "eccentric breaks" to the whole arm. This second phase establishes **osteokinematic control of the arm** along with arthrokinematic control at the glenohumeral joint. The final or third stage is resistance at the wrist doing eccentric breaks into functional movements. The position of the clinician's hands is the same (around the humeral head and at the wrist), and perturbations are applied only at the wrist into functional positions. The hand around the glenohumeral joint only palpates to ensure minimal translation is occurring at the glenohumeral joint. The result should be eccentric movement of the arm with minimal translation at the glenohumeral joint, which mimics normal arthrokinematic control at the glenohumeral joint and osteokinematic control of the arm. Once co-contraction and coupling are obtained, functional isometrics can be started. If the patient is having difficulty engaging different muscles (e.g., different parts of the deltoid—anterior deltoid often does not engage or contract following injury to the anterior shoulder), electrical stimulation may be used (Figure 6-25).

If the patient complains of pain in the shoulder, ice can be applied to give some relief. In addition, active exercise to the other joints of the arm, cervical spine, trunk and pelvis, and the rest of the body may be instituted to ensure involvement of the whole kinetic chain.

As the patient improves (as evidenced by decreased pain and discomfort), isotonic exercises, especially flexion and extension, can be initiated (usually by the third or fourth day), again below shoulder level and with no lateral rotation beyond 0°, within the pain-free and controllable range. By the fourth day, medial and lateral rotation to 0° with the arm in the adducted position may be performed very carefully. For the lateral rotators, only very careful isometrics should be performed, to prevent excessive stress to the healing tissues. By the fifth day, the patient may begin assisted abduction. To achieve proper scapular and humeral control, exercises are used when appropriate and when strength and pain allow.[134] Once the pain has

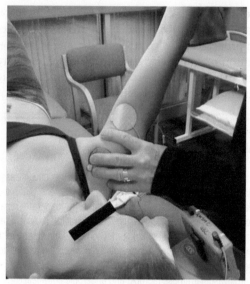

Figure 6-25 Electrical stimulation of anterior deltoid.

diminished and as the patient is weaned from the sling, the clinician can follow the treatment concepts for rehabilitation of shoulder instability described later in the chapter.

PITFALLS OF TREATMENT FOR SHOULDER INSTABILITY AND IMPINGEMENT MANAGEMENT

As with any treatment, the clinician must be aware of common pitfalls. If the following mistakes are kept in mind, the rehabilitation program will have every chance of success.

1. *Failure to perform a complete and thorough assessment.* The assessment must involve the shoulder complex, trunk, pelvic core, and lower kinetic extremity to determine which structures are weak and which are tight and to check for incorrect movement patterns.[85,135]

2. *Failure to assess and address scapulohumeral dysfunction.* The clinician must remember that scapular motion is dynamic for the most part and that the scapula constantly moves, even as it functions as a stable base from which most of the glenohumeral muscles originate. Proximal stability (i.e., scapular control) must be achieved early in the rehabilitation process, before distal mobility (i.e., glenohumeral movement) is encouraged.[47,85] Coordinated scapulohumeral movement is affected by muscle length, muscle strength (especially eccentric muscle strength), capsular tightness, the type of muscle contraction (e.g., isometric, concentric, eccentric, econcentric), timing, and pain. Scapular movement itself is affected by gravity, altered posture, tight muscles, whether the activity is an open or closed kinetic chain, the amount of load the arm lifts, and the speed of arm movement. The clinician must keep all these issues in mind when progressing activity.

3. *Failure to understand the mechanics and demands of the activities to which the patient is returning.* The clinician must have a clear picture of these activities, whether they involve sports or are part of the

individual's everyday life, such as work or recreational activites.[85] Driving is obviously not the same as throwing. Although patients may present with similar types of painful movement, the clinician must be able to assess the problem with a clear understanding of the demands of the activities the patient wants to accomplish. The practitioner must understand that an injury in one part of the body may cause an alteration in another part (i.e., alteration in shoulder mechanics, movement patterns, and how they are accomplished). The shoulder is a link in a kinetic chain of movement.[2-4,85] This kinetic chain allows the generation, summation, transfer, and regulation of forces from the foot to the hand during everyday activity.[2-4,47,81,85] Although individual muscles are the early emphasis in rehabilitation, eventually, as the patient progresses, the whole body must be integrated with shoulder movement patterns (i.e., so that the lower extremity and "core" drive the shoulder).

4. *Failure to deal with any hypomobility early in the treatment to ensure that the joint can regain normal arthrokinematic movement.*[85] Particular attention should be paid to tightness of the posterior glenohumeral capsule, restricted glenohumeral medial rotation (GIRD) or imbalance between the medial (internal) and lateral rotation ROM,[3] tightness of the pectoralis minor and pectoralis major muscles, tightness of the

inferior glenohumeral ligament (caudal glide of the glenohumeral joint), and hypomobility in the thoracic spine and ribs.[3] Treatment of structures must ensure proper movement patterns. Testing for tight anterior structures may be accomplished by doing the Mattison 20 cm test and the horizontal extension test. For the **Mattison 20 cm test**, the patient lies supine while the examiner places one hand over the humeral head to palpate humeral head anterior movement with the patient's arm in 90° abduction. The clinician, using the other hand, medially rotates the patient's arm over the clinician's arm (Figure 6-26). Normally, the patient's hand should be within 20 cm (horizontally) of the ASIS on the same side without the humeral head projecting anteriorly. For the **horizontal extension test**, the patient again lies supine with the arm abducted to 90°. The examiner is positioned such that the elbow of one hand lies over the humeral head to prevent it translating forward. While holding the humeral head down, the examiner horizontally extends the patient's arm (Figure 6-27). The examiner should normally be able to horizontally extend the arm at least 20° to 30° without the humeral head translating anteriorly.

5. *Failure to make sure that stretches are performed properly.* Although stretching may be necessary to restore normal arthrokinematics in a joint, it should not compromise other structures (e.g., scapular stabilizers)

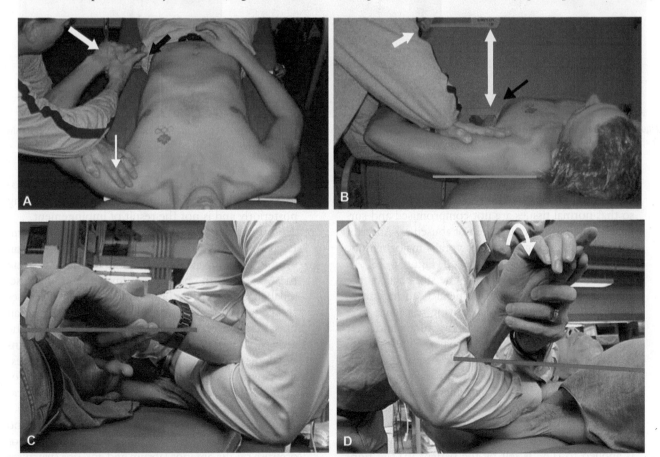

Figure 6-26 Mattison 20 cm test. **A,** Medial rotation of the patient's arm over the clinician's arm. Note how the clinician is holding the humeral head down with his hand. **B,** The distance from the patient's wrist to the ASIS is measured. **C,** Negative test. **D,** Positive test.

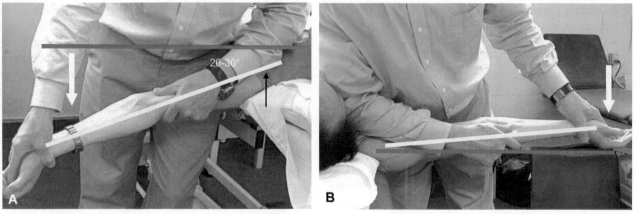

Figure 6-27 Horizontal extension test. Note how the examiner is using his elbow to prevent anterior movement of the humeral head in the glenoid. **A,** Normal. **B,** Restricted movement.

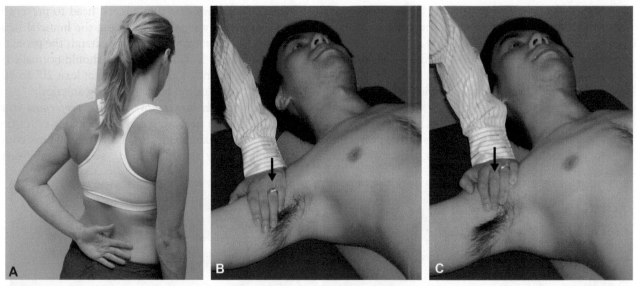

Figure 6-28 Stretching pectoral muscles. **A,** Doorway stretch (shoulder should not hike up) for pectoralis major. **B,** Clinician stretching pectoralis major (push down on head of humerus). **C,** Clinician stretching pectoralis minor (push down on coracoid process).

or reinforce faulty movement patterns. The clinician should teach the patient how to do stretches correctly so that normal tissues are not compromised and surgically repaired structures are not abused.[3,85] Anterior stretching involving a tight pectoralis major may be done by doing a "doorway" stretch (Figure 6-28, *A*). Pectoralis major and minor may be stretched by the clinician ensuring that the humeral head and scapula do not tilt forward and by giving resistance over the coracoid process for pectoralis minor and over the humeral head for pectoralis major (Figures 6-28, *B* and *C*, respectively). Posterior scapular stretching should be performed in three positions—at nipple-diaphragm line, shoulder-acromion line, and chin-mouth (Figure 6-29). Traction stretching (Figure 6-30) can be used to stretch the whole upper kinetic chain, but the clinician must ensure stress is applied to (i.e., is felt by the patient in) the tight structures. The sleeper stretch and modified sleeper stretch (Figure 6-31) are two examples of stretches for a tight posterior glenohumeral joint capsule, provided the clinician is sure the stretching is occurring posteriorly and is not the result of impingement.

6. *Failure to control pain, fatigue, and painful movement.* Exercises must be virtually pain free (pain is less than 4 on a 0 to 10 pain scale [0 being no pain; 10 being the worst pain the patient can imagine]). Otherwise, rehabilitation will be compromised. Ideally, exercises should be performed in a pain-free ROM. The clinician must design exercises that enable the patient to do the activity without pain. It is important to watch for signs of fatigue and to terminate the exercise before excessive fatigue leads to incorrect movement patterns. For example, early activity or overactivity of the upper trapezius is an early sign of fatigue in shoulder exercises.

7. *Failure to correct poor posture.* A normal posture (i.e., no rounded shoulders) is important for reducing anterior pressure on the anterior labrum and anterior structures of the shoulder both statically and dynamically, so the clinician must watch the patient closely to ensure correct

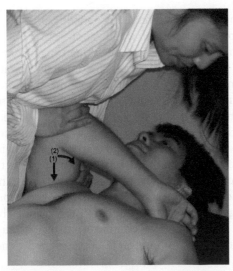

Figure 6-29 Stretching the posterior capsule of the glenohumeral joint. The clinician forward flexes the arm to 90° and then pushes the humeral head backward by pushing down on the elbow. While pushing down, the clinician carefully adducts the arm, increasing the tension on the posterior capsule. The stretch is performed at the nipple-diaphragm line, shoulder acromion line, and chin-mouth line, and the patient should feel the stretch posteriorly.

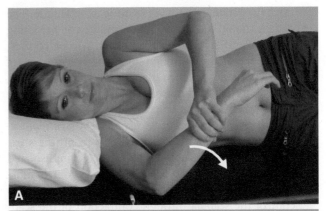

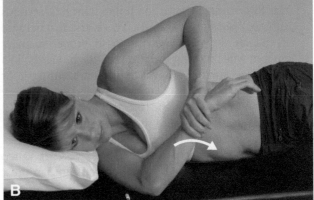

Figure 6-31 A, Sleeper stretch. **B,** Modified sleeper stretch.

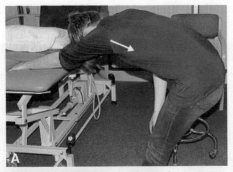

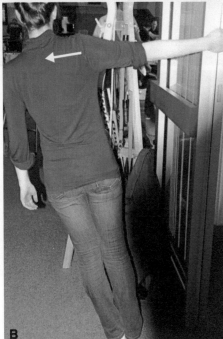

Figure 6-30 Self-traction stretch. **A,** In elevated forward flexion. **B,** In abduction. Patient should relax muscles around glenohumeral joint as much as possible while doing the stretch.

posture and muscle action during movement. The clinician must make sure the patient can maintain a neutral pelvis position (i.e., patient can hold the neutral pelvis statically and dynamically by ensuring correct alignment of the pelvis and spine), proper trunk alignment, rib mobility, and scapular positioning. The clinician should also teach the patient to maintain the correct shoulder position by discouraging exercises that cause rounding of the shoulders (e.g., scapular dumping).

8. *Failure to control for fatigue and compensating postures.* The number of repetitions a patient is asked to do should be based on the number the patient can do correctly with control. The clinician should be specific in the instructions regarding the number of repetitions or sets the clinician wants the patient to complete. Normally, a specific number of repetitions should not be given; rather, the clinician should watch for and

Indicators of Fatigue or Loss of Control or that Load Being Used is Too Great

- Erratic movement
- Incorrect movement patterns
- Breath holding
- Inability to "hit" target
- Phasic movements
- Instability jog or catching movement
- Trick movements, loss of control of the scapular base
- Facial signs of fatigue

teach the patient to be aware of evidence of fatigue. The patient should recognize fatigue and its compensating postures and stop when they occur. Motor control, muscle memory, the firing (contraction) sequences of muscles (stabilizers, then mobilizers), fatigue patterns, and muscle and cardiovascular endurance all play major roles in the rehabilitation process.

9. *Failure to note habitual exercises performed in compensatory postures.* Many clinicians tend to progress exercise routines too quickly, before achieving isolated muscle control, especially of the scapular control muscles. Scapular control implies that the patient is able to control the scapula through contraction of the scapular force couple (lower and upper trapezius, serratus anterior) (see Figure 6-2, *A*). This is essential because it enables the patient to establish proper scapular rhythm while moving the arm (i.e., the humerus) in a controlled fashion. Many activities start with little or no weight, often with gravity eliminated or only very small amounts of weight (0.5 to 0.8 kg [1 to 2 lb]). Progression in resistance should be small. No advantage is gained from lifting heavy weights.

10. *Failure to select appropriate (low risk) exercises.* When asking the patient to do exercises, the clinician must remember to correct the patient's posture, ensure scapular control or stabilization, ensure functional isometric exercises are performed in uncompromising positions, and retrain co-contraction or arthrokinematic control at the glenohumeral joint. Speed of movement should only come toward the end of treatment and should not be a major focus until the functional phase. Initially the goal should be to use low-risk exercises that use the rotator cuff to compress the head of the humerus into the glenoid, such as two-hand stick drills (narrow and wide handle), medial and lateral rotation, and wiper drills (Figure 6-32). Such exercises may include rhythmic stabilization and co-contraction using the supine or lateral Hawkins position (i.e., placing the glenoid under the humerus) (see Figure 6-22, *A* and *B*).[2-4,85] Hawkins drills can include, in the Hawkins positions, small circles, bilateral open and closed gate, scapular movements on a stable arm, one and two arm punch outs, and table and floor push ups with a plus to flys and arm scissors and, as the patient progresses, core exercises—scapular push ups, wall or floor planks (hold core while allowing scapula to move in and out of winging), lateral plank, and V-plank (Figure 6-33).

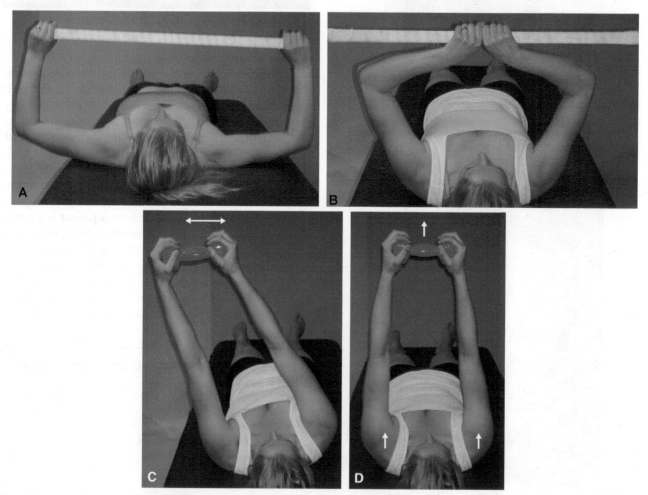

Figure 6-32 Low-risk exercises. **A,** Stick drill–wide hands (power square position). **B,** Stick drill–narrow hands. **C,** Supine wiper drill (can go side to side and up and down to 90°). **D,** "Reach for ceiling" then do circles while maintaining reach. (All exercises can be done in the three zones - i.e., level of diaphragm, shoulder, and forehead.)

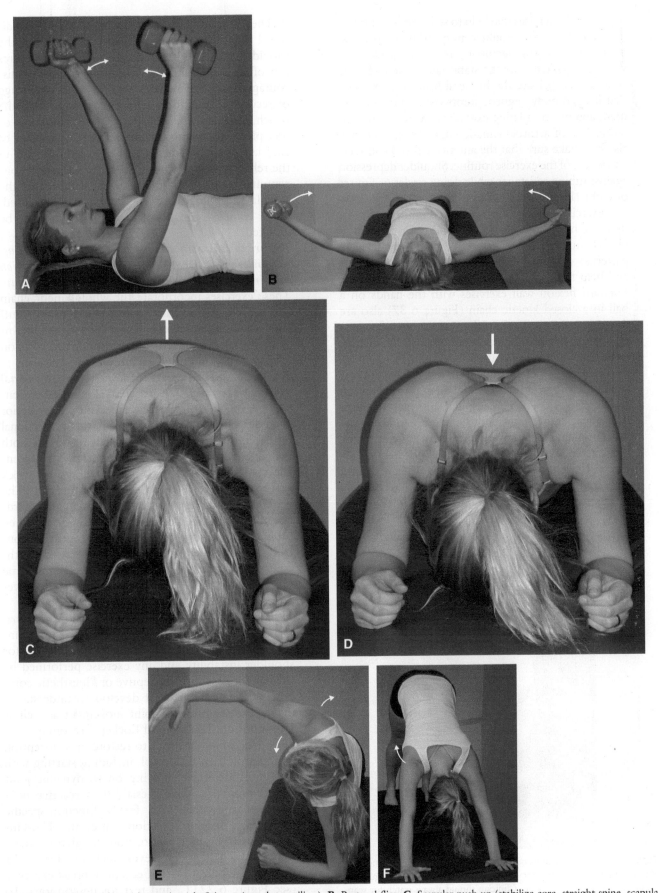

Figure 6-33 Advanced low-risk exercises. **A,** Scissors (punch to ceiling). **B,** Pectoral flies. **C,** Scapular push up (stabilize core, straight spine, scapula should be flat against ribs). **D,** Scapular push up down (relax). Note how scapula wing away from ribs. **E,** Lateral plank with arm motion. Note how left humerus is compressed into glenoid. Motion of right arm and trunk allows arthrokinematic slide at left glenohumeral joint. **F,** "V" plank. Patient can roll back and forth over shoulder again allowing arthrokinematic sliding at the glenohumeral joint.

Low-risk exercises that help to stabilize the humeral head and keep the shoulder away from compromising pinching or impingement postures are preferable. While the patient does the stabilization exercises, the clinician can palpate the humeral head to make sure that it is properly aligned, compressing into the glenoid, and not translating excessively which would indicate loss of arthrokinematic control. The clinician also can make sure that the anterior deltoid contracts and is part of the exercise routine. Shoulder depression against tubing resistance while doing circles or figures of eight (Figure 6-34) is another example of a low-risk exercise. Punch out exercises (Figure 6-35, *A*), dynamic hug (Figure 6-35, *B*), and push ups with a plus (Figure 6-35, *C*) along with PNF exercises (D2 patterns) (Figure 6-36) work the serratus anterior and help to ensure minimal upper trapezius activity. Forward flexion wall exercises with the hands on a ball in a closed kinetic chain (Figure 6-37) also are low-risk exercises. The clinician's repertoire of rotator cuff exercises must include more than simple medial and lateral rotation in neutral.

The empty can position puts the glenohumeral joint in a compromising impingement posture and in the anterior tipped (i.e., scapular anti-tilt) position. The classic empty can strengthening exercise actually is an impingement posture and is not functional for most activities.[136] This exercise does not help to reestablish scapulohumeral rhythm and often is painful early in the rehabilitation process, leading to counterproductive exercises.

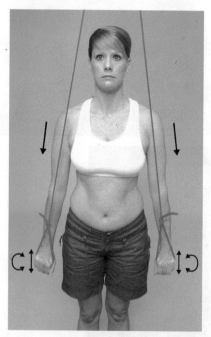

Figure 6-34 Shoulder depression (i.e., dynamic caudal glide) using tubing. Example exercises include having a patient do circles or figures of eight or write his or her name. Clinician should always watch for scapular control.

The clinician should always be aware that traditional weight room exercises used to strengthen the shoulder musculature and surrounding structures can often compound an injury and should be discouraged until the person is in the functional stage of recovery. Traditional gym exercises, such as the bench press and military press, may compound or precipitate shoulder problems. A common mistake of clinicians is to introduce these exercises too early in the rehabilitation program. Early rehabilitation concentrates on training the individual stabilizers of the scapula and humerus. Once this has been achieved, more complex functional motor patterns can be initiated.

11. *Failure to create an exercise program or to make use of functional patterns in later stages of rehabilitation that integrate lower extremity and trunk movements.* These exercises incorporate the whole kinetic chain and are complementary to traditional rotator cuff and scapulohumeral exercises.[2-4,48,82] Examples include the lunge walk with and without trunk rotation (Figure 6-38) and using "lift and chop" patterns.

12. *Failure to rehabilitate the deceleration (eccentric) component of shoulder activity.* Controlled eccentric lengthening of muscles, especially the posterior shoulder muscles, is essential for proper functional return to activity. The patient needs to control both the concentric and, even more important, the eccentric components (i.e., eccentric braking and shock absorption, especially for the posterior muscles). The patient must be able to control movement regardless of its direction. This is especially important when tubing is used. If the patient has to eccentrically control the shortening of the tubing as well as its lengthening (concentric movement), the exercises become more difficult, the patient will be able to do fewer repetitions, and control will improve more quickly.

13. *Failure to address proprioception (static) and kinesthesia (dynamic).* Proprioception is an important and integral part of the rehabilitation process for shoulder instability and any exercise performed by the patient has a proprioceptive or kinesthetic component. The patient must develop an understanding of the sensation of joint movement as well as joint position. Lephart and Kocker[137] recommended a progression of activities to restore proprioception and neuromuscular control, including starting with joint position sense, moving on to dynamic joint stabilization (i.e., kinesthesia), then reactive neuromuscular control, and finally function-specific exercises. For joint position sense, the Hawkins position can be used to position the glenohumeral joint with the patient's eyes open or closed, for rhythmic stabilization and eccentric break exercises (see Figure 6-22, *C*, and text for description). To do these exercises, the clinician positions the patient

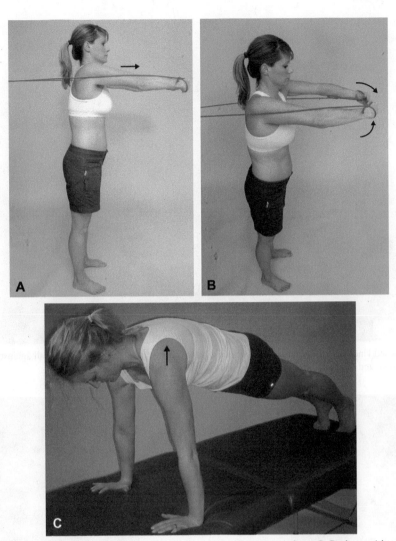

Figure 6-35 Exercises for serratus anterior. **A**, Punch out. **B**, Dynamic hug. **C**, Push up with a plus.

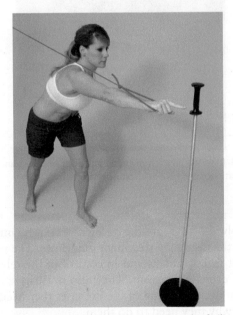

Figure 6-36 Exercise for proprioceptive neuromuscular facilitation (e.g., D2 pattern) using tubing in a lunge position. Note patient aiming for a target, which will help to give an indication of onset of fatigue. If the patient cannot consistently hit the target, he or she is fatigued or the resistance is too great.

and then says, "Don't let me move you," while applying co-contraction forces at the joint, along with eccentric breaking forces on the arm. PNF exercises can be used for dynamic joint stabilization and joint loading with closed kinetic chain exercise (Figure 6-39). To train reactive neuromuscular control, plyometrics, throwing and catching, balance drills, and "falls" (Figure 6-40) all play a role later in the rehabilitation process. For functional motor patterns, PNF (acceleration and deceleration), Body Blade® and Boing® exercises (Figure 6-41), and actual controlled functional activities can be used.

14. *Failure to take the time to work one on one with the patient.* Clinicians must make sure the patient performs the proper movement patterns and controls posture, and they must assist with the timing and sequencing with compensatory motions. This is performed by using individualized, accommodating resistance through all parts of the ROM.

15. *Failure to integrate the patient into the treatment program.* The clinician must convince the patients that their efforts play a crucial role in the rehabilitation process. Treatment for shoulder instability

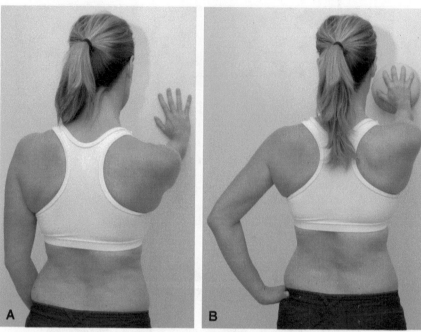

Figure 6-37 Forward flexion closed kinetic chain exercises. **A**, Without a ball against wall (stable). **B**, With a ball against wall (unstable). Patient can be told to retract, elevate, depress, and protract the scapula while pushing against wall or ball.

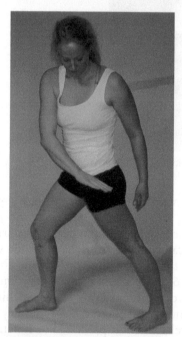

Figure 6-38 Lunge walk with "lift and chop" patterned movement. Patient does lunge as arm goes through PNF pattern, stopping at ASIS bilaterally.

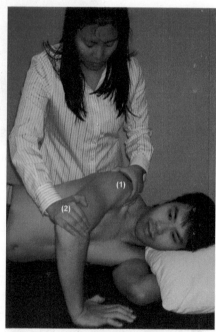

Figure 6-39 Joint stabilization in closed kinetic chain. Resistance for arthrokinematic control (*1*) or osteokinematic control (*2*).

The Patient as "Quarterback"

- Follow clinician instructions
- Ensure correct posture before beginning
- Stabilize the "core," then the scapula before beginning
- Start with "power square" position in supine
- Watch for compensating postures and stop when they occur
- Be sure movement pattern is performed correctly
- Stop when fatigued
- Ask clinician questions if you do not understand

will not succeed unless the patients are actively involved—"they are the quarterback!" who must follow the instability treatment guidelines. The patients must feel confident and in control of the rehabilitation exercise program. They also must have a thorough understanding of the exercises they need to do and why they need to do them.

16. *Failure to use caution when using exercise machines.*[48] Generally machines use long lever arms; this makes controlling the motion difficult and increases the risk of a joint shear, especially if the patient has not

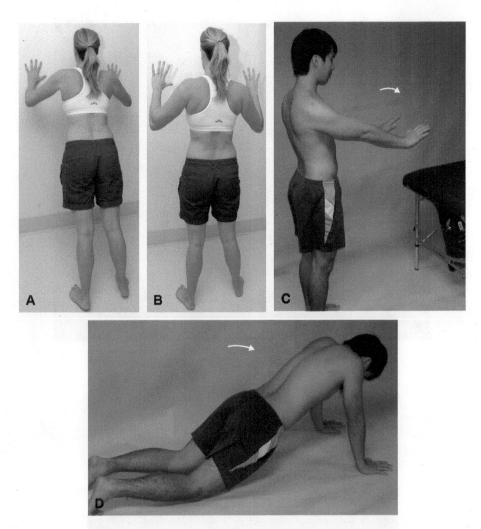

Figure 6-40 Proprioceptive exercises. **A,** Wall push up. **B,** Wall fall: the patient falls forward and catches himself/herself. This can be performed with the eyes closed. **C,** Table fall. **D,** Floor fall.

gained arthrokinematic control. Exercises performed on these machines often are not functional and only work isolated parts of the kinetic chain. In addition, they often emphasize anterior muscle groups rather than posterior muscle groups, which are often more important, especially with anterior instability.

17. *Failure to maintain or restore an appropriate fitness level.* Patients must be encouraged to maintain or do activity during their recovery from injury. Depending on the fitness level of the individual, this may involve low-level activities or higher-level activities within the confines of what the injury will allow them to do. Activities such as walking ("taking the shoulder for a walk"), water activities (walking in water with breast stroke action), and using an upper body exerciser (UBE) (Figure 6-42) to "bicycle the shoulder" are all activities that can help to maintain some aerobic activity and contribute to the feeling of well-being. Improving fitness will also enable the patient to recover from an exercise regime more quickly.

CONSERVATIVE TREATMENT OF INSTABILITY

For proper conservative treatment of impingement or instability syndromes, patients must understand the problem and must recognize that the outcome depends on their compliance with the clinician's instructions about what they should and should not do. The physician will prescribe rest, anti-inflammatory medication, pain-relieving medication, and physical therapy in the early stages. However, in most cases, sound rehabilitation is the key to resolution of these problems.

If the problem is one of atraumatic instability, the rehabilitation process follows a course that ensures that the exercises activate the appropriate muscle or muscle groups in the proper sequence and that functional control is achieved (see Volume 2 of this series, *Scientific Foundations and Principles of Practice in Musculoskeletal Rehabilitation,* Chapter 19).

Although many modalities may be used to treat instability and impingement, the clinician's primary concern is to restore normal shoulder mechanics and function by

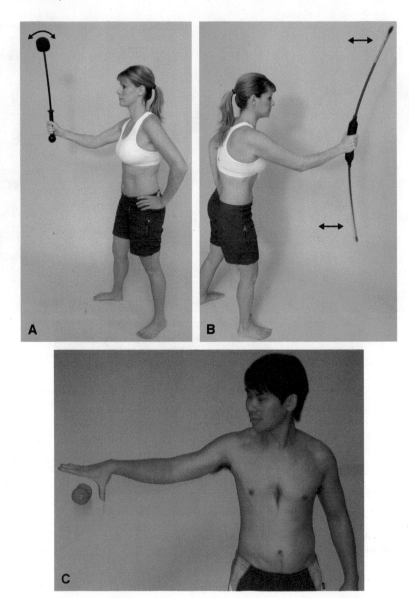

Figure 6-41 Proprioceptive drills using (**A**) Boing, (**B**) Body Blade, and (**C**) Dumbbell drop and catch.

Stabilization Training Sequence

Stages	Steps	Purpose
Stage 1	1.1	Reduce pain
	1.2	Allow freedom of movement (normal arthrokinematic movement)
Stage 2	2.1	Ensure proper muscle function
	2.2	Ensure proper muscle recruitment and motor patterns
	2.3	Correct muscle imbalances
Stage 3	3.1	Correct endurance discrepancies
	3.2	Correct strength discrepancies
Stage 4	4.1	Retrain proprioception and kinesthesia
Stage 5	5.1	Re-educate the muscle stabilizers statically
	5.2	Teach advanced static stabilization exercises
	5.3	Re-educate the muscle stabilizers dynamically
	5.4	Teach advanced dynamic stabilization exercises
	5.5	Teach functional stabilization
Stage 6	6.1	Restore or maintain fitness throughout program

restoring the muscles and improving their coordinated action, contraction sequence, strength, endurance, and proprioceptive or kinesthetic control.[2-4,47,85]

In the early stages of rehabilitation, the emphasis is on scapular control, humeral head stabilization, and restoring the coordinated action of the force couples of the scapulothoracic and glenohumeral joints.[35,85,134,138] This should include integration of the lower limb and trunk as early as possible. Examples of glenohumeral force couples include the subscapularis muscle (a primary stabilizer following anterior dislocation), counterbalanced by the infraspinatus and teres minor muscles, and the deltoid moving the humerus while the supraspinatus, infraspinatus, teres minor, and subscapularis muscles compress the humeral head into the glenoid.[30] By establishing strength and neuromuscular control of these force couples, the patient will regain control of humeral head translation (i.e., arthrokinematic control) during dynamic movement.[79]

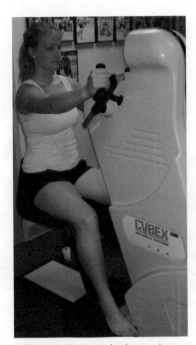

Figure 6-42 Upper body exerciser.

Proper rehabilitation of instability of the shoulder involves controlled aggressiveness in terms of pushing the patient and pushing the envelope of progression for the patient as much as possible, while making sure the patient can control the movement and do it correctly. Because corrective movement depends on force generation and coordinated action of the muscles, as well as freedom of joint movement, the clinician must ensure that patients work only in the ROM in which they are able to control the movement and to do the movement correctly (i.e., using correct movement patterns). This is demonstrated by patients working at a speed at which they demonstrate movement control through precise, smooth (nonjerky) movement patterns, although part of the later rehabilitation continuum involves ensuring that patients progress to functional speeds and loads. With instability, the clinician is concerned with dysfunction that is primarily a motor control problem. The stabilization regimen is a multifaceted program that corrects impairment by improving neuromuscular control and coordination of specific muscles and movements of the shoulder. At the same time, the clinician must work to correct the mechanical factors that predispose or contribute to the abnormal movement patterns. This requires active participation and "buy in" by the patient and an accurate diagnosis by the clinician to determine what restrictions are present; that is, what muscles are at fault and which movements are being done incorrectly. This education and exercise program involves maximum psychological concentration on the part of the patient and very specific movement patterns at minimal speed in a range in which the patient has control. Throughout the process, the principles of specificity apply (see the Principles of Specificity Related to Sports and Rehabilitation box on p. 209). Stabilization

is best achieved by isometric (co-contraction) exercises for static stabilization and concentric-eccentric exercises for dynamic stabilization.

The following steps are not necessarily sequential, but the clinician must consider each one to obtain optimum treatment outcomes. For example, with anterior instability, the clinician may treat the anterior glenohumeral joint for pain (step 1.1) while at the same time, treating the scapula by ensuring isolated contraction of the lower trapezius (step 2.1).

Step 1.1: Reduce Pain (Aim: Pain Control)

The first step is to relieve pain or at least diminish it because the aim is to establish pain control.[85] Instability training may be fatiguing, but it should not be painful. Generally, pain should be kept below a 4 on a 0 to 10 visual analogue scale or at a level that ensures control throughout the exercise (Figure 6-43). This can be accomplished through the use of pain-relieving modalities (e.g., ice, transcutaneous electronic nerve stimulation [TENS], interferential therapy) or by positioning the shoulder in the resting position (see Figure 6-11, *A*). Other approaches that have a role in pain management include modified traction (e.g., shaking out the arm and "throwing" the arm [Figure 6-44]), glenohumeral compression activities, using a sling, nonsteroidal anti-inflammatory drugs (NSAIDs), and gentle mobilizations.[2-4] Exercises should be low risk (i.e., isometric or slow speed) starting from a stabilized or the resting position and ensuring humeral head compression in the glenoid.

Rest from activity is relative and implies decreased length, intensity, and/or frequency of activity. It seldom means total rest. It is important to "take the shoulder for a walk" for 30 minutes each day, which implies moving the shoulder (e.g., swinging the arms while walking).

Step 1.2: Allow Freedom of Movement (Aim: To Restore Normal Arthrokinematic and Osteokinematic Movement)

The clinician should address any movement restriction in any of the joints, muscles, or inert tissues of the shoulder complex, including the spine and ribs. This often is necessary to restore normal arthrokinematic movement in the glenohumeral joint (i.e., allowing the humeral head to centralize in the glenoid cavity), acromioclavicular joint, sternoclavicular joint, scapulothoracic "joint," and thoracic

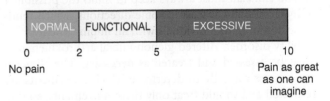

Figure 6-43 Pain-monitoring system (visual analogue scale).

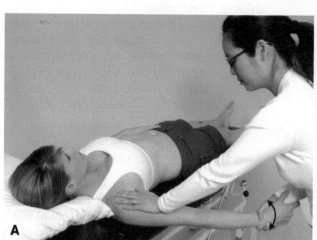
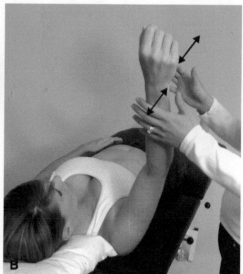

Figure 6-44 A, Shaking the arm. **B**, Throwing the arm.

spine and upper ribs.[21,85] The clinician should check for loss of medial (internal) rotation (Mattison 20 cm test) (see Figure 6-26), restriction of the inferior glenohumeral ligament (decreased inferior glide at the glenohumeral joint), a tight posteroinferior capsule (causes the humeral head to migrate anteriorly and superiorly[2]), and any loss of range due to tightness of the pectoralis major and/or pectoralis minor. Restricted rib motion can limit end ranges of shoulder motion. All have the potential of being tight.[2-4]

A tight posterior capsule, which is often seen with instability, can be suspected if, in supine, there is a loss of medial rotation at the glenohumeral joint, tight anterior chest muscles, restricted shoulder extension performed with the elbow at the nipple-diaphragm line, clavicle-shoulder, and/or chin-forehead (three positions), decreased inferior glide, and restriction at arm 90°-90° (arm forward flexed to 90° and elbow bent to 90°), followed by medial rotation.

Tight Structures Seen in Shoulder Instability and Impingement

- Pectoralis major and/or minor
- Subscapularis
- Posteroinferior capsule
- Ribs
- Thoracic spine

The clinician must always keep in mind the possibility of hypermobility at least in some directions, which tends to be common in individuals with an impingement or instability disorder. Altered glenohumeral arthrokinematics must be assessed and treated as necessary. The clinician must assess carefully to determine which movements are restricted and should treat only these movements, so that

the joint play mobilization techniques to stretch the capsule are effective.[138-142] As the circle concept of movement implies, if the joint is hypermobile in one direction, it may be hypomobile in the opposite direction. With anterior instability, the posteroinferior capsule tends to be tight and therefore requires mobilization, whereas the anterior capsule is hypermobile and requires protection. The clinician should always check the ribs (Figure 6-45) and upper thoracic spine because these are commonly tight with associated chronic shoulder problems.

Active-assisted exercises using a rigid bar (i.e., a T bar, L bar, wand, or stick) may be used to increase ROM.[8,93,138] Stretching of the posterior structures can be accomplished using a stick (Figure 6-46), with stretches performed in different ROMs of shoulder abduction. In the United States, it is currently popular to use a sleeper, modified sleeper, or rollover sleeper stretch or doorway stretch (see Figures 6-28 and 6-31). If the sleeper stretch is to be used, the clinician must ensure the patient feels the stress or stretch posteriorly. Many patients feel pain anteriorly when doing the sleeper stretch, indicating a compromising position with the tissues being impinged anteriorly. Traction stretch (see Figure 6-30) in several positions of abduction will also gain medial rotation.

Posterior stretching may also be accomplished by forward flexing the arm and then pushing the humerus posteriorly (see Figure 6-29). The technique may also be performed actively by having the patient resist as the clinician pushes the humerus posteriorly. Humeral head depression (Figure 6-47) is an effective technique for ensuring inferior glide of the humeral head if excursion of the humeral head under the acromion is restricted.[143] It also poses less risk of compromising the medial scapular stabilizers. Other posterior stretch techniques include anterior chest eccentric breaks and anterior–posterior traction scoop.

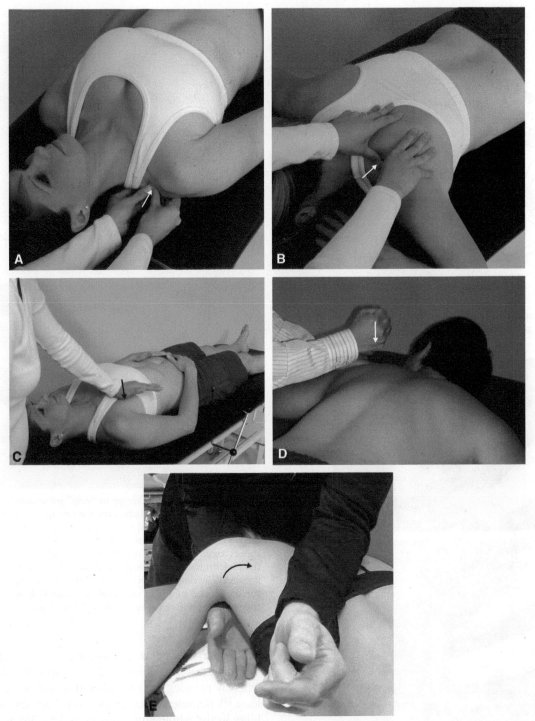

Figure 6-45 Checking the mobility of the ribs. **A,** First rib with patient in the supine position. **B,** First rib with patient in the prone position. **C,** Other ribs. **D,** Gentle "pounding" ribs feeling resistance to movement. **E,** Extension and rotation of thoracic spine and ribs.

Following anterior surgery, the clinician should not stretch or stress the anterior capsule in the early stages of recovery. In most postoperative programs, stretching of vulnerable tissues is contraindicated for the first 6 weeks. In these cases, it is important to follow the surgeon's protocols. In nonsurgical cases, stretching should be performed only in hypomobile directions using precise positions and complete control. Restriction may be the

result of inert tissue tightness or muscle tightness, and different techniques are used to address these two problems. If the patient has signs of muscle tightness (most commonly, the pectoralis minor and subscapularis),[86] the clinician may use muscle energy techniques, hold-relax, or active release techniques or passive (anterior chest) stretching (Figure 6-48). Trigger point therapy, another muscle technique, can be used effectively to increase

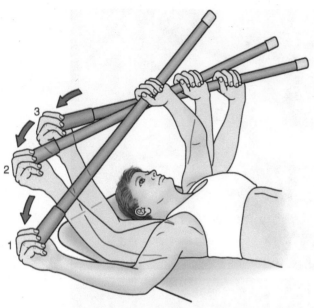

Figure 6-46 A stick can be used to increase the ROM in the glenohumeral joint by going through different parts of the ROM.

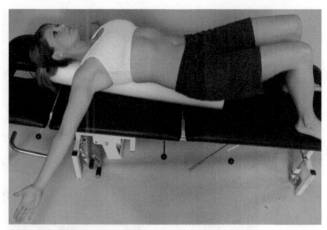

Figure 6-48 Stretching the anterior structures of the shoulder and trunk on a foam roll ("open book" stretch).

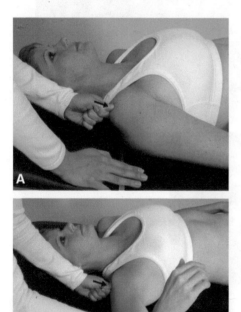

Figure 6-47 Humeral head depression. **A,** Arm by the side. **B,** Arm in 90° abduction.

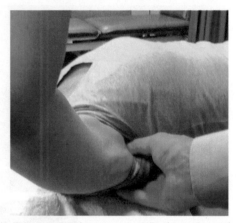

Figure 6-49 Trigger point therapy to "strip" subscapularis. The clinician holds the arm in slight abduction and forward flexion. Using the thumb (or middle and ring fingers) of the other hand, the clinician palpates for the trigger points on the striations of subscapularis. The clinician then applies trigger point pressure with the thumb while with the other hand the clinician resists the patient isometrically holding the arm in various postures. The clinician then eccentrically breaks the postural holds. The clinician does 3 to 5 hold and break positions while applying different trigger point pressure for each of the hold positions

range with isolated muscle tightness (e.g., the subscapularis) (Figure 6-49). Restriction or loss of abduction, inferior humeral glide, or medial or lateral rotation of the shoulder may also need to be addressed.[85]

Clinicians must also consider the effect of crossed syndromes (Figure 6-50) on the mobility and strength of muscles about the shoulder. **Janda's "upper crossed"**

syndrome showed that muscles (primarily postural) on one diagonal at a joint could be tight and hypertonic, whereas muscles on the other diagonal were weak and long.[144] Because similar cross syndromes can affect flexibility in the whole kinetic chain, inflexibility in the upper and lower kinetic chains may need to be addressed.[85] The clinician should assess for and treat any tight lower kinetic chain structures, including the Achilles-calf musculature, hamstrings, hip flexors, abductors, and extensors. Tight trunk flexors and abnormal gait patterns must also be considered.[85]

Pendular exercises (e.g., the Codman pendular arm swing exercises) may be used initially (see Figure 6-20), provided the exercises are pain free and the patient can control the movement (start with small pendular exercises progressing to scapular and humeral muscle control

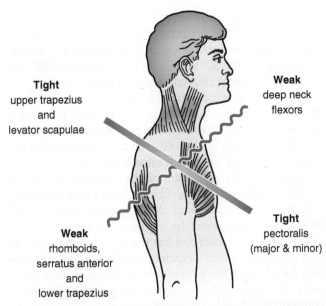

Tight
upper trapezius
and
levator scapulae

Weak
deep neck
flexors

Weak
rhomboids,
serratus anterior
and
lower trapezius

Tight
pectoralis
(major & minor)

Figure 6-50 Upper crossed syndrome. (From Magee DJ: *Orthopedic physical assessment*, ed 6, p 165, Philadelphia, 2014, Saunders/Elsevier.)

with circles). Caution is required with pendular exercises, especially after arthroscopic surgery, because they apply gravity traction to the repaired vulnerable structures. The clinician may also try modified Codman exercises, which eliminate gravity traction by having the patient roll a ball on a low chair or table with the elbow extended (see Figure 6-20, *C*). This prevents inferior translation and caudal traction on the glenohumeral joint. Anterior translation of the humeral head (common in active lateral rotation) must be avoided, especially in patients with anterior instability.[145] The clinician must not allow scapular hitching (i.e., upward movement) or dumping (i.e., downward tilting of the glenoid) with any assisted exercises. The arm may be swung horizontally in a variety of planes. These exercises are useful in the early stages to maintain ROM, but compensated shoulder postures must be avoided because some reports have indicated that in pathological shoulder conditions, the upper trapezius and supraspinatus are less likely to relax.[146] Shoulder depression exercises using tubing (e.g., dynamic caudal glide) help to improve range, enhance scapular control, and promote coordinated scapulohumeral and glenohumeral activity.

Step 2.1: Ensure Proper Muscle Function (Aim: To Ensure All Muscles Contract Individually)

Ensuring Proper Muscle Function

- Start by positioning the muscle in the "muscle test" position
- Use low (10% to 30% MVC) isometric contraction
- STOP as soon as fatigue is evident
- Work muscle in inner range of movement

This stage involves restoring individual muscle function to ensure proper muscle recruitment or proper activation of the muscle. Proper contraction of the scapular force couple, including the lower trapezius with the serratus anterior, requires special attention. If the patient does appropriate exercises and compensatory postures are not allowed, these muscles will contract or "turn on." The upper trapezius and latissimus dorsi can dominate in compensatory postures, causing an incorrect movement pattern. For example, with a Kibler type III dyskinesia of the scapula, the upper trapezius, levator scapulae, and posterior deltoid do not function in concert most of the time, resulting in the postural deformity.[2-4,86] Biofeedback may be used to teach the patient to contract the desired muscle and to "turn off" the unwanted compensatory muscle contraction.

To encourage isolated muscle contractions (i.e., specificity), the patient is positioned in the "muscle test" position for that muscle.[43-45] The clinician positions the patient so as to isolate the muscle and then asks the patient to hold the position against minimal clinician resistance to ensure that the desired isometric contraction is achieved. The patient contracts the muscle only to 10% to 30% of the MVC to ensure an isolated contraction of the muscle while the clinician watches for no compensatory contraction of other muscles. Functional activation may be tested by doing "open shutter" and supine and standing "streamline" exercises, "four corner" drills, and PNF diagonals (Figure 6-51).

During these early stages of treatment, it is important that the clinician watch for the first sign of fatigue and stop the patient when it appears. Signs of fatigue are shaking when doing movement, not being consistently able to hit a target, loss of or change in segmental colinear posture, inability to hold proper functional posture, or contraction

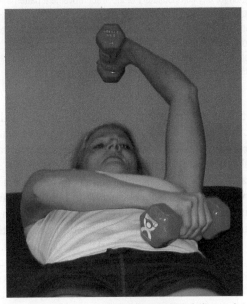

Figure 6-51 Functional activation exercise. PNF D2 diagonal patterns.

of compensatory muscles. Early on, patients commonly find contracting the isolated muscles difficult and in some cases, impossible—these people need electrical stimulation to the muscles to "reboot" them, and they frequently show psychological fatigue, which mirrors physiological fatigue.

If inferior instability is present, the scapula must be able to stabilize both statically and dynamically, the humeral head must be balanced in terms of ROM (e.g., medial and lateral rotation should be close to equal), compression of the humeral head by the rotator cuff must be evident, and the patient must be able to contract the anterior and posterior deltoid muscles simultaneously.

Postural correction is an essential component of this step. The clinician should determine whether the patient can achieve the neutral pelvis position (i.e., stabilize the core) and hold the position during both static and dynamic activities. As the patient begins to assume and hold the neutral pelvis position (i.e., demonstrating a stable core), the posture will begin to correct. If the connection is slow or the patient appears to be having problems, the clinician must look for potential restrictive and weak cross syndromes that are limiting the return to normal posture and stretch (e.g., pectoralis minor, hip flexors) and strengthen these components (e.g., abdominal flexors, scapular control muscles).

Step 2.2: Ensure Proper Muscle Recruitment and Motor Patterns (Aim: To Ensure All Muscles Contract When They Should)

Ensuring Proper Muscle Recruitment and Motor Patterns

- When muscle can be recruited, the aim is then to ensure the muscle contracts when it is supposed to
- Make sure the patterns of movement are correct
- Watch for any compensatory or incorrect movement patterns
- Start with low-load isotonics and progress to eccentric (for muscle shock absorption and braking functions) and concentric (for correct movement) loaded exercises
- Can initiate proprioceptive exercises at this point keeping in mind the different proprioceptive receptors to be stimulated

---

At this stage, treatment is directed primarily at the stabilizer muscles of the scapula, followed by the stabilizers of the glenohumeral joint, because these muscles maintain the normal relationship between the glenohumeral and scapulothoracic joints. The scapular stabilizers provide a stable base for the arm, preserve deltoid fiber length so that acromiohumeral length is maintained, and help control impingement of the rotator cuff. Proper activation and functioning of the scapular stabilizers is essential (see Table 5-1).[49,85,147] The clinician must ensure that scapular substitution patterns are not occurring and that the stabilizer muscles contract before the mobilizer muscles.[148] For example, when the patient abducts the arm to 30°, the scapula should stabilize

and "lock in" in this phase of scapulohumeral rhythm. In the first phase of arm abduction (0° to 30°), no or minimal scapular movement should occur. If the scapula keeps moving during the first 30° of abduction, the scapular stabilizers are not functioning properly and the mobilizers are dominating or the exercise is too advanced (i.e., too hard) for the patient. In the second phase (30° to 90°), the scapula should rotate but show minimal protraction or elevation. In the third phase (90° to 180°), lateral rotation to the humerus is necessary along with some elevation.

In scaption (i.e., the plane of the scapula), scapulohumeral rhythm is slightly different, with more individual variation in the movement. More scapular rotation and protraction often occur. In scaption, less lateral rotation of the humerus occurs and less stress is placed on the tissues of the shoulder. Therefore scaption is a good position for working the patient initially because there tends to be less pain with movement and scaption is a more common functional movement pattern.

If the patient is having difficulty determining how to contract individual muscles, electrical stimulation or biofeedback may be used.[149] Useful scapular control exercises include retraction and depression of the scapula, as well as elevation and protraction. These involve individual exercises for the three parts of the trapezius muscle, serratus anterior, rhomboids, and levator scapulae. Exercises for the scapular control muscles include scapular squeezes or pinch, thumb tubes in the three positions starting in the "power square" (90°-90°) position for the middle and lower trapezius, dynamic hug and punch outs for the serratus anterior, shoulder depression with tubing and press down exercises (Figure 6-52),[85] and V-plank exercises (see Figure 6-33, *F*) for compression of the humeral head into the glenoid.

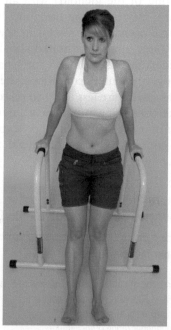

Figure 6-52 Press down exercise for shoulder depression using bars.

At this step, force-couple training also plays a predominant role. Force-couple training involves recruitment of the muscles, along with synchronized action of the muscles using loaded and unloaded activities. Co-contraction (i.e., arthrokinematic stabilization) with rhythmic stabilizations has a stabilizing and stiffening effect, adds compression for joint position sense, and tends to be done isometrically.[85] Coordinated coactivation results in less torque or sheer loads on the glenohumeral joint on the shoulder and increased joint control. Co-contraction primarily works the small (inner cone) muscles (i.e., the rotator cuff) of the joint. An example is rhythmic stabilization to the humeral head in the Hawkins punch out position (see Figure 6-22, *A*) and scapular movements on a stable arm (e.g., closed kinetic chain scapular "clock" exercises—the patient moves the scapula through the different hours of a clock while stabilizing the hand against the wall). These exercises also help emphasize the rotator cuff, stabilize the glenohumeral joint by compressing the humeral head in the glenoid, and reduce deltoid activation.[48,85]

Closed kinetic chain activities in the shoulder (e.g., rhythmic stabilization) are more stable, involve less translation, provide static stability, and are often used with coactivation.[85] Closed kinetic chain activities provide motion control, sequencing, and improved proprioception and often are more functional.[48] Exercises include weight shifts with the hand on a stable or unstable surface, rotator cuff clock exercises, and wall washes ("wax on, wax off") exercises (Figure 6-53), and "wiper" and "Spiderman" (see Figure 6-21, *D*) exercises.[48]

Once scapular control has been achieved, humeral control exercises can be instituted for the rotator cuff and deltoid. These help to prevent humeral head migration and to restore voluntary arthrokinematic control of the humeral head through rotator cuff coactivation (especially of the supraspinatus and subscapularis) and stabilization, as well as activation of the biceps and triceps (Figure 6-54) and pectoralis major.[134-137,149] These exercises also can be used later in the rehabilitation program, as long as the patient has no impingement signs and good scapular control.

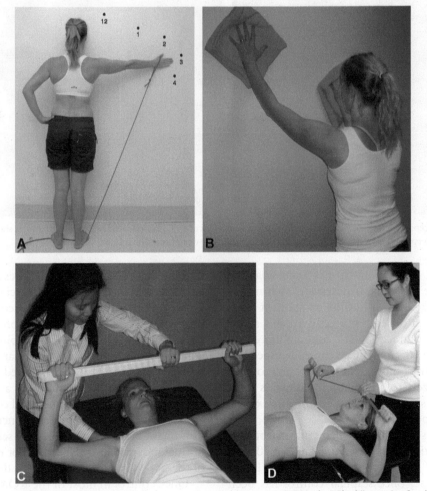

Figure 6-53 Exercises for proprioception, motion-controlled sequencing, and increasing ROM. **A,** "Clock" exercise for the scapula with the arm in abduction. **B,** Wall washes ("wax on, wax off"). **C,** Rhythmic stabilization with a stick in power square position. Note how clinician is palpating for arthrokinematic control of patient's right shoulder. **D,** Rhythmic stabilization with thumb tube in power square position. Clinician is applying perturbations to tube.

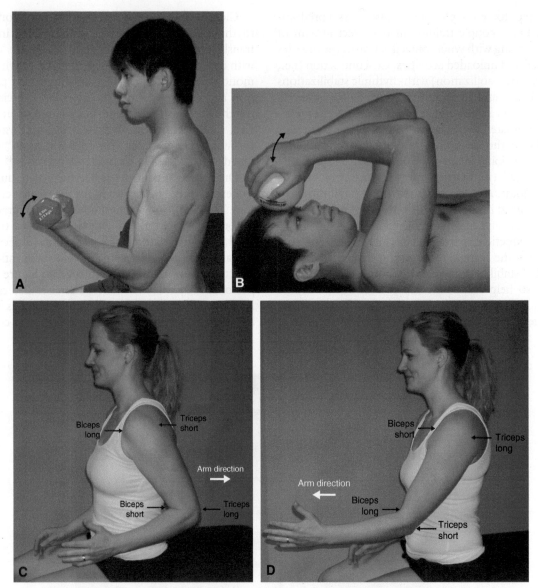

Figure 6-54 Biceps and triceps exercises. **A**, Biceps curls. **B**, Skull crushers (triceps). **C**, Econcentric biceps and triceps in shoulder extension. **D**, Econcentric biceps and triceps into forward flexion. Doing C and D together would result in a functional arm pump.

The patient must concentrate to make sure that the movements are done correctly. If necessary, each movement should be broken down into its component parts so that the patient can do each correctly. At this stage, maximum strength contractions are contraindicated. A contraction of 10% to 30% of MVC at controlled speeds is the aim to ensure correct movement patterns and to keep fatigue of the stabilizers to a minimum. Fatigue is most evidenced by muscle substitution (e.g., contraction of the upper trapezius and posterior deltoid).

Short arc exercises (in this case, in a pain-free range) into scaption, abduction, and forward flexion to 30° initially and then to 90° can be prescribed, especially in the initial treatment phase, once scapular control has been achieved. If scapular control has not been achieved, these exercises should be limited to 30°. Once the patient is able to control motion up to the horizontal plane, movement

to full elevation can begin. Exercises above 90° should be performed in lateral rotation to facilitate clearance of the greater tuberosity under the coracoacromial ligament.[52] Tubing exercises, if performed properly, are effective. In most cases, when and how tubing is used should be controlled unless the patient has learned to do the tubing exercises correctly. To be performed correctly, tubing exercises should be performed only at the speed at which the patient has complete functional control of the activity. If functional control is lost, dysfunctional compensatory movement patterns result (usually seen in winging or abnormal movement of the scapula or excessive contraction of the upper trapezius or posterior deltoid).

Once control in most of the ROM has been achieved, diagonal PNF exercises may be used to teach control and stabilization throughout the ROM. The shoulder D2 pattern (flexion, abduction, and lateral rotation) is especially useful for instability. Full range should not be attempted in patients with signs of impingement or those showing apprehension.[93,134,150,151] Techniques such as slow reversals, contract-relax, rhythmic stabilization, and timing for emphasis are useful for treating instability by increasing awareness of movement, stimulating appropriate weak muscles, and strengthening weak patterns.[93,95,145] Tubing exercises using these patterns have also been found to be effective, provided they are performed with control.

Once the muscles can contract in the correct sequence, the primary shoulder accelerators or movers of the glenohumeral joint (i.e., pectoralis major, anterior deltoid, latissimus dorsi, teres major, biceps, and pectoralis minor) are trained concentrically, whereas the primary decelerators (i.e., infraspinatus, teres minor, supraspinatus, posterior deltoid, and triceps) and scapular stabilizers are trained eccentrically. Concentric and econcentric exercises of the biceps and triceps should begin as the patient progresses toward more functional movement. *Econcentric* or *pseudo-isometric* exercise is so named because commonly during function these two-joint muscles are lengthening over one joint while they shorten over the other joint. For example, when swinging the arms into extension with bent elbows during running, the biceps is lengthening over the shoulder but is shortening at the elbow as the elbow flexes (see Figure 6-54, *C* and *D*). Thus, to ensure correct movement patterns, two-joint muscles need to be trained to function econcentrically.

Step 2.3: Correct Muscle Imbalances (Aim: To Ensure Correct Force-Couple Action)

Correcting Muscle Imbalances

- Ensure joint can move through full ROM by stretching tight structures and allowing lengthened structures to tighten
- Correct any unbalanced cross syndromes
- Ensure near-equal right and left body strength and endurance
- Correct any kinetic chain movement imbalances that involve injured structures
- Proprioceptive (static) and kinesthetic (dynamic) exercises keeping in mind the different proprioceptive receptors to be stimulated and whether they function statically or dynamically

To correct muscle imbalances, any lengthened muscles must be exercised in the inner range to shorten them, and short muscles must be stretched to lengthen them. The clinician must make sure that strength and endurance are equal between the left and right sides for what the patient wants to do and that any strength and/or endurance discrepancies are corrected.[152] For example, with the humeral control muscles, a good relationship should exist between the medial and lateral rotators, between the flexors and extensors, and between the abductors and adductors, which will lead to many exercises being performed bilaterally.[152] Cross syndromes with their strong and tight muscles on one diagonal and weak and long muscles on the other diagonal must also be addressed.[144] People with anterior shoulder instability commonly demonstrate overactivity of the upper trapezius and underactivity of the serratus anterior. A standard push up "with a plus" (this implies scapula is fully protracted) has been reported to be a good exercise to accentuate the serratus anterior while minimizing the upper trapezius, thus reversing this abnormal movement pattern.[152] Isokinetic tests have shown that medial-to-lateral rotation strength ratios should be approximately 3:2, extension-to-flexion strength ratios should be 5:4, and adduction-to-abduction strength ratios should be 2:1.[113,137]

Muscle balance does not necessarily imply maximum strength of the muscles. Rather, it implies that the force couples are able to work in a coordinated fashion and with sufficient strength and endurance to do the correct motor patterns during activity. The "mover" muscles must have the strength and endurance to move an object concentrically one or more times, and the "stabilizer" muscles must have the strength and endurance to stabilize isometrically (statically) and eccentrically (during dynamic movement or as a shock absorber) in the correct movement pattern.[85,153] Eccentric control in throwing activities is more important than concentric control, and if eccentric fatigue occurs, injury is more likely.[154] Tubing may be used provided the resistance and speed of contraction are carefully controlled. The shoulder should not be overloaded, and the patient must understand that the exercises can be done only at the speed at which control and correct movement (i.e., smooth, coordinated movement) are demonstrated. If ROM is a problem, pulleys or T bar routines may be used as active-assisted exercises to help to increase the ROM and control large lever forces.[155,156]

Because synchronization of shoulder movement is important during normal activities, the patient must develop neuromuscular functional control. Therefore any treatment program must ensure good muscle balance between the agonist and antagonist and enable the patient to work at properly controlled speeds. This control eventually must be demonstrated at functional speeds. Too often, the clinician rehabilitates the patient only to have the patient return, complaining of problems when performing the activity. The problem commonly is lack of control at functional speeds.

Step 3.1: Correct Endurance Deficiencies (Aim: To Ensure Sufficient Muscle Endurance to Do Activity and Minimize the Likelihood of Injury)

The clinician must take extreme care in choosing the type of strengthening program to which the patient is exposed, especially if the rotator cuff or biceps muscles are

Correcting Endurance Discrepancies

- Use low load, high repetitions
- Patient must be able to control the pelvis (neutral pelvis), thorax (alignment), and scapula (dynamic stabilization)
- Need to build up endurance to delay fatigue with "built in protection" factor
- Ensure correct movement patterns
- Watch for compensatory postures
- Work at only speeds at which the patient can control the movement (i.e., can do the movement correctly)

involved. Because instability often has an overuse component, unsuitable exercises or too many exercises may aggravate the condition. The quality of the exercises is more important than the quantity. That being said, endurance plays a significant role in instability training because incorrect movement patterns are more likely to be seen with fatigue.

Once scapular control is achieved and the patient can control active exercises, progression to free weights (2.3 kg [5 lb] or less for up to 30 repetitions) and tubing exercises may be initiated, in the range in which the patient is able to control the movement.[157] Pappas et al.[157] found that weights heavier than 2.3 kg (5 lb) tended to precipitate loss of muscle balance in the shoulder. Initially, this movement may occur over 10° to 30° (i.e., a short arc). Once control is demonstrated by smooth, coordinated movement with minimal or no evidence of pain and discomfort, the exercises can be progressed into greater ROMs. The clinician must monitor the exercises to make sure the patient can do them correctly without fatigue, to provide a baseline for improving endurance. For example, if a patient can do four repetitions correctly, this is the starting point for the exercises. The aim is to increase the number of repetitions to a level that meets the patient's eventual functional needs plus a built-in protection (BIP) factor. If a patient needs to do 30 repetitions in a 15-minute period, the aim is to get the patient to be able to do the 30 repetitions in 15 minutes with a 10% to 15% cushion (*the BIP factor*) (i.e., 33 to 35 repetitions), so that there is less chance of injury due to fatigue. It is essential that the patient demonstrate control in terms of scapular stabilization, movement pattern, strength, endurance, and movement direction when progressing into greater ROMs. Exercises such as controlled tubing routines and wall dribbles (Figure 6-55) can enhance endurance.[149]

Step 3.2: Correct Strength Deficiencies (Aim: To Ensure Sufficient Muscle Strength to Do Activity and Minimize the Likelihood of Injury or Reinjury)

To improve strength, the patient initially should use low repetitions with high-load contractions. Active and resisted exercises may include progressive resisted exercises with minimal weight at the beginning, working up to

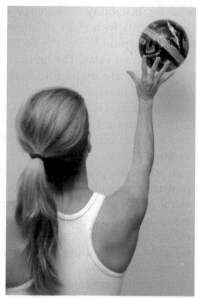

Figure 6-55 Wall dribbles used for proprioception and endurance.

Correcting Strength Discrepancies

- Start with isometric exercises moving on to concentric, eccentric, and econcentric exercises
- Use concentric exercises to ensure correct movement patterns
- Watch for compensatory postures
- Use eccentric breaks to retrain muscle shock absorption and braking action
- Use econcentric exercises to strengthen and increase endurance of two-joint muscles

heavier weights or using various commercial exercise machines, keeping in mind the limitations of these devices (Table 6-3).[149,158]

Once the scapular stabilizers are functioning correctly, the glenohumeral stabilizers may be strengthened. Common exercises for strengthening the glenohumeral stabilizers include those involving the supraspinatus and deltoid ("open can" exercises or prone horizontal abduction at 100° with full lateral rotation),[136] subscapularis (medial rotation, side lying, eccentric breaks), infraspinatus and teres minor (side lying lateral rotation at 0° to 45° abduction, eccentric breaks) (Figure 6-56), biceps (flexion), and triceps (extension).[159,160] Strengthening of the scapular control muscles, along with the supraspinatus, infraspinatus, teres minor, biceps, and all three parts of the deltoid should be stressed.[143,145,146]

Eccentric exercises for the scapular and humeral control muscles help improve their strength and endurance for decelerating the arm and for shock absorption.[30,162] Closed-chain shoulder activities should be encouraged when the patient has attained suitable strength and control. Open-chain activities may begin

TABLE **6-3**

Correcting Strength Deficiencies

Muscle	Exercise
Supraspinatus	Side lying, 45° abduction[159] Full can at 90° elevation in scaption[126]
Subscapularis	Side lying, 45° abduction[159] Lift off (Gerber push)[126]
Infraspinatus	Side lying, 0° to 45° lateral rotation[159] Sitting, lateral rotation of the arm from −45° to 0° (multiple angles)[126]
Teres minor	Side lying, 0° to 45° and lateral rotation
Biceps	Yergason's drill (Yergason's test used as an exercise) Speed's drill (Speed's test used as an exercise) Arm pumping
Upper trapezius	Military press[159]
Middle trapezius	T exercise: Scapular retraction with the arm at 90° abduction in the prone position
Lower trapezius	Y exercise: Scapular retraction with the arm abducted to 120° in the prone position, Spiderman exercise
Serratus anterior	Wall walks, dynamic hug, V-plank
Deltoid	Side lying, 45° abduction[159]
Rhomboids	With shoulder abduction at 90°, the patient resists forward flexion of the arm[126] (also exercises the posterior deltoid)

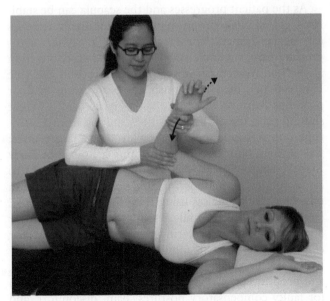

Figure 6-56 Lateral rotation eccentric break. Patient laterally rotates the arm and clinician eccentrically "breaks" the contraction into medial rotation.

early with high repetitions using low weights, as long as the patient can control the movement. High-risk activities (e.g., dead lifts, military presses, hands behind head "lats" for latissimus dorsi and shrugs with weights in the hands) should be avoided if scapular protraction occurs because they can cause harmful sheer forces and lead to lack of control.[150] Similarly, daily activities such as sleeping in a supine position with the hand under the pillow or over the head, fixing the hair, reaching into the back of a car from the front seat, leaning back on the arms while sitting for long periods, and putting on a backpack should be discouraged because of the stress they place on the anterior capsule.

In terms of strength about the shoulder, adduction should be the strongest, followed by extension, flexion, abduction, medial rotation, and lateral rotation. It is especially important to strengthen the medial humeral rotators (i.e., subscapularis, pectoralis major, and latissimus dorsi) and the scapular control muscles, especially the serratus anterior and lower and middle trapezius muscles, all of which show marked weakness when impingement or instability is demonstrated.[35]

Controlled pulleys or tubing may be used in the pain-free ROM for abduction, scaption (thumbs up), and forward flexion with the palm supinated. Supinating the palm causes lateral rotation of the humerus and moves the shoulder out of the impingement position. Such movement in standing may provide gravity assistance to humeral depression.[162] Strengthening exercises should progress from isometric pain-free activity to isotonic pain-free activity.

As the patient progresses through the strengthening regime, special attention must be paid to two-joint muscles because these are the muscles most commonly injured during activity. Functionally, these muscles are moving two joints at the same time and should be exercised this way (i.e., econcentrically).

Step 4.1: Retrain Proprioception and Kinesthesia (Aim: To Ensure Voluntary Control and Awareness of Movement)

Retraining Proprioception and Kinesthesia

- Remember that proprioceptive receptors are stimulated only with specific actions (e.g., muscle spindle–muscle stretch; Golgi tendon organs–muscle contraction; Golgi ligament endings–end range stretch)
- Start with slow, precise movements
- Stop when fatigue evident
- Ensure correct movement patterns
- Watch for incorrect compensatory postures
- Break complex movement patterns down into simple components

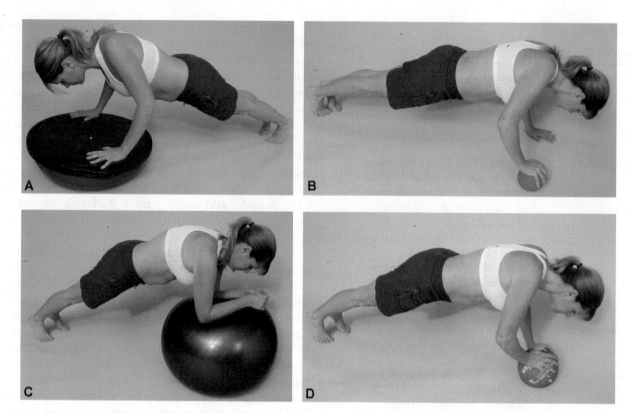

Figure 6-57 Push up on **(A)** a Bosu Ball®, **(B)** small ball using one hand, **(C)** big ball, and **(D)** small ball using two hands for proprioception.

In reality, any exercise can be used for proprioceptive or kinesthetic training because they all have a proprioceptive or kinesthetic effect. However, to specifically target individual proprioceptive receptors, exercises have to be individualized. As soon as the patient has gained scapular control, proprioceptive or kinesthetic training can be instituted to restore proprioceptive deficits.[163] Proprioceptive and kinesthetic training involves gaining voluntary control of different movement patterns, increasing the patient's awareness of correct movement patterns, and establishing automatic control of movements. Proprioceptive and kinesthetic exercises may involve closed kinetic chain weight shift, recovery phase closed kinetic chain exercises, and concentric as well as eccentric motion, movement in different parts of the ROM, and activities at different speeds.

In closed-chain activities, the distal segment is fixed or the patient holds on to an immovable object so that fixation feedback is possible, thus providing better proprioception, co-contraction, and stabilization.[164] Examples include arm wall slides into abduction, flexion diagonal patterns, and "wax on, wax off" routines (i.e., wall washes).[86,87] Dips and many proprioceptive control activities (e.g., balance board, Bosu Ball®, or using different size balls) are considered closed-chain activities (Figure 6-57). Overuse injuries are less likely to occur during closed-chain activities. Closed-chain activities for the shoulder should be primarily eccentric to reduce the effects of gravity and inertia. These activities tend to compress the joint, increasing stability,

and may be used in the reverse origin insertion mode. For example, although the latissimus dorsi is viewed as an extensor and medial rotator of the shoulder, it may also be used as a trunk extensor. The clinician should look at each exercise to determine which proprioceptive or kinesthetic receptors he or she wants to stimulate (e.g., different parts of the ROM, different speeds, acceleration or deceleration) and design the exercises to meet that goal.

As the patient progresses and the scapula can be stabilized, closed-chain proprioceptive or kinesthetic activities can be performed. These can include push ups (progressing from rhythmic stabilization) and co-contraction at the joint; wall push ups progressing to wall falls (see Figure 6-40), then table push ups progressing to floor push ups (with or without a ball) (Figure 6-57); weight shifting from the push up position, shifting from a quadruped to a tripod position; ball rolling; target drills; wall washes; balancing on balls; using a Boing® or Body Blade®, dumbbell and ball drops (see Figure 6-41) to cause sudden alterations in joint position; sitting push ups; Profitter® exercises using the hands; use of an UBE (see Figure 6-42) or similar cycling device for the upper limb; hand balancing or using a balance board; hand stair climbing; and hand treadmill walking.* All of these activities are excellent for improving strength, endurance, and proprioception, but the clinician must always watch for faulty compensatory postures, pain, discomfort, and

*Refs. 30, 85, 87, 138, 158, 160, 161, 165, 166.

fatigue resulting in loss of scapular and/or humeral control, leading to compensatory patterns.

Open kinetic chain activities may be used, but they are not as effective, and they do not provide the same stability. However, they are often more functional. They must also be done with good posture. Shoulder dumps and punch outs with weight (e.g., 3 sets of 20) are some open kinetic chain activities that simulate a shoulder function.[85]

Step 5.1: Reeducate the Stability Muscles Statically (Aim: To Ensure Isometric Positioning for Form and Skill Execution)

Stage 5, consisting of five parts, is where true integrated stabilization training begins. The previous parts are individual parts of a stabilization training program that must be addressed before functional integrated stabilization training can begin.

Reeducating the Muscle Stabilizers Statically

- To begin, clinician must ensure the patient has control of the pelvis, thorax, and scapula
- Clinician places the patient in the correct position and asks the patient to hold the contraction isometrically (statically)
- Basic movements can be broken into segments and isometric hold exercises performed in each segment to establish isometric control in different positions
- Initially the contraction is submaximal
- Resistance to holding the correct position is started close to the joint (proximal) and moved distally as the patient demonstrates isometric stabilization of the joint
- Clinician watches for correct force-couple activation
- Co-activation or co-contraction used to ensure arthrokinematic control of the joint—*resistance is given at the joint*
- Closed kinetic chain activities are used to assist joint stabilization (aids compression at the joint and stress distribution)
- Positions close to the close-packed position provide more stability
- Clinician must stop exercise if fatigue or compensatory postures are evident

Once the patient has gained control of the shoulder segments (e.g., the scapulothoracic and glenohumeral joints) through isolated contraction of muscles, ensuring proper muscle function and recruitment in isolation, true integrated stabilization training can be initiated. First, the clinician must ensure that the stabilizer muscles function statically. Part of this training will have been accomplished during training of the individual stabilizer muscles. This stage also involves maintaining a stable scapula, along with correct posture (i.e., stable pelvis, or core), while doing controlled movements of the arm below 30° abduction initially (above 30°, the scapula will rotate) and then progressing to full ROM. To reeducate the stabilization muscles statically, the clinician must be concerned

primarily with positioning the arm in different positions. The exercises must be performed isometrically in specific positions with control. The focus of muscle reeducation moves from proximal (i.e., ensuring a stable scapula proximally with correct posture) to distal (while allowing distal movement). Static force-couple action ensures that the muscles work in a coordinated fashion to produce a smooth, coordinated isometric hold both when the upper extremity is loaded (in close pack, or closed kinetic chain) and unloaded (in open pack, or open kinetic chain). Rhythmic stabilization and closed kinetic chain isometric scapular stabilization on a balance board or ball are examples of static stabilization exercises.

Step 5.2: Advanced Static Stabilization Exercises (Aim: Isometric Positioning for Activity-Specific Skills)

Teaching Advanced Static Stabilization Exercises

- Clinician places the patient in the desired position and asks the patient to hold the contraction isometrically (statically) (e.g., start position, follow-through position, mechanism of injury)
- Movements can be broken into segments and isometric hold exercises performed in each segment to establish isometric control in different positions
- Resistance to holding the correct position is given distally to gain static osteokinematic control while maintaining arthrokinematic control at the joint
- Clinician watches for correct force-couple activation
- Move from closed kinetic chain to open kinetic chain activities
- Stronger contractions used to stimulate isometric activation of whole kinetic chain
- Clinician must stop exercise if fatigue or compensatory postures are evident

In advanced static stabilization exercises, the patient works to stabilize the scapula statically in positions above 30°, most commonly in open kinetic chain.[85] The patient may be taken into the position of the mechanism of injury to do rhythmic stabilization exercises or taken into positions related to function, working from submaximal to maximal isometric effort to ensure control of different positions. The clinician can have the patient do isometric hold or eccentric break activities of the medial and lateral rotators in various positions of glenohumeral abduction, scaption, and forward flexion. Rhythmic stabilization with compression with the glenoid under the humeral head in the Hawkins position (see Figure 6-22), "throwing the arm," resisted isometric PNF D1 and D2 patterns, and rhythmic stabilization of the medial and lateral rotators in various postures from low risk to high risk should be attempted. To accomplish this, the patient's arm is taken into the desired position and the patient is asked to hold the position while the clinician applies perturbations to the arm and affected joint. For example, the clinician can place the patient's shoulder in the position close to the mechanism of injury and then ask the patient to statically stabilize the shoulder while doing rhythmic stabilizations. Wall falls, table falls, and floor falls from the knees are progressions, and balancing on different balance devices are closed kinetic chain examples of this.

Step 5.3: Dynamic Stabilization Exercises (Aim: Dynamic Form and Execution with Voluntary Control)

Re-educating the Muscle Stabilizers Dynamically

- Training correct (specific) movement patterns with voluntary concentric and eccentric control
- Need to ensure proximal stability with distal mobility involving the whole kinetic chain
- Want to establish voluntary control of functional movement patterns
- Clinician watches for correct force-couple activation
- Resistance movement is given distally to gain dynamic osteokinematic control while maintaining dynamic arthrokinematic control
- Clinician watches for correct force-couple activation
- Open kinetic chain activities
- Clinician must stop exercise if fatigue or compensatory postures are evident

---

Dynamic stabilization exercises involve movement of the joints of the shoulder girdle performed slowly and in control above 30° abduction. This involves controlled eccentric movement of the scapula while the arm moves. When the clinician teaches dynamic stabilization exercises, the focus is on correct movement patterns. The clinician must make sure that the patient has voluntary control and that agonist and antagonist activities are performed involving both concentric and eccentric exercises. Exercises such as bent-over rowing, "lawn mower" pulls using tubing, dumbbell or tubing punch outs, and lunges with dumbbell or tubing reaches are examples of open kinetic chain dynamic stabilization exercises (Figure 6-58).[87,153]

Step 5.4: Advanced Dynamic Stabilization (Aim: Dynamic Form and Execution of Activity-Specific Skills)

Advanced dynamic stabilization involves faster movements and the whole kinetic chain, including multidimensional activities. These exercises should stress functional diagonal patterns that the patient will use when he or she returns to previous activities. They may include exercises against gravity, exercises in water, the use of free weights or tubing, isokinetic exercises, PNF

Teaching Advanced Dynamic Stabilization Exercises

- Training control in activity-specific movement (diagonal) patterns
- Multidirectional stability activities
- Progressive eccentric exercises at functional speeds
- Need to ensure proximal stability with distal mobility involving the whole kinetic chain
- Clinician watches for correct force-couple activation
- Resistance movement is given distally to gain dynamic osteokinematic control while maintaining dynamic arthrokinematic control in diagonal patterns
- Clinician watches for correct force-couple activation
- Open kinetic chain activities
- Clinician must stop exercise if fatigue or compensatory postures are evident

---

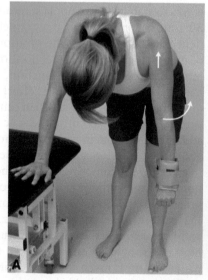 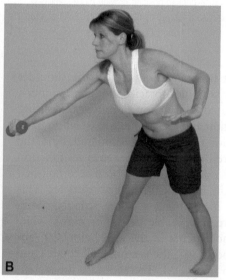

Figure 6-58 Examples of open kinetic chain dynamic stabilization exercises. **A,** Bent-over rowing. **B,** Lunges with dumbbell reaches.

patterns, and medicine ball and plyometric activities. Clock drills and reach-and-stretch (target) drills are examples of these exercises. Oblique or torsional movement, along with plyometrics and eccentric deceleration or braking, plays a major role.

The clinician should keep in mind the rules of specificity and the specific requirements of the patient in the rehabilitation program. Open-chain activity is a concentric movement against gravity with no fixation feedback. Injury to the shoulder from overuse is most likely to occur during open-chain activities and is often the result of loss of functional control of the scapula, the humerus, or both. Consequently, the clinician must make sure the patient has good scapular and humeral control before progressing to open kinetic chain exercises.[164] Open-chain activities include free weight exercises, which often are combined with proprioceptive activities (i.e., eyes open or closed, positioning or mirroring) to teach "free hand" feedback.

Step 5.5: Functional Stabilization (Aim: Functional Form and Skill Execution)

In the final stage of the stabilization program, the clinician teaches the patient functional stabilization, in which functional activities are broken down into their component parts so that the patient can develop particular motor skills that he or she will need in everyday life.[98,167,168] Patients are asked to perform specific, synchronized, multidirectional skilled pattern sequences (Figure 6-59). Eccentric patterns and power development are emphasized to develop the braking action and shock absorption of the muscles to protect the glenohumeral joint and the ability to control movement at functional speeds. All activities should involve most if not all of the whole kinetic chain.

Teaching Functional Stabilization

- Training synchronized skilled movement sequences and activity-specific skills
- Clinician must watch for *patient carriage* (e.g., weight shift, weight acceptance, movement symmetry, appropriate limb braking), *control* (e.g., smooth, automatic, and unrestricted execution and movement with proper form and skill), and *confidence*
- Clinician watches for correct force-couple activation
- Clinician must stop exercise if fatigue, apprehension, or compensatory postures occur
- Teach injury or reinjury prevention strategies

Open-chain activities using devices, such as the Body Blade® and Boing® activities, plyometrics, and the use of a medicine ball are helpful in later stages of rehabilitation to teach functional stabilization and control.

Plyometric programs for the upper limb (Figure 6-60) are designed to increase the excitability of the neurological receptors and improve the reaction of the neuromuscular system.[85,126] The patient must be taught to accept greater loads (the clinician must keep in mind that with plyometrics, the rate of stretch rather than the length of stretch

---

Criteria for Return to Activity[85,167,168]

- Little or no pain
- No or minimal apprehension
- Functional ROM with involvement of the whole kinetic chain
- Near-normal strength (80% to 90%)
- Normal movement patterns
- Normal functional ability
- Able to perform the skills the patient wants to resume
- Appropriate level of fitness
- Appropriate patient expectations

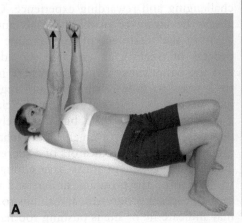

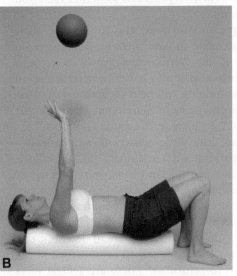

Figure 6-59 Multidirectional instability exercises. **A,** Punch out on roll. **B,** Ball toss on a roll.

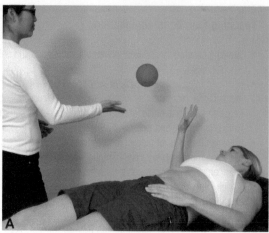 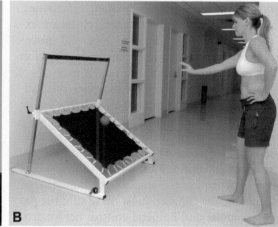

Figure 6-60 Plyometric exercises. **A,** Ball throw. **B,** Plyoback exercises using a weighted ball.

is important).[169,170] Activities using a 0.9- to 1.8-kg (2 to 4 lb) ball (e.g., medicine ball or Plyoball), a bounce-back device (Plyoback™) or partner, or tubing (progressing from slow to fast sets) can be effective.

Step 6.1: Fitness Aim: To Restore or Maintain Fitness throughout Program

While the patient's shoulder is being rehabilitated, the clinician must keep in mind that the patient at some point will be returning to activity. A program to maintain or restore cardiovascular fitness should be instituted and should be as specific as possible to the patient's occupation or activity. Little good is achieved if the shoulder is rehabilitated and the patient is cleared medically to participate in activities or return to work, if patients do not have the cardiovascular fitness or activity-specific fitness to compete or to do their job. This process is sometimes referred to as *work hardening.*

To keep the patients involved and to enhance their recovery, it is imperative to have them work to maintain their fitness level if they have been active or to work to improve their fitness level if they have not been active. In both cases, fitness training will help their recovery physiologically and psychologically. Activity may be as simple as asking them to "go for a walk around the block" for someone who has done little activity to someone doing a vigorous workout on a stationary bike or elliptical apparatus. This stage can, in reality, start presurgery or postsurgery using lower limb activities that will not stress the patient's shoulder. Most commonly, patients are started with activity at about 60% of their maximum heart rate working up over time to 75% to 85%, but this will depend on their level of fitness to begin with and the activity they want to return to. There are several ways patients' target heart rate can be calculated, but probably the easiest is (220−age)×percentage of maximum heart

rate. This will give a target heart rate for training. If the activity is going to take place in water (e.g., running in water), then the target heart rate should be 10 to 13 beats less than the target heart rate calculated above because of the increased stress placed on the heart due to water resistance.

Fitness training may be modified based on what the clinician is trying to accomplish and based on the activity the individual wants to return to. For example, initially the desire may simply be to establish a good aerobic base, which will enhance the patient's recovery from exercise. Depending on the activity the individual wants to return to, the clinician may initiate different exercise regimes which may tax the alactic anaerobic system (ATP-PC system), lactic anaerobic system (glycolysis), and/or the aerobic system, each of which have their own special characteristics.

SUMMARY

Rehabilitation of the unstable shoulder can be both a challenging and rewarding experience. Clinicians must always be aware of possible pitfalls and special concerns in the treatment of the unstable shoulder. The process of treating an unstable shoulder takes time, and the patient may require anywhere from 6 months to 2 years to fully rehabilitate and regain the preinjury or preoperative status. The clinician may devise a sterling treatment plan, but ultimately the patient's dedication to and involvement in the rehabilitation program are the main predicators of a successful outcome. Therefore the patient must have enough information to "buy into" the program, understand what to expect as the program progresses, and things to watch for that may indicate he or she is pushing too hard or not hard enough, as well as having realistic expectations as to the outcomes.

REFERENCES

1. Reid DC: *Sports injury: assessment and rehabilitation*, New York, 1992, Churchill Livingstone.
2. Burkhart S, Morgan CD, Kibler WB: The disabled throwing shoulder: spectrum of pathology. I. Pathoanatomy and low mechanics, *Arthroscopy* 19:209–420, 2003.
3. Burkhart S, Morgan CD, Kibler WB: The disabled throwing shoulder: spectrum of pathology. II. Evaluation and treatment of SLAP lesions in throwers, *Arthroscopy* 19:531–539, 2003.
4. Burkhart S, Morgan CD, Kibler WB: The disabled throwing shoulder: spectrum of pathology. III. The SICK scapula: scapular dyskinesis, the kinetic chain and rehabilitation, *Arthroscopy* 19:641–661, 2003.
5. Cleeman E, Flatow EL: Classification and diagnosis of impingement and rotator cuff lesions in athletes, *Sports Med Arthrosc Rev* 8:141–157, 2000.
6. Reid DC: The shoulder girdle: its structure and function as a unit in abduction, *J Chart Soc Physiother* 55:5–59, 1969.
7. Neer CS: Impingement lesions, *Clin Orthop Relat Res* 173:70–77, 1983.
8. Burkhead W, Rockwood C: Treatment of instability of the shoulder with an exercise program, *J Bone Joint Surg Am* 70:890–896, 1992.
9. Tehvanzadeh J, Ken R, Amster J: Magnetic resonance imaging of tendon and ligament abnormalities. Part I. Spine and upper extremities, *Skeletal Radiol* 21(15):1992.
10. Kunkel SS, Hawkins RJ: Open repair of the rotator cuff. In Andrews JR, Wilk KE, editors: *The athlete's shoulder*, New York, 1994, Churchill Livingstone.
11. Jobe F, Kvitne R: Shoulder pain in the overhead athlete: the relationship of anterior instability and rotator cuff impingement, *Orthop Rev* 18:963–975, 1989.
12. Wickiewicz TL, Pagnani MJ, Kennedy K: Rehabilitation of the unstable shoulder, *Sports Med Arthrosc Rev* 1:227–235, 1993.
13. Warner JJ: The gross anatomy of the joint surfaces, ligaments, labrum and capsule. In Matsen FA, Fu FH, Hawkins RJ, editors: *The shoulder: a balance of mobility and stability*, Rosemont, IL, 1993, American Academy of Orthopedic Surgeons.
14. Mallon W, Brown H, Vogler J, et al: Radiographic and geometric anatomy of the scapula, *Clin Orthop Relat Res* 277:142–154, 1992.
15. Lo IKY, Parten PM, Burkhart SS: The inverted pear glenoid: an indicator of significant glenoid bone loss, *Arthroscopy* 20(2):169–174, 2004.
16. Bowen MK, Warren RF: Ligamentous control of shoulder stability based on selective cutting and static translation experiments, *Clin Sports Med* 10:757–782, 1991.
17. Howell SM, Galinat BJ: The glenoid-labrum socket: a constrained articular surface, *Clin Orthop Relat Res* 243:122–125, 1983.
18. Browne A, Hoffmeyer P, An K, et al: The influence of atmospheric pressure on shoulder stability, *Orthop Trans* 14:259–263, 1990.
19. Lew WD, Lewis JL, Craig EV: Stabilization by capsule, ligaments and labrum: stability at the extremes of motion. In Matsen FA, Fu FH, Hawkins RJ, editors: *The shoulder: a balance of mobility and stability*, Rosemont, 1993, American Academy of Orthopedic Surgeons.
20. Travlos J, Goldberg I, Boome RS: Brachial plexus lesions associated with dislocated shoulders, *J Bone Joint Surg Br* 72:68–71, 1990.
21. Matsen FA, Chebli C, Lippitt S: Principles for the evaluation and management of shoulder instability, *J Bone Joint Surg Am* 88:648–659, 2006.
22. Simonet WT, Colfield RH: *Prognosis in anterior shoulder dislocation*, Maui, March 20-25, 1993, Paper presented at the Joint Meeting of the American Orthopaedic Society for Sports Medicine and the Japanese Orthopaedic Society for Sports Medicine.
23. Rowe CR: Recurrent transient anterior subluxation of the shoulder: the "dead arm" syndrome, *Clin Orthop Relat Res* 223:11–19, 1987.
24. Zarins B, McMahon MS, Rowe CR: Diagnosis and treatment of traumatic anterior instability of the shoulder, *Clin Orthop Relat Res* 291:75–84, 1993.
25. Silliman JF, Hawkins RJ: Current concepts and recent advances in the athlete's shoulder, *Clin Sports Med* 10:693–705, 1991.
26. Pollock RG, Bigliani LU: Glenohumeral instability: evaluation and treatment, *J Am Acad Orthop Surg* 1:24–32, 1993.
27. Williams MM, Snyder SJ, Buford D: The Buford complex—the "cord-like" middle glenohumeral ligament and absent anteroposterior labrum complex: a normal anatomic capsulolabral variant, *Arthroscopy* 10(3):241–247, 1994.
28. Shortt CP, Morrison WB, Shah SH, et al: Association of glenoid morphology and anterosuperior labral variation, *J Comput Assist Tomogr* 33(4):584–586, 2009.
29. Burkhart SS, De Beer JF: Traumatic glenohumeral bone defects and their relationship to failure of arthroscopic Bankart repairs: significance of the inverted-pear glenoid and the humeral engaging Hill-Sachs lesion, *Arthroscopy* 16(7):677–694, 2000.
30. Speer KP, Garrett WE: Muscular control of motion and stability about the pectoral girdle. In Matsen FA, Fu FH, Hawkins RJ, editors: *The shoulder: a balance of mobility and stability*, Rosemont, 1993, American Academy of Orthopedic Surgeons.
31. Rodowsky MW, Harner CD, Fu FH: FH: The role of the long head of the biceps muscle and superior glenoid labrum in anterior stability of the shoulder, *Am J Sports Med* 22:121–130, 1994.
32. Matsen FA, Harryman DT, Sidles JA: Mechanics of glenohumeral instability, *Clin Sports Med* 10:783–788, 1991.
33. Habermeyer P, Schmuller U, Wiedemann E: The intra-articular pressure of the shoulder: an experimental study on the role of the glenoid labrum in stabilizing the joint, *Arthroscopy* 8:166–172, 1992.
34. Henry JH, Genung JA: Natural history of glenohumeral dislocation revisited, *Am J Sports Med* 10:135–141, 1982.
35. Bradley JP, Tibone JE: Electromyographic analysis of muscle action about the shoulder, *Clin Sports Med* 10:789–805, 1991.
36. Rowe CR, Patel D, Southmayd WW: The Bankart procedure: a long term end result study, *J Bone Joint Surg Am* 60:1–16, 1978.
37. Akeson WH, Amiel D, Abel MF, et al: Effects of immobilization on joints, *Clin Orthop Relat Res* 219:28–37, 1987.
38. Reid DC: Focusing the diagnosis of shoulder pain: pearl of practice, *Phys Sports Med* 22(6):28–45, 1994.
39. Neer CS: Anterior acromioplasty for chronic impingement syndrome in the shoulder: a preliminary report, *J Bone Joint Surg Am* 54:41–50, 1972.
40. McFarland EG, Maffulli N, Del Buono A, et al: Impingement is not impingement: the case for calling it "rotator cuff disease," *Muscles Ligaments Tendons J* 3(3):196–200, 2013.
41. Solem-Bertoft E, Thuomas KA, Westerberg CE: The influence of scapular retraction and protraction on the width of the subacromial space: an MRI study, *Clin Orthop Relat Res* 296:99–103, 1993.
42. Reid DC: A practical approach to the painful shoulder, *Can J Contin Med Educ* 3(6):29–31, 1991.
43. Clarkson HM, Gilewich GB: *Musculoskeletal assessment: joint range of motion and manual muscle strength*, Baltimore, 1989, Williams & Wilkins.
44. Hislop HJ, Montgomery J: *Daniel's and Worthingham's muscle testing: technique of manual examination*, Philadelphia, 1995, WB Saunders.
45. Kendall HO, Kendall FP, Boynton DA: *Posture and pain*, Huntington, 1970, Robert E Krieger.
46. Parni RM, Voight M: The role of the scapula, *J Orthop Sports Phys Ther* 18:386–391, 1993.
47. Kibler WB: Management of the scapula in glenohumeral instability, *Tech Shoulder Elbow Surg* 4:89–98, 2003.
48. Kibler WB, McMullen JB: *Accelerated postoperative shoulder rehabilitation. Orthopedic knowledge update: shoulder and elbow*, Rosemont, 2002, American Academy of Orthopedic Surgeons.
49. Manska RC, Rieman MP, Stovak ML: Nonoperative and operative management of snapping scapula, *Am J Sports Med* 32:1554–1565, 2004.
50. Bullock MP, Foster NE, Wright CC: Shoulder impingement: the effect of sitting posture on shoulder pain and range of motion, *Man Ther* 10:28–37, 2005.
51. Magee DJ: *Orthopedic physical assessment*, ed 6, Philadelphia, 2014, WB Saunders.
52. Pink MM, Jobe FW: Biomechanics of swimming. In Zachazewski JE, Magee DJ, Quillen WS, editors: *Athletic injuries and rehabilitation*, Philadelphia, 1996, WB Saunders.
53. Hegedus EJ: Which physical examinationtests provide clinicians with the most value when examining the shoulder? Update of a systematic review with meta-analysis of individual tests, *Br J Sports Med* 46:964–978, 2012.
54. Boileau P, Zumstein M, Balg F, et al: The unstable painful shoulder (UPS) as a cause of pain from unrecognized anteroinferior instability in the young athlete, *J Shoulder Elbow Surg* 20:98–106, 2011.
55. Ren H, Bicknell RT: From the unstable painful shoulder to multidirectional instability in the young athlete, *Clin Sports Med* 32:815–823, 2013.
56. Poppen N, Walker P: Normal and abnormal motion of the shoulder, *J Bone Joint Surg Am* 58:195–201, 1976.
57. Ciullo JV: Swimmer's shoulder, *Clin Sports Med* 5:115–137, 1986.
58. Okoro T, Reddy VRM, Pimpelnarkar A: Coracoid impingement syndrome—a literature review, *Curr Rev Musculoskelet Med* 2:51–55, 2009.
59. Freehill MQ: Coracoid impingement: diagnosis and treatment, *J Am Acad Orthop Surg* 19:161–167, 2011.
60. Brown GA, Tan JL, Kirkley A: The lax shoulder in females, *Orthop Rehabil Res* 372:110–122, 2000.
61. McClusky CM: Classification and diagnosis of glenohumeral instability in athletes, *Sports Med Arthosc Rev* 8:158–169, 2000.
62. Jobe FW, Kritue RS, Giangarra CE: Shoulder pain in the overhead or throwing athlete: the relationship of anterior instability and rotator cuff impingement, *Orthop Rev* 18:963–975, 1989.
63. Rockwood CA: Subluxation and dislocations about the shoulder. In Rockwood CA, Green DP, editors: *Fractures in adults*, ed 2, Baltimore, 1984, Lippincott.
64. Jobe CM: Superior glenoid impingement, *Orthop Clin North Am* 28:137–143, 1997.
65. Ketola S, Lehtinen J, Arnala I, et al: Does athroscopic acromioplasty provide any additional value in the treatment of shoulder impingement syndrome? *J Bone Joint Surg Br* 91:1326–1334, 2009.
66. Ketola S, Lehtinen J, Rousi T, et al: No evidence of long-term benefits of arthroscopic acromioplasty in the treatment of shoulder impingement syndrome, *Bone Joint Res* 2:132–139, 2013.
67. Holmgren T, Hallgren HB, Oberg B, et al: Effect of a specific exercise strategy on the need for surgeryin patients with subacromial impingement syndrome: a randomized controlled study, *BMJ* 344,2012, e787.

68. Eid AS, Dwyer AJ, Chambler AF: Mid-term results of athroscopic subacromial decompression in patients with or without partial thickness rotator cuff tears, *Int J Shoulder Surg* 6(3):86–88, 2012.

69. Ketola S, Lehtinen J, Nissinen M, et al: Arthroscopic decompression with acromioplasty and structured exercise was no more effective and was more expensive than exercise alone, *J Bone Joint Surg Am* 92:1999, 2010.

70. Haahr JP, Ostergaard S, Dalsgaard J, et al: Exercises versus arthroscopic decompression in patients with subacromial impingement—a randomized control study, *Ann Rheum Dis* 64:760–764, 2005.

71. Singh HP, Mehta SS, Pandey R: A preoperative scoring system to select patients for arthroscopic subacromial decompression, *J Shoulder Elbow Surg* 23:1251–1256, 2014.

72. Freehill MQ: Coracoid impingement: diagnosis and treatment, *J Am Acad Orthop Surg* 19(4):191–197, 2011.

73. Apiegl UJ, Warth RJ, Millett PJ: Symptomatic internal impingement of the shoulder in overhead athletes, *Sports Med Arthrosc* 22(2):120–129, 2014.

74. Riebel GD, McCabe JB: Anterior shoulder dislocation: a review of reduction techniques, *Am J Emerg Med* 9:180–188, 1991.

75. Flatlow EL, Miller SR, Neer CS: Chronic anterior dislocation of the shoulder, *J Shoulder Elbow Surg* 2:210, 1993.

76. Soslowsky L, Flatlow E, Bigliani L, et al: Articular geometry of the glenohumeral joint, *Clin Orthop Relat Res* 285:181–190, 1992.

77. Pagnani MJ, Warren RF: The pathophysiology of anterior shoulder instability, *Sports Med Arthrosc Rev* 1:177189, 1993.

78. Neer CS, Forster CR: Inferior capsular shifts for involuntary inferior and multi-directional instability of the shoulder, *J Bone Joint Surg Am* 62:897–908, 1980.

79. Harryman D, Sidles J, Clark J, et al: Translation of the humeral head on the glenoid with passive glenohumeral motion, *J Bone Joint Surg Am* 72:1334–1343, 1990.

80. Hawkins RJ, Mohtadi NG: Clinical evaluation of shoulder instability, *Clin J Sports Med* 1:59–64, 1991.

81. Kibler WB: Evaluation of sports demands as a diagnostic tool in shoulder disorders. In Matsen FA, Fu FH, Hawkins RJ, editors: *The shoulder: a balance of mobility and stability*, Rosemont, 1993, American Academy of Orthopedic Surgeons.

82. Symeonides PP: The significance of the subscapularis muscle in the pathogenesis of recurrent dislocation of the shoulder, *J Bone Joint Surg Br* 54:476–483, 1972.

83. Howell S, Galinat B, Renzi A, et al: Normal and abnormal mechanism of the glenohumeral joint in the horizontal plane, *J Bone Joint Surg Am* 70:227–232, 1988.

84. O'Driscoll SW: Atraumatic instability: pathology and pathogenesis. In Matsen FA, Fu FH, Hawkins RJ, editors: *The shoulder: a balance of mobility and stability*, Rosemont, 1993, American Academy of Orthopedic Surgeons.

85. Kibler WB, McMullen J, Uhl T: Shoulder rehabilitation strategies, guidelines and practice, *Oper Tech Sports Med* 8:258–267, 2000.

86. Kibler WB, McMullen J: Scapular dyskinesis and its relation to shoulder pain, *J Am Acad Orthop Surg* 11:143–151, 2003.

87. Kibler WB, McMullen J, Uhl T: Shoulder rehabilitation strategies, guidelines and practice, *Orthop Clin North Am* 32:527–538, 2001.

88. Gibson K, Growse A, Korda L, et al: The effectiveness of rehabilitation for non-operative management of shoulder instability—a systematic review, *J Hand Surg* 17:229–242, 2004.

89. Desmenles F, Cote CH, Fremont P: Therapeutic exercise of orthopedic manual therapy for impingement syndrome: a systematic review, *Am J Sports Med* 13:176–182, 2003.

90. Green S, Buchbinder R, Hetrick S: Physiotherapy interventions for shoulder pain, *Cochrane Library* 2:1–82, 2004.

91. Rowe CR, Pierce DS, Clark JG: Voluntary dislocation of the shoulder: a preliminary report on a clinical, electromyographic, and psychiatric study of twenty-six patients, *J Bone Joint Surg* 55:445–460, 1973.

92. Cooper RA, Brems JJ: The inferior capsular shift procedure for multidirectional instability of the shoulder, *J Bone Joint Surg Am* 74:1516–1521, 1992.

93. Loeb PE, Andrews JR, Wilk KE: Arthroscopic debridement of rotator cuff injuries. In Andrews JR, Wilk KE, editors: *The athlete's shoulder*, New York, 1994, Churchill Livingstone.

94. Neviaser R, Neviaser T, Neviaser J: Concurrent rupture of the rotator cuff and anterior dislocation in the older patient, *J Bone Joint Surg Am* 70:1308–1311, 1988.

95. Mohtadi NG: Advances in the understanding of anterior instability of the shoulder, *Clin Sports Med* 10:863–870, 1991.

96. Wolf EM, Cheng JC, Dickson K: Humeral avulsion of the glenohumeral ligaments as a cause of anterior shoulder instability, *Arthroscopy* 11(5):600–607, 1995.

97. Cain P, Mutschler T, Fu F: Anterior stability of the glenohumeral joint: a dynamic model, *Am J Sports Med* 15:144–148, 1987.

98. Hayes K, Callanan M, Walton J, et al: Shoulder instability: management and rehabilitation, *J Orthop Sports Phys Ther* 32:497509, 2002.

99. Rowe CR: Prognosis in dislocations of the shoulder, *J Bone Joint Surg Am* 38:957–977, 1956.

100. Bowen MK, Warren RF: Surgical approaches to posterior instability of the shoulder, *Oper Tech Sports Med* 1:301–310, 1993.

101. van Kampen DA, van den Berg T, van der Woude HJ, et al: Diagnostic value of patient characteristics, history and six clinical tests for traumatic anterior shoulder instability, *J Shoulder Elbow Surg* 22(10):131–139, 2013.

102. Ropars M, Fournier A, Campillo B, et al: Clinical assessment of external rotation for the diagnosis of anterior shoulder hyperlaxity, *Orthop Traumatol Surg Res* 96(suppl 8):S84–S87, 2010.

103. Fuchs B, Jost B, Gerber C: Posterior-inferior capsular shift for the treatment of recurrent voluntary posterior subluxation of the shoulder, *J Bone Joint Surg Am* 82:16–25, 2000.

104. Hawkins RH: Glenoid osteotomy for recurrent posterior subluxation of the shoulder: assessment by computed axial tomography, *J Shoulder Elbow Surg* 5:393–400, 1996.

105. Provencher MT, Bell SJ, Menzel KA, et al: Arthroscopic treatment of posterior shoulder instability. Results of 33 cases, *Am J Sports Med* 33:1463–1471, 2005.

106. Higgs GB, Weinstein D, Flatlow EL: Evaluation and treatment of acute anterior glenohumeral dislocations, *Sports Med Arthrosc Rev* 1:190–201, 1993.

107. Videman T: Connective tissue and immobilization: key factors in musculoskeletal degeneration? *Clin Orthop Relat Res* 221:26–32, 1987.

108. Donatelli R, Owens-Burkhart H: Effects of immobilization on the extensibility of periarticular connective tissue, *J Orthop Sports Phys Ther* 3:67–72, 1981.

109. Mascarenhas R, Rusen J, Saltzman BM, et al: Management of humeral and glenoid bone loss in recurrent glenohumeral instability, *Adv Orthop* 640952,2014.

110. Wolf E, Pollack M, Smalley C: Hill-Sachs "Remplissage": an arthroscopic solution for the engaging Hill-Sachs lesion, *Arthroscopy* 23(6):e1–e2, 2007.

111. Purchase RJ, Wolf EM, Hobgood ER, et al: Hill-Sach "Remplissage": an arthroscopic solution for the engaging Hill-Sach lesion, *Arthroscopy* 24(6):723–726, 2008.

112. van der Zwaag HM, Brand R, Obermann WR, et al: Glenohumeral osteoarthrosis after Putti-Platt repair, *J Shoulder Elbow Surg* 8(3):252–258, 1999.

113. Reid DC, Saboe L, Burnham R: Current research of selected shoulder problems. In Donatelli R, editor: *Physical therapy of the shoulder*, New York, 1987, Churchill Livingstone.

114. Hovelius L, Akermark C, Albrektsson B, et al: Bristow-Latarjet procedure for recurrent anterior dislocation of the shoulder, *Acta Orthop Scand* 54:284–290, 1983.

115. Hehne HJ, Hubner H: Die Behandlung des Rezidivieremden Schulter Luxation nach Putti-Platt-Bankart and Eden-Hybinette-Lange, *Orthop Prax* 16:331–335, 1980.

116. Torg JS, Balduini FC, Bonci C, et al: A modified Bristow-Helfet-May procedure for recurrent dislocation and subluxation of the shoulder: report of 212 cases, *J Bone Joint Surg Am* 69:904–913, 1987.

117. Du Toit GT, Roux D: Recurrent dislocation of the shoulder: a 24 year study of the Johannesburg stapling operation, *J Bone Joint Surg Am* 38:1–12, 1956.

118. Sisk TD, Boyd HB: Management of recurrent anterior dislocation of the shoulder: Du Toit type or staple capsulorrhaphy, *Clin Orthop Relat Res* 103:150–154, 1974.

119. Bankart ASB: Recurrent or habitual dislocation of the shoulder, *Br Med J* 2:1132–1133, 1923.

120. Hovelius L, Thorling J, Fredin H: Recurrent anterior dislocations of the shoulder: results after the Bankart and Putti-Platt operations, *J Bone Joint Surg Am* 61:566–569, 1979.

121. Osmond-Clarke H: Habitual dislocation of the shoulder: the Putti-Platt operation, *J Bone Joint Surg Br* 30:19–25, 1948.

122. Collins KA, Capito C, Cross M: The use of Putti-Platt procedure in the treatment of recurrent anterior dislocation with reference to the young athlete, *Am J Sports Med* 14(5):380–382, 1986.

123. Magnuson PB, Stack K: Recurrent dislocation of the shoulder, *JAMA* 123:889–892, 1943.

124. Karadimas J, Rentis G, Varouchas G: Repair of recurrent anterior dislocation of the shoulder using transfer of the subscapularis tendon, *J Bone Joint Surg Am* 62:1147–1149, 1980.

125. Rockwood CA: Subluxations and dislocations about the shoulder. In Rockwood C.A., Green D.P., editors: Fractures, vol 1, Philadelphia, 1975, JB Lippincott.

126. Matsen FA, Tomas SC, Rockwood CA: Anterior glenohumeral instability. In Rockwood C.A., Matsen F.A., editors: *The shoulder*, vol 1, Philadelphia, 1990, WB Saunders.

127. Banas MP, Dalldorf PG, DeHaven KE: The Allman modification of the Bristow procedure for recurrent anterior glenohumeral instability, *Sports Med Arthrosc Rev* 1:242–249, 1993.

128. Liu SH, Henry MH: Anterior shoulder instability, *Clin Orthop Relat Res* 323:327–337, 1996.

129. Balg F, Boileau P: The instability severity index score. A simple preoperative score to select patients for arthroscopic or open shoulder stabilization, *J Bone Joint Surg Br* 89:1470–1477, 2007.

130. Caspair RB, Beach WR: Arthroscopic anterior shoulder capsulorrhaphy, *Sports Med Arthrosc Rev* 1:237–242, 1993.

131. Ryu RK: Open versus arthroscopic stabilization for traumatic anterior shoulder instability, *Sports Med Arthrosc Rev* 12:90–98, 2004.

132. Griesser MJ, Harris JD, McCoy B, et al: Complications and re-operations after Bristow-Latarjet shoulder stabilization: a systematic review, *J Shoulder Elbow Surg* 22(2):286–292, 2013.

133. Warner JJP, Marks PH: Management of complications of surgery for anterior shoulder instability, *Sports Med Arthrosc Rev* 1:272–292, 1993.

134. Wilk KE: Current concepts in the rehabilitation of athletic shoulder injuries. In Andrews JR, Wilk KE, editors: *The athlete's shoulder*, New York, 1994, Churchill Livingstone.

135. Kelly BT, Kadrmas WR, Speer KP: The manual muscle examination for rotator cuff strength, *Am J Sports Med* 24:581–588, 1996.

136. Thigpen CA, Padum DA, Morgan N, et al: Scapular kinematics during supraspeculative rehabilitation exercises: a comparison of full-can versus empty-can techniques, *Am J Sports Med* 34:644–652, 2006.

137. Lephart SM, Kocker MS: The role of exercise in the prevention of shoulder disorders. In Matsen FA, Fu FH, Hawkins RJ, editors: *The shoulder: a balance of mobility and stability*, Rosemont, 1993, American Academy of Orthopedic Surgeons.

138. Dickoff-Hoffman SA: Neuromuscular control exercises for shoulder instability. In Andrews JR, Wilk KE, editors: *The athlete's shoulder*, New York, 1994, Churchill Livingstone.

139. Quillen WS, Halle JS, Rouillier LH: Manual therapy: mobilization of the motion-restricted shoulder, *J Sports Rehab* 1:237–248, 1992.

140. Maitland GD: *Peripheral manipulation*, ed 3, London, 1991, Butterworth.

141. Kaltenborn FM: *Mobilization of the extremity joints: examination and basic treatment techniques*, Oslo, 1980, Olaf Norles Bokhandel.

142. Lee D: *A workbook of manual therapy techniques for the upper extremity*, Delta, 1989, DOPC.

143. Flatow EL, Soslowsky LJ, Ticker JB, et al: Excursion of the rotator cuff under the acromion: patterns of subacromial content, *Am J Sports Med* 22:779–788, 1994.

144. Janda V: Muscles and motor control in cervicogenic disorders: assessment and management. In Grant R, editor: *Physical therapy of the cervical and thoracic spine*, New York, 1994, Churchill-Livingstone.

145. Lazarus MD: *Acute and chronic dislocations of the shoulder. Orthopedic knowledge update: shoulder and elbow*, Rosemont, 2002, American Academy of Orthopedic Surgeons.

146. Ellsworth AA, Mullaney M, Tyler TF, et al: Electromyography of selected shoulder musculature during unweighted and weighted pendulum exercises, *J Sports Phys Ther* 1:73–79, 2006.

147. Myers JB, Ju YY, Hwang JH, et al: Reflexive muscle activation alternations in a shoulder with anterior glenohumeral instability, *Am J Sports Med* 32:1013–1021, 2004.

148. Babyar SR: Excessive scapular motion in individuals recovering from painful shoulders: causes and treatment strategies, *Phys Ther* 76(3):226–238, 1996.

149. Wilk KE, Macrina LC, Reinhold MM: Non-operative rehabilitation for traumatic and non-traumatic glenohumeral instability, *North Am J Sports Phys Ther* 1:16–31, 2006.

150. Sutter JS: Conservative treatment of shoulder instability. In Andrews JR, Wilk KE, editors: *The athlete's shoulder*, New York, 1994, Churchill Livingstone.

151. Wilk KE, Arrigo C: Current concepts in the rehabilitation of the athletic shoulder, *J Orthop Sports Phys Ther* 18:365–378, 1993.

152. Ludewig PM, Hoff MS, Osowski EO, et al: Relative balance of serratus anterior and upper trapezius muscle activity during push-up exercises, *Am J Sports Med* 32:484–493, 2004.

153. Warner JJ, Micheli LJ, Arslaman LE, et al: Patterns of flexibility, laxity and strength in normal shoulder and shoulder with instability and impingement, *Am J Sports Med* 18:366–375, 1990.

154. Glousman R, Jobe FW, Tibone JE, et al: Dynamic electromyographic analysis of the throwing shoulder with glenohumeral instability, *J Bone Joint Surg Am* 70:220–226, 1988.

155. Blackburn TA: Throwing injuries to the shoulder. In Donatelli R, editor: *Physical therapy to the shoulder*, New York, 1987, Churchill Livingstone.

156. Middleton K: Rehabilitation following shoulder arthroscopy, *Sports Med Update* 4:10–13, 1989.

157. Pappas AM, Zawacki RM, McCarthy CF: Rehabilitation of the pitching shoulder, *Am J Sports Med* 13:223–235, 1985.

158. Taylor NF, Dodd KJ, Damiano DL: Progressive resistance exercises in physical therapy: a summary of systematic reviews, *Phys Ther* 85:1208–1223, 2005.

159. Horrigan JM, Shellock FG, Mink JH, et al: Magnetic resonance imaging evaluation of muscle usage associated with 3 exercises for rotator cuff rehabilitation, *Med Sci Sports Exerc* 31:1361–1366, 1999.

160. Reinold MM, Wilk KE, Fleisig GS, et al: Electromyographic analysis of the rotator cuff and deltoid musculature during common shoulder external rotation exercises, *J Orthop Sports Phys Ther* 34:385–394, 2004.

161. Bennett JG, Marous NA: The decelerator mechanism: eccentric muscular contraction applications at the shoulder. In Andrews JR, Wilk KE, editors: *The athlete's shoulder*, New York, 1994, Churchill Livingstone.

162. Keirns MA: Conservative management of shoulder impingement. In Andrews JR, Wilk KE, editors: *The athlete's shoulder*, New York, 1994, Churchill Livingstone.

163. Potzl W, Thorwesten L, Gotze C, et al: Proprioception of the shoulder joint after surgical repair for instability: a long term follow-up study, *Am J Sports Med* 32:425–430, 2004.

164. Cipriani D: Open and closed chain rehabilitation for the shoulder complex. In Andrews JR, Wilk KE, editors: *The athlete's shoulder*, New York, 1994, Churchill Livingstone.

165. Davies GJ, Dickoff-Hoffman S: Neuromuscular testing and rehabilitation of the shoulder complex, *J Orthop Sports Phys Ther* 18:449–458, 1993.

166. Borsa PA, Lephart SM, Kocher MS, et al: Functional assessment and rehabilitation of shoulder proprioception for glenohumeral instability, *J Sports Rehab* 3:84–104, 1994.

167. McCarty EC, Ritchie P, Gill HS, et al: Shoulder instability: return to play, *Sports Med* 23:335–351, 2004.

168. Park HB, Lin SK, Yokota A, et al: Return to play for rotator cuff injuries and superior labrum anterior posterior (SLAP) lesions, *Sports Med* 23:321–334, 2004.

169. Wilk KE, Voight ML: Plyometrics for the shoulder complex. In Andrews JR, Wilk KE, editors: *The athlete's shoulder*, New York, 1994, Churchill Livingstone.

170. Gambetta V: Conditioning of the shoulder complex. In Andrews JR, Wilk KE, editors: *The athlete's shoulder*, New York, 1994, Churchill Livingstone.

CHAPTER 7

Rotator Cuff Pathology

JUDY C. CHEPEHA, MARTIN J. BOULIANE, DAVID M. SHEPS

INTRODUCTION

Shoulder pain is well established as one of the most common musculoskeletal complaints managed by physicians and physical therapists.[1-3] Up to half the population experiences at least one episode of shoulder pain per year,[3] and nearly 50% of patients have some type of rotator cuff disease.[1] Conditions affecting the rotator cuff include tendinopathy of one or more of the muscles of the rotator cuff, partial-thickness tears, and full-thickness tears.[4] Rotator cuff injuries affect individuals across the life span—they are common in young, overhead athletes, as well as in individuals 65 years and older.[5-7] The prevalence of rotator cuff tendinopathy is reported at approximately 30% of all shoulder-related disorders.[8] Studies specific to rotator cuff tears have reported incidence rates between 13% and 32%, with a significant increase in occurrence as an individual ages.[9,10] Kibler et al.[11] suggested that more than 50% of individuals older than 60 years of age have at least a partial-thickness tear of their rotator cuff and that this estimate may be low because a large number of individuals are asymptomatic.[12,13] Rotator cuff disease tends to progress over time, becoming more painful and/or involving more muscles.[14] Because of the current aging population, and that many older individuals are maintaining an active lifestyle, the incidence of symptomatic rotator cuff pathology is expected to grow.

Rotator cuff disease manifests itself clinically in a variety of ways; however, most patients complain of pain worsened with overhead activities, and exhibit strength deficits and functional impairment(s).[9,15,16] These symptoms can cause significant disruption of an individual's physical functioning within activities of daily life (ADL), work, and recreational activities, as well as negatively affect the individual's mental health and social participation.[17] The effect that rotator cuff pathology has on a patient's quality of life and resulting impairment has been compared with that of congestive heart failure, diabetes, myocardial infarction, and depression.[18]

Physical therapy, consisting of cryotherapy, therapeutic exercise, manual therapy, and electrical modalities, is the usual first course of treatment for rotator cuff-related pathology. Surgical intervention is generally considered only after a failed course of appropriate, conservative treatment lasting at least 3 months.

Clinical Note

Rotator cuff surgery should only be considered after at least 3 months of appropriate conservative treatment.

ROTATOR CUFF ANATOMY

Successful treatment of the patient with rotator cuff disease begins with a thorough understanding of the anatomy of the rotator cuff and its adjacent structures. Advances in basic science and surgical technology over the past decade have improved knowledge regarding the osseous and soft-tissue structures of the shoulder and have led to a better understanding of the role these tissues play in normal and abnormal shoulder function.

Rotator Cuff Muscles

- Supraspinatus
- Infraspinatus
- Subscapularis
- Teres minor

The four muscles that constitute the rotator cuff (supraspinatus, infraspinatus, teres minor, and subscapular muscles) arise from the scapula, a bone stabilized by different muscles, and converge with the articular capsule, coracohumeral ligament, and glenohumeral ligaments, to attach on the tuberosities of the humerus (Figure 7-1).[19-21] The supraspinatus muscle arises from the supraspinatus fossa on the upper one third of the posterior scapula. It passes beneath the acromion and the acromioclavicular joint and attaches to the superior aspect of the greater tuberosity. It is innervated by the suprascapular nerve after

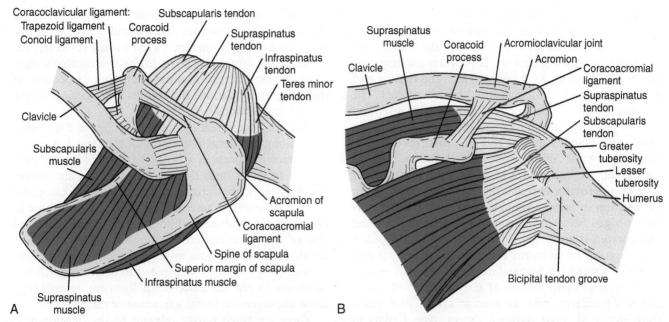

Figure 7-1 A, Superior view of the rotator cuff musculature as it courses anteriorly underneath the coracoacromial arch to insert on the greater tuberosity. **B,** Anterior view of the shoulder reveals the subscapularis, which is the only anterior rotator cuff muscle inserting on the lesser tuberosity. It rotates the humerus medially (internally) and provides dynamic anterior stability to the shoulder. (From Firestein GS, Budd RC, Harris ED et al: *Kelley's textbook of rheumatology,* ed 8, Philadelphia, 2008, Saunders/Elsevier.)

it passes through the suprascapular notch. The infraspinatus muscle arises from the infraspinatus fossa on the lower two thirds of the posterior scapula and attaches to the posterolateral aspect of the greater tuberosity. It is innervated by the suprascapular nerve after it passes through the spinoglenoid notch. Despite their distinct attachment sites, the tendons of supraspinatus and infraspinatus join together to form a single tendon, approximately 15 mm proximal to the insertion points on the greater tuberosity.[22] The teres minor muscle, innervated by a branch of the axillary nerve, arises from the lower lateral aspect of the scapula and attaches to the lower aspect of the greater tuberosity. The subscapularis muscle arises from the anterior aspect of the scapula and attaches over much of the lesser tuberosity. It is innervated by the upper and lower subscapular nerves. The tendons of supraspinatus and subscapularis, along with the superior glenohumeral and coracohumeral ligaments, form a sheath that encapsulates and stabilizes the biceps tendon as it enters the bicipital groove. Part of the supraspinatus tendon forms the roof, whereas the subscapularis tendon forms the sheath floor. Tearing or rupture of the anterior supraspinatus or superior subscapularis muscle can cause injury to the biceps "sling" and lead to instability of the long head of biceps.[23–25] The rotator cuff insertions form a horseshoe pattern that tapers away from the anatomic neck inferiorly. The superior insertion is tendinous, becoming more muscular inferiorly.[26] This continuous cuff around the humeral head allows the muscles to provide an infinite variety of moments to rotate the humerus and to oppose unwanted components of the deltoid and pectoralis muscle forces. Research related to the insertional anatomy

of the rotator cuff tendons, known as the **rotator cuff footprint**, has helped to improve diagnosis of rotator cuff tears and assist surgeons in surgical repair.[26,27]

The long head of the biceps tendon is an important part of the rotator cuff complex; so much so, it is sometimes referred to as the fifth rotator cuff tendon (Figure 7-2).[28] It attaches to the supraglenoid tubercle of the scapula and travels between the subscapularis and supraspinatus muscles, exiting the shoulder through the bicipital groove under the transverse humeral ligament, finally attaching to its muscle in the proximal arm. Tension in the long head of the biceps tendon assists the rotator cuff in compression of the humeral head into the glenoid and guides the head of the humerus as it is elevated.[24,25,29]

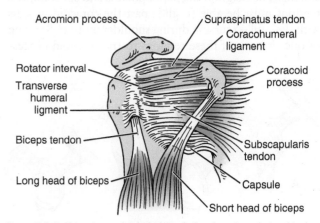

Figure 7-2 Rotator interval (*dashed lines*) showing the relationship between the supraspinatus tendon, long head of biceps, subscapularis tendon, and the coracohumeral ligament. (From Magee DJ: *Orthopedic physical assessment,* ed 6, p 255, St Louis, 2014, Saunders/Elsevier.)

The coracoacromial arch refers to the inferiorly concave surface consisting of the anterior undersurface of the acromion, the coracoid process, and the coracoacromial ligament (see Figure 5-6). It provides a strong ceiling for the shoulder joint, along which the rotator cuff tendons must glide during all shoulder movements. The coracoacromial arch has received considerable attention over the years because of its anatomic relationship to the rotator cuff tendons and the role its structures may play in causing rotator cuff injury.[30-33] Investigations[34,35] have highlighted the importance of contact and load transfer between the rotator cuff and the coracoacromial arch in the function of normal shoulders. Because there is normally no gap between the superior rotator cuff and the coracoacromial arch, the slightest amount of superior translation of the humerus compresses the rotator cuff tendons between the humeral head and the arch, resulting in impingement. Bigliani et al.[32] studied 140 shoulders in 71 cadavers with an average age of 74.4 years. They identified three acromial shapes: type I (flat) in 17%, type II (curved) in 43%, and type III (hooked) in 40%. Of the shoulders, 33% had full-thickness tears, 73% of which were seen in association with a type III acromion; 24% with type II; and 3% with type I (Figure 7-3). The clinical significance of this relatively small difference is unknown and controversial because other authors have discovered no significant association between acromial morphology and rotator cuff pathology.[36-38] A fourth type has been added to the classification as convex or upturned, but has no correlation to impingement. However, a significant correlation between age and rotator cuff tears was noted, with older patients more likely to have type II and III acromion.[36,38] These findings suggest that correlations between acromial morphology and rotator cuff tears may be exaggerated because of the confounding variable of age.

The coracoid process acts as the medial attachment site for both the coracohumeral and coracoacromial ligaments. The neighboring supraspinatus and subscapularis tendons must be able to glide past the coracoid process with their full excursion during shoulder motion. Scarring of one or both of these tendons to the coracoid process can inhibit passive and active shoulder motion. Although the coracoid process does not normally contact the anterior subscapularis tendon, forced medial (internal) rotation of the arm, particularly in the presence of a tight posterior capsule, can produce such contact because of the obligate translation, and lead to impingement of the rotator cuff tendons.[34,39]

The coracoacromial ligament (see Figure 5-6) originates along the distal two thirds of the lateral aspect of the coracoid process as a broad ligament. It passes posteriorly to insert onto the anteromedial and anteroinferior surfaces of the acromion. Spur formation can occur preferentially on the anterolateral band and contribute to impingement syndrome, although it has been suggested that substantial alterations in morphological and biomechanical properties occur in the coracoacromial ligament during aging.[40] Studies are needed to determine whether variations in the coracoacromial ligament morphology cause impingement or are a function of the problem.

There are three bursae relevant to the development of shoulder pain and rotator cuff disease: subacromial, subdeltoid, and subcoracoid (Figure 7-4). The subacromial bursa occupies a space above the rotator cuff and under the acromion. It is a synovium-lined cavity that acts as a gliding surface in two locations: (1) between the rotator cuff tendons and the coracoacromial arch and (2) between the deltoid muscle and the rotator cuff tendon. The subdeltoid bursa is an independent structure located on the deep surface of the deltoid muscle. The subacromial and subdeltoid bursae act together and extend as far medially as the coracoid process. The subcoracoid bursa is located inferior to the coracoid process between the subscapularis tendon and the conjoined tendon of the coracobrachialis muscle and short head of the biceps muscle. Subacromial "disease" encompasses a spectrum of pathologies ranging from bursitis to adhesion formation. Rotator cuff tears are often associated with subacromial bursitis, and this bursitis can lead to the formation of adhesions, which then contribute to rotator cuff impingement. Machida et al.[41] studied 18 patients with shoulder pain and found that subacromial bursa adhesions increased impingement between the acromion process and the rotator cuff insertion.

Anatomical consideration should also be given to the proximal portion of the rotator cuff muscles on the scapula and the relationship between the rotator cuff origins and the scapulothoracic articulation. The scapula, which is stabilized by muscles, provides a stable base for the controlled movements of the humeral head in the glenoid fossa. The muscles that attach to and stabilize the scapula (i.e., trapezius, rhomboids, latissimus dorsi, serratus anterior, levator scapulae, and pectoralis minor) aid in the positioning of the glenoid fossa to accommodate the head of the humerus (Figure 7-5). Scapular dysfunction, from altered muscle balance and/or instability, is one of the contributing factors of rotator cuff injury, especially in the young, active patient population.

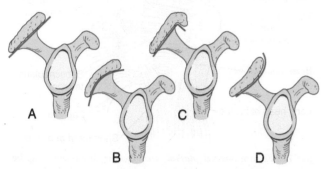

Figure 7-3 Acromion morphology. **A,** Type I (*flat*). **B,** Type II (*curved*). **C,** Type III (*hooked*). **D,** Convex (upturned). (From Magee DJ: *Orthopedic physical assessment,* ed 6, p 257, St Louis, 2014, Saunders/Elsevier.)

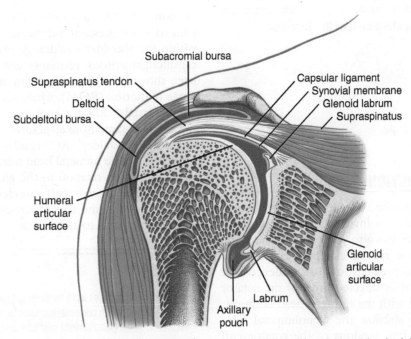

Figure 7-4 Anterior view of a frontal plane cross section of the right glenohumeral joint. Note the subacromial and subdeltoid bursa within the subacromial space. Bursa and synovial lining are depicted in blue. The deltoid and supraspinatus muscles are also shown. (From Neuman DA: *Kinesiology of the musculoskeletal system: foundations for rehabilitation*, ed 2, p 143, St. Louis, 2010, Mosby/Elsevier.)

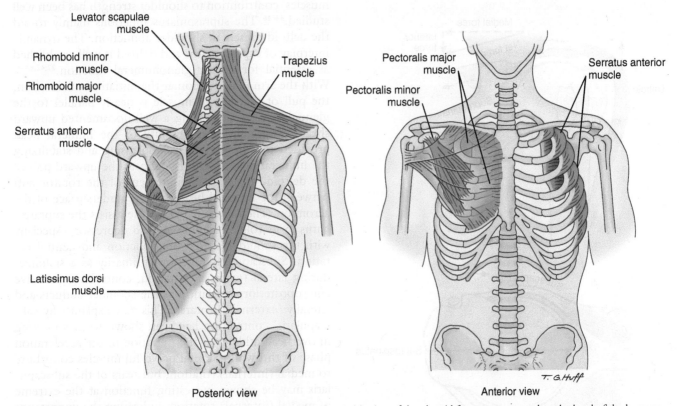

Figure 7-5 The muscles that attach to and stabilize the scapula aid in the positioning of the glenoid fossa to accommodate the head of the humerus. Note that if the elbow is braced, the rotator cuff muscles (supraspinatus, subscapularis, infraspinatus, and teres minor), teres major, deltoid, and pectoralis major can also move the scapula by "reverse origin-insertion."

Muscles Controlling the Movement of the Scapula

- Trapezius (three parts)
- Rhomboids
- Serratus anterior
- Levator scapula
- Pectoralis minor
- Latissimus dorsi (inferior angle)

ROTATOR CUFF FUNCTION

The term *rotator cuff* may be a misnomer because its role relative to shoulder function involves not only joint rotation and muscle force but also joint compression and stability. In the past, the rotator cuff has been referred to as a humeral head depressor; however, evidence now indicates that the inferiorly directed force of the rotator cuff is small compared with the humeral head compressive force it exerts to stabilize the glenohumeral joint (Figure 7-6).[42,43] The four tendons of the rotator cuff perform as a unit, precisely centering the humeral head through compression (called concavity compression) into the glenoid cavity to improve stability, resist translation, and provide rotation about the three major axes

of motion.[42-44] Joint stability, through the rotator cuff's concavity-compression mechanism, is provided mostly within the shoulder's midrange positions, where passive capsuloligamentous restraints are lax; however, it has been shown to also be important at the end of shoulder range of motion (ROM), where forces acting on the joint are increased.[45] Rotator cuff compression acts to protect the capsuloligamentous structures in extreme positions by limiting the shoulder's ROM and reducing strain on these structures.[43] The humeral head maintains a relatively constant position in relation to the glenoid during shoulder rotation. The rotator cuff muscles are closer than any other muscles to the axes of rotation and therefore have shorter lever arms to affect rotation.

Clinical Note

The rotator cuff muscles work as a unit to center the humeral head in the glenoid cavity through compression, to improve stability at the joint, resist translation at the glenohumeral interface, and provide rotation.

The amount of force that can be generated by a rotator cuff muscle is determined by its size, health or condition, and joint position. The individual rotator cuff muscles' contribution to shoulder strength has been well studied.[44-46] The supraspinatus functions mainly to aid the deltoid muscle in shoulder abduction. The dynamic interplay of supraspinatus and deltoid is well established as essential for proper glenohumeral function.[22,42,44-46] With the arm in adduction at the initiation of elevation, the pull of the deltoid muscle is nearly parallel to the glenoid surface, producing a well-documented upward shear component. The stability of the humeral head provided by supraspinatus compressing and stabilizing the humeral head inferiorly opposes the upward pull of the deltoid, avoiding impingement of the rotator cuff between the humeral head and the undersurface of the acromion. The infraspinatus muscle assists the supraspinatus in its role as a humeral head depressor, especially with the shoulder at 90° of abduction and neutral rotation. Subscapularis functions primarily as a stabilizer during lateral (external) rotation, controlling excessive anteroposterior translation as the shoulder abducts and laterally (externally) rotates. This may explain why subscapularis' contraction has been shown to be so strong in overhead athletes at the initiation of the acceleration phase of throwing. Several powerful muscles contribute to medial (internal) rotation, but tears of the subscapularis may be shown by testing function at the extreme of medial (internal) rotation, indicating the importance of this muscle at this end ROM. Patients who have sustained subscapularis tears feel the loss of joint compression and stabilization normally provided by this portion of the rotator cuff. The infraspinatus and teres minor are the only two muscles that produce lateral (external)

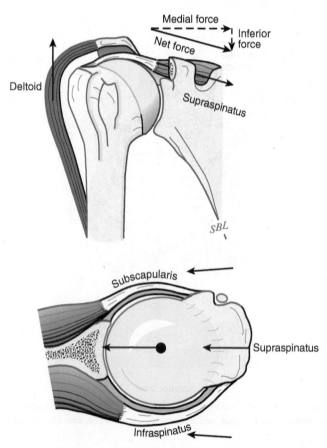

Figure 7-6 Concavity compression of the rotator cuff. (Modified from Matsen FA III, Lippitt SB: *Shoulder surgery: principles and procedures*, p. 85, Philadelphia, 2004, WB Saunders.)

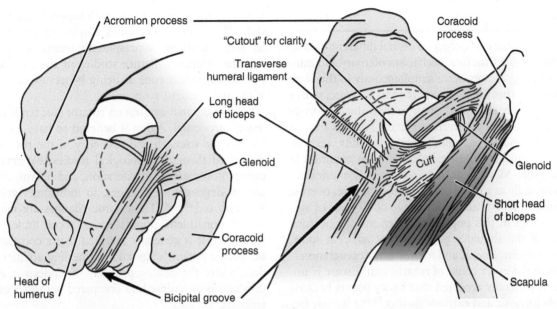

Figure 7-7 The biceps apparatus. (From Magee DJ: *Orthopedic physical assessment*, ed 6, p 254, St Louis, 2014, Saunders/Elsevier.)

rotation, and large tears in this region of the rotator cuff have profound effects on a patient's motion and strength.

The long head of biceps is often considered a functional part of the rotator cuff complex due, in part, to its intimate anatomical relationship with the rotator cuff tendons at the glenohumeral joint (Figure 7-7).[23,29] Its superior-anterior location assists the superior-posterior rotator cuff tendons in stabilizing the glenohumeral joint through humeral head compression, especially into forward elevation. The importance of the relationship between the rotator cuff and long head of biceps is evidenced through injury to one or both of these tissues. Greater than 90% of patients with a diagnosis of biceps tendinitis were found to have underlying shoulder impingement and/or instability believed to be the cause of irritation of the biceps tendon.[47] Lesions of the superior labrum, anterior to posterior (i.e., a SLAP lesion), and adjoining biceps anchor have received considerable attention over the past two decades, including work that has demonstrated a high incidence of rotator cuff tears in overhead athletes with superior labral defects (see Figure 5-27).[48-50] Rotator cuff tears were discovered in 31% of throwers with type II SLAP lesions: 38% of these were full thickness, and 62% were partial thickness. Finally, biceps were found to have an increased tendon-tension force in the presence of a large rotator cuff tear, suggesting the increase of its role in restraining superior humeral head translation to compensate for the rotator cuff failure.[25]

It is important to remember that the shoulder joint differs from single axis joints, such as the knee, in that it functions in the absence of a fixed axis. In a specified position, activation of a muscle creates a unique set of rotational moments. For example, the anterior deltoid can produce moments in forward flexion, medial (internal) rotation, and horizontal adduction. If forward elevation is to occur without rotation, the cross-body and medial (internal) rotation moments of the anterior deltoid must be neutralized by other muscles, such as the posterior deltoid and infraspinatus. As another example, use of the latissimus dorsi in a movement of pure medial (internal) rotation requires that its adduction moment be neutralized by the superior rotator cuff and deltoid. Conversely, use of the latissimus dorsi in a movement of pure adduction requires that its medial (internal) rotation moment be neutralized by the posterior rotator cuff and posterior deltoid muscles.[51]

The timing and magnitude of these balancing muscle effects must be precisely coordinated to avoid unwanted directions of humeral motion. Therefore, the simplified view of muscles functioning in isolation or as part of "force couples" must be replaced with the understanding that all shoulder girdle muscles function together in a precisely coordinated way: opposing muscles canceling out undesired elements and leaving only the net torque that is needed to produce the desired action. This degree of coordination requires a fine-tuned strategy of muscle activation or motor engram that must be established before the motion is carried out. The rotator cuff muscles are critical elements of this shoulder balance equation.

Functions of the Rotator Cuff

- Rotation of the humerus relative to the scapula
- Compression of the humeral head into the glenoid fossa, providing a critical stabilizing mechanism known as concavity compression
- Provision of muscle balance and force

ETIOLOGY

Injury to the rotator cuff occurs via several different mechanisms. Often, more than one mechanism of injury and multiple contributing factors occur simultaneously in the same patient. Injuries that are traumatic tend to be acute, with a well-defined mechanism, and occur in individuals younger than 40 years of age. Concurrent clinical findings such as glenohumeral and/or scapulothoracic instability, secondary impingement, and muscle imbalances are common in this population. More frequently, rotator cuff injuries occur atraumatically as a result of multiple, repetitive, overuse mechanisms, in individuals over the age of 40 years of age. Clinical findings in this population often include postural alterations of the shoulder girdle and/or adjacent spine, subacromial impingement, and rotator cuff degeneration.

Although the exact cause of rotator cuff disease is unknown, it is generally accepted that injury occurs because of multiple intrinsic and extrinsic factors.[52–54] Intrinsic factors include traumatic, reactive, or degenerative changes that originate within the tendon from inferior tissue mechanical properties, direct tendon overload, intrinsic degeneration, or other insult. Extrinsic mechanisms are those that damage the tendon through external forces such as compression against surrounding tissue.[55]

The proposed causes of intrinsic degeneration are primarily the vascular supply of the rotator cuff tendon, aging, and tensile overload. Several researchers have suggested that hypovascularity within the area of greatest impingement (i.e., Codman's critical zone) is the main reason why rotator cuff tears occur in this region (Figure 7-8).[56,57]

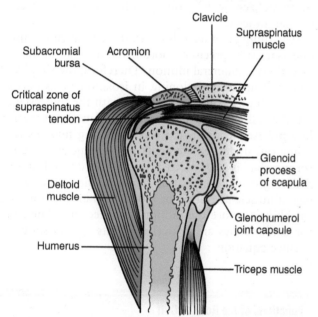

Figure 7-8 The "critical zone." Note the close relationship of the supraspinatus tendon and subacromial bursa to the humeral head and acromion, making an exact clinical diagnosis very difficult. (From Foley BA, Christopher TQ: Injection therapy of bursitis and tendinitis. In Roberts JR, Hedges JR, editors: *Clinical procedures in emergency medicine*, ed 5, Philadelphia, 2010, Saunders/Elsevier.)

Evidence has emerged that both supports and refutes this claim.[58–61] Cadaveric studies confirmed this hypovascular area within the supraspinatus tendon's critical zone, whereas microvasculature studies of the rotator cuff revealed the critical zone as being hypervascular in patients with impingement syndrome.

The effect that age has on rotator cuff tendons is much less controversial. Aging is believed to have a negative effect on the strength and resiliency of the rotator cuff, as evidenced through histological studies that reveal calcification, fibrovascular proliferation, and microtears, suggestive of degenerative changes, in individuals greater than 40 years old.[40,53,60] These same changes are rarely noted in the nonathletic population of those under 40 years. Moreover, it is generally accepted that a correlation exists between a patient's age and the healing abilities of a tendon, where the healing property of tendons of elderly individuals is diminished, as compared with that of younger tendons.[61]

Tension overload is another intrinsic factor found to contribute to rotator cuff injury. Studies have attempted to distinguish specific mechanisms that may contribute to tension overload injuries. One study reported that if the joint and bursal sides of the supraspinatus tendon are subjected to similar loads, the joint side will be more susceptible to failure.[62] Methods to measure intratendinous strain using magnetic resonance imaging have discovered that intratendinous strain fields increased with increasing glenohumeral joint angle, but the strain did not change between the articular and bursal sides.[63] These findings suggest that individuals, such as overhead throwing athletes or those working overhead, may be at risk of articular-sided rotator cuff tears from tendon overload because the joint side of the tendon may be closer to its failure strain during these activities.

Extrinsic factors that contribute to rotator cuff pathology include anatomical findings such as narrowing within the coracoacromial arch or other osseous or soft-tissue changes that result in anterior, external mechanical impingement of the rotator cuff tendons (Figure 7-9). Numerous studies have confirmed that abnormal soft-tissue and bony anatomy surrounding the rotator cuff affect the incidence of pathology; however, the degree to which anatomical variations *cause* rotator cuff injury is less clear.[30,33,34,39] Osteoarthritis of the acromioclavicular joint as well as changes to the coracoacromial ligament have also been implicated as extrinsic factors that could cause anterior impingement and mechanical irritation of the rotator cuff tendons.[38] Internal impingement can occur posteriorly, between the posterior-superior labrum and the posterior rotator cuff tendons (Figure 7-10).[5,50] This is a common problem in overhead throwing athletes because of the tremendous amount of stress placed on the rotator cuff as the athlete accelerates and decelerates the arm during the throwing motion. The rotator cuff muscles must counteract these forces, especially during the

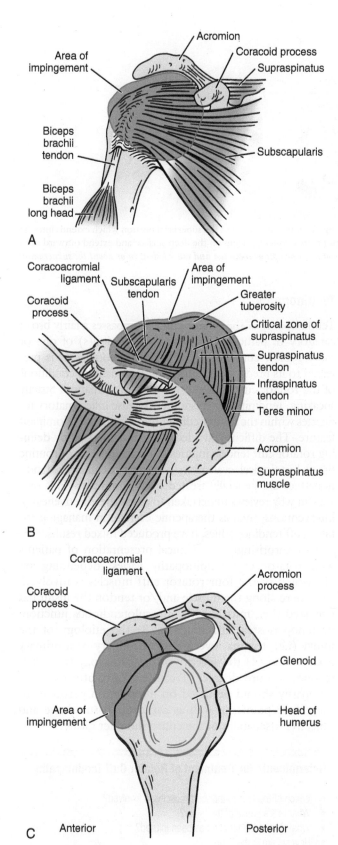

Figure 7-9 Impingement zone. **A,** Anterior view. **B,** Superior view. **C,** Lateral view. (From Magee DJ: *Orthopedic physical assessment,* ed 6, p 316, St Louis, 2014, Saunders/Elsevier.)

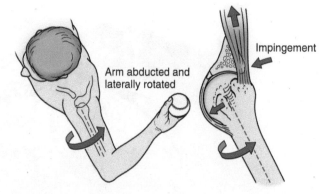

Figure 7-10 Internal impingement of the undersurface of the rotator cuff against the posterior aspect of the labrum in maximum lateral rotation and abduction. (From Magee DJ: *Orthopedic physical assessment,* ed 6, p 318, St Louis, 2014, Saunders/Elsevier.)

deceleration phase, to keep the humeral head centered in the glenoid. Thus, repetitive throwing motion can lead to repetitive microtrauma or impingement on the posterior glenoid margin, usually involving the undersurface of the posterior half of the supraspinatus and the superior half of the infraspinatus. With repeated injury, articular-sided partial-thickness tears can develop.[5,6,50]

Finally, glenohumeral instability and altered scapulothoracic motion must also be considered as possible extrinsic factors leading to rotator cuff injury. Whether instability is due to a structural defect, such as a torn labrum or from muscle imbalance and altered kinematics, the resultant increased translation at the glenohumeral joint affects the integrity of the rotator cuff through either direct compression and/or increased demand on the rotator cuff to stabilize the humeral head on an unstable glenoid.

Pain in the shoulder exists as a vicious cycle of instability, impingement, weakness, and inflammation: all signs and symptoms associated with rotator cuff pathology. Clinicians must have a clear understanding of the multiple etiological factors that can contribute to rotator cuff injuries, and identify clinical findings associated with the cause of the injury, in addition to those resulting from the injury process. Failure to recognize and address *both* of these etiological factors will affect patient outcomes and possibly lead to recurrent rotator cuff injury.

ROTATOR CUFF INJURIES

Optimal functioning of the rotator cuff occurs if all of its muscles are healthy, intact, and well conditioned, and if there is a normal amount of capsular laxity present at the glenohumeral joint, a smooth contour of the undersurface of the coracoacromial arch, a thin, lubricating bursa, and concentricity of the glenohumeral joint and rotator cuff and coracoacromial spheres of rotation.[19–21,34] Given its intricate anatomy and complex role, it is easy to understand why injuries are so common in the rotator cuff.

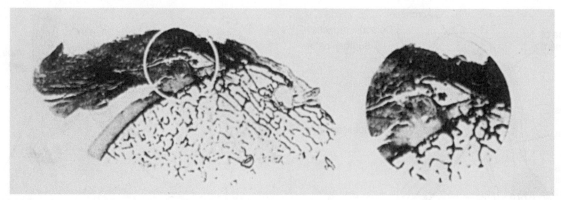

Figure 7-11 Codman's illustration of "a rim rent where all the tendon is torn away from the sulcus except the superficial portion which extends into the periosteum." These photomicrographs provide a convincing argument that cuff tears frequently begin on the deep surface and extend outward until they become full-thickness defects. (From Codman EA: *The shoulder: rupture of the supraspinatus tendon and other lesions in or about the subacromial bursa*, Malabar, 1984, Robert E. Krieger.)

Pathology of the rotator cuff includes a spectrum of injuries, ranging from minor tendinitis to various degrees of partial- and full-thickness tearing. Authors dating back to the 1930s have proposed terms and classification systems to help describe the different types of rotator cuff disease. Codman, considered a pioneer in the realm of rotator cuff injuries, described four different lesions of the supraspinatus tendon, including what he described as a "condition of great clinical importance"—partial tears or "rim rents" (Figure 7-11).[64] The Neer three-stage classification of subacromial impingement lesions has been used extensively to describe injury in this area.[30] Stage I refers to reversible edema and hemorrhage within the rotator cuff and is typically seen in patients under 25 years of age. Stage II occurs with repeated inflammation and results in fibrosis and tendinosis of the rotator cuff, typically in patients 25 to 40 years of age. Stage III occurs with further degeneration of the rotator cuff and adjacent osseous tissue(s) and results in partial or complete tears in individuals older than 40 years of age. Newer classification systems have focused on describing tears of the rotator cuff. Ellman[65] graded partial-thickness tears into three types according to depth. Grade 1 is noted as less than 3 mm deep; grade 2, 3 to 6 mm deep; and grade 3, greater than 6 mm deep. He also included information on the location of the tear, identifying bursal surface, articular surface, or interstitial tears. Fukuda[7] labeled rotator cuff injuries as grade 1, a subacromial bursitis or tendinitis (a "pretear"); grade 2, a partial-thickness tear (involving at least one-quarter thickness of the supraspinatus tendon); and grade 3, a full-thickness tear. Fukuda also classified the location of partial-thickness tears as bursal-side tears, intratendinous tears, and joint-sided tears. Snyder[66] described a classification based on tear location and severity: articular and bursal for partial-thickness tears, named "A" and "B," and "C" for complete tears. Degree of damage is labeled from zero (normal tendon) to four (very severe partial-thickness tear).

Tendinopathy

Tendinopathy of the rotator cuff encompasses a fairly broad category of pathology involving the tendon(s) of one or more rotator cuff muscles. The term *tendinopathy* is preferred to its predecessor, tendinitis, as it includes conditions of the rotator cuff with and without inflammation. Strictly speaking, tendinitis is a misnomer because inflammatory infiltrates within the rotator cuff tendon are not a predominant feature. The difficulty in adequately and consistently defining rotator cuff tendon injuries stems from a lack of routine tissue histological evaluation because patients with tendinopathies are generally treated nonoperatively.[67] This may explain why reviews undertaken to assess the effectiveness of interventions, such as therapeutic exercise in managing rotator cuff tendinopathies, have produced mixed results.[68-72]

Not surprisingly, the clinical presentation of patients with rotator cuff tendinopathy varies, depending on (1) which of the four rotator cuff muscles is involved, (2) where along the muscle and/or tendon the insult has occurred (i.e., muscle belly, musculotendinous junction, or tenoperiosteal attachment), (3) the etiology of the injury (i.e., trauma, overuse, or secondary to a primary injury), and (4) the severity of the pathology (i.e., first, second, or third degree). Treatment of rotator cuff tendinopathy should be based on information pertinent to these four points, as well as a thorough subjective and objective assessment of the entire shoulder girdle.

Determinants for Treatment of Rotator Cuff Tendinopathy

- Which of the four rotator cuff muscles is involved?
- What is the cause of the injury?
- What part of the tendon has been injured?
- How severe is the injury?

The majority of patients with rotator cuff tendinopathy describe shoulder pain as aggravated with overhead activities and relieved with rest. ROM is generally preserved, with possible decrease at the extremes of motion. Resisted strength testing reproduces pain and, depending on the severity of tendon injury, possible weakness. Patients' chief complaints are usually related to diminished function lasting longer than 3 months.[68] Tendinopathy of the rotator cuff has been shown to demonstrate similar pathological changes to tendon disorders in other areas of the body in which loaded (i.e., against gravity or resistance) exercise has proven beneficial. Littlewood et al.[68,73] evaluated the effectiveness of loaded exercise programs for rotator cuff tendinopathy and concluded that the role of loaded exercise in treating rotator cuff tendinopathy was promising, but it required further high-quality research.

Impingement Syndromes

The term *impingement syndrome* was popularized by Neer in 1972, in an evaluation he performed on 100 dissected scapulae.[74] He described 11 as having a "characteristic ridge of proliferative spurs and excrescences on the undersurface of the anterior process of the acromion," which he attributed to repeated contact or impingement of the rotator cuff and the humeral head, with traction of the coracoacromial ligament (Figure 7-12). Of special interest was his discovery that the anterior lip and undersurface of the anterior third of the acromion were involved in all cases. In this region, the supraspinatus tendon inserts onto the greater tuberosity, lying anterior to the coracoacromial arch with the shoulder in the neutral position. With forward flexion, the structures must pass beneath the arch, providing the opportunity for impingement. This early description of shoulder impingement syndrome is now commonly referred to as *primary impingement* because the primary cause of the resultant impingement is the actual abutting of soft-tissue structures (e.g., the rotator cuff and glenoid labrum) and bony prominences (e.g., the acromion and coracoid process). Static factors believed to cause impingement include abnormalities of the coracoacromial arch that may lead to areas of higher than normal compression of the rotator cuff.

The shape of the acromion has been implicated as one cause of mechanical impingement of the supraspinatus tendon. Bigliani et al.[32] studied the relationship between acromion shape and external impingement by comparing the shape of the acromion to full-thickness supraspinatus tears in cadaveric specimens. Their results concluded that there are three distinct acromion shapes: flat (type I), curved (type II), and hooked (type III). Type II and type III acromion shapes had the strongest correlation with full-thickness tears, leading the authors to conclude that rotator cuff disease is influenced by acromion shape (see Figure 7-3).

Importantly, subacromial impingement is not always the sole cause of rotator cuff disease; in fact, it is more accurately described as the phenomenon that occurs because of the more probable causes of aging and physical loading of the shoulder and arm (Figure 7-13). The process of aging causes degeneration in the rotator cuff, particularly at its insertion points, which leads to fiber thickening and the formation of granulation tissue. The damaged rotator cuff then malfunctions, leading to further disorders in the subacromial area. Excessive loading of the rotator cuff may occur either through a static or "structural" (e.g., hooked acromion) mechanism, or dynamically because of the humeral head and rotator cuff moving against an unyielding structure. Current evidence indicates that both static and dynamic factors act upon the rotator cuff, leading to eventual rotator cuff disease.[33,62] With dynamic causes, the coracoacromial arch and other subacromial structures initially may be normal; however, abnormal motion of the humeral head and the rotator cuff relative to the scapula is the cause of the impingement, leading to sometimes permanent structural changes.[39,75,76] This type of anterior, external impingement is known as *secondary impingement* because the impingement is secondary to the underlying instability and pathology. A third type of impingement, termed *posterior internal impingement*, occurs with the shoulder in 90° of abduction and lateral (external) rotation, and involves compression of the undersurface of the posterior rotator cuff tendons against the posterior-superior glenoid rim (see Figure 7-10). This type of impingement commonly affects individuals involved in overhead work or throwing sports.[28,75]

Rotator Cuff Tears

Rotator cuff tears are among the most common conditions affecting the shoulder, accounting for 4.5 million physician visits in the United States per year.[77] They may

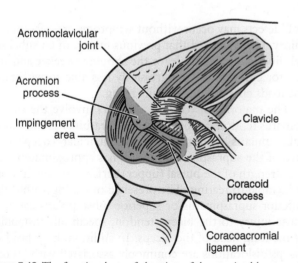

Figure 7-12 The functional arc of elevation of the proximal humerus is forward, as proposed by Neer. The greater tuberosity impinges against the anterior one third of the acromial surface. This critical area comprises the supraspinatus and bicipital tendons and the subacromial bursa. (From Magee DJ: *Orthopedic physical assessment*, ed 6, p 317, St Louis, 2014, Saunders/Elsevier.)

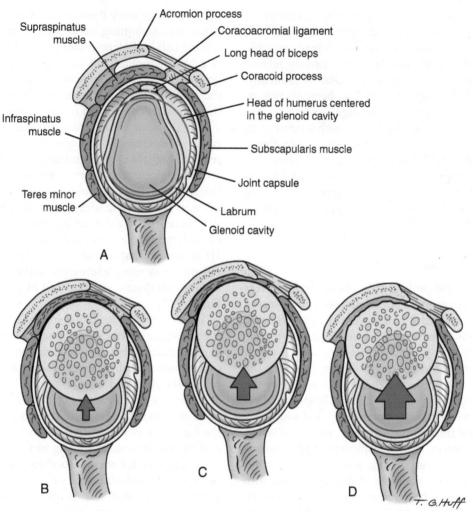

Figure 7-13 Rotator cuff degeneration. **A,** Normal relationships of the cuff and the coracoacromial arch. **B,** Upward displacement of the head, which squeezes the cuff against the acromion and the coracoacromial ligament. **C,** Greater contact and abrasion give rise to a traction spur in the coracoacromial ligament. **D,** Still greater upward displacement, resulting in abrasion of the humeral articular cartilage and cuff tear arthropathy.

be classified as partial or full thickness, acute, chronic, or acute on chronic, and traumatic or atraumatic or degenerative. Tears can range from mild microtearing to total absence of one or more of the rotator cuff tendons. In a young, active patient, rotator cuff tears are almost always the result of a traumatic insult and may occur in combination with other injuries such as an avulsion fracture of the greater tuberosity or injury to the glenoid labrum (Figure 7-14). Degenerative rotator cuff failure, associated with the older individual, typically begins with a partial-thickness defect on the deep undersurface of the supraspinatus as it attaches to the greater tuberosity (Figure 7-15).[78,79] A common misdiagnosis of shoulder pain (e.g., tendinitis, bursitis, and impingement syndrome) may actually represent failure of the deep surface fibers of the rotator cuff. The degree to which the intact fibers may hypertrophy, strengthen, or adapt to stabilize the tear and take up the function of the damaged fibers is unknown. Pettersson[80] used the term *creeping tendon ruptures* to describe a condition in which major rotator

cuff defects may occur without symptoms or a recognized injury. He suggested that previous minor, often subclinical, fiber failure could leave the shoulder weaker and the rotator cuff tendons progressively less able to withstand the loads encountered in daily living.

The majority of rotator cuff tears involve the supraspinatus tendon, followed by the infraspinatus and upper subscapularis tendons.[52,54,78] The articular (deep) surface of the supraspinatus tendon has approximately half the strength of the bursal (upper) surface, making it more vulnerable to tearing. The presence of tearing within the anterior supraspinatus or superior subscapularis can also cause injury to the biceps tendon, specifically instability of the long head of the biceps. In addition, long head of biceps dislocations are commonly associated with lesions of the rotator cuff.[29,47,81]

The reported incidence of rotator cuff tears ranges anywhere from 13% to 32%; however, the actual frequency of all tears is unknown because partial-thickness tears are poorly defined and can occur without symptoms.[4,10,82]

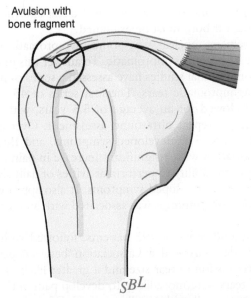

Avulsion with
bone fragment

SBL

Figure 7-14 Partial-thickness cuff tear with avulsion of a bony fragment from the tuberosity. (From Matsen FA III, Lippitt SB, Sidles JA, et al: *Practical evaluation and management of the shoulder*, Philadelphia, 1994, WB Saunders.)

One group of authors,[82] studying the role age plays in the prevalence of rotator cuff tears, noted that the incidence in cadavers younger than 60 was 6%, compared with cadavers older than 60 years, where it was 30%. Partial-thickness tears appear approximately twice as often as full-thickness defects and can occur on the bursal side, on the articular side, or in the intratendinous region of the rotator cuff. Bursal-sided tears are reported to produce the most severe symptoms due in part to the large number of pain receptors in bursal tissue and the location of the tear within the subacromial space.[7,62,83]

Massive rotator cuff tears are reported as ranging from 10% to 40% of all rotator cuff tears[84] and defined as tears larger than 5 cm in combined areas or a tear involving two or more tendons.[85] The conditions that lead to a massive tear of the rotator cuff are diverse, and its presentation is similarly diverse. A common feature of the shoulder with a massive rotator cuff tear is the subsequent upward migration of the humeral head, which develops over time because of the shear forces created by muscles such as deltoid (Figure 7-16). These tears can cause an uncoupling of forces across the glenohumeral joint and result in unstable shoulder kinematics. Patients typically present with pain, periscapular atrophy, and significant weakness. Rotator cuff tear arthropathy is a pathological condition of the glenohumeral joint in which chronic rotator cuff tearing is associated with structural glenohumeral joint destruction.[86] The joint destruction involves humeral head erosion or collapse, and in some patients, glenoid erosion (Figure 7-17). Rotator cuff tear arthropathy does not include rotator cuff disease in which proximal migration of the humeral head is present without advanced structural changes in the joint surfaces. After a massive rotator cuff tear, the shoulder joint is progressively affected by the profoundly altered biomechanical and biological changes. The corresponding morphological changes were recognized as early as the mid-1800s, when tear-associated joint destruction was compared with localized destructive arthritis. The term *rotator cuff tear arthropathy* was first used by Neer in 1977 to describe shoulder joint destruction secondary to rotator cuff tearing.[87]

Natural History of Rotator Cuff Tears

Natural history refers to the progression of change of the rotator cuff over time in the absence of medical intervention. An understanding of natural history allows for the development of prevention and treatment programs and allows the clinician to inform the patient about what may happen should the disorder go untreated.[88]

As previously noted, rotator cuff tears may be either asymptomatic or symptomatic, and appear to increase in prevalence with increasing age.[89] Approximately 50% of

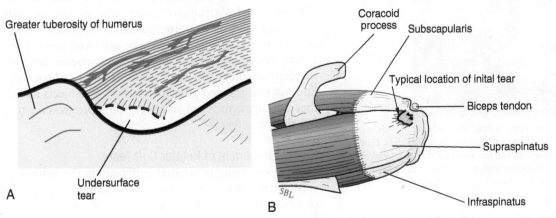

Greater tuberosity of humerus

Undersurface tear

A

Coracoid process

Subscapularis

Typical location of inital tear

Biceps tendon

Supraspinatus

Infraspinatus

SBL

B

Figure 7-15 In degenerative cuff disease, the tendon fibers fail a few at a time, usually starting at the deep surface of the supraspinatus near its insertion, close to the long head of the biceps. **A,** Anterior view. **B,** Posterior view. (From Matsen FA III, Lippitt SB, Sidles JA, et al: *Practical evaluation and management of the shoulder*, Philadelphia, 1994, WB Saunders.)

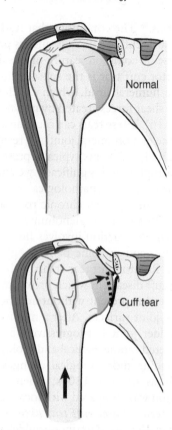

Figure 7-16 In chronic cuff deficiency, erosion of the upper glenoid may leave the shoulder with a permanent tendency toward superior subluxation that cannot be reversed by cuff repair surgery. (From Matsen FA III, Lippitt SB, Sidles JA, et al: *Practical evaluation and management of the shoulder*, Philadelphia, 1994, WB Saunders.)

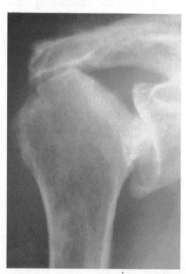

Figure 7-17 Collapse of the humeral head in combination with massive cuff deficiency because of cuff tear arthropathy. (From Walch G, Edwards TB, Boulahia A, et al: Arthroscopic tenotomy of the long head of the biceps in the treatment of rotator cuff tears: clinical and radiographic results of 307 cases, *J Shoulder Elbow Surg* 14(3):238-246, 2005.)

asymptomatic, untraumatized shoulders, belonging to patients between 60 and 90 years of age, were reported as having partial- or full-thickness rotator cuff defects.[12,89–91] Thus, when describing the natural history of rotator cuff

tears, the course of the asymptomatic tear and the symptomatic tear both must be examined.

It remains unclear why some asymptomatic rotator cuff tears become symptomatic. To answer this question, two longitudinal studies have assessed a series of patients with asymptomatic tears. The first series of 45 patients were followed for an average of 5.5 years, with 23 returning for repeat ultrasound assessment. Over a mean of 2.8 years, 51% developed symptoms, and there was an association with a significant increase in pain and decrease in the ability to perform activities of daily living in patients who developed symptoms. It also appeared that the onset of symptoms was associated with an increase in tear size.[14]

A second series of 195 patients, followed with ultrasound, demonstrated an association between pain and the progression in tear size and a greater likelihood that larger tears were more likely to develop pain in the short term compared with smaller tears.[92] Of note, both of these studies examined individuals with a symptomatic rotator cuff tear in the contralateral shoulder. The authors acknowledged that there may have been differences between the patient population studied and individuals without involvement of the contralateral shoulder.

No longitudinal studies exist that examine the untreated symptomatic rotator cuff tear. A series of 59 shoulders receiving nonoperative treatment and followed with serial magnetic resonance imaging suggested that full-thickness tears were more likely to progress in size compared with partial-thickness tears, and that this rate of progression was more prevalent after 18 months than it was during the first 18 months. Additionally, the authors also demonstrated greater progression in individuals over 60, atrophy only with full-thickness tears, and a 17% rate of development or progression of fatty infiltration.[93]

Increased use of diagnostic imaging, such as magnetic resonance imaging and arthrography, over the past decade has identified a seemingly "normal" indicator of aging tissue. Furthermore, rotator cuff defects have been found to be compatible with normal, painless, functional activity. Yamanaka and Matsumato[94] used arthrography to study the progression of 40 untreated partial-thickness tears in asymptomatic patients with a mean age of 61 years. Their 1-year results revealed overall improvements in their subjects' shoulder function scores, despite arthrography findings that showed greater than 50% of subjects had either an enlargement of their tear or a progression to a full-thickness tear.

General Treatment of Rotator Cuff Tears

The management of rotator cuff tears is the subject of substantial debate among clinicians and researchers. In a number of studies, the clinical results of rotator cuff repairs in symptomatic patients, who were followed for as long as 10 years, were good to excellent in a high percentage of cases, even though rerupture of the rotator cuff was known to occur in 20% to 65% of cases.[94–97] Interestingly, a massive, irreparable rotator cuff tear is not incompatible with good overhead function. Observations such as these have made clinical decision making relative to the treatment of symptomatic rotator cuff tears challenging. Historically, treatments have consisted of rehabilitation and surgical repair such as subacromial decompression without repair, tendon transfers, and tendon substitution techniques. The most commonly reported prognostic factors for rotator cuff repair are patient age, chronicity of tear, and size of tear.[28,97–100] Rerupture is clearly a major concern in these patient populations, and it has been correlated with tear size, tear chronicity, and patient satisfaction.

Some current controversies in the management of rotator cuff tears include the role of rehabilitation, the indications for and timing of surgical repair, the method of surgical repair, and the management of irreparable defects. Important factors that must be considered in the decision between surgical and conservative management of a patient with a symptomatic, full-thickness rotator cuff tear are the patient's age and expected activity level and whether muscle or tissue retraction and rotator cuff muscle atrophy and fatty replacement are present.[100–102] Surgery is almost always suggested for patients in the fourth or fifth decade of life who have suffered a traumatic injury that resulted in a full-thickness tear. Patients in the sixth, seventh, or eighth decade of life may or may not be well suited for surgical repair, depending on the chronicity of the tear and the quality of the remaining tendon and muscle tissue, as well as other health issues.[97,98] If the tissue is less than optimal, failure to heal is a significant possibility. Most patients in the older age groups are more interested in eliminating shoulder pain and achieving a functional ROM than in having powerful overhead use of the arm. However, the average age of the general population is increasing, and a sizable proportion of these individuals are remaining active. Therefore, the clinician is likely to be faced with challenging questions about the best way to manage rotator cuff tears and maximize a patient's functional goals and requirements.

CLINICAL PRESENTATION OF ROTATOR CUFF PATHOLOGY

Rotator cuff pathology manifests itself clinically in a variety of ways, depending on the type and severity of pathology, as well as the individual patient characteristics (i.e., concurrent injuries, co-morbidities, and activity level). Common complaints include pain worsened with overhead activities, strength limitations, and functional impairments. Limitations in mobility are related to muscle weakness; therefore, active ROM is usually affected more than passive ROM is. Pain is reported at the end point of motion and is generally greater in abduction and lateral (external) rotation planes of motion. Patients with subacromial impingement or rotator cuff tears, however, may present with limitations in both active and passive ROM because of altered anatomy and/or biomechanics of the shoulder girdle. Patients with subacromial impingement also may possess a characteristic painful arc of movement between 60° and 120° of abduction (Figure 7-18). Patients with rotator cuff tendinopathies and partial-thickness tears tend to have more pain because of the intact sensory components, as compared with patients with full-thickness tears. Functional impairments commonly described by this patient population include difficulty with reaching overhead and behind one's back, lifting (especially with an extended elbow), and lying on the affected shoulder.

Weakness and pain are the primary causes of functional limitations associated with rotator cuff pathology. The degenerative tendon fibers may be weakened and may fail without a specific clinical manifestation.[40,53,54] Patients with partial-thickness tears have substantially more pain on resisted muscle action than those with full-thickness tears have, again because of the often intact nervous tissue, and bursal-sided tears seem to be more symptomatic than deeper tears because of the resultant problems with roughness of the articulation between the upper surface of the rotator cuff and the undersurface of the coracoacromial arch.[62,83,103] Some authors and clinicians believe that a subacromial injection of local anesthetic can be used to differentiate weakness caused by painful inhibition from weakness caused by a tendon defect.[104]

Rotator cuff tears may cause shoulder instability because of a loss of efficient centering of the humeral head in the glenoid. Acute tears of the subscapularis, although less common, may contribute to recurrent anterior instability. Chronic loss of the normal compressive effect of the rotator cuff mechanism and of the stabilizing effect of the superior rotator cuff tendon interposed between the humeral head and the coracoacromial arch may contribute to superior glenohumeral instability (and secondary impingement).[105]

Patients with rotator cuff tears frequently complain of a symptomatic crepitus during passive glenohumeral ROM. This roughness often is caused by bursal hypertrophy, secondary changes in the undersurface of the coracoacromial arch, loss of integrity of the upper aspect of the rotator cuff tendons, or degenerative changes in the tuberosities of the humerus.[28,34,78,103] These factors culminate in a condition known as **subacromial abrasion** (Figure 7-19). Neer et al.[87] used the term *rotator cuff tear arthropathy* to describe a similar phenomenon, which they believed was a cause of this roughness associated with rotator cuff defects.

Patient History

Clinical evaluation of the patient with suspected rotator cuff pathology begins with a detailed medical history, as well as a comprehensive objective examination of the shoulder girdle and adjacent spine and ribs. Shoulder pain can be caused by injury to the osseous and/or soft tissue of the

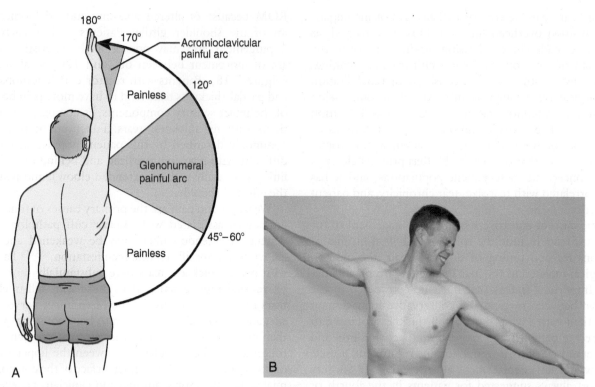

Figure 7-18 Painful arc in the shoulder. **A,** Painful arc of the glenohumeral joint. In the case of acromioclavicular joint problems only, the range of 170° to 180° would elicit pain. **B,** Note the impingement causing pain on the right at approximately 85°. (From Magee DJ: *Orthopedic physical assessment*, ed 6, p 273, St Louis, 2014, Saunders/Elsevier. **A,** Modified from Hawkins RJ, Hobeika PE: Impingement syndrome in the athletic shoulder, *Clin Sports Med* 2:391-405, 1983.)

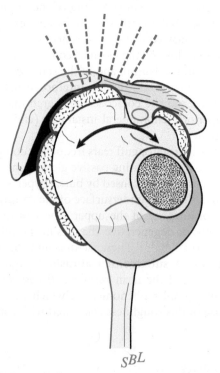

Figure 7-19 Abrasion sign. Symptomatic subacromial crepitance on rotation of the arm elevated to 90° with respect to the thorax, a position in which the capsule and ligaments are normally not under tension. (Modified from Rockwood CA, Matsen FA, editors: *The shoulder*, p 824, Philadelphia, 1998, WB Saunders; Matsen FA III, Lippitt SB, Sidles JA, et al: *Practical evaluation and management of the shoulder*, Philadelphia, 1994, WB Saunders.)

glenohumeral joint, dysfunction about the scapulothoracic region, or it may originate within the cervical or thoracic spine regions. Clinicians must be cognizant of primary and secondary causes of rotator cuff pathology and include all suspected regions within a patient's assessment. The subjective history should follow a systematic approach, similar to all other musculoskeletal assessments, with particular attention given to the following factors.

Patient Profile

Factors such as patient age, occupation, and activity level are key in understanding the etiology and pattern of rotator cuff injuries. Injuries are common in young, active individuals, as well as in patients over 65 years of age who possess normal, degenerative processes at the glenohumeral joint. Younger patients with rotator cuff injuries are often involved in some type of overhead sport or an occupation that places excessive force and repetitive demand on the shoulder, especially during overhead activities. The rotator cuff is particularly susceptible to conditions such as subacromial impingement and partial tears in patients over 50 years of age, where normal degeneration of the shoulder joint occurs. The prevalence of subacromial impingement and rotator cuff tears has been shown to increase significantly in this population, but it is not limited to older adults—partial-thickness tears are also reported in younger athletes.[5] Age does, however, seem to be most consistently related to the incidence of full-thickness tears, with older patients being significantly more affected.[12,16,79] Activities that are repetitive and occur overhead, place individuals at greater risk of rotator cuff injury. These include daily life, work, and/or recreational activities. Minagwa et al.[10] performed a population study that showed an increased prevalence of full-thickness tears in people who performed heavy labor. The nature of work performed may also influence frequency of partial-thickness tears, but no studies have looked at this as a risk factor.

Mechanism of Injury

Rotator cuff injuries can occur as a result of an acute traumatic mechanism, such as a fall on an outstretched hand ("FOOSH" injury), or they can be atraumatic in nature, often because of repetitive overload or degeneration. Many patients possess a combination of mechanisms ("acute on chronic"), describing one incident that caused the eventual injury on a shoulder that was previously injured to a lesser degree and/or was always "sore." The literature indicates that a memorable incident of trauma is related to degree of tearing. Of patients with a full-thickness tear, 65% were able to describe a defined incident that caused their shoulder injury, whereas only 47% of patients with partial tears, and 37% with tendinitis were able to recall a specific onset.[7] Differences between grades of lesion and mechanism have also been reported: patients with a well-defined injury more often had full tears (65%), versus 53.3% of patients with partial tears, who had no episodic injury.[95]

Aggravating and Easing Factors

Information related to what aggravates and eases a patient's injured shoulder is helpful in establishing the type and degree of rotator cuff pathology involved. In addition, these factors form important, patient-directed functional outcome measures. Typical aggravating factors include movements and positions that place the arm overhead and behind the plane of the body. Both of these positions are made worse if load is added to the arm and the elbow is extended, resulting in greater leverage forces directed on the shoulder joint. Activities performed in abduction are worse than flexion and scaption (i.e., movement in the scapular plane), and most patients with rotator cuff pathology describe impingement-type symptoms when their arm is medially (internally) rotated and elevated to around 90° of elevation, especially in combination with horizontal adduction.

Pain

Pain almost certainly accompanies the patient with rotator cuff pathology. It typically presents in the anterolateral aspect of the shoulder with a common referral pattern to the deltoid insertion point. A deep ache that intensifies to a sharp pain when the arm is placed in aggravating positions is commonly noted in this patient population. Night pain is also a common complaint for both partial-thickness and full-thickness tears, with pretears and partial-thickness tears generally more painful than full-thickness tears are.[7] Pain is a strong motivator for patients seeking care and the most common symptom of a rotator cuff tear.[15] Radicular pain is not indicative of rotator cuff pathology, and if reported, it should direct the clinician to perform a cervical spine examination.

Function and Health-Related Quality of Life

Rotator cuff disease has a high incidence rate, and active individuals are often affected.[106] As noted, common clinical features are pain at rest and at night, motion loss, and weakness.[26,33,51] These symptoms can lead to disruption of activities of daily living, work, and leisure, with overall poor quality-of-life experience.[17] The functional disability of rotator cuff injuries affects not just the physical aspect of a patient's life but also the mental and social aspects.[17,18] Therefore, clinicians should include outcome measures related to upper-extremity functional capacity and quality-of-life measures to understand and monitor the level of effect a rotator cuff injury has on the patient's livelihood.

Physical Examination

The objective physical examination of the patient with suspected rotator cuff pathology should include the entire shoulder girdle, as well as the proximal (cervical and thoracic spine), ribs, and distal segments (elbow, wrist, and hand) of the upper-extremity kinetic chain. Diagnostic imaging (i.e., ultrasound and magnetic resonance imaging) and arthroscopic surgery may or may not be included in the diagnostic procedure. Objective assessment of the shoulder consists of a series of tests that measure how the shoulder and related tissue(s) move, as well as "special tests" designed to discern the type and severity of rotator cuff involvement. Despite this systematic approach, accurate diagnosis of an injured rotator cuff is notoriously difficult. Partial-thickness tearing is especially troublesome to diagnose because its signs and symptoms mimic those of other shoulder conditions such as rotator cuff tendinopathy, impingement syndromes, and atraumatic instability.[107-109] Open surgery is considered the gold standard for rotator cuff disease diagnosis; however, this is clearly impractical for use in every patient with suspected pathology. Magnetic resonance imaging and ultrasound are considered reference standards.[110] However, there is uncertainty regarding the accuracy of these tests in identifying conditions such as partial-thickness tears.[107] Special tests for the rotator cuff, although easy to apply and inexpensive,[110] generally have high sensitivity but low specificity.[109,111,112] Most research into the diagnosis of rotator cuff pathology concludes that no single test (physical or imaging) is accurate on its own,[113] reinforcing the importance of considering all components of the patient's assessment (i.e., subjective, objective, and imaging tests) when determining a patient's diagnosis.[114]

Observation

Observation starts at the beginning of the patient-clinician interaction and continues throughout the entire examination. The patient should be observed at rest and with movement, from the anterior, lateral, and posterior views (Figure 7-20). Ideally, the patient should be observed in positions he or she reports as aggravating, as well as while performing his or her functional activities. Careful inspection of the scapulothoracic region and adjacent spine and ribs is important because these regions may play a role in the cause and effect of the rotator cuff pathology. In the young patient, there may be evidence of scapular dyskinesis or muscle imbalance seen, specifically the lower trapezius (i.e., decreased) and the upper trapezius muscles (i.e., increased) (Figure 7-21). The older patient with rotator cuff disease may have an altered or reversed scapulohumeral rhythm because of significant rotator cuff weakness and/or pain, and this may be in combination with muscle atrophy of one or more of the rotator cuff muscles. The thoracic and lumbar spine regions may be important to inspect depending on the patient's history and/or initial presentation. The young, athletic patient with suspected rotator cuff pathology should be carefully observed for postural abnormalities of the spine and hypomobility of the ribs and lower kinetic chain that may be contributing factors to his or her shoulder injury. Postural abnormalities such as shoulder girdle rounding, chin poking, and thoracic spine kyphosis are common in older patients with shoulder pain.

Mobility

Mobility testing assesses several components involved in movement: a patient's willingness to move, joint range,

and muscle power.[115] Active and passive ROM testing of the scapulothoracic and glenohumeral joints, as well as selective testing of tissue known to be tight in this population, should all be included in this portion of the examination. Because the primary tissue at fault (i.e., rotator cuff) is contractile, active ROM should be affected more than passive ROM is; however, this will depend on whether the tissue surrounding the rotator cuff is involved (i.e., coracoacromial arch). Common limitations include: (1) glenohumeral abduction affected more than flexion, (2) greater than 90° elevation positions affected more than those less than 90°, and (3) active ROM affected more than passive ROM. Patients with impingement or acute rotator cuff pathology may demonstrate a painful arc of movement from approximately 60° to 120° of abduction and a compensatory shoulder hike pattern (i.e., reversed scapulohumeral rhythm). Overhead athletes with an injured rotator cuff should be carefully assessed for deficits of medial (internal) rotation ROM at 90° of abduction, particularly of their dominant shoulder (Figure 7-22). Loss of this movement, with a concurrent increase in lateral (external) rotation ROM, is believed to occur as a result of osseous and soft-tissue changes about the shoulder, and it has been linked to shoulder pathology.[50,116,117]

Limitations in movement about the shoulder can occur as a result of different mechanisms. They can be as a direct result of the injured rotator cuff, as seen in the patient with decreased abduction from a supraspinatus tear, or a painful arc of motion in the patient with subacromial impingement. Motion can also be altered because of a compensation pattern adopted by the patient to avoid pain, impingement, or instability at the glenohumeral joint.

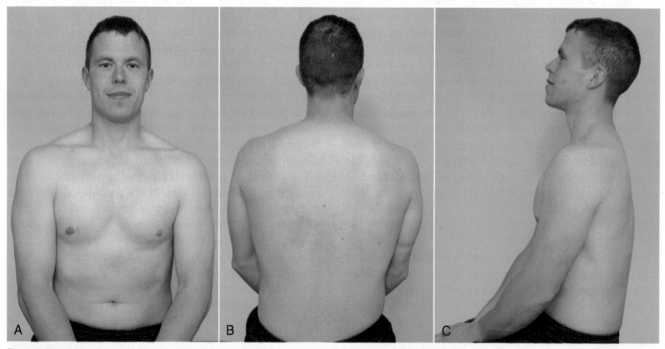

Figure 7-20 Views of the shoulder. **A,** Anterior. **B,** Posterior. **C,** Side. (From Magee DJ: *Orthopedic physical assessment,* ed 6, p 265, St Louis, 2014, Saunders/Elsevier.)

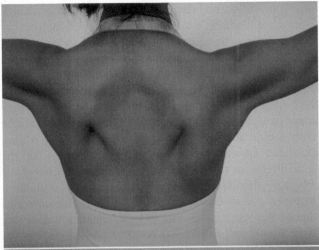

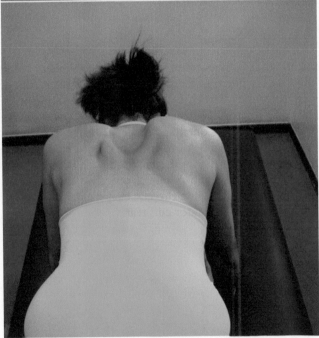

Figure 7-21 Imbalance pattern of the upper and lower trapezius. Note the overdevelopment of the upper trapezius and lower trapezius working to prevent rotary winging. (From Magee DJ: *Orthopedic physical assessment*, ed 6, p 269, St Louis, 2014, Saunders/Elsevier.)

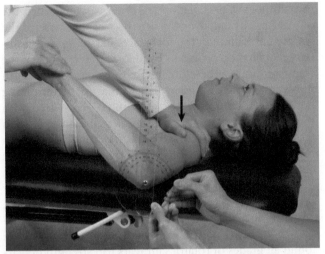

Figure 7-22 Glenohumeral medial rotation passive ROM measurement using stabilization of the scapula by holding the coracoid process and the scapula down. (From Magee DJ: *Orthopedic physical assessment*, ed 6, p 277, St Louis, 2014, Saunders/Elsevier.)

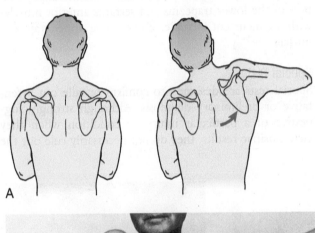

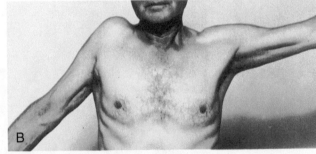

Figure 7-23 Reverse scapulohumeral rhythm (notice shoulder hiking) and excessive scapular movement. Examples include **A,** frozen shoulder or **B,** tear of rotator cuff. (**A,** From Magee DJ: *Orthopedic physical assessment*, ed 6, p 276, St Louis, 2014, Saunders/Elsevier. **B,** From Beetham WP, Polley HF, Slocum CH et al: *Physical examination of the joints*, p. 41, Philadelphia, 1965, WB Saunders.)

An example of this is the patient who uses a reversed scapulohumeral rhythm (i.e., shoulder hike) to elevate his or her arm because of significant rotator cuff weakness or the patient who uses scapular retraction instead of lateral (external) rotation to avoid painful motion or instability at the glenohumeral joint (Figure 7-23). Finally, abnormal ROM may be part of the contributing cause of the rotator cuff pathology. Common clinical features associated with patients with rotator cuff pathology include scapular instability (i.e., in the young patient) and decreased thoracic spine extension (i.e., in the older patient). Distal ROM alterations such as decreased hip and trunk rotation can affect the efficiency of the kinetic chain and have a detrimental effect on the shoulder and rotator cuff in individuals who use their arm in overhead positions.[118] Clinicians must be aware of all of the interrelationships of the kinetic chain during shoulder movement and be careful to differentiate which of the three categories the limitation falls into for successful treatment planning.

Strength

Strength testing should include the muscles of the entire shoulder girdle, not just the rotator cuff. Muscles that attach to and control the stability and movement of the scapulothoracic articulation are often weakened because of rotator cuff injury or they are part of the cause of the rotator cuff failure in the first place. Furthermore, shoulder rehabilitation programs emphasize the strength of the scapular muscles; therefore, establishing baseline strength measures of these muscles is essential for determining outcome. Rotator cuff strength should be assessed with the glenohumeral joint in neutral, as well as in abduction (at 90°), if pain allows. In young, athletic individuals with rotator cuff pathology, information related to the rotator cuff muscles' endurance, as well as strength, may prove more useful. Most patients with rotator cuff pathology present with weakness of lateral (external) rotation (i.e., primarily infraspinatus) and abduction (i.e., supraspinatus) movements of the glenohumeral joint.[115] McCabe found all grades of rotator cuff tears had strength deficits in most movements, but 10° abduction showed a distinction between partial and full thickness—full-thickness tears had a greater loss of strength.[16] The most common finding relative to the scapulothoracic joint includes weakness of the lower trapezius and serratus anterior muscles with a concurrent increase of overactive upper trapezius muscle.[119,120]

Special Tests

Special tests are designed to confirm or rule out a tentative or preliminary diagnosis. Although strongly suggestive of a particular injury or condition when they yield positive results, they do not necessarily rule out the injury or condition when a negative result is obtained. Ever since Codman's original description of rotator cuff disease, special tests have been developed to identify lesions of the rotator cuff. Tests most commonly included in the shoulder examination of a patient with suspected rotator cuff pathology are those that measure rotator cuff integrity (e.g., empty can test) and detect impingement (e.g., Neer test) (Figure 7-24). Shoulder instability tests should also be included when examining a young, overhead athlete. A comprehensive description of the special tests for the shoulder may be found in *Orthopedic Physical Assessment*.[115] Systematic reviews evaluating many of the special tests used to diagnose rotator cuff disease have found the tests to be adequate at ruling out rotator cuff lesions but less accurate for ruling them in (Table 7-1).[4,109,110,121–123]

Diagnostic Imaging

Although the importance of a thorough history and physical examination for a patient with suspected rotator cuff pathology cannot be understated, the suspicion of an acute rotator cuff tear or the failure of nonoperative treatment supports obtaining objective imaging of the rotator cuff. Imaging helps to confirm or refute a suspected diagnosis, and it assists the clinician with planning further nonoperative and potential operative management. Imaging may also assist the clinician in better assessing the prognosis of a rotator cuff tear.

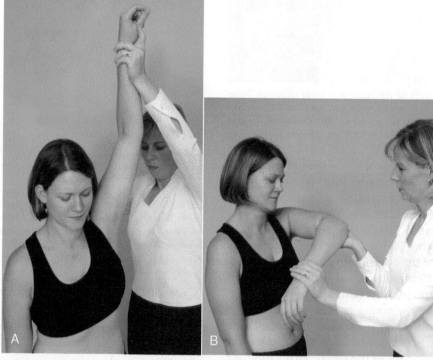

Figure 7-24 Impingement sign. **A,** A positive Neer impingement sign is present if pain and its resulting facial expression are produced when the examiner forcibly flexes the arm forward, jamming the greater tuberosity against the anteroinferior surface of the acromion. **B,** An alternative method (Hawkins-Kennedy impingement test) demonstrates the impingement sign by forcibly medially rotating the proximal humerus when the arm is forward flexed to 90°. (From Magee DJ: *Orthopedic physical assessment*, ed 6, p 318, St Louis, 2014, Saunders/Elsevier.)

TABLE **7-1**

Sensitivity and Specificity of Special Tests for Diagnosis of Rotator Cuff Pathology

Test	Sensitivity	Specificity
Neer's	0.89	0.32
Hawkin's	0.92	0.2
Jobe	0.84	0.58
Empty can	0.89	0.5

Data from Dinnes J, Loveman E, McIntyre L et al: The effectiveness of diagnostic tests for the assessment of shoulder pain due to soft tissue disorders: a systematic review, *Health Technol Assess* 7:iii, 1-166, 2003.

TABLE **7-2**

Sensitivity and Specificity of Diagnostic Tests

Test	Sensitivity	Specificity
MRI: FTT	0.89	0.93
MRI: PTT	0.9	0.44
US: FTT	0.87	0.96
US: PTT	0.67	0.9

MRI, Magnetic resonance imaging; *US,* ultrasound; *FTT,* full-thickness tears; *PTT,* partial-thickness tears

Data from Dinnes J, Loveman E, McIntyre L et al: The effectiveness of diagnostic tests for the assessment of shoulder pain due to soft tissue disorders: a systematic review, *Health Technol Assess* 7:iii, 1-166, 2003.

Many imaging options exist, including x-rays, arthrography, computed tomography arthrography, ultrasound, and magnetic resonance imaging without or with contrast. However, it is critically important to assess imaging in the context of clinical findings. Imaging is highly sensitive, and management based solely on imaging findings may lead to unnecessary or overtreatment.[124]

Multiple studies exist assessing the accuracy of the various imaging modalities for rotator cuff tears. Regional variations exist in the preference of one modality over the other, with computed tomography arthrography being more prominent in Europe than in North America. Studies assessing the accuracy of imaging compared with surgical findings generally provide the highest level of evidence; however, the assessment of atrophy and fatty infiltration cannot be done surgically, which is why these studies provide a measure that is less defined.

Studies with a higher level of evidence exist for the assessment of ultrasound and magnetic resonance imaging, compared with surgical findings, as well as for the comparison of ultrasound, magnetic resonance imaging and magnetic resonance imaging with contrast, and surgical findings. The literature does demonstrate a trend for imaging to define full-thickness tears better, compared with partial-thickness tears and tendinosis, with the accuracy of ultrasound and magnetic resonance imaging decreasing with tears that are less severe. As with all imaging, the results require interpretation and are thus dependent on the skill and experience of the interpreter.

For the evaluation of the rotator cuff specifically, ultrasound should be considered as the imaging modality of choice for the initial detection of full- and partial-thickness rotator cuff tears in patients with a history and clinical findings that do not suggest any other intra-articular disorder.[125] Magnetic resonance imaging may be reserved for cases with equivocal findings and in patients with involvement of anatomical structures not well defined by ultrasound.[126] Ultrasound has the advantage of being noninvasive, well tolerated, inexpensive with minimal risk, and it can be used for bilateral comparisons. However, it does not reveal pathological conditions in bone or intra-articular lesions, and there is a significant

learning curve before obtaining adequate results.[127] In most cases, the use of both modalities is redundant, and their use in combination with the use of magnetic resonance imaging with contrast should be reserved for cases where the desired information can only be provided by the specific modality or combination of modalities.

All of these tests, however, have limitations when compared with the gold standard of arthroscopic surgery. Magnetic resonance imaging has fairly high sensitivity and specificity for full-thickness tears, but for partial-thickness tears, sensitivity is much lower with continued high specificity.[109] Although magnetic resonance imaging is acceptable for ruling in any rotator cuff tears, cost and wait times for testing are additional issues.[108] Ultrasound is also more accurate for full-thickness tears but only fair for evaluating partial-thickness tears (Table 7-2).[109]

TREATMENT OF ROTATOR CUFF PATHOLOGY

Treatment of the patient with rotator cuff pathology is based upon the specific nature of the injury or condition, as well as the individual patient's goals and functional requirements. Care must be taken to understand and address the underlying pathology, as well as the causal factors that led to or are secondarily contributing to the injury. Finally, treatment plans should be based upon information obtained from the patient history and physical examination.

The initial treatment of most rotator cuff injuries, including partial-thickness and some full-thickness tears, is nonoperative. The literature, however, is diverse with respect to best practice recommendations, specifically regarding which patients require surgical intervention and when and what nonoperative interventions are most effective in managing the various rotator cuff pathologies.

Operative versus Nonoperative Management

As mentioned, the majority of rotator cuff injuries benefit from nonoperative management for a period of at least 3 months, before surgical consideration. Exceptions to this include an acute, traumatic tear, especially in a young, active individual or chronic full-thickness tears in patients younger than 65 years of age.[99,101,128] Early operative intervention may also be considered in cases with mitigating factors such as severe recalcitrant pain, inability to work because of symptoms, or timing of surgery according to the start or end of an athlete's season to minimize time lost for recovery.[28] Comparative outcome studies of operative versus nonoperative interventions in rotator cuff patients have yielded inconclusive results. Seida et al.[69] studied the benefits and harm of conservative and surgical treatments on clinically important outcomes in adults with full- and partial-thickness rotator cuff tears. They identified five studies in their review that compared nonoperative with operative treatments. Four of these studies included physical therapy (treatment components not specified) with or without the addition of steroid injections, oral medications, activity modification, or manual therapy.[102,128–130] One study examined the use of shockwave therapy.[131] All study groups showed statistically significant improvements regardless of the intervention; however, the reviewers noted that the evidence was too limited to draw conclusions regarding comparative effectiveness. Decisions regarding which patients with rotator cuff pathology ultimately require surgery and at what stage remain unclear.

Nonoperative Management

The state of evidence, relative to physical therapy management of patients with rotator cuff disease, is limited and of low-moderate methodological quality.[68,102,128–130,132–134] Very little evidence exists to support its effectiveness in treating patients with rotator cuff injuries. Reports of treatment programs are inconsistent and often lacking in detail regarding specific interventions, exercise dosage parameters, and treatment delivery methods. In fact, "physical therapy" is often labeled as the intervention with no further description provided. Very little work has examined the effect of physical therapy on specific rotator cuff pathologies. Most studies combine tendinopathies, impingement syndromes, partial-thickness tears, and full-thickness tears within their study populations, despite evidence that some rotator cuff injuries (i.e., full-thickness tears) require surgical repair.[69,84,85] Conversely, some studies investigate a specific physical therapy intervention (e.g., laser) but have applied it to a heterogeneous sample of patients with varying types of shoulder pathologies.[69,71] Despite this, physical therapy remains a mainstay of treatment for rotator cuff injuries, and clinicians should continue to deliver treatments grounded in general shoulder rehabilitation principles. Goals of treatment include (1) protecting and encouraging optimal healing of the injured rotator cuff muscle or tendon(s) and surrounding tissue, (2) educating patients (including how to avoid repeated injury), (3) managing pain, (4) restoring normal mobility or tissue length of the shoulder girdle and adjacent kinetic

chain segments, (5) restoring normal strength with emphasis on the affected and nonaffected rotator cuff muscles and scapular stabilization muscles, (6) including or encouraging a component of aerobic exercise to the overall treatment, and (7) educating patients on modifying work and recreational activities that may interfere with achievement of the optimum outcome.

Pain is a powerful inhibitor of muscle activation at the shoulder. This is particularly problematic given the number of muscles that act to coordinate shoulder girdle motion, stability, and function. Efforts should be taken to relieve or manage pain in the patient with rotator cuff pathology. This can be accomplished through the use of pain-relieving modalities, patient education, and active exercise. Complete rest from activity is seldom recommended; instead, exercises should be modified by reducing the intensity and/or frequency and altering factors such as arm position (e.g., neutral versus overhead), leverage (e.g., bent elbow versus straight elbow), and degree of motion (e.g., small arc versus large arc exercises). Ideally, exercises should be done within a pain-free ROM, and patients should be instructed on how to manage and monitor pain responses.

Rotator cuff injuries are commonly associated with local and distant deficits in flexibility, strength, and muscle balance that can affect the entire kinetic chain. For example, poor upper-body or trunk posture is often observed in individuals with chronic rotator cuff impingement syndrome. Exercises to correct poor posture should be implemented early in the rehabilitation process, and patients should be instructed that all subsequent exercises begin with establishing "proper posture." Reduced hip and lumbar spine flexibility (i.e., rotation) can lead to increased stress on the shoulder of an overhead athlete. To maintain the maximum force output, the athlete compensates for the loss of hip and trunk flexibility by overextending his or her shoulder into greater degrees of abduction and lateral (external) rotation—a position known to stress the rotator cuff. A breakdown or deficit of any part of the kinetic chain may cause shoulder injury or may occur because of the injury. Regardless, all deficits of the kinetic chain should be noted on assessment and incorporated into the overall treatment plan.

The stabilizing muscles of the scapula should always be included in a strengthening program for the rotator cuff. Scapular winging, abnormal periscapular muscle recruitment, and disruption of the scapulohumeral rhythm are all common in patients with rotator cuff pathology.[116,135] The lower trapezius and serratus anterior muscles are often affected and become "underactive," whereas the upper trapezius compensates and becomes "overactive." The resultant loss of scapular control can contribute to or worsen shoulder impingement, acromioclavicular dysfunction, and rotator cuff disease.[135,136] Proper shoulder rehabilitation should include careful evaluation and treatment of any abnormalities in this region. Patients should be first taught how to perform an isolated contraction of the weakened scapular muscle(s), followed by a sequence of progressions that encourage the muscle(s) to work in a coordinated, synchronous manner with other scapular muscles, postural trunk muscles, and finally muscles of the glenohumeral joint and arm. Proximal stability (i.e., scapular control) must be achieved early in the rehabilitation process, before distal mobility (i.e., glenohumeral and arm movement) is encouraged.

It is important to remember that activation of the rotator cuff muscles involves a concentric movement, whereas stabilization is both static (i.e., isometric) and dynamic (primarily eccentric). Exercise programs should reflect all three of these types of muscle contractions. As previously mentioned, patients must be taught to stabilize their scapula while performing rotator cuff exercises, to ensure a proper base of support for the working muscles. Initially, rotator cuff exercises should be performed with minimal resistance in low-risk positions (i.e., neutral position with a 90° bent elbow) that encourage proper muscle firing without compensation, pain, and/or impingement (Figure 7-25). When appropriate, progressions toward more complex, functional movement patterns that

incorporate the rotator cuff should be initiated. Examples include increasing the amount of glenohumeral elevation, eventually performing rotation in overhead positions; increasing volume and resistance; incorporating muscles and joints from the rest of the upper kinetic chain (e.g., proprioceptive neuromuscular facilitation [PNF] patterns); altering the body's base of support to engage the trunk and lower kinetic chain (e.g., sitting on a physioball, standing on one leg); and proprioception and balance types of exercises (e.g., Body Blade® and closed kinetic chain exercises). The patient's signs and symptoms, as well as his or her ability to perform the exercise(s) properly, are always the best guide for progressing to more challenging levels. The goals of rehabilitation for a patient with a symptomatic, full-thickness rotator cuff tear are a combination of education about activity modification, pain management, and ROM and strengthening exercises that focus on the remaining muscles of the rotator cuff and the supporting musculature.[137,138]

The shoulder complex, particularly the glenohumeral joint, is prone to stiffness after trauma, injury, or immobilization.[139] Early intervention through a combination of gentle stretching and joint mobilization techniques may

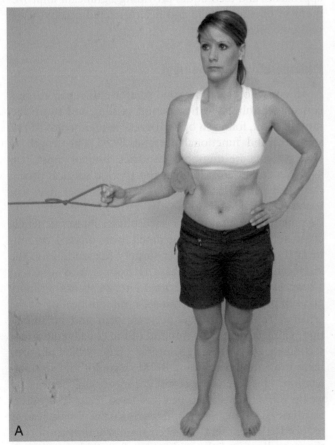 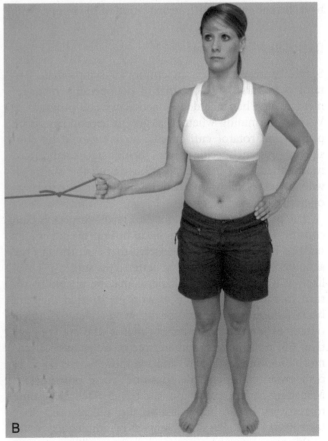

Figure 7-25 Examples of tubing exercises into medial rotation, with the arm at the side, both with (**A**) and without (**B**) a towel at the elbow. Note that the clinician should be cautious in using a towel to hold the elbow against the side. If the patient does not have good control of the scapula, stabilization through the elbow occurs, and using a towel reinforces the incorrect pattern.

prevent this restriction, reduce associated pain, and allow the shoulder to function normally. Special consideration must be given to the adaptive tightening of the gleno-humeral posterior capsule, which presents clinically as a medial (internal) rotation ROM deficit, and to the anterior shoulder muscles (e.g., pectoralis minor), which also tend to shorten because of postural and scapular malpositioning.[116,117,140] The sleeper stretch (for posterior capsule tightness) (see Figure 6-31) and the open book stretch (for pectoralis minor tightness) are two examples of appropriate stretches that may be useful with this patient population. Exercises such as the pendular arm swing and the active-assist stick or cane may be used initially to increase ROM. Once a patient is able to actively move his or her shoulder with proper scapulohumeral rhythm (i.e., no upper trapezius shoulder hiking) and minimal pain, he or she should be progressed to active ROM exercises. Eventually, patients with rotator cuff pathology should be performing a variety of ROM exercises—in both open and closed chain positions, with and without load—that mimic functional movement patterns (see Figure 6-37). The goal of nonsurgical treatment of partial-thickness tears specifically is to ensure that the scar collagen that forms in the defect becomes as supple as a normal tendon. If this does not happen, scar contracture tends to concentrate the load of the rotator cuff on the scar, leading to recurrence and further propagation of the injury.[141,142]

Operative Management

Surgical intervention is an option for symptomatic rotator cuff tears that fail a trial of nonoperative management, which has included an active exercise program.[143] When determining whether surgery is appropriate, both patient and rotator cuff–specific factors should be considered. Patient-specific factors include age, medical comorbidities, worker compensation status, and ability or willingness to follow instructions and participate in postoperative physical therapy.

The primary goal of rotator cuff repair surgery is pain control, and although function can be improved, patients need to be appropriately counseled that even though the shoulder will be significantly better after surgery, it will likely still not be normal. Patients may be unable to return to their previous line of work or sport if they are heavy laborers or overhead or throwing athletes. Surgical outcomes tend to be better in patients who are younger than 65, nonsmokers, and are free of other medical comorbidities such as diabetes and osteoporosis.[143-148] Worker compensation patients demonstrate worse outcomes.[149] Managing patient expectations in terms of length of time to recovery is also important because full recovery may take up to 1 year. Physical therapy is recommended to aid in this recovery, and patients who are unwilling or noncompliant in following postoperative instructions should be counseled to avoid surgical management.

Rotator cuff–specific factors to be considered include tear size, chronicity, and status of the rotator cuff musculature. Large, retracted tears that are associated with significant atrophy of the involved muscles have a worse prognosis with surgical intervention.[143,148,150] For acute traumatic tears, early surgical management should be considered, providing the absence of muscle atrophy and retraction.[143,151]

Surgical repair of the torn rotator cuff can be performed through an arthroscopic, mini-open, or an open approach. The repair involves securing the torn edge of the rotator cuff back down to its native insertion on the proximal humerus. The tendon can be reattached using suture anchors or through transosseous tunnels with heavy suture material. Tears can be repaired either through a formal open incision, a smaller mini-open approach, or an all-arthroscopic technique. Over the past decade, the latter technique has significantly increased in popularity. At the time of surgery, concomitant pathology of the long head of biceps, labrum, and acromioclavicular joint can be treated if warranted. At present, evidence is lacking for routine subacromial decompression or removal of bone from the undersurface of the anterolateral acromion.[152] Furthermore, the type of surgical repair that has the best outcome has yet to be elucidated, with all approaches and techniques providing significant improvement in disease-specific and health-related quality-of-life outcome measures.[153-155]

Postoperative Management

A patient who has undergone rotator cuff repair surgery is managed initially with a period of sling and swath immobilization, followed by a progressive regimen of ROM, strength, and functional exercises.[155-157] The length of time patients are immobilized varies, but for most, it is 4 to 6 weeks, depending on the specific surgical procedure and patient adherence.[156] Most postoperative protocols are divided into phases with specific goals and treatment interventions for each phase. Phases generally coincide with tissue-healing timeframes: phase I extends from 0 to 4 to 6 weeks after surgery (depending on the immobilization period); phase II from 4 to 6 weeks to 12 weeks; and phase III from 12 to 24 weeks. Primary goals of phase I are to encourage optimum healing of the repaired rotator cuff and decrease pain and inflammation. Clinicians must be mindful of the equally important secondary goals during this initial phase, which are protecting glenohumeral joint ROM, scapulothoracic stabilization, kinetic chain exercises, and general health and wellness. Patients should be considered ready to progress to phase II of their rehabilitation if pain is significantly reduced at rest, there has been no disruption to normal tissue healing, and the patient has been able to manage the exercises within phase I. The goals of phase II, following rotator cuff repair, include increasing glenohumeral joint ROM and shoulder girdle strength, while still protecting the healing rotator cuff tissue. During this stage of recovery, patients should begin to resume normal ADL and should be able to engage in increased integration of the whole kinetic chain. Clinicians must remain careful not to disrupt the repair through aggressive stretching or loading of the healing tissue during phase II. By the end of phase II, it is expected that most patients will be able to achieve approximately 120° of active shoulder elevation in either flexion or scaption and about 40° of lateral (external) rotation. Active ROM should be achieved with minimal or no pain and with proper scapulohumeral rhythm.

The primary goals of phase III are directed primarily toward improving strength and endurance of the shoulder girdle. Full, functional ROM of the glenohumeral joint and the entire upper-extremity kinetic chain is also expected by the end of this stage of rehabilitation. The majority of patients achieve these goals and are able to use their affected arm in most to all ADL by 6 months' time. The decision regarding when to return to heavy work and/or overhead sporting activities is generally at the discretion of the surgeon and physical therapist; however, most patients resume these high-demand activities sometime between 6 and 9 months.

REFERENCES

1. Kooijman M, Swinkels I, Dijk CV, et al: Patients with shoulder syndromes in general and physiotherapy practice: an observational study, *BMC Musculoskelet Disord* 14:128–137, 2013.
2. Arce G, Bak K, Bain G, et al: Management of disorders of the rotator cuff: proceedings of the ISAKOS upper extremity committee consensus meeting, *Arthroscopy* 29:1840–1850, 2013.
3. Luime JJ, Koes BW, Heridriksen IJ, et al: The prevalence and incidence of shoulder pain in the general population: a systematic review, *Scand J Rheumatol* 33:73–81, 2004.
4. Hermans J, Luime JJ, Meuffels DE, et al: Does this patient with shoulder pain have rotator cuff disease? The rational clinical examination, a systematic review, *JAMA* 310:837–847, 2013.
5. Dodson CC, Brockmeier SF, Altchek DW: Partial-thickness rotator cuff tears in throwing athletes, *Oper Tech Sports Med* 15:124–131, 2007.
6. Kaplan LD, Flanigan DC, Norwig J, et al: Prevalence and variance of shoulder injuries in elite collegiate football players, *Am J Sports Med* 33:1142–1146, 2005.
7. Fukuda H: Partial-thickness rotator cuff tears: a modern view on Codman's classic, *J Shoulder Elbow Surg* 9:163–168, 2000.
8. Van der Windt DA, Koes BW, Boeke AJ, et al: Shoulder disorders in general practice: prognostic indicators of outcome, *Br J Gen Pract* 46:519–523, 1996.
9. Shin KM: Partial-thickness rotator cuff tears, *Korean J Pain* 24:69–73, 2011.
10. Minagawa H, Yamamoto N, Abe H, et al: Prevalence of symptomatic and asymptomatic rotator cuff tears in the general population: from mass-screening in one village, *J Orthop Med* 10:8–12, 2013.
11. Kibler W, Warme B, Sciascia A, et al: Nonacute shoulder injuries. In Kibler W, editor: *Orthopedic knowledge update: sports medicine*, Rosemont, 2009, American Academy of Orthopedic Surgeons.
12. Milgrom C, Schaffer M, Gilbert S, van Holsbeeck M: Rotator cuff changes in asymptomatic adults: the effect of age, hand dominance and gender, *J Bone Joint Surg Br* 77:296–298, 1995.
13. Tempelhof S, Rupp S, Seil R: Age-related prevalence of rotator cuff tears in asymptomatic shoulders, *J Shoulder Elbow Surg* 8:296–299, 1999.
14. Yamaguchi K, Tetro AM, Blam O, et al: Natural history of asymptomatic rotator cuff tears: a longitudinal analysis of asymptomatic tears detected sonographically, *J Shoulder Elbow Surg* 10:199–203, 2001.
15. Itoi E: Rotator cuff tear: physical examination and conservative treatment, *J Orthop Sci* 18:197–204, 2013.
16. McCabe RA, Nicholas SJ, Montgomery KD, et al: The effect of rotator cuff tear size on shoulder strength and range of motion, *J Orthop Sports Phys Ther* 35:130–135, 2005.
17. Piitulainen K, Ylinen J, Kautiainen H, et al: The relationship between functional disability and health related quality of life in patients with a rotator cuff tear, *Disabil Rehabil* 34:2071–2075, 2012.
18. Mighell M: Massive irreparable rotator cuff tears. In Frankle M, editor: *Rotator cuff deficiency of the shoulder*, New York, 2008, Thieme Medical.
19. Harryman DT, Clark Jr. JM: Anatomy of the rotator cuff. In Burkhead WZ, editor: *Rotator cuff disorders*, Philadelphia, 1996, Williams & Wilkins.
20. Warner JJ: The gross anatomy of the joint surfaces, ligaments, labrum and capsule. In Matsen FA, Fu FH, Hawkins RJ, editors: *The shoulder: a balance of mobility and stability*, Rosemont, 1993, American Academy of Orthopedic Surgeons.
21. De Franco MJ, Cole BJ: Current perspectives on rotator cuff anatomy, *Arthroscopy* 25:305–320, 2009.
22. Clark JM, Harryman II DT: Tendons, ligaments and capsule of the rotator cuff. Gross and microscopic anatomy, *J Bone Joint Surg Am* 74:713–725, 1992.
23. Vangsness CT, Jorgenson SS, Watson T, et al: The origin of the long head of the biceps from the scapula and glenoid labrum, *J Bone Joint Surg Br* 76:951–954, 1994.
24. Rodowsky MW, Harner CD, Fu FH: The role of the long head of the biceps muscle and superior glenoid labrum in anterior stability of the shoulder, *Am J Sports Med* 22:121–130, 1994.
25. Itoi E, Kuechle DK, Newman SR, et al: Stabilizing function of the biceps in stable and unstable shoulders, *J Bone Joint Surg Br* 75:546–550, 1993.
26. Dugas JR, Campbell DA, Warren RF, et al: Anatomy and dimensions of rotator cuff insertions, *J Shoulder Elbow Surg* 11:498–503, 2002.
27. Ruotolo C, Fow JE, Nottage WM: The supraspinatus footprint: an anatomic study of the supraspinatus insertion, *Arthroscopy* 20:246–249, 2004.
28. Browning DG, Desai MM: Rotator cuff injuries and treatment, *Prim Care* 31:807–829, 2004.
29. Yamaguchi K, Riew KD, Galatz CM: Biceps function in normal and rotator cuff deficient shoulders: an EMG analysis, *Orthop Trans* 18:191, 1994.
30. Neer II CS: Impingement lesions, *Clin Orthop* 173:70–77, 1983.
31. Gschwend N, Ivosevik-Radovanovi D, Patte D: Rotator cuff tear-relationship between clinical and anatomopathological findings, *Arch Orthop Trauma Surg* 107:7–15, 1988.
32. Bigliani LU, Morrison D, April E: The morphology of the acromion and rotator cuff impingement, *Orthop Trans* 10:228–235, 1986.
33. Bigliani LU, Ticker JB, Flatow EL, et al: The relationship of acromial architecture to rotator cuff disease, *Clin Sports Med* 10:823–838, 1991.
34. Ardic F, Kahraman Y, Kacar M, et al: Shoulder impingement syndrome: relationships between clinical, functional, and radiological findings, *Am J Phys Med Rehabil* 85:53–60, 2006.
35. Ludewig PM, Braman JP: Shoulder impingement: biomechanical considerations in rehabilitation, *Man Ther* 16:33–39, 2011.
36. Morrison D, Bigliani L: The clinical significance of variations in acromial morphology, *Orthop Trans* 11:234–242, 1987.
37. Zuckerman JD, Kummer FJ, Cuomo F, et al: Interobserver reliability of acromial morphology classification: an anatomic study, *J Shoulder Elbow Surg* 6:286–287, 1997.
38. Cuomo F, Kummer FJ, Zuckerman JD, et al: The influence of acromioclavicular joint morphology on rotator cuff tears, *J Shoulder Elbow Surg* 7:555–559, 1998.
39. Fu FH, Harner CD, Klein AH: Shoulder impingement syndrome: a critical review, *Clin Orthop* 269:162–173, 1991.
40. Hashimoto T, Nobuhara K: Pathologic evidence of degeneration as a primary cause of rotator cuff tear, *Clin Orthop Relat Res* 415:111–120, 2003.
41. Machida A, Sugamoto K, Miyamoto T, et al: Adhesion of the subacromial bursa may cause subacromial impingement in patients with rotator cuff tears: pressure measurements in 18 patients, *Acta Orthop Scand* 75:109–113, 2004.
42. Soslowsky LJ, Carpenter JE, Buccieri JS, et al: Biomechanics of the rotator cuff, *Orthop Clin North Am* 28:17–30, 1997.
43. Labriola JE, Lee TQ, Debski RE, et al: Stability and instability of the glenohumeral joint: the role of shoulder muscles, *J Shoulder Elbow Surg* 14:32S–38S, 2005.
44. Wuelker N, Wirth CJ, Plitz W, et al: A dynamic shoulder model: reliability testing and muscle force study, *J Biomech* 28:489–499, 1995.
45. Morrey BF, Itoi E, An K: Biomechanics of the shoulder. In Rockwood CA, Matsen FA, editors: *The shoulder*, Philadelphia, 1998, WB Saunders.
46. Bradley JP, Tibone JE: Electromyographic analysis of muscle action about the shoulder, *Clin Sports Med* 10:789–805, 1991.
47. Habermeyer P, Walch G: The biceps tendon and rotator cuff disease. In Burkhead WZ Jr., editors: *Rotator cuff disorders*, Media, 1996, Williams & Wilkins.
48. Snyder SJ, Karzel RP, Del Pizzo W: SLAP lesions of the shoulder, *Arthroscopy* 6:274–279, 1990.
49. Andrews J, Carson W, McLeod W: Glenoid labrum tears related to the long head of the biceps, *Am J Sports Med* 13:337–341, 1985.

50. Burkhart SS, Morgan CD, Kibler WB: The disabled throwing shoulder: spectrum of pathology part II: evaluation and treatment of SLAP lesions in throwers, *Arthroscopy* 19:531–539, 2003.

51. Sharkey NA, Marder RA, Hanson PB: The entire rotator cuff contributes to elevation of the arm, *J Orthop Res* 12:699–708, 1994.

52. Mehta S, Gimbel JA, Soslowsky LJ: Etiologic and pathogenetic factors for rotator cuff tendinopathy, *Clin Sports Med* 22:791–812, 2003.

53. Matsen FA III: Rotator cuff failure, *N Engl J Med* 358:2138–2147, 2008.

54. Wolf AB, Sethi P, Sutton KM, et al: Partial-thickness rotator cuff tears, *J Am Acad Orthop Surg* 14:715–725, 2006.

55. Gramstad G, Yamaguchi K: Anatomy, pathogenesis, natural history and nonsurgical treatment of rotator cuff disorders. In Galatz L, editor: *Orthopedic knowledge update: shoulder and elbow*, Rosemont, 2007, American Academy of Orthopedic Surgeons.

56. Chansky HA, Iannotti JP: The vascularity of the rotator cuff, *Clin Sports Med* 10:807–922, 1991.

57. Ling SC, Chen CF, Wan RX: A study on the vascular supply of the supraspinatus tendon, *Surg Radiol Anat* 12:161–165, 1990.

58. Lohr JF, Uhthoff HK: The microvascular pattern of the supraspinatus tendon, *Clin Orthop* 254:35–38, 1990.

59. Rathbun JB, Macnab I: The microvascular pattern of the rotator cuff, *J Bone Joint Surg Br* 52:540–553, 1970.

60. Kumagai J, Sarkar K, Uhthoff HK: The collagen types in the attachment zone of rotator cuff tendons in the elderly: an immunohistochemical study, *J Rheumatol* 21:2096–2100, 1994.

61. Nakajima T: Histologic and biomechanical characteristics of the supraspinatus tendon: reference to rotator cuff tearing, *J Shoulder Elbow Surg* 3:79–87, 1994.

62. Ishii H, Brunet JA, Welsh RP, et al: Bursal reactions in rotator cuff tearing, the impingement syndrome and calcifying tendonitis, *J Shoulder Elbow Surg* 6:131–136, 1997.

63. Bey MJ, Song HK, Wehrli FW, et al: Intratendinous strain fields of the intact supraspinatus tendon: the effect of glenohumeral joint position and tendon region, *J Orthop Res* 20:869–874, 2002.

64. Codman EA: Rupture of the supraspinatus tendon and other lesions in or about the subacromial bursa. In Codman EA, editor: *The shoulder*, Boston, 1934, Thomas Todd.

65. Ellman H: Diagnosis and treatment of incomplete rotator cuff tears, *Clin Orthop Relat Res* 254:64–74, 1990.

66. Snyder SJ: Arthroscopic classification of rotator cuff lesions and surgical decision making. In Snyder SJ, editor: *Shoulder arthroscopy*, ed 2, Philadelphia, 2003, Lippincott Williams & Wilkins.

67. Lewis J: Rotator cuff tendinopathy, *Br J Sports Med* 43:236–241, 2009.

68. Littlewood C, Ashton J, Chance-Larsen K, et al: Exercise for rotator cuff tendinopathy: a systematic review, *Physiotherapy* 98:101–109, 2012.

69. Seida JC, LeBlanc C, Schouten JR, et al: Systematic review: nonoperative and operative treatments for rotator cuff tears, *Ann Intern Med* 153:246–255, 2010.

70. Desmeules F, Cote C, Fremont P: Therapeutic exercise and orthopedic manual therapy for impingement syndrome: a systematic review, *Clin J Sports Med* 13:176–182, 2003.

71. Grant H, Arthur A, Pichora D: Evaluations of interventions for rotator cuff pathology, *J Hand Ther* 17:274–299, 2004.

72. Johansson K, Oberg B, Adolfsson L, et al: A combination of systematic review and clinicians' beliefs in interventions for subacromial pain, *Br J Gen Pract* 52:145–152, 2002.

73. Littlewood C, Malliaras P, Mawson S, et al: Development of a self-managed loaded exercise programme for rotator cuff tendinopathy, *Physiotherapy* 99:358–362, 2013.

74. Neer CS II: Anterior acromioplasty for the chronic impingement syndrome in the shoulder. A preliminary report, *J Bone Joint Surg Am* 54:41–50, 1972.

75. Jobe F, Kvitne R: Shoulder pain in the overhead athlete: the relationship of anterior instability and rotator cuff impingement, *Orthop Rev* 18:963–975, 1989.

76. Kvitne RS, Jobe FW: The diagnosis and treatment of anterior instability in the throwing athlete, *Clin Orthop* 291:107–123, 1993.

77. Jain NB, Higgins LD, Losina E, et al: Epidemiology of musculoskeletal upper extremity ambulatory surgery in the United States, *BMC Musculoskelet Disord* 15:4–7, 2014.

78. Iannotti JP: Lesions of the rotator cuff: pathology and pathogenesis. In Matsen FA, Fu FH, Hawkins RJ, editors: *The shoulder: a balance of mobility and stability*, Rosemont, 1993, American Academy of Orthopedic Surgeons.

79. Matava MJ, Purcell DB, Rudzki JR: Partial-thickness rotator cuff tears, *Am J Sports Med* 33:1405–1417, 2005.

80. Pettersson G: Rupture of the tendon aponeurosis of the shoulder joint in anterior-inferior dislocation, *Acta Chir Scand Suppl* 77:1–87, 1942.

81. Smith MA, Smith WT: Rotator cuff tears, *Orthop Nurs* 29:319–322, 2010.

82. Lehman C, Cuomo F, Kummer FJ, et al: The incidence of full thickness rotator cuff tears in a large cadaveric population, *Bull Hosp Joint Dis* 54:30–31, 1995.

83. Norwood LA, Barrack R: Clinical presentation of complete tears of the rotator cuff, *J Bone Joint Surg Am* 71:499–505, 1989.

84. Bedi A, Dines J, Warren RF, et al: Massive tears of the rotator cuff, *J Bone Joint Surg Am* 92:1894–1908, 2010.

85. Gerber C, Fuchs B, Hodler J: The results of repair of massive tears of the rotator cuff, *J Bone Joint Surg Am* 82:505–515, 2000.

86. Visotsky JL, Basamania C, Seebauer L, et al: Cuff tear arthropathy: pathogenesis, classification and algorithm for treatment, *J Bone Joint Surg Am* 86:35–40, 2004.

87. Neer CS II, Craig EV, Fukuda H: Cuff-tear arthropathy, *J Bone Joint Surg Am* 65:1232–1244, 1983.

88. Weiss NS: *Clinical epidemiology: the study of the outcome of illness*, Oxford, 2006, Oxford University Press.

89. Tempelhof S, Rupp S, Seil R: Age-related prevalence of rotator cuff tears in asymptomatic shoulders, *J Shoulder Elbow Surg* 8:296–299, 1999.

90. Sher JS, Uribe JW, Posada A, et al: Abnormal findings on magnetic resonance images of asymptomatic shoulders, *J Bone Joint Surg Am* 77:10–15, 1995.

91. Yamaguchi K, Sher JS, Andersen WK: Glenohumeral motion in patients with rotator cuff tears: a comparison of asymptomatic and symptomatic shoulders, *J Shoulder Elbow Surg* 9:6–11, 2000.

92. Mall NA, Kim HM, Keener JD, et al: Symptomatic progression of asymptomatic rotator cuff tears: a prospective study of clinical and sonographic variables, *J Bone Joint Surg Am* 92:2623–2633, 2010.

93. Maman E, Harris C, White L, et al: Outcome of nonoperative treatment of symptomatic rotator cuff tears monitored by magnetic resonance imaging, *J Bone Joint Surg Am* 91A:1898–1906, 2009.

94. Yamanaka K, Matsumoto T: The joint side tear of the rotator cuff: a follow-up study by arthrography, *Clin Orthop* 304:68–73, 1994.

95. Fukuda H: The management of partial thickness tears of the rotator cuff, *J Bone Joint Surg Br* 85:3–11, 2003.

96. Baysal D, Balyk R: Functional outcome and health-related quality of life after surgical repair of full thickness rotator cuff tear using a mini-open technique, *Am J Sports Med* 33:1346–1355, 2005.

97. Harryman DT, Hettrich CM: A prospective, multipractice investigation of patients with full thickness rotator cuff tears: the importance of comorbidities, practice and other covariables on self-assessed shoulder function and health status, *J Bone Joint Surg Am* 85:690–696, 2003.

98. Williams GR, Rockwood CA, Bigliani LU, et al: Rotator cuff tears: why do we repair them? *J Bone Joint Surg Am* 86:2764–2776, 2004.

99. Tashjian RZ: Epidemiology, natural history, and indications for treatment of rotator cuff tears, *Clin Sports Med* 31:589–604, 2012.

100. Wu XL, Briggs L, Murrell GAC: Intraoperative determinants of rotator cuff repair integrity: an analysis of 500 consecutive repairs, *Am J Sports Med* 40:2771–2776, 2012.

101. Franceschi F, Papalia R, Del Buono A, et al: Repair of partial tears of the rotator cuff, *Sports Med Arthro Rev* 19:401–408, 2011.

102. Vad VB, Warren RF, Altchek DW, et al: Negative prognostic factors in managing massive rotator cuff tears, *Clin J Sport Med* 12:151–157, 2002.

103. Millstein MS, Snyder SJ: Arthroscopic evaluation and management of rotator cuff tears, *Orthop Clin North Am* 34:507–520, 2003.

104. Ben-Yishay A, Zuckerman JD, Gallagher M, et al: Pain inhibition of shoulder strength in patients with impingement syndrome, *Orthopedics* 17:685–688, 1994.

105. Gomberawalla MM, Sekiya JK: Rotator cuff tear and glenohumeral instability: a systematic review, *Clin Orthop Relat Res* 472:2448–2456, 2014.

106. De Witte PB, Henseler JF, Nagels J, et al: The Western Ontario Rotator Cuff Index in rotator cuff disease patients: a comprehensive reliability and responsiveness validation study, *Am J Sports Med* 40:1611–1619, 2012.

107. Xiao J, Cui GQ, Wang JQ: Diagnosis of bursal-side partial-thickness rotator cuff tears, *Orthop Surg* 2:260–265, 2010.

108. Ekeberg OM, Bautz-Holter E, Juel NG, et al: Clinical, socio-demographic and radiological predictors of short-term outcome in rotator cuff disease, *BMC Musculoskelet Disord* 11:239–247, 2010.

109. Dinnes J, Loveman E, McIntyre L, et al: The effectiveness of diagnostic tests for the assessment of shoulder pain due to soft tissue disorders: a systematic review, *Health Technol Assess* 7(iii):1–166, 2003.

110. Hanchard CA, Nigel R, Lenza M, et al: Physical tests for shoulder impingements and local lesions of bursa, tendon or labrum that may accompany impingement, *CDSR* 4:2013 Apr 30, CD007427.

111. Castoldi F, Bionna D, Hertel R: External rotation lag sign revisited: accuracy for diagnosis of full thickness supraspinatus tear, *J Shoulder Elbow Surg* 18:529–534, 2009.

112. Park H, Yokota A, Gill H, et al: Diagnostic accuracy of clinical tests for the different degrees of subacromial impingement syndrome, *J Bone Joint Surg Am* 87:1446–1455, 2005.

113. Millican J, Murrell G: Can handheld dynamometers diagnose partial-thickness rotator cuff tears? *Br Elbow Shoulder Soc* 4:100–105, 2012.

114. Litaker D, Pioro M, El Bilbeisi H, et al: Returning to the bedside: using the history and physical examination

to identify rotator cuff tears, *J Am Geriatr Soc* 48:1633–1637, 2000.

115. Magee DJ: *Orthopedic physical assessment*, ed 6, St. Louis, 2014, Saunders/Elsevier.

116. Burkhart SS, Morgan CD, Kibler WB: The disabled throwing shoulder: spectrum of pathology part III—the SICK scapula, scapular dyskinesis, the kinetic chain and rehabilitation, *Arthroscopy* 19:641–661, 2003.

117. Myers JB, Laudner KG, Pasquale MR, et al: Glenohumeral range of motion deficits and posterior shoulder tightness in throwers with pathologic internal impingement, *Am J Sports Med* 34:385–391, 2006.

118. Sauers EL, Huxel Bliven KC, Johnson MP, et al: Hip and glenohumeral rotational range of motion in healthy professional baseball pitchers and position players, *Am J Sports Med* 42:430–436, 2014.

119. Huang HY, Lin JJ, Guo YL, et al: EMG biofeedback effectiveness to alter muscle activity pattern and scapular kinematics in subjects with and without shoulder impingement, *J Electromyogr Kinesiol* 23:267–274, 2013.

120. Merolla G, De Santis E, Campi F, et al: Supraspinatus and infraspinatus weakness in overhead athletes with scapular dyskinesis: strength assessment before and after restoration of scapular musculature balance, *Musculoskelet Surg* 94:119–125, 2010.

121. Beaudril J, Nizard R, Thomas T, et al: Contribution of clinical tests to the diagnosis of rotator cuff disease: a systematic literature review, *Joint Bone Spine* 76:15–19, 2009.

122. Hegedus EJ, Goode A, Campbell S, et al: Physical examination tests of the shoulder: a systematic review with meta-analysis of individual tests, *Br J Sports Med* 42:80–92, 2008.

123. Hughes P, Taylor N, Green RA: Most clinical tests cannot accurately diagnose rotator cuff pathology: a systematic review, *Aust J Physiother* 54:159–170, 2008.

124. Miller M, Flatow E, et al: Biomechanics of the coracoacromial arch and rotator cuff; kinematics and contact of the subacromial space. In Iannotti JP, editor: *The rotator cuff: current concepts and complex problems*, Rosemont, 1998, American Academy of Orthopedic Surgeons.

125. Fotiadou AN, Vlychou M, Papadopoulos P, et al: Ultrasonography of symptomatic rotator cuff tears compared with MR imaging and surgery, *Eur J Radiol* 68:174–179, 2008.

126. Vlychou M, Dailiana Z: Symptomatic partial rotator cuff tears: diagnostic performance of ultrasound and magnetic resonance imaging with surgical correlation, *Acta Radiol* 50:101–105, 2009.

127. Moosmayer S, Lund G, Seljom U, et al: Comparison between surgery and physiotherapy in the treatment of small and medium-sized tears of the rotator cuff, *J Bone Joint Surg Br* 92:83–91, 2010.

128. Lunn JV, Castellanos-Rosas J, Tavernier T, et al: A novel lesion of the infraspinatus characterized by musculotendinous disruption, edema, and late fatty infiltration, *J Shoulder Elbow Surg* 17:546–553, 2008.

129. Yamada N, Hamada K, Nakajima, et al: Comparison of conservative and operative treatments of massive rotator cuff tears, *Tokai J Exp Clin Med* 25:151–163, 2000.

130. De Carli A, Vulpiani M, Russo A, et al: Reparable rotator cuff tears: surgery vs. shock wave therapy, *J Orthop Traumatol* 7:S51, 2006.

131. Ellenbecker TS, Cools A: Rehabilitation of shoulder impingement syndrome and rotator cuff injuries: an evidence-based review, *Br J Sports Med* 44:319–327, 2010.

132. Hayes K, Ginn KA, Walton JR, et al: A randomised clinical trial evaluating the efficacy of physiotherapy after rotator cuff repair, *Austr J Physiother* 50:77–83, 2004.

133. Ainsworth R, Lewis JS: Exercise therapy for the conservative management of full thickness tears of the rotator cuff: a systematic review, *Br J Sports Med* 41:200–210, 2007.

134. Kibler WB, McMullen J: Scapular dyskinesis and its relation to shoulder pain, *J Am Acad Orthop Surg* 11:142–151, 2003.

135. Kibler WB, Sciascia A: Current concepts: scapular dyskinesis, *Br J Sports Med* 44:300–305, 2010.

136. Neri BR, Chan KW, Kwon YW: Management of massive and irreparable rotator cuff tears, *J Shoulder Elbow Surg* 18:808–818, 2009.

137. Ainsworth R: Physiotherapy rehabilitation in patients with massive, irreparable rotator cuff tears, *Musculoskelet Care* 4:140–151, 2006.

138. Tauro JC: Stiffness and rotator cuff tears: incidence, arthroscopic findings, and treatment results, *Arthroscopy* 22:581–586, 2006.

139. Rubin BD, Kibler WB: Fundamental principles of shoulder rehabilitation: conservative to postoperative management, *Arthroscopy* 18:29–39, 2002.

140. Bytomski JR, Black D: Conservative treatment of rotator cuff injuries, *J Surg Orthop Adv* 15:126–131, 2006.

141. Andrews JR: Diagnosis and treatment of chronic painful shoulder: review of nonsurgical interventions, *Arthroscopy* 21:333–347, 2005.

142. Tashjian RZ: Epidemiology, natural history, and indications for treatment of rotator cuff tears, *Clin Sports Med* 31:589–604, 2012.

143. Oh JH, Kim SH, Kang JY, et al: Effect of age on functional and structural outcome after rotator cuff repair, *Am J Sports Med* 38:672–678, 2010.

144. Favard L, Bacle G, Berhouet J: Rotator cuff repair, *Joint Bone Spine* 74:551–557, 2007.

145. Mallon WJ, Misamore G, Snead DS, et al: The impact of preoperative smoking habits on the results of rotator cuff repair, *J Shoulder Elbow Surg* 13:129–132, 2004.

146. Clement ND, Hallett A, MacDonald D, et al: Does diabetes affect outcomes after arthroscopic rotator cuff repair? *J Bone Joint Surg Br* 92:1112–1117, 2010.

147. Chung SW, Oh JH, Gong HS, et al: Factors affecting rotator cuff healing after arthroscopic repair: osteoporosis as one of the independent risk factors, *Am J Sports Med* 39:2099–2107, 2011.

148. Frank Henn III R, Kang L, Tashjian RZ, et al: Patients with workers' compensation claims have worse outcomes after rotator cuff repair, *J Bone Joint Surg Am* 90:2105–2113, 2008.

149. Wu XL, Briggs L, Murrell GAC: Intraoperative determinants of rotator cuff repair integrity: an analysis of 500 consecutive repairs, *Am J Sports Med* 40:2771–2776, 2012.

150. Hantes ME, Karidakis GK, Vlychou M, et al: A comparison of early versus delayed repair of traumatic rotator cuff tears, *Knee Surg Sports Traumatol Arthrosc* 19:1766–1770, 2011.

151. Shi LL, Edwards B: The role of acromioplasty for the management of rotator cuff problems: where is the evidence? *Adv Orthop* 2012:467–475, 2012.

152. Sheibani-Rad S, Giveans MR, Arnoczky SP, et al: Arthroscopic single-row versus double-row rotator cuff repair: a meta-analysis of the randomized clinical trials, *Arthroscopy* 29:343–348, 2013.

153. Nho SJ, Shindle MK, Sherman SL, et al: Systematic review of arthroscopic rotator cuff repair and mini-open rotator cuff repair, *J Bone Joint Surg Am* 89:127–136, 2007.

154. van der Zwaal P, Bregje JW, Nieuwenhuijse MJ, et al: Clinical outcome in all-arthroscopic versus mini-open rotator cuff repair in small to medium-sized tears: a randomized controlled trial in 100 patients with 1-year follow-up, *Arthroscopy* 29:266–273, 2013.

155. Ghodadra NS, Provencher MT, Verma NN, et al: Open, mini-open, and all-arthroscopic rotator cuff repair surgery: indications and implications for rehabilitation, *J Orthop Sports Phys Ther* 39:81–89, 2009.

156. Jackins S: Postoperative shoulder rehabilitation, *Phys Med Rehabil Clin North Am* 15:643–682, 2004.

157. Millett PJ, Wilcox RB, O'Holleran JD, et al: Rehabilitation of the rotator cuff: an evaluation-based approach, *J Am Acad Orthop Surg* 14:599–609, 2006.

CHAPTER 8

Shoulder Arthroplasty

TIMOTHY F. TYLER, THOMAS F. HOBSON, STEPHEN J. NICHOLAS, NEIL S. ROTH

INTRODUCTION

According to the American Academy of Orthopaedic Surgeons, approximately 4 million people in the United States seek medical care each year for shoulder problems. These conditions range from injuries, such as dislocations and fractures, to chronic debilitating diseases, such as arthritis. Shoulder arthroplasty has been available to patients with severe, chronic, debilitating shoulder pathology since the early 1960s (Figure 8-1).[1-3] Like other joint replacement surgeries, it is designed to remove diseased portions of bone and joint and replace them with a prosthesis, thereby reducing the friction caused by disease and improving range of motion (ROM), eliminating the associated pain.

PREVALENCE OF SHOULDER ARTHROPLASTY

The prevalence of total shoulder arthroplasty in the United States is less than that of total hip or knee arthroplasty but more than total elbow replacements. Shoulder arthroplasty has become the treatment of choice for many patients with a glenohumeral articular disease. The frequency of shoulder arthroplasties has increased substantially, from approximately 10,000 in 1990 to 20,000 in 2000.[4] From 1990 to 1993, fewer than 5000 total shoulder arthroplasties were performed each year in this country; in comparison, combined hip and knee replacement operations exceeded 500,000 per year. According to an orthopedic news source, the prevalence of total shoulder arthroplasty in 1998 was 15,266, of which 8556 were hemiarthroplasties and 6710 were total shoulder athroplasties.[5] As the average age of the population increases and the outcome of shoulder arthroplasty continues to improve, the prevalence of this procedure will continue to rise.

ANATOMY AND JOINT DESIGN

Because of its anatomy and design, the glenohumeral joint does not lend itself to mechanical overload and cartilaginous breakdown. This non–weight-bearing joint is a ball and socket joint. The top of the humerus widens and forms the humeral head, which fits into a shallow socket of the scapula (glenoid fossa). During motion the humeral head moves upon the glenoid fossa, providing a wide ROM. Because of the fit of these two bones, very little surface area of the bones is actually in contact at any given moment, which may contribute to site-specific cartilage breakdown. The stability of the glenohumeral joint relies primarily on the joint capsule and the rotator cuff musculature. The tendons of the rotator cuff help create dynamic stability to the glenohumeral joint by connecting the humerus to the scapula. The primary force producer of the glenohumeral joint is the large deltoid muscle, which creates a force couple with the rotator cuff to allow normal kinematics to occur.

A layer of articular cartilage covers the head of the humerus and the surface of the glenoid fossa; in a healthy joint, this cartilaginous layer protects the bones against friction during movement. In addition, the glenoid labrum surrounds the periphery of the glenoid fossa and provides a slightly deeper socket for the humeral head to rest in. The joint capsule is lined with a synovial membrane, which provides synovial fluid to help reduce friction. In a normal glenohumeral joint, these parts work together to provide stability during a wide ROM. When any of these joint surfaces become diseased, the normally smooth surface becomes rough, causing friction and pain (Figure 8-2). Arthritis leads to the breakdown of cartilage, allowing the bones to rub against each other. When this happens, scar tissue and bone spurs may also develop, leading to further pain and stiffness.

INDICATIONS FOR SHOULDER ARTHROPLASTY

Many different conditions can affect the glenohumeral joint and lead to a discussion about total shoulder replacement. (A hemiarthroplasty replaces the humeral head only, whereas a total shoulder arthroplasty involves replacing the glenoid fossa as well.) Some of these

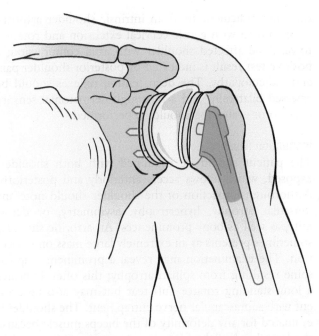

Figure 8-1 Components of a total shoulder arthroplasty.

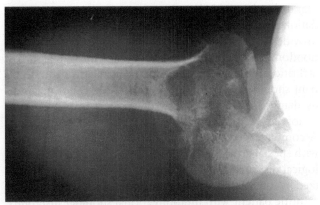

Figure 8-3 Proximal humeral fracture requiring shoulder arthroplasty.

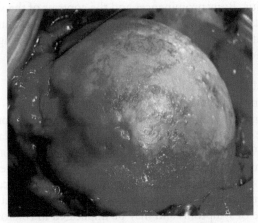

Figure 8-2 Humeral head with severe degenerative disease.

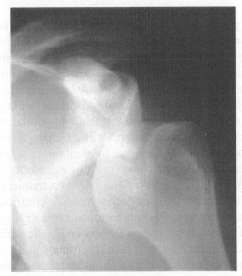

Figure 8-4 Inferior glenohumeral dislocation.

conditions include rheumatoid arthritis, osteoarthritis, rotator cuff arthropathy, avascular necrosis, fractures of the shoulder region, and a failed shoulder prosthesis (from a previous joint replacement).[6-9] Some proximal humeral fractures (e.g., displaced anatomical neck fractures, four-part fractures, fracture-dislocations, and head-splitting fractures) are also indications for shoulder replacement (Figure 8-3).[10-13]

Deterioration of the glenohumeral joint after capsulorrhaphy for recurrent instability is more common in athletes; this condition arises more commonly after surgical procedures such as Bristow, Magnuson-Stack, and Putti-Platt and less commonly after the Bankart and capsular shift procedures.

Pain relief is the primary indication for total shoulder arthroplasty. Most surgeons are cautious about recommending shoulder replacement for improved ROM and function. However, the most common reason for total shoulder arthroplasty is arthritis. Because arthritis causes the cartilage to break down, it can cause a number of associated problems, such as scar formation and osteophytes. Posttraumatic arthritis is a form of osteoarthritis that develops after an injury, such as a fracture or dislocation of the shoulder (Figure 8-4). Arthritis also can develop after a rotator cuff tear. Rheumatoid arthritis is a systemic inflammatory condition of the joint lining that can affect people of any age and that usually affects multiple joints on both sides of the body.

EVALUATION OF THE ARTHRITIC SHOULDER

History

Total shoulder arthroplasty has become the treatment of choice for most glenohumeral arthritides. A systematic, reproducible approach to each patient ensures comprehensive information gathering and therefore the proper diagnosis and choice of surgical procedure. Initially the patient's age, hand dominance, occupation, athletic activities, medical history, and family history are recorded.

Hand dominance is important to treatment recommendations because the dominant arm of an active individual provides a different therapeutic challenge than the nondominant shoulder of a sedentary individual. Most arthritic shoulders and rotator cuff tears affect the dominant shoulder.[14] Although a patient's age is not necessarily diagnostic, full-thickness rotator cuff tears are found almost exclusively in patients more than 50 years of age. A complete general medical history should be obtained, with special attention given to any systemic or rheumatological disorders. In addition, a family history of generalized ligamentous laxity is important in the treatment of an arthritic patient with multidirectional shoulder instability. A previous incident of trauma can be the precursor of an arthritic shoulder; this can be an important piece of information in presurgical planning.

The patient's chief shoulder complaint usually consists of some element of pain, weakness, or loss of motion. Documenting the pattern of these symptoms is important, most notably the duration, severity, provocation, and location. Shoulder arthritis can arise from a traumatic event, but it often is atraumatic in origin, arising from repetitive loading. Severe night pain and pain at rest are common complaints in patients with mechanical shoulder pathology and usually are due to glenohumeral arthritis; however, infection and tumor must be ruled out.

Weakness of the affected shoulder is a frequent complaint, but splinting from pain commonly contributes to this lack of strength. Patients with concomitant large rotator cuff tears often report weakness or fatigue with overhead use, but they also can have surprisingly good motion and function once the arthritic shoulder has been replaced. Patients also may complain of "crackling" in their shoulders with motion; this can be due to a variety of disorders, including full-thickness tears (which produce crepitus when the greater tuberosity comes into contact with the undersurface of the acromion), glenohumeral osteoarthritis, and acromioclavicular (AC) arthritis. However, when the "crackling" is accompanied by severe pain on movement, glenohumeral osteoarthritis needs to be ruled out.

Physical Examination

Physical examination of the arthritic shoulder should proceed in an organized, reproducible manner. The examination consists of five basic parts: inspection, palpation, ROM, strength testing, and provocative tests. The shoulder often is the site of referred pain, commonly from the cervical spine. Therefore the cervical spine must be thoroughly examined for any coexisting or referred pathology. Often a patient with shoulder arthritis has some degree of cervical spine arthritis and some degree of referred pain to the shoulder. The cervical spine is brought through an ROM, including flexion, extension, and lateral rotation. Pain and crepitation with motion should be noted. Spurling's test, which is effective in distinguishing cervi-

cal spine radiculopathy from intrinsic shoulder arthritis, is performed with gentle cervical extension and rotation toward the affected shoulder with axial compression; a positive test result is indicated by posterior shoulder pain and radiculopathy. The deep tendon reflexes should be assessed bilaterally, and a thorough dermatomal sensory and motor evaluation should be performed.

Inspection (Observation)
The patient should be examined with both shoulders exposed, which allows access anteriorly and posteriorly. A thorough inspection of the shoulder should note any muscular atrophy, hypertrophy, asymmetry, or deformity, as well as bony prominences. An arthritic shoulder sometimes presents as an extremely large mass on inspection. The examination may reveal a prominent scapular spine resulting from spinati atrophy; this often indicates a long-standing rotator cuff tear but may also be present with suprascapular nerve entrapment. The shoulder is evaluated for any deformity of the biceps muscle because the long head of the biceps tendon often is ruptured in patients with rotator cuff disease and severe glenohumeral arthritis. Bony prominences and the contour of the shoulder also are noted because a patient with glenohumeral arthritis loses normal contour and shows squaring and anterior fullness.

Palpation
Palpation around the shoulder joint should be done systematically so that each muscle, joint, and bony prominence is evaluated. The sternoclavicular joint; the clavicle; the AC joint; the anterior, lateral, and posterior acromion; the anterior and posterior joint lines; and the biceps tendon each should be tested for discrete tenderness. Localized tenderness over the AC joint often is overlooked as a source of symptoms and may be implicated in rotator cuff pathology or degenerative joint disease. Pain often is elicited by palpation of the greater tuberosity with rotator cuff pathology, but it also may be due to glenohumeral arthritis, and the finding should be correlated with rotational radiographs of the humerus (Figure 8-5). Tenderness in the bicipital groove may be present with involvement of the biceps tendon and can be implicated in both rotator cuff pathology and glenohumeral instability. Anterior and posterior joint line tenderness may be present with glenohumeral instability, whereas posterior joint line tenderness commonly is noted in patients with glenohumeral arthritis.

Range of Motion
The general motion of the shoulder complex is observed for glenohumeral rhythm, scapulothoracic motion, and overall synchrony of motion. The American Shoulder and Elbow Surgeons professional organization currently recommends that four functionally necessary arcs of motion be measured both actively and passively: total elevation, lateral rotation at neutral abduction, lateral rotation

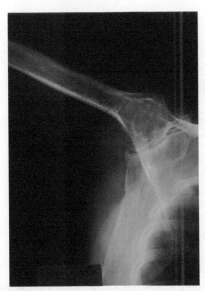

Figure 8-5 Radiograph confirming the diagnosis of severe glenohumeral arthritis.

at 90° abduction, and medial rotation.[15,16] Patients with limited motion in a single or multiple planes must be examined carefully to differentiate the possible etiologies, such as a rotator cuff tear, adhesive capsulitis, and glenohumeral arthritis.

In this patient population, total elevation, including both glenohumeral and scapulothoracic motion, may be more reproducibly measured than attempting to isolate glenohumeral motion and is more functionally relevant. However, both measurements are important for determining which joint is contributing to a functional loss. Passive elevation is more accurately measured in the supine position, whereas active elevation is measured erect. Lateral rotation is tested with the arm at the side, the patient supine (to eliminate trunk rotation), and with the arm at 90° abduction.

Functional rotation ranges of motion are also documented. Functional medial rotation is measured according to the highest vertebral level an upright patient can reach with the thumb. Apley's scratch test evaluates the available functional lateral rotation ROM.

Strength Testing

The strength and integrity of joints, muscles, and tendons are important aspects of surgical planning. Manual strength testing may be difficult to assess quantitatively because of coexistent pain. Crepitation with motion from the glenohumeral joint, subacromial space, or scapulothoracic joint should be noted. Manual muscle testing of the supraspinatus is performed with the arm in 90° forward elevation and 20° medial rotation with the elbows extended (i.e., the empty can test). Manual muscle testing in lateral rotation is performed with the elbow flexed and the arm at the side to prevent deltoid contribution; weakness in this position is a common finding with a tear involving the infraspinatus tendon. Weakness in lateral rotation at neutral may indicate

a long-standing rotator cuff tear,[17] and with concomitant weakness in shoulder abduction it shows a statistically significant correlation with the size of the tear.[18]

Manual muscle testing of the shoulder in lateral rotation above 45° abduction is performed primarily to assess the teres minor. Patients with large or massive tears involving the infraspinatus often are unable to maintain the arm in lateral rotation at neutral and when the arm is abducted. The lateral rotation lag sign is designed to test the integrity of the supraspinatus and infraspinatus tendons; it is performed by passively flexing the elbow to 90° and the shoulder to 20° elevation and near maximum lateral rotation. The patient then is asked to maintain this position while the clinician releases the wrist; a positive result is a lag or angular drop.[19] The drop sign is designed to assess infraspinatus function; for this test, the patient is seated with his or her back to the clinician, who holds the affected arm at 90° elevation and maximum lateral rotation with the elbow at 90° flexion. The patient is asked to maintain this position while the physician supports the elbow and releases the wrist; the result is positive if a lag occurs.

Patients with subscapularis tears have an increased passive lateral rotation ROM and weakness of medial rotation. The competence of the subscapularis muscle can be assessed using the lift-off test, which has been shown to be both sensitive and specific for a tear in the subscapularis tendon. Originally the lift-off test was determined to be positive (i.e., poor subscapularis function) when a patient could not lift the hand posteriorly off the lumbar region; however, the test was modified to achieve even greater sensitivity for subscapularis tears.[20] In the modified lift-off test, the examiner places the arm in maximum medial rotation by passively lifting the patient's arm posteriorly off the lumbar region; the test result is positive (poor subscapularis function) if the patient is unable to maintain that position and the arm falls or "springs back" onto the back.

The internal (medial) rotation lag sign is used to assess subscapularis competency. It is similar to the modified lift-off test except that the examiner releases the wrist at maximum internal (medial) rotation, maintains support of the elbow, and then measures the lag between the maximum internal (medial) rotation position and the lag position (Figure 8-6).

The abdominal compression test (Figure 8-7) also is used to assess subscapularis weakness or deficiency, especially when passive medial rotation is difficult to perform during the lift-off test or internal rotation lag sign. A positive abdominal compression test is indicated by an inability to keep the palm of the hand compressed against the abdomen while bringing the elbow anterior to the scapular plane. A side-to-side difference between the affected and unaffected shoulders during the abdominal compression test may indicate subtle subscapularis weakness or a tear and warrants further investigation. Medial rotation strength and integrity must be taken into consideration during surgery for proper intraoperative muscle balancing.[21]

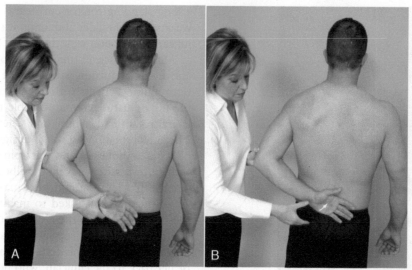

Figure 8-6 Internal (medial) rotation lag sign (also called the subscapularis spring back or lag test). **A**, Start position. **B**, Patient is unable to hold the start position and hand springs back toward the lower back. (From Magee DJ: *Orthopedic physical assessment*, ed 6, p 339, St Louis, 2014, Elsevier/Saunders.)

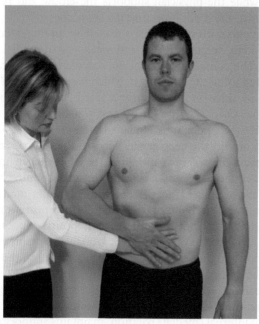

Figure 8-7 Abdominal compression test. (From Magee DJ: *Orthopedic physical assessment*, ed 6, p 334, St Louis, 2014, Elsevier/Saunders.)

To ensure maximum shoulder function after arthroplasty, a thorough assessment of shoulder motion and strength must include evaluation of the scapular muscle stabilizers. Some of the key muscles tested before shoulder arthroplasty that may affect the final outcome include the serratus anterior, trapezius, and rhomboids. Weakness in the serratus anterior muscle can cause scapular winging and disruption of the synchronous glenohumeral motion. Scapular winging, which can be detected by having the patient flex to 90° or do a wall push up, is commonly the result of a palsy of the long thoracic nerve. Trapezius muscle function is tested with a shoulder shrug, and weakness or atrophy of this muscle may be due to a palsy

of the spinal accessory nerve. The motor strength of the rhomboid muscles is tested with the patient prone, shoulder abducted 90°, and arms extended.

When assessing function in shoulder arthritis and arthroplasty patients, the clinician should be aware of the possible existence of contractures as well as generalized ligamentous laxity. In addition, identification of a pattern of instability or contracture is a key component in planning for a shoulder arthroplasty.[16,22] The presence of glenohumeral instability affects the surgical procedure. For example, if excessive posterior laxity and anterior contracture are factors, a posterior capsulorrhaphy and anterior capsular releases can be performed. Conversely, if the patient has anterior laxity, precise soft tissue balancing and prosthetic positioning are needed to prevent functional deficits.

DIAGNOSTIC MODALITIES

Imaging studies, such as radiographs, computed tomography (CT), arthrography, and magnetic resonance imaging (MRI), are used to confirm and further define the pathological process. Early in the development of glenohumeral arthrosis, subtle radiographic findings may suggest the diagnosis when the symptoms are mild. Later in the progression of joint destruction, imaging studies are crucial to the planning of prosthetic arthroplasty. Subsequent to arthroplasty, imaging studies can identify coexisting or potential problems that might correlate with the clinical outcome.

Plain Radiographs

Plain radiographs or x-rays are part of a comprehensive history and physical examination for a patient with shoulder arthritis. All patients should have anteroposterior

(AP) views in the scapular plane in neutral, medial, and lateral rotation, a lateral view in the scapular plane, and an axillary view. Although these radiographs usually are normal in early rotator cuff disease or glenohumeral instability, they are essential to the diagnosis of glenohumeral arthritis, tumors, fractures, or dislocations. Cervical spine films should be ordered for patients with concomitant neck and shoulder pain.

With more advanced glenohumeral arthritis and rotator cuff disease, AP radiographs may demonstrate degenerative changes of the greater tuberosity, AC joint, or anterior acromion, as well as the glenohumeral joint. Radiographic criteria for evidence of a rotator cuff tear, such as the acromiohumeral interval, can also be assessed on the AP view; a decrease of more than 7 mm is considered abnormal and suggestive of chronic cuff pathology.[23] Rotational AP views are valuable for detecting calcium deposits in the rotator cuff. The lateral rotation AP view shows the greater tuberosity in profile, which may reveal sclerosis, cysts, or excrescences. These tests are included for a complete evaluation of the surgical candidate and to allow the surgeon to visualize any other pathology or conditions that may be encountered before the start of the surgical procedure.

Axillary radiographs are useful for demonstrating glenoid degenerative changes or fractures associated with instability, as well as posterior dislocations that may be overlooked on routine AP views. Special views to visualize the AC joint often are obtained using an underpenetrated, or soft tissue, technique in the AP and cephalic tilt AP views. These views often demonstrate osteolysis of the distal clavicle, arthritic changes, and inferior osteophyte formation, as well as fractures. Although patients have shoulder arthroplasty primarily for pain relief, the arthritic changes on radiographs and degree of degeneration can be key factors in the decision on whether to have surgery. Changes visualized on the radiographs can also assist the clinical evaluation in determining the source of pain if no degenerative changes appear on the radiographs.

Key Factors That Determine the Need for Arthroplasty

- Pain
- Arthritic changes on radiographs (decreased joint space, decreased acromiohumeral interval, degenerative changes to greater tuberosity, acromion, osteophytes, subchondral sclerosis, bone deformation)[24,25]
- Degree of degeneration

Arthrography

Long considered the gold standard for imaging full-thickness rotator cuff tears, the arthrogram is an invasive procedure with significant risks, such as infection, allergic reaction, radiation exposure, and pain. Double contrast arthrography is inexpensive and easily performed; how-

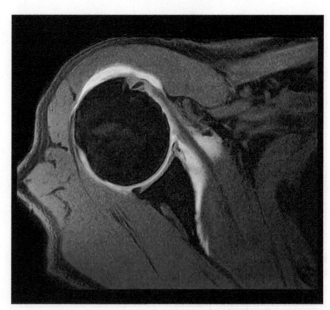

Figure 8-8 Infiltration of dye into the subscapularis fossa indicates a possible rotator cuff tear.

ever, it has a limited ability to diagnose partial cuff tears accurately and provide information about their size and location. Despite this, arthrography remains an excellent modality for diagnosing full-thickness rotator cuff tears that may accompany glenohumeral arthrosis (Figure 8-8).

Computed Tomography

When an arthritic patient is suspected of having glenohumeral instability, CT images can be obtained to delineate bony and soft tissue intra-articular pathology. CT images also can be useful in a standardized technique to determine the humeral torsion angle and landmarks that can be used during surgery.[26,27] Three-dimensional CT scans (Figure 8-9) can further delineate complex proximal humeral fractures and assist planning for a hemiarthroplasty.[28,29] Hernigou et al.[26] found that retroversion with CT is more accurate than palpating the epicondylar axis or using the forearm as a goniometer during surgery. CT is useful for measuring the amount of rotation of the humerus with a malunited fracture or severe arthritic deformity.

Magnetic Resonance Imaging

MRI is an excellent, noninvasive, radiation-sparing modality that is useful in the diagnosis of rotator cuff pathology and glenohumeral instability but is not always necessary for patients with shoulder arthritis. Soini et al.[30] demonstrated that in severely destroyed rheumatoid shoulders scheduled for arthroplasty, MRI soft tissue findings were not consistent with tissue changes at the time of surgery. The integrity of tendons could not readily be elucidated with MRI because of an inflammatory process and scarred

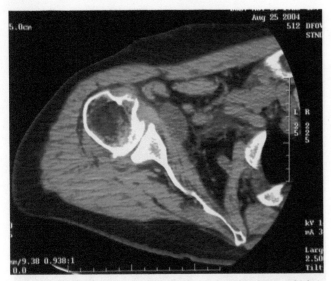

Figure 8-9 CT scan showing signs of glenohumeral arthritis, which is important in preoperative planning.

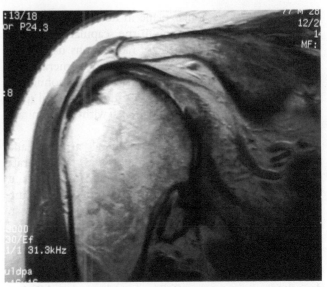

Figure 8-11 MRI demonstrating humeral head migration superiorly with rotator cuff arthropathy.

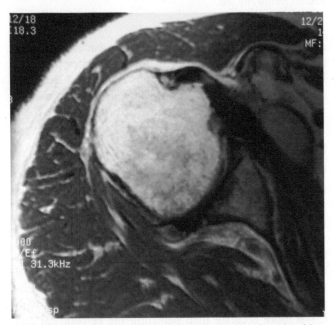

Figure 8-10 MRI scan showing increased signal in the glenoid and humeral head in addition to joint space narrowing; these findings indicate severe degenerative disease.

tissues. Often, during surgery, the changes were difficult to categorize. MRI scans of severely destroyed rheumatoid shoulders before arthroplasty were shown to be of only minor importance. However, this may not be true for patients with osteoarthritis of the glenohumeral joint (Figures 8-10 and 8-11).

Other Modalities

When systemic disorders are suspected, routine blood tests to evaluate for rheumatological disorders, infection, and tumors should be considered. A complete blood count with differential, sedimentation rate, C-reactive protein

level, chemistry profile, latex fixation test, serum protein electrophoresis, and an acid phosphatase level should be obtained as part of preoperative testing (Table 8-1). This panel allows the surgeon to rule out any other significant factors and pathology and provides a baseline for comparison after surgery, if necessary.

YOUNG SHOULDER ARTHROPLASTY PATIENTS

Shoulder arthroplasty is becoming more common in young patients. Although trauma to the glenohumeral joint is associated with a dislocation episode, little is known about the incidence of shoulder arthroplasty in patients with shoulder instability. The long time span between dislocation and the development of arthritis makes determining any cause and effect relationship difficult.

Severe damage to the humeral head cartilage can occur after a dislocation. Taylor and Arciero[31] reported on 63 young patients under 24 years of age with first-time, traumatic anterior shoulder dislocations who were evaluated arthroscopically within 10 days of dislocation. Fifty-seven patients had Hill-Sachs lesions. However, osteochondral lesions of the humeral head were identified in 34 patients, and chondral lesions were noted in an additional 24, providing evidence that humeral head damage occurs. Hovelius et al.[32] followed 245 patients 10 years after primary anterior dislocations of the shoulder. The patients' ages at the time of dislocation ranged from 12 to 40 years. Radiographs taken on 185 shoulders at the time of primary dislocation demonstrated a Hill-Sachs lesion in 99 shoulders. This finding was associated with a significantly worse prognosis with regard to recurrent instability but had no effect on the development of arthritis. Radiographs made for 208 shoulders at the 10-year follow-up examination were evaluated for

TABLE 8-1

Preoperative Laboratory Tests with Normal Ranges

CBC with Differential and PLT		Complete Metabolic Panel	
WBC	3.8-10.83/µL	Glucose	65-139 mg/dL
RBC	3.80-5.106/µL	Sodium	135-146 mmol/L
Hemoglobin	11.7-15.5 g/dL	Potassium	3.5-5.3 mmol/L
Hematocrit	35%-45%	Chloride	98-110 mmol/L
MCV	80-100 fL	Carbon dioxide	21-33 mmol/L
MCH	27-33 pg	Urea nitrogen	7-25 mg/dL
MCHC	32-36 g/dL	Creatinine	0.5-1.2 mg/dL
RDW	11%-15%	BUN/creatinine ratio	6-25
PLT	140-4003/µL	Calcium	8.5-10.4 mg/dL
MPV	7.5-11.5 fL	Protein, total	6.0-8.3 g/dL
Total neutrophils, %	38%-80%	Albumin	3.5-4.9 g/dL
Total lymphocytes, %	15%-49%	Globulin, calculated	2.2-4.2 g/dL
Monocytes, %	0%-13%	A/G ratio	0.8-2
Eosinophils, %	0%-8%	Bilirubin, total	0.2-1.3 mg/dL
Basophils, %	0%-2%	Alkaline phosphatase	20-125 units/L
Neutrophils, absolute	1500-7800 cells/µL	AST	2-35 units/L
Lymphocytes, absolute	850-3900/µL	ALT	2-40 units/L
Monocytes, absolute	200-950 cells/µL		
Eosinophils, absolute	15-550 cells/µL		
Basophils, absolute	0-200 cells/µL		

ALT, Alanine aminotransferase; *AST,* aspartate aminotransferase; *BUN,* blood urea nitrogen; *CBC,* complete blood count; *fL,* fluid liter; *MCH,* mean corpuscular hemoglobin; *MCHC,* mean corpuscular hemoglobin concentration; *MCV,* mean corpuscular volume; *MPV,* mean platelet volume; *PLT,* platelet count; *RBC,* red blood cell; *RDW,* red cell distribution width; *WBC,* white blood cell.

posttraumatic dislocation arthritis. Twenty-three shoulders (11%) had mild arthritis, and 18 (9%) had moderate or severe arthritis. No further instability was reported in some of the shoulders that had arthritis.

The most defining study to date was published by Marx et al.,[33] who used a case-control study to examine whether shoulder dislocation was associated with the development of arthrosis. Patients with osteoarthrosis who had undergone hemiarthroplasty or total shoulder arthroplasty were asked whether they had ever sustained a shoulder dislocation. Ninety-one patients who had undergone shoulder arthroplasty and 282 control subjects responded. The authors concluded that the risk of developing severe arthrosis of the shoulder is 10 to 20 times greater for individuals who have had a dislocation of the shoulder. It is evident that some degree of chondral injury and hemarthrosis may be associated with a shoulder dislocation and is not beneficial to the glenohumeral joint. Whether the hemarthrosis predisposes this patient population to arthritis and an eventual shoulder arthroplasty remains unclear.

One thing that is clear is the effect of overconstraining the glenohumeral joint during surgery for shoulder instability. Sperling et al.[34] reported on the intermediate to long-term results of shoulder arthroplasty performed to treat osteoarthritis after instability surgery in 33 patients with glenohumeral arthritis. The mean age at the time of the shoulder arthroplasty was 46 years. Twenty-one patients who had a total shoulder arthroplasty and 10 who had a hemiarthroplasty were followed for a minimum of 2 years. Shoulder arthroplasty was associated with significant pain relief and significant improvement in lateral rotation and active abduction. Interestingly no significant difference was seen between the hemiarthroplasty group and the total shoulder arthroplasty group with regard to postoperative lateral rotation, active abduction, or pain. This study suggests that shoulder arthroplasty for the treatment of osteoarthritis of the glenohumeral joint after instability surgery in a group of young patients provides pain relief and improved motion. However, it may be associated with a higher incidence of revision surgery. Three patients in the hemiarthroplasty group and eight patients in the total shoulder arthroplasty group underwent revision surgery. In contrast, this was not the case in a series of 22 shoulder arthroplasties followed up over an average of 6 years. Burroughs et al.[35] reported no evidence of accelerated deterioration of shoulder function, and only two patients underwent revision surgery.

Given this conflict in the literature, little information is available to guide clinical decision making with regard to shoulder arthroplasty after instability surgery. The management of these patients requires a thorough preoperative evaluation and a careful review of diagnostic modalities. The severity of glenoid wear should be assessed using CT scans to determine the need for glenoid bone grafting. In addition, the surgeon should obtain the previous operative reports to determine the type of stabilization performed; this allows the surgeon to recognize frequently distorted anatomy and facilitates safe, effective soft tissue releases. The decision to proceed with a shoulder arthroplasty in a patient who has had a previous stabilization procedure should be made with caution. The surgeon should be prepared to address associated soft tissue contracture and potential bone deficiency.

Shoulder arthroplasty in the young patient for osteoarthritis of the glenohumeral joint after instability surgery provides satisfactory pain relief and improvement in motion but may be associated with a high rate of revision surgery and unsatisfactory results as a result of implant failure, instability, and painful glenoid arthritis.[35]

PREOPERATIVE REHABILITATION

Accepting differences in expectations, patient goals, physician goals, and physical therapist goals is essential. The physical therapist ideally should meet with the patient and the patient's caregiver before the surgery. At this time the rehabilitation team can set reasonable goals for both early and eventual outcomes (Table 8-2). At this point, when the patients are not under the influence of pain medications, feeling ill, or experiencing pain, they can better

TABLE 8-2

Rehabilitation Guidelines after Shoulder Arthroplasty

Immediate Postoperative Phase (Days 0 to 7)	
Goals	Patient understands surgery, precautions, and pain-relief methods
	Protect the surgery
	Improve ROM at shoulder and maintain ROM of proximal and distal joints
	Improve scapular stability
PROM	Pendulums, CPM (facility dependent)
	PROM flexion and lateral rotation (if allowed) by therapist
AAROM	Pulleys for sagittal plane flexion and scaption
	Cane exercises for flexion and lateral rotation
AROM	AROM of hand, wrist, elbow, scapula, and cervical spine
	Gripping
Patient education	Sling use (full time for community activities, as needed at home) or as instructed by physician
	Arm can be used for light, waist-level activity
	Patient understands that activity should not increase pain level drastically
	Patient should ice shoulder to reduce pain
	Patient should sleep sitting up (in chair)
Precautions	Do not force lateral rotation
	No medial rotation isometrics, isokinetics (no medial rotation muscle activation)
	Exercises should not cause severe pain
	Watch for and minimize muscle guarding
Early Postoperative Phase (Weeks 1 to 6)	
Goals	Continue to restore motion, scapular stability
	Begin light rotator cuff activation
	Continue pain modulation
PROM	Pendulums for warm-up and pain modulation
AAROM	Pulleys for sagittal plane flexion, medial rotation, and scaption
	Cane exercises for flexion, horizontal adduction and abduction, and punches
AROM	Continue cervical, scapular, elbow, wrist, and hand motion
	Continue gripping
	Begin submaximum isometrics for external rotators (i.e., pushing against towel or ball on wall)
	Begin submaximum isometrics for deltoid if no pain is present
	Begin upper body exercises at 4 weeks (shoulder flexion below 80°)
	Begin serratus strengthening if done below 90° shoulder flexion (punches, dynamic hugs, scaption)
Patient education	No heavy pushing, pulling, or lifting for 6 weeks
	No weight bearing for 6 months
Precautions	Patient feels fine, but healing is not complete. *Protect the joint.*
Intermediate Postoperative Phase (Weeks 6 to 12)	
Goals	Ensure stable prosthesis and joint stability
	ROM goals, active and passive
	Minimal pain
	Begin improving strength and endurance
	Improve function

(Continued)

TABLE 8-2

Rehabilitation Guidelines after Shoulder Arthroplasty—cont'd

Intermediate Postoperative Phase (Weeks 6 to 12) *cont'd*

PROM	Mobilizations as needed Posterior capsule stretching/sleeper stretch
AAROM	As needed (cane, pulleys) Posterior capsule stretching/sleeper stretch
AROM	Muscle activation exercises: • Dusting • Active lateral rotation/medial rotation within pain-free motion Open chain stability exercises: • Flexbar 0°, then 45°, and finally 90°, as tolerated • Body Blade at 0° • Rhythmic stabilizations (at 8 to 10 weeks, higher level patients) Closed chain stability exercises: • Ball stabilization • Perturbation training with therapist • PWB through shoulder Strengthening exercises: • Medial rotation/lateral rotation pain free (e.g., with Thera-Band) • Side-lying lateral rotation with weight • Lateral rotation at 45° with elbow supported (8-9 weeks) • Prone extension • Prone horizontal abduction • Biceps and triceps curls • Anterior deltoid strengthening • Strengthening of all scapular muscles (e.g., punches, lower and middle traps, rows, extensions with Thera-Band)
Patient education	No heavy lifting No sports
Precautions	Do not initiate base strengthening until pain is minimal

Return to Activity Phase (Weeks 12 to 24)

Goals	Full ROM in all planes Strength 80% or greater of uninvolved side Improved endurance and neuromuscular control Patient confident in shoulder Full return to activity
PROM/ AAROM	PROM as needed
AROM	Strength testing: • Isokinetic Continue activation, stability, and strength exercises; progress as tolerated: • Lateral rotation 90/90 • Overhead wall taps • Light ball toss; chest pass, overhead • Plyometrics up to 90/90 position Functional exercises: • Thera-Band golf/tennis • Golf chipping and putting • Breast stroke
Patient education	Patient very familiar with HEP to maximize strength and ROM gains
Precautions	Avoid increasing inflammation Do not strengthen in abduction Do not strengthen with high weights; use low weights and medium repetitions Use caution with overhead activity until all pain has resolved If pain requires use of treatments, reduce exercise or intensity of ADLs

AAROM, active-assisted range of motion; *ADLs,* activities of daily living; *AROM,* active range of motion; *CPM,* continuous passive motion; *HEP,* home exercise program; *PROM,* Passive range of motion; *PWB,* partial weight bearing; *ROM,* range of motion.

comprehend the rehabilitation program, precautions, and expectations. This allows the patient and physical therapist to establish a relationship that will foster better cooperation during the sometimes painful and frustrating rehabilitation process. After the educational process, the preoperative assessment should include the available ROM, strength, and the presence of visible atrophy, sensation, pain, and functional evaluation.

The educational process is essential for informing the patient of the risks and complications of surgery and anesthesia.[36] These risks for shoulder replacement surgery include injury to nerves and blood vessels, stiffness or instability of the shoulder joint, loosening of the prosthetic parts (requiring additional surgery), tearing of a rotator cuff tendon, and fracture of the humerus. In addition, total shoulder replacement carries with it the normal risks of any elective surgery, such as complications from anesthesia, excessive bleeding, infection, blood clots, and ultimately death.[37-39] The surgical procedure and the components of shoulder arthroplasty also are explained.

The educational process is essential for informing the patient of the restriction on the use of the shoulder and the impact on activities of daily living for at least the next 6 weeks. Because the subscapularis muscle is cut to expose the shoulder joint, no active medial rotation motion is permitted. For the patient, this means no violent squeezing, hugging, or slamming of car doors. However, the patient should be encouraged to use the upper extremity for light functional activities such as eating, brushing the teeth, or putting on a hat; the patient should avoid lifting anything heavier than 0.91 kg (2 lb). The patient also should be instructed to avoid immobilization.

The importance of a postoperative rehabilitation program is reviewed, and the importance of the first 6 weeks of rehabilitation also is emphasized. The immediate and early program is geared toward regaining the motion achieved at the time of surgery. The patient needs to appreciate that this time frame is the most important period of the rehabilitation process, a period in which significant changes and gains in ROM and maintaining optimum neuromuscular function can be accomplished. The home environment is discussed to determine whether the patient is one of approximately 50% of patients who require home nursing assistance, home physical therapy, or, infrequently, discharge to an extended care facility after hospitalization. In addition, special considerations need to be identified for patients who require assistive devices for ambulation, the visually impaired, or those who use wheelchairs.

Patient and family education is essential for achieving consistently good outcomes after shoulder arthroplasty. It is essential that family members be made aware of restrictions on activity and the importance of frequent home exercise. The patient and caregivers must understand that being active, but using only the arms at the side, does not replace stretching overhead to prevent contracture or stiffness. The recommendation for long-term active ROM exercise is 5 times a day for the first 6 weeks, 2 times a day for the next 6 weeks or until goals are achieved, then once a day for a lifetime. Patients who are involved and enthusiastic about their management tend to recover and regain shoulder function rapidly.[40]

Clinical Note

The patient must take an active role because the patient is the most valuable member of the multidisciplinary team.

Risks and Complications of Arthroplasty[37-39]

- Injuries to nerves and blood vessels
- Glenohumeral joint stiffness
- Glenohumeral or scapular instability
- Loosening of prosthesis
- Additional surgery
- Rotator cuff tear
- Humeral fracture
- Ectopic ossification
- Excessive bleeding
- Infection
- Blood clots
- Death

Although age is not a limiting factor, the patient must be able to cooperate in a postoperative rehabilitation program, which is crucial to the success of the surgery.[40] Patients are expected to obtain medical clearance from their primary care physician with regard to any systemic medical conditions, along with preoperative testing (e.g., laboratory tests, electrocardiography [ECG]). Patients should discontinue nonsteroidal anti-inflammatory medications or aspirin-containing medications 7 to 10 days before the scheduled surgery to minimize postoperative bleeding and complications with coagulation. For total shoulder arthroplasty, 1 unit of autologous blood may be donated in anticipation of the surgery, which can result in a blood loss of 1 to 2 units, especially in complicated cases.

The clinical examination includes shoulder ROM and strength measurements. Limited abduction and lateral rotation movements and decreased rotator cuff muscle strength are common.[40-42] Preoperative motions that should be measured include forward elevation, lateral rotation in a supine position, and medial rotation with the hand reaching up the back. Deficits of active versus passive motion also provide information about the function of the rotator cuff, and these data are supplemented with manual muscle testing of abduction and lateral rotation strength against resistance.

A demonstration of therapeutic exercises by a physical therapist can be part of the preparation for the surgical procedure. Preoperative demonstration of therapeutic exercises in the rehabilitation program is associated with better patient understanding and a more rapid progression after surgery.[40] Unfortunately, most insurance companies do not provide for preoperative therapy or a preoperative home health assessment, despite their intuitive benefits.

HEMIARTHROPLASTY VERSUS TOTAL SHOULDER ARTHROPLASTY

Arthroplasty is the most definitive method for managing the pain associated with severe glenohumeral arthritis. Since 1893 when the first shoulder replacement was performed, shoulder arthroplasty has continued to improve with advances in component materials, instrumentation, and surgical techniques.[1] Good candidates for shoulder arthroplasty are older patients who will place minimal demands on the shoulder and have no rotator cuff damage. A total shoulder arthroplasty involves the replacement of both sides of the glenohumeral joint (the humerus and glenoid).[22] A hemiarthroplasty replaces the humeral head only and is the treatment of choice when replacement of the glenoid is not advised.[43] The decision is made based on the nature and degree of the patient's arthritis. Individuals who should not have shoulder arthroplasty at all are contact athletes and heavy laborers. They are not good candidates for shoulder replacement because of the long-term demands they place on the shoulder. In addition, total shoulder arthroplasty is not always appropriate for patients with large, inoperable rotator cuff tears. Because the rotator cuff muscles hold the humeral head tightly to the glenoid, these massive tears would allow excessive movement of the humeral component, leading to abnormal loading and loosening of the glenoid component.[44] Hemiarthroplasty is recommended for patients with isolated humeral head arthritis and normal glenoid cartilage. Patients with poor glenoid bone quality need to consider a hemiarthroplasty. Patients with an active infection in the shoulder joint should not have shoulder arthroplasty.[45]

Patients Unsuitable for Shoulder Arthroplasty

- Athletes in contact sports
- Heavy laborers
- Patients with large, inoperable rotator cuff tears
- Patients with an active infection

Another subset of patients in whom primary hemiarthroplasty is indicated are patients with proximal humeral fractures. Hemiarthroplasty has become the gold standard for the treatment of such fractures when the humeral head is deemed to be nonviable or not amenable to reconstruction with internal fixation techniques.[46] The current indications for primary hemiarthroplasty

include a displaced and translated four-part fracture, with or without associated dislocation of the humeral head, and a head-splitting fracture with involvement of more than 40% of the articular surface.[46] Outcomes with this procedure have been mixed. The shoulder usually is free of pain, but the overall functional result at 1 year varies in terms of ROM, function, and power. A better functional outcome can be anticipated for a younger individual than for elderly patients.[47] However, total shoulder arthroplasty should be considered in these cases; Carroll et al.[48] reported on long-term follow-up of 16 patients after conversion of painful hemiarthroplasty to total shoulder arthroplasty. The authors concluded that revision of a failed hemiarthroplasty to a total shoulder arthroplasty is a salvage procedure, and the results are inferior to those of primary total shoulder arthroplasty. Recently, in patients with rotator cuff arthropathy, a "reverse" shoulder prosthesis was attempted. The premise is that a "reverse" shoulder prosthesis resists glenohumeral subluxation and potential component loosening by preventing superior displacement of the humeral head (Figure 8-12).[49-53] Modern implant designs emphasize a medial center of rotation to recruit more deltoid muscle fibers which aid with active elevation.[54] In a 10-year follow-up study performed by Guery et al.,[55] survival rates for the prosthesis were 91% and 84% among 80 patients with mostly massive rotator cuff tears. However, the authors also found that the protheses were prone to functional deterioration over time; a statistic they attributed to aseptic glenoid loosening.

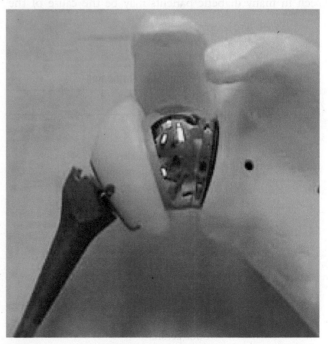

Figure 8-12 Example of a reverse total shoulder replacement prosthesis. (From Harman M, Frankle M, Vasey M et al: Initial glenoid component fixation in "reverse" total shoulder arthroplasty: a biomechanical evaluation, *J Shoulder Elbow Surg* 14[1 suppl S]:162S-167S, 2005.)

FACTORS ASSOCIATED WITH SUCCESSFUL OUTCOMES

The outcome of a shoulder arthroplasty can never be predicted with certainty; however, a number of preoperative, intrasurgical, and rehabilitative factors are associated with a successful outcome.[16] Factors observed at the time of surgery, such as the quality of the cartilage, bone, and rotator cuff, are a recognized influence on the result of arthroplasty, but preoperative information also is associated with greater improvement in patient-assessed function after shoulder arthroplasty (Table 8-3). Preoperative decision making by patients and their surgeons can influence the final outcome. It was found that higher surgeon and hospital case volumes led to improved perioperative metrics with all shoulder arthroplasty procedures, including reverse total shoulder arthroplasty.[56] The success of shoulder arthroplasty also depends on postoperative rehabilitation.[15,36,40,57,58]

The first preoperative predictor of outcome is the presence of systemic disease. Numerous research studies have demonstrated that patients with Parkinson's disease, systemic lupus erythematosus (SLE), and rheumatoid arthritis have poorer outcomes after shoulder arthroplasty.[59-61] In the case of SLE and rheumatoid arthritis, the soft tissues needed for muscle balancing may be severely compromised. The tissue also may have become friable and thin because of excessive use of steroids.[62] In addition, patients with preexisting diabetes are at a higher risk for perioperative morbidity and mortality following shoulder arthroplasty.[63] The progressive multisystem involvement seen in many diabetic patients may be the cause of the higher perioperative mortality encountered in patients with this condition.

Hettrich et al.[64] examined preoperative factors associated with improvements in shoulder function after hemiarthroplasty in 71 shoulders. These researchers were able to demonstrate that shoulders with rheumatoid arthritis, capsulorrhaphy arthropathy, and rotator cuff tear arthropathy had the least functional improvement, whereas those with osteonecrosis or primary and secondary degenerative joint disease had the greatest improvement. The patient's age and gender did not significantly affect the outcome. Shoulders that had not had previous surgery had greater functional improvement than those that had had previous surgery. These results were supported by Kay and Amstutz,[65] who found better results in patients with osteonecrosis compared with those who had a fracture. Trail and Nuttall[66] found that an intact rotator cuff was associated with a better outcome in patients with rheumatoid arthritis. Levy and Copeland[67] found poorer outcomes in patients with cuff tear arthropathy and posttraumatic arthropathy than in those with other diagnoses. As these studies show, patient selection plays an important role in determining the final outcome. In a recent study, Bot et al.[68] noted that patients with preoperative psychological illness were found to be at an increased risk for perioperative morbidity and posthospitalization care following shoulder arthroplasty.

Preoperative ROM can also have an effect on the postoperative outcome. Iannotti and Norris[69] found that patients with less than 10° of passive lateral rotation before surgery had substantially less improvement in lateral rotation after hemiarthroplasty. Thirteen of 128 shoulders had a repairable full-thickness tear of the supraspinatus tendon, but these tears did not affect the overall outcome, decrease in pain, or patient satisfaction. The authors' experience has been that patients scheduled for shoulder arthroplasty who lack passive medial rotation and have a tight posterior capsule have a very difficult time regaining the motion postoperatively and report poorer outcomes. Surgeons and patients thinking of shoulder arthroplasty need to consider identifying these preoperative factors.

Shoulder arthroplasty is considered among the most technically demanding of the current joint replacement procedures because of the glenohumeral joint's lack of intrinsic stability.[21] The tension of the rotator cuff and glenohumeral capsule must be balanced for mobility and stability. The surgeon is faced with many decisions regarding the choice of implant, implant fixation, soft tissue management, and options for glenoid resurfacing.[70,71] In general, if the precise cause of the arthritic condition has been identified, the choices become more straightforward. For advanced osteoarthritis of the shoulder joint in an older patient with asymmetrical posterior erosion of the glenoid, total shoulder arthroplasty renders the best relief of pain and improvement in motion. Similarly, for

TABLE 8-3

Factors Associated with Successful Outcomes

Stage	Factors
Preoperative	Cartilage quality
	Bone quality
	Rotator cuff quality
	Glenohumeral instability
	Systemic disease
	Posterior glenoid wear
	Heterotropic ossification
Intrasurgical	Soft tissue balancing
	Prosthetic component positioning
	Intraoperative fracture
	Nerve injury
	Infection
	Inadequate range of motion
Postoperative	Infection
	Contracture
	Lack of range of motion
	Inadequate strength recovery
	Prosthetic component loosening

advanced rheumatoid arthritis in a patient with an intact rotator cuff, total shoulder arthroplasty results in the best pain relief. If the rotator cuff is deficient and irreparable, an anatomically sized humeral head replacement is appropriate.

Many types of implants are available. Biomechanical and anatomical studies suggest that a better technical result can be achieved with the most recent implant design, which is able to recreate accurately the proximal anatomy of the humerus.[72,73] Nevertheless, complications are inevitable in shoulder replacement surgery (incidence of approximately 14%). Numerous intraoperative complications have been identified. In order of decreasing frequency, they include instability, rotator cuff tear, ectopic ossification, glenoid component loosening, intraoperative fracture, nerve injury, infection, and humeral component loosening.[16,36,74,75] Successful treatment of these surgical difficulties requires careful identification and surgical planning, and the surgeon must always keep in mind that the etiology often is multifactorial.

OPERATIVE TECHNIQUE FOR TOTAL SHOULDER REPLACEMENT

Patient Positioning

Appropriate patient positioning is essential in total shoulder surgery. The patient is placed in a modified beach chair position with a headrest that allows access to the superior part of the table (Figure 8-13). The head of the table should be raised to approximately 25° to 30° to reduce venous pressure, and an arm board should be used on the side of the table that will be raised and lowered as necessary throughout the procedure. A mild sedative and an interscalene block are administered.[76]

Incision and Exposure

The first step is to demarcate all bony landmarks, including the clavicle, and the coracoid process. The incision will be made from the lateral aspect of the coracoid process at the level of the clavicle and extend in line with the deltoid toward the midaspect of the humeral shaft and along the deltopectoral groove. The subcutaneous flaps are dissected from the deltoid fascia to expose the deltoid and pectoralis major muscles. The skin is retracted with self-retaining retractors, and the deltopectoral interval is developed. The pectoralis major is retracted medially, and the deltoid is retracted laterally. The cephalic vein, which delineates the deltopectoral groove, is retracted either medially or laterally (preferably laterally) because this minimizes bleeding from the deltoid muscle or cephalic vein (Figure 8-14). The upper 1 to 2 cm (0.5 to 1 inch) of the pectoralis major tendon is released. The interval between the deltoid, the coracobrachialis, and the short head of the biceps is developed, and a retractor is placed deep to it. The superior portion of the subacromial space is exposed, and the anterior aspect of the coracoacromial ligament is resected. The subscapularis major tendon is identified, as are both the superior and inferior margins of the muscle. The tendon is divided just medial to the bicipital grove and is removed from the lesser tuberosity. Care is taken to avoid the axillary nerve. The subscapularis muscle is retracted medially, exposing the articular surface of the humeral head. As a unit, the capsule and subscapularis tendon are taken laterally off the lateral aspect of the humerus (Figure 8-15). Care must be taken to avoid the axillary nerve during this approach. Lateral rotation of the humerus at this point is helpful for protecting the axillary nerve.[77]

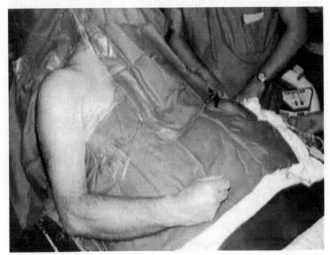

Figure 8-13 Patient is placed in a modified beach chair position for shoulder arthroplasty.

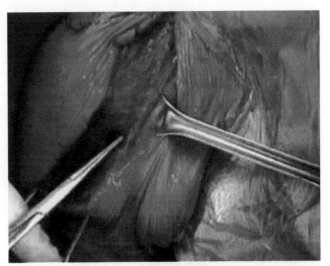

Figure 8-14 Pectoralis major is retracted medially, and the deltoid is retracted laterally. The cephalic vein, which delineates the deltopectoral groove, is retracted to minimize bleeding.

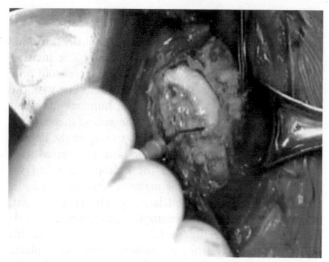

Figure 8-15 Capsule and subscapularis tendon are reflected, and the humeral head is exposed.

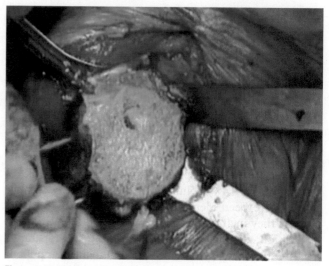

Figure 8-17 Humeral head is removed.

Preparation of the Humerus

Once the subscapularis and capsule have been retracted sufficiently, the arm is placed into extension and lateral rotation to facilitate dislocation of the humeral head. Once the humeral head has been dislocated, arthritic osteophytes are removed so that the anatomical neck of the humerus junction of the articular cartilage and the cortical bone can be identified. An intramedullary reamer (drill) is placed just posterior to the bicipital groove, and a starter hole is made. Sequential reaming then is performed, using a tapered reamer in the intramedullary canal.

The humeral head is then resected with a cutting block technique (Figure 8-16). The cut is made with proper retroversion, which is 20° to 40° retroversion. The resected head is removed (Figure 8-17) and used to size the prosthesis appropriately.[10]

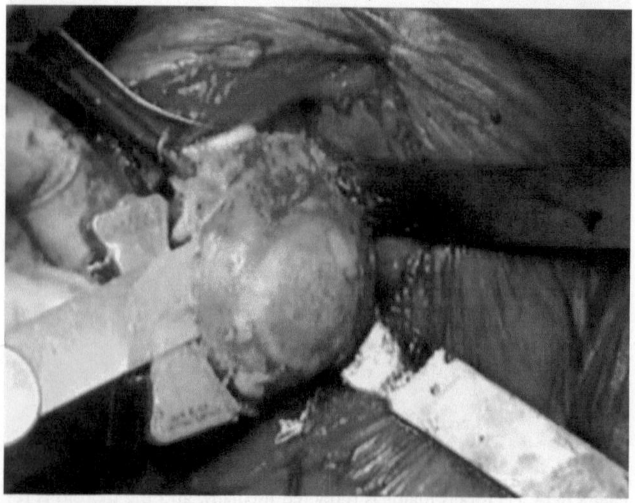

A provisional humeral stem is used and correlated to the last size of the largest reamer used initially. Retroversion is additionally checked at this point. It is critical that the humeral head be centered relative to the rotator cuff.[43] Many of the current prostheses allow offset head placement; this allows the margin of the humeral head to rest immediately adjacent to the rotator cuff insertion superiorly on the greater tuberosity and slightly overhang the calcar spur medially. ROM could be limited postoperatively if the humeral component is placed too low. If the humeral component is placed too high, the rotator cuff muscles will be under too much tension, and loosening of the glenoid component may occur.[78]

Preparation of the Glenoid

Preparation of the glenoid is essential to a successful outcome in total shoulder arthroplasty. It is essential that the surgeon have a good understanding of the patient's glenoid anatomy before implantation of the component; this involves using either an axillary radiograph of the glenoid or a CT or MRI scan to assess for anterior and posterior wear. It is important to identify the center of the glenoid cavity. Osteophytes that may be obstructing the center of the glenoid need to be removed. If an inadequate or deformed glenoid prevents proper placement of the glenoid component, the surgeon should consider performing a hemiarthroplasty rather than a total shoulder arthroplasty. Any cartilage remaining on the glenoid should be removed, and the glenoid must be sized appropriately.

A centering hole should be made in the glenoid (Figure 8-18). Whether a keeled or pegged glenoid component is used depends on the surgeon's preference.[79] Regardless of the type of component chosen, the appropriate placement for drilling and reaming into the glenoid must be followed. Reaming to the appropriate depth is critical, as is taking care not to remove a

Figure 8-16 Humeral head is resected using a cutting block and oscillating saw.

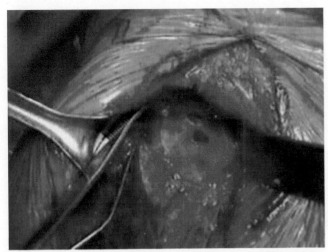

Figure 8-18 Centering and pegged glenoid holes are drilled into the glenoid.

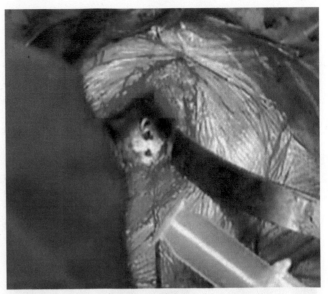

Figure 8-19 Glenoid prosthesis is inserted.

substantial amount of subcortical bone, because this could affect glenoid stability and long-term preservation of the arthroplasty.[80] Reaming is performed by hand and a drill is not used so as to preserve as much subcortical bone as possible. The glenoid then is sized. The optimum glenoid component should not overhang any perimeter of the glenoid.[81]

The humeral head prosthesis is then selected. The prosthesis should be sized according to the removed humeral head. Standard offset heads may be used. The humeral head and its stem as well as the glenoid are then tried together. The joint is reduced and put through a ROM.

Implantation of the Prosthesis

The glenoid component is implanted first. Cement is introduced into the keel or peg holes with a pressurized syringe. The cement is placed, pressurized, and held. The glenoid prosthesis then is inserted and impacted with pressure, which is maintained until the cement has hardened (Figure 8-19). Excess cement is removed.

The humeral component then is prepared for implantation. The surgeon's preference determines whether a press fit or cement is used. Often cement is placed circumferentially around the collar proximally instead of being packed completely into the intramedullary canal.[82]

Various trials should allow for a humeral head that permits 50% of the head to be subluxed posteriorly and inferiorly and to fall back into place once the pressure is released. A prosthetic component that is too large will overstuff the glenohumeral joint and will not allow proper soft tissue balancing.[83]

Before inserting and cementing the final humeral component, the surgeon makes several suture holes through the anterior neck of the proximal humerus. Heavy braided #2 sutures should be passed before cement fixation of the humeral shaft. The suture holes are used to reattach the

subscapularis tendon; they often are best placed medially against the neck of the humerus, which effectively lengthens the tendon and thus prevents it from being overtightened.[84] If a cement restrictor plug is used, the proper canal diameter must be determined so that the appropriate-sized cement restrictor can be placed. Before cementing, the intramedullary canal should be thoroughly cleaned and dried. The cement is injected into the humeral canal and finger packed to pressurize it thoroughly. Once the final sizing has been done, the prosthesis is placed and held in position until the cement has dried fully. Bireduction is performed with a modular head. Once the proper sizing has been performed, the humeral taper stem should be thoroughly cleaned and dried. After the proper humeral head has been selected, the humeral head is applied and impacted appropriately (Figure 8-20). The joint then is brought through ROM, and stability is assessed.

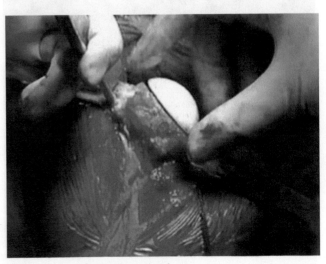

Figure 8-20 Humeral head is replaced.

Closure

The wound is irrigated copiously. Then, beginning inferiorly, the subscapularis is reattached using the sutures that were passed before cementing of the humeral shaft. A Hemovac drain is placed deep to prevent hemarthrosis. Care is taken to avoid all neurovascular structures upon closure. The deltoid and subcutaneous layers are closed, with the subarticular stitches close to the skin (Figure 8-21). Steri-Strips and a sterile dressing are applied. A postoperative radiograph is then taken (Figure 8-22). The patient is kept in a sling and swath until interscalene anesthesia has worn off, and perioperative antibiotics are continued for 24 to 48 hours. Major complications that can arise before discharge include neurovascular injuries and dislocation.

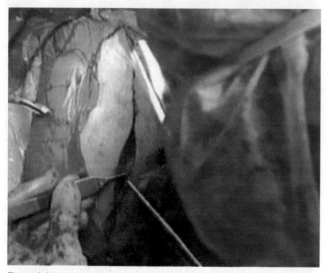

Figure 8-21 Deltoid and subcutaneous layers are closed, with the subarticular stitches close to the skin. Steri-Strips and a sterile dressing are applied.

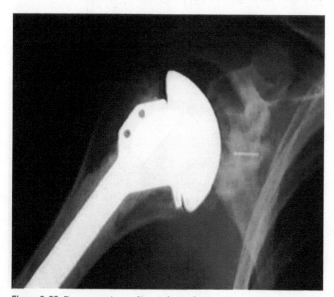

Figure 8-22 Postoperative radiograph is taken.

READMISSION

Readmission rates for shoulder arthroplasty have not been closely evaluated in very many studies. Fehringer et al.[85] assessed the Veterans Association population for postoperative complications and found that 14-day readmission rates and 30-day mortality rates in total shoulder arthroplasty incidence compared favorably with knee and hip arthroploasty. Mahoney et al.[86] found that the readmission rate for all arthroplasties was 5.9%. For hemiarthroplasty, total shoulder arthroplasty, and reverse total shoulder arthroplasty, 90-day readmission rates were 8.8%, 4.5%, and 6.6%, respectively. Thirty-day readmission rates were significantly more common for hemiarthroplasty and reverse total shoulder arthroplasty.[86]

POSTOPERATIVE REHABILITATION

A successful outcome for total shoulder arthroplasty depends on a well-designed and well-executed physical therapy program. For maximum benefit, the program usually is initiated immediately after surgery and follows a logical pattern of joint mobilization and stretching, followed by muscle strengthening. This design attempts to balance the need to obtain and maintain motion with the need to allow adequate soft tissue healing. Overly protective rehabilitation can result in stiffness, whereas overly aggressive therapy could compromise healing of the subscapularis and rotator cuff musculature and therefore shoulder stability and function.[87]

Immediate Postoperative Phase (Days 0 to 7)

The rehabilitation process should start as soon after surgery as the surgeon allows. Many surgeons begin at least some passive mobility on the same day as surgery, while the patient is still under the influence of a regional nerve block. At the authors' hospital, continuous passive motion is not used for the shoulder; however, some surgeons may prescribe this modality. The patient is seen in the hospital for 2 to 4 days after surgery. Immediate postoperative care involves monitoring pain management and evaluating vital signs and the neurovascular status of the operated arm, as well as caring for the surgical wound site. Pain control is essential during hospitalization. The authors use a regional block to provide effective pain relief for approximately 12 hours. Patients can use an indwelling patient-controlled analgesia (PCA) pump at home for the first 24 hours, but most surgeons want to avoid the extra risk for infection.[88]

After the surgery, the surgeon delineates the extent of soft tissue damage and repair for the physical therapist because these factors determine when exercises can begin. For example, a Z-plasty lengthening, which sometimes is performed on the subscapularis if a long-standing medial rotation contracture is present, may limit the amount of lateral rotation allowed. Also, a massive rotator cuff repair may delay active lateral rotation for up to 8 weeks. Finally, the authors find it extremely useful for the surgeon to inform the physical therapist of the motion achieved at the end of the case.[15,87]

Early mobilization is essential to prevent the formation of adhesions and capsular contracture, especially if a complete capsular release was performed at the time of surgery. Early mobilization exercises (e.g., pendulum exercises) are recommended to relieve pain and prevent adhesion formation. Pendulum exercises produce minimal muscle activity and are considered a safe exercise during this period. The authors have even found that having the patient rest the hand on a physioball and perform pendular exercises makes the patient feel more relaxed and in control (Figure 8-23). Active-assisted shoulder flexion also is initiated at this time in the hospital bed (Figure 8-24). In fact, the electronic bed can be raised or lowered to use the influence of gravity to the patient's benefit. During this period, elbow and wrist ROM and gripping exercises are encouraged.

Milestones the authors look to achieve for discharge and progression to the next rehabilitation phase are (1) review with the patient the surgical procedure, precautions, and expectations during rehabilitation, (2) provide some pain relief, (3) ensure the patient's independence in performing exercises, and (4) accomplish initial ROM goals. With mobilization of the soft tissues, capsular releases, and proper component placement, the hospital therapy goals of 140° of forward elevation and 40° of lateral rotation before discharge can be achieved in many patients.

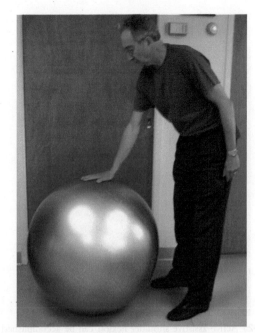

Figure 8-23 Example of the pendulum exercise in the supported position.

Immediate Postoperative Phase Milestones

- Review surgical procedure with patient
- Review precautions and expectations during rehabilitation
- Provide pain relief
- Help patient attain independence in performing exercises
- Achieve initial ROM goals (140° forward flexion, 40° lateral rotation)

Early Postoperative Phase (Weeks 1 to 6)

The early postoperative phase focuses on returning motion, restoring scapular stability, and initiating rotator cuff muscle activation. Active-assisted ROM (AAROM) should be initiated, using a pulley for sagittal plane flexion and scapular plane elevation. In addition, a cane, golf club, or umbrella can be used to help the patient regain flexion, abduction, adduction, and lateral rotation at 0°, 45°, and 90° abduction. An early series of exercises the authors prefer is using the cane supine three different ways for a total of 90 repetitions of horizontal adduction, serratus supine, and flexion (Figures 8-25 and 8-26). Unfortunately, the authors have not found a preferred method of AAROM

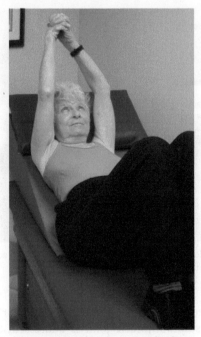

Figure 8-24 Active-assisted shoulder flexion can be done anywhere with the use of the uninvolved upper extremity.

for medial rotation with a cane, nor have they found the towel stretch to be useful for regaining medial rotation ROM. The authors' preferred method is to have the patient use pulleys in the standing position (Figure 8-27) or to perform the sleeper stretch (Figure 8-28) after 6 to 8 weeks of healing.

Joint mobilization and passive ROM can be important adjuncts if ROM difficulties occur. As mentioned, passive motion exercises, such as pendulum exercises, are good for pain relief and preventing the formation of adhesions.

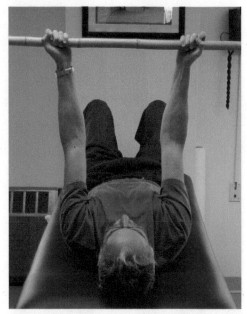

Figure 8-25 Active-assistive shoulder flexion can be accomplished with the use of a cane or stick.

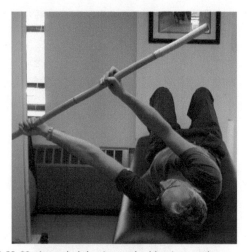

Figure 8-26 Horizontal abduction and adduction can be accomplished with the use of a cane or stick.

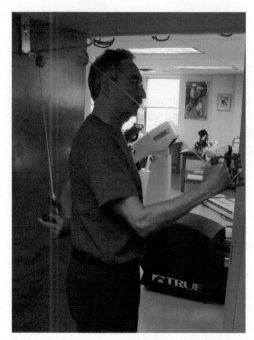

Figure 8-27 Use of pulleys to regain functional medial (internal) rotation ROM.

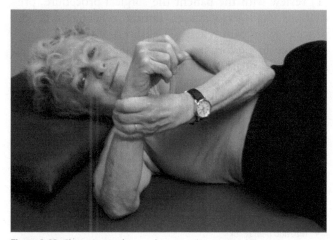

Figure 8-28 Sleeper stretch.

At this time, the mobility of the sternoclavicular joint, AC joint, and scapulothoracic joint is addressed, and these joints are mobilized if indicated. Once the milestone of mobility of these proximal joints has been reached, manual scapular stabilization is initiated. In the side-lying position, manual resistance can be applied to the scapula to resist elevation, depression, protraction, and retraction. The authors have found that pain can be a limiting factor when starting scapular stabilization and rotator cuff isometrics. However, submaximum pain-free isometrics for lateral rotation can be started as early as 7 days after surgery provided there is no rotator cuff involvement (Figure 8-29).

Isometric deltoid activity may also be initiated during this phase, provided pain is not a limiting factor. An arm

upper body ergometer (UBE) using light resistance can be beneficial at this time (4 weeks) to facilitate ROM and initiate active muscular control of the shoulder. The axis of rotation of the UBE should remain below the level of the shoulder joint so that forward flexion is not forced above 80°. The authors also stress the retro component of performing the UBE. By performing retro UBE (going backward), the authors hypothesize, the patient mobilizes the scapula and encourages proper posture.

Early strengthening of the serratus anterior muscle also is encouraged, provided the arm is maintained slightly below 90° of shoulder flexion and movement is pain free. Subsequent atrophy of the serratus anterior muscle, as a result of disuse, may allow the scapula to rest in a downwardly rotated position, causing inferior border

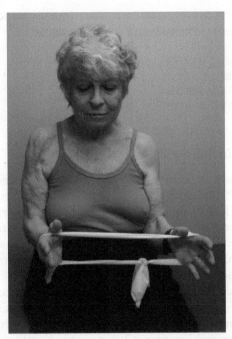

Figure 8-29 Early lateral (external) rotation strengthening.

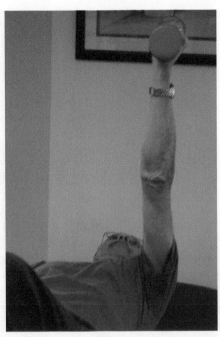

Figure 8-30 Serratus anterior strengthening in the supine position.

prominence. Decker et al.[89] used electromyography (EMG) to determine which exercises consistently elicited the highest percentage of the maximum voluntary contraction (MVC) of the serratus anterior. They found that the serratus anterior punch out, scaption, dynamic hug, knee push up plus, and push up plus exercises consistently elicited greater than 20% MVC. Most important, they determined that the push up plus and the dynamic hug exercises maintained the greatest percentage of the MVC and maintained the scapula in an upwardly rotated position. Although the early postoperative phase is too early in the rehabilitation process to perform these late exercises, Decker et al.[89] highlighted the serratus anterior punch out as a valuable exercise. Performed in a controlled, supervised setting, this is an excellent choice to initiate early serratus anterior neuromuscular reeducation (Figure 8-30). Progression to the more challenging serratus anterior strengthening exercises can be considered during the intermediate phase of rehabilitation, keeping in mind that the patient is instructed to avoid heavy pushing, pulling, and lifting for the first 6 weeks, and no upper extremity weight-bearing activities are allowed for 3 months.

A delicate balance exists between pushing patients too hard and progressing them as planned. Too often the patient may feel better rather than worse during this early protective phase; therefore the clinician must always respect the laws of tissue healing.

Milestones the authors look to achieve for progression to the next rehabilitation period are (1) toleration of submaximum isometrics of the rotator cuff muscles at 0° abduction; (2) attaining symmetrical mobility of the sternoclavicular, AC, and scapulothoracic joints; and (3) protraction,

retraction, elevation, and depression of the scapula against submaximum manual resistance. Adequate passive ROM in flexion, abduction, adduction, and medial rotation at 45° abduction (50% to 75% of the uninvolved side) also should be attained before the patient is progressed.

Early Postoperative Phase Milestones

- Ability to tolerate submaximum rotator cuff isometrics at 0°
- Symmetrical mobility of sternoclavicular, acromioclavicular, and scapulothoracic joints
- Ability to protract, retract, elevate, and depress scapula against submaximum manual resistance
- Adequate passive ROM (50% to 75% of uninvolved side) at 45° abduction

Intermediate Postoperative Phase (Weeks 6 to 12)

During the intermediate postoperative phase of rehabilitation, the patient attempts to regain all available ROM, including passive medial rotation. Initiation of passive lateral rotation ROM at 0°, 45°, and 90° abduction and stretching beyond neutral rotation position are emphasized. Advancement to terminal ranges in all planes of motion is advocated unless otherwise specified by the referring surgeon. Medial rotation submaximum resistive exercise progressions also are initiated during this phase. A traditional rotator cuff isotonic exercise program is started, which includes side-lying lateral rotation, prone extensions, and prone horizontal abduction (which may need to be limited between neutral to the scapular plane position initially, with progression to the coronal plane

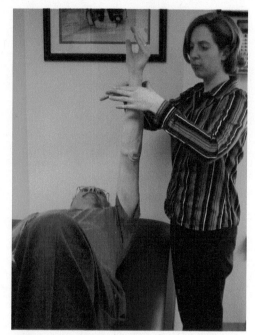

Figure 8-31 Rhythmic stabilization in open kinetic chain.

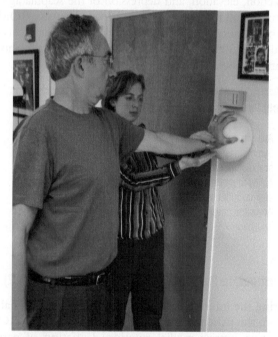

Figure 8-32 Rhythmic stabilization in closed kinetic chain.

as ROM improves). Biceps and triceps curls in the standing position with glenohumeral joint rotation in a neutral resting position are begun. In addition, oscillation exercises with Flexbar or a Body Blade can begin. Rhythmic stabilization in open kinetic chain (Figure 8-31) and closed kinetic chain (Figure 8-32) environments can begin, with caution in shoulder arthroplasty patients who will be placing higher demands on the shoulder.

> **Intermediate Postoperative Phase Milestones**
>
> - Regaining of full ROM
> - Rotator cuff isotonic exercise program
> - Oscillation exercises
> - Open and closed kinetic chain exercises

Return to Activity Phase (Weeks 12 to 24)

The return to activity phase is the stage of rehabilitation in which clinicians begin "to lose" their patients. Often patients lose focus, exhaust insurance coverage, or neglect the importance of fine-tuning the shoulder's function before fully returning to their lifestyle. This phase is designed to prepare patients to return without hesitation to full participation in all activities.

Milestones to complete this phase successfully include (1) acceptable (functional) pain-free ROM and (2) isokinetic or handheld dynamometry strength testing demonstrating less than a 20% deficit in shoulder flexion, abduction, and medial rotation. A deficit greater than 20% may still exist, depending on rotator cuff integrity at the time of surgery. Although not always considered as such, inadequate ROM is a complication that can occur after total shoulder arthroplasty. Acceptable ROM after shoulder arthroplasty has been defined as forward elevation to 140° to 160°, lateral rotation with the arm at the side to 40° to 60°, full extension, and 70° of medial rotation with the arm at 90° in the coronal plane. Inadequate ROM may be due to insufficient soft tissue release or joint overstuffing.

> **Return to Activity Phase Milestones**
>
> - Functional, pain-free ROM
> - No more than 20% strength deficit
> - Patient has confidence in shoulder

In this phase, the patient continues to work in functional positions, including plyometrics and strengthening at 90° abduction, and gradually returns to full activity, provided the individual is pain free, has nearly full ROM in all planes, confidence in the shoulder, and 85% to 90% of the strength of the opposite side for the motions of internal and lateral rotation. The patient acquires confidence by being able to perform pain-free functional movement in the person's usual activities. In the authors' experience, recreational athletes require 1 to 2 months more to allow the shoulder to accommodate to the sports-specific motion. The authors currently use the American Shoulder and Elbow Surgeons Shoulder Evaluation Form to standardize the documentation of pain, motion, strength, stability, and function. However, enough data have not been gathered to determine a criterion score for return to sports after shoulder arthroplasty. In a review article by Healy et al.,[90] 35 members of the American Shoulder and Elbow Surgeons Society were surveyed about their recommendations for athletics and sports participation for their patients who had shoulder replacement surgery. The surgeons were asked to rate 42 athletic activities as recommended or allowed, allowed with experience, no opinion, and not recommended. The 35 responses were analyzed to obtain a consensus recommendation for each activity. If a valid percentage was not achieved for either a positive or negative recommendation, no conclusion was provided for those activities. These recommendations are presented in Table 8-4.

These rehabilitation guidelines are a continuum of rehabilitation phases based on the effect of surgery on the tissue and surrounding structures. Scientific rationale is applied whenever possible, but as surgical procedures evolve, so must rehabilitation procedures. However, these guidelines are by no means set in stone, nor is every exercise distinct to that phase (see Table 8-2). The goals and exercises must be modified based on the performer, pathology, and performance demands. No exercise prescription should be viewed as protocol, but as a guideline upon which to base rehabilitation.

Key Points in Rehabilitation

- Goals and exercises must be modified based on the individual, pathology, performance demand, and functional outcome the individual hopes to achieve
- No exercise prescription should be viewed as a protocol but instead as a guideline based on individual patient needs and desires for a good functional outcome

OUTCOMES OF SHOULDER ARTHROPLASTY

Diagnosis of the correct indication for shoulder arthroplasty, the preoperative planning, and the postoperative rehabilitation program are essential for a good functional outcome and the keys to physical activity after shoulder arthroplasty. Although the optimum method for measuring the outcome in patients with shoulder arthroplasty has yet to be defined, the ideal assessment should include measures of general health, a shoulder-specific assessment, and an assessment specific to the disease state for which the shoulder arthroplasty was indicated.[91] Each of these levels of sensitivity offers a different perspective on the outcome of shoulder arthroplasty until the ideal universal outcome tool is developed.

Overall, shoulder arthroplasty has been shown to provide predictable pain relief and functional improvement in patients with glenohumeral degenerative arthritis and an intact rotator cuff.[92-94] Norris and Iannotti[95] reported on 133 total shoulder replacements and 43 hemiarthroplasties at an average follow-up of 46 months. They found no differences in postoperative pain, function, American Shoulder and Elbow Surgeons scores, or ROM. Also, no differences were seen between total shoulder arthroplasty and hemiarthroplasty in patients with repairable rotator cuff tears. Total shoulder arthroplasty and hemiarthroplasty for the treatment of primary osteoarthritis result in good or excellent pain relief, improved function, and patient satisfaction in 95% of cases. Boyd et al.[96] compared 64 patients who had hemiarthroplasty with 146 patients who had total shoulder arthroplasty in a retrospective review with a mean follow-up of 44 months. They found similar outcomes in terms of patients' functional improvement. No difference in

TABLE 8-4

Activity after Total Shoulder Arthroplasty: 1999 American Shoulder and Elbow Surgeons Survey

Recommended or Allowed	Allowed with Experience	Not Recommended	No Conclusion
• Cross-country skiing	• Golf	• Football	• High-impact aerobics
• NordicTrack	• Ice skating	• Gymnastics	• Baseball, softball
• Speed walking and jogging	• Shooting	• Hockey	• Fencing
• Swimming	• Downhill skiing	• Rock climbing	• Handball
• Doubles tennis			• Horseback riding
• Low-impact aerobics			• Lacrosse
• Bicycling (road and stationary)			• Racquetball, squash
• Bowling			• Skating (roller, inline)
• Canoeing			• Rowing
• Croquet			• Soccer
• Shuffleboard			• Tennis, singles
• Horseshoes			• Volleyball
• Dancing (ballroom, square, and jazz)			• Weight training

From Healy WL, Iorio R, Lemos MJ: Athletic activity after joint replacement, *Am J Sports Med* 29:377-388, 2001.

overall patient outcomes was observed between hemiarthroplasty and total shoulder arthroplasty.

Secondary to improvements in design and implant survivorship, total shoulder arthroplasty patients strive to return to higher levels of function and sports activity. In a case series conducted in 2010, 100 consecutive patients with unilateral total shoulder arthroplasty were followed for at least 1 year. Of the 55 patients who played sports before shoulder disease, 89% were still playing at a mean follow-up of 2.8 years, whereas more than two thirds (69.4%) reached the same level of intensity as before the shoulder pathology.[97] McCarty et al.[98] exhibited similar findings among 75 patients followed for a minimum of 2 years. Of the 48 patients who stated one of the reasons they opted for surgery was to return to sport, 71% demonstrated an improvement in their ability to play their sport and 50% increased their respective frequency of participation postoperatively (Figure 8-33). Jensen and Rockwood[99] retrospectively evaluated 24 golfers with shoulder replacements and found 23 players (96%) were able to resume playing golf. Three of these patients had bilateral shoulder arthroplasty. Among the 26 shoulder replacements in 24 patients, 6 were hemiarthroplasties and 20 were total shoulder arthroplasties. Of the 18 patients who were able to report a preoperative handicap, an average improvement of five strokes was reported after the operation.

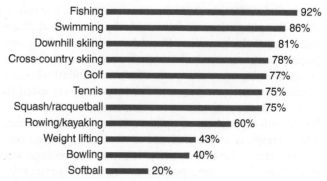

Figure 8-33 Sports participation after shoulder replacement surgery. (From McCarty EC, Marx RG, Maerz D et al: Sports participation after shoulder replacement surgery, *Am J Sports Med* 36(8):1579, 2008.)

SUMMARY

The success of shoulder arthroplasty depends on proper patient selection through a comprehensive history and physical examination, appropriate use of diagnostic modalities, good surgical skill, and effective rehabilitation. A thorough understanding of the pitfalls and complications that can affect patients undergoing shoulder arthroplasty is essential to a successful outcome. Technical advances in shoulder arthroplasty have allowed surgeons the use of this procedure with confidence and have helped optimize results.

REFERENCES

1. Lugli T: Artificial shoulder joint by Pean (1893): the facts of an exceptional intervention and the prosthetic method, *Clin Orthop Relat Res* 133:215–218, 1978.
2. Cofield RH: Status of total shoulder arthroplasty, *Arch Surg* 112:1088–1091, 1977.
3. Bankes MJ, Emery RJ: Pioneers of shoulder replacement: Themistocles Gluck and Jules Emile Pean, *J Shoulder Elbow Surg* 4:259–262, 1995.
4. American Academy of Orthopaedic Surgeons: *Arthroplasty and total joint replacement procedures: 1991 to 2000*, Rosemont, 2005, American Academy of Orthopaedic Surgeons.
5. Healy WL, Iorio R, Lemos MJ: Athletic activity after joint replacement, *Am J Sports Med* 29:377–388, 2001.
6. Rodosky MW, Bigliani LU: Indications for glenoid resurfacing in shoulder arthroplasty, *J Shoulder Elbow Surg* 5:231–248, 1996.
7. Fenlin JM, Frieman BG: Indications, technique, and results of total shoulder arthroplasty in osteoarthritis, *Orthop Clin North Am* 29:423–434, 1998.
8. Waldman BJ, Figgie MP: Indications, technique, and results of total shoulder arthroplasty in rheumatoid arthritis, *Orthop Clin North Am* 29:435–444, 1998.
9. Hattrup SJ: Indications, technique, and results of shoulder arthroplasty in osteonecrosis, *Orthop Clin North Am* 29:445–451, 1998.
10. Bos G, Sim F, Pritchard D, et al: Prosthetic replacement of the proximal humerus, *Clin Orthop Relat Res* 224:178–191, 1987.
11. Boileau P, Trojani C, Walch G, et al: Shoulder arthroplasty for the treatment of the sequelae of fractures of the proximal humerus, *J Shoulder Elbow Surg* 10:299–308, 2001.
12. Brems JJ: Shoulder arthroplasty in the face of acute fracture: puzzle pieces, *J Arthroplasty* 17(suppl 1): 32–35, 2002.

13. Antuna SA, Sperling JW, Sanchez-Sotelo J, et al: Shoulder arthroplasty for proximal humeral nonunions, *J Shoulder Elbow Surg* 11:114–121, 2002.
14. Neer CS: Shoulder arthroplasty today, *Orthopade* 20:320–321, 1991.
15. Brown DD, Friedman RJ: Postoperative rehabilitation following total shoulder arthroplasty, *Orthop Clin North Am* 29:535–547, 1998.
16. Cuomo F, Checroun A: Avoiding pitfalls and complications in total shoulder arthroplasty, *Orthop Clin North Am* 29:507–518, 1998.
17. Neer CS, Flatow EL, Lech O: Tears of the rotator cuff: long term results of anterior acromioplasty and repair, *Orthop Trans* 12:735, 1988.
18. Hawkins RJ, Misamore GW, Hobeika PE: Surgery for full thickness rotator cuff tears, *J Bone Joint Surg Am* 67:1349–1355, 1985.
19. Hertel R, Ballmer F, Lombert SM, et al: Lag signs in the diagnosis of rotator cuff rupture, *J Shoulder Elbow Surg* 5:307–313, 1996.
20. Gerber C, Krushell RJ: Isolated tears of the subscapularis muscle: clinical features in sixteen cases, *J Bone Joint Surg Br* 73:389–394, 1991.
21. Gerber A, Ghalambor N, Warner JJ: Instability of shoulder arthroplasty: balancing mobility and stability, *Orthop Clin North Am* 32:661–670, 2001.
22. Zuckerman JD, Cuomo F: Glenohumeral arthroplasty: a critical review of indications and preoperative considerations, *Bull Hosp Joint Dis* 52:21–30, 1993.
23. Norwood LA, Barrack R, Jacobson KE: Clinical presentation of complete tears of the rotator cuff, *J Bone Joint Surg Am* 71:499–505, 1989.
24. Millett PJ, Gobezie R, Boykin RB: Shoulder osteoarthritis: diagnosis and management, *Am Fam Physician* 78:605–611, 2008.

25. Kircher J, Morhard M, Magosch P, et al: How much are radiological parameters related to clinical symptoms and function in osteoarthritis of the shoulder? *Int Orthop* 34:677–681, 2009.
26. Hernigou P, Duparc F, Hernigou A: Determining humeral retroversion with computed tomography, *J Bone Joint Surg Am* 84:1753–1762, 2002.
27. Hernigou P, Duparc F, Filali C: Humeral retroversion and shoulder prosthesis, *Rev Chir Orthop Reparatrice Appar Mot* 81:419–427, 1995.
28. Kuhlman JE, Fishman EK, Ney DR, et al: Complex shoulder trauma: three dimensional CT imaging, *Orthopedics* 11:1561–1563, 1988.
29. Couteau B, Mansat P, Mansat M, et al: In vivo characterization of glenoid with use of computed tomography, *J Shoulder Elbow Surg* 10:116–122, 2001.
30. Soini I, Belt EA, Niemitukia L, et al: Magnetic resonance imaging of the rotator cuff in destroyed rheumatoid shoulder: comparison with findings during shoulder replacement, *Acta Radiol* l45:434–439, 2004.
31. Taylor DC, Arciero RA: Pathologic changes associated with shoulder dislocations: arthroscopic and physical examination findings in first-time, traumatic anterior dislocations, *Am J Sports Med* 25:306–311, 1997.
32. Hovelius L, Augustini BG, Fredin H, et al: Primary anterior dislocation of the shoulder in young patients: a ten-year prospective study, *J Bone Joint Surg Am* 78:1677–1684, 1996.
33. Marx RG, McCarty EC, Montemurno TD, et al: Development of arthrosis following dislocation of the shoulder: a case-control study, *J Shoulder Elbow Surg* 11:1–5, 2002.
34. Sperling JW, Antuna SA, Sanchez-Sotelo J, et al: Shoulder arthroplasty for arthritis after instability surgery, *J Bone Joint Surg Am* 84:1775–1781, 2002.

35. Burroughs PL, Gearen PF, Petty WR, et al: Shoulder arthroplasty in the young patient, *J Arthroplasty* 18:792–798, 2003.

36. Wirth MA, Rockwood CA: Complications of shoulder arthroplasty, *Clin Orthop Relat Res* 307:47–69, 1994.

37. Arcand M, Burkhead WZ, Zeman C: Pulmonary embolism caused by thrombosis of the axillary vein after shoulder arthroplasty, *J Shoulder Elbow Surg* 6:486–490, 1997.

38. Saleem A, Markel DC: Fatal pulmonary embolus after shoulder arthroplasty, *J Arthroplasty* 16:400–403, 2001.

39. Lynch NM, Cofield RH, Silbert PL, et al: Neurologic complications after total shoulder arthroplasty, *J Shoulder Elbow Surg* 5:53–61, 1996.

40. Brems JJ: Rehabilitation following total shoulder arthroplasty, *Clin Orthop Relat Res* 307:70–85, 1994.

41. Gallagher LL: When your patient has a shoulder arthroplasty: here's how to help, *Nursing* 10:46–49, 1980.

42. Matsen FA: Early effectiveness of shoulder arthroplasty for patients who have primary glenohumeral degenerative joint disease, *J Bone Joint Surg Am* 78:260–264, 1996.

43. Cofield RH, Frankle MA, Zuckerman JD: Humeral head replacement for glenohumeral arthritis, *Semin Arthroplasty* 6:214–221, 1995.

44. Nwakama AC, Cofield RH, Kavanagh BF, et al: Semiconstrained total shoulder arthroplasty for glenohumeral arthritis and massive rotator cuff tearing, *J Shoulder Elbow Surg* 9:302–307, 2000.

45. Smith KL, Matsen FA: Total shoulder arthroplasty versus hemiarthroplasty: current trends, *Orthop Clin North Am* 29:491–506, 1998.

46. Robinson CM, Page RS, Hill RMF, et al: Primary hemiarthroplasty for treatment of proximal humeral fractures, *J Bone Joint Surg Am* 85:1215–1223, 2003.

47. Edwards TB, Kadakia NR, Boulahia A, et al: A comparison of hemiarthroplasty and total shoulder arthroplasty in the treatment of primary glenohumeral osteoarthritis: results of a multicenter study, *J Shoulder Elbow Surg* 12:207–213, 2003.

48. Carroll RM, Izquierdo R, Vazquez M, et al: Conversion of painful hemiarthroplasty to total shoulder arthroplasty: long-term results, *J Shoulder Elbow Surg* 13:599–603, 2004.

49. Sirveaux F, Favard L, Oudet D, et al: Grammont inverted total shoulder arthroplasty in the treatment of glenohumeral osteoarthritis with massive rupture of the cuff: results of a multicentre study of 80 shoulders, *J Bone Joint Surg Br* 86:388–395, 2004.

50. Rittmeister M, Kerschbaumer F: Grammont reverse total shoulder arthroplasty in patients with rheumatoid arthritis and nonreconstructible rotator cuff lesions, *J Shoulder Elbow Surg* 10:17–22, 2001.

51. Franklin JL, Barrett WP, Jackins SE, et al: Glenoid loosening in total shoulder arthroplasty: association with rotator cuff deficiency, *J Arthroplasty* 3:39–46, 1988.

52. Boulahia A, Edwards TB, Walch G, et al: Early results of a reverse design prosthesis in the treatment of arthritis of the shoulder in elderly patients with a large rotator cuff tear, *Orthopedics* 25:129–133, 2002.

53. Harman M, Frankle M, Vasey M, et al: Initial glenoid component fixation in "reverse" total shoulder arthroplasty: a biomechanical evaluation, *J Shoulder Elbow Surg* 14(suppl S):162S–167S, 2005.

54. Boileau P, Watkinson DJ, Hatzidakis AM, et al: Grammont reverse prosthesis: design, rationale, and biomechanics, *J Shoulder Elbow Surg* 14(suppl S):147S–161S, 2005.

55. Guery J, Favard L, Sirveaux F, et al: Reverse total shoulder arthroplasty. Survivorship analysis of eighty replacements followed for five to ten years, *J Bone Joint Surg Am* 88:1742–1747, 2006.

56. Singh A, Yian EH, Dillon MT, et al: The effect of surgeon and hospital voume on shoulder arthroplasty perioperative quality metrics, *J Shoulder Elbow Surg* 23:1187–1194, 2014.

57. Boardman ND, Cofield RH, Bengtson KA, et al: Rehabilitation after total shoulder arthroplasty, *J Arthroplasty* 16:483–486, 2001.

58. Deuschle JA, Romeo AA: Understanding shoulder arthroplasty, *Orthop Nurs* 17:7–15, 1998.

59. Boyd AD, Thornhill TS: Surgical treatment of osteoarthritis of the shoulder, *Rheum Dis Clin North Am* 14:591–611, 1988.

60. Sojbjerg JO, Frich LH, Johannsen HV, et al: Late results of total shoulder replacement in patients with rheumatoid arthritis, *Clin Orthop Relat Res* 366:39–45, 1999.

61. Lehtinen JT, Belt EA, Kauppi MJ, et al: Bone destruction, upward migration, and medialisation of rheumatoid shoulder: a 15 year follow up study, *Ann Rheum Dis* 60:322–326, 2001.

62. Cameron B, Galatz L, Williams GR: Factors affecting the outcome of total shoulder arthroplasty, *Am J Orthop* 30:613–623, 2001.

63. Ponce BA, Menendez ME, Oladeji LO, et al: Diabetes as a risk factor for poorer early postoperative outcomes after shoulder arthroplasty, *J Shoulder Elbow Surg* 23:671–678, 2014.

64. Hettrich CM, Weldon E, Boorman RS, et al: Preoperative factors associated with improvements in shoulder function after humeral hemiarthroplasty, *J Bone Joint Surg Am* 86:1446–1451, 2004.

65. Kay SP, Amstutz HC: Shoulder hemiarthroplasty at UCLA, *Clin Orthop Relat Res* 228:42–48, 1988.

66. Trail IA, Nuttall D: The results of shoulder arthroplasty in patients with rheumatoid arthritis, *J Bone Joint Surg Br* 84:1121–1125, 2002.

67. Levy O, Copeland SA: Cementless surface replacement arthroplasty (Copeland CSRA) for osteoarthritis of the shoulder, *J Shoulder Elbow Surg* 13:266–271, 2004.

68. Bot AGJ, Menendex ME, Neuhaus V, et al: The influence of psychiatric comorbidity on perioperative outcomes after shoulder arthroplasty, *J Shoulder Elbow Surg* 23:519–527, 2014.

69. Iannotti JP, Norris TR: Influence of preoperative factors on outcome of shoulder arthroplasty for glenohumeral osteoarthritis, *J Bone Joint Surg Am* 85:251–258, 2003.

70. Kelly JD, Norris TR: Decision making in glenohumeral arthroplasty, *J Arthroplasty* 18:75–82, 2003.

71. Friedman RJ: Biomechanics of total shoulder arthroplasty: a preoperative and postoperative analysis, *Semin Arthroplasty* 6:222–232, 1995.

72. Fenlin JM, Ramsey ML, Allardyce TJ, et al: Modular total shoulder replacement: design rationale, indications, and results, *Clin Orthop Relat Res* 307:37–46, 1994.

73. McCullagh PJ: Biomechanics and design of shoulder arthroplasty, *Proc Inst Mech Eng H* 209:207–213, 1995.

74. Cofield RH, Edgerton BC: Total shoulder arthroplasty: complications and revision surgery, *Instr Course Lect* 39:449–462, 1990.

75. Brems JJ: Complications of shoulder arthroplasty: infections, instability, and loosening, *Instr Course Lect* 51:29–39, 2002.

76. Tetzlaff JE, Yoon HJ, Brems J: Interscalene brachial plexus block for shoulder surgery, *Reg Anesth* 19:339–343, 1994.

77. Romeo AA: Total shoulder arthroplasty: pearls and pitfalls in surgical technique, *Semin Arthroplasty* 6:265–272, 1995.

78. Friedman RJ: Humeral technique in total shoulder arthroplasty, *Orthop Clin North Am* 29:393–402, 1998.

79. Lacroix D, Murphy LA, Prendergast PJ: Three-dimensional finite element analysis of glenoid replacement prostheses: a comparison of keeled and pegged anchorage systems, *J Biomech Eng* 122:430–436, 2000.

80. Ibarra C, Dines DM, McLaughlin JA: Glenoid replacement in total shoulder arthroplasty, *Orthop Clin North Am* 29:403–413, 1998.

81. Churchill RS, Brems JJ, Kotschi H: Glenoid size, inclination, and version: an anatomic study, *J Shoulder Elbow Surg* 10:327–332, 2001.

82. Boileau P, Avidor C, Krishnan SG, et al: Cemented polyethylene versus uncemented metal-backed glenoid components in total shoulder arthroplasty: a prospective, double-blind, randomized study, *J Shoulder Elbow Surg* 11:351–359, 2002.

83. Vaesel MT, Olsen BS, Sojbjerg JO, et al: Humeral head size in shoulder arthroplasty: a kinematic study, *J Shoulder Elbow Surg* 6:549–555, 1997.

84. Ibarra C, Craig EV: Soft-tissue balancing in total shoulder arthroplasty, *Orthop Clin North Am* 29:415–422, 1998.

85. Fehringer EV, Mikuls TR, Michaud KD, et al: Shoulder arthroplaties have fewer complications than hip or knee arthroplasties in US veterans, *Clin Orthop Rel Res* 468:717–722, 2010.

86. Mahoney A, Bosco JA, Zuckerman JD: Readmission after shoulder arthroplasty, *J Shoulder Elbow Surg* 23:377–381, 2014.

87. Jackins S: Postoperative shoulder rehabilitation, *Phys Med Rehabil Clin North Am* 5:643–682, 2004.

88. Maurer K, Ekatodramis G, Hodler J, et al: Bilateral continuous interscalene block of brachial plexus for analgesia after bilateral shoulder arthroplasty, *Anesthesiology* 96:762–764, 2002.

89. Decker MJ, Hintermeister RA, Faber KJ, et al: Serratus anterior muscle activity during selected rehabilitation exercises, *Am J Sports Med* 27784–27791: 1999.

90. Healy WL, Iorio R, Lemos MJ: Athletic activity after joint replacement, *Am J Sports Med* 29:377–388, 2001.

91. Jain N, Pietrobon R, Hocker S, et al: The relationship between surgeon and hospital volume and outcomes for shoulder arthroplasty, *J Bone Joint Surg Am* 86:496–505, 2004.

92. Barrett WP, Franklin JL, Jackins SE, et al: Total shoulder arthroplasty, *J Bone Joint Surg Am* 69:865–872, 1987.

93. Matsoukis J, Tabib W, Guiffault P, et al: Shoulder arthroplasty in patients with a prior anterior shoulder dislocation. Results of a multicenter study, *J Bone Joint Surg Am* 85:1417–1424, 2003.

94. Cofield RH: Total shoulder arthroplasty with the Neer prosthesis, *J Bone Joint Surg Am* 66:899–906, 1984.

95. Norris TR, Iannotti JP: Functional outcome after shoulder arthroplasty for primary osteoarthritis: a multicenter study, *J Shoulder Elbow Surg* 11:130–135, 2002.

96. Boyd Jr. AD, Thomas WH, Scott RD, et al: Total shoulder arthroplasty versus hemiarthroplasty. Indications for glenoid resurfacing, *J Arthroplasty* 5:329–336, 1990.

97. Schumann K, Flury MP, Schwyzer HK, et al: Sports activity after anatomical total shoulder arthroplasty, *Am J Sports Med* 38:2097–2105, 2010.

98. McCarty EC, Marx RG, Maerz D, et al: Sports participation after shoulder replacement surgery, *Am J Sports Med* 36:1577–1581, 2008.

99. Jensen KL, Rockwood CA: Shoulder arthroplasty in recreational golfers, *J Shoulder Elbow Surg* 7:362–367, 1998.

CHAPTER 9

Elbow

KEVIN E. WILK, CHRISTOPHER A. ARRIGO, MARC R. SAFRAN, STEVEN A. AVILES

INTRODUCTION

Elbow injuries affect patients of all ages and activity levels. Whether caused by acute trauma or chronic overuse, elbow pathology can result in significant pain and disability. Because the elbow positions the hand for use, normal elbow motion, strength, and stability are essential not only for activities of daily living (ADLs) but also for higher level professional and athletic skills. Appropriate diagnosis and treatment require a detailed understanding of the normal anatomy of the elbow and the pathophysiology of injuries that affect the joint and its surrounding tissues. Symptoms can arise from abnormalities in bone, cartilage, muscles, tendons, ligaments, and/or neurovascular structures. The clinician should consider the functional expectations of the individual patient when determining the most appropriate course of treatment. Many patients can be managed successfully with medications, physical therapy, and other nonsurgical approaches. However, depending on the specific pathology and the response to conservative care, some patients require surgical treatment.

FUNCTIONAL ANATOMY AND BIOMECHANICS

The anatomical structures of the elbow must provide stability through a complex range of motions. Normal elbow function, whether for ADLs or high-level activities, requires motion through both flexion/extension and pronation/supination. The dynamic stability seen in the normal elbow depends on varying contributions from the osseous, ligamentous, and other soft tissue structures about the elbow.

Bony Anatomy

The ulnohumeral joint acts primarily as a hinge joint and provides most of the anteroposterior stability to the elbow.[1] In addition, it is a major contributor to varus-valgus stability, particularly near full extension and with higher degrees of flexion. The normal carrying angle across the elbow joint is 11° to 16° of valgus (Figure 9-1).[2] Pronation and supination are provided by the articulation of the proximal radius with the capitellum of the distal humerus and proximal ulna (Figure 9-2). The radial head acts as a secondary restraint to valgus stress when the medial ligaments of the elbow have been injured.[3,4]

Range of Motion

Normal range of motion (ROM) at the elbow is full extension to 140° of flexion with 75° of pronation and 85° of supination.[5] The basic functional goals and tasks of ADLs generally can be accomplished with a ROM of 30° to 130° of elbow extension to flexion and approximately 50° of pronation/supination.[6] However, for many high-level and athletic goals, the functionally acceptable ROM may be different. For instance, a gymnast or power lifter will not tolerate any less than full extension because of the weight that must be borne by the upper extremity. Baseball pitchers, on the other hand, can throw effectively with a flexion contracture exceeding 20° and only 100° of elbow flexion.

Ulnar/Medial Ligament Complex

The medial ligament, or ulnar collateral ligament (UCL), is the ligamentous complex on the medial aspect of the elbow between the distal humerus and the proximal ulna (Figure 9-3). Its anterior portion, the anterior oblique ligament (AOL), is the elbow's primary restraint against valgus stress, especially the forces associated with throwing.[3,4,7,8] The AOL consists of an anterior band, which is taut between 0° and 60° of flexion, and a posterior band, which is taut from 60° to 120° of elbow flexion.[8,9] The anterior band is primarily responsible for stability against valgus stresses at 30°, 60°, and 90° of flexion, making it the most important component in resisting the valgus forces associated with overhead sports activities. The posterior band of the AOL begins as a secondary restraint to valgus stability at 30° and 90° and is a primary restraint to valgus force at 120° of flexion.[7] The posterior oblique ligament forms the floor of the cubital tunnel and plays a bigger role as a restraint against valgus stress at higher degrees of flexion. The role of the transverse ligament (Cooper's ligament) in elbow stability remains unclear,

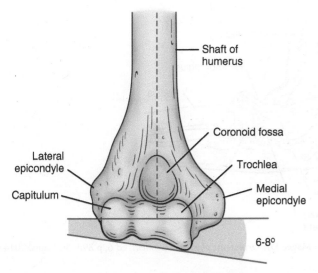

Figure 9-1 Anatomy of the distal humerus showing how the bony anatomy contributes to the overall valgus alignment of the elbow. There is approximately 6° to 8° of valgus tilt of the distal humeral articulation with respect to the long axis of the humerus.

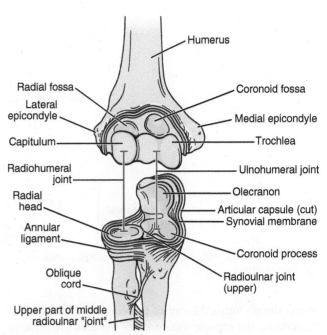

Figure 9-2 Anterior view of the right elbow, disarticulated to expose the ulnohumeral and radiohumeral joints. The margin of the proximal radioulnar joint is shown within the elbow's capsule. (From Magee DJ: *Orthopedic physical assessment*, ed 6, p 389, St. Louis, 2014, Saunders/Elsevier.)

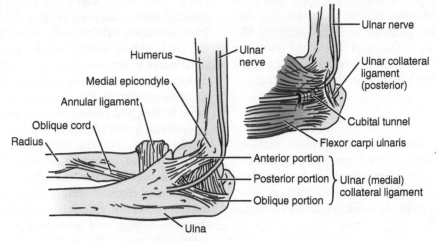

Figure 9-3 The ulnar (medial) collateral ligament complex of the elbow. Note the passage of the ulnar nerve through the cubital tunnel. (From Magee DJ: *Orthopedic physical assessment*, ed 6, p 390, St. Louis, 2014, Elsevier/Saunders.)

because this ligament originates from and inserts into the olecranon.

Lateral Ligament Complex

The lateral ligament complex consists primarily of the lateral ulnar collateral ligament (LUCL), the lateral radial collateral ligament (RCL), and the annular ligament (AL) (Figure 9-4). The LUCL, first described by Morrey and An,[9] originates from the lateral epicondyle. It passes over the AL and then begins to blend with the AL distally, where it inserts onto the supinator crest of the ulna. O'Driscoll et al.[10,11] have suggested that the LUCL is the essential structure that prevents posterolateral rotatory

instability. However, other studies have indicated that many components of the lateral ligament complex contribute to the prevention of posterolateral instability. Isolated sectioning of the LUCL distal to the AL results only in minor laxity. In contrast, significant rotatory instability is observed with more proximal transection of the LUCL and RCL.[12] Most likely all the components of the lateral ligament complex act together to prevent rotatory instability, but the LUCL clearly is the major contributor.

Capsule

The anterior capsule originates from the distal humerus proximal to the radial and coronoid fossae. It then

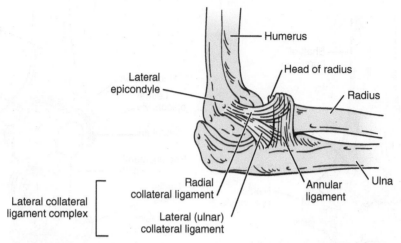

Figure 9-4 The lateral (radial) collateral ligament complex of the elbow. (From Magee DJ: *Orthopedic physical assessment*, ed 6, p 390, St. Louis, 2014, Elsevier/Saunders.)

inserts distally onto the rim of the coronoid and the AL. Posteriorly, the capsule incorporates the area proximal to the olecranon process. It attaches distally along the articular margin of the sigmoid notch and the proximal aspect of the olecranon fossa.[13] In terms of elbow stability, most of the literature has focused on the osseous articulation and ligaments. However, the anterior capsule apparently does make a significant contribution as well. The anterior capsule has been shown in a cadaveric study to contribute 38% of the resistance to valgus force and 32% of the resistance to varus force in full extension.[14] The posterior capsule's contribution to stability has not been well documented.

Muscles

The muscles about the elbow also provide stability. Because of the conformity of the elbow joint, the muscles about the elbow provide dynamic stability by compressing the joint surfaces through muscular contraction.[13,15–17] The muscles also may passively assist in stability by means of a "bulk effect."[13,18]

PATHOPHYSIOLOGY AND PATHOMECHANICS

The elbow can be subjected to numerous external forces in activities that place high loads on it, especially during sports. The elbow of the athletes doing overhead activities is subjected to major valgus forces and as a result is at risk for specific elbow injuries. Sports such as baseball, football, tennis, volleyball, golf, and water polo are most commonly associated with both acute and chronic elbow pathologies. Overhead throwing athletes are predisposed to overuse syndromes secondary to the repetitive, high-velocity stresses placed on the elbow during these high-velocity activities. The highest stress at the elbow occurs during the late cocking and acceleration phases of the throwing cycle.[19] Studies have indicated that the valgus stress at the elbow during the acceleration phase of

throwing can be as high as 64 N-m, which exceeds the ultimate tensile strength of the UCL.[20] These supraphysiological stresses create the potential for injuries that can typically be determined based on the pathophysiology of the forces applied to the elbow complex. These include traction or tensile forces on the medial-sided structures, compression of the lateral side of the elbow, and medially directed shear posteriorly (Figure 9-5).[21,22] Overhead athletes commonly exhibit both chronic and acute injuries to the UCL with or without medial epicondylitis, as well as ulnar nerve symptoms. Laterally, compression leads to radiocapitellar degeneration and loose bodies, and posterior shear forces may lead to olecranon osteophyte formation, loose bodies, and olecranon stress fractures.

Golf and tennis players have a high incidence of medial and lateral epicondylitis. Gymnasts can develop radiocapitellar overload, including osteochondritis dissecans, and posterior impingement secondary to weight bearing on an extended elbow.[23] Weight lifters and shot-putters may develop posterior elbow compressive injuries, including chondral damage and loose bodies, in addition to being susceptible to developing triceps injuries.[24]

Acute injuries, such as fractures and dislocations, can occur as a result of a fall on an outstretched hand (**FOOSH injury**) or direct trauma. These occur in sports as well as in everyday activities.

FRACTURES AND DISLOCATIONS

Dislocations

The elbow is the second most commonly dislocated major joint in the body and the most frequently dislocated joint in children.[25] Elbow dislocation is most often produced with high-energy mechanisms of injury. It usually results from a FOOSH, which imparts a combination of axial compression, supination, and valgus stress to the elbow dislocating the bony elements of the joint.[26]

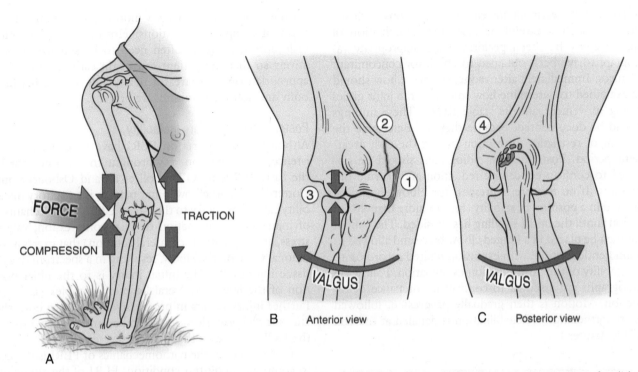

Figure 9-5 Valgus overload to the elbow. **A,** Mechanism of injury. **B,** Anterior view. **C,** Posterior view. Injury may lead to (1) stretching of medial collateral ligament, (2) stress on epicondylar growth plate (pitcher's or little leaguer's elbow), (3) compression at radiohumeral joint, or (4) compression of the olecranon in the fossa, which may lead to osteophyte and loose body formation. (From Magee DJ: *Orthopedic physical assessment*, ed 6, p 391, St. Louis, 2014, Saunders/Elsevier.)

No single classification system is used consistently for elbow dislocations. They generally are described according to the direction and degree of displacement, whether associated fractures are present, and the acuity or chronicity of the injury.

Elbow Dislocations

- The elbow is the second most frequently dislocated major joint
- Elbow dislocations are the most common dislocation in pediatric patients

O'Driscoll et al.[27] described the most common mechanism of acute elbow instability as posterolateral rotatory instability (PLRI). This instability involves a complex pattern of injury that involves rotational displacement of the ulna on the trochlea and subluxation or dislocation of the radius posteriorly from the capitellum, while the radius and ulna maintain their normal relationship to each other. The full spectrum of injury seen with an elbow dislocation can be understood as a disruption of the circle of soft tissue and bone that begins on the lateral side of the elbow and progresses medially (circle of Horii).[26] Stage 1 involves partial or complete disruption of the LUCL, resulting in posterolateral rotatory subluxation. In stage 2, additional disruption occurs anteriorly and posteriorly, resulting in an incomplete posterolateral dislocation, or

"perched" dislocation. More severe injury results in stage 3A, in which all soft tissues except the UCL have been disrupted and the elbow is stable only in pronation. In stage 3B the UCL has been disrupted, and in stage 3C the entire distal humerus has been stripped of soft tissues, resulting in stability only with flexion greater than 90°. Josefsson et al.[25,28] in his series, however, reported that all simple elbow dislocations (i.e., those not associated with fracture) involved injury to the UCL.

In children, elbow dislocations are associated with fractures in up to 50% of cases, especially fractures of the radial head, neck, and medial or lateral epicondyle.[29] Elbow dislocations in children may involve avulsion of the medial epicondyle apophysis instead of direct injury to the ligaments because the physis is weaker than the ligaments. The avulsed fragment may be nondisplaced or displaced a few millimeters; or worse, it may be even more displaced and become incarcerated in the joint. Avulsions of the medial epicondyle may occur in up to 30% of children with dislocations.[30-32]

Injury to the musculotendinous origins of the wrist flexors and/or extensors is not uncommon in elbow dislocations. Other concomitant injuries include radial head and neck fractures, which may occur in 5% to 10% of elbow dislocations, and olecranon fractures.[33] It is important that the examiner identify coronoid fractures, because the prognosis for recurrent elbow instability is directly affected by the amount of the coronoid involved (see discussion later in this chapter).

The initial treatment for elbow dislocations is closed reduction after a careful neurovascular examination of the extremity has been performed and appropriate radiographs have been obtained to check for concomitant fractures. Immediately after reduction, the elbow should be examined to determine how smoothly the joint glides during movement and its stable ROM. These findings should be documented, because they will determine the amount of restriction of motion during the early treatment period. Postreduction radiographs should be obtained to confirm concentric reduction and to rule out fractures. If no fracture is present, the elbow should be splinted in a position of stability (but no more than 90° of flexion) until the initial swelling has subsided. The patient can then be placed in a hinged elbow brace and allowed to begin gentle motion, with extension limited according to the stability of the postreduction examination. Follow-up radiographs are essential to confirm maintenance of reduction. Motion is then gradually progressed, followed by strengthening.[34] (Rehabilitation is detailed at the end of this chapter.)

Postreduction Elbow Assessment

- The postreduction stable ROM and gliding smoothness determine the amount of motion allowed in early treatment

---

Follow-up is important. Long-term follow-up studies have reported that persistent valgus laxity after elbow dislocation is associated with poorer overall clinical and radiographic results compared with elbows without increased valgus laxity after elbow dislocation.[35] Furthermore, chronic problems related to PLRI may occur; therefore care must be taken to evaluate the patient for this problem.

It is helpful to distinguish simple from complex elbow dislocations. Simple dislocations are not associated with fractures, whereas complex dislocations result in an associated elbow fracture. Simple dislocations rarely require surgical treatment, and recurrent instability is extremely rare (fewer than 2%).[36] Josefsson et al.[28] compared the operative and nonoperative treatment of simple dislocations. In a prospective trial, they found that elbows treated nonoperatively actually had a slightly improved ROM and better subjective results than those treated operatively.

Early ROM is essential to achieve a good outcome. Posttraumatic stiffness is the most common complication. Mehlhoff et al.[37] and Protzman[31] reported that a shorter immobilization time significantly correlated with better outcomes. Regardless, most patients commonly have at least 10° of flexion contracture. For this reason, some surgeons advocate early surgical repair or reconstruction of the injured ligament or ligaments after unstable elbow dislocations to allow for aggressive early ROM.[38]

The same principle of early motion applies in the treatment of complex dislocations. However, with complex dislocations, fractures often need to be stabilized operatively so that the patient can begin early motion. The appropriate operative treatment depends on exactly which bony and soft tissue injuries are present.

Posterolateral Rotatory Instability

Although case reports on PLRI have long been in existence, the condition was brought to the forefront in the early 1990s by O'Driscoll et al. and Osbourne and Cotterill.[27,39] This elbow injury pattern is a rotatory instability caused by injury to the lateral UCL. The mechanism of injury is a combination of axial compression, valgus stress, and supination (or lateral rotation) that exerts a rotational force on the elbow, resulting in a spectrum of soft tissue injuries.[26,27] The initial injury is to the ulnar portion of the lateral collateral ligament complex (LCLC). Further injury results in progressive damage to both the anterior and posterior capsule and eventually may involve the UCL complex if the injury is severe enough.[10,26,27]

Understanding the pathomechanics of PLRI is the key to comprehending this condition. PLRI of the elbow results from a rotatory subluxation of the radius and ulna (which move together as a unit) relative to the distal humerus. Because the AL remains intact in this injury, the radioulnar joint maintains its normal relationship, and the proximal radius and ulna therefore move together in a "coupled" motion. Most give credit to Osbourne and Cotterill[39] as the first investigators to fully appreciate the importance of the lateral ligament complex of the elbow in recurrent instability and to describe the findings of PLRI. Although much of the initial literature by O'Driscoll and the laboratory at the Mayo Clinic reported the results of biomechanical studies demonstrating that the primary stabilizer in PLRI is the LUCL, much of the recent literature suggests that the injury may not be to the LUCL alone.[10,26,27,40] According to some reports, the RCL and anteroposterior capsule serve as secondary stabilizing restraints and are also involved in PLRI of the elbow. However, clinically, it is known that elbow dislocations and injury to the LCLC occur as the primary injury and PLRI is most commonly seen after an elbow dislocation. Subsequent research by other investigators has suggested that isolated injury to the LUCL alone may not be enough to produce PLRI.[12,13,41] Some suggest that the complex works in a Y configuration and that a proximal injury, near the epicondyle, as seen clinically, can and does produce PLRI.[42]

The diagnosis of PLRI is much more elusive than other ligament injuries, including injuries of the UCL. It requires a careful history and physical examination to discern its presence. The clinician must be diligent with the assessment and maintain a high degree of suspicion in patients with vague reports of elbow discomfort. Patients with PLRI frequently report that they have painful sensations of clicking, snapping, clunking, locking, dislocating, or giving way. The position of the hand during maneuvers that elicit these symptoms is critical, because the symptoms of PLRI often are produced when the patient extends the elbow with the forearm supinated.[27] Examples include using the hands to get out of a chair with the forearms maximally supinated or doing a push-up in full supination.[43]

The standard preliminary physical examination of the elbow is generally unremarkable with regard to strength, ROM, and tenderness. The diagnosis requires a provocative test of stability described by O'Driscoll, called the **lateral pivot-shift test of the elbow**.[27] This pivot-shift test is performed with the patient supine and the examiner standing above the patient's head (Figure 9-6). The affected extremity is brought above the patient's head into

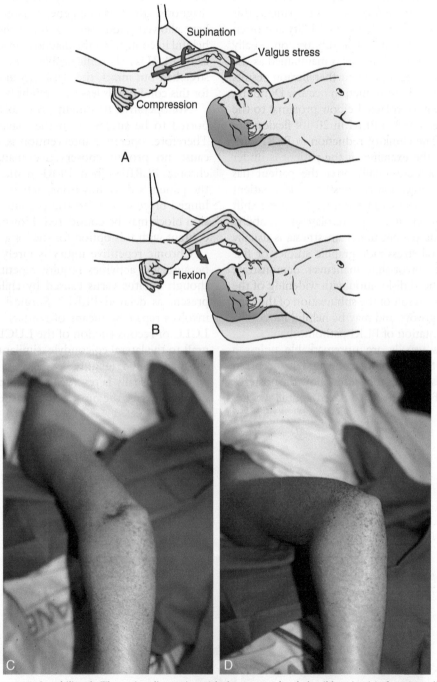

Figure 9-6 Posterolateral rotatory instability. **A,** The patient lies supine with the arm overhead. A mild supination force is applied to the forearm at the wrist. The patient's elbow is then flexed with a valgus stress, and compression is applied to the elbow. **B,** If the examiner continues flexing the elbow at about 40° to 70°, subluxation and a clunk on reduction when the elbow is extended may occur, although usually only in an unconscious patient. **C,** The radial out of anatomical position; this leads to a fullness with dimpling proximal to the radial head. **D,** The same patient as in **C**; as the elbow is brought into flexion, the radial head reduces, eliminating the fullness and dimpling. (**A** and **B** from Magee DJ: *Orthopedic physical assessment,* ed 6, p 405, St Louis, 2014, Saunders/Elsevier.)

forward elevation, and the shoulder is placed in full lateral rotation to stabilize the humerus for the test. The patient's forearm is held in maximal supination, with the examiner using one hand to grasp the wrist distally. A valgus force is applied with the examiner's other hand as the elbow is slowly flexed from a starting position of full extension. The combination of supination and valgus force results in an axial joint compression, which produces a posterolateral rotatory subluxation of the combined radius and ulna relative to the humerus. In an unanesthetized patient, this maneuver reproduces the sensation of instability and often elicits apprehension or guarding. The subluxation usually is maximized in extension and usually is maintained as the elbow reaches 40° of flexion, and further flexion results in a sudden clunk when joint reduction occurs. Dimpling of the skin along the posterolateral elbow proximal to the radial head can be seen with a PLRI in 20° of flexion before the reduction. The clunk of reduction in PLRI generally is felt only by the examiner if the patient is under general anesthesia or occasionally after the patient has had an intra-articular injection of anesthetic. If a patient displays apprehension or guarding during the pivot-shift maneuver, confirmation of the posterolateral instability by examination of the patient under anesthesia is usually recommended. Lateral stress radiographic studies or fluoroscopy during the pivot-shift maneuver demonstrate posterolateral radial head dislocation with widening of the ulnohumeral joint as a result of the subluxation of the ulna out of the trochlear groove and may be helpful for confirmation and documentation of PLRI pathomechanics.

Plain radiographs usually are unremarkable unless a bony avulsion off the lateral epicondyle has occurred (Figure 9-7, *A*). Stress radiographs often show the posterolateral subluxation if the patient is relaxed and allows the

application of the forces necessary (Figure 9-7, *B*). Positive lateral stress radiographs will show that the ulna is rotated off the distal humerus with slight gapping of the ulnohumeral joint and that the radial head is rotated with the ulna so that the radial head rests posterior to the capitellum. The normal radioulnar relationship differentiates PLRI from radial head subluxation or dislocation in which the radial head is displaced but the ulnohumeral joint is entirely normal. Although arthrography has not been shown to aid in diagnosis, advances in magnetic resonance imaging (MRI) have allowed good visualization of the LCLC and can be helpful in confirming the diagnosis in some cases.[44] Yet, because PLRI is a dynamic problem and the ligament may be stretched but intact, the sensitivity and specificity of MRI for this condition is less than might be preferred.

Nonoperative treatment protocols have not been reported to be successful in the management of PLRI.[45] Therefore, operative intervention is often necessary because no proven conservative management exists for chronic PLRI.[1] When PLRI markedly interferes with the patient's daily functions, activity modification and a hinged brace with a forearm pronation and elbow extension block may be considered. However, few patients are content with this option for the long term.

Chronic repetitive injury is rarely the cause of PLRI because few activities require repetitive varus stress, although cubitus varus caused by childhood trauma may present as delayed PLRI.[46] Surgical treatment of PLRI involves repair by means of reattachment of the avulsed LCLC or reconstruction of the LUCL with a free tendon graft to the lateral epicondyle, similar to reconstruction of the medial UCL (Figure 9-8, *A*).

Repair usually is reserved for acute avulsions from the distal humerus, the most common site of LUCL injury in

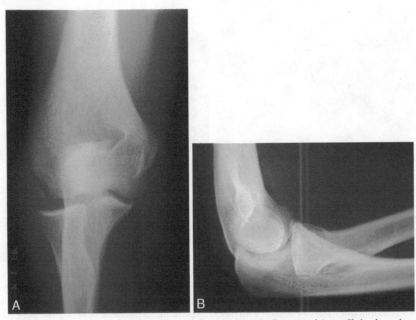

Figure 9-7 Radiographs of patients with posterolateral rotatory instability (PLRI). **A,** Bony avulsion off the lateral epicondyle, leading to PLRI. **B,** Stress radiograph showing the radial head posteriorly subluxated and the ulnohumeral joint slightly widened.

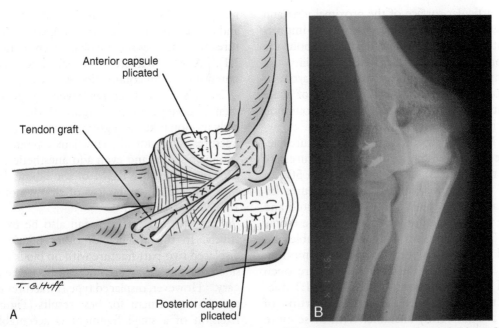

Figure 9-8 PLRI surgical repair and reconstruction. **A,** Schematic representation of PLRI reconstruction using a free graft. The graft is woven through bony tunnels. The bony avulsion of the origin of the lateral collateral ligament (LCL) has been reattached with suture anchors. **B,** Radiograph of the patient in Figure 9-7, *A.*

PLRI bone (Figure 9-8, *B*).[47-49] Because the AL is intact in these patients, radioulnar dislocation does not occur, and surgery to this ligament is not indicated. Ligament reconstruction usually is required in adults, particularly in chronic cases of PLRI. This is done through the same incision as the repair. Ligamentous reconstruction is used to replicate LUCL anatomy using a free tendon graft through bony tunnels in the distal humerus and ulna. Modifications of the technique originally described by O'Driscoll include making the distal connecting tunnels perpendicular to the isometric point of the lateral epicondyle and using the interference screw technique.[46]

Overall, surgical results have been fairly good. Osborne and Cotterill[39] reported excellent results in eight patients with transosseous repair, and Nestor et al.[48] reported excellent results in three patients. Sanchez-Sotelo et al.[49] reported a 90% success rate in restoring stability in the absence of arthritis or radial head fracture at an average follow-up of 6 years, with 60% of patients exhibiting excellent results and 40% continuing to have pain or some loss of motion. The overall patient satisfaction rate was 86%.[49] Lee and Teo[50] had 80% good to excellent results and 100% stability at follow-up, and all 10 patients were satisfied with the surgical reconstruction. Olsen and Søjbjerg[51] used a triceps graft and had 94% satisfactory results and 78% stability at nearly 4 years' follow-up.

Fractures

As with dislocations, the most common complication after elbow fractures is posttraumatic stiffness. The key to minimizing stiffness is early motion. For this reason the goal with elbow fracture surgery is rigid fixation. Rigid fixation allows early motion to be started as part of the rehabilitation process. Some fractures may be considered stable and do not require surgery; however, early motion still is essential to obtain a good result. One of the most important factors is anatomical restoration of articular surface congruity to reduce the risk of posttraumatic degenerative arthritis.

Clinical Point

- In the elbow, the key to minimizing stiffness is early controlled motion

Despite the best treatment, some elbow injuries still have poor outcomes. This is at least partly related to the severity of the trauma to the articular cartilage at the time of the initial injury. The term **terrible triad** of the elbow, coined by Hotchkiss, refers to a high-energy injury that results in elbow dislocation, radial head fracture, and coronoid fracture.[52] Triad injuries require treatment of each component to improve the likelihood of success, because failure to address all three parts of the triad leads to an extremely poor outcome. However, even with aggressive operative treatment to provide anatomical reduction and stable internal fixation, the results may still be poor. These patients are prone to early recurrent instability, chronic instability, and posttraumatic arthritis.[53]

Coronoid Fractures

Coronoid fractures are most commonly seen with high-energy injuries. The coronoid forms a significant portion of the articular surface of the proximal ulna and acts as an anterior buttress. It also serves as an important attachment site for muscles and ligaments about the elbow. The coronoid is essential for elbow stability and is the most important part of the ulnohumeral articulation.[54] Coronoid fractures occur in 2% to 15% of acute elbow dislocations.[33,36,55] Coronoid fracture nonunion may result in chronic recurrent elbow dislocation.

Regan and Morrey[56] classified coronoid fractures according to the size of the fragment: type I fractures are tip avulsions; type II fractures involve less than 50% of the height of the coronoid; and type III fractures involve more than 50% of the height of the coronoid and frequently are accompanied by instability of the elbow (Figure 9-9). Type I fractures generally are stable and can be treated as simple dislocations with early motion. Many type II fractures are unstable and require open reduction and internal fixation (ORIF). Type III fractures involve the insertion of the anterior portion of the UCL and are inherently unstable. With these more severe injuries, ORIF or a hinged external fixator may be required to maintain reduction of these coronoid fractures.

Radial Head Fractures

Radial head fractures are very common injuries and are often seen in association with other elbow injuries. These injuries usually occur as a result of a FOOSH, which transmits force to the elbow. They can also occur in conjunction with elbow dislocations. The radial head plays an important role as a secondary elbow stabilizer for valgus stress, and it also facilitates pronation and supination of the forearm. Mason[57] divided these injuries into nondisplaced fractures involving less than 25% of the radial head (type I); two-part displaced fractures or fractures that are marginally displaced, including angulation, impaction, and depression fractures (type II); and comminuted fractures and fractures that involve the entire radial head (type III).[57] A type IV fracture is usually described as a comminuted fracture in conjunction with elbow dislocation.

Nondisplaced fractures (type I) generally can be treated nonoperatively (Figure 9-10, *A*). Once again, early motion is key to a good outcome with these "stable" fractures. Occasionally, clinicians aspirate the hematoma within the joint and even add anesthetic to reduce pain, allowing for earlier ROM of the elbow. However, even with early ROM, some loss of elbow motion (averaging 10°) can be expected.[58]

Some type II fractures can also be treated nonoperatively. In the absence of other injuries, a minimally displaced two-part fracture with no block to ROM is considered a stable fracture and can be treated without surgery.[59] However, displaced type II fractures usually require operative treatment for best results (Figure 9-10, *B*).[60] Excision of a small fragment is acceptable, but larger fragments should be internally fixed.[61] All radial head fractures require careful evaluation of the elbow and the distal radioulnar joint (DRUJ) for any associated injuries. If pain or instability is present at the DRUJ, excision of a significant portion of the radial head is contraindicated. Such an injury, known as an **Essex-Lopresti injury**, can result in proximal migration of the radius after excision of the radial head.[62] In the absence of associated injuries, type III fractures can be treated with excision of the radial head. If a DRUJ injury has occurred, the surgeon must either attempt to reduce and fix the fracture fragments to retain the radial head or replace it with a prosthetic radial head (Figure 9-10, *C*).[53] With interosseous ligament injury and/or DRUJ injury, radial head replacement is mandatory if the radial head cannot be fixed. Temporary radial head replacement, such as with a Silastic implant that is removed later, has fallen out of favor because late displacement after removal of the prosthesis, even after a year, has been reported.[63–65]

Surgery for radial head fractures should be carried out within the first 48 hours or after 3 to 4 weeks, because surgery performed between 2 days and 3 weeks is associated with a higher risk of myositis ossificans.

In skeletally immature patients, most radial head and neck fractures can be treated nonoperatively. In the young throwing athlete, valgus forces at the elbow can result in a physeal fracture at the radial neck. Radiographs generally show an abnormal fat pad sign, which signifies an effusion. With significantly displaced fractures, operative treatment can be considered; however, in younger children, most proximal radial fractures can be successfully treated nonoperatively.

Olecranon Fractures

Because of its subcutaneous location in the posterior elbow, the olecranon is at risk of fracture as a result of

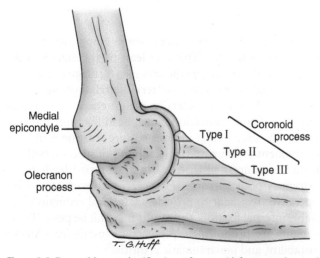

Figure 9-9 Regan-Morrey classification of coronoid fractures. A type I fracture involves the tip of the coronoid. A type II fracture involves less than 50% of the coronoid tip; this usually correlates to a line drawn parallel to the shaft of the ulna from the tip of the olecranon. A type III fracture involves more than 50% of the coronoid.

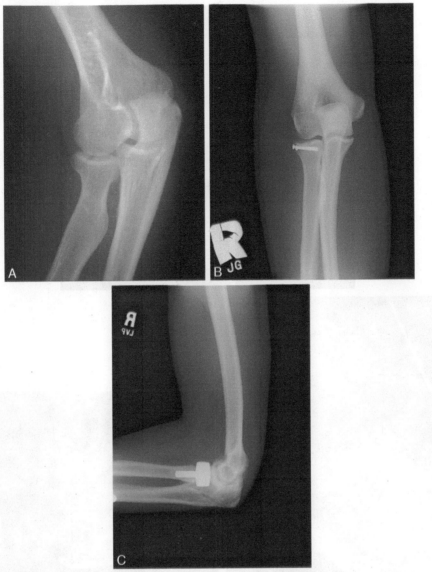

Figure 9-10 Radial head fractures. **A,** Nondisplaced radial head fracture that was treated nonoperatively. **B,** Radial head fracture treated with internal fixation using two screws. **C,** Radiograph of a patient who had a comminuted radial head fracture; treatment required prosthetic replacement of the radial head.

falls, direct blows, or dislocations. By definition, the olecranon is the proximal articulating part of the ulna, and this part of the ulna is critical in serving as the final link in the transmission of force from the triceps mechanism to enable elbow extension. Olecranon fractures usually are intra-articular. Displaced fractures may result in ulnohumeral instability and incongruity of the articular surface. Loss of more than 50% of the olecranon articular surface is associated with a 50% loss of stability.[14,66] In addition, the superior pull of the triceps on the proximal olecranon tends to displace the fracture and prevent healing (Figure 9-11, *A*). For these reasons only nondisplaced fractures can be treated nonoperatively, and even these fractures require follow-up radiographic evaluation to ensure that displacement has not occurred after the initial injury. For most olecranon fractures, ORIF is the recom-

mended treatment.[53] Tension band techniques generally are used for transverse fractures (Figure 9-11, *B*). Other options include screw fixation and other tension band variations. Comminuted and more proximal fractures may require plate fixation (Figure 9-11, *C*). Excision of the proximal fragment and triceps reattachment is an option in an elderly patient with poor bone quality, but this technique should be avoided in younger, active patients because it can lead to elbow instability.

Distal Humeral Fractures
Significant energy is required to cause a distal humeral fracture in young patients. These injuries may be intra-articular or extra-articular. Much of the distal humerus is covered with articular cartilage. The trochlea articulates with the proximal ulna, and the capitellum, with

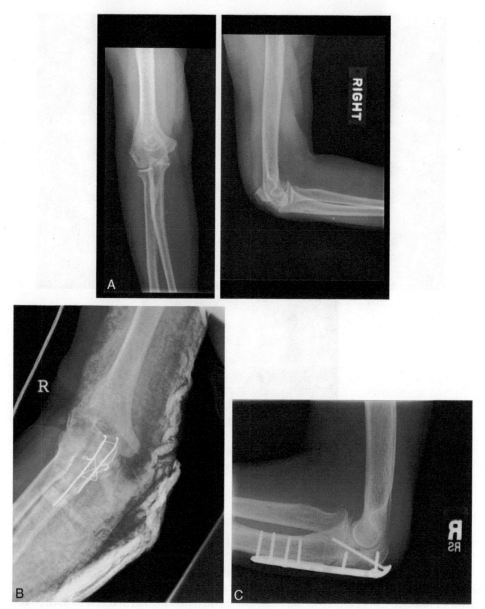

Figure 9-11 Olecranon fracture. **A,** Displaced olecranon fracture. This intra-articular fracture is displaced because of the pull of the triceps. **B,** Radiograph of a patient treated with tension band wiring for a simple olecranon fracture. **C,** Radiograph of a patient with a comminuted olecranon fracture treated with plates and screws.

the radius. As a result, many distal humeral fractures are intra-articular. The goal of treatment, as with other elbow fractures, is congruent reduction of the articular surfaces and stable fixation of the fracture to allow early motion. Displaced and intra-articular distal humeral fractures generally require ORIF for optimal results.[67] Some extra-articular, nondisplaced, and avulsion fractures can be treated nonoperatively, but these are less common. Very comminuted fractures in older patients who place less demands on the elbow may be treated with noncustom total elbow replacements.[68] Most distal humeral fractures in healthy, active adults are treated with operative fixation and early motion rehabilitation (Figure 9-12). These fractures generally have a high incidence of elbow

stiffness, fixation failure, malunion, nonunion, infection, and ulnar nerve injury.

Supracondylar humeral fractures are the second most common fracture in pediatric patients.[69] These injuries usually are the result of a fall onto an outstretched hand or a direct blow to the back of the elbow. They can be treated with closed reduction and casting if the fracture can be maintained in the appropriate position without compromising the neurovasculature structures of the elbow. Otherwise, temporary pin fixation, percutaneously or open, may be indicated. These are important injuries, because complications may occur, such as compartment syndrome, brachial artery laceration or thrombosis, loss of motion, cubitus varus, and nerve injury.

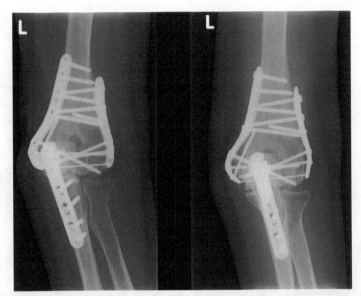

Figure 9-12 Radiograph of a patient who had open reduction and internal fixation for a comminuted distal humeral fracture.

ELBOW ARTHRITIS

The treatment of elbow arthritis is similar to the treatment of arthritis of other joints. Elbow arthritis generally can be categorized as inflammatory arthritis, posttraumatic arthritis, or osteoarthritis. Primary degenerative arthritis of the elbow is relatively uncommon compared with other joints such as the hip, knee, ankle, and shoulder. Rheumatoid arthritis commonly affects the elbow, and posttraumatic sequelae are a more common cause of arthritis of the elbow. The presenting symptom is usually pain, but it can be accompanied by stiffness or loss of motion, weakness, and/or instability. Treatment is dictated by the severity of the symptoms, the etiology, and the patient's age. The initial treatment is generally conservative. However, when pathology and symptoms are severe, operative intervention is indicated. Significant advances have been made in recent years in the surgical treatment of arthritis of the elbow, most notably in arthroscopic techniques.[70–73]

Rheumatoid arthritis is the most common form of inflammatory arthritis. Although other joints are more commonly affected, rheumatoid arthritis of the elbow is often marked by severe pain and disability. Bone loss and articular destruction cause instability at the ulnohumeral articulation. Surgical treatment, often total elbow arthroplasty (TEA), is frequently necessary and can be quite successful at relieving pain and restoring function.[70,74]

Posttraumatic elbow arthritis can result from any insult to the articular cartilage or bony anatomy but most often is seen after intra-articular distal humeral fractures. Stiffness is often present and may occur secondary to associated heterotopic ossification. Osteoarthritis is found almost exclusively in men who have a history of heavy labor or athletic use of the arm, such as weight lifters and throwing athletes. Limitation of ROM, especially a flexion contracture, is common.[70]

Nonoperative treatment for elbow arthritis consists of medications, injections, and physical therapy. Operative treatment should be considered for patients with debilitating and persistent symptoms. Arthroscopic techniques include synovectomy, debridement of impinging osteophytes, loose body removal, and contracture release. Although technically a bit more demanding, arthroscopic excision of the radial head may also be performed. Many think that arthroscopic synovectomy is more complete and effective than an open technique. However, the procedure is technically demanding, and the neurovascular structures are at risk because of their proximity during surgical intervention.[71,72] Open synovectomy, with or without excision of the radial head, is an established procedure for rheumatoid arthritis of the elbow. Open osteotomy or debridement of impinging osteophytes can also be done to reduce pain and improve ROM.[70]

Arthrodesis is poorly tolerated because elbow ROM is essential for use of the hand.[70] It is indicated only for salvage situations when TEA is contraindicated.

Total Elbow Replacement

Total elbow replacement may be performed because of arthritic changes or as a primary treatment for difficult distal humeral fractures in older patients. TEA is an excellent surgical intervention that produces reliable results in a certain subgroup of patients with advanced degenerative changes.[73] Patients with rheumatoid arthritis generally have excellent and reliable pain relief and, because of their relatively low functional demands, tend not to have problems with early loosening or failure of the prosthesis (Figure 9-13).[74] For other elderly patients with low to moderate functional expectations, TEA offers reliable pain relief with medium-term results similar to those for hip and knee arthroplasty.[75] Many now advocate the use

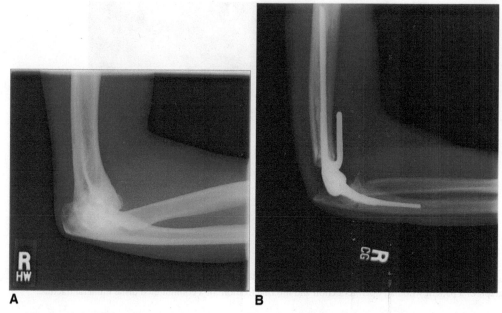

Figure 9-13 Rheumatoid arthritis. **A,** Radiograph of a patient with severe rheumatoid arthritis of the elbow. **B,** Postoperative radiograph after a total elbow arthroplasty for the rheumatoid arthritis.

of TEA as an acute surgical treatment for elderly patients with comminuted osteoporotic elbow fractures, contending that the results are similar to or better than those obtained with ORIF.[68,76-78]

Unfortunately, in younger, more active patients, early failure, including loosening of the prosthesis, limits the use of TEA. The treatment of young patients with high functional expectations and severe elbow arthritis is both difficult and controversial. The results with TEA are inferior to those seen in older, more sedentary patients.[75] However, alternatives such as interposition arthroplasty and resection arthroplasty give less reliable and less sustainable results. In young, active patients who want surgery for painful arthritic changes but who do not want fusion (i.e., arthrodesis) of the elbow, arthroscopy and distraction interposition arthroplasty are currently the only viable alternatives. With either procedure, particularly distraction arthroplasty, limited postoperative goals and expectations should be stressed.[79] With interposition arthroplasty, the arthritic surfaces are conservatively removed and replaced by fascia lata soft tissue. Studies report about 70% satisfactory results (i.e., for pain and function) at 5-year follow-up[79] and 40% at follow-up of more than 20 years.[80] In addition, the role of arthroscopy in the treatment of advanced elbow arthritis needs to be more clearly defined.

OVERUSE INJURIES OF THE ELBOW

Anterior Elbow

Climber's Elbow

The term *climber's elbow* refers to a strain of the brachialis tendon.[81] It usually is seen in association with repetitive pull-ups, hyperextension, or repeated forceful supination or from violent extension against a forceful contraction.[24] Rock climbers are susceptible to this injury as a result of repetitive weight bearing through the upper extremities.[82] Patients typically have pain with extension or resisted flexion and supination. The rule for successful management of this injury is slow and steady improvement with nonoperative treatment. Resolution of the symptoms is obtained with rest and anti-inflammatory treatment. Early rehabilitation should focus on regaining ROM before eccentric strengthening is initiated.

Distal Biceps Tendonitis and Tendon Rupture

Tendonitis at the distal biceps insertion is an uncommon overuse syndrome. It is seen in association with activities similar to those that produce climber's elbow. It also results in pain with resisted flexion and supination, which can be elicited during the physical examination. Rest and conservative care generally result in gradual resolution of symptoms. Surgical treatment is generally not indicated.

Distal biceps tendon rupture is uncommon but is seen more often than biceps tendinopathy, in which the torn end of the biceps, through an acute event without prodromal (i.e., early) symptoms, usually reveals chronic tendinopathy. Distal biceps tendon rupture represents only 3% of all biceps ruptures, with an incidence that has been estimated at 1.2 per 100,000 people per year.[83,84] It typically affects the dominant arm of middle-aged men. Smoking may be a risk factor for this injury.[83] The mechanism is a sudden, forceful overload with the elbow in midflexion. Although degenerative changes in the tendon predispose it to rupture, most patients have no history of prior pain or prodromal symptoms. These individuals present with localized pain and tenderness at the bicipital tuberosity, proximal displacement of the biceps tendon with a bulge in the distal arm, inability to palpate the taut tendon within the antecubital fossa, and marked weakness of forearm supination and elbow flexion (often associated with increased pain) (Figure 9-14). The pain and tenderness identified after the acute rupture quickly subside, but a dull ache may persist for weeks. Ecchymosis is usually present in the antecubital fossa, and sometimes above and below the elbow, starting 2 to days 3 after the injury.

The two proposed mechanisms of attritional rupture are due to a relatively poor vascular supply and/or a mechanical impingement against the bicipital tuberosity. Both of these mechanisms appear to play a role in the pathophysiology.[85] Partial ruptures have been documented, although they are less common than complete ruptures.[86-88] Partial tears can be managed conservatively and frequently have good outcomes, particularly if less than 50% of the tendon is damaged.

Muscle-tendon junction injuries are highly uncommon. Their presentation is similar to a complete or partial distal biceps avulsion, although the tendon can typically still be felt in the cubital fossa. MRI may confuse the picture, suggesting that the tendon is torn. These injuries do well with relative rest initially, followed by rehabilitation.[89]

MRI is the imaging modality of choice for the diagnosis of partial tears,[90] but it is rarely needed for the diagnosis of complete tears of the distal biceps tendon. Complete tears should be managed with surgical repair; inferior results have been documented with nonoperative treatment of these injuries.[91,92] Patients who do not undergo surgical repair have significant limitations in terms of strength and ability to perform certain activities. Nonanatomical tendon reinsertion also gives inferior results compared with anatomical reinsertion. Rantanen and Orava[93] found that for both acute and chronic injuries, nonanatomical reinsertion gave good to excellent results in 60% of patients compared with 90% who had anatomical reinsertion.[93]

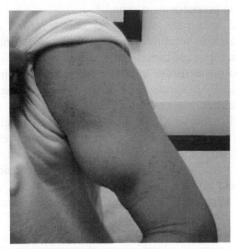

Figure 9-14 Patient with a distal biceps rupture; note the proximal migration and muscle bulge in the arm that are associated with this injury.

Only 14% of the patients treated nonoperatively had a good to excellent result, and the main complaint was loss of strength, or muscular endurance, with elbow flexion (30% loss of strength) and/or supination (40% loss of strength).[91,93] Recently, it was reported that following conservative treatment of distal biceps tendon rupture resulted in a 60% decrease in supination strength with the forearm in a neutral position. This strength loss was not different between dominant and nondominant arms.[94]

Distal Biceps Tendon Repair

Initially, the biceps tendon was repaired with a one-incision technique. However, the exposure required to repair the biceps tendon avulsion to the radial tuberosity with bone tunnels put the radial nerve at risk, and several cases of radial nerve injuries have been reported.[95] For this reason, a two-incision technique was devised so that bone tunnels could be made with the arm in full pronation. This forearm rotation pushed the nerve out of the way, reducing the risk of nerve injury. With the advent of new devices, such as suture anchors, the EndoButton, and interference screws, exposure of the proximal radius can be limited, reducing the risk to the nerve with a one-incision technique.[96,97] However, concerns still exist with the use of the one-incision technique with bone anchors; for example, the anchors may back out, and the tendon may heal onto the bone.

Overall, the results of distal biceps tendon repair using either one or two incisions have not been shown to be different, and the technique used generally is based on the surgeon's preference.

The method of anatomical reinsertion is controversial. The two-incision bone tunnel technique produces reliable results but has a relatively higher risk of radioulnar synostosis (fusion).[98,99] However, modification of the Boyd-Anderson technique so that contact with the ulna is avoided has reduced this uncommon complication.[95] Traditionally, the one-incision technique has been associated with more neurological complications, because it required more extensive dissection, particularly movement of the posterior interosseous nerve. More recently, however, many authors have recommended a one-incision technique that does not require bone tunnels and thus can be performed with less dissection, theoretically reducing the risk of nerve injury. Both suture anchors and EndoButton techniques have been described, with good early results with the one-incision technique.[100-105] Overall, anatomical repair restores strength and function in more than 90% of patients, regardless of the technique used.[93]

The general recommendation is to perform distal biceps reattachment acutely. Chronic biceps tendon ruptures require a more extensive approach.[96,106] A distal biceps rupture is considered chronic if it is not treated within 4 weeks, although excellent results have been obtained after anatomical reinsertion 3 years after injury.[107] The key to success in delayed surgery is the status of the lacertus fibrosus (i.e., the bicipital aponeurosis). If it is intact, the tendon will retract only to the level just proximal to the antecubital fossa. The amount of muscle shortening is not very significant, and delayed repair is easily attainable. However, if the lacertus fibrosus is torn, the tendon may "slingshot" into the arm; significant muscle shortening may occur, along with scarring within the arm; and delayed primary reattachment may be difficult. In such cases, allograft reconstruction may be attempted to bridge the gap between the shortened muscle and the bicipital tuberosity. However, this is a salvage procedure, and although the condition is often improved, the patient is unlikely to regain full strength. Reports have identified a range of 13% to 50% deficit in flexion and supination strength in these cases.[106] The rerupture rate of distally repaired biceps tendon has been found to be low at 1.5% and usually occurs within the first 3 weeks.[108]

Pronator Syndrome

Pronator syndrome is proximal entrapment neuropathy of the median nerve. Pronator syndrome must be distinguished clinically from carpal tunnel syndrome (CTS; distal median nerve entrapment), which is, by far, the most common entrapment neuropathy of the median nerve. An understanding of pronator syndrome is important, because this condition frequently is misdiagnosed, and many patients undergo unsuccessful operations before the correct diagnosis is made.[109]

Four anatomical sites of compression of the median nerve can be found in the elbow region.[110] When a supracondylar process is present at the distal medial humerus (1% of the population), compression can occur under the ligament of Struthers, which originates at the supracondylar process and attaches to the medial epicondyle. At the elbow, the median nerve passes under the bicipital aponeurosis, the second possible location of compression. It then passes between the humeral (superficial) and ulnar (deep) heads of the pronator teres muscle, where compression also commonly occurs. Finally, the nerve passes under the fibrous arch of the flexor digitorum superficialis muscle.

Sites of Compression of the Median Nerve at the Elbow

- Under the ligament of Struthers
- Bicipital aponeurosis
- Pronator teres muscle
- Flexor digitorum superficialis muscle

Although conflicting reports have emerged, the most common site of compression in pronator syndrome is between the two heads of the pronator teres, resulting in its nomenclature.[111] Entrapment at the bicipital aponeurosis and at the arch of the flexor digitorum superficialis is also common.[110,111] Compression caused by the ligament of Struthers is rare.

Clinically, pronator syndrome is seen in patients who engage in repetitive pronation and supination activities, including pitching, rowing, weight training, archery, and racquet sports.[110,112] It occurs most commonly in women in their 40s. Patients most often report activity-related pain in the anterior aspect of the elbow and forearm. A patient may have a history of a direct blow to the forearm, or repetitive trauma may be the cause; however, in most patients the cause is unknown. In contrast to CTS, patients do not usually experience nocturnal symptoms. The pain with pronator syndrome may be described as a dull pain or an ache in the proximal anterior forearm just distal to the antecubital fossa, and it may radiate distally to the wrist. Pronator syndrome symptoms rarely radiate proximally. Paresthesias are common in the median nerve distribution, and unlike with CTS, numbness may be present over the thenar eminence in the distribution of the palmar cutaneous branch of the median nerve.[112-116]

Tenderness over the pronator muscle mass is typically found on examination.[117] Weakness, if present, is usually subtle. A complete examination should include evaluation for Tinel's sign, Phalen's sign, and the carpal tunnel compression test to assess for CTS. Provocative tests that have been described for localizing pathology to a specific anatomical structure should also be performed: resisted forearm pronation and elbow extension for the pronator teres, active supination against resistance with the elbow flexed for the bicipital aponeurosis, and resisted flexion of the long finger for the arch of the flexor digitorum superficialis.[116-118]

When evaluating a patient with possible pronator syndrome, the clinician must consider all potential sites of nerve compression from the cervical spine to the wrist. Also, median nerve compression at more than one location (the so-called **double crush phenomenon**) is not uncommon.[109] Electrodiagnostic studies are rarely helpful in the diagnosis of pronator syndrome. However, they can help confirm an alternative or concurrent diagnosis, such as CTS. Nerve conduction studies are most often normal in pronator syndrome.[116]

Initial treatment should be nonoperative, consisting of activity modification, rest, immobilization, anti-inflammatory medications, physical therapy, and in some cases, local cortisone injections. Conservative management usually is successful, but if it fails or if significant abnormalities are noted on nerve conduction studies, the median nerve should be decompressed surgically.[115] Because assessing for sites of significant compression is difficult even intraoperatively, consideration should be given to releasing all the potential sites of compression. The outcomes of surgical treatment generally are good, with reports of a greater than 90% satisfactory outcomes rate.[117]

Annular Ligament Disruption

AL disruption is a rare cause of popping or snapping pain in the anterior elbow. It is associated with injury to the radial head, either subluxation or dislocation, and it often is seen in throwing athletes, who report popping symptoms with pronation and supination. A complete disruption in a symptomatic patient is treated with surgical repair.[24] One report has described arthroscopic and histological findings of loose, degenerative AL tissue in two brothers who were overhead throwing athletes and who had snapping elbow pain.[119]

Heterotopic Ossification

Pathological bone formation in nonosseous tissues, usually referred to as **heterotopic ossification** (HO), is most often seen as a result of elbow trauma,[120] although it also can be seen in association with burns, head trauma, and genetic disorders.[121-123] Although sometimes asymptomatic, HO can often progress to disabling pain and stiffness. Despite aggressive therapy, nonoperative treatment generally does not reverse the progression of decreased motion. Fortunately, recent results of surgical excision of HO have shown consistently good outcomes with minimal recurrence and complications.[124]

In susceptible individuals, the process likely begins soon after injury. Symptoms of swelling, erythema, and pain may be present in just a few weeks, and elbow stiffness starts 1 to 4 months after the initial injury. Limitation of active and passive ROM often progresses despite aggressive therapy.[125] The ectopic bone formation usually stabilizes after 3 to 9 months. Morrey et al.[6] have demonstrated that most ADLs can be performed with a 100° arc of elbow motion from 30° to 130° of elbow flexion (i.e., normal elbow functional ROM). However, each patient's ROM goals should be assessed based on the individual's professional and recreational activities.

In most cases, the diagnosis, location, and maturity of the HO can be assessed with plain radiographs. Computed tomography (CT) scans can also be helpful in certain cases, especially for preoperative planning. Classification systems for HO are based on location and functional limitation. The most common location about the elbow is posterolateral, but HO can involve almost any part of the elbow.[120]

Initial treatment should involve aggressive therapy to maintain as much motion as possible and minimize progression to ankylosis. Most surgeons recommend both active and passive ROM exercises, although this is somewhat controversial.[124] When elbow stiffness becomes severe enough to limit recreational or daily activities, surgical excision should be considered. Associated nerve compression, most commonly of the ulnar nerve, can develop secondary to ectopic bone and generally should be treated with surgery to prevent the development of a permanent nerve lesion. Furthermore, it recently was found that with long-standing loss of elbow motion, ulnar nerve dysfunction may occur once the patient regains elbow motion. For this reason, ulnar nerve transposition should be considered in conjunction with procedures to gain ROM, even if no ulnar nerve symptoms are present preoperatively, if large gains in elbow motion are expected.[126]

Because of concerns about recurrence, it has long been suggested that HO excision not be undertaken before 1 year after injury. However, multiple reports have demonstrated good results and low recurrence rates with HO excision as early as 3 to 6 months after injury.[127-130] Consideration should be given to prophylaxis after HO excision (e.g., indomethacin or radiation) to prevent recurrence.

Medial Elbow

Medial Epicondylar Physeal Injury

In the adolescent elbow, the medial epicondylar apophysis is the weakest portion of the medial stabilizing structures. As a result, injury to the medial epicondylar apophysis is common in the skeletally immature elbow. This may be manifested by inflammation of the apophyseal growth plate or progress to avulsion fractures of the medial epicondyle. Medial epicondylar avulsion fractures are much more common than UCL injuries in the immature elbow and are the most common fractures in the immature throwing athlete. This fracture is seen in association with elbow dislocation, and the displaced fragment of the medial epicondyle occasionally can become trapped in the joint, preventing reduction. In throwing athletes, this injury generally occurs during an especially hard pitch or throw when valgus stress is coupled with flexor/pronator muscle contraction. However, a less stressful throw or a FOOSH may also result in a medial epicondylar avulsion fracture. These patients have acute onset of medial elbow pain and, occasionally, associated ulnar nerve paresthesias.[131,132] Although some may have prodromal symptoms of medial epicondylar apophysitis, this is not frequently the case. Patients with medial apophysitis complain of pain on throwing and a decrease in throwing distance, accuracy, and velocity. On examination, these children have tenderness over the medial epicondyle and pain with resisted elbow flexion and pronation. Frequently, they have a flexion contracture of approximately 15°, attributable to muscular and capsular tightness.

Radiographs are necessary to confirm the diagnosis, and as is always the case with children, comparison views are important (Figure 9-15). Assessment of apophyseal thickness is important for apophysitis or nondisplaced fractures. This measurement varies by individual and skeletal maturity, which is why the comparison view of the nonaffected elbow is important. With apophysitis, the growth plate can be widened and occasionally fragmented.

The treatment of the inflamed apophysis is rest from throwing for 4 to 6 weeks, application of ice (care must be taken to protect the ulnar nerve from thermal injury), and nonsteroidal medication to reduce the pain and acute inflammation. After the symptoms subside, a rehabilitation program is instituted consisting of stretching to eliminate

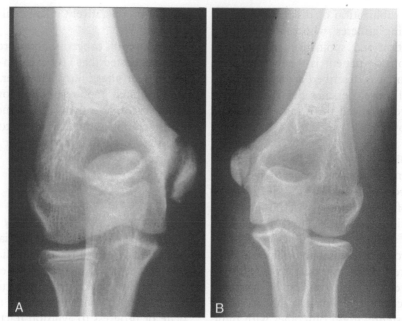

Figure 9-15 Medial epicondylar physeal injury. **A,** Anteroposterior radiograph of the elbow of a 13-year-old boy who plays baseball in several leagues year round. The medial physis appears slightly widened. **B,** The contralateral elbow; clearly the injured elbow has significant widening compared with the normal elbow.

the flexion contracture and strengthening of the muscles that cross the elbow joint, followed by transitioning to functional activities.

Clinical Point - Yellow Flag!

- Whenever ice is applied around the elbow as a treatment, care must be taken to ensure nerves, especially the ulnar nerve, are protected from hypothermic injury

---

Most avulsion injuries can be treated nonoperatively. Certainly in nondisplaced and minimally displaced fractures (the amount of displacement is controversial), when the elbow is stable to valgus stress testing, the condition should be treated conservatively with a short course of immobilization, activity restriction for 2 to 3 weeks, and a gradual return to ROM exercises, strengthening, and functional activities. Absolute indications for surgery include incarceration of a fragment of the medial epicondyle in the joint and complete ulnar nerve dysfunction. Incomplete ulnar nerve deficits generally resolve with conservative treatment.[132]

The treatment of displaced fractures is more controversial. Surgery may be necessary to reduce and fix some displaced fractures. However, historically surgeons have found that even widely displaced fractures have good results with nonoperative treatment. Josefsson and Danielsson[133] reported good to excellent results at long-term follow-up in 56 patients treated nonoperatively with widely displaced medial epicondyle fractures. Although more than half of the patients had a persistent fibrous nonunion, their outcome was as good as that in patients

whose fractures healed. Other authors advocate operative treatment for displaced fractures.[1,134,135] They argue that, especially in high-level throwing athletes, no significant displacement should be tolerated (Figure 9-16). However, the benefit of operative over nonoperative treatment for displaced fractures has not been clearly demonstrated. The senior surgical author of this chapter usually treats avulsions that are more than 5 mm (0.2 inch) displaced in the dominant arm of throwing athletes, and those that are 1 cm (0.5 inch) or more displaced in all other individuals surgically.

Medial Epicondylitis

Medial epicondylitis, or **golfer's elbow**, is a term for tendinosis at the common medial flexor/pronator origin. Specifically, the origins of the flexor carpi radialis and the pronator teres are most affected. Medial epicondylitis is much less common than lateral epicondylitis. Young to middle-aged athletes involved in golf, tennis, and overhead throwing are most commonly affected. In fact, medial epicondylitis is more common in professional tennis players than lateral epicondylitis. The repetitive valgus stress of these activities subjects these muscles to injury and chronic inflammation.[19,24]

The peak incidence of medial epicondylitis occurs in the fourth and fifth decades of life.[136] Occasionally, affected patients note medial elbow swelling and medial elbow pain that is worse with gripping, batting, hitting a serve in tennis, and/or throwing. Patients present with medial elbow pain and often symptoms of ulnar nerve irritation. Examination reveals tenderness over the medial epicondyle and slightly distal and lateral in the tendon of the pronator teres, as well as pain with resisted pronation

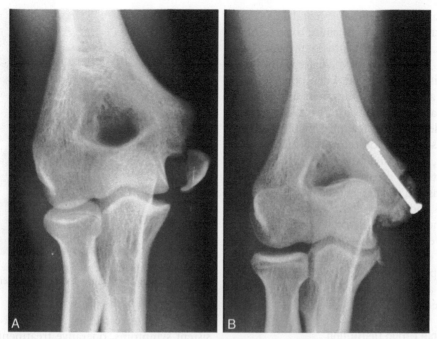

Figure 9-16 Medial epicondylar avulsion fracture. **A,** Radiograph of a 15-year-old baseball player with a medial epicondylar avulsion fracture. **B,** Postoperative radiograph showing a screw in the medial epicondyle to reduce and fix the fracture.

and/or wrist flexion (Figure 9-17). Careful assessment for UCL instability and ulnar nerve symptoms is required, because medial epicondylitis may occur in conjunction with these problems. Radiographs usually are normal. MRI is not usually necessary for the diagnosis of medial epicondylitis, but the changes seen are consistent with a tendinosis, or they may be more extensive and include muscular and/or bony edema.

Treatment is generally nonoperative, including rest and anti-inflammatory medications with a gradual return to stretching and eccentric strengthening of the involved muscles. In more than 80% of patients, symptoms resolve with conservative treatment and the patient is able to return

to the sport or activity.[19] Cortisone injections may be of benefit as an adjunct to rehabilitation.[137] Rehabilitation includes application of ice, anti-inflammatory medications, and stretching and strengthening of the flexor/pronator muscle group. A counterforce brace may be beneficial in patients who are rehabilitating but still involved in activities that may aggravate the symptoms.

If the condition does not respond to an appropriate trial of nonoperative treatment, surgery may be required. Surgical intervention involves excision of the abnormal degenerative tissue at the common flexor/pronator origin and reapproximation of the remaining healthy tissue. Unfortunately, the surgery for medial epicondylitis

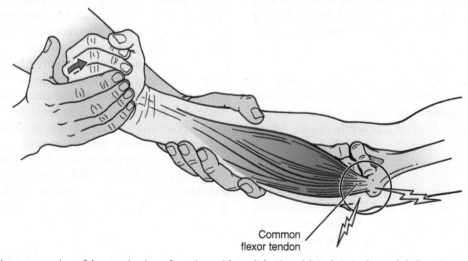

Common
flexor tendon

Figure 9-17 Schematic representation of the examination of a patient with medial epicondylitis. Pain in the medial elbow is reproduced by having the patient resist wrist flexion with the elbow extended. (Redrawn from Esch JC, Baker CL: *Arthroscopic surgery (surgical arthroscopy): the shoulder and elbow*, Philadelphia, 1993, JB Lippincott.)

is not as successful as that for lateral epicondylitis. Part of the reason for decreased success is failure to recognize concomitant disease. Ulnar neuropathy is present 40% to 60% of the time. The success of medial epicondylitis debridement is significantly reduced when concomitant ulnar neuropathy is a factor.[138,139] Vangsness and Jobe[140] reported 34 of 35 patients had good to excellent results after surgical debridement and reapproximation of the flexor/pronator musculature for refractory medial epicondylitis. However, Gabel and Morrey[138] showed that 96% of patients treated for medial epicondylitis without ulnar nerve symptoms had good to excellent results, compared with only 40% good to excellent results in patients with concomitant moderate to severe ulnar neuropathy requiring ulnar nerve decompression or transposition at the time of medial epicondylitis surgery. Furthermore, one needs to be suspicious of UCL instability in throwing athletes, and the appropriate workup needs to be performed in these patients.[22]

Flexor/Pronator Muscle Group Disruption

Complete disruption of the flexor/pronator muscle origin is rare. It generally occurs during the acceleration and follow-through stages of throwing in an overhead athlete or in conjunction with dislocation of the elbow. This disruption usually occurs as a result of forceful extension of the elbow and pronation of the forearm or forceful valgus stress. Patients generally present after an acute onset of medial-sided elbow pain during a throw or pitch.[19,141,142] Clinically, disruption of the flexor/pronator muscle origin must be distinguished from a UCL injury, because the two structures frequently are injured concomitantly.[142] Patients with an isolated flexor/pronator rupture have tenderness over the anterior half of the medial epicondyle, which can be distinguished from the more posterior tenderness seen with UCL injury.[143] A muscular bulge may be present in the medial forearm from muscular contraction, as well as pain and/or weakness of wrist flexion and/or pronation. MRI is usually helpful for confirming the diagnosis (Figure 9-18). Although some authors recommend a trial of nonoperative treatment, most advocate surgical repair for complete ruptures because of the significant contribution of the flexor/pronator muscles to dynamic elbow stability and their important contributions to wrist strength. Repair is technically difficult, and results are inconsistent. Athletes frequently cannot return to compete at the same level.[24]

Snapping Triceps

Snapping symptoms at the medial elbow can be caused by dislocation of the medial head of the triceps tendon over the medial epicondyle during elbow flexion, which often produces ulnar nerve symptoms and can be seen in association with ulnar nerve subluxation.[144,145] Underlying anatomical abnormalities are generally present.[146] Snapping of the lateral triceps tendon over the lateral epicondyle

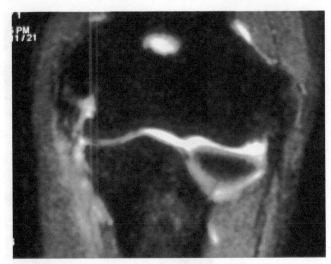

Figure 9-18 MRI scan of a patient with an acute flexor/pronator muscle strain with edema of the muscles and some edema about the tendon.

has also been described, although it is rare.[147] For persistent symptoms, operative treatment may be necessary. This most commonly involves anterior transposition of the ulnar nerve and correction of the underlying anatomical abnormality that resulted in dislocation of the tendon.

Ulnar Collateral Ligament Injury

Overhead throwing athletes subject their elbows to severe and repetitive valgus stress. The UCL, particularly the anterior band of the AOL of the UCL complex, which is the primary soft tissue restraint to valgus stress, is commonly injured. Chronic UCL insufficiency results from microscopic tears and attenuation.[148] Patients report pain and soreness in the medial elbow with throwing, usually in the late cocking or early acceleration phases or with ball release. Specifically, the athletes note that they are unable to throw more than 60% to 75% of maximal effort. Acute rupture can also occur with or without chronic changes. Most acute UCL ruptures (i.e., 87%) occur midsubstance.[141] Ulnar and humeral avulsions are much less common. Athletes often report an episode of sudden onset of pain and "giving way" during throwing. The most common situation is an acute exacerbation of a chronically injured ligament. Associated ulnar neuropathy is quite common, and patients may report pain or numbness in the ulnar nerve distribution. Associated pathology, such as loose bodies, osteophytes, and a flexion contracture, can also produce symptoms.

Patients generally have point tenderness at the insertion of the UCL approximately 2 cm (1 inch) distal to the medial epicondyle. The UCL is the most important static stabilizer to valgus stress between 30° to 120° of elbow flexion.[7] Therefore the appropriate position in which to assess for UCL insufficiency is midrange of elbow flexion. The valgus stress test has been described with the elbow at 30° flexion (Figure 9-19, *A*). The **milking maneuver** (Figure 9-19, *B*)[149] and its modification (Figure 9-19, *C*)[21] assess for valgus laxity at a higher degree of flexion. In

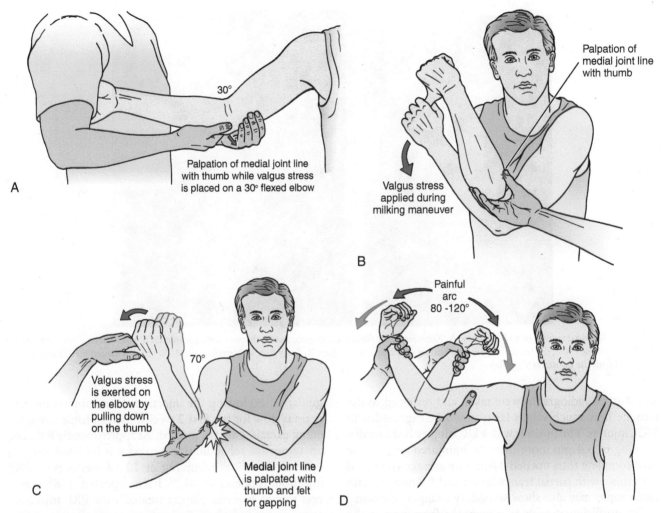

Figure 9-19 Examination of the ulnar collateral ligament (UCL). **A,** Schematic representation of the classic examination of the elbow for UCL injury. The elbow is at 30° flexion, and the hand is positioned between the examiner's elbow and body. The examiner exerts a valgus force on the elbow with one hand while palpating for medial joint opening with the other hand. **B,** The milking maneuver. The patient grabs the thumb on the arm with the affected elbow by passing the other hand beneath the affected elbow. This locks the shoulder, thereby reducing the effect of shoulder rotation and motion, which may confuse the examination. The examiner palpates the medial joint as the patient pulls on the thumb, exerting a valgus force on the elbow. Note that the elbow is in a high degree of flexion, greater than the angle at which a person throws; it also is flexed to the point that bony anatomy contributes to valgus stability of the elbow. **C,** Modified milking maneuver, in which the patient's elbow is flexed approximately 70° and the shoulder is adducted and slightly forward elevated. The examiner pulls on the patient's thumb, exerting the valgus stress with the shoulder locked in lateral rotation, and palpates the medial joint with the other hand. **D,** Schematic representation of the moving valgus stress test. The shoulder is brought into abduction and lateral rotation. The elbow is flexed and extended. The patient should reproducibly note pain in a particular degree of elbow flexion (80° to 120°). (**A** and **B** Redrawn from Selby RM, Safran MR, O'Brien SJ: Elbow injuries. In Johnson DH, Pedowitz RA, editors: *Practical orthopaedic sports medicine and arthroscopy,* Philadelphia, 2007, Kluwer/Lippincott Williams & Wilkins; **C** and **D** Redrawn from Safran MR: Injury to the ulnar collateral ligament: diagnosis and treatment, *Sports Med Arthrosc Rev* 11:19-20, 2003.)

this test the patient's arm is stabilized proximally and the thumb is pulled laterally, imparting a valgus stress to the elbow in 70° to 90° flexion, while the examiner palpates the medial joint line for opening. O'Driscoll et al.[150] described an alternative way to assess for valgus instability, which they called the **moving valgus stress test** (Figure 9-19, *D*). In this test the elbow is brought from full flexion into extension with constant valgus force reproducing the patient's medial pain, although the pain from the UCL usually is reproducibly present between 80° and 120° of elbow flexion. The differential diagnosis includes medial epicondylitis and flexor/pronator origin rupture.

Stress radiographs can be helpful for demonstrating UCL insufficiency.[22] These radiographs can be done with manual stress,[151] with a Telos device,[152,153] or by gravity.[154] With the elbow flexed approximately 20° to 45°, an anteroposterior radiograph is taken while a valgus stress is applied. With UCL insufficiency, gapping at the medial joint line exceeds that of the contralateral normal side (Figure 9-20). Recently, it was reported that gravity valgus stress radiography found similar findings with use of a Telos device while testing 57 patients with medial elbow pain.[154] In a retrospective review of 273 baseball players who had undergone UCL reconstruction, bilateral static

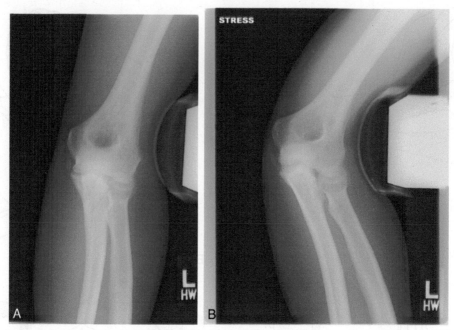

Figure 9-20 Stress x-ray films of a UCL injury. **A,** Nonstress x-ray film of a collegiate javelin thrower with chronic UCL insufficiency. Note the calcific change within the UCL, the result of attempted healing of the ligament injury. **B,** X-ray film with stress applied. Note the widened medial joint space, compared with the nonstress x-ray film.

elbow stress radiographs were taken and reviewed to determine how much valgus laxity could be expected with UCL injuries. The thrower with a UCL injury had a medial opening of 0.4 mm more than the uninjured side. Those with complete tears opened 0.6 mm on average compared with those with partial tears who opened 0.1 mm.[155] Plain radiographs may also show secondary changes of chronic UCL insufficiency, such as osteophyte formation at the medial joint, loose bodies, sclerosis, radiocapitellar degeneration, or osteophytes of the olecranon. MRI can be helpful for detecting a torn UCL and for defining associated pathology. However, a MR arthrogram is even more sensitive (97%) at detecting UCL injury.[156,157] Arthroscopy is limited as a diagnostic tool because most of the anterior oblique portion of the UCL is not visualized arthroscopically. However, dynamic testing demonstrating gapping of the ulnohumeral joint when valgus stress is applied in 70° of elbow flexion and forearm pronation is consistent with UCL injury.[158,159] Diagnostic ultrasonography also has been used to detect UCL injury by demonstrating changes both within the ligament and with medial joint opening with valgus stress, although it continues to be used only sparingly at this time.[160,161]

The initial treatment of UCL injury is generally nonoperative[22] and consists of rest from the overhead sports, anti-inflammatory medications, and physical therapy. One report indicates that about half of these patients were treated successfully without surgery and were able to return to the same level of athletic activity.[162] The patient with a UCL sprain can also be treated with a PRP injection followed by appropriate rehabilitation. The PRP injection is usually performed under ultrasound guidance. Following the injection the rehabilitation program is slow for the first 2 weeks, then isotonic strengthening exercises are performed. At approximately 8 weeks, an aggressive rehabilitation program is initiated with an interval throwing beginning at 12-14 weeks post PRP injection. Podesta et al.[163] have reported a 88% success rate in baseball players treated with PRP injection. Surgery was indicated if symptoms recur after an appropriate trial of nonoperative treatment. Surgical treatment of an UCL injury also should be considered with acute ruptures in high-level throwing athletes, with significant chronic instability, and after debridement of UCL calcification. A concern after surgery is always the level of performance that the athlete will return to. Recently, it has been reported that in Major League Baseball pitchers, the mean percentage change in velocity of pitches thrown by players who underwent UCL reconstruction was not significantly different compared with that of players in a control group. Mean innings pitched were statistically different only for the year of injury and first postinjury year. There were also no statistically significant differences between the two groups with regard to performance measurements, including earned run average, batting average against, walks per 9 innings, and walks plus hits per inning pitched.[164]

Surgery for Ulnar Collateral Ligament Deficiency

When conservative treatment of UCL injuries fails, surgical options must be considered.[22] Elbow arthroscopy is used to treat complex elbow pathology. Although complications with elbow arthroscopy are rare, they can be described as both minor and major. In a series of 417 patients receiving elbow arthroscopy, 37 (8.9%) minor complications developed, compared with 20 major complications (4.8%). These complications included superficial and deep infections, HO, and nerve complications.[165] Surgical treatment of the UCL depends on several variables. Currently, the mainstay of surgical treatment is UCL reconstruction. Primary repair of acute ruptures of the UCL had been advocated for years; however, this has changed because of the overall consistently better results obtained with ligamentous reconstruction.[21,22] Although most tears are midsubstance (87%), some are avulsion injuries, and all are considered amenable to suture repair, particularly in younger throwers with less intrasubstance ligamentous change.[141,166] This was the treatment of choice until 1992, when Conway et al.[141] reviewed their results with repair and reconstruction. They recommended reconstruction, citing the finding that overhead athletes performed significantly worse with repair than with reconstruction. They noted that repair should be considered only if the tear was a proximal avulsion, if the procedure was performed soon after injury, if the rest of the ligament was undamaged, and if no ulnar nerve symptoms were present. Repair of most injuries usually involves repair of tissue that frequently is chronically injured and therefore not ideal tissue, unless in a young athlete. Reconstruction, therefore, has become the treatment of choice for UCL deficiency.

A newer type of surgical repair for the UCL has been performed at the lead chapter author's (Dr. Kevin Wilk's) sports medicine center in Birmingham, AL and will be described later in this chapter.

UCL reconstruction with a free tendon graft is the procedure generally performed for acute rupture in overhead sports athletes and for chronic UCL instability and elbow pain with UCL instability. The procedure has evolved considerably over the years.[22] Azar et al.[156] reported that 81% of patients were able to return to the same level of sports after UCL reconstruction, compared with 63% with primary repair.

Several graft options are available. A palmaris longus autograft is most often used, but other sources of autograft and even allograft can be used for anatomical reconstruction. Sources of grafts include the ipsilateral or contralateral palmaris longus, a fourth toe extensor, a hamstring tendon, a strip of Achilles tendon, the plantaris tendon, and an allograft (e.g., hamstring and posterior or anterior tibialis tendon), although palmaris longus and hamstring grafts currently are used most often.[22] A variety of fixation techniques can be used, including bone tunnels, the docking procedure, and placement of interference screws (Figure 9-21).[167,168]

Although originally recommended with UCL reconstruction,[169] routine ulnar nerve transposition is not performed routinely in conjunction with UCL reconstruction, except by a few surgeons, because of the high rate of complications (21%).[141,156] If significant ulnar nerve symptoms are present, ulnar nerve transposition is performed at the same time as the reconstruction.

As the reconstruction procedure has evolved, the rate of operative success has reliably and reproducibly improved. Over the past several years, successful outcomes have been reported to be between 79% and 97%, with success defined as the patient returning to play at the same level or better than before the injury.[22,156,167,170–172] Long-term follow-up of UCL reconstruction in baseball players indicates that most patients were satisfied, with few reports of persistent elbow pain or limitations of function. During their baseball career, most of these athletes were able to return to the same or higher level of competition in less than 1 year, with acceptable career longevity and retirement typically for reasons other than the elbow.[173] However, recent research suggests that the return to the same or higher level may not be as good as originally thought in professional baseball players.[174] To achieve this level of success all sources of pathology need to be addressed. Medial epicondylitis may also be present. In addition, concomitant valgus extension overload can result in olecranon osteophytes or loose bodies that need to be removed. Osbahr et al.[175] reported that the results of UCL reconstruction were not as good if there was posteromedial chondromalacia of the elbow. If clinically present, associated ulnar neuritis, as noted previously, is addressed through nerve transposition.

Repair of the UCL has been performed in the past with mixed results. Dr. Jeffrey Dugas (Birmingham, AL) has developed the following surgical technique to repair the UCL and use an augmentation tape to provide additional strength.[176] Direct or side-to-side repair of the UCL has a history dating back to the original series published by Conway et al.[141] In that series, only 2 of 9 major league pitchers returned to competition after UCL repair. Subsequent to that, Azar et al.[156] reported on similarly poor outcomes with direct repair of the ligament. In 2008, Savoie et al.[166] reported on a series of overhead athletes using direct repair of the UCL to bone using modern anchor and suture technology, with 95% success at minimum one-year follow up. In 2013, a novel technique of direct repair of the ligament with augmentation using an ultra-strong collagen coated tape was first performed at the main author's institution. Biomechanically, this construct has been shown to allow for less gap formation than standard UCL reconstruction at time-zero in cadaveric specimens, with no difference in ultimate failure load.[176] The clinical outcomes of these procedures have been very encouraging, with shorter recovery time back to competition (approximately 6 months) than standard UCL reconstruction techniques (approximately 12 months). The author indicates they are currently using this technique for many end-avulsions and partial-thickness tears of the UCL, particularly in high school and collegiate throwers. Further experience with this technique may allow for expansion of the indications, however at this point we feel

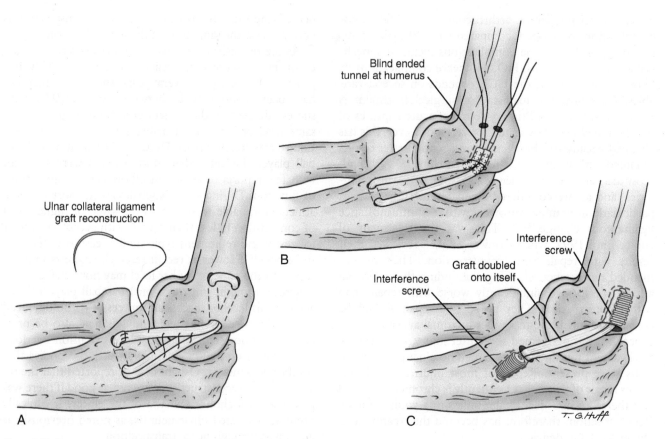

Figure 9-21 Reconstruction of the UCL. **A,** Classic three-ply UCL reconstruction. Two holes are drilled to make a tunnel in the ulna, and three holes are drilled to make two tunnels on the humeral side. This figure-of-eight appearance of the free tendon graft allows the tendon to have three strands at the medial elbow. **B,** Schematic representation of the docking technique of UCL reconstruction. The ulnar tunnel is made in the same way as for the classic technique, but a single, blind-end tunnel is used on the humeral side. This technique results in only two strands of tendon across the medial elbow, but it has two advantages: the graft is easier to tighten/tension, and the risk of medial epicondylar fracture is reduced. **C,** Interference screw technique of UCL reconstruction. Two strands are brought across the medial elbow, and both ends are fixed with interference screws in blind-end tunnels. This technique reduces the risk of tunnel fracture and, for the ulnar side, helps reduce injury to the ulnar nerve. (Redrawn from Safran MR: Injury to the ulnar collateral ligament: diagnosis and treatment, *Sports Med Arthrosc Rev* 11:21-22, 2003.)

that any tissue deficiency (e.g., bone within the ligament, poor quality tissue from chronic overuse) still warrants standard UCL reconstruction using tendon autograft.

Ulnar Nerve Injuries

After CTS, ulnar nerve compression at the elbow is the most common compressive neuropathy of the upper extremity.[177] It is frequently seen in the general population but is even more common in overhead athletes. This medial elbow pathology seen in throwing athletes is associated with ulnar nerve symptoms approximately 50% of the time.[19] The ulnar nerve is susceptible to injury because of (1) the tight path it follows, which changes its dimensions with elbow flexion and extension; (2) its subcutaneous location; and (3) the considerable excursion required of it to accommodate the full motion of not only the elbow but also the shoulder (Figure 9-22, *A*). Proximally, the ulnar nerve can be compressed by the intermuscular septum or by a hypertrophied medial head of the triceps. At the cubital tunnel, nerve irritation and injury can result from osteophytes, loose bodies, a thickened retinacu-

lum, or an inflamed UCL, especially with elbow flexion (Figure 9-22, *B*). The most common site of ulnar nerve compression is distal, between the two heads of the flexor carpi ulnaris (Figure 9-22, *C*).[1]

Both physiological and pathological factors contribute to irritation and compression of the ulnar nerve. Compression, either alone or in combination with other causes, can result in ulnar nerve irritation. With the elbow in full flexion, the confines of the cubital tunnel become restrictive and the retinaculum becomes taut, compressing the nerve. Flexion of the elbow and wrist extension increase the normal pressure on the ulnar nerve threefold. In overhead throwing, the pressure on the nerve has been demonstrated to be up to six times greater than normal.[178] The confines of the cubital tunnel may be reduced by scarring of the UCL to the floor of the cubital tunnel or by osteophytes of the medial ulna at the olecranon or distal humerus (see Figure 9-22, *C*). The cumulative effect of repeated and prolonged pressure elevations is nerve ischemia and fibrosis. This pathology can be exacerbated when it occurs in association with ulnar nerve subluxation or dislocation.

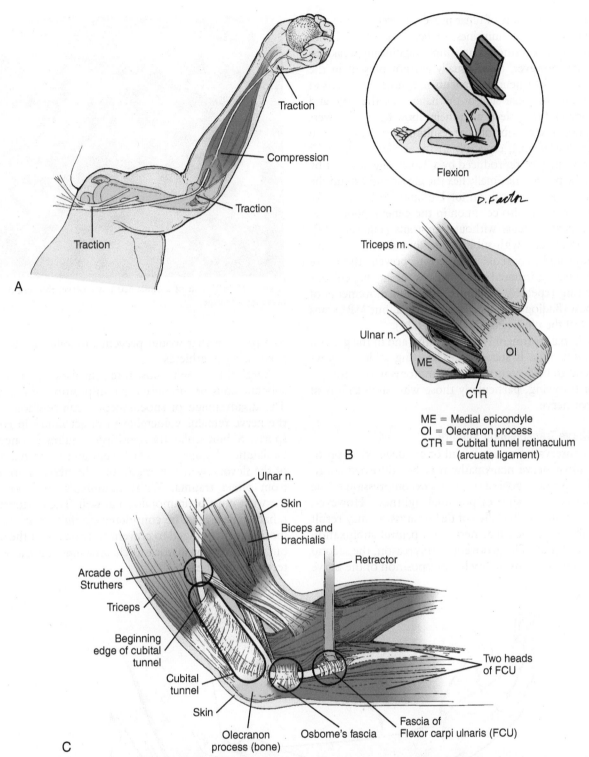

Figure 9-22 Ulnar nerve injury. **A,** Multiple sites of stress to the ulnar nerve in the throwing athlete. **B,** Elbow flexion leads to compression of the ulnar nerve within the cubital tunnel. Anything that occupies space in the tunnel (e.g., osteophytes, thickened retinaculum or ligament) can increase compression on the nerve. *ME,* Medial epicondyle; *OI,* olecranon process; *CTR,* cubital tunnel retinaculum (arcuate ligament). **C,** Multiple sites of compression where the ulnar nerve may become entrapped about the elbow. The fascia forming the roof of the cubital tunnel is sometimes called the cubital tunnel retinaculum. (**A** and **C** from Miller MD, Howard RF, Plancher KD: *Surgical atlas of sports medicine,* Philadelphia, 2003, Saunders; **B** modified from O'Driscoll SW, Horii E, Carmichael SW, Morrey BF: The cubital tunnel and ulnar neuropathy, *J Bone Joint Surg Br* 75:615, 1991. Copyright Mayo Foundation.)

The first symptoms of ulnar nerve involvement are medial elbow pain and clumsiness or heaviness of the hand. Subsequently, paresthesias and more significant weakness can ensue; however, these usually are not present in the athlete with ulnar neuritis. Patients may note numbness at night along the ulnar side of the hand (i.e., the little and ring fingers) if they sleep with their elbow bent. Throwers usually note loss of control. The results of nerve conduction tests can be normal, especially in the earlier stages.[1,19,179] Symptoms may be reproduced by a Tinel's sign and/or by having the patient maximally flex the elbow and extend the wrist and hold that position for 1 minute. Subluxation of the ulnar nerve is also common in the general population and frequently occurs without symptoms (Figure 9-23). Overhead athletes with subluxating ulnar nerves can have symptoms and may require surgery to prevent the nerve from becoming irritated as it traverses the medial epicondyle during repetitive flexion to extension movements of the elbow. Radiographs usually are normal, but MRI scans may reveal the ulnar neuritis (Figure 9-24).

The initial treatment is nonoperative and in the general population often is successful. Throwing athletes, however, tend to have recurrence of symptoms upon resumption of throwing, particularly those with subluxation of the ulnar nerve.

Ulnar Nerve Transposition Surgery

When conservative measures fail or are deemed inappropriate, ulnar nerve neuropathy may be addressed surgically. The primary goal of surgery is decompression of the ulnar nerve at all sites of potential tightness. However, addressing all possible sites of decompression may result in instability of the ulnar nerve and painful subluxation of the nerve out of its groove. For this reason, the second goal is to prevent instability by transposition of the nerve

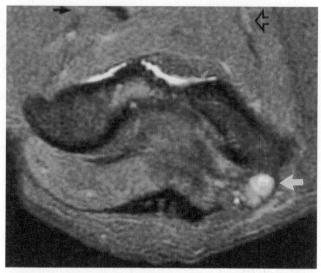

Figure 9-24 MRI scan of an inflamed ulnar nerve, showing the white nerve on T2 image.

to a position that would prevent instability if necessary, particularly in athletes.

Surgical treatment most often involves either anterior subcutaneous or submuscular transposition of the nerve. The disadvantage of subcutaneous transposition is that the nerve remains vulnerable to direct injury in contact sports. Submuscular transposition requires a longer rehabilitation because of detachment and reapproximation of the flexor/pronator origin, but the nerve is protected from direct trauma. With submuscular transpositions, the wrist must be immobilized as well. The postoperative rehabilitation must be considered carefully, because early motion is encouraged to prevent scarring about the nerve, but the flexor/pronator muscle attachment must be protected until it heals.

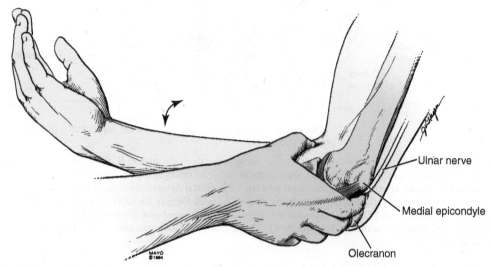

Figure 9-23 Examination for a subluxing ulnar nerve. The ulnar nerve is palpated as the elbow is flexed and extended. The nerve tends to slip out of the ulnar groove in higher degrees of elbow flexion (the more unstable the nerve, the less flexion is needed to sublux the nerve). (Modified from Morrey BF: *The elbow and its disorders,* ed 2, Philadelphia, 1993, Saunders.)

Simple decompression and medial epicondylectomy are thought to produce poor results in the throwing athlete because of the risk of UCL injury and subluxation of the nerve.[19] However, simple decompression may be a reasonable alternative in nonthrowing athletes. Two recent prospective studies reported similar results for simple decompression and anterior submuscular decompression.[180,181] The preference of the senior surgical author of this chapter is to perform submuscular transposition in athletes at risk for direct trauma to the area of the nerve (e.g., football and rugby players) and subcutaneous transposition in all others.

Posterior Elbow

Olecranon Apophysitis/Stress Fracture

In the adolescent athlete, the olecranon physeal plate is susceptible to injury, especially with overhead throwing.[24] The repetitive pull of the triceps tendon can lead to olecranon apophysitis and physeal widening.[182,183] These injuries tend to occur in adolescents and may also be the result of valgus extension overload (discussed later in this chapter). These patients report pain on resisted elbow extension and tenderness over the olecranon. Widening of the olecranon apophysis is visible on radiographs, and the findings should be confirmed by comparison with radiographs of the contralateral elbow (Figure 9-25, *A*). Recently a new classification system for olecranon stress fractures has been developed. This classification system has devised five different types, including physeal, classic, transitional, sclerotic, and distal stress fractures. The physeal type was further separated into stages 1 to 4 based on severity. The mean age for each type identified was as follows: physeal, 14.1 years; classic, 18.6 years; transitional, 16.9 years; sclerotic, 18.0 years; and distal, 19.6 years. Among baseball-related elbow disorders, the incidence of olecranon stress fractures was 5.4%.[184] An MRI can help confirm the diagnosis when radiographs are not conclusive (Figure 9-25, *B*).

When the apophysis is widened but not separated or avulsed, the initial treatment is rest from the offending activity, gentle ROM and flexibility exercises, and progression to strengthening. Ice and nonsteroidal anti-inflammatory drugs (NSAIDs) are useful if acute inflammation is present. If the child is in severe pain, a short course of immobilization in a splint or cast may be beneficial.[185] If separation of the secondary growth center has occurred or if the adolescent has pain despite conservative management because of lack of fusion of the physis, internal fixation is recommended (Figure 9-26, *A*). Surgical intervention to promote fusion of the apophysis may require internal fixation with a screw, in addition to bone grafting, because of the high incidence of fibrous union when bone grafting is not used (Figure 9-26, *B*).[183,186,187] Left untreated, apophysitis of the olecranon may result in an incompletely fused

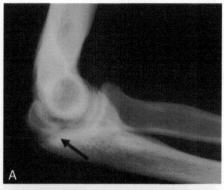

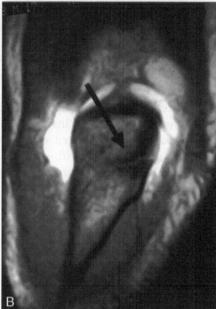

Figure 9-25 A, Olecranon stress fracture on a lateral x-ray film. **B,** MRI scan of a patient with an olecranon stress fracture.

olecranon apophysis, which may fracture as a result of direct trauma when the patient is older.[183,187-189]

In mature athletes, posterior elbow pain may represent an occult (or stress) fracture of the olecranon. This type of fracture, which is most common in baseball players, javelin throwers, shot-putters, and gymnasts, can be associated with valgus extension overload syndrome (discussed later in this chapter). If radiographs are inconclusive, a bone scan or MRI may be necessary for diagnosis. Most of these injuries heal with rest from the offending activity. Surgery is rarely necessary.[186,190-193]

Triceps Tendonitis and Tendon Rupture

Tendonitis of the triceps insertion at the olecranon is most often seen in weight lifters. It also occurs with other sports in which large forces are required in elbow extension, such as shot put, javelin, and football. In addition, the problem has affected participants in motocross racing and BMX cycling, because the riders absorb the force of landing with the arms.[1] Patients have pain at the triceps insertion that is worsened by resisted active elbow extension and throwing. On examination these

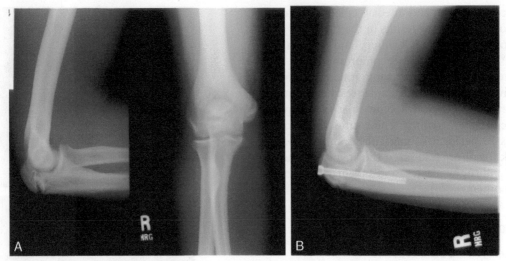

Figure 9-26 **A,** X-ray film of an unfused olecranon apophysis, which was treated with intramedullary screw fixation (**B**).

individuals have tenderness at the tip of the olecranon and slightly proximal to the triceps insertion point. The pain may be accentuated by resisted elbow extension and full elbow flexion combined with shoulder flexion. This problem may be acute or chronic. Treatment is conservative. Corticosteroid injections into the tendon are contraindicated because of the risk of tendon rupture.[194]

Triceps tendon rupture is rare, the least common of all tendon ruptures in the body, although it has been reported in weight lifters and football players.[195,196] In many cases, it is associated with corticosteroid injections or oral anabolic steroids.[197] It commonly involves avulsion with a bony fragment as a result of a decelerating counterforce during active extension of the elbow or a direct blow. Patients with this injury usually are unable to extend the elbow against gravity and have a palpable defect in the tendon proximal to the olecranon (Figure 9-27).

In the intact tendon, squeezing the triceps will result in extension of the elbow, whereas with triceps rupture, this does not occur. This injury rarely occurs at the musculotendinous junction. A small fleck of bone off the olecranon is classically seen on radiographs (Figure 9-28). MRI is rarely necessary to make the diagnosis but can confirm it. Treatment for complete ruptures is acute surgical repair, which gives consistently good results compared with the universally poor results seen with nonoperative treatment.[195,198,199]

Valgus Extension Overload Syndrome (VEOS)

Overhead throwing athletes are at risk for specific elbow pathology that occurs secondary to the repetitive valgus stresses involved in throwing, which causes the olecranon to be repeatedly and forcefully driven into the olecranon fossa. A valgus stress typically causes shearing posteriorly, resulting in impingement of the posteromedial olecranon against the lateral aspect of the medial wall of the olecranon fossa (see Figure 9-5, *B*). Ahmad et al.[200] demonstrated that UCL injury results in contact alterations in

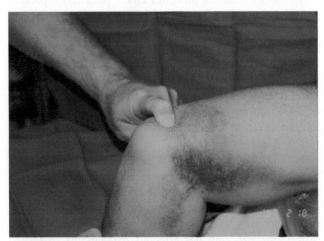

Figure 9-27 Photograph from the operating room with a patient in the prone position. This patient has a triceps tendon rupture, as evidenced by the palpable defect just proximal to the olecranon. Ecchymosis also is present, because the injury occurred only a few days before the patient underwent surgical repair.

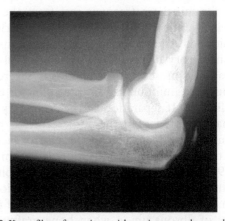

Figure 9-28 X-ray film of a patient with a triceps tendon avulsion. Note the small fleck of bone just proximal to the olecranon; this is a common finding in this rare injury.

the posterior compartment that lead to osteophyte formation. This suggests that osteophyte formation may result from subtle UCL injury or increased valgus laxity as a result of increased shear forces to the posteromedial elbow. Compounding this posterior impingement is the bony hypertrophic narrowing of the olecranon fossa and hypertrophy of the proximal ulna that occurs in overhead athletes who have been involved in the activity since childhood. Moreover, the repeated high-extension velocities produced during overhead athletic activities may result in impaction of the olecranon tip within the fossa, producing localized inflammation, chondromalacia, and further osteophyte formation. With persistent impaction and shear forces, the osteophytes may break off and become loose bodies within the joint.[201,202] These loose bodies can get caught in the joint surfaces and damage the articular cartilage.

Individuals with valgus extension overload syndrome (VEOS) have posterior elbow pain, pain with forced extension of the elbow, and occasionally, locking caused by loose bodies. On examination the patient may have a flexion contracture, swelling of the joint, and pain on forced extension of the elbow that is exacerbated by applying a valgus force to the extended elbow.[22,202] It is important that the examiner evaluate the integrity and tenderness of the UCL, because studies have reported that 42% of patients who undergo surgery for VEOS require a second operation, and 25% of these patients required reconstruction of the UCL as a result of valgus instability.[202,203]

Initial conservative treatment should focus on strengthening of the flexor/pronator muscle group while reducing inflammation. This is achieved through relative rest, application of ice, and use of NSAIDs. However, surgery is often required if loose bodies are present. Furthermore, our experience has been that patients with posteromedial osteophytes on the olecranon tend not to respond to therapy and require surgery to remove the osteophytes.[21,22,202] Nonetheless, surgery usually is indicated if 6 to 12 weeks of conservative management does not lead to improvement.

Surgery for Valgus Extension Overload Syndrome (VEOS)

VEOS surgery involves the removal of loose bodies, which can be done arthroscopically. The osteophytes on the proximal medial olecranon also are debrided, but the surgeon must take care not to remove any normal olecranon because this may create a risk of UCL injury by eliminating the proximal olecranon's function as a secondary stabilizer to valgus stress. Most authors recommend arthroscopic over open techniques for the removal of osteophytes and loose bodies (Figure 9-29)[202–206] because arthroscopic procedures have proven to be safe and effective. Because VEOS often is associated with UCL injury, the surgeon must carefully assess for evidence of valgus instability when a patient presents with VEOS.

It is unclear whether debridement uncovered a UCL injury or laxity or whether removal of the osteophytes

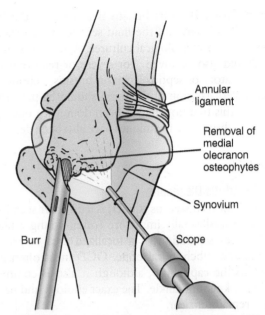

Figure 9-29 Schematic representation of arthroscopic excision of the posterior olecranon osteophytes seen in valgus extension overload syndrome (VEOS). (Redrawn from Selby RM, Safran MR, O'Brien SJ: Elbow injuries. In Johnson DH, Pedowitz RA, editors: *Practical orthopaedic sports medicine and arthroscopy,* Philadelphia, 2007, Kluwer/Lippincott Williams & Wilkins.)

increased stress on the UCL, leading to injury.[200,207–209] Removal of just the loose bodies and the osteophytes is recommended when the UCL is intact; however, removal of more than just the osteophytes, as was recommended in the 1980s and 1990s, is no longer recommended. Removal of too much olecranon may put the UCL at risk by increasing the stress on the ligament with throwing, possibly leading to UCL injury.[199,206–209] However, some believe that concurrent but untreated chronic UCL injury probably is responsible for the relatively high reoperation rate when only the posterior osteophytes and loose bodies are addressed.[1]

Olecranon Bursitis

The olecranon bursa, normally a subcutaneous potential space over the olecranon, can become inflamed or infected. This is a common problem both in the general population and in some athletes. Direct or repetitive trauma over the olecranon is the most common cause of olecranon bursitis.[24] This is seen frequently in football and rugby players, especially those who play on artificial turf.[210] Patients have swelling, fluctuance, and pain over the olecranon. If the bursa is infected, fever and surrounding erythema may be prominent. Nonseptic bursitis generally can be treated conservatively with protection (i.e., not resting on the elbow, use of a clean elbow pad), a compressive dressing, and occasionally NSAIDs. If the bursitis is severe, therapeutic aspiration with or without injection of a corticosteroid can be performed, although reaccumulation of fluid is common and the risk of introducing an infection arises. If septic bursitis is a concern, the bursa should be aspirated and the fluid sent for Gram staining and standard bacteriological cultures. Appropriate antibiotics should also be given. For severe or recurrent cases of inflammatory or septic olecranon bursitis, debridement and complete excision of the bursa should be performed. Although this traditionally has been done with open procedures, arthroscopic techniques have also been described.

Lateral Elbow

Osteochondritis Dissecans

Osteochondritis dissecans (OCD) is a disorder seen in the elbow of the skeletally immature (often young athletes) that involves separation of a localized area of articular cartilage and subchondral bone. OCD most often is localized to the capitellum, although it also is commonly seen in the knee and ankle. The exact etiology and natural history remain unclear.

OCD needs to be distinguished from Panner's disease. Panner's disease is a focal osteonecrosis of the entire capitellum that is not specifically associated with a history of trauma. It generally affects boys 7 to 12 years of age, and the peak incidence is age 9 years. It is a self-limited disease that can almost always be treated nonoperatively and rarely results in significant morbidity.[211-213]

In contrast, OCD is generally seen in a slightly older age group and is associated with a history of repetitive trauma and overuse. It usually presents in athletes between 10 and 21 years of age, with a peak range between 13 and 16 years. It most commonly affects the capitellum of the dominant arm of patients who participate in sports such as baseball, gymnastics, weight lifting, racquet sports, and cheerleading.[211-213] Kida et al.[214] assessed 2433 baseball players in junior high and high school using diagnostic ultrasound with further examination with radiographs. OCD of the humeral capitellum was found in 3.4% of elbows. Players with a lesion began playing baseball at an earlier age, had a longer duration of competitive play, and had more present and past elbow pain compared with players without a lesion.[214]

The exact etiology of OCD is unknown. The association with a history of overuse in throwing athletes and gymnasts supports the theory of repetitive microtrauma as an etiological factor.[211,212,215] Biomechanical studies have indicated that the radiocapitellar joint acts as a secondary stabilizer of the elbow and receives a large proportion of forces transmitted across the elbow with axial compression.[216] Microtrauma in these patients can lead to fatigue fracture of the subchondral bone. During the reparative process, repetitive stress could inhibit healing and lead to fragmentation of the involved segment of subchondral bone and articular cartilage.

Ischemia also appears to play a role in the pathophysiology of OCD.[217,218] The distal humerus, specifically the capitellum, has been reported to have a tenuous vascular supply.[217] In fact, the histopathology of OCD is consistent with osteonecrosis of the subchondral bone.[219] Therefore repetitive microtrauma in a genetically predisposed individual results in vascular insufficiency and necrosis of the bone at the subchondral plate. The resorption of the bone under the articular cartilage puts the chondral surface at risk of collapse as a result of stresses and loss of underlying support, which leads to loose bodies.

Patients with OCD most often have pain of insidious onset that is activity related.[132] They have tenderness laterally over the elbow and often have limitation of full extension. Flexion contractures of 5° to 23° have been reported. Mechanical symptoms and swelling are common.[132] The **active compression test** may result in pain when the extended elbow is pronated and supinated. Radiographs may show the classic findings of radiolucency and rarefaction of the capitellum with flattening or irregularity of the articular surface (Figure 9-30, *A*). Loose bodies may also be present in the elbow joint. Further imaging should involve MRI, which can help define both the size and stability of the lesion (Figure 9-30, *B* and *C*). MR arthrography can be helpful as well,[211] and ultrasound has been reported to be useful in the evaluation of the elbow for OCD.

Both MRI and arthroscopic classification schemes have been used in an attempt to differentiate lesions that are stable, those that are unstable but attached, and those that are detached or loose.[106,220] Stable lesions with intact cartilage are managed conservatively. The initial treatment is rest with avoidance of sports or other aggravating activities for 3 to 6 weeks. When symptoms resolve, stretching and gradual strengthening should be initiated to restore maximal functional ability of the elbow. Some clinicians have recommended unloading-type braces to protect the radiocapitellar joint and help reduce stresses during healing. Return to unrestricted activities usually is not allowed before 3 to 6 months. Healing evident on a radiograph usually lags behind the clinical resolution of symptoms.[1,132]

Indications for surgical intervention include evidence of loose bodies; unstable lesions where the overlying articular cartilage is not intact, either partially or completely; and failure of prolonged conservative treatment.[132,211,213] If loose bodies are present, the recommended treatment is removal of the fragment or fragments, usually arthroscopically. Arthroscopy is the most direct and reliable way to assess the integrity of the articular cartilage and the stability of lesions. The most appropriate treatment for unstable but attached lesions remains controversial. Most surgeons advocate excision of the unstable fragment, debridement, and possible microfracture of the exposed bony bed.[211] Others, such as the lead surgical author of this chapter, recommend fixation of the fragment whenever possible.[215,221,222]

Bauer et al.[223] reported an average 23-year follow-up on 31 patients who underwent open fragment excision, loose body removal, and debridement. The results showed significant resultant morbidity, with 40% of the patients

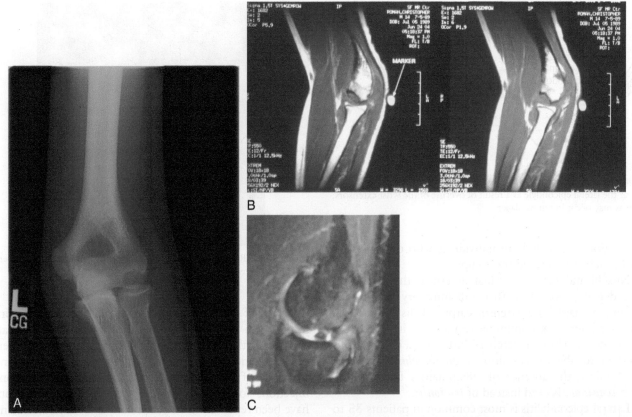

Figure 9-30 Osteochondritis dissecans (OCD). **A,** X-ray film of a 14-year-old male baseball player with OCD of the capitellum. **B,** MRI scan of the same boy. The lesion was partly detached and ultimately was repaired surgically. **C,** MRI scan of the elbow of a 16-year-old gymnast with OCD and an apparent loose body.

reporting pain and 60% showing radiographic evidence of degenerative joint disease. Subsequent studies have reported improved but variable short-term outcomes with arthroscopic techniques.[220,224] Takeda et al.[225] recently reported a 57-month follow-up on 11 baseball players who underwent open bone grafting and wire fixation of OCD lesions that had failed conservative treatment. Of the 11 players, 9 had excellent results and returned to their previous level of activity. Removal of lesions that are repairable, therefore, may result in premature arthritis of the elbow and poor function in the long term. Repair of the fragments, when possible, appears to produce a better long-term outcome.

Overall, it appears that regardless of treatment, larger lesions carry a significantly worse prognosis with a higher incidence of persistent pain and the development of degenerative changes.[226] For lesions that do not involve a bony fragment to fix, some recommend debridement and microfracture of the bony bed. Others have tried osteochondral autograft plugs, particularly when the lateral column is involved in the lesion. Early experience with the osteochondral plugs is encouraging.[227,228]

Radiocapitellar Degeneration

As previously discussed, radiocapitellar degeneration most often occurs with UCL insufficiency.[22] Incompetence of the medial stabilizing structures (UCL) results in increased force at the radiocapitellar joint, which leads to softening and degeneration of the articular cartilage. Osteochondral loose bodies are common and often cause mechanical symptoms and pain.[24] Eventually, degenerative arthritis of the radiocapitellar joint may develop. Tenderness at the lateral elbow that is worsened by pronation and supination of the elbow is a common finding on examination. Arthroscopic surgery is effective for removing loose bodies but cannot reverse the changes in the articular cartilage. In athletes the symptoms usually recur when the individual returns to the same level of throwing, especially if the UCL instability has not been corrected. For constant pain caused by radiocapitellar arthritis, radial head excision, using either open or arthroscopic techniques, often is successful. Some clinicians also advocate isolated radiocapitellar arthroplasty.

Lateral Epicondylitis

Lateral epicondylitis, or **tennis elbow,** is by far the most common overuse injury of the elbow. It is approximately seven times more common than medial epicondylitis.[136,229] It is commonly seen in tennis players and other athletes, although 95% of individuals with tennis elbow do not play tennis (Figure 9-31). Lateral epicondylitis, or more appropriately, epicondylosis, is very common in the general

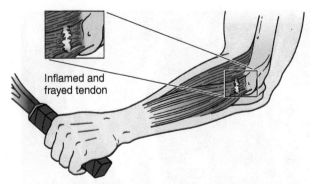

Figure 9-31 Lateral epicondylitis, a tendinosis of the wrist extensor muscles at the lateral epicondyle as a result of overuse of the wrist extensors, such as may occur in tennis players.

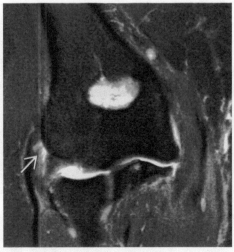

Figure 9-32 MRI scan of a patient with epicondylosis of the wrist extensors at the lateral epicondyle.

population, particularly in individuals who do repetitive work, such as typing on the computer.

Nirschl and Pettrone[230] first described this condition as a degenerative more than inflammatory process involving primarily the extensor carpi radialis brevis. The extensor digitorum communis can also be involved to a lesser degree. These researchers' histological observations led them to label the condition *angiofibroblastic hyperplasia*.[230] Given the absence of inflammatory findings, the term *tendinosis* is used instead of *tendonitis*.

Lateral epicondylitis is most common in patients 35 to 50 years of age and is associated with higher levels and frequency of activity.[24] Poor conditioning and poor technique likely exacerbate the problem in many tennis players, and certainly many racquet factors have been attributed to tennis elbow, including heavy racquets, metal racquets, stiffer racquets, incorrect grip size, and string tension. As many as half of club tennis players older than age 30 have had tennis elbow.[230,231] Patients initially report activity-related lateral elbow pain, often a dull, aching, lateral pain, and may show weakness of grip strength. Symptoms can progress to pain at rest in the more severe stages and difficulty holding a cup, lifting a milk carton, shaking hands or opening a door, or engaging in any activity that requires holding the wrist in its functional position (slightly extended) while loading the wrist.[24] On examination patients have tenderness approximately 1 to 2 cm (0.5 to 1 inch) distal to the lateral epicondyle and pain with passive wrist flexion, with resisted active wrist extension, and during grasping or lifting. Radiographs often are normal but may show a spur at the lateral epicondyle or calcification of the common extensor tendon.[1,229,231] MRI is rarely necessary but can reveal changes consistent with a tendinosis of the extensor muscles at the elbow (Figure 9-32).

Initial treatment is typically nonoperative. Of patients, 95% improve with conservative treatment.[231] Rest (i.e., avoidance of the stress or overuse) must be combined with a program that reestablishes the patient's strength, flexibility, and endurance. Counterforce bracing is thought to reduce the load at the lateral epicondyle by preventing the forearm muscles from fully expanding or changing the

direction of musculotendinous pull.[229] Corticosteroid injections can be helpful and are a common form of treatment by orthopedic surgeons. A survey of 400 members of the American Academy of Orthopaedic Surgeons found that 93% of its membership had administered cortisone injections for tennis elbow.[232] Corticosteroid injections have been reported to be particularly effective in reducing symptoms, allowing the patient to perform rehabilitation exercises, but repeated injections (i.e., more than three in a 1-year period) are not recommended.[233] A recent randomized study showed a short-term benefit to iontophoresis of dexamethasone in patients with severe lateral epicondylitis.[234] Other research suggests that topical nitric oxide, metalloprotease inhibitors, and botulinum toxin may be beneficial.[235–237] Shock wave therapy has not been shown to be beneficial.[238] Blood injections and platelet-rich plasma (PRP) injections recently have been reported to be beneficial in small case series.[239,240] Additionally, a recent larger sample randomized controlled trial of 230 patients found meaningful improvements with leukocyte-enriched PRP injection at 24 weeks compared with a control group.[241] Recreational tennis players should be encouraged to seek professional instruction, because improper technique often contributes to the problem.[24]

Surgery for Lateral Epicondylitis

If 6 months of nonoperative treatment for lateral epicondylitis fails to result in satisfactory improvement, surgery is indicated.[1,24] Lateral epicondylitis can be treated percutaneously, by an open technique, or arthroscopically. A detailed review is beyond the scope of this chapter but can be found in the literature.[242] Only one paper in the literature compares the three main procedures for tennis elbow: percutaneous release, the open procedure described by Nirschl and Ashman,[231] and arthroscopic release. None of the three was found to be superior.[243] A systematic review also did not reveal any difference between the different procedures, but this may be due to the limited number of quality studies in the literature.[242] The principal goals generally are to remove abnormal, degenerative tissue at the origin of the extensor carpi radialis brevis and to encourage healing with minimal disruption of normal stabilizing structures (Figure 9-33). Outcomes after surgical treatment are excellent. According to Nirschl and Ashman,[231] 85% of patients experience complete pain relief and full return of strength. Similar outcomes have been noted with arthroscopic release. In addition, concomitant intra-articular problems may be identified and treated arthroscopically that might not be seen with an open approach.[242,244] Arthroscopy for lateral epicondylitis provides significant improvements in pain and functional recovery up to 3 months after surgery. However, it takes more than 6 months for pain scales to decrease to normal levels.[245]

Extensor/Supinator Muscular Disruption

Lateral muscle disruption is rare. It has been reported in patients who have had repeated corticosteroid injections for lateral epicondylitis.[233] Patients report an acute onset of pain associated with a snap that results in weakness of wrist extension and forearm supination. For complete or near-complete injuries, surgical repair is recommended.[1]

Radial Nerve Entrapment

For some time, it has been accepted that certain cases of persistent tennis elbow represent radial or posterior interosseous nerve compression, the so-called **radial tunnel syndrome.**[246] The radial tunnel is defined by the bony and soft tissue structures that surround the radial nerve and its posterior interosseous branch as they travel through the proximal forearm. Nerve compression in this area most commonly occurs at the **arcade of Frohse,** the tendinous proximal edge of the supinator muscle. Other potential sites of compression include the proximal edge of the extensor carpi radialis brevis, branches of the radial artery, and fibrous bands.[247,248]

When persistent forearm pain and tenderness are associated with muscle weakness in the distribution of the posterior interosseous nerve, nerve entrapment in the radial tunnel is the likely etiology. The tenderness associated with radial nerve entrapment is more distal and medial than that seen in lateral epicondylitis. That is, it is located more over the muscular area of the proximal forearm.[24] Nonoperative management is typically successful in treating this problem.[1] Cases that do not respond to conservative treatment may require surgical decompression.[24] However, many cases of persistent or recurrent tennis elbow are not associated with objective neurological deficits. These cases most likely do not represent a true entrapment neuropathy, and practitioners should be cautious about recommending surgical decompression.[248,249]

CONSERVATIVE THERAPY AND MODALITIES

Ice and Nonsteroidal Anti-inflammatory Medications

Nonoperative treatment of elbow injuries usually involves multiple approaches. Ice is often recommended, especially in the acute period, because it has minimal risks and may provide symptomatic relief of swelling and pain. NSAIDs also are used as a first-line medical treatment for painful and inflammatory conditions about the elbow. They are most often administered topically or orally, although intramuscular injection is also available. For lateral elbow pain, topical NSAIDs have shown a significant effect, compared with placebo, for short-term pain relief and patient satisfaction.[250] Oral NSAIDs are also often used, although the benefit is not as well documented and the adverse effects are more significant. Long-term oral use of NSAIDs can be associated with adverse effects on the gastrointestinal and renal systems. Fortunately, these complications are uncommon with short-term use in medically healthy patients when taken with food.

Therapeutic Ultrasound

Therapeutic ultrasound has been used as a treatment for chronic musculotendinous problems. Phonophoresis involves the addition of a gel containing a corticosteroid to the ultrasound treatment. In one study, therapeutic ultrasound was reported to achieve short-term improvement in pain and pressure tolerance in patients with tendonitis, but adding phonophoresis did not provide any additional benefit.[251]

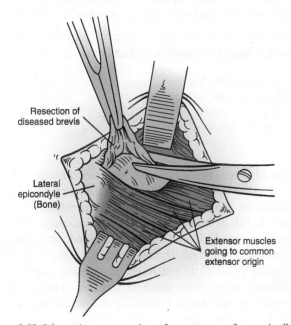

Resection of diseased brevis

Lateral epicondyle (Bone)

Extensor muscles going to common extensor origin

Figure 9-33 Schematic representation of open surgery for tennis elbow with excision of the degenerative tissue. (Redrawn from Safran MR: Elbow tendinopathy: surgical repair of the epicondylitides. In Craig E, editor: *Clinical orthopaedics,* p 279, Philadelphia, 1999, Lippincott Williams & Wilkins.)

High-Voltage Electrical Stimulation

Electrical stimulation frequently has been used as a treatment for various musculoskeletal conditions. Specifically, it often is used to treat nerve and tendon injuries of the upper extremity, and some evidence in animal models indicates that it may help stimulate nerve repair. However, no human clinical studies have demonstrated a significant effect in the treatment of nerve or tendon injuries.[252]

Transverse Friction Massage

Transverse friction massage has been suggested as a physical therapy modality for tendonitis pain. However, the controlled studies that have been reported have not shown a significant effect. One study looked at lateral epicondylitis and showed no difference in terms of pain relief, grip strength, or functional status compared with other physical therapy modalities.[253] **Scar massage** is a gentle transverse friction massage.

Cortisone Injections

Local corticosteroid injections are commonly used to treat a variety of chronic musculoskeletal problems. They have been used extensively to treat lateral epicondylitis. Smidt et al.[233] did an extensive review of the literature on the use of corticosteroid injections for this condition. They found a statistically significant short-term effect for pain, grip strength, and global improvement; however, no medium- or long-term effect could be demonstrated.[233] The most commonly cited complication of corticosteroid injection was tendon rupture.[254] Although some have attempted to use cortisone injections as a treatment, most use cortisone, such as oral NSAIDs, as an adjunct, to make it more tolerable for patients to do their rehabilitation.

GENERAL REHABILITATION GUIDELINES

Rehabilitation after elbow injury or elbow surgery follows a sequential and progressive multiphased approach. The ultimate goal of elbow rehabilitation is to return patients to their previous functional level as quickly and safely as possible. The following sections provide an overview of the rehabilitation process after elbow injury and surgery. Rehabilitation protocols for specific pathologies are then presented.

Four Phases of Elbow Rehabilitation

- Phase I: immediate motion phase
- Phase II: intermediate phase (full ROM, minimal pain, good muscle strength)
- Phase III: advanced strengthening phase
- Phase IV: return to activity phase

Phase I: Immediate Motion Phase

The first phase of elbow rehabilitation is the immediate motion phase. The goals of this phase are to minimize the effects of immobilization, reestablish pain-free ROM, reduce pain and inflammation, and retard muscular atrophy. Early ROM activities are performed to nourish the articular cartilage and assist in the synthesis, alignment, and organization of collagen tissue.[255-263] ROM activities are performed for all planes of elbow and wrist motions to prevent the formation of scar tissue and adhesions. Active-assisted and passive ROM exercises are performed for the ulnohumeral joint to restore flexion/extension, as well as supination/pronation for the radiohumeral and radioulnar joints. The reestablishment of either full elbow extension or preinjury motion is the primary goal of early ROM activities to minimize the occurrence of elbow flexion contractures.[263-265] Preoperative elbow motion must be carefully assessed and recorded. Patients should be asked whether they have had full elbow extension in the past 2 to 3 years. Postoperative ROM often is related to preoperative motion, especially with UCL reconstruction. Elbow flexion contractures can be a deleterious side effect of surgery for the overhead athlete. The elbow is predisposed to flexion contractures because of the intimate congruency of the joint articulations, the tightness of the joint capsule, and the tendency of the anterior capsule to develop adhesions after injury.[262] The brachialis muscle also attaches to the capsule and crosses the elbow joint before becoming a tendinous structure. Injury to the elbow may cause excessive scar tissue formation of the brachialis muscle and to the adjacent tissues, which may require functional splinting of the elbow.[262]

Phase I: Goals of Immediate Motion Phase

- Minimize the effects of immobilization
- Reestablish pain-free ROM
- Reduce pain and inflammation
- Reduce muscle atrophy

In addition to ROM exercises, joint mobilizations may be performed as tolerated to minimize the occurrence of joint contractures. Posterior glides with oscillations are performed at end ROM to help regain full elbow extension. Initially grade I and grade II mobilizations are used, with progression to aggressive mobilization techniques (grade III/III+ and grade IV/IV+) at end ROM during later stages of rehabilitation, when symptoms have subsided. Joint mobilization must include the radiocapitellar and radioulnar joints.

If the patient continues to have difficulty achieving full extension using ROM and mobilization techniques, a low load–long duration (L3D) stretch (also called *collagen creep* or *plastic flow stretch*) may be performed to produce a deformation or creep of the collagen tissue, resulting in tissue elongation.[265-268] We have found this technique to be extremely beneficial for regaining full elbow extension. The patient lies supine with a towel or foam roll placed under the distal brachium to act as a cushion and fulcrum. Light-resistance exercise tubing is applied to the wrist and secured to the table or to a dumbbell on the ground (Figure 9-34). The patient is instructed to relax as much as possible for 12 to 15 minutes. The patient performs this type of exercise at home periodically during the day, totaling 60 minutes of stretching per day. The resistance applied should be low enough in magnitude to enable the patient to perform the stretch for the entire duration without pain or muscle spasm. The technique should impart a low load but a long duration stretch.

The aggressiveness of stretching and mobilization techniques is dictated by the healing constraints of the involved tissues, the specific pathology or surgical technique, and the amount of motion and end feel. If the patient has decreased motion and a pathologically hard end feel without pain, aggressive stretching and mobilization techniques may be used. Conversely, a patient who has pain before resistance or an empty end feel must be progressed slowly with gentle stretching.

Another goal of phase I is to reduce the patient's pain and inflammation. Grade I and grade II mobilization techniques are used to neuromodulate pain by stimulating type I and type II articular receptors.[269,270] Cryotherapy and high-voltage stimulation may be performed as required to further assist in reducing pain and inflammation. Once the acute inflammatory response has subsided, moist heat, warm whirlpool, and therapeutic ultrasound may be used at the onset of treatment to prepare the tissue for stretching and improve the extensibility of the capsule and musculotendinous structures. In addition, joint mobilization glides are increased to grade III/III+ and grade IV/IV+ mobilizations.

The early phase of rehabilitation also focuses on voluntary activation of muscle and the retardation of muscular atrophy. Nonpainful, submaximal isometrics are performed initially for the elbow flexors and extensors, as well as for the wrist flexor, extensor, pronator, and supinator muscle groups. Shoulder isometrics may also be performed during this phase, but care must be taken to avoid medial (internal) and lateral (external) shoulder rotation exercises if these are painful. Alternating rhythmic stabilization drills for shoulder flexion/extension/horizontal abduction/adduction, shoulder medial/lateral rotation, and elbow flexion/extension/supination/pronation are performed to begin reestablishing proprioception and neuromuscular control of the upper extremity.

Phase II: Intermediate Phase (Full ROM, Minimal Pain, Good Muscle Strength)

Phase II, the intermediate phase, is initiated when the patient exhibits full ROM, minimal pain and tenderness, and a good (4/5) manual muscle test of the elbow flexor and extensor musculature. The emphasis in this phase includes enhancing elbow and upper extremity mobility, improving muscular strength and endurance, and reestablishing neuromuscular control of the elbow complex.

Stretching exercises are continued to maintain full elbow and wrist ROM. Mobilization techniques may be progressed to more aggressive grade III techniques as needed to apply a stretch to the capsular tissue at end range. Flexibility is progressed during this phase to focus on wrist flexion, extension, and forearm pronation and supination. Elbow extension and forearm pronation flexibility is specifically emphasized in throwing athletes so that they can perform efficiently. Shoulder flexibility is also maintained in athletes, with emphasis on medial and lateral rotation at 90° of abduction, flexion, and horizontal adduction. In particular, shoulder lateral rotation at 90° of abduction is emphasized because even a slight loss of lateral rotation may result in increased strain on the medial elbow structures during the overhead throwing motion. Medial rotation motion should also be diligently performed.

Wilk et al.[271] has reported that bilateral differences in shoulder total rotation and flexion had a significant effect on the risk for elbow injuries in pitchers. Pitchers with deficits of greater than 5° in total rotation in their throwing shoulders had a 2.6 times greater risk for injury. Pitchers with a deficit of greater than 5° in flexion of the throwing shoulder had 2.8 times greater risk for injury.

Strengthening exercises are progressed during this phase to include isotonic contractions, beginning concentrically and progressing to include eccentric contractions. Emphasis is placed on elbow flexion and extension, wrist flexion and extension, and forearm pronation and supination. The glenohumeral and scapulothoracic muscles are placed on a progressive resistance program during the later stages of phase II, emphasizing strengthening the shoulder lateral rotators and scapular muscles. A complete upper extremity strengthening program, such as the thrower's 10 program (Figure 9-35), may be performed.

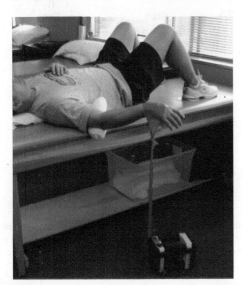

Figure 9-34 Low load–long duration (L3D technique) stretching to improve elbow extension. A low-intensity stretch is applied for 10 to 12 minutes. Note that the elbow is pronated and the shoulder is internally rotated to lock the humerus and prevent compensation.

1A. Diagonal D2 Extension Pattern: Involved hand grips tubing handle overhead and out to the side. Pull tubing down and across the body to the opposite side of leg. During the motion, lead with the thumb.

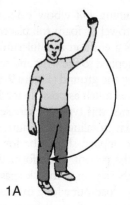

1B. Diagonal D2 Flexion Pattern: Gripping tubing handle in hand of involved arm, begin with arm out from side 45° and palm facing backward. While turning palm forward, proceed to flex elbow and bring arm up and over involved shoulder. Reverse to take arm to starting position while turning the palm down. Note: D2 flexion pattern is the reverse of the D2 extension pattern.

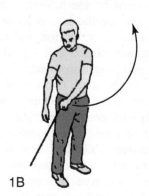

2A. Lateral (External) Rotation at 0° Abduction: Stand with involved elbow fixed at side, elbow at 90° and involved arm across front of body. Grip tubing handle while the other end of tubing is fixed. Rotate arm out, keeping elbow at side leading with the thumb. Return to start position moving slowly and in a controlled fashion.

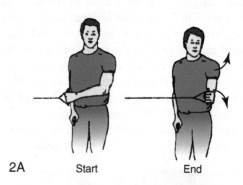

2B. Medial (Internal) Rotation at 0° Abduction: Standing with elbow at side fixed at 90° and shoulder rotated out. Grip tubing handle with thumb out while other end of tubing is fixed. Pull arm across body keeping elbow at side leading with thumb. Return to start position moving slowly and in a controlled fashion.

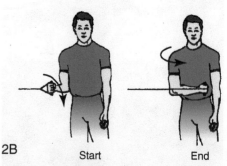

Figure 9-35 The thrower's exercise program. This program is designed to exercise the major muscles necessary for throwing. The goal is to establish an organized, concise exercise program. All exercises included are specific to the thrower and are designed to improve the strength, power, and endurance of the shoulder complex musculature along with elbow "2 joint" muscles. (Modified from Wilk KE, Reinold MR, Andrews JR: *The athlete's shoulder*, ed 2, New York, 2009, Churchill Livingstone/Elsevier.)

(Continued)

2C. Lateral (External) Rotation at 90°
Abduction: Stand with shoulder abducted to 90°. Grip tubing handle while the other end is fixed straight ahead, slightly lower than the shoulder. Keeping shoulder abducted, rotate shoulder back keeping elbow at 90°. Return hand to start position. Start at slow speed. As control achieved, do rotations faster.

2D. Medial (Internal) Rotation at 90°
Abduction: Stand with shoulder abducted to 90°, laterally rotated 90° and elbow bentto 90°. Keeping shoulder abducted, rotate shoulder forward, keeping elbow bent at 90°.Return hand to start position.Start at slow speed. As control achieved, do rotations faster.

2E. Sidelying Lateral (External) Rotation: Lie onuninvolved side, with involved arm at side of body and elbow bent to 90°. Keeping the elbow of involved arm fixed to side, raise arm and lower slowly.

3. Shoulder Abduction to 90°: Stand with arm at side, elbow straight, and palm against side. Raise arm to the side, palm down, until arm reaches 90° (shoulder level). Be sure to engage scapula before beginning.

4. Scaption, Lateral (External) Rotation: Stand with elbow straight and thumb up. Raise arm to shoulder level at 30° angle in front of body (scaption). Do not go above shoulder height. Be sure to engage scapula before beginning.

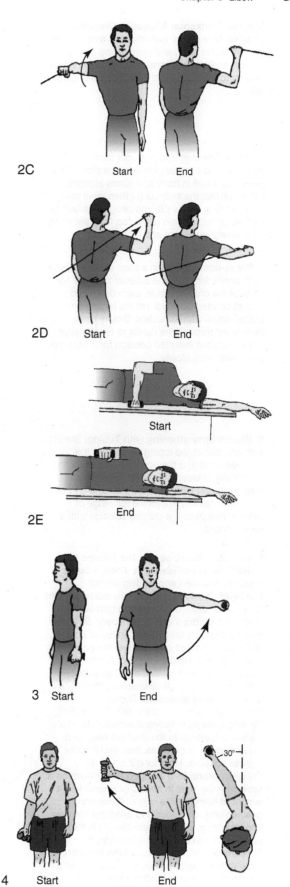

Figure 9-35 Cont'd

5. Prone Horizontal Abduction (Neutral): Lie on table, face down, with involved arm hanging straight to the floor, and palm facing down. Engage scapula and raise arm out to the side, parallel to the floor. Hold 2 seconds and lower slowly.

6. Prone Rowing: Lying on your stomach with your involved arm hanging over the side of the table, dumbbell in hand and elbow straight. Slowly retract the scapula (A) then raise the arm, bending elbow (B), and bring dumbbell as high as possible. Hold at the top for 2 seconds, then slowly lower arm and then release scapula.

7. Press-ups: Seated on a chair or table, place both hands firmly on the sides of the chair (or arms of the chair) or table, palm down and fingers pointed outward. Hands should be placed equal with shoulders. Slowly push downward through the hands to elevate your body. Hold the elevated position for 2 seconds and lower body slowly.

8. Biceps Strengthening with Tubing: Stand with one end of the tubing securely in the involved hand and the opposite end under the foot of the involved side while controlling tension. Assist with the opposite hand so that the arm is flexed through the full range of motion. Return to the starting position with a slow 5 count.

9. Dumbbell Exercises for the Triceps and Wrist Extensors/Flexors: *A. Triceps curls:* Raise the involved arm holding weight overhead. Provide support at the elbow with the uninvolved hand. Straighten the arm overhead. Hold for 2 seconds and lower slowly. ***B. Wrist flexion:*** Support the forearm on leg or on a table with the hand off the edge, the palm facing upward. Hold a weight or hammer in the involved hand and lower it as far as possible, then curl it up as high as possible. Hold for a 2 count. ***C. Wrist extension:*** Support the forearm on leg or on a table with the hand off the edge, the palm facing downward. Hold a weight or hammer in the involved hand and lower it as far as possible, then curl it up as high as possible. Hold for a 2 count. ***D. Forearm pronation:*** Support the forearm on a table with the wrist in neutral position. Hold a weight or hammer in a normal hammering position and roll the wrist to bring the hammer into pronation as far as possible. Hold for a 2 count. Raise to the starting position. ***E. Forearm supination:*** Support the forearm on a table with the wrist in neutral position. Hold a weight or hammer in a normal hammering position and roll the wrist to bring the hammer into full supination. Hold for a 2 count. Raise back to the starting position.

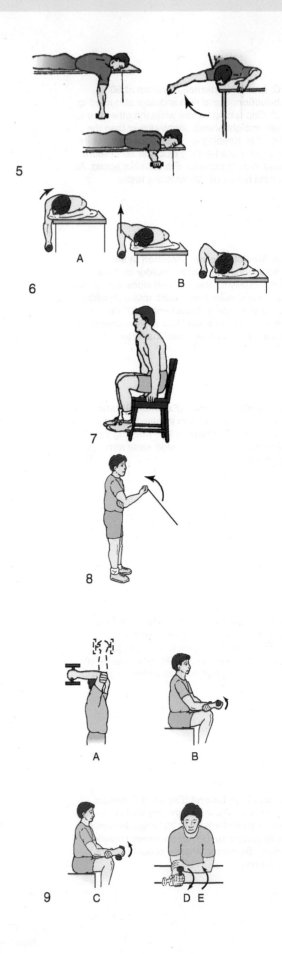

Figure 9-35 Cont'd

10. Serratus Anterior Strengthening (Push Up with "+"): Start with a push up away from the wall (wall push up). Gradually progress to the tabletop (table push up) and eventually to the floor (floor push up) as tolerable. Push up in any of the 3 positions as far as possible without hunching the shoulders.

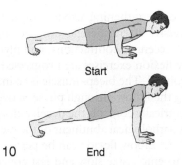

Start

10   End

Figure 9-35 Cont'd

Neuromuscular control exercises are initiated in this phase to enhance the muscles' ability to control the elbow joint during athletic activities. These exercises include proprioceptive neuromuscular facilitation exercises with rhythmic stabilizations (Figure 9-36) and slow reversal manual resistance elbow/wrist flexion drills (Figure 9-37).

Phase II: Goals of Intermediate Phase (Full ROM, Minimal Pain, Good Muscle Strength)

- Enhance elbow and upper extremity mobility
- Improve muscle strength and endurance
- Re-establish neuromuscular control

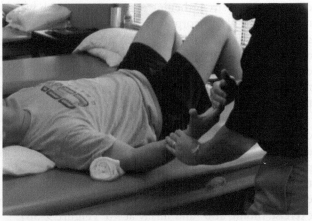

Figure 9-37 PNF exercise drills that include slow reversal of manual resistance.

Phase III: Advanced Strengthening Phase

The third phase of elbow rehabilitation involves a progression of activities to prepare the patient or athlete for high-level stress situations or participation in sports. The goals of this phase are to gradually increase strength, power, endurance, and neuromuscular control to prepare for a gradual return to sports. Specific criteria that must be met before this phase is entered include full, nonpainful ROM; absence of pain or tenderness; and strength that is 70% of the contralateral extremity.

Phase III: Goals of Advanced Strengthening Phase

- Increase strength to functional levels
- Increase power to functional levels
- Increase endurance to functional levels
- Increase neuromuscular control

Criteria for Progression to Phase III

- Full, pain-free ROM
- No pain
- No tenderness
- Strength at least 70% of contralateral limb

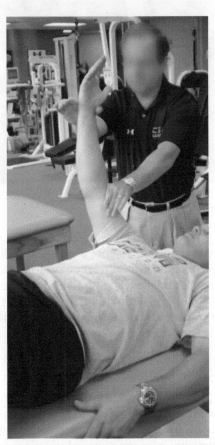

Figure 9-36 Proprioceptive neuromuscular facilitation (PNF) exercises to the elbow to enhance elbow stability.

Advanced strengthening activities during this phase include aggressive strengthening exercises that emphasize high speed, eccentric contractions, and plyometric activities. Elbow flexion exercises are progressed to emphasize eccentric control. The biceps muscle is an important stabilizer during the follow-through phase of overhead throwing; it eccentrically controls the deceleration of the elbow, preventing pathological abutment of the olecranon within the fossa.[272,273] Elbow flexion can be performed with elastic tubing to emphasize slow and fast concentric and eccentric contractions. Manual resistance may be applied for concentric and eccentric contractions of the elbow flexors. Aggressive strengthening exercises done with weight machines are also incorporated during this phase. These most commonly begin with bench press, seated rowing, and front latissimus dorsi pull-downs. The triceps is exercised primarily with a concentric contraction because of the acceleration (i.e., muscle shortening) activity of the triceps during the acceleration phase of throwing.

Neuromuscular control exercises are progressed to include side-lying lateral (external) rotation with manual resistance. Concentric and eccentric lateral rotation is performed against the clinician's resistance with the addition of rhythmic stabilizations. This manual resistance exercise may be progressed to standing lateral rotation with exercise tubing at 0° and finally at 90° (Figure 9-38).

Plyometric drills can be an extremely beneficial form of functional exercise for training the elbow in overhead athletes.[263,274] Plyometric exercises are performed using a weighted medicine ball during the later stages of phase III to train the shoulder and elbow to develop and withstand high levels of stress. Plyometric exercises initially are performed with two hands performing a chest pass, side-to-side throw, and overhead soccer throw. These may be progressed to include one-handed activities such as 90/90 throws (Figure 9-39), external and internal rotation

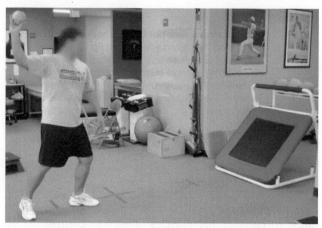

Figure 9-39 Plyometric drills: one-handed baseball throw at 90° abduction.

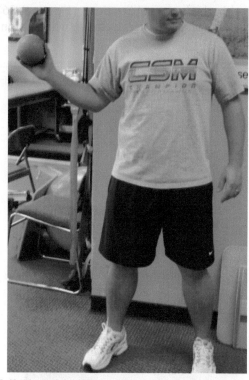

Figure 9-40 Plyometric drills: one-handed medial rotation side throws at 0° abduction.

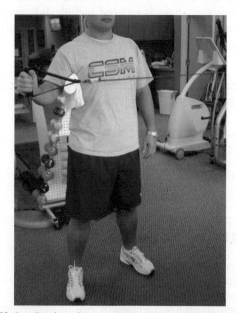

Figure 9-38 Standing lateral rotation with exercise tubing at 0° abduction.

throws at 0° abduction (Figure 9-40), and wall dribbles. Specific plyometric drills for the forearm musculature include wrist flexion flips (Figure 9-41) and extension grips (Figure 9-42). Wrist flexion flips and extension grips are important components of an elbow rehabilitation program because they emphasize the forearm and hand musculature.

Phase IV: Return to Activity Phase

The final phase of elbow rehabilitation is the return to activity phase. It allows the patient to progressively return to full activity or, for the overhead athlete, the ability to return to competition using an interval athletic program be it throwing, tennis, golf, swimming, volleyball, and so on.[275]

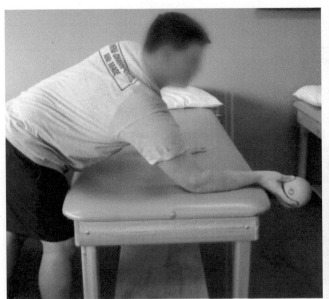 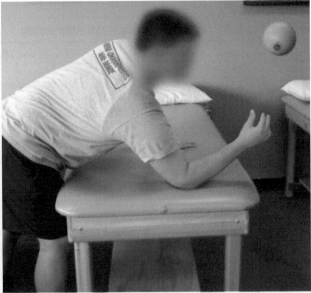

Figure 9-41 Plyometric drills: wrist flexion ball flips.

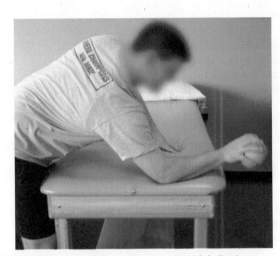

Figure 9-42 Plyometric drills: wrist extension with ball grips.

Phase IV: Goal of Return to Activity Phase

- Program geared to individual functional needs
- Return to full activity

Criteria for Progression to Phase IV

- Full ROM
- No pain or tenderness
- Satisfactory isokinetic test
- Satisfactory clinical examination

Before being allowed to begin the return to activity phase of rehabilitation, patients must exhibit full ROM and have no pain or tenderness. They also must have a satisfactory isokinetic test and a satisfactory clinical examination.

Isokinetic testing is commonly used to determine the readiness of the athlete to begin an interval sports program.[275] Athletes routinely are tested at 180° and 300°/sec (degrees per second). The bilateral comparison at 180°/sec indicates the dominant arm's elbow flexion to be 10% to 20% stronger and the dominant extensors 5% to 15% stronger than the nondominant arm.

Upon achieving the previously mentioned criteria for returning to sports, a formal interval sports program as described by Reinold et al. can begin.[275] For the overhead thrower, a long toss interval throwing program begins at 13.7 m (45 feet) and gradually progresses to 36.6 or 54.9 m (120 or 180 feet) (player and position dependent) (Table 9-1).[276] Throwing should be performed without pain or a significant increase in symptoms. We believe it is important for the overhead patient or athlete to perform stretching and an abbreviated strengthening program before and after performing the interval sports program. Typically, overhead throwers warm up, stretch, and perform one set of their exercise program before throwing, followed by two additional sets of exercises following throwing.[275] This not only provides an adequate warm-up but also ensures maintenance of necessary ROM and flexibility of the shoulder joint. The next day, the thrower exercises the scapular muscles and external rotators and performs a core stabilization program.

After completing a long toss program, pitchers progress to phase II of the throwing program, throwing off of a mound.[275] In phase II the number of throws, intensity, and type of pitch are progressed to gradually increase stress on the elbow and shoulder joints.[275] Generally, the pitcher begins at 50% intensity and gradually progresses to 75%, 90%, and 100% over 4 to 6 weeks. Breaking balls are initiated once the pitcher can throw 40 to 50 pitches with at least 80% intensity with no symptoms.

TABLE **9-1**

Postoperative Rehabilitation Following Elbow Arthroscopy

Initial phase (week 1)	*Goals:* achieve full wrist and elbow ROM; reduce swelling and pain; retard muscle atrophy.
	1. Day of surgery
	  • Begin gently moving elbow in bulky dressing
	2. Postoperative days 1-2
	  • Remove bulky dressing, and replace with elastic bandages
	  • Immediate postoperative hand, wrist, and elbow exercises:
	    o Putty/grip strengthening
	    o Wrist flexor stretching
	    o Wrist extensor stretching
	    o Wrist curls
	    o Reverse wrist curls
	    o Neutral wrist curls
	    o Forearm pronation/supination
	    o AA/AROM elbow extension/flexion
	3. Postoperative days 3-7
	  • Begin PROM elbow extension/flexion (motion to tolerance)
	  • Begin progressive resistance (PRE) exercises with 0.5-kg (1-pound) weight:
	    o Wrist curls
	    o Reverse wrist curls
	    o Neutral wrist curls
	    o Forearm pronation/supination
	    o Broomstick rollup

Intermediate phase (weeks 2-4)	*Goals:* improve muscular strength and endurance; normalize joint arthrokinematics.
	1. Week 2: ROM exercises (overpressure into extension)
	  • Add biceps curls and triceps extension
	  • Continue to progress PRE weight and repetitions as tolerable
	2. Week 3
	  • Initiate eccentric exercises for biceps and triceps
	  • Initiate exercises for rotator cuff:
	    o Lateral (external) rotators
	    o Medial (internal) rotators
	    o Deltoid
	    o Supraspinatus
	    o Scapulothoracic strengthening

Advanced phase (weeks 4-8)	*Goal:* prepare patient for return to functional activities.
	Criteria for progression to advanced phase:
	  • Full, pain-free ROM
	  • No pain or tenderness
	  • Isokinetic test that fulfills criteria for throwing
	  • Satisfactory clinical examination
	1. Weeks 4-6
	  • Continue maintenance program, emphasizing muscular strength, endurance, and flexibility
	  • Initiate interval throwing program phase

ROM, Range of motion; *AA/AROM,* active assisted and active range of motion; *PROM,* passive range of motion; *PRE,* progressive resistance exercises.

SPECIFIC REHABILITATION GUIDELINES

Tendinopathy

The treatment of tendinopathy is based on a careful examination to determine the exact pathology present. Often practitioners diagnose patients as having "tendonitis" only to discover later that the tendon actually had undergone a degenerative process, or *tendinosis.*[230,231] The treatments for tendonitis and tendinosis are dramatically different.

The treatment for tendonitis typically is targeted at reducing inflammation and pain. This is accomplished through reduction in activities, anti-inflammatory medications, cryotherapy, iontophoresis, light exercise, and stretching.

The treatment for tendinosis focuses on increasing circulation to promote collagen synthesis. This includes application of heat, class IV deep tissue LASER, ultrasound, stretching, eccentric exercises, transverse friction massage, and soft tissue mobilization.

Medial Epicondylitis

The treatment of medial epicondylitis should focus first on reducing pain and inflammation and then on increasing strength. Heat therapy followed by stretching and light strengthening is the hallmark of treatment for this condition. The session is finished with cryotherapy and electrical stimulation to decrease inflammation and pain. A gradual increase in stretching and strengthening should be attempted, with care taken not to exacerbate the patient's symptoms. If exacerbation occurs, a step back should be taken in the program, and the patient should be readvanced more slowly.

In some cases, medial epicondylitis is treated with surgical debridement. Rehabilitation after surgery may be aggressive, because the flexor/pronator mass has not been stripped from the medial epicondyle. The patient is placed in a protective posterior splint for 10 to 14 days to allow the soft tissues to heal. Once the splint is removed, ROM of the elbow is allowed immediately in all directions, including elbow flexion and extension and forearm supination and pronation. Full motion should be obtained by 4 weeks. Light isometric exercise (i.e., 10%-40% of the maximum voluntary contraction [MVC]) can be performed immediately after surgery. Once full motion has been obtained, strengthening may begin. Strengthening begins with isometric exercises and progresses to concentric and then eccentric exercises. Plyometric exercises are the final step.

As with all surgical procedures at the elbow, scar massage is incorporated at 2 to 3 weeks and nerve glides (i.e., neurodynamic techniques such as "flossing") commence when adequate motion is established. In addition, transverse friction massage can be performed over the debrided and released tendon.

In some cases, the surgeon may choose to detach the flexor/pronator mass in the process of debridement. In these patients, active wrist extension and flexion should be prevented for 4 weeks. Although full passive motion is allowed, it should be done gently and only in the presence of the clinician for the first 4 weeks.

Lateral Epicondylitis

A principal aspect of conservative treatment for lateral epicondylitis is therapy. Despite the misnomer, lateral epicondylitis is not a disease of inflammation but rather a disease of degeneration. Usually little or no swelling is present; therefore heat therapy should begin each treatment session. Stretching of the extensor mass with wrist flexion is an important component of treatment. This may be done in conjunction with soft tissue mobilization. If the

stretching and mobilization are well tolerated, isotonic eccentric strengthening exercises for the lateral extensor muscle mass may be attempted. The patient also should perform shoulder and scapular flexibility and strengthening exercises during the rehabilitation program.

Conservative measures should be attempted for at least 6 months before surgical intervention is considered. Rehabilitation after surgical debridement primarily depends on whether the surgeon chooses to detach and reattach the extensor mass during surgery. If the extensor mass is detached during the procedure, active wrist extension and flexion should be prevented for 4 weeks. Although full passive motion is allowed, it should be done gently and only in the presence of the therapist for the first 4 weeks.

Caution with Elbow Surgery/Rehabilitation

- If the flexor or extensor muscle mass is detached during surgery, active wrist movement is prevented for 4 weeks to allow sufficient time for healing

---

The posterior splint is removed at 10 to 14 days. Elbow flexion and extension and forearm supination and pronation are allowed immediately after removal of the splint. Care should be taken to perform supination and pronation gently. Cold therapy and electrical stimulation are instituted to reduce swelling and pain after sessions. Scar massage may begin at 2 to 3 weeks, and nerve glides may commence when adequate motion has been obtained. Full active motion at the elbow and wrist may begin at 4 weeks. If full motion already has been restored as a result of the passive motion instituted earlier, strengthening exercises may begin. Isometric exercises are succeeded by concentric exercises, which are followed by eccentric exercises. If the flexor mass was not detached, full motion of the elbow and wrist is allowed once the splint has been removed.

Ulnar Neuropathy

Therapy aimed at treating ulnar neuropathy depends on the pathology present. The nerve may be stretched secondary to instability at the elbow joint or compressed secondary to hypertrophy of surrounding soft tissue structures, or the condition may be a result of compression secondary to fibrous bands anywhere along the path of the ulnar nerve. This compression usually is observed in extremes of flexion or extension. The initial goal should be to bring the pain under control. This may involve the use of a nighttime splint with the elbow in 45° flexion to prevent recurrent compression and further damage. A full-time splint is not advised because elbow stiffness may develop. If stability is a concern, strengthening exercises also should be performed, focusing on the elbow flexors and extensors. In other patients, particularly those with a large muscle mass, this may be contraindicated because the musculature may be a contributing factor to the problem.

All patients with ulnar neuropathy have nerve irritation that may result in scar formation. For this reason, nerve glides may be helpful in breaking scar tissue enveloping the nerve and possibly causing compression. The glides should be done gently at first using distal stretching techniques, graduating to more aggressive proximal stretching. This helps prevent a traction neuropraxia.

In the athlete, ulnar neuropathy often is a sequela of some other pathology and will not improve unless the underlying pathological condition is addressed. Numerous theories have been advanced on the cause of ulnar neuropathy of the elbow in throwing athletes. Ulnar nerve changes can result from tensile forces, compressive forces, or nerve instability. As noted previously, any one or a combination of these mechanisms may be responsible for ulnar nerve symptoms.

Ulnar neuropathy has three stages. The first stage is marked by the acute onset of radicular symptoms. The second stage is manifested by a recurrence of symptoms as the patient attempts to return to competition. The third stage is associated with persistent motor weakness and sensory changes. If the patient first seeks treatment in the third stage of injury, conservative management may not be effective.

Nonoperative treatment of ulnar neuropathy focuses on reducing ulnar nerve irritation, enhancing dynamic medial joint stability, and gradually returning the patient to previous levels and types of activities. NSAIDs often are prescribed, and rehabilitation includes an iontophoresis disposable patch and cryotherapy. With a diagnosis of ulnar neuropathy, throwing patients are instructed to discontinue throwing activities for at least 4 weeks, depending on the severity and chronicity of symptoms. The patient progresses through the immediate motion and intermediate phases over 4 to 6 weeks, with emphasis on eccentric and dynamic stabilization drills. Plyometric exercises are used to facilitate further dynamic stabilization of the medial elbow. The patient is allowed to begin an interval throwing program when full, pain-free ROM and muscle performance are present without neurological symptoms, and the individual may gradually return to activity if progression through the interval throwing program does not reveal neurological symptoms.

Ulnar Collateral Ligament Injury

Isolated UCL injuries usually are the result of chronic degeneration in repetitive movement overhead athletes. Pain and inflammation usually are present, as is loss of muscle strength throughout the extremity. Because instability may be present, a brace to protect against varus and valgus stresses may be helpful. The athlete must be instructed not to perform the throwing motion or

to throw a ball until adequate healing time has elapsed (to control and limit valgus stress on the UCL). The first goal of treatment is to establish a painless ROM. The clinician begins with passive and active-assisted motion. Motion should be restored in a painless fashion to allow the ligament proper time to heal. Elbow flexion and extension ROM does not create deleterious stress on the UCL and is actually beneficial for ligament healing. Motion begins in a pain-free arc, and ROM is increased as tolerance allows. The patient progresses to active ROM after full motion has been established with the previous measures. Elbow flexion and extension and forearm supination and pronation are addressed, as are all wrist movements.

Gradual strengthening should begin with isometric exercises of the elbow and wrist. A shoulder program should be implemented to normalize ROM and flexibility and to improve shoulder strength.

Light isotonic exercises at the elbow and wrist are started around weeks 3 to 4, after full motion has been established. The goal is to increase wrist flexor and pronator strength to assist in elbow stability. This is continued until weeks 6 to 7. At this point, plyometric exercises are initiated slowly. Once full motion, full strength, and dynamic stability have returned and the patient is symptom free, the patient may begin an interval throwing program. Upon satisfactory completion of the interval throwing program (i.e., pain-free throwing at full velocity), the patient may return to high-level activity. To assist in pain-free throwing and sports, the overhead athlete should undergo a biomechanical evaluation to determine whether improper throwing mechanics are a factor or whether any biomechanical faults need to be corrected to help control the forces applied to the elbow joint.

Osteochondritis Dissecans (OCD)

In OCD, conservative measures typically are reserved for nondisplaced lesions. In the painful elbow associated with this lesion, a brief period of immobilization (i.e., up to 3 weeks) can be beneficial. Used in association with cryotherapy and NSAIDs, immobilization can help limit the inflammatory process. At the end of the immobilization period, ROM exercises can begin. When motion returns, strengthening may begin with isometric exercises. Care must be taken to avoid compressive forces on the radiocapitellar joint. Progression to isotonic exercises may begin with the same limitations. Sequential MRI and bone scans are obtained to assess the progression of healing. If healing does not progress, conservative measures should be abandoned in favor of surgical intervention. If the bone scans show evidence that the elbow is attempting to heal or is making progress, exercises that create stress in the radiocapitellar joint must be avoided to prevent detachment or collapse of the fragment.

Medial Epicondylar Apophyseal Injury (Little Leaguer's Elbow)

Medial epicondylar apophyseal injury is the result of abnormal stress to the epicondylar growth plate (apophysis) caused by excessive traction stresses. A rehabilitation protocol similar to that for a UCL strain is used for medial epicondylar apophyseal injuries. Reducing pain and restoring motion are the initial priorities. When pain dissipates and motion returns, gradual strengthening may commence. One goal is to begin heavy lifting and plyometrics by 14 weeks. In milder cases, such as nondisplaced injuries, a more aggressive rehabilitation protocol may be used. An interval throwing program is the last step of the rehabilitation process.

Ulnar Nerve Transposition

The goal of rehabilitation for ulnar nerve transposition is to return motion, function, and strength while minimizing pain and preventing failure of the surgery and complications, including adhesions to the nerve. A splint is applied immediately postoperatively with elbow flexion at 45°. This is left in place until approximately the tenth postoperative day to allow the soft tissues to heal and to enable some scar tissue to form and further secure the ulnar nerve in its new location. As with most rehabilitation around the elbow, the initial goal is to restore motion while minimizing pain.

Several techniques can be used for ulnar nerve decompression. Decompression in situ decompresses the ulnar nerve only at a specific site of compression, and no transposition takes place. In general, the ulnar nerve is quite stable and is not at risk for subluxation. For this reason, immediate active motion and passive motion are allowed. Motion should be fully restored by 4 weeks after surgery. Once motion has been restored, nerve glides are commenced to prevent scar adherence to the nerve. Isometric strengthening exercises may begin as well.

If a medial epicondylectomy or submuscular transposition is performed, active motion of the wrist should be avoided for 4 weeks to prevent flexor muscle mass avulsion. Although full passive motion of the wrist is allowed, it should be done gently and only in the presence of a clinician for the first 4 weeks. Full active and passive motion at the elbow may begin when the splint is removed, but care should be taken to be gentle with forearm supination and pronation. Scar massage may begin at 2 to 3 weeks, and nerve glides may commence when adequate motion has been obtained. Full active motion at the elbow and wrist may begin at 4 weeks. If full motion has already been restored, strengthening exercises may begin at 6 weeks. Isometrics may graduate to isotonic exercises. Plyometric exercises follow next. If the goal is to return a throwing athlete to his or her sport, an interval throwing program

may commence by week 8. Return to competition may begin around week 12.

With a subcutaneous transposition, the flexor/pronator mass is not disrupted. The ulnar nerve is kept in place with a fascial sling. The splint is removed in 14 days, and this initial 2 weeks should be sufficient time for the soft tissues to heal. Once the splint has been removed, unlimited motion at the elbow and wrist may begin. Motion should be restored by 4 weeks. Once motion has been restored, strengthening can begin, in the same fashion as described previously. Nerve glides may begin when adequate motion has been restored. As described, scar massage may begin at 2 to 3 weeks.

Cryotherapy and electrical stimulation are encouraged in the initial stages to help minimize inflammation while motion exercises are performed; however, the nerve must be protected from thermal injury (particularly important with subcutaneous transpositions). Table 9-2 outlines a postsurgical treatment protocol.

Arthroscopic Excision of Osteophytes

Osteophytes most often appear on the olecranon in the posterior elbow, but they also may appear anteriorly on the coronoid. Throwing athletes may develop posteromedial olecranon osteophytes associated with VEOS.

Direct posterior osteophytes on the olecranon may limit extension of the elbow. Depending on the duration and magnitude of osteophyte formation, the resultant loss of motion may cause contracture of the anterior capsule. Therefore, even with surgical excision of the osteophytes, return of full extension may be a challenge, especially if no concomitant anterior capsule release is performed. Rehabilitation focuses on return of motion, particularly extension. The general rehabilitation guidelines for the elbow should be followed. However, less emphasis is placed on strengthening and more emphasis is placed on ROM exercises. Instability should not be expected with this procedure; therefore the clinician can be more aggressive with motion exercises, provided they do not result in increased inflammation. Control of inflammation and pain is crucial to this process, because pain markedly limits the amount of stretching a patient can tolerate. NSAIDs, cryotherapy, and high-voltage electrical stimulation all play roles in pain control. Once motion has been restored, strengthening may commence on a more aggressive basis. It is important to note that restoration of full extension may not be possible; therefore communication between the surgeon and clinicians is important to clarify the realistic goals of the surgical intervention.

Anterior coronoid osteophyte formation has a similar pathology. Full flexion is limited because of a bony blockage of motion anteriorly. This also results in soft tissue contractures. Therefore, even after the bone is removed, the motion in flexion is difficult to restore. Rehabilitation is similar to that described earlier, although more aggressive flexion exercises are instituted.

TABLE **9-2**

Postoperative Rehabilitation after Ulnar Nerve Transposition

Phase I: immediate postoperative phase (weeks 0-2)	*Goals:* allow soft tissue healing of relocated nerve; reduce pain and inflammation; retard muscular atrophy. **1.** Week 1 • Posterior splint at 90° elbow flexion with wrist free for motion (sling for comfort) • Compression dressing • Exercises such as gripping exercises, wrist ROM, shoulder isometrics **2.** Week 2 • Remove posterior splint for exercise and bathing • Progress elbow ROM (PROM 150° to 120°) • Initiate elbow and wrist isometrics • Continue shoulder isometrics
Phase II: intermediate phase (weeks 3-7)	*Goals:* restore full, pain-free ROM; improve strength, power, and endurance of upper extremity musculature; gradually increase functional demands. **1.** Week 3 • Discontinue posterior splint • Progress elbow ROM, emphasizing full extension • Initiate flexibility exercises for wrist extension/flexion, forearm supination/pronation, and elbow extension/flexion • Initiate strengthening exercises for wrist extension/flexion, forearm supination/pronation, elbow extensors/flexors, and a shoulder program • Initiate nerve glide (flossing) techniques combining movements at the shoulder, elbow, wrist and fingers simultaneously **2.** Week 6 • Continue all exercises previously listed • Initiate light sports activities
Phase III: advanced strengthening phase (weeks 8-12)	*Goals:* increase strength, power, and endurance; gradually initiate sports activities. **1.** Week 8 • Initiate eccentric exercise program • Initiate plyometric exercise drills • Continue shoulder and elbow strengthening and flexibility exercises • Initiate interval throwing program
Phase IV: return to activity phase (weeks 12-16)	*Goal:* gradually return to sporting/functional activities. **1.** Week 12 • Return to competitive throwing • Initiate thrower's 10 exercise program (see Figure 9-35)

ROM, Range of motion; *PROM,* passive range of motion.

Throwing athletes can develop posteromedial osteophytes of the olecranon. This condition is different from the posterior osteophytes mentioned previously. One fourth of throwing athletes require instability surgery after excision of posteromedial osteophytes of the olecranon.[202] It is unclear whether a subtle preexisting instability caused these osteophytes and their removal unmasked the true nature of the injury or whether removal of the osteophytes was the primary pathology leading to instability. Regardless, this surgery is associated with instability, a factor that needs to be addressed in the rehabilitation process. Care must be taken to avoid valgus stress on the elbow. Medial and lateral rotation exercises of the shoulder should be avoided until 6 weeks after the operation. Thrower's isotonic exercises may begin at week 6, and an interval throwing program may begin by week 10.

Ulnar Collateral Ligament Reconstruction

Surgical reconstruction of the UCL attempts to restore the stabilizing functions of the anterior bundle of the UCL.[276] The palmaris longus or gracilis graft source is taken and passed in a figure-of-eight pattern through drill holes in the sublime tubercle of the ulna and the medial epicondyle.[276] An ulnar nerve transposition may be performed at the same time.[275]

The rehabilitation program the authors currently use after UCL reconstruction is outlined in Table 9-3. The patient is placed in a posterior splint with the elbow immobilized at 90° flexion for the first 7 days after surgery. This allows adequate healing of the UCL graft and soft tissue slings involved in the nerve transposition. The patient is allowed to perform wrist ROM and gripping and submaximal isometrics for the wrist and elbow. The

TABLE **9-3**

Postoperative Rehabilitation after Ulnar Collateral Ligament Reconstruction Using an Autogenous Palmaris Longus Graft

Phase I: immediate postoperative phase (weeks 0-3)	*Goals:* protect healing tissue; reduce pain and inflammation; retard muscle atrophy; protect graft site to allow healing.

1. Postoperative week 1
  - Brace: posterior splint at 90° elbow flexion
  - ROM: wrist AROM extension/flexion immediately postoperative
  - Elbow ROM: day 1
  - Elbow postoperative compression dressing: 5-7 days
  - Wrist (graft site) compression dressing: 7-10 days as needed
  - Exercises:
    - Gripping exercises
    - Wrist ROM
    - Shoulder isometrics (no lateral [external] rotation of the shoulder)
    - Biceps isometrics
  - Cryotherapy: to elbow joint and to graft site at the wrist

2. Postoperative week 2
  - Brace: elbow ROM 25° to 100° (gradually increase ROM by 5° extension/10° flexion per week)
  - Exercises:
    - Continue all exercises previously listed
    - Perform elbow ROM in brace (30° to 105°)
    - Initiate elbow extension isometrics
    - Continue wrist ROM exercises
    - Initiate light scar mobilization over distal incision (graft)
  - Cryotherapy: continue ice to elbow and graft site

3. Postoperative week 3
  - Brace: elbow ROM 15° to 115°
  - Exercises:
    - Continue all exercises previously listed
    - Perform elbow ROM in brace
    - Initiate active ROM for wrist and elbow (no resistance)
    - Initiate light wrist flexion and stretching
    - Initiate active ROM for the shoulder:
      - "Full can" exercises
      - Lateral raises
      - Lateral rotation/medial rotation exercises with tubing
      - Elbow flexion/extension
  - Initiate light scapular strengthening exercises.
  - May incorporate bicycle workouts for lower extremity strength and endurance

Phase II: intermediate phase (weeks 4-7)	*Goals:* gradually advance to full ROM; promote healing of repaired tissue; regain and improve muscle strength; restore full function of graft site.

1. Week 4
  - Brace: elbow ROM 0° to 125°
  - Exercises:
    - Begin light resistance exercises for the arm (0.5 kg [1 pound]):
      - Wrist curls, wrist extensions, forearm pronation and supination
      - Elbow extension/flexion
  - Progress shoulder program; emphasize rotator cuff and scapular strengthening.
  - Initiate shoulder strengthening with light dumbbells.

2. Week 5
  - ROM: elbow ROM 0° to 135°
  - Discontinue brace.
  - Continue all exercises:
    - Progress all shoulder and upper extremity exercises (progress weight 0.5 kg [1 pound])

3. Week 6
  - AROM: 0° to 145° without brace (i.e., full ROM)
  - Exercises:
    - Initiate thrower's 10 program
    - Progress elbow strengthening exercises
    - Initiate shoulder lateral rotation strengthening
    - Progress shoulder program

(Continued)

TABLE **9-3**

Postoperative Rehabilitation after Ulnar Collateral Ligament Reconstruction Using an Autogenous Palmaris Longus Graft—Cont'd

	4. Week 7
	• Exercises:
	  o Progress thrower's 10 program (progress weights)
	  o Initiate proprioceptive neuromuscular facilitation (PNF) diagonal patterns (light)

Phase III: advanced strengthening phase (weeks 8-14)	*Goals:* increase strength, power, and endurance; maintain full elbow ROM; gradually initiate sports/functional activities (specificity).
	1. Week 8
	• Exercises:
	  o Initiate eccentric elbow flexion/extension
	  o Continue shoulder program (thrower's 10 program)
	  o Initiate manual resistance PNF diagonal patterns
	  o Initiate plyometric exercise program (two-handed plyometrics close to the body only):
	    – Chest pass
	    – Side throw close to the body
	  o Continue calf and hamstring stretching
	2. Week 10
	• Exercises:
	  o Continue all exercises listed previously
	  o Advance plyometrics to two-handed drills away from the body:
	    – Side-to-side throws
	    – Soccer throws
	    – Side throws
	3. Weeks 12-14
	• Continue all exercises
	• Initiate strengthening exercises on isotonic machines (if desired):
	  o Bench press (seated)
	  o Latissimus dorsi pull-down
	• Initiate golf, swimming
	• Initiate interval hitting program

Phase IV: return to activity phase (weeks 14-32)	*Goals:* continue to increase strength, power, and endurance of upper extremity musculature. Gradually return to sports/functional activities.
	1. Week 14
	• Exercises:
	  o Continue strengthening program
	  o Emphasize elbow and wrist strengthening and flexibility exercises
	  o Maintain full elbow ROM
	  o Initiate one-handed plyometric throwing (stationary throws)
	  o Initiate one-handed wall dribble
	  o Initiate one-handed baseball throws into wall
	2. Week 16
	• Exercises:
	  o Initiate interval throwing program (phase I) (long toss program)
	  o Continue thrower's 10 program and plyometrics
	  o Continue stretching before and after throwing
	3. Week 22-24
	• Exercises:
	  o Progress to phase II throwing (once phase I has been successfully completed)
	4. Week 30-32
	• Exercises:
	  o Gradually progress to competitive throwing/sports
	  o Functional activities

ROM, Range of motion; *AROM,* active range of motion.

patient is progressed from the posterior splint to an elbow ROM brace, which is adjusted to allow elbow ROM of 30° to 100° flexion. Motion is increased by 5° of elbow extension and 10° of elbow flexion thereafter to restore full ROM (0° to 145°) by the end of weeks 5 to 6. The brace is discontinued by weeks 5 to 6.

Isometric exercises are progressed to include light resistance isotonic exercises at week 4 and the full thrower's 10 program by week 6. Progressive resistance exercises are incorporated at weeks 8 to 9. Emphasis again is placed on developing dynamic stabilization of the medial elbow. Because of the anatomical orientation of the flexor carpi ulnaris and flexor digitorum superficialis muscles overlying the UCL, isotonic and stabilization activities for these muscles may assist the UCL in stabilizing valgus stress at the medial elbow.[277] For this reason, concentric strengthening of these muscles is performed.

Aggressive exercises involving eccentric and plyometric contractions are included in the advanced phase, usually weeks 9 to 14. Two-handed plyometric drills are performed by week 10, one-handed drills by weeks 12 to 14. An interval throwing program is allowed by week 16. In most cases, throwing from a mound is progressed within 4 to 6 weeks after initiation of an interval throwing program, and return to competitive throwing is permitted at approximately 9 months after surgery. The actual rate of progression of the throwing program should be individualized to each athlete and adjusted based on symptoms, mechanics, and desired goals.

Lateral Collateral Ligament Complex Reconstruction

Lateral-side instability of the elbow usually is the result of a sudden traumatic injury rather than a chronic repetitive injury. It results in varus instability and a PLRI that can be promoted with forearm supination. For this reason, special attention to elbow rotation is emphasized during the rehabilitation.

Initially, the postoperative elbow is placed in a splint with 90° of flexion and mild pronation. The splint is removed at the end of the first week (we immobilize for 2-4 weeks, depending on the type of activity to which the patient will return), and a brace is used that incorporates an extension block of 30° and a flexion block of 100°. Extension is increased by 5° per week, and flexion is increased by 10° per week. Supination encourages the radial head to sublux laterally, potentially stretching the graft. Therefore supination is restricted for 3 weeks. Active supination is allowed when the elbow passes 90° of flexion. Once supination is obtained at greater than 90° of elbow flexion, supination may be attempted in extension. Full motion about the elbow should be obtained by 6 weeks. Shoulder forward elevation and abduction may be treated aggressively for motion restriction, but medial and lateral rotation are limited to active motion only. Passive and active-assisted motion of the shoulder for rotation re-

quires torque through the elbow and should be avoided until week 9.

Isometric strengthening exercises of the elbow and wrist are initiated once the splint has been removed. Lateral and medial rotation strength exercises for the shoulder are avoided until 9 weeks after surgery, because these motions put the graft at risk. Light isotonic exercises may begin about the elbow and wrist at week 6. At week 9, an aggressive strengthening regimen may commence, including eccentric contraction exercises and plyometrics.

Nerve glides (e.g., flossing) and scar massage are important to prevent pain from adherent scar after surgery. Scar massage should begin at 2 weeks, and nerve glides should commence once the appropriate motion has returned.

Total Elbow Arthroplasty

The complexity of TEA depends on the disease requiring the prosthesis, the type of prosthesis to be implanted, and the presence of soft tissue constraints. Despite these variables, the rehabilitation regimens for most total elbow arthroplasties remain relatively similar. The most popular prosthesis is a linked, semiconstrained prosthesis with joint stability that is quite solid. On the first postoperative day, the elbow is elevated to minimize soft tissue swelling. Motion in all directions may begin on postoperative day 1. Elbow flexion and extension and forearm pronation and supination may begin and can be progressed as tolerated. Lifting is limited to less than 0.5 kg (1 pound) for the first 3 months. To preserve the viability of the prosthesis, the patient is limited to lifting less than 4.5 kg (10 pounds) at one time and no more than 0.9 kg (2 pounds) repetitively in the affected arm.

Soft tissue mobilization, cryotherapy, and electrical stimulation help minimize inflammation. Scar massage and nerve glides help reduce the likelihood of problems associated with scar formation.

Arthroscopic Arthrolysis

Loss of motion is a difficult problem associated with injuries of the elbow. It can be a result of soft tissue contracture or HO associated with the injury. Often, the motion cannot be regained through conservative measures alone, and surgical intervention is necessary. The surgeon should inform the therapist of what motion has been obtained in the operating room so that realistic goals can be set.

Motion and pain control are at the forefront of rehabilitation for this procedure. HO represents a difficult rehabilitation problem. It has been reported that passive stretching outside the painless arc of motion may cause the generation of ectopic bone in patients with burns or brain injuries.[278] Whether this literature, in a rather unique population, is relevant to other patients with HO is unclear; however, caution is advised, and aggressive passive motion exercises should not be performed. The goal is to obtain full motion by 4 weeks. The most beneficial means of achieving this goal has been the L3D technique described earlier. As with all the motion exercises, the stretching should not cause pain.

With arthrolysis for soft tissue contractures, the clinician may be more aggressive with motion exercises. Although the risk of generating HO may be in question, other problems may arise with aggressive rehabilitation. Aggressive motion can create an inflammatory cascade and generate pain that could inhibit progress, which would be self-defeating. The goal of establishing full motion at 4 weeks does not change with soft tissue contractures.

As with the other protocols, pain should be treated with cryotherapy, high-voltage electrical stimulation, and gentle soft tissue mobilization. Heat and therapeutic ultrasound may be used once the initial swelling from surgery has dissipated. These are used before motion exercises to "warm up" the joint.

Strengthening exercises should begin after motion has been established. There are no contraindications to an aggressive approach to strengthening once motion has been restored. Isometric exercises are begun and progressed to plyometrics in the usual fashion. Regardless of the origin of the contracture, stretching should be continued for 4 to 6 months after activities are resumed to prevent return of the contracture.

Fractures

The complexity of the fracture and the degree of stability after internal fixation can vary considerably in the elbow. Communication between the surgeon and all members of the rehabilitation team is essential to determine the aggressiveness of the rehabilitation process. Several different fractures about the elbow merit attention. The goal of rehabilitation after a fracture is to facilitate osseous healing, restore full motion and strength, and gradually return the individual to functional activities. With an elbow fracture (whether treated surgically or nonoperatively), the goal is to minimize immobilization to prevent loss of motion. Loss of motion is more common in adults than in children after an elbow fracture.

Radial Head and Neck Fractures

When fractures of the radial head and neck are nondisplaced, the injury may be treated conservatively and motion should be initiated immediately. Unlimited passive and active motion is the priority. This is achieved through the use of stretching techniques, as well as techniques for reducing swelling and pain, which have been mentioned earlier. The goal is to reestablish motion by 4 weeks. Strengthening about the elbow and wrist may begin once full motion has been established.

Valgus stress should be avoided until the fracture has healed.

With displaced or angulated fractures, internal fixation may be necessary. In some cases, the fracture is beyond repair and requires replacement with a metal implant. With stable fixation or an implant, the elbow is placed in a posterior splint at 45° to 90° of elbow flexion for 10 days. Once the splint has been removed, motion exercises are initiated without limitation. Full elbow flexion and extension and forearm supination and pronation should be obtained by 4 to 6 weeks. Often patients present with mechanical blocks to motion. This may result in soft tissue contractures. With these patients, the goals for motion may be more limited. Valgus stress is avoided in patients with internal fixation until the fracture has healed. This is not necessary when a radial head prosthesis is used. Once full motion has been achieved, strengthening of the elbow and wrist may commence. If swelling and pain persist, cryotherapy and electrical stimulation may be used to limit these symptoms.

Olecranon Fractures

For most olecranon fractures, the treatment of choice is open reduction and internal fixation. Several fixation techniques yield a stable fracture, and rehabilitation should not have to be altered because of the type of fixation. Traditionally, a posterior splint is used for 7 to 10 days to allow the soft tissues to heal. The length of immobilization depends on the patient's variables (e.g., age, osseous status, health, desired goals, healing response). Once the splint has been removed, unlimited passive motion may begin. Active forearm pronation and supination and elbow flexion are allowed, but active extension is avoided for 6 weeks. Full motion in all directions should be achieved by 6 weeks. Gentle active extension may be initiated, and strengthening of the elbow and wrist in all directions may begin at 8 weeks.

As with all fracture fixations at the elbow, cryotherapy and electrical stimulation should be used to reduce pain and swelling. Scar massage should be initiated at 2 weeks, and nerve glides should be used when possible.

Distal Humeral Fractures

Distal humeral fractures usually require open reduction and internal fixation. If the surgeon has difficulty with stability, a hinged external fixator that allows elbow flexion and extension may be used, although this is not common. After fixation, a splint is used for 10 to 14 days. Once the splint has been removed, gentle passive motion at the elbow and wrist may begin. Pain and swelling are limiting factors in restoring motion to the elbow; therefore cryotherapy and electrical stimulation are crucial to this process. The clinician must take care with cryotherapy to avoid nerve injury, because ulnar nerve transposition is a routine part of distal humeral fixation.

Active motion at the elbow and wrist may begin at 6 weeks. Once full motion has been established and bony healing is apparent, strengthening may begin. Strengthening should be limited to pain-free exercises. It begins with isotonic exercises and gradually progresses to plyometrics.

Coronoid Fractures and Elbow Dislocation

After reduction of a dislocated elbow, the patient is temporarily immobilized to allow healing of the injured capsule. The length of immobilization varies, depending on the required use of the elbow for ADL or work activities, the type of sport or activity the patient takes part in, whether it is the dominant or nondominant elbow, the patient's age, and whether concomitant lesions are present. Coronoid fractures (see Figure 9-9) often put the patient at risk for future elbow instability. For this reason, the rehabilitation protocols for elbow dislocation and coronoid fractures are similar. The priority is to restore motion quickly while guarding against instability. The patient is placed in a posterior splint for 10 to 14 days in a position that allows no visible subluxation on radiographs. In the initial evaluation, the stable ROM is determined. The elbow will sublux with further extension; therefore parameters are set so that the initial restrictions do not permit extension beyond this point. When the splint is removed, a dynamic elbow brace that prevents valgus and varus forces is used. This splint should also have a variable locking mechanism that blocks various degrees of extension. The clinician may work on elbow flexion and forearm pronation without limitation. Passive extension may be increased by 10° every week until full extension is obtained. The patient should be closely watched for any evidence of subluxation. Often, with elbow dislocations, either the UCL or the LUCL may rupture. If the LUCL ruptures, supination should be limited for at least 3 weeks after removal of the splint. The goal is to restore motion by 8 weeks.

Motion of the wrist should be instituted immediately. Upon removal of the splint, control of pain and swelling must be established immediately to aid in the restoration of motion. As mentioned earlier, cryotherapy and electrical stimulation are beneficial. Gentle soft tissue mobilization also may help.

Strengthening may begin at 8 weeks. If the expected motion has not been achieved, strengthening should be delayed until the desired motion is obtained. Strengthening is performed in the usual fashion.

If the patient's clinical picture requires operative intervention, rehabilitation should be dictated by the procedure performed. LCL reconstruction, UCL reconstruction, and radial head fixation are common surgical procedures. If a coronoid fracture is present and fixed, it should not change the protocol; the other fixations present should guide the treatment.

SUMMARY

The elbow is a complex joint, and our understanding of it continues to evolve. The elbow is important for positioning the hand in space and for the specialized functions demanded of athletes and the everyday requirements of the general population. Many injuries and pathological conditions can affect the elbow and its associated bony and soft tissue. The rehabilitation of these injuries, as well as conservative and surgical treatments, has been reviewed, although the depth of these discussions has had to conform to the limitations on the length of the chapter. Clearly, the anatomy and biomechanics of the elbow guide our understanding of the pathophysiology of elbow injury and pain and help direct the treatment of elbow conditions. However, the elbow's response to trauma, even iatrogenic trauma, can be tricky, because stiffness or loss of motion is a common problem after such challenges.

REFERENCES

1. Safran MR, Bradley J: Elbow injuries. In Fu FH, Stone DA, editors: *Sports injuries: mechanisms, prevention and treatment*, ed 2, Philadelphia, 2001, Lippincott Williams & Wilkins.
2. Keats TE, Diamond AE: Normal axial relationships of the major joints, *Radiology* 87:904–907, 1966.
3. Hotchkiss RN, Weiland AJ: Valgus stability of the elbow, *J Orthop Res* 5:372–377, 1987.
4. Morrey BF, Tanaka S, An KN: Valgus stability of the elbow: a definition of primary and secondary constraints, *Clin Orthop Relat Res* 265:187–195, 1991.
5. Surgeons of the AAOS: *Joint motion: method of measuring and recording*, Chicago, 1981, American Academy of Orthopedic Surgeons.
6. Morrey BF, Askew LJ, Chao EY: A biomechanical study of normal functional elbow motion, *J Bone Joint Surg Am* 63:872–877, 1981.
7. Callaway GH, Field LD, Deng XH, et al: Biomechanical evaluation of the medial collateral ligament of the elbow, *J Bone Joint Surg Am* 79:1223–1231, 1997.
8. Regan WD, Korinek SL, Morrey BF, An KN: Biomechanical study of ligaments around the elbow joint, *Clin Orthop Relat Res* 271:170–179, 1991.
9. Morrey BF, An KN: Functional anatomy of the ligaments of the elbow, *Clin Orthop Relat Res* 201:84–90, 1985.
10. O'Driscoll SW, Morrey BF, Korinek SL, An KN: The pathoanatomy of posterolateral rotatory instability of the elbow, *Trans Orthop Res Soc* 15:6, 1990.
11. O'Driscoll SW, Horii E, Morrey BF, Carmichael SW: Anatomy of the ulnar part of the lateral collateral ligament of the elbow, *Clin Anat* 5:296–303, 1992.
12. Olsen BS, Søjbjerg JO, Dalstra M, Sneppen O: Kinematics of the lateral ligamentous constraints of the elbow joint, *J Shoulder Elbow Surg* 5:333–341, 1996.
13. Safran MR, Baillargeon D: Soft-tissue stabilizers of the elbow, *J Shoulder Elbow Surg* 14(1 suppl S):179S–185S, 2005.
14. Morrey BF, An KN: Articular and ligamentous contributions to the stability of the elbow joint, *Am J Sports Med* 11:315–319, 1983.
15. An KN, Hui FC, Morrey BF, et al: Muscles across the elbow joint: a biomechanical analysis, *J Biomech* 14:659–669, 1981.

16. Park MC, Ahmad CS: Dynamic contributions of the flexor-pronator mass to elbow valgus stability, *J Bone Joint Surg Am* 86:2268–2274, 2004.

17. Seiber K, Gupta R, McGarry MH, et al: The role of elbow musculature and forearm rotation in elbow stability. In Paper presented at the Orthopaedic Research Society Meeting, Chicago, IL, March 20–22, 2006.

18. Safran MR, McGarry MH, Shin S, et al: Effects of elbow flexion and forearm rotation on valgus laxity of the elbow, *J Bone Joint Surg Am* 87:2065–2074, 2005.

19. Chen FS, Rokito AS, Jobe FW: Medial elbow problems in the overhead-throwing athlete, *J Am Acad Orthop Surg* 9:99–113, 2001.

20. Fleisig GS, Andrews JR, Dillman CJ, Escamilla RF: Kinetics of baseball pitching with implications about injury mechanisms, *Am J Sports Med* 23:233–239, 1995.

21. Safran MR: Ulnar collateral ligament injury in the overhead athlete: diagnosis and treatment, *Clin Sports Med* 23:643–663, 2004.

22. Safran MR, Ahmad C, El Attrache N: Ulnar collateral ligament injuries of the elbow: current concepts, *Arthroscopy* 21:1381–1395, 2005.

23. Loftice J, Fleisig GS, Zheng N, Andrews JR: Biomechanics of the elbow in sports, *Clin Sports Med* 23:519–530, 2004.

24. Safran MR: Elbow injuries in athletes, *Clin Orthop Relat Res* 310:257–277, 1995.

25. Josefsson PO, Johnell O, Gentz CF: Long-term sequelae of simple dislocation of the elbow, *J Bone Joint Surg Am* 66:927–930, 1984.

26. O'Driscoll SW, Morrey BF, Korinek S, An KN: Elbow subluxation and dislocation: a spectrum of instability, *Clin Orthop Relat Res* 280:186–197, 1992.

27. O'Driscoll SW, Bell DF, Morrey BF: Posterolateral rotatory instability of the elbow, *J Bone Joint Surg Am* 73:440–446, 1991.

28. Josefsson PO, Gentz CF, Johnell O, Wendeberg B: Surgical versus non-surgical treatment of ligamentous injuries following dislocation of the elbow joint: a prospective randomized study, *J Bone Joint Surg Am* 69:605–608, 1987.

29. Beaty JH: Fractures and dislocations about the elbow in children, *Instr Course Lect* 16:373–384, 1992.

30. Nevaisier JS, Wickstrom JK: Dislocations of the elbow: a retrospective study of 115 patients, *South Med J* 70:172–173, 1977.

31. Protzman RR: Dislocation of the elbow joint, *J Bone Joint Surg Am* 60:539–541, 1978.

32. Roberts PH: Dislocation of the elbow, *Br J Surg* 56:806–815, 1969.

33. Linscheid RL, O'Driscoll SW: Elbow dislocations. In Morrey BF, editor: *The elbow and its disorders*, ed 2, Philadelphia, 1993, WB Saunders.

34. Cohen MS, Hastings H: Acute elbow dislocation: evaluation and management, *J Am Acad Orthop Surg* 6:15–23, 1998.

35. Eygendaal D, Verdegaal SH, Obermann WR, et al: Posterolateral dislocation of the elbow joint: relationship to medial instability, *J Bone Joint Surg Am* 82:555–560, 2000.

36. Linscheid RL, Wheeler DK: Elbow dislocations, *JAMA* 194:1171–1176, 1965.

37. Mehlhoff TL, Noble PC, Bennett JB, Tullos HS: Simple dislocation of the elbow in the adult: results after closed treatment, *J Bone Joint Surg Am* 70:244–249, 1988.

38. Mehta JA, Bain GI: Elbow dislocations in adults and children, *Clin Sports Med* 23:609–627, 2004.

39. Osbourne G, Cotterill P: Recurrent dislocation of the elbow, *J Bone Joint Surg Br* 48:340–346, 1966.

40. Olsen BS, Søjbjerg JO, Nielsen KK, et al: Posterolateral elbow joint stability: the basic kinematics, *J Shoulder Elbow Surg* 7:19–29, 1998.

41. Dunning CE, Zarzour ZD, Patterson SD, et al: Ligamentous stabilizers against posterolateral rotatory instability of the elbow, *J Bone Joint Surg Am* 83:1823–1828, 2001.

42. Seki A, Olsen BS, Jensen SL, et al: Functional anatomy of the lateral collateral ligament complex of the elbow: configuration of Y and its role, *J Shoulder Elbow Surg* 11:53–59, 2002.

43. Regan W, Lapner PC: Prospective evaluation of two diagnostic apprehension signs for posterolateral instability of the elbow, *J Shoulder Elbow Surg* 15:344–346, 2006.

44. Potter HG, Weiland AJ, Schatz JA, et al: Posterolateral rotatory instability of the elbow: usefulness of MR imaging in diagnosis, *Radiology* 204:185–189, 1997.

45. Morrey BF, O'Driscoll SW: Lateral collateral ligament injury. In Morrey BF, editor: *The elbow and its disorders*, ed 2, Philadelphia, 1993, WB Saunders.

46. O'Driscoll SW, Spinner RJ, McKee MD, et al: Tardy posterolateral rotatory instability of the elbow due to cubitus varus, *J Bone Joint Surg Am* 83:1358–1369, 2001.

47. Imatani J, Hashizume H, Ogura T, et al: Acute posterolateral rotatory subluxation of the elbow joint: a case report, *Am J Sports Med* 25:77–80, 1997.

48. Nestor BJ, O'Driscoll SW, Morrey BF: Ligamentous reconstruction for posterolateral rotatory instability of the elbow, *J Bone Joint Surg Am* 74:1235–1241, 1992.

49. Sanchez-Sotelo J, Morrey BF, O'Driscoll SW: Ligamentous repair and reconstruction for posterolateral rotatory instability of the elbow, *J Bone Joint Surg Br* 87:54–61, 2005.

50. Lee BP, Teo LH: Surgical reconstruction for posterolateral rotatory instability of the elbow, *J Shoulder Elbow Surg* 12:476–479, 2003.

51. Olsen BS, Søjbjerg JO: The treatment of recurrent posterolateral instability of the elbow, *J Bone Joint Surg Br* 85:342–346, 2003.

52. Hotchkiss RN, Green DP: Fractures and dislocations of the elbow. In Rockwood CA, Green DP, Bucholz RW, editors: *Rockwood and Green's fractures in adults*, ed 3, New York, 1991, JB Lippincott.

53. Browner B, Jupiter J, Levine A, Trafton PG, editors: *Skeletal trauma*, Philadelphia, 2003, WB Saunders.

54. Morrey BF, editor: *The elbow and its disorders*, Philadelphia, 1993, Saunders.

55. Selesnick FH, Dolitsky B, Haskell SS: Fracture of the coronoid process requiring open reduction with internal fixation, *J Bone Joint Surg Am* 66:1304–1305, 1984.

56. Regan W, Morrey BF: Fractures of the coronoid process of the ulna, *J Bone Joint Surg Am* 71:1348–1354, 1989.

57. Mason JA: Some observations on fractures of the head of the radius with a review of 100 cases, *Br J Surg* 42(172):123–132, 1954.

58. Mason JA, Shutkin NM: Immediate active motion in the treatment of fractures of the head and neck of the radius, *Surg Gynecol Obstet* 76:731, 1943.

59. Hamilton C: Traumatic elbow injuries in the athlete. In Arendt E, editor: *Orthopaedic knowledge update: sports medicine*, ed 2, Rosemont, IL, 1999, American Academy of Orthopaedic Surgeons.

60. Esser RD, Davis S, Taavao T: Fractures of the radial head treated by internal fixation: late results in 26 cases, *J Orthop Trauma* 9:318–323, 1995.

61. Hotchkiss RN: Displaced fractures of the radial head: internal fixation or excision? *J Am Acad Orthop Surg* 5:1–10, 1997.

62. Essex-Lopresti P: Fractures of the radial head with distal radio-ulnar dislocation: report of two cases, *J Bone Joint Surg Br* 33:244–247, 1951.

63. Bain GI, Ashwood N, Baird R, Unni R: Management of Mason type III radial head fractures with a titanium prosthesis, ligament repair and early mobilization: surgical technique, *J Bone Joint Surg Am* 87(suppl 1, part 1):136–147, 2005.

64. Ikeda M, Sugiyama K, Kang C, et al: Comminuted fractures of the radial head: comparison of resection and internal fixation, *J Bone Joint Surg Am* 87:76–84, 2005.

65. Sowa DT, Hotchkiss RN, Weiland AJ: Symptomatic proximal translation of the radius following radial head resection, *Clin Orthop Relat Res* 317:106–113, 1995.

66. An KN, Morrey BR, Chao EY: The effect of partial removal of proximal ulna on elbow constraint, *Clin Orthop Relat Res* 209:270–279, 1986.

67. Boyer MI, Galatz LM, Borrelli J, et al: Intra-articular fractures of the upper extremity: new concepts in surgical treatment, *Instr Course Lect* 52:591–605, 2003.

68. Kamineni S, Morrey BF: Distal humeral fractures treated with noncustom total elbow replacement, *J Bone Joint Surg Am* 86:940–947, 2004.

69. Hanlan CR, Estes WL: Fractures in childhood: a statistical analysis, *Am J Surg* 87:312–323, 1954.

70. O'Driscoll SW: Elbow arthritis: treatment options, *J Am Acad Orthop Surg* 1:106–116, 1993.

71. O'Driscoll SW: Arthroscopic treatment for osteoarthritis of the elbow, *Orthop Clin North Am* 26:691–706, 1995.

72. Steinmann SP, King GJ, Savoie FH: American academy of orthopaedic surgeons: arthroscopic treatment of the arthritic elbow, *J Bone Joint Surg Am* 87:2114–2121, 2005.

73. Little CP, Graham AJ, Carr AJ: Total elbow arthroplasty: a systematic review of the literature in the English language until the end of 2003, *J Bone Joint Surg Br* 87:437–444, 2005.

74. Little CP, Graham AJ, Karatzas G, et al: Outcomes of total elbow arthroplasty for rheumatoid arthritis: comparative study of three implants, *J Bone Joint Surg Am* 87:2439–2448, 2005.

75. Chafik D, Lee TQ, Gupta R: Total elbow arthroplasty: current indications, factors affecting outcomes, and follow-up results, *Am J Orthop* 33:496–503, 2004.

76. Armstrong AD, Yamaguchi K: Total elbow arthroplasty and distal humerus elbow fractures, *Hand Clin* 20:475–483, 2004.

77. McCarty LP, Ring D, Jupiter JB: Management of distal humerus fractures, *Am J Orthop* 34:430–438, 2005.

78. Muller LP, Kamineni S, Rommens PM, Morrey BF: Primary total elbow replacement for fractures of the distal humerus, *Oper Orthop Traumatol* 17:119–142, 2005.

79. Cheng SL, Morrey BF: Treatment of the mobile, painful arthritic elbow by distraction interposition arthroplasty, *J Bone Joint Surg Br* 82:233–238, 2000.

80. Fernandez-Palazzi F, Rodriguez J, Oliver G: Elbow interposition arthroplasty in children and adolescents: long-term follow-up, *Int Orthop*, 2007 (Epub ahead of print).

81. Bollen SR: Soft tissue injury in extreme rock climbers, *Br J Sports Med* 22:145–147, 1988.

82. Haas JC, Meyers MC: Rock climbing injuries, *Sports Med* 20:199–205, 1995.

83. Gilcreest EL: The common syndrome of rupture dislocation and elongation of the long head of the biceps brachii: an analysis of 100 cases, *Surg Gynecol Obstet* 58:322, 1934.

84. Safran MR, Graham SM: Distal biceps tendon ruptures: incidence, demographics, and the effect of smoking, *Clin Orthop Relat Res* 404:275–283, 2002.

85. Seiler JG III, Parker LM, Chamberland PD, Sherbourne GM, et al: The distal biceps tendon: two potential mechanisms involved in its rupture—arterial supply and mechanical impingement, *J Shoulder Elbow Surg* 4:149–156, 1995.

86. Bourne MH, Morrey BF: Partial rupture of the distal biceps tendon, *Clin Orthop Relat Res* 271:143–148, 1991.

87. Durr HR, Stabler A, Pfahler M, et al: Partial rupture of the distal biceps tendon, *Clin Orthop Relat Res* 374:195–200, 2000.

88. Rokito AS, McLaughlin JA, Gallagher MA, Zuckerman JD: Partial rupture of the distal biceps tendon, *J Shoulder Elbow Surg* 5:73–75, 1996.

89. Safran MR, Schamblin M: Injuries of the musculotendinous junction of the distal biceps, *J Shoulder Elbow Surg* 16:208–212, 2007.

90. Falchook FS, Zlatkin MB, Erbacher GE, et al: Rupture of the distal biceps tendon: evaluation with MR imaging, *Radiology* 190:659–663, 1994.

91. Baker BE, Bierwagen D: Rupture of the distal tendon of the biceps brachii: operative versus non-operative treatment, *J Bone Joint Surg Am* 67:414–417, 1985.

92. Morrey BF, Askew LJ, An KN, Dobyns JH: Rupture of the distal tendon of the biceps brachii: a biomechanical study, *J Bone Joint Surg Am* 67:418–421, 1985.

93. Rantanen J, Orava S: Rupture of the distal biceps tendon: a report of 19 patients treated with anatomic reinsertion and a meta-analysis of 147 cases found in the literature, *Am J Sports Med* 27:128–132, 1999.

94. Schmidt C, Brown BT, Sawardeker PJ, et al: Factors affecting supination strength after a distal biceps rupture, *J Shoulder Elbow Surg* 23:68–75, 2014.

95. Kelly EW, Morrey BF, O'Driscoll SW: Complications of repair of the distal biceps tendon with the modified two-incision technique, *J Bone Joint Surg Am* 82:1575–1581, 2000.

96. Morrey BF: Distal biceps tendon rupture. In Morrey BF, editor: *Masters techniques in orthopaedic surgery: the elbow*, ed 2, Philadelphia, 2002, Lippincott Williams & Wilkins.

97. Safran MR: Management of distal biceps tendon ruptures: single versus two incision technique, *Op Tech Orthop* 5:248–253, 1995.

98. D'Alessandro DF, Shields CL, Tibone JE, Chandler RW: Repair of distal biceps tendon ruptures in athletes, *Am J Sports Med* 21:114–119, 1993.

99. Davison BL, Engber WD, Tigert LJ: Long term evaluation of repaired distal biceps brachii tendon ruptures, *Clin Orthop Relat Res* 333:186–191, 1996.

100. Bain GI, Prem H, Heptinstall RJ, et al: Repair of distal biceps tendon rupture: a new technique using the EndoButton, *J Shoulder Elbow Surg* 9:120–126, 2000.

101. El-Hawary R, Macdermid JC, Faber KJ, et al: Distal biceps tendon repair: comparison of surgical techniques, *J Hand Surg Am* 28:496–502, 2003.

102. Greenberg JA, Fernandez JJ, Wang T, Turner C: EndoButton-assisted repair of distal biceps tendon ruptures, *J Shoulder Elbow Surg* 12:484–490, 2003.

103. Lintner S, Fischer T: Repair of the distal biceps tendon using suture anchors and an anterior approach, *Clin Orthop Relat Res* 322:116–119, 1996.

104. Ozyurekoglu T, Tsai TM: Ruptures of the distal biceps brachii tendon: results of three surgical techniques, *Hand Surg* 8:65–73, 2003.

105. Pereira DS, Kvitne RS, Liang M, et al: Surgical repair of distal biceps tendon ruptures: a biomechanical comparison of two techniques, *Am J Sports Med* 30:432–436, 2002.

106. Sanchez-Sotelo J, Morrey BF, Adams RA, O'Driscoll SW: Reconstruction of chronic ruptures of the distal biceps tendon with use of an Achilles tendon allograft, *J Bone Joint Surg Am* 84:999–1005, 2002.

107. Dobbie RP: Avulsion of the lower biceps brachii tendon: analysis of 51 previously reported cases, *Am J Surg* 51:661, 1941.

108. Hinchey JW, Aronowitz JG, Sanchez-Sotelo J, Morrey BF: Re-rupture rate of primarily repaired distal biceps tendon, *J Shoulder Elbow Surg* 23:850–854, 2014.

109. Rehak D: Overuse injuries in the upper extremity: pronator syndrome, *Clin Sports Med* 20:1–11, 2001.

110. McCue FC, Baumgarten TE: Median nerve entrapment at the elbow in athletes, *Op Tech Sports Med* 4:21–27, 1996.

111. Szabo R: Entrapment and compression neuropathies. In Green DP, Hotchkiss RN, Pederson WC, editors: *Operative hand surgery*, New York, 1998, Churchill Livingstone.

112. Hartz CR, Linscheid RL, Gramse RR, Daube JR: The pronator teres syndrome: compressive neuropathy of the median nerve, *J Bone Joint Surg Am* 63:885–890, 1981.

113. Olehnik WK, Mankske PR, Szerzinski J: Median nerve compression in the proximal forearm, *J Hand Surg Am* 19:121–126, 1994.

114. Johnson RK, Spinner M, Shrewsbury MM: Median nerve entrapment syndrome in the proximal forearm, *J Hand Surg Am* 4:48–51, 1979.

115. Posner M: Compressive neuropathies of the median and radial nerves at the elbow, *Clin Sports Med* 9:343–363, 1990.

116. Spinner M, Linschied RL: Nerve entrapment syndromes. In Morrey BF, editor: *The elbow and its disorders*, Philadelphia, 1993, WB Saunders.

117. Stern PJ: Pronator syndrome. In Gelberman RH, editor: *Operative nerve repair and reconstruction*, Philadelphia, 1991, Lippincott Williams & Wilkins.

118. Idler RS, Strickland JW, Creighton JJ: Pronator syndrome, *Indiana Med* 84:124–127, 1991.

119. Aoki M, Okamura K, Yamashita T: Snapping annular ligament of the elbow joint in the throwing arms of young brothers, *Arthroscopy* 19:E89–E92, 2003.

120. Ilahi OA, Strausser DW, Gabel GT: Post-traumatic heterotopic ossification about the elbow, *Orthopedics* 21:265–268, 1998.

121. Chua KS, Kong KH: Acquired heterotopic ossification in the settings of cerebral anoxia and alternative therapy: two cases, *Brain Inj* 17:535–544, 2003.

122. de Palma L, Rapali S, Paladini P, Ventura A: Elbow heterotopic ossification in head-trauma patients: diagnosis and treatment, *Orthopedics* 25:665–668, 2002.

123. Melamed E, Robinson D, Halperin N, et al: Brain injury–related heterotopic bone formation: treatment strategy and results, *Am J Phys Med Rehabil* 81:670–674, 2002.

124. Viola RW, Hastings H: Treatment of ectopic ossification about the elbow, *Clin Orthop Relat Res* 370:65–86, 2000.

125. Bruno RJ, Lee ML, Strauch RJ, Rosenwasser MP: Posttraumatic elbow stiffness: evaluation and management, *J Am Acad Orthop Surg* 10:106–116, 2002.

126. O'Driscoll SW: Personal communication, 2006.

127. Garland DE: Early excision of heterotopic ossification about the elbow followed by radiation therapy, *J Bone Joint Surg Am* 80:453–454, 1998.

128. Moritomo H, Tada K, Yoshida T: Early, wide excision of heterotopic ossification in the medial elbow, *J Shoulder Elbow Surg* 10:164–168, 2001.

129. Park MJ, Kim HG, Lee JY: Surgical treatment of post-traumatic stiffness of the elbow, *J Bone Joint Surg Br* 86:1158–1162, 2004.

130. Yang SC, Chen AC, Chao EK, et al: Early surgical management for heterotopic ossification about the elbow presenting as limited range of motion associated with ulnar neuropathy, *Chang Gung Med J* 25:245–252, 2002.

131. Kocher MS, Waters PM, Micheli LJ: Upper extremity injuries in the paediatric athlete, *Sports Med* 30:117–135, 2000.

132. Rudzki JR, Paletta GA: Juvenile and adolescent elbow injuries in sports, *Clin Sports Med* 23:581–608, 2004.

133. Josefsson PO, Danielsson LG: Epicondylar elbow fracture in children: 35-year follow-up of 56 unreduced cases, *Acta Orthop Scand* 57:313–315, 1986.

134. Fowles JV, Slimane N, Kassab MT: Elbow dislocation with avulsion of the medial humeral epicondyle, *J Bone Joint Surg Br* 72:102–104, 1990.

135. Ireland ML, Andrews JR: Shoulder and elbow injuries in the young athlete, *Clin Sports Med* 7:473–494, 1988.

136. Leach RE, Miller JK: Lateral and medial epicondylitis of the elbow, *Clin Sports Med* 6:259–272, 1987.

137. Stahl S, Kaufman T: Efficacy of an injection of steroids for medial epicondylitis: a prospective study of 60 elbows, *J Bone Joint Surg Am* 79:1648–1652, 1997.

138. Gabel GTR, Morrey BF: Operative treatment of medial epicondylitis: influence of concomitant ulnar neuropathy at the elbow, *J Bone Joint Surg Am* 77:1065–1069, 1995.

139. Kurvers H, Verhaar J: The results of operative treatment of medial epicondylitis, *J Bone Joint Surg Am* 77:1374–1379, 1995.

140. Vangsness CT, Jobe FW: Surgical treatment of medial epicondylitis: results in 35 elbows, *J Bone Joint Surg Br* 73:409–411, 1991.

141. Conway JE, Jobe FW, Glousman RE, Pink M: Medial instability of the elbow in throwing athletes: treatment by repair or reconstruction of the ulnar collateral ligament, *J Bone Joint Surg Am* 74:67–83, 1992.

142. Norwood LA, Shook JA, Andrews JR: Acute medial elbow ruptures, *Am J Sports Med* 9:16–19, 1981.

143. Schickendantz MS: Diagnosis and treatment of elbow disorders in the overhead athlete, *Hand Clin* 18:65–75, 2002.

144. Spinner RJ, Goldner RD: Snapping of the medial head of the triceps and recurrent dislocation of the ulnar nerve: anatomical and dynamic factors, *J Bone Joint Surg Am* 80:239–247, 1998.

145. Yiannakopoulos CK: Imaging diagnosis of the snapping triceps syndrome, *Radiology* 225:607–608, 2002.

146. Spinner RJ, An KN, Kim KJ, et al: Medial or lateral dislocation (snapping) of a portion of the distal triceps: a biomechanical, anatomic explanation, *J Shoulder Elbow Surg* 10:561–567, 2001.

147. Spinner RJ, Goldner RD, Fada RA, Sotereanos DG: Snapping of the triceps tendon over the lateral epicondyle, *J Hand Surg Am* 24:381–385, 1999.

148. Kandemir U, Fu FH, McMahon PJ: Elbow injuries, *Curr Opin Rheumatol* 14:160–167, 2002.

149. Veltri D, O'Brien S, Field LD, et al: The milking maneuver: a new test to evaluate the MCL of the elbow in the throwing athlete. In Transactions of the Open Meeting of the American Shoulder and Elbow Surgeons, February 17, 1994. New Orleans.

150. O'Driscoll SW, Lawton RL, Smith AM: The "moving valgus stress test" for medial collateral ligament tears of the elbow, *Am J Sports Med* 33:231–239, 2005.

151. Lee GA, Katz SD, Lazarus MD: Elbow valgus stress radiography in an uninjured population, *Am J Sports Med* 26:425–427, 1998.

152. Conway JE, Jobe FW, Glousman RE, Pink M: Medial instability of the elbow in throwing athletes, *J Bone Joint Surg Am* 74:67–83, 1992.

153. Ellenbecker TS, Mattalino AH, Elam EA, Caplinger RA: Medial elbow joint laxity in professional baseball pitchers. A bilateral comparison using stress radiography, *Am J Sports Med* 26:420–424, 1998.

154. Harada M, Takahara M, Maruyama M, et al: Assessment of medial elbow laxity by gravity stress radiography: comparison of valgus stress radiography with gravity and a Telos stress device, *J Shoulder Elbow Surg* 23:561–566, 2014.

155. Bruce JR, Hess R, Joyner P, Andrews JR: How much valgus instability can be expected with ulnar

collateral ligament (UCL) injuries? A review of 273 baseball players with UCL injuries, *J Shoulder Elbow Surg* 23:1521–1526, 2014.

156. Azar FM, Andrews JR, Wilk KE, Groh D: Operative treatment of ulnar collateral ligament injuries of the elbow in athletes, *Am J Sports Med* 28:16–23, 2000.

157. Timmerman LA, Schwartz ML, Andrews JR: Preoperative evaluation of the ulnar collateral ligament by magnetic resonance imaging and computed tomography arthrography: evaluation in 25 baseball players with surgical confirmation, *Am J Sports Med* 22:26–31, 1994.

158. Field LD, Altchek DW: Evaluation of the arthroscopic valgus instability test of the elbow, *Am J Sports Med* 24:177–181, 1996.

159. Timmerman LA, Andrews JR: Histology and arthroscopic anatomy of the ulnar collateral ligament of the elbow, *Am J Sports Med* 22:667–673, 1994.

160. Nazarian LN, McShane JM, Ciccotti MG, et al: Dynamic US of the anterior band of the ulnar collateral ligament of the elbow in asymptomatic major league baseball pitchers, *Radiology* 227:149–154, 2003.

161. Sasaki J, Takahara M, Ogino T, et al: Ultrasonographic assessment of the ulnar collateral ligament and medial elbow laxity in college baseball players, *J Bone Joint Surg Am* 84:525–531, 2002.

162. Rettig AC, Sherrill C, Snead DS, et al: Nonoperative treatment of ulnar collateral ligament injuries in throwing athletes, *Am J Sports Med* 29:15–17, 2001.

163. Podesta L, Crow SA, Volkmer D, et al: Treatment of partial ulnar collateral ligament tears in the elbow with platelet-rich plasma, *Am J Sports Med* 41(7):1689–1694, 2013.

164. Jiang JJ, Leland M: Analysis of pitching velocity in major league baseball players before and after ulnar collateral ligament reconstruction, *Am J Sports Med* 42(2):880–885, 2014.

165. Nelson GN, Wu T, Galatz LM, et al: Elbow arthroscopy: early complications and associated risk factors, *J Shoulder Elbow Surg* 23:273–278, 2014.

166. Savoie 3rd FH, Trenhaile SW, Roberts J, et al: Primary repair of ulnar collateral ligament injuries of the elbow in young athletes: a case series of injuries to the proximal and distal ends of the ligament, *Am J Sports Med* 36(6):1066–1072, 2008.

167. Rohrbough JT, Altchek DW, Hyman J, et al: Medial collateral ligament reconstruction of the elbow using the docking technique, *Am J Sports Med* 30:541–548, 2002.

168. Ahmad CS, Lee TQ, ElAttrache NS: Biomechanical evaluation of a new ulnar collateral ligament reconstruction technique with interference screw fixation, *Am J Sports Med* 31:332–337, 2003.

169. Jobe FW, Stark H, Lombardo SJ: Reconstruction of the ulnar collateral ligament in athletes, *J Bone Joint Surg Am* 68:1158–1163, 1986.

170. Thompson WH, Jobe FW, Yocum LA, Pink M: Ulnar collateral ligament reconstruction in athletes: muscle splitting approach without transposition of the ulnar nerve, *J Shoulder Elbow Surg* 10:152–157, 2001.

171. Cain EL, Andrews JR, Dugas JR, et al: Outcome of ulnar collateral ligament reconstruction of the elbow: minimum 2-year follow-up. In Transactions of the 28th Annual Meeting of the American Orthopaedic Society for Sports Medicine vol 28, 2002, p 173.

172. Paletta GA, Wright RW: The docking procedure for elbow MCL reconstruction: 2-year follow-up in elite throwers. In Transactions of the 28th Annual Meeting of the American Orthopaedic Society for Sports Medicine vol 28, 2002, p 172.

173. Osbahr DC, Cain EL, Raines T, et al: Long-term outcomes after ulnar collateral ligament reconstruction in competitive baseball players. Minimum 10-year follow-up, *Am J Sports Med* 42(6):1333–1342, 2014.

174. Cohen SB, Sheridan S, Ciccotti MG: Return to sports for professional baseball players after surgery of the shoulder or elbow, *Sports Health* 3(1):105–111, 2011.

175. Osbahr DC, Dines JS, Rosenbaum AJ, et al: Does posteromedial chondromalacia reduce rate of return to play after ulnar collateral ligament reconstruction? *Clin Orthop Relat Res* 470(6):1558–1564, 2012.

176. Dugas JR, Walters BW, Chronister JA, et al: A biomechanical comparison of UCL repair with internal bracing vs modified Jobe reconstruction, *Am J Sports Med*, 2015 in-press.

177. Bartels RH: History of the surgical treatment of ulnar nerve compression at the elbow, *Neurosurgery* 49(2):391–399, 2001. discussion, 399-400.

178. Pechan J, Julis I: The pressure measurement in the ulnar nerve: a contribution to the pathophysiology of the cubital tunnel syndrome, *J Biomech* 8:75–79, 1975.

179. Arle JE, Zager EL: Surgical treatment of common entrapment neuropathies in the upper limbs, *Muscle Nerve* 23(8):1160–1174, 2000.

180. Bartels RH, Verhagen WI, van der Wilt RJ, et al: Prospective randomized controlled study comparing simple decompression versus anterior subcutaneous transposition for idiopathic neuropathy of the ulnar nerve at the elbow. Part 1, *Neurosurgery* 56:522–530, 2005. discussion, 522-530.

181. Gervasio O, Gambardella G, Zaccone C, Branca D: Simple decompression versus anterior submuscular transposition of the ulnar nerve in severe cubital tunnel syndrome: a prospective randomized study, *Neurosurgery* 56:108–117, 2005.

182. Micheli LJ: The traction apophyses, *Clin Sports Med* 6:389, 1987.

183. Torg JS, Moyer RA: Non-union of a stress fracture through the olecranon epiphyseal plate observed in adolescent baseball pitcher. A case report, *J Bone Joint Surg Am* 59:264–265, 1977.

184. Furushima K, Itoh Y, Iwabu S, et al: Classification of olecranon stress fractures in baseball players, *Am J Sports Med* 42(6):1343–1351, 2014.

185. Parr TJ, Burns TC: Overuse injuries of the olecranon in adolescents, *Orthopedics* 26:1143–1146, 2003.

186. Hulkko A, Orava S, Nikula P: Stress fractures of the olecranon in javelin throwers, *Int J Sports Med* 7:210–213, 1986.

187. Kovach J, Baker BE, Mosher JE: Fracture separation of the olecranon ossification center in adults, *Am J Sports Med* 13:105–111, 1985.

188. Lowery WE, Kurzweil PR, Forman SK, Morrison DS: Persistence of the olecranon physis: a cause of "little league elbow,", *J Shoulder Elbow Surg* 4:143–147, 1995.

189. Skak SV: Fracture of the olecranon through a persistent physis in an adult: a case report, *J Bone Joint Surg Am* 75:272–275, 1993.

190. Iwamoto J, Takeda T: Stress fractures in athletes: review of 196 cases, *J Orthop Sci* 8:273–278, 2003.

191. Maffulli N, Chan D, Aldridge MJ: Overuse injuries of the olecranon in young gymnasts, *J Bone Joint Surg Br* 74:305–308, 1992.

192. Nakaji N, Fujioka H, Nagura I, et al: Stress fracture of the olecranon in an adult baseball player, *Knee Surg Sports Traumatol Arthrosc* 14:390–393, 2006.

193. Suzuki K, Minami A, Suenaga N, Kondoh M: Oblique stress fracture of the olecranon in baseball pitchers, *J Shoulder Elbow Surg* 6:491–494, 1997.

194. Gabel GT: Acute and chronic tendinopathies at the elbow, *Curr Opin Rheumatol* 11:138–143, 1999.

195. Mair SD, Isbell WM, Gill TJ, et al: Triceps tendon ruptures in professional football players, *Am J Sports Med* 32:431–434, 2004.

196. Sollender JL, Rayan GM, Barden GA: Triceps tendon rupture in weight lifters, *J Shoulder Elbow Surg* 7:151–153, 1998.

197. Lambert MI, St Clair Gibson A, Noakes TD: Rupture of the triceps tendon associated with steroid injections, *Am J Sports Med* 23:778, 1995.

198. van Riet RP, Morrey BF, Ho E, O'Driscoll SW: Surgical treatment of distal triceps ruptures, *J Bone Joint Surg Am* 85:1961–1967, 2003.

199. Weistroffer JK, Mills WJ, Shin AY: Recurrent rupture of the triceps tendon repaired with hamstring tendon autograft augmentation: a case report and repair technique, *J Shoulder Elbow Surg* 12:193–196, 2003.

200. Ahmad CS, Park MC, ElAttrache NS: Elbow medial ulnar collateral ligament insufficiency alters posteromedial olecranon contact, *Am J Sports Med* 32:1607–1612, 2004.

201. Ahmad CS, ElAttrache NS: Valgus extension overload syndrome and stress injury of the olecranon, *Clin Sports Med* 23:665–676, 2004.

202. Eygendaal D, Safran MR: Posteromedial elbow problems in the adult athlete, *Br J Sports Med* 40:430–434, 2006.

203. Andrews JR, Timmerman LA: Outcome of elbow surgery in professional baseball players, *Am J Sports Med* 23(4):407–413, 1995.

204. McGinty JB: Arthroscopic removal of loose bodies, *Orthop Clin North Am* 13:313–328, 1982.

205. Ogilvie-Harris DJ, Gordon R, MacKay M: Arthroscopic treatment for posterior impingement in degenerative arthritis of the elbow, *Arthroscopy* 11:437–443, 1995.

206. Redden JF, Stanley D: Arthroscopic fenestration of the olecranon fossa in the treatment of osteoarthritis of the elbow, *Arthroscopy* 9:14–16, 1993.

207. Andrews JR, Heggland EJH, Fleisig GS, Zheng N: Relationship of ulnar collateral ligament strain to amount of medial olecranon osteotomy, *Am J Sports Med* 29:716–721, 2001.

208. Kamineni S, ElAttrache NS, O'Driscoll SW, et al: Medial collateral ligament strain with partial posteromedial olecranon resection: a biomechanical study, *J Bone Joint Surg Am* 86:2424–2430, 2004.

209. Kamineni S, Hirahara H, Pomianowski S, et al: Partial posteromedial olecranon resection: a kinematic study, *J Bone Joint Surg Am* 85:1005–1011, 2003.

210. Reilly JP, Nicholas JA: The chronically inflamed bursa, *Clin Sports Med* 6:345–370, 1987.

211. Bradley JP, Petrie RS: Osteochondritis dissecans of the humeral capitellum: diagnosis and treatment, *Clin Sports Med* 20:565–590, 2001.

212. Pappas A: Osteochondritis dissecans, *Clin Orthop* 158:59–69, 1981.

213. Yadao MA, Field LD, Savoie FH: Osteochondritis dissecans of the elbow, *Instr Course Lect* 53:599–606, 2004.

214. Kida Y, Morihara T, Kotoura Y, et al: Prevalence and clinical characteristics of osteochondritis dissecans of the humeral capitellum among adolescent baseball players, *Am J Sports Med* 42(8):1963–1971, 2014.

215. Jackson DW, Silvino N, Reiman P: Osteochondritis in the female gymnast's elbow, *Arthroscopy* 5:129–136, 1989.

216. Schenck RC, Athanasiou KA, Constantinides G, Gomez E: A biomechanical analysis of articular cartilage of the human elbow and a potential relationship to osteochondritis dissecans, *Clin Orthop* 299:305–312, 1994.

217. Haraldsson S: On osteochondrosis deformans juvenilis capituli humeri, including investigation of intra-osseous vasculature in distal humerus, *Acta Orthop Scand* 38(suppl):1–232, 1959.

218. Takahara M, Shundo M, Kondo M, et al: Early detection of osteochondritis dissecans of the capitellum in young baseball players: report of three cases, *J Bone Joint Surg Am* 80:892–897, 1998.

219. Kusumi T, Ishibashi Y, Tsuda E, et al: Osteochondritis dissecans of the elbow: histopathological assessment

of the articular cartilage and subchondral bone with emphasis on their damage and repair, *Pathol Int* 56:604–612, 2006.

220. Baumgarten TE, Andrews JR, Satterwhite YE: The arthroscopic classification and treatment of osteochondritis dissecans of the capitellum, *Am J Sports Med* 26:520–523, 1998.

221. Harada M, Ogino T, Takahara M, et al: Fragment fixation with a bone graft and dynamic staples for osteochondritis dissecans of the humeral capitellum, *J Shoulder Elbow Surg* 11:368–372, 2002.

222. Kiyoshige Y, Takagi M, Yuasa K, Hamasaki M: Closed-wedge osteotomy for osteochondritis dissecans of the capitellum, *Am J Sports Med* 28:534–537, 2000.

223. Bauer M, Jonsson K, Josefsson PO, Linden B: Osteochondritis dissecans of the elbow: a long-term follow-up study, *Clin Orthop* 284:156–160, 1992.

224. Ruch DS, Cory JW, Poehling GG: The arthroscopic management of osteochondritis dissecans of the adolescent elbow, *Arthroscopy* 14:797–803, 1998.

225. Takeda H, Watarai K, Matsushita T, et al: A surgical treatment for unstable osteochondritis dissecans lesions of the humeral capitellum in adolescent baseball players, *Am J Sports Med* 30:713–717, 2002.

226. Takahara M, Ogino T, Sasaki I, et al: Long term outcome of osteochondritis dissecans of the humeral capitellum, *Clin Orthop Relat Res* 363:108–115, 1999.

227. Iwasaki N, Kato H, Ishikawa J, et al: Autologous osteochondral mosaicplasty for capitellar osteochondritis dissecans in teen-aged patients, *Am J Sports Med* 34:1233–1239, 2006.

228. Yamamoto Y, Ishibashi Y, Tsuda E, et al: Osteochondral autograft transplantation for osteochondritis dissecans of the elbow in juvenile baseball players: minimum 2-year follow-up, *Am J Sports Med* 34:714–720, 2006.

229. Whaley AL, Baker CL: Lateral epicondylitis, *Clin Sports Med* 23:677–691, 2004.

230. Nirschl RP, Pettrone FA: Tennis elbow: the surgical treatment of lateral epicondylitis, *J Bone Joint Surg Am* 61:832–839, 1979.

231. Nirschl RP, Ashman ES: Elbow tendinopathy: tennis elbow, *Clin Sports Med* 22:813–836, 2003.

232. Hill JJ, Trapp RG, Colliver JA: Survey on the use of corticosteroid injections by orthopedists, *Cont Orthop* 18:39–45, 1989.

233. Smidt N, Assendelft WJ, van der Windt DA, et al: Corticosteroid injections for lateral epicondylitis: a systematic review, *Pain* 96:23–40, 2002.

234. Nirschl RP, Rodin DM, Ochiai DH, et al: Iontophoretic administration of dexamethasone sodium phosphate for acute epicondylitis: a randomized, double-blinded, placebo-controlled study, *Am J Sports Med* 31:189–195, 2003.

235. Paoloni JA, Appleyard RC, Nelson J, Murrell GA: Topical nitric oxide application in the treatment of chronic extensor tendinosis at the elbow: a randomized, double-blinded, placebo-controlled clinical trial, *Am J Sports Med* 31:915–920, 2003.

236. Placzek R, Drescher W, Deuretzbacher G, et al: Treatment of chronic radial epicondylitis with botulinum toxin A: a double-blind, placebo-controlled, randomized multicenter study, *J Bone Joint Surg Am* 89:255–260, 2007.

237. Wong SM, Hui AC, Tong PY, et al: Treatment of lateral epicondylitis with botulinum toxin: a randomized, double-blind, placebo-controlled trial, *Ann Intern Med* 143:793–797, 2005.

238. Haake M, Konig IR, Decker T, et al: Extracorporeal shock wave therapy in the treatment of lateral epicondylitis: a randomized multicenter trial, *J Bone Joint Surg Am* 84:1982–1991, 2002.

239. Edwards SG, Calandruccio JH: Autologous blood injections for refractory lateral epicondylitis, *J Hand Surg Am* 28:272–278, 2003.

240. Mishra A, Pavelko T: Treatment of chronic elbow tendinosis with buffered platelet-rich plasma, *Am J Sports Med* 34:1774–1778, 2006.

241. Mishra AK, Skrepnik NV, Edwards SG, et al: Efficacy of platelet-rich plasma fo chronic tennis elbow. A double-blind, prospective, multicenter, randomized controlled trial of 230 patients, *Am J Sports Med* 4(2):463–471, 2014.

242. Lo M, Safran MR: Surgical management of lateral epicondylitis: a systematic review, *Clin Orthop Relat Res* 463:98–106, 2007.

243. Szabo SJ, Savoie FH, Field LD, et al: Tendinosis of the extensor carpi radialis brevis: an evaluation of three methods of operative treatment, *J Shoulder Elbow Surg* 15:721–727, 2006.

244. Baker CL, Murphy KP, Gottlob CA, Curd DT: Arthroscopic classification and treatment of lateral epicondylitis: 2-year clinical results, *J Shoulder Elbow Surg* 9:475–482, 2000.

245. Oki G, Iba K, Sasaki K, et al: Time to functional recovery after arthroscopic surgery for tennis elbow, *J Shoulder Elbow Surg* 23:1527–1531, 2014.

246. Roles NC, Maudsley RH: Radial tunnel syndrome: resistant tennis elbow as a nerve entrapment, *J Bone Joint Surg Br* 54:499–508, 1972.

247. Lister GD, Belsole RB, Kleinert HE: The radial tunnel syndrome, *J Hand Surg Am* 4:52–59, 1979.

248. Rosenbaum R: Surgical treatment for radial tunnel syndrome, *J Hand Surg Am* 24:1345–1346, 1999.

249. Rosenbaum R: Disputed radial tunnel syndrome, *Muscle Nerve* 22:960–967, 1999.

250. Green S, Buchbinder R, Barnsley L, et al: Non-steroidal anti-inflammatory drugs (NSAIDs) for treating lateral elbow pain in adults, *Cochrane Database Syst Rev* 2:CD003686, 2002.

251. Klaiman MD, Shrader JA, Danoff JV, et al: Phonophoresis versus ultrasound in the treatment of common musculoskeletal conditions, *Med Sci Sports Exerc* 30:1349–1355, 1998.

252. Fehlings DL, Kirsch S, McComas A, et al: Evaluation of therapeutic electrical stimulation to improve muscle strength and function in children with types II/III spinal muscular atrophy, *Dev Med Child Neurol* 44:741–744, 2002.

253. Brosseau L, Casimiro L, Milne S, et al: Deep transverse friction massage for treating tendonitis, *Cochrane Database Syst Rev* 4:CD003528, 2002.

254. Nichols AW: Complications associated with the use of corticosteroids in the treatment of athletic injuries, *Clin J Sport Med* 15:E370, 2005.

255. Coutts R, Rothe C, Kaita J: The role of continuous passive motion in the rehabilitation of the total knee patient, *Clin Orthop Relat Res* 159:126–132, 1981.

256. Dehne E, Tory R: The treatment of joint injuries by immediate mobilization based upon the spiral adaptation concept, *Clin Orthop Relat Res* 77:218–232, 1971.

257. Haggmark T, Eriksson E: Cylinder or mobile cast brace after knee ligament surgery: a clinical analysis and morphologic and enzymatic studies of changes of the quadriceps muscle, *Am J Sports Med* 7:48–56, 1979.

258. Noyes FR, Mangine RE, Barber SE: Early knee motion after open and arthroscopic anterior cruciate ligament reconstruction, *Am J Sports Med* 15:149–160, 1987.

259. Perkins G: Rest and motion, *J Bone Joint Surg Br* 35:521–539, 1954.

260. Salter RB, Hamilton HW, Wedge JH: Clinical application of basic research on continuous passive motion on healing of full thickness defects in articular cartilage, *J Bone Joint Surg Am* 62:1232–1251, 1980.

261. Salter RB, Hamilton HW, Wedge JH: Clinical application of basic research on continuous passive motion for disorders and injuries of synovial joints: a preliminary report of a feasibility study, *J Orthop Res* 1:325–342, 1984.

262. Tipton CM, Mathies RD, Martin RF: Influence of age and sex on strength of bone-ligament junctions in knee joints in rats, *J Bone Joint Surg Am* 60:230–236, 1978.

263. Wilk KE, Arrigo C, Andrews JR: Rehabilitation of the elbow in the throwing athlete, *J Orthop Sports Phys Ther* 17(6):305–317, 1993.

264. Akeson WH, Amiel D, Woo SLY: Immobilization effects on synovial joints: the pathomechanics of joint contracture, *Biorheology* 17:95–107, 1980.

265. Green DP, McCoy H: Turnbuckle orthotic correction of elbow flexion contractures, *J Bone Joint Surg Am* 61:1092, 1979.

266. Nirschl RP, Morrey BF: Rehabilitation. In Morrey BF, editor: *The elbow and its disorders*, Philadelphia, 1985, WB Saunders.

267. Kottke FJ, Pauley DL, Ptak RA: The rationale of prolonged stretching for connective tissue, *Arch Phys Med Rehabil* 47:345–352, 1966.

268. Sapega AA, Quedenfeld TC, Moyer RA, Butler RA: Biophysical factors in range of motion exercise, *Arch Phys Med Rehabil* 57:122–126, 1976.

269. Warren CG, Lehmann JF, Koblanski JN: Elongation of rat tail tendon: effect of load and temperature, *Arch Phys Med Rehabil* 52:465–474, 1971.

270. Warren CG, Lehmann JF, Koblanski JN: Heat and stretch procedures: an evaluation using rat tail tendon, *Arch Phys Med Rehabil* 57:122–126, 1976.

271. Wilk KE, Macrina LC, Fleisig GS, et al: Deficits in glenohumeral passive range of motion increase reisk of elbow injury in professional baseball pitchers. A prospective study, *Am J Sports Med* 42(9):2075–2081, 2014.

272. Fleisig GS, Escamilla RF: Biomechanics of the elbow in the throwing athlete, *Op Tech Sports Med* 4(2):62–68, 1996.

273. Wyke BD: The neurology of joints, *Ann R Coll Surg Engl* 41:25–29, 1966.

274. Andrews JR, Frank W: Valgus extension overload in the pitching elbow. In Andrews JR, Zarins B, Carson WB, editors: *Injuries to the throwing arm*, Philadelphia, 1985, WB Saunders.

275. Reinold MM, Wilk KE, Reed J, et al: Internal sport programs: guidelines for baseball, tennis, and golf, *J Orthop Sports Phys Ther* 32:293–298, 2002.

276. Andrews JR, Jelsma RD, Joyse ME, Timmerman LA: Open surgical procedures for injuries to the elbow in throwers, *Op Tech Sports Med* 4(2):109–113, 1996.

277. Davidson PA, Pink M, Perry J: Functional anatomy of the flexor pronator muscle group in relation to the medial collateral ligament of the elbow, *Am J Sports Med* 23:245–250, 1995.

278. Crawford CM, Varghese G, Mani MM, Neff JR: Heterotopic ossification: are range of motion exercises contraindicated? *J Burn Care Rehabil* 7:323–327, 1986.

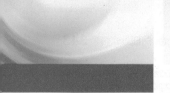

CHAPTER 10

Hand, Wrist, and Digit Injuries

JENNIFER B. GREEN, CHARLES DEVEIKAS, HELEN E. RANGER, JOANNE G. DRAGHETTI,
LINDSAY C. GROAT, EVAN D. SCHUMER, BRUCE M.LESLIE

*"Most of the fundamental ideas of science are essentially simple, and may, as a
rule, be expressed in a language comprehensible to everyone."*

Albert Einstein

INTRODUCTION

The hand is one of the preeminent tools of human beings. The hand allows an individual to touch and take hold, but the anatomy allows much more than gross grasp and coarse sensation. The structure of the hand allows a musician to play with different shades of meaning; it allows an artist to apply subtle shades of texture; it allows a parent to convey meaning by touching a child. The hand can convey all these emotions. The inability to accomplish gross grasp and coarse sensation or the subtleties in these higher functions can affect the ultimate outcome of the patient.

The anatomy of the wrist and hand is not too difficult to understand. However, its compact nature and precision create a complexity in which subtle changes in the way tissues move in relation to one another can have a dramatic effect on function. Seemingly simple injuries that ultimately prevent tendon gliding can severely affect the ability to flex or extend the digits. Wounds that heal by secondary intention may be acceptable in some areas but in others may greatly diminish the ability to feel and move.

Insight into hand function arises from an understanding of the way in which anatomy, biomechanics, physiology, and wound healing work together to allow the hand to perform a myriad of tasks. This knowledge then needs to be tempered by the patient's expectations, needs, and socialization. An operation to restore hand function in one patient may be totally unacceptable to another patient. Each intervention needs to be customized to the individual patient.

Hand rehabilitation plays a critical role in restoring upper extremity function. The therapist is a crucial member of a team whose ultimate goal is to improve hand function. Not only does the therapist assist in promoting the restoration of the soft tissues to maximize function, in many cases the therapist is in the best position to recognize the patient's goals and needs. A good hand therapist is not only knowledgeable of upper extremity anatomy but also recognizes the social and psychological implications of the original injury and subsequent treatment.

This chapter presents a fundamental approach to the diagnosis and classification of wrist and hand injuries. It also includes treatment and rehabilitation guidelines for bone and soft tissue injuries of the hand.

FRACTURE INJURIES OF THE HAND

Phalangeal Fractures

General Considerations

Phalangeal and metacarpal fractures are among the most common skeletal injuries. In one large series of 11,000 fractures, these two injuries accounted for 10% of the total.[1] Modes of injury are predictable based on population age groups. Children and young adults are usually injured in sports-related activities. Young and middle-aged men are prone to work-related injury. Elderly patients are vulnerable to hand trauma from falls or accidents.[2] Unfortunately, these fractures frequently are treated as a trivial malady by both patients and health care providers. This can lead to a profound loss of digital and hand function, either from neglect or, worse still, from poorly executed treatment.

The force required to fracture one of the phalangeal bones also damages the soft tissue structures of the digit. This can lead to significant scarring and fibrosis in the postinjury period. Function can best be restored with early intervention by the treating physician and by allowing the patient to begin rehabilitation of the digit as soon as stability permits. Studies have reported that immobilization for longer than 3 weeks leads to loss of total active range of motion (AROM).[3] Before the 20th century, treatment of phalangeal fractures was limited to nonoperative methods. Today, most of these fractures can be successfully treated in this fashion because most fractures are functionally stable either before or after closed reduction.

Indications for surgical intervention for phalangeal fractures include angulation more than 25° to prevent compromised digit flexion and extension[4]; malrotation; bone loss; open fracture; intra-articular fracture with displacement; associated soft tissue injury (skin, vessel, tendon, nerve); and multiple trauma to the upper extremity. The treating physician must also take into consideration the patient's age, occupation, ability to cooperate with the postoperative regimen, and the surgeon's experience and skill.

Indications for Surgery for Phalangeal Fractures

- Angulation greater than 25° and/or malrotation
- Bone loss
- Open fracture
- Intra-articular fracture with displacement
- Associated soft tissue injury
- Multiple trauma to the upper extremity

Anatomy

The proximal and middle phalanges are similar in their osseous anatomy. The distal phalanx is different in shape and in the specialized attachment of the nail bed to the dorsal periosteal surface. The soft tissue envelope can greatly affect the stability of the fracture, treatment of the injury, and the ultimate outcome. In the digits are found the osteocutaneous ligaments of Cleland and Grayson. These can serve to stabilize the bone and prevent fracture displacement. The ligaments can prevent closed reduction of a fracture if they are interposed between the displaced fragments. The proximal interphalangeal (PIP) joint and distal interphalangeal (DIP) joint are highly constrained hinged joints that do not tolerate even a small amount of fracture displacement. The metacarpophalangeal (MCP) joint has a less constrained configuration that allows for more lateral motion, some rotation, and slightly more forgiveness in terms of fracture displacement.

Injury Classification

Shaft fractures can be classified by their location, that is, in the neck, the midshaft, or the base of the bone. They can be further classified according to the fracture geometry; for example, the fracture may be spiral, transverse, short or long oblique, or comminuted. This characteristic can predict fracture stability and can help determine the best type of surgical treatment if fracture stabilization is required. The fracture can be further classified as open or closed, which is less than intuitive during the examination

of a crushed distal phalanx and a nail bed injury that, for all intents and purposes, is an open injury.

Diagnosis and Medical Treatment
Fractures of the Distal Phalanx

Tuft Fractures. Tuft fractures are the most common fractures of the fingers[5] and are frequently the result of a crushing injury. A crush injury may result in comminuted fractures that fail to unite. Nonunion, however, does not usually lead to instability because the bone fragments are held tightly to the pulp tissue of the fingertip. An associated laceration of the nail matrix may be seen. Splinting for 1 to 2 weeks for comfort, with a rapid return to function, is the usual treatment course for this injury (Figure 10-1).

Repair of the nail bed is warranted if the injury causes wide displacement of that tissue. Replacement of the nail plate, if it still exists, creates a template for the nail bed to heal, provides protection for the sensitive tissues of the fingertip, and also serves as a splint for the underlying distal phalanx. Despite adequate treatment, the end result of this injury may be some loss of motion, decreased sensation, and chronic mild pain. These unfortunate sequelae are exacerbated by prolonged immobilization. In the case of the index finger, the phenomenon of *bypassing* (i.e., using a different finger) may be observed and should be addressed early in the course of treatment.

Shaft Fractures. Shaft fractures are either longitudinal or, more commonly, transverse in orientation. If displacement or angulation is present, they often are easily repaired. Displacement signifies an injury of the nail bed or germinal matrix, as well, which, if left untreated, can lead to nail plate deformity. If the dorsal cortex of the bone can be realigned and the overlying nail plate is also intact, the matrix will be sandwiched into the correct orientation for healing, and no further treatment likely is necessary. Displaced fractures are easily treated with a longitudinally oriented Kirschner wire (K-wire) or headless screw (Figure 10-2).

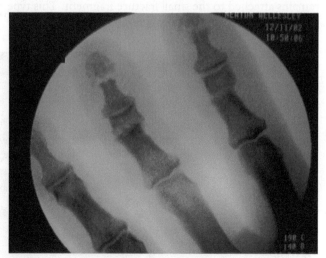

Figure 10-1 Snow blower injury, which resulted in multiple tuft fractures and fractures of the middle phalanx with overlying soft tissue trauma.

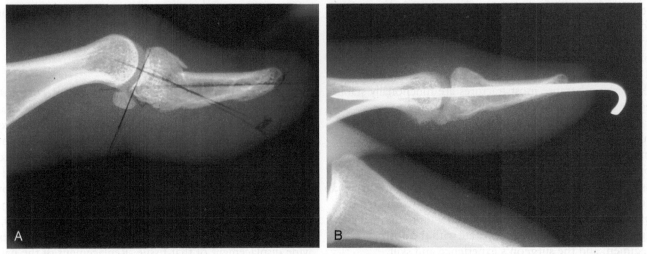

Figure 10-2 A, Angulated shaft fracture of the distal phalanx; the fracture has created a deformity of the digit that will affect the growth of the nail. **B,** Correction of the shaft fracture with a pin, which holds the bone aligned for 3 weeks. The pin subsequently was removed in the outpatient setting.

Intra-articular Fractures. Intra-articular fractures in adults usually involve either the volar or dorsal lip at the end of the bone. In children, an epiphyseal separation also may occur. Dorsal rim fractures usually are associated with a terminal tendon avulsion injury (sometimes called a *bony mallet injury*). If the dorsal fragment of bone is small enough, no volar translation of the distal phalanx occurs at the joint surface, and the injury can be treated in the same way as a soft tissue mallet injury, only with splinting. However, the larger the fragment, the greater is the potential that the flexor digitorum profundus (FDP) tendon, which is still attached to the volar fragment, will translate the distal fragment palmarly. This can be a subtle finding on the lateral x-ray film, and the possibility must always be considered with a fracture fragment of more than 30% of the joint surface. In such cases operative intervention to restore joint alignment is indicated (Figure 10-3).

Volar Lip Fractures. Volar lip fractures are also tendon avulsion injuries. In these fractures, the FDP tendon remains attached to the small fracture fragment. This type of injury is also known as a *rugger Jersey finger* or *sweater finger* because it commonly occurs when gripping to tackle an opponent in football or rugby. Unlike its counterpart on the extensor surface, these flexor tendon injuries frequently require surgery because the flexor tendon retracts toward the palm after injury, pulling the fracture fragment along with it. In these cases, if the fragment is more than a few millimeters in size, it is usually caught and held in place under one of the distal annular pulleys. The fragment usually can easily be found there and reattached surgically with a screw, suture anchor, or suture over a button.

Fractures of the Proximal and Middle Phalanges

Shaft Fractures. A direct blow frequently causes transverse fractures to the shaft, whereas twisting injuries cause spiral or oblique fractures. Whether or not displacement of the fracture occurs is determined by the location of the fracture and the influence of the intrinsic and extrinsic forces at that specific site.

Fractures of the proximal phalanx, when displaced, fall into apex volar angulation. This occurs because the insertion of interosseous muscles on the proximal fragment

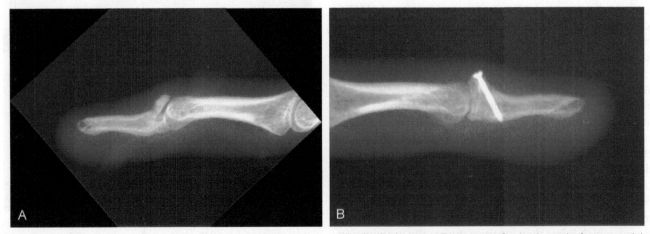

Figure 10-3 A, Bony mallet injury in which a large fracture fragment has caused volar displacement. **B,** Operative fixation is required to restore joint congruency. In the preoperative x-ray film, note that despite the splint, the joint is not congruent because of the volar translation of the distal fragment.

flexes the MCP joint while the pull of the lateral bands and central slip extends the distal fracture fragment.

Fractures of the middle phalanx are affected more by the pull of the central slip insertion and the flexor digitorum superficialis (FDS) tendon and therefore tend to angulate apex dorsally when they are displaced.

Rotational malalignment is poorly tolerated and is best assessed with active flexion of the digit, which may require digital block anesthesia for comfort. Tenodesis is preferable to passive motion for assessment of this type of deformity. Patients sometimes use the adjacent digits to "capture" the fractured finger, thus limiting their deformity. Care must be taken to observe for this during the examination to evaluate the true extent of digital scissoring from malrotation (Figure 10-4).

The majority of proximal and middle phalanx fractures are stable or will be stable after closed reduction, which often is the first course of treatment considered for these injuries. Significant stripping of the soft tissue from the bone makes reduction easier, but the fracture will be more unstable in the long run, often requiring implant augmentation. If closed reduction is not possible, the reason may be a bony spike caught on the soft tissue envelope. Most surgeons prefer to gain anatomical alignment of these fractures,[6,7] because any degree of malrotation and angulation over 25° can negatively affect hand function.[8,9] Closed treatment can be accomplished with digital block anesthesia in the office or operating room. Immediate postreduction x-ray films should be obtained, before immobilization, to confirm the reduction and stability. If satisfactory alignment is achieved, the usual treatment protocol is intrinsic plus splinting for 2 to 3 weeks, with weekly confirmatory x-ray films, followed by range of motion (ROM) with the affected finger buddy-taped. Dynamic or static progressive splinting and formal therapy are initiated at week 5 if motion fails to return toward normal.

K-wire fixation is used if there is loss of reduction, comminution, or inability to hold the initial reduction. The wires can be placed down the intramedullary shaft or across the fracture to affix adjacent cortices. In this way, transverse, oblique, and spiral fractures are all amenable to this treatment. Frequently K-wire fixation can be accomplished without a skin incision if the fracture is reducible by closed means. Intraoperative fluoroscopy is essential for proper pin placement and confirmation of the reduction in multiple planes. Midlateral placement of the pin or pins prevents interference with the flexor and extensor tendons and the neurovascular structures. Two pins are required for stability unless an intramedullary pin is used. The pins usually are removed at 3 weeks, when fracture tenderness subsides, to allow resumption of motion and stretching of the scar tissue (Figure 10-5).

Open reduction may be required even in simple fracture patterns if intervening soft tissue or a hematoma prevents reduction. In addition, comminution or an open fracture with bone loss may require open reduction for bone grafting or the application of stabilizing plates. K-wire fixation may be an acceptable alternative in some open cases. Long oblique and spiral fractures, however, are highly amenable to interfragmentary screw fixation. These fracture patterns may allow anatomical reduction and early return to motion with little interference from overlying gliding structures. Transverse and short oblique fractures cannot be treated with interfragmentary screws and must be held with a plate. Plates also can bridge gaps in the bone or secure a bone graft to the reduced fracture fragments and allow early motion. The downside to plate fixation in the phalanges is that scar adherence may cause the plate to interfere with tendon gliding. Also, some patients complain of persistent pain at the plate site, requiring removal of the hardware once the fracture is healed (Figure 10-6). External fixation currently is used less often, but indications for its use still exist (Figure 10-7).

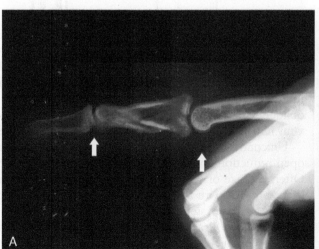
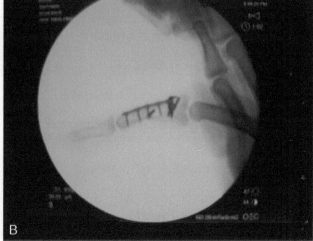

Figure 10-4 A, In the preoperative x-ray film, the distal aspect of the proximal phalanx is a perfect lateral, as evidenced by the complete overlap of the two condyles. This should also be true of the distal aspect of the middle phalanx; however, the fracture has caused a rotational deformity. **B,** A lateral fluoroscopic view obtained in the operating room shows the correction of the rotational deformity.

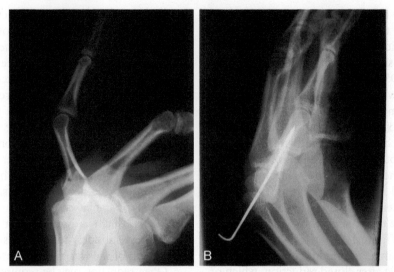

Figure 10-5 A, Low-energy transverse fracture of the proximal phalanx results in volar apex angulation. **B,** This simple fracture pattern requires only closed reduction and pinning to obtain anatomical alignment of the bone and to correct the secondary deformity at the MCP and PIP joints seen in the preoperative x-ray film.

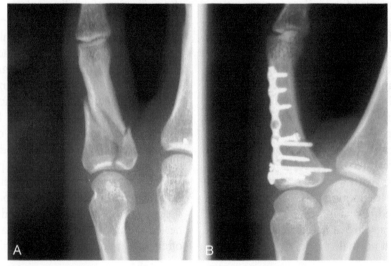

Figure 10-6 A, Markedly unstable, comminuted, intra-articular fracture of the proximal phalanx. **B,** Plate fixation was required to obtain alignment and stability. Active range of motion was started on postoperative day 5.

Indications for External Fixation of a Fracture

- Fractures with marked comminution and soft tissue injury or that have been contaminated
- Fractures with significant soft tissue injury in which further dissection may compromise digit viability
- Fractures with a segmental defect in which length needs to be preserved until formal open reduction and internal fixation (ORIF) is done
- Temporary stability in a patient with multiple injuries

Articular and Periarticular Fractures

Unicondylar Fractures. Unicondylar fractures of the phalanges occur from a shearing force and tend to be unstable, falling into a shortened and malrotated position.

This injury, although subtle, causes pain, deformity, and loss of motion. The collateral ligament remains attached to the fragment, causing it to rotate, creating an angular deformity and intra-articular incongruity. Often the fracture malalignment is best appreciated on a true lateral or oblique x-ray film because, on an anteroposterior (AP) x-ray film, it may appear only mildly gapped (Figure 10-8).

Unicondylar fractures are treated surgically because open reduction and fragment stabilization are required. Often the size of the fragments prevents the use of anything but a K-wire for fixation (Figure 10-9), but occasionally a larger fragment can be fixed with a screw.

Bicondylar Fractures. A bicondylar fracture occurs when a compressive load to the digit splits the head of the phalanx into two pieces and further separates it from the shaft. Each condylar piece is held by the collateral

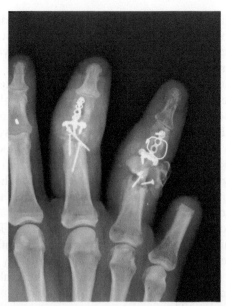

Figure 10-7 Roller crush injury with extensive soft tissue and bony damage. The patient was a poor candidate for internal fixation; he presented with open wounds, infection, and unstable fixation. External fixation was the ideal treatment in this case because it allowed the soft tissues to heal and the infection to resolve, and it permitted eventual bone grafting and stabilization, which facilitated bony union.

ligament, which tends to separate and rotate them apart. These injuries usually require open reduction and internal fixation (ORIF); K-wires often are used, but they do not allow early motion. Newly devised plates allow early motion but can be difficult to use.

Pilon fractures occur with an axial load to the digit. Fracture of the dorsal and volar lip of the middle phalanx occurs, with loss of congruency and stability of the PIP joint. Dynamic external fixation uses ligamentotaxis (i.e., the use of the ligament to reduce the fracture) to restore overall joint alignment. The dynamic nature of the fixator

allows early motion to promote joint congruency and cartilage health (Figure 10-10).

Rehabilitation Principles and Considerations for Hand Fractures

Fracture healing is the regeneration of mineralized tissue, which results in the restoration of bony mechanical strength. The primary concern during rehabilitation and before motion is initiated is the stability of the fracture. The ultimate goals of rehabilitation are (1) to produce pain-free, functional motion and strength and (2) to restore and optimize soft tissue balance and glide without disrupting the healing tissues.

The progression of rehabilitation is based on the stages of soft tissue and bony healing. Two well-documented progressions of fracture healing, described as primary and secondary healing, have been classified based on both the approximation and motion between the bone fragments.

Progression of Fracture Healing

- Primary healing
- Secondary healing

Primary Healing. Primary healing occurs when the fracture fragments are aligned and compressed so that no motion is allowed between the fragments. Motionless fixation of the fracture fragments is achieved through open reduction and internal fixation. The fixation hardware acts as a support matrix to provide immediate strength at the fracture site. Calcification and remodeling of the tissues, which are required for true fracture strength, generally take 6 weeks. Primary healing allows for early therapeutic intervention to initiate motion and soft tissue glide, to control edema, to address wounds, and to restore normal

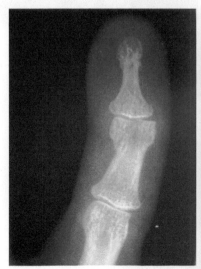
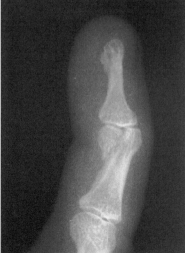

Figure 10-8 The displacement seen with a unicondylar fracture of the phalanx is not as easily appreciated in the AP view as in the oblique view. The articular incongruity and instability of the fracture require operative treatment.

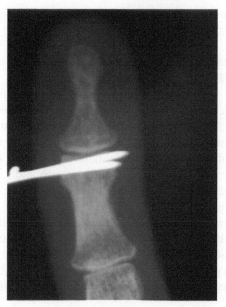

Figure 10-9 Fixation of a unicondylar fracture with K-wires.

neurological input to prevent guarding or avoidance of use. Primary healing does not allow for early strengthening because true fracture strength is not achieved until week 6 or later.[10,11]

Secondary Healing. Secondary healing takes place when the fracture fragments are approximated but not compressed, leaving a slight gap and/or potential for motion. Bone healing occurs through progressive stages in which callus formation is a precursor to bone.[10,11] Fractures primarily managed by closed reduction heal in these stages. Closed reduction is achieved through casting and semirigid fixation, such as K-wires, external fixators, and intramedullary pins.

Secondary healing progresses in three stages. The first stage, which lasts approximately 2 weeks, is the inflammatory stage. During this stage, high cellular activity occurs, which is required for ultimate healing. The healing tissues are at their weakest and are vulnerable to mechanical disruption. The fracture site requires protection and

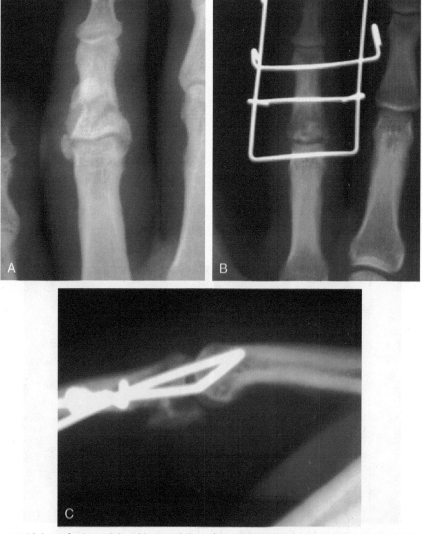

Figure 10-10 A, Pilon fracture with loss of volar and dorsal bony stability of the middle phalanx at the PIP joint. **B** and **C,** It is critical to obtain PIP joint alignment and to begin motion early. This can be accomplished with dynamic fixators through ligamentotaxis.

immobilization by means of splinting or casting during the inflammatory stage.[10,11]

The second stage, the repair stage, occurs during weeks 2 through 4. During this stage, soft callus forms and stabilizes the fracture site. Splint protection continues, and controlled motion, tendon gliding, and edema management are initiated.[10,11]

During the third stage, which can last from weeks 4 to 6 up to 2 years, remodeling of the fracture progresses. During this stage, restoration of bone strength occurs. At this point, the tissues have regained enough strength to tolerate passive range of motion (PROM), stretching, splinting for motion, strengthening, and return to preinjury function. In general, as with primary healing, fractures progressing through the stages of secondary healing should not be subjected to strengthening exercises until weeks 6 to 8, when healing is confirmed (Figure 10-11).

Factors that can impede healing should be considered before increased demand is placed on a fracture through stretching, strengthening, or high demand activity. These include infection, prolonged steroid use, diabetes, anemia, osteopenia, and use of alcohol, nicotine, or caffeine.[12–16] Fracture healing is a dynamic process in which healing stages are progressive but overlap. Special care must be taken with patients with multiple trauma, in whom multiple fixation methods are used and who may have fractures that are progressing through both primary and secondary healing. Multiple trauma also causes significant soft tissue damage. Attention should be given to soft tissue healing, which takes place in a well-documented, staged healing process.[11,17–21] In devising a therapeutic approach and initiating therapy, clinicians involved in the rehabilitation of patients with these types of fractures should pay close attention to differences in the healing time frames for the various tissues involved.

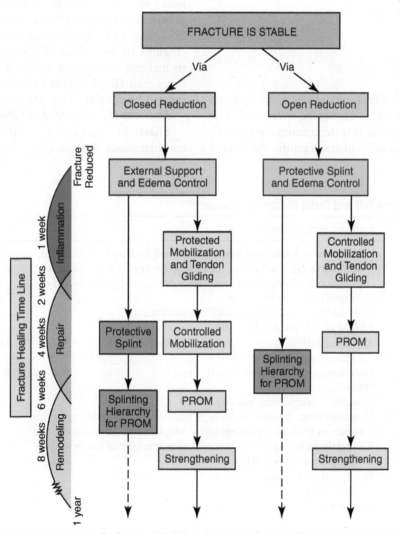

Figure 10-11 Algorithm for therapeutic management of a fracture. *PROM,* passive range of motion. (From LaStayo PC, Winters KM, Hardy M: Fracture healing: bone healing, fracture management and current concepts related to the hand, *J Hand Ther* 16:90, Copyright © Paul LaStayo, PhD, PT, CHT, 2003.)

Factors That Delay Healing

- Infection
- Prolonged steroid use
- Diabetes
- Anemia
- Osteopenia
- Use of alcohol, nicotine, or caffeine

The combined impact of soft tissue injury and the effects of immobilization creates challenges for both the treating physician and the therapist. Immobilization can cause a reduction in spacing and lubrication among collagen fibers, leading to reduced soft tissue gliding, shortening, and contracture development.[22] Muscle atrophy, with decreased extensibility and motion loss, is another documented effect of immobilization.[23]

Effects of Prolonged Immobilization

- Reduced soft tissue glide
- Soft tissue contracture
- Muscle atrophy
- Motion loss

The importance of direct communication between the surgeon and the therapist cannot be overstated. The most important information that determines the rehabilitation strategy is the stability of the fracture. Additional information that is significant for determining a therapeutic approach includes the type and location of the fracture and the fixation method or methods used to stabilize it.

Fractures of the Distal Phalanx. Rehabilitation guidelines for fractures of the distal phalanx can be found in Table 10-1. Therapeutic considerations are presented, taking into account the stage of healing and whether the fracture has been fixated (Figure 10-12).

Mallet Finger. Treatment of a bony mallet injury consists of continuous splint immobilization of the DIP joint in extension for 6 to 8 weeks (Figure 10-13). Care should be taken to avoid skin blanching on the dorsum of the finger with forced hyperextension. The remaining joints of the finger are left free. Immobilization promotes healing and scarring of the terminal tendon. Skin checks should be performed during the immobilization period to prevent complications from skin breakdown. Care should be taken to keep the DIP joint in full extension during skin checks.

Gentle active motion is initiated around week 8. Splinting is continued when the patient is not exercising. Blocking exercises (i.e., limited movement at one joint) should be avoided until week 10 to protect the oblique retinacular ligament (ORL) from stretching (the ORL assists in DIP extension with the PIP in extension) (Figures 10-14 and 10-15). Stretching and strengthening to increase motion are initiated at week 12. If a lag of more than 10° persists at week 8, continuous static splinting can be continued through week 16.[24]

Fractures of the Proximal and Middle Phalanges

Shaft Fractures. Table 10-2 presents details and considerations the clinician should keep in mind when

TABLE **10-1**

Rehabilitation Guidelines for Tuft and Distal Phalanx Fractures[24–27]

Healing Stages	Fractures Without Fixation	Fractures with Fixation
Stage I: Inflammatory stage (weeks 0 to 2)	Wound care and dressing changes: If the nail bed has been repaired, sterile dressing changes may be required every 24 hours using a gauze-covered petroleum or nonstick dressing (e.g., Xeroform or Adaptic) over the injury site Static and resting splint with DIP immobilization AROM of PIP and MCP joints	Fixation for 3 weeks Static resting splint to protect the fixation
Stage II: Fibroplasia and repair stage (weeks 2 to 4)	AROM of DIP joint Edema management is required Light functional tasks may be performed Splint is discontinued Protective padding with silicone is used Desensitization: Because of the high number of nerve endings in this region of the finger, patients often complain of cold sensitivity and hypesthesia for a prolonged period after this type of injury Blocking exercises for DIP joint	AROM of uninvolved joints Week 3: Progress as stage II of tuft fracture without fixation
Stage III: Remodeling and maturation stage (weeks 4 to 6+)	Functional progression Strengthening Splinting to increase motion	Functional progression Strengthening Splinting to increase motion

DIP, Distal interphalangeal; *AROM,* active range of motion; *PIP,* proximal interphalangeal; *MCP,* metacarpophalangeal.

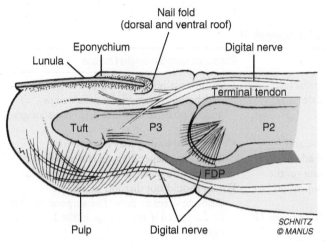

Figure 10-12 Schematic of the distal phalanx. The distal phalanx often is referred to as *P3*, the middle phalanx as *P2*, and the proximal phalanx *(not shown)* as *P1*. *FDP,* flexor digitorum profundus. (From Cannon NM: Rehabilitation approaches for distal and middle phalanx fractures of the hand, *J Hand Ther* 16:105-116, 2003.)

working with patients who have sustained proximal and middle phalanx fractures (Figures 10-16 to 10-18).

Articular and Periarticular Fractures. Initiation of motion after ORIF or percutaneous pinning of unicondylar and bicondylar fractures depends on the stability of the fragments after surgery.

With an early AROM program, a forearm-based dorsal block splint is fabricated for protection and worn for up to 6 weeks. Positioning within the splint may vary, depending on the injured structures and the surgical repair procedure. An AROM program begins on postoperative days 3 to 5, with the affected finger buddy-taped to the adjacent finger or fingers to prevent lateral or rotary stresses to the joint. Motion parameters differ, depending on the stability of the fracture and bony fixation. Limitations in both terminal flexion and extension may be necessary to protect the healing structures. Advancement in 10° increments per week should be done if the initial motion has been restricted. PROM, stretching, splinting for motion,

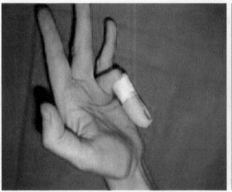

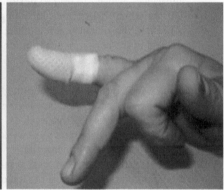

Figure 10-13 Custom splint for mallet finger. Similar prefabricated splints are available in a variety of designs and in the choice of thermoplastic materials used. A variation of the design shown is a simple clamshell splint in which thin perforated splinting material is brought up and around the tip of the finger, providing both dorsal and volar support to the DIP in extension. Although the middle phalanx is enclosed in the splint, the PIP joint is left free to move. If splinting materials are not available, a similar splint can be formed using aluminum strips covered with foam. In each case, strapping or tape around the middle phalanx portion of the splint is required for stability. Maintaining skin integrity is a prime concern with any type of splint. (From Tocco S, Boccolari P, Landi A et al: Effectiveness of cast immobilization in comparison to the gold standard self-removal orthotic intervention for closed mallet fingers: A randomized clinical trial, *J Hand Ther* 26:191-201, 2013.)

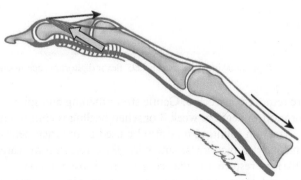

Figure 10-14 The ORL *(arrow)* arises from the volar lateral ridge of the distal tip of the middle phalanx and courses distally and dorsally to attach to the terminal tendon. (Redrawn from Tubiana R: *The hand,* Philadelphia, 1981, WB Saunders.)

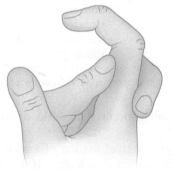

Figure 10-15 Blocking of the metacarpophalangeal (MCP) joint in extension. **Note:** If the proximal interphalangeal (PIP) joint is blocked in extension and the distal interphalangeal (DIP) joint is flexed, a stretch is placed on the oblique retinacular ligament (ORL) which should be avoided until week 10. (From Skirven TM, Osterman AL, Fedorczyk JM: *Rehabilitation of the hand and upper extremity,* ed 6, Philadelphia, Mosby, 2011.)

TABLE **10-2**

Rehabilitation Guidelines for Fractures of the Proximal and Middle Phalanges[27-30]

Healing Stages	Fractures with Rigid Fixation	Fractures with Semirigid Fixation
Stage I: Inflammatory stage (weeks 0 to 2)	AROM is initiated on postoperative day 5 (pain level should be kept under 5 on a 1-10 pain scale) Edema management Soft tissue mobilization Splinting is done in the intrinsic plus position and includes the adjacent finger or fingers for added stability (hand or forearm based, depending on the fracture's site and stability and the patient profile) (see Figure 10-16) In the intrinsic plus position (MCP joint: 70° flexion; IP joints, straight): • Intrinsic muscles are placed at rest, reducing forces to the proximal phalanx • The extensor hood glides distally, providing compressive stability to a fracture of the proximal phalanx • The IP joints are held in extension, reducing force imbalances, which can lead to flexion contracture • The periarticular structures, including the MCP collaterals, the IP collaterals, and the PIP volar plate, are held in the optimum position for preventing flexion contracture	Fixation usually is removed at 3-4 weeks; midshaft fractures of the proximal or middle phalanx may take 1-2 weeks longer to heal Casting or splinting may be used for 3-6 weeks, depending on the stability of the fracture in the intrinsic plus position Forces should not disrupt, loosen, or dislodge wires or pins. The surgeon should be contacted if any change in the hardware occurs
Stage II: Fibroplasia and repair stage (weeks 2 to 4)	Tendon gliding exercises Blocking for differential flexor tendon gliding and extensor tendon excursion (see Figure 10-17) Light functional tasks begin at week 4 Protective splinting continues until week 6 Protective splinting or buddy taping for sports or high-level activity may be indicated until week 8, depending on the stability of the fracture	After 3-6 weeks of immobilization in a cast or splint: • AROM is initiated (with fractures of the middle phalanx, the pull of the FDS can put stress on the fracture fragments; therefore *gentle* AROM is indicated) • Protective splint in the intrinsic plus position is fabricated for wear between exercises and is used until week 6-8 • Light functional tasks are begun at week 4
Stage III: Remodeling and maturation stage (weeks 4 to 6+)	Functional progression Stretching Strengthening begins after fracture healing is confirmed at 6-8 weeks Splinting to increase motion (see Figure 10-18) Dynamic and/or static progressive splinting can be initiated at week 6 when healing is confirmed. Studies have shown the positive effects of prolonged stretching of a stiff joint and presented considerations for choosing dynamic versus static progressive splinting[31-34]	Functional progression Stretching Strengthening begins after fracture healing is confirmed at 6-8 weeks Splinting to increase motion

AROM, Active range of motion; *MCP*, metacarpophalangeal; *IP*, interphalangeal; *PIP*, proximal interphalangeal; *FDS*, flexor digitorum superficialis.

and strengthening occur at 8 weeks or when healing is confirmed.[30]

With hinged external fixation of a pilon fracture, motion is initiated within 3 to 5 days. If the external fixator does not lock into extension, a static resting extension finger splint is fabricated, and the patient wears it at all times when not exercising. The resting splint is removed for AROM exercises in the clinic and 3 to 5 times daily as a home program (Figure 10-19). External fixators generally

are removed at week 6. Gentle strengthening and splinting for motion begin at week 8 or when healing is confirmed.

Traction splinting may also be used in the treatment of unicondylar, bicondylar, and pilon fractures. In some cases, ORIF to restore articular congruency is used in combination with traction splinting. The traction splint is fabricated using an outrigger. Outriggers can be custom fabricated or prefabricated. The finger is attached to the outrigger, which is designed to provide consistent traction to the PIP joint

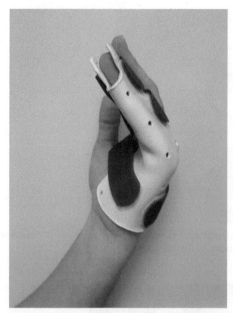

Figure 10-16 Hand-based ulnar gutter static resting splint in the intrinsic plus position: MCP joints in 70° flexion; PIP and DIP joints, extended.

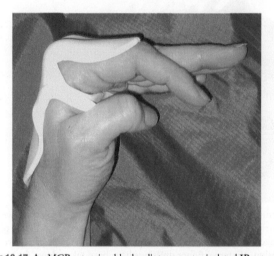

Figure 10-17 An MCP extension block splint promotes isolated IP extension.

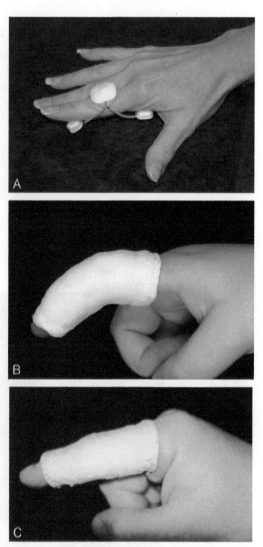

Figure 10-18 Rehabilitation for proximal phalangeal fractures. Dynamic splinting (**A**), serial casting (**B**), and static progressive splinting (**C**) can be used to regain PIP extension and IP flexion. (**A,** From Canale ST, Beaty JH: *Campbell's operative orthopaedics,* ed 12, Philadelphia, 2013, Mosby. **B,** From Tang JB, Amadio PC, Guimberteau JC et al: *Tendon surgery of the hand,* Philadelphia, 2012, Saunders. **C,** From Freeland AE, Hardy MA, Singletary S: Rehabilitation for proximal phalangeal fractures, *J Hand Ther* 16:129-142, 2003.)

through an arc of motion. The traction reduces the fracture fragments through ligamentotaxis and restores optimal joint space for tissue healing and gliding (Figure 10-20). The optimal traction and motion parameters vary, depending on the fracture. Imaging and a tension gauge are used to measure appropriate traction on the tissues within a safe range. The splint usually is removed at week 6. After removal of the splint, a program of edema management, AROM and PROM exercises, differential tendon gliding, and stretching is initiated. Gentle strengthening and splinting for motion begins at week 8 or when healing is confirmed.[30] Management of fractures with external fixators or traction splinting requires direct, consistent communication with the physician. The risk of infection is a complication with external fixation or traction splinting.

Complications of fractures of the proximal and middle phalanges include soft tissue adherence of the flexor and extensor tendons. Moreover, the imbalance in strength between the flexor and extensor tendon forces creates an initial extensor lag (inability to fully extend actively). This lag can lead to a chronic flexion contracture of the PIP joint (Figure 10-21).[30]

Metacarpal Fractures

General Considerations

The metacarpals support the phalanges, ensuring the proper length for optimal function and balance between the extrinsic and intrinsic tendons of the hand. They also provide for the origin of the intrinsic muscles and the mobility

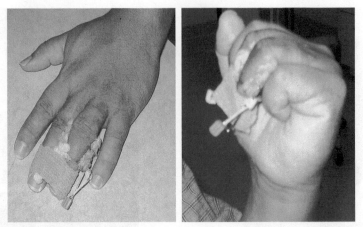

Figure 10-19 A pilon fracture of the ring finger is stabilized with finger-based dynamic external fixation, which allows for active PIP flexion and extension at day 3. The ring finger is buddy-taped to the long finger to provide increased stability to the PIP joint.

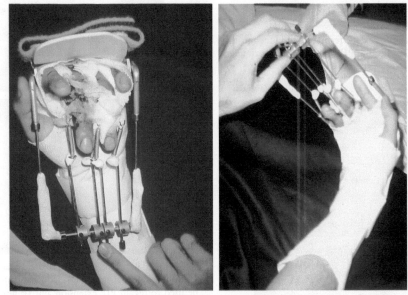

Figure 10-20 Custom-fabricated traction splint for traumatic PIP intra-articular fractures of the middle and ring fingers. This type of splint allows flexion and extension of the PIP joints. The fingers are attached to a custom-made outrigger by means of springs, which are hooked to surgically placed K-wires that exit through the skin from the middle phalanx, providing consistent traction through the available range of motion. The patient rests at night against the dorsal protective hood with the PIP and DIP strapped into extension. (External finger dressings have been taken down for clarity.)

obtained at the carpometacarpal and metacarpophalangeal joints. A change in the normal length and alignment of the metacarpals as a result of injury must be recognized and treated to prevent a loss in hand function. Fractures of the metacarpals account for up to one third of hand fractures, and fifth metacarpal fractures account for more than 50% of metacarpal fractures.[35] The goal of treatment is to regain stability with enough osseous length for correct tendon balance and to prevent the complications of soft tissue injury, tendon adhesion, and malalignment.

Anatomy

The anatomy of the metacarpals, specifically their articulations and muscle attachments, directly affects the injury pattern and the management of these fractures. The index and middle finger metacarpals articulate with the trapezoid and capitate bones, respectively. These carpometacarpal (CMC) joints have very little motion. The ulnar two metacarpals articulate with the hamate bone, which, with its relatively flat articular surface, allows for substantial motion both in flexion and extension and to a lesser degree in rotation. Because these metacarpals align with a joint allowing considerable motion in the plane of flexion and extension, more fracture malalignment can be accepted on this side of the hand. Deformity is much more obvious and difficult to compensate for in the two radial metacarpals, where little to no motion occurs at the CMC joints.

The deforming forces that displace metacarpal fractures are related to the crossing extrinsic tendons and the attachments of the intrinsic musculature. The intrinsic hand muscles, including the palmar and dorsal interossei, originate on the metacarpal shafts. The lumbrical muscles,

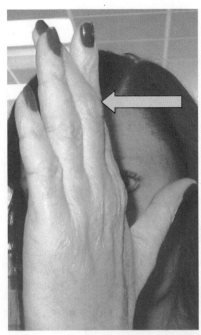

Figure 10-21 Flexion contracture of the long finger PIP joint.

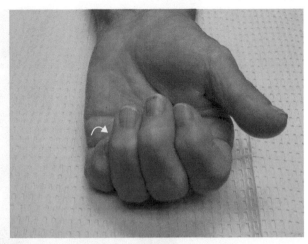

Figure 10-22 Malrotation of the little finger, caused by a metacarpal fracture, is best appreciated during active finger flexion. (From Skirven TM, Osterman AL, Fedorczyk JM: *Rehabilitation of the hand and upper extremity,* ed 6, Philadelphia, 2011, Mosby.)

originating from the tendons of the flexor digitorum profundi and the interossei, are the primary flexors of the MCP joint. The metacarpal bones act as a fulcrum for digital motion by stabilizing the phalanges against the pull of the flexor and extensor tendons. When these bones are fractured, the resulting disruption causes an imbalance in these forces, leading to specific patterns of deformity.

Diagnosis

Fractures of the metacarpal shaft generally are caused by a fall or direct blow to the hand. Neck fractures, particularly those of the fourth and fifth metacarpals, are the result of an axial load, such as when a fist strikes a hard surface. Areas of edema, ecchymosis, and tenderness should alert the examiner to the potential for an underlying fracture and should be thoroughly examined. Clinical suspicion should be increased if the patient has a gross deformity over the dorsum of the hand, loss of normal knuckle height or contour, and an alteration in the rotational alignment of the digits.

Rotational malalignment is best appreciated in digital flexion, and the injured finger or fingers should be examined under AROM, with use of a digital block if pain is limiting the evaluation (Figure 10-22). PROM is not reliable because the examiner may inadvertently alter the digital rotation while flexing the digit. Tenodesis active motion is better than PROM for an uncooperative patient who cannot actively range the digits. The clinician also must ensure the patient does not use an adjacent finger to "capture" and hold the affected digit "in alignment." The results of the examination should be compared with the findings for the contralateral hand. Plain x-ray films, including AP, lateral, and oblique views, are necessary to evaluate most metacarpal fractures, and special views occasionally are required (e.g., Brewerton, 20° pronation).

Injury Classification and Medical Treatment

General Principles. Metacarpal fractures usually are discussed in terms of the location of the fracture, the pattern of the fracture, and the resulting deformity. Fractures can occur at the level of the metacarpal base, shaft, neck, or head. The pattern that results usually is secondary to the mechanism of injury; the fracture may be transverse, oblique, spiral, or comminuted (Figure 10-23). A direct blow usually produces a transverse fracture, whereas torsion of the digit causes a spiral or oblique fracture. Comminuted fractures result from higher energy injuries. Fracture deformity is described relative to changes in angulation, rotation, or length. Malrotation is problematic because, if not corrected, it may interfere with flexion of the adjacent fingers (referred to as *scissoring*). Malrotation of as little as 5° may cause 1.5 cm (0.6 inch) of digital overlap with flexion of the fingers.[36,37] An uncorrected angular deformity of the metacarpal shaft (usually a flexion deformity) not only results in a cosmetic concern; if severe enough, it may cause hyperextension at the MCP joint with resultant flexion at the PIP joint (e.g., clawing) (Figure 10-24). Metacarpal fractures with significant shortening may cause an imbalance of the intrinsic and extrinsic tendons with subsequent loss of full motion.

Management Approach. The management of a patient with a metacarpal fracture depends on a variety of factors. The location of the fracture, degree of displacement, angulation, and rotation all influence the acceptability of fracture alignment and also predict the likelihood that the injury will proceed to further displacement. The patient's age, occupation, general health, and concomitant injuries also must be considered.

Transverse fractures with minimal displacement usually have little potential for further displacement and are relatively stable. Treatment usually is nonoperative, consisting of immobilization in a plaster splint or cast for 3 to 4 weeks.[38] Displaced and unstable transverse fractures can be treated

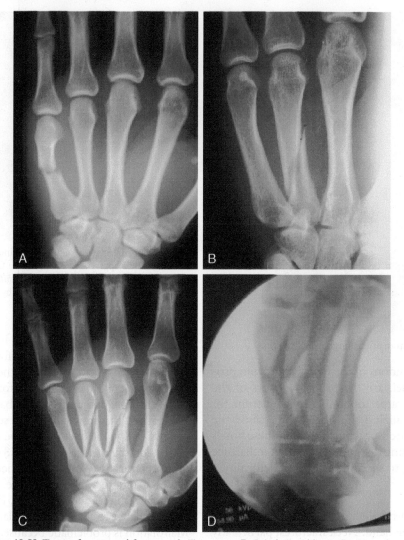

Figure 10-23 Types of metacarpal fractures. **A,** Transverse. **B,** Spiral. **C,** Oblique. **D,** Comminuted.

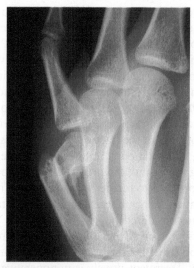

Figure 10-24 Oblique x-ray film showing the secondary claw deformity that occurs at the MCP joint as a result of a flexion deformity of the metacarpal shaft at the site of the fracture.

with closed reduction and splinting or closed reduction and percutaneous pin fixation, depending on the perceived fracture stability at the time of evaluation and reduction.

Oblique and spiral fractures with a minimal amount of shortening and no malrotation can be treated nonoperatively with casting or splinting. If any malrotation or significant shortening is present, open reduction and fixation with interfragmentary lag screws is indicated. Short fracture lines may need the additional stability of a dorsal plate for resistance to torsional and bending stresses. Fractures of the index and small finger metacarpals have less inherent stability because they lack the suspensory effect of the intermetacarpal ligaments; therefore these fractures may benefit from the added stability of plate fixation.

Specific Metacarpal Fractures

Metacarpal Head Fractures. Fractures of the metacarpal head are a rare injury. They often are the result of an axial load or direct trauma, and they generally are intra-articular. These fractures can be classified in terms of their descriptive characteristics: epiphyseal, ligamentous avulsion, osteochondral, comminuted, and compression fractures. Treatment of metacarpal head fractures is individually based on the type of fracture and the degree of displacement. Nondisplaced fractures are stable and can be treated with a short course of immobilization. Noncomminuted fractures with more than 1 mm of articular displacement or with joint surface involvement greater than 25% likely will require operative fixation in the form of ORIF using K-wires, interfragmentary screws, or headless screws.[39] Fractures that involve ligamentous avulsion and displaced osteochondral fragments can also be treated with open reduction and internal fixation (Figure 10-25). Comminuted intra-articular metacarpal fractures usually are the result of a higher energy injury. This makes them difficult to manage because of the surrounding soft tissue injury, the degree of bone loss, and the presence of small bony fragments. Treatment options include immobilization, ligamentotaxis through placement of an external fixator, or primary or secondary joint arthroplasty if the degree of bone loss and fragmentation prevents adequate reduction and stabilization.

Metacarpal Neck Fractures. Fractures of the metacarpal neck are common and usually occur in the ring and small fingers. The mechanism of injury commonly involves a flexed MCP joint striking a solid object, causing a neck fracture with apex dorsal angulation. This pattern of angulation occurs because the traumatic impact causes volar comminution at the level of the neck and also because the intrinsic muscles maintain the metacarpal head in a flexed position, leading to apex dorsal angulation. The CMC joints in the ring and small fingers allow more mobility than the CMC joints in the index and middle fingers, and they therefore compensate for a larger degree of angular deformity. The amount of angulation that

can be tolerated without functional impairment varies throughout the orthopedic literature, ranging from 20° to 60° in the small metacarpal and 10° to 40° in the ring metacarpal.[40-42] Malrotation of a metacarpal neck fracture cannot be tolerated because it will affect the flexion ability of the other fingers and impair the ability to grip.

Treatment of metacarpal neck fractures depends on the stability of the fracture and whether a reduction will hold the fracture within the acceptable range of alignment. Closed reduction may be attempted, with subsequent immobilization. If the fracture remains reduced and stable and has no associated malrotation, immobilization may be the definitive treatment. If the reduction cannot be maintained because of fracture instability or comminution or if an unacceptable degree of angulation or rotation is present, closed reduction and fixation with K-wires or open reduction with plate and screw constructs may be necessary (Figure 10-26).

Metacarpal Shaft Fractures. Fractures of the metacarpal shaft are common injuries, and the management of these fractures must take into account several factors, including the fracture pattern, the degree of displacement, and the overall stability of the fracture.

Transverse fractures usually are caused by a direct blow or an axial load. Because of the deforming force of the intrinsic muscles, these fractures tend to fall into apex dorsal angulation. As with metacarpal neck fractures, a certain degree of angulation can be tolerated without compromising hand function. More deformity is tolerated in the small and ring finger metacarpals because of the larger degree of motion at their CMC joints. Angulation of the index and middle metacarpal shafts is not as well tolerated because of the limited motion at these CMC joints. The acceptable degree of angulation is the subject of debate in orthopedic literature. The acceptable degree of angulation for the ring and small finger metacarpals ranges from less

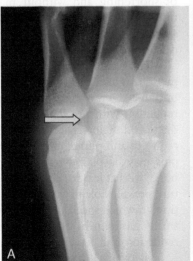 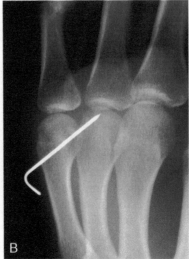

Figure 10-25 Osteochondral avulsion fracture (**A**) involving the ulnar collateral ligament and part of the articular surface in a thin section of bone fixed with a K-wire (**B**).

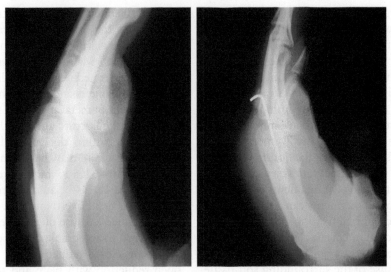

Figure 10-26 Preoperative and postoperative lateral x-ray films of a transverse displaced fracture of the fifth metacarpal. Note that in the preoperative view *(left)*, the metacarpal head does not align with the other metacarpals nor along the shaft of the fifth metacarpal, as it does in the postoperative view *(right)* after reduction and pinning.

than 20° to 40°, whereas the acceptable angulation for the index and middle metacarpals ranges from 0° to 10°.[38,43,44] Excess angulation causes prominence of the metacarpal head in the palm, which can make gripping uncomfortable; it also results in hyperextension of the MCP joint, causing limited MCP joint flexion and loss of grip.

Oblique and spiral fractures typically are caused by a torsional load. If these fractures are unstable, they tend to cause a rotational deformity. The presence of any degree of malrotation, regardless of the specific metacarpal involved, warrants reduction and stabilization; otherwise, the fingers will overlap, causing problems with digital flexion.

Comminuted fractures usually are caused by a high-energy force and often are associated with significant soft tissue injury. The clinician must include the integrity of the skin and soft tissue envelope as part of the treatment algorithm when determining management options. Comminuted fractures tend to cause shortening of the metacarpal because of the multiple small bone fragments and the overall unstable fracture pattern. Shortening of the metacarpals results in an imbalance of forces and compromised function of the flexor and extensor mechanisms. For every 2 mm of shortening, a 7° extensor lag of the MCP joint results.[45] The degree of acceptable shortening for metacarpal fractures is somewhat controversial, ranging from 3 to 6 mm in the orthopedic literature.[46-48]

Management of metacarpal shaft fractures is based on the degree of displacement, including angulation, malrotation, and shortening, and the stability of the fracture. In essence, the clinician needs to determine whether the fracture is acceptably aligned and whether it is likely to remain that way if treated by closed techniques.

For minimally displaced, stable fractures, nonoperative management with cast or splint immobilization is adequate treatment. However, surgical intervention is warranted if the fracture is unstable, if the resulting deformity compromises function, and in some cases when the concomitant injury necessitates correction. The surgical options for shaft fractures include transosseous percutaneous or open K-wire fixation, cerclage wires, intramedullary wire fixation, interfragmentary screws, plate fixation, and external fixation (Figure 10-27).

Transverse fractures with minimal displacement usually have little potential to further displace and are relatively stable. Treatment usually is nonoperative, consisting of immobilization in a plaster splint or cast for 3 to 4 weeks.[38] If the degree of angulation is unacceptable or the reduction cannot be maintained by nonoperative methods, operative fixation is warranted.

Oblique and spiral fractures with a minimal amount of shortening and without malrotation can be treated nonoperatively with casting or splinting. If malrotation, significant shortening, or instability is present, open reduction and fixation are necessary.

Metacarpal shaft fractures with significant displacement, angulation, rotation, or shortening that are still unstable after reduction attempts require either closed reduction with percutaneous pin placement or open reduction and internal fixation. Fractures may be closed, reduced, and pinned directly through the fracture site, or pins may be placed transversely through the metacarpal bone, with at least one proximal and one distal to the fracture site. Flexible intramedullary nail fixation is also an option, in which special rods or K-wires are placed through a small incision near the base of the metacarpal. The closed reduction and fixation technique is beneficial because it is less invasive than open management; however, controlling the rotation of the distal fragment is difficult with this method. Open reduction allows direct control of the

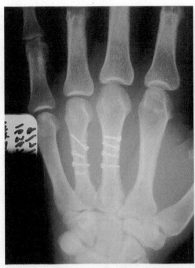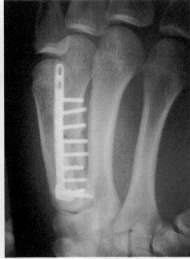

Figure 10-27 Previously seen as Figure 10-23, *C* and *D*, these oblique and comminuted fractures were treated with different operative techniques. The long oblique fractures *(left)* are amenable to interfragmentary screw fixation, which allows early range of motion with little interference from hardware. The more unstable comminuted fracture *(right)* requires the plate for rigidity. This allows early range of motion, but the hardware sometimes interferes with gliding structures.

bone and the potential for perfect anatomical restoration, albeit at the cost of increased trauma to the soft tissue envelope in the surgical approach. Also, rigid fixation may be obtained with interfragmentary compression screws or a plate and screw construct, allowing for earlier return to motion. With an open fracture or an injury with significant bone loss or contamination of the soft tissue envelope surrounding the metacarpal shaft, the best course of action is to rigidly stabilize the skeleton with the least trauma to the surrounding soft tissues. Often this can be accomplished most readily with external fixation.

Metacarpal Base Fractures. Fractures of the base of the metacarpal are often intra-articular and frequently are associated with subluxation or frank dislocation of the CMC joint. This fracture pattern is far less common in the index and middle finger metacarpals because of the tight bony geometry and firm ligamentous support at these CMC joints. On the ulnar side of the hand, an axially directed force causes a fracture of the metacarpal base, along with a proximal and dorsal subluxation of the fourth and fifth metacarpals relative to their articulation with the hamate. This fracture-dislocation can be difficult to visualize on plain AP or lateral x-ray films, and suspicion for this injury should alert the clinician to the need for 30° rotated x-ray views or possibly a computed tomography (CT) scan. This fracture is inherently unstable, and if it goes unrecognized or ignored, it may result in articular surface incongruity and possibly weakened grip strength and arthrosis.[49] These fractures may be treated with closed reduction and percutaneous pinning, but if reduction is difficult or inadequate, ORIF is indicated (Figure 10-28).

Thumb Metacarpal Fractures. The thumb accounts for 40% of hand function, and total disability of the thumb

results in a loss of 22% of bodily function.[50] Fractures of the thumb metacarpal are common, accounting for 25% of all metacarpal fractures.[51] Thumb metacarpal fractures have the same type of classification and management options as the other types of metacarpal fractures, and the treatment of head, neck, and shaft fractures usually is similar to that for the digits. More angulation and rotation are tolerated in thumb metacarpal shaft fractures because of the large degree of compensatory motion at the thumb CMC joint.

Fractures of the thumb metacarpal base deserve unique consideration because of the frequency of intra-articular extension and the association of these fractures with CMC joint subluxation or frank dislocation. In order of increasing fracture fragmentation and instability, these fractures are **Bennett's fracture**, **Rolando's fracture**, and intra-articular comminuted fractures. The mechanism of injury is the same; all are the result of an axial load applied through a partially flexed metacarpal shaft. Bennett's fracture is a two-part fracture involving an avulsion of the thumb metacarpal from the volar ulnar aspect of the metacarpal base. The ligament attached to this fragment, the volar oblique ligament, keeps the small avulsed fracture fragment aligned to the joint while the remainder of the metacarpal shaft is subluxed. The deforming forces that create the subluxation include the thumb extensors, the abductor pollicis longus (APL), and the adductor pollicis longus. The pull of these muscles results in a dorsal, radial, and proximal subluxation of the thumb metacarpal shaft. Rolando's fracture is similar to Bennett's fracture, except that the metacarpal is broken into three pieces instead of two. An intra-articular comminuted fracture has additional fracture components and therefore is more difficult to treat. Because of strong deforming forces and bony

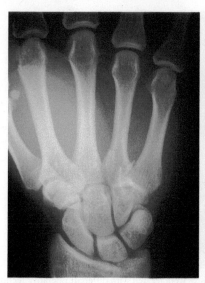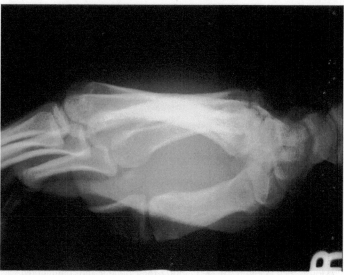

Figure 10-28 AP and lateral x-ray views of a fracture-dislocation of the fifth CMC joint. On the AP view, note the inability to see the joint space between the base of the metacarpal and the hamate, as well as the loss of the normal height cascade of the metacarpals. The lateral view shows the dorsal displacement of the base of the fifth metacarpal compared with the rest of the hand.

instability, these injuries tend to displace and therefore require operative fixation. The disrupted articular congruity may hasten the onset of post traumatic arthritis, which can lead to pain and functional compromise.

Thumb metacarpal fractures often are difficult to manage because of the degree of displacement and the involvement of the articular surface. The degree of articular incongruity that is acceptable without predisposing a patient to symptomatic post traumatic arthritis is the subject of controversy. Some authors believe that the articular surface must be restored as anatomically as possible (within 1 mm),[52,53] whereas others believe that good outcomes result with articular surface incongruity up to 2 mm.[54] When closed reduction can produce restoration of the articular surface, K-wires may be used to secure the reduction. If the articular surface remains significantly displaced after attempted reduction, open reduction and fixation are indicated to maintain length, using lag screws, plates, K-wires, or possibly an external fixator.

Rehabilitation of Metacarpal Fractures

Therapeutic intervention for metacarpal fractures differs, depending on the location and stability of the fracture. The progression of rehabilitation is determined by bony healing (see Figure 10-11). The major complication of these fractures is adherence of soft tissues as a result of injury, immobilization, and persistent edema. Soft tissues can adhere to extrinsic tendons, intrinsic muscles, and periarticular structures. Reduction of soft tissue glide can result in a lag and contractures at the MCP joint and secondarily at the PIP joint. The primary goals of rehabilitation are to restore and optimize soft tissue balance and glide, allowing pain-free motion and strength, while protecting the healing tissues (Tables 10-3 and 10-4).

Splinting Guidelines. Splinting is an essential element of the optimal management of metacarpal fractures. Guidelines for appropriate splinting vary, depending on the particular metacarpal fractured.

TABLE **10-3**

Rehabilitation Guidelines for Fractures of the Second Through Fifth Metacarpals[27,30,55–57]

Healing Stages	Fractures with Rigid Fixation*	Fractures with Semirigid Fixation†
Stage I: Inflammatory stage (weeks 0 to 2)	AROM tendon gliding exercises are initiated on postoperative day 5 (pain level should be kept under 5 on a 1-10 pain scale) Edema management Soft tissue mobilization Scar management with silicone Splinting	Casting or splinting for 3-6 weeks, depending on fracture stability, in the forearm-based intrinsic plus position

(Continued)

TABLE **10-3**

Rehabilitation Guidelines for Fractures of the Second Through Fifth Metacarpals—Cont'd

Healing Stages	Fractures with Rigid Fixation*	Fractures with Semirigid Fixation†
Stage II: Fibroplasia and repair stage (weeks 2 to 4)	Gentle blocking for flexor and extensor pull-through, including isolated EDC exercises and soft tissue mobilization of the scar	After 3-6 weeks of immobilization in a cast or splint: • AROM and tendon gliding are started • Gentle blocking and isolated EDC pull-through exercises are started • Protective hand-based splint in the intrinsic plus position (IP joints may or may not be included) is fabricated for use between exercises and is worn until week 6-8 • Hand-based ulnar gutter or radial gutter splint that leaves the MCP joints free is indicated for stable shaft and base fractures
Stage III: Remodeling and maturation stage (weeks 4 to 6+)	Week 4: Splint is reduced to a hand-based protective splint for use between exercises; it is worn until week 6 Protective splint for sports or high-level activity may be worn until week 8: • Protective, hand-based ulnar gutter or radial gutter splint with MCP joints included at 70° to 90° flexion, IP joints free • Hand-based ulnar gutter or radial gutter splint with MCP joints free is indicated for stable shaft and base fractures Light functional tasks are initiated Functional progression: high-level activities may be limited until week 8 Stretching begins for all tissues, including the intrinsics Strengthening begins after fracture healing is confirmed at weeks 6-8 Splinting to increase motion begins at weeks 6-8	Protective splint for sports or high-level activity may be worn until week 8 Light functional tasks begin at week 4 Functional progression: high-level activities may be limited until week 8 Stretching, including intrinsic stretching Splinting to increase motion begins at week 6, when healing is confirmed Strengthening begins after fracture healing is confirmed at weeks 6-8

AROM, Active range of motion; *EDC*, extensor digitorum communis; *IP*, interphalangeal; *MCP*, metacarpophalangeal.

*Fixation may or may not be removed.

†Fixation is removed at 3-4 weeks.

TABLE **10-4**

Rehabilitation Guidelines for Fractures of the First Metacarpal[27,30,55–57]

Healing Stages	Fractures with Rigid Fixation*	Fractures with Semirigid Fixation†
Stage I: Inflammatory stage (weeks 0 to 2)	Head and shaft fractures: AROM of the thumb IP joint and tendon gliding exercises of the FPL and EPL are initiated on postoperative day 5 if the surgeon has confirmed the stability of the fracture. The pain level should be kept under 5 on a 1-10 scale IP joint should not be moved if the fracture is unstable Base fractures: IP joint is immobilized for 2 weeks to prevent stress force to the CMC joint unless stability is confirmed by the surgeon Splinting (see splinting guidelines for thumb metacarpal fractures)	Casting or splinting for 3-6 weeks, depending on fracture stability, in a forearm-based opponens splint or thumb spica cast

(Continued)

TABLE **10-4**

Rehabilitation Guidelines for Fractures of the First Metacarpal—Cont'd

Healing Stages	Fractures with Rigid Fixation*	Fractures with Semirigid Fixation†
Stage II: Fibroplasia and repair stage (weeks 2 to 4)	AROM of IP joint continues or is initiated, based on fracture stability and stress-loading considerations for the CMC joint (with base fractures)	After 3-6 weeks of immobilization with a cast or splint: • AROM and tendon gliding: Blocking and isolated EPL and FPL pull-through exercises • Protective, hand-based short opponens splint with the IP joint free, to be used between exercises and worn until weeks 6-8
Stage III: Remodeling and maturation stage (weeks 4 to 6+)	Stable fractures: Splint may be reduced to a hand-based short opponens protective splint that is used between exercises and worn until weeks 6-8 Protective splinting for sports or high-level activity may be indicated until week 8 Light functional tasks are initiated Splinting for motion begins at week 6 Strengthening begins when healing is confirmed at approximately weeks 6-8 Functional progression	Light functional tasks begin at week 4 Functional progression Stretching Splinting to increase motion begins at week 6 Strengthening begins after fracture healing is confirmed at weeks 6-8

AROM, Active range of motion; *IP,* interphalangeal; *FPL,* flexor pollicis longus; *EPL,* extensor pollicis longus; *CMC,* carpometacarpal.

*Fixation may or may not be removed.
†Fixation is removed at 3-4 weeks.

Guidelines for Splinting Fractures of the Second through Fifth Metacarpals[26,30,56,58]

- The splint design is based on the location and stability of the fracture and the patient profile, including the individual's compliance with fracture healing precautions and activity level (Figures 10-29 and 10-30)
- The adjacent digit is included for added stabilization and to prevent rotational forces
- A circumferential splint is used (e.g., ulnar or radial gutter splint)
- For fractures of the metacarpal head, the forearm-based intrinsic plus position is used (i.e., wrist, 0° to 20° extension; MCP joints, 70° to 90° flexion; interphalangeal [IP] joints, 0° extension)*
- For fractures of the metacarpal neck, shaft, or base, a forearm-based splint is used with the wrist in 0° to 20° extension, the MCP joints flexed 70° to 90°, and the IP joints left free[30,56]
- For a stable shaft fracture, a three-point stabilization splint is used. This is a hand-based circumferential splint with counterforces that stabilize the fracture site. The involved finger is buddy-taped to the adjacent finger to prevent rotational forces to the fracture site[58]

*The intrinsic plus position (MCP joint flexed 70°, IP joints in 0° extension) allows the intrinsic muscles to relax, reducing forces on the proximal phalanx. The extensor hood glides distally, providing compressive stability to the metacarpal head fracture. The IP joints are held in extension, reducing force imbalances, which can lead to flexion contractures. The periarticular structures, including the MCP joint collaterals, the IP collaterals, and the PIP volar plate, are held in the optimum position to prevent a flexion contracture.[26]

Guidelines for Splinting Fractures of the First Metacarpal[26,30,55,56]

- The splint design is based on the location and stability of the fracture and the patient profile, including the individual's compliance with fracture healing precautions and activity level
- The design should prevent first web contracture
- The splint is circumferential, passing around the thumb, and is forearm based, as in a long-opponens splint
- For fractures of the head, shaft, or base, a long-opponens splint that includes the IP joint is used. IP motion is allowed after fracture stability has been confirmed by imaging

LIGAMENT INJURIES OF THE HAND

Ligament Injuries of the Digits

General Considerations

Stretching and tearing of the soft tissue constraints of the PIP joint are the most common ligamentous injuries in the hand. Sports, industrial mishaps, falls, and motor vehicle accidents account for most of these injuries.

Complete digital dislocations are quite painful, and the deformity is obvious enough that patients usually seek acute treatment; however, follow-up care for these injuries is surprisingly limited. Often patients are seen months later with chronic joint contractures, loss of tendon excursion, and swelling. By this time, they may require extensive therapy or even surgery. In the more

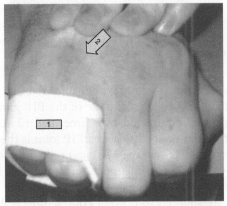

Figure 10-29 *1,* A flexion strap can be made to hold the IPs in flexion. The patient is asked to extend the MCP joints, which encourages isolated pull-through of the extensor digitorum communis (EDC). *2,* Applying pressure on the dorsum of the hand, pushing distally, while the exercise is performed encourages further separation from the scar tissue.

acute stage, therapeutic intervention for these injuries is far simpler and more effective. Prompt treatment and immediate follow-up care are particularly important in a patient with an injury to the ulnar collateral ligament to the thumb (see later discussion). In the acute stage, the thumb may be quite swollen and ecchymotic, but no obvious deformity may be present, and in these injuries the acute symptoms improve over several days to a week. Unfortunately, if the ligament remains incompetent and untreated, a chronic painful condition develops perhaps months to years later, as does the potential for arthritis at the MCP joint.[59]

Anatomy

The PIP joint is a constrained hinge joint with tight articular congruency. The proximal phalanx is cam shaped and composed of a bicondylar head with a central groove. The double concave middle phalanx is divided in the midline by a bony tongue that guides the joint through its eccentric arc of motion (Figure 10-31).

The main lateral stabilizer of the joint is the proper collateral ligament, which is 2 to 3 mm thick. This ligament originates at the head of the proximal phalanx and inserts into the base of the middle phalanx. The proper collateral ligament is connected to the volar plate by the shroudlike fibers of the accessory collateral ligament. The collateral ligaments and the volar plate combine to act as a three-sided box that stabilizes the PIP joint through its arc, resisting hyperextension and lateral forces (Figure 10-32). In extension, the volar plate is tight and the collateral ligaments are relatively lax. As the joint flexes, the collateral ligaments are tightened over the bulge of the condyles; as a result, the base of the middle phalanx is firmly seated against the proximal phalanx.

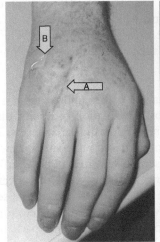
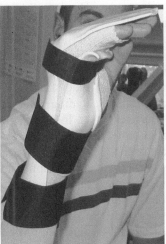
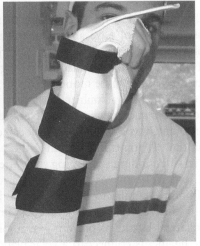

Figure 10-30 Postoperative management of open reduction and internal fixation of a fourth metacarpal neck fracture (**A**) and pinning of a fifth metacarpal head fracture on day 5 after cast removal (**B**). A custom-made, protective, forearm-based splint is fabricated to put the long, ring, and little fingers in the intrinsic plus positions; this allows active flexion and extension within the splint and prevents adherence of soft tissue structures. The design of this splint provides circumferential, maximum protection for healing fractures. The patient straps the fingers into the hood or roof of the splint for sleeping. A similar, hand-based version can be fabricated if less protection is needed.

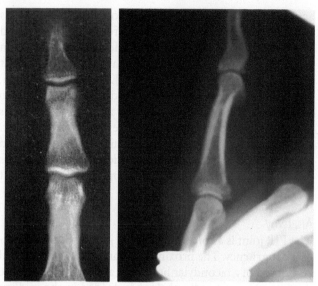

Figure 10-31 AP and lateral x-ray films of the PIP joint. The cam shape of the proximal phalanx is apparent on the lateral view. The tight, bony geometry of the joint can be appreciated on both views.

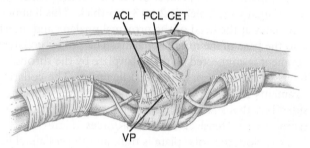

Figure 10-32 Lateral view of the PIP joint. The proper collateral ligament (*PCL*), accessory collateral ligament (*ACL*), volar plate (*VP*), and dorsal capsule with the central extensor tendon (*CET*) provide support to the PIP joint. Note that the ACL inserts into the volar plate, and the PCL travels distally and volarly to insert onto the bone of the middle phalanx. (From Skirven TM, Osterman AL, Fedorczyk JM: *Rehabilitation of the hand and upper extremity,* ed 6, Philadelphia, Mosby, 2011.)

The MCP joint has less bony constraint than the PIP joint because it does not have an intercondylar groove. The PIP joint is considered a "sloppy hinge" joint with only a small amount of motion outside of the sagittal plane (flexion/extension). Far more motion exists in the MCP joint for coronal plane (radioulnar deviation) and transaxial motion (pronation/supination). Despite the lack of bony constraint, the MCP joint is dislocated less frequently than the PIP joint. Its location at the base of the fingers and its surrounding supporting structures serve to protect the joint. The overall ligamentous arrangement of the MCP joint is similar to that of the PIP joint with certain subtle differences. Radial and ulnar proper and accessory collateral ligaments prevent lateral joint movement. These ligaments connect to a volar plate ligament that forms the stabilizing element to hyperextension on the volar portion of the joint.

The main differences in the ligamentous support structures of the MCP and PIP joints are (1) the volar plate

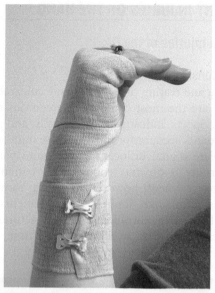

Figure 10-33 The *intrinsic plus position* of splinting. Positioning the IP joints in extension and flexing the MCP joints to 70° or more prevents the development of contractures.

of the MCP joint is highly mobile and does not become contracted, unlike the volar plate of the PIP joint, which easily becomes contracted over time, and (2) the distal insertion of the volar plate at the PIP joint is the weakest attachment, whereas in the MCP joint the weakest area of attachment is the proximal portion. Both of these points are clinically relevant. The first is that the position in which patients are splinted to prevent contractures is flexion of the MCP and extension of the PIP joints (Figure 10-33). The second is that dorsal dislocations of the PIP joint rarely interpose the volar plate into the joint, whereas this is more of a concern in the MCP joint.

Injury Classification

Displacement of the MCP or PIP joint can occur in any of three directions, which are referenced by the position of the distal bone: volar, lateral, or dorsal. The direction of displacement aids the classification of the injury.

Diagnosis

Radiographic analysis of the injured digit is instrumental in the diagnostic evaluation of a joint dislocation or subluxation. Standard AP and lateral views of the digit are always warranted. Because the lateral view often is the most helpful, it is important to avoid overlap of the other digits in obtaining this view. Loss of concentric reduction of the joint can be subtle and can be seen only on a perfect lateral view of the joint; therefore the clinician must not settle for inferior x-ray films, particularly in type III injuries (Table 10-5), in which treatment might be affected by joint reduction.

It is important that the examiner first determine whether the digit is currently reduced. If the joint is anatomically located, the examiner should determine whether

TABLE 10-5

Nonoperative Rehabilitation Guidelines for Dorsal Dislocation of the PIP Joint[27-29,70,71]

	TYPES OF DORSAL DISLOCATION			
	Type I	Type II	Type III (Stable)	Type III (Unstable)
Pathology	Disruption of the volar plate from the middle phalanx Minor disruption of collateral ligaments Joint is stable	Avulsion of the volar plate Major disruption of collateral ligaments Bayoneting of middle phalanx dorsally on top of proximal phalanx Unstable joint	Fragment is less than 30%-40% of the articular surface Collateral ligament remains attached to larger shaft of middle phalanx but is not attached to small fracture fragment After reduction joint is stable	Fragment is more than 30%-40% of the articular surface Collateral ligament remains attached to smaller shaft of the volar fracture fragment No ligament support to the dorsally displaced midphalanx With concentric reduction, PIP joint is stable in flexion

Healing Stages

	Type I	Type II	Type III (Stable)	Type III (Unstable)
Stage I: Inflammatory stage (weeks 0 to 2)	Static IP extension splinting	Static IP extension splinting Alternative: Dorsal block splint at 30° flexion, progressed 10° weekly to week 3-4 Adjacent digit is included and buddy-taped Full motion within the splint is allowed	Hand-based dorsal block splint at 10° to 45° PIP flexion (usually 30°) for 4 weeks, progressed 10° of extension weekly Adjacent digit is included and buddy-taped to prevent lateral stress to the joint Buddy taping ROM within the splint Dorsal block splinting continues Edema management techniques should not place lateral stress on the PIP joint If Coban wrap is used, use 5 cm (2 inches) and make a sleeve that can be removed easily	Hand-based dorsal block splint with PIP joint in flexion to weeks 4-6 When x-ray films confirm a stable PIP flexion position, 5° to 10° is added to the flexion angle to protect the reduction Adjacent digit is included and buddy-taped to prevent lateral stress to the joint Buddy taping ROM within the splint Dorsal block splinting continues Edema management techniques should not place lateral stress on the PIP joint If Coban wrap is used, use 5 cm (2 inches) and make a sleeve that can be removed easily
Stage II: Fibroplasia and repair stage (weeks 2 to 6)	Buddy taping for 2-6 weeks to protect against hyperextension AROM Blocking exercises Edema management with Coban or a compression sleeve Soft tissue mobilization	Buddy taping for 2-12 weeks to protect against hyperextension and lateral stress AROM Blocking exercises and tendon gliding exercises Edema management with Coban or a compression sleeve Soft tissue mobilization Static IP extension splint is worn at night		
Stage III: Remodeling and maturation stage (weeks 6 to 8+)	Strengthening as tolerated at weeks 6-8	Splinting for motion as tolerated at weeks 6-8 Strengthening as tolerated at weeks 8-12 Night static splint continues	Buddy taping for up to 12 weeks for protection Blocking exercises to maintain ORL length Tendon gliding exercises Edema management with Coban or a compression sleeve Soft tissue mobilization Static IP extension splint is worn at night Strengthening is begun at week 12+ as tolerated	Buddy taping for up to 12 weeks for protection Blocking exercises to maintain ORL length Tendon gliding exercises Edema management with Coban or a compression sleeve Soft tissue mobilization Static IP extension splint is worn at night Strengthening is begun at week 12+ as tolerated

PIP, Proximal interphalangeal; *IP*, interphalangeal; *ROM*, range of motion; *AROM*, active range of motion; *ORL*, oblique retinacular ligament.

AROM in flexion and extension causes joint instability and, if so, at what point in the arc of motion. If the joint is stable throughout AROM, passive stability is tested. Each collateral ligament is gently stressed, and the examiner looks for pain and instability.

Medical Treatment

Volar dislocation of the PIP joint is an extremely rare injury. The mechanism usually involves rotation and axial loading of a partly flexed digit. This results in the rupture of at least one of the collateral ligaments and part of the volar plate. The middle phalanx then displaces volarly, causing the distal aspect of the proximal phalanx to move dorsally through the extensor mechanism. This most often occurs with the proximal phalanx rupturing through the interval between the central slip and one of the lateral bands. Less often, the proximal phalanx moves directly dorsally, disrupting the attachment of the central slip on the base of the middle phalanx (Figure 10-34). The latter mechanism produces loss in continuity of the extensor mechanism, which results in a closed boutonniere deformity. After reduction of the joint, the clinician must be sure to evaluate the extensor function at the PIP joint and treat any loss accordingly with extension splinting, as a closed boutonniere injury would be treated. Closed reduction of a volar dislocation can be difficult, especially when the proximal phalanx protrudes through the interval between the central slip and the lateral band. Flexion of the MCP and interphalangeal (IP) joints with the wrist held in extension to relax the extensor apparatus may allow manipulation and closed reduction; otherwise, an open reduction may be required. Once the joint has been reduced, assuming that the extensor mechanism is intact, the ligaments should fall back into anatomical alignment without the need for surgical intervention. Management therefore is aimed at regaining motion and limiting scar formation while protecting the joint from additional injury.

Lateral dislocation of the PIP joint constitutes a rupture of one of the collateral ligaments and at least a partial tearing of the volar plate. The diagnosis is confirmed with stress testing of the joint that indicates more than 20° of deformity.[60] With reduction of the joint, the collateral ligaments and volar plate return to their anatomical locations. By virtue of its bony congruency, the joint should allow for AROM without instability that enables the patient to begin a protected therapy program. The most common complication of this injury is not late instability but rather arthrofibrosis with loss of joint motion. Therefore it is imperative to begin regaining motion, reducing swelling, and manipulating the scar process early to achieve the best possible outcome for the patient.

Dorsal dislocation is the most common of the three types of PIP injuries and occurs when a longitudinal force coupled with some extension is applied to the digit. Basketballs and footballs are frequently the culprits in this injury mechanism. The distal aspect of the volar plate is disrupted, and the interval between the accessory and proper collateral ligaments is torn, allowing the middle phalanx to ride dorsally up on the proximal phalanx. The injury is further classified into three categories that depict increasing energy and further damage and instability of the joint.

In a type I injury (see Table 10-5), hyperextension results in the avulsion of the volar plate from the middle phalanx and a minor longitudinal split in the collateral ligaments. In severe cases, the middle phalanx may be locked in 70° of hyperextension.

A type II injury involves an avulsion of the volar plate plus a major bilateral collateral ligament tear that allows complete bayoneting (overriding) of the middle phalanx on top of the proximal phalanx (Figure 10-35).

When the longitudinal force is great enough to produce shearing of the volar rim of the middle phalanx, a fracture-dislocation occurs. This is a type III injury, which differs from the previous two patterns. As the middle phalanx begins to ride dorsally over the proximal phalanx, the volar rim is fractured off. This type III injury is subclassified simply into two types, stable (type IIIA) and unstable (type IIIB) (Figure 10-36). In a stable dorsal fracture-dislocation of the PIP joint, the fracture fragment is small (i.e., less than 30% to 40% of the articular contour of the joint). In this case the collateral ligaments are not attached to the small fracture fragment but remain

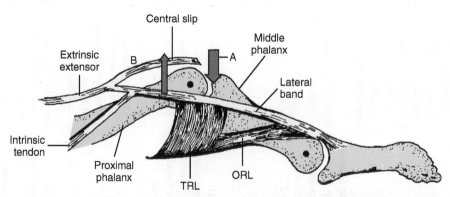

Figure 10-34 Anterior proximal interphalangeal joint dislocation. **A,** Anterior translation of middle phalanx. **B,** Proximal phalanx gets caught between the central slip and the lateral band, which usually is not disrupted from the middle phalanx as depicted here. *TRL,* Transverse retinacular ligament; *ORL,* oblique retinacular ligament. (From Coons MS, Green SM: Boutonniere deformity, *Hand Clin* 11:389, 1995.)

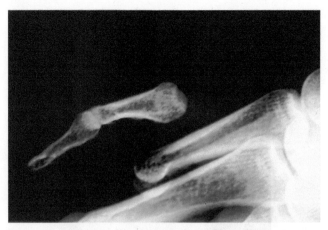

Figure 10-35 Lateral x-ray film of a type II dorsal dislocation of the PIP joint, showing complete overlapping of the bones. This often is an open injury.

attached to the larger shaft fracture. An unstable dorsal fracture-dislocation involves a disruption of more than 40% of the joint. In this instance the collateral ligaments remain with the volar fracture segment. The dorsally displaced shaft no longer has any soft tissue constraint or bony buttress to contain the joint (Figure 10-37).

Type I and type II dorsal PIP dislocations are stable injuries (type II requires reduction). The patient may be splinted for comfort for up to 2 weeks and must take care to avoid excessive flexion of the IP joints, which could promote the formation of a flexion contracture. ROM with the affected finger buddy-taped is then begun, and therapy is initiated to control edema, reduce scar formation, and gain motion.

Type III dorsal dislocations with fracture of the volar rim of the middle phalanx are higher energy injuries. In the stable subtype (type IIIA), the joint is congruent on a lateral x-ray film. The patient is treated with 1 to 2 weeks of immobilization. If a small amount of joint incongruence is present, the joint can be flexed slightly to obtain alignment in a dorsal block splint. ROM with the finger buddy-taped for protection is begun after the period of immobilization.

Multiple treatment options are available for type III dorsal dislocations with a large, unstable fracture fragment (type IIIB). These include a dorsal block splint, ORIF, a dynamic external fixator, volar plate arthroplasty, fusion, silicone arthroplasty, and hemihamate reconstruction of the PIP joint, using bone obtained from the patient's joint between the hamate and the metacarpal.[2]

A dorsal block splint is used if the dislocated joint can be concentrically reduced by some degree of flexion. Beyond this, the joint remains stable in any amount of further flexion. The clinician confirms the position of the stable concentric reduction and creates a splint adding 5° to 10° of further flexion for safety. Extension to this point is allowed with full active flexion. Each week, the splint is adjusted to increase the extension 10°, and x-ray films are taken to confirm that the reduction is maintained (Figure 10-38).

Open reduction and internal fixation is a technically demanding procedure because the bone fragment to be fixed is quite small and frequently more comminuted than it appears on x-ray films. However, if the fragment can be fixed with a screw, rehabilitation can be started much sooner, and the best results are obtained (Figure 10-39).

Dynamic external fixation uses forces to counteract those that displace the intra-articular fracture.[61] The attachment of rubber bands or other dynamic traction forces to pins implanted temporarily into the bone reduces the joint while allowing it to move through an arc of motion to prevent contracture and to facilitate healing of the cartilage (Figure 10-40).[62] Therapy is provided throughout the immediate postoperative period to prevent tendon adherence and joint contracture. The device usually is removed 4 to 6 weeks later, when the joint is stable enough to move without fear of late dislocation.

Volar plate arthroplasty is a technique for inserting the torn distal end of the volar plate into the fractured base of the middle phalanx to reestablish ligamentous attachment to the base of the middle phalanx. The volar plate serves to prevent hyperextension of the joint and to provide a smooth contour for the joint for motion; also, over time,

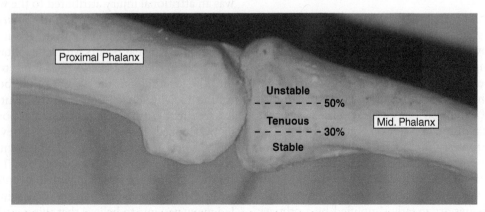

Figure 10-36 The level of the fracture determines the stability of the joint. A large fracture fragment causes a loss of volar support at the PIP joint. With a large volar fragment of bone, the insertions of the collateral ligaments are still attached to the fragment. This leaves the shaft of the middle phalanx without the support of the collateral ligaments or the volar bone at the PIP joint.

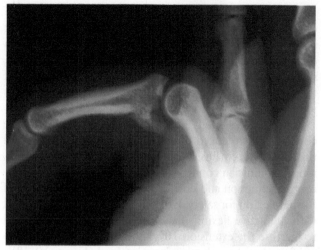

Figure 10-37 Clinical example of a type IIIB fracture-dislocation of the PIP joint. In this case, because the fracture fragment is large, the joint no longer remains congruently aligned. This can be appreciated by the V shape formed by the intact middle phalanx and the proximal phalangeal head.

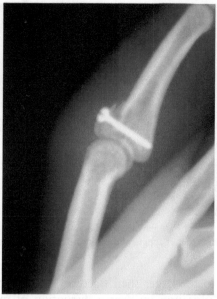

Figure 10-39 In this rare case of a volar fracture-dislocation, the insertion of the central slip has avulsed, which allows the middle phalanx to sublux on the proximal phalanx. Screw fixation allows concentric joint reduction and immediate return to motion.

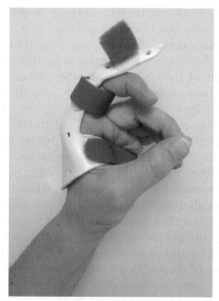

Figure 10-38 A dorsal block splint can be used to allow motion within the stable range for types IIIA and IIIB dorsal fracture-dislocations at the PIP joint.

it has been shown to metaplase (convert) into a more normal-appearing bony joint surface.[63] In the immediate postoperative period, the joint must be protected from extension, which can tear the repair apart. To regain motion, AROM of extension can be attempted at 4 weeks and PROM of extension at 6 weeks (Figure 10-41).

Silicone arthroplasty is a viable primary option for an older patient with an already arthritic PIP joint who has sustained an unstable fracture-dislocation of the PIP joint.[64] In this case, rehabilitation, return to function, and pain issues are greatly simplified by a primary arthroplasty of the joint (Figure 10-42). The caveat with this procedure is the index finger; in this digit, forces from lateral pinch with the thumb are too great for a silicone arthroplasty, which will fail. In this unique situation a primary fusion of the PIP joint might be the better course, if the patient's MCP function is adequate. Therapy proceeds as for a primary arthroplasty performed from the volar approach (the extensor mechanism is spared, but the collateral ligaments have been resected or, in this case, torn).[64]

Collateral Ligament Injuries of the Thumb

General Considerations

Injury to the ligaments of the thumb occur most commonly at the MCP joint in ball-handling sports and, even more frequently, from falls during skiing; this injury therefore generally is called *skier's thumb*. In the 18th and 19th centuries, tearing of the ulnar collateral ligament was an attritional injury attributed to the work of Scottish game wardens and was known as *gamekeeper's thumb*. This often is how a hyperextension, abduction, and radial deviation event that occurs with ball contact or a fall with a ski pole in the hand allows the thumb to strike directly into the ground with the weight of the body forcing the thumb radially. Radial collateral ligament injuries occur less frequently, usually in ball-handling sports, and are easily overlooked. Either type of injury, if severe, causes significant bruising and swelling. The patient also may have considerable pain that lasts several days. The pain usually resolves, as does the swelling, with local anti-inflammatory treatment. The rapid resolution of swelling and pain has led many patients to believe that this is a trivial injury that does not require treatment. Unfortunately, this belief can lead to poor outcomes, including chronic laxity, pain, and the onset of MCP joint arthrosis (Figure 10-43).[59]

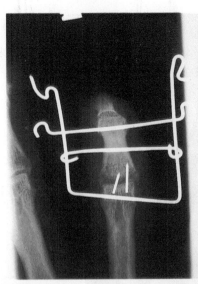
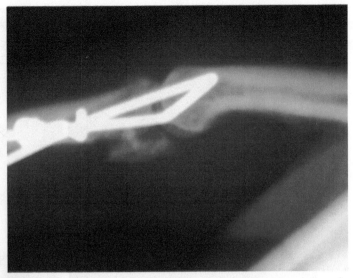

Figure 10-40 Ligamentotaxis can be used to regain joint congruency and allow for motion. This prevents joint subluxation and allows fractures of the middle phalanx to remodel using the intact proximal phalanx as a template during the healing process.

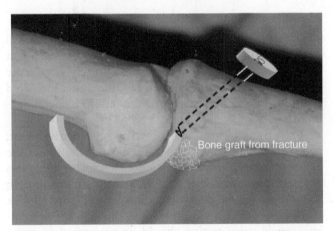

Bone graft from fracture

Figure 10-41 Representation of a volar plate arthroplasty. In this operation the volar plate is detached distally and reinserted into the fracture site to reestablish the smooth contour of the joint. The fibrocartilage of the volar plate metaplases into bone, reestablishing a bony joint with a concentric rim for the phalangeal head.

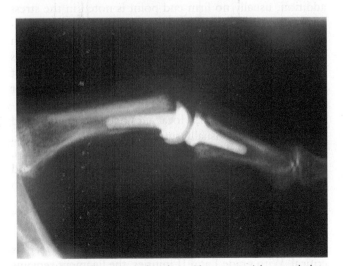

Figure 10-42 Replacement arthroplasty. Newer materials recently have become available that may outlast silicone, particularly for higher demand patients. (Courtesy B.M. Leslie, MD.)

Anatomy

The MCP joint of the thumb is primarily designed to allow flexion and extension. However, some degree of abduction and adduction, as well as rotation, can occur. The shape of the joint is condyloid, with the proximal phalanx behaving like an inverted golf tee sitting on a golf ball (i.e., the metacarpal head). Some people have far more round metacarpal heads than others; therefore the amount of flexion and extension at the joint varies considerably from patient to patient. Radial and ulnar deviation (abduction/adduction) and rotation are limited by both static and dynamic constraints. The primary stabilizers to ulnar and radial motion are the proper collateral ligaments, which originate at the lateral condyles of the metacarpal head dorsal to the axis of rotation. These ligaments pass obliquely and distally to insert on the proximal phalanx volar (anterior) to the axis of rotation. Along the volar aspect of the proper collateral ligament is a shroud-like attachment, the accessory collateral ligament, which connects the proper collateral ligament to the volar plate of the joint. This arrangement creates a three-sided box configuration between the two collateral ligaments and the intervening volar plate, similar to that seen at the PIP joint in the digits (see Figure 10-32). Dynamic support of the joint is created by the adductor pollicis muscle, which inserts into the ulnar sesamoid at the base of the MCP joint, and the flexor pollicis brevis and abductor pollicis brevis (APB) muscles, which insert onto the radial sesamoid bone at the base of the MCP joint. These muscles are intrinsic to the thumb, and they flex the MCP joint and extend the IP joint by way of attachments to the extensor mechanism. They also create dynamic stability to radial and ulnar stress, respectively.

Injury Classification

Collateral ligament injuries of the thumb can be classified in the same way as ligamentous injuries to other parts of the body, such as the ankle and knee. Grade I

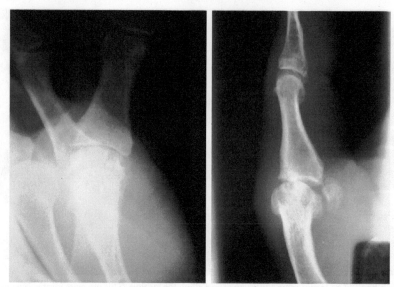

Figure 10-43 AP and lateral x-ray films showing chronic laxity of the ulnar collateral ligament of the thumb at the MCP joint. Note the radial deviation of the thumb at rest, as well as the volar subluxation of the joint. These factors, in addition to some rotational malalignment, have created the incongruence that has caused joint destruction.

injuries consist of stretching of the collagen fibers within the ligaments without macroscopic fiber tearing. Grade II injuries involve further deformity of the collagen fibers, with tearing of some portion of the ligament, but overall continuity remains. Grade III injuries are the most severe and show disruption of the collagen fibers, which results in discontinuity of the ligament.

In addition to the tearing of the collateral ligament, the dorsal capsule and the volar plate on the same side as the ligament injury usually are also partly disrupted. Furthermore, the ligament may avulse a portion of the proximal phalanx at its insertion. The fracture fragment usually does not represent a large segment of the articular surface, but on rare occasions it may be as large as 10% of the joint. The clinician cannot assume that the ligament is attached to the small fragment of bone. The presence of a nondisplaced small fracture fragment does not exclude the possibility of a displaced ligament; studies have reported that the two can be present simultaneously.[65]

When the injury involves the ulnar collateral ligament (UCL) at the MCP of the thumb, a unique situation can arise with grade III injuries. As was first described in 1962, the adductor aponeurosis can be interposed between the distal end of the avulsed ligament and the proximal phalanx, holding it in a displaced position.[66] This is known as a *Stener lesion,* and it has important implications in both diagnosis and treatment (Figure 10-44).

Diagnosis

Diagnosis begins with the history and careful attention to the mechanism of injury. The amount of swelling and ecchymosis can alert the examiner to the degree of damage to the soft tissues. If the injury is more chronic and the swelling has receded, the resting posture of the thumb (i.e., both its angle and its rotational alignment) provides clues to the amount of ligamentous disruption.

With a grade III UCL injury, the thumb rests in radial deviation. Also, because of the loss of the ulnar ligament and dorsal capsular support, the thumb tends to rotate around the intact radial collateral ligament in a supinated position. In a complete tear of the radial collateral ligament, the opposite is found.

Tenderness to palpation is noted over the torn ligament, and swelling and induration are present at the site of the ligament injury. With a Stener lesion, a palpable hard mass is felt that is asymmetrical to the patient's other thumb; this is the displaced distal end of the UCL (Figure 10-45). If x-ray films have confirmed that no fracture is present, gentle stress testing should be performed to assess ligament competence. It is imperative to differentiate a grade III injury from either a grade I or grade II tear. A grade III injury shows 30° more instability to radial stress testing than is seen on the patient's opposite side. In addition, usually no firm end point is noted in the stress test.[67,68] Testing should be done with the joint in full extension and in 30° flexion. Clinicians should practice on normal thumbs to get an idea of what a normal end feel is like. Patients often contract the muscles to guard against the pain of stress testing. The clinician must be alert for this, and if the patient is too uncomfortable to reliably relax for the examination, a local anesthetic injected around the torn ligament usually suffices to allow stress testing. Stress x-ray films have little use in the diagnostic process. Alternative imaging studies, including ultrasound and magnetic resonance imaging (MRI), can be performed to delineate the position of the ligament.

Medical Treatment

Differentiation of partial and complete ligament tears is critical. With grade I and II injuries, the ligament remains in its anatomically correct position. In this situation, protection of the ligament with a thumb spica cast for

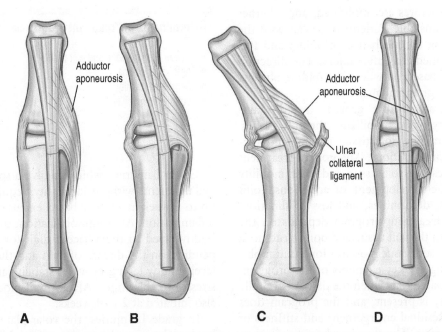

A   B   C   D

Figure 10-44 Stener lesion: Diagram of the displacement of the ulnar collateral ligament of the thumb metacarpophalangeal joint. **A,** Normal relationship, with the ulnar ligament covered by the adductor aponeurosis. **B,** With slight radial angulation, the proximal margin of the aponeurosis slides distally, leaving part of the ligament uncovered. **C,** With major radial angulation, the ulnar ligament ruptures at its distal insertion. With this degree of angulation, the aponeurosis has displaced distal to the rupture, allowing the ligament to escape from beneath it. **D,** As the joint is realigned, the proximal edge of the adductor aponeurosis sweeps the free end of the ligament proximally and farther from its insertion. This is the Stener lesion. Unless surgically restored, the ulnar ligament will not heal properly and will be unstable to lateral stress. (From Chang J, Neligan PC: *Plastic surgery*, vol 6, *Hand and upper limb*, ed 3, London, 2013, Saunders.)

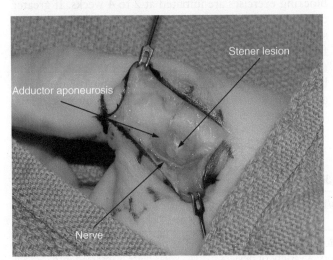

Figure 10-45 Surgical view of a Stener lesion. The ulnar collateral ligament has been torn from its distal insertion on the proximal phalanx. It now is reflected back on itself, resting superficial and proximal to the adductor aponeurosis (it normally is located deep to this structure). Note the nerve encountered during this surgical approach; injury to or irritation of this nerve can result in postoperative symptoms.

In a ligament tear, the torn tissue generally avulses from the bone and can be directly repaired with sutures through drill holes or with the use of small bone anchors. The volar plate and dorsal capsule are repaired at the same time.[69] Four to six weeks of casting is completed before therapy commences.

If a small fracture fragment is associated with the avulsion, the surgeon may choose to discard the fragment and repair the ligament into the cancellous bony bed. However, if the fracture fragment represents a substantial portion of the joint surface, direct repair of the bone with small screw fixation is preferable. It is critical that the tiny sensory nerve branches be protected in the dissection because these can be a source of debilitating pain postoperatively. Even under the gentlest of circumstances, therapists frequently must spend time desensitizing these nerves from the traction endured during the procedure.

Rehabilitation of Proximal Interphalangeal Joint Injuries and Ulnar Collateral Ligament Injuries of the Thumb

Proximal Interphalangeal Joint Injuries

Both the tight articular congruency of the PIP joint and the soft tissue constraints that surround it contribute to the joint's stability. The soft tissue stabilizers include the joint capsule, the proper and accessory collateral ligaments, the volar plate, and the flexor and extensor tendons.

The rehabilitation treatment strategy takes into consideration the direction and type of fracture–dislocation,

4 to 6 weeks, followed by a return to motion rehabilitation program, generally leads to excellent results. In the case of complete ligament disruption, the question arises whether the ligament is anatomically positioned and will heal under conservative management. Clearly, if a Stener lesion can be felt, the answer is no, and some clinicians believe that it is best to surgically fix all grade III injuries so that a displaced ligament is never missed.

which soft tissue structures are implicated, and whether the joint is stable or unstable. Patients often can assist the clinician by describing the mechanism of injury and PIP joint positioning immediately after injury. The direction of the dislocation is based on where the middle phalanx sits in relation to the proximal phalanx.

Rehabilitation strategies are geared toward maintaining joint stability while mobilizing the soft tissues. Restoring and optimizing soft tissue gliding and mechanics are prime considerations. The goal of treatment is to regain and preserve soft tissue and joint mobility while preventing the development of adhesions, joint flexion contractures, deformities, and loss of function. Progression of the treatment program depends on the healing stages of both the soft tissue and bony structures; edema management, soft tissue mobilization, joint mobilization, and splinting are key elements of the program. Strengthening is initiated only when the tissues have fully healed, no instability is present, and the program does not provoke pain. Residual enlargement and stiffness of the PIP joint is common. The clinician should explain to the patient that management of these injuries can take 6 months to 1 year.

Dorsal Dislocation. Rehabilitation guidelines for dorsal dislocations are based on the stability of the joint, the classification type, and nonoperative and postoperative treatment. Soft tissues injured in dorsal dislocations include the collateral ligaments and the volar plate (Table 10-6).

Lateral Dislocation. Rehabilitation for lateral dislocations is based on the degree of injury to the collateral ligaments and volar plate. The Bowers classification system divides soft issue injuries into three grades.[71]

Determinants of Treatment Progression

- Tissue healing (bone and soft tissue)
- Amount of edema
- Degree of stability
- Soft tissue mobility
- Joint mobility
- Pain

Grade I injuries, which involve a sprain to the collateral ligaments without instability, require immobilization up to 1 week in a finger-based extension splint to reduce inflammation. After immobilization, the affected finger is buddy-taped to the adjacent digit for 2 to 4 weeks, depending on the degree of pain and the patient's activity level. Buddy taping provides stability and prevents lateral stresses to the finger. AROM and blocking exercises are also initiated at 2 to 4 weeks.

In grade II injuries, the volar plate remains attached but may be injured, and the collateral ligaments are completely disrupted. Treatment varies, depending on the amount of disruption to the volar plate. Treatment consists of immobilization for 1 to 2 weeks with the finger splinted in 10° to 20° of PIP flexion for pain tolerance. Buddy taping for 8 to 12 weeks follows, and AROM and blocking exercises are initiated at 2 to 4 weeks. If greater disruption of the volar plate is present and the joint is unstable, an extension block splint is fabricated at 0° to 45° flexion. The degree of flexion depends on the stability of the joint, which is determined by imaging. The extension block splint is advanced into extension by 10° per week, and joint reduction should be confirmed by x-ray films.

TABLE **10-6**

Postoperative Rehabilitation Guidelines for Dislocation of the PIP Joint[27–29,70–72]

	Open Reduction and Internal Fixation	External Fixation/Traction Splinting (Weeks 0-6)	Volar Plate Arthroplasty
Special considerations	Hand therapy may or may not be initiated until weeks 4-6, depending on the stability of the reduction	A risk for infection exists with the use of external fixators; a variety of devices can be used for external fixation: • Commercially available finger-based hinge devices • Surgeon-fabricated finger-based fixators using K-wires and elastics • Traction splinting fabricated by a hand therapist (Designs vary. Forearm based. Finger is attached to an outrigger providing consistent traction through a safe arc of motion.) Positioning in the splint varies, depending on the injury classification or the direction of dislocation and implicated structures[73]	The torn distal end of the volar plate is inserted into the fractured base of the middle phalanx to reestablish ligamentous attachment to the base of the middle phalanx

(Continued)

TABLE **10-6**

Postoperative Rehabilitation Guidelines for Dislocation of the PIP Joint—Cont'd

	Open Reduction and Internal Fixation	External Fixation/Traction Splinting (Weeks 0-6)	Volar Plate Arthroplasty
Healing Stages			
Stage I: Inflammatory stage (weeks 0 to 2)	Immobilization is achieved in a forearm-based dorsal protective cast or splint that includes the full hand Gentle AROM with buddy taping may be initiated only if the reduction is stable Positioning in the splint may vary, depending on the implicated structures and surgical procedure	*External fixation:* • Immobilization for 3 days • At days 3-5, AROM is initiated within a safe range determined by the physician • Static protective splinting at night if the device does not lock • Resting PIP position is determined by the physician *Traction splinting:* • Initiation of motion varies from day 1 to week 3, depending on the stability of the fracture and the implicated structures • AROM of the PIP joint within a safe arc of motion is begun, and DIP blocking exercises are initiated • Dorsal block splint is worn, resting the finger in MCP flexion, the PIP joint in the safe amount of extension as determined by the physician, and the DIP joint in extension, until AROM is initiated and also at night until week 6 • Patient is taught to monitor for signs of infection and to modify activities	Immobilization in a cast for 2-4 weeks
Stage II: Fibroplasia and repair stage (weeks 2 to 6)	Gentle AROM with the finger buddy-taped to the adjacent finger Edema management techniques should not put lateral stress on the PIP joint If Coban wrap is used, use 5 cm (2 inches) and make a sleeve that can be removed easily Gentle tendon gliding exercises	*External fixation:* • AROM within the device continues • Blocking initiated with emphasis on DIP flexion *Traction splinting:* • AROM of the PIP joint within a safe arc of motion and DIP blocking exercises are begun or continued	Hand-based dorsal block splint with the PIP joint in 30° flexion is fabricated at weeks 2-4, and extension is increased 10° per week *Or* the digit may remain immobilized, depending on the stability of the repair The finger is buddy-taped to the adjacent digit Edema management techniques should not put lateral stress on the PIP joint If Coban wrap is used, use 5 cm (2 inches) and make a sleeve that can be easily removed Blocking, full tendon gliding, and stretching are initiated at weeks 4-6
Stage III: Remodeling and maturation stage (weeks 6 to 8+)	PROM Stretching Blocking and tendon gliding Splinting for motion Functional progression Gentle strengthening at week 8, respecting tissue tolerance and pain	Device is removed Edema management Full tendon gliding and blocking exercises are initiated The finger is buddy-taped to the adjacent digit to protect soft tissue healing Strengthening begins at weeks 8-12, respecting tissue tolerance and pain Splinting for motion Functional progression	Buddy taping continues Splinting for motion is done, respecting tissue tolerance Strengthening begins at weeks 8-12, respecting tissue tolerance and pain Functional progression

AROM, active range of motion; *PIP*, proximal interphalangeal; *DIP*, distal interphalangeal; *MCP*, metacarpophalangeal; *PROM*, passive range of motion

Active flexion and extension into the block is completed after an initial week of immobilization. After removal of the extension block splint, the finger is buddy-taped for 8 to 12 weeks to protect the joint.

Grade III injuries are associated with complete disruption of both the collateral ligaments and volar plate; these injuries may require surgical intervention for stabilization. Postoperative rehabilitation is similar to that for grade II injuries (see Table 10-6).

Volar (Anterior) Dislocation. Volar dislocation injuries are rare. The soft tissue structures injured in volar dislocations are the collateral ligaments, the volar plate, and the extensor mechanism, including the central slip and lateral bands. Bony involvement can include middle phalanx dorsal lip fractures at the insertion of the central slip.[29,74]

Initial rehabilitation for nonoperative volar dislocations consists of immobilization in a finger-based extension splint with the DIP free for 6 to 8 weeks to protect soft tissue healing (Figure 10-46). AROM of the DIP maintains soft tissue gliding and appropriate positioning of the lateral bands dorsal to the joint axis. The PIP joint is then mobilized at 6 to 8 weeks. Buddy taping is used for 6 to 12 weeks to protect the joint.[29] A PIP extension splint can be worn at night to prevent periarticular soft tissue shortening and can be used for up to 3 to 6 months. An extension block splint with the MCP joints in flexion can help the patient perform blocking exercises to promote pull-through and glide of the extensor mechanism. If the collateral ligaments and volar plate have been completely disrupted, surgical intervention is necessary.

Ulnar Collateral Ligament Injuries of the Thumb

The rehabilitation strategy for the thumb is based on the degree of injury to the ulnar collateral ligament and/or the volar plate, which renders the joint stable or unstable. The degree of ligamentous injury has been classified into three grades. Rehabilitation strategies are geared toward maintaining thumb MCP joint stability while mobilizing the soft tissues to prevent the development of adhesions,

flexion contractures, and loss of function. Progression of the therapy program depends on the stages of healing. Emphasis is placed on avoiding lateral and radial stresses to the MCP joint in the initial stages of healing. Terminal thumb abduction should be initially avoided. Force transmission to the MCP joint through pinching and pulling activities, in which the thumb tip is engaged, should also be modified and/or avoided to reduce demands on the healing tissues.

Consideration should be given to protecting the IP joint from hyperextension, which can place stress on the MCP joint. Edema management, soft tissue mobilization, joint mobilization, and splinting are key elements of the program. Care should be taken with cast or splint designs to protect the ligament while preventing a thumb adduction contracture. Strengthening of the thumb is initiated only when the soft tissues have fully healed, no instability is present, and the program does not provoke pain and/or an inflammatory response. Residual problems include stiffness at both the MCP and IP joints (Table 10-7).

TENDON INJURIES OF THE HAND

Flexor Tendon Injury

General Considerations

Tendon injuries are common, although the exact incidence is unknown. Patients with a tendon injury face months of profound physical, emotional, and socioeconomic hurdles. These hurdles arise under the best of circumstances, such as when the injury is recognized early and treated appropriately. Unfortunately, many pitfalls can lead to a poor result after a tendon injury, with profound repercussions that can affect the patient's ability to return to gainful employment and to use the hand for activities of daily living.

Tendon injuries often are the result of a sharp instrument coming into contact with the digit, hand, or wrist. This can occur accidentally at work or in the home or sometimes deliberately, as in an altercation or self-inflicted wound. In the case of an accidental injury, the nondominant hand frequently is hurt because the individual is wielding the knife in the dominant hand when the accident occurs. The opposite is true for a person who uses the hand to protect himself or herself from an assailant; these individuals reflexively use the dominant limb to ward off the knife assault.

Spontaneous tendon ruptures can occur without any preceding trauma. The most common cause of this type of tendon injury is rheumatoid arthritis, although other conditions, such as chronic tenosynovitis, partial flexor tendon lacerations, and attrition of the flexor tendons over bony prominences or hardware from previous surgery, may result in the same type of atraumatic tendon rupture (Figure 10-47). Timely recognition, diagnosis, and direct repair are important to increase the chances of restoring function.

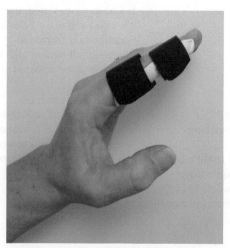

Figure 10-46 Static PIP and DIP extension splint.

TABLE **10-7**

Rehabilitation of Ulnar Collateral Ligament Injuries of the Thumb[27,56,65–67]

	Grade I	Grade II	Grade III
Description	Ligamentous stretching without tearing	Ligamentous tearing without complete disruption	Ligamentous disruption. Surgical repair or reconstruction
Healing Stages			
Stage I: Inflammatory stage (weeks 0 to 2)	Splinting at all times for weeks 0-4. Splint design may vary, depending on the surgeon's preference: • Hand-based short opponens splint with MCP joint in slight flexion, with or without a dorsal hood extending to the thumb tip that allows IP flexion while restricting hyperextension • Thumb spica cast or splint	Weeks 0-4: Thumb spica cast or splint at all times; IP joint may be included or free	Weeks 0-6: Casting
Stage II: Fibroplasia and repair stage (weeks 2 to 6)	Splint immobilization continues until weeks 4-6 Functional use is progressed, with modifications to avoid heavy pinching, pulling, and grasping	Weeks 4-6: Thumb spica cast is reduced to a hand-based short opponens splint that leaves the IP joint free; a dorsal hood prevents hyperextension of the IP joint. The splint must be worn between exercises. Splinting time frames vary, depending on stability and pain at the MCP joint; the splint can be worn up to week 12 for protection Week 6: • AROM • Soft tissue mobilization • Edema management	Weeks 0-6: Casting
Stage III: Remodeling and maturation stage (weeks 6 to 8+)	Week 8: Strengthening to tissue tolerance, focusing on the abductor pollicis brevis, flexor pollicis brevis, and adductor pollicis brevis	Splinting continues Blocking exercises for tendon gliding Light functional tasks Joint mobilization, respecting tissue tolerance Strengthening begins at week 12, respecting tissue tolerance and pain Full pinching and pulling activities at weeks 12-16, as tolerated	Progression to hand-based thumb splint with IP joint free; worn between exercises Splint worn up to weeks 8-12 Straight plane flexion and extension AROM Radial stress (terminal abduction) to the MCP joint must be avoided. Soft tissue and scar mobilization Edema management Blocking for tendon excursion Weeks 8+: Unrestricted AROM, PROM, gentle stretching Strengthening and return to full pinching and pulling activities at weeks 12-16

MCP, Metacarpophalangeal; *IP,* interphalangeal; *AROM,* active range of motion; *PROM,* passive range of motion.

Avulsion injuries to the flexor tendons usually are caused by a closed traumatic injury to the finger. These tend to occur during athletic events, and unfortunately, the diagnosis often is missed initially, which can lead to permanent disability. Avulsion injuries of the flexor digitorum superficialis tendons are rare compared with disruption of the flexor digitorum profundus tendons.

The ability of a tendon to heal and the degree to which adhesions develop in the area of the healing tendon depend on factors that relate to the injury and the surgical repair. The goal of tendon repair is based on establishing a strong enough repair to enable the patient to begin early protected motion while achieving the repair without inducing excessive scarring. Crush injuries and aggressive handling

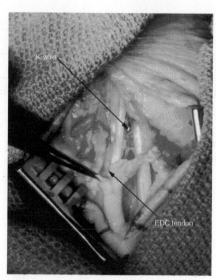

Figure 10-47 Rupture of a tendon from attrition over prominent hardware. The extensor digitorum communis (EDC) tendon to the index finger ruptured over the K-wire when the wire backed out of the bone. Side-to-side tendon repair produced an excellent result.

of the tendon sheath and tendon during surgery increase the chances of scar formation. Tendon ischemia, tendon immobilization, and gapping at the repair site also contribute to the formation of excursion-restricting adhesions.

After tendon repair, healing progresses through several stages. The first stage involves an inflammatory response. During this stage, the strength of the tendon repair relies primarily on the strength of the sutures in place, with the fibrin clot (between the tendon ends) offering a small contribution. The second stage is the fibroblast-producing stage. The strength of the tendon increases rapidly during this stage as granulation tissue forms at the site of the repair. The final stage is the remodeling stage, in which collagen synthesis continues and the repaired tendon becomes progressively stronger. This restorative progression is important because it is the physiological basis for the protected therapy program, which prevents the formation of adhesions while caring for the still mending tendon.[75,76]

Anatomy

The tendons for the flexor muscle groups insert distally on the metacarpals and phalanges to provide wrist and finger flexion. The forearm flexor muscles that power these tendons originate on the medial aspect of the elbow and are divided into three anatomical layers. The superficial layer of muscles consists of the pronator teres, flexor carpi radialis (FCR), flexor carpi ulnaris (FCU), and palmaris longus (PL). The intermediate muscle group is the flexor digitorum superficialis (FDS). The deep muscle group consists of the flexor digitorum profundus (FDP) and the flexor pollicis longus (FPL). The FDS tendons arise from individual muscle bundles and act independently to provide flexion of the PIP joints. This is in contrast to the FDP tendons, which arise from a common muscle, simultaneously flexing the DIP joints of the four digits. Each digit therefore has two flexors that originate in the forearm, and the thumb

has one. Every one of these nine tendons travels through the forearm and enters the wrist through the carpal tunnel beneath the transverse carpal ligament. The tendons continue in the palmar aspect of the hand, with the FDS tendons traveling anterior to the FDP tendons. They remain in this configuration until they enter their individual digits, through the digital sheath at the A1 pulley (Figure 10-48). At this point, the FDS tendon divides into two slips, traveling dorsally and on either side of the FDP tendon. The split FDS fibers rejoin, now dorsal to the FDP tendon, and insert along the proximal half of the middle phalanx, functioning to flex the PIP joint. The FDP tendons pass through the FDS bifurcation (*Camper's chiasm*) and insert on the distal phalanx, providing flexion of the DIP joint (Figure 10-49).

In the digits, the flexor tendons are enclosed in synovial sheaths. These sheaths provide a smooth synovial lining for tendon nutrition and to reduce the work of gliding. An intricate pulley system exists to create an efficient flexor mechanism by maintaining the tendons in close contact with the phalanges and preventing bowstringing of the tendons with the flexion motion. The A1, A3, and A5 annular pulleys arise from the volar plates of the MCP joints, the PIP joints, and the DIP joints, respectively. The A2 and A4 pulleys are functionally the most important pulleys, arising from the periosteum of the proximal half of the proximal phalanx (A2) and the midportion of the middle phalanx (A4). Also present are the thinner, less substantial cruciate pulleys: C1 (between A2 and A3), C2 (between A3 and A4), and C3 (between A4 and A5). These pulleys allow the annular pulleys to approximate each other during flexion (see Figure 10-49).

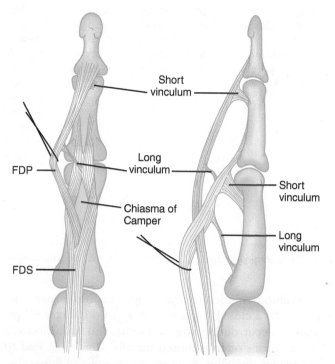

Figure 10-48 Anatomy of the flexor tendon. *FDS,* flexor digitorum superficialis; *FDP,* flexor digitorum profundus. (Redrawn from Schneider LH: *Flexor tendon injuries,* Boston, 1985, Little, Brown.)

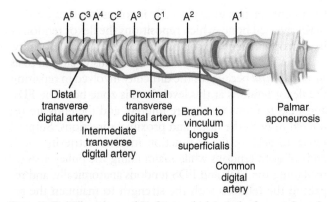

Figure 10-49 Pulley system of the finger, which includes five annular pulleys (A1-A5) and three cruciform pulleys (C1-C3). (From Skirven TM, Osterman AL, Fedorczyk J et al, editors: *Rehabilitation of the hand and upper extremity*, ed 6, Philadelphia, 2011, Mosby.)

Injury or disruption of these tendons anywhere along their course causes functional impairment of the distally involved joints.

Injury Classification

Flexor tendon injuries have been divided into zones over the volar aspect of the hand and wrist, based on differing anatomical characteristics. Zone I, the most distal zone, includes the area distal to the insertion of the FDS on the proximal phalanx. Zone II encompasses the area from the proximal border of zone I to the level of the distal palmar crease, which is the beginning of the flexor tendon sheath. This zone has been known historically as *no man's land* because of the complexity of the flexor tendons and fibro-osseous sheath anatomy in this region, which has led to poorer outcomes after tendon repairs. Zone III represents the area between the start of the fibro-osseous tendon sheath and the distal edge of the transverse carpal ligament. This also happens to be the area of the lumbrical muscle origin. The carpal tunnel region is zone IV, and proximal to the transverse carpal ligament is zone V. The thumb has its own zone distribution: zone T-I is distal to the DIP joint, zone T-II is between the MCP and IP joints, and zone T-III is proximal to the MCP volar flexion crease (Figure 10-50).

Diagnosis

A complete examination of the involved extremity must be performed to evaluate the extent of injury. In the inspection of the upper extremity, the examiner should note the posture of the hand. The presence of an abnormal cascade because of a digit resting in extension and an inability to perform specific flexion motor tests should alert the examiner to possible tendon injury. Specifically, when examining for a potential FDS injury, the examiner must hold the other digits in extension at the tips to prevent flexion of the injured digit through its possibly intact FDP tendon. Likewise, when examining for a FDP injury, the examiner must allow the patient to flex all the fingertips freely because the muscle for DIP flexion is not independent. Sensory evaluation can identify injuries to the digital

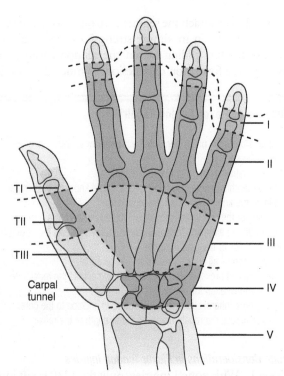

Figure 10-50 Flexor tendon zones: Fingers I, II, III, IV, V; Thumb TI, TII, TIII.

nerves, which may accompany trauma to a flexor tendon. It is important that the clinician recognize concomitant nerve injuries because nerve and vascular injuries affect the approach to operative management.

Medical Treatment

Before surgery is performed on an injured flexor tendon, relevant factors such as timing, prognosis, and concomitant injuries must be considered because they may affect the approach to surgical management. In the past a flexor tendon injury was considered a surgical emergency. This is no longer true, given current evidence that delayed primary flexor tendon repair leads to results that are equal to or better than those obtained with immediate repair.[77] With increasing delay, however, repair of the tendons at the appropriate length becomes more difficult because the tendon ends begin to deteriorate, and the flexor tendon/muscle system shortens.[77] The preferable course, therefore, is to perform the repair within a reasonable period. In most cases the time elapsed before myostatic contraction makes primary repairs technically difficult or impossible to achieve is thought to be 3 weeks.

Any concomitant injuries must be taken into consideration at the time of surgery. A contaminated wound or an injury with significant skin loss usually is a contraindication to repair of an injured flexor tendon. Associated fractures and neurovascular injuries are not a contraindication, and treating these injuries may actually be useful in maintaining stability and adequate perfusion of the tendon as it goes through the reparative process.

The main goals in performing a flexor tendon repair are (1) to retrieve both the proximal and distal ends of the tendons, (2) to reattach the segments to one another in such a way as to maintain maximum strength of the repair and allow easy tendon gliding within the tendon sheath, and (3) prevent the formation of adhesions as much as possible.

Principles of Flexor Tendon Repair[78,79]

- Repair strength is proportional to the number of strands that cross the repair site
- Repairs usually rupture at the suture knots
- The preferable course is to have as few suture knots as possible and to keep the knots away from the repair site
- Gapping at the repair site should be avoided because it is a major contributor to adhesion formation and negatively affects the strength and stiffness of the tendon repair
- Tension across all suture strands should be equal
- Equal tension prevents asymmetrical loading across the repair site, which can weaken the repair
- Use of a peripheral circumferential suture in addition to the core sutures across the repair increases the strength of the repair

---

Zone Considerations in Flexor Tendon Injuries

Zone I. With zone I injuries, only the FDP is cut, and locating the proximal end of the FDP tendon is relatively simple. A primary end-to-end suture repair can be performed if adequate length of the distal portion of the tendon is left. If the distal portion is short or nonexistent, the proximal tendon end may be attached directly to the bone of the distal phalanx either by a suture anchor within the bone or by sutures pulled through the bone and tied over a button on the dorsal aspect of the distal phalanx.

Avulsion of the FDP usually results from forced extension of a flexed digit, which causes the profundus tendon to pull away at its insertion on the distal phalanx. This injury has a high incidence among young, male athletes, and the ring finger is involved in more than 75% of cases.[80] This injury should be suspected if a patient has tenderness and swelling over the volar aspect of the finger and is unable to flex the DIP joint.

Three types of avulsion injuries can occur at the level of the profundus tendon.[81] In type I injuries the proximal portion of the tendon retracts into the palm. This end should be retrieved and reattached to the distal segment before muscle contracture occurs, resulting in shortening of the flexor system and making primary repair impossible. Surgical repair should take place within 7 to 10 days.

With type II injuries the proximal segment of tendon retracts to the level of the PIP joint and is held in place by an intact vinculum (small blood vessel to the tendon). Because this muscle-tendon unit has less of a tendency to shorten, surgical repair of this tendon injury is not as emergent as a type I injury. However, the clinician must keep in mind that if the vinculum breaks, the type II injury becomes a type I injury and requires repair within 7 to 10 days.

Type III injuries involve an avulsion of the large bony fragment to which the FDP attaches. The bone fragment tends to prevent proximal retraction of the tendon, and

treatment for this injury usually involves internal fixation of the avulsed bone, which repositions the flexor tendon at its appropriate length, correcting the extension deformity.

Zone II. Zone II injuries were previously referred to as *no man's land* because of the difficulty involved in repairing the flexor tendons at this level. In this zone both the FDP and FDS tendons usually are injured, and the ends are retracted in both the distal and proximal directions. Surgical repair to achieve flexor function involves retrieving both ends of both tendons while maintaining the pulley system, realigning the FDP and FDS tendons anatomically, and repairing the tendons with the strength to maintain the repair without generating increased formation of adhesions.

Zone III. Zone III injuries occur in the region just distal to the carpal tunnel. Both the FDP and FDS tendons travel in this region, and either one or both tendons may be injured. Primary repair of the tendon ends has a good prognosis in this region.

Zone IV. In zone IV the carpal tunnel, the FDP and FDS tendons travel together, along with the median nerve. Laceration at this level may result in injury to one or multiple tendons and to the median nerve. A thorough neurovascular examination must be performed to determine the extent of tendon and nerve damage, and primary repair should be performed before muscle contractures occur.

Zone V. In zone V (i.e., the wrist and forearm), the tendons originate from their musculotendinous junctions and travel together toward their insertion sites. They are less constrained in this region, and tendon repair tends to have a favorable prognosis. However, these injuries may be complicated by multiple tendon lacerations or accompanying neurovascular injury.

The Thumb. Flexor tendon repair of the thumb follows the same principles as tendon injury in the digits, even though the thumb has only one flexor tendon and three pulleys. The lacerated proximal portion of the FPL may be located within the thumb, or it may have retracted into the thenar eminence or the carpal tunnel, making retrieval more complicated. The proximal section should be located, retrieved, and then sutured to the distal section of tendon.

Complications

Surgical repair of flexor tendons often is successful at restoring tendon function; however, the procedure is not without associated complications. The most significant complication is rupture of the flexor tendon at the repair site. If this is recognized, treatment involves reexploration of the area and repair at the earliest possible time. Flexion contractures at the DIP or PIP joints are frequent complications of repair of flexor tendon injuries. If noted early, alteration of therapy strategies may help reverse these contractures. The development of tendon adhesions is another frustrating complication of flexor tendon repairs. The formation of adhesions prevents functional excursion of the tendon within the sheath, resulting in decreased motion of the involved digit. A tenolysis procedure may be performed to remove adhesions once a plateau has been reached in therapy.

Extensor Tendon Injury

General Considerations

The extensor mechanism of the hand is a unique system that relies on an intricate link between the **radial nerve–innervated extrinsic extensor system**, which originates in the forearm, and the **ulnar nerve–innervated intrinsic system**, which originates in the hand.

Injury to the extensor tendon mechanism occurs more frequently than flexor tendon injury because of the more superficial anatomical location of these tendons. This injury should be recognized and taken seriously because a very delicate balance is achieved within the extensor mechanism. Injury that compromises length, alignment, or stability disrupts this equilibrium, and repair must be meticulous to reestablish the balance of function.

Anatomy

The extrinsic extensor muscles located in the forearm and inserting into the phalanges include the extensor pollicis longus (EPL), extensor pollicis brevis (EPB), extensor indicis proprius (EIP), and extensor digiti minimi (EDM). The tendons arising from these muscle bellies have an independent origin and action. The extensor digitorum communis (EDC) is the common origin of four independent tendons. These become the primary extensor component of the four digits. The intrinsic muscle contribution to the extensor system consists of four dorsal interossei, three palmar interossei, and four lumbrical muscles. These intrinsic muscles function to flex the MCP joints of the four digits and extend the PIP and DIP joints.

The extensor tendons leave the forearm and enter the hand through six dorsal compartments at the level of the wrist and are secured by the extensor retinaculum. This retinaculum functions to prevent bowstringing of the tendons, causing close approximation of the tendon to the bone and allowing efficient extension. As the tendons enter the hand and travel dorsal to the metacarpals, the EDC tendons, despite originating as independent tendons, become interconnected by the juncturae tendinum. This interconnection results in some codependence and shared extensor activity by these four digits. As the tendons continue to travel distally toward the fingers, they become centrally located over their respective metacarpal heads. They extend the proximal phalanx by way of a sling mechanism and are stabilized in this central position by the sagittal bands, which run on both sides of the tendon and insert on the volar plate of the MCP joint. As the tendons travel distally along the proximal phalanx (never inserting into that bone), they divide into three slips. The central slip crosses the PIP joint and inserts on the proximal portion of the middle phalanx. The lateral slips travel along both sides of the PIP and the middle phalanx (Figure 10-51).

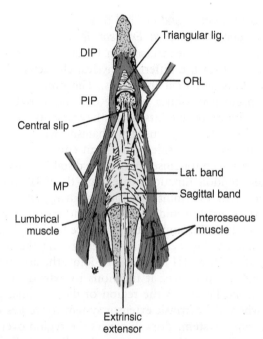

Figure 10-51 Dorsal view of the extensor mechanism. *DIP*, distal interphalangeal joint; *PIP*, proximal interphalangeal joint; *MP*, metacarpophalangeal joint; *ORL*, oblique retinacular ligament. (From Coons MS, Green SM: Boutonniere deformity, *Hand Clin* 11:387-402, 1995.)

In the region of the proximal phalanx, the intrinsic muscle tendons begin their contribution to the extensor mechanism. The lumbrical and the palmar and dorsal interossei tendons converge to form the lateral bands, which travel on either side of the proximal phalanx. A portion of the lateral bands joins with the extensor tendon at the PIP joint to insert as a central slip. The remainder contributes fibers that travel on both sides of the middle phalanx and insert into the dorsum of the distal phalanx as the terminal tendon. Because the intrinsic tendons are located volar to the axis of rotation of the MCP joints and dorsal to the axis of rotation of the PIP and DIP joints, the intrinsic muscles function to flex the MCP joint and extend the PIP and DIP joints. In summary, the central slip insertion on the middle phalanx is a convergence of the extrinsic extensor tendon, lumbrical tendon, and interossei tendon. Portions of these tendons travel distally to form the lateral bands, which then converge to form the terminal tendon, inserting on the proximal aspect of the distal phalanx.

The anatomy of the extensor mechanism of the thumb is somewhat different than that of the fingers. The extrinsic tendons enter the hand via the extensor retinaculum in the wrist. The EPB inserts at the base of the proximal phalanx, and the EPL inserts at the base of the distal phalanx. The EPL is stabilized in its central position over the thumb MCP joint by sagittal bands. The intrinsic extensor component to the thumb comes from the ulnar nerve–innervated adductor pollicis, which functions to adduct the thumb, flex the thumb MCP joint, and extend the thumb IP joint.

Injury Classification and Medical Treatment

Zone Considerations in Extensor Tendon Injuries. The extensor tendon mechanism can be divided into eight zones based on the differing physical characteristics of the tendons and their insertions. The even-numbered zones occur over bones, and the odd-numbered zones are positioned over joints. Zone I represents the most distal aspect of the extensor mechanism, where the lateral bands on either side of the digit converge to form the terminal tendon, inserting on the distal phalanx. The terminal tendon functions to extend the DIP joint in concert with PIP joint extension. Moving proximally, zone II covers the middle phalanx, the area where the two lateral bands join together, and are held in place by the triangular ligament just before forming the terminal tendon. Zone III is at the PIP joint, the area where the central slip inserts; it functions to extend the PIP joint. Zone IV covers the region of the proximal phalanx, where the extrinsic extensor system converges with the intrinsic system. Zone V covers the region over the MCP joint, where the extensor tendons lie centrally over the joint, stabilized by the sagittal bands. Zone VI exists over the metacarpal bones, where the extensor communis tendons are interconnected by the juncturae tendinum. In zone VII, at the level of the wrist joint, the tendons lie within the tenosynovium, covered by the extensor retinaculum. Zone VIII is the most proximal zone, containing the extensor tendons at their musculotendinous junctions. Zone IX consists of the proximal one half of the forearm above the musculotendinous junction (Figure 10-52).

Zone I (Mallet Finger Deformities).

Zone I injuries create a *mallet finger deformity* (Figure 10-53). These injuries result in disruption of the extensor tendon at the level of the DIP joint, caused by a closed avulsion injury, an open skin and tendon injury, or a fracture of the proximal portion of the distal phalanx, where the terminal tendon of the extensor system inserts. Closed injuries occur more often, usually when sudden flexion of the extended digit ruptures the tendon from its bony insertion – or the bony insertion site, with the tendon attached, may avulse from the distal phalanx. Open injuries may be lacerations or crush injuries that disrupt the extensor tendon.

Upon physical examination, the distal phalanx is found to be in some degree of flexion, and the patient is unable to actively extend the distal portion of the injured finger. Hyperextension of the PIP joint may be present, secondary to the unopposed tension of the central slip combined with volar plate laxity, resulting in a *swan neck deformity.*

Mallet finger deformities have been classified according to the cause of the deformity because this assists in the determination of the treatment plan. The goal of management is to restore tendon continuity with maximum return to function.

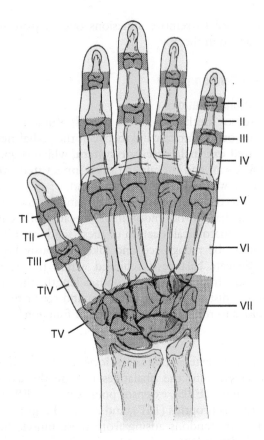

Figure 10-52 Extensor tendon zones. (From Trumble TE et al, editors: *Core knowledge in orthopaedics: hand, elbow, and shoulder*, Philadelphia, 2006, Mosby.)

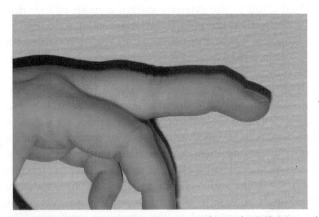

Figure 10-53 Mallet injury. Note the extensor lag at the DIP joint and the mild hyperextension at the PIP joint (swan neck deformity).

A *type I mallet finger injury* is the result of closed or blunt trauma, with or without a small avulsion fracture. This is the most common type of injury, and splinting of the DIP in extension is the optimum treatment option. Hyperextension should be avoided because this may cause ischemia of the thin dorsal skin. The patient wears a splint continuously for a minimum of 6 weeks, followed by 2 weeks of nighttime splinting.[82] This usually results in excellent recovery. On rare occasions, if a patient is unable to wear a splint, a K-wire may be placed across the DIP joint to maintain the joint in extension.

A *type II mallet deformity* results from a laceration at the level of or just proximal to the DIP joint, causing disruption of the extensor tendon. Given the numerous attachments of the extensor tendon to the digit, very little retraction of the proximal end occurs, and in this situation the tendon should be primarily repaired. The extensor tendon at this level is broad and thin, and repair should consist of a running suture that reapproximates the skin and tendon simultaneously. After repair, a splint should be worn to maintain the DIP in an extended position for 6 weeks.

A *type III mallet deformity* is caused by a deep abrasion to the distal aspect of the finger, resulting in loss of skin, subcutaneous tissue, and tendon substance. Given the nature of this injury, reconstructive surgery is needed for soft tissue coverage, and tendon reconstruction with a free tendon graft should be the treatment of choice. The loss of tendon substance, resulting in loss of extensor tendon length, impairs the surgeon's ability to restore function of the extensor mechanism using primary repair.

Type IV mallet deformities are further subdivided into three groups. Type IV-A deformities result from a transepiphyseal fracture in children. Because the extensor tendon is attached to the epiphysis, a mallet finger deformity results secondary to the fracture. Closed reduction of the fracture corrects this deformity. Continuous splinting of the DIP in extension for 3 to 4 weeks usually produces union of the fracture and resolution of the deformity. Type IV-B deformities are caused by a hyperflexion injury with a fracture that compromises 20% to 50% of the dorsal articular surface. A hyperextension injury that causes a fracture with a bone fragment larger than 50% of the dorsal articular surface results in a type IV-C mallet finger deformity. Because of the largely compromised articular surface in these injuries, they often are associated with volar subluxation of the distal phalanx relative to the proximal phalanx. In both type IV-B and IV-C injuries, the mallet deformity results because the extensor tendon remains attached to the fractured segment of bone.

For fractures that have subluxed anteriorly, operative management is recommended to achieve an accurate reduction of the fracture and to restore articular congruity (see Figure 10-3). Surgery restores the extensor tendon length and resolves the mallet deformity. For fractures that are not subluxed, splinting of the DIP in extension for 6 weeks results in fracture union and remodeling of the articular surface, with subsequent resolution of the mallet deformity.

Mallet thumb, or injury to the extensor mechanism of the thumb in zone I, at the level of the IP joint is a rare injury, which may be caused by a closed rupture of the EPL insertion or a laceration of the tendon at this level. A closed injury should be treated with IP extension splinting

for 6 to 8 weeks. An open laceration is best treated by primary repair, with sutures incorporating both skin and tendon.

Zone II. Zone II injuries of the fingers and thumb occur at the level of the middle phalanx and usually result from a laceration or crush injury that leads to disruption of the extensor tendon. Partial lacerations, in which less than 50% of the tendon is disrupted, are common in this region because of the broad, curved shape of the tendon as it lies against the phalanx. If a partial laceration occurs, treatment involves wound care and splinting for 7 to 10 days. If the laceration causes more extensive tendon damage, the distal and proximal tendon ends should be primarily repaired, followed by extension splinting.

Zone III. Zone III injuries occur at the level of the PIP joint, with disruption to the central slip. If allowed to progress, these injuries cause the classic boutonniere deformity (i.e., hyperflexion of the PIP joint and subsequent hyperextension at the DIP joint). Loss of extension at the PIP joint may not result immediately because the lateral bands retain the ability to extend this joint. However, over time, the head of the proximal phalanx buttonholes through the defect created by the ruptured central slip, and the lateral bands migrate anteriorly below the axis of rotation of the PIP joint, converting them from PIP extensors to PIP flexors. This causes loss of extension at the PIP joint, and a flexion deformity results. At the same time, the more anterior position of the lateral bands at the level of the PIP joint causes increased tension along these bands, which is transmitted to the terminal tendon and leads to hyperextension of the DIP joint. This injury may result from either a laceration of the central slip or closed trauma with acute forceful flexion of the PIP joint, causing avulsion of the central slip. Correction of this deformity requires reestablishment of the tendon balance and the tendon length relationship between the central slip and the lateral bands. If a closed rupture has occurred, the PIP can be splinted, gradually progressing to full extension. This allows reapproximation and healing of the ends of the central slip. A K-wire across the extended PIP joint can achieve the same goal. If the central slip is injured by an acute laceration, primary repair of this tendon should be performed.

Zone III injuries of the thumb at the level of the MCP joint may involve one or both of the thumb extensor tendons. If only the EPB is injured, thumb extension at the MCP joint likely will be retained because the EPL remains functional. If the EPL is disrupted, an extension lag across both the MCP and IP joints results. Primary repair is usually indicated for laceration injuries within this zone.

Zone IV. Zone IV injuries occur at the level of the proximal phalanx. In this region, the lateral bands contribute significantly to the extensor function and offer protection against complete lacerations of the central tendon. Therefore injury in this zone usually results in partial lacerations; however, this diagnosis can be made only under direct visualization of the tendon. If the tendon is partly lacerated, splinting the PIP for 3 to 4 weeks is adequate treatment.[83] If laceration of a lateral band is diagnosed, primary repair may be performed, followed by early protected motion. For complete lacerations of the extensor tendon, primary repair should be undertaken, followed by 4 to 6 weeks of PIP extension splinting. Preserving appropriate tendon length during this repair is crucial, so that the balance between the central tendon and the lateral bands is maintained.

Zone V. Many types of injuries involving the extensor mechanism can occur in zone V, at the level of the MCP joint. Open wounds often occur at this level and are of special concern given the proximity of the MCP joint to the surface of the skin. If a patient uses a fist to strike someone in the mouth, a fight bite may result, which is a contaminated open wound most likely communicating with the MCP joint. Immediate debridement, irrigation, and antibiotic therapy must be started. Partial tendon injuries usually are associated with this type of wound, but if a complete tendon injury does occur, then either a primary or secondary repair may be performed, depending on the status of the wound. If a clean laceration occurs at the level of the MCP joint, primary repair of the tendon may be performed.

The sagittal bands, which are found on both sides of the extensor tendon at the level of the MCP joint, are vulnerable to injury in zone V. The sagittal bands centralize the extensor tendon over the MCP joint. Injuries to these bands may be caused by a laceration, or the bands may be ruptured by a forceful blow of the clenched fist against a hard surface. Prompt recognition of this injury allows for treatment by extension splinting. If this is not successful, repair of the sagittal bands may be undertaken at a later date to prevent subluxation and to improve extensor function at the MCP joint.

Zone V injuries of the thumb occur at the level of the CMC joint and commonly involve lacerations of the EPB and APL tendons. Injuries in this region must be carefully evaluated for possible compromise of the radial artery and the radial nerve sensory branches. The proximal segment of the APL may retract in this region, therefore retrieval of this tendon and primary repair should be performed.

Zone VI. Injuries in zone VI occur at the level of the metacarpals, where the tendons for the EDC, extensor indicis proprius, and extensor digiti minimi are located. Tendon lacerations, either partial or complete, are difficult to diagnose at this level because full active extension may not be completely lost; extensor action may be transmitted through the juncturae tendinae, or redundant tendon function may be present (in the case of the index and small fingers). To test for independent tendon function on the physical examination, the examiner should hold all digits except the one being examined in flexion at the MCP joints to prevent any possible contribution of the juncturae tendinum from confounding the examination.[84] Ideally, the diagnosis for this injury should be made under direct visualization. Tendons in this region are thicker and more oval and can support a stronger core suture for use in primary repair. After repair, postoperative management includes splinting for 4 to 6 weeks. If an EDC tendon is involved, all fingers should be splinted; if an extensor indicis proprius tendon was injured, only the specific index finger needs splinting.

Zone VII. Zone VII injuries occur at the level of the wrist and usually involve injury to the extensor retinaculum. The wrist and finger extensor tendons coexist in this region, and the chance of multiple tendon injuries is high. Injury may result from lacerations, tendon ruptures after fracture, or tendon dislocation after injury to the retinaculum. The distal and proximal ends of the injured tendons retract in this area, making primary repair of these injuries more complicated. If multiple tendons are lacerated, the appropriate proximal and distal regions must be retrieved and anatomically matched and then primarily repaired. Damage to the retinaculum also complicates injury in this zone. This structure is necessary to prevent bowstringing of the extensor tendons, as they function to extend the wrist and the fingers. Part of the retinaculum may be resected to allow adequate exposure and retrieval of the tendons, but the retinaculum should not be fully excised, and its function should be preserved. However, tendon healing at this level is often associated with the formation of adhesions to the overlying retinaculum.[85] Measures attempted to prevent adhesion formation include early dynamic splinting.

Zone VIII. Tendon injuries in the distal forearm, zone VIII, usually occur at the musculotendinous junction and may be caused by a laceration or rupture. Primary repair of these injuries is difficult because, although the distal tendon segment retains suture well, the proximal muscle region does not. Options for restoring adequate extensor function in this type of injury are side-to-side suture repairs or tendon transfers.

Zone IX. Zone IX injuries occur in the proximal forearm and usually are caused by a penetrating wound. Injury at this level is complicated by the multiple structures present and vulnerable. Muscle transection or nerve injury may result in functional impairment. A careful, thorough physical examination must be performed, and often surgical exploration is undertaken for diagnosis. If the muscle is found to be damaged, it is repaired primarily or, if the muscle defect is too extensive, tendon grafting may be performed.

Rehabilitation Principles and Considerations for Tendon Injuries

Flexor Tendon Injuries of the Hand

Numerous articles and studies have been written about the rehabilitation of flexor tendon injuries. Despite the wealth of information available to clinicians, determining which approach to choose can be confusing and difficult.

Effects of Early, Controlled Force on a Repaired Flexor Tendon

- More rapid recovery of tensile strength
- Fewer adhesions
- Improved tendon excursion
- Less gapping at the repair site

Several studies provide evidence that incremental stress and tendon excursion increase the rate at which the repair site achieves normal tensile strength and reduce the amount of scar adhesion. A variety of postoperative flexor tendon protocols have been designed to provide the optimal amount of tension loading at the precise time in the patient's treatment.[10,87,88] Early mobilization, either passive or active, starting within the first week of the repair, has been reported to produce excellent results compared with postoperative immobilization.[88] Early passive mobilization (EPM) consists of passive flexion with active extension within the confines of a protective splint. Early active mobilization (EAM) consists of active flexion and extension of the involved finger within certain parameters of a protective splint.[87-90] Recent literature has also emphasized the importance of the positions of the adjacent fingers on the tendon gliding and excursion of the repaired flexor tendon on the operative digit.[91]

Despite the benefits of these early mobilization programs, questions remain as to how much motion should be allowed and when to begin. If early active motion is too aggressive, it may cause gap formation or even rupture the repaired tendon. However, traditional early passive motion protocols may not provide enough tendon gliding within the tendon sheath to prevent scar adhesions.[92]

Selection of a Treatment Protocol. The postoperative treatment protocol and guidelines chosen to guide rehabilitation decisions and interventions are critically important. Surgical repairs and treatment protocols can vary greatly. Communication between the surgeon and therapist is vital to ensure the most successful outcome for the patient. It is important that the therapist know the type of flexor tendon repair and suture technique performed before initiating a rehabilitation protocol. The combination of advanced suture techniques and immediate passive mobilization has reduced adhesions and repair site gaps and increased tendon excursion. Recent methods of core suture techniques offer greater tensile strength to the tendon at the time of the repair and improve strength up to 6 weeks postoperatively.[93] Stronger suture techniques designed for active motion have also been developed, but it is critical that the therapist know what type of repair was performed before initiating early EAM protocols.

Several factors can affect the strength of a flexor tendon repair, such as the suture caliber, the number of strands crossing a repair, and the type of suture loops used. A suture caliber of 3-0 is recommended over 4-0, and a four-strand repair is thought to be better than a two-strand repair. Also, some surgeons believe that locking suture loops that hold the tendon on either side are best for enhancing the strength of the repair.[94,95] It has become accepted that four- or six-strand flexor tendon repair methods, combined with a strong epitendinous suture, should be sufficiently strong to withstand light active forces through healing.[96]

Factors Affecting the Strength of a Tendon Repair

- Suture caliber (e.g., 3-0)
- Number of suture strands that cross the repair (four to six)
- Type of suture loops

Another important consideration for therapists treating patients with flexor tendon repairs is how much friction is present and how well the tendon glides. In an injured finger, joint stiffness caused by diffuse swelling or soft tissue restrictions becomes a major factor, and significant tendon force is needed to overcome it. Other sources that cause resistance to motion within the tendon sheath include damage to the pulley system, tendon sheath, or gliding surfaces of the tendon, all of which can cause adhesions to form later during the healing process.[94]

Sources of Resistance to Tendon Motion

- Swelling
- Scarring (adhesions)
- Joint stiffness (hypomobility)
- Damage to the pulley system
- Damage to the tendon sheath
- Damage to the tendon gliding surfaces

The effects of drag and other viscous effects on a joint significantly affect the outcome of a tendon repair. Gentle passive motion of the involved finger joints should be performed at slow speeds to eliminate the potential for viscoelastic forces. Passive motion serves to release and reduce fluid around a joint, which reduces the resistance to motion.[96] Passive joint motion also enhances the motion of the tendons with respect to one another. Passive flexion of the DIP joint produces excursion of the FDP in relation to the FDS of 1 to 2 mm for every 10° of motion, and passive flexion of the PIP joint produces 1.5 mm of tendon excursion between the two tendons for every 10° of joint flexion.[97]

An extremely swollen finger will have a significant increase in friction, which can affect tendon gliding. Any degree of joint excursion will require significantly more force, posing the danger of gapping at the tendon repair site. Discrepancy in the literature exists about the acceptable amount of gapping at the repair site. Gaps also cause increased friction, and gaps of 3 mm or more can block tendon motion, causing the tendon to rupture or adhesions to form.[94,97]

Most protocols developed for both EPM and EAM recommend that treatment begin 24 to 48 hours after surgery to prevent adhesion formation and joint contracture. Recently some experts have said that starting passive motion the day after surgery may hurt the final result because the gliding resistance of the tendon is high during this time because of swelling. Starting early motion the day after surgery can be associated with an increased risk of inducing fresh bleeding, which can lead to adhesions; therefore some recommend waiting 3 to 5 days before initiating treatment to prevent joint stiffness and scar formation. The consensus for all tendon rehabilitation is that treatment should begin early, no later than 3 to 5 days after surgery, to prevent joint stiffness and adhesions.[94,98] One of the benefits of early mobilization is an increase in tensile strength, which is achieved by stimulating maturation of the tendon wound and remodeling the scar tissue. This process prevents "softening" of the tendon, which can occur after day 5 if the tendon has been immobile, causing the tendon to be weaker during this time frame.[86,99] Clinicians must evaluate each patient and determine with the patient's surgeon the most appropriate time to begin treatment.

A third consideration in treating flexor tendon injuries involves the position of the wrist and its relationship to the finger flexors. Internal flexor tendon loading is greatly influenced by wrist position. Tendon loading occurs during wrist flexion because passive finger extension causes the tendon to move distally. Internal tendon loading also occurs during wrist extension with passive finger flexion as the tendon is pulled proximally. The tenodesis effect of wrist extension with finger flexion and wrist flexion with finger extension enhances tendon excursion. This concept has been incorporated into both EPM and EAM tendon rehabilitation protocols.[100,101] A study by Savage[102] reported that a position of wrist extension and MCP joint flexion produces the least tension in a repaired flexor tendon during active finger flexion.

It also is important that the clinician know the zone or location of the injury and repair because this affects the patient's treatment. The flexor tendons are divided into five zones, which were described previously. Treatment protocols vary, depending on the zone of the injury and repair. The literature primarily focuses on zone II flexor tendon injuries. This zone has the highest probability of developing adhesions because the FDP travels through the FDS at Camper's chiasm, and the two tendons are located within one flexor tendon sheath.

Other important considerations are associated injuries, patient compliance, and the timing of surgery. The presence of associated injuries, such as digital nerve or artery lacerations, significant soft tissue loss, and dislocations or fractures, also influences the course of treatment for a flexor tendon injury. Clinicians may need to alter rehabilitation protocols to accommodate these injuries. The patient's ability to understand a rehabilitation program and to follow it faithfully is critical to a successful recovery.

Rehabilitation protocols are valuable guidelines, but each patient must be evaluated independently to determine the most suitable treatment regimen and the ways it might need to be altered to best serve the individual.

Early Passive Mobilization. Immobilization protocols have largely been abandoned in favor of early mobilization programs, which have resulted in much better motion and greater function. Occasionally, a young child or patient who is unable to participate appropriately with an early mobilization program is a candidate for an immobilization program, which usually consists of 4 weeks of immobilization in a plaster cast or protective splint before initiation of passive and AROM exercises. Patients can begin gentle resistance at 8 weeks and progress with a strengthening program at 10 weeks, with no restrictions by 12 weeks. Unfortunately, some patients treated with immobilization programs may not achieve full motion and have some residual limitations, depending on the location and nature of the injury.

One of the original controlled motion protocols developed by Kleinert for flexor tendon repairs consisted of a dorsal block splint with the wrist positioned at 40° flexion and the MCP joints in 40° to 60° flexion. The injured finger was held in flexion by a rubber band attached from the fingernail to a bandage or strap at the wrist level. Patients were instructed to actively extend against the rubber band up to the dorsal hood of the splint and then relax the finger, allowing the rubber band to passively flex the digit. Active flexion of the finger was not permitted for 4 weeks. After 4 weeks in the dorsal protective splint, patients were instructed to begin active flexion and extension exercises.[103] Modifications of the Kleinert traction approach include a palmar bar with pulley to increase DIP joint flexion. Although results using the rubber bands, or Kleinert method (Figure 10-54), were much better than

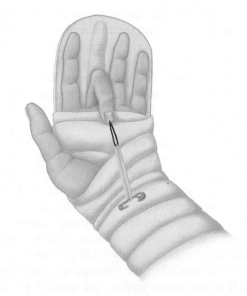

Figure 10-54 Kleinert splinting protocol. (From Canale ST, Beaty JH: *Campbell's operative orthopaedics*, ed 12, Philadelphia, 2013, Mosby.)

the immobilization programs, some patients developed flexion contractures at the PIP joint from being held in flexion by the rubber band traction.

In the 1970s, Duran and Houser presented a controlled passive motion method that has been modified over the years. It has become the basis for EPM protocols used today by many clinicians and surgeons. Duran used a dorsal block splint similar to that described previously, but, instead of a rubber band positioning the finger in flexion, the fingers were held in the splint with the PIP and DIP joints held in neutral (0°) with a Velcro strap, up against the hood of the dorsal block splint. The patient was instructed to remove the Velcro strap and perform three passive exercises within the confines of the splint. The first exercise was isolated passive DIP flexion, which allowed the FDP to independently glide from the FDS. The second exercise was passive flexion and extension of the PIP joint with the MCP in flexion in the splint, which allowed the FDS and FDP to move away from the damaged tendon sheath. The third exercise was full composite passive flexion of the MCP, PIP, and DIP joints, alternated with passive extension of the IP joints while the MCP joint was blocked in flexion (Figure 10-55).[104]

Modified Duran protocols incorporate active finger extension to meet the confines of the dorsal block splint, after passive flexion and extension of the finger. Active flexion of the finger is contraindicated for 3½ to 4 weeks after surgery. Proponents of the modified Duran method believe that it is less likely to cause flexion contractures at the IP joints than the Kleinert method and

that the involved finger is protected better with a Velcro strap when the patient is not exercising. In recent years clinicians have combined some components of early active motion with the modified Duran protocol.[96,105,106] Modified Duran flexor tendon protocols are used to treat zone I and zone II flexor tendon injuries and may vary slightly among clinicians, surgeons, and clinics; this is the reason good communication with the surgeon and a thorough knowledge of the patient's injury and repair are important. (The modified Duran program with place and hold guidelines are presented in Table 10-8.)

Early Active Mobilization. Early mobilization programs originally focused on EPM. It is now widely accepted that tensile strength at the repair site increases when tendons are mobilized early. Despite improved results with EPM, some patients with zone I and zone II flexor tendon repairs still fail to achieve normal range of motion. This has led to the desire for rehabilitation algorithms that would allow for safe, early active mobilization. Suture techniques have been designed to minimize repair site gapping, which can lead to adhesions and tendon rupture but allow some early active motion. Repair site strength is directly related to the number of suture strands crossing the tendon laceration; however, as the number of sutures increases, so does repair site volume and the work for tendon gliding. The suture technique used by surgeons may vary, and debate continues as to whether four-, six-, or eight-strand repairs are best.[93-95] Strickland[97] has determined that a four-strand core suture plus a strong peripheral suture can withstand the stress of gentle early active motion.

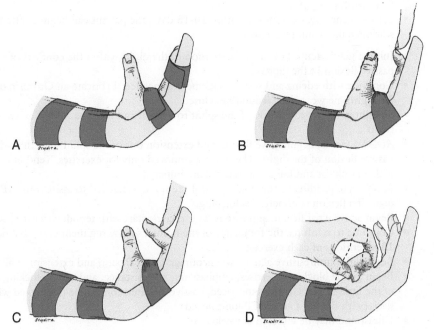

Figure 10-55 Duran protocol. **A,** Right hand in dorsal block splint. **B,** Exercise 1: passive flexion of the distal interphalangeal (DIP) joint (*right hand illustrated*). **C,** Exercise 2: passive flexion-extension of the proximal interphalangeal (PIP) joint (*right hand illustrated*). **D,** Exercise 3: Composite passive flexion of metacarpophalangeal (MCP) joint along with PIP and DIP joints followed by passive extension of PIP and DIP joints while MCP joint held in flexion (*left hand illustrated*). (From Strickland WJ: Biologic rationale, clinical application, and results of early motion following flexor tendon repair, *J Hand Ther* 2:78, 1989.)

TABLE **10-8**

Flexor Tendon Repairs in Zones I and II: Modified Duran Program with Place and Hold

Time Frame	Program Considerations

0 to 5 days	• Inspect the wound. Apply a nonrestrictive sterile dressing (e.g., Xeroform or Adaptic); if bleeding occurs, combine with light gauze. Instruct the patient in all precautions:
	  ○ Avoid all active finger or wrist flexion.
	  ○ Avoid functional use of the injured hand and avoid lifting with the involved extremity.
	  ○ Avoid fully extending the fingers and wrist.
	• *Splint:* Fabricate a dorsal block protective splint (position may vary slightly, depending on surgeon's preference): 20° to 30° wrist flexion, 50° to 70° MCP finger flexion, 0° IP finger extension. (If a digital nerve repair was performed, the PIP joint should be in slight flexion to protect the nerve repair.)
	• *Exercise program:* The protocol may vary depending on the type of repair, the surgeon's preference, and the patient's age and compliance. The following is a modified Duran protocol with a place and hold component (four strand repair):
	  ○ Instruct the patient in *gentle passive flexion* of each digit at the MCP joint, the PIP joint, and the DIP joint, and in *active extension* within the confines of the splint. The splint should be worn at all times and during exercises; only the top strap is removed to complete the exercises. The exercises should be performed 10 times for each digit once an hour if the patient is very restricted in passive flexion; otherwise, the exercises should be performed 5-6 times a day for 3½ weeks after surgery.
	  ○ Apply compressive wrap (e.g., Coban) to reduce swelling: instruct the patient in edema management, ice packs, and elevation. The patient should be assisted by another person in applying the Coban.
	• *Early AROM/place and hold:* In addition to the previous program, the following can be initiated within 5 days after surgery *only* with reliable patients who have full passive flexion and decreased edema. The therapist needs to know whether the procedure was at least a four-strand repair of the flexor tendon before initiating place and hold:
	  ○ Place and hold should be done after passive flexion of the digits within the confines of the splint. Passively place the patient's finger in a partly flexed position and have the patient hold this position with minimum tension for 3 seconds. During weeks 2 and 3, place and hold can progress with the finger held in more flexion, again using minimum tension to hold.
	• Sutures generally are removed within 10-15 days; the patient can begin gentle massage to the scar once the wound has closed.

3½ to 4½ weeks	• Initiate gentle active flexion and extension of the digits within the confines of the splint after passive flexion of the digits. • Continue with edema and scar management as needed. Fabricate an Otoform or elastomer mold for nighttime wear if the wound has closed. • Straighten the wrist position of the splint to neutral and increase MCP flexion, if needed, to 60° to 70°. • At 4-4½ weeks, begin active flexion and extension out of the splint with the wrist in neutral after passive flexion of the digits. The splint is removed only for exercises. Tendon gliding exercises with a hook fist and full composite fist are initiated. • Apply foam padding to the dorsal part of the splint as needed to assist with PIP extension of the digits if a flexion contracture is forming. • Begin active wrist flexion and extension exercises; start with tenodesis wrist motion. • Continue to reinforce the frequency of the home exercise regimen: every 1-2 hours, 10 repetitions of each exercise. • Begin light, nonresistive activity to encourage finger flexion and extension while in therapy. • Begin gentle blocking exercises, emphasizing no resistance, and avoid blocking to the DIP joint of the little finger. Gentle, supervised, passive IP extension can be performed with the tendon on slack (with the wrist and MCP joint flexed). • Ultrasound may be initiated at weeks 4-6.

(Continued)

TABLE **10-8**

Flexor Tendon Repairs in Zones I and II: Modified Duran Program with Place and Hold—cont'd

Time Frame	Program Considerations
6 to 8 weeks	• Depending on the patient's judgment and activity level, the dorsal block protective splint may be discharged. The patient may need the splint for protection only in certain situations; otherwise, it should be kept off. • The patient can begin to use the injured hand for light ADLs (e.g., buttoning a shirt, washing the face). *Emphasize:* o No heavy gripping or squeezing o No lifting o No using the hand for pushing or pulling (e.g., opening doors) • Begin light resistive exercises and activities (e.g., squeeze soft putty, sponge, or light grippers). Some patients may benefit from a resting splint at night to gradually increase finger and wrist extension. • Aggressive scar management is continued. • Gradually increase resistance for strengthening program (moderate resistance). • Dynamic or static progressive PIP extension splinting or casting may be necessary. • Evaluate grip strength at weeks 8-10 after surgery, depending on the level of scar tissue present.
10 to 12 weeks	• Continue with strengthening program and progress as tolerated or as needed. • The patient can return to all normal activities, including heavy work or sports, as tolerated. Most patients should be on a home program by week 12; however, treatment may vary for patients with complex injuries or complications.

MCP, Metacarpophalangeal; *IP,* interphalangeal; *PIP,* proximal interphalangeal; *DIP,* distal interphalangeal; *AROM,* active range of motion; *ADLs,* activities of daily living.

Trends over the past decade have been moving toward EAM programs that allow active flexion and extension of the involved fingers within the first 3 to 5 days. In 2004, Gail N. Groth presented the **Pyramid of Progressive Force Application**.[101] Progressive force application to the healing flexor tendon juncture is theorized as a series of eight specific rehabilitation exercise levels. These exercises are conceptualized in a pyramid format with the base of the pyramid signifying the lowest level of force across the juncture as well as exercises that are performed with the highest frequency (Figure 10-56). Loads rise as the pyramid builds, although the frequency of prescription decreases. Patients begin force application at the lowest level progressing upward only as determined necessary, reaching maximum loads (i.e., the pinnacle of the pyramid) on an infrequent basis. The uniqueness of this approach lies in the prescription of specific levels of load according to tendon performance rather than uniqueness in the exercises themselves.[101]

A concept known as **place and hold** is included in this category of EAM, in which the involved finger is passively flexed to a certain position and the patient is asked to hold it there through active contraction of that muscle. Evans and Thompson[96] studied the forces applied to a tendon with minimal active muscle-tendon tension (MAMTT) and developed guidelines for joint angles and force application with an adequate safety margin. Their study showed that, as the angle of joint flexion increases, the amount of force required also increases. They devised a protocol for treating flexor tendon repairs, recommending a position of place and hold with the wrist in 20° extension, the MCP joint in 83° flexion, the PIP joint

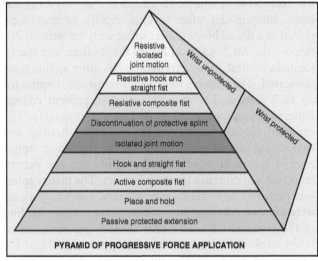

Figure 10-56 Pyramid of progressive force application. (Modified from Groth G: Pyramid of progressive force exercises to the injured flexor tendon, *J Hand Ther* 17:31-42, 2004.)

in 75° flexion, and the DIP joints in 40° flexion, using a Haldex pinch gauge and string held perpendicular to the digit to measure external force during the active hold position. According to this protocol, the patient should apply only 15 to 20 g of force to hold the position.

This method of treatment has been modified by various clinicians and treatment centers, and EAM protocols have emerged with varying degrees of motion involving the digits and wrist. Incorporating tenodesis, wrist and finger motion has become standard treatment along with decreasing the degree of wrist flexion in the dorsal block splint. The Indiana Hand Center[107,108] has devised an EAM protocol using a tenodesis wrist hinge splint that allows wrist flexion but blocks wrist extension at 30°; the MCP joints are blocked with a dorsal hood at 60° flexion. The patient wears this splint for exercise only and wears a dorsal protective block splint when not exercising. The patient is instructed to passively flex the involved finger into full composite flexion and then to bring the wrist up to extension. The patient is instructed to actively hold the flexed position of the finger with a minimal amount of tension for a few seconds. The patient then relaxes the muscle contraction and allows the wrist to drop into flexion and the fingers to extend to the dorsal hood of the splint (Figure 10-57).[107,108] This method should be used only by an experienced clinician who can evaluate a patient to determine whether the individual is an appropriate candidate for this type of synergistic protocol. EAM programs should be used with patients who are very compliant and can fully understand the program and its precautions.

Zones I and II. Gratton[106] described an uncomplicated method of splinting and an EAM program, which took place in Great Britain, for the treatment of zone I and zone II flexor tendon repairs. This protocol was devised with the goal of producing a treatment program that could be used for difficult cases and for patients who were less compliant or unable to attend therapy on a regular basis. Immediately after surgical repair, patients were placed in a dorsal block plaster splint with the wrist in 20° flexion, the MCP joints in 80° to 90° flexion, and the IP joints in neutral (0° in extension). No other splints were fabricated. The patients were admitted to the hospital for up to 3 days, and they wore a sling to prevent edema. Patients began motion 24 to 48 hours after surgery. The program consisted of passive flexion, active flexion, and two repetitions of active extension in the plaster splint every 4 hours. If joint stiffness was present, the patient increased the exercises to every 2 hours. The plaster splint was removed at 5 weeks after surgery, and the patients were allowed AROM; they worked toward active loading of the tendon at 8 weeks after surgery and returned to heavy work at 12 weeks. With this approach, 49% of the patients achieved an excellent outcome, 36% achieved a good outcome, and 7% had tendon ruptures.[106]

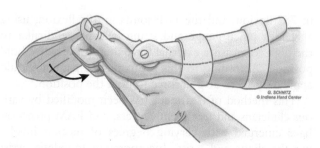

Figure 10-57 Indiana protocol with a hinge splint allows for active wrist extension combined with passive finger flexion. (From Cannon N: Post flexor tendon repair motion protocol, *Indiana Hand Center Newsletter* 1:13, 1993.)

Protocols vary from clinic to clinic because each clinic develops an individualized approach, which often depends on the surgeons' and therapists' preferences and expertise. A survey of 191 therapists revealed that 33% used some type of active finger flexion exercise within the first operative week. Only 5.5% of the therapists used the tenodesis hinge splint, but most of the therapists reported using a Kleinert type or Duran type of protocol, and 89.6% used some type of dorsal protective splint. More than half of those surveyed reported that their patients had experienced a tendon rupture, but this was less likely to occur in patients whose therapists saw them more frequently.[109]

Hold for Flexor Tendon Repairs in Zones I and II. Evans[110] has devised a postoperative program for treating FDP injuries in zone I that have undergone tendon to tendon or tendon to bone repair, using a technique consisting of limited DIP extension and active flexion. In addition to the dorsal block splint, the patient wears an individual static dorsal splint that positions the DIP joint in 40° to 45° flexion. This prevents the loss of DIP joint flexion that commonly occurs with zone I lacerations. The splint is taped in place to hold the DIP securely flexed, but the PIP joint is not included.

Evans' protocol includes the use of passive flexion/active extension exercises and an active exercise component known as *immediate active short arc motion* (SAM). After gentle passive exercises, the therapist removes the patient's splint and positions the patient with the wrist in 20° extension, the MCP joints in 75° to 80° flexion, the PIP joints in 70° to 75° flexion, and the DIP joints in 40° flexion (SAM position). The patient is instructed to gently hold this position to create minimum active tension in the flexor system. The force of flexion is measured with a Haldex pinch gauge, as described earlier with the MAMTT program. The therapist also performs wrist tenodesis exercises with the patient by passively holding the digits into a composite fist and simultaneously extending the wrist to 30° to 40°. The wrist then is passively flexed to 60° while the digits are allowed to extend through tenodesis action. The patient follows this exercise regimen for 3 to 4 weeks before full AROM and traditional tendon gliding exercises are begun. This protocol was developed with a defined safety margin for the active short arc motion.[110] Many clinicians and clinics have incorporated these concepts and modified them, depending on their level of experience, the surgeon's preference, and the individual patient's status. Table 10-9 details this type of protocol.

Zones III to V. Injuries in zones III to V are also treated with the modified Duran protocol or EPM. Flexor tendon repairs in zone IV and proximally, which include the wrist and forearm, generally result in better range of motion in the digits than repairs distal to this area. Peritendinous scar adhesions are less likely to form in these regions. The tensile strength of repaired tendons in zone IV and proximally is substantial enough to tolerate AROM exercises starting at 3 weeks after surgery. AROM of the digits can begin in the dorsal block splint at 3 weeks after surgery

TABLE **10-9**

Flexor Digitorum Profundus Repairs in Zone I (Tendon to Bone): Modified Early Mobilization Program

Time Frame	Program Considerations
0 to 5 days	• *Splint:* Fabricate a static dorsal block splint: Wrist, 0-20° flexion; MCP joints, 30° to 50° flexion; IP joints extended. The DIP joint may be positioned in flexion up to 45° by the surgeon to prevent stress on the repair. Based on the surgeon's guidelines, the dorsal block splint may be padded, or a separate finger splint may be taped dorsally over the involved digit, positioning the DIP joint in flexion. • *Exercise program:* Instruct the patient in the following: passive flexion of all finger joints within the splint; passive DIP flexion to 75° within a static finger splint and dorsal block splint; active extension of the IP joints within the splint with the MCP blocked in full passive flexion. Exercises are performed as 10 repetitions, 5-6 times a day. • Initiate edema management.
1 to 2 weeks	• In addition to the previously described exercises, DIP extension is progressed in the splint weekly to tissue tolerance or to the surgeon's guidelines. Begin scar management when appropriate. • Begin passive modified hook position (hook with the MCP joints resting on the hood of the splint with full IP flexion to tolerance). • Begin modified place and hold within the splint once edema has decreased and full passive motion has been achieved. Passively flex the PIP joint of the affected finger while holding the uninvolved fingers to the hood of the splint to encourage differential FDS gliding from the FDP. Instruct the patient to gently contract to hold the PIP joint in this flexed position with minimum tension for 3 seconds. • These exercises should be performed in the clinic by the therapist: Remove the patient's splint. Passively extend the patient's wrist to 30° to 40° with the fingers passively held in composite flexion. Passively flex the wrist to 60° with passive hook fisting of the fingers.
3 to 4 weeks	• Continue as previously described. The individual finger splint or DIP extension block can be discarded. The patient can begin full composite flexion with place and hold with the wrist positioned in slight flexion to neutral. • Begin active finger flexion and extension with the wrist in slight flexion to neutral; also begin active hook fisting with the wrist in slight flexion to neutral. • Instruct the patient in active tenodesis wrist exercises.
4 to 6 weeks	• Gentle blocking exercises are initiated, with care taken not to apply resistance during flexion while blocking. • Instruct the patient in full active wrist flexion and extension; begin passive finger extension with the MCP joints flexed and then progress to stretching and splinting to restore motion if needed. • Low-intensity ultrasound (3 MHz) is initiated if appropriate.
6 to 8 weeks	• The dorsal block splint is discharged unless the patient needs splinting for protection in certain environments. Instruct the patient to use the affected hand for light ADLs but to avoid lifting, gripping, or heavy activities. Begin gentle resistance.
8 weeks	• Progress with the strengthening program as needed and tolerated. The patient can begin resisted blocking exercises to increase IP flexion.

MCP, Metacarpophalangeal; *IP,* interphalangeal; *DIP,* distal interphalangeal; *FDS,* flexor digitorum superficialis; *FDP,* flexor digitorum profundus; *PIP,* proximal interphalangeal; *ADLs,* activities of daily living.

and gentle blocking exercises of the PIP and DIP joints at 4 weeks. Unrestricted AROM of the wrist and fingers can begin at 4 to 4½ weeks after surgery, and gentle resistance can be initiated at 6 weeks, progressing with strengthening at 8 to 10 weeks; most patients are discharged at 12 weeks after surgery. Patients may develop extrinsic flexor tightness with repairs in these zones. The dorsal block splint is discontinued at 6 weeks, and a full extension resting splint may be indicated if extrinsic flexor tightness is present.[111,112]

Anatomical structures that may be involved with a laceration to the wrist and forearm include the FDS, FDP, FPL, PL, FCR, FCU, the medial nerve, the ulnar nerve, the radial artery, and/or the ulnar artery. All these structures must be repaired to ensure a positive functional outcome

for the patient.[111] If an injury in zone IV or V involves a median and/or ulnar nerve repair, the wrist should be positioned in approximately 30° flexion in the dorsal block splint and, starting at 3 weeks after surgery, the amount of wrist extension should be increased by 10° each week. If the ulnar nerve has been repaired, the MCP joints must be positioned in flexion to prevent hyperextension and clawing of the digits. If the median nerve has been repaired, adding a thumb component to the dorsal block splint is recommended to prevent shortening of the first web space and to maintain abduction.[113] If repairs in zone V are the tendon to tendon type, early active motion can be initiated and can follow the zone II protocol. However, if repairs in zone V are at the musculotendinous junction, active motion should be delayed until 3 to 4 weeks after surgery.

Flexor Pollicis Longus Injuries of the Thumb

Surgical repairs of the FPL tendon can be challenging because the proximal end of the lacerated FPL tendon retracts more proximally than a lacerated digital flexor tendon, which is restrained by its interconnections. Delaying surgery even up to 48 hours can make pulling out the proximal tendon to its original length difficult because muscle shortening can occur quickly. Unfortunately, increased tension of the FPL tendon from muscle shortening puts the patient at risk of rupturing the tendon and/or of developing thumb IP flexion contractures. Tendon retraction can be addressed during surgery by lengthening the FPL tendon within the muscle with transverse divisions or Z-lengthening of the tendon at the musculotendinous junction, which reduces FPL tension.[114]

Factors that affect the outcome of FPL injuries include retraction of the proximal tendon, the zone of injury, and postoperative management. Patients with proximal stump retraction have a higher incidence of unsatisfactory results. FPL lacerations in zone II can involve the A1 pulley, which is important for FPL function because it prevents the tendon from bowstringing. Excessive scarring in this area can lead to loss of tendon gliding. A study by Kasashima et al.[115] showed that passive flexion and active extension exercises using rubber band traction significantly reduced the risk of unsatisfactory results in patients with FPL repairs, particularly in those with a zone II laceration or retraction of the proximal tendon stump.

Many of the concepts and methods discussed for postoperative management of finger flexor tendon repairs apply to repairs of the FPL. Therapists and surgeons may use immobilization or EPM or EAM protocols, depending on their experience, preference, the type of repair, and the patient's age and compliance. Splint position and treatment protocols can vary; therefore communication is essential between the surgeon and the therapist.

Young children or patients who are noncompliant may benefit from an immobilization program. Cooperation is reported to be poor in children younger than 5 years of age, and some advocate immobilizing these injuries in an above-the-elbow cast (with the wrist and the MCP and IP joints in flexion and the thumb abducted) for 4 to 6 weeks, at which time motion can begin. No significant formation of adhesions was found using this method with this age group.[116] Older children and adults involved in an immobilization program after FPL repair generally are splinted with a forearm-based dorsal protective splint with the wrist in approximately 15° to 25° flexion, the thumb abducted, the CMC joint in 10° flexion, and the MCP joint in 20° to 30° flexion.

The thumb IP joint is in neutral, although this position could vary, depending on the type of repair and the amount of tension on the FPL tendon (Figure 10-58). If tendon shortening occurred or if approximating the tendon ends was difficult, the IP joint may need to be positioned in slight flexion.[112] Patients are immobilized for 4 weeks and then can begin gentle AROM exercises.

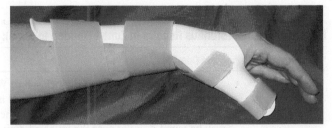

Figure 10-58 Dorsal protective splint for a flexor pollicis longus repair. The wrist is held in flexion, and the thumb is also placed in flexion to protect the healing tendon repair.

Proponents of the Kleinert method use rubber band traction to position the thumb in flexion for active extension/passive flexion exercises for the first 3 to 4 weeks before starting active thumb flexion.[115] The modified Duran protocol is also used for FPL repairs, and the patient is instructed to passively flex the thumb and then actively extend to the confines of the dorsal block splint for the first 3 to 4 weeks after surgery. As described earlier, with finger flexor tendon rehabilitation, some protocols treating FPL repairs combine elements of the modified Duran method with a place and hold component. The Evans MAMTT technique recommends using an active hold component with the thumb positioned in 15° of CMC joint flexion, 45° of MCP joint flexion, and 40° of IP joint flexion with an external force of 15 to 20 g, measured with a Haldex pinch gauge and string held perpendicular to the thumb.[96] Table 10-10 details the guidelines and most widely used protocols for the postoperative management and rehabilitation of FPL injuries in zones I and II.

Elliot and Southgate[114] have reported an EAM regimen for FPL repairs in zones I and II performed with a four-strand core suture with a Silfverskiöld circumferential suture. They recommended splinting the patient with the wrist in 10° extension and 10° ulnar deviation, the thumb abducted to 30°, the CMC joint flexed to 10°, the MCP joint flexed to 30°, and the IP joint at 0° extension. The patient is positioned in ulnar deviation at the wrist to reduce the turning angle of the FPL as it passes from the carpal tunnel into the thenar muscles. All remaining digits are also strapped into the dorsal hood of the splint with the fingers in neutral. The rationale for splinting the fingers is to prevent inadvertent increased strain on the FPL tendon with free finger motion.[114] This protocol is detailed in Table 10-11.

Extensor Tendon Injuries of the Hand

Extensor tendon rehabilitation involves many of the same concepts that apply to flexor tendon rehabilitation. Communication between the surgeon and the therapist is crucial, and the therapist must have a thorough understanding of the patient's injury and the type of surgical repair performed. Just as flexor tendon management has moved from immobilization toward EPM and EAM, so has the management of extensor tendons.[88] A variety of

TABLE **10-10**

Flexor Pollicis Longus Repairs in Zones I and II: Guidelines for Kleinert, Modified Duran, and Place and Hold Programs

Time Frame	Program Considerations

0 to 1 week	• *Splint:* Fabricate a dorsal protective splint: wrist, 15° to 30° flexion; CMC joint, 0° to 10° flexion; MCP joint, 20° to 30° flexion; IP joint, 0° (unless otherwise specified by the physician) to position in flexion.
	• *Exercise program:* Begin postoperative day 2-5; communicate with surgeon to determine the most appropriate program for the specific patient:
	  ○ Modified Duran: Begin passive flexion of the IP, MCP, and CMC joints and allow active extension to meet the confines of the splint.
	  ○ Kleinert traction: Begin passive flexion with a rubber band and active extension against the rubber band traction to meet the confines of the splint.
	  ○ PROM and AROM to all noninvolved digits, with care taken not to actively flex the thumb. Instruct the patient to avoid all functional use of the injured thumb at this time (i.e., no lifting or gripping with the noninvolved digits). Instruct the patients to do the exercises frequently (i.e., 10 repetitions every 1-2 hours).
	  ○ Place and hold should begin only with the physician's orders and once edema has diminished and the patient demonstrates good passive thumb flexion. Instruct the patient to place the thumb in limited flexion, exert a minimum amount of tension, and hold the position for 2-3 seconds. The degree of restriction of motion may be determined by the surgeon.
	• Begin edema management and scar management when the incision has healed.

3 to 4 weeks	• Discharge Kleinert rubber band traction unless the patient does not have full passive flexion. Continue with modified Duran exercises. Progress to place and hold with full range of motion. • Begin active thumb flexion in the splint with caution because FPL repairs have a higher rate of rupture. The wrist position of the splint may be changed to neutral.
4 to 6 weeks	• AROM of the thumb out of the splint, AROM of the wrist. • No resistance or gripping is allowed; light, functional, nonresistive activity of the thumb is allowed at week 6. • Ultrasound can be used at weeks 4-6 if indicated. • Gentle IP joint blocking with no resistance can begin.
6 to 8 weeks	• Dorsal block splint is discontinued unless protection is needed in a high-risk environment or circumstance. • Minimal resistance with a soft sponge or putty can begin. • Light functional use but no forceful pinching or gripping is allowed. • Progress with strengthening activities over 8-12 weeks.

CMC, Carpometacarpal; *MCP,* metacarpophalangeal; *IP,* interphalangeal; *FPL,* flexor pollicis longus; *PROM,* passive range of motion; *AROM,* active range of motion.

early motion protocols have been developed for zones III through VII, including thumb zones T-I to T-III.

The strength of the repaired tendon, the ability of the tendon to glide, and tendon excursion in relation to the position of the wrist all affect the treatment of extensor tendon repairs. The extensor tendon is smaller and flatter than the flexor tendon and therefore is not as suitable for more complicated, multistrand suture techniques. However, some suture techniques have been developed for extensor tendon repairs that allow for early controlled motion (ECM).[117]

Factors That Affect the Strength of a Repaired Extensor Tendon

• Ability of the tendon to glide
• Tendon excursion in relation to wrist position
• Wrist position
• Metacarpophalangeal joint position

Studies done by Newport and Tucker[117] have reported that finger extension strength varies significantly, depending on the wrist and MCP joint positions, because of the tenodesis effect the wrist has on the extensor tendons. The extensor tendons have less excursion than the flexor tendons because of the linkage between them known as the *juncturae tendinae.*[117] Evans and Burkhalter[118] have determined that 5 mm of EDC excursion is generated when the MCP joints of the index and middle fingers are flexed to 30° and when the MCP joints of the ring and little fingers are flexed to 40°. This amount of gliding is considered to be sufficient to prevent the formation of adhesions after an extensor tendon repair.[118]

Zones I and II (Mallet Finger Injuries). Mallet finger injuries involve a disruption of the terminal tendon and are treated with immobilization by splinting the DIP joint of the finger in 0° extension. The length of time in the splint depends on the classification of the injury (see previous descriptions of the four types of mallet injuries). Closed mallet injuries without fractures are treated by

TABLE **10-11**

Flexor Pollicis Longus Repairs in Zones I and II: Guidelines for the Elliot and Southgate Program[114]

Time Frame	Program Considerations
Week 1	• Instruct the patient to actively flex and extend the fingers only 25% of their full motion • Limit active flexion of the thumb to touching the tip of the middle finger • After 1 week the patient can passively flex the fingers fully
Week 2	• Increase finger active range of motion to 50% • Limit active flexion of the thumb to touching the tip of the ring finger • Begin passive flexion of the thumb
Week 3	• Full active range of motion of the fingers is allowed • Full active flexion of the thumb is allowed*

*The authors did not discuss resistive activity, strengthening exercises, and functional activity; however, they concluded that the repair they chose was strong enough to allow early active mobilization and to avoid the risk of rupture.

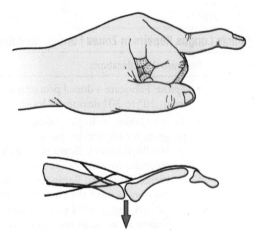

Figure 10-59 Swan neck deformity. Note the hyperextension at the proximal interphalangeal joint. (From Magee DJ: *Orthopedic physical assessment,* ed 6, p 440, St. Louis, 2014, Saunders/Elsevier.)

splinting the DIP joint in extension with a stack splint, a custom-molded thermoplastic splint, or aluminum foam splint. The splint should not interfere with PIP flexion and should be checked regularly to ensure proper positioning, especially if the swelling in the patient's finger is declining. Proper alignment at 0° extension is important because it prevents hyperextension of the DIP joint, which can cause blanching of the dorsal skin and lead to skin necrosis. The patient wears the splint continuously for 6 to 7 weeks; then gentle AROM can begin. If an extension lag occurs at the DIP joint, the splint may need to be applied for an additional 2 to 4 weeks. Patients are gradually weaned out of the splint during the day, although they may need to continue with night splinting if a lag persists. Open lacerations to a terminal tendon or those with associated fractures may be repaired and the DIP joint pinned in extension with a K-wire. Patients are instructed in AROM at approximately 6 weeks after surgery but continue to wear a static extension splint for several more weeks between exercises and at night.[119]

Swan neck deformities, which cause hyperextension of the PIP joint with flexion of the DIP joint, can occur if a significant mallet injury goes untreated (Figure 10-59). This deformity occurs as a result of unopposed tension of the central slip, dorsal migration of the lateral bands, and laxity of the volar plate. Swan neck deformities can be treated with a figure-of-eight splint that allows for PIP flexion but blocks hyperextension of the PIP joint. Splinting helps with functional grasp and prevents the finger from locking in hyperextension, but this is not a long-term or permanent solution for severe deformities, which may require surgical intervention (Figure 10-60).

Zones III and IV. Zone III extensor tendon injuries occur at the PIP joint and involve the central slip. Zone IV extensor tendon injuries occur at the level of the proximal phalanx and involve the lateral bands. If these injuries go untreated, a boutonniere deformity can develop, causing flexion of the PIP joint and hyperextension of the DIP joint. Early intervention is important to prevent a flexion contracture of the PIP joint. If a closed rupture has occurred, the recommended course is to splint only the PIP joint in full extension and leave the DIP joint free to move. The patient is instructed to passively and actively flex the DIP joint with the PIP splint on. This allows the lateral bands, which have migrated anteriorly, to return to their proper anatomical position and also assists the central slip in moving distally to heal in the correct position. Closed boutonniere injuries are splinted anywhere from 2 to 6 weeks, depending on the severity of the injury. Patients should be checked frequently and instructed to remove the splint to perform gentle AROM, with active-assistive extension exercises. Passive PIP joint flexion should be avoided for 6 weeks. The patient may be weaned out of the splint gradually to wearing it at night as needed.[119]

Complete extensor tendon lacerations in zones III and IV are treated with surgical intervention. Postoperative treatment consists of immobilization (Table 10-12), ECM (Table 10-13), or EAM protocols.

Immobilization After Extensor Tendon Repair. Immobilization is considered the "safest" treatment because it limits motion altogether, thereby minimizing tension on the repaired tendon; however, it unfortunately leads to adhesion formation, loss of joint flexion, and extensor tendon lag. Despite these disadvantages, immobilization programs may be most appropriate for young children or for patients who are unable to comply with ECM methods.[117]

Effect of Immobilization on a Repaired Extensor Tendon

- Limit movement
- Lead to the formation of adhesions
- Decrease joint tension on the tendon
- Lead to extensor tendon lag

Early Controlled Motion After Extensor Tendon Repair. ECM programs that incorporate various combinations of dynamic splinting and tendon gliding, when used after extensor tendon repair, have resulted in significant improvements in the outcome of these injuries. ECM

programs for extensor tendon repairs limit active flexion but allow passive extension of the digit, provided by rubber band traction attached to an outrigger (Figure 10-61). Based on the same rationale as that for flexor tendon studies, controlled stress combined with early motion has been shown to have a positive outcome on the healing extensor tendon.[120] Studies have reported that the protocol presented in Table 10-13, using a hand-based dynamic splint with ECM for repairs in zones III and IV, provides excellent results with fewer treatment visits and a shorter duration of treatment.[121,122]

Extensor tendon repairs in zones III and IV can also be treated with a dynamic extension assist splint with a

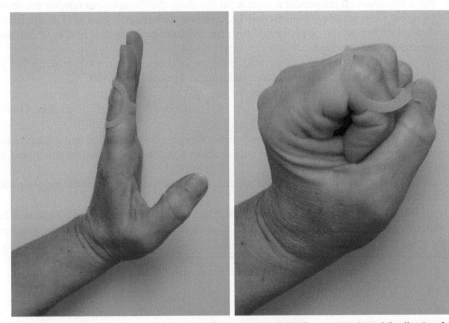

Figure 10-60 Figure-of-eight splint (Oval 8 Splint) for a swan neck deformity prevents PIP hyperextension while allowing full PIP and DIP flexion.

TABLE 10-12

Extensor Tendon Repairs in Zones III and IV: Immobilization Protocol

Time Frame	Program Considerations
0 to 1 week	• *Splint:* PIP joint in 0° extension; if only zone III was repaired, leave the MCP and DIP joints free. If zone IV repair or lateral bands were involved, include the DIP joint in the splint at 0° extension for 4-6 weeks. • *Exercise program:* Begin 10-14 days after repair. If zone III was repaired, instruct the patient to actively flex the DIP joint every 2 hours. • Manage edema.
3 to 6 weeks	• Isometric extensor exercises can begin with the splint on; continue with DIP flexion exercises. • At weeks 4-6, remove the splint to begin gentle AROM exercises (hook and composite fist) but instruct the patient to wear the splint between exercise sessions. • Begin scar management if needed.
6 to 8 weeks	• Progress with gentle AROM and AAROM to increase flexion; progress to gentle flexion exercises. Incorporate a dynamic flexion splint, if needed, and alternate with the extension splint. • Begin resistive activity and progress as needed.

PIP, Proximal interphalangeal; *MCP,* metacarpophalangeal; *DIP,* distal interphalangeal; *AROM,* active range of motion; *AAROM,* active-assisted range of motion.

TABLE **10-13**

Extensor Tendon Repairs in Zones III and IV: Early Controlled Motion with Dynamic Splinting

Time Frame	Program Considerations

0 to 1 week	• *Splint:*
	   ○ Fabricate a dorsal hand-based splint with the wrist free, the MCP joint in 0° to 20° flexion (surgeon's preference), and a Velcro strap around the proximal phalanx.
	   ○ Apply dynamic traction to hold the PIP joint in 0° extension or slight hyperextension (surgeon's preference). The DIP joint is left free.
	   ○ Apply a stop bead to the dynamic traction to limit PIP flexion (which is determined by surgeon) (see Figure 10-61).
	 • *Exercise program:*
	   ○ Allow the patient to actively flex the PIP joint against the rubber band traction, with limited flexion because of the stop bead (generally 30° if the repair is strong) and with passive extension back to neutral through dynamic traction.
	   ○ Zone III repairs: If the patient is reliable, in the clinic the therapist can remove the strap around the proximal phalanx and perform limited MCP flexion with the PIP joint held in 0° extension.
	   ○ Active DIP flexion can be performed with the PIP joint positioned or held in 0° extension. Begin edema management if indicated.
	   ○ Week 2: With the physician's approval, adjust the stop bead to allow 40° of active PIP joint flexion. Continue with active flexion, passive extension, and previous exercises.
	 • Begin scar management when incision heals.

3 weeks	• With the surgeon's approval, adjust the stop bead to allow 50° of active PIP flexion. Continue with previous exercises.
4 to 6 weeks	• Discharge dynamic traction. Instruct the patient to begin active extension and full active flexion exercises (composite fist, hook fist). Educate the patient about light use of the hand for functional, nonresistive, light tasks at week 6. • Begin blocking exercises to increase PIP flexion. Continue use of the static extension splint at night and for protection between exercises if needed.
6 to 8 weeks	• Begin PROM or dynamic flexion splinting or strap to increase flexion only if no extensor lag is present. • Continue use of the night extension splint if needed. Begin resistive flexion exercises and progress with strengthening program.

MCP, Metacarpophalangeal; *PIP,* proximal interphalangeal; *DIP,* distal interphalangeal; *PROM,* passive range of motion.

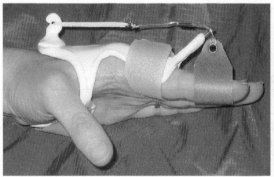 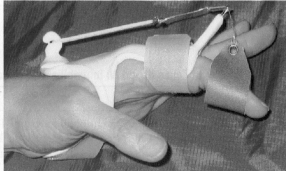

Figure 10-61 Hand-based dynamic extension splint for extensor tendon repairs in zones III and IV.

spring coil, referred to as a modified Wynn Parry splint or Capener splint. The advantages of this splint are that it is finger based and low profile, and it allows the MCP joint to be free.[123] The disadvantages are that it requires a longer splinting period before AROM out of the splint begins; it can be difficult to fit, especially if edema is present; it can cause pressure sores; and the duration of the treatment is longer than with dynamic splinting.

Early Active Motion for a Zone III Extensor Tendon Repair. Evans and Thompson[124] have defined the parameters for an early active SAM protocol for a repaired central slip. The patient begins controlled active finger extension and limited flexion within 24 to 48 hours immediately after surgery. These researchers showed that 30° of PIP active motion allows 3.75 mm of EDC excursion. This provides enough gliding to allow healing but prevents the formation of adhesions in zones III and IV. The patient is splinted with the PIP and DIP joints in 0° extension and wears the splint at all times except when exercising. The patient uses two other static volar splints for an exercise program. One splint limits PIP flexion to 30° and DIP flexion to 20° to 25°. The patient is allowed to perform active extension of the digit and then flexes to meet the splint, but the MCP joint must be positioned in 0° extension and the wrist in 30° flexion. The second exercise splint positions the PIP joint in extension and allows DIP flexion. If the lateral bands have been repaired, DIP flexion is limited to 30°; if the lateral bands are not involved, the DIP is allowed to flex fully. The patient is instructed to perform each exercise 20 times every hour.[124,125]

Two weeks after surgery, if no extensor lag is present, the exercise splint that limits PIP flexion is adjusted to limit PIP flexion to 40°; 3 weeks after surgery, it can be adjusted to 50°; by the end of the fourth week, it can be adjusted up to 70° to 80° of PIP flexion if no extension lag exists. Patients can begin composite flexion exercises and gentle strengthening at 5 weeks after surgery, and some are discharged at 6 weeks after surgery. If the PIP joint is stiff, intermittent flexion splinting is recommended at approximately 4 weeks, alternating with night static extension splinting, which may need to continue for 5 to 6 weeks after surgery.[124,125] Evans[96] also recommended the MAMTT technique combined with dynamic splinting for more proximal extensor tendon zones.

Early Protected Motion with Passive Flexion. Crosby and Wehbe[126] advocate an early protected motion program that combines dynamic splinting with early passive flexion. This method is recommended for extensor tendon repairs in zones III to VII and all thumb zones (T-I to T-III), as well as in zones VI and VII. Their study included incomplete, complete, and complex extensor tendon lacerations. Surgical repairs were performed with mattress, figure-of-eight, or modified Kessler sutures, depending on the level of repair and the thickness of the tendon. Repairs in zones III and IV were treated with a dorsal hand-based dynamic splint with the MCP joint at 0° extension and the PIP joint held in 0° extension with traction from the splint. Some patients were allowed to flex the PIP joint with no limitations in the splint. In other patients, PIP flexion was limited with a block, as determined by the surgeon based on the integrity and status of the repair. Patients were instructed to perform, on an hourly basis, active hook fisting within the confines of the splint, allowing the dynamic traction to passively extend the finger back to extension.[126]

This protocol introduced the concept of tendon mobilization, performed by the clinician, which involves holding the affected digit and the wrist in maximum extension while passively ranging only one joint at a time. The PIP joint is passively flexed to its specified block while the MCP and DIP joints and the wrist are all held in maximum extension. If there is no flexion block, the clinician applies gentle gradual force until full range of motion is obtained or until resistance or pain is encountered.[126]

Dynamic splinting and tendon mobilization are initiated 1 to 5 days after surgery. After 4 weeks, the patient is instructed in AROM and tendon gliding exercises and weaned out of the splint over a few days. If an extension lag is present, the patient uses a static volar splint for extension. After removal of the splint, the patient begins a gentle, graded strengthening program. Grip and pinch strength are measured at 8 weeks after surgery with a Jamar Dynamometer and pinch meter. A flexion strap is used at 8 weeks if IP flexion is limited.[126]

This method is used with extensor tendon repairs performed in zones V through VII. These patients are splinted with a dorsal forearm-based dynamic splint that positions the wrist in 20° extension and holds the MCP joints at 0° extension with dynamic traction. The use and degree of MCP joint flexion blocks are determined at the time of surgery, depending on the strength of the repair and how well the tendon is able to glide without tension. These zones are also treated with an early protected mobilization program, and excellent to good results have been reported.[126]

Zones V to VIII

Immobilization Program. Zone V involves the area over the MCP joint, and zone VI is located over the dorsal aspect of the metacarpals. Zones VII and VIII, which are found at the extensor retinaculum and the musculotendinous junction, often are associated with scar adhesions that lead to extrinsic tightness and loss of finger flexion. Debate exists over whether patients treated with immobilization in zones V to VIII may not do as well as with ECM, resulting in extensor tendon lag and limited flexion. Proponents of immobilization programs for extensor tendon zones V to VIII report that equally good functional results can be achieved using static splints that are simpler, less labor intensive, and less expensive than programs that use dynamic splinting.[127] Many experts seem to agree that immobilization methods may be indicated for young children or noncompliant patients.

The position for immobilization depends on the level and complexity of the injury and whether other associated structures have been involved. The patient generally is splinted with the wrist in 30° extension and the MCP joints in 20° to 30° flexion. The IP joints may be included at neutral or left free to move. Patients who are allowed to actively flex and extend the IP joints without compromising the repair do better than patients whose IP joints are splinted.[127] Three to 4 weeks after surgery, the patient can remove the splint only for gentle AROM exercises, with the wrist extended during finger flexion and care taken to avoid full wrist and finger composite flexion. Tenodesis exercises for the wrist can begin 4 to 6 weeks after surgery, with composite AROM of the wrist and fingers at 6 weeks after surgery. Gentle passive finger flexion can be initiated at 4 to 6 weeks after surgery, or gentle dynamic splinting alternating with extension splinting may be used if needed. A gentle strengthening program can begin at 6 weeks and progress to 8 weeks after surgery.[125]

Early Controlled Motion. Early motion protocols consisting of dynamic splinting and tendon gliding have become widely accepted and successful in treating zones V to VIII (Table 10-14). Protocols for treatment vary, depending on the position of the wrist and the MCP joints; they also may be determined by the surgeon at the time of surgery based on the status of the repair. More proximal zones often can tolerate more composite flexion within the confines of the dynamic splint, especially if the wrist is extended beyond 20° extension (Figure 10-62).

However, excessive wrist extension may cause the extensors to buckle in the more proximal zones and interfere with tendon gliding.[117]

Chow et al.[120] presented a study of ECM for extensor zones IV through VII. The authors used a dorsal forearm-based splint with dynamic traction to passively extend the MCP joint to 0° extension, allowed limited MCP flexion, and provided unrestricted active flexion of the PIP and DIP joints. During the first week after surgery, the MCP joint of the involved finger was allowed to flex to 30°; during the second week, this was increased to 45°; during the third week, to 60°, and during the fourth and fifth weeks, full flexion was allowed with the splint on. Patients were instructed to actively flex within the confines of the splint 10 times every hour. The splint was discontinued by the end of the fifth week, and AROM out of the splint was initiated. Resistive exercises and strength were not discussed in this study, but patients had no restrictions after 8 weeks.[120]

Some protocols advocate positioning the MCP joint in 0° extension, whereas others suggest blocking the MCP

TABLE 10-14

Extensor Tendon Repairs in Zones V to VIII: Early Controlled Motion with Dynamic Splinting

Time Frame	Program Considerations

0 to 1 week	• *Splint:*
	  ○ Fabricate a dorsal forearm-based dynamic splint with the wrist in 20° extension and the MCP joints in 0° to 20° flexion (depending on the surgeon's preference and the repair performed).
	  ○ The surgeon may order an MCP flexion block, or the MCP joint may be allowed to flex fully. The IP joints may be unrestricted, or the surgeon may request that loops from dynamic traction support them in neutral position. Adjacent fingers may or may not be included, depending on the level and location of the injury.
	  ○ Some surgeons may request a separate volar resting splint that blocks MCP flexion and supports the IP joints in extension. This splint is worn with the dorsal dynamic splint for exercises (see Figure 10-62).
	  ○ Some patients may find sleeping while wearing the dorsal forearm-based dynamic splint difficult; these patients may benefit from wearing a volar static resting splint at night, which positions the wrist and fingers in extension. (The IP joints may or may not be included in the splint, depending on the repair zone and the surgeon's orders.)
	• *Exercise program:*
	  ○ Begin active MCP flexion within the confines of the splint with passive MCP extension through the dynamic traction of the splint. If loops are not restricting IP motion, the patient is instructed to perform active flexion and extension of the PIP and DIP joints in the splint (i.e., active hook fisting) 10 times every hour.
	• Begin edema management.

2 to 3 weeks	• Continue with the previous exercises. The therapist can begin gentle passive IP flexion with the MCP joints and wrist in extension. • Begin scar management when appropriate.
4 to 6 weeks	• The patient can begin AROM and tendon gliding out of the splint, taking care with full composite wrist and finger flexion. Instruct the patient to keep the wrist extended with gentle finger flexion. • The patient can also begin tenodesis wrist and finger motion. Continue use of the night static extension splint if extension lag is present. Gradually wean the patient out of the dynamic extension splint for daytime.
6 to 8 weeks	• Full wrist and finger composite flexion and extension can be performed. The patient should wean out of the dynamic splint and continue with a night static splint if needed. • Instruct the patient in gentle PROM exercises. A dynamic flexion splint or strap can be used if flexion is limited. • Begin a gentle strengthening program and progress as needed. No restrictions are necessary after 10-12 weeks.

MCP, Metacarpophalangeal; *IP*, interphalangeal; *PIP*, proximal interphalangeal; *DIP*, distal interphalangeal; *AROM*, active range of motion; *PROM*, passive range of motion.

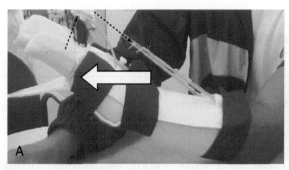 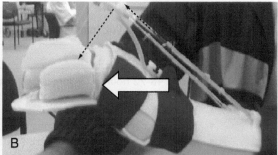

Figure 10-62 A, Dynamic forearm-based extension splint with elastic band assistance for passive finger extension. **B,** This splint allows active MCP flexion into a volar resting splint, blocking MCP flexion to approximately 30° for zone V extensor tendon repairs in the index, long, ring, and little fingers. The injuries, caused by a table saw accident, required open reduction and internal fixation of metacarpal fractures in the index, ring, and long fingers. The PIP and DIP joints are held in extension in finger troughs, which are attached to the elastics by opaque fishing line *(dotted lines and arrows).*

joints at 5° to 10° flexion to prevent hyperextension and extensor activity, which has been detected through electromyographical (EMG) studies when the extensor tendons are at rest in 0° extension.[122] Active MCP flexion may also be limited with early motion protocols, depending on the repair and the ability of the tendon to glide freely.[126]

Immediate Controlled Active Motion for Zones IV to VII After Extensor Tendon Repair. Early mobilization programs vary among clinicians, surgeons, and clinics, depending on their experience level, the patient's presentation, and the extent of the injury. Just as there are trends toward early active flexion with flexor tendon rehabilitation, a trend has arisen for early active extension after extensor tendon repairs.

Immediate controlled active motion (ICAM) has been used to treat extensor tendon repairs in zones IV to VII. Howell et al.[128] designed an EAM program that consists of three phases and uses a low profile, two-part splint. The patient wears two static splints. One is a static volar wrist cock-up splint that positions the wrist in 20° to 25° extension. The second splint, called the ICAM yoke splint, links the injured digit to the noninjured digits to unload the repair and harness extension forces during active motion. The yoke is positioned across the proximal phalanges of the fingers and allows active flexion and extension of the fingers but positions the involved MCP joint in 15° to 20° more extension relative to the uninjured MCP joints (Figure 10-63).[128] The EAM program consists of three phases (Table 10-15). The authors had a 30% noncompliance rate, but they did not know of any complications or ruptured tendons. One hundred and forty patients completed the program. Categorization of an excellent outcome was based on the occurrence of no extensor lag or loss of terminal flexion. Of the 140 patients, 81% of the patients had no extensor lag and 79% of the patients had no loss of terminal flexion. The timing of strengthening and resistive exercises was not discussed, but grip strength was reported to be 85% of the opposite, uninjured hand at the time of discharge, which averaged 7 weeks after surgery.[128]

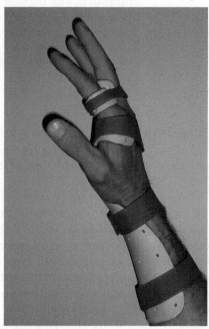

Figure 10-63 The immediate controlled active motion (ICAM) splint (third version) with wrist positioned in 20° to 25° extension. The yoke component positions the involved MP joint in 20° to 25° hyperextension relative to the MP joints of the noninjured digits. (From Howell JW, Merritt WH, Robinson SJ: Immediate controlled active motion following zone 4-7 extensor tendon repair, *J Hand Ther* 18:183, 2005.)

Rehabilitation of the Extensor Pollicis Longus in the Thumb

Immobilization Program After Extensor Pollicis Longus Tendon Repair. EPL tendon repairs can be treated with immobilization or ECM programs. Treatment programs vary, depending on the level of injury, the clinician's expertise, and the individual patient. Injuries in zone T-I are referred to as a *mallet thumb* and can be treated by splinting the IP joint of the thumb in 0° extension for 6 to 8 weeks for a closed injury or 5 to 6 weeks for an open repair. Gentle AROM can begin after the immobilization period, using caution if an extensor lag is present, and the

TABLE **10-15**

Extensor Tendon Repairs in Zones IV to VIII: Immediate Controlled Active Motion

Time Frame	Program Considerations
Phase 1 (0 to 21 days)	• Within 48-72 hours after surgery, splints are fabricated and the ICAM program begins. • The patient begins full active composite finger flexion and extension within the confines of the splint. • The splint must be worn at all times. • The patient is instructed in edema and scar management.
Phase 2 (22 to 35 days)	• Before the patient can begin phase 2, full active motion must be achieved within the limits of the ICAM splint. The patient continues to wear the ICAM yoke splint, but the wrist splint is removed to begin AROM exercises to the wrist with the finger held in a relaxed position. • The patient is instructed to wear the wrist splint and yoke if doing medium to heavy activity. If no extension lag is present, the patient progresses to wrist flexion with finger fisting in the yoke and wrist extension with finger extension. • Once the wrist is moving freely, the patient can discontinue the wrist splint for light tasks but should be instructed to wear the wrist splint and yoke if performing medium to heavy tasks.
Phase 3 (36 to 49 days)	• The wrist splint is discharged. • To prepare the patient for yoke-off activity, the yoke is removed for AROM of the digits. • The finger yoke or a buddy strap is worn during activities. • Full composite wrist and finger flexion and extension without the splints should be achieved during phase 3.

ICAM, Immediate controlled active motion; *AROM,* active range of motion.

patient continues to wear a static extension splint between exercises and at night. Patients can progress in active IP joint flexion slowly and begin resistive exercises at 6 to 8 weeks.[125]

Zone T-II injuries are also treated by immobilizing the MCP and IP joints in 0° extension in a hand-based splint with the thumb in radial extension. Limited AROM begins at 3 to 4 weeks, and over the next 3 weeks, the patient can increase joint motion gradually. If an extension lag is present, an extension splint should be used. Patients should use the splint for protection between exercises for a total of 6 weeks.[120]

EPL repairs in zones T-III and T-IV are treated by splinting the thumb MCP joint at 0° extension and slight abduction with the wrist in 30° extension for 3 to 4 weeks before starting AROM exercises. The MCP joint may become restricted from hyperextension or from prolonged splinting in extension, requiring dynamic flexion splinting at 4 to 6 weeks. Injuries in zone V are susceptible to the formation of dense adhesions, which can limit the excursion of the EPL at the retinacular level. Extension contractures of the thumb MCP joint, thumb web space contracture, and restrictions in the joint capsule and on tendon gliding are all problems that can occur at this level with immobilization.[125]

Immobilization programs can result in loss of thumb motion after repair of the EPL tendon. Scar tissue causes the extensor tendon to adhere to bone or skin. In addition, the scar tissue causes a thickening of the dorsal joint capsule. Even if no actual injury has occurred to the dorsal joint capsule, it can play a role in the loss of motion at these levels. The potential for loss of IP joint motion is greatest for zone T-I injuries, and loss of MCP joint motion is greatest for zone T-III injuries, which can be caused by tendon tethering. Scar tethering of the small branches of the superficial radial nerve of the thumb not only results in loss of thumb IP motion but also can cause dorsal thumb pain.[114]

Early Mobilization Programs After Extensor Pollicis Longus Tendon Repair. Early mobilization programs have been designed to reduce the potential for loss of thumb motion caused by scar formation and decreased tendon gliding. Most early mobilization programs used to treat EPL tendon repairs involve the use of a dynamic extension splint that allows for active flexion and provides passive extension of the thumb to neutral. This splint is used for approximately 4 weeks and then can be removed so that the patient can begin AROM out of the splint. Graded strengthening exercises begin at 6 to 8 weeks after surgery, and a static extension splint may be necessary if an extensor lag is present. The amount of active thumb IP or MCP flexion may be determined at the time of surgery and may depend on the level of injury. Protocols can vary among clinicians, surgeons, and clinics, depending on the surgical repair, the clinician's experience, and the patient's presentation.

Elliot and Southgate[114] have described an early mobilization program for EPL repairs in zones T-I to T-IV that allows the IP joint to be free in zones T-II to T-IV and to partly flex in zone T-I. Patients underwent primary repair, and splinting and exercises began 3 to 4 days after surgery using the protocol (Table 10-16).[114]

Early Active Motion to Zones T-IV to T-V After Extensor Tendon Repair. For extensor tendon repairs in zones T-IV and T-V, Evans[125] described the use of a dorsal forearm-based dynamic extension splint and a volar component that

TABLE **10-16**

Extensor Pollicis Longus Repairs in Zones T-I to T-IV: Early Controlled Motion with Dynamic Splinting

Time Frame	Program Considerations

0 to 1 week	• *Splint:*
	  o Zones T-II to T-IV are splinted with a forearm-based dynamic extension splint with the wrist in 30° extension and the thumb MCP joint held in neutral by the dynamic traction with the loop supporting the proximal phalanx. The IP joint is free to move. Only partial MCP flexion is allowed in the splint.
	  o Zone I is splinted in the same way except the traction loop should support the IP joint in neutral; it also should restrict full IP active flexion slightly but allow passive extension of the MCP and IP joints with dynamic traction.
	• *Exercise program:*
	  o Injuries in zones II through IV allow partial MCP active flexion with the IP joint held in extension within the confines of the splint. Full MCP flexion is restricted for the first 2 weeks. The dynamic traction passively extends the MCP joint back to neutral. Instruct the patient to perform exercises 10 times every hour.
	  o Also instruct the patient to manually support the MCP joint in neutral and actively flex and extend the IP joint of the thumb 10 times every hour.
	  o Rehabilitation of zone I repairs follows the same regimen of active MCP flexion except that the patient is allowed only slight flexion of the IP joint.
	• Begin edema management.

2 weeks	• Patients with repairs in zones II through IV are allowed to synchronously flex the MCP and IP joints of the thumb in the splint to oppose the tip of the middle finger. Patients with a zone I repair do the same, but full IP flexion is restricted. • Continue previous exercises. • Begin scar management if needed.
3 weeks	• Patients with repairs in zones II through IV are allowed to flex and oppose the thumb MCP and IP joints in the splint to oppose the tip of the ring finger. • The regimen for zone I repairs is the same, although with limited IP flexion.
4 to 5 weeks	• Patients with repairs in zones II through IV are allowed to flex and oppose the thumb MCP and IP joints in the splint to the base of the little finger. The regimen for zone I repairs is the same, although with the IP joint restricted from full flexion. • The splint is worn at all times until the end of the fourth week. The patient then can begin AROM of the MCP and IP joints out of the splint. • Ultrasound is initiated at 4 weeks if needed. • The patient can wear the splint only for protection during the fifth and sixth weeks at night and in crowded places.
6 to 12 weeks	• PROM can begin at 7 weeks. Begin gentle resistive flexion exercises and progress to 8 weeks. Patients can return to driving at 8 weeks. • No restrictions are necessary at 12 weeks.

MCP, Metacarpophalangeal; *IP,* interphalangeal; *AROM,* active range of motion; *PROM,* passive range of motion.

supports the MCP joint in neutral and the wrist in extension, with a cutaway at the IP joint that enables the dynamic traction to support it in neutral (0° extension) but allows the IP joint to flex only 60°. The author added the component of active hold (MAMTT), which is done after protected passive exercise. The patient's wrist is placed in 20° flexion while the CMC, MCP, and IP joints are held in extension, and the patient is asked to gently maintain this position. The patient can come out of the splint for exercises during the third and fourth weeks but must continue to wear the splint for protection. Composite thumb flexion and opposition exercises are initiated by the fifth week, and resistive exercises can begin at 6 to 8 weeks.[125]

SPECIFIC INJURIES OF THE WRIST

Radial Fractures

General Considerations
Distal radial fractures are extremely common and account for about 10% to 25% of all fractures,[129] and about 17% of all fractures treated in the emergency department. In the United States, 1 person in 500 is treated each year for a distal radial fracture. These also are the most common physeal fractures in children. There is a bimodal preponderance of immature patients with physeal injuries and older patients with osteoporotic bone (6 to 10 and 60 to 69 years of age).[130]

The alignment requirements for a good functional outcome are still a subject of controversy for the fracture named after Abraham Colles, who said, "[despite] the distortion... the limb will at some remote period again enjoy perfect freedom in all its motions and be completely exempt from pain.[131] It is remarkable that this common fracture remains one of the most challenging of all fractures [with] no consensus regarding description, outcome, or treatment."[132]

Anatomy

The distal radius consists of two intra-articular surfaces with three concave facets. The resting plateau for the carpal bones is the radiocarpal joint, which consists of two concave surfaces: the scaphoid and lunate fossae (Figure 10-64). The scaphoid fossa is a concave triangular space with the radial styloid as its apex. A ridge running dorsally to palmarly separates it from the lunate fossa. The lunate fossa is concave in both dorsal to palmar and radial to ulnar directions, making it more of a quadrangular space than the scaphoid fossa. The lunate therefore is nearly always congruently aligned within the joint, unlike the scaphoid, which can easily become incongruent within its fossa when it is rotated out of position.

The second intra-articular component, which is often overlooked in the evaluation of distal radial fractures, is the distal radioulnar joint. It consists of a concave fossa, the sigmoid notch, which has well-defined distal, dorsal, and palmar margins. This joint allows the radius, along with the attached hand, to rotate about the stationary ulnar head in pronation and supination.

Injury Classification

Any classification system ought to accomplish several tasks. It should make organizing data and communicating the information to other health care providers simple; in addition, it should provide insight into the treatment of and prognosis for the injury. At best, the system enables the user to better understand the injury by clearly explaining the mechanism, graphically depicting the fracture fragments, or revealing the concomitant injuries.

Over the years, multiple systems have been devised to categorize wrist fractures. Some are based on historical eponyms (a person's name), others on the mechanism of injury, and still others on the number of fracture fragments and the location of the fracture. Many of these systems remain in use today, and each has its strengths and weaknesses. Although it is tempting to choose one that works well, clinicians should examine and develop an understanding of several to gain the knowledge that each imparts.

Of all the fracture classification systems, those based on eponyms impart the least insight; they require the health care provider to memorize a fracture pattern and assign a name to it. Frequently misnamed by the casual user, the systems impart limited information as to prognosis and treatment.

The most common eponyms used to describe distal radial fractures are *Colles' fracture*, *Barton's fracture*, *Smith's fracture*, and *Chauffeur's fracture*. Colles' fracture is a transverse metaphyseal fracture with dorsal comminution that results in radial shortening, dorsal tilt, and loss of radial height. Classically, it does not enter the radiocarpal joint but may enter the distal radioulnar joint. Barton's fracture is a shear-type fracture that involves either the volar or dorsal rim of the radius. Smith described three fractures that are in essence either Colles' or Barton's fractures.

Archetype classification systems work by organizing known fracture patterns from simple into more intricate models with a concomitantly worse prognosis and more complex treatment algorithms. The *Frykman classification system* is an excellent example.[133] This system, which was based on biomechanical and clinical studies, was presented in 1967 (Figure 10-65). It distinguishes between extra-articular radial fractures and three types of intra-articular radial fractures (radiocarpal, distal radioulnar, and radiocarpal–distal radioulnar fractures). This leads to four possible fracture patterns; however, each pattern is further differentiated based on whether the ulnar styloid is also fractured. The fractures get more intricate as the system progresses from type I to type VIII, with worsening prognoses. The strength of this system is that it reveals multiple intra-articular fracture patterns and the importance of the ulnar styloid (and ulnar carpal ligaments) to the prognosis for the injury. Its weakness lies in the fact that not all fractures within one class behave the same way. In other words, the treatment and prognosis for a minimally displaced intra-articular fracture of the radiocarpal joint are very different from the treatment and prognosis for a fracture in the same location that is massively comminuted and displaced.

Melone's classification system,[134] introduced in 1984, identifies four possible major fracture fragments of the radius: the radial styloid, the radial shaft, and the medial

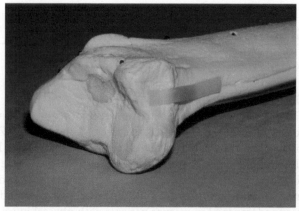

Figure 10-64 Model of the distal radius showing both the distal radioulnar joint and the radiocarpal joint. The radiocarpal joint has a fossa for the lunate and one for the scaphoid.

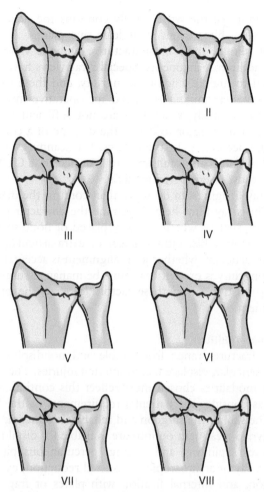

Figure 10-65 Frykman classification of distal radial fractures: types I to VIII. The higher numbers in the classification system indicate a poorer prognosis. (From Frykman G: Fracture of the distal radius including sequelae—shoulder-hand-finger syndrome, disturbance in the distal radio-ulnar joint and impairment of nerve function. A clinical and experimental study. *Acta Orthop Scand* 108: 1-155, 1967.)

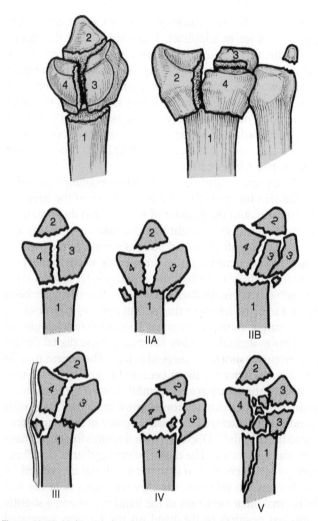

Figure 10-66 Melone's classification of distal radial fractures. (From Fernandez DL, Wolfe SW: Distal radius fractures. In Green DP, Hotchkiss RN, Pederson WC, Wolfe SW, editors: *Green's operative hand surgery*, ed 5, Philadelphia, 2005, Churchill Livingstone.)

aspect of the radius (the lunate facet), which frequently is split coronally into two fragments (Figure 10-66). Fractures can have one component or all four, and they become more complex and worsen prognostically as the number of fragments increases. This system of categorizing complex fractures has regained popularity with the advent of newer, more aggressive open fixation techniques. Its strength lies in its accurate depiction of complex fracture patterns and its emphasis on the lunate facet fragments, which affect the distal radioulnar articulation and therefore subsequently affect forearm rotation.

Fernandez[135] described a fracture classification system based on the mechanism of the injury. This system links the pattern of the break to the forces that caused it to occur. For instance, a shearing mechanism results in an unstable, oblique fracture off the volar or dorsal rim of the radius that requires open reduction and internal fixation. Although this system can be cumbersome, it relates the force that caused the injury to the relative stability of the fracture and makes treatment recommendations. This train

of thought should start the clinician thinking about what other soft tissue injuries occurred with the osseous insult that will affect the overall outcome for the patient.

Diagnosis

The diagnosis of wrist fractures begins with a careful history to discover the mechanism of damage to the bone and the surrounding soft tissue envelope and to uncover any previous wrist injuries and concurrent damage. Likewise, it is important to get to know some things about the patient that will help determine the approach to this specific wound and to treatment in general. Important questions include: What does the patient do for work and hobbies? Which is the dominant hand? Does the patient live alone or with family and friends? What other health concerns does the patient have that may affect treatment?

The physical examination is conducted not only on the fractured wrist but on the entire upper extremity and any other body part the patient may have injured. Special consideration is warranted with patients who have fallen without an obvious reason (e.g., they cannot remember slipping on ice or tripping). This should alert the examiner to the fact that the patient may have passed out briefly because of cardiac or neurological reasons that require further workup. Patients often are not forthcoming with this information. For them, it is a momentary blackout of memory, often filled in with the assumption that they simply tripped over something but cannot recall what it was. At this point, it is frequently helpful to note whether anyone else witnessed the injury.

The extremity then should be gently examined to evaluate the skin integrity, the overall alignment of the hand on the forearm, and the amount of swelling and discoloration. All these factors give insight into the amount of energy absorbed by the soft tissue and bone as a result of the trauma. Vascular and neurological examinations need to be performed carefully to verify brisk capillary refill in each digit and subjectively normal sensation. Wrist fractures have been known to cause injury to the median nerve or to worsen or create carpal tunnel syndrome. This possibility should be carefully evaluated. Tendon function for the digital flexors and extensors should be checked as well. The patient may be reluctant to move the digits because the gliding of the tendons past the injury zone is painful; however, the clinician must remember that tendon rupture can occur even with nondisplaced fractures, especially rupture of the long extensor to the thumb.[136] Displaced wrist fractures frequently have a similar appearance. The classic "silver (or dinner) fork" deformity has been used to describe the dorsal tilt created by the fracture. In addition, the clinician might note the loss of normal ulnar deviation of the hand at rest and a slightly pronated position of the hand on the forearm compared with the opposite side. If the swelling is not substantial, the distal ulna will look much more prominent because the radius has shortened and the ulna has not (Figure 10-67). Gentle palpation causes pain at the fracture site, and a palpable area of cortical incongruity and crepitus often is noted.

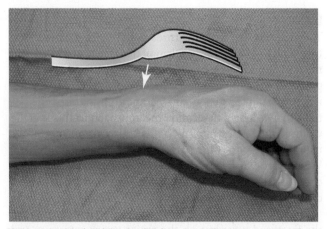

Figure 10-67 Displaced distal radial fracture (Colles fracture) with a classic "silver fork" or "dinner fork" deformity. Note the pronation and dorsal angulation of the hand on the forearm.

Imaging of the wrist usually confirms the diagnosis. Plain x-ray films taken in at least two planes, AP and lateral, should show most fractures. Oblique views can show additional fragments. Special x-ray views have been created to highlight joint incongruity, and these can be useful in determining the need for operative intervention. Occasionally, x-ray films are not sufficient to find an occult fracture or to depict the damage of a complex fracture accurately. In these cases, CT scanning can aid the clinician. If an occult fracture is suspected, a CT scan, MRI study, or bone scan is useful.

X-ray imaging can do more than confirm the diagnosis. The x-ray films help determine the character of the fracture, such as whether it is displaced or nondisplaced, stable or unstable, intra-articular or extra-articular, and, if intra-articular, whether joint alignment is acceptable or a incongruity is present that must be managed surgically. Determination of all these factors leads to the proper treatment.

Medical Treatment

Wrist fractures range from stable and nondisplaced to intra-articular, displaced, comminuted injuries. The treatment modalities chosen must reflect this continuum, as well as consider the patient's requirements of the hand and the skill of the surgeon and rehabilitation team.

Myriad treatment options are available for distal radial fractures. Splinting and casting, percutaneous pinning with x-ray or arthroscopically assisted reduction, external fixation, and internal fixation with plates or fragment-specific fixation devices are all currently in use. Recent advances in fragment-specific fixation and plate design, with the introduction of locking plates, has allowed hand surgeons to surgically repair extremely comminuted fractures in which such repair might not have been previously attempted.

When the clinician is deciding among this variety of options, clearly experience, preference, and the availability of equipment have an impact; however, certain principles guide treatment. The clinician must first determine whether the fracture is acceptably aligned. Knirk and Jupiter[137] reported that 90% of patients who had a healed intra-articular distal radial fracture with more than 1 mm of step-off went on to have symptomatic arthritis in the radiocarpal joint.[137] Multiple studies of extra-articular fractures have been done to determine the biomechanical changes that result from displacement. One study reported that a 12° loss of palmar tilt increases the ulnar load by 35%.[138] Another study reported that a loss in radial length of 2.5 mm increases the load on the ulna by almost 45%.[139] Increased ulnar loading is presumed to lead to an increased incidence of ulnar-sided wrist pain. Other effects of radial malunion include secondary midcarpal alignment changes and the possibility of early onset of degenerative joint changes in both the radiocarpal and distal radioulnar joints.[140]

If the fracture currently is acceptably aligned, the clinician must try to determine whether it is likely to stay in that satisfactory position as it heals. Good epidemiological studies are available describing what usually constitutes a stable fracture. The amount of displacement and comminution of the fracture and the patient's age are excellent predictors of subsequent redisplacement despite what initially might be a perfect closed reduction.[141–143]

If an injury requires operative intervention, either to prevent loss of reduction or to treat bony incongruence that cannot be resolved by closed methods, the surgeon must choose the method of treatment. Surgeons must have in their arsenal as many tactics or techniques as possible from which to choose. The surgeon must perform the appropriate surgery for the fracture *and the patient* to obtain the best outcome.

Pin Fixation. Pin fixation is percutaneous surgery that requires no dissection and causes very little additional soft tissue swelling. It relies on relatively good bone to hold the fixation around the pins and cannot correct extensively comminuted intra-articular fractures, nor can it reliably correct all of the volar tilt. This technique is most useful in older patients with shortened, dorsally tilted, minimally comminuted fractures because it holds better than a cast and does not require formal surgical dissection. Pin fixation also is useful in young patients with open growth plates who require reduction. With careful application of the pins, the growth plate can be avoided, and the small amount of volar tilt correction can usually be counted on to remodel with normal bone growth over time. Intrafocal dorsal pin application corrects length and volar tilt, and the addition of supplemental radial styloid K-wires provides stability. Pins require casting for supplemental stability; therefore motion cannot begin for 6 weeks or longer until the bone unites and the cast is removed. Pins are easily removed in the office and leave little scarring (Figure 10-68).

External Fixation. External fixation is a technique that uses ligamentotaxis to pull the fracture fragments into better alignment. The surgeon dissects and drills threaded pins into the radius proximal to the fracture and into the index finger metacarpal distal to the fracture and spanning the carpal joint. The surgeon attaches to these pins a mechanical frame with gears, which can be used to apply traction in different directions to pull on the hand to reduce the fracture fragments. This technique has recently begun to fall out of favor among hand surgeons as improved internal fixation technologies have become available. It still has a variety of indications that make it the procedure of choice. For fractures with extensive bone disruption, plate application may not be possible. Also, crush injuries may damage the soft tissue envelope such that the surgeon does not want to dissect extensively to apply a plate and screws to obtain rigid fixation. In this case an external fixator is the ideal choice. Finger motion should be started early because a potential drawback of the technique is stiff fingers as a result of overdistraction with the device. However, wrist motion must wait for removal of the device.

Internal Fixation. Internal fixation with a single locking plate and screws or with multiple small fragment-specific fixation components has been the most recent advance in the treatment of distal radial fractures. Previous attempts to apply plates to the distal radius had not been entirely successful because of the poor quality of the distal bone and the subsequent inability of the screws to obtain purchase and any type of holding strength. The new designs have successfully addressed these concerns and enabled anatomical repair of markedly comminuted unstable fractures in a stable configuration. The techniques differ in dissection and complexity, with the locking plate being far simpler to apply. However, in some instances the single locking plate will not obtain anatomical fixation of the joint surface, and the individual

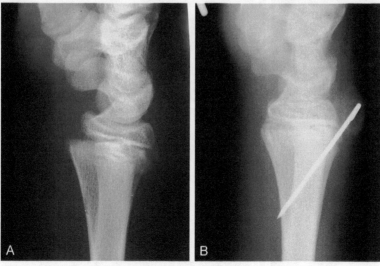

Figure 10-68 A, X-ray film of a displaced Salter II fracture. **B,** The fracture was treated with closed reduction and percutaneous pin fixation. The pin avoids the growth plate but helps maintain alignment while healing occurs in a cast over a few weeks.

fracture fragments need to be addressed and repaired with the fragment-specific technique. These approaches require a surgeon who is experienced and comfortable with operating around the wrist. They should result in a stable reduction that allows motion in the early postoperative period. Ideally, because both the dissection and the initial injury will cause scarring, aggressive therapy to obtain mobility should be started in the first 7 to 10 days (Figures 10-69 and 10-70).

Complications. Treatment of distal radius fractures, both operatively and nonoperatively, has associated complications. Tendon irritation and rupture can occur secondary to plate position for operatively treated fractures. Tendon rupture, specifically EPL, has also been associated with nonoperative management of these fractures.[129] **Carpal tunnel syndrome** and **complex regional pain syndrome** are examples of nerve dysfunction that can result from operative and nonoperative management of wrist fractures and should be recognized and treated adequately to improve patient outcomes.[129]

As the operative techniques evolve, so must the rehabilitation protocols. New expectations for recovery of function in these injuries are being developed. Along the way, pitfalls and setbacks undoubtedly will be encountered and must be overcome. Hand surgeons and therapists must work more closely than ever to accomplish these tasks.

Scaphoid Fractures

General Considerations

The scaphoid is the most commonly fractured carpal bone, accounting for nearly 80% of all wrist bone injuries.[144]

Fractures of the other carpal bones are much more rare, accounting for about 1.1% of all fractures.[145] The mechanism usually is a fall onto an outstretched hand (FOOSH injury), which creates a forced dorsiflexion of the wrist. The injured person may not have much pain, thinking the injury is little more than a sprain. Frequently, little swelling or ecchymosis is present except in the anatomical snuffbox. Young men are the most frequently affected. The injury can be associated with ligamentous injuries of the wrist, particularly scapholunate dissociations[146] or perilunate dislocations.[140]

Anatomy

The carpus consists of eight bones that are best thought of biomechanically as existing in two rows. The scaphoid traverses and links the two rows. This unique feature makes fractures of the scaphoid particularly important because the injury, in essence, unlinks the two rows, allowing them to function independently. It has been reported that, over time, chronic scaphoid fracture nonunions produce arthritis of the wrist in a reproducible and predictable pattern.[147,148]

The scaphoid is the most mobile bone in the wrist, bridging the midcarpal joint and providing three planes of motion. It is subject to the same deforming forces that cross the midcarpal joint, which in the fractured state causes the distal pole to flex with the distal carpal row, whereas the proximal pole tends to extend with the lunate and triquetrum. This creates foreshortening of the bone and the "humpback," or flexion, deformity. Simulated wrist motion has shown that healing of a 5° flexion deformity of the scaphoid leads to a 24% loss of wrist extension.[149]

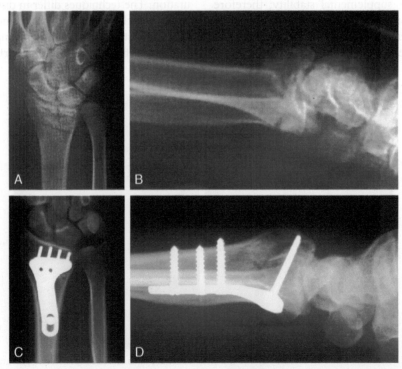

Figure 10-69 A and **B,** Comminuted intra-articular radial fracture. **C** and **D,** The fracture is repaired with a fixed-angle locking plate.

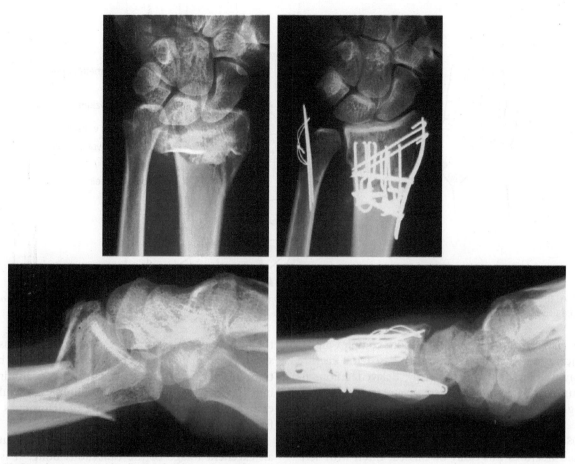

Figure 10-70 Complex intra-articular distal radial fracture. The fracture is treated with fragment-specific fixation. Anatomical restoration can be obtained, but this technique requires more extensive dissection than the fixed-angle volar plate.

The shape of the scaphoid is complex, and its orientation makes visualizing fracture lines with plain x-ray films difficult. The bone is described in thirds: the distal tubercle; the midportion, or waist; and the proximal pole. The scaphoid has multiple ligamentous attachments, both intrinsic (within the carpus) and extrinsic (between the radius or metacarpals and carpus). The scaphoid is nearly entirely covered with articular cartilage, which means that few areas are available for vessels to enter the bone. The blood supply is quite tenuous, which directly affects the bone's ability to heal. The scaphoid receives blood through a set of dorsal and volar arteries. The most important of these is the scaphoid branches of the radial artery, which enter the bone dorsally through foramina at the scaphoid waist. These dorsal ridge vessels supply blood to the proximal half of the bone. Because they enter the waist or distal third of the scaphoid, retrograde flow is required for blood to reach the proximal portions of the bone. This means that the proximal one third of the scaphoid is analogous to the femoral head or the talus in that it has little or no direct vascular input and it receives its blood through intraosseous flow. A fracture that displaces the waist or especially the proximal pole can disrupt this blood supply and prevent fracture healing or cause avascular necrosis of the proximal portion of the bone. The second group of vessels arises from the palmar branches of the radial artery and enters the distal end of the scaphoid. The scaphoid tubercle and the distal 20% to 30% of the bone are perfused by this arterial leash. The increased supply of blood at the distal pole of the scaphoid helps account for its more rapid fracture healing (Figure 10-71).

Injury Classification

The *Russe classification system*[150] is relatively straightforward and is based on the relationship of the fracture line to the long axis of the scaphoid bone. The horizontal oblique and transverse fracture types are considered stable and are not expected to displace with immobilization. The third type, the vertical oblique fracture, is considered far more unstable and requires longer immobilization with a higher potential for late instability.

Critical Elements in the Classification of a Scaphoid Fracture

- Location of the fracture
- Chronicity of the fracture
- Type of fracture (i.e., displaced or nondisplaced)
- Fracture pattern (i.e., stable or unstable)

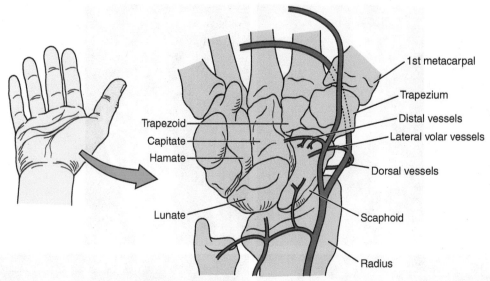

Figure 10-71 Blood supply to the scaphoid bone. Note how the blood supply to the scaphoid enters the bone proximally and distally in most people. If avascular necrosis occurs, it is primarily seen in the proximal fragment.

The *Herbert classification*[151] is a more complex alphanumeric system that rates the injury based on fracture anatomy, stability, and history (e.g., delayed union, fibrous union). By combining these several factors, a prognostic grade can be assigned to each injury.

Diagnosis

Scaphoid fractures can easily be missed, often with serious consequences; therefore it is imperative that clinicians have a high index of suspicion for this fracture in making the diagnosis. The patient's age (the fracture is uncommon in very young patients) and the mechanism of trauma should alert the clinician to the possibility the injury exists. Any tenderness on careful examination at the anatomical snuffbox should be presumed to indicate a scaphoid fracture until proven otherwise.

Radiographic imaging is the mainstay in confirming the diagnosis. However, plain films frequently can fail to detect acute nondisplaced fractures. Initial x-ray films should include a posteroanterior (PA) view, a PA view with ulnar deviation to extend the bone in a plane more parallel with the x-ray film, and lateral and oblique views (Figure 10-72). If the clinical examination leads to a high level of suspicion for a fracture but the plain films are negative, the patient should be treated with cast immobilization and the plain films repeated in 2 to 3 weeks. At that time, resorption of bone around the fracture line may be sufficient to allow positive identification of the injury on plain x-ray films. If an urgent need exists to rule out the fracture before 2 to 3 weeks has elapsed (e.g., professional athletes), imaging with MRI or a thin slice CT scan can be performed. The cost of these imaging modalities may make them prohibitive for routine applications.

CT scanning gives the highest resolution images of the bone and the trabeculae and is useful for evaluating

the healing of treated fractures. It frequently is used after surgery or cast immobilization to confirm that bridging trabeculae are crossing the fracture site, indicating healing. In chronic nonunion, CT scanning is useful preoperatively to plan for bone grafting of deformities that are frequently encountered.

MRI does not depict the cortical bone well, but it gives an excellent image of the cancellous bone. It is both a highly sensitive and specific method of detecting occult scaphoid fractures. With gadolinium contrast, MRI is the best means of evaluating the blood supply to the proximal pole of the scaphoid if avascular necrosis is suspected.

Medical Treatment

For an acute, nondisplaced scaphoid fracture, treatment traditionally has consisted of cast immobilization. Healing time depends on the level of the fracture; distal fractures heal most quickly, and those that are most proximal take longest. Proximal fractures sometimes require 3 to 6 months of immobilization to heal, whereas fractures of the distal third generally heal in 6 to 8 weeks. Some studies have reported a slightly faster time to union if the initial casting is done above the elbow for the first several weeks.[152]

More recent techniques have become available that allow limited incision or even percutaneous compression screw placement in the scaphoid (Figure 10-73), which can obviate the need for prolonged cast immobilization while the fracture heals.[153] This has the obvious benefit of returning patients to work or sports much more quickly.

In one study in which 12 athletes were treated surgically for minimally displaced or nondisplaced fractures, the average time for return to sports was within 6 weeks. Only one fracture in the study failed to unite.[154] A recent meta-analysis also determined that surgical management for nondisplaced and minimally displaced scaphoid fractures gave better patient results with respect to functional

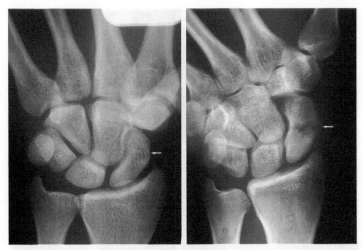

Figure 10-72 An AP x-ray film may fail to show a scaphoid fracture *(arrows).* Ulnar deviation extends the bone and may help reveal the fracture.

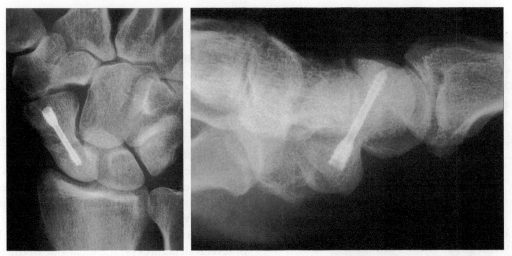

Figure 10-73 Percutaneous compression screw fixation of a scaphoid fracture. This allows early removal from a cast and return to function.

outcome and time off work, although there was an increased risk of complications.[155]

Fractures that are unstable and/or displaced are associated with a nonunion rate of 50% and an avascular necrosis rate of 55%; these fractures therefore need to be treated operatively.[156,157] Displacement (and subsequent instability) is considered present if a gap of more than 1 mm is present at any point along the fracture, if the scapholunate angle exceeds 60°, or if the radiolunate angle is more than 15°.[158] If the fracture is acute and does not require bone grafting, a limited approach from either a volar or a dorsal direction (i.e., manipulation of the fragments into alignment and placement of a compression screw) can be used. However, if the fracture requires bone grafting or cannot be manipulated into alignment, a more traditional open reduction and internal fixation should be performed. For waist and midthird fractures, a volar approach may be favored, as this typically requires less dissection, while still allowing enough screw threads to pass the fracture site (Figure 10-74). Unfortunately, with the

volar approach, it is more difficult to place the screw in line with the central axis of the scaphoid, although this does not seem to affect healing. A recent cadaveric study has reported that the percutaneous transtrapezial volar approach to the scaphoid may have the benefit of placing the screw more in line with the central axis of the scaphoid, which theoretically may affect healing.[159] With proximal third fractures, a dorsal approach is recommended, as this approach allows the screw to be placed for optimum compression of the usually small proximal fragment.[160]

Nonunions of the scaphoid that have not progressed to arthritis and do not require any type of salvage surgery require operative treatment to achieve a bony union. The fracture needs to be opened, bone grafted, and then rigidly fixed so that it can heal.[161,162] With fractures of the proximal third of the scaphoid or if sclerosis of the proximal pole of the bone is seen on plain x-ray films, the surgeon must consider that the blood supply to the proximal fracture fragment may have been disrupted. A preoperative

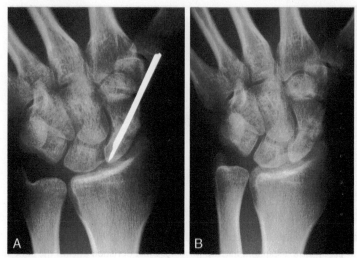

Figure 10-74 **A,** AP x-ray films of a chronic scaphoid nonunion that was treated with bone grafting and pins. **B,** After the fracture healed, the pins were removed.

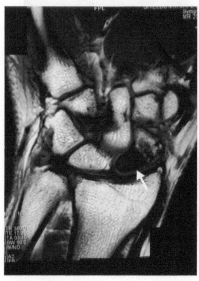

Figure 10-75 MRI scan of the scaphoid showing avascular changes in the proximal pole *(arrow).*

MRI scan should help determine whether this is the case (Figure 10-75). If, in fact, the bone is avascular, a vascularized bone grafting procedure may be chosen in an effort to increase the likelihood of successful union.[163,164] This procedure is more technically demanding than traditional fracture repair. A dorsal approach is used, and a segment of bone with its intact blood vessel is elevated from the radius and directly inserted into the scaphoid.

The treatment of scaphoid fractures that have gone unrecognized is a problem that frequently plagues clinicians. Some studies[165] have suggested that a scaphoid fracture that is left untreated for longer than 4 weeks is at increased risk of nonunion. For this reason, fractures of the scaphoid that are delayed in coming to treatment should be considered more readily for operative repair.[165]

Triangular Fibrocartilage Complex (TFCC) Injuries

General Considerations

A common problem clinicians encounter in patients is ulnar-sided wrist pain. Previously considered the "low back pain" of the upper extremity, this is an area of exciting new developments and understanding. Although still a significant diagnostic challenge, a better understanding of the anatomy and biomechanics of the ulnar side of the wrist has enabled clinicians to more accurately screen and treat patients with injuries that previously might have meant vocational retraining or limited sports activity.

The triangular fibrocartilage complex (TFCC) is one of several structures on the ulnar side of the wrist that can be injured, leading to debilitating pain and mechanical changes. Discussion of the more than three dozen recognized causes of ulnar-sided wrist pain is beyond the scope of this text. However, by understanding the function and pathology of the TFCC, the clinician can develop an appreciation of one common cause of ulnar-sided wrist pain and gain knowledge of some of the other structures in which injury can lead to pathology on the ulnar side of the wrist.[166]

Anatomy

The TFCC is described as a composite of ligaments and fibrocartilage that originates from the ulnar border of the distal radius at the articular surface. It inserts onto the base of the ulnar styloid and the fovea of the ulnar head.[167] This horizontal portion, considered the TFCC, or the articular disc proper, is fibrocartilaginous and relatively avascular. The periphery of this horizontal portion is composed of highly vascular ligaments, both dorsally and volarly, that connect the distal radius and ulna. These radioulnar ligaments are oriented perpendicular to the long axis of the forearm. In contrast with this are additional

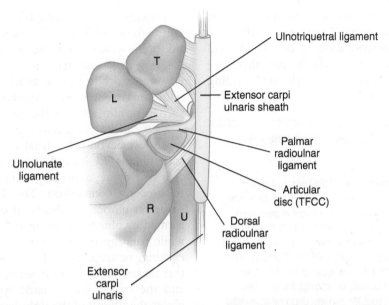

Figure 10-76 Ulnocarpal joint and triangular fibrocartilage complex (TFCC). Triquetrum (*T*), lunate (*L*), ulna (*U*), radius (*R*). (From Skirven TM, Osterman AL, Fedorczyk JM: *Rehabilitation of the hand and upper extremity*, ed 6, Philadelphia, 2011, Mosby.)

ligaments still considered part of the TFCC that arise from the base of the ulnar styloid to insert on the lunate, triquetrum, hamate, and base of the fifth metacarpal (Figure 10-76).[168] The distinct anatomical structures composed of differing biomaterial and oriented in several planes should alert the reader that the TFCC is both complex and multifunctional.

As the forearm moves through pronation and supination, the TFCC ligaments stabilize the distal radioulnar joint. As it arcs over the ulna in pronation, the radius becomes shorter relative to the ulna, resulting in positive ulnar variance, while in supination the radius is out at its maximum length relative to the ulna, resulting in a relative negative ulnar variance. These changes in relative ulnar height in relation to the carpus produce significant changes in the load borne by the TFCC.[169-176]

Major Roles of the Triangular Fibrocartilage Complex

- The triangular fibrocartilage complex (TFCC) creates a shock absorber for the ulnar carpus. The ulnar side of the lunate and the triquetrum do not articulate with the ulna, as the scaphoid and lunate do with the radius. The TFCC transfers about 20% of the axial load between the hand and the forearm.
- The dorsal and volar radioulnar ligaments are the primary stabilizers of the distal radioulnar joint. This arrangement allows stable pronation and supination of the forearm. The ligaments become taut at the end range of rotation in either direction.
- The ligaments that arise from the ulna and insert onto the lunate, triquetrum, hamate, and fifth metacarpal serve as stabilizers for the ulnar carpus. Their function is similar to that of the extrinsic wrist ligaments on the radial side of the wrist.

Injury Classification

In 1989, a classification system was devised that described TFCC lesions based on the mechanism of injury, the location of the injury, and the involvement of surrounding structures. This system is widely accepted as the standard for describing these injuries.[177]

Lesions of the TFCC are divided into two major types, traumatic and degenerative (Table 10-17). Traumatic (type I) lesions have four subtypes based on the location of the injury in the TFCC. Degenerative

TABLE **10-17**

Classification of Triangular Fibrocartilage Complex (TFCC) Tears

Type	Subclassification
Type I: Traumatic	IA: Central perforation IB: Ulnar avulsion (with or without a styloid fracture) IC: Volar tear ID: Radial avulsion
Type II: Degenerative	IIA: TFCC wear IIB: TFCC wear plus lunate or ulnar articular wear (chondromalacia) IIC: TFCC perforation plus lunate or ulnar chondromalacia IID: TFCC perforation plus chondromalacia plus lunotriquetral ligament tear IIE: TFCC perforation, chondromalacia, lunotriquetral ligament tear, and ulnocarpal arthritis

lesions are the result of chronic loading on the ulnar side of the wrist (ulnar carpal impaction syndrome). This leads to chronic deterioration of the TFCC and surrounding structures. These lesions are therefore subclassified by the extent of injury to the surrounding bones and ligaments.

Classification of Traumatic Lesions of the Triangular Fibrocartilage Complex

- *Type IA* lesions consist of a perforation of the horizontal portion of the triangular fibrocartilage complex (TFCC) in its avascular region. The tear usually is 1-2 mm wide, anterior to dorsal in orientation, and about 3 mm ulnar to the radial side attachment of the TFCC proper. These lesions cause mechanical pain on the ulnar side of the wrist but are not usually associated with instability (Figure 10-77).
- *Type IB* tears represent injury to the dorsal aspect of the TFCC or its insertion into the ulna. These tears may be accompanied by an ulnar styloid fracture, and they are frequently seen with displaced distal radial fractures. Type IB lesions can cause instability at the distal radioulnar joint.
- *Type IC* injuries are tears of the anterior aspect of the TFCC at its periphery. The lesion often occurs with avulsion of the attachment of the TFCC to the lunate or the triquetrum. This can result in ulnocarpal instability, which is manifested as palmar translocation of the ulnar carpus.
- *Type ID* lesions are traumatic avulsions of the ligament proper from its origin at the radius just distal to the sigmoid notch (Figure 10-78).

Diagnosis

Patients often are seen months after the initial symptoms have started. They frequently cannot remember any specific trauma. When an injury is recalled, it is regularly a fall onto a pronated and outstretched hand or a traction or rotation injury. We have treated several patients injured by rotating power tools that became bound and forcibly rotated the forearm. They also have treated several golfers who injured the nondominant wrist when they inadvertently struck a tree root or made a deep divot.

Patients generally complain of ulnar-sided wrist pain, although not all can readily localize the pain to the ulnar side of the wrist without the prompting of an examination. Clicking and mechanical symptoms are sometimes encountered but are not nearly as reliable as pain. The symptoms seem most evident with rotational activities such as turning a key or the steering wheel of a car.

Pain can be elicited in the ulnar-sided snuffbox, the space just beyond the distal ulna between the extensor carpi ulnaris (ECU) and FCU tendons. This is a sensitive area to palpate, and the patient's opposite wrist should be used for comparison. The **TFCC load test** is used to detect ulnocarpal abutment or TFCC tears. It is performed by ulnarly deviating and axially loading the wrist while rotating the forearm. A positive test elicits pain, clicking, or crepitus.[178] The **ulnomeniscal dorsal glide test** increases the motion between the ulna, the TFCC, and the triquetrum to elicit symptoms. The examiner places the thumb of the right hand on the dorsum of the right ulnar head of the patient; the radial aspect of the examiner's right index finger PIP joint then rests on the patient's pisiform. The examiner compresses the pisotriquetral joint dorsally while pushing the ulnar head volarly by reproducing a key pinch maneuver. This increases the stress on the TFCC and ulnocarpal ligaments and should produce pain if a lesion or laxity is present in this region.[179] Evaluation of the distal radioulnar joint for laxity may reveal torn ligaments of the TFCC. This can be accomplished by moving/gliding the distal ulna head while stabilizing the radius in neutral rotation, pronation, and supination and comparing the findings to those of the patient's opposite wrist.

Imaging studies should always be part of the workup of ulnar-sided wrist pain. These begin with a series of plain x-ray films, including a PA and a gripping PA view taken in neutral rotation, as well as lateral views. These films aid the evaluation for distal radioulnar joint arthritis, ulnar variance, lesions consistent with ulnar abutment syndrome, ulnar styloid fractures, and wrist instability consistent with intrinsic ligament lesions.

However useful x-ray films are, they fail to visualize the ligaments of the wrist. Therefore other diagnostic imaging modalities are used if questions remain as to the diagnosis of the patient's ulnar-sided wrist pain. Wrist arthrography is useful for assessing the integrity of the TFCC complex and the other intrinsic ligaments of the wrist, including the lunotriquetral joint. Arthrography is accomplished by injecting dye into the radiocarpal joint and radiographically looking for leaks of the contrast material into the other compartments of the wrist, each of which should be watertight. If no contrast is seen to leak, the examination is repeated by injecting dye into the distal radioulnar joint and then the midcarpal joint and looking for dye leaking back into the radiocarpal joint. This three-phase arthrogram is more sensitive than a single-phase study for detecting small ligament tears (Figure 10-79).

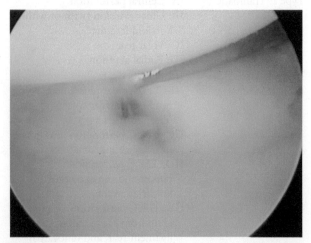

Figure 10-77 Arthroscopic view of a type IA tear in the TFCC (indicated by the probe).

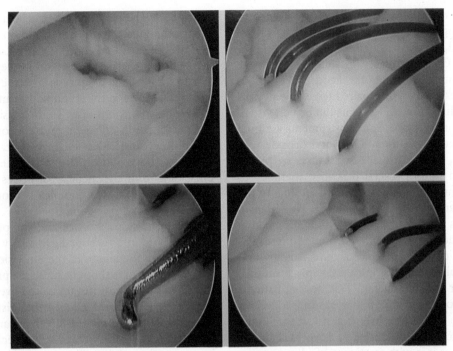

Figure 10-78 Peripheral TFCC tear (i.e., type ID lesion). Tears such as this cause instability and require fixation, which can be done arthroscopically.

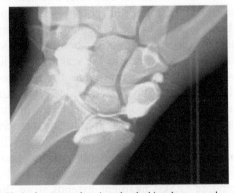

Figure 10-79 Arthrogram showing dye leaking between the radiocarpal joint and the distal radioulnar joint, an indication of a TFCC tear.

MRI, both with and without arthrographic dye injection, has also been used to visualize the ligaments of the wrist, including the TFCC. It has proved to be a highly sensitive modality, with up to 95% correlation with arthroscopic findings when positive.[180] However, it is not as useful in patients in which the MRI is found to be normal. In this case Skahen et al.[181] reported its sensitivity to be 44% and the specificity only 75%. These same authors reported that the clinical examination could be more sensitive than MRI, with up to a 95% correlation with arthroscopic findings. Therefore a patient with a strongly positive clinical examination should not be assumed to have an intact ligament if the MRI results are normal. As the clinician gains more experience and confidence in wrist examination, the need for MRI for correlation diminishes.

Medical Treatment

The treatment of acute TFCC lesions initially is conservative. Long arm cast immobilization is used if the patient does not have a fracture of the ulnar styloid or instability of the distal radioulnar joint. If the tear is peripheral and acute, the highly vascular tissue is likely to scar together over a 4- to 6-week period. If the tear is more central, it is not expected to heal, although the synovitis associated with it may diminish and the symptoms of wrist pain may abate. Central tears do not cause instability and require treatment only if they are painful. Patients who present acutely but have instability of the distal radioulnar joint should undergo ligament repair.

When conservative treatment fails or a patient presents months after the onset of injury, arthroscopic evaluation is the gold standard for diagnosis of TFCC pathology. This modality also affords the possibility of treatment. Open treatment of TFCC tears is possible but creates more scarring postoperatively, and visualization of the ligament structure may not be as good as can be obtained arthroscopically.

Central (type IA) tears of the TFCC do not cause instability as long as the outer third of the TFCC remains intact. In patients with ulnar neutral or negative variance, debridement of the central tear to a stable rim of tissue (leaving at least 2 mm of the volar and dorsal ligaments of the TFCC) should resolve the pain. Several studies have reported that, with ulnar positive variance, simple ligament debridement will fail to give long-term pain relief in many patients, and the procedure should be combined with ulnar recession either in the form of a wafer-type procedure or formal ulnar shortening.[182,183] Postoperatively, no immobilization is required, and patients are encouraged to begin using the hand and wrist immediately. Pain relief is fairly rapid, usually within a few weeks.

Peripheral TFCC tears can cause instability and a change in the load distribution between the hand and the forearm. These injuries need to be repaired to restore normal mechanics and reduce pain. TFCC tears can be best visualized through the arthroscope. Small instruments are used to remove inflamed synovium and scar and debride torn ligaments to fresh, healing tissue. Also, sutures are placed arthroscopically in one of several described methods to recreate the preinjury anatomy (see Figure 10-78). In the case of ID-type tears in which the ligament is avulsed from the radius, sutures are passed through drill holes made in the radius to reattach the TFCC to its point of origin. IC-type tears can be difficult to repair arthroscopically and may require a small open incision to safely place sutures. After suture repair of a peripheral TFCC lesion, patients are immobilized for the first 3 to 4 weeks in a long arm cast, followed by a well-molded short arm cast that limits forearm rotation for an additional 2 to 3 weeks. Pain relief is not as rapid as it is with treatment of IA-type tears. Immobilization can lead to stiffness and loss of strength, which respond well to therapy. Studies report that 95% of patients who undergo surgery for a torn TFCC return to work and sports, and grip strength can be expected to return to 85% of normal.[183]

Scapholunate Dissociation

General Considerations

Instability of the scaphoid and lunate secondary to a traumatic ligamentous disruption has been described many times, beginning with Vaughan-Jackson and Russell in 1949.[184,185] The characteristic symptoms of pain, clicking, and loss of motion at the radioscaphoid joint, along with the radiographic findings of scaphoid flexion, pronation, and lunate extension, have been well documented. Despite this, patients frequently fail to be diagnosed with this injury until months or often years after the onset. This can have unfortunate consequences in that the instability, given enough time, causes arthritic changes. This has been clearly borne out in the hand literature and is referred to as **scapholunate advanced collapse**.[186,187] With an understanding of the relevant anatomy, common mechanisms of injury, and clinical signs and symptoms, clinicians can be more prepared to make the diagnosis in patients at an earlier stage, perhaps preventing or at least delaying the onset of painful arthrosis of the wrist.

Anatomy

The wrist joint is made up of eight bones, best thought of biomechanically to exist in two rows. The lunate is located in the center of the proximal carpal row and articulates distally with the capitate, which is in the center of the distal carpal row. The scaphoid bone articulates with the radial side of the lunate and is the single bone in the wrist that bridges the proximal and distal rows. Both scaphoid and lunate bones move on the radius in their respective fossae. What is important to note is that the lunate fossa has a spherical shape and the scaphoid has an elliptical shape.

The ligaments of the wrist are considered intrinsic ligaments if they both begin and end on carpal bones. In contrast, extrinsic wrist ligaments attach on one side to the carpal bone and on the other side to the radius, the ulna, or one of the metacarpal bones of the hand. The scapholunate ligament complex is thought to have both intrinsic and extrinsic components.

The intrinsic portion of the complex consists of the scapholunate interosseous ligament, which connects the radial side of the lunate to the ulnar side of the scaphoid. This component is thought to be the primary stabilizer of the SL joint and contributes to the overall stability of the carpus.[188] It is composed of three distinct regions. The thick dorsal portion is the strongest and is composed of short transverse fibers that are biomechanically the most important for stability. The proximal section is composed primarily of fibrocartilage and is the least important stabilizer of the three sections. The volar ligament is thinner than the dorsal ligament and consists of obliquely oriented fibers that allow some movement to account for the differences in the arcs of motion between the scaphoid and lunate. Isolated cutting of the scapholunate ligament in cadaver models has not caused instability patterns that mimic those seen clinically, which has lead clinicians to believe that more than an isolated injury to the intrinsic ligament is needed to produce a scapholunate dissociation.[189]

The extrinsic portion of the scapholunate ligament complex is made up of ligaments that originate from the radius and insert on various carpal bones. The radioscaphocapitate (RSC) ligament extends from the radial styloid through a small groove on the volar aspect of the scaphoid to insert onto the palmar portion of the capitate. It serves as a rotational fulcrum around which the scaphoid can revolve. The long radiolunate ligament runs parallel and just ulnar to the RSC ligament from the radius to the volar radial portion of the lunate. The short radiolunate ligament originates from the palmar portion of the radius and inserts onto the palmar portion of the lunate. Both the intrinsic and extrinsic ligaments described can be partly visualized during routine wrist arthroscopy.

On the dorsal surface of the wrist capsule are some thickenings considered to be ligamentous; these provide additional stability to the wrist. They are not easily seen during routine wrist arthroscopy. The dorsal radiocarpal (DRC) ligament originates on the dorsal radial portion of the radius and runs ulnarly and distally to insert onto the lunate, lunotriquetral ligament, and dorsal portion of the triquetrum. The dorsal intercarpal (DIC) ligament originates from the triquetrum and runs radially and distally to insert onto the lunate, scaphoid, and dorsal aspect of the trapezium (Figure 10-80).

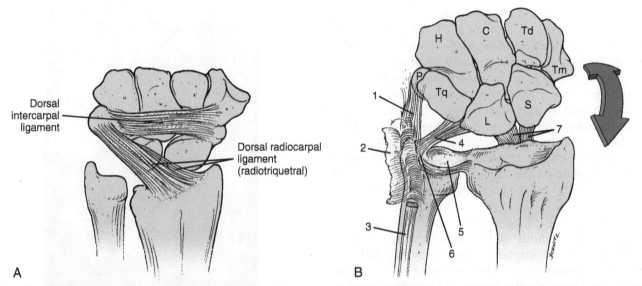

Figure 10-80 A, Posterior (dorsal) aspect of the wrist. **B,** Anterior (volar) aspect of the wrist. *1,* Ulnar collateral ligament; *2,* retinacular sheath; *3,* tendon of extensor carpi ulnaris; *4,* ulnolunate ligament; *5,* triangular fibrocartilage complex (TFCC); *6,* ulnocarpal meniscus homologue; *7,* palmar radioscaphoid lunate ligament. *P,* Pisiform; *H,* hamate; *C,* capitate; *Td,* trapezoid; *Tm,* trapezium; *Tq,* triquetrum; *L,* lunate; *S,* scaphoid. (From Fess E, Gettle K, Philips C, Janson J: *Hand and upper extremity splinting principles and methods,* ed 3, St Louis, 2005, Mosby.)

The importance of understanding the complexity of the extrinsic ligaments is twofold. First, these ligaments are used or reconstructed in the soft tissue operations that have been developed to treat scapholunate dissociation injuries. Second, some have reported that injury to the extrinsic ligaments is required to produce the radiographic results seen clinically in patients with scapholunate dissociation patterns.[190]

Injury Classification

Classification of scapholunate dissociative injuries can be based on several factors: the time since the injury, the presence or absence of radiographic abnormalities, the extent of ligamentous disruption, and the presence of additional carpal abnormalities or arthritic changes.

Injuries sustained within 6 weeks of diagnosis are classified as acute. Those that have happened beyond 6 weeks but before degenerative changes in the wrist have occurred are considered to be subacute. After degenerative changes have taken place within the wrist, the injury is best thought of as chronic and the treatment options differ considerably.

The chronic condition of scapholunate dissociation is referred to as **scapholunate advanced collapse,** or a **SLAC wrist.** It is a progression of arthrosis that occurs in the wrist because of the scapholunate instability and rotatory subluxation of the scaphoid. The arthritic changes begin at the radial styloid and progress into the radioscaphoid articulation. Over time, the midcarpal joints become arthritic, specifically in the scaphocapitate and lunocapitate joints. The radiolunate joint is spared in all but the most severe cases of pancarpal arthritis.

The injury is also classified according to whether it is apparent on x-ray films at rest or requires some provocative maneuver. With a less severe ligament injury, a stress x-ray film is required to uncover the changes caused by the instability. The stress can be created by asking the patient to tightly grip and/or ulnarly deviate the hand on the PA view. A wrist that can be seen to be unstable at rest is classified as having static instability, whereas a wrist that requires stress to uncover the instability is considered dynamically unstable. A third group is thought to exist: those that are predynamically unstable. In this case the wrist cannot be shown to be unstable radiographically by any means, but the patient is clinically believed to have the beginnings of instability secondary to ligamentous injury.

Diagnosis

The typical patient describes the mechanism as a FOOSH (Fall On an OutStretched Hand) injury, which causes a dorsiflexion and pronation injury at the wrist. A less common mechanism of injury is a rotational injury to the hand and wrist from a twisting force. Pain and swelling often are not severe and generally subside with rest after a few days. Frequently, little ecchymosis or edema is present, and no obvious deformity makes the diagnosis clearer to the patient, sports trainers, or coaches or to the uninitiated health care worker. Because these patients often do not seek treatment in the acute phase, they may not recall the inciting injury when, at some later time, they present for evaluation of the wrist pain.

Physical findings are related to the degree of instability of the scaphoid. In the least severe cases, pain is present over the dorsal scapholunate ligament and the radioscaphoid joint. Dorsal wrist pain usually can be elicited by applying dorsal pressure to the volar pole of the scaphoid. In addition, pain often is elicited at the anatomical snuffbox secondary to synovitis of the radial side of the wrist joint.

The stability of the scaphoid can be checked in the manner described by Watson et al.[191]; dorsal pressure is applied to the volar pole of the scaphoid while the wrist is moved from ulnar to radial deviation in an effort to sublux the proximal pole of the scaphoid out over the dorsal rim of the radius. This is known as a **scaphoid shift test**, and it can produce pain either from the instability or from compression of the scaphoid in its fossa in the presence of chronic synovitis. In a patient with an unstable injury, a discernable, painful clunk occurs when the examiner releases pressure on the scaphoid, allowing the subluxed proximal pole to reduce back into the scaphoid fossa of the radius.

A patient with long-standing instability who has progressed to arthritis of the joint may have a fixed subluxation of the scaphoid. This can be palpated as a firm dorsal prominence at the distal edge of the radius. Severe limitation of wrist motion and significant tenderness are indicative of the degenerative changes that have occurred at the radiocarpal joint. Osteophyte formation on the radial side of the wrist can lead to a deformity that is observable and palpable.

Plain x-ray films are the most important imaging study and should accompany the history and physical examination whenever a ligamentous injury of the wrist is suspected. Many articles have been devoted to the way the x-ray films should be obtained. It has been our practice to obtain a PA, a clenched fist PA, and a lateral view. In obtaining the PA films, a foam block is used that elevates the ulnar side of the wrist 10° to 15°, which allows a more perpendicular view of the scapholunate articulation. Abnormalities seen on the PA films include a widened scapholunate gap, usually greater than 3 mm in adults. The clinician can see signs of the flexed scaphoid by noting its loss of length and the appearance of the "signet ring sign," which is indicative of the cortical projection of the distal pole seen through the long axis of the bone as it becomes more vertical (Figure 10-81).[192]

The lateral projection views require more experience to read but generally provide even more information than the PA views. The scaphoid flexes and creates a bigger angle in relation to the long axis of the radius. In addition, the lunate tends to extend, pointing dorsally and translating volarly. The angle between the axial long axis of the lunate and scaphoid normally is 30° to 60°, with the average being 47°. As the scaphoid flexes and the lunate extends, that angle increases to more than 60° and often approaches 90° (Figure 10-82).

Clinicians occasionally can see the proximal pole of the scaphoid sitting dorsal to the center of its fossa on the radius. As the lunate extends, the capitate translates proximally and dorsally, and the normal collinear relationship of the radius, lunate, and capitate is disrupted.

Arthrography can confirm loss of the watertight compartment between the midcarpal and radiocarpal joints. This indicates a tear of some portion of the scapholunate

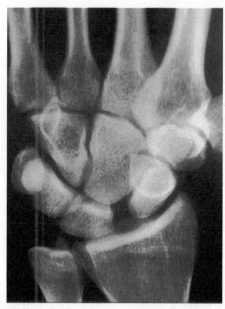

Figure 10-81 AP x-ray film of a wrist with a scapholunate tear. The scaphoid is flexed and shortened, and the lunate is extended. A gap is created between the scaphoid and the lunate as the scaphoid rotates away from the lunate. The scaphoid no longer lies correctly in its fossa in the radius, and over time this will cause joint degeneration.

interosseous ligament. Communication can be seen if a small perforation exists in the membranous portion of the ligament; this perforation is not biomechanically important, but it increases the potential for false positive results. In addition, some tears flow only unidirectionally; therefore, if the dye is injected into only one compartment, it may fail to reveal a substantial tear, leading to false negative results. Detection can be improved by injecting dye into all three compartments of the wrist over the course of the test.[193]

MRI can visualize the different sections of the scapholunate ligament. Edema, thickening, tortuosity (twisting), and lengthening of the ligament indicate injury and possible disruption. Joint fluid flow through the ligament indicates a tear as much as arthrography does, without the need for an injection before the examination. In addition, the MRI can help visualize the bony alterations between the radius, capitate, lunate, and scaphoid that occur with scapholunate instability.

Medical Treatment

With acute or subacute injuries in which the scaphoid flexion deformity is still flexible and no joint destruction has occurred, the preferable course is to attempt a soft tissue reconstruction of the wrist. This retains the most mobility of the radiocarpal and midcarpal joints while attempting to regain stability. By restoring appropriate carpal alignment and improving the kinematics of the wrist, the surgeon attempts to prevent or delay the onset of arthritic changes that would occur if no treatment were given.

Many surgical solutions have been proposed for acute and subacute scapholunate dissociation. Many surgeons

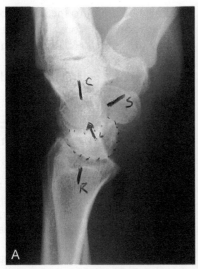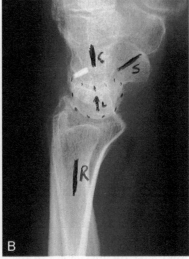

Figure 10-82 A, Lateral x-ray film of a patient with a scapholunate dissociation. The lunate is tilted dorsally, and the scapholunate angle is nearing 90°. **B,** Lateral x-ray film of the same patient after repair of the ligament and capsulodesis of the scaphoid. The lunate is no longer tilting backward, and the scaphoid is more extended. This creates a more normal angle between the two (approximately 45°). *R,* radius; *L,* lunate; *S,* scaphoid; *C,* capitate.

attempt to restore the normal anatomy by repairing the scapholunate interosseous ligament back to the ulnar side of the scaphoid from which it usually detaches. This can be done through bone tunnels drilled into the scaphoid or with various suture anchors. However, this repair does not address the flexion and rotation deformity of the scaphoid. To do so, ligamentous tissue from the dorsal capsule of the wrist is rerouted to the distal pole of the scaphoid to act as a tether that prevents the scaphoid from flexing and rotating.

Additional soft tissue repairs have been created using various tendons, including the extensor carpi radialis longus (ECRL) and FCR ligaments. Tunnels are drilled through the scaphoid in a dorsal-volar direction, allowing one of these tendons to be passed through the bone, in an attempt to correct the position of the scaphoid in relation to the lunate.

The alternative to soft tissue procedures is partial wrist fusion or proximal row carpectomy. The scaphotrapezio-trapezoid (STT) fusion has been advocated in cases that have not progressed to arthritis at the radiocarpal joint. The scaphoid is brought out of its flexed position and locked in place by its fusion across the midcarpal row. This allows motion to continue at the radiocarpal joint. Criticism of this procedure relates to the increased load borne on the radial side of the wrist between the scaphoid and radius after the fusion, in the area at risk for arthritic changes secondary to the initial injury.

If arthritis has developed within the radioscaphoid joint but left the midcarpal joint intact, a proximal row carpectomy can be considered. In this instance the scaphoid, lunate, and triquetrum are excised, allowing the capitate to articulate in the lunate fossa of the radius. This changes the wrist from a complex link joint to a simple hinge joint with concomitant loss of motion. This

procedure is criticized for the fact that the capitate is not an exact fit in the lunate fossa of the radius and that the relative shortening of the wrist leads to some weakness of grip.

As arthritis progresses in chronic scapholunate instability, the midcarpal joint between the scaphoid, lunate, and capitate is affected. In many surgeons' eyes, this midcarpal arthrosis, especially of the proximal capitate, is a contraindication to the proximal row carpectomy. In this case they favor removal of the arthritic scaphoid and fusion of the ulnar midcarpal joint (four-corner fusion). This stabilizes the midcarpal joint in the absence of the scaphoid. Again, the link joint has been turned into a hinge joint, with subsequent sacrifice of 30% to 50% of flexion and extension, as well as radioulnar deviation. The operation succeeds because, despite the progression of arthritis with scapholunate advance collapse, the surface between the lunate and the radius usually is preserved. This occurs because the radiolunate articulation is spherical; therefore, when the lunate tips backward because of ligament instability, the congruency between the two bones is maintained. This is not true of the radioscaphoid fossa, which is elliptical and becomes incongruous and eventually arthritic, as the scaphoid flexes and pronates.

Rehabilitation Principles and Considerations for Wrist Injuries

Rehabilitation of wrist injuries requires an understanding of carpal anatomy, force distribution, and wrist kinematics.[194] An optimally aligned, stable but mobile wrist is capable of the precise interaction needed between bone and soft tissues to produce pain-free, functional motion. Restoration of alignment, stability, and pain-free motion poses a challenge to the treating clinician.

Distal Radial Fractures

Understanding normal force distributions at the wrist and the impact of altered mechanics is essential in initiating therapy regimens. When the distal ulna is equal in length to the distal radius, this is termed **ulnar neutral variance**. Changes from ulnar neutral variance can occur as a result of injury, and they alter the mechanics of the wrist joint (Figure 10-83). Shortening of the distal radius during fracture healing, with no change in the position of the ulna, results in **ulnar positive variance**. This change increases the force distributed to the ulna and potentially results in ulnar-sided wrist pain.[175,200–203]

In a typical ulnar neutral wrist, 80% of the force is borne by the radius, with only 20% through the ulnocarpal joint. However, even a small change in height results in the ulna absorbing 40% of the load if the ulna is 2 mm ulnar positive or 4% of the load if it is 2 mm ulnar negative.[139,175,203–205] Loading the wrist, which occurs during weight bearing and gripping, places stress on the primary ligamentous stabilizers of the wrist. Evaluation for ligamentous injury should be considered in the event of persistent pain with loading of the wrist.[206] The **push-off test** measures upper extremity weight bearing, using a grip dynamometer,

and may be useful to measure progress as patients recover strength and heal from their wrist injuries.[207]

For the clinician charged with the rehabilitative management of a patient with a wrist injury and pain, the key considerations regarding force distribution at the wrist are summarized below.

The dynamics of wrist motion are important for the rehabilitation strategy. Wrist kinematics is described by the direction in which the proximal carpal row moves.[208,209] Normal kinematics and wrist motion are detailed in Table 10-18. Normal values for AROM at the wrist compared with what is needed for light activities of daily living (ADL) tasks are presented in Table 10-19. Of note, 40% to 60% of wrist flexion and extension occurs at the radiocarpal joint, and the remaining motion occurs at the midcarpal joint. As well, 60% of radial and ulnar deviation occurs at the midcarpal joint and 40% at the radiocarpal joint.[210,211]

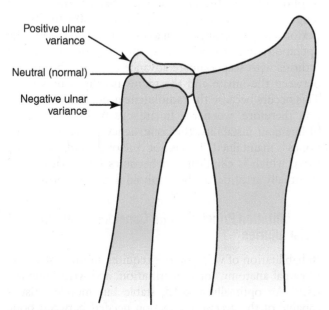

Figure 10-83 Differences in ulnar variance. (Redrawn from Frykman GK, Krop WE: Fractures and traumatic conditions of the wrist. In Hunter JM, Mackin EJ, Callahan AD, editors: *Rehabilitation of the hand: surgery and therapy*, ed 4, p 325, St Louis, 1995, Mosby.)

Positive ulnar variance

Neutral (normal)

Negative ulnar variance

TABLE 10-18

Normal Wrist Kinematics and Motion

Physiological Motion	Carpal Movement
Wrist flexion	The proximal carpal row shifts dorsally in relation to the radius
Wrist extension	The proximal carpal row shifts volarly in relation to the radius
Ulnar deviation	The proximal carpal row extends and shifts radially
Radial deviation	The proximal carpal row flexes and shifts ulnarly

TABLE 10-19

Degrees of Normal Active Range of Motion Compared with Active Motion Used in Light Activities of Daily Living (ADLs)[212,213]

Active Motion	Normal (degrees)	Light ADLs (degrees)
Wrist flexion	80	30-40
Wrist extension	70	30-40
Ulnar deviation	30	20
Radial deviation	20	20
Pronation	80-90	40-50
Supination	80-90	60

In a postoperative or postinjury therapy regimen, the clinician should consider the ultimate goals for motion and strength. Joint mobilization should focus on restoring normal kinematics.[214,215] Surgical procedures with any partial fusion of the wrist reduce motion 40% to 60%. However, most ADLs can be completed without full motion. Optimizing pain-free motion is essential. The clinician must perform a realistic evaluation of the patient's needs and expectations.

Newer philosophies for therapeutic intervention consist of an accelerated rehabilitation program. A recent study has reported that patients who underwent ORIF of a distal radius fracture, with stable fixation, had better mobility, strength, and DASH scores in the early postoperative period, after engaging in a rehabilitation protocol that emphasized early motion and strengthening.[216] Another newer philosophy is that there may be a role for wrist proprioception reeducation in the therapeutic plan for recovering wrist function and stability and preventing further injury.[217] The literature in this field is growing, and early success is promising.

Although some literature fails to support a therapist-governed exercise program as being more beneficial than a home exercise program,[218] it is clear that some patients benefit from having the motivation and supervision of a trained therapist.

In summary, the wrist is a complex structure with key specific considerations for the treating clinician. Direct communication between the surgeon and the therapist is essential. The overall rehabilitation strategy must account for the type and location of injury, possible concomitant ligament disruption, fixation methods used for fracture stabilization, overall fracture stability, and joint alignment (Figure 10-84). Table 10-20 presents rehabilitation

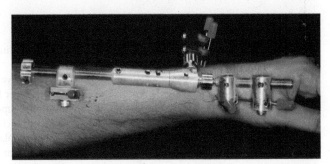

Figure 10-84 Use of an external fixator to stabilize a distal radial fracture. (From Slutsky DJ: Nonbridging external fixation of intra-articular distal radius fractures, *Hand Clin* 21:381-94, 2005.)

TABLE 10-20

Rehabilitation Guidelines for Wrist Fractures[27,219–225]

	Closed Reduction	External Fixation	ORIF with Plate and Screws	ORIF with Fixed-Angle Locking Plate
Description	• Fracture is manually reduced • Reduction is maintained in cast support for 6 weeks	• Fracture is reduced through distraction provided by external fixation in which pins are inserted into the radial shaft proximal to the fracture and distal to the fracture in the second metacarpal • Fixation is removed at 6 weeks	• Fragments require internal stabilization to hold reduction and achieve alignment • Plate and screws still allow slight motion at the fracture site • Casting is required for additional stability for 6 weeks	• Fragments require internal stabilization to hold reduction • Technique provides optimal anatomical realignment and stabilization of the fracture fragment • Procedure allows for early motion

(Continued)

TABLE **10-20**

Rehabilitation Guidelines for Wrist Fractures—cont'd

	Closed Reduction	External Fixation	ORIF with Plate and Screws	ORIF with Fixed-Angle Locking Plate
Healing Stages				
Stage I: Inflammatory stage (weeks 0 to 2)	• Casting; elbow may or may not be included in the cast • AROM of the uninvolved joints, with emphasis on the fingers and shoulder • Tendon gliding exercises • Blocking exercises to maintain flexor tendon gliding and encourage extensor tendon gliding • Edema management of the fingers with Coban • Soft tissue mobilization of the fingers	• AROM of the uninvolved joints: emphasis on the fingers and shoulder • Tendon gliding exercises • Blocking exercises to maintain flexor tendon gliding and encourage extensor tendon gliding • Edema management with Coban or a compression sleeve • Soft tissue mobilization	• Casting • AROM of the uninvolved joints; emphasis on the fingers and shoulder • Tendon gliding exercises • Blocking exercises to maintain flexor tendon gliding and encourage extensor tendon gliding • Edema management of the fingers with Coban	• Splinting between exercises and at night • AROM of the wrist and forearm (per physician guidelines) • AROM of the uninvolved joints; emphasis on the fingers and shoulder • Tendon gliding exercises to prevent adhesions • Blocking exercises to maintain flexor tendon gliding and encourage extensor tendon gliding • Scar management • Soft tissue mobilization • Edema management • Activity modification: no lifting, pulling, or pushing
Stage II: Fibroplasia and repair stage (weeks 2 to 6)	• As above • Nerve symptoms, color changes, and extreme swelling should be reported to physician because they may indicate the cast is too tight	• As above • Stretch to thumb web space • Median nerve symptoms or findings should be reported to the physician; distraction placed by the fixator may compromise the nerve	• As above • Nerve symptoms, color changes, and extreme swelling should be reported to physician because they may indicate the cast is too tight or that an infection may have developed	• As above • Stretch to thumb web space • Progress to PROM, gentle stretching at weeks 3-4 • Progress to light activities
Stage III: Remodeling and maturation stage (weeks 6 to 8+)	• Joint mobilization • Stretching • Splinting for motion • Static wrist splint for comfort during the day and support at night, worn for 2 weeks • Strengthening as tolerated at weeks 6-8 • Functional progression	• Joint mobilization • Stretching • Splinting for motion • Strengthening at weeks 8-12 as tolerated • Static wrist splint for comfort, to be worn during the day and at night as necessary • Functional progression • After removal of the fixator, structures shift slightly because the distraction from the fixator has been removed; patient's performance may be reduced as the tissues adjust	• Joint mobilization • Stretching • Splinting for motion • Strengthening at weeks 8-12 as tolerated • Static wrist splint for comfort to be worn during the day and at night as necessary • Functional progression • New onset of pain with active finger or thumb flexion and extension may be a sign of soft tissue shearing against the hardware and should be reported to the physician	• Joint mobilization • Stretching • Splinting for motion • Strengthening at weeks 8-12 as tolerated • Static resting splint usually is discontinued • Functional progression • New onset of pain with active finger or thumb flexion and extension may be a sign of soft tissue shearing against the hardware and should be reported to the physician

ORIF, Open reduction and internal fixation; *AROM,* active range of motion; *PROM,* passive range of motion.

strategies the clinician can use with patients who have suffered a wrist injury. Successful therapeutic intervention and its progression must incorporate all stages of the healing process.

Scaphoid Fractures

Rehabilitation of scaphoid fractures depends on the location and healing of the fracture. General casting guidelines for nondisplaced fractures at the distal pole is 4 to 8 weeks in a thumb spica cast. Midscaphoid (waist) fractures are immobilized longer (6 to 12 weeks). Proximal pole fractures are protected the longest (12 to 20 weeks).[152] During the casting phase, emphasis is placed on maintaining normal ROM of the fingers. After the cast is removed, the goals of therapy are joint mobilization and strengthening at the wrist and fingers.

Compression screw fixation of scaphoid fractures allows for earlier motion and return to activities. Generally, the thumb and wrist are immobilized for 1 to 4 weeks after compression screw fixation of minimally displaced fractures. After the cast has been removed, gentle motion is initiated. Weight bearing, gripping, and loading of the wrist should be avoided for the first 3 weeks. Between weeks 3 and 6, return to sports with casting or splinting is possible. Strengthening is initiated at week 8, after fracture healing allows for an increased demand. After 8 weeks, return to normal activities generally is permissible.

Displaced fractures that require ORIF are immobilized for 4 to 12 weeks, depending on the type of fixation. After the cast has been removed, active motion begins. If the scaphoid vascular supply is a concern, no weight bearing or strengthening can begin until CT scanning has confirmed fracture healing. Return to sports usually begins at 4 to 6 months.

Complications from scaphoid fractures include nonunion and malunion. Either of these causes kinematic disturbance within the wrist that can cause pain, instability, loss of motion, and eventually arthritic degeneration.[152,222,226–228]

Triangular Fibrocartilage Complex (TFCC) Injuries

Splinting in an ulnar gutter splint for stable TFCC sprains and strains to prevent ulnar deviation can be helpful for reducing inflammation and preventing repetitive stress to the region. Activity modification is essential. Activities that require ulnar deviation or forceful gripping should be avoided. Splinting during these activities prevents the incriminating wrist motions of ulnar deviation with or without terminal wrist flexion and extension. The splint often acts as a reminder to the patient to avoid the positions or activities that irritate the TFCC. Weight bearing, such as yoga or cycling, should be avoided regardless of the wrist position used. A splinting approach is used until the pain diminishes (approximately 4 to 6 weeks), at which time a strengthening to tolerance regimen can be initiated in all wrist positions. As previously mentioned, if pain persists

after a 4-week period of splinting and activity modification, the patient should return to the referring physician.

Cast immobilization in a long arm cast as an initial treatment for peripheral and central tears has been reviewed previously and is used for 4 to 6 weeks. After cast immobilization, the goal of therapeutic strategies is restoration of pain-free motion and function. Strengthening is initiated when full AROM has returned. Weight bearing is avoided for 6 to 12 weeks and should be pain free before the patient returns to aggressive weight-bearing activities. If pain limits progression of the rehabilitation course, further evaluation is required.

Debridement of the central portion of the TFCC requires little or no immobilization. The patient wears a wrist or ulnar gutter splint for 1 week when not exercising. Occasionally, the splint time is extended to respect patient comfort. AROM is initiated during the first week to pain tolerance. At 2 to 4 weeks, light functional tasks can be resumed with limited ulnar deviation and weight bearing. Strengthening and functional progression begin at 6 to 8 weeks, during which a gradual return of ulnar deviation and weight-bearing activities is initiated. If pain limits progression of the therapeutic intervention, a mechanical issue (e.g., positive ulnar variance) may be contributing to the patient's pain and TFCC irritation.

Repair of the peripheral portion of the TFCC is treated with an initial casting period of 3 to 4 weeks in a long arm cast, followed by a short arm cast for an additional 2 to 3 weeks. Casting times can vary. At 6 to 8 weeks, restoration of motion begins with the initiation of AROM. Ulnar deviation and forearm rotation are avoided. A wrist or ulnar gutter splint is worn between exercises and at night for comfort. Progression of motion, including forearm rotation and ulnar deviation, occurs between 8 and 12 weeks. Strengthening is initiated at week 12, with a gradual return to sports and weight-bearing activities as tolerated.[229,230]

Scapholunate Dissociation

As noted, surgical solutions for scapholunate dissociation include both soft tissue repairs or reconstructions and fusions. The period of cast immobilization after soft tissue repairs or reconstructions varies and can last up to 12 weeks.[210]

After cast immobilization, an AROM program is initiated, as well as scar management, edema control, and activity modification, avoiding weight bearing and gripping. At 12 weeks, gentle stretching and strengthening and functional progression are begun. A wrist splint can be worn for comfort. Taking care to avoid stretching out the repair is a prime postoperative concern. Motion limitations of approximately 30° of flexion and 50° of extension are to be expected in procedures such as the Blatt technique,[231] in which a portion of the dorsal wrist capsule is used to correct the rotation and flexion deformity of the scaphoid (Figure 10-85). Return to high-demand activities and/or competitive sports occurs at 6 to 9 months after surgery.[210,231]

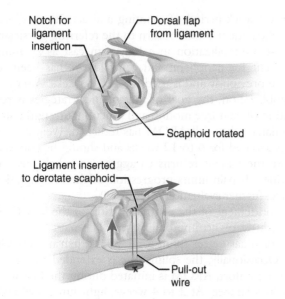

Figure 10-85 Blatt capsulodesis. (From Canale ST, Beatty JH: *Campbell's operative orthopaedics*, vol. 6, ed 12, Philadelphia, 2013, Mosby.)

The surgical fusion procedures (proximal row carpectomy, STT fusion, and four-corner fusion) follow a similar rehabilitative course (Figure 10-86). The wrist is immobilized for up to 6 to 12 weeks. After immobilization, AROM is initiated, along with scar management, edema control, and activity modification and splinting for comfort. At 12 weeks, stretching, strengthening, and functional progression begin. A reduction in motion is to be expected. Return to high-demand function and competitive sports may occur at 6 to 9 months after surgery.

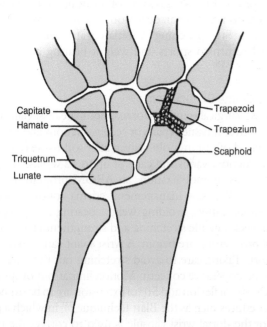

Figure 10-86 STT joint fusion with pinning and bone grafting. (From Frykman GK, Krop WE: Fractures and traumatic conditions of the wrist. In Hunter JM, Mackin EJ, Callahan AD, editors: *Rehabilitation of the hand: surgery and therapy*, ed 4, p 330, St Louis, 1995, Mosby.)

Persistent problems with scapholunate dissociation can include wrist pain despite surgical intervention to correct the instability.

TENDONITIS, TENOSYNOVITIS, AND ENTRAPMENT

Trigger Finger or Thumb (Stenosing Tenosynovitis)

General Considerations
Stenosing tenosynovitis of the digits and thumb, also known as *trigger finger* and *trigger thumb*, is a common cause of hand pain and dysfunction. The problem arises from a size disparity between the flexor tendon and the annular pulley portion of the tendon sheath through which the tendon should glide smoothly. The two types of stenosing tenosynovitis are nodular stenosing tenosynovitis and diffuse stenosing tenosynovitis. Patients present with a catching or snapping sensation (which often is quite painful) that occurs with finger or thumb motion. If this problem progresses, the affected finger or thumb may become locked in flexion and the patient may lose the ability to actively extend the digit. Treatment of this disability ranges from conservative nonoperative management to surgical release of the constrictive A1 pulley.

Anatomy
The flexor tendons are enveloped in a synovial sheath that glides through a series of pulleys, which function to keep the tendon closely apposed to the bone during bending. Damage to critical portions of the pulley system leads to bowstringing of the tendon away from the bone, which causes finger flexion contracture and loss of motion (Figure 10-87). The two types of pulleys in the flexor system are the annular pulleys and the cruciate pulleys. Two annular pulleys (A2 and A4; see Figure 10-49) cover the flexor tendons over the proximal and middle phalanges and are the most critical in preventing bowstringing. The three remaining annular pulleys (A1, A3, and A5) are closely associated with the volar plates of the MCP joint, the PIP joint, and the DIP joint, respectively. The three cruciate pulleys (C1, C2, and C3) provide additional support to the flexor tendon as it crosses the MCP, PIP, and DIP joints, but they are more flexible by design than the annular pulleys (Figure 10-88).

Pathophysiology
During finger flexion, the annular pulleys are under the greatest degree of stress from the flexor tendons. Flexion of the proximal phalanx, especially with power gripping, induces high angular loads across the most proximal pulley (the A1 pulley). Hypertrophy of the A1 pulley occurs in response to the increased stress. Microscopic examination of an A1 pulley involved in trigger digits shows degeneration, cyst formation, fiber splitting, and the

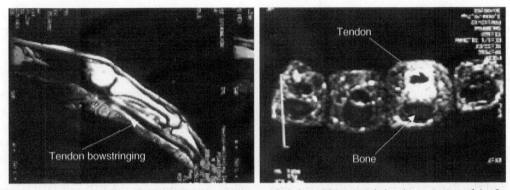

Figure 10-87 MRI scan of a closed rupture of the A2 pulley over the proximal phalanx. This injury led to bowstringing of the flexor tendon *(black structure)* away from the bone.

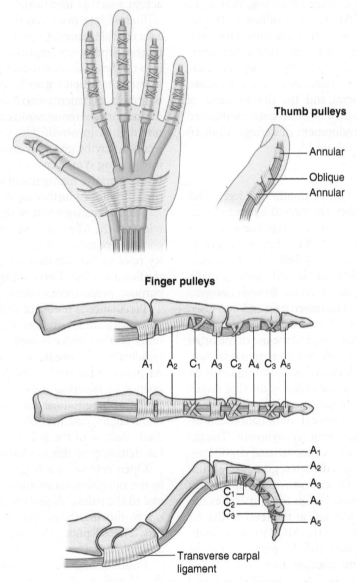

Figure 10-88 Synovial sheaths and retinacular and annular pulleys of the fingers and thumb. (Redrawn from Chase RA: *Atlas of hand surgery*, vol 2, Philadelphia, 1984, WB Saunders.)

presence of inflammatory cells. Inflammation and thickening also occur in the associated area of the flexor tendon. In nodular stenosing tenosynovitis, the thickening of the flexor tendon occurs in a localized area, just distal to the A1 pulley, where the increased friction between the pulley and tendon causes a thickened nodule to form. In diffuse stenosing tenosynovitis, the inflammation in the flexor tendon is not localized but rather extends beyond the region of the A1 pulley. No discrete nodule develops in this form of trigger finger. In both types of stenosing tenosynovitis, because of the inflammation noted in both the A1 pulley and the flexor tendon, a size disproportion develops, and the flexor tendon is no longer able to glide smoothly through the pulley. The patient experiences this as a snapping sensation when attempting to extend the affected finger. The etiology of this process is unclear, but it may be associated with repetitive activity that causes trauma to the hands. Activities that require increased finger flexor activity, such as cutting or sewing, may exert excessive stress across the A1 pulley, resulting in the inflammatory process of stenosing tenosynovitis. However, in most cases of trigger finger or thumb, no inciting activity can be identified. The majority of trigger digit cases are thought to be idiopathic in nature, but there is a known relationship between diabetes and the development of trigger digits, and there is also a more recently established association between the development of a trigger digit after a surgical carpal tunnel release.[232]

Diagnosis

Patients with a triggering finger or thumb may feel a click or snapping sensation as they attempt to extend the affected digit from a flexed position. Although the pathology of this process usually occurs at the A1 pulley, at the level of the MCP joint, the patient generally believes the mechanical problem exists at the level of the PIP joint. Initially, this triggering may not be painful. As the stenosis becomes worse, the patient may report increased pain and decreased ability to actively extend the affected digit. The digit may become locked in a flexed position, and the use of the other hand to passively extend the digit may be required to "unlock" the flexed digit. The thumb is the most frequently affected digit, followed in declining order by the ring finger, the middle finger, the small finger, and the index finger.

The medical history and physical examination can assist with the diagnosis of stenosing tenosynovitis. Trigger digits have been associated with other medical conditions, including rheumatoid arthritis, diabetes, gout, carpal tunnel syndrome, De Quervain's tenosynovitis, Dupuytren's contracture, and hypertension.[233] On the physical examination, the patient has tenderness at the level of the A1 pulley over the palmar aspect of the MCP joint. A catching sensation may be felt over the A1 pulley when the patient is asked to extend the affected digit from a flexed position. In severe cases the patient is unable to extend the digit. A tender nodule sometimes may be palpable on the flexor tendon at the level of the A1 pulley. This is as-

sociated with the nodular type of stenosing tenosynovitis. Usually the diagnosis of trigger digit can be based on the history and physical examination.

Medical Treatment

Treatment for stenosing tenosynovitis ranges from nonoperative management to splinting and cortisone injections to surgical management, including release of the A1 pulley. If a patient presents with a mild form of trigger finger or thumb, initial management may consist of splinting the MCP joint of the involved digit. The splint should allow free motion at the PIP and DIP joints.[234] Splinting has been successful, mostly in the four fingers, excluding the thumb, and in fingers that have mild triggering. However, the patient may need to spend up to 4 months in the splint. Because of this, patients may be less compliant with this treatment regimen. This method is an alternative for patients with mild disease who are hesitant to accept a steroid injection.

Steroid injections into the flexor tendon sheaths can be a successful treatment option for some patients with trigger fingers. Studies have reported that corticosteroid injections into the flexor tendon sheath tend to be more successful in women, in patients who have had symptoms for less than 6 months, in patients who have the nodular rather than the diffuse form of tenosynovitis, and in patients in whom only one digit is involved.[235,236] Usually two corticosteroid injections may be given for an attempt at successful therapy; if triggering symptoms continue or recur after three injections, operative management should be considered because the efficiency of further injections seems to decrease.[235]

Surgical management of stenosing tenosynovitis involves release of the A1 pulley, resulting in the return of the smooth gliding mechanism of the flexor tendon. Opening the pulley resolves the size disproportion between the pulley and the flexor tendon. Two different techniques are used for this purpose: percutaneous release and open release.

Percutaneous release of a trigger digit can be done in the office with administration of a local anesthetic. A needle or other cutting device is used to transect the A1 pulley longitudinally. The needle is placed through the skin into the A1 pulley at the level of the metacarpal head. The pulley is opened by sweeping the needle or cutting device back and forth in a longitudinal direction. After the cutting utensil is removed, the patient is asked to flex and extend the affected digit. Release of the pulley is confirmed when the patient can demonstrate this motion without any triggering.

Open release of a trigger digit typically is performed in the operating room and involves a skin incision proximal to the palmar digital crease. Blunt dissection is carried out by moving the neurovascular structures out of harm's way. The A1 pulley then is longitudinally transected with a scalpel or scissor tips under direct visualization.

Possible complications associated with surgical release of the A1 pulley include injury to the closely associated digital nerves. These nerves travel parallel to the flexor tendon on either side of the A1 pulley in the fingers. In the thumb, however, the radial digital nerve crosses from the ulnar to the radial side of the digit at the level of the palmar digital crease, just proximal to the A1 pulley. The proximity of these digital nerves to the A1 pulley, especially in the thumb, puts the nerves at risk during pulley transection. Inadvertent release of the A2 pulley, resulting in bowstringing of the flexor tendon, has been reported with both open and percutaneous techniques.[237] Incomplete release of the A1 pulley and injury to the underlying flexor tendon can occur and seem to be more prevalent with the percutaneous technique.[238]

For the most part, surgical management of this problem results in successful resolution of symptoms, and the chance of recurrence is low.

De Quervain's Disease

General Considerations

De Quervain's disease is a stenosing tenosynovitis of the first dorsal compartment in the wrist. It causes pain over the radial aspect of the wrist that worsens with thumb motion as well as wrist radial and ulnar deviation.

Anatomy

Extension of the wrist, fingers, and thumb is controlled by a group of muscles that originate in the proximal half of the forearm. The tendons of these muscles course over the dorsal aspect of the wrist and hand before inserting on their target of motion. As these tendons approach the wrist, their outer covering forms a synovial sheath, which provides lubrication for the tendons as they glide back and forth. As the extensor tendons cross the dorsal aspect of the wrist, they are covered by the extensor retinaculum, a ligamentous structure that prevents bowstringing of the extensor tendons, allowing the tendons to stay closely approximated to the bones despite changes in wrist position.

The extensor retinaculum also organizes the tendons into six distinct anatomical compartments. The first compartment lies over the radial aspect of the wrist and contains the multiple slips of the APL and EPB tendons, both of which control thumb motion (Figure 10-89). The APL inserts on the dorsal base of the thumb metacarpal. The EPB inserts at the proximal dorsal aspect of the first phalanx of the thumb. Pathology of these tendons is the cause of de Quervain's tenosynovitis. The second dorsal compartment contains the ECRL and extensor carpi radialis brevis (ECRB) tendons, which provide wrist extension and radial deviation of the hand. The third compartment contains the EPL tendon, which extends the distal joint of the thumb. This tendon travels ulnar to Lister's tubercle and can be ruptured in distal radial fractures, particularly those that are nondisplaced. The fourth compartment contains the EDC and extensor indicis proprius (EIP) tendons, which control finger extension. The fifth compartment contains the extensor digiti minimi tendon, which extends the small finger, in combination with EDC to the small finger. The sixth compartment contains the ECU tendon, which extends and ulnarly deviates the wrist and hand.

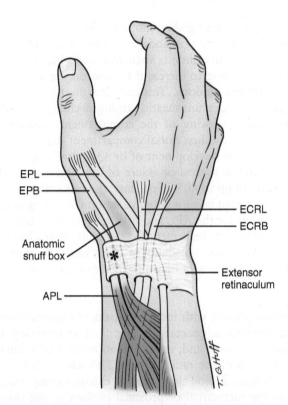

Figure 10-89 De Quervain's disease. Tenosynovitis (*) of tendons of abductor pollicis longus (APL) and extensor pollicis brevis (EPB). *ECRB*, extensor carpi radialis brevis; *ECRL*, extensor carpi radialis longus; *EPL*, extensor pollicis longus.

Also relevant to the anatomy of the dorsal wrist is the presence of the radial artery and branches of the radial sensory nerve that travel close to the first dorsal compartment. The radial artery travels from the volar to the dorsal wrist through the anatomical snuffbox. The tendons of the first dorsal compartment (APL and EPB) form the volar border of this space, and the EPL tendon forms its dorsal portion. The radial artery lies deep to these tendons as it moves to pass between the heads of the first dorsal interosseous muscle on its way to become the deep palmar arch. Branches of the radial sensory nerve lie superficial to the first dorsal compartment, providing sensation in this region. Just volar to the first dorsal compartment tendons, in the subcutaneous layer reside the terminal branches of the lateral antebrachial cutaneous nerve. Either nerve can easily be injured in the surgical approach to release the first extensor compartment, resulting in a painful neuroma.

Pathophysiology

Normally, the extensor tendons glide smoothly through the fibro-osseous compartments of the extensor retinaculum with finger and thumb motion. De Quervain's disease is a stenosing tenosynovitis that occurs because of a thickening of the tendons in the first dorsal compartment and a narrowing of the compartment itself. This disproportion in size between the tendon and the canal results in the loss of the smooth gliding motion, which leads to significant pain with any wrist and thumb movement. The cause may be repetitive thumb abduction and ulnar deviation motions, leading to increased tension on the first dorsal compartment tendons. This increases the friction at the extensor retinaculum sheath, causing swelling of the tendons and narrowing of the compartment. Anatomical variations of the first dorsal compartment may also contribute to the development of de Quervain's disease, as well as to the success or failure of the treatment of this disorder. In up to 80% of patients, the first compartment may be divided by a longitudinal septum, resulting in separate canals for the APL and EPB tendons.[239,240] Separate canals may even be present for the multiple tendon slips of the APL. The possibility of these variations must be recognized because it may influence management.

Diagnosis

Patients present with increasing pain of insidious onset. The tenderness generally is described as involving the thumb and wrist and, on examination, may be localized to the area of the radial styloid. This pain radiates in a longitudinal fashion along the first extensor compartment from the metacarpal or proximal phalanx of the thumb onto the distal third of the forearm. Aching usually accompanies thumb motions, as well as grasping with the thumb and ulnar deviation of the wrist.

Examination of a patient with de Quervain's disease may demonstrate tenderness with palpation at the radial styloid and pain with active or passive stretching of the APL and EPB tendons. Finkelstein's test is pathognomonic for the diagnosis of de Quervain's tenosynovitis. This test is performed by passively adducting the patient's thumb into the palm of the patient's hand and then providing an ulnar deviation force to the wrist. Replication of the patient's pain with this action is a positive **Finkelstein's sign** and leads to the diagnosis of de Quervain's disease (Figure 10-90). The clinician must take care to rule out arthrosis of the thumb as the primary source of pain because this condition can easily mimic or even coexist with de Quervain's tenosynovitis.

Medical Treatment

The management of de Quervain's stenosing tenosynovitis ranges from immobilization to steroid injection therapy to an operative procedure. Immobilization in a cast or a splint may be attempted for a patient who is hesitant about having an injection or undergoing an operative procedure. This may alleviate symptoms for a short period, but pain tends to recur after the cast is removed. Overall, the failure rate for immobilization alone is 70%.[241]

A corticosteroid injection is a useful treatment option for patients with de Quervain's tenosynovitis. An injection is given into the two separate tendon sheaths of the first dorsal compartment, which is located approximately 1 cm (0.4 inch) proximal to the radial styloid. It is important to recognize that subdivisions may be present in the first dorsal compartment; therefore some of the injection solution should be redirected in a more dorsal direction to permeate a separate EPB sheath. The success rate for alleviating de Quervain's disease with corticosteroid injections can be as high as 80% after two injections.[239]

If nonoperative management has been unsuccessful for a patient with de Quervain's tenosynovitis, a surgical procedure may be necessary to release the stenotic fibro-osseous canal and restore smooth gliding of the tendons through the first dorsal compartment. The procedure involves incising the extensor retinaculum that covers the first dorsal compartment, and allowing decompression of the residing tendons. It is important to visualize the compartment fully and to incise any septa that may be subdividing the compartment. Each tendon slip should be identified and proven to glide smoothly before the procedure is completed. Some surgeons elect to widen and repair the extensor retinaculum, whereas others simply leave the compartment open after the release. A tenosynovectomy of the tendons can be performed at the time of surgery.

Complications

Both the operative and nonoperative management of de Quervain's disease can have complications. Corticosteroid injections have been associated with depigmentation in the area of the injection, fat necrosis, and subcutaneous

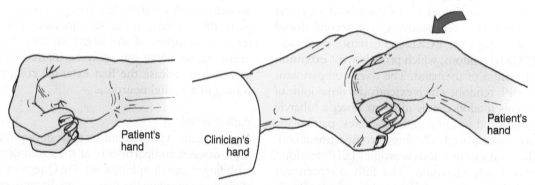

Figure 10-90 The Finkelstein maneuver is performed by placing the patient's thumb inside the palm and then gently deviating the wrist ulnarly. This maneuver causes severe discomfort in a patient with de Quervain's tenosynovitis. (From Magee DJ: *Orthopedic physical assessment*, ed 6, p 472, St. Louis, 2014, Saunders/Elsevier.)

atrophy. Also, the risk of infection or nerve injury, although remote, is still present.

Operative treatment for de Quervain's disease risks injury to the lateral antebrachial cutaneous or superficial sensory branch of the radial nerve because they both lie close to the tendons and can easily be injured in the surgical approach. If these branches are not identified and preserved, injury may result in a painful neuroma. Incomplete release of the first dorsal compartment leads to ongoing painful symptoms. Incomplete release most often results from failure to recognize a septum separating the APL and EPB tendons into different compartments or multiple compartments for the slips of the APL tendons. Failure to release this separate subsheath has been associated with persistent pain and unfavorable outcomes.[242] Persistent pain also may be the result of a secondary diagnosis (e.g., arthritis of the CMC joints) that was overlooked during the patient's workup. A more major complication of surgical release of the first compartment without its repair is the painful volar subluxation of the tendons from their usual position with wrist and thumb motion. This causes a painful snapping of the tendons as they slip volarly away from the radius. This generally requires reconstruction of a retinacular sling for tendon stabilization.

Carpal Tunnel Syndrome

General Considerations

According to Kerwin et al., carpal tunnel syndrome is the most frequently encountered peripheral compressive neuropathy.[243] Because of the frequency of this condition in the United States, approximately **500,000** operations to decompress the median nerve are performed each year.[244]

To understand carpal tunnel syndrome, it is necessary to appreciate the response of a peripheral nerve to injury, specifically the effect of compression and ischemia. Then the clinical manifestations that enable diagnosis and treatment will become clear.

Peripheral Nerves. Peripheral nerves consist of cell bodies that project axons to the extremities. The cell body resides in the anterior horn of the spinal cord for motor neurons and in the dorsal root ganglion for sensory neurons. Axons are surrounded by an outer layer, called *myelin,* which is produced by Schwann cells. Together, the axon and the surrounding Schwann cells constitute what is commonly referred to as a nerve.

The myelin sheath produced by the Schwann cells functions as insulation so that the axons can more efficiently transmit electrical impulses, a phenomenon known as *saltatory conduction*. These nerve fibers transfer sensory information from the periphery to the cell body in the dorsal root ganglion (i.e., afferent conduction). They also conduct motor orders from the brain and spinal cord to the extremities to dictate muscle function (i.e., efferent conduction).

Microscopically, the smallest unit of the nerve is a fiber called a *fascicle*. These fibers are often bundled together in groups that are surrounded by a strong connective tissue layer called the *perineurium*. Groups of fascicles, each bundled within its perineurial sleeve, travel together within a loose connective tissue known as the *internal epineurium*. This material is believed to function as a mechanical insulator to shock and pressure, and different nerves have various amounts of internal epineurium. The groups of fascicles lying in the internal epineurium are ultimately surrounded by the external epineurium, which defines the periphery of the nerve (Figure 10-91).

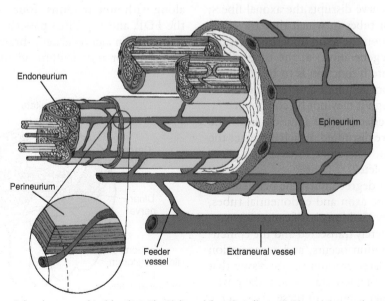

Figure 10-91 Cross section of a peripheral nerve and its blood supply. (Adapted from Lundborg G: Nerve injury and repair, Edinburgh, 1988, Churchill Livingstone. In Magee DJ, Zachazewski JE, Quillen WS, editors: *Scientific foundations and principles of practice in musculoskeletal rehabilitation*, p 178, St Louis, 2007, Saunders.)

The blood supply to the peripheral nerves runs from superficial epineurium to the deep endoneurial layer. A plexus of vessels runs longitudinally with the nerve at the level of the epineurium. These vessels send perforating arterioles into the perineurium. At the level of the endoneurium is a thin capillary network that is supplied by the vessels of the perineurial matrix. For the median nerve, the blood supply arises from branches from the radial and ulnar arteries. Nutrient vessels from these two major arteries accompany the median nerve through the carpal tunnel.

Peripheral nerves are subjected to different types of injury mechanisms, including compression, ischemia, stretching, chemical injury, and complete transection. Injuries to peripheral nerves are commonly classified by one of two systems. The simpler system, devised by Seddon,[245] describes three levels of nerve injury: the neuropraxia, the axonotmesis, and the neurotmesis. Sunderland[246] subsequently devised a more complex classification that describes injuries in terms of degrees, ranging from first degree (least severe) to fifth degree (most severe). Sunderland's system, although more involved to learn, appears to correlate better with clinical and pathological findings.

A first-degree Sunderland injury (classified as a neuropraxia by Seddon) is localized damage to the myelin sheath without injury to the axon. In this situation, the electrical impulses carrying the sensory and motor information are temporarily interrupted, but the nerve fiber architecture remains intact. This is a reversible injury, with full recovery of nerve function anticipated within 3 months. Most patients with carpal tunnel syndrome fall into this category.

A second-degree Sunderland injury (Seddon classification: axonotmesis) involves injury to the axon. Traction or a severe crush to the nerve disrupts the axonal fibers; however, the endoneurial tubes in which they travel remain intact. In this situation the axon undergoes degeneration (i.e., wallerian degeneration) at the time of the injury and must regenerate if function is to be regained. Surgical intervention is not required and return of function is anticipated, although it may not be complete.

In third-degree Sunderland nerve injuries, both the axon and endoneurium are disrupted, which increases the difficulty of regeneration. Therefore recovery of nerve function usually is incomplete.

In a Sunderland fourth-degree injury, the perineurium is disrupted along with the axon and endoneurial tubes, and in a fifth-degree injury (Seddon classification: neurotmesis), the nerve is completely transected and the epineurium is cleaved. Degeneration occurs, and regeneration is limited because of the large amount of scar tissue that forms and, in the case of complete transection, the physical separation of the cut nerve ends. In these cases, nerve damage is irreversible and surgical nerve repair is necessary to regain function.

Compression Injury. Carpal tunnel syndrome is a chronic compressive injury to the median nerve caused by increased pressure within the carpal canal at the wrist. Compression causes mechanical deformation of the nerve. Chronically this pressure compromises the neural blood flow, resulting in nerve ischemia. This creates an inflammatory response within the nerve. The connective tissue of the endoneurium and perineurium becomes edematous and eventually fibrotic. Demyelination occurs, resulting in less efficient signal conduction and compromised nerve function. If compression continues, axonal degeneration can occur. This manifests itself clinically on a continuum, depending on the degree of nerve damage. Initially a patient may complain of pain and sensory disturbances ranging from intermittent paresthesia to constant numbness. With progression of the compression, the patient loses the ability of two-point discrimination. Symptoms of motor disturbance may begin as pain and progress to muscle atrophy as more diffuse nerve damage occurs.

Anatomy

The carpal tunnel (Figure 10-92) is a relatively rigid structure, open ended at both the proximal and distal margins, which allows structures to pass through it from the forearm to the hand. The carpal bones border the tunnel on the dorsal, radial, and ulnar sides. The ulnar border consists of the hook of the hamate, triquetrum, and pisiform. The scaphoid and trapezium make up the radial border. The volar surface or roof of the tunnel is the flexor retinaculum, which extends from the distal radius to the metacarpal bases. The flexor retinaculum is made up of three structures: the deep forearm fascia, the transverse carpal ligament, and the aponeurosis between the thenar and hypothenar muscles. The median nerve, along with nine tendons (four from the FDS, four from the FDP, and the FPL) pass through the carpal tunnel. The median nerve usually branches at the distal edge of the flexor retinaculum, giving rise to the recurrent

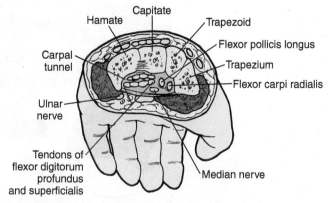

Figure 10-92 Cross section of the wrist showing the carpal tunnel. (From Magee DJ: *Orthopedic physical assessment*, ed 6, p 447, St. Louis, 2014, Saunders/Elsevier.)

motor branch, which supplies the APB muscle and the digital nerves to the radial three and one-half fingers. Variability in the anatomy of both the median nerve and the branch point of the recurrent motor nerve are common and must be considered during surgical treatment of carpal tunnel syndrome. In most cases the recurrent motor nerve branches distal to the distal edge of the flexor retinaculum (extraligamentous), putting it at low risk during carpal tunnel releases.

Etiology

Several possible reasons can account for the development of increased pressure within the carpal tunnel.

Conditions that alter fluid balance in the body may cause increased edema and pressure within the carpal tunnel, resulting in compression of the median nerve. Pregnancy, hypothyroidism, renal disease, and hemodialysis all have been associated with the onset of symptoms. Inflammatory conditions, such as rheumatoid arthritis, lupus, and infection, may also cause increased pressure within the carpal tunnel. Traumatic injuries such as distal radial fractures or carpal dislocations can directly injure the nerve and lead to increased pressure in the carpal tunnel. Space-occupying lesions, arthritic spurs, or ganglions also can compress the median nerve at the wrist.

Neuropathic factors, such as diabetes, alcoholism, or nutritional deficiency, may affect the median nerve directly without ever altering the fluid pressure within the carpal canal. It is imperative that, during the workup, the clinician differentiate these intrinsic nerve processes from extrinsic pressure that is compromising median nerve function.

Despite this list of multiple etiologies, which is far from complete, most cases of carpal tunnel syndrome are idiopathic. Patients with this type of carpal tunnel syndrome usually are women between the ages of 40 and 60, and in half of the cases, the carpal tunnel syndrome is bilateral.[247] Currently, the cause of the nerve compression in this situation is unclear. It may be associated with hormonal factors, changes in the tenosynovium in a person with an anatomically small tunnel, or vascular sclerosis. A well-established myth exists that carpal tunnel syndrome is directly correlated to the workplace environment and is associated with repetitive motion, typing, and work activities. There is little scientific evidence to support this popular belief.[248]

Determining the etiology of the carpal tunnel syndrome is important because the etiology influences the treatment options. If carpal tunnel syndrome results from an underlying disorder, resolution of the condition sometimes can alleviate the median nerve dysfunction. For example, if carpal tunnel syndrome results from the fluid shifts induced by pregnancy, operative treatment usually can be avoided. Delivery of the child frequently resolves the compression quite quickly; therefore steps to alleviate symptoms during the pregnancy may be all that is required.

Diagnosis

The diagnosis of carpal tunnel syndrome is made primarily on the patient's experience of symptoms. However, a number of physical examination findings, if positive, can help confirm the diagnosis.

A patient usually presents with a complaint of pain and/or paresthesia along the median nerve sensory distribution in the hand. This encompasses the palmar aspect of the thumb, index finger, middle finger, and the radial border of the ring finger. Symptoms increase insidiously over time from activity-related paresthesia and pain to constant, unrelenting numbness. Patients complain that these usually are worse at night, and this is believed to be related to the flexed position of the wrists during sleep, resulting in narrowing of the carpal tunnel and increased pressure on the median nerve.[249] Patients report worsening of symptoms during activities that cause prolonged wrist flexion or wrist extension, such as driving and talking on the telephone. If compression continues, weakness and atrophy of the thenar muscles may develop, resulting in loss of dexterity, difficulty grasping and holding objects, and an overall compromise in hand function.

The patient's history is critical in making the diagnosis. Provocative clinical tests, such as **Durkan's carpal compression test** (compression directly over the carpal tunnel), **Phalen's wrist flexion test** (wrist flexion for 60 seconds), and **Tinel's nerve percussion test** (tapping along the course of the median nerve), attempt to reproduce symptoms in the median nerve. Reproduction of the pain, numbness, or tingling is considered a positive finding and supports the diagnosis of carpal tunnel syndrome. However, if the tests are negative, this does not rule out the condition. Threshold sensory tests using Semmes-Weinstein monofilaments can elucidate the degree of sensibility the patient has lost secondary to nerve compression.

Electrodiagnostic tests (e.g., nerve conduction) and electromyographic studies provide objective evidence of impaired nerve conduction and intrinsic muscle function, which can be useful adjuncts to the clinical examination. These tests establish nerve conduction velocity, latency, and intrinsic muscle activity. They are helpful in isolating the location of a nerve lesion or injury and the degree of conduction block. This is important in cases in which the compression of the median nerve occurs at a level more proximal than the carpal canal.

Medical Treatment

Treatment options for carpal tunnel syndrome are varied, ranging from noninvasive splinting and cortisone injections to operative release of the transverse carpal ligament either by open or endoscopic techniques. Initially, attempts at nonoperative management are emphasized. The use of splints to maintain the wrist in a neutral position, which reduces the pressure in the carpal canal, is a standard option for patients with low-grade symptoms. The patient may wear the splint at night while asleep or during activities that provoke symptoms.

If wrist splints are unsuccessful, a steroid injection into the carpal tunnel is another treatment option. This reduces the inflammation in the carpal tunnel, creating more space for the median nerve. In a select group of patients this results in complete alleviation of symptoms; however, 50% to 70% of patients have a return of their symptoms months after the injection. Care must be taken during the procedure to avoid needle injury or, even worse, injection into the nerve, which has long-term negative effects.

Surgical management of carpal tunnel syndrome is useful for patients who have thenar muscle weakness, who have failed nonoperative therapy, or who have numbness and tingling that is constant and no longer intermittent. Operative management consists of opening the roof of the carpal tunnel by incising the flexor retinaculum. This allows the carpal canal to increase its volume, relieving the pressure on the median nerve. Currently, two major surgical options are available. The first is the open release procedure, and the second is the endoscopic release procedure. Both accomplish the same goal, incising the transverse retinacular ligament to release the carpal tunnel.

The open carpal tunnel release begins with a vertical skin incision at the proximal aspect of the palm. Dissection continues through the subcutaneous tissue and the palmar fascia, ultimately leading to transection of the transverse carpal ligament. Care must be taken to preserve all cutaneous nerve branches and to visualize and preserve any branches of the median nerve, specifically the recurrent motor branch, which innervates the thenar muscles. Possible postoperative problems associated with open carpal tunnel release are scar tenderness and pillar pain. **Pillar pain**, which is discomfort that extends along the thenar and hypothenar borders of the hand, may be related to the release of the thenar-hypothenar fascia, which is necessary to reach the transverse carpal ligament through the open approach. If this develops, pillar pain typically resolves by 3 months.

With endoscopic carpal tunnel release, the palmar incision and dissection are avoided. Instead, an endoscope and cutting instrument are placed into the carpal canal and used to visualize and transect the transverse carpal ligament from its undersurface (Figure 10-93). During this procedure, care must be taken to avoid injury to the recurrent motor branch of the median nerve because this nerve occasionally has an anomalous course. The procedure is technically demanding and, in the hands of

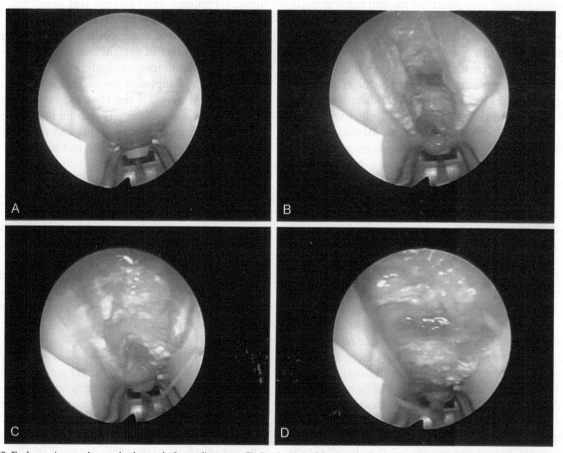

Figure 10-93 Endoscopic carpal tunnel release. **A,** Intact ligament. **B,** Partly incised ligament. **C** and **D,** Ligament is completely divided and "pops" widely apart. The overlying normal muscle and fascia are left intact.

an inexperienced surgeon, poses risks to neurovascular and tendinous structures.[250] Some studies have reported that postoperatively, patients have fewer complaints of discomfort, and they return to work sooner than with the open procedure.[251] Although outcomes at 3 months for both procedures are the same.

Each technique has its advocates. However, the final result with either procedure, the transection of the transverse carpal ligament, releases the pressure within the canal and alleviates the patient's symptoms of pain and paresthesia. A recent study has reported that 88% of patients were satisfied with their outcomes of open carpal tunnel release at a minimum of 10 years.[252]

Rehabilitation Principles and Considerations for Tendonitis, Tenosynovitis, and Entrapment

Trigger Finger

Rehabilitation for trigger digit begins after the involved digit is splinted in extension and if the patient experiences pain or stiffness, or both. It is important that the splint allow free motion at the PIP and DIP joints, with a hooked flexed position and full extension (Figure 10-94). Flexion of the IP joint with the MCP joint extended allows the flexor tendon to glide without stressing the A1 pulley. Splinting in extension prevents PIP flexion contractures and assists maximal glide of the flexor tendons.[234] The splint should be hand based and can be limited to the involved digit. A recent study published in the *Journal of Hand Therapy* demonstrated an 87% success rate with the use of a trigger splint.[253] Although there were limitations to this study, this treatment option may be beneficial to some patients.

Postoperative referral for therapy is indicated if pain, diminished AROM, scar adhesion, and tissue tightness persist. After inflammation has diminished, night extension splinting is implemented to aid in prolonged stretching of the flexors, if shortening has occurred. Emphasis is placed on differential flexor tendon gliding with blocking

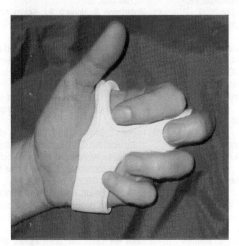

Figure 10-94 Anterior (volar) based trigger finger splint. The MCP is supported in extension, allowing PIP and DIP flexion. An alternative dorsal splint can be made, depending on the patient's preference.

exercises. Edema and scar management, to improve gliding of the soft tissues, is often necessary. Strengthening and prolonged grasp activities are avoided until full healing and the return of pain-free motion have been achieved.

De Quervain's Disease

In the early treatment of de Quervain's disease, intervention through immobilization may be initiated in the acute inflammatory cycle. In this case a thumb spica splint with the IP joint free reduces stress to the tendons by resting the tissues. Soft tissue mobilization may help reduce inflammation and tissue guarding. Extensive patient education is essential to protect the tissues from overuse. Splinting can be attempted for 4 to 6 weeks. Once the patient has reduced pain from splinting, education for positioning of the thumb and wrist during ADLs is important to avoid further recurrence of the pain.

There is some evidence that modalities such as iontophoresis, noxious level stimulation, and transverse friction massage may be useful in treating tendinopathies such as de Quervain's tenosynovitis. These may help to alleviate pain and allow the treating clinician to progress patients to eccentric exercises and strengthening protocols.[254]

Patients should be advised to modify activities after a corticosteroid injection for 1 to 2 weeks. These patients may also benefit from wearing a thumb spica splint for 1 to 2 weeks after the injection.

Postoperatively, emphasis should be placed on differential tendon gliding, edema and scar management, and modalities to improve soft tissue glide. Desensitization for nerve irritability is often also needed. Strengthening and prolonged pinching are avoided until healing is complete and the patient is pain free.

Carpal Tunnel Syndrome

Nonsurgical intervention for carpal tunnel syndrome consists of splinting the wrist in a neutral position, tendon and nerve gliding exercises, and extensive patient education, including activity and work site modification and positions to avoid to prevent irritation of the median nerve. Splints are worn at night to prevent the wrist from resting in flexion and/or extension.[249] Splinting may also be recommended for day use if the symptoms are not improving. Patients may benefit from wearing a splint for 1 to 2 weeks after a corticosteroid injection.

Postoperative referral to therapy is indicated if pain, hypersensitivity, AROM deficits, and reduced soft tissue mobilization, including scar tissue, persist. Emphasis is placed on scar management, differential tendon gliding exercises, and modalities (ultrasound) to improve the soft tissue mobility and function. Acetic acid iontophoresis is a treatment modality that may be beneficial for helping patients recover function that is lost secondary to impairment caused by recalcitrant scar tissue.[255] Desensitization is included if nerve irritability is present. Activity modification (e.g., avoiding prolonged grasping) is indicated if inflammation is present.

REFERENCES

1. Emmet E, Breck LW: A review of analysis of 11,000 fractures seen in a private practice of orthopaedic surgery, 1937-1956, *J Bone Joint Surg Am* 40:1169–1175, 1958.
2. Meals C, Meals R: Hand Fractures: a review of current treatment strategies, *J Hand Surg* 38A:1021–1031, 2013.
3. Strickland JW, Steichen JB, Kleinman WB: Phalangeal fractures: factors influencing digital performance, *Orthop Rev* 11:39–50, 1982.
4. Coonrad RW, Pohlman MH: Impacted fractures of the proximal phalanx, *J Bone Joint Surg Am* 51:1291–1296, 1969.
5. Schneider LH: Fractures of the distal phalanx, *Hand Clin* 4:537–547, 1988.
6. Kilbourne BC: Management of complicated hand fractures, *Surg Clin North Am* 8:201–213, 1968.
7. Lamphier TA: Improper reduction of fractures of the proximal phalanges of fingers, *Am J Surg* 94:926–930, 1957.
8. Buehler U, Gupta A, Ruf S: Corrective osteotomy for post-traumatic malunion of the phalanges in the hand, *J Hand Surg Br* 21:33–42, 1996.
9. Green DP: Complications of phalangeal and metacarpal fractures, *Hand Clin* 2:307–328, 1986.
10. McKibbin B: The biology of fracture healing in long bones, *J Bone Joint Surg Br* 60:150–162, 1978.
11. LaStayo PC, Winters KM, Hardy M: Fracture healing: bone healing, fracture management and current concepts related to the hand, *J Hand Ther* 16:81–93, 2003.
12. Herbsman H, Powers JC, Hirschman A, Shaftan GW: Retardation of fracture healing in experimental diabetes, *J Surg Res* 8:424–431, 1968.
13. Hogevold HE, Grogaard B, Reikeras O: Effects of short-term treatment with corticosteroids and indomethacin on bone healing: a mechanical study of osteotomies in rats, *Acta Othop Scand* 63:607–611, 1992.
14. Krop P: Fractures: general principles of surgical management. In Hunter JM, Mackin EJ, Callahan AD, editors: *Rehabilitation of the hand: surgery and therapy*, ed 4., St Louis, 1995, Mosby.
15. Slade JF, Chou KH: Bony tissue repair, *J Hand Ther* 11:118–123, 1998.
16. Brown CW: The rate of pseudarthrosis (surgical nonunion) in patients who are smokers and patients who are non-smokers: a comparison study, *Spine* 1:942–943, 1986.
17. Liu SH, Yang RS, al-Shaikh R, Lane JM: Collagen in tendon, ligament and bone healing: a current review, *Clin Orthop Relat Res* 318:265–278, 1995.
18. Simmons D: Fracture healing perspectives, *Clin Orthop Relat Res* 200:100–110, 1985.
19. Davidson JM: Wound repair, *J Hand Ther* 11:80–93, 1998.
20. Hardy MA: The biology of scar formation, *Phys Ther* 69:1014–1024, 1989.
21. Smith KL, Dean SJ: Tissue repair of the epidermis and dermis, *J Hand Ther* 11:95–105, 1998.
22. Akeson WH, Amiel D, Mechanic GL, et al: Collagen cross-linking alterations in joint contractures: change in reducible cross-links in per articular connective tissue collagen after nine weeks of immobilization, *Connect Tissue Res* 5:15–19, 1977.
23. Booth FW: Physiologic and biochemical effects of immobilization on muscle, *Clin Orthop Relat Res* 219:15–20, 1987.
24. Cannon NM: Rehabilitation approaches for distal and middle phalanx fractures of the hand, *J Hand Ther* 16:105–116, 2003.
25. Zoot E: Understanding the perionychium, *J Hand Ther* 13:269–275, 2000.
26. Freeland AE, Hardy MA, Singletary S: Rehabilitation for proximal phalangeal fractures, *J Hand Ther* 16:129–142, 2003.
27. Harris BA, Dyrek DA: A model of orthopaedic dysfunction for clinical decision making in physical therapy practice, *Phys Ther* 69:548–553, 1989.
28. Belsky MR, Eaton RG, Lane LB: Closed reduction and internal fixation of proximal phalangeal fractures, *J Hand Surg Am* 9:725–729, 1984.
29. Chichalkar SJ, Gan BS: Management of proximal interphalangeal joint fractures and dislocations, *J Hand Ther* 16:117–128, 2003.
30. Colditz JC: Functional fracture bracing. In Hunter JM, Mackin EJ, Callahan AD, editors: *Rehabilitation of the hand: surgery and therapy*, ed 4., St Louis, 1995, Mosby.
31. Flowers K: A proposed decision hierarchy for splinting the stiff joint, with emphasis on force application parameters, *J Hand Ther* 15:158–162, 2002.
32. Flowers K, LaStayo P: Effect of total end range time on improving passive range of motion, *J Hand Ther* 7:150–157, 1994.
33. Schultz-Johnson K: Static progressive splinting, *J Hand Ther* 15:163–178, 2002.
34. Michlovitz SL, Harris BA, Watkins MP: Therapy intervention for improving joint range of motion: a systemic review, *J Hand Ther* 17:118–131, 2004.
35. Greene TL: Metacarpal fractures. In American Society for the Surgery of the Hand, editors: *Hand surgery update*, Rosemont, IL, 1996, American Academy of Orthopaedic Surgery.
36. Royle SG: Rotational deformity following metacarpal fracture, *J Hand Surg Br* 15:124–125, 1990.
37. Freeland AE, Jabaley ME, Hughes JL: *Stable fixation of the hand and wrist*, New York, 1986, Springer.
38. Opgrande JD, Westphal SA: Fractures of the hand, *Orthop Clin North Am* 14:779–792, 1983.
39. Stern P: Fractures of the metacarpals and phalanges. In Green DP, Hotchkiss RN, Pederson WC, Wolfe SW, editors: *Green's operative hand surgery*, ed 5 Philadelphia, 2005, Churchill Livingstone.
40. Hunter JM, Cowan NJ: Fifth metacarpal fractures in a compensation clinic population, *J Bone Joint Surg Am* 52:1159–1165, 1970.
41. Birndorf MS, Daley R, Greenwald DP: Metacarpal fracture angulation: decreased flexor mechanical efficiency in human hands, *Plast Reconstr Surg* 99:1079–1083, 1997.
42. Lee SG, Jupiter J: Phalangeal and metacarpal fractures of the hand, *Hand Clin* 16:323–332, 2000.
43. Flatt A: *The care of minor hand injuries*, ed 3, St Louis, 1972, Mosby.
44. Peimer CA, Smith RJ: Injuries to the metacarpal bones and joints, *Adv Surg* 2:341–374, 1977.
45. Strauch RJ, Rosenwasser MP, Lunt JG: Metacarpal shaft fractures: the effect of shortening on the extensor tendon mechanism, *J Hand Surg Am* 23:519–523, 1998.
46. Burkhalter WE: Hand fractures, *Instr Course Lect* 34:249–253, 1990.
47. Brown PW: The management of phalangeal and metacarpal fracture, *Surg Clin North Am* 53:1393–1437, 1973.
48. Workman CE: Metacarpal fractures, *Mo Med* 61:687–690, 1964.
49. Bora FWJ, Didizian NH: Treatment of injuries to the carpometacarpal joint of the little finger, *J Bone Joint Surg Am* 56:1459–1463, 1974.
50. Carlsen B, Moran S: Thumb trauma: Bennett fractures, Rolando fractures, and ulnar collateral ligament injuries, *J Hand Surg Am* 34:945–952, 2009.
51. Gedda KO, Moberg E: Open reduction and osteosynthesis of the so-called Bennett's fracture in the carpometacarpal joint of the thumb, *Acta Orthop Scand* 22:249–257, 1953.
52. Timmenga EJF, Blokhuis TJ, Maas M, Raaijmakers ELFB: Long term evaluation of Bennett's fracture: a comparison between open and closed reduction, *J Hand Surg Br* 19:373–377, 1994.
53. Thurston AJ, Dempsey SM: Bennett's fracture: a medium to long-term review, *Aust N Z J Surg* 63:120–123, 1993.
54. Cullen JP, Parentis MA, Chinchilli VM, Pellegrini VD: Simulated Bennett fracture treated with closed reduction and percutaneous pinning, *J Bone Joint Surg Am* 79:413–420, 1997.
55. Rettig AC, Ryan R, Shelbourne KD, et al: Metacarpal fractures in the athlete, *Am J Sports Med* 7:567–572, 1989.
56. McNemar TB, Howell JW, Chang E: Management of metacarpal fractures, *J Hand Ther* 16:143–151, 2003.
57. Singletary S, Freeland AE, Jarrett CA: Metacarpal fractures in athletes: treatment, rehabilitation and early return to play, *J Hand Ther* 16:171–179, 2003.
58. Sorensen JS, Freund KG, Kejla G: Functional fracture bracing in metacarpal fractures: the Galveston metacarpal brace versus a plaster of paris bandage in a prospective study, *J Hand Ther* 6:263–265, 1993.
59. Bowers WH, Hurst LC: Gamekeeper's thumb: evaluation by arthrography and stress roentgenography, *J Bone Joint Surg Am* 59:519–524, 1977.
60. Kiefhaber TR, Stern PJ, Grood ES: Lateral stability of the proximal interphalangeal joint, *J Hand Surg Am* 11:661–669, 1986.
61. Schenck RR: Dynamic traction and early passive movement for fractures of the proximal interphalangeal joint, *J Hand Surg Am* 11:850–858, 1986.
62. Salter RB, Simmonds DF, Malcolm BW, et al: The biologic effect of continuous passive motion on the healing of full thickness defects in articular cartilage, *J Bone Joint Surg Am* 62:1232–1251, 1980.
63. Eaton FG, Malerich MM: Volar plate arthroplasty of the proximal interphalangeal joint: a review of 10 years' experience, *J Hand Surg Am* 5:260–268, 1980.
64. Swanson AB, Maupin BK, Gajjar NV, Swanson GD: Flexible implant arthroplasty in the proximal interphalangeal joint of the hand, *J Hand Surg Am* 10:796–805, 1985.
65. Hintermann B, Holzach PJ, Schütz M, Matter P: Skiers thumb: the significance of bony injuries, *Am J Sports Med* 21:800–804, 1993.
66. Stener B: Displacement of the ruptured ulnar collateral ligament of the metacarpalphalangeal joint of the thumb: a clinical and anatomical study, *J Bone Joint Surg Br* 44:869–879, 1962.
67. Palmer AK, Louis DS: Assessing ulnar instability of the MCP joint of the thumb, *J Hand Surg Am* 3:542–546, 1978.
68. Heyman P, Gelberman RH, Duncan K, et al: Injuries of the ulnar collateral ligament of the thumb in MCP joint: biomechanical and prospective clinical studies on the usefulness of valgus stress testing, *Clin Orthop Relat Res* 292:165–171, 1993.
69. Rhee P, Jones DB, Kakar S: Management of thumb metacarpophalangeal ulnar collateral ligament injuries, *J Bone Joint Surg Am* 94:2005–2012, 2012.
70. Eaton RG, Littler JW: Joint injuries and their sequelae, *Clin Plast Surg* 3:85–98, 1976.
71. Bowers WH: Sprains and joint injuries in the hand, *Hand Clin* 2:93–98, 1986.

72. Dennys LJ, Hurst LN, Cox J: Management of proximal interphalangeal joint fractures using a new dynamic traction splint and early active motion, *J Hand Ther* 5:16–24, 1992.

73. Feldscher SB, Blank JE: Management of a proximal interphalangeal joint fracture dislocation with a compass proximal interphalangeal joint hinge and therapy: a case report, *J Hand Ther* 15:266–273, 2002.

74. Spinner M, Choi BY: Anterior dislocation of the proximal interphalangeal joint: cause of rupture of the central slip of the extensor mechanism, *J Bone Joint Surg Am* 52:1329–1336, 1970.

75. Manske PR, Gelberman RH, Vande Berg JS, Lesker PA: Intrinsic flexor tendon repair, *J Bone Joint Surg Am* 66:385–396, 1984.

76. Gelberman RH, Manske PR, Akeson WH, et al: Flexor tendon repair, *J Orthop Res* 4:119–128, 1986.

77. Gelberman RH, Siegel DB, Woo SL, et al: Healing of digital flexor tendons: importance of interval from injury to repair—a biomechanical, biochemical and morphological study in dogs, *J Bone Joint Surg Am* 73:66–75, 1991.

78. Boyer M: Flexor tendon injury. In Green DP, Hotchkiss RN, Pederson WC, Wolfe SW, editors: *Green's operative hand surgery*, ed 5., Philadelphia, 2005, Churchill Livingstone.

79. Gelberman RH, Boyer MI, Brodt MD, et al: The effect of gap formation at the repair site on the strength and excursion of intrasynovial flexor tendons, *J Bone Joint Surg Am* 81:975–982, 1999.

80. Manske PR, Lesker PA: Avulsion of the ring finger digitorum profundus tendon: an experimental study, *Hand* 10:52–55, 1978.

81. Leddy JP: Avulsion of the flexor digitorum profundus, *Hand Clin* 1:77–83, 1985.

82. Scott S: Closed injuries to the extension mechanism of the digits, *Hand Clin* 16:367–373, 2000.

83. Blair WF, Steyers CM: Extensor tendon injuries, *Orthop Clin North Am* 23:141–148, 1992.

84. Newport ML: Extensor tendon injuries in the hand, *J Am Acad Orthop Surg* 5:59–66, 1997.

85. Lovett WL, McCalla MA: Management and rehabilitation of extensor tendon injuries, *Orthop Clin North Am* 14:819–826, 1983.

86. Gelberman RH, Botte MJ, Spiegelman JH, Akeson WH: The excursion and deformation of repaired flexor tendons treated with protected early motion, *J Hand Surg Am* 11:106–110, 1986.

87. Strickland WJ, Glogoval SV: Digital function following flexor tendon repair in zone II: a comparison of immobilization and controlled passive motion techniques, *J Hand Surg* 5:537–543, 1980.

88. Evans R: Managing the injured tendon: current concepts, *J Hand Ther* 25:173–190, 2012.

89. Strickland WJ: Biologic rationale, clinical application, and results of early motion following flexor tendon repair, *J Hand Ther* 2:71–83, 1989.

90. Pettengill KM: The evolution of early mobilization of the repaired flexor tendon, *J Hand Ther* 18:157–168, 2005.

91. Korstanje J, Soeters JN, Schreuders TA, et al: Ultrasonographic assessment of flexor tendon mobilization: effect of different protocols on tendon excursion, *J Bone Joint Surg Am* 94:394–402, 2012.

92. Tanaka T, Amadio PC, Chunfeng Z, et al: Flexor digitorum profundus tendon tension during finger manipulation: a study in human cadaver hands, *J Hand Ther* 18:330–338, 2005.

93. Boyer MI, Goldfarb CA, Gelberman RH: Recent progress in flexor tendon healing: the modulation of tendon healing with rehabilitation variables, *J Hand Ther* 18:80–85, 2005.

94. Amadio PC: Friction of the gliding surface: implications for tendon surgery and rehabilitation, *J Hand Ther* 18:112–119, 2005.

95. Thurman RT, Tremble TE, Hanel DP, et al: Two-, four-, and six-strand zone II flexor tendon repairs: an in situ biomechanical comparison using a cadaver model, *J Hand Surg Am* 23:261–265, 1998.

96. Evans RB, Thompson DE: The application of force to the healing tendon, *J Hand Ther* 6:266–284, 1993.

97. Strickland JW: The scientific basis for advances in flexor tendon surgery, *J Hand Ther* 18:94–110, 2005.

98. Chenfeng Z, Anuadio PC, Tanaka T, et al: Short term assessment of optimal timing for postoperative rehabilitation after flexor digitorum profundus tendon repair in a canine model, *J Hand Ther* 18:322–329, 2005.

99. Gelberman RH, Manske PR: Factors influencing flexor tendon adhesions, *Hand Clin* 1:35–42, 1985.

100. Horii E, Ling GT, Cooney WP, et al: Comparative flexor tendon excursion after passive mobilization: an in vitro study, *J Hand Surg* 17:559–566, 1992.

101. Groth GN: Pyramid of progressive force exercises to the injured flexor tendon, *J Hand Ther* 17:31–42, 2004.

102. Savage R: The influence of wrist position on the minimum force required for active movement of the interphalangeal joints, *J Hand Surg Br* 13:262–268, 1988.

103. Lister GD, Kleinert HE, Kutz JE, Atasoy E: Primary flexor tendon repair followed by immediate controlled mobilization, *J Hand Surg Am* 2:441–451, 1977.

104. Duran RJ, Houser RG: Controlled passive motion following tendon repair in zones I and II. In Hunter JM, Schneider LH, editors: *AAOS symposium on tendon surgery of the hand*, St Louis, 1975, Mosby.

105. Groth GN, Bechtold LL, Young VT: Early active mobilization for flexor tendons repaired using the double loop locking suture technique, *J Hand Ther* 8:206–211, 1995.

106. Gratton P: Early active mobilization after flexor tendon repair, *J Hand Ther* 6:285–289, 1993.

107. Strickland JW: Flexor tendon repair: Indiana method, *Indiana Hand Center News* 1:1–12, 1993.

108. Strickland JW: Development of flexor tendon surgery: twenty-five years of progress, *J Hand Surg* 25:214–235, 2000.

109. Groth GN: Current practice patterns of flexor tendon rehabilitation, *J Hand Ther* 19:169–174, 2005.

110. Evans RB: Zone I flexor tendon rehabilitation with limited extension and active flexion, *J Hand Ther* 18:128–140, 2005.

111. Cannon, NM: Tendon injuries. In Malick MH, Kasch MC, editors: *Manual on management of specific hand problems*, Pittsburgh, 1984, AREN Publications.

112. Athwal GS, Wolfe SW: Treatment of acute flexor tendon injury: zones III-V, *Hand Clin* 21:181–186, 2005.

113. Colditz JC: Splinting the hand with a peripheral nerve injury. In Hunter JM, Mackin EJ, Callahan AD, editors: *Rehabilitation of the hand: surgery and therapy*, St Louis, 1995, Mosby.

114. Elliot D, Southgate CM: New concepts in managing the long tendons of the thumb after primary repair, *J Hand Ther* 18:141–156, 2005.

115. Kasashima T, Kato H, Minami A: Factors influencing prognosis after direct repair of the flexor policies bogus tendon: multivariate regression modal analysis, *Hand Surg* 7:171–176, 2002.

116. Fitoussi F, Mazda K, Frajman JM, et al: Repair of the flexor policies longus tendon in children, *J Bone Joint Surg Br* 82:1177–1180, 2000.

117. Newport ML, Tucker RL: New perspectives on extensor tendon repair and implications for rehabilitation, *J Hand Ther* 18:175–181, 2005.

118. Evans RB, Burkhalter WE: A study of the dynamic anatomy of extensor tendons and implications for treatment, *J Hand Surg* 11:74–79, 1986.

119. Rosenthal LA: The extensor tendons: anatomy and management. In Hunter JM, Mackin EJ, Callahan AD, editors: *Rehabilitation of the hand: surgery and therapy*, St Louis, 1995, Mosby.

120. Chow JA, Dowelle S, Thomes LJ, et al: A comparison of results of extensor tendon repair followed by early controlled mobilization versus static immobilization, *J Hand Surg Br* 14:18–20, 1989.

121. Walsh MT, Rinehimer W, Muntzer E: Early controlled motion with dynamic splinting versus static splinting for zones III and IV extensor tendon lacerations: a preliminary report, *J Hand Ther* 7:232–236, 1994.

122. Thomes LJ, Thomes BJ: Early mobilization method for surgically repaired zone III extensor tendons, *J Hand Ther* 5:195–198, 1995.

123. Maddy LS, Meyerdierks EM: Dynamic extension assist splinting of acute central slip lacerations, *J Hand Ther* 10:206–212, 1997.

124. Evans RB, Thompson DE: An analysis of factors that support early active short arc motion of the repaired central slip, *J Hand Ther* 5:187–201, 1992.

125. Evans RB: An update on extensor tendon management. In Hunter JM, Mackin EJ, Callahan AK, editors: *Rehabilitation of the hand: surgery and therapy*, St Louis, 1995, Mosby.

126. Crosby CA, Wehbe MA: Early protected motion after extensor tendon repair, *J Hand Surg Am* 24:1061–1070, 1999.

127. Slater RR, Bynum DK: Simplified functional splinting after extensor tenorrhaphy, *J Hand Surg Am* 22:445–451, 1997.

128. Howell JW, Merritt WH, Robinson SJ: Immediate controlled active motion following zone 4-7 extensor tendon repair, *J Hand Ther* 18:182–190, 2005.

129. Meyer C, Chang J, Stern P, et al: Complications of distal radial and scaphoid fracture treatment, *J Bone Joint Surg Am* 95:1517–1526, 2013.

130. Owen RA, Melton LJ, Johnson KA, et al: Incidence of Colles' fractures in a North American community, *Am J Public Health* 72:605–607, 1952.

131. Colles A: The classic: on the fracture of the carpal extremity of the radius, *Edinburgh Med Surg J* 1814, *Clin Orthop* 83:3–5, 1972.

132. Jupiter J: Fractures of the distal end of the radius, *J Bone Joint Surg Am* 73:461–469, 1991.

133. Frykman G: Fracture of the distal radius including sequelae: shoulder-hand-finger syndrome, disturbance in the distal radioulnar joint and impairment of nerve function—a clinical and experimental study, *Acta Orthop Scand (Supp)* 108:1–153, 1967.

134. Melone CP: Articular fractures of the distal radius, *Orthop Clin North Am* 15:217–236, 1984.

135. Fernandez DL: Fracture of the distal radius: operative treatment, *Instr Course Lect* 42:73–88, 1993.

136. Skoff HD: Post fracture extensor policies longus tenosynovitis and tendon rupture: a scientific study and personal series, *Am J Orthop* 32:245–247, 2003.

137. Knirk JL, Jupiter JB: Intra-articular fractures of the distal end of the radius in young adults, *J Bone Joint Surg Am* 68:647–659, 1986.

138. Short WH, Palmer AK, Werner FW, Murphy DJ: A biomechanical study of distal radius fractures, *J Hand Surg Am* 12:529–534, 1987.

139. Palmer AK, Werner FW: Biomechanics of the distal radioulnar joint, *Clin Orthop* 187:26–35, 1984.

140. Taleisnik J, Watson HK: Midcarpal instability caused by malunited fractures of the distal radius, *J Hand Surg Am* 9:350–357, 1984.

141. Cooney WP, Linscheid RL, Dobyns JH: External pin fixation for unstable Colles' fractures, *J Bone Joint Surg Am* 61:840–845, 1979.

142. Vaughan PA, Lui SM, Harrington IJ, Maistrelli GL: Treatment of unstable fractures of the distal end radius by external fixation, *J Bone Joint Surg Br* 67:385–389, 1985.

143. Solgaard S: Early displacement of distal radius fractures, *Acta Orthop Scand* 57:229–231, 1986.

144. Dunn AW: Fractures and dislocation of the carpus, *Surg Clin North Am* 52:1513–1538, 1972.

145. Suh N, Ek ET, Wolfe SW: Carpal fractures, *J Hand Surg Am* 39:785–791, 2014.

146. Black DM, Watson HK, Vender MI: Scapholunate gap with scaphoid nonunions, *Clin Orthop Relat Res* 224:1987. 205-20-9.

147. Ruby LK, Stinson J, Belsky MR: The natural history of scaphoid nonunion: a review of 55 cases, *J Bone Joint Surg Am* 67:428–432, 1985.

148. Mack GR, Bosse MJ, Gelberman RH, Yu E: The natural history of scaphoid nonunion, *J Bone Joint Surg Am* 66:504–509, 1984.

149. Burgess RC: The effect of a simulated scaphoid malunion on wrist motion, *J Hand Surg Am* 12:774–776, 1987.

150. Russe O: Fracture of the carpal navicular: diagnosis, nonoperative treatment and operative treatment, *J Bone Joint Surg Am* 42:759–768, 1960.

151. Herbert TJ: *The fractured scaphoid*, St Louis, 1990, Quality Medical Publishing.

152. Gellman H, Caputo RJ, Carter V, et al: Comparison of short and long thumb spica casts for nondisplaced fractures of the carpal scaphoid, *J Bone Joint Surg Am* 71:354–357, 1989.

153. Slade JF, Moore AE: Dorsal percutaneous fixation of stable, unstable, and displaced scaphoid fractures and selected nonunions, *Atlas of Hand Clinics* 8:1–18, 2003.

154. Rettig AC, Kollias SC: Internal fixation of acute stable scaphoid fractures in the athlete, *Am J Sports Med* 24:182–186, 1996.

155. Buijze GA, Doornberg JN, Ham JS, et al: Surgical compared with conservative treatment for acute nondisplaced or minimally displaced scaphoid fractures, *J Bone Joint Surg Am* 92:1534–1544, 2010.

156. Szabo RM, Manske D: Displaced fractures of the scaphoid, *Clin Orthop Relat Res* 230:30–38, 1988.

157. Dabezies EF: Injuries to the carpus: fractures of the scaphoid, *Orthopedics* 5:1510–1515, 1982.

158. Cooney WP: Fractures of the scaphoid: a rational approach to management, *Clin Orthop Relat Res* 149:90–97, 1980.

159. Meermans G, Van Glabbeek F, Braem MJ, et al: Comparison of two percutaneous volar approaches for screw fixation of scaphoid waist fractures, *J Bone Joint Surg Am* 96:1369–1376, 2014.

160. Stark HH: Treatment of nonunited fractures of the scaphoid by iliac bone grafts and Kirschner wire fixation, *J Bone Joint Surg Am* 70:982–991, 1988.

161. Fernandez DL: A technique for anterior wedge-shaped grafts for scaphoid nonunions with carpal instability, *J Hand Surg Am* 9:733–777, 1984.

162. Cooney WP, Linscheid RL, Dobyns JH, Wood MB: Scaphoid nonunion: role of anterior interpositional bone grafts, *J Hand Surg Am* 13:635–650, 1988.

163. Zaidemberg C, Siebert JW, Angrigiani C: A new vascularized bone graft for scaphoid nonunion, *J Hand Surg Am* 16:474–478, 1991.

164. Sheetz KK, Bishop AT, Berger RA: The arterial blood supply of the distal radius and ulna and its potential use in vascularized pedicled bone grafts, *J Hand Surg Am* 20:902–914, 1995.

165. Langhoff O, Andersen IL: Consequences of late immobilization of scaphoid fractures, *J Hand Surg Br* 13:77–79, 1988.

166. Sachar K: Ulnar-sided wrist pain: Evaluation and treatment of triangular fibrocartilage complex tears, ulnocarpal impaction syndrome, lunotriquetral tears, *J Hand Surg Am* 37:1489–1500, 2012.

167. Dailey SW, Palmer AK: The role of arthroscopy in the evaluation and treatment of triangular fibrocartilage complex injuries in athletes, *Hand Clin* 16:461–476, 2000.

168. Ishii S, Palmer AK, Werner FW: An anatomical study of the ligamentous structure of the triangular fibrocartilage complex, *J Hand Surg Am* 23:977–985, 1998.

169. Bowers WH: Problems of the distal radioulnar joint, *Adv Orthop Surg* 7:289–303, 1984.

170. Bowers WH: The distal radioulnar joint. In Green D.P., editor: Operative hand surgery, vol 2, New York, 1988, Churchill Livingstone.

171. Palmer AK: The distal radioulnar joint. In Lichtman DM, editor: *The wrist and its disorders*, Philadelphia, 1988, WB Saunders.

172. Palmer AK: The distal radioulnar joint. In Talesnik J, editor: *Hand clinics: management of wrist problem*, Philadelphia, 1987, WB Saunders.

173. Palmer AK, Werner FW: Biomechanics of the distal radioulnar joint, *Clin Orthop Relat Res* 187:26–34, 1984.

174. Palmer AK, Werner FW: The triangular fibrocartilage complex of the wrist anatomy and function, *J Hand Surg* 6:153–162, 1981.

175. Werner FW, Glisson RR, Murphy DJ, Painter AK: Force transmission through the distal radioulnar carpal joint: effect of ulnar lengthening and shortening, *Handchirurgie, Mikrochirurgie, Plastische Chirureie* 18:304–308, 1986.

176. Ekenstam F, Palmer AK, Glisson RR: The load on the radius and ulna in different positions of the wrist and forearm, *Acta Ortho Scand* 55:363–365, 1984.

177. Palmer AK: Triangular fibrocartilage complex lesions: a classification, *J Hand Surg Am* 14:594–606, 1989.

178. Lipshultz T, Osternman AL: New methods in the evaluation of chronic wrist pain, *Univ Penn Orthop J* 6:37–40, 1990.

179. Skirven T: Clinical examination of the wrist, *J Hand Ther* 9:96–107, 1996.

180. Golumbi CN, Firooznin H, Melone CP, et al: Tears of the triangular fibrocartilage of the wrist: MR imaging, *Radiology* 173:731–733, 1989.

181. Skahen JR, Palmer AK, Levinsohn EM, et al: Magnetic resonance imaging of the triangular fibrocartilage complex, *J Hand Surg* 15:552–557, 1990.

182. Trumble TE, Gilbert M, Vedder N: Ulnar shortening combined with arthroscopic repairs in the delayed management of a triangular fibrocartilage complex tear, *J Hand Surg Am* 22:807–813, 1997.

183. Cooney WP, Linscheid RL, Dobyns JH: Triangular fibrocartilage tears, *J Hand Surg Am* 19:143–154, 1994.

184. Vaughan-Jackson OJ: A case of recurrent subluxation of the carpal scaphoid, *J Bone Joint Surg Br* 31:532–533, 1949.

185. Russell TB: Intercarpal dislocations and fractures-dislocations, *J Bone Joint Surg Br* 31:524–531, 1949.

186. Watson HK, Ballet FL: The SLAC wrist: scapholunate advanced pattern of degenerative arthritis, *J Hand Surg Am* 9:358–365, 1984.

187. Sebald JR, Dobyns JH, Linscheid RL: The natural history of collapse deformities of the wrist, *Clin Orthop Relat Res* 104:140–148, 1974.

188. Kitay A, Wolfe S: Scapholunate instability: current concepts in diagnosis and management, *J Hand Surg Am* 37:2175–2196, 2012.

189. Berger RA, Blair WF, Crownshield RD, Flatt AE: The scapholunate ligament, *J Hand Surg Am* 7:87–91, 1982.

190. Kozin SH: The role of arthroscopy in scapholunate instability, *Hand Clin* 15:435–444, 1999.

191. Watson HK, Ashmead D, Makhlouf MV: Examination of the scaphoid, *J Hand Surg* 5:320–327, 1980.

192. Cautilli GP, Wehbe MA: Scapholunate distance and cortical ring sign, *J Hand Surg Am* 16:501–503, 1991.

193. Levinsohn EM, Rosen ID, Palmer AK: Wrist arthrography: value of the three-compartment injection method, *Skeletal Radiol* 16:539–544, 1987.

194. Berger RA: The anatomy and bare biomechanics of the wrist joint, *J Hand Ther* 9:84–93, 1996.

195. Greenspan ID: Nociceptors and the peripheral nervous system's role in pain, *J Hand Ther* 10:78–85, 1997.

196. Manning DC: Reflex sympathetic dystrophy, sympathetically maintained pain, and complex regional pain syndrome, *J Hand Ther* 13:260–268, 2000.

197. Robinson AJ: Central nervous system pathways for pain transmission and pain control: issues relevant to the practicing clinician, *J Hand Ther* 10:64–77, 1997.

198. DePalma MT, Weiss CS: Psychological influences on pain perception and nonpharmacologic approaches to the treatment of pain, *J Hand Ther* 10:183–191, 1997.

199. Hardy MA, Hardy SG: Reflex sympathetic dystrophy: the clinician's perspective, *J Hand Ther* 10:137–150, 1997.

200. Palmer AK: The distal radioulnar joint: anatomy, biomechanics, and triangular fibrocartilage complex abnormalities, *Hand Clin* 3:31–40, 1987.

201. Veigas SF, Patterson R, Peterson P, et al: The effects of various load paths and different loads on the load transfer characteristics of the wrist, *J Hand Surg Am* 14:458–465, 1989.

202. Veigas SF, Tencer AF, Cantrell J, et al: Load transfer characteristics of the wrist. I. The normal joint, *J Hand Surg Am* 12:971–978, 1987.

203. Werner FW, Palmer AK, Fortino MD, Short WH: Force transmission through the distal ulna: effect of ulna variance, lunate fossa angulation, and radial and palmar tilt of the distal radius, *J Hand Surg Am* 17:423–428, 1992.

204. Gelberman RH, Bauman TD, Menon J, Akeson WH: The vascularity of the lunate bone and Kienbock's disease, *J Hand Surg* 5:272–278, 1980.

205. Botte MJ, Gelberman RH: Fractures of the carpus, excluding the scaphoid, *Hand Clin* 3:149–161, 1987.

206. Friedman SL, Pahner AK, Short WH, et al: The change in ulnar variance with grip, *J Hand Surg Am* 18:713–716, 1993.

207. Vincent JI, MacDermid JC, Michlovitz SL, et al: The push-off test: development of a simple, reliable test of upper extremity weight bearing capability, *J Hand Ther* 27:185–191, 2014.

208. Linscheid RL: Kinematic considerations of the wrist, *Clin Orthop Relat Res* 202:27–39, 1986.

209. Ruby LK, Cooney WP, An KN, et al: Relative motions of selected carpal bones: a kinematic analysis of the normal wrist, *J Hand Surg Am* 13:1–10, 1988.

210. Wright TW, Michlovitz SL: Management of carpal instabilities, *J Hand Ther* 9:148–156, 1990.

211. Bednar JM, Osterman AL: Carpal instability: evaluation and treatment, *J Am Acad Orthop Surg* 1:10–17, 1993.

212. Ryu JY, Cooney WP, Askew LJ, et al: Functional ranges of motion of the wrist joint, *J Hand Surg Am* 16:409–419, 1991.

213. Safee-Rad R, Shwedyk E, Quanbury AO, Cooper JE: Normal functional range of motion of upper limb joints during performance of three feeding activities, *Arch Phys Med Rehabil* 71:505–509, 1990.

214. Maitland G: *Peripheral manipulation*, London, 1980, Butterworth.

215. Myers R: *Saunders manual of physical therapy practice*, Philadelphia, 1995, WB Saunders.

216. Brehmer JL, Husband JB: Accelerated rehabilitation compared with a standard protocol after distal radial fractures treated with volar open reduction and internal fixation, *J Bone Joint Surg Am* 96:1621–1630, 2014.

217. Hagert E: Proprioception of the wrist joint: a review of current concepts and possible implications on the rehabilitation of the wrist, *J Hand Ther* 23:2–17, 2010.

218. Valdes K, Naughton N, Michlovitz S: Therapist supervised clinic based therapy versus instruction in a home program following distal radius fracture: a systematic review, *J Hand Ther* 27:165–174, 2014.

219. Raskin KB: Management of fractures of the distal radius: surgeon's perspective, *J Hand Ther* 12:92–98, 1999.

220. Fryknruin GK, Kropp WE: Fractures and traumatic conditions of the wrist. In Hunter JM, Mackin EJ, Callahan AD, editors: *Rehabilitation of the hand: surgery and therapy*, St Louis, 1995, Mosby.

221. Hurov J: Fractures of the distal radius: what are the expectations of therapy? A two year retrospective study, *J Hand Ther* 10:269–276, 1997.

222. Jabaley ME, Wegner EE: Principles of internal fixation as applied to the hand and wrist, *J Hand Ther* 16:95–104, 2003.

223. Lasseter GF, Carter PR: Management of distal radius fractures, *J Hand Ther* 9:114–128, 1996.

224. Michlovitz SL, LaStayo PC, Alzner S, Watson E: Distal radius fractures: therapy practice patterns, *J Hand Ther* 14:249–257, 2001.

225. Weinstock TB: Management of fractures of the distal radius: therapist's commentary, *J Hand Ther* 12:99–102, 1999.

226. Whipple TL: Arthroscopic management of the athlete. I. Internal fixation of scaphoid fractures. II. Triangular fibrocartilage tears, *J Hand Ther* 4:57–63, 1991.

227. Brach P: An update on the management of carpal fractures, *J Hand Ther* 16:152–160, 2003.

228. Prosser R, Herbert T: The management of carpal fractures and dislocations, *J Hand Ther* 9:139–147, 1996.

229. Lucio BT: Management of isolated triangular fibrocartilage complex perforations of the wrist, *J Hand Ther* 4:162–168, 1991.

230. Jaffe R, Chidgey LK, LaStayo PC: The distal radioulnar joint: anatomy and management of disorders, *J Hand Ther* 9:129–138, 1996.

231. Blatt G: Capsulodesis in reconstructive hand surgery, *Hand Clin* 3:81–102, 1987.

232. Gancarczyk S, Strauch R: Carpal tunnel syndrome and trigger digit: Common diagnoses that occur "hand in hand,", *J Hand Surg Am* 38:1635–1637, 2013.

233. Lapidus PW: Stenosing tenovaginitis of the wrist and fingers, *Clin Orthop* 83:87–90, 1972.

234. Evans RB, Hunter JM, Burkhalter WE: Conservative management of the trigger finger: a new approach, *J Hand Ther* 1:59–68, 1988.

235. Newport ML, Lane LB, Stuchin SA: Treatment of trigger finger by steroid injection, *J Hand Surg Am* 15:748–750, 1990.

236. Freiberg A, Mulholland RS, Levine R: Nonoperative treatment of trigger fingers and thumb, *J Hand Surg Am* 14:553–558, 1989.

237. Heithoff SJ, Millender LH, Helman J: Bowstringing as complication of trigger finger release, *J Hand Surg Am* 13:507–570, 1988.

238. Bain GI, Turnbull J, Charles MN, et al: Percutaneous A1 pulley release: a cadaveric study, *J Hand Surg Am* 20:781–784, 1995.

239. Harvey FJ: Surgical or nonsurgical treatment of De Quervain's disease, *J Hand Surg Am* 15:83–87, 1990.

240. Jackson WT: Anatomical variations in the first extensor compartment of the wrist, *J Bone Joint Surg Am* 68:923–926, 1986.

241. Weiss AP, Akelman E, Tabatabai M: Treatment of De Quervain's disease, *J Hand Surg Am* 19:595–598, 1994.

242. McAuliffe JA: Tendon disorders of the hand and wrist, *J Hand Surg Am* 35:846–853, 2010.

243. Kerwin G, Williams CS, Seiler JG: The pathophysiology of carpal tunnel syndrome, *Hand Clin* 12:243–251, 1996.

244. Palmar DH: Social and economic costs of carpal tunnel surgery, *Instr Course Lect* 44:167–172, 1995.

245. Seddon H, editor: *Surgical disorders of the peripheral nerves*, ed 2., Edinburgh, 1972, Churchill Livingstone.

246. Sunderland S: *Nerves and nerve injuries*, Edinburgh, 1978, Churchill Livingstone.

247. Phalen GS: The carpal-tunnel syndrome: clinical evaluation of 598 hands, *Clin Orthop Relat Res* 83:29–40, 1972.

248. Koo JT, Szabo RM: Compression neuropathies of the median nerve, *J Am Soc Surg Hand* 4:156–175, 2004.

249. Gelherniari RH, Hergenroeder PT, Hargens AR, et al: The carpal tunnel syndrome: a study of carpal tunnel pressures, *J Bone Joint Surg Am* 63:380–383, 1981.

250. Abrams R: Endoscopic versus open carpal tunnel release, *J Hand Surg Am* 34:535–539, 2009.

251. Trumble T: Single portal endoscopic carpal tunnel release compared to open release, *J Bone Joint Surg Am* 84:1107–1115, 2002.

252. Louie DL, Earp BE, Collins JE, et al: Outcomes of open carpal tunnel release at a minimum of ten years, *J Bone Joint Surg Am* 95:1067–1073, 2013.

253. Valdes K: A retrospective review to determine the long-term efficacy of orthotic devices for trigger finger, *J Hand Ther* 25:89–96, 2012.

254. Fedorczyk JM: Tendinopathies of the elbow, wrist, and hand: histopathology and clinical considerations, *J Hand Ther* 25:191–201, 2012.

255. Dardas A, Bae GH, Yule A, et al: Acetic acid iontophoresis for recalcitrant scarring in post-operative hand patients, *J Hand Ther* 27:44–48, 2014.

CHAPTER 11

The Thoracic Ring Approach™
A Whole Person Framework to Assess and Treat the Thoracic Spine and Rib Cage

LINDA-JOY (LJ) LEE*

INTRODUCTION: THE NEED FOR A BROADER VIEW OF THE THORAX

The thoracic spine is the largest region of the vertebral column and trunk, comprising approximately 20% of overall body length, compared with 12% for the lumbar spine and 8% for the cervical spine.[1] The complex arrangement of thoracic vertebrae, intervertebral discs, ribs, cartilage, sternum, and manubrium, together with the internal cavity created by the skeletal frame, defines what is called the thorax.[1] Clinicians have long recognized that the thoracic spine can be the silent but underlying cause, or **driver**, for problems elsewhere in the body. Most commonly, the hypothesis is that a stiff thorax creates excessive forces and pain in adjacent areas such as the lumbar spine, neck, and shoulder girdle.[2–4] The thoracic structures can also be a source of referred pain in neighboring regions.[5,6]

A challenge for clinicians is how to determine when treatment to the thorax will resolve symptoms either locally or distally. Research on the benefits of thoracic spine treatment is limited and provides conflicting insight into when treatment will improve outcomes. For example, although some patients with neck pain have experienced positive outcomes with thoracic spine manipulation or mobilization treatment, approximately one third of patients in both groups experienced adverse responses, including aggravation of symptoms, muscle spasm,

and headache.[3] These data are consistent with clinical experiences. That is, although some patients benefit from treatment to the thorax, others do not. Furthermore, treatment of the thorax may aggravate symptoms or cause other adverse experiences such as nausea and sympathetic nervous system symptoms. It is therefore proposed that to make wise clinical decisions regarding when and how to treat the thoracic spine and ribs, a broader lens is needed.

Broadening our view of the thorax is required on multiple levels. First, the thoracic spine, ribs and their associated articulations need to be assessed and treated within the context of the three-dimensional "thoracic ring" wherever there are anterior attachments.[7–10] Second, it is necessary to consider other types of dysfunction in the thorax beyond the problems of stiffness and referred pain. Evidence supports that the thorax is inherently flexible,[9,11–14] and the presentation of decreased mobility reflects a loss of optimal neuromuscular control and imbalanced muscular forces around and between the thoracic rings.[9,15–19] A broader view of dysfunction in the thorax provides insight into the role of the thorax in whole body function and how the thorax can be the driver for more varied and distal problems, including incontinence, pelvic organ prolapse, groin pain, knee pain, Achilles tendinopathy, headaches, and sympathetic system sensitization.[15–19] Thus the thoracic rings need to be assessed within the context of the

---

*The author, editors, and publisher wish to acknowledge Diane Lee for her contributions on this topic in the previous edition.

whole person and whole body function. That is, to determine whether treatment of the thorax will positively affect a patient's problem, it is necessary to understand and assess the connections between the thorax and the rest of the body and to recognize the potential role of emotional and psychosocial features. Finally, treatment of the thorax needs to expand beyond techniques that aim to increase mobility to incorporate training optimal neuromuscular control and muscle balance around and between the thoracic rings for optimal movement, load transfer, and respiration.

It has been more than a decade since the original proposals about the importance of neuromuscular control in the thorax were made.[7,20] Since that time, there has been extensive development of the clinical ideas, techniques, and clinical reasoning approach to assess and treat the thorax. There has also been greater research interest around the thorax, which has informed and refined the developing clinical ideas. The Thoracic Ring Approach™[17,18] incorporates the most current research and extensive clinical experiences, providing a range of assessment and treatment techniques for the thoracic rings, along with a clinical reasoning framework to determine whether the dysfunctional thorax, whether painful or pain free, is the true underlying cause or driver of the patient's problems. Even if the thorax is painful, if it is not the driver, then treatment applied to the thorax will not provide optimal clinical outcomes and may exacerbate symptoms. With thorax-driven problems, whether it be pain anywhere in the body, disability, or decreased performance, treatment to the thorax will be the most efficient and effective way to address the patient's nonoptimal experience of his or her body and restore optimal function and performance in a meaningful way. The aim of this chapter is to introduce key concepts and the assessment framework to determine whether the thorax is a driver and then discuss principles and techniques to effectively treat thoracic ring drivers.

CONNECTING THE THORACIC SPINE AND RIB CAGE: EVIDENCE FOR "THORACIC RINGS"

In both the research and clinical realms, the thoracic spine is commonly considered in isolation from the ribs and rib cage, with separate assessment and treatment techniques for each.[21-24] However, anatomical[1] and recent biomechanical data[25,26] support that it is most accurate to view the thoracic spine and rib cage as an integrated complex rather than as separate. Multiple articulations and strong ligaments connect the ribs to their related thoracic spinal segment.[1] In cadaveric studies, if these connections are disrupted by removing the ribs or preserving only posterior stubs of the ribs, the axis of rotation of the thoracic vertebral segment is significantly displaced anteriorly to a location in front of the vertebral body or in the anterior portion of the vertebral body,

respectively. Both of these locations would cause shear and endanger the integrity of the spinal cord. Therefore, data from thoracic specimens without an intact rib cage slice should be considered inaccurate.[25] Measurement of the integrated thoracic ring in vivo is challenging, but recent data support that during functional movements, the thoracic spine and ribs move as an integrated three-dimensional complex. For example, small changes in thoracic spine alignment in the sagittal plane (i.e., flexion/extension) create three-dimensional changes in the shape of the rib cage at multiple levels.[26]

Thus, the evidence supports that wherever anterior attachments are present, it is most accurate to define the functional spinal unit (FSU) of the thorax as a **thoracic ring**.[7-10,15,16,25,26] For example, the fifth thoracic ring is comprised of the right and left fifth ribs, their anterior attachments to the sternum, the T4 and T5 thoracic vertebrae, and the T4-T5 intervertebral disc.[7-10,18] The thorax is thus composed of a "stack" of 10 thoracic rings (rings 1-10) and the thoracolumbar region (made up of T11 and T12 vertebrae and the 11th and 12th ribs). The thoracolumbar region is functionally more similar to the lumbar spine and thus will not be covered in this chapter. For the rest of the thorax, given the integrated nature of the thoracic spine and rib cage, there is a need for manual assessment and treatment techniques for the entire thoracic ring.

Manual Techniques to Assess and Treat the Thoracic Rings

Thoracic Ring Approach[17,18] techniques use palpation points and forces applied around the anterior, lateral, and posterior rib cage to assess and treat the three-dimensional thoracic rings (Figure 11-1).[7,8,10,16-18] Because of the strong anatomical connections, motion detected at the lateral ribs reflects vertebral motion, and forces applied to the side of the ring affect the vertebral segment as well as the ribs (i.e., the entire ring).[27] Thoracic "ring palpation"[7,8,10,16-18] is applied farthest from the axis of rotation of the thoracic segment and where greater amplitude of motion can be detected compared with palpation points centrally at the vertebra. There is also less muscle bulk over the sides of the rings compared with the posterior aspect of the ring (and over the transverse processes of the vertebrae), providing less confounding input from changes in muscle activity when analyzing ring motion during functional tasks. Thoracic ring techniques facilitate assessment of inter-ring (i.e., segmental) position, motion and control during functional tasks, as well as analysis of multiple rings and inter-regional relationships simultaneously. For example, palpation at the lateral aspect of rings 3, 4, and 5 reflects motion of the T2 to T5 vertebral segments and their related ribs (right and left third, fourth, and fifth ribs). Treatment can be applied

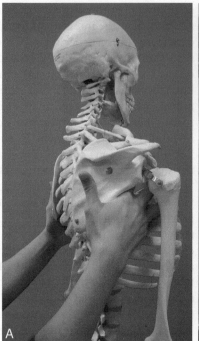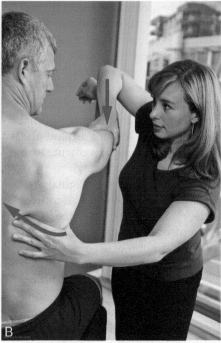

Figure 11-1 A, Hand position illustrating technique for Thoracic Ring Assessment and Correction of the upper thoracic rings (from the Thoracic Ring Approach). Because of differences in anatomy, ring palpation techniques change when moving from the upper thoracic rings to the lower thoracic rings. **B,** Lower thoracic ring correction technique during resisted arm flexion (*vertical arrow*) to determine whether restoring optimal biomechanics and neuromuscular control to the thoracic ring will result in positive change for the meaningful task and support a hypothesis that the thoracic ring is the driver for the patient's shoulder problem. Note the change in orientation of the correcting left hand to match the angle of the lower rings (*lower arrow*). (Copyright LJ Lee Physiotherapist Corp.)

to several sequential thoracic rings at once, so that dysfunction at several vertebral segments and ribs can be addressed simultaneously (Figure 11-2).

It is a well-accepted principle in manual therapy that findings from articular accessory glides should be interpreted in reference to the starting position of the segment. For example, if the C5 segment is in a position of right side bending/right rotation, this affects findings for the amplitude of motion found on examination of both the right and left zygapophyseal joint glides. It is proposed that similarly, the position of the three-dimensional thoracic ring must be considered when interpreting the findings from established articular mobility assessment techniques of the thoracic spine and rib articulations. Without consideration of the thoracic ring positions, articular mobility may be evaluated as restricted, but when thoracic ring position is aligned into a neutral position, articular mobility is restored as symmetrical and equal to levels above and below. If treatment techniques for the thorax are chosen based on articular findings without incorporating findings from the thoracic ring assessment, the potential for less effective treatment choices is greater.

In relation to the challenging question of when treating the thorax will positively improve a patient's problem or not, a significant benefit of thoracic ring palpation and "thoracic ring correction" techniques[7,8,16-18] is that they

provide a method of evaluating the connections between a dysfunctional thoracic ring and whole body function across postural and movement tasks.[8,16,18,28] In this way, the clinician can evaluate the effect of temporarily providing optimal thoracic ring function on the rest of the body and on other painful structures, which forms a key part of the clinical reasoning process to decide whether or not the thorax is the true underlying driver for the patient's problem.

However, before the assessment framework to determine whether the thorax is the driver is discussed, it is necessary to broaden one's understanding of the role of the thorax in whole body function and what the most common underlying impairments in the thorax are.

OPTIMAL FUNCTION OF THE THORACIC RINGS: STIFF AND STABLE, OR NEEDING FINE CONTROL?

The thoracic spine has long been characterized as an inherently stiff and stable structure because of the rib cage.[4,29,30] However, minimal data support this belief. Although the rib cage does increase the stiffness of the thoracic spine and increases the critical buckling load sustainable by the osseoligamentous thoracolumbar spine by a factor of 3 or 4, these loads are still well below those

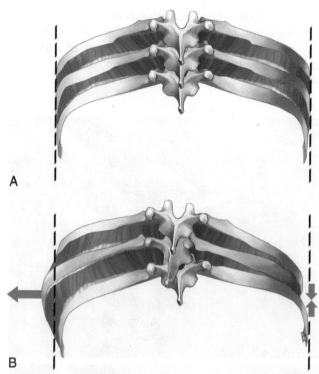

for control of upright posture and respiration, requires complex coordination of muscle activity by the central nervous system (CNS) to meet the demands of stability and movement. For example, during tasks that create perturbations to the thorax in the sagittal plane (flexion/ extension), the deep multifidus and superficial longissimus muscles are similarly recruited to control challenges to stability. In contrast, when challenges to stability occur in the transverse plane, the CNS controls the deep multifidus and superficial longissimus muscles differentially. Differential control of these two layers of thoracic paraspinal muscles is apparent only in the plane in which the thorax has the greatest movement, in the transverse plane, for control of opposite rotational perturbations.[32-34]

These data are consistent with clinical proposals that the most common direction for poor control in the thorax is related to control of rotational forces.[4,7,15-17,28] Because of the coupling of lateral translation with rotation,[11,12] functionally, a loss of rotational control can also be manifested as poor control of lateral translation forces.[7,8] Similarly, loss of rotational control can be coupled with loss of lateral bending control (i.e., control of coronal plane motion).

Shifting from the paradigm that the thorax is stiff and requiring mobilization to one where the thorax is flexible and requiring optimal neuromuscular control provides greater insight into why the thorax can drive distal problems. This is because the paradigm moves away from conceptualizing the thorax as a static, stiff box to being a **dynamic stack of 10 rings**, much like a Slinky or a shock-absorbing spring. When there is loss of optimal sequencing, force modulation, and synergy between the muscles around the thoracic ring, between the 10 thoracic rings, and between the rings and other regions of the body, there are many possible consequences throughout the whole body. These consequences can result in nonoptimal loading of multiple different structures and regions of the body that can drive conditions as diverse as hip osteoarthritis, impingement and groin pain, pelvic girdle and low back pain, incontinence and prolapse, patellofemoral pain, Achilles tendinopathy, lack of "core stability," headaches, and shoulder impingement. Furthermore, because of the anatomical relationships to the sympathetic chain and innervation of the viscera, the dysfunction of the thoracic rings can drive other nonoptimal experiences such as sensitization of the sympathetic nervous system and gastrointestinal symptoms.

Clinical Example: Potential Mechanisms by Which Nonoptimal Neuromuscular Function of Thoracic Rings Can Drive Distal Problems

Suppose one considers the possible effect when there is nonoptimal neuromuscular control and altered muscle balance related to the fourth thoracic ring during a squat, resulting in left translation and right rotation of the

Figure 11-2 A, "Stacked" thoracic rings. When neuromuscular forces are balanced around and between the thoracic rings, optimal alignment is supported and provides a base from which to initiate movement. There is sufficient space between the thoracic rings. Although not all depicted here, optimal alignment of the thoracic rings is supported by balance between the deep and superficial muscles attaching to the rings. Note that the top vertebra is missing from the superior thoracic ring. If this figure depicts rings 3, 4, and 5, the related vertebral segments include T2 to T5. Less muscle bulk over the sides of the rings compared with the posterior aspect of the ring facilitates more accurate analysis of ring motion during functional tasks. **B,** "Unstacked" thoracic rings. When force vectors around the thoracic rings are unbalanced, there are multiple patterns of thoracic ring dysfunction that can occur. This figure depicts one potential pattern of nonoptimal inter-ring relationships. Compression between the upper and lower rings on the right creates left translation of the middle ring, which is coupled with right rotation. Compression of the rings also creates side bending, which is coupled with rotation. These inter-ring relationships can be assessed simultaneously using thoracic ring palpation techniques. Findings from manual assessment of the posterior joints of the thoracic spine and rib cage need to be interpreted in reference to the position and behavior of the related thoracic ring. (Copyright LJ Lee Physiotherapist Corp.)

that the spine is exposed to in normal function.[31] Support from neuromuscular forces is essential. Biomechanical data show that the intact thorax is mobile in all planes.[11-13] In contrast to the limited rotation of lumbar spine segments, the primary movement of the thorax is rotation (transverse plane motion), followed by lateral bending (coronal plane motion), with significantly less flexion and extension range of motion.[11-14] Thus the evidence supports that the thorax is inherently *flexible*.

Each typical thoracic ring has 13 articulations,[1] and in total, the 136 joints of the thorax provide significant mobility. The capacity for movement within and between the segments of the thorax, along with the requirements

fourth ring (upper thorax) upon initiation of the squat motion. This movement of the fourth thoracic ring creates both a lateral and rotational perturbation to the trunk. To counter this perturbation, activity in the right external oblique and left internal oblique muscles may increase, resulting in asymmetrical abdominal wall activation and potentially an opposite rotation in the lower thorax. Commonly, the pelvis and hips counter-rotate to compensate for the rotation of the upper thorax, so the pelvis rotates to the left and the right hip moves forward. The twist in the thorax alters all muscle relationships around the thorax, affecting scapular, neck, and head neuromuscular control and position. Because all abdominal muscles are innervated from the lower thorax (T7 to L1/L2), the twist of the thorax may further contribute to abdominal wall dys-synergies via neural mechanisms. Excessive and asymmetrical contraction of the superficial muscles such as the external obliques (EO), changes in diaphragm activity (attaches to the lower six thoracic rings), and depression of the scapulae restrict mobility and compress the thorax, affecting the balance between intrathoracic and intra-abdominal pressure, and create increased pressure in the lower abdomen (a "pressure belly"). In response to the increase in intra-abdominal pressure, the pelvic floor muscles can become hypertonic, contributing to pain syndromes and/or stress urinary incontinence (SUI). Interestingly, the EO attaches as high as the fifth thoracic ring, and increased resting activity of the EO and pelvic floor muscles occurs in subgroups of women with SUI.[35]

Left lateral translation of the fourth thoracic ring also results in a left translation of the upper thorax and affects the position of the center of mass over the feet, which, in turn, affects control of postural equilibrium and alters medial-lateral forces all the way down the kinetic chain to the feet, altering muscle activation and loading patterns. For example, left translation of the trunk often correlates with decreased right gluteus medius and maximus muscle activity as a result of decreased weight bearing on the right leg. When combined with compensatory pelvis rotation, this creates an altered axis of movement and control of the right hip, providing a biologically plausible mechanism to explain thoracic driven hip impingement and groin pain. In these subgroups the hip symptoms do not resolve without treatment to change neuromuscular control of the driving thoracic rings. Figures 11-1, 11-3, 11-4, and 11-5 show clinical examples of thorax driven shoulder pain, abdominal wall dysfunction, low back pain, and foot pain.

The previous example is simplified to illustrate the effect of nonoptimal muscle synergies around the fourth thoracic ring. It is also common to find patterns of excessive compression between the thoracic rings and hypertonicity of the intercostals at different points around the 3-dimensional ring that create a loss of the ability to dissociate movement of each ring relative to the other rings, creating **"glued ring complexes"**. The nonoptimal muscle patterns around two to three rings (or more)

creates an "unstacked" multiring complex that is unable to behave optimally across a variety of tasks. The rings may be held as a unit in various patterns of rotation/ lateral translation/ side bending and/or compression (see Figure 11-2). These patterns of nonoptimal muscle

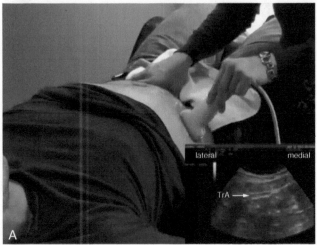

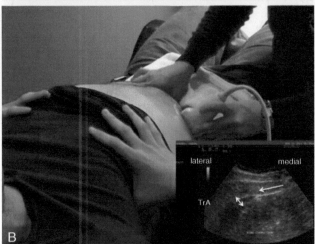

Figure 11-3 The thoracic rings are a common underlying cause for dys-synergies of the abdominal wall, inability to recruit transversus abdominis (TrA) and/or pelvic floor muscles, asymmetry of transversus abdominis muscle and pelvic floor contraction, and/or hypertonicity and asymmetry of the superficial and deep layers of the abdominal wall and/or the pelvic floor. **A**, With verbal cues designed to elicit a bilateral (symmetrical) contraction of transversus abdominis muscle, there is a response from the left transversus abdominis (not shown) but no response on the right. Note inset ultrasound image and arrow indicating transversus abdominis layer; with cues there is no change in the architecture of the transversus abdominis muscle. Changing cues and effort and paying more attention to the right side do not change the ability to recruit the right transversus abdominis muscle. **B**, When the driving thoracic rings are corrected (third/fourth), the same cues result in immediate recruitment of the right transversus abdominis muscle in a symmetrical manner with the left transversus abdominis—symmetry of recruitment is restored. Inset shows response of right transversus abdominis; note the increase in width of the TrA layer and the lateral slide of the muscle (indicated by arrows). In thoracic driven abdominal wall dysfunction, transversus abdominis muscle contraction occurs in response to a cue directed to control of the thoracic rings, *not* in response to abdominal wall cues. (Copyright LJ Lee Physiotherapist Corp.)

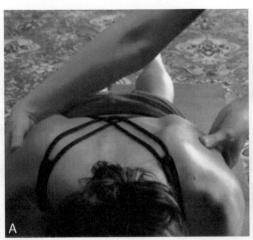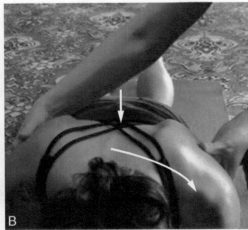

Figure 11-4 Assessment of thoracic ring control during the plank task. Patient reported an inability to do plank exercises because of difficulty breathing and low back pain during this task. **A,** With correction of upper thoracic rings (3 and 4), there was no low back pain and the patient was able to breathe and feel her abdominal and pelvic floor muscles contract. **B,** The change in thoracic and lumbar spine position is shown once the correction to the upper thoracic rings is released. The upper rings translate to the left and rotate right (*horizontal arrow*). This imparts a rotation, extension, and anterior translation load to the lumbar spine (*vertical arrow*). This patient also reported an inability to feel a pelvic floor muscle contraction without thoracic ring correction that was fully restored with the correction. (Copyright LJ Lee Physiotherapist Corp.)

activity and hypertonicity create a significant loss of variability in available options for movement of the thoracic rings, and the more rings that are held together and function as one unit, the greater the loss of options and the greater impact on mobility of the thoracic rings. These glued ring complexes are common, and therefore it is advisable that the clinician always palpate and determine thoracic ring behavior relative to the ring above and the ring below in order to implement treatment that will restore optimal relationships between the thoracic rings. When intercostal hypertonicity is present, assessment and treatment of the two related sequential thoracic rings is essential (these complexes are annotated as "Ring 4/3 correction," indicating that the fourth ring is relatively left translated and the third ring relatively right translated).

ASSESSMENT: DETERMINING WHETHER THE THORAX IS THE DRIVER FOR THE PATIENT'S PROBLEM

The previous section illustrates that a patient with a dysfunctional thorax can present with a wide variety of symptoms and functional problems. Location of pain or tissue changes do not always correlate to the primary underlying cause of the problem. Thoracic pain can be driven from dysfunction in the thorax or from elsewhere in the body, such as the foot or pelvis. Similarly, the presence of dysfunction in the thorax is insufficient to make a clinical decision to treat the thoracic rings. In every patient, there are multiple different impairments that can be identified throughout the body. Therefore a whole body assessment paradigm is required to determine how a dysfunctional thorax relates to the presenting problem.

Meaningful Task Analysis (MTA) was initially proposed as an assessment framework to determine whether dysfunction in the thorax was the *underlying cause,* or *driver,* of the patient's problem[28] and is thus the assessment framework to find thoracic drivers within the Thoracic Ring Approach.[17,18] The principles of MTA are also part of the Integrated Systems Model for Disability and Pain (ISM)[36] and have been further developed in the ConnectTherapy™ Model.[37,38]

MTA incorporates not only the biomechanical features of a task but also the emotional, cognitive, social, and contextual features related to a specific problematic or goal-related movement. Meaningful tasks are determined from the patient's story and direct the choice of screening tasks analyzed in the objective assessment. A **"meaningful task"** is one in which symptoms such as pain or other nonoptimal sensorial experiences, such as decreased power, decreased ease of movement, altered breathing, or incontinence, occur.

Many meaningful tasks are complex, multiplanar, multijoint movements. The purpose behind **"meaningful screening tasks"** is to use related simple movements that enable accurate manual assessment of joint and muscle function throughout the body during functional movements. To determine whether the thorax is the driver, thoracic ring function is assessed and manual thoracic ring corrections are applied to evaluate their impact on task performance and patient experience. Ideally, the screening tasks chosen closely resemble the meaningful task from multiple aspects, including biomechanical, emotional, and contextual features. The complexity of the screening task used depends on practitioner skill; more skilled practitioners can use more complex movements as screening tasks. In the early stages of thoracic ring skill acquisition,

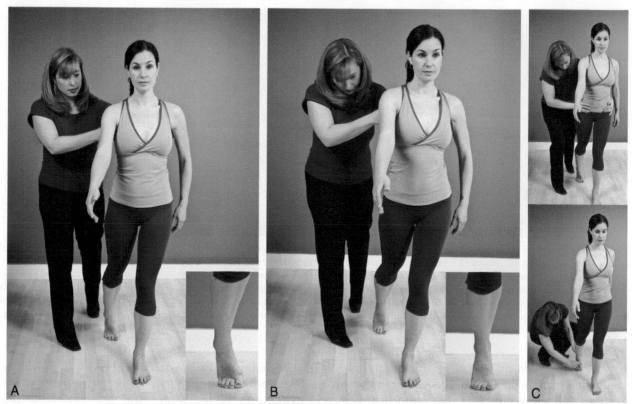

Figure 11-5 Meaningful Task Analysis (MTA).[28] To find the driver for the patient's foot pain related to push-off during running, a step forward task is used as a meaningful screening task. Multiple areas of nonoptimal alignment, biomechanics, and/or control (nonoptimal load transfer [NOLT]) are identified during the task. **A,** During left step forward, the right foot demonstrates lateral weight bearing on push-off, with varus forces at the ankle. At initiation of the step forward, the fourth thoracic ring is felt to translate left, creating a segmental right rotation. Optimally, the upper thorax should rotate left, and therefore the movement of the fourth thoracic ring is nonoptimal. The resultant left shift of the thorax over the base of support requires the compensatory varus at the ankle to neutralize the center of mass over the base of support. On loading of the left leg, the left side of the pelvis loses segmental control and "unlocks" (palpation not shown; the innominate anteriorly rotates relative to the sacrum, a less optimal position to transfer loads in the pelvis). Inset shows a close up of the impact of the early left translation of the fourth thoracic ring on the right foot. **B,** Correction of the fourth thoracic ring during the left step forward task results in optimal weight bearing through the right ankle and foot during push-off and reduction of the patient's symptoms. The left side of the pelvis no longer loses segmental control (palpation not shown). The starting position of the thoracic rings needs to be corrected by stacking them into optimal inter-ring relationships in standing posture; then optimal movement and control are manually facilitated during the task. The thorax can drive distal problems in the hip, knee, ankle, and foot because of rotational mechanisms and the effect that lateral translation of the thorax has on the center of mass relative to the base of support. Inset shows close-up of the right foot at push-off in response to the fourth thoracic ring correction. Note the significantly improved position. Application of thoracic ring correction techniques during functional movement analysis allows evaluation of the potential impact that treating specific levels of the thorax will have on symptoms, task performance, and other problematic areas in the kinetic chain. **C,** The impact of corrections to other areas of NOLT is assessed and compared with the impact of the thoracic ring correction. Upper panel demonstrates correction of pelvis alignment with bilateral anterior compression, and lower panel demonstrates a correction of the right ankle/foot. The thoracic ring correction resulted in the best change in task performance, the most positive change on all areas of NOLT, and optimized load transfer through the right foot (area of symptoms) and pelvis. (Copyright LJ Lee Physiotherapist Corp.)

simpler, "building block" or component movements of the meaningful task are used to rule in or rule out a thoracic ring driver. Correction of the hypothesized driver can then be performed in the more complex meaningful task to provide further confirmation. In some situations, the meaningful task is simple enough to be used itself (Figure 11-6).

For any task that is chosen for assessment, the clinician uses observation and palpation skills to determine whether the current strategy being used is optimal or nonoptimal, considering task requirements and individual characteristics of the patient. The ability to function optimally across the diverse spectrum of human activity

requires that one can access and choose multiple strategies. The CNS needs to have the ability to match the strategy to the specific demands of the task whether that task is sitting at a desk or running a marathon. Clinically, it is common for patients to lose movement options and variability. That is, they have fewer strategies to choose from, or they "get stuck" in one or two strategies that they apply across multiple tasks. In some cases, the strategy is appropriate for the task, but in other tasks, the same strategy causes pain or other nonoptimal sensorial experiences, along with disability or loss of performance.

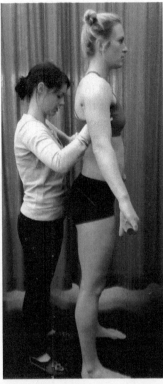
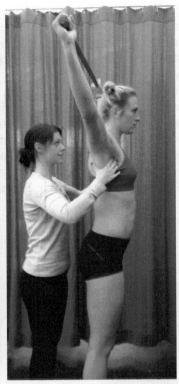
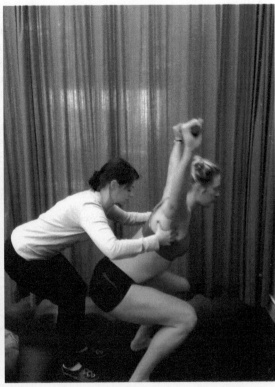

Figure 11-6 Meaningful Task Analysis (MTA)—overhead squat with dowel. In this case the meaningful task (MT) is simple enough relative to the clinician's skills to be able to use the MT to assess for nonoptimal load transfer (NOLT) of the thoracic rings and perform corrections to find the driver. The panels from left to right show therapist hand and body position to assess rings 4/3 during the MT. (Copyright LJ Lee Physiotherapist Corp.)

When the CNS is successful at planning an optimal strategy for matching task demands:

1. Motion of all joint complexes is controlled with optimal axes of rotation, while allowing the necessary range of motion required for the task, without rigidity.
2. Spinal posture and orientation are controlled both within and between regions and appropriate for the demands of the task.
3. Postural equilibrium is maintained.
4. Respiration, continence, and other systems are supported and not compromised (e.g., vascular system is not compromised by musculoskeletal structures during movement).
5. Intra-abdominal and intrathoracic pressure are sufficient and balanced.
6. Desired qualitative and quantitative features are present.

In addition, there is enough movement (i.e., give) in the system to dampen and control multiple predictable and unpredictable challenges such as internal or external perturbations, varying loads, and risk in potentially changing environments.[39-41] Therefore, the clinician can determine whether a strategy is optimal based on the ability of the patient to demonstrate these features during any task. Failure to maintain any of these features is an indication that the patient is using a **nonoptimal strategy** for the task. The clinician must determine how the nonoptimal strategy and the nonoptimal sensorial experience are connected.

Correction of the "primary driver" will result in positive changes in all nonoptimal features identified during task performance and a positive sensorial experience.

Signs of Optimal Strategies for Meaningful Task Analysis

Optimal strategies for function and performance support optimal function of multiple systems (Figure 11-7) and will do the following:

- Balance mobility and control of all joints in the body. Joint motion will be controlled without rigidity and optimal axis of motion maintained. This equates to optimal load transfer (OLT).
- Control spinal posture and orientation and maintain postural equilibrium under varying loads.
- Maintain sufficient intra-abdominal pressure (IAP) that is balanced with intrathoracic pressure ("pressure belly" is a sign of an imbalance, excessive IAP).
- Allow the rib cage to expand for optimal respiration.
- Support other systems such as vascular function and continence.
- Allow sufficient mobility to dampen and react to perturbation forces. This is the "give" in the system.
- Create desired qualitative and quantitative features related to function and performance goals, "beautiful movement."
- Support positive experiences of the body (e.g., Center Circle, the Patient Experience).

Nonoptimal strategies affect multiple systems; therefore there are multiple possible signs of nonoptimal strategies. When the driver is corrected, all these signs should show positive change.

In some cases, patients may be choosing a nonoptimal strategy related to performance or one that causes nonoptimal loading of some structures but offloads other structures that are the priority for the nervous system to support. For example, a nonoptimal strategy may be appropriate when there is tissue injury and the state of healing is currently associated with inflammation (e.g., acute ankle sprain, muscle tear or strain, inflamed nerve or organ). In these cases, the nonoptimal strategy is appropriate or adaptive in the short term but would be in inappropriate in the long term. Therefore, a clinical reasoning process that considers all influences on the patient's current strategy for posture and movement and his or her current experience allows the clinician to decide appropriate treatment intervention for each individual at different stages of the rehabilitation process (see Figure 11-7).

As noted previously, dysfunction in any region or system can be the underlying cause for the whole body nonoptimal strategy and patient experience. Thus, any positive findings for dysfunction in a region may be a sign indicating that the region is a driver or that it is a "victim," a consequence rather than the cause. To determine whether an area is a driver, the relationship of regional dysfunction

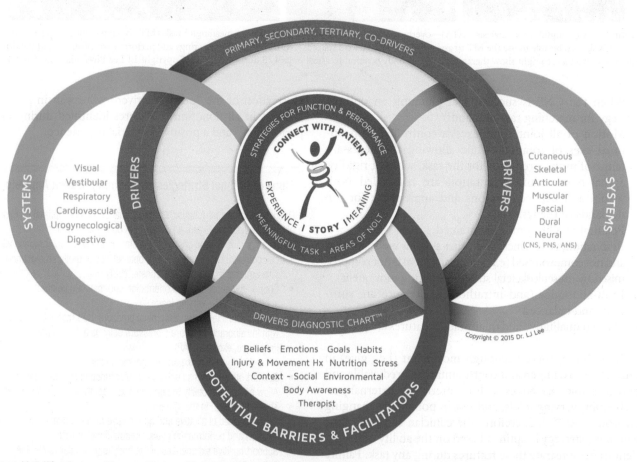

Figure 11-7 The ConnectTherapy Circles of Influence™ is a tool to facilitate organization of knowledge and information from multiple domains and determine the most relevant influencers on the patient's current (1) experience of his or her body and (2) strategies for function and performance. The circles represent influences both intrinsic and extrinsic to the patient; the amount of overlap and linking between the different circles can change over time and help the clinician adjust priorities and choose appropriate interventions. The Circles of Influence illustrate the construct of connectedness that is central to ConnectTherapy. *Hx,* History; *CNS,* central nervous system; *PNS,* peripheral nervous system; *ANS,* autonomic nervous system. (Copyright LJ Lee Physiotherapist Corp.)

to whole body function and patient experience needs to be assessed and determined. This is accomplished by implementing a series of clinical tests governed by a robust clinical reasoning process. The ConnectTherapy Drivers Diagnostics Chart™[37,38] for MTA and provides a clinical reasoning algorithm that facilitates an understanding of the connections between all dysfunctional regions of the body and is used to determine which areas are the underlying problems, or drivers, for the patient's problem. In complex or chronic problems, there is often more than a single **"primary driver"**, with several areas contributing to the problem, either as a **"secondary driver"** or **"tertiary driver"** or two dysfunctional areas equally contributing as co-drivers. It is beyond the scope of this chapter to cover the full depth of this diagnostic process; however, the process to rule in or rule out the thoracic rings as a primary driver is described here to illustrate the basic clinical reasoning principles involved.

In summary, the clinical decision as to whether the thorax should be treated, and which specific thoracic rings to treat, is determined by assessing and manually modifying thoracic ring behavior during meaningful screening tasks. For example, for a runner who experiences lateral foot pain on the push-off phase of gait, a relevant screening task is a step forward task (see Figure 11-5). If nonoptimal alignment, biomechanics, movement, or control of any thoracic rings occurs during the task, a thoracic ring correction is performed, whereby optimal thoracic ring alignment, biomechanics, movement, and control are provided through gentle but specific manual facilitation at the specific ring level.[7,8,17,18,28] Ring correction involves different hand position and direction of force input depending on whether the upper or lower rings are being corrected.[7,17,18] The reference for what is optimal behavior for the thoracic rings is based on the task requirements and the patient's individual architectural features. If the thoracic ring correction (1) positively changes the ease of task performance, (2) positively changes the meaningful experience/symptoms during task performance, and (3) optimizes transfer of loads and neuromuscular function in other areas of the body, then there is support for the hypothesis of a thoracic ring driver. To further strengthen the hypothesis, manual corrections are also applied to other areas of **nonoptimal load transfer (NOLT)** identified and their impact compared with the thoracic ring correction. In the case of a primary thoracic ring driver, corrections to other areas either have a negative effect or not as positive an effect as the thoracic ring correction.[7,8,16–18,28] If manual correction to a different area of the body results in a greater improvement in task performance and patient experience and automatically fully restores optimal behavior of the thoracic rings, then the thorax is *not* the primary driver for the patient's problem, and even if there is dysfunction in the thorax present, it should not be treated.

Clinical Findings That Support the Hypothesis of a Thoracic Ring Driver Underlying the Patient's Problem

- Specific thoracic rings demonstrate nonoptimal Alignment, Biomechanics/movement, and/or motor Control (ABCs) = nonoptimal load transfer (NOLT) *early* during the meaningful task (MT) or meaningful screening task; often starts in nonoptimal alignment before movement.
- Manual correction of the specific thoracic rings (to provide optimal ABCs) creates a significant positive change in the following:
  - Performance of the task, both subjectively and objectively (i.e., range of motion, strength, ease of movement increase)
  - The patient's experience of his or her body during the task
  - The meaningful complaint
  - Automatic improvement or full correction of multiple other areas of NOLT identified during the MT
- Manual correction of other areas of NOLT in the body (e.g., pelvis, foot, hip, neck) do not create as positive a change, make the specific thoracic rings' function worse, or make the task performance and experience worse.
- Manual correction of the specific thoracic rings results in positive changes in other signs of nonoptimal strategies (e.g., improves ease of breathing, decreases pressure belly, improves pelvic floor muscle contraction, etc.).

Analysis of Thoracic Ring Function in Common Screening Tasks

Optimal function of the thoracic rings supports optimal function of multiple systems and structures for optimal health of the whole person across a wide variety of postures and functional tasks. It is therefore important to understand what optimal thoracic ring behavior is across different functional tasks as a reference point in the assessment process. This section describes thoracic ring function and assessment across several screening tasks relevant to common meaningful tasks for patients, but many other tasks can be used based on the clinical context (see Figures 11-1, 11-4, 11-5, and 11-6). The aim is to provide reference principles that can then be applied to more complex and diverse meaningful tasks based on what is known from research and clinical experience. The clinical reasoning process described earlier to determine whether the thorax is the primary driver for the patient's problem applies to all of the tasks described next.

Standing Posture

The way patients hold themselves in space can provide insight on many levels, including habitual patterns, the degree of pain, and the patient's emotional status. For some patients, standing is their *meaningful task;* that is, they experience their symptoms when they are standing, especially during prolonged standing. For these patients, more time is spent analyzing standing posture and performing manual corrections to different body regions, including the thoracic rings, in order to find the driver for the problem. If standing is not the patient's meaningful task, the findings in standing serve as a reference and starting point for movement into the screening task/meaningful task. In this case, the impact of corrections on standing posture is less important than the impact these corrections have during performance of the screening task. It is also important to recognize that asymmetry in postural findings is common and not always relevant to the problem the patient experiences during his or her meaningful task.

If the individual identifies particular postures as painful or aggravating to his or her symptoms, those specific postures are assessed and the findings compared with standing posture. It is most relevant to assess how a patient habitually assumes his or her posture, rather than changing foot position or giving cues before the initial evaluation of the habitual posture is completed. In patients who have ongoing or recurrent pain, the posture assumed often puts excessive forces through structures that are painful, perpetuating the generation of nociceptive input. In other cases, the alignment assumed may be ideal in terms of the position of the bones, but the muscle strategy (i.e., *how* the patient attained the ideal alignment) is not optimal, resulting in excessive compression, repetitive microtrauma, and pain. Conversely, in acute pain states, the posture the patient chooses often is one that results in the most relief and unloading of the painful structure or structures.

Nonoptimal alignment of the thorax is a sign of a nonoptimal strategy for the task of standing and will be linked to asymmetrical and nonoptimal patterns of muscle activity (i.e., resting tone) throughout the body. Several questions should be considered when analyzing posture. How is the thorax aligned? What muscles are being used? How does the muscle activity relate to the resultant posture? Why are those muscles being used? What is the impact of the resultant forces (e.g., line of gravity, compression from muscle activity) on the joints as a result of the combination of alignment and muscle patterns? How does this relate to the pain-generating structure?

In assessing alignment of the thorax, the relationship of the thorax relative to other regions (i.e., inter-regional relationships) is determined first, and these findings are correlated with intrathoracic findings (inter-ring alignment) as determined by thoracic ring palpation techniques (Figure 11-8). Optimal strategies support the thoracic rings in a centered position in all planes related to one another, and as a whole, the thorax is centered under the head, over the pelvis and in relation to the base of support (i.e., the feet). In the sagittal plane, the manubriosternal (MS) junction will be vertically aligned over the pubic symphysis (PS) for neutral anteroposterior (AP) alignment of the thorax over the pelvis.

Optimal postural strategies place the joints in a neutral position, where compression forces are best distributed; however, the ability to maintain this position relies on complex feedback and feedforward mechanisms to modulate and maintain muscle activity at multiple levels.

Multiple patterns of nonoptimal alignment are possible, creating various presentations in altered multisegmental curves of the thoracic spine, which correlate to the sum of all segmental alterations in rotation, side bending, and translation (i.e., lateral, anterior, posterior) of the 10 thoracic rings (see Figure 11-2). In volume 1 of this series (*Orthopedic Physical Assessment*), several categories of deviation from optimal alignment are described.[42] Excessive thoracic kyphosis and loss of kyphosis (lordosis) are two common presentations. Commonly, these patterns are perceived to be solely related to thoracic spine alignment, with segments excessively flexed (kyphosis) or extended (lordosis). This belief is in conflict with the evidence that there is minimal flexion and extension of the thoracic vertebrae. In contrast, the greatest neutral zone exists for rotation and side bending.[11-14] Data support that increased kyphosis or lordosis of the thoracic spine is more related to the degree of posterior and anterior translation of the thorax relative to the pelvis.[43] Furthermore, although the altered position is most obvious in the sagittal plane, there are actually three-dimensional, multiplanar alterations in the alignment of the thoracic rings, which is more consistent with the large available motion in the neutral zone related to the transverse and coronal planes. It is the author's clinical experience that a combination of lateral translation, rotation, side bending, and compression, along with posterior translation (kyphosis) or anterior translation (lordosis) of the thoracic rings relative to the pelvis and/or feet, underlies the observed, seemingly sagittal plane altered alignment. Therefore these postures are best corrected by addressing the lateral translation/rotational/side bending components first using thoracic ring correction techniques, which then frees up motion in the neutral zone to allow correction of the AP translation relative to neighboring regions. Thoracic ring correction techniques are used to determine whether specific levels in the thorax are the driver for the inability of the patient to correct the AP thoracopelvic translational relationship. If corrections to specific thoracic rings creates optimal alignment and loading of all other areas in the thorax and in the rest of the body, then those specific thoracic rings are the driver for the patient's problem in the meaningful task of standing.

Seated Trunk Rotation

In contrast to the limited rotation of lumbar spine segments,[44] the primary movement of the thorax is rotation, and control of rotational forces is essential for functional activities. It, therefore, is an important movement to assess in patients with thoracic pain or dysfunction and is a key screening task related to any meaningful activity that requires trunk rotation. Furthermore, because of the relatively large amplitude of motion of the rings and marked change in trunk rotation range of motion when the "driving" thoracic ring(s) are corrected in this activity, trunk rotation

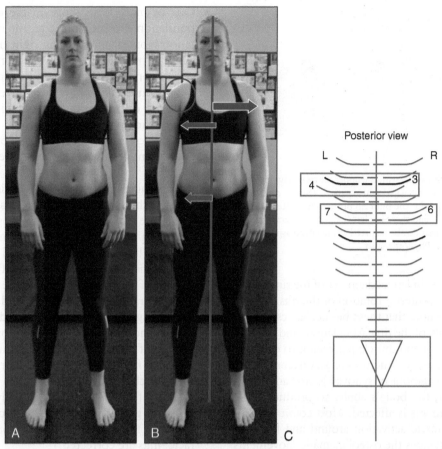

Figure 11-8 Analysis of strategy for standing posture. **A** and **B,** Inter-regional relationships are sometimes more obvious when viewed from the anterior aspect. Note that if a line is drawn vertically from a midpoint between the feet (the base of support), the thorax is left translated relative to the pelvis and relative to the base of support. Note also the asymmetry in the abdominal wall resting tone and infrasternal angle. Visually there is an appearance that the upper thorax is left rotated, but palpation reveals right rotation and left translation of the upper thoracic rings. The visual impression of left rotation comes from the right shoulder position being anterior, which is related to the shoulder girdle being in a left intrashoulder girdle torsion. **C,** Manual palpation of the rings provides more detail about inter-ring relationships and position of the rings relative to the base of support. This schematic represents ring alignment from the *posterior* aspect of the same patient. The vertical blue line represents the midline relative to the base of support. As indicated by the blue rectangular boxes, there are several rings translated left/rotated right relative to midline in the upper thorax (rings 2, 3, 4), with the fourth ring translation amplitude the greatest. Ring 3 and ring 5 are therefore right translated relative to the fourth ring when considering inter-ring relationships. The lower rings (7, 6) are slightly translated right relative to midline but significantly right translated relative to the upper rings, and they could be hypothesized as the body's attempt to compensate for the upper ring left translation. However, without performing ring corrections to determine the primary driver in the thorax, it is not possible to confirm this hypothesis. The pelvis is also slightly translated right of midline. Ring corrections are performed based on the inter-ring relationships. In this patient, if standing was the meaningful task, the impact of several different ring corrections would be compared with each other: correction of rings 4/3, correction of rings 4/5, correction of rings 5/6, and correction of rings 7/6. If the meaningful task was not standing, ring corrections would not be performed until assessment of ring nonoptimal load transfer (NOLT) during a relevant screening task was performed. The rings identified as showing NOLT on the dynamic task would then direct which rings to correct. (Copyright LJ Lee Physiotherapist Corp.)

provides the clinician with good opportunity to acquire and hone his or her thoracic ring palpation and correction skills.

During trunk rotation, motion of each thoracic ring contributes to the total range of motion, with somewhat greater contributions from the upper thoracic rings.[14] With right rotation of the trunk, the osteokinematics of the typical thoracic ring (between the third to seventh thoracic ring) have been described as follows: for the fifth thoracic ring, the T4 vertebra rotates and side flexes to the right and translates to the left relative to T5; the right fifth rib posteriorly rotates and translates anteromedially relative to the T5 transverse process; and the left fifth rib anteriorly rotates and translates posterolaterally relative to the T5 transverse process.[45] These movements are osteokinematic

(i.e., movements of the bones) and require concurrent accessory movements at all joints (i.e., arthrokinematics) of the functional thoracic ring. In addition, a contralateral translation (i.e., left translation) of the entire ring complex occurs that is palpable as inter-ring motion (Figure 11-9).[7,8,10,17,18] However, there should not be a large shift of the entire thorax to the left or right relative to the pelvis base. These same biomechanics occur in the lower thoracic rings (Figure 11-10), but the direction of coupled side flexion can be ipsilateral or contralateral given the increased flexibility from greater cartilaginous attachments anteriorly and a decrease in size of the rib head articulation with the superior vertebra.[45] Furthermore, because of the more planar articulations of the costotransverse joints,

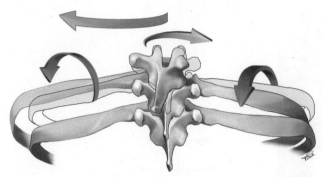

Figure 11-9 Two "thoracic rings," with the upper thoracic ring depicting the osteokinematics that occur with right rotation. During right rotation, the vertebra rotates right, the right rib posteriorly rotates, and the left rib anteriorly rotates,[45] and there is a left (i.e., contralateral) translation of the thoracic ring that can be palpated at the lateral aspect of the ring.[7,8] (Copyright LJ Lee Physiotherapist Corp.)

there is greater change in lateral diameter of the rings associated with anterior/posterior rotation of the ribs.

It is important to note that these biomechanics require intact passive integrity of the ring articulations and optimal neuromuscular control and muscle patterning to occur. If trauma disrupts the passive structures (e.g., vertebral body, disc, ligaments, cartilaginous or synovial joints) anteriorly, posteriorly, or both, the body's ability to produce these physiological movements is affected. Most commonly, altered patterns of muscle activation around and between the thoracic rings changes the osteokinematic movements and therefore the arthrokinematic movements produced during trunk rotation also changes.

In addition to assessing overall range of rotation motion in each direction, the examiner should note whether asymmetry of range is present. If rotation is restricted bilaterally, it is often easiest to find the best ring correction that changes the most restricted direction of rotation and then confirm that the same ring correction also improves the other direction of rotation. The examiner uses thoracic ring palpation and spans two to three rings concurrently (i.e., anterolaterally and laterally along the sides of the rings from rings 2-10) to identify any rings that NOLT during trunk rotation. The upper rings can also be palpated anteriorly, just lateral to the costochondral joints. NOLT is generally defined for any region of the body with nonoptimal alignment, biomechanics, and/or control relative to what is optimal for performance of a task or activity. Therefore, for the task of right trunk rotation, several possibilities of NOLT for the thoracic rings can occur:

1. An unstacked complex of two or more rings maintain their nonoptimal inter-ring relationships (see Figure 11-2) and are unable to dissociate to create optimal ring osteokinematics. They may remain in their nonoptimal alignment and not move, or as a complex, they may translate to the left or right.
2. One or more rings do not move in synchrony with the rings above and below, which can be palpated as a loss of contralateral inter-ring translation and the associated intraring biomechanics.

3. One or more rings move in the opposite pattern of translation and rotation (e.g., the ring displays left rotation biomechanics during right trunk rotation), palpated as prominence of the ring on the ipsilateral side of rotation (i.e., right side in example).
4. One or more rings move excessively into the optimal direction of translation but out of synchrony in relation to the rings above and below.
5. Excessive compression between two or more thoracic rings at different points around the three-dimensional ring.

The examiner notes all rings that display NOLT during the task and then systematically performs thoracic ring corrections at those levels. Two sequential rings are first "stacked" or aligned in neutral and then gentle manual facilitation of optimal ring biomechanics is performed while the patient repeats the difficult rotation movement. The examiner assesses the impact of the ring correction on the following:

1. Rotation range of motion (It should markedly increase if the driving rings are being corrected; see Figure 11-10.)
2. Ease of movement and any symptoms
3. NOLT of other rings (These should significantly improve or fully correct when the primary driving rings are corrected.)
4. NOLT of other areas of the body (e.g., pelvis, hip, shoulder girdle, neck) (These should significantly improve or fully correct when the primary driving thoracic rings are corrected.)

The impact of ring corrections at all levels displaying NOLT during the task are compared, and the correction with most positive changes is then compared with corrections of other regions of the body (e.g., cervical spine, scapula, glenohumeral joint, pelvis, and foot as described later). If the specific thoracic ring correction provides the most positive changes compared with all other corrections, it indicates the specific thoracic ring levels that are the primary drivers for the task of trunk rotation. If the patient's meaningful task is a more complex task requiring rotation, the examiner then applies the same ring correction during the more complex task to confirm that similar positive changes in task performance, patient experience, and other areas of NOLT occur.

Further tests of the driving thoracic ring(s) are then performed to determine the treatment techniques and progressive exercise plan required (see Treatment section later in this chapter), but the clinician has confirmed which specific ring(s) need to be addressed to restore full functional trunk rotation. Note that if motion of the ring can be fully restored with gentle manual correction, joint fixations and articular fibrosis are ruled out.

Single-Arm Lift

The **single-arm lift (SAL) test** has previously been described as the "sitting arm lift"[7,8,10]; The name has now been changed because it is useful to perform in standing, sitting, and other postures related to the patient's meaningful task (Figures 11-11 and 11-12). The **prone arm lift (PAL)**

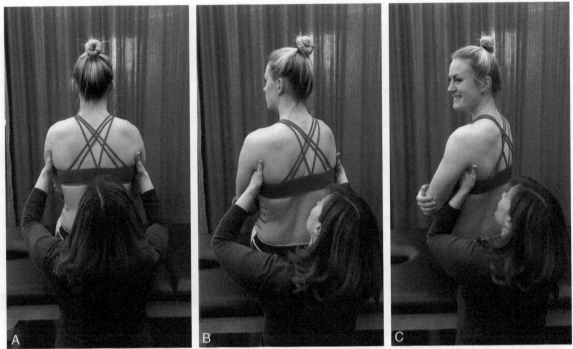

Figure 11-10 Seated trunk rotation with thoracic ring palpation and correction. **A,** Clinician's hand position for palpation of the third and fourth thoracic rings. The palpation is performed along the distal end of flat fingers; there is no pressure posteriorly from the heel of the hand or palm. **B,** The patient left rotates; the clinician notes the range of motion and any nonoptimal load transfer (NOLT) of the upper thoracic rings during the movement. The patient then returns to neutral. **C,** Left rotation with correction of the fourth thoracic ring on the left and the third thoracic ring on the right and facilitation of optimal biomechanics for the task. Note the increased range of motion and positive patient experience resulting from this ring correction. (Copyright LJ Lee Physiotherapist Corp.)

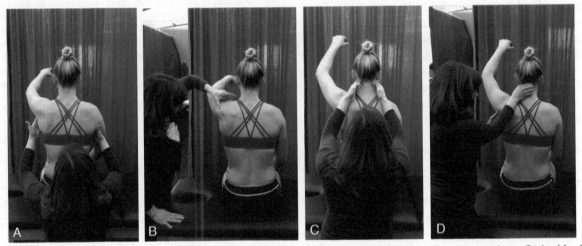

Figure 11-11 Single-arm lift (SAL) in sitting. Palpation for areas of nonoptimal load transfer (NOLT) in the upper quadrant. Optimal load transfer for each region for the task is the reference for determining whether NOLT is occurring. **A,** Palpation of several upper thoracic rings for any loss of neutral ring alignment. There should be no translations of any ring along any axis and no rotation or side bending occurring until the end range of movement. **B,** Palpation of the glenohumeral joint. The humeral head is palpated anteriorly and posteriorly just inferior to the acromion process. The position of the humeral head is noted at rest and during the SAL. The humeral head should remain centered in the glenoid fossa; note any anterior or superior translations during the task. **C,** Bilateral palpation of the articular pillars of the cervical spine is performed to monitor loss of neutral lordosis and any lateral translation or rotation of the cervical segments. As with the thorax, a small amount of extension, rotation, or lateral bending occurs at the very end of arm elevation, but this should be shared throughout the midcervical spine rather than occur excessively at one level. **D,** The clinician performs a correction at C0-C1 with one hand while monitoring the impact of the correction on left translation (NOLT) of the upper thoracic rings with the other hand. (Copyright LJ Lee Physiotherapist Corp.)

and the SAL were originally developed as tests for segmental control in the thorax[8,20] based on the principles of the **active straight-leg raise (ASLR) test,**[46-48] a validated test of failed load transfer in the pelvic girdle in pregnancy-related pelvic girdle pain. As arm function is also supported by optimal load transfer through multiple regions in the upper quadrant, the SAL and PAL tests were soon further developed to include evaluation and manual corrections of NOLT (previously described as "failed load transfer") in other regions of the upper quadrant, including the cervical spine, scapula, and glenohumeral joint to guide the clinician in determining where to focus treatment in patients with upper quadrant symptoms.[8,10] This clinical reasoning process formed the basis for finding the driver in MTA, which recognizes that any task is a whole body task and that the driver for the patient's problem could be in any region, both locally or distally to the problem site. For example, although the ASLR has been researched as a test for patients with pelvic girdle pain, if there is loss of optimal strategies for control of the thoracic rings, thoracic dysfunction could be the driver of a positive ASLR test, "unlocking" of the sacroiliac joints during one leg loading, and pelvic girdle pain.[16]

Because any unilateral limb movement creates a rotational or lateral translation perturbation to the thorax, a single-arm or single-leg lift can highlight the presence of poor strategies for rotational control of the thoracic rings, indicated by the presence of lateral translation or rotation of the ring(s) on loading. When optimal strategies are used, during the SAL, all the thoracic rings will be aligned and stacked in a neutral position relative to the pelvis and the feet, with sufficient space between the rings. There will be no translations (i.e., anterior, posterior, or lateral), rotations, side bending, or increased vertical compression between the rings. During the last stage of full arm elevation, all levels of the thorax should move into extension, ipsilateral rotation, and side bending, with more movement in the upper thorax than in the lower portion. These movements should not occur through range.

The clinician instructs the patient to lift one arm (usually the pain-free side first if ipsilateral symptoms are present), with the arm straight, into elevation through shoulder flexion and then to lower the arm. Next, the patient is instructed to lift the other arm and lower it. The patient then is asked, "Does one arm feel heavier to lift than the other or different to lift than the other?" The clinician notes whether symptoms are produced and also observes which arm looks as if it requires more effort to lift. With regard to effort, the key part of the range to note is from the initiation of movement to the first 70° to 90° of flexion. If one arm is heavier or requires more effort to lift, *finding the driver analysis* is performed using the positive (i.e., the heavy) arm. The assessment and clinical reasoning process to find the driver for the positive SAL is the same as that described earlier for trunk rotation and follows the principles previously outlined. Figures 11-11 and 11-12 illustrate corrections of other regions that can be compared with thoracic ring corrections when ruling in or ruling out a thoracic ring driver for this task.

Neurodynamic Tests and The Thoracic Rings

Because of connections between the nervous system and the thorax, thoracic ring dysfunction can play a role in distal symptoms in the legs or arms. To assess the impact of the thoracic rings on distal symptoms, thoracic ring assessment and correction techniques are applied to neu-

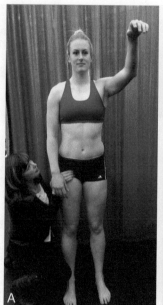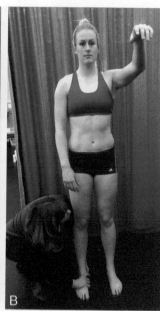

Figure 11-12 Single-arm lift (SAL) performed in standing. This position may be more relevant to the patient's meaningful task and is also an easier position to evaluate the impact of distal areas of nonoptimal load transfer (NOLT) on the ability to perform the task. In relation to testing the hypothesis of a thoracic ring driver for the SAL task, the impact of each of these distal corrections is compared with the impact of the best thoracic ring correction. **A,** The right hip is corrected by applying gentle posterosuperior distraction to the ischial tuberosity to create space to glide the femoral head posteriorly and center the femoral head. The correction is maintained while the SAL is repeated and the impact of the hip correction is compared with other corrections. **B,** The right ankle and foot are corrected by neutralizing perpendicular compression forces across the joints of the foot and creating a more optimal foot "pyramid" by aligning the bones of the foot. When in an optimal pyramid, there will be equal weight bearing on the medial and lateral columns of the foot. The foot correction is maintained while the SAL task is performed and the impact noted. (Copyright LJ Lee Physiotherapist Corp.)

rodynamic tests such as the slump and upper limb neurodynamic tests.[49,50]

Slump Test. The slump test is described in *Orthopedic Physical Asssessment*[42] and by Butler.[49,50] Using thoracic ring palpation, the clinician assesses the thorax and identifies any rings that demonstrate NOLT (i.e., excessive or asymmetrical compression, lateral translation or rotation, side flexion) as the patient moves into the slump position while extending the knee and then dorsiflexing the ankle (Figure 11-13). The side of knee extension and ankle dorsiflexion that reproduce the patient's symptoms is noted, along with any asymmetry or restriction of range of leg movement. The thoracic rings should be in neutral alignment with respect to translation/rotation/side bending and remain stacked throughout the slump test, while moving into flexion and posterior translation. If any thoracic rings demonstrate NOLT during any component of the slump test, the patient is asked to return to the neutral starting position. The clinician then performs thoracic ring corrections and maintains optimal alignment of the ring(s) as the patient repeats the slump test and lower extremity movements that reproduced the symptoms. If

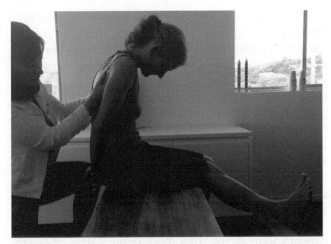

Figure 11-13 Neurodynamics and thoracic ring function: the slump test. The clinician spans several rings with his or her hands to determine whether nonoptimal load transfer (NOLT) occurs as the patient performs the slump test. The overall range of motion of the slump test (i.e., the amount of leg extension and ankle dorsiflexion) is noted, and all thoracic rings are palpated to identify any levels displaying nonoptimal alignment, biomechanics, or control during the task (NOLT). Timing of NOLT relative to initiation of the slump movement is noted, and the rings displaying NOLT the earliest are corrected first while the slump test is repeated. The impact of the correction on leg extension range of motion and on the patient's symptoms are then noted. (Copyright LJ Lee Physiotherapist Corp.)

correction of any of the identified thoracic rings reduces the symptoms and increases the range of motion of the lower extremity movements, the ring or ring complex should be considered a driver for altered neurodynamic function. These findings are compared with the drivers found in MTA; if the same thoracic rings are found to be the driver in MTA, it indicates that treatment to the thoracic rings will address the patient's problem and restore altered neurodynamic function.

Upper Limb Neurodynamic Test. The upper thorax is often involved when the upper limb neurodynamic test result is positive, although all rings should be assessed. The upper limb neurodynamic test as described by Butler[49,50] and in *Orthopedic Physical Assessment*[42] is performed. The clinician then repeats the positive variation of the test (ULNT1 [median], ULNT2 [median], ULNT2 [radial], ULNT3 [ulnar]) while palpating the lateral border of the rings to feel for any lateral translation or other NOLT (Figure 11-14). The ideal response is neutral alignment of all the thoracic rings (until very end range movement) and, specifically, no movement or loss of alignment at one level compared with the rest of the rib cage. The arm is returned to the starting position, and the clinician corrects the ring of interest while the neurodynamic test is repeated. If correction of the thoracic ring reduces the symptoms and increases the

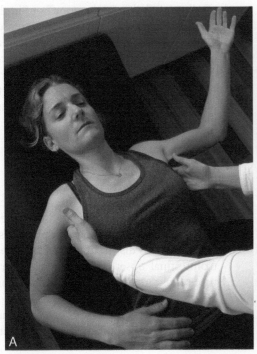
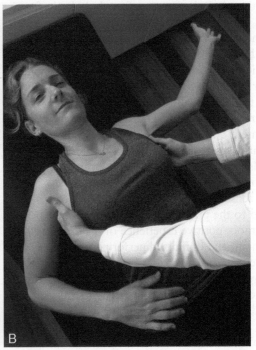

Figure 11-14 Neurodynamics and thoracic ring function: upper limb neurodynamic test. The clinician performs the variations of the upper limb neurodynamic test to determine which variation is positive for symptom reproduction and restricted motion compared with the other side. **A,** Several thoracic rings are then palpated laterally while the positive test is repeated. **B,** If lateral translation or other types of nonoptimal load transfer are palpated of one or more thoracic rings during the test, the clinician returns to the start position and performs a thoracic ring correction and maintains optimal ring alignment while the test is repeated. A significant increase in range of motion and/or decrease in symptoms supports that the thoracic ring(s) may be a driver for the restriction in the neurodynamic test. (Copyright LJ Lee Physiotherapist Corp.)

range of motion of the arm movements, treatment of the thoracic ring should be included to alleviate the distal arm symptoms. These findings are compared with the drivers found in MTA; if the same thoracic rings are found to be the driver in MTA, it indicates that treatment to the thoracic rings will address the patient's problem and restore altered neurodynamic function.

When doing both the slump test and the upper limb neurodynamic tests, thoracic ring correction may only partially improve findings, which indicates that there are neural system vectors connected to the thoracic ring and related to specific ranges of the neurodynamic test. Treatment, in this instance, involves performing "sliders" or other nerve gliding techniques while maintaining the thoracic rings corrected and stacked.

TREATMENT: SUPPORTING OPTIMAL HEALTH | CHANGE STRATEGIES FOR WHOLE BODY FUNCTION AND PERFORMANCE TO CREATE POSITIVE EXPERIENCES OF THE BODY

General Principles

Regardless of where the patient's symptoms present, the indication to treat the thorax, and specific levels of the thorax, is that specific thoracic ring(s) are shown to be a "driver" for the patient's problem in MTA. This provides a clinical rationale that treatment to the thoracic rings will result in positive clinical outcomes for whole body function and will create positive change in the patient's experience of their body. Changing the patient's experience of his or her body during MTA illustrates for the patient how dysfunction of the driver is connected to the problem and is the starting point for educating the patient on how treatment to the driver will resolve the symptoms. When patients experience significant change in symptoms and ease of movement during MTA, new synaptic connections and neural pathways are created.[51] This creates change at multiple levels, not only physically, but emotionally and cognitively, and sets up the potential for training new brain maps. A new sensorial experience during MTA opens the patient's mind to the possibilities and potential that he or she has for a more positive experience of his or her body, better movement, and optimized performance.

If one takes the broader view that "pain is an opinion on the organism's state of health rather than a mere reflexive response to injury,"[52] one needs to alter his or her focus and consider what it means to be "in health" and not only what it means to be "in pain." The World Health Assembly has defined *health* as "a state of complete physical, mental, and social well-being and not merely the absence of disease or infirmity."[53] Restoring health is about more than removing disease; similarly, creating optimal strategies for function and performance is about more than removing pain.

What it means to be "in health" is individually defined. Therefore, changing one's focus from removing pain to restoring optimal health and optimal strategies for function and performance is intrinsically linked to the patient's values and goals. The role of the clinician is to best facilitate and empower patients on their journey to achieve their personal optimal health and function. To do this effectively, one needs to understand not only the patient's pain but also the patient as a person. Jones and Rivett[54] refer to this as "understanding both the problem and the person."

This paradigm requires clinicians to broaden their perspectives and skill sets, and also opens up a wider range of potential and possibility for effecting change.

Ultimately, the goal of treatment is to facilitate the patient's journey toward a more optimal state of health. Changing the way the patient lives and moves in his or her body supports this overarching goal. Any type of treatment intervention should, therefore, support these two interconnected aims:

1. *To teach and train more optimal strategies for posture, movement, and performance.* This requires establishing new brain maps and consolidating new whole body movement patterns into unconscious and automatic behaviors. Training optimal strategies creates maximum efficiency and synergy within and between systems in the body so that the patient experiences ease of movement, confidence in his or her body, and a sense of grace and power during movement. Optimal strategies create beautiful, fluid movement. Athletes will often describe the feeling of "being in the zone" or "in the flow" that comes when a state of relaxed, but intense, movement is attained during periods of high performance.

2. *To change the way the patient experiences his or her body from negative to positive experiences.* Negative experiences include pain and discomfort, as well as other nonpainful but undesired symptoms such as the following:
   - Stiffness
   - Loss of ease of movement
   - Incontinence
   - Feeling of heaviness or pressure
   - Sensation of one side of the body "feeling wrong" or "feeling twisted" compared with the other side
   - Difficulty breathing in certain positions or tasks
   - Other systems disturbances, such as bloating or gastrointestinal upset, hyperhidrosis, altered temperature regulation, paresthesias, altered balance

Research from the pain sciences has established that pain is an output based on multiple different inputs, and the same can be said of other undesirable, negative sensorial experiences of the body. How the clinician focuses the patient's attention can have a significant effect on these experiences. This may be as simple as changing the patient's focus to positive constructs, such as a newly found ease of movement and lighter limbs when walking up stairs.

So how does one facilitate change? How much change is possible? There are many factors that influence the answers to these questions, and they are individually determined. Letting go of old postural and movement strategies and replacing them with new ones requires a multidimensional treatment approach that has an impact on emotional, social, environmental, and cognitive dimensions along with physical factors. The ConnectTherapy Circles of Influence™55 (see Figure 11-7) is a tool that provides a broad framework to organize knowledge from multiple domains and determine the most relevant influencers, both intrinsic and extrinsic, on the patient's current (1) experience of his or her body and (2) strategies for function and performance. The Circles of Influence represent both intrinsic and extrinsic influences to the patient; the amount of overlap and linking between the different circles can change over time and help the clinician adjust priorities and choose appropriate interventions. Impairments related to the underlying drivers are a strong influencer, and it is proposed that the "Primary Driver" is the "way in" to making change in the nervous system, because it has not only physical but also emotional and cognitive impact as a result of use of MTA. Therefore, a key construct of ConnectTherapy and the Thoracic Ring Approach is that if the patient has a primary thoracic ring driver for his or her loss of function and current problem, then treating the thoracic ring driver is the most efficient and effective pathway to reach the goal of restoring optimal health.

TREATING THE THORACIC RING DRIVER

To effectively treat the thoracic rings, the underlying impairments specific to the driving ring(s) must be determined. Although it is widely held that the most common impairment in the thorax is stiffness, resulting from the presence of the rib cage,[4,29,30] minimal data support this belief. As highlighted in previous sections of this chapter, taken as a whole, the evidence supports that the thorax is inherently flexible in nature.[9,11-13] Clinically, multiple patterns of nonoptimal sequencing, force modulation, and synergy between the muscles around the thoracic ring(s), between the 10 thoracic rings, and between the rings and other regions of the body have been observed.[7,16-18] These nonoptimal neuromuscular forces create the appearance of stiffness that is not related to true articular restriction. This proposal is consistent with studies that demonstrate that mobilization and manipulation techniques effect change via neurophysiological mechanisms that alter muscle tone and activity.[56]

Therefore, it is essential that treatment of the thoracic ring driver support the overall goal of creating more optimal patterns of muscle recruitment and muscle balance related to the thoracic rings during function. This is addressed through a multimodal treatment program, ensuring that any cognitive or emotional components are addressed along with physical impairments. In general terms, treatment interventions can be categorized into two objectives (Figure 11-15):

1. *Down-train the existing nonoptimal strategy and create options to set the stage for learning new strategies for posture and movement.* This is accomplished by treating underlying impairments related to the thoracic ring driver and addressing any barriers such as cognitive or emotional factors (see *Potential Barriers & Facilitators* circle within Circles of Influence - Figure 11-7).

2. *Support, teach, and train a new, more optimal strategy for posture and movement.* Exercises are designed

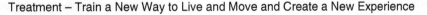

Treatment – Train a New Way to Live and Move and Create a New Experience

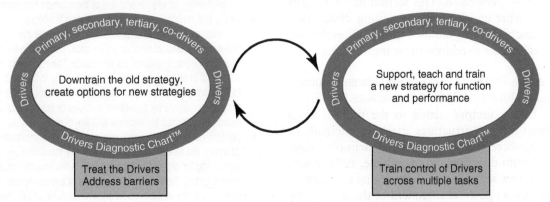

Figure 11-15 Treatment principles for the Thoracic Ring Approach and ConnectTherapy. Treatment interventions for the thoracic ring driver fall into two interconnected objectives that positively influence outcomes in the other. Down-training nonoptimal strategies is best achieved by treating system impairments related to the Primary Driver (see Circles of Influence [see Figure 11-7] where the *Drivers* circle and *Systems* circle intersect). Addressing current barriers, both extrinsic and intrinsic to the patient, will facilitate the rehabilitation process (see *Potential Barriers and Facilitators* circle). New, more optimal strategies are taught by focusing exercise and movement training to the primary driver across a variety of tasks. (Copyright LJ Lee Physiotherapist Corp.)

to train new patterns of neuromuscular activity, balance muscular synergies, and build capacity (strength, endurance) for more optimal control and movement of the driving thoracic ring(s) across a wide variety of movements and loading contexts. To enhance retention of new brain maps, it is important to train control of the thoracic ring driver across multiple tasks and movement patterns to support increased movement variability. The patient's goals and meaningful task also guide exercise prescription, along with the multitude of different movements required for daily function.

These two objectives are not linear; they are interconnected such that success in one domain positively influences outcomes in the other. The treatment program can be conceptualized into three phases that are really part of a continuum of progressive input and reevaluation to move the patient from early rehabilitation to discharge. As the patient progresses from phase 1 to phase 3, there is less reliance on hands-on treatment from the clinician and more active mechanisms for the patient to be self-sufficient in self-treating his or her thoracic ring driver.

Down-Train the Nonoptimal Strategy and Create Options to Train a New Strategy for Posture and Movement

Barriers to training new strategies for movement and control of the driving thoracic rings can originate in multiple different systems. It is common to find impairments that create nonoptimal force vectors around the thoracic rings that reduce mobility and/or reduce options for movement between the rings and between the rings and other regions. Loss of integrity in different systems may present as excessive movement or restricted movement depending on how the neuromuscular system compensates for the loss of integrity.

Therefore, to design the most effective treatment program, further assessment of the specific driving thoracic ring needs to be performed. This section describes tests to determine what impairments are causing dysfunction of the thoracic rings and outlines specific thoracic ring treatment techniques to address those impairments.

Tests for Vectors That Limit Dissociation between Thoracic Rings, Reduce Movement Options, and Reduce Mobility

Nonoptimal force vectors related to the thoracic rings can arise from multiple structures attaching externally or internally anywhere around the three-dimensional ring. Vectors have both direction and magnitude, and the sum of all force vectors acting on the thoracic ring at any point in time determines postural alignment of the ring(s) and behavior of the rings during movement. Most common vectors are related to hypertonic muscles, whereby increased resting tone in muscles attaching to the thoracic ring(s) prevents optimal ring movement (i.e., osteokinematics), dissociation between thoracic rings, and loss of optimal coordination between the thoracic rings and

other regions of the body during function. Hypertonicity in muscles reflects altered neural drive and is therefore an impairment of the neural system and is most effectively addressed using techniques that effect change via neurophysiological mechanisms. Other types of neural system impairments, for example, those related to nerve injury, are possible but less common than neuromuscular vectors.

Impairments in other systems can also create nonoptimal vectors on the thoracic rings, such as adhesions or fibrosis related to the visceral system, muscular system, fascial system (including superficial and deep fascia), dural system, cutaneous system, and articular system (see *Systems Circles* in the Circles of Influence - Figure 11-7).

"Thoracic ring vector analysis"[57] assesses the location and type of system vectors. This technique can be performed in any position and also more statically or through movement ("dynamic vector analysis"). The driving rings (usually two sequential thoracic rings) are manually corrected and stacked into optimal alignment in all planes and dimensions, and the location and quality of the resistance to the correction are evaluated. Different system impairments have characteristic qualities of resistance. Combined with anatomical knowledge, a hypothesis can be made about the type of impairment affecting the thoracic ring, which is confirmed by palpation of the relevant structure while changing the degree of thoracic ring correction and noting if changes in tension in the palpated structure correlate with changes in the degree of thoracic ring correction performed.

Assessment of System Impairments: Thoracic Ring Vector Analysis

- Manually correct and stack the driving thoracic rings in a position related to the meaningful task, and note the following:
  - Quality of the resistance
  - Location of the resistance (relate to anatomy)
  - Point in the neutral zone where the resistance occurs (i.e., beginning, middle, or end feel of the thoracic ring correction)
- As the first resistance to the ring correction is encountered, consider the anatomy of different structures attaching to the thoracic ring and make a hypothesis of what structure could be creating the resistance given the characteristics of the resistance. The most common vectors are neural in origin, presenting as hypertonicity in muscles attaching to the driving thoracic ring(s); these have an elastic quality to the resistance. Palpate for hypertonic fascicles or fascial restriction in muscles that match the location and line of pull that is felt.
- Confirm neuromuscular and myofascial vectors. Increase and decrease the amount of correction on the thoracic rings while monitoring for change in tone/tension in the muscle hypothesized to be creating the vector. If the muscle is a relevant vector to treat, tone/resistance in the muscle should increase and decrease as the degree of thoracic ring correction is increased and decreased.
- Confirm articular vectors with passive accessory vertebral movements (PAVMs), and relate findings to the starting position of the thoracic ring. If PAVM findings change with correction of the ring, it is unlikely to be a true articular impairment; rather, the decreased movement is related to altered neuromuscular forces changing the joint glide findings.

- Neuromuscular vectors (neural impairment creating hypertonicity or excessive activity in muscles attaching to the driving thoracic rings) have an elastic quality to their resistance and typically occur at the beginning and throughout the neutral zone. The line of pull of the resistance is related to the angle and location of the muscle attachment. As vectors are released, the resistance is felt at a later point in the neutral zone.

- Visceral vectors create a resistance from deep inside the thoracic rings, are less linear in quality, and can feel like a broader fullness inside the ring preventing motion anywhere around the inner cavity of the chest. Different viscera create characteristic qualities dependent on their structure; programs such as the visceral curriculum with the Barral Institute (www.barralinstitute.com) provide the practitioner with more specific assessment and treatment skills for visceral system vectors.

- Myofascial vectors resulting from adhesions or lack of sliding of muscle and/or fascial interfaces can occur in any part of the neutral zone and are more easily detected once neuromuscular vectors are released. Myofascial vectors have a fibrotic, scar tissue–like quality and can have a sheet-like dimension to the resistance felt. Similar to neuromuscular vectors, their location is dependent on orientation and direction of specific muscle attachments and fascial planes.

- Articular vectors can result from capsular fibrosis (as consequence of a joint effusion) or joint ankylosis (related to a pathological condition such as ankylosing spondylitis) of the costotransverse and/or zygapophyseal joints. The location of articular vectors is therefore at the most posterior aspect of the thoracic rings and are best assessed after neuromuscular, visceral, and myofascial vectors are released. Articular vectors reduce the size of the neutral zone, but they do not affect the quality of the neutral zone until the end; that is, articular vectors create resistance late in the neutral zone with a firm end feel. They are confirmed with passive accessory joint glides (see volume 1 of this series, *Orthopedic Physical Assessment*[42]).

Treat the Underlying Impairments Related to the Thoracic Ring Driver

Specific treatment to the structures identified as creating the resistance can then be applied. Tools such as specific myofascial and neuromuscular release, dry needling (Figure 11-16), muscle energy, **Release with Awareness (RWA)**,[10,58,59] mobilization, and manipulation can be successful in addressing these impairments (Table 11-1). However, multiple vectors are usually present concurrently, and accurate identification of vectors around the thoracic ring requires a more advanced level of skill. A novel treatment technique, the thoracic ring stack and breathe technique,[57] provides a method to simultaneously release multiple different vectors around and between the thoracic rings. Given the anatomical complexity of possible vectors attaching to the thoracic rings, the stack and breathe technique provides an efficient and effective route of addressing multiple vectors on the rings and can be progressed to dynamic contexts to combine release and neuromuscular training (Figure 11-17).[57]

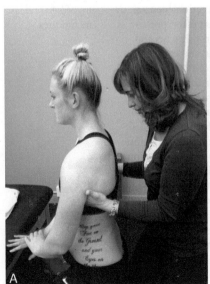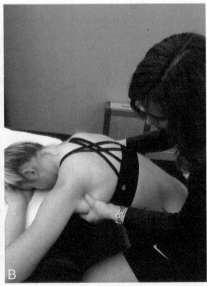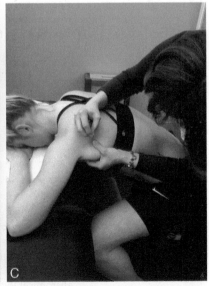

Figure 11-16 Dry needling can be a useful adjunct to release neuromuscular vectors related to the thoracic rings. In cases of long-standing altered alignment and movement patterns in the thoracic rings, muscle adaptation, asymmetries, and imbalances are often present in neighboring regions. For example, in upper thoracic ring drivers, it is common to also find nonoptimal vectors in the shoulder girdle muscles that create vertical compression forces on the rings. To determine the most relevant shoulder girdle muscles to release, the driving thoracic rings are first stacked (**A**) and then the patient positioned such that shoulder range of motion is increased to engage vectors related to the shoulder girdle and the rings. Manual palpation while maintaining the stacked rings identifies hypertonic fascicles in the most relevant muscles (**B**). Once identified, specific neuromuscular release techniques can be applied to the muscle, in this case dry needling to specific fascicles of the left latissimus dorsi (**C**). (Copyright LJ Lee Physiotherapist Corp.)

TABLE **11-1**

Potential System Vectors and Treatment to Restore Mobility of the Thoracic Ring

Type of Vector/System	Location of Resistance around Ring	Quality of Resistance	Point in Neutral Zone Related to Ring Correction	Treatment Techniques
Neuromuscular (neural)	Anywhere around the three-dimensional ring related to anatomical muscular attachments Muscles like the diaphragm create vectors from inside the ring	Elastic resistance that can be modulated with speed of correction force application; has a linear line of pull that is consistent with anatomy of hypertonic muscle fascicle orientation	Present throughout the neutral zone, commonly early and felt at initiation of ring correction Onset of resistance becomes later during ring correction as more vectors are released Resistance from vectors can change dependent on task and position of body/orientation of thoracic rings relative to upper and lower extremities, lumbopelvic region	• Stack and breathe[57] • Stack and breathe combined with specific muscle release • Release with Awareness (RWA)[10] to specific muscles • Breath work (focused, vary positions to address different vectors) • Manipulation • Oscillatory mobilization • Dry needling • Acupuncture • Muscle energy
Visceral	Resistance felt within the rings, at any point around the three-dimensional ring depending on anatomical attachments of related viscera	Less linear, more general fullness deep inside the ring	Throughout the neutral zone, can be felt at any point during ring correction Can change dependent on task and position of body	• Stack and breathe[57] • Visceral techniques • Breath work (use inversion postures to change relationship of viscera to gravity and the diaphragm)
Myofascial	Anywhere around the three-dimensional ring related to anatomical muscular and fascial attachments	Fibrous quality that can be linear or sheet-like and does not change with speed of application of ring correction	Can be felt at any point in the ring correction/neutral zone; often present later in the neutral zone and easiest to discern quality once neuromuscular and/or visceral vectors are released Can change dependent on task and position of body/orientation of thoracic rings relative to upper and lower extremities, lumbopelvic region	• Stack and release[57] • Specific fascial or myofascial release techniques
Articular	Farthest posterior aspect of rings, close to midline (related to anatomical location of zygapophyseal and costotransverse joints)	Firm end feel; rapid increase in resistance to movement that does not change with speed	Occurs at end of neutral zone/ring correction and easiest to identify once other types of vectors are released Presence of vector does not change relative to body position or task	• Specific end range sustained joint mobilization

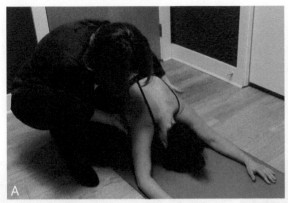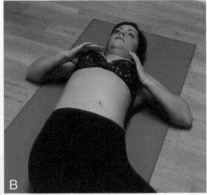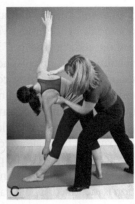

Figure 11-17 Thoracic ring stack and breathe.[57] This technique can be performed by the therapist in combination with specific muscle releases (e.g., the serratus anterior) or taught to patients as a self-release technique. The driving thoracic rings are corrected and manually controlled while different breathing patterns and movements of the trunk and extremities are used to tension different vectors acting on the rings. Over multiple cycles of deep breaths and through movement, the relevant vectors are released, creating a platform to train new muscle recruitment patterns. **A,** Thoracic ring stack and breathe of rings 3/4 while moving through child's pose to release vectors between the shoulder girdle/arms and the driving thoracic rings. **B,** Self-stack and breathe of rings 3/4. The patient self-corrects two sequential thoracic rings on opposite sides and uses a bent knee lift or head lift to check that he or she has corrected the desired rings (i.e., the effort to lift the leg or the head should be easier with the driving ring corrected). Over several breath cycles, the patient maintains the ring correction and moves the pelvis/hips into rotation to release vectors between the driving thoracic rings and the lumbopelvic–hip region. **C,** Dynamic thoracic ring stack and breathe. The driving thoracic rings are corrected while the patient moves into a functional task and breathes in different patterns. The clinician can modify this to become a training exercise for thoracic ring control by modulating the degree of support and correction provided, giving primarily sensory input and less manual correction support so that the patient actively controls the thoracic rings during movement. (Copyright LJ Lee Physiotherapist Corp.)

Clinical Reasoning to Decide Which Neuromuscular Vectors are Relevant to Treat

- Patients presents with many hypertonic and overactive muscles in the trunk. The most clinically relevant muscles to release are the following:
  - Those who display increased tone at rest and further *increase* in tone when correction of the thoracic ring driver is performed
  - Those who display early or dominant activity during meaningful screening task analysis and the timing of muscle activation correlates to nonoptimal load transfer (NOLT) of the driving thoracic ring
- Muscles that exhibit *reduced* tone or activity when the driving thoracic rings are corrected are muscles that are active to counter the forces created by the driving ring and do not need to be treated. Treating these muscles have the potential to make the driver worse. For example, in the case of a fourth thoracic ring driver translating left and rotating right, activity in the lower right external oblique (EO) muscle increases to counter the right rotation and can be the source of a runner's "stitch." Releasing the right EO muscle will enhance the right rotation force generated from the fourth thoracic ring driver and will not effectively treat the problem.

Benefits of Thoracic Ring Stack and Breathe Treatment Technique

- It simultaneously releases multiple vectors three-dimensionally around the driving thoracic rings.
- Clinician can control and maintain optimal relationships between two sequential rings (i.e., three vertebrae) and release vectors between "glued" rings, thereby preventing inadvertently making one ring more nonoptimal while correcting a ring above or below that is held by intercostal tone

- Treatment efficacy is not dependent on accurate identification of location and type of vector.
- It can be combined with specific neuromuscular release and myofascial release (ring stack and release).
- It indirectly releases visceral vectors (i.e., diaphragmatic movement creates movement of the viscera).
- It can be used in any position and dynamically with multiple movement variations (see Figure 11-17) to release vectors between the thoracic rings and other regions to combine release and exercise training for integrated treatment.

Thoracic Ring Stack and Breathe: Basic Technique

Patient Position. Multiple positions and postures are used related to different aims. In irritable, sensitized systems, supine is chosen. Supine also provides a position of greater mechanical advantage to release stronger vectors around the rings, but different vectors may be present in upright postures such as sitting or standing. It is usually necessary as treatment progresses to use postures and movements of the trunk and extremities in order to release longer vectors between the thoracic rings and the lumbopelvic–hip region, the upper extremities, and the lower extremities. Determine a loading task that is relatively heavy or has decreased ease compared with the other side (e.g., bent knee lift, SAL, head lift).

Technique. The two sequential thoracic rings identified as the primary driver are fully corrected and aligned in three dimensions, stacking them so that the intraring and inter-ring rotation/sidebending/translation are neutralized and the center of each ring is aligned with the midline of the body. This is done by gently introducing a vector of correction and adjusting the next input for correction based on the response felt in the rings. Verbal cues are used to facilitate relaxation and "letting go" of specific muscles to facilitate correction of the rings. Once the clinician has stacked the rings, accuracy of the ring correction should be checked by ensuring it improves a loading task such as limb movement, a squat, a head lift, or a bent knee lift. The position of the rings is then maintained while deep breaths are cued into different patterns (i.e., lateral costal, apical, belly breath, breath between the scapulae). The pattern of breathing that creates the greatest pull and resistance to maintaining the ring correction is identified. The breath pattern is repeated over three to four deep breaths while the ring correction is maintained throughout. As the muscles release around the rings, the resistance to correction will decrease. The correction pressure is gently released and ring alignment, inter-ring neutral zone glide, and control of the ring are reassessed during the screening task or meaningful task.

Multiple variations of the stack and breathe technique can be used depending on the phase of treatment (see "Support, Teach, and Train a New Strategy" later in this chapter), the specific vectors affecting the rings, the need to release longer vectors between the driving rings and other regions, and treatment aims (see Figure 11-17). These include the following:

1. "Releasing of the vectors" between the rings and other regions: upper extremities, lower extremities, lumbopelvic–hip complex, head and neck. Movement of the limbs or trunk is induced to engage new vectors, that is, until the point where increased resistance to the thoracic ring correction is felt. Movement is then paused, and stack and breathe is performed in the new position until the vectors release and then greater range of movement is performed to engage the next vectors. Movements are chosen related to goals for exercise training and functional tasks; releases are graded to allow for training new strategies for control as new range of motion is gained.

Variations of Thoracic Ring Stack and Breathe Technique to Release Longer Vectors and Visceral Vectors

- Supine, knees move to right or left to induce rotation of the lumbopelvic–hip complex relative to the rings, repeat to the other side for balance (see Figure 11-17, *B*)
- Sitting with head rotation; both right and left rotation
- Supine knees bent to legs straight
- On decline bench or inversion table to alter relationship of viscera to diaphragm motion
- High kneeling → 4 point → child's pose (see Figure 11-17, *A*)
- Hands on wall → increase arm elevation range of motion with sequential releases, change shoulder abduction/adduction, use internal/external rotation to engage different vectors
- Forward fold

- Downward dog in yoga, starting with table dog (Figure 11-18) and progressing to modified downward dog (Figure 11-19), then to weight bearing on bent elbows instead of hands (dolphin pose in yoga, Figure 11-20)
- Unilateral high kneeling lunge ± trunk rotation
- Through any meaningful task (dynamic ring stack and breathe) (see Figure 11-17, *C*)

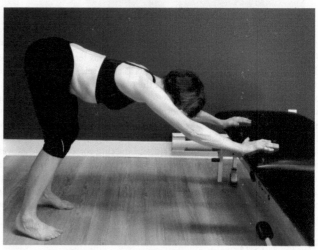

Figure 11-18 "Table dog" exercise, a phase 2 exercise to train control of the thoracic rings in neutral while dissociating and integrating with shoulder girdle control in closed-chain positions. The thoracic ring stack and breathe technique can be performed by stacking the driving rings in standing and maintaining their position while the patient moves into the position. As resistance to ring correction is noted, the movement is paused and breathing and manual release are used to release specific vectors before moving into range requiring greater shoulder elevation. Once vectors are released, the patient is able to train control of the rings in this exercise. (Copyright LJ Lee Physiotherapist Corp.)

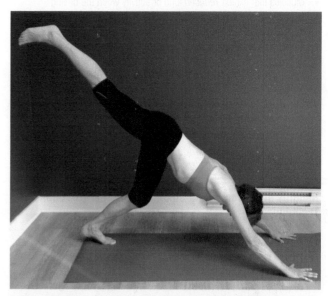

Figure 11-19 Three-point modified downward dog. To increase the challenge to thoracic ring control, one leg is extended from the downward dog position. This is a closed-chain phase 2 inversion exercise. (Copyright LJ Lee Physiotherapist Corp.)

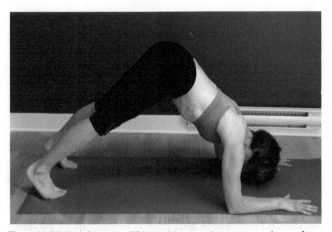

Figure 11-20 Dolphin pose. This position requires greater release of vectors between the thoracic rings and the upper extremities. The thoracic ring stack and breathe technique can be used to release vectors with the forearms in a similar position on the wall before progressing the release and then training into this position. (Copyright LJ Lee Physiotherapist Corp.)

2. "Self-stack and breathe." Patients are taught in supine how to self-correct their driving rings and use trunk rotation and lower extremity movements to self-release vectors as part of their self-management strategies and in preparation for training exercises.
3. "Stack and breathe combined with manual release." The stack and breathe technique can be combined with the manual release of specific vectors using trigger point pressure and patient cues for muscles such as the intercostals, serratus anterior, pectoralis minor, external oblique, and shoulder girdle muscles affected by altered ring function and position. The rings are maintained in their stacked position while hypertonic bands are palpated. The patient is made aware of holding patterns and is taught how to decrease activity in these hypertonic muscles; in this way the patient learns how to down-train the key muscles that are part of the old strategy. Myofascial release can also be added as the hypertonic fascicles decrease in tone (stack and release).
4. "Dynamic stack and breathe." This combines release and training of new strategies simultaneously, as partial or full correction of thoracic rings is maintained during dynamic movement. This can also facilitate strength and endurance training in superficial muscles that have deficits from long-standing altered ring function, which then facilitates recruitment of segmental ring control muscles.

Specific Neuromuscular Vector Releases

The thoracic ring stack and breathe technique and its variations are very effective at releasing vectors around the thoracic rings. However, after treating a patient with the stack and breathe technique, there may be one or two more dominant vectors related to specific muscles. As long as intercostal hypertonicity and glued rings have been released to dissociate the driving rings, then specific muscle releases can be performed. Techniques can include dry needling, Release with Awareness,[10,58,59] manipulation, mobilization, and other types of release techniques that create a change in muscle tone via neurophysiological mechanisms.

Release with Awareness

The principles of the Release with Awareness technique,[10,58,59] as they are applied to the thorax and scapula, are as follows:

1. The driving thoracic rings are manually stacked to identify the most relevant muscles to release. The area of increased tone (i.e., hypertonic fascicle or trigger point) is palpated with gentle pressure.
2. To release the erector spinae muscles, the driving ring is positioned so as to shorten the origin and insertion of the specific fascicle of the erector spinae muscle that is hypertonic (e.g., spinalis, longissimus, iliocostalis). For scapular release, the scapula is moved to shorten the origin and insertion of the hypertonic muscle. As the clinician passively shortens the muscle, the afferent input from the primary annulospiral ending in the intrafusal muscle spindle decreases, and the spinal cord responds by decreasing the efferent output to the extrafusal muscle fiber. This is felt as a "softening of tone" in the trigger point. The clinician waits for this to occur (up to 30-45 seconds).
3. The clinician cues the patient to "release," or soften, the muscle with verbal and manual cues to "let go." This step is critical to the awareness training, and it is the point where learning occurs.
4. The scapula or thoracic ring is moved in various combinations to maximally release the muscle as the clinician cues the patient (with words and touch) to be aware of the softening and release. The key is to use words that encourage the patient to let go and stop holding rather than to "do something." As greater release occurs, the clinician can increase the amount of correction of the driving thoracic rings, and new vectors will be engaged.

   If there is a specific muscle that creates recurring vectors on a driving thoracic ring, home exercises for self-release with awareness can be designed and prescribed for specific muscles around the thoracic ring, such as the pectoralis minor, the intercostals, latissimus dorsi, and serratus anterior muscles.
5. The patients' homework is to recreate this sensation of letting go. As they practice at home, they quickly remember and learn how to stop bracing. They also learn that they can control and reduce the pain when the bracing is decreased. This is positive reinforcement for changing their nonoptimal strategy.

Manipulation and the Thorax

Manipulation, or high-velocity low-amplitude thrust (HVLAT) techniques, are often used in the thorax. Notably, the thorax has been reported to be the most commonly manipulated area of the spine,[60] and there is increasing research interest in the effectiveness of thoracic manipulation in the treatment of pain in neighboring regions, such as for patients with neck pain[3] and shoulder pain.[2] Manipulation to the thoracic spine is perceived to be significantly safer than manipulation to the cervical spine, and as such, it is being considered as an alternative treatment for neck pain in place of cervical spine thrust manipulation. However, serious adverse effects from thoracic manipulation, including herniation of thoracic discs,[61] epidural bruising,[62] and esophageal rupture,[63] have been reported in the literature. It is the author's clinical experience that adverse responses to thoracic manipulation occur when excessive posterior translation is used as a manipulation vector. Instead, the primary vector for thoracic spine facet joint manipulation should be in a cranial direction, with a slight posterior vector to gap the joint. Posterior translation in the thoracic spine has no bony barrier and therefore excessive amplitude or force combined with posterior translation is likely to injure the thoracic disc.

In terms of the clinical decision as to *when* to manipulate the thorax and *what levels* to manipulate, the clinical reasoning approach of the Thoracic Ring Approach supports that the thoracic joints should be manipulated only if the thorax is the driver for the patient's problem as assessed with MTA. Thoracic manipulation affects change in muscle tone (i.e., neuromuscular vectors) via neurophysiological mechanisms and, therefore, will most likely result in changes in muscles innervated by the thoracic segment being manipulated. As discussed earlier, there are many nonoptimal vectors that can affect the driving thoracic ring, but not all of these muscles receive their innervation from the thorax. These muscles include the thoracic erector spinae (T1-T12), the intercostals (T1-T12), and the abdominal muscles (T7-L1). Many patients have experienced the significant change in trunk rotation range of motion when the large thoracic longissimus and the abdominal muscles decrease in resting tone after a manipulation. However, if thoracic ring vector analysis indicates that the strongest vectors around the ring are around the lateral and anterior aspect of the ring(s), then release of the posterior erector spinae vectors via upper thoracic spine manipulation has the potential to relatively enhance the effect of lateral and anterior vectors, thereby making the thoracic rings functionally worse and increasing symptoms. Furthermore, in terms of intercostal tone, because of their complex neural drive related to breathing, manipulation of the related vertebral segment may or may not change intercostal tone around the entire thoracic ring. Vector analysis of the two sequential rings is required to determine whether the manipulation produced the desired release effect. If thoracic ring vector analysis is used consistently as a premanipulation and postmanipulation test, over time, the skilled practitioner will acquire a library of "characteristic vector resistance patterns" that are effectively released by

manipulation and those that are not. In this way, the chance of adverse reactions will be decreased, and more effective treatment choices can be made based on a collection of clinical tests and a clinical reasoning process.

Tests for Integrity of Systems Related to the Thoracic Ring

If the patient's story and injury history suggest that there may be loss of integrity in any system, specific tests for integrity need to be performed. The nature and degree of loss of integrity will inform expectations about rate of recovery, grading, and progressing treatment, and potential for future recurrences and thus is important to establish early on in the process.

Passive Integrity of the Articular System

Tests for integrity of the articular system are also known as passive stability tests. In the presence of underlying loss of passive integrity, different patterns of neuromuscular compensation are possible. Depending on how the nervous system modulates resting muscle tone and alters recruitment patterns to support deficiency in articular structures, patients may present with either increased or decreased mobility when doing active range of motion tests and/or passive articular mobility tests. In cases in which neuromuscular vectors are present, these must first be released before performing stability tests in order to get a valid test result. Hypertonic muscles can result in a false-negative finding (e.g., consider the case of hamstring spasm with an underlying third degree anterior cruciate ligament [ACL] tear).

Once hypertonic muscles are released or relaxed, several signs are consistent with a loss of passive integrity of the anterior or posterior articulations of the thoracic ring:

- Marked altered positional findings (nonoptimal alignment) of the thoracic ring or specific bones of the thoracic ring relative to the ring above and below, especially in translational components (posterior, anterior, or lateral translation)
- Excessive movement of the ring or bones of the ring on active and passive mobility tests

However, it is important to recognize that significant loss of optimal neuromuscular control and decreased muscular capacity in the segmental muscles around the ring can also be consistent with the aforementioned findings. If the patient's story is not consistent with injury to the articular structures, then the likely underlying impairment is one of neuromuscular control and/or muscle capacity (e.g., cross-sectional area, endurance, and/or strength).

To rule in or rule out a loss of passive integrity, specific articular integrity tests are performed; these have been described elsewhere.[22,64] These are tests of multiple articular structures to resist translation in nonphysiological planes. An analysis of the amplitude and quality of both the neutral and elastic zones of motion is performed with the joints and rings initially in a neutral position (i.e., not rotated, flexed or extended). An increase in the size of the neutral zone combined with a soft end feel are characteristic of a segment with a loss of integrity in the passive system (see volume 2 of this series, *Scientific Foundations and Principles of Practice in Musculoskeletal Rehabilitation*, Chapters 19 and 24). The specific structures affected depend on the direction of the translation applied. If an increased neutral zone and soft end feel are noted with the joint in a neutral position, a loss of passive integrity in structures related to the directional restraints is supported. The tests can be repeated with the facet joints in the close packed position (i.e., full extension) or under full posterior ligamentous tension (i.e., full flexion), in which the size of the neutral zone should be markedly reduced and the end feel firm. The presence of an increased neutral zone and soft end feel in full extension or flexion confirms that more significant laxity exists in the articular (and connecting fascial) support system (i.e., a loss of passive integrity).

Data from resection studies indicate the importance of the thoracic disc as a key restraint for passive stability, along with the costovertebral joints.[9,30,65] Notably, at the segmental level, loss of rib articulations does not affect mobility until the disc is also resected.[66] These findings have implications for treatment decisions involving interventions such as prolotherapy to the facet joints and costotransverse joints (discussed later). A specific adaptation of the initially proposed lateral translation stability test[22,64] assesses lateral integrity of the posterior structures of the thoracic ring and is designed to bias forces through the head of the rib into the thoracic intervertebral disc (Figure 11-21).

A dynamic component can be added to any of the passive articular integrity tests in several ways. In the sitting position, the patient can be asked to lift the arms against the clinician's resistance. The stability test is repeated while the muscles are active. If the segmental deep and multisegmental superficial muscles are working synergistically, the results of the stability test will be negative (i.e., translation is controlled). If the deep segmental muscles of the ring are not working appropriately, even with contraction of the superficial muscles, the result of the stability test is positive (i.e., translation is not controlled). Once the patient has been taught how to recruit the deep segmental stabilizing muscles, the stability test can be repeated with a precontraction of the segmental muscles in any position. With a low-force contraction of the local stabilizing muscles (i.e., 10%-20% of the maximum voluntary contraction), the neutral zone should be reduced to zero and produce a solid resistance to the translation applied in the stability test. This resistance to translation suggests a good prognosis for recovery of dynamic control of the thoracic ring even in the presence of decreased passive integrity. A progressive training program for tho-

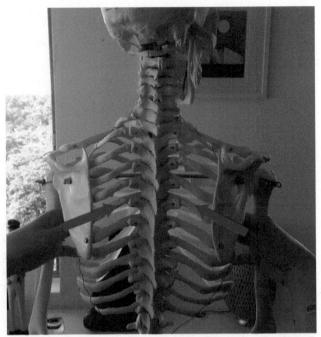

Figure 11-21 Intraring integrity with a focus on posterior articular structures: lateral translation. Patient position: Compare findings in both sitting and prone. Clinician position and palpation: At the ring of interest, the left hand translates the left half of the ring (i.e., left rib) medially into the rib–vertebrae–disc interface at the spinal segment and stabilizes the segment (*left arrow*). The other hand translates the right half of the ring (i.e., right rib) medially into the rib–vertebrae–disc interface (left translation) (*right arrow*) and notes any increase in amplitude of the neutral zone or soft end feel. The test is repeated with the right hand stabilizing the right half of the ring segment and the left hand testing the amplitude and quality of the end feel to right translation. (Copyright LJ Lee Physiotherapist Corp.)

racic ring control across a variety of movement tasks and contexts is essential for successful return to activities (see later discussion). However, given the presence of the underlying loss of passive integrity, this subgroup of patients is more likely to experience recurrent episodes of pain and dysfunction, depending on their activities and postures, and intermittent treatment may be necessary to settle flare-ups.

Treatment of Thoracic Ring Driver with an Underlying Loss of Passive Articular Integrity

DOWN-TRAIN THE OLD STRATEGY, CREATE OPTIONS FOR NEW STRATEGIES, ADDRESS BARRIERS
- Systems Circle—Neural
  - Release hypertonic muscles around the thoracic ring creating excessive compression on articular structures.
- Systems Circle—Articular
  - Perform specific articular integrity tests.
  - Teach recruitment of deep segmental ring muscles and determine their ability to control positive articular integrity tests.

SUPPORT, TEACH, AND TRAIN A NEW STRATEGY FOR FUNCTION AND PERFORMANCE

- Tape the driving rings.
- Systems Circle—Neural and Muscular
  - Train control of the thoracic ring across multiple tasks and in diverse contexts (Table 11-2).
- Circles of Influence—Potential Barriers and Facilitators
  - Educate about potential activities and postures that could overload patient's capacity to control the underlying loss of integrity.
  - Provide self-management strategies, including self-release and reset exercises; self-check movements help determine whether and when they need to seek treatment.

If the neutral zone does not change with segmental muscle contraction, the clinician has several scenarios to consider. First, the patient may not be sufficiently recruiting the segmental muscles. Second, the segmental muscles (e.g., multifidus and intercostals) may have insufficient

bulk to produce a sufficient increase in tension in the fascial system to change the resistance to translation. Change in fascial tension is one mechanism by which the muscle system changes compression across joints.[67-69] In this case, a palpable decrease in the bulk and resting tone of the segmental muscles will be noted. Again, a well-designed and prescribed training program is an essential component for successful treatment. As the exercise rehabilitation program is progressed and muscle bulk increases, the resultant increased fascial tension may increase passive support sufficiently to produce a negative result on the stability test.

Prolotherapy has been proposed to be a tool for remediation of significant passive articular deficiencies. One *note of caution* in these cases is to consider that of the posterior articulations, the thoracic intervertebral disc, and the costovertebral articulations provide the most significant contribution to passive stability.[30,65,66] If prolotherapy is performed to the zygapophyseal and costotransverse joints

TABLE **11-2**

Exercise Categories for Thoracic Ring Exercise Progressions and Program Design

Exercise Category	Description and Exercise Examples
Segmental control *Intraring and inter-ring*	Deep muscles; optimal recruitment evidenced by change in ring position and control in response to verbal cues and without superficial muscle activity (establish in *Phase 1*).
Inter-regional control *Thoracic rings—head/neck*	*Phase 2:* Maintain neutral thoracic ring stacking and dissociate from head movements (e.g., seated head rotation, side flexion) *Phase 3:* Concurrent movement of thoracic rings and head into ipsilateral and contralateral rotation patterns; more complex loading between thoracic rings and head in rotation (e.g., triangle pose in yoga)
Inter-regional control *Thoracic rings—shoulder girdle: open kinetic chain*	*Phase 2:* Maintain neutral thoracic ring stacking and dissociate from shoulder girdle movement (e.g., supine horizontal shoulder abduction, triceps extensions, bilateral elevation) *Phase 3:* Dissociate thoracic ring control from shoulder girdle in rotation/side flexion/lateral translation patterns; both congruent and incongruent from other region (e.g., bow and arrow with pulley, lateral medicine ball throws)
Inter-regional control *Thoracic rings—shoulder girdle: closed kinetic chain*	*Phase 2:* Maintain neutral thoracic ring stacking with upper extremity weight bearing: wall lands, wall ball roll-outs (Figure 11-24) wall push-ups, bench push-ups; include movements that require movement of neutral thoracic rings through fixed weight-bearing arm (e.g., 4-point kneeling transition to modified downward dog in yoga (Figure 11-22), then moving in and out of plank—dynamic) *Phase 3:* Dissociate thoracic ring control from shoulder girdle in rotation/side flexion/lateral translation patterns (e.g., wall "plank" open into unilateral wall side "plank") Inversion postures are key to train vertical loading capacity in the thorax (e.g., downward dog modified with knees bent → wall handstands → handstand push-ups on wall)
Inter-regional control *Thoracic rings-lumbopelvic-hip (trunk control)*	*Phase 2:* Maintain neutral trunk position during lower extremity challenges (e.g., squats, split squats, forward-backward lunges → progress to deep lateral lunges, diagonal lunges, star lunges) → progress to combined upper/lower extremity challenges (e.g., pulley reach patterns, unilateral pulley resistance to forward lunges, front medicine ball throws) *Phase 3:* Dissociate thoracic ring control in rotation/side flexion patterns—both congruent and incongruent from other region (e.g., walking lunges with contralateral trunk rotation, rotational pulley patterns [e.g., wood chop])
Postural equilibrium *Thoracic rings—feet (base of support)*	Use challenges to postural equilibrium and trunk control in coronal plane (i.e., lateral perturbations) while ensuring optimal thoracic ring alignment and control (e.g., asymmetrical resistance with tubing or pulley applied to the trunk/ upper extremity/ lower extremity during sagittal plane movements like forward lunges, deep lateral lunges, star lunges, lateral hops)
Thoracic spring	Ensure thoracic ring control while maintaining vertical space and without bracing or rigidity: jump squats, front-back hops, lateral hops, skipping

when the disc is the most significant underlying impairment, the existing loss of disc integrity will be functionally amplified as a result of the relative increase in passive support to the other structures. In this case, symptoms will be exacerbated and functional ability diminished. Therefore, careful consideration of the structures involved is needed before implementation of tools such as prolotherapy.

Surgical intervention in the thorax is indicated only in extreme and severe cases when cord compromise is a risk.

Articular Fixation of the Costotransverse or Zygapophyseal Joints

When a force is applied to the joints of the thorax sufficient to stretch or tear the articular ligaments, the muscles respond to prevent dislocation and further trauma to the joint. The resulting spasm may fix the joint in an abnormal resting position, and marked asymmetry may be present. This type of articular "fixation"[70] can occur in any movement direction. It is common with trauma involving excessive rotation of the unrestrained thorax or when rotation of the thorax is forced against a fixed rib cage (e.g., seat belt injury). Another common scenario is an impact force to a specific rib, such as can occur in contact sports. This results in a fixation of the costotransverse joint.

The degree of underlying loss of integrity of the articular structures is variable and can be minimal or significant, but the consistent presenting feature is excessive compression from neuromuscular vectors, and the clinician will note marked altered positional findings and joint restriction. Resistance on thoracic ring vector analysis depends on whether the zygapophyseal (facet) or costotransverse joint is fixated. If the facet joint is fixated, the clinician can initiate ring correction via motion of the rib, but as the vertebral component is engaged, there will be a rapid increase in resistance from the farthest posteromedial aspect of the ring on one side of the ring. If the costotransverse joint is fixated, there will be early and rapid increase in resistance to ring correction on one half of the ring, again coming from the posterior aspect of the ring on one side. On passive mobility testing, the neutral zone of movement cannot be felt, and a hard, nonbony end feel is present.

Initial treatment must include techniques to release the neuromuscular vectors and restore articular mobility; high-velocity low-amplitude manipulation (grade 5 mobilization) treatment (HVLAT)[22] techniques to gap the specific fixated joint can provide an effective neurophysiological release. Treatment for this patient that focuses on exercise without first addressing the fixation of the joint tends to be ineffective and commonly increases symptoms. Conversely, if treatment includes only manual therapy (i.e., joint mobilization, manipulation, or muscle energy techniques), relief tends to be temporary, and dependence on the health care practitioner to provide the manual correction is common. This impairment requires a multimodal therapeutic approach to management that includes manual therapy to decompress and align the thoracic rings. It is essential that release techniques be followed by assessment of articular integrity, taping to support the thoracic ring, and training for neuromuscular control and capacity (i.e., endurance and strength) across a variety of functional tasks (see later discussion).

Anterior Joints of the Thoracic Ring

Anteriorly, the costochondral and sternochondral joints can become excessively loaded and a source of localized anterior chest pain. Consider the impact on these joints when there are asymmetrical rotational and compressive loads related to nonoptimal function of the three-dimensional thoracic ring. Altered forces between the rings and the shoulder girdle can also medially compress the anterior joints, and the combination of medial compression and rotational torque through the ring can exhaust the adaptive potential of these structures under loads and create an acutely painful articulation. Treatment of these cases involves the approach as outlined earlier, that is, a clinical reasoning process to determine where the underlying driver is and then treatment to the driver to restore more optimal loading through the anterior articulations. It is important to note that the driving thoracic rings may be one or more levels above or below the painful level; thus the function of the entire thorax needs to be considered in the context of the meaningful task in order to determine which thoracic rings to treat.

The anterior articulations can also be damaged by blunt force injury, creating a loss of passive integrity. Acute management of these injuries is essential to prevent a chronic passive integrity problem. These joints may be fixated or subluxed as a result of the trauma, but they are not treated with manipulation. Instead, thoracic ring vector analysis and the ring stack and breathe technique are used to release neuromuscular vectors around the three-dimensional ring and restore optimal relationships between the ring and the rings above and below. Balancing forces around the ring creates an optimal position for the injured anterior structures to heal. Tape is used to support the anterior joints and thoracic ring in optimal alignment to reduce stress on the injured structures and optimize formation of a functional scar.

SUPPORT, TEACH, AND TRAIN A NEW STRATEGY FOR MOVEMENT AND CONTROL OF THE THORACIC RINGS ACROSS MULTIPLE TASKS

Evaluation of neuromuscular strategies for the thorax needs to include segmental control (i.e., intraring and inter-ring), inter-regional control, and control of postural equilibrium.[9,39] As patients learn how to release and down-train specific muscles around the thoracic rings, skills needed to recruit new muscles are taught concurrently. Exercise prescription is based on control impairments found on assessment. Based on anatomical attachments and research from other areas of the spine, it has been proposed that the deep segmental muscles such as thoracic multifidus/rotatores and the intercostals are architecturally suited to control intraring and inter-ring motion.[71] These clinical proposals are consistent with studies showing that the CNS exhibits differential control of the deep and superficial thoracic paraspinal muscles for control of opposite rotational perturbations.[32-34] Imagery, visualization, and sensory cues combined with specific thoracic ring taping (Figure 11-23) are used to decrease activity in hypertonic, overactive muscles around the thoracic ring, and facilitate recruitment of the deep ring control muscles. This new strategy for thoracic ring control is progressively integrated across a variety of movement patterns and relevant loads to increase capacity and robustness, and to train synergistic patterns with superficial, multisegmental muscles connecting the thoracic rings to other regions.[7,10,17,18,20,28]

Movement patterns and exercises for the thoracic rings can be organized into different categories (see Table 11-2). As the rehabilitation program is progressed, the clinician should ensure that multiple categories of exercises are incorporated to ensure there is diversity in challenges to thoracic ring loading and control. Task variability enhances retention and consolidation of new brain maps.

Training new strategies for thoracic ring control and movement is organized into three phases of treatment progression. Each phase has different features and aims as outlined here.

Phase 1: Establish A New Strategy to Control the Driving Thoracic Rings - Optimize Recruitment Between Deep and Superficial Thoracic Ring Muscles

Principle: Train a new strategy for control of the driver by creating awareness of previous non-optimal neuromuscular patterns and teaching new recruitment patterns around the driver. Find the best "ring stack" cue or combination of cues that changes control of the rings during the initiation of simple, low load tasks so that the patient can compare the impact of the old strategy to the new strategy. Best positions are those where the thorax is symmetrical (e.g., supine lying). Side lying is too challenging for early progressions due to lateral translation forces on the rings.

- Phase 1 should last approximately the first 1 to 2 weeks.
- Release nonoptimal vectors on the driving rings.
- Establish whether any underlying loss of passive integrity is present.
- Address other barriers (e.g., sympathetic system sensitization can be treated with acupuncture and breathing exercises to increase parasympathetic system activity).
- Teach self-release techniques (e.g., self-stack and breathe, specific muscle release techniques).
- Establish best "ring stack" cue. This best "driver cue" results in a more optimal balance of deep and superficial muscle activity around the driving thoracic rings. Determine best position to practice the "ring stack" cue for intraring and inter-ring control in simple tasks that will act as a "Cue Check" for the patient (discussed later). (SAL, squat, one leg standing, supine bent knee fall-outs, supine arm abduction). This cue may need to be modified over the first few sessions as the patient learns and adapts.
- Train awareness and confidence in ability to release vectors and activate deep ring muscles to change the patient's subjective effort in simple task performance; use sensory feedback and mirrors.
- Train endurance of the new ring control strategy (best "Driver Cue") (aim for 3 sets of 10-15 repetitions, practice twice a day).

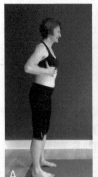
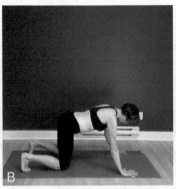
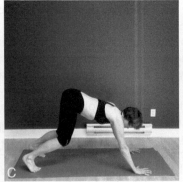
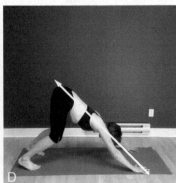

Figure 11-22 Examples of phase 2 exercises to train control of the thoracic rings in neutral while dissociating and integrating with shoulder girdle control in closed-chain and inversion postures. Inversion postures are essential to increase the ability to sustain vertical loading in the thorax. Note that the thoracic ring stack and breathe technique can be performed by the therapist in any of these positions by maintaining full correction of the driving rings and pausing to perform release and breathing at points through range when new or stronger vectors are felt on the rings. **A,** The patient provides sensory input to facilitate the best phase 1 "ring stack" cue before starting the movement; this cue is maintained throughout the exercise. **B,** Four-point kneeling provides a starting position to transition into the modified downward dog pose. **C,** Controlling neutral alignment of the thoracic rings is facilitated by thinking of "space" and "length" between the sides of the driving rings while the rings move in relation to the fixed hands. This requires coordination of ring control and shoulder girdle control. **D,** Modified downward dog. The knees are flexed and the femoral heads seated. The patient thinks of pushing their rings away from the hands in a line toward the hips (*blue arrow*); the thorax is not allowed to drop into anterior translation or extension. (Copyright LJ Lee Physiotherapist Corp.)

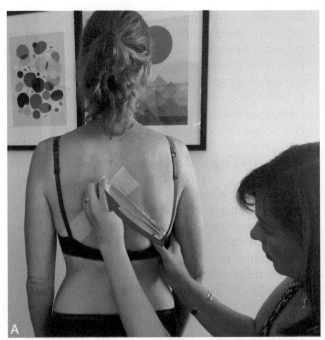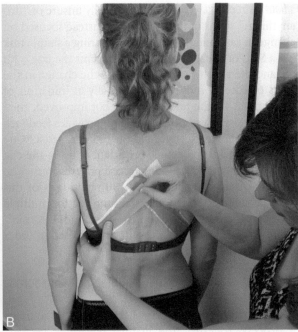

Figure 11-23 Lower thoracic ring taping. Supportive tape can be applied in a variety of directions to provide both proprioceptive input and mechanical support to the driving ring(s). Here, the eighth ring is corrected from a right lateral translation/left rotated position via the right eighth rib while the ninth ring is corrected from a relative left lateral translation/right rotated position via the left ninth rib. **A,** White COVER-ROLL® tape is applied along the line of both rings to ensure appropriate placement of the leukotape and to guide the direction of the force application. The clinician's right hand provides a gentle force to craniomedially translate the ring to the left along the line of the rib to facilitate optimal biomechanics of the ring *(blue arrow)* as LEUKOTAPE® is applied to support the ring in this position. The entire ring can be corrected in this way only in the absence of a significant loss of integrity in the passive system in one of the articulations of the ring. **B,** The process is repeated for the left ninth ring. It is essential that nonoptimal vectors around the ring and related to the 9/8 ring complex be released before the tape is applied. Otherwise, taping may make symptoms worse. The relevant screening task should be repeated after the tape is applied to ensure that the correct level has been taped and that sufficient support has been provided (i.e., the task movement should be easier after application of the tape). (Copyright LJ Lee Physiotherapist Corp.)

- Support with ring taping. Scapula taping in addition to ring taping is helpful when large shoulder girdle muscle bulk creates excessive compression on the rings.
- Integrate best "ring stack" (driver) cues into daily activities (e.g., walking), and integrate postural education cues.

Phase 1 Cueing. After releasing vectors around the driving thoracic rings, reassess for NOLT during a simple loading task (SAL, squat, one leg standing). Determine how many repetitions can be performed without NOLT. If NOLT of the driver (thoracic rings) still occurs after release of vectors (e.g., within 0-20 repetitions), this indicates that the patient needs to be taught a new neuromuscular strategy for ring control. NOLT may recur due to insufficient recruitment of the deep segmental ring muscles, or due to a return of the non-optimal patterns of excessive superficial muscle activity.

Provide sensory/proprioceptive input into the lateral aspect of the rings with gentle vertical decompression of the rings, or sink deep into the segmental multifidus muscle posteriorly next to the spinous process and provide a cranial pressure. Try different *verbal cues or images,* and assess the response of the thoracic rings to the cues:

- "Imagine a hook attaching to your vertebra and a string gently lifting the vertebra 1 mm off the rest of the spine."
- "Think of the sides of the rings floating up and apart—space between the rings right where you feel my fingers."
- "Keep the sides of the body long, like you are opening space between the slinky of your rib cage from my fingers."
- "Imagine balloons inflating in your armpits to float your shoulder girdle."
- "Imagine space opening between the back of your rings and your shoulder blades."

The clinician palpates the driving rings and monitors the response to different cues. The key indicator that there is a more optimal recruitment pattern between the deep and superficial muscles around the thoracic ring(s) is that the thoracic rings of interest correct and stack with the cue without bracing or superficial muscle recruitment, and without breath holding.

Patient Instructions. The patient is usually unsure of "doing anything," so his or her attention is instead focused on the change in ease of task performance during a simple task such as a SAL or squat. The patient performs the task with no cue and then with the cue and notes the change in the lightness or ease of movement, especially at initiation of the movement. (If the task effort has not improved, then the patient finesses his or her cue). This provides feedback that the cue is being effective, and the task is called a "Cue Check." The goal is to become proficient at using the cue to stack the rings as a base for exercise progressions. The patient is advised to practice 10 to 30 repetitions of this "ring stack" cue and to try to sustain the cue for multiple breaths with each repetition (up to 10 seconds). A minimum of two sessions of practice a day are advised in order to consolidate the skill in 7 to 14 days.

Phase 2: Control of Neutral Thoracic Ring Stacking across Multiple Tasks

As the patient moves from phase 1 to phase 2 of the treatment process, together, the manual release of vectors, supportive taping, education, and home exercise practice for better thoracic ring control create positive change in both symptoms and function. However, progression of the exercise program is essential to ensure sufficient capacity for thoracic ring control and loading across multiple tasks.

If dysfunction of the thoracic rings has been present for any significant period of time, alterations in strength and synergies of muscles between the driving thoracic rings and connected regions will be present. For example, if the upper thoracic rings have functioned in left translation/right rotation, muscles on both sides of the shoulder girdle will have adapted. As old nonoptimal patterns are removed, weakness in specific shoulder girdle muscles will become evident and need to be addressed. Exercises that train maintenance of thoracic ring control with shoulder girdle dissociation, both in open- and closed-chain progressions, provide an intermediate step to more complex movements. These types of building block movements are characteristic of phase 2 treatment progression.

Furthermore, the clinician needs to be mindful that the changes being made to thoracic ring alignment and control change loading throughout the kinetic chain, and many other structures are being loaded in a new way. These structures require a graded training program for positive adaptation to occur. Consider, for example, the loads through the Achilles tendon pre– and post–thoracic ring treatment in the scenario in Figure 11-5, where medial-lateral forces through the lower limb are significantly altered by changes in the thorax. Therefore, an understanding of the connections between thoracic ring function and the rest of the body inform the clinician's advice to patients about how to progress training loads and return to activities.

In phase 2, the focus is on training control of neutral thoracic ring alignment with upper and lower extremity dissociation and perturbation patterns, progressing from simple to complex movement patterns and from sagittal plane movements to movements outside the sagittal plane. For thoracic ring drivers, lateral perturbation forces will create the greatest challenge to rotational control. As patients progress through phase 2, there should be increasing variability in movement patterns and challenges to thoracic ring control to include all categories of exercises (see Table 11-2 and Figures 11-18, 11-19, 11-20, 11-22, and 11-24). Timing and speed of progression to phase 3 levels of exercise may vary for different categories of exercise (e.g., open kinetic chain versus closed kinetic chain), but the aim is to progress all categories to more three-dimensional, whole body movement patterns that require thoracic ring control during trunk rotation patterns relative to other regions (Figure 11-25). Several examples are provided in Table 11-2.

Principles for Phase 2 Exercise Prescription.

- Focus is on inter-regional control and establishing ability to control stacked thoracic rings (in neutral) during movements that require dissociation from other regions.
- Initially, the clinician decides whether the patient can perform higher repetitions with upper or lower extremity dissociation challenges (e.g., squat versus bilateral arm elevation in supine) and trains these patterns separately to build endurance in thoracic ring control and new superficial muscle movement patterns.
- Establish "*self-check*" movements. These are simple movements that the patient can perform to check the current status of their driver. The self-check task provides the patient with a way to self-evaluate the impact of any exercise or activity on their driver, as well as determine when he or she needs to do self-release of vectors on his or her driver. A reduction in ease of motion or range of motion of the self-check movement indicates a return of nonoptimal strategies and related vectors on the driving thoracic rings. Self-checks are any movement or task that the patient can feel a difference pre– and post–thoracic ring release and are used throughout phase 2 and phase 3 whenever new, more challenging exercises are added. Self-check tasks must be sensitive to changes in the status of the driver and this change must be detectable by the patient. Some options include the following:
  - Head rotation (in cases when the thoracic rings are the driver for neck function)
  - Forward arm reach with shoulder protraction (note ease of scapular glide and feel for "sticky shoulder blade")
  - Trunk rotation (with or without a deep breath at end range)
  - Right versus left SAL
- Once the first phase 2 exercise progression is trained to the point where the patient finds it easy

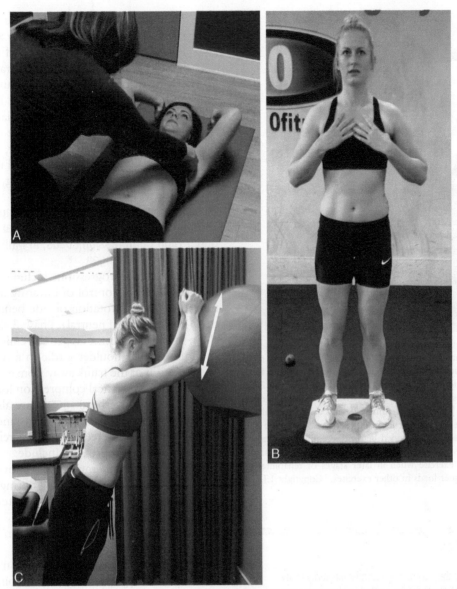

Figure 11-24 Examples of phase 2 exercises: training control of neutral alignment of the thoracic rings. **A,** Unweighted triceps extensions are a very early phase 2 exercise to train dissociation of the shoulder girdle with neutral thoracic ring stacking. The clinician monitors control of the driving ring(s) and provides sensory input, cues and partial corrections to facilitate optimal control during the exercise. **B,** The patient is self-palpating and cueing her thoracic ring control while balancing on a rocker board set to create sagittal plane challenges. This can be progressed to performing squats on the rocker board. **C,** Swiss ball roll-outs on the wall are an example of an intermediate phase 2 exercise for inter-regional control between the thoracic rings and the shoulder girdle in a closed-chain loading. The rings are kept stacked while the shoulders are flexed and extended to roll the ball up and down the wall (*double arrow*). This exercise prevents scapular muscle bracing as closed-chain loads are added. (Copyright LJ Lee Physiotherapist Corp.)

to perform 3 sets of 15 repetitions with good thoracic ring control, this exercise is a likely candidate to become the first "reset" exercise that will be used during the next progressions. A *reset exercise* is an exercise in which the patient demonstrates the ability to use the new, more optimal neuromuscular strategy for control of the driver, with ease and with a high number of repetitions. The active use of the new strategy creates an automatic release of nonoptimal vectors. Reset exercises are performed interspersed with other exercises when new progres-

sions are added to the exercise program as the patient learns to implement the new strategy for ring control in the new exercises. If there is a negative change to the self-check after performing a new exercise, the patient can perform the reset exercise to release the nonoptimal vectors or strategies that have returned during the preceding exercise. After a reset exercise is performed, the clinician will find the thoracic rings more stacked and fewer nonoptimal vectors on ring vector analysis, and the patient will feel a positive effect on the self-check.

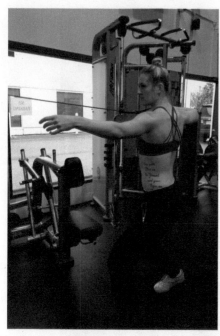

Figure 11-25 "Bow and arrow" is an example of a phase 3 exercise because it requires optimal *control of rotation* through the thoracic rings and the shoulder girdle with *dissociation of the shoulder girdle* from the thoracic rings. Patients may progress from phase 2 to phase 3 exercises at different rates for the different categories. For example, open kinetic chain shoulder girdle–thoracic ring exercises can commonly be progressed faster than closed kinetic chain exercises. Therefore this bow and arrow exercise is often added before the equivalent phase 3 closed-chain exercise is added. Many patients find the bow and arrow exercise a good reset exercise when in later stages of rehabilitation and progressing to higher loads in other exercises. (Copyright LJ Lee Physiotherapist Corp.)

Reset Exercise Criteria

- Any exercise where the patient demonstrates the ability to use the new, optimal strategies for ring control with ease and minimal concentration.
- Patient must be able to perform high repetitions with optimal strategy (3 sets of 10-15 repetitions).
- If self-check movement becomes restricted, performing one set of 10 repetitions of the reset exercise decreases nonoptimal vectors on the thoracic rings and improves the ease and range of motion of the self-check movement.

Reset exercises create an automatic release of vectors because the new, more optimal strategy for thoracic ring control is being used. They empower patients to self-release, self-monitor, and explore exercise progressions with confidence. Reset exercises should be progressed in complexity as the patient progresses through phases 2 and 3 (i.e., as the patient masters using the optimal strategy for thoracic ring control in more challenging exercises, those exercises become options to be used as reset exercises).

- A variety of Phase 2 exercise progression options are listed in Table 11-2.
- Unstable surfaces can be used to progress any exercise and "thoracic spring" category of exercises should be added in phase 2.

- Manual release techniques are progressed from static positions to *dynamic ring vector analysis and release*, where the ring stack and breathe technique is performed in the midst of training exercises to release through relevant ranges and integrate release and training simultaneously (see Figure 11-17, C).
- The clinician can provide partial ring corrections during movement to train more optimal superficial muscle patterning/recruitment, which will conversely support better segmental ring control.
- Continue to support with taping.

Phase 3: Control Thoracic Ring Stacking and Movement Through Rotation and Side Bending Range of Motion; Under High Compression Loads; In Multiplanar Perturbation Challenges

Phase 3 exercise progressions include any movement or task that requires control of intraring and inter-ring motion during trunk rotation or side bending range of motion (moving out of neutral). Phase 3 also includes closed chain tasks through the upper extremity that require dissociation of the shoulder girdle in a rotation movement (e.g. rotation of the trunk away from a fixed arm). Higher loads, especially vertical compression loads with overhead weight (such as overhead squats) are also a Phase 3 exercise. For inversion exercises, handstands and handstand push-ups are considered Phase 3 exercises. Principles for Phase 3 exercise progression include:

- Use multijoint, multiplanar movements that challenge thoracic ring control during rotational movements between regions (i.e., inter-regional control of rotation).
- Add lateral challenges to postural equilibrium and thoracic spring exercises.
- Add more complex whole body movement patterns and training specific to the meaningful task or sport activity.
- Continue to use dynamic ring vector analysis and release and taping, and progress reset exercises to more complex movement patterns in which the patient can still maintain optimal control of the driving thoracic rings.

OUTCOME MEASURES AND THE THORACIC RING APPROACH

Because dysfunction of the thoracic rings can be the underlying driver for a diverse range of symptoms and problems, the choice of outcome measures is based on what tools are available and shown to be best suited to measure change in the meaningful complaint and impairment. For example, when treating a patient with thoracic driven neck pain the Neck Disability Index (NDI)[72] can be used. When treating a patient with thoracic driven adductor tendinopathy, adductor squeeze pressure measures with a blood pressure cuff (mm Hg) can track change. For all patients, a meaningful measure is provided by the Patient-Specific Functional Scale (PSFS),[73] whereby the patient ranks his or her ability to perform the desired meaningful task on a scale of 0 to 10 (0 = no ability to perform the meaningful task; 10 = full return to meaningful task/activity).

SUMMARY

Shifting from the paradigm that the thorax is stiff and requires mobilization to one where the thorax is flexible and requires optimal neuromuscular control provides greater insight into why the thorax can drive distal problems. This paradigm shift moves away from conceptualizing the thorax as a static, stiff box to being a dynamic stack of 10 rings, much like a Slinky or a shock-absorbing spring. When there is loss of optimal sequencing, force modulation, and synergy between the muscles around the thoracic ring; between the 10 thoracic rings; and between the rings and other regions of the body, there are many possible consequences throughout the whole body.

The Thoracic Ring Approach[17,18] incorporates current research on the thorax and provides innovative clinical assessment and treatment skills for the thorax, as well as a clinical reasoning framework that considers the multiple connections between the thorax and other regions of the body. Patients present with nonoptimal strategies for their meaningful task that are linked to nonoptimal experiences of their body. In thorax-driven cases, treating the thoracic ring(s) in the context of a biopsychosocial model that recognizes both intrinsic and extrinsic influences on the patient provides the pathway to change these nonoptimal strategies and create a positive experience of movement, reconceptualize pain, and support optimal strategies for function and performance for the whole person.

REFERENCES

1. Standring S: *Gray's anatomy: the anatomical basis of clinical practice*, ed 40, Edinburgh, 2008, Churchill Livingstone.
2. Bergman GJD, Winters JC, van der Heijden GJM, et al: Groningen Manipulation Study. The effect of manipulation of the structures of the shoulder girdle as additional treatment for symptom relief and for prevention of chronicity or recurrence of shoulder symptoms. Design of a randomized controlled trial within a comprehensive prognostic cohort study, *J Manipulative Physiol Ther* 25:543–549, 2002.
3. Cleland JA, Glynn P, Whitman JM, et al: Short-term effects of thrust versus nonthrust mobilization/manipulation directed at the thoracic spine in patients with neck pain: a randomized clinical trial, *Phys Ther* 87:431–440, 2007.
4. McConnell J: The use of taping for pain relief in the management of spinal pain. In Boyling JD, Jull GA, editors: *Grieve's modern manual therapy: the vertebral column*, 3 ed., Edinburgh, 2005, Elsevier Churchill Livingstone.
5. Kellgren JP: On the distribution of pain arising from deep somatic structures with charts of segmental pain areas, *Clin Sci* 4:35–46, 1939.
6. Feinstein B, Langton JN, Jameson RM, Schiller F: Experiments on pain referred from deep somatic tissues, *J Bone Joint Surg Am* 36:981–997, 1954.
7. Lee LJ: *Thoracic stabilization and the functional upper limb: restoring stability with mobility, course notes*, 2003. Vancouver, BC.
8. Lee LJ: *A clinical test for failed load transfer in the upper quadrant: how to direct treatment decisions for the thoracic spine, cervical spine, and shoulder complex.* In Proceedings of the 2005 orthopaedic symposium of the Canadian Physiotherapy Association. 2005 London, Ontario, Canada.
9. Lee LJ: *Motor control and kinematics of the thorax in pain-free function*, Australia, 2013, University of Queensland.
10. Lee LJ, Lee DG: An integrated multimodal approach to the thoracic spine and ribs. In Magee DJ, Zachazewski JE, Quillen WS, editors: *Pathology and intervention in musculoskeletal rehabilitation*, St. Louis, 2008, Elsevier.

11. Lovett R: The mechanism of the normal spine and its relation to scoliosis, *Boston Med Surg J* 153:349–358, 1905.
12. Gregersen GG, Lucas DB: An in vivo study of the axial rotation of the human thoracolumbar spine, *J Bone Joint Surg Am* 49:247–262, 1967.
13. Watkins R IV, Watkins R III, Williams L, et al: Stability provided by the sternum and rib cage in the thoracic spine, *Spine* 30:1283–1286, 2005.
14. Willems JM, Jull G, J KF: An in vivo study of the primary and coupled rotations of the thoracic spine, *Clinical Biomech* 11:311–316, 1996.
15. Lee LJ: Is it time for a closer look at the thorax? *Musculoskeletal Physiotherapy Australia In Touch Magazine* 1:13–16, 2008.
16. Lee LJ: *The role of the thorax in pelvic girdle pain.* In 6th interdisciplinary world congress on low back and pelvic pain, Barcelona, Spain. November 7–10, 2007.
17. Lee LJ: *Discover the role of the thorax in total body function: introduction to the Thorax 'Ring Approach', course notes*, 2011. Bergen, Norway.
18. Lee LJ: *The essential role of the thorax in whole body function and the "Thoracic Ring Approach"*, Assessment and Treatment Videos, 2012, Linda-Joy Lee Physiotherapist Corp. www.ljlee.ca.
19. Lee LJ: Thoracic ring control: a missing link? *Musculoskeletal Physiotherapy Australia In Touch Magazine* 4:13–16, 2013.
20. Lee LJ: Restoring force closure/motor control of the thorax. In Lee DG, editor: *The thorax: an integrated approach*, White Rock, BC, 2003, Diane G. Lee Physiotherapist Corporation.
21. Giles LGF, Singer KP: *The clinical anatomy and management of thoracic spine pain, The clinical anatomy and management of back pain series*, Oxford, 2000, Butterworth-Heinemann.
22. Lee DG: *Manual therapy for the thorax*, DOPC, British Columbia, 1994, Diane G. Lee Physiotherapist Corp.
23. Maitland GD: *Vertebral manipulation*, London, 1964, Butterworths.
24. Mitchell FL, Mitchell PKG: *The muscle energy manual—evaluation and treatment of the thoracic spine, lumbar spine and rib cage*, ed 2, East Lansing, Michigan, 2002, MET press.

25. Molnar S, Mano S, Kiss L, Csernatony Z: Ex vivo and in vitro determination of the axial rotational axis of the human thoracic spine, *Spine* 31:E984–E991, 2006.
26. Lee LJ, Chang AT, Coppieters MW, Hodges PW: Changes in sitting posture induce multiplanar changes in chest wall shape and motion with breathing, *Respir Physiol Neurobiol* 170:236–245, 2010.
27. Keene C: Some experiments on the mechanical rotation of the normal spine, *J Bone Joint Surg* s2-4:69–79, 1906.
28. Lee LJ: *The essential role of the thorax in restoring optimal function.* Keynote presentation at *the 2008 orthopaedic symposium of the Canadian Physiotherapy Association*, Montreal, Canada, 2008.
29. Geelhoed MA, McGaugh J, Brewer PA, Murphy D: A new model to facilitate palpation of the level of the transverse processes of the thoracic spine, *J Orthop Sports Phys Ther* 36:876–881, 2006.
30. Takeuchi T, Abumi K, Shono Y, et al: Biomechanical role of the intervertebral disc and costovertebral joint in stability of the thoracic spine, a canine model study, *Spine* 24:1414–1420, 1999.
31. Andriacchi T, Schultz A, Belytschko T, Galante J: A model for studies of mechanical interactions between the human spine and rib cage, *J Biomech* 7:497–507, 1974.
32. Lee LJ, Coppieters MW, Hodges PW: Differential activation of the thoracic multifidus and longissimus thoracis during trunk rotation, *Spine* 30:870–876, 2005.
33. Lee LJ, Coppieters MW, Hodges PW: Anticipatory postural adjustments to arm movement reveal complex control of paraspinal muscles in the thorax, *J Electromyogr Kinesiol* 19:46–54, 2009.
34. Lee LJ, Coppieters MW, Hodges PW: En bloc control of deep and superficial thoracic muscles in sagittal loading and unloading of the trunk, *Gait Posture* 33:588–593, 2011.
35. Smith MD, Coppieters MW, Hodges PW: Postural response of the pelvic floor and abdominal muscles in women with and without incontinence, *Neurourol Urodyn* 26:377–385, 2007.
36. Lee LJ, Lee DG: Clinical practice—the reality for clinicians. In Lee DG, editor: *The pelvic girdle*, 4 ed., Edinburgh, 2011, Elsevier.

37. Lee LJ: *ConnectTherapy.* Available at https://ljlee. ca/teaching-models/connecttherapy. Accessed January 15, 2015.

38. Lee LJ: *The ConnectTherapy Series: build your clinical expertise I the Thoracic Ring Approach™ and ConnectTherapy™,* January 2015. Vancouver, BC.

39. Hodges PW: *Neuromechanical control of the spine,* PhD thesis, Stockholm, Sweden, 2003, Karolinska Institutet.

40. Hodges PW, Cholewicki JJ: Functional control of the spine. In Vleeming A, Mooney V, Stoeckart R, editors: *Movement, stability and lumbopelvic pain,* ed 2 Edinburgh, 2007, Churchill Livingstone/Elsevier.

41. Reeves NP, Narendra KS, Cholewicki J: Spine stability: the six blind men and the elephant, *Clin Biomech* 22:266–274, 2007.

42. Magee DJ: *Orthopedic physical assessment,* ed 6, St. Louis, 2014, Saunders/Elsevier.

43. Harrison DE, Cailliet R, Harrison DD, Janik TJ: How do anterior/posterior translations of the thoracic cage affect the sagittal lumbar spine, pelvic tilt, and thoracic kyphosis? *Eur Spine J* 11:287–293, 2002.

44. Bogduk N: *Clinical anatomy of the lumbar spine and sacrum,* London, UK, 2005, Churchill Livingstone/Elsevier.

45. Lee DG: Biomechanics of the thorax: a clinical model of in vivo function, *J Man Manip Ther* 1:13–21, 1993.

46. Mens JM, Vleeming A, Snijders CJ, et al: The active straight leg raising test and mobility of the pelvic joints, *Eur Spine J* 8:468–473, 1999.

47. Mens JM, Vleeming A, Snijders CJ, et al: Validity of the active straight leg raise test for measuring disease severity in patients with posterior pelvic pain after pregnancy, *Spine* 27:196–200, 2002.

48. Mens JM, Vleeming A, Snijders CJ, et al: Reliability and validity of the active straight leg raise test in posterior pelvic pain since pregnancy, *Spine* 26:1167–1171, 2001.

49. Butler DS: *The sensitive nervous system,* Unley, South Australia, 2000, Noigroup Publications.

50. Butler DS: *Mobilisation of the nervous system,* Edinburgh, 1991, Churchill Livingstone.

51. Siegel DJ: *Mindful therapist: a clinician's guide to mindsight and neural integration,* New York, 2010, WW Norton & Company, Inc..

52. Doidge N: *The brain that changes itself. Stories of personal triumph from the frontiers of brain science,* New York, 2007, Penguin Books.

53. World Health Organization: *Constitution of the World Health Organization.* Available at: http://www.who.int/governance/eb/who_constitution_en.pdf?ua = 1.

54. Jones MA, Rivett D: Introduction to clinical reasoning. In Jones MA, Rivett DA, editors: *Clinical reasoning for manual therapists,* Edinburgh, 2004, Elsevier.

55. Lee LJ: Circles of Influence. Available at: https://ljlee.ca/teaching-models/circles-influence/. Retrieved January 15, 2015.

56. Bialosky JE, Bishop MD, Price DD, et al: The mechanisms of manual therapy in the treatment of musculoskeletal pain: a comprehensive model, *Man Ther* 14:531–538, 2009.

57. Lee LJ: *Discover the thorax—level 1: inter-ring rotational control for optimal trunk function, course notes,* 2009. Vancouver, BC.

58. Lee DG, Lee LJ: *An integrated approach to the assessment and treatment of the lumbopelvic-hip region,* Vancouver, BC, Canada, 2004, Diane G. Lee Physiotherapist Corp. and LJPT Consulting.

59. Lee DG, Lee LJ: Techniques and tools for addressing barriers in the lumbopelvic-hip complex. In Lee DG, editor: *The pelvic girdle,* 4 ed., Edinburgh, 2011, Elsevier.

60. Adams G, Sim J: A survey of manual therapists' practice of and attitudes towards manipulation and its complications, *Physiother Res Int* 3:206–227, 1998.

61. Lanska DJ, Lanska MJ, Fenstermaker R, et al: Thoracic disk herniation associated with chiropractic spinal manipulation, *Arch Neurol* 44:996–997, 1987.

62. Domenicucci M, Ramieri A, Salvati M, et al: Cervicothoracic epidural hematoma after chiropractic spinal manipulation therapy: case report and review of the literature, *J Neurosurg* 7:571–574, 2007.

63. Sozio MS, Cave M: Boerhaave's syndrome following chiropractic manipulation, *Am Surg* 74:428–429, 2008.

64. Lowcock J: Thoracic joint stability and clinical stress tests, *Canadian Orthopaedic Manipulative Physiotherapists, Orthopaedic Division of the Canadian Physiotherapy Association Newsletter.* 15, 1990.

65. Oda I, Abumi K, Lu D, et al: Biomechanical role of the posterior elements, costovertebral joints, and rib cage in the stability of the thoracic spine, *Spine* 21:1423–1429, 1996.

66. Feiertag MA, Horton WC, Norman JT, et al: The effect of different surgical releases on thoracic spinal motion. A cadaveric study, *Spine* 20:1604–1611, 1995.

67. Hodges PW, Richardson CA: Feedforward contraction of transversus abdominis is not influenced by the direction of arm movement, *Exp Brain Res* 114:362–370, 1997.

68. Hodges P, Kaigle Holm A, Holm S, et al: Intervertebral stiffness of the spine is increased by evoked contraction of transversus abdominis and the diaphragm: in vivo porcine studies, *Spine* 28:2594–2601, 2003.

69. Barker PJ, Guggenheimer KT, Grkovic I, et al: Effects of tensioning the lumbar fasciae on segmental stiffness during flexion and extension: Young Investigator Award winner, *Spine* 31:397–405, 2006.

70. Lee DG: Rotational instability of the midthoracic spine: assessment and management, *Man Ther* 1:234–241, 1996.

71. Perret C, Robert J: Electromyographic responses of paraspinal muscles to postural disturbance with special reference to scoliotic children, *J Manip Physiol Ther* 27:375–380, 2004.

72. Vernon H, Mior S: The neck disability index: a study of reliability and validity, *J Manipulative Physiol Ther* 14:409–415, 1991.

73. Stratford P: Assessing disability and change on individual patients: a report of a patient specific measure, *Physiother Can* 47:258–263, 1995.

CHAPTER 12

Low Back Pain
Disability and Diagnostic Issues

MARK D. BISHOP, TREVOR A. LENTZ, STEVEN Z. GEORGE

INTRODUCTION

This chapter presents a current and practical approach to the diagnosis of low back pain (LBP). It discusses the etiology, epidemiology, course, and societal impact of LBP so as to give the clinician a context for understanding the importance of effective LBP management. The chapter also presents a model for management of LBP that emphasizes a psychologically informed classification approach. This approach involves the identification of red flags, screening for yellow flags, as well as specific subgroups of patients with LBP.

RISK AND ETIOLOGY OF INCIDENT LOW BACK PAIN

Definitive causes of LBP represent a "holy grail" for clinicians and researchers working in spine care. Evidence indicates that identifiable causes exist for specific lumbar conditions. Most notable is the line of research involving intervertebral disc degeneration. However, evidence also suggests that single, definite causes of clinical LBP remain elusive. This point was illustrated in a meta-analysis investigating incident LBP rates and risk factors associated with these rates.[1] The literature search in this meta-analysis was limited to 41 prospective studies that investigated reports of first-time LBP or LBP after a pain-free state. Results were similar for occupational or community-based samples and indicated that the pooled incident rate was approximately 25%. There was wide variation in the physical and psychosocial factors that were predictive of incident LBP but little consistency in these predictors. In fact, the only consistent finding was that a prior episode of LBP was predictive of LBP after a pain-free state.

In an attempt to provide additional guidance on causes and risk factors for LBP in this chapter, the authors have limited their narrative review to factors that have a theoretically plausible link to the development of LBP. Furthermore, the authors have emphasized results from two commonly implemented study designs that are used to investigate causes of LBP: epidemiological and monozygotic twin studies. In epidemiological studies,[2] cause can be inferred if the proposed causative factor meets all five criteria presented in Table 12-1. If the proposed causative factor does not meet all five criteria, it is not likely to cause LBP.

Monozygotic twin studies can also be used to infer causes of LBP because they control for potential confounding factors by matching participants on gender, age, genotype, and childhood environments.[3] Using this methodology, groups of twins who have discordance on the factor of interest are recruited and statistically compared for differences in the prevalence of LBP. For example, in this study design, LBP prevalence would be compared in monozygotic twins who differed in smoking status to determine whether smoking was a likely cause of LBP.[4]

Genetics

When genetic causes of LBP are considered, research has focused on allele (i.e., certain inherited characteristics) variations that adversely affect the quality of the intervertebral discs. A direct pathway involves polymorphisms that affect intervertebral disc composition, resulting in an increased probability of disc degeneration. Polymorphisms in the collagen IX,[5,6] aggrecan,[7] vitamin D receptor,[8,9] and matrix metalloproteinase-3[10] genes all have been associated with the development of intervertebral disc degeneration in humans. For example, one case-control study found that a specific variation in one of three collagen IX genes was present in 12.2% of patients with intervertebral disc degeneration but in only 4.7% of control patients. This difference was statistically significant ($p < 0.001$) and suggested that a polymorphism in one of the collagen IX genes increased the risk of disc degeneration by approximately 3 times.[6] Another study demonstrated that patients with a specific polymorphism in the vitamin D receptor gene were more likely to experience annular tears.[8]

TABLE **12-1**

Determining the Cause of Low Back Pain from Epidemiological Studies

Criteria	Definition
Theoretically plausible	The factor of interest has a reasonable biological, anatomical, biomechanical, or physiological causal link with low back pain
Significant and meaningful association	The factor of interest has a consistent, statistically significant, and strong association (i.e., odds or relative risk ratios greater than 2) with low back pain as reported across several studies
Monotonic dose-response relationship	Low back pain increases in prevalence as the factor of interest increases in magnitude
Temporality	The factor of interest is present before the onset of low back pain
Reversibility	Low back pain decreases in prevalence when the factor of interest is stopped or is no longer present

Data from Leboeuf-Yde C: Body weight and low back pain: a systematic literature review of 56 journal articles reporting on 65 epidemiologic studies, *Spine* 25:226-237, 2000.

An indirect pathway for a genetic cause of LBP involves polymorphisms that adversely affect the inflammatory cascade by creating excessive amounts of proinflammatory cytokines (i.e., interleukin-1, interleukin-6, interleukin-8, and tumor necrosis factor-α), and/or creating limited amounts of cytokines that mediate the inflammatory response (i.e., interleukin receptor antagonists). Proinflammatory cytokines are produced when intervertebral discs are damaged,[11,12] and these substances can irritate nerve roots without concurrent mechanical compression.[13,14] Therefore it has been hypothesized that polymorphisms in genes that produce proinflammatory or inflammation-mediating cytokines have the potential to cause intervertebral disc degeneration, LBP, and/or sciatica.[15-17] Research supports this hypothesis because a cluster polymorphism in the interleukin-1 gene locus has been associated with increased odds of disc degeneration.[16] Specifically, patients who were heterozygous (odds ratio [OR], 2.2; 95% confidence interval [CI], 1.1 to 4.5) or homozygous (OR, 3.5; 95% CI, 1.0 to 11.9) for the interleukin-1αT[889] allele were more likely to have a specific sign of degeneration (i.e., disc bulge) when compared with those homozygous for the interleukin-1αC[889] allele.[16] Monozygotic twin studies corroborate these findings by investigating the broad role that heredity plays, without investigating the effect of specific genes. It has been estimated that heredity for lumbar disc degeneration is approximately 74% (95% CI, 64% to 81%).[18] In a study by Battie et al.,[19] heredity explained the largest amount of variance in disc degeneration in a multivariate model also containing age and physical loading. When predicting variance in disc degeneration from monozygotic twins at levels T12 to L4, the addition of physical loading explained 7% of the variance, age explained 9% of the variance, and familial aggregation explained 61%, and a similar pattern was noticed for levels L4 to S1.[19] A systematic review of studies of LBP based on twin studies concluded that these effects of genetics were higher for chronic LBP compared with acute LBP.[20]

Collectively the studies suggest genetic factors play an important role in the development of lumbar disc degeneration. However, the clinician must interpret these studies with caution because the presence of lumbar disc degeneration does not automatically preclude clinical presentation of LBP.[3] In fact, a monozygotic twin study published in 1989 suggested that the overall genetic influence on clinical LBP may be low.[21] In this study, the heredity estimates for LBP were low: 20.8% for sciatica and 10.6% for hospitalizations due to disc herniation.[21] Studies linking specific genetic factors to LBP have recently been reported in the literature, and cluster polymorphisms in the aforementioned interleukin-1 gene locus were associated with increased prevalence of LBP in the past year, increased number of days experiencing LBP, and increased pain intensity with LBP.[17] Another study involving a single polymorphism of the interleukin-6 gene locus demonstrated that a specific genotype was more likely to be associated with sciatica (OR, 5.4; 95% CI, 1.5 to 19.2).[15] These studies demonstrate a promising start on confirming a genetic link to clinical presentation of LBP, but these results should be viewed with caution because they conflict with what was reported in the better controlled twin study[21] and they involved small sample sizes with imprecise estimates of the influence genetic factors had on LBP.

Genetic factors seem to play an important role in the development of disc degeneration, but their role in the cause of clinical LBP is not as clear (Table 12-2). This is an area of current interest in the scientific literature, and there are likely to be many advances made in the next few years. The clinician should realize that genetic factors do not appear to play a purely Mendelian role in the development of LBP. In fact, there is already some evidence in the literature that indicates how complex the relationship may be between genetic factors, nongenetic factors, and clinical LBP. A monozygotic twin study modeled the influence of genes and the environment to predict what was the strongest component in the development of LBP.[22] The results suggested that shared environment was the

TABLE **12-2**

Summary of Possible Causative Factors in Low Back Pain

Criteria	Genetic	Physical Loading	Smoking	Obesity	Psychological and Psychosocial	Alcohol
Significant and meaningful association	?	?	N	N	?	N
Monotonic dose-response relationship	?	?	N	N	?	N
Temporality	Y	?	N	N	Y	N
Reversibility	?	N	N	N	N	N

?, Preliminary or inconsistent evidence supporting this factor; N, Consistent evidence against this factor; Y, Consistent evidence supporting this factor.

strongest component until age 15, and after 15, the effect of non-shared environment increased, as did nonadditive genetic effects. The authors of this study estimated the age-adjusted heredity for LBP to be 44% (95% CI, 37% to 50%) for males and 40% (95% CI, 34% to 46%) for females and concluded, "As people grow older, the effect of the non-shared environment increases and non-additive genetic effects become more evident, indicating an increasing degree of genetic interaction as age increases."[22] Another study demonstrated that a polymorphism in the collagen IX gene was more likely to be associated with lumbar disc degeneration for obese subjects.[23] Clearly, more research is needed to elucidate the relationships between genetic factors, nongenetic factors, and their role in the development of LBP.

Physical Loading

In the peer-reviewed literature, relations between physical loading factors, intervertebral disc degeneration, and LBP have been extensively investigated. Common examples of physical loading factors that have been studied include materials handling, postural loading, vehicular vibration, and type and/or amount of exercise. The common way these factors are theorized to cause LBP is that excessive or repeated loads cause macro or micro tissue damage, respectively, to spinal structures. This tissue damage then accelerates degenerative changes to spinal structures, eventually causing LBP. For example, basic studies have suggested that intervertebral disc degeneration results from increased intradiscal pressure and/or ligamentous creep following physical loading.[24-28]

The clinical evidence presented on physical loading factors and lumbar disc degeneration is paradoxical because some studies have demonstrated a positive association between the two factors[29-33] and other studies have not.[34-36] In these studies, many potential confounding factors were not adequately controlled, which limits their comparison and interpretability. As a result, this review is focused on studies of monozygotic twins that differed in amounts of physical loading. In a study of monozygotic twins that differed in occupational and leisure time activities, Battie et al.[19] found that physical loading explained only small amounts of variance in disc degeneration: 7% (occupational physical loading) and 2% (leisure time physical loading) for the upper and lower lumbar spine, respectively. In other monozygotic twin studies, there was no difference in lumbar disc degeneration for twins who differed on resistance or endurance training.[32] However, it should be noted that the same study did find evidence for increased disc degeneration in the lower thoracic (T6 to T12) spine for twins participating in resistance training.[32] Twins who differed in whole-body vibration through lifetime exposure to motorized vehicles did not have measurable differences in lumbar disc degeneration.[29] Therefore it appears that physical loading has a minimal effect on lumbar disc degeneration when these better controlled clinical studies are considered.[3]

In contrast to the association for disc degeneration, the evidence presented on physical loading factors and the clinical presentation of LBP suggests a positive association between the two.[37-43] However, it is not clear if this is a causal relationship. For example, a study in a machinery manufacturing plant compared LBP prevalence between 69 workers involved with manual handling and 51 involved in machinery operation.[43] The workers involved with manual handling were more likely to have experienced LBP in the past year (63.8% versus 37.3%, $p < 0.01$).[43] However, it is not possible to determine if the jobs caused the differences in the LBP because the study was cross sectional and lacked the necessary temporal requirement for inferring cause. Other examples in the literature that meet the temporal requirement for causality appear to have inconsistent results. A 3-year study of LBP incidence and prevalence in a cohort of 288 scaffolders found that none of the physical loading factors (i.e., high manual handling of materials, high strenuous arm movements, and high awkward back postures) were associated with onset of LBP.[38] In contrast, a study found policemen wearing body armor (weighing approximately 8.5 kg [18.7 lb]) were more likely to have LBP when compared with those not wearing body armor.[37] A likely reason for the inconsistency in the literature is that these studies often did not adequately control for confounding factors with the potential to influence associations between physical factors and LBP. Another likely reason for the inconsistency is that many different occupations have been studied, and standard definitions for job demands are not universally applied. Therefore it appears that more rigorous studies are necessary before it can be determined if physical factors definitively cause LBP (see Table 12-2) or if the causality of physical factors is occupation specific.

Smoking

Smoking has been hypothesized to be a causative factor in LBP, and one theory suggests that smoking adversely affects the blood supply to the lumbar spine (i.e., abdominal aorta, lumbar artery, and middle sacral artery) through functional vasoconstriction (immediate effect) and cardiovascular disease (long-term effect).[44,45] It has been suggested that either of these mechanisms could cause LBP. For example, functional vasoconstriction could cause LBP through ischemia, and cardiovascular disease could cause LBP by limiting the blood supply to lumbar structures, accelerating degeneration of the lumbar intervertebral disc and/or spinal structures. The importance of an oxygen gradient for the intervertebral disc was confirmed in a statistical model,[46] and an acute smoking test has been shown to adversely affect the diffusion of nutrients into the disc in an animal model.[47] Another way smoking has been linked to lumbar disc degeneration is through nicotine exposure. In basic studies, direct nicotine exposure to intervertebral discs caused morphological changes (i.e., disruptions in cell proliferation and architecture) that were indicative of early degenerative changes.[48,49]

Support for a link between the effects of smoking, disc degeneration, and LBP is consistently found in smaller-scale studies ($n < 200$) involving postmortem examinations of patients.[50-52] In one study, atherosclerosis of the abdominal aorta and stenosis of the ostia of the lumbar and middle sacral arteries were significantly associated with lumbar disc degeneration, which was independent of the age of the subject.[51] In addition, lumbar and middle sacral arteries were significantly more likely to be missing or occluded in patients who had reported a history of low back symptoms during their lifetime.[52] Occluded lumbar and middle sacral arteries were more common in those having had a history of LBP that lasted 3 months or more, with an OR of 8.5 (95% CI, 2.9 to 24.0), adjusted for age and sex.[50]

Support for a link between effects of smoking, disc degeneration, and LBP can also be found in population-based studies. For example, a prospective cohort of 606 subjects was followed, and those who developed calcifications in the posterior wall of the abdominal aorta were twice as likely to develop intervertebral disc degeneration (OR, 2.0; 95% CI, 1.2 to 3.5).[52] In the same study, subjects with grade 3 (severe) posterior aortic calcification were more likely to report LBP during adult life (OR, 1.6; 95% CI, 1.1 to 2.2).[53] In a different population-based study of 29,244 subjects, habitual smokers (defined as at least one cigarette/day) reported 57% prevalence of LBP in the past year, whereas only 40% of nonsmokers (defined as those that had never smoked) reported LBP in the past year (OR, 2.0; 95% CI, 1.9 to 2.1).[45]

Habitual smoking was also associated with a longer duration of LBP, with an OR of 1.4 (95% CI, 1.3 to 1.6) for 1 to 7 days of LBP and increasing to an OR of 3.0 (95% CI, 2.8 to 3.3) for more than 30 days of LBP.[45]

However, support for a smoking link to LBP diminishes when studies of monozygotic twins are considered. Differences in LBP were either minimal or not observed when monozygotic twins who smoked and did not smoke were compared.[4,19,45] In one specific twin study, 53% of smokers reported LBP and 52% of the nonsmokers reported LBP, a difference that was not statistically significant.[45] Further evidence against smoking as a cause of LBP was demonstrated in this same study, which reported no clear dose-response association between smoking and LBP for number of cigarettes smoked or number of years smoked; smoking cessation was not associated with lower prevalence of LBP, and there were no differences in LBP for smokers based on body mass index (BMI).[45] Additional work in 2006 indicated that in a longitudinal cohort of twins discordant for back pain, there were only very weak, nonsignificant effects related to smoking.[54] A 1999 systematic literature review of 47 epidemiological studies had similar conclusions, finding statistically significant associations between LBP and smoking in only 51% of the studies, and rate ratios reported were generally below 2.0 (indication of a noncausal association).[44] In addition, the systematic literature review found no clear evidence of a dose-response association between smoking and LBP, and no true data supporting temporality or reversibility of smoking and LBP.[44] Thus there does not appear to be substantive evidence to support smoking as a definitive cause of LBP (see Table 12-2).

Obesity

People who are obese do have more LBP. For example, the results of a meta-analysis that pooled the results of 35 studies indicated that compared with people with normal BMI, overweight and obese people had an increased prevalence of LBP in the past 12 months (OR, 1.3; 95% CI, 1.1 to 1.5), seeking care for LBP (OR, 1.6; 95% CI, 1.5 to 1.7), and chronic LBP (OR, 1.4; 95% CI, 1.3 to 1.6).[55] However, the studies included in that particular analysis were cross sectional and as such were unable to identify obesity as a cause of LBP. When cohort studies were analyzed, there was a small increase in the incidence of LBP in the past 12 months (OR, 1.5; 95% CI, 1.2 to 1.9).[55] Obesity has been hypothesized to be a cause of LBP by increasing the mechanical demands (i.e., via compressive or shear forces) on lumbar anatomy.[2,56] Obesity is also hypothesized to be an indirect cause of LBP because it may represent a proxy measure for another more difficult to measure factor (i.e., lifestyle) that is actually the "true cause" of LBP (Figure 12-1).[2,56] There is evidence to suggest that biochemical and metabolic changes related to increased adiposity might also play a role.[57]

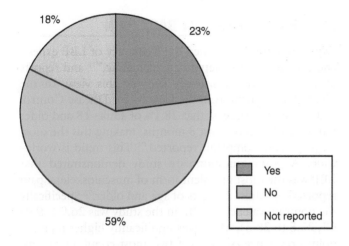

Yes = Significant, positive association between body weight and LBP variable

No = No significant, positive association between body weight and low back pain (LBP) variable

Not reported = No association reported in study

Figure 12-1 Statistically significant associations reported in the literature between body weight measures and variables related to low back pain. (Adapted from Leboeuf-Yde C: Body weight and low back pain: a systematic literature review of 56 journal articles reporting on 65 epidemiologic studies, *Spine* 25:226-237, 2000.)

Evidence against obesity as a cause of LBP is demonstrated in a study that investigated monozygotic twins who differed in BMI. In that study, there was no association between obesity and LBP in the past year with the OR for LBP being 0.9 (95% CI, 0.7 to 1.2) for an underweight category, 1.1 (95% CI, 0.8 to 1.5) for an overweight category, and 1.1 (95% CI, 0.5 to 2.0) for a heavy overweight category.[56] The lack of a consistent dose-response curve is another indication that obesity is not a cause of LBP. Positive monotonic dose-response curves (i.e., higher weight associated with more LBP) have been reported in the literature[58,59]; however, other shaped dose-response curves have also been reported.[56,60] Furthermore, there are no studies reported in the literature to suggest that temporality or reversibility exists with regard to obesity and LBP.[2] Collectively the peer-review literature does not appear to support obesity as a definitive cause of LBP (see Table 12-2).

Obesity does not appear to be causative of LBP (see Table 12-2), but there is some evidence that suggests obesity is associated with longer duration of LBP. In one study, LBP lasting greater than 30 days was consistently associated with BMI categories, for example, the OR for the underweight category was 0.7, the OR for the overweight category was 1.6, and the OR for the heavy overweight category was 1.7.[56] The authors did not report the 95% CI for the ORs in the text, but they did indicate that there were significant differences between the underweight and heavy overweight categories.[56] In a separate

study in an occupational setting, obesity was a significant prognostic factor (OR, 1.68; 95% CI, 1.01 to 2.81) in a multivariate model for determining patients receiving compensation 3 months following a low back injury.[61] This evidence is preliminary, but it suggests although *obesity may not cause LBP*, it may have a *meaningful impact on how long LBP persists*.

Psychological and Psychosocial Factors

Psychological and/or psychosocial distress are thought to be causative of LBP through two pathways.[62] The first pathway involves the notion that psychological distress can lead to a situation in which the nervous system is "sensitized," making it more likely to receive a nonnoxious peripheral stimuli as painful. The second pathway relates to the notion that patients with psychological distress also have a tendency to somatize their symptoms.[63] Therefore certain patients who are distressed may express their psychological symptoms as LBP. Here, evidence is presented from prospective studies that considered whether psychological and/or psychosocial factors were associated with or causative of LBP.

In a U.K. study of 1638 adults who were not currently experiencing LBP, a validated measure of psychological distress (i.e., the General Health Questionnaire, which primarily focuses on symptoms of anxiety and depression) was predictive of new episodes of LBP during the next 12 months.[62] Specifically the OR for those with higher psychological distress (i.e., patients in upper third of General Health Questionnaire versus those in the lower third) was 1.8 (95% CI, 1.4 to 2.4).[62] This factor remained predictive even when potential confounders, such as poor physical health, history of LBP, employment status, age, sex, and social status, were considered.[62] A prospective study of 403 volunteers with no prior history of "serious" LBP demonstrated that psychological distress (i.e., a combination of somatic perception and depressive symptoms) was significantly predictive of a "serious" first-time episode of LBP, whereas only somatic perception was predictive of "any" first-time episode of LBP.[64]

In another U.K. study of 1412 workers not currently experiencing LBP, psychosocial factors related to the workplace were predictive of new episodes of LBP.[65] Patients who were slightly dissatisfied (OR, 1.7; 95% CI, 1.2 to 2.4) or severely dissatisfied (OR, 2.0; 95% CI, 1.2 to 3.3) with their job were more likely to experience an episode of LBP in the 12-month study period. Patients who perceived their income to be severely inadequate were also more likely (OR, 3.6; 95% CI, 1.8 to 7.2) to experience an episode of LBP during the 12-month study period.[65] The psychosocial factors remained predictive, even after controlling for the potential confounder of general psychological distress.[65] Further evidence suggesting psychological factors precede LBP can be found in an intriguing study that reported that discography in asymptomatic patients with psychological distress resulted in reports of significant back pain for at least 1 year after injection, whereas subjects with normal psychometric test results reported no long-term back pain after discography.[66]

This smaller body of literature suggests that psychological and psychosocial factors are associated with new episodes of LBP.[62,64-66] The influence of these factors has been estimated to account for approximately 16% of new episodes of LBP in the general population[62] and up to 25% of new episodes in the working population.[65] However, these factors still cannot be seen as causative of LBP due to the fact that the number of prospective cohort reports remains relatively small, the magnitude of the reported associations is not consistently higher than 2.0, a clear monotonic dose-response curve has not been reported, and studies of reversibility have not been reported (see Table 12-2).

Therefore, psychological and psychosocial factors may not cause LBP, but like obesity, they do appear to have a meaningful effect on the duration of LBP. Several prospective studies have documented that psychological and/or psychosocial distress during acute LBP episodes significantly increased the probability of experiencing chronic LBP.[67,68] The OR for high levels of psychological distress predicting chronic LBP was 3.3 (95% CI, 1.5 to 7.2) in a group of 180 patients followed for a year in the United Kingdom.[68] The identification of psychological and/or psychosocial distress factors (i.e., "yellow flags") is an *important part of the differential diagnosis of LBP because of their strong link to development of chronic LBP*. A specific strategy for identifying specific psychological factors will be discussed later in this chapter.

Alcohol

Alcohol has been hypothesized to contribute to LBP by a direct route, involving uncoordinated movements that damage spinal structures, or by indirect routes, involving the development of co-morbidities that cause LBP.[69] Alcohol has not been thoroughly investigated as a cause of LBP in the peer-reviewed literature. For example, a systematic review identified only nine potential studies that focused on alcohol and LBP, and none of them were prospective in nature.[69] When these studies were reviewed collectively, none reported statistically significant associations between increased alcohol consumption and LBP.[69] For example, one study found similar LBP rates between moderate (OR, 0.88; 95% CI, 0.79 to 0.99) and excessive (OR, 0.72; 95% CI, 0.62 to 0.85) alcohol consumption.[59] Because of the limited number of reports and concerns with the methodology of the studies that were reported in the literature, the author of the systematic review concluded that alcohol did not appear to be a cause of LBP (see Table 12-2).[69]

EPIDEMIOLOGY OF LOW BACK PAIN

Expert opinion has likened the frequency of LBP experienced by modern society to an "epidemic,"[70] and reports in the literature consistently support this view. In the United States, data from the Centers for Disease Control and Prevention suggest that 28.1% of adults 18 and older reported LBP in the past 3 months, making this the most frequent pain complaint reported.[71] This trend is worldwide. A postal questionnaire study demonstrated that LBP was the most prevalent form of musculoskeletal pain reported by adults 25 years of age and older.[72] Specifically the point prevalence of LBP in the study was 26.9% (95% CI, 25.5 to 28.3), which was significantly higher than the point prevalence of the next two most common categories: shoulder pain at 20.9% (95% CI, 19.6 to 22.2) and neck pain at 20.6% (95% CI, 19.3 to 21.9).[72] Although it is clear that individuals in all strata of society commonly experience LBP, its prevalence does appear to vary based on factors such as sex, age, occupation, and socioeconomic status.

Women tend to have a higher prevalence of LBP than men, although the differences reported vary in magnitude.[72-76] For example, in the previously mentioned Dutch study, the point prevalence for women was 28.1% (95% CI, 26.1 to 30.1) and for men it was 25.6% (95% CI, 23.5 to 27.7). In a study involving Arabic subjects, the difference in overall prevalence was larger, reported as 56.1% for males and 73.8% in females. An increase in age is also associated with higher prevalence of LBP. In a Greek population-based study, the odds of experiencing any LBP in the past month were significantly higher for those aged 46 to 65 (OR, 1.82; 95% CI, 1.38 to 2.38) and 66+ (OR, 2.7; 95% CI, 1.85 to 3.93) years, when compared with those 45 years old and younger.[77] In a Danish study of 12- to 41-year-olds, the prevalence of LBP in the past year increased from 7% for 12-year-olds to 56% for 41-year-olds.[74] A separate epidemiological review suggests that this trend in increasing prevalence of LBP continues past 41 and peaks in the sixth decade of life.[78] After the sixth decade, the prevalence of LBP appears to level and eventually decline in the later decades (Figure 12-2).[72]

Occupational differences in LBP prevalence are demonstrated in a study of Chinese workers. A 50% annual prevalence rate of LBP (defined as lasting 24 hours or more) was reported, but this rate was significantly higher for garment workers than teachers (74% versus 40%).[39] In a study involving 1562 Canadian utility workers, lifetime and point prevalence of LBP were 60% and 11%, respectively.[41] In this same sample, LBP prevalence was significantly higher in workers who had jobs that were physically demanding or involved heavy lifting.[41] In a group of 288 scaffolders who were followed for 3 years, 60% experienced LBP in the past year and the prevalence was significantly associated with high material handling

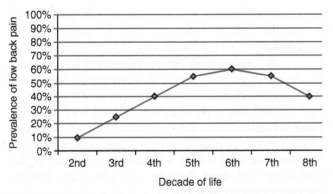

Figure 12-2 Qualitative composite of 1-year LBP prevalence through the second to eighth decades of life.[72,74,78]

or job demand.[38] It is interesting to note that although differences exist between different occupational groups, similar LBP prevalence rates have been reported between working and nonworking groups.[75] Results of a global study of occupational LBP in 187 countries indicated that the relative risk of LBP was highest for workers in agriculture, forestry, and fishing (OR, 3.7; 95% CI, 2.6, 5.3) compared with clerical workers.[79]

Specific socioeconomic factors appear to be associated with the prevalence of LBP. In the previously mentioned Greek study, being married resulted in an OR of 1.53 (95% CI, 1.15 to 2.03) for experiencing LBP in the past month,[77] and a study of Canadian utility workers found a similar association between LBP and marriage.[41] In addition, lower educational levels have been linked with higher prevalence of LBP,[72,73] and social classes involving unskilled occupations have been weakly linked with a higher prevalence of LBP.[65]

The differences in reported LBP prevalence rates for specific factors (i.e., sex and age) can be confusing to interpret. It is important for the clinician to realize that these prevalence estimates vary in a large part because of methodological differences between studies.[70] For example, it is common for epidemiological studies to differ on sampling methods, populations sampled, response rates, definitions of LBP, and measurement techniques. All of these factors have the potential to influence the prevalence estimate reported in a study. This fact is best demonstrated when systematic reviews of prevalence studies are attempted. One systematic review of LBP prevalence found only 30 of 56 identified studies were homogeneous and methodologically sound enough for pooling. Once pooled, the prevalence estimates continued to have wide intervals, for example, LBP point prevalence was estimated at 12% to 33%, 1-year prevalence was estimated at 22% to 65%, and lifetime LBP prevalence was estimated at 11% to 84%.[80] Although LBP clearly is a common experience, improving the precision of prevalence estimates is a goal of future epidemiological research.

Given its overall prevalence, it is not surprising that LBP is a common reason to seek health care. In a Finnish study, pain was the primary reason for visiting a physician in 40% of reviewed cases, and LBP was the most common source of pain.[81] In the United States, LBP is the second most common reason to visit a physician, behind the common cold.[82] Patients commonly seek health care from traditional medical providers, such as general practice (i.e., primary care) physicians, orthopedic physicians, and physical therapists.[82-84] LBP is also one of the most common reasons to seek health care from complementary and alternative medical (CAM) providers.[85] The 2007 National Health Interview Survey indicated that 38% of adults in the United States sought interventions from a CAM provider and that LBP was the most common disorder for which intervention was sought.[86]

The clinician should be aware that a patient with LBP could be using some form of CAM treatment during the episode of care. This issue is relevant because evidence suggests that only 38.5% of patients discussed their CAM treatment with their traditional medical provider and 46.0% used a CAM treatment for a principal medical condition without input from either type of provider.[85] The clinician managing the patient with LBP should determine what type of CAM treatments are currently being used because this will allow appropriate coordination of the patient's subsequent therapy.

Clinicians must also recognize that not all who experience LBP seek health care. In fact, several studies involving general practice and occupational settings reported that only 25% to 50% of individuals who experience LBP actually sought health care.[72,83,87] These studies found that high amounts of disability and pain were the primary differences between patients seeking health care and those not seeking health care.[72,83,87,88] Specifically women and men with high disability were more likely to seek health care for LBP compared with individuals of the same sex with low disability, with the ORs being 7.4 (95% CI, 5.0 to 11.0) and 4.9 (95% CI, 3.3 to 7.1), respectively.[88] Women and men with high pain intensity were also more likely to seek health care for LBP, compared with individuals of the same sex with low pain intensity, with the OR being 3.7 (95% CI, 2.2 to 6.0) and 1.7 (95% CI, 1.1 to 2.8), respectively.[88] Another study suggested that patients from unskilled, manual occupations (OR, 4.8; 95% CI, 2.0 to 11.5) were more likely to seek health care for LBP, as were those who perceived their income to be inadequate (OR, 3.6; 95% CI, 1.8 to 7.2).[65]

COURSE OF LOW BACK PAIN

The course of LBP has been described as consisting of acute, subacute, and chronic phases, with temporal definitions typically associated with each phase. Different operational definitions have been reported in the literature, but a commonly accepted definition for the acute phase is between 0 and 1 month since the episode of LBP, the subacute phase is between 2 and 3 months since episode of LBP, and the chronic phase is greater than 3 months since episode of LBP. The prognosis of LBP appears to be favorable, predictable, and static when these temporal definitions are used (Figure 12-3, *A*). For example, up to 90% of patients with LBP are expected to be pain free or show dramatic improvement during the acute phase, and only approximately 10% of patients are expected to report LBP that continues into the chronic phase.

Because LBP is often recurrent in nature, exclusive use of temporal definitions to describe its course has been challenged in the literature.[89,90] The primary argument is that when LBP is recurrent, the time to improvement from a single episode does not accurately describe its outcome. This issue is perhaps best summarized by Von Korff et al.[90]: "*For example, a person experiencing recurrent episodes of back pain on half the days in a year might appear to have a favorable outcome of each episode, but an unfavorable outcome across episodes. For this reason, the outcome of a recurrent pain condition is more appropriately assessed by the total time with pain across episodes and the characteristic severity of those episodes than by the duration of a single episode*" (p. 855).

This is not purely an academic issue because the prognosis of LBP changes when the influence of recurrence is considered. Of patients with acute LBP who were followed for 1 year, 65% reported one or more additional episodes.[91] In that same study, 2 months was the me-

dian time to another episode of LBP and 60 days was the median time to experience LBP in the year. Other studies have reported lower, but still substantial, recurrence rates ranging from 20% to 35% (6 and 22 months)[92] to 45% (4 years). Von Korff[89] has suggested operational definitions to standardize the description of the course of LBP for clinicians and researchers (Table 12-3). Although these definitions have not been universally adopted, preliminary evidence exists to support their construct validity because patients classified with chronic LBP had higher pain scores and social disability and were more likely to use medication to treat LBP.[93]

When these other factors are considered, the prognosis for LBP becomes less favorable and more variable (Figure 12-3, *B*). At 1-year follow-up of primary care back patients, 69% of patients with recent onset (i.e., within the past 6 months) of LBP reported having pain in the last month.[90] Only 21% of these patients were pain free at 1 year, with 55% reporting low disability and pain intensity, 10% reporting low disability and high pain intensity, and 14% reporting high disability with varying amounts of pain intensity.[90] Similar trends were noted for the 82% of patients with prevalent (i.e., onset longer than the past 6 months) LBP that reported having pain in the last month.[90] At 1-year follow-up, only 12% were pain free, with 52% reporting low disability and pain intensity, 16% reporting low disability and high

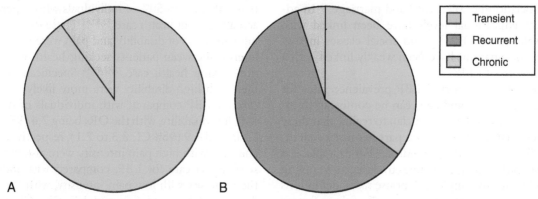

Figure 12-3 **A,** Traditional course of low back pain. **B,** Evidence-based course of low back pain.

TABLE **12-3**

Standard Definitions for Manifestations of Low Back Pain

Descriptor	Operational Definition for an Episode of Low Back Pain
Transient back pain	Present for no more than 90 consecutive days and does not recur over a 12-month period
Recurrent back pain	Present for fewer than half the days in a 12-month period and occurs in multiple episodes over the year
Chronic back pain	Present for at least half the days in a 12-month period in single or multiple episodes
Acute back pain	Recent and sudden in onset and does not meet the previously defined criteria for recurrent or chronic pain
First onset	First occurrence in the patient's lifetime
Flare-up	Distinct phase of pain (with definable beginning and end points) superimposed on a chronic or recurrent course; a period when the pain is markedly more severe than is usual for the patient

Data from Von Korff M: Studying the natural history of back pain, *Spine* 19:2041S-2046S, 1994.

pain intensity, and 20% reporting high disability with varying amounts of pain intensity.[90] These results are further supported by a systematic review that pooled results from 11 longitudinal studies of the course of LBP. The pooled estimates for the proportion of patients with ongoing pain were 80% at 1 month, 67% at 3 months, and 57% at 6 months, and 65% of patients continue to experience pain at 1 year.[94]

This line of research suggests that the clinician obtaining a history from a patient with LBP must ask the patient to describe the course of the back pain in more than just temporal terms associated with the most recent episode that led to the present episode of health care. Other pertinent historical factors include number of previous episodes, the severity of the present episode, the number of days with LBP in the past year, and the amount of interference with daily activities.[89,95]

Important Historical Questions Related to the Course of Low Back Pain[89,95]

- How long has the present episode of low back pain bothered you?
- How many previous episodes of low back pain have you experienced?
- How many days have you had low back pain in the past year?
- How severe is your present episode of low back pain?
- How much does low back pain interfere with your daily activities?

SOCIETAL IMPACT OF LOW BACK PAIN

Given that LBP is a common experience and can be chronic or recurrent in nature, it is not surprising that it is a significant cause of disability and cost to society, and this cost seems to be increasing exponentially over the past three decades.[70,96-99] In the general population, 53% of adults had experienced some disability from LBP during a 6-month period.[99] Chronic LBP substantially influences the capacity to work and has been associated with the inability to obtain or maintain employment[97] and to reduced productivity at work.[98]

LBP is included in a top 10 list for most costly physical ailments.[78] LBP related to occupational settings appears to have made an especially large impact on society. It has been estimated that at least 33% of all health care and indemnity costs under workers' compensation are accounted for by LBP.[100] The cost of lost work productivity due to the most common chronic pain conditions (including LBP, headache, arthritis, and an "other" category) has been estimated at $61.2 billion per year.[98] Of specific pain categories studied, chronic LBP accounted for the most lost productivity time (5.2 hours/wk).[98]

Other estimates of annual health care expenditure for chronic LBP are excessive, especially when compared with other chronic pain conditions. For example, the 1993 direct health care cost estimates were $1 billion dollars for headache[101] and $33 billion for LBP.[102] Indirect cost estimates demonstrated a similar discrepancy, with estimates exceeding $13 billion for headache[101] and $50 billion for LBP.[102] Interestingly the excessive costs associated with disability from LBP did not appear to be evenly distributed.[103] For example, Williams et al.[104] found that health care costs were disproportionate, with 20% of the claimants disabled for 16 weeks or more accounting for 60% of the health care costs. Other authors have reported similar disproportionate patient-cost associations in LBP.[105-107] From 1997 to 2006, health care expenditures for the management of spine conditions increased from 82% to $85 billion.[108]

Therefore, the excessive and increasing societal cost of LBP does not appear to be due to an increase in the condition because a study that used consistent methodology showed similar prevalence rates over different time periods.[109] Instead, the increased cost seems to be associated with the way LBP has traditionally been managed.[70] Clinicians working in progressive environments must be aware that a priority of their treatment is the effective reduction of LBP for the minority of individuals who eventually experience chronic symptoms and accrue exorbitant health care costs.[110-115]

BIOPSYCHOSOCIAL MODEL OF LOW BACK PAIN

Currently there is very little evidence to support a single "magic bullet" cause of LBP (see Table 12-2). The conceptualization of LBP as a distinct and specific disease may be the most direct explanation for difficulty identifying causative factors of LBP.[113] Instead of a specific disease, LBP may be best conceptualized as an illness, one which is characterized and influenced by input from different factors across multiple domains.[113] This realization has led to the implementation of a comprehensive model that describes the development of LBP.

In 1987, Gordon Waddell first proposed a model that considered the simultaneous influence of physical, psychological, and social factors in the development of LBP.[113] The exact parameters of this "biopsychosocial" model have been modified over time, but it remains the currently accepted model of LBP for research and clinical practice (Figure 12-4). The advantage of using this model in clinical practice is that it accounts for all the previously described considerations relating to etiology, epidemiology, course, and societal impact of LBP. Quite simply, a biopsychosocial model regards LBP as an illness, which is a more accurate representation of the clinical presentation. In addition, a task force charged in part to develop diagnostic criteria for LBP by the National Institutes of Health reported that developing pathoanatomic diagnostic criteria for LBP was unfeasible at present.[116] Therefore a biopsychosocial model of LBP is this chapter's framework for discussing the management of LBP.

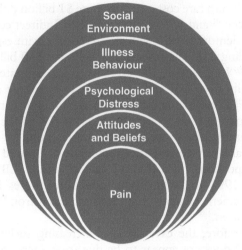

Figure 12-4 Biopsychosocial model of low back pain. (From Waddell G: 1987 Volvo Award in Clinical Sciences: a new clinical model for the treatment of low-back pain, *Spine*, 12:632-644, 1987.)

DIFFERENTIAL DIAGNOSIS OF LOW BACK PAIN

The tasks of the clinician are straightforward when a biopsychosocial model is used for differential diagnosis and classification of patients with LBP. The specific tasks are described in detail, after a brief review of anatomical causes of LBP and imaging of the lumbar spine.

POTENTIAL PAIN GENERATORS IN THE LUMBAR SPINE

Any innervated structure in the lumbar spine can cause symptoms of LBP and referred pain into the extremity or extremities. For example, Kuslich et al.[117] present data from 193 consecutive patients with back pain who were progressively anesthetized and the structures of the lumbar spine stimulated by either blunt mechanical force from a surgical tool or low-power cautery. Only stimulation of the posterior dura and nerve roots by mechanical or thermal stimuli gave patients the sensation of leg pain in this investigation (Table 12-4). In comparison, after Kellgren[118] injected the intraspinous ligaments with saline, subjects reported aching pain in the buttock and leg from a variety of segmental levels, implying that somatic musculoskeletal structures could also refer pain into the extremity (Figure 12-5).

Potential Generators of Low Back Pain[117-119]

- Muscles
- Ligaments
- Dura mater
- Nerve roots
- Zygapophyseal joints
- Annulus fibrosus
- Thoracolumbar fascia
- Vertebrae

TABLE 12-4

Percentage of Patients Reporting Pain and Pain Location after Stimulation of Different Lumbar Tissues

Anatomical Structure	Number Tested	Percentage Reporting Pain (%)	Pain Location
Lumbar fascia	193	17	Back
Paravertebral muscle	193	41	Back
Supraspinous ligament	193	25	Back
Lamina	193	10	Back
Facet capsule	192	30	Back, buttock
Ligamentum flavum	167	0	—
Posterior dura	92	23	Buttock, leg
Compressed nerve root	167	99	Buttock, leg, foot
Normal nerve root	55	11	Buttock, leg
Central annulus	183	74	Back
Lateral annulus	144	71	Back
Nucleus	176	0	—
Vertebral end plate	109	61	Back

Data from Kuslich SD, Ulstrom CL, Michael CJ: The tissue origin of low back pain and sciatica: a report of pain response to tissue stimulation during operations on the lumbar spine using local anesthesia, *Orthop Clin North Am* 22:181-187, 1991.

The quality of pain reported by the patient may help to differentiate whether the source of the pain is related to a somatic musculoskeletal structure or if the pain is radicular in origin. *Radicular pain* is a sharp, shooting pain in the leg in a defined band less than 4 cm wide[120] either superficial or "deep in the leg,"[120,121] whereas *somatic pain* is poorly localized and reported as aching. However, it is unlikely that compression of the nerve root is the primary causative mechanism. Compression of nerve root tissue causes radiculopathy; that is, radiating paresthesia, numbness, weakness, or a combination of symptoms but not pain.[120] It is only when a previously damaged nerve root is compressed[117,120] that the characteristic pain is elicited. Consequently, a patient may not always present with radiculopathy *and* radicular pain.

Radicular Pain, Radiculopathy, and Somatic Pain

- *Radicular pain:* Sharp, shooting, superficial, or deep pain into the leg in a defined band less than 4 cm (1.6 inches) wide
- *Radiculopathy:* Radiating paresthesia, numbness in a dermatome, weakness (myotome), or a combination of these; however, the patient does not experience pain
- *Somatic pain:* Poorly localized, aching pain

Inflammation of the dural sleeve and nerve root is implicated in the genesis of the initial radicular symptoms. Although the source of the inflammation is not obvious,

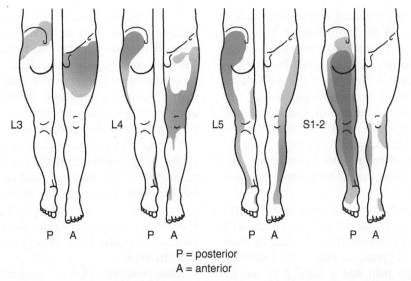

P = posterior
A = anterior

Figure 12-5 Distribution of pain from the interspinous ligament, which has been injected with saline. (From Kellgren J: On the distribution of pain arising from deep somatic structures with charts of the segmental areas, *Clin Sci* 4:35-46, 1939.)

exposure to nuclear material of the intervertebral disc may cause a chemical inflammatory response in the dural and nerve root tissue and eventual fibrosis of the perineural tissues.[120,122] Subsequent compression of the damaged neural tissue will generate radicular symptoms. For example, Kuslich et al.[117] demonstrated that mechanical deformation of perineural scar tissue evoked no pain response, but stimulation of the nerve root at the point of compression produced radicular symptoms.

In the absence of extrusion of nucleus pulposis material into the spinal canal, a precursor inflammatory response may result from traumatic compression.[123] Animal models also suggest that compression of the nerve root tissue eventually generates local edema and ischemia of the nerve root and ganglion.[124,125] Therefore any of the pathologies that cause prolonged nerve root compression may eventually result in damage to the nerve root or ganglion. After this damage occurs, further compression may then result in complaints of radicular pain.

SPECIFIC SOMATIC PAIN GENERATORS

Contractile Tissue

Available literature suggests that paraspinal muscles of patients with LBP are dysfunctional. Studies have demonstrated muscle atrophy,[126-128] reduced activity during trunk movements,[129,130] decreased muscle strength,[131,132] and increased trunk muscular fatigability[133,134] in patients with LBP. The studies that demonstrate decreased muscle performance associated with LBP support a model of muscle deficiency in lumbar dysfunction, rather than a muscle spasm model.[135] Atrophy of the paraspinal muscles has been documented in those patients with short duration[128] and chronic[126] LBP. The atrophy appears specific to multifidus muscle, suggesting a mechanism other than

disuse to explain the atrophy noted.[135] Hides et al.[128] have suggested that reflex inhibition is a likely cause of atrophy in lumbar paraspinal muscles. Experimental support for this theoretical construct is offered in a porcine model in which rapid inhibition of the deep paraspinal muscles occurs after distention of the zygapophyseal joints by injection with saline solution.[136] However, this theory has been challenged given the lack of association between paraspinal muscle asymmetry with LBP severity, disability, or frequency of episodes.[137]

Characteristics of Paraspinal and Trunk Muscles in Patients with Low Back Pain

- Atrophy
- Reduced activity during trunk movements
- Decreased muscle strength
- Increased fatigability
- Change in percentage of fiber types

In addition to deep muscle atrophy, patients with LBP have a significantly higher proportion of type IIB (i.e., fast-twitch glycolytic) fibers than the slow-twitch type I fibers[134] in the posterior trunk muscles. Duration of LBP symptoms has been shown to be significantly associated with a higher proportion of type II fibers, such that the longer the duration of pain, the more glycolytic the paraspinal fiber composition.[134] This finding may provide some explanation for the increase in fatigability noted in patients with LBP. These muscular performance changes may contribute to LBP by decreasing the muscular support of the lumbar spine, placing increased stress on the noncontractile structures.

The disorders that affect predominantly the musculature of the lumbar spine include muscle strain injury, spasm or guarding, and myofascial complaints, such as trigger points. Muscles of the lumbar spine have been demonstrated to act as primary sources of back and buttock pain in experiments using saline distention of a muscle[119] and mechanical stimulation.[117,118] However, consistent with studies of noncontractile tissues, the magnitude of muscle damage does not match well with ratings of pain intensity. In an experimental study using eccentric exercise to induce muscle damage, pain intensity had very weak, nonsignificant correlations with the area of muscle damage determined using magnetic resonance imaging (MRI).[138]

Evidence that increased muscle activity occurs in the muscles in response to pain has been shown in patients with temporomandibular dysfunction,[139] healthy subjects chewing gum,[140] and patients with cervical dysfunction.[141,142] Subjects with pain and a history of cervical soft-tissue injury have lower blood flow in the muscles on the painful side relative to the nonpainful side, when compared with control subjects.[143] The differences in blood flow were pronounced at low-level muscle contractions. The impaired circulation probably contributes to muscle pain by causing an accumulation of metabolites producing pain and a further disturbance of the circulation in a vicious circle.[144] Although this phenomenon has not been demonstrated in the lumbar spine, it is conceivable that similar increases in muscle activity and changes in circulation might occur.

Noncontractile Tissue

Kellgren[118,119] demonstrated that noncontractile tissue, such as fascia, ligaments, and the periostium, are viable sources of LBP. Research by Kuslich et al.[117] supports these early observations and provides additional insight into components of the intervertebral disc as direct sources of pain (see Table 12-4).

Discogenic Pain

Mechanical stimulation of the outer annulus fibrosis causes central back pain, not leg pain,[117,120] and the innervation of the outer annulus fibrosis has been well documented. Therefore the intervertebral disc should be considered a cause of back pain. In addition, changes in the intervertebral disc contribute to other conditions that subsequently result in somatic or radicular pain.

Only the outer third of the annulus is innervated. Torsional injury is thought to occur to the outer annulus fibrosis particularly when the torsion is coupled with lumbar flexion.[145,146] Bogduk[147] has suggested that this mechanism be considered similar to a ligamentous sprain injury because fibers of the outer annulus might be traumatized.

Alternatively, pain response from outer annulus fibrosis may be elicited with exposure of nociceptive endings in the annulus fibrosis to material from the nucleus pulposis or breakdown products from nuclear degradation.

The specific mechanism of degeneration is not well understood but may be related to genetic factors (see 'Genetics' in the section "Risk and etiology of incident low back pain"). In vitro evidence suggests that changes in compressive stress on the disc (such as occurs with disruption of the annulus or minor vertebral body damage) within the nucleus will disrupt cellular metabolism throughout the disc, progressively deteriorating the matrix.[148] Radial fissures developing in the inner two thirds of the annulus will eventually reach the innervated outer third.[146,149,150] As the innervated outer third of the annulus becomes disrupted, comes in contact with nuclear material, or both, the patient will complain of backache but is not likely to have radicular pain or signs of radiculopathy because there is no prolapse or herniation of disc material.

Disc prolapse can occur gradually when discs are subjected to repetitive compression and flexion loading,[148] but radial fissuring in the annulus must precede disc prolapse.[151] Milette et al.[152] report that disc bulges and disc protrusions do not differ significantly in internal architecture, based on the findings of discography. A bulge in the disc that occurs as the annulus weakens may impinge on neural structures within the spinal canal. Eventually herniation of disc material will occur, that is, when radial fissures reach the periphery of the disc and nuclear material may be herniated into the spinal canal.[148,149] The chemical irritation of the nerve root or ganglion will lead to subsequent radicular pain. However, not only nuclear material is herniated. Lebkowski and Dzieciol[153] examined specimens of herniated disc material from 187 patients and reported that in 29% of the cases, the herniation was primarily annular material. This finding may explain the lack of radicular symptoms in some cases of disc herniation (i.e., the nerve root is predominantly exposed to annular not nuclear material).

Ligament and Fascia

Kuslich et al.[117] demonstrated that both the supraspinous and interspinous ligaments might be a source of central LBP, whereas Kellgren[118] reported back and leg pain in subjects in whom the interspinous ligament had been injected. However, the prevalence of specific sprain injury to the interspinous ligament is likely to be very low. The common tendon of the longissimus thoracis muscle[154,155] and the long dorsal sacroiliac ligament[156] are also ligamentous sources of pain, particularly pain to palpation around the posterior iliac spine. In addition, the thoracolumbar fascia might be a source of pain. Little data have been identified regarding diagnosis of ligamentous or fascial injury in the low back; however, one might speculate that sprain injuries to these structures would have a similar mechanism of injury in the trunk as in the extremities. Alternatively, pain might arise after prolonged stress on ligamentous tissue related to postural changes or movement impairments.[157]

Zygapophysial Joints (Facet Joint Syndrome)

The prevalence of zygapophysial involvement in the genesis of LBP may be as high as 25%.[158] The zygapophysial joints have been identified as a source of back and leg pain by generating pain in healthy subjects,[159] reproducing pain in patients,[117] and by relieving pain with injection in certain patients.[160]

El-Bohy et al.[161] demonstrated the potential for capsular sprain injury of the zygapophysial joint, and fractures, capsular tears, and damage to the articular cartilage have been documented on postmortem studies.[162] Degenerative arthritis of the zygaphophysial joints is another possible cause of pain. However, not all arthritis is painful because radiographic changes of osteoarthritis are equally common in patients with and without LBP.[163] Other theories regarding the genesis of lumbar pain from the zygapophysial joint include meniscoid entrapment,[164] synovial impingement,[160,164] and mechanical injury to the joint's capsule.[165] Unfortunately, there is no definitive way to identify the zygapophysial joint as the source of LBP and lower extremity pain from history or clinical findings.[160,166,167] For example, Marks[168] reported that pain radiating to the buttock or trochanteric region occurred mostly from the L4 and L5 levels and that groin pain was produced from L2 to L5, but no consistent pain pattern has been identified related to the joints. This work is supported by that of O'Neill et al., who also identified referral of pain from zygapophysial joints into the groin and anterior thigh.[169] Diagnosis of the zygapophysial joint as the source of LBP is based on controlled diagnostic blocks of the joint or its nerve supply.[160,166,167]

Vertebrae

The vertebral body is involved in several painful conditions, such as Paget's disease,[170] primary or secondary tumors,[170,171] and fracture. The posterior elements of the vertebrae can be affected similarly to the vertebral body; however, several lesions are peculiar to the posterior elements. Increased lumbar lordosis or hyperextension trauma may result in impact of the spinous process or lamina of articulating vertebrae. This may result in periostitis of the spinous process or lamina or inflammation of the interspinous ligament.

Spondylolysis is a defect of the pars articularis often related to fatigue fracture,[172] although there may be some predisposition to development of the condition related to weakness in the pars interarticularis.[173] The location of a pars defect is related to activities in which the patient is involved. For example, fast bowling in cricket is associated with unilateral defects, whereas soccer players develop more bilateral defects.[172] Likewise, the incidence of spondylolysis is related to activity. In gymnastics the incidence of a pars defect is 11% in females,[174] whereas the incidence in university-aged athletes playing American football may be as high as 15%.

The prevalence of spondylolysis in asymptomatic adult subjects ranges from 6%[175] to 9.7%.[176] Libson et al.[176] compared 938 asymptomatic individuals to 662 subjects with LBP and determined the overall incidence of spondylolysis to be equivalent (9.7%) for both groups. However, these authors did indicate that a bilateral defect is more likely to be associated with a complaint of pain. These data suggest that a pars defect itself may not be the source of pain. Rather the defect compromises the arthokinematics of intervertebral motion such that increased stress is placed on other structures of the posterior vertebral arch, such as the ligaments or paraspinal muscles.

Spondylolisthesis is anterior displacement of one vertebra over another.[177] Spondylolisthesis usually results from spondylolysis after the normal resistance to forward displacement of the vertebra is disrupted because of fracture or elongation of the pars interarticularis.[178] Narrowing of the spinal canal will occur if posterior elements also slide forward. Szyprt et al.[179] demonstrated that a pars defect was associated with a prevalence of disc degeneration greater than that seen in a normal aging population.

With enough anterior slippage, the central spinal canal and the structures within may become compromised. However, slips present in juvenile or adolescent patients may autofuse or ankylose once the patient reaches skeletal maturity and remain asymptomatic throughout life.[180] Frennered et al.[181] performed follow-up with juvenile patients with spondylolisthesis after a mean time of 7 years. Thirty percent of the patients had surgery after 3.7 years, whereas 83% of the nonoperatively treated patients were rated excellent or good. These authors were unable to predict progression of slip or need for future operative treatment from findings at the initial consultation.[181] Beutler et al.[182] followed juvenile patients who had lesions of the pars identified using radiography, for 45 years. Patients with unilateral defects never experienced slippage over the course of the study, with 30% of the defects healing. Of the patients with bilateral defects, 81% progressed to spondylolisthesis. Progression of spondylolisthesis was greatest in the first decade after identification (i.e., in the teens) with subsequent slowing with each subsequent decade. There was no association of slip progression and LBP.[182]

Other vertebral anomalies, such as transitional lumbar vertebrae (TLV) or spina bifida occulta (SBO), have been associated with increased severity of LBP,[183] but the overall evidence for such an association is equivocal.[184] In a series of 4000 individuals, Tini et al.[185] demonstrated no association between LBP and the presence of a TLV. Peterson et al.[186] found similar results—352 patients with LBP had no difference in self-report of pain or disability based on TLV status.

Other reports indicated that TLV increased nerve root symptoms, whereas SBO did not.[183] Patients with nerve root symptoms and a TLV have a greater incidence of disc prolapse than those without a TLV for the vertebral level directly above the TLV.[187] In addition, spinal stenosis in the absence of spondylolisthesis is more likely to occur at the level above a TLV.[187] However, it is important to note that radiographic evidence of a vertebral anomaly does not necessarily indicate a greater likelihood of LBP.

LUMBAR SPINE IMAGING

The advent of stronger magnets used in MRI has resulted in finer resolution of subsequent image reconstructions of the target tissue. For example, researchers at the University of Florida have successfully obtained MR images and spectra from single neurons.[188] One might expect that improving the resolution of imaging technology increased the likelihood of detecting a link between pathology and pain in the lumbar spine. Realistically, the determination of a pathoanatomic origin of LBP is made difficult by the rate of false-positive findings on imaging studies (i.e., subjects without LBP showing abnormal findings).

The reported rates of these false-positive findings appear to vary. For example, Stadnik et al.[189] report that 81% of asymptomatic patients had evidence of a disc bulge and that radial annular tears might be found in 56% of asymptomatic patients, whereas Jensen et al.[190] reported in their study that 52% of subjects without pain had a bulge at one level, and 27% showed disc protrusion, and 14% had evidence of disruption of the outer annulus. Evidence of herniation of disc material is shown on computerized tomography (CT) scan,[163] MRI,[191] and myelography,[192] in 20% to 76% of persons with no sciatica.

Nondisc pathology is also often identified in patients without back pain. Some 13%[192,193] to 19%[190] of asymptomatic patients have evidence of Schmorl's nodes. SBO (26%) and osteophyte formation (47%) may be present in individuals without the symptoms of back pain,[193] as is stenotic change.[194] In addition, the prevalence of all identified conditions increases with age. Autopsy studies on a large number of subjects have found disc degeneration, facet joint osteoarthritis, or osteophytes in 90% to 100% of subjects over age 64.[195] Using MRI, researchers have identified central stenosis in as many as 21% of asymptomatic subjects over age 60 and 80% of subjects over age 70.[194] Likewise the prevalence of disc bulges increases but not that of protrusions.[190] Other vertebral anomalies, such as SBO and TLV, also occur in people without pain. For example, 12% of high school- and college-aged males without LBP have evidence of SBO without LBP,[196] and the incidence of TLV may be as high as 30%, regardless of whether the person has LBP.[197]

Thus, the association between clinical complaints and concurrent "pathological" radiological findings must be considered cautiously. This association also appears to apply to the predictive ability of imaging. Savage et al.[36] reported that 32% of asymptomatic subjects had "abnormal" lumbar spines (i.e., evidence of disc degeneration, disc bulging or protrusion, facet hypertrophy, or nerve root compression). To obfuscate matters, only 47% of subjects who were experiencing LBP had an abnormality identified.[36] When those subjects without LBP but with abnormal findings on imaging were followed for 12 months, 13 subjects experienced LBP for the first time; however, there were no changes in the MRI appearances of their lumbar spines that these authors could identify that accounted for the onset of LBP.[36] Therefore pain developed in the absence of any associated change in the radiographic appearance of the spine.

In contrast, Elffering[198] reported that over the course of 5 years, identified disc herniations progressed to degenerative disc disease while the patients remained asymptomatic, indicating that pathology progressed in the absence of any associated pain response. In addition, Boos et al.[199] also followed asymptomatic patients with a disc herniation for 5 years and determined that physical job characteristics and psychological aspects of work were more powerful than MRI-identified disc abnormalities in predicting the need for medical consultation related to LBP.

Multiple potential pathoanatomical pain generators have been identified in the lumbar spine by diagnostic imaging. However, the reality is that the ability of the clinician to identify specific anatomical lesions causing the pain is limited, even with the best available imaging studies. In fact, it has been estimated that the specific anatomical lesion causing LBP is unidentifiable 80% to 85% of the time.[200] On top of this, reviews and editorials have indicated that unnecessary imaging is associated with higher rates of spinal surgery, contributes to additional harm from radiation exposure, and does not improve outcomes in patients without serious pathology.[201]

However, the utility of imaging of the lumbar spine does increase when the clinician is suspicious of a serious pathology or nerve root compression. For example, radiography is indicated when the clinician suspects a compression fracture or neoplasm. Likewise, ultrasound of the abdomen is the currently accepted gold standard for identification of abdominal aneurysm.[202] Imaging studies may also be appropriate if the patient fails to improve with conservative therapy or shows progression of neurological involvement. These assertions of focused imaging in the diagnostic process of LBP are supported by a longitudinal study that found limited accuracy of "common" MRI findings (i.e., disc desiccation, bulges, loss of height) but improved accuracy when less common MRI findings (i.e., central stenosis and nerve root compression) were considered.[203]

MANAGEMENT OF LOW BACK PAIN

Figure 12-6 summarizes the specific management process presented in this chapter. The primary task of the

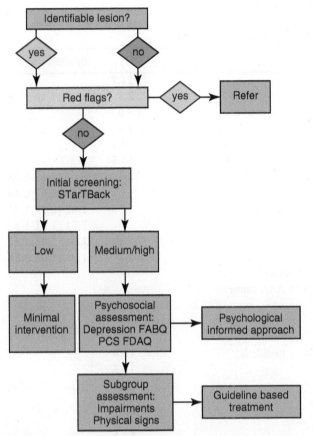

Figure 12-6 Proposed conceptual model for the diagnosis and management of low back pain. *FABQ,* Fear-Avoidance Beliefs Questionnaire; *PCS,* Pain Catastrophizing Scale; *FDAQ,* Fear of Daily Activities Questionnaire.

clinician is to identify red flags that may indicate a serious pathology, mimicking the symptoms of LBP, that should be referred to a specialist. Red flag identification is accomplished through the patient history or appropriate laboratory studies. Once systemic pathology has been eliminated as a potential source of LBP, the secondary task is to identify yellow flags that are predictive of the development of chronic LBP. Once factors that affect the prognosis have been identified, the tertiary task is to recognize the subgroup classification associated with the optimum treatment outcome.

Identification of Red Flags

The clinician must first determine whether the LBP symptoms arise from a serious pathology of another source (Table 12-5). This procedure should take little time for most patients, and a high number of "positive" findings is not expected. However, the clinician must remain diligent in performing this part of the diagnostic process because the consequences of failing to identify serious pathology are potentially severe for the patient.

Deyo et al.[204] have suggested a set of historical questions that can be used in screening for serious pathology in patients with LBP. These cover topics such as a history of cancer, unexplained weight loss, failure of rest to relieve

pain, and a history of fevers or chills, intravenous drug use, and/or recent urinary tract infection.[204] Additional screening questions should be specific for urinary retention and saddle anesthesia, osteoporosis, and/or history of compression fracture.[204] If necessary, a review of pertinent medical history in first-order relatives may give insight into possible spondyloarthropathies, if these are suspected in a particular patient.

Red Flags for Low Back Pain

- Abdominal aortic aneurysm
- Kidney disease
- Liver disease
- Duodenal ulcers
- Pancreatitis
- Endometriosis
- Cancer
- Cauda equina syndrome
- Spondyloarthropathies
- Fractures
- Infection

Abdominal Aortic Aneurysm

An abdominal aortic aneurysm (AAA) is a pathological dilatation of the abdominal aorta below the renal arteries to a diameter greater than 3.0 cm (1.2 inches). AAAs are found in 4% to 8% of older men and 0.5% to 1.5% of older women.[205-208] Feilding et al.[209] reported that the most common symptoms reported by patients on the first presentation with AAA are abdominal pain and backache. Age, smoking, sex, and family history are the most significant AAA risk factors. In fact, Lederle et al.[207] indicated that the excess prevalence associated with smoking (i.e., 100 cigarettes lifetime) accounted for 75% of all AAAs of 4.0 cm or larger. Table 12-5 lists the ORs associated with these individual risk factors for AAA.

Fielding et al.[209] indicated that diagnosis could be made by careful routine palpation. Deep and careful palpation should be performed to the left of the midline, keeping the hands steady in one position until the aortic pulse is felt, and then carefully evaluating the lateral extent of the pulse with the pads of the fingers.[210] Physical findings may include a tender, palpable, pulsatile abdominal mass.[209] However, the reported sensitivity and specificity of palpation vary dramatically.[211] For example, detection of AAA by palpation improves in thinner patients[210] and in the presence of recognizable risk factors.[202,210]

Despite the support for palpation, abdominal ultrasound remains the gold standard for identification of AAA.[202] Specifically, the clinician should consider the possibility of rupture of an AAA in a male patient over the age of 60 years who smokes and presents with sudden onset of back and/or loin pain.[212]

TABLE **12-5**

Red Flag Pathology and Associated Likelihood and Odds Ratios Indicative of Serious Disease

Condition	Findings	LR	OR (95% CI)
Cancer[171]	Previous history of cancer	14.7	
	Age >50	2.7	
	Failure to respond to conservative intervention	3.0	
	ESR ≥20 mm/h	2.4	
	ESR ≥50 mm/h	19.2	
	ESR ≥100 mm/h	55.5	
Aneurysm (≥4 cm [1.6 inches])[205]	Smoking (100 cigarettes lifetime)		5.07 (4.13-6.21)
	Female		0.18 (0.07-0.48)
	Non-Caucasian		1.02 (0.77-1.35)
	Age		1.71 (1.61-1.82)
	Family history		1.94 (1.63-2.32)
Aneurysm[209]	Positive palpation examination: Abdominal girth ≤100 cm (39.4 inches) Each 1 cm (0.5 inches) increase in AAA diameter	3.2	1.95 (1.06-3.58)
Compression fracture[171,237]	Age >70	11.2	
	Female	—	
	Corticosteroid use	48.5	
	Trauma (significant in young, minor in elderly)	10.0	
	2 of 4	15.5	
	3 of 4	218.3	
Spinal infection[171,222,239]	Fever: tuberculous osteomyelitis	13.5	
	Fever: pyogenic osteomyelitis	25.0	
	Fever: spinal epidural abscess	41.5	
General red flag history[240]	Sleep problems (wakes from sleep, uses medication, cannot sleep)	3.8	
	Unable to urinate	3.0	
	Unable to hold urine	1.4	
	Current smoker	3.3	

AAA, Abdominal aortic aneurysm; *CI*, confidence interval; *ESR*, erythrocyte sedimentation rate; *LR*, likelihood ratio; *OR*, odds ratio.

Back pain is a common historical complaint in a variety of conditions affecting the kidney. LBP (71.3%) was the most common discomfort reported by patients with polycystic kidney disease (PKD) during the course of their disease, with abdominal pain the second most common. These complaints were recorded by 42% of patients before diagnosis of PKD.[213] In addition, 26% of patients with PKD in a study by Bajwa et al.[213] reported back pain radiating to the hips or legs. Central back and flank pain has been described by patients in renal failure[214] and with viral infection.[215]

Massive liver cysts may also result in LBP from the effect of changes in posture as cysts grow, enlarging the abdomen.[213] Duodenal ulcers[216] may refer pain into the upper lumbar spine, and abdominal pain and LBP are the primary historical complaints of patients with pancreatitis[217] and endometriosis.[218]

Cancer
Although spinal cord compression is a complication of malignancy that affects the quality of life of an estimated 12,700 new patients each year,[219] the prevalence of cancer

related to back pain is likely to be low in primary care settings. Deyo and Diehl[171] reported a prevalence of cancer-related back pain in primary care patients of 0.66%. This is similar to the prevalence reported for academic multidisciplinary spine centers (0.69%) and higher than that noted (0.12%) in private practice multidisciplinary spine centers.[220] Deyo and Diehl[171] have presented several historical and laboratory findings associated with cancer-related back pain. These authors outline a strategy whereby key historical findings (i.e., age over 50, previous history of cancer, unexplained weight loss, and failure to respond to conservative intervention) are supported by key laboratory tests (erythrocyte sedimentation rate [ESR]).[171] Subsequent investigation has supported the key historical findings of night pain, aching character of symptom manifestation, and unexplained weight loss originally reported.[220] Cancers of the skin may also be implicated in local tenderness over the tissues of the lumbar spine. Ogboli et al.[221] reported that six different types of common skin tumors may present as areas that are tender when palpated.

The positive likelihood ratios for cancer screening using selected historical and laboratory findings are presented in Table 12-5. It has been suggested that prompt spinal imaging might be indicated for those patients having two or more historical findings and an ESR ≥20 mm/h.[171] It should also be noted that Hollingworth et al.[222] indicated that the benefits of using MR imaging for screening rather than x-ray did not justify the increased costs.

Cauda Equina Syndrome

Compression of the cauda equina of any cause (e.g., trauma, central disc protrusion, hemorrhage, or tumor) requires immediate surgical referral.[204] Fortunately the incidence and prevalence of this condition are very low. Johnsson et al.[223] report the population incidence of the syndrome to be 0.03% in Denmark and 0.005% in Sweden.[224,225]

The most consistent findings in cauda equina syndrome are urinary retention and sensory changes on the buttocks, thighs, and peritoneum "saddle anaesthesia."[226] Loss of anal sphincter tone is present in 60% to 80% of cases.[227] Urinary retention is also common in simple nerve root compression syndromes with no relation to true cauda equina syndrome.[227]

Spondyloarthropathies

The prevalence of spondyloarthropathies is estimated to be 1% to 2% of the population. Spondyloarthropathies are related inflammatory spinal arthropathies characterized by sacroiliac involvement and a relationship to HLA-B27 but distinct from rheumatoid arthritis. This group of conditions includes ankylosing spondylitis (AS), reactive arthritis (including Reiter's syndrome), psoriatic arthritis, arthritis associated with bowel disease (i.e., enteropathic arthritis), juvenile spondyloarthropathy, and a set of unspecified spondyloarthropathies. The diagnostic criteria recommended by the Assessment of Spondyloarthritis International Society are listed in Box 12-1.[228]

AS is considered the most common of the spondyloarthropathies. Connective tissue changes occur as subchondral tissue thickens and eventually is replaced by fibrocartilage and finally bone. AS affects men more than women, beginning with complaints of back pain and stiffness in early adulthood. The final diagnosis often is not made until the patient is older because the earlier symptoms are minimal. Neck pain and stiffness are associated with advanced disease. Historical findings include reports of insidious onset back pain that is worse with inactivity and improves with exercise. These complaints are not particularly specific; however, association with a family history of spondyloarthropathy, acute anterior uveitis (iritis), and impaired trunk mobility or chest expansion strengthens the clinical picture. Clinical diagnosis is further supported by radiographic evidence of sacroiliitis, which is considered the hallmark of AS. MRI can be helpful in detecting early change in the spine, but the increased cost may limit its routine use.

BOX 12-1

Assessment of Spondyloarthritis International Society Classification Criteria

AXIAL SPONDYLOARTHRITIS

Criterion: In patients with >3 months' back pain and age <45 years
Sacroiliitis on imaging
AND 1 or more features
OR HLA-B27 AND 2 or more features

Features of Spondyloarthropathies:
- Inflammatory back pain
- Arthritis
- Enthesitis (heel) (inflammation where tendons insert)
- Uveitis (inflammation of the uvea in the eye)
- Dactylitis (inflammation of an entire finger or toe)
- Psoriasis
- Crohn's disease and colitis
- Good response to NSAIDs
- Family history of spondyloarthritis
- HLA-B27
- Elevated C-reactive protein

HLA-B27, human leukocyte antigen-B27; NSAIDs, non-steroidal anti-inflammatory drugs.
Data from Mease P: Psoriatic arthritis and spondyloarthritis assessment and management update, *Curr Opin Rheumatology* 25(3):287-296, 2013.

Reactive arthritis is an episode of aseptic, acute, asymmetric peripheral arthritis occurring within 1 month of a primary infection elsewhere in the body. It is frequently associated with one or more extra-articular features, such as conjunctivitis or acute iritis, enthesitis at the Achilles tendon or plantar fascia, mucocutaneous lesions, urethritis, and carditis.[229] The combination of arthritis, conjunctivitis, and urethritis has been called Reiter's syndrome, but most patients with reactive arthritis do not present with this triad.[229]

Psoriasis is a common skin disease (1% to 3% prevalence)[230,231] in Caucasian adults that affects men and women equally. The disease is less common in other ethnic groups, such as Native Americans (0.3%).[230] Approximately 10%[230] to 30%[232,233] of patients with psoriasis have associated inflammatory arthritis. Skin lesions usually appear before the arthritis in approximately 50% of patients with psoriatic arthritis. The arthritis usually begins between 30 and 50 years of age, but it can also begin in childhood. When searching for psoriasis, the skin check should not be limited to the extremities but should also include the scalp, ears, umbilicus, pelvic area, perineum, natal cleft, palms, soles, and nails. Nail involvement is often a useful clue in diagnosis of psoriatic arthritis.[231] Gladman[234] suggests that psoriatic arthritis may be distinguished from the other spondyloarthropathies by the presence of asymmetrical, peripheral arthritis, asymmetrical spinal involvement, and lower level of pain.

Enteropathic arthritis refers to inflammatory arthritic conditions associated with bowel disorders, such as

Crohn's disease and ulcerative colitis. de Vlam et al.[235] reported that 39% of consecutive patients with ulcerative colitis or Crohn's disease had enteropathic arthritis and 90% met the criteria for spondyloarthropathy. Peripheral arthritis tends to be more frequent in enteropathic arthritis than AS.[235]

Fractures

Compression fractures usually occur in osteoporotic bone, most frequently at T8, T12, L1, and L5.[236] Historical findings that increase the probability of compression fracture are reported in Table 12-5. The patient is often older without a history of specific spinal trauma but with other clinical features of osteoporosis, such as kyphosis or a previous history of wrist and hip fractures.[236] The patient will often report pain after a seemingly simple maneuver, such as a cough or opening a window. In addition, some compression fractures occur spontaneously while the patient is lying in bed.[236] Deyo et al.[204] recommend that a patient on long-term corticosteroid therapy who is complaining of spine pain should be considered to have a fracture until proven otherwise because this historical finding greatly affects the probability of compression fracture. This observation has been supported in a primary care study in which Henschke et al.[237] investigated a combination of four red flags (i.e., age >70 years, female, corticosteroid use, and history of trauma). Two positive of four red flags resulted in an increase in the suspicion of fracture (likelihood ratio [LR]+15.5; 95% CI, 8.5 to 28.4). Three red flags of four yielded a large LR+ (LR+ 218.3; 95% CI, 45.6 to 953.8), but the authors encouraged caution when interpreting this result because of the extremely large CI (see Table 12-5).

Spinal Infections

Fever of unknown origin is defined as a temperature higher than 38.3 °C (101 °F).[238] Urinary tract infections, indwelling urinary catheters, skin infections, and injection sites for intravenous drugs have been identified as potential sites from which a spinal infection develops in approximately 40% of patients with osteomyelitis.[239] Fewer than 2% of patients with back pain attending a primary care clinic presented with fever,[171] indicating that there are very few false positives when associating fever to infection in patients with LBP (see Table 12-5).

Red Flag Summary

Roach et al.[240] collected demographic and clinical information from 174 patients with LBP to examine the sensitivity and specificity of historical questions to identify patients with serious pathology in the lumbar spine. These authors classified serious pathology to include osteoporotic fracture, tumor, infection, and surgical management of spinal stenosis or disc herniation. The historical questions with the best positive LRs were related to the inability to urinate or hold urine, sleep disturbances, and current smoking history (see Table 12-5).[240] It should be noted that although these questions had very high specificity (i.e., high true negative), they also had a very low true positive rate. The implication of this relationship is that many of the patients with serious pathology (as defined by Roach et al.[240]) did not answer "yes" to the historical questions.

Identification of Yellow Flags

Once red flags have been considered, the clinician may decide that referral to another specialist is necessary before conservative rehabilitation is deemed appropriate. This outcome must always be considered, but it is not a frequent outcome for most practice areas. More often the clinician proceeds to screen for yellow flags, the second step of the differential diagnosis and classification approach.

Yellow Flags for Low Back Pain

- Depression
- Fear-avoidance beliefs
- Pain catastrophizing

Yellow flags represent psychological constructs with documented influences on pain, treatment participation, and outcomes.[241] In general terms, the identification of yellow flags allows the clinician to determine the potential for a psychological influence on a patient's clinical presentation of LBP. The rationale for considering yellow flags in the differential diagnosis and classification of LBP is summarized in the *New Zealand Acute Low Back Pain Guide*[242]: "The goal of identifying yellow flags is to find factors that can be influenced positively to facilitate recovery and prevent or reduce long-term disability and work loss. This includes identifying both the frequent unintentional learning or emotional barriers and the less common intentional barriers to improvement."

Waddell et al.[243,244] first described signs believed to be associated with aspects of distress and abnormal illness behavior that could lead to increasing amounts of disability. These signs were described as nonorganic and have been investigated in prospective studies predicting return to work status. Several studies have demonstrated that the presence of nonorganic signs were predictive of a delayed return to work,[245-248] whereas other studies have reported that nonorganic signs were not predictive of return to work.[249,250] Fritz et al.[251] investigated nonorganic signs as a screening tool for predicting return to work and presented strong evidence indicating high false-positive rates are a consistent problem with nonorganic signs (Table 12-6). For example, even under the best condition reported in the literature (−LR, 0.48), the posttest probability only decreases from 50% to 32% for predicting

TABLE **12-6**

Lack of Evidence for Use of Nonorganic Signs to Screen for Return to Work

Author	Sample Description	Nonorganic Signs for Positive Finding	Outcome Determination	Negative LR
Bradish et al.[249]	Work-related LBP	Three or more	Return to at least part-time work	0.60
Werneke et al.[250]	Nonworking or partly disabled patients with LBP	One or more	Return to work or improved work status	0.59
Kummel[247]	Work-related LBP	Three or more	Return to at least part-time work	0.48
Karas et al.[246]	Work-related LBP	Three or more	Return to at least part-time work	0.77
Fritz et al.[251]	Work-related LBP	Two or more	Return to full-time work	0.75

LBP, Low back pain; *LR*, likelihood ratio.

Data from Fritz JM, Wainner RS, Hicks GE: The use of nonorganic signs and symptoms as a screening tool for return-to-work in patients with acute low back pain, *Spine* 25:1925-1931, 2000.

inability to return to work based on two or fewer nonorganic signs. Collectively, this evidence suggests clinicians should consider methods other than nonorganic signs when screening for psychological influence.

Screening for Yellow Flags

Screening tools have been developed in an effort to better identify patients at risk for poor outcomes due to psychological distress following an episode of LBP. Some tools are designed to identify patient subgroups for the purposes of treatment allocation,[252-254] whereas others are used to identify those at risk for poor functional or pain-related outcomes.[255-258] Two common multifactorial screening tools for the assessment of yellow flags in patients with LBP are the Örebro Musculoskeletal Pain Screening Questionnaire (ÖMPSQ) and the Subgroups for Targeted Treatment (STarT) Back Tool, or SBT.

The ÖMPSQ is a 25-item yellow flag screening tool that predicts long-term disability and the inability to return to work.[257] Originally developed to predict sick leave outcomes in occupational LBP, the ÖMPSQ has been adopted as a subgrouping tool in clinical practice. High-risk cutoff scores have been reported in the literature for a variety of patient populations.[259-264] A systematic review concluded the ÖMPSQ had a moderate ability to predict long-term pain, disability, and sick leave outcomes.[265] A short-form of the ÖMPSQ was developed in a primary care sample with good correlation to information obtained from the original questionnaire. A cutoff of 50 on the short form identified 83% of patients accumulating more than 14 days of sick leave.[258]

In contrast to the ÖMPSQ, which was originally developed as a prognostic tool, the SBT was designed as a subgrouping tool to identify treatment-modifiable indicators associated with low, medium, and high risk of poor functional outcomes. The SBT is a brief, nine-item questionnaire consisting of physical and psychosocial subscales appropriate for use across the spectrum of patients with nonspecific LBP.[266] The psychosocial subscale comprises individual items from single-construct questionnaires representing modifiable psychosocial factors shown to predict poor functional or pain-related outcomes. Physical and psychosocial subscales are combined to provide an overall risk assessment. In a randomized, clinical trial, Hill et al.[254] demonstrated superior improvements in disability, generic health benefits, and cost savings with stratified care as the result of SBT screening. Studies using the SBT in outpatient physical therapy support its validity for identifying patients at risk of poor outcomes.[267,268] The SBT provides comparable measurement properties to the ÖMPSQ, yet offers the advantages of being shorter and easier to score.[269]

Figure 12-6 outlines the integration of the SBT into a clinical decision-making algorithm. Overall scores of ≤3 indicate a low-risk category. Overall scores >3 but <4 on the psychosocial subscale indicate medium risk. Psychosocial subscale scores ≥4 indicate high risk.[266] Because prognosis for patients in the low-risk group is generally favorable, minimal intervention is suggested. For patients in the medium- or high-risk categories, a more thorough assessment of psychological factors is suggested before initiation of treatment. This assessment allows the clinician to more thoroughly evaluate specific psychological constructs involved in the development and maintenance of chronic LBP. Furthermore, this assessment provides direction for psychologically informed interventions that may improve outcomes for patients in medium- or high-risk categories.[254] A comprehensive review of specific psychological constructs is beyond the scope of this chapter; however, interested readers are referred to reviews by Pincus.[270,271]

Assessment of Yellow Flags

Typically, self-report questionnaires are used to more thoroughly assess common psychological influences involved with LBP that are general (depression) or specific (fear-avoidance beliefs, activity-specific fear, pain catastrophizing) in nature.

Depression

Depression is a commonly experienced illness or mood state, with a wide variety of symptoms ranging from loss of appetite to suicidal thoughts.[272] Depression is commonly experienced in the general population, but it appears to be more commonly experienced in conjunction with chronic LBP.[273-275] A Canadian population-based study estimated the general rate of major depression to be 5.9% for pain-free individuals and 19.8% for individuals with chronic LBP.[274] Other studies have reported depression prevalence rates of up to 32% for individuals with chronic LBP.[276,277] Based on this epidemiological information, the authors felt that routine screening for depression should be part of the clinical diagnosis of LBP.

Studies have linked depressive symptoms with increased pain intensity, disability, medication use, satisfaction with care, and unemployment in patients seeking care for LBP.[264,278,279] Depression is also predictive of poor functional and pain-related outcomes. For example, Melloh et al.[280] found that depression and maladaptive cognitions predicted the development of persistent pain following an acute episode of LBP. In a study of patients undergoing physical therapy, George et al.[281] found depressive symptoms were the strongest contributors to baseline pain and function and were predictive of pain intensity ratings and functional status at discharge. They also found patients with higher levels of depression had a longer duration of treatment and more clinic visits compared with patients with normal depressive symptoms.

Despite this evidence of its deleterious influence on LBP, depression does not appear to be adequately screened for in practice settings that commonly examine patients with LBP. For example, depressive symptoms were not identified in 35% to 75% of patients seeking treatment from primary care physicians,[272,282] 63% of spine surgeons indicated that they only occasionally or never screen use psychological tests,[283] and surveys of physical therapy practice do not mention psychological screening as part of normal practice patterns.[284-286]

Effective screening for depression involves more than just generating a clinical impression that the patient is depressed. Separate studies involving spine surgeons[283] and physical therapists[275] have demonstrated that clinical impressions are

not sensitive enough to detect depression in patients with LBP. Instead, it appears to be more effective to use self-report questionnaires (e.g., Zung Self-Rating Depression Scale, Beck's Depression Inventory, or the Depression Anxiety Stress Scales) to screen for depression. However, these questionnaires often contain more than 20 items, which may place a burden on the patient and clinician.

Any dialogue between mental health and spine clinicians should determine whether depressed patients should be treated concurrently. In our opinion, examples of **inappropriate treatment** of a depressed patient by a spine clinician include (1) a patient in whom low back symptoms represent only somatic complaints, without associated physical impairment, and (2) a patient whose depressive symptoms are severe or extreme and include suicidal thoughts.

Evidence suggests that using two specific questions from the **Primary Care Evaluation of Mental Disorders** patient questionnaire can effectively screen for depression in primary care settings.[287] The questions are (1) "During the past month, have you often been bothered by feeling down, depressed, or hopeless?" and (2) "During the past month, have you often been bothered by little interest or pleasure in doing things?" The patient responds to the questions with "yes" or "no," and the number of yes items are totaled, giving a potential range of 0 to 2. A study involving LBP suggests that these two questions also accurately identified depression in patients seeking physical therapy treatment for LBP (Table 12-7).[275] Studies indicate a single question from the **Subjective Health Complaints (SHC) Inventory** (*"To what extent have you been affected by depression/low mood during the last month?"*) has sufficient sensitivity (0.79 to 0.95) and negative predictive value (89% to 99%) to screen for depressive symptoms.[288,289]

Fear-Avoidance Beliefs

Fear-avoidance beliefs are a measure of patients' beliefs and attitudes toward LBP.[290] Specifically, fear-avoidance

TABLE **12-7**

Accuracy of Screening for Depression Using Two Questions from the Primary Care Evaluation of Mental Disorders Patient Questionnaire

	Mild Depression	Moderate Depression	Severe Depression	Extreme Depression
One Question Result				
Positive LR	3.40 (2.40, 4.82)	2.76 (2.10, 3.62)	2.44 (1.91, 3.12)	2.25 (1.71, 2.96)
Negative LR	0.37 (0.26, 0.51)	0.29 (0.18, 0.49)	0.25 (0.11, 0.55)	0.23 (0.06, 0.84)
Two Questions Result				
Positive LR	5.40 (3.10, 9.42)	4.61 (3.0, 7.0)	4.32 (3.0, 6.1)	3.89 (2.80, 5.40)
Negative LR	0.55 (0.44, 0.67)	0.43 (0.30, 0.60)	0.28 (0.14, 0.53)	0.18 (0.05, 0.66)

LR, Likelihood ratio.

Modified from Haggman S, Maher CG, Refshauge KM: Screening for symptoms of depression by physical therapists managing low back pain, *Phys Ther* 84:1157-1166, 2004; and Whooley MA, Avins AL, Miranda J et al: Case-finding instruments for depression: two questions are as good as many, *J Gen Intern Med* 12:439-445, 1997.

beliefs are a composite measure of the patient's fear related to LBP, how physical activity and work affect LBP, and how LBP should be managed.[290-292] Theoretically, patients with elevated fear-avoidance beliefs are more likely to use an avoidance response to their LBP, resulting in the development of an exaggerated pain perception and chronic disability.[290] Prospective studies have supported the validity of fear-avoidance beliefs because they are predictive of the development of chronic LBP,[293-296] poor work-related outcomes,[297,298] reduced function,[299,300] and higher health care use.[301]

As a result of this evidence, identification of elevated fear-avoidance beliefs has been suggested as an important component in the diagnosis of LBP. The **Fear-Avoidance Beliefs Questionnaire (FABQ)** is commonly used to assess fear-avoidance beliefs in patients with LBP.[292] The FABQ has 16 items that are scored on a scale ranging from 0 (strongly disagree) to 6 (strongly agree). The individual items are then summed to generate an estimate of fear-avoidance beliefs, and higher numbers on the FABQ indicate increased levels of fear-avoidance beliefs. Two subscales are contained within the FABQ: a seven-item (items 6, 7, 9-12, and 15) work subscale (FABQ-W; score range 0 to 42) for fear-avoidance beliefs about work and a four-item (items 2-5) physical activity subscale (FABQ-PA; score range 0 to 24) for fear-avoidance beliefs about physical activity. Several studies indicate that the FABQ is a reliable, valid, and/or responsive measure,[292,302-304] suggesting it is appropriate for use in clinical settings.

Evidence suggests the FABQ-W can be used effectively in occupational LBP.[305] A study of patients with acute, work-related LBP who were evaluated for demographic, physical, and psychosocial factors found that the FABQ-W was the strongest predictor for return to work at 4 weeks.[293] Patients who scored greater than 34 on the FABQ-W were less likely to return to work by 4 weeks (+LR, 3.33; 95% CI, 1.65 to 6.77). In contrast, patients who scored less than 29 on the FABQ-W were less likely to return to work (−LR, 0.08; 95% CI, 0.01 to 0.54). In another study of work-related musculoskeletal disorders, Holden et al.[306] showed an FABQ-W score of ≤27.5 had maximum sensitivity (100%), whereas an FABQ-W score of >39.5 had maximum specificity (81.9%) for identifying patients at risk for poor return to work outcomes. Although the FABQ-W may be most effective in predicting functional and work-related outcomes in patients with occupational LBP, a study by George et al.[307] suggests the FABQ-W may also be useful for identifying patients at risk for higher disability as the result of nonoccupational LBP in physical therapy settings. This study found patients scoring above a previously established cutoff score (>29) on the FABQ-W had higher disability scores and were less likely to show improvements in disability at 6 months. Further analysis in this cohort found FABQ-W scores <5 might be useful in identifying patients most likely to show improve-

ments in disability at 6 months. Conversely, FABQ-W scores >20 were associated with the highest positive likelihood ratios (2.3 to 5.1) for showing no improvements in disability at 6 months.[307] Unfortunately, similar cutoff scores have not been reported for the FABQ-PA, making assessment of fear-avoidance beliefs related to physical activity difficult. It has been suggested that a score higher than 14 indicates an elevated FABQ-PA,[292,308] but studies have not supported the predictive utility of this cutoff for identifying patients likely to experience poor functional outcomes.[293,307]

Activity-Specific Fear

Many studies have examined the relationship between fear-avoidance beliefs and actual physical capacity in patients with chronic LBP with variable results.[309-314] One potential explanation for this variability is the differential demands of individual tasks used in each study to measure physical capacity. For instance, pain-related fear may influence tasks that require maximum effort more significantly than tasks that require submaximal effort.[315] As a result, general fear-avoidance belief measures (e.g., FABQ) may not be sensitive enough to predict fear-related functional limitations equally across tasks. In these cases, activity-specific fear may be a stronger predictor of clinical outcomes.

Beneciuk et al.[316] provide empirical support for assessing general and activity-specific fear separately. In a study of patients with LBP seeking physical therapy, they found patients with high specific fear and patients with high general fear and high catastrophizing comprised two distinct groups. Interestingly, patients reporting elevated levels of specific activity-related fear did not demonstrate elevated levels of general pain-related fear beliefs or catastrophizing, supporting the differential assessment of general and activity-specific fear. Furthermore, the authors found a subgroup by time interaction, suggesting different types of fear may be differentially associated with clinical outcomes. Further evidence to support consideration of activity-specific fear is provided by Demoulin et al.,[315] who found poor associations between general and activity-specific measures of pain-related fear. These findings suggest general and activity-specific fear measures may be evaluating distinct fear-related constructs.[315]

Activity-specific fear measures have been proposed (1) to more adequately assess the influence of fear on function and (2) to direct in vivo graded exposure paradigms.[317] The **Photograph Series of Daily Activities (PHODA)** is an assessment tool for activity-specific fear commonly used in the development of graded exposure paradigms. It includes 100 photographs of common activities patients may encounter in their daily life, from household chores to physical exercise. Patients report concern for harming their back when engaging in each activity from 0 (not harmful) to 100 (extremely harmful). An electronic, 40-question version of the PHODA (PHODA-SeV) has demonstrated good construct validity, with overall PHODA-SeV scores moderately correlated with self-reported pain severity and fear of movement/(re)injury.[318] Leeuw et al. also reported that patients who received graded exposure in vivo aimed at reducing the perceived harmfulness of activities had significantly lower PHODA-SeV scores after treatment than patients receiving graded activity that did not address these assumptions.[318]

The **Fear of Daily Activities Questionnaire (FDAQ)** is another activity-specific fear assessment tool designed for use in clinical practice.[319] The FDAQ lists 10 activities that patients commonly report fear of performing due to LBP. Patients can also list two additional open-ended responses and rate their fear for performing those activities. Patients rate each FDAQ item on a numeric rating scale from 0 (no fear) to 100 (maximal fear). The FDAQ is scored by totaling the Numerical Rating Scale (NRS) ratings for the 10 standard activities and divided by 10. Like the PHODA, the FDAQ was primarily designed to guide physical therapy interventions supplemented with graded exposure. Currently, there is limited support for the predictive validity of the FDAQ for pain-related outcomes; however, strong associations with concurrent disability suggest fear of specific activities may contribute to the disablement process in LBP. Furthermore, changes in fear of specific activities were shown to predict change in disability after 4 weeks of physical therapy.[319] These findings provide empirical support for the incorporation of both general beliefs about pain-related fear and beliefs about specific activities in the assessment of LBP.[319,320]

Pain Catastrophizing

Pain catastrophizing is a negative cognition related to the belief that the experienced pain will inevitably result in the worst possible outcome.[321] Pain catastrophizing is believed to be a multidimensional construct comprising rumination, helplessness, and pessimism.[321] A practical example might help to illustrate the concept of pain catastrophizing. A patient with elevated pain catastrophizing would expect to have severe pain for the rest of his or her life, even if his LBP were mild in severity and was being treated appropriately.

Pain catastrophizing has also been linked to the development and maintenance of chronic pain. Most of the literature documenting the unique influence of pain catastrophizing on chronic pain is cross sectional,[322-325] but there are some prospective studies that provide supporting evidence. For example, frequent pain catastrophizing during acute LBP was predictive of self-reported disability 6 months[67] and 1 year later,[326] even after considering select historical and clinical predictors. In a systematic

review, pain catastrophizing at baseline predicted disability at follow-up in four studies and pain at follow-up in two studies.[327] Three studies found no predictive effect of catastrophizing. In another systematic review, 66% ($n = 8$) of studies that investigated self-reported outcome measures found catastrophizing to be associated with pain and disability at follow-up in acute, subacute, and chronic LBP patients.[328] In studies that applied cutoff values, 83% ($n = 5$) found that patients with high levels of pain catastrophizing experienced worse clinical outcomes compared with patients with low levels of pain catastrophizing.[327]

Pain catastrophizing can be measured by the **Pain Catastrophizing Scale (PCS)**, which is a 13-item scale that assesses the degree of catastrophic cognitions a patient experiences while in pain.[329] The scale ranges from 1 (not at all) to 4 (always), and an example of an item is, "I worry all the time about whether the pain will end." In clinical settings, the PCS is commonly reported as a whole number by summing all 13 items (range, 0 to 52). Psychometric studies suggest acceptable levels of reliability and validity.[322,329] Factor analysis suggests a hierarchical factor structure, with three individual subscales of the PCS (i.e., rumination, magnification, and pessimism) contributing to an overall factor of pain catastrophizing.[322,329] Accordingly, the PCS offers multidimensional measurement of catastrophizing, whereas other common measures of catastrophizing (e.g., **Pain-Related Self-Statement Scale [PRSS]** or **Coping Strategies Questionnaire [CSQ]**) assess the construct unidimensionally.[327] Prediction of pain and disability with PCS is supported analytically[327,328]; however, few cutoffs have been reported in the peer-reviewed literature for use of the PCS to predict the clinical outcome of LBP. Of the cutoffs reported, many of the values are based on normative distributions.[330-332] For example, Linton et al.[331] established a cutoff of >23 for high versus low catastrophizing based on a quartile split and found higher disability in patients with a combination of high depression and high catastrophizing. Franklin et al.[330] found higher opioid use with elevated levels on a PCS; however, they used cutoffs based on a shortened version of the PCS.

Yellow Flag Summary

The consideration of yellow flags is an important part of the diagnostic process of LBP because it alerts the clinician to patients (1) who may be appropriate for referral because of depression or (2) who need treatment modifications to decrease risk of experiencing chronic disability. Specific education and exercise philosophies, more commonly referred to as psychologically informed practice approaches, have been proposed to address elevated psychosocial factors.[291] These approaches may be especially warranted for patients who score high on individual psychosocial or yellow flag screening measures. A detailed discussion of these approaches is beyond the scope of this chapter; however, they have been described in the literature, for example, synthesized in a 2011 Special Issue of *Physical Therapy*,[333,334] and results from randomized trials demonstrating efficacy of psychologically informed practice.[254,308,335]

SUMMARY

In 2014, the National Institutes of Health Pain Consortium convened a taskforce that was charged to develop research standards for LBP.[116] As part of that process, the group concluded that a pathophysiological diagnosis of LBP was unfeasible. Therefore, the primary way for the clinician to proceed is to first rule out "red flags," then screen for "yellow flags" and assess yellow flags in greater detail if indicated by the screening. After this, the next task is to determine the appropriate patient treatment strategy. Treatment strategies may include psychologically informed approaches when appropriate and/or assignment to a treatment subgroup classification (i.e., the subgroup that maximizes the probability of a favorable outcome). A review of treatment strategies and classification systems is beyond the scope of this chapter. Readers are referred to clinical practice guidelines for the treatment of LBP established by the Orthopedic Section of the American Physical Therapy Association.[336]

CASE EXAMPLES FOR DIAGNOSING LOW BACK PAIN

Case Example 1

A 62-year-old patient presents with complaints of nonspecific central LBP. He is unable to describe a mechanism of injury but relates that the pain has gradually worsened over several months. Furthermore, he describes his current pain as a constant, deep ache. During the history, the patient indicates that he has a previous history of cancer.

Cancer is a potential cause of LBP for this patient. The LRs from Table 12-5 are used to estimate the probability that this patient has cancer. In general, a 0.66% probability exists that cancer is a source of back pain (this estimate is based on a previously reported prevalence study[171]). The +LR that a patient over age 50 has cancer as a source of LBP is 2.7. Figure 12-7 shows a graphic method used to estimate the effect the patient's age has on the probability that cancer is a source of LBP. The Y-axis on the left side of the graph is the pretest probability in percentage. The line begins at 0.66%, crosses the central Y-axis (representing the LR) at 2.7, and as a result, intersects the right axis at approximately 2% (see Figure 12-7, *A*). Two percent is the new (post-test) probability that the patient has cancer

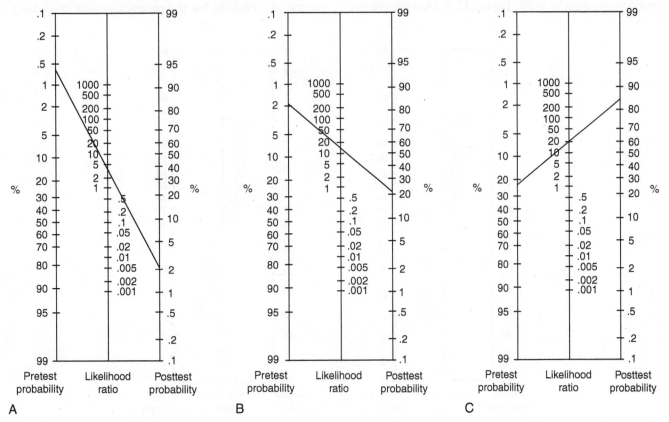

A   B   C

Figure 12-7 A, The probability of cancer for this patient increases from 0.66% to approximately 2% because he is over 50 years of age. **B,** The probability of cancer for this patient increases from 2% to approximately 22% because he has a previous history of cancer. **C,** The probability of cancer for this patient increases from 22% to greater than 80% based on erythrocyte sedimentation rate results.

(the actual calculated value is 1.8%). The previous history of cancer (+LR, 14.7) is considered in Figure 12-7, *B* and the resultant posttest probability of cancer has increased to 22%. Blood work is ordered for this patient, and it shows an ESR of 60 mm/h (+LR, 19.2) (see Figure 12-7, *C*); the resultant posttest probability of cancer has increased to greater than 80%. At this point, the most appropriate course of action for this patient is referral to an oncologist.

This example also provides specific detail on how to estimate the influence of examination findings on pretext to posttest probabilities using likelihood ratios.

Case Example 2

A 45-year-old patient presents to a clinic with complaints of LBP. Patients examined in this clinic are routinely screened for depression with the two previously described questions from the Primary Care Evaluation of Mental Disorders patient questionnaire.

The LRs from Table 12-7 were used to estimate the probability that this patient has severe depression. In general, approximately a 20% probability exists that patients with back pain also have major depression (this estimate is based on a previously reported prevalence study[274]).

The −LR that a patient with one negative response has severe depression is 0.29. Figure 12-8 shows a graphic method used to estimate the effect that one negative response has on the probability of having severe depression. The Y-axis on the left side of the graph is the pretest probability in percentage. The line begins at 20%, crosses the central Y-axis (representing the LR) at 0.29, and as a result, intersects the right axis at approximately 5% (see Figure 12-8, *A*). Five percent is the new (posttest) probability that the patient has severe depression (the actual calculated value is 5.8%). The most appropriate course of action in this scenario would be to continue the examination of this patient, with lowered suspicion of severe depression.

In contrast, the +LR that a patient with two positive responses has severe depression is 4.32 (see Table 12-5). Figure 12-8, *B* demonstrates that two positive responses raise the posttest probability of having severe depression from 20% to approximately 50% (the actual calculated value is 51.9%). The most appropriate course of action in this scenario would be to consider the patient for referral or further workup for depression, depending on the expertise of the clinician.

Case Example 3

A 34-year-old patient injured his back at work and is examined 7 days after the injury. As part of the examination process, the clinician has the patient complete the FABQ.

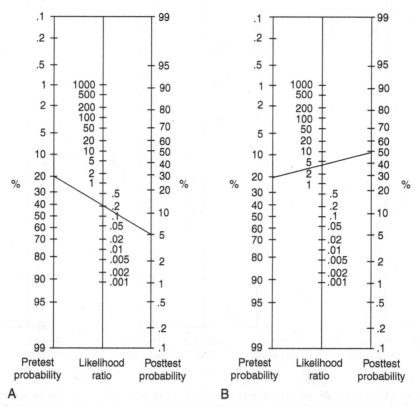

Figure 12-8 A, The probability of severe depression decreases from 20% to approximately 5% with one negative response to the two-question depression screening instrument. **B,** The probability of severe depression increases from 20% to approximately 50% with two positive responses to the two-question depression screening instrument.

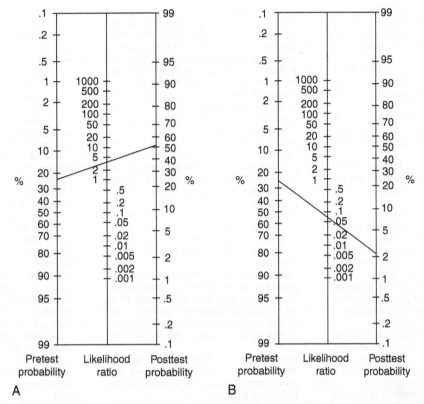

Figure 12-9 A, The probability of not returning to work increases from 25% to approximately 52% with a positive FABQ-W. **B,** The probability of not returning to work decreases from 25% to approximately 2.5% with a negative FABQ-W.

Then, estimates of whether the patient will return to work in 4 weeks can be generated. The LRs from the study[293] cited in the text were used to estimate the probability that this patient would *not* return to work. The clinician estimates that a 25% probability exists that patients with back pain will not return to work (this estimate is based on a clinic's database).

In the first scenario, the patient has an FABW-W score of 38, and the associated +LR is 3.33. Figure 12-9 shows a graphic method used to estimate the effect this FABQ score has on the probability of not returning to work in 4 weeks. The Y-axis on the left side of the graph is the pretest probability in percentage. The line begins at 25%, crosses the central Y-axis (representing the LR) at 3.33, and as a result, intersects the right axis at approximately 52% (see Figure 12-9, *A*). Fifty-two percent is the new (post-test)

probability that the patient will not return to work in 4 weeks (the actual calculated value is 52.6%). The most appropriate course of action in this scenario would be a management strategy that optimized the likelihood of returning to work. For example, interventions that addressed elevated fear-avoidance beliefs and/or early involvement of case management might be considered.

In the second scenario of this case, the patient has an FABQ-W score of 17, and the associated −LR is 0.08. Figure 12-9, *B* shows that the posttest probability of not returning to work has decreased from 25% to approximately 2.5% (the actual calculated value is 2.6%). The most appropriate course of action in this scenario would be to continue the examination process in anticipation of a favorable outcome.

REFERENCES

1. Taylor JB, Goode AP, George SZ, et al: Incidence and risk factors for first-time incident low back pain: a systematic review and meta-analysis, *Spine J* 14:2299–2319, 2014.
2. Leboeuf-Yde C: Body weight and low back pain: a systematic literature review of 56 journal articles reporting on 65 epidemiologic studies, *Spine* 25:226–237, 2000.
3. Battie MC, Videman T, Parent E: Lumbar disc degeneration: epidemiology and genetic influences, *Spine* 29:2679–2690, 2004.
4. Battie MC, Videman T, Gill K, et al: 1991 Volvo award in clinical sciences: smoking and lumbar intervertebral disc degeneration—an MRI study of identical twins, *Spine* 16:1015–1021, 1991.
5. Annunen S, Paassilta P, Lohiniva J, et al: An allele of COL9A2 associated with intervertebral disc disease, *Science* 285:409–412, 1999.
6. Paassilta P, Lohiniva J, Goring HH, et al: Identification of a novel common genetic risk factor for lumbar disk disease, *JAMA* 285:1843–1849, 2001.
7. Kawaguchi Y, Osada R, Kanamori M, et al: Association between an aggrecan gene polymorphism and lumbar disc degeneration, *Spine* 24:2456–2460, 1999.
8. Videman T, Gibbons LE, Battie MC, et al: The relative roles of intragenic polymorphisms of the vitamin D receptor gene in lumbar spine degeneration and bone density, *Spine* 26:E7–E12, 2001.
9. Videman T, Leppavuori J, Kaprio J, et al: Intragenic polymorphisms of the vitamin D receptor gene associated with intervertebral disc degeneration, *Spine* 23:2477–2485, 1998.
10. Takahashi M, Haro H, Wakabayashi Y, et al: The association of degeneration of the intervertebral disc with 5a/6a polymorphism in the promoter of the human matrix metalloproteinase-3 gene, *J Bone Joint Surg Br* 83:491–495, 2001.
11. Burke JG, Watson RW, McCormack D et al: Intervertebral discs which cause low back pain secrete high levels of proinflammatory mediators, *J Bone Joint Surg Br* 84:196–201, 200.

12. Kang JD, Georgescu HI, McIntyre-Larkin L, et al: Herniated lumbar intervertebral discs spontaneously produce matrix metalloproteinases, nitric oxide, interleukin-6, and prostaglandin E2, *Spine* 21:271–277, 1996.

13. McCarron RF, Wimpee MW, Hudkins PG, et al: The inflammatory effect of nucleus pulposus: a possible element in the pathogenesis of low-back pain, *Spine* 12:760–764, 1987.

14. Takebayashi T, Cavanaugh JM, Cuneyt OA, et al: Effect of nucleus pulposus on the neural activity of dorsal root ganglion, *Spine* 26:940–945, 2001.

15. Noponen-Hietala N, Virtanen I, Karttunen R, et al: Genetic variations in IL6 associated with intervertebral disc disease characterized by sciatica, *Pain* 114:186–194, 2005.

16. Solovieva S, Kouhia S, Leino-Arjas P, et al: Interleukin 1 polymorphisms and intervertebral disc degeneration, *Epidemiology* 15:626–633, 2004.

17. Solovieva S, Leino-Arjas P, Saarela J, et al: Possible association of interleukin 1 gene locus polymorphisms with low back pain, *Pain* 109:8–19, 2004.

18. Sambrook PN, MacGregor AJ, Spector TD: Genetic influences on cervical and lumbar disc degeneration: a magnetic resonance imaging study in twins, *Arthritis Rheumatol* 42:366–372, 1999.

19. Battie MC, Videman T, Gibbons LE, et al: 1995 Volvo award in clinical sciences: determinants of lumbar disc degeneration—a study relating lifetime exposures and magnetic resonance imaging findings in identical twins, *Spine* 20:2601–2612, 1995.

20. Ferreira PH, Beckenkamp P, Maher CG, et al: Nature or nurture in low back pain? Results of a systematic review of studies based on twin samples, *Eur J Pain* 17:957–971, 2013.

21. Heikkila JK, Koskenvuo M, Heliovaara M, et al: Genetic and environmental factors in sciatica: evidence from a nationwide panel of 9365 adult twin pairs, *Ann Med* 21:393–398, 1989.

22. Hestbaek L, Iachine IA, Leboeuf-Yde C, et al: Heredity of low back pain in a young population: a classical twin study, *Twin Res* 7:16–26, 2004.

23. Solovieva S, Lohiniva J, Leino-Arjas P, et al: COL9A3 gene polymorphism and obesity in intervertebral disc degeneration of the lumbar spine: evidence of gene-environment interaction, *Spine* 27:2691–2696, 2002.

24. Ekstrom L, Holm S, Holm AK, et al: In vivo porcine intradiscal pressure as a function of external loading, *J Spinal Disord Tech* 17:312–316, 2004.

25. Holm S, Holm AK, Ekstrom L, et al: Experimental disc degeneration due to endplate injury, *J Spinal Disord Tech* 17:64–71, 2004.

26. Kaapa E, Holm S, Han X, et al: Collagens in the injured porcine intervertebral disc, *J Orthop Res* 12:93–102, 1994.

27. Kaigle A, Ekstrom L, Holm S, et al: In vivo dynamic stiffness of the porcine lumbar spine exposed to cyclic loading: influence of load and degeneration, *J Spinal Disord* 11:65–70, 1998.

28. Keller TS, Holm SH, Hansson TH, et al: 1990 Volvo award in experimental studies: the dependence of intervertebral disc mechanical properties on physiologic conditions, *Spine* 15:751–761, 1990.

29. Battie MC, Videman T, Gibbons LE, et al: Occupational driving and lumbar disc degeneration: a case-control study, *Lancet* 360:1369–1374, 2002.

30. Luoma K, Riihimaki H, Raininko R, et al: Lumbar disc degeneration in relation to occupation, *Scand J Work Environ Health* 24:358–366, 1998.

31. Luoma K, Vehmas T, Riihimaki H, et al: Disc height and signal intensity of the nucleus pulposus on magnetic resonance imaging as indicators of lumbar disc degeneration, *Spine* 26:680–686, 2001.

32. Videman T, Battie MC, Gibbons LE, et al: Lifetime exercise and disk degeneration: an MRI study of monozygotic twins, *Med Sci Sports Exerc* 29:1350–1356, 1997.

33. Videman T, Sarna S, Battie MC, et al: The long-term effects of physical loading and exercise lifestyles on back-related symptoms, disability, and spinal pathology among men, *Spine* 20:699–709, 1995.

34. Frymoyer JW, Newberg A, Pope MH, et al: Spine radiographs in patients with low-back pain: an epidemiological study in men, *J Bone Joint Surg Am* 66:1048–1055, 1984.

35. Hirsch C: Studies on the pathology of low back pain, *J Bone Joint Surg Br* 41:237–243, 1959.

36. Savage RA, Whitehouse GH, Roberts N: The relationship between the magnetic resonance imaging appearance of the lumbar spine and low back pain, age and occupation in males, *Eur Spine J* 6:106–114, 1997.

37. Burton AK, Tillotson KM, Symonds TL, et al: Occupational risk factors for the first-onset and subsequent course of low back trouble: a study of serving police officers, *Spine* 21:2612–2620, 1996.

38. Elders LA, Burdorf A: Prevalence, incidence, and recurrence of low back pain in scaffolders during a 3-year follow-up study, *Spine* 29:E101–E106, 2004.

39. Jin K, Sorock GS, Courtney TK: Prevalence of low back pain in three occupational groups in Shanghai, People's Republic of China, *J Safety Res* 35:23–28, 2004.

40. Kaneda K, Shirai Y, Miyamoto M: An epidemiological study on occupational low back pain among people who work in construction, *J Nippon Med Sch* 68:310–317, 2001.

41. Lee P, Helewa A, Goldsmith CH, et al: Low back pain: prevalence and risk factors in an industrial setting, *J Rheumatol* 28:346–351, 2001.

42. Smedley J, Egger P, Cooper C, et al: Prospective cohort study of predictors of incident low back pain in nurses, *Br Med J* 314:1225–1228, 1997.

43. Xiao GB, Dempsey PG, Lei L, et al: Study on musculoskeletal disorders in a machinery manufacturing plant, *J Occup Environ Med* 46:341–346, 2004.

44. Leboeuf-Yde C: Smoking and low back pain: a systematic literature review of 41 journal articles reporting 47 epidemiologic studies, *Spine* 24:1463–1470, 1999.

45. Leboeuf-Yde C, Kyvik KO, Bruun NH: Low back pain and lifestyle. I. Smoking: information from a population-based sample of 29,424 twins, *Spine* 23:2207–2213, 1998.

46. Stairmand JW, Holm S, Urban JP: Factors influencing oxygen concentration gradients in the intervertebral disc: a theoretical analysis, *Spine* 16:444–449, 1991.

47. Holm S, Nachemson A: Nutrition of the intervertebral disc: acute effects of cigarette smoking—an experimental animal study, *Ups J Med Sci* 93:91–99, 1988.

48. Akmal M, Kesani A, Anand B, et al: Effect of nicotine on spinal disc cells: a cellular mechanism for disc degeneration, *Spine* 29:568–575, 2004.

49. Kim KS, Yoon ST, Park JS, et al: Inhibition of proteoglycan and type II collagen synthesis of disc nucleus cells by nicotine, *J Neurosurg Spine* 99:291–297, 2003.

50. Kauppila LI: Prevalence of stenotic changes in arteries supplying the lumbar spine: a postmortem angiographic study on 140 subjects, *Ann Rheum Dis* 56:591–595, 1997.

51. Kauppila LI, Penttila A, Karhunen PJ, et al: Lumbar disc degeneration and atherosclerosis of the abdominal aorta, *Spine* 19:923–929, 1994.

52. Kauppila LI, Tallroth K: Postmortem angiographic findings for arteries supplying the lumbar spine: their relationship to low-back symptoms, *J Spinal Disord* 6:124–129, 1993.

53. Kauppila LI, McAlindon T, Evans S, et al: Disc degeneration/back pain and calcification of the abdominal aorta: a 25-year follow-up study in Framingham, *Spine* 22:1642–1647, 1997.

54. Hestbaek L, Leboeuf-Yde C, Kyvik KO: Are lifestyle-factors in adolescence predictors for adult low back pain? A cross-sectional and prospective study of young twins, *BMC Musculoskelet Disord* 7:27, 2006.

55. Shiri R, Karppinen J, Leino-Arjas P, et al: The association between obesity and low back pain: a meta-analysis, *Am J Epidemiol* 171:135–154, 2010.

56. Leboeuf-Yde C, Kyvik KO, Bruun NH: Low back pain and lifestyle. II. Obesity: information from a population-based sample of 29,424 twin subjects, *Spine* 24:779–783, 1999.

57. Samartzis D, Karppinen J, Cheung JP, et al: Disk degeneration and low back pain: are they fat-related conditions? *Global Spine J* 3:133–144, 2013.

58. Deyo RA, Bass JE: Lifestyle and low-back pain: the influence of smoking and obesity, *Spine* 14:501–506, 1989.

59. Wright D, Barrow S, Fisher AD, et al: Influence of physical, psychological and behavioural factors on consultations for back pain, *Br J Rheumatol* 34:156–161, 1995.

60. Rissanen A, Heliovaara M, Knekt P, et al: Risk of disability and mortality due to overweight in a Finnish population, *Br Med J* 301:835–837, 1990.

61. Fransen M, Woodward M, Norton R, et al: Risk factors associated with the transition from acute to chronic occupational back pain, *Spine* 27:92–98, 2002.

62. Croft PR, Papageorgiou AC, Ferry S, et al: Psychologic distress and low back pain: evidence from a prospective study in the general population, *Spine* 20:2731–2737, 1995.

63. Craig TK, Boardman AP, Mills K, et al: The South London Somatisation Study. I. Longitudinal course and the influence of early life experiences, *Br J Psychiatry* 163:579–588, 1993.

64. Mannion AF, Dolan P, Adams MA: Psychological questionnaires: do "abnormal" scores precede or follow first-time low back pain? *Spine* 21:2603–2611, 1996.

65. Papageorgiou AC, Macfarlane GJ, Thomas E, et al: Psychosocial factors in the workplace: do they predict new episodes of low back pain? Evidence from the South Manchester Back Pain Study, *Spine* 22:1137–1142, 1997.

66. Carragee EJ, Chen Y, Tanner CM, et al: Can discography cause long-term back symptoms in previously asymptomatic subjects? *Spine* 25:1803–1808, 2000.

67. Picavet HS, Vlaeyen JW, Schouten JS: Pain catastrophizing and kinesiophobia: predictors of chronic low back pain, *Am J Epidemiol* 156:1028–1034, 2002.

68. Thomas E, Silman AJ, Croft PR, et al: Predicting who develops chronic low back pain in primary care: a prospective study, *Br Med J* 318:1662–1667, 1999.

69. Leboeuf-Yde C: Alcohol and low-back pain: a systematic literature review, *J Manip Physiol Ther* 23:343–346, 2000.

70. Waddell G: Low back pain: a twentieth century health care enigma, *Spine* 21:2820–2825, 1996.

71. IOM (Institute of Medicine): *Relieving pain in America: A blueprint for transforming prevention, care, education, and research*, Washington, DC, 2011, The National Academies Press.

72. Picavet HS, Schouten JS: Musculoskeletal pain in the Netherlands: prevalences, consequences and risk groups, the DMC(3)-study, *Pain* 102:167–178, 2003.

73. Bener A, Alwash R, Gaber T, et al: Obesity and low back pain, *Coll Antropol* 27:95–104, 2003.

74. Leboeuf-Yde C, Kyvik KO: At what age does low back pain become a common problem? A study of 29,424 individuals aged 12-41 years, *Spine* 23:228–234, 1998.

75. Picavet HS, Schouten JS, Smit HA: Prevalence and consequences of low back problems in The Netherlands, working vs non-working population: the MORGEN-Study, monitoring project on risk factors for chronic disease, *Public Health* 113:73–77, 1999.

76. Santos-Eggimann B, Wietlisbach V, Rickenbach M, et al: One-year prevalence of low back pain in two Swiss regions: estimates from the population participating in the 1992-1993 MONICA project, *Spine* 25:2473–2479, 2000.

77. Stranjalis G, Tsamandouraki K, Sakas DE, et al: Low back pain in a representative sample of Greek population: analysis according to personal and socioeconomic characteristics, *Spine* 29:1355–1360, 2004.

78. Goetzel RZ, Hawkins K, Ozminkowski RJ, et al: The health and productivity cost burden of the "top 10" physical and mental health conditions affecting six large US employers in 1999, *J Occup Environ Med* 45:5–14, 2003.

79. Driscoll T, Jacklyn G, Orchard J, et al: The global burden of occupationally related low back pain: estimates from the Global Burden of Disease 2010 study, *Ann Rheum Dis* 73:975–981, 2014.

80. Walker BF: The prevalence of low back pain: a systematic review of the literature from 1966 to 1998, *J Spinal Disord* 13:205–217, 2000.

81. Mantyselka P, Kumpusalo E, Ahonen R, et al: Pain as a reason to visit the doctor: a study in Finnish primary health care, *Pain* 89:175–180, 2001.

82. Deyo RA, Phillips WR: Low back pain: a primary care challenge, *Spine* 21:2826–2832, 1996.

83. Cote P, Cassidy JD, Carroll L: The treatment of neck and low back pain: who seeks care? Who goes where? *Med Care* 39:956–967, 2001.

84. Vingard E, Mortimer M, Wiktorin C, et al: Seeking care for low back pain in the general population: a two-year follow-up study—results from the MUSIC-Norrtalje Study, *Spine* 27:2159–2165, 2002.

85. Eisenberg DM, Davis RB, Ettner SL, et al: Trends in alternative medicine use in the United States, 1990-1997: results of a follow-up national survey, *JAMA* 280:1569–1575, 1998.

86. Barnes PM: Bloom B, Nahin RL: Complementary and alternative medicine use among adults and children: United States, 2007, *Natl Health Stat Report* 1–23: 2008.

87. IJzelenberg W, Burdorf A: Patterns of care for low back pain in a working population, *Spine* 29:1362–1368, 2004.

88. Mortimer M, Ahlberg G: To seek or not to seek? Care-seeking behaviour among people with low-back pain, *Scand J Public Health* 31:194–203, 2003.

89. Von Korff M: Studying the natural history of back pain, *Spine* 19:2041S–2046S, 1994.

90. Von Korff M, Deyo RA, Cherkin D, et al: Back pain in primary care: outcomes at 1 year, *Spine* 18:855–862, 1993.

91. Bergquist-Ullman M, Larsson U: Acute low back pain in industry: a controlled prospective study with special reference to therapy and confounding factors, *Acta Orthop Scand* 170:1–117, 1977.

92. Carey TS, Garrett JM, Jackman A, et al: Recurrence and care seeking after acute back pain: results of a long-term follow-up study, North Carolina Back Pain Project, *Med Care* 37:157–164, 1999.

93. McGorry RW, Webster BS, Snook SH, et al: The relation between pain intensity, disability, and the episodic nature of chronic and recurrent low back pain, *Spine* 25:834–841, 2000.

94. Itz CJ, Geurts JW, van Kleef M, et al: Clinical course of non-specific low back pain: a systematic review of prospective cohort studies set in primary care, *Eur J Pain* 17:5–15, 2013.

95. Von Korff M, Dworkin SF, Le Resche L: Graded chronic pain status: an epidemiologic evaluation, *Pain* 40:279–291, 1990.

96. Andersson HI, Ejlertsson G, Leden I, et al: Chronic pain in a geographically defined general population: studies of differences in age, gender, social class, and pain localization, *Clin J Pain* 9:174–182, 1993.

97. Stang P, Von Korff M, Galer BS: Reduced labor force participation among primary care patients with headache, *J Gen Intern Med* 13:296–302, 1998.

98. Stewart WF, Ricci JA, Chee E, et al: Lost productive time and cost due to common pain conditions in the US workforce, *JAMA* 290:2443–2454, 2003.

99. Walker BF, Muller R, Grant WD: Low back pain in Australian adults: prevalence and associated disability, *J Manip Physiol Ther* 27:238–244, 2004.

100. Andersson GB, Pope MH, Frymoyer JW, et al: *Occupational low back pain: assessment, treatment, and prevention*, St Louis, 1995, Mosby.

101. Hu XH, Markson LE, Lipton RB, et al: Burden of migraine in the United States: disability and economic costs, *Arch Intern Med* 159:813–818, 1999.

102. Frymoyer J, Durett C: The economics of spinal disorders. In Frymoyer J, editor: The adult spine, Philadelphia, 1997, Lippincott-Raven.

103. Spitzer WO: Magnitude of the problem, *Spine* 12S:12–25, 1987.

104. Williams DA, Feuerstein M, Durbin D, et al: Health care and indemnity costs across the natural history of disability in occupational low back pain, *Spine* 23:2329–2336, 1998.

105. Hashemi L, Webster BS, Clancy EA: Trends in disability duration and cost of workers' compensation low back pain claims (1988-1996), *J Occup Environ Med* 40:1110–1119, 1998.

106. Hashemi L, Webster BS, Clancy EA, et al: Length of disability and cost of workers' compensation low back pain claims, *J Occup Environ Med* 39:937–945, 1997.

107. Snook SH: The costs of back pain in industry, *Occup Med* 3:1–5, 1988.

108. Martin BI, Turner JA, Mirza SK, et al: Trends in health care expenditures, utilization, and health status among US adults with spine problems, 1997-2006, *Spine (Phila PA 1976)* 34:2077–2084, 2009.

109. Leino PI, Berg MA, Puska P: Is back pain increasing? Results from national surveys in Finland during 1978/9-1992, *Scand J Rheumatol* 23:269–276, 1994.

110. Burton AK, Erg E: Back injury and work loss: biomechanical and psychosocial influences, *Spine* 22:2575–2580, 1997.

111. Frank JW, Brooker AS, DeMaio SE, et al: Disability resulting from occupational low back pain. II. What do we know about secondary prevention?: a review of the scientific evidence on prevention after disability begins, *Spine* 21:2918–2929, 1996.

112. Frank JW, Sinclair S, Hogg-Johnson S, et al: Preventing disability form work-related low-back pain: new evidence gives new hope—if we can just get all the players onside, *CMAJ* 158:1625–1631, 1998.

113. Waddell G: 1987 Volvo award in clinical sciences: a new clinical model for the treatment of low-back pain, *Spine* 12:632–644, 1987.

114. Waddell G: Low back disability: a syndrome of Western civilization, *Neurosurg Clin North Am* 2:719–738, 1991.

115. Webster BS, Snook SH: The cost of 1989 workers' compensation low back pain claims, *Spine* 19:1111–1115, 1994.

116. Deyo RA, Dworkin SF, Amtmann D, et al: Focus article: report of the NIH task force on research standards for chronic low back pain, *Eur Spine J* 23:2028–2045, 2014.

117. Kuslich SD, Ulstrom CL, Michael CJ: The tissue origin of low back pain and sciatica: a report of pain response to tissue stimulation during operations on the lumbar spine using local anesthesia, *Orthop Clin North Am* 22:181–187, 1991.

118. Kellgren J: On the distribution of pain arising from deep somatic structures with charts of the segmental areas, *Clin Sci* 4:35–46, 1939.

119. Kellgren J: Observations on the referred pain arising from the muscles, *Clin Sci* 3:175–190, 1938.

120. Smyth MJ, Wright V: Sciatica and the intervertebral disc: an experimental study, *J Bone Joint Surg Am* 40:1401–1418, 1958.

121. Bove GM, Zaheen A, Bajwa ZH: Subjective nature of lower limb radicular pain, *J Manip Physiol Ther* 28:12–14, 2005.

122. Ido K, Urushidani H: Fibrous adhesive entrapment of lumbosacral nerve roots as a cause of sciatica, *Spinal Cord* 39:269–273, 2001.

123. Chung SK, Lee SH, Kim DY, et al: Treatment of lower lumbar radiculopathy caused by osteoporotic compression fracture: the role of vertebroplasty, *J Spinal Disord Tech* 15:461–468, 2002.

124. Igarashi T, Yabuki S, Kikuchi S, et al: Effect of acute nerve root compression on endoneurial fluid pressure and blood flow in rat dorsal root ganglia, *J Orthop Res* 23:420–424, 2005.

125. Kobayashi S, Yoshizawa H, Yamada S: Pathology of lumbar nerve root compression. Part 1. Intraradicular inflammatory changes induced by mechanical compression, *J Orthop Res* 22:170–179, 2004.

126. Danneels LA, Vanderstraeten GG, Cambier DC, et al: CT imaging of trunk muscles in chronic low back pain patients and healthy control subjects, *Eur Spine J* 9:266–272, 2000.

127. Hides JA, Richardson CA, Jull GA: Multifidus muscle recovery is not automatic after resolution of acute, first-episode low back pain, *Spine* 21:2763–2769, 1996.

128. Hides JA, Stokes MJ, Saide M, et al: Evidence of lumbar multifidus muscle wasting ipsilateral to symptoms in patients with acute/subacute low back pain, *Spine* 19:165–172, 1994.

129. Sihvonen T, Huttunen M, Makkonen M, et al: Functional changes in back muscle activity correlate with pain intensity and prediction of low back pain during pregnancy, *Arch Phys Med Rehabil* 79:1210–1212, 1998.

130. Sihvonen T, Partanen J, Hanninen O, et al: Electric behavior of low back muscles during lumbar pelvic rhythm in low back pain patients and healthy controls, *Arch Phys Med Rehabil* 72:1080–1087, 1991.

131. Cassisi JE, Robinson ME, O'Conner P, et al: Trunk strength and lumbar paraspinal muscle activity during isometric exercise in chronic low-back pain patients and controls, *Spine* 18:245–251, 1993.

132. Mooney V, Gulick J, Perlman M, et al: Relationships between myoelectric activity, strength, and MRI of lumbar extensor muscles in back pain patients and normal subjects, *J Spinal Disord* 10:348–356, 1997.

133. Latimer J, Maher CG, Refshauge K, et al: The reliability and validity of the Biering-Sorensen test in asymptomatic subjects and subjects reporting current or previous nonspecific low back pain, *Spine* 24:2085–2089, 1999.

134. Mannion AF, Weber BR, Dvorak J, et al: Fibre type characteristics of the lumbar paraspinal muscles in normal healthy subjects and in patients with low back pain, *J Orthop Res* 15:881–887, 1997.

135. Fryer G, Morris T, Gibbons P: Paraspinal muscles and intervertebral dysfunction. Part 2, *J Manip Physiol Ther* 27:348–357, 2004.

136. Indahl A, Kaigle AM, Reikeras O, et al: Interaction between the porcine lumbar intervertebral disc,

zygapophysial joints, and paraspinal muscles, *Spine* 22:2834–2840, 1997.

137. Fortin M, Yuan Y, Battie MC: Factors associated with paraspinal muscle asymmetry in size and composition in a general population sample of men, *Phys Ther* 93:1540–1550, 2013.

138. Bishop MD, Horn ME, Lott DJ, et al: Magnitude of spinal muscle damage is not statistically associated with exercise-induced low back pain intensity, *Spine J* 11:1135–1142, 2011.

139. Glaros AG, Glass EG, Brockman D: Electromyographic data from TMD patients with myofascial pain and from matched control subjects: evidence for statistical, not clinical, significance, *J Orofac Pain* 11:125–129, 1997.

140. Christensen LV, Tran KT, Mohamed SE: Gum chewing and jaw muscle fatigue and pains, *J Oral Rehabil* 23:424–437, 1996.

141. Fredin Y, Elbert J, Britschgi N, et al: A decreased ability to relax between repetitive muscle contractions in patients with chronic symptoms after whiplash trauma of the neck, *J Musculoskelet Pain* 5:55–70, 1997.

142. Vasseljen Jr. O, Westgaard RH: Can stress-related shoulder and neck pain develop independently of muscle activity? *Pain* 64:221–230, 1996.

143. Larsson SE, Cai H, Oberg PA: Continuous percutaneous measurement by laser-Doppler flowmetry of skeletal muscle microcirculation at varying levels of contraction force determined electromyographically, *Eur J Appl Physiol Occup Physiol* 66:477–482, 1993.

144. Larsson R, Oberg PA, Larsson SE: Changes of trapezius muscle blood flow and electromyography in chronic neck pain due to trapezius myalgia, *Pain* 79:45–50, 1999.

145. Farfan HF: The torsional injury of the lumbar spine, *Spine* 9:53, 1984.

146. Steffen T, Baramki HG, Rubin R, et al: Lumbar intradiscal pressure measured in the anterior and posterolateral annular regions during asymmetrical loading, *Clin Biomech* 13:495–505, 1998.

147. Bogduk N: *Clinical anatomy of the lumbar spine and sacrum*, ed 3, New York, 1997, Churchill Livingstone.

148. Adams MA, Freeman BJ, Morrison HP, et al: Mechanical initiation of intervertebral disc degeneration, *Spine* 25:1625–1636, 2000.

149. Adams MA, Hutton WC: Gradual disc prolapse, *Spine* 10:524–531, 1985.

150. Farfan HF, Huberdeau RM, Dubow HI: Lumbar intervertebral disc degeneration: the influence of geometrical features on the pattern of disc degeneration—a post mortem study, *J Bone Joint Surg Am* 54:492–510, 1972.

151. Brinckmann P, Porter RW: A laboratory model of lumbar disc protrusion: fissure and fragment, *Spine* 19:228–235, 1994.

152. Milette PC, Fontaine S, Lepanto L, et al: Differentiating lumbar disc protrusions, disc bulges, and discs with normal contour but abnormal signal intensity: magnetic resonance imaging with discographic correlations, *Spine* 24:44–53, 1999.

153. Lebkowski WJ, Dzieciol J: Degenerated lumbar intervertebral disc: a morphological study, *Pol J Pathol* 53:83–86, 2002.

154. Macintosh JE, Bogduk N: 1987 Volvo Award in Basic Science: the morphology of the lumbar erector spinae, *Spine* 12:658–668, 1987.

155. Macintosh JE, Bogduk N: The attachments of the lumbar erector spinae, *Spine* 16:783–792, 1991.

156. Vleeming A, Pool-Goudzwaard AL, Hammudoghlu D, et al: The function of the long dorsal sacroiliac ligament: its implication for understanding low back pain, *Spine* 21:556–562, 1996.

157. Maluf KS, Sahrmann SA, Van Dillen LR: Use of a classification system to guide nonsurgical management of a patient with chronic low back pain, *Phys Ther* 80:1097–1111, 2000.

158. Manchikanti L, Boswell MV, Singh V, et al: Prevalence of facet joint pain in chronic spinal pain of cervical, thoracic, and lumbar regions, *BMC Musculoskelet Disord* 5:15, 2004.

159. McCall IW, Park WM, O'Brien JP: Induced pain referral from posterior lumbar elements in normal subjects, *Spine* 4:441–446, 1979.

160. Derby R, Bogduk N, Schwarzer AC: Precision percutaneous blocking procedures for localizing spinal pain. Part 1. The posterior lumbar compartment, *Pain Digest* 3:89–100, 1993.

161. El-Bohy AA, Yang KH, King AI: Experimental verification of facet load transmission by direct measurement of facet lamina contact pressure, *J Biomech* 22:931–941, 1989.

162. Twomey LT, Taylor JR, Taylor MM: Unsuspected damage to lumbar zygapophyseal (facet) joints after motor-vehicle accidents, *Med J Aust* 151:210–217, 1989.

163. Wiesel SW, Tsourmas N, Feffer HL, et al: A study of computer-assisted tomography. I. The incidence of positive CAT scans in an asymptomatic group of patients, *Spine* 9:549–551, 1984.

164. Bogduk N, Jull GA: The theoretical pathology of the acute locked back: a basis for manipulative therapy, *Man Med* 1:78–82, 1985.

165. Ashton IK, Ashton BA, Gibson SJ, et al: Morphological basis for back pain: the demonstration of nerve fibers and neuropeptides in the lumbar facet joint capsule but not in ligamentum flavum, *J Orthop Res* 10:72–78, 1992.

166. Jackson RP, Jacobs RR, Montesano PX: 1988 Volvo Award in Clinical Sciences: facet joint injection in low-back pain—a prospective statistical study, *Spine* 13:966–971, 1988.

167. Schwarzer AC, Aprill CN, Derby R, et al: Clinical features of patients with pain stemming from the lumbar zygapophysial joints: is the lumbar facet syndrome a clinical entity? *Spine* 19:1132–1137, 1994.

168. Marks R: Distribution of pain provoked from lumbar facet joints and related structures during diagnostic spinal infiltration, *Pain* 39:37–40, 1989.

169. O'Neill S, Graven-Nielsen T, Manniche C, et al: Ultrasound guided, painful electrical stimulation of lumbar facet joint structures: an experimental model of acute low back pain, *Pain* 144:76–83, 2009.

170. Hadjipavlou AG, Gaitanis LN, Katonis PG, et al: Paget's disease of the spine and its management, *Eur Spine J* 10:370–384, 2001.

171. Deyo RA, Diehl AK: Cancer as a cause of back pain: frequency, clinical presentation, and diagnostic strategies, *J Gen Intern Med* 3:230–238, 1988.

172. Gregory PL, Batt ME, Kerslake RW: Comparing spondylolysis in cricketers and soccer players, *Br J Sports Med* 38:737–742, 2004.

173. Hensinger RN: Spondylolysis and spondylolisthesis in children and adolescents, *J Bone Joint Surg Am* 71:1098–1107, 1989.

174. Jackson DW, Wiltse LL, Cirincoine RJ: Spondylolysis in the female gymnast, *Clin Orthop Relat Res* 117:68–73, 1976.

175. Jones DM, Tearse DS, el Khoury GY, et al: Radiographic abnormalities of the lumbar spine in college football players: a comparative analysis, *Am J Sports Med* 27:335–338, 1999.

176. Libson E, Bloom RA, Dinari G: Symptomatic and asymptomatic spondylolysis and spondylolisthesis in young adults, *Int Orthop* 6:259–261, 1982.

177. Iwamoto J, Takeda T, Wakano K: Returning athletes with severe low back pain and spondylolysis to original sporting activities with conservative treatment, *Scand J Med Sci Sports* 14:346–351, 2004.

178. Lonstein JE: Spondylolisthesis in children: cause, natural history, and management, *Spine* 24:2640–2648, 1999.

179. Szypryt EP, Twining P, Mulholland RC, et al: The prevalence of disc degeneration associated with neural arch defects of the lumbar spine assessed by magnetic resonance imaging, *Spine* 14:977–981, 1989.

180. Harris IE, Weinstein SL: Long-term follow-up of patients with grade III and IV spondylolisthesis: treatment with and without posterior fusion, *J Bone Joint Surg Am* 69:960–969, 1987.

181. Frennered AK, Danielson BI, Nachemson AL: Natural history of symptomatic isthmic low-grade spondylolisthesis in children and adolescents: a seven-year follow-up study, *J Pediatr Orthop* 11:209–213, 1991.

182. Beutler W, Fredrickson B, Murtland A, et al: The natural history of spondylolysis and spondylolisthesis: 45-year follow-up evaluation, *Spine* 28:1027–1035, 2003.

183. Taskaynatan MA, Izci Y, Ozgul A, et al: Clinical significance of congenital lumbosacral malformations in young male population with prolonged low back pain, *Spine* 30:E210–E213, 2005.

184. Hughes RJ, Saifuddin A: Imaging of lumbosacral transitional vertebrae, *Clin Radiol* 59:984–991, 2004.

185. Tini PG, Wieser C, Zinn WM: The transitional vertebra of the lumbosacral spine: its radiological classification, incidence, prevalence, and clinical significance, *Rheumatol Rehabil* 16:180–185, 1977.

186. Peterson CK, Bolton J, Hsu W, et al: A cross-sectional study comparing pain and disability levels in patients with low back pain with and without transitional lumbosacral vertebrae, *J Manip Physiol Ther* 28:570–574, 2005.

187. Otani K, Konno S, Kikuchi S: Lumbosacral transitional vertebrae and nerve-root symptoms, *J Bone Joint Surg Br* 83:1137–1140, 2001.

188. Grant SC, Aiken NR, Plant HD, et al: NMR spectroscopy of single neurons, *Magn Reson Med* 44:19–22, 2000.

189. Stadnik TW, Lee RR, Coen HL, et al: Annular tears and disk herniation: prevalence and contrast enhancement on MR images in the absence of low back pain or sciatica, *Radiology* 206:49–55, 1998.

190. Jensen MC, Brant-Zawadzki MN, Obuchowski N, et al: Magnetic resonance imaging of the lumbar spine in people without back pain, *N Engl J Med* 331:69–73, 1994.

191. Boden SD, Davis DO, Dina TS, et al: Abnormal magnetic-resonance scans of the lumbar spine in asymptomatic subjects: a prospective investigation, *J Bone Joint Surg Am* 72:403–408, 1990.

192. Hitselberger WE, Witten RM: Abnormal myelograms in asymptomatic patients, *J Neurosurg* 28:204–206, 1968.

193. Torgerson WR, Dotter WE: Comparative roentgenographic study of the asymptomatic and symptomatic lumbar spine, *J Bone Joint Surg Am* 58:850–853, 1976.

194. Sasaki K: Magnetic resonance imaging findings of the lumbar root pathway in patients over 50 years old, *Eur Spine J* 4:71–76, 1995.

195. Videman T, Nurminen M, Troup JD: 1990 Volvo Award in Clinical Sciences: lumbar spinal pathology in cadaveric material in relation to history of back pain, occupation, and physical loading, *Spine* 15:728–740, 1990.

196. Iwamoto J, Abe H, Tsukimura Y, et al: Relationship between radiographic abnormalities of lumbar spine and incidence of low back pain in high school and college football players: a prospective study, *Am J Sports Med* 32:781–786, 2004.

197. Luoma K, Vehmas T, Raininko R, et al: Lumbosacral transitional vertebra: relation to disc degeneration and low back pain, *Spine* 29:200–205, 2004.

198. Elfering A, Semmer N, Birkhofer D, et al: Risk factors for lumbar disc degeneration: a 5-year prospective MRI study in asymptomatic individuals, *Spine* 27:125–134, 2002.

199. Boos N, Semmer N, Elfering A, et al: Natural history of individuals with asymptomatic disc abnormalities in magnetic resonance imaging: predictors of low back pain–related medical consultation and work incapacity, *Spine* 25:1484–1492, 2000.

200. White III AA, Gordon SL: Synopsis: workshop on idiopathic low-back pain, *Spine* 7:141–149, 1982.

201. Chou R, Fu R, Carrino JA, et al: Imaging strategies for low-back pain: systematic review and meta-analysis, *Lancet* 373:463–472, 2009.

202. Lederle FA, Simel DL: The rational clinical examination: does this patient have abdominal aortic aneurysm? *JAMA* 281:77–82, 1999.

203. Jarvik JJ, Hollingworth W, Heagerty P, et al: The longitudinal assessment of imaging and disability of the back (LAIDBack) study: baseline data, *Spine* 26:1158–1166; 2001.

204. Deyo RA, Rainville J, Kent DL: What can the history and physical examination tell us about low back pain? *JAMA* 268:760–765, 1992.

205. Collin J: The epidemiology of abdominal aortic aneurysm, *Br J Hosp Med* 40:64–67, 1988.

206. Lederle FA, Johnson GR, Wilson SE: Abdominal aortic aneurysm in women, *J Vasc Surg* 34:122–126, 2001.

207. Lederle FA, Johnson GR, Wilson SE, et al: The aneurysm detection and management study screening program: validation cohort and final results, Aneurysm Detection and Management Veterans Affairs Cooperative Study Investigators, *Arch Intern Med* 160:1425–1430, 2000.

208. Vardulaki KA, Walker NM, Couto E, et al: Late results concerning feasibility and compliance from a randomized trial of ultrasonographic screening for abdominal aortic aneurysm, *Br J Surg* 89:861–864, 2002.

209. Fielding JW, Black J, Ashton F, et al: Diagnosis and management of 528 abdominal aortic aneurysms, *Br Med J* 283:355–359, 1981.

210. Fink HA, Lederle FA, Roth CS, et al: The accuracy of physical examination to detect abdominal aortic aneurysm, *Arch Intern Med* 160:833–836, 2000.

211. Lynch RM: Accuracy of abdominal examination in the diagnosis of non-ruptured abdominal aortic aneurysm, *Accid Emerg Nurs* 12:99–107, 2004.

212. Duthie JJ: Screening for abdominal aortic aneurysm, *Lancet* 2:1319, 1988.

213. Bajwa ZH, Sial KA, Malik AB, et al: Pain patterns in patients with polycystic kidney disease, *Kidney Int* 66:1561–1569, 2004.

214. Delanaye P, Bovy C, de Leval L, et al: Back pain and renal failure, *Lancet* 364:1992, 2004.

215. Settergren B: Clinical aspects of nephropathia epidemica (Puumala virus infection) in Europe: a review, *Scand J Infect Dis* 32:125–132, 2000.

216. Weiss DJ, Conliffe T, Tata N: Low back pain caused by a duodenal ulcer, *Arch Phys Med Rehabil* 79:1137–1139, 1998.

217. Duffy JP, Reber HA: Surgical treatment of chronic pancreatitis, *J Hepatobiliary Pancreat Surg* 9:659–668, 2002.

218. Wellbery C: Diagnosis and treatment of endometriosis, *Am Fam Physician* 60:1753–1758, 1999.

219. Abrahm JL: Assessment and treatment of patients with malignant spinal cord compression, *J Support Oncol* 2:377–388, 2004 391.

220. Slipman CW, Patel RK, Botwin K, et al: Epidemiology of spine tumors presenting to musculoskeletal physiatrists, *Arch Phys Med Rehabil* 84:492–495, 2003.

221. Ogboli MI, Ilchyshyn A, Walker RS, et al: Glomus tumor as a cause of chronic low back pain: case report, *Spine* 28:E146–E147, 2003.

222. Hollingworth W, Gray DT, Martin BI, et al: Rapid magnetic resonance imaging for diagnosing cancer-related low back pain, *J Gen Intern Med* 18:303–312, 2003.

223. Johnsson KE, Sass M: Cauda equina syndrome in lumbar spinal stenosis: case report and incidence in Jutland, Denmark, *J Spinal Disord Tech* 17:334–335, 2004.

224. Ahn NU, Ahn UM, Nallamshetty L, et al: Cauda equina syndrome in ankylosing spondylitis (the CES-AS syndrome): meta-analysis of outcomes after medical and surgical treatments, *J Spinal Disord* 14:427–433, 2001.

225. Johnsson KE: Lumbar spinal stenosis: a retrospective study of 163 cases in southern Sweden, *Acta Orthop Scand* 66:403–405, 1995.

226. Kostuik JP, Harrington I, Alexander D, et al: Cauda equina syndrome and lumbar disc herniation, *J Bone Joint Surg Am* 68:386–391, 1986.

227. Perner A, Andersen JT, Juhler M: Lower urinary tract symptoms in lumbar root compression syndromes: a prospective survey, *Spine* 22:2693–2697, 1997.

228. Mease P: Psoriatic arthritis and spondyloarthritis assessment and management update, *Curr Opin Rheumatol* 25(3):287–296, 2013.

229. Keat A: Reactive arthritis, *Adv Exp Med Biol* 455:201–206, 1999.

230. Hohler T, Marker-Hermann E: Psoriatic arthritis: clinical aspects, genetics, and the role of T cells, *Curr Opin Rheumatol* 13:273–279, 2001.

231. Nigam P, Singh D, Matreja VS, et al: Psoriatic arthritis: a clinico-radiological study, *J Dermatol* 7:55–59, 1980.

232. Zachariae H: Prevalence of joint disease in patients with psoriasis: implications for therapy, *Am J Clin Dermatol* 4:441–447, 2003.

233. Zachariae H, Zachariae R, Blomqvist K, et al: Quality of life and prevalence of arthritis reported by 5,795 members of the Nordic Psoriasis Associations, data from the Nordic Quality of Life Study, *Acta Derm Venereol* 82:108–113, 2002.

234. Gladman DD: Clinical aspects of the spondyloarthropathies, *Am J Med Sci* 316:234–238, 1998.

235. De Vlam K, Mielants H, Cuvelier C, et al: Spondyloarthropathy is underestimated in inflammatory bowel disease: prevalence and HLA association, *J Rheumatol* 27:2860–2865, 2000.

236. Patel U, Skingle S, Campbell G, et al: Clinical profile of acute vertebral compression fractures in osteoporosis, *Br J Rheumatol* 30:418–421, 2005.

237. Henschke N, Maher CG, Refshauge KM, et al: Prevalence of and screening for serious spinal pathology in patients presenting to primary care settings with acute low back pain, *Arthritis Rheum* 60:3072–3080, 2009.

238. Petersdorf R, Beeson P: Fever of unexplained origin: report on 100 cases, *Medicine* 4:1–30, 1961.

239. Waldvogel F, Vasey H: Osteomyelitis: the past decade, *N Engl J Med* 303:360–370, 1980.

240. Roach K, Brown M, Ricker E, et al: The use of patient symptoms to screen for serious back problems, *J Orthop Sports Phys Ther* 21:2–6, 1995.

241. Main CJ, Foster N, Buchbinder R: How important are back pain beliefs and expectations for satisfactory recovery from back pain? *Best Pract Res Clin Rheumatol* 24:205–217, 2010.

242. Accident Compensation Corporation (ACC) and National Health Committee: *New Zealand Acute Low Back Pain Guide*, Wellington, New Zealand, 1997.

243. Waddell G, Main CJ, Morris EW, et al: Chronic low-back pain, psychologic distress, and illness behavior, *Spine* 9:209–213, 1984.

244. Waddell G, McCulloch JA, Kummel E, et al: Nonorganic physical signs in low-back pain, *Spine* 5:117–125, 1980.

245. Gaines Jr. WG, Hegmann KT: Effectiveness of Waddell's nonorganic signs in predicting a delayed return to regular work in patients experiencing acute occupational low back pain, *Spine* 24:396–400, 1999.

246. Karas R, McIntosh G, Hall H, et al: The relationship between nonorganic signs and centralization of symptoms in the prediction of return to work for patients with low back pain, *Phys Ther* 77:354–360, 1997.

247. Kummel BM: Nonorganic signs of significance in low back pain, *Spine* 21:1077–1081, 1996.

248. Lancourt J, Kettelhut M: Predicting return to work for lower back pain patients receiving workers' compensation, *Spine* 17:629–640, 1992.

249. Bradish CF, Lloyd GJ, Aldam CH, et al: Do nonorganic signs help to predict the return to activity of patients with low-back pain? *Spine* 13:557–560, 1988.

250. Werneke MW, Harris DE, Lichter RL: Clinical effectiveness of behavioral signs for screening chronic low-back pain patients in a work-oriented physical rehabilitation program, *Spine* 18:2412–2418, 1993.

251. Fritz JM, Wainner RS, Hicks GE: The use of nonorganic signs and symptoms as a screening tool for return-to-work in patients with acute low back pain, *Spine* 25:1925–1931, 2000.

252. Childs JD, Fritz JM, Flynn TW, et al: A clinical prediction rule to identify patients with low back pain most likely to benefit from spinal manipulation: a validation study, *Ann Intern Med* 141:920–928, 2004.

253. Hicks GE, Fritz J: M, Delitto A et al: Preliminary development of a clinical prediction rule for determining which patients with low back pain will respond to a stabilization exercise program, *Arch Phys Med Rehabil* 86:1753–1762, 2005.

254. Hill JC, Whitehurst DG, Lewis M, et al: Comparison of stratified primary care management for low back pain with current best practice (STarT Back): a randomised controlled trial, *Lancet* 378:1560–1571, 2011.

255. Dionne CE, Bourbonnais R, Fremont P, et al: A clinical return-to-work rule for patients with back pain, *CMAJ* 172:1559–1567, 2005.

256. Duijts SF, Kant IJ, Landeweerd JA, et al: Prediction of sickness absence: development of a screening instrument, *Occup Environ Med* 63:564–569, 2006.

257. Linton SJ, Hallden K: Can we screen for problematic back pain? A screening questionnaire for predicting outcome in acute and subacute back pain, *Clin J Pain* 14:209–215, 1998.

258. Linton SJ, Nicholas M, MacDonald S: Development of a short form of the Orebro Musculoskeletal Pain Screening Questionnaire, *Spine (Phila PA 1976)* 36:1891–1895, 2011.

259. Dunstan DA, Covic T, Tyson GA, et al: Does the Orebro Musculoskeletal Pain Questionnaire predict outcomes following a work-related compensable injury? *Int J Rehabil Res* 28:369–370, 2005.

260. Gabel CP, Burkett B, Neller A, et al: Can long-term impairment in general practitioner whiplash patients be predicted using screening and patient-reported outcomes? *Int J Rehabil Res* 31:79–80, 2008.

261. Heneweer H, Aufdemkampe G, van Tulder MW, et al: Psychosocial variables in patients with (sub)acute low back pain: an inception cohort in primary care physical therapy in The Netherlands, *Spine (Phila PA 1976)* 32:586–592, 2007.

262. Linton SJ, Boersma K: Early identification of patients at risk of developing a persistent back problem: the predictive validity of the Orebro Musculoskeletal Pain Questionnaire, *Clin J Pain* 19:80–86, 2003.

263. Margison DA, French DJ: Predicting treatment failure in the subacute injury phase using the Orebro Musculoskeletal Pain Questionnaire: an

observational prospective study in a workers' compensation system, *J Occup Environ Med* 49:59–67, 2007.

264. Nordeman L, Gunnarsson R, Mannerkorpi K: Prognostic factors for work ability in women with chronic low back pain consulting primary health care: a 2-year prospective longitudinal cohort study, *Clin J Pain* 30:391–398, 2014.

265. Hockings RL, McAuley JH, Maher CG: A systematic review of the predictive ability of the Orebro Musculoskeletal Pain Questionnaire, *Spine (Phila PA 1976)* 33:E494–E500, 2008.

266. Hill JC, Dunn KM, Lewis M, et al: A primary care back pain screening tool: identifying patient subgroups for initial treatment, *Arthritis Rheum* 59:632–641, 2008.

267. Beneciuk JM, Bishop MD, Fritz JM, et al: The STarT back screening tool and individual psychological measures: evaluation of prognostic capabilities for low back pain clinical outcomes in outpatient physical therapy settings, *Phys Ther* 93:321–333, 2013.

268. Fritz JM, Beneciuk JM, George SZ: Relationship between categorization with the STarT back screening tool and prognosis for people receiving physical therapy for low back pain, *Phys Ther* 91:722–732, 2011.

269. Hill JC, Dunn KM, Main CJ, et al: Subgrouping low back pain: a comparison of the STarT back tool with the Orebro Musculoskeletal Pain Screening Questionnaire, *Eur J Pain* 14:83–89, 2010.

270. Pincus T, Burton AK, Vogel S, et al: A systematic review of psychological factors as predictors of chronicity/disability in prospective cohorts of low back pain, *Spine* 27:E109–E120, 2002.

271. Pincus T, Vlaeyen JW, Kendall NA, et al: Cognitive-behavioral therapy and psychosocial factors in low back pain: directions for the future, *Spine* 27:E133–E138, 2002.

272. Pignone MP, Gaynes BN, Rushton JL, et al: Screening for depression in adults: a summary of the evidence for the US Preventive Services Task Force, *Ann Intern Med* 136:765–776, 2002.

273. Atkinson JH, Slater MA, Patterson TL, et al: Prevalence, onset, and risk of psychiatric disorders in men with chronic low back pain: a controlled study, *Pain* 45:111–121, 1991.

274. Currie SR, Wang J: Chronic back pain and major depression in the general Canadian population, *Pain* 107:54–60, 2004.

275. Haggman S, Maher CG, Refshauge KM: Screening for symptoms of depression by physical therapists managing low back pain, *Phys Ther* 84:1157–1166, 2004.

276. Antunes RS, de Macedo BG, Amaral TS, et al: Pain, kinesiophobia and quality of life in chronic low back pain and depression, *Acta Ortop Bras* 21:27–29, 2013.

277. de Moraes Vieira EB, de Goes SM, Damiani LP, et al: Self-efficacy and fear avoidance beliefs in chronic low back pain patients: coexistence and associated factors, *Pain Manag Nurs* 15:593–602, 2014.

278. Henschke N, Wouda L, Maher CG, et al: Determinants of patient satisfaction 1 year after presenting to primary care with acute low back pain, *Clin J Pain* 29:512–517, 2013.

279. Sullivan MJ, Reesor K, Mikail S, et al: The treatment of depression in chronic low back pain: review and recommendations, *Pain* 50:5–13, 1992.

280. Melloh M, Elfering A, Egli PC, et al: Predicting the transition from acute to persistent low back pain, *Occup Med (Lond)* 61:127–131, 2011.

281. George SZ, Coronado RA, Beneciuk JM, et al: Depressive symptoms, anatomical region, and clinical outcomes for patients seeking outpatient physical therapy for musculoskeletal pain, *Phys Ther* 91:358–372, 2011.

282. Spitzer RL, Williams JB, Kroenke K, et al: Utility of a new procedure for diagnosing mental disorders in primary care: the PRIME-MD 1000 study, *JAMA* 272:1749–1756, 1994.

283. Grevitt M, Pande K, O'Dowd J, et al: Do first impressions count?: a comparison of subjective and psychologic assessment of spinal patients, *Eur Spine J* 7:218–223, 1998.

284. Battie MC, Cherkin DC, Dunn R, et al: Managing low back pain: attitudes and treatment preferences of physical therapists, *Phys Ther* 74:219–226, 1994.

285. Foster NE, Thompson KA, Baxter GD, et al: Management of nonspecific low back pain by physiotherapists in Britain and Ireland: a descriptive questionnaire of current clinical practice, *Spine* 24:1332–1342, 1999.

286. Li LC, Bombardier C: Physical therapy management of low back pain: an exploratory survey of therapist approaches, *Phys Ther* 81:1018–1028, 2001.

287. Whooley MA, Avins AL, Miranda J, et al: Case-finding instruments for depression: two questions are as good as many, *J Gen Intern Med* 12:439–445, 1997.

288. Reme SE, Eriksen HR: Is one question enough to screen for depression? *Scand J Public Health* 38:618–624, 2010.

289. Reme SE, Lie SA, Eriksen HR: Are 2 questions enough to screen for depression and anxiety in patients with chronic low back pain? *Spine (Phila PA 1976)* 39:E455–E462, 2014.

290. Lethem J, Slade PD, Troup JDG, et al: Outline of a fear-avoidance model of exaggerated pain perception. Part I, *Behav Res Ther* 21:401–408, 1983.

291. Vlaeyen JW, Linton SJ: Fear-avoidance and its consequences in chronic musculoskeletal pain: a state of the art, *Pain* 85:317–332, 2000.

292. Waddell G, Newton M, Henderson I, et al: A Fear-Avoidance Beliefs Questionnaire (FABQ) and the role of fear-avoidance beliefs in chronic low back pain and disability, *Pain* 52:157–168, 1993.

293. Fritz JM, George SZ: Identifying psychosocial variables in patients with acute work-related low back pain: the importance of fear-avoidance beliefs, *Phys Ther* 82:973–983, 2002.

294. Fritz JM, George SZ, Delitto A: The role of fear avoidance beliefs in acute low back pain: relationships with current and future disability and work status, *Pain* 94:7–15, 2001.

295. Klenerman L, Slade PD, Stanley IM, et al: The prediction of chronicity in patients with an acute attack of low back pain in a general practice setting, *Spine* 20:478–484, 1995.

296. Sieben JM, Vlaeyen JW, Tuerlinckx S, et al: Pain-related fear in acute low back pain: the first two weeks of a new episode, *Eur J Pain* 6:229–237, 2002.

297. Hiebert R, Campello MA, Weiser S, et al: Predictors of short-term work-related disability among active duty US Navy personnel: a cohort study in patients with acute and subacute low back pain, *Spine J* 12:806–816, 2012.

298. Wertli MM, Rasmussen-Barr E, Weiser S, et al: The role of fear avoidance beliefs as a prognostic factor for outcome in patients with nonspecific low back pain: a systematic review, *Spine J* 14:816–836, 2014.

299. Hart DL, Werneke MW, Deutscher D, et al: Using intake and change in multiple psychosocial measures to predict functional status outcomes in people with lumbar spine syndromes: a preliminary analysis, *Phys Ther* 91:1812–1825, 2011.

300. Sindhu BS, Lehman LA, Tarima S, et al: Influence of fear-avoidance beliefs on functional status outcomes for people with musculoskeletal conditions of the shoulder, *Phys Ther* 92:992–1005, 2012.

301. Keeley P, Creed F, Tomenson B, et al: Psychosocial predictors of health-related quality of life and health service utilisation in people with chronic low back pain, *Pain* 135:142–150, 2008.

302. George SZ, Fritz JM, McNeil DW: Fear-avoidance beliefs as measured by the fear-avoidance beliefs questionnaire: change in fear-avoidance beliefs is predictive of change in self-report of disability and pain intensity for patients with acute low back pain, *Clin J Pain* 22:197–203, 2006.

303. Holm I, Friis A, Storheim K, et al: Measuring self-reported functional status and pain in patients with chronic low back pain by postal questionnaires: a reliability study, *Spine* 28:828–833, 2003.

304. Pfingsten M, Kroner-Herwig B, Leibing E, et al: Validation of the German version of the Fear-Avoidance Beliefs Questionnaire (FABQ), *Eur J Pain* 4:259–266, 2000.

305. Cleland JA, Fritz JM, Brennan GP: Predictive validity of initial fear avoidance beliefs in patients with low back pain receiving physical therapy: is the FABQ a useful screening tool for identifying patients at risk for a poor recovery? *Eur Spine J* 17:70–79, 2008.

306. Holden J, Davidson M, Tam J: Can the Fear-Avoidance Beliefs Questionnaire predict work status in people with work-related musculoskeletal disorders? *J Back Musculoskelet Rehabil* 23:201–208, 2010.

307. George SZ, Fritz JM, Childs JD: Investigation of elevated fear-avoidance beliefs for patients with low back pain: a secondary analysis involving patients enrolled in physical therapy clinical trials, *J Orthop Sports Phys Ther* 38:50–58, 2008.

308. Burton AK, Waddell G, Tillotson KM, Summerton N: Information and advice to patients with back pain can have a positive effect: a randomized controlled trial of a novel educational booklet in primary care, *Spine* 24:2484–2491, 1999.

309. Al-Obaidi SM, Al-Zoabi B, Al-Shuwaie N, et al: The influence of pain and pain-related fear and disability beliefs on walking velocity in chronic low back pain, *Int J Rehabil Res* 26:101–108, 2003.

310. Lariviere C, Bilodeau M, Forget R, et al: Poor back muscle endurance is related to pain catastrophizing in patients with chronic low back pain, *Spine (Phila PA 1976)* 35:E1178–E1186, 2010.

311. Smeets RJ, van Geel KD, Verbunt JA: Is the fear avoidance model associated with the reduced level of aerobic fitness in patients with chronic low back pain? *Arch Phys Med Rehabil* 90:109–117, 2009.

312. Thomas JS, France CR: Pain-related fear is associated with avoidance of spinal motion during recovery from low back pain, *Spine (Phila PA 1976)* 32:E460–E466, 2007.

313. Thomas JS, France CR, Lavender SA, et al: Effects of fear of movement on spine velocity and acceleration after recovery from low back pain, *Spine (Phila PA 1976)* 33:564–570, 2008.

314. Verbunt JA, Seelen HA, Vlaeyen JW, et al: Fear of injury and physical deconditioning in patients with chronic low back pain, *Arch Phys Med Rehabil* 84:1227–1232, 2003.

315. Demoulin C, Huijnen IP, Somville PR, et al: Relationship between different measures of pain-related fear and physical capacity of the spine in patients with chronic low back pain, *Spine J* 13:1039–1047, 2013.

316. Beneciuk JM, Robinson ME, George SZ: Low back pain subgroups using fear-avoidance model measures: results of a cluster analysis, *Clin J Pain* 28:658–666, 2012.

317. Pincus T, Smeets RJ, Simmonds MJ, et al: The fear avoidance model disentangled: improving the clinical

utility of the fear avoidance model, *Clin J Pain* 26:739–746, 2010.

318. Leeuw M, Goossens ME, van Breukelen GJ, et al: Measuring perceived harmfulness of physical activities in patients with chronic low back pain: the Photograph Series of Daily Activities—short electronic version, *J Pain* 8:840–849, 2007.

319. George SZ, Valencia C, Zeppieri Jr. G, et al: Development of a self-report measure of fearful activities for patients with low back pain: the fear of daily activities questionnaire, *Phys Ther* 89:969–979, 2009.

320. Leeuw M, Goossens ME, Linton SJ, et al: The fear-avoidance model of musculoskeletal pain: current state of scientific evidence, *J Behav Med* 30:77–94, 2007.

321. Sullivan MJ, Thorn B, Haythornthwaite JA, et al: Theoretical perspectives on the relation between catastrophizing and pain, *Clin J Pain* 17:52–64, 2001.

322. Pain catastrophizing and general health status in a large Dutch community sample, *Pain* 99:367–376, 2002.

323. Severeijns R, Vlaeyen JW, van den Hout MA, et al: Pain catastrophizing predicts pain intensity, disability, and psychological distress independent of the level of physical impairment, *Clin J Pain* 17:165–172, 2001.

324. Sullivan MJ, Stanish W, Sullivan ME, et al: Differential predictors of pain and disability in patients with whiplash injuries, *Pain Res Manag* 7:68–74, 2002.

325. Sullivan MJ, Stanish W, Waite H, et al: Catastrophizing, pain, and disability in patients with soft-tissue injuries, *Pain* 77:253–260, 1998.

326. Burton AK, Tillotson KM, Main CJ, et al: Psychosocial predictors of outcome in acute and subchronic low back trouble, *Spine* 20:722–728, 1995.

327. Wertli MM, Eugster R, Held U, et al: Catastrophizing-a prognostic factor for outcome in patients with low back pain: a systematic review, *Spine J* 2014.

328. Wertli MM, Burgstaller JM, Weiser S, et al: Influence of catastrophizing on treatment outcome in patients with nonspecific low back pain: a systematic review, *Spine (Phila PA 1976)* 39:263–273, 2014.

329. Sullivan MJL, Bishop SR, Pivik J: The pain catastrophizing scale: development and validation, *Psychol Assess* 7:524–532, 1995.

330. Franklin GM, Rahman EA, Turner JA, et al: Opioid use for chronic low back pain: a prospective, population-based study among injured workers in Washington state, 2002-2005, *Clin J Pain* 25:743–751, 2009.

331. Linton SJ, Nicholas MK, MacDonald S, et al: The role of depression and catastrophizing in musculoskeletal pain, *Eur J Pain* 15:416–422, 2011.

332. Turner JA, Franklin G, Fulton-Kehoe D, et al: ISSLS prize winner: early predictors of chronic work disability: a prospective, population-based study of workers with back injuries, *Spine (Phila PA 1976)* 33:2809–2818, 2008.

333. Main CJ, George SZ: Psychologically informed practice for management of low back pain: future directions in practice and research, *Phys Ther* 91:820–824, 2011.

334. Nicholas MK, George SZ: Psychologically informed interventions for low back pain: an update for physical therapists, *Phys Ther* 91:765–776, 2011.

335. George SZ, Fritz JM, Bialosky JE, et al: The effect of a fear-avoidance-based physical therapy intervention for patients with acute low back pain: results of a randomized clinical trial, *Spine* 28:2551–2560, 2003.

336. Delitto A, George SZ, Van Dillen LR, et al: Low back pain, *J Orthop Sports Phys Ther* 42:A1–A57, 2012.

CHAPTER 13

Lumbar Spine
Treatment of Hypomobility and Disc Conditions

JIM MEADOWS, DAVID J. MAGEE

INTRODUCTION

Manual therapy techniques (i.e., spinal mobilization and spinal manipulation) play a major role in the treatment of low back pain. This chapter discusses the use of manual therapy, particularly specific and indirect segmental techniques for lumbopelvic pain. In the context of this chapter, **mobilization** is defined as a series of rhythmical or nonrhythmical movements of the joints' articular surfaces that are applied by the clinician but are within the patient's control to stop (through muscle contraction). Similarly, **manipulation** is defined as a single, high-velocity, low-amplitude thrust technique that is intended to abolish the barrier to movement and is not within the patient's control (i.e., it happens too quickly for the patient to react).

Characteristics of Hypomobility Dysfunction

- Altered patterns of movement
- Decreased range of motion
- Tissue or joint swelling
- Altered joint play
- Abnormal end feel
- Tight, short muscles
- Inhibition of antagonists

For the most part, the manual therapy techniques applied in the treatment of lumbar hypomobility are used to reduce pain and increase range of movement. They also may be used to reduce reflex inhibition of the musculature that supports the spine. The exact mechanism of these effects is presently unknown. However, two primary models are used to explain the effects of spinal mobilization and manipulation: the neurophysiological model and pathomechanical model.

Neurophysiological Model

According to the neurophysiological model, segmental hypomobility occurs as a result of a neurophysiological processing problem in the control system; this processing problem is caused by pain, which produces protective muscle spasm and instability. In this context, the term *control system* refers to the concept set forth by Panjabi[1-3] and involves neural control (through the central and peripheral nervous systems) as well as the passive structures around the joints (i.e., ligaments, capsules, and discs) and active components (i.e., muscles). It also refers to control of the arthrokinematic movements (e.g., spin, slide, roll).[4-6] Inadequate control of the joint leads to changes in muscle tone which, in turn, result in more pain and reduced range of motion, a somewhat circuitous model.

Manual therapy techniques, such as mobilization and manipulation, in the neurophysiological model, provide a sensory stimulus that affects one or more of the joint mechanoreceptors, muscle spindle systems, or Golgi tendon organs, resulting in reduced muscle tone, increased range of motion, and decreased pain.[6] These changes are produced through neurophysiological pain and mechanoreceptor modulation at the spinal cord level (summation or gating) and/or by activating descending pathways.

Pathomechanical Model

The pathomechanical model is based on the premise that the primary dysfunction is essentially the result of a structural breakdown of one or more spinal segments, which allows the articulations to jam, fixate, lock, or sublux. In this context, a *spinal segment* is the trijoint complex (i.e., two vertebrae, the zygapophyseal joints, and the disc). The result of the structural breakdown is a pathomechanical hypomobility that limits movement in one or more directions. Pain is caused by mechanical stress; this stress can occur to the affected joint, or it may occur at another location as a result of excess stress on some other, remote tissue, possibly resulting in hypermobility of the remote tissue because of the pathomechanical hypomobility of the specific segment in question. In the pathomechanical model, manual treatment mechanically mobilizes the hypomobile joint to relieve the stress on the painful structure while protecting the hypermobile structures.[7]

Both the neurophysiological and pathomechanical models are able to explain clinical observations (i.e., pain, restricted or excessive movement), and each of the two models can be used in isolation. However, they are more useful to clinicians if they are combined.

Manual therapy techniques have been shown to produce both neurophysiological and mechanical effects on the segmental tissues.[4,8–15] In acute pain states, particularly with spasm or nonreflexive muscle guarding, overly aggressive manual therapy techniques (e.g., Maitland grade 3+ and grade 4+) can, and usually do, aggravate the condition by exacerbating existing inflammation (see Volume 2 in this series, *Scientific Foundations and Principles of Practice in Musculoskeletal Rehabilitation*, Chapter 24). In these cases, more gentle manual therapy techniques (e.g., Maitland grade 1 and grade 2) are used to reduce the pain through neurophysiological modulation.[16] These gentle techniques do not (or should not) directly engage the pathological or anatomical barrier (i.e., end of range of motion) or cause any discomfort. They can be considered *pain-dominant* techniques. If pain is not the predominant clinical feature and if its onset follows the clinician's perception of the pathological barrier to passive movement (*restriction-dominant* condition), a technique that directly stresses the pathological barrier (e.g., Maitland grade 3+ and grade 4+ and minithrusts) is the treatment of choice. For pathomechanical or pericapsular hypomobility (i.e., stiff, inextensible articular tissues), manipulation and mobilization, respectively, may be more efficient and effective.

For the purposes of manual therapy, pathological barriers can be divided into muscle, collagen, or inert tissue related, as well as neurological barriers. Muscle barriers occur as a result of injury to contract out tissue (i.e., muscle), or they are the result of protective muscle spasm. Examples of a muscle barrier include hypertonicity of a muscle, muscle spasm, and adaptive shortening of the muscle.[17] In these cases, the end feel is muscle spasm or, as Cyriax described it, a "vibrant twang" or "mushy" tissue stretch (i.e., a tight muscle).[18–21] Collagen and inert tissue barriers occur as a result of injury to inert tissue (e.g., the capsule and ligaments) and other collagen in or adjacent to the joint, including scar tissue. In these cases, the end feel is capsular (e.g., a capsular pattern), soft capsular (e.g., synovitis or soft tissue edema), springy block (e.g., meniscus), or bone to bone (e.g., osteophyte formation). Inert tissue barriers

may be articular or periarticular. Neurological barriers are primarily the result of pain causing an empty end feel or one with neurological signs (e.g., tingling, numbness, "pins and needles", painless weakness).

MANUAL THERAPY FOR LUMBAR INTERVERTEBRAL DISC HERNIATION

In addition to addressing pain and segmental pathomechanics, manual therapy techniques (especially manipulation) may be used as an intervention for lumbar intervertebral disc herniation. Probably the greatest proponent of manipulative therapy for the treatment of disc herniation was James Cyriax.[18–21] However, his advocacy of this approach was not based so much on existing pathology but on the clinical model he proposed. This model essentially held that facet joint syndrome (and other, similar pathomechanical conditions) and sacroiliac joint dysfunction were extremely rare and that most low back pain was caused by varying degrees of disc pathology (i.e., protrusion, prolapse, extrusion, or sequestration).

Currently spinal manipulation in the treatment of disc herniation is used primarily by chiropractors and it tends to be avoided by the medical, osteopathic, and physical therapy professions. The contention that manipulative techniques affect the intervertebral disc is not controversial; what is open to question is whether the effect is beneficial or harmful. In a cadaveric study, Sheng et al.[22] found that rotation manipulation combined with compression increased intradiscal pressure and rotation manipulation combined with traction reduced it. Two magnetic resonance imaging (MRI) and clinical outcome studies of patients with lumbar disc herniation found that spinal manipulation combined with traction, physical therapy (undefined), and exercises[23] or spinal manipulation alone[24] resulted in a significant improvement in clinical symptoms, function, and MRI findings.

Most of the evidence for the efficacy of manipulation in the treatment of disc herniation is anecdotal or comes from case reports[25]; however, the use of spinal manipulation for lumbar disc herniation appears to have some degree of effectiveness.[26,27] Chiropractic reports provide examples of cases of lumbosacral disc herniations that were more lateral, causing back and leg pain with sensory deficit (confirmed by MRI), and that were treated successfully by manipulation.[28–30] Some case reports even indicate the successful use of manipulation in patients with established cauda equina lesions, a condition most clinicians consider an absolute contraindication to manual therapy.[31–34]

Many other reports show harmful effects from spinal manipulation with a disc herniation. According to Assendelft,[35] disc herniation, aggravation of disc herniation, and cauda equina syndrome (CES) are the most common serious complications of lumbar spinal manipulation, accounting for more than 20% of all serious complications of manipulation in all spinal regions, making possible disc herniation the second most serious complication after neurovascular injury subsequent to manipulation of the cervical spine.

A literature review by Haldeman and Rubinstein[36] that covered the years 1911 to 1989 found only 10 cases of CES after spinal manipulative therapy (SMT). Their review also reported on three new cases that were related at least temporally to SMT. In the three new cases, neither the treating clinician nor the emergency department physician recognized the onset of the problem.[36] A number of other cases of CES have been reported since 1989. In an unusual case, the disc fragment did not fragment but bulged onto the artery that supplied the conus (i.e., caudal narrowing area of the spinal canal).[37] Li[38] reported five cases of CES or conus medullaris syndrome (CMS), all of which occurred after spinal manipulation, some of them immediately after the manipulation. Powell et al.[39] listed six risk factors for spinal manipulation, one of which was the presence of a herniated nucleus pulposus.

Therefore, it cannot be argued that SMT does not result in CES or CMS syndrome in some cases; however, the incidence of these syndromes as adverse effects of SMT is believed to be very low, somewhere in the range of 0.5 to 1 per 1 million manipulations.[34,40]

For most clinicians, the risk (however low) of very serious complications, unproven efficacy, and inexperience in the use of manipulation for disc herniation are factors that cause them to avoid using these techniques. Most clinicians also have the advantage of working in a system that encourages referral of difficult cases for further investigation and the availability of other treatment methods that do not carry the same degree of risk. Consequently, for the most part, clinicians tend to view the presence of an established disc herniation as a contraindication to most forms of manual therapy.

TRACTION FOR DISC HERNIATIONS (VERTEBRAL AXIAL DECOMPRESSION THERAPY)

In contrast to manipulation, spinal traction is used quite frequently in the treatment of disc herniation. Since the age of Hippocrates, practitioners have known about the application of longitudinal force to the axis of the spine to provide facet joint distraction, reduction of disc protrusion, soft tissue elongation, muscle relaxation, and patient mobilization. Spinal traction has been heavily explored as a therapeutic option in musculoskeletal medicine since the late 18th century. It enjoyed a renewed popularity in the 1950s and 1960s based on James Cyriax's findings on the efficacy of spinal traction for the treatment of discogenic back and leg pain.[19] Saunders[41] further popularized the use of intermittent spinal traction in the 1980s and 1990s through the development of improved stabilization belts and split table technology. In the 2000s, as a result of improved pneumatic instrumentation, an enhanced form of vertebral axial spinal decompression (VAX-D) is being widely used in the management of disc conditions. Advances in imaging and microinstrumentation have

fueled a growing body of clinical evidence that spinal decompression and/or traction should be considered a front-line intervention for these conditions.[42–44]

Vertebral axial decompression therapy uses a computer-driven table to apply traction to the lumbar spine. It is postulated that this traction technique may effect decompression of the disc. Experimental results have been encouraging,[45,46] but the lack of scientific evidence based on well-designed studies has led several groups to question its effectiveness.[45–49]

SELECTION OF A LUMBAR SPINE MANUAL THERAPY TECHNIQUE

The primary use of manual therapy is in the treatment of segmental dysfunction or hypomobility. In this context, "segmental dysfunction" means injury or abnormal movement in the trijoint complex, which consists of the two zygapophyseal joints and the disc. The technique selected must be specific to the pathological barrier associated with the dysfunction. If pain, spasm, or hypertonicity (or all three) is the principal problem, a neurophysiological technique is indicated; however, if inextensibility of pericapsular tissues or pathomechanical hypomobility is the chief problem, a restriction-dominant technique is the preferred choice. If the joint must be stretched or if it is fixed (jammed or subluxed) and the hypomobility is pathomechanical, the joint needs to be manipulated with a sudden, low-amplitude force. The following information is based on the clinical experience of the chapter's first author, Jim Meadows.

A number of factors must be considered in the selection of a manual technique. Two of these have already been discussed: the level of pain (i.e., pain dominant or restriction dominant) and the condition itself (i.e., disc herniation, pericapsular restriction, pathomechanical hypomobility). In addition, the dose of the treatment, which is actually a subset of the previous considerations, must be selected.

Causes of Hypomobility

MYOFASCIAL CAUSES
- Adaptive shortening or hypertonicity of muscles
- Posttraumatic adhesions
- Scarring

PERICAPSULAR CAUSES
- Damage to capsule or ligament
- Adhesions
- Scarring
- Arthritis or arthrosis
- Fibrosis
- Tissue adaptation

PATHOMECHANICAL CAUSES (JOINT TRAUMA)
- Macrotrauma
- Microtrauma

Causes of a Pathological (Restrictive) Barrier

- Trauma (macrotrauma or microtrauma)
- Inflammatory response
- Muscle spasm
- Edema
- Pain
- Tissue alterations (e.g., adaptive shortening)

Important Factors in the Mobilization Process

- Presenting condition or tissue disorder (contractile?, inert [collagen]?, neurological?)
- Quality of the movement present
- Resistance felt (i.e., type of barrier, end feel)
- Pathological state of the tissues (i.e., acute, subacute, chronic; stage of healing)
- Symptoms elicited before, during, and after treatment (i.e., pain dominant or restriction dominant pattern)
- Indications for treatment (i.e., pain-dominant or restriction dominant pattern)
- Treatment parameters (e.g., grade of technique, positioning of patient)
- Cautions and contraindications to use of certain techniques
- Patient's use of any medications (e.g., nonsteroidal anti-inflammatory drugs [NSAIDs]) that may affect treatment
- Methods of testing for instability and vascular insufficiency
- Need for adjunctive treatment (e.g., exercise, electrophysical agent)
- Need to reassess

Probably the most common method used to discuss doses of manual treatment is the Maitland grading system.[16,50,51] This system has undergone many refinements over the years; however, for the purposes of this chapter, the grades can be divided into two categories: those that have mainly a neurophysiological effect and those that have a mechanical effect on the pathological barrier. Figure 13-1 depicts the simplest interpretation of this system. Purists may take issue with this interpretation, but it presents all that is required to discuss grading techniques for the purposes of this chapter.

As Figure 13-1 shows, grade 1 and grade 2 techniques are unquestionably neurophysiological in effect because they do not approach the end of the available range of movement, and they should not produce pain or discomfort. Technically, grade 3 and grade 4 techniques are also subbarrier because they should reach the end of range but not stress the tissues at end range. Minithrusts and grade 5 (manipulation) techniques would be applied at the barrier. If pain is experienced before or at the same time tissue resistance is encountered, a subbarrier technique is indicated. If any attempt at reaching the pathological barrier produces or increases pain, the condition is in a subacute stage or almost certainly in the acute phase. However, in clinical practice, clinicians commonly tend to push into the barrier; when this happens, these techniques more properly should be labeled grade 3+ and grade 4+ techniques. Regardless of

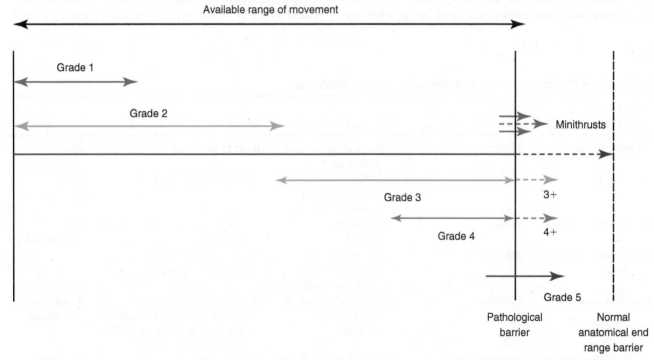

Figure 13-1 Maitland grades of movement used in lumbar mobilization techniques. As the diagram shows, grade 1 and grade 2 techniques are definitely neurophysiological because they do not approach the end of the available range of movement, and they should not produce pain or discomfort. Technically, grade 3 and grade 4 techniques are also subbarrier because they should reach the end of the available range but not stress it. However, in clinical practice, clinicians commonly tend to push into the barrier. When this happens, these techniques are more properly labeled grade 3+ and grade 4+. Regardless of the grade of the technique, all mobilizations have an oscillatory component. Oscillation prevents neurophysiological accommodation to the input, which would attenuate the pain-reduction effect of the technique. (Data from Maitland GD: *Vertebral manipulation*, London, 1986, Butterworth.)

the grade of technique used, all mobilizations include an oscillatory component, which prevents neurophysiological accommodation to the input from attenuating the pain-reduction effect of the technique.

Clinicians commonly use terms such as *acute, subacute,* and *nonacute* in nontemporal terms to depict how painful and irritable (i.e., acute) the condition is. Semantics, definitions, and communication, as well as a common level of understanding, are critical among clinicians, and this is often a problem in manual therapy. Terms must be standardized, and associating the onset of pain with the onset of the symptoms can do this. Table 13-1 is an attempt to "quasi-quantify" the relationship of pain to the end feel to enable the clinician to determine whether the problem is pain dominant or restriction dominant.

True constant pain must be considered to possibly indicate visceral or certain types of bone pathology that are not usually amenable to manual therapy techniques. Pain that is unrelieved by rest and generally considered an indication of inflammation should actually be called *variable pain* because it is affected by varying mechanical stresses and therefore variable rather than constant. In actuality this is high-level, continuous pain that may be treated by manual therapy techniques (see Table 13-1).

To summarize, the choice of manual therapy techniques depends on the dominant tissue type barrier. In addition, whether pain or restriction predominates or whether the problem is pericapsular or pathomechanical, the clinician must consider whether the patient's personal attributes (e.g., emotional liability, psychological well-being) might be

affecting the condition. Ultimately, all of these factors must be assessed to optimize the use of manual therapy techniques. Patient selection is a critical concern for therapeutic success. In addition, the clinician must ensure that informed consent is obtained before any treatment is provided.

Informed Consent Process

- Discuss the proposed technique and reason it is deemed the best choice
- Discuss possible alternatives
- Discuss both the benefits and risks of the technique
- Have information sheets available for the patient, or note how the information was given; include the time and date it was provided (i.e., documentation)
- Allow the patient to ask questions (if necessary, prompt the person)
- Obtain the patient's written consent

Patient Selection

Not all patients are suited for manual therapy. The list of patients who fall into this category is longer for some professions than for others. For example, physical therapists generally lack enthusiasm for manual treatment of a disc herniation, whereas chiropractors frequently use manipulation for this condition. For most physical therapists, the patients suited for manual therapy are those suffering from a biomechanical segmental dysfunction (or its peripheral equivalent). For the purposes of this chapter, manual therapy as described is used for a very specific type of mechanical low back pain.

TABLE 13-1

Relationship of Pain to End Feel, Presumptive Pathology, and Treatment

Pain and Tissue Resistance (End Feel)	Acuteness or "Irritability" Level	Presumptive Pathology	Treatment	Dominance
All pain, no resistance	Hyperacute	Almost always serious pathology	Refer to physician	Pain dominant
Constant pain*	Hyperacute	Significant inflammation or serious pathology	No manual treatment	Pain dominant
Pain before resistance	Acute	Inflammation, very irritable	Low-dose subbarrier techniques (grade 1)	Pain dominant
Pain simultaneous with resistance	Subacute	Moderate or mild inflammation, moderately irritable	Higher-dose subbarrier techniques (grade 2)	
Pain after resistance	Nonacute	Mechanical pathology; may be slightly irritable	Barrier techniques (grade 3/3+ or grade 4/4+), either mobilization or manipulation, depending on end feel	Restriction dominant
No pain, all resistance	Stiff or jammed	Mechanical pathology with no irritability	Barrier techniques (grade 3/3+ or grade 4/4+), either mobilization or manipulation grades, depending on end feel	Restriction dominant

*Constant pain implies pain that is always present and does not change with movement or weight bearing.

Mechanical Low Back Pain: Two Theoretical Models

The term *mechanical low back pain* is a way of saying that the problem encountered does not lend itself to a true medical diagnosis. Although the average clinical presentation of a patient with this condition is fairly easy to recognize, the explanations given for the underlying pathology are controversial and contentious. In general, a patient with pathomechanical segmental dysfunction (i.e., caused by hypomobility) displays the clinical findings listed in Table 13-2.[51-53]

The clinical findings in Table 13-2 are the criteria used to diagnose pathomechanical segmental dysfunction (i.e., hypomobility), which can be addressed with mobilization techniques. In contrast, neurophysiological segmental dysfunction (i.e., instability), which often accompanies or results from hypomobility, is not amenable to mobilization therapy because it involves excessive motion, not reduced motion. However, conditions involving excessive motion are amenable to stabilization training (see Chapter 14 and Volume 2 of this series, *Scientific Foundation and Principles of Practice in Musculoskeletal Rehabilitation,* Chapter 19).

Two primary theories have been proposed for this apparent dichotomy. One theory holds that in patients with the clinical profile previously described, two distinct dysfunctions are present at different joints or different segments, one being hypomobile and the other unstable. According to the other theory, only one dysfunction is present, but its characteristics change from time to time, with painful episodes interrupting longer periods of pain-free function. The affected segment undergoes a form of phase transition. A *phase transition* can be defined as a clinical episode in which a profound change occurs in symptom behavior and manifestation with little change in the physical composition of the segment. Regardless of which theory is preferred, it must be understood that a theory or explanation is not required to be the "truth"; rather, its function is to offer a conceptualization of what is happening so that the user of the model can visualize events. Theories are used, consciously or unconsciously, all of the time. The following model of phase transition fits the observations concerning the presentation of biomechanical back pain and its response to various treatments at least as well if not better than most other models, but it is not necessarily true.

As mentioned, a phase transition is considered to have occurred when a radical change in the behavioral characteristics of a substance or system occurs without a similar change in the composition of the substance or system. This concept has been taken from physics. It describes a major change in the thermodynamics of a system in which essentially the same substance has completely different behavioral characteristics. For example, consider the change from water to ice—ice cannot put out fire until it changes to water; ice is extremely slippery, water considerably less so. Although in the strictest sense the term *phase transition* is used to describe fundamental property changes in a thermodynamic system, it might be used to good effect to describe a model of biomechanical dysfunction of the lumbar spine.

If the patient is experiencing a "phase" that may best be described as a lack of spinal stability and control, this phase is relatively painless and mobile, and it leaves the patient fully functional but with symptoms indicating that the patient cannot control the movement. Assessment during this unstable phase reveals abnormally pliable tissue compliance (i.e., instability) and hypermobility. If a phase transition occurs, passive physiological mobility tests will demonstrate hypomobility and will be painful; however, all of the characteristics of subluxation-fixation and the stability test results will be negative. In effect, the segment goes from the matrix of instability to hyperstability and from a painless state to a painful state. It undergoes transition from one phase to another and back again as effective forces are applied. Therefore, using the phase transition model for segmental dysfunction, an unstable segment oscillates between a pain-free phase, which is its unstable ground state, and a painful phase, in which its instability allows the joint to fix at one end of its range and either become painful itself or cause pain at another joint that is stressed by the hypomobility. Therefore treatment focuses on the phase in which patients find themselves at the time of treatment. If the painful, hypomobile phase is encountered, manual therapy to move the joint and relieve the pain is required. If the unstable phase is to be treated, stability therapy and movement reeducation can be used.

To determine the motion state dysfunction at the segment, the clinician must perform a detailed biomechanical

TABLE 13-2

Signs and Symptoms of Segmental Dysfunction

Neurophysiological Segmental Dysfunction (Hypermobility and Instability)	Pathomechanical Segmental Dysfunction (Hypomobility)
• Asynchronous movement	• Altered patterns of movement
• Increased range of motion	
• Joint swelling	• Decreased range of motion when joint is painful
• Altered joint play	
• Late muscle spasm	• Tissue or joint swelling
• Abnormal end feel	• Altered joint play
• Pain localized to back	• Abnormal end feel
• Seldom pain referral	• Tight (hypertonic) muscles (postural)
• Painful episode related to load, speed of movements, muscle fatigue	• Inhibition of antagonists
	• Moderate nonneuropathic pain
• No incapacitation deformity	• Possibly referral of pain to buttock
• Possible instability jog (muscle twitch)	• Minor or unknown trigger to painful episodes

examination. This examination must determine four important factors:

1. Is a movement dysfunction present?
2. If a movement dysfunction is present, is it one of hypomobility, hypermobility, or instability?
3. If the dysfunction is a hypomobility dysfunction, is it articular or extraarticular in origin?
4. If the hypomobility dysfunction is articular in origin, is it pericapsular or pathomechanical?

Only after these determinations have been made, can a specific treatment be applied to a specific segment in a specific direction. Some schools of thought hold that it is unnecessary to be specific about the segment to be mobilized. The intervention discussion in this chapter focuses on specific treatments. However, some discussion of the nonspecific approach is needed, because it is rapidly becoming *the* method of treatment, especially in the United States.

The use of nonspecific manual treatment by physical therapists was first popularized by Cyriax in the 1950s, and this approach still has its adherents.[19] A disc herniation model was used, and it was thought that large-amplitude regional techniques using strong traction would have a beneficial effect on the disc lesion. The differential diagnostic examination afforded limited specificity as to the segment requiring treatment, and absolutely no attempt was made to make the treatment technique specific. In 2002 Flynn et al.[54] resurrected this idea, using clinical prediction rules to determine which patients would benefit from manipulative therapy of the lumbar spine. The study came up with a five-point clinical prediction rule that gave a likelihood of success of 45% to 90% if four out of five points were evident.

Flynn's Clinical Prediction Rules[54]

- Recent onset of symptoms (<16 days)
- No fear-avoidance beliefs (i.e., Fear-Avoidance Beliefs Questionnaire [FABQ] score < 19)
- Lumbar hypomobility in at least one segment
- Good medial rotation range of motion in at least one hip (>35°)
- No symptoms distal to the knee

The manipulation used in the study was not only nonspecific to any segment, but it also had been used previously to manipulate the sacroiliac joint. Flynn et al.[54] further made the point that segmental specificity was not necessary for a technique to be effective (a point borne out by the longevity of the Cyriax techniques and other studies).[19-21] However, clinical reasons exist for making both the thought processes involved in the determination of treatment and the technique itself more specific. The previous discussion is entirely about effectiveness. It does not address other issues, such as safety and ways to treat patients who do not meet four of the five criteria described by Flynn et al.[54]

Nonspecific techniques do not pretend to safeguard segments that may not be able to withstand the forces involved in manual treatment if they are not specifically locked. For example, in the cervical spine, the vertebral artery is at risk unless the technique's effect is minimized throughout the neck, especially if rotational techniques are used. Although the clinical prediction rule may help to include patients in the manipulation group, it does not do much about excluding those who are marginal or who should not be manipulated because of unrelated but significant pathologies. This oversimplification of a very complex system (i.e., the patient) allows newcomers to manual therapy to assume that all that is required is that the patient match a few points on a list. As much as Flynn et al.[54] speak out against an algorithmic approach, it is the way clinicians tend to think, and it provides a stronger rationale for doing what clinicians do than simply following a clinical prediction rule.

Biomechanical Segmental Assessment

To determine whether a specific manual treatment should be performed for pathomechanical dysfunction, the clinician must perform a passive biomechanical segmental assessment that uses passive physiological intervertebral movements (PPIVMs), followed by passive arthrokinematic (accessory) intervertebral movements (PAIVMs). Figure 13-2 presents a simple algorithm of the examination.

Using PPIVMs and PAIVMs, the clinician can determine a number of findings that will guide the use of manual therapy techniques for the hypomobile joint or segment. A pericapsular restriction is indicated by restriction on PPIVM tests associated with restriction on PAIVM tests, with both types of movements showing the hard capsular end feel of stiffness. A pathomechanical hypomobility may be determined by the PPIVM tests associated with restriction on the PAIVM tests, with both showing a pathomechanical end feel. For a hypermobile joint or segment, using the phase transition model, the presence of an instability requires treatment of the instability because this is the phase the back condition exhibits.

Before the definitive technique can be applied, the clinician may and probably will encounter one or more pathological barriers between the initial hands-on end feel once the patient has been positioned for treatment. The end feel will vary, depending on the pathological barrier encountered. To briefly review barrier end feels, an inextensibility of the pericapsular tissues produces a predominantly hard capsular end feel, and a subluxation produces a hard, jammed end feel. Increased muscle tone can produce a variety of end feels, depending on the degree of hypertonicity and its effect. A minor degree of hypertonicity may produce only an increased drag on the way to the definitive end feel, whereas a greater amount of hypertonicity can cause an almost capsular end feel but

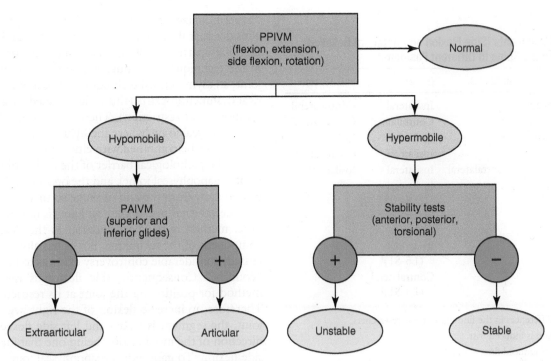

Figure 13-2 Algorithm for the passive biomechanical segmental assessment.

with a "lively resilience" (Cyriax's "vibrant twang").[19] If the hypertonus alters the biomechanics of the segment by acting as an "abnormal ligament," it can cause the joint to jam, resulting in a pathomechanical end feel similar to that of a subluxed joint. In all cases, light hold-relax, contract-relax, or muscle energy techniques can reduce the hypertonus and drastically alter the end feel.

Another pathological barrier is soreness, which often is first encountered once the segment is positioned near its abnormal end of range. The patient may complain of soreness, or the clinician may feel the patient's reaction to the position (this is not acute pain, and certainly no spasm accompanies the pain).

For manual therapy techniques to succeed, each of these pathological barriers must be addressed as it is met. Mild degrees of soreness can be reduced or eliminated with grade 3 or grade 4 oscillatory techniques that do not produce pain; hypertonus can be addressed with muscle relaxation techniques, including hold-relax, contract-relax, and muscle energy and active release techniques; pericapsular restrictions are best treated with a grade 3+ or grade 4+ mobilization; and subluxations are treated with manipulation or with minithrusts, if manipulation is not chosen. Usually multiple pathological barriers are met at each treatment. The positioning causes some minor soreness, which is relieved by a grade 3 or grade 4 mobilization, and muscle tone (normal or high) may then be encountered and reduced. Finally the definitive pathological barrier is met and treated with a grade 3+ or 4+ mobilization or manipulation (minithrusts if manipulation is not an option). This approach is more effective because it eliminates the inappropriate use of manual therapy techniques, such as ballistic stretching of muscle (which occurs if grade 4+ techniques are used on hypertonic muscles) and incorrect manipulative methods for extensive capsular tightening.

Positioning and Treatment

When deciding how to position the patient for the most effective use of manual therapy techniques, the clinician first must consider whether the hypomobility occurs into flexion or extension and whether it is at the right or the left zygapophyseal joint. If side flexion is considered in terms of flexion or extension of the zygapophyseal joint, rather than the segment's movement as a whole, right side flexion is seen by most authors as causing the right joint to extend and the left to flex. If rotation is considered instead of side flexion, the issue of which joint flexes and which extends becomes much more problematic; considerable controversy exists about the coupling that occurs with rotation, and there is almost no agreement on which direction of side flexion couples with a specific direction of rotation (Table 13-3). A study using live subjects found that coupling depended not only on whether it occurred at the lumbar spine but also at which specific level[55-57]; a cadaveric study found that at L5-S1, the coupling changed, depending on whether it was initiated by rotation or by side flexion.[50]

In addition to the lack of consensus among experts and research studies on this point, the indisputable fact is that patients do not have normal or even optimum biomechanics; therefore a discussion of normal movement may be irrelevant. The most useful course is to ignore rotation

TABLE 13-3

Coupled Movements (Side Flexion and Rotation) Believed to Occur in the Spine in Different Positions*

Author	In Neutral	In Flexion	In Extension
MacConnaill		Ipsilateral	Contralateral
Farfan		Contralateral	Contralateral
Kaltenborn		Ipsilateral	Ipsilateral
Grieve		Ipsilateral	Contralateral
Fryette	Contralateral	Ipsilateral	Ipsilateral
Pearcy		Ipsilateral (L5-S1) Contralateral (L4,5)	
Oxland		Ipsilateral (L5-S1)[†] Contralateral (L5-S1)[‡]	

*Note the differences in the findings of these researchers.

[†]If side flexion is induced first.

[‡]If rotation is induced first.

From Magee DJ: *Orthopedic physical assessment,* ed 6, p 573, St Louis, 2014, Elsevier/Saunders.

and use side flexion as the coupling model because side flexion does not interfere with the way the joint moves; it moves down with ipsilateral (same) side flexion and up with contralateral (opposite) side flexion (Table 13-4).

If the clinical requirement for treating the patient is to increase flexion of the right zygapophyseal joint, the whole segment could be mobilized into left side flexion. However, this carries the risk that the mobilization will

TABLE 13-4

Positioning for Flexion and Extension of the Zygapophyseal (Facet) Joints

Position	Flexion or Extension Side	Extremity of Position
Flexion	Bilateral flexion	Moderate
Extension	Bilateral extension	Moderate
Right side flexion	Right extension	Moderate
	Left flexion	Moderate
Left side flexion	Left extension	Moderate
	Right flexion	Moderate
Flexion and right side flexion	Left flexion	End range
Flexion and left side flexion	Right flexion	End range
Extension and right side flexion	Right extension	End range
Extension and left side flexion	Left extension	End range

"hypermobilize" the left joint. The clinician must also consider that if this joint has been overstressed by its hypomobile partner, it should be protected from the force of the technique. To reduce the stresses on the opposite joint, an asymmetrical technique is chosen if an asymmetrical dysfunction exists (this is determined by asymmetrical movement restriction). Therefore flexion of the right zygapophyseal joint (where the hypomobility dysfunction exists) must be combined with either rotation or side flexion to the pathological barrier of the target joint (i.e., the right zygapophyseal joint), and the opposite joint must be moved away from the end of range so that the unaffected side (i.e., the left zygapophyseal joint) is not stressed. The usual method is to select rotation as the discriminative component of the technique, but as has already been discussed, considerable controversy exists as to how rotation "couples." Consequently, side flexion is the preferred method for positioning the joint at its restrictive barrier. Therefore, to increase flexion of the right zygapophyseal joint, the segment is flexed and left side flexed with the direction of the mobilization being one that increases left side flexion. To gain right zygapophyseal joint extension, the segment is extended and right side flexed, and the technique is into right side flexion. The hypomobility can be treated with the patient lying on either the right or left side.

"Barriering" (Locking)

If acute pain is not a factor, standard positioning can be used to mobilize a stiff or subluxed joint. When standard positioning is used, the spine is not locked specifically above and below the target segment to keep it in neutral because there is no point in doing so. This is analogous to mobilizing the elbow to regain the last 10° of extension from the biomechanically neutral position. The effort of moving through 60° would be wasted to get to the point where treatment was needed.

If standard positioning is not used, the spine is positioned so that the target joint is moved as close to the end of its reduced physiological (or osteokinematic) range of motion as possible from above and below. This is more properly called *"barriering,"* rather than locking, because the latter implies moving nontarget segments to block their motion while retaining the neutral position of the target segment. After the spine has been put in its end range of the movement to be recovered, the segments that will be levered through are "unbarriered" by passively moving them away from the end of range so that they are protected to some degree from the force of the mobilization.

Another variation in positioning is locking down to the affected segment (i.e., locking all the segments above the target joint), leaving the target joint in neutral to "barrier" it against the abnormal restriction. This positioning technique (Figure 13-3) is used when pain is to be treated with subbarrier or pain-dominant techniques (i.e., grade

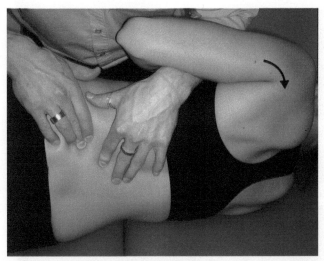

Figure 13-3 Positioning for a target segment. The clinician's right hand is pulling the pelvis forward while fingers of the clinician's left hand are palpating the spinal segment being mobilized.

1 and grade 2) or when very specific positioning is required to protect an irritable or vulnerable segment above or below the segment.

Mobilization Using the "Pelvis Upward" or "Pelvis Downward" Technique

The mobilization or thrust force is generated through the pelvis. Clinicians can achieve this either by using the strength of their arm (if the patient is relatively small and light) or, more usually, by exploiting gravity through the use of controlled body weight. The force is directed through the uppermost innominate, rocking the pelvic girdle on its opposite trochanter and causing side flexion of the lumbar spine. Imagine the patient lying on the left side. If the pelvis is rocked down toward the feet, left side flexion of the spine results (Figure 13-4, A). If the pelvis is tipped up toward the head, right side flexion occurs (Figure 13-4, B).

Rocking the "pelvis upward" requires positioning by arm strength and is a somewhat more complicated technique. However, it is generally a more specific technique, and the lead author's experience is that most clinicians are more comfortable using it to deliver the sudden, sharp thrust demanded for manipulation. The "pelvis downward" technique allows the clinician to use body weight; therefore it is easier to maintain for longer periods and is better used for mobilizations.

In the following treatment descriptions, the L3-4 segment is used as an example; however, these techniques may be used throughout the lumbar spine and even into the lower thoracic region.

Left Flexion Hypomobility: "Pelvis Downward" Technique

The patient lies on the right side. The patient's hips are flexed while the target segment (e.g., L3-4) is palpated to ensure that the flexion movement goes at least through this segment (Figure 13-5, A). The segment is bilaterally flexed at this point. The patient's lower leg can then be extended so that the patient's thighs are not parallel to each other; this allows rotation of the patient's pelvis when rotation locking is required for the segments below L3-4 (Figure 13-5, B).

The segment is now flexed and right side flexed from above; the patient's upper arm is allowed to lie forward in front of the body (this allows the side flexion to be induced into flexion), and the patient's lower arm is pulled caudally and parallel to the bed while the clinician palpates the L3-4 segment to ensure that the side flexion or flexion movement is carried through this segment (Figure 13-5, C). The clinician need not be concerned if the segments below are also moving because these will be unflexed later.

The patient's upper arm can now be moved back onto the patient's side without fear of extending the spine, provided the movement is produced at the patient's shoulder and not at the trunk. The patient's lower thigh is pushed backward so that the segments below L3-4 are extended while the clinician palpates L3-4 to ensure that this segment remains in flexion (Figure 13-5, D). At this point, the lower segments are in side flexion but away from their

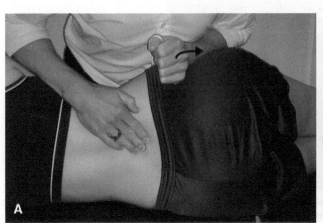

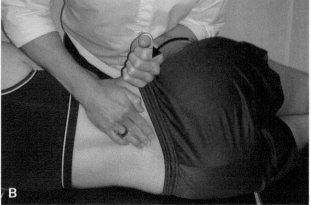

Figure 13-4 A, "Pelvis downward" technique. **B,** "Pelvis upward" technique. Note: The fingers of the clinician's right hand are palpating for movement at the spinal segment.

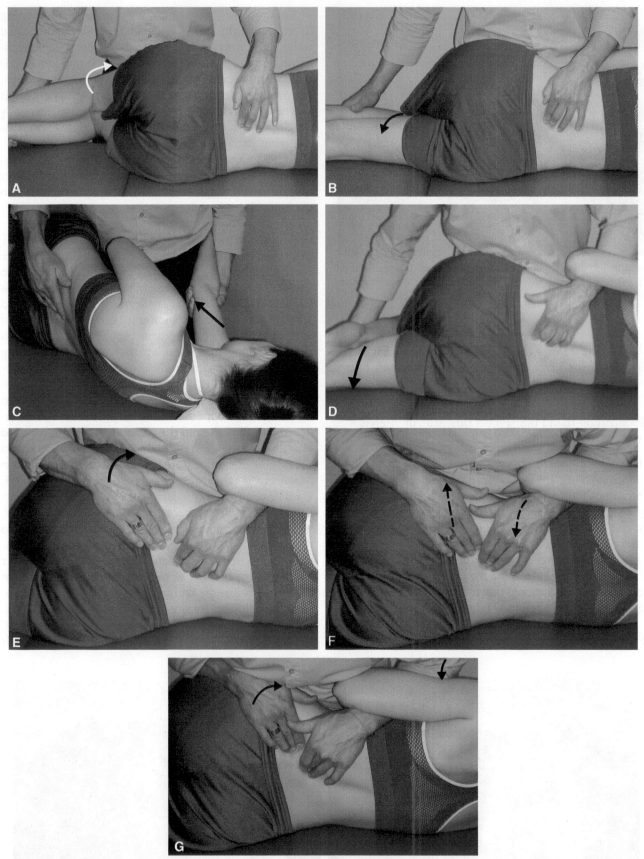

Figure 13-5 Left flexion hypomobility: "pelvis downward" technique. **A,** Bilateral flexion. **B,** Lower leg extension. **C,** Arm is pulled caudally, causing trunk flexion, left side flexion. **D,** Extension of segments below target segment. **E,** Locking of lower segments. **F,** Mobilization of L3-4. **G,** Locking of segments above and below the target segment. Note: The clinician's fingers on the spine are palpating for movement at the spinal segment.

flexion barrier, whereas the target segment is fully flexed and right side flexed, meaning that the left zygapophyseal joint is fully flexed, at least as far as its restriction allows. In essence it is at its abnormal pathological barrier and ready to be mobilized or manipulated.

To safeguard the patient's lower segments a little more, the patient's lower segments are rotated to lock them. This is accomplished by rotating the patient's pelvis forward toward the clinician while L3-4 is palpated to ensure that the rotation does not go through this segment (Figure 13-5, *E*). If rotation in the segment occurs, coupled side flexion will alter the position and perhaps undo the previously induced side flexion, depending on the direction of coupling at this segment. The rotation should be as pure (i.e., axial) as possible to minimize the coupled side flexion, although this must occur to some degree, if not at this point, then when the treatment technique is applied.

The segments below the target segment are now locked away from a flexion or extension pathological barrier (at least as much as the clinician is able to do), the segments above the target are locked in flexion and right side flexion (however, because the mobilization force going through the segments is subsequent to that going through the target segment, it should be minimal if the appropriate force is applied), and the target segment's left zygapophyseal joint is at its flexion barrier and ready to be mobilized (Figure 13-5, *F*).

The clinician "snuggles" against the patient's abdomen, linking the clinician's cranial arm with the patient's upper arm, and palpates the target segment while pulling the patient toward the clinician. The flexor aspect of the clinician's caudal forearm makes contact with the soft part of the patient's innominate between the trochanter and the crest, approximately over the piriformis muscle belly, and pulls the patient's pelvis forward. The patient now is logrolled into the clinician and is stable (Figure 13-5, *G*). The patient's pelvis then is independently rotated forward, which sequentially rotates each spinal segment to the left (i.e., the lower vertebra is rotating to the right, of course, but the segment is rotating to the left), until slight movement is felt at the target segment. This is then undone by reversing the pelvic rotation, leaving the target segment unrotated.

The clinician's chest is then lowered onto the forearm, which rests on the patient's pelvis, and the clinician applies body weight onto the arm by gently lunging from the left leg. The final direction of the technique is against the worst end feel but is roughly in a sagittal plane. Whether a single thrust, multiple minithrusts, or prolonged grade 3+ or grade 4+ techniques are used depends entirely on the pathological barrier to be mobilized and the clinician's decision whether to manipulate, taking into account cautions and contraindications.

Left Flexion Hypomobility: "Pelvis Upward" Technique

The same hypomobility can be mobilized with the patient lying on the left side. One side may be chosen over the other because of the clinician's preference or the patient's requirements. For example, if a left rotatory instability is present at L5-S1 or L4-5 (or any segment below the target segment), the patient's pelvis cannot be pulled forward if the patient is lying on the left side because this would produce right rotation; because of the right rotatory instability, locking could not be achieved. Similarly, if attempts at locking the lower segments with rotation produce discomfort to the point where the patient will not tolerate the attempt, an alternative position must be used.

With the patient in the left side lying position, the lumbar spine is flexed from below by flexing the patient's hips (Figure 13-6, *A*) and the patient's legs are taken from the parallel orientation by extending the lower leg in the same manner as for the previous technique. However, another method now must be used to produce flexion and right side flexion from above. The patient's upper arm is allowed to hang forward to bias the trunk to flexion in the same manner as before, but now the patient's lower arm is pulled cranially and parallel to the bed to produce right side flexion and flexion (Figure 13-6, *B*).

The clinician brings the patient's lower arm back onto the patient's side. The clinician's cranial arm is linked through and the clinician palpates the segment in the same manner as in Figure 13-5 as the patient's lower thigh is extended until the segments below the target segment are moved out of flexion and then rotated to lock them.

The patient is logrolled into the clinician in the same manner as in the previous technique, but the clinician now pulls the patient's pelvis upward, away from the table, rocking it onto the cranial side of the patient's trochanter and thereby producing side flexion to the right (Figure 13-6, *C*). The clinician holds the pelvis in that position by applying controlled body weight through the forearm. The mobilization or thrust is achieved using graded amounts of body weight to the patient's pelvis. Because the pelvis is already prerocked, the clinician's "drops" (i.e., the controlled body weight through the clinician's forearm to the patient's pelvis) do not have to deliberately produce side flexion but can be more or less straight downward, which is far easier.

Left Extension Hypomobility: "Pelvis Downward" Technique

The patient lies on the left side with the hips extended as the clinician palpates the target segment (L3-4 in this case) to ensure that the extension movement runs through the segment (Figure 13-7, *A*). The patient's hip is then flexed to allow pelvic rotation, and the clinician makes sure that the target segment does not flex to take the legs out of their parallel orientation.

The patient's upper arm then is positioned behind the patient so that the side flexion is induced into extension (Figure 13-7, *B*). The patient's lower arm is pulled caudally but away from the bed to right side flex and extend the spine (Figure 13-7, *C*).

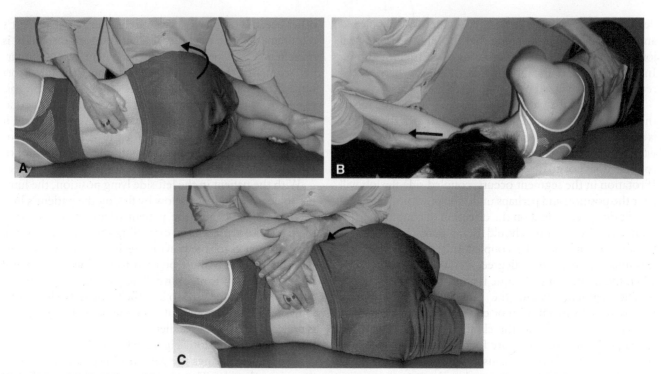

Figure 13-6 Left flexion hypomobility: "pelvis upward" technique. **A,** Flexing the lumbar spine. **B,** Lower arm is pulled cranially. **C,** Rocking the pelvis upward. Note: The fingers of the clinician's right hand are palpating for movement at the spinal segment.

The patient's upper arm is now moved back onto the patient's side, and the patient's lower thigh is pulled forward to flex the segments below L3-4 while the clinician palpates L3-4 to make sure this segment remains in extension (Figure 13-7, *D*). At this point, the lower segments are away from their extension barrier but in side flexion, whereas the target segment is fully extended and left side flexed, meaning that the left zygapophyseal joint is fully extended at least as far as its restriction allows. The L3-4 left zygapophyseal joint is now at its abnormal pathological barrier and ready to be mobilized or manipulated.

The patient is now logrolled toward the clinician, locking the lower segments with axial rotation (Figure 13-7, *E*), and the clinician applies a caudal force to the patient's innominate, with the forearm resting on the innominate, to rock the pelvis downward over the trochanter.

Right Extension Hypomobility: "Pelvis Upward" Technique
As in the previous description, the target segment needs to be extended and right side flexed; however, the patient now is lying on the left side. Again, the clinician's preference or the patient's requirements determine which side lying position is used. For example, if a left rotatory instability is present at L5-S1 or L4-5 (or any segment below the target segment), the patient's pelvis cannot be pulled forward if the patient is lying on the right side because this would produce left rotation; because of the left rotatory instability, locking could not be achieved. Similarly, if attempts at locking the lower segments with left rotation produce discomfort to the point where the patient will not tolerate the attempt, an alternative position must be used.

With the patient in the right side lying position, the patient's lumbar spine is extended from below by extending the patient's hips, and the legs are taken from their parallel orientation by flexing the patient's lower leg in the same manner as for the previous technique (see Figure 13-7, *A* which shows the opposite side). However, now another method must be used to produce extension and right side flexion from above. The patient's upper arm is positioned behind the patient to bias the trunk to extension in the same manner as before, but now the patient's lower arm is pulled cranially and upward toward the ceiling, away from the bed, to produce right side flexion (Figure 13-8, *A*).

The clinician brings the patient's lower arm back to the patient's side. The clinician's cranial arm is linked through the patient's upper arm and the clinician palpates the target segment as the patient's lower thigh is flexed until the segments below the target segment are moved out of extension. These segments are then rotated forward (i.e., right rotation) to lock them (Figure 13-8, *B*). The patient is logrolled into the clinician in the same manner as in the previous technique, but now the clinician pulls the patient's pelvis upward, away from the table, rocking it onto the cranial side of the trochanter, thereby producing side flexion to the right. The clinician holds the patient's pelvis in this position by applying controlled body weight through the forearm (Figure 13-8, *C*). The mobilization or thrust is achieved using graded amounts of the clinician's body weight to the patient's pelvis; because the patient's pelvis is already prerocked, the clinician's "drops" do not have to deliberately produce side flexion but can be more or less straight downward, which is far easier.

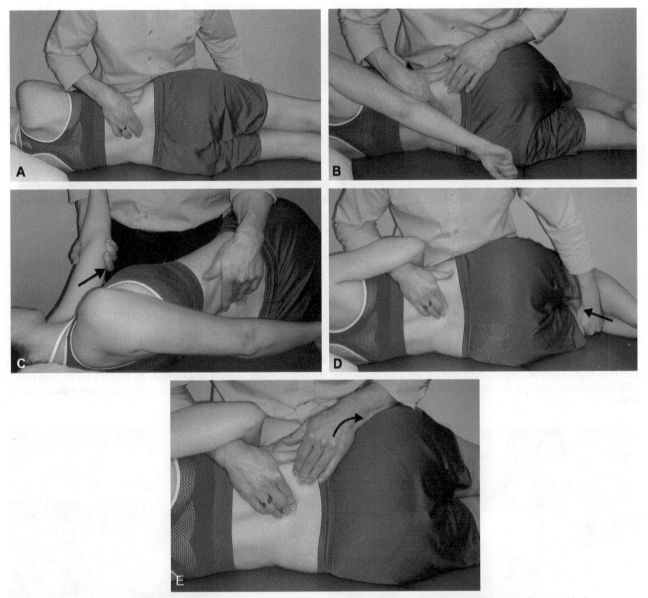

Figure 13-7 Right extension hypomobility: "pelvis downward" technique. **A,** Extension of L3-4. **B,** Patient's arm is drawn behind to encourage extension. **C,** Lower arm is pulled caudally. **D,** Flexing segments below L3-4. **E,** Extension mobilization, pelvis down technique. Note: The fingers of the clinician's right hand are palpating for movement at the appropriate spinal segment.

Superior Vertebrae Hypomobility: "Rotation Lock"

If a problem above the target segment must be treated (e.g., instability or discomfort with side flexion barriering such that either side flexion or the flexion or extension pathological barriers cannot be achieved), the vertebrae may be locked by means of rotation, provided the rotation does not enter the target segment. This technique is also useful when a considerable size discrepancy exists between the clinician and the patient because rotation is easier to achieve. Side flexion requires more clinician upper body strength than does rotation, and it is not as easy to use specifically. However, care must be taken to avoid rotating through the segment (if the clinician wants to avoid issues with the coupling theory). The rotation may be combined with either flexion or extension, and the choice depends on the condition of the segments to be locked. For example, if a painful extension hypermobility exists, it can be avoided by locking the segments with rotation and flexion; because the lock does not enter the target segment, it does not matter whether flexion, extension, or right or left rotation is used.

For the lock with rotation technique, the patient lies on one side. The clinician then barriers the target segment from below through flexion or extension, as required by the dysfunction, in the manner already described. The patient's lower arm is now pulled anteriorly, away from the body, which rotates the patient's trunk around the vertical axis of the body (Figure 13-9, *A*). *If the patient is lying on the left side, right rotation occurs; if the patient is lying on the right side, left rotation occurs.*

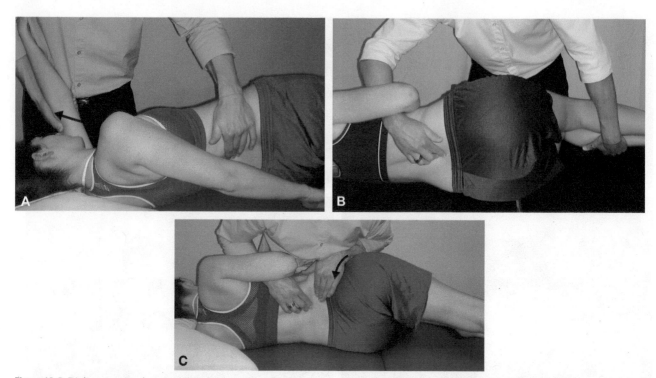

Figure 13-8 Right extension hypomobility: "pelvis upward" technique. **A,** Arm is pulled cranially and upward. **B,** Patient's lower thigh is flexed. **C,** Right side flexion, pelvis up technique. Note: The clinician's fingers on the spine are palpating for movement at the appropriate segment and when it stops.

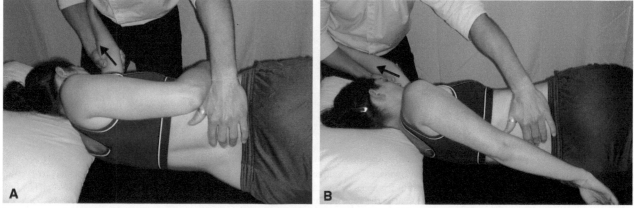

Figure 13-9 Superior vertebrae hypomobility: "rotation lock." **A,** Patient's lower arm is pulled anteriorly, causing right rotation. **B,** Extension rotation. Note: The fingers of the clinician's left hand are palpating for movement at the appropriate segment and when it stops.

To bias the rotation to flexion, the patient's upper arm is allowed to hang forward in front of the body, and the patient's lower arm is pulled parallel to the bed. If extension rotation is required, the patient's upper arm is positioned behind the patient, and the patient's lower arm is pulled away from the body but toward the ceiling (Figure 13-9, *B*).

CAUTIONS (YELLOW FLAGS) AND CONTRAINDICATIONS (RED FLAGS) TO MANUAL THERAPY

The risk of serious adverse effects from manipulative therapy (and presumably mobilization) to the lumbar spine is considered very low.[34,58–64] However, the actual risk is not well understood. In a review of the literature, Assendelft et al.[35] found 61 cases of either cauda equine syndrome or lumbar disc herniation after manipulation, approximately 21% of all serious complications in this review. Another review of the literature for the years 1911 to 1989 found only 10 cases of CES related to manipulative treatment.[36]

Some clinicians may believe that only one contraindication exists to manual treatment of the spine, intolerance to the technique, and that all other considerations are "detail." However, the detail is important. Presumably, manipulation carries a higher threat to the patient in that the force is sudden and not under the patient's control;

therefore any unfortunate effect occurs without warning if the detail has not been recognized before the technique is applied. This is not to say that mobilization does not carry some degree of risk. Indeed, any treatment that is completely without risk is almost certainly without benefit. Any adverse effects from mobilization are likely to be less drastic (i.e., are less likely to cause fracture and bleeding) than manipulative techniques, especially in the lumbar spine, where injuries to the arterial system seem not to occur unless a predisposition exists. Therefore all general contraindications to manipulation and mobilization must be considered as either absolute or relative contraindications.

Absolute contraindications are those that scream "don't touch me," and this demand must be obeyed by all clinicians who care anything about the patient's and their own well-being, at least until adequate objective diagnostic imaging and other medical tests have ruled out any risk. For example, multiple sclerosis produces spinal cord signs and symptoms, but it is not necessarily a contraindication to manual therapy. Examples of absolute contraindications include instability, fractures, acute pain, severe osteoporosis, bleeding disorders, acute CES, spinal cord compromise, severe rheumatoid arthritis, a suggestion of cancer or visceral disease, and a truly disoriented or psychotic patient.

Relative contraindications are those that are contraindications for some clinicians, usually the newcomer to manual therapy, but not for the more experienced manual therapist; however, even these require extreme caution. Relative contraindications include pregnancy, spinal stenosis, spondylolisthesis in a nontarget segment, a patient with a history of cancer who has had a recent clear screening test, equivocating signs of disc herniation, atypical patterns, neurological signs and symptoms, collagenous disease, and a history of poor response to manual techniques.

The main risks are misdiagnosis of cancer (especially prostatic or metastatic) and enlargement of a disc herniation with or without cauda equina compression, but other conditions must be considered. Table 13-5 lists contraindications and the possible problems that may arise if these risks are realized.

clinician becomes more experienced and confident with both examination and treatment techniques. The profile of the patient with mechanical back pain has been described numerous times, even in this chapter. Flynn et al.[54] looked at factors that would determine which patients would have a greater chance of a successful outcome from manipulation, and Fritz et al.[49] investigated factors that would reduce that chance. Between the two studies, a shorter duration of symptoms, minimum referred pain, restricted range of motion in the lumbar spine, and normal hip rotation range of motion indicated a better chance of a successful outcome, particularly when these factors were clustered in the individual patient. In effect, these criteria suggest the standard patient with mechanical low back pain who does not have more complex problems or contraindicating signs or symptoms. It is reasonable to suppose that these factors similarly would point to a successful outcome for mobilization and that they would also indicate patients with a greater likelihood of responding well to manual treatment in general.

High-Risk Indicators in Spinal Mobilization

General indicators of high risk in the mobilization of the lumbar spine, especially manipulation, include suggestions of disc herniation and cauda equina syndrome:

- Radicular pain, especially bilateral
- Paresthesia, especially bilateral
- Severe somatic sciatica, especially bilateral
- Motor paresis, especially multisegmental and bilateral
- Sensory paresis, especially multisegmental and bilateral
- Saddle paresthesia
- Saddle anesthesia
- Segmental or multisegmental hyporeflexia or areflexia
- High frequency, low-volume bladder
- Bladder incontinence
- Lack of rectal expulsive power
- L1 or L2 palsy
- Exacerbations related to diet
- Hematuria
- Severe leg pain without straight leg raising (SLR) limitation
- Severe limitation of range of motion
- Deviation with radicular pain

Clinical Note

Clinicians must understand that mere lists are not the same as being faced with problematic conditions, and the clinician must be more adept at recognizing presentations that preclude manual therapy than at performing manual therapy.

Signs of an Enlarging Disc Herniation

- Peripheralization of symptoms
- Bilateral symptoms
- Appearance of radicular pain
- Appearance of neurological signs
- Numbness that replaces paresthesia
- Increase in the severity of the articular signs
- Appearance of urinary retention or incontinence signs
- Decrease in the straight leg raise or prone knee bending

For the newcomer to manual therapy, the wise course is to develop a clear understanding of the indications for manipulation and to avoid treating any patient who does not fall within these strict parameters, at least until the

TABLE 13-5

Contraindications and Cautions to Lumbar Manipulation and Mobilization

Cautions and Contraindications	Characteristics and Potential Problems
Neoplastic disease	Medical diagnosis: possibility of fracture
Cauda equina signs and symptoms	Bilateral, multisegmental lower motor neuron signs and symptoms, including bladder dysfunction: possibility of serious compression damage and permanent palsy
Spinal cord signs and symptoms	Multisegmental upper motor neuron signs and symptoms: possibility of serious compression damage and permanent deficit
Nonmechanical causes	Minimal musculoskeletal signs and symptoms: wasted effort and delay in getting appropriate care
Trilevel segmental signs	Disc compression (can affect a maximum of two levels of the nerve root): possibility of neoplastic disease, spondylolisthesis, or cauda equina compression
Neuropathic pain	Nerve root damage or severe inflammation
Sign of the buttock	Empty end feel on hip flexion; painful weakness of hip extension; limited straight leg raising, trunk flexion, and hip flexion; noncapsular pattern of hip restriction; swollen buttock: Possible serious disease (e.g., sacral fracture, neoplasm, infection)
Various serious pathologies	Empty end feel and severe multidirectional spasm
Adverse joint environment	Spasm: acute inflammation, fracture
Acute fracture or dislocation	Immediate onset of posttraumatic pain and loss of function
Bone disease	Deep pain and relatively minimal musculoskeletal signs: wasted effort and possibility of a fracture
Acute rheumatoid arthritis episode	Medical diagnosis: possibility of increased tissue damage and severe exacerbation
Infective arthritis	Severe inflammation and reddening: delay in getting appropriate medical care
Emotionally dependent patient	Seeks manipulation: long-term dependency without much hope of benefit
Chronic pain or fibromyalgia-type syndromes	Inadequate signs to explain the patient's widespread symptoms: long-term dependency without much hope of benefit
Rheumatoid arthritis	Medical diagnosis: possibility of increased tissue damage and severe exacerbation
Osteoporosis	Medical diagnosis: fracture
Spinal nerve (root) compression	Segmental neurological signs: probable wasted effort and possibility of increasing the compression
Spondylolisthesis	Radiographic evidence: exacerbation of signs and symptoms
Hypermobility	Clinical finding: increased hypermobility and pain
Acute pain states	Onset of pain before or simultaneous with tissue resistance: possibility of severe exacerbation
Pregnancy	Risk of ligamentous damage as a result of relaxing effect and risk of coincident miscarriage
Repeated steroid injections	Tearing of collagen tissue
Long-term systemic steroid use	Tearing of collagen tissue and fracture
History of neoplastic disease	Risk of recurrence
Distal pain on movement	Acute root compression or severe joint inflammation
Nuclear prolapse or meniscoid entrapment	Springy end feel
Central or lateral stenosis	Paresthesia that dominates pain

SUMMARY

Manual therapy for mechanical low back pain, particularly lumbar hypomobility, is reasonably well established, both from a research perspective and as a standard of care for clinical treatment. The risk is low and the benefits, at least over the short term, are great, as long as appropriate inclusion and exclusion criteria are met. This means that before applying any technique, clinicians must have exercised competent diagnostic skills to rule out medical conditions that would contraindicate a particular type of manual treatment.

REFERENCES

1. Panjabi M: Low back pain and spinal instability. In Weinstein JN, Gordon SL, editors: *Low back pain: a scientific and clinical overview*, Rosemont, 1996, American Academy of Orthopedic Surgeons.
2. Panjabi MM: The stabilizing system of the spine. I. Function, dysfunction, adaptation, and enhancement, *J Spinal Disord* 5:383–389, 1992.
3. Panjabi MM: The stabilizing system of the spine. II Neutral zone and instability hypothesis, *J Spinal Disord* 5:390–396, 1992.
4. Colloca CJ, Keller TS, Gunzburg R: Biomechanical and neurophysiological responses to spinal manipulation in patients with lumbar radiculopathy, *J Manip Physiol Ther* 27:1–15, 2004.
5. Hegedus EJ, Goode A, Butler RJ, et al: The neurophysiological effects of a single session of spinal joint mobilization: does the effect last, *J Manip Physiol Ther* 19(3):143–151, 2011.
6. Bialosky JE, Bishop MD, Price DD, et al: The mechanisms of manual therapy in the treatment of musculoskeletal pain: a comprehensive model, *Man Ther* 14(5):531–538, 2009.
7. Hertel J: Functional anatomy, pathomechanics and pathophysiology of lateral ankle instability, *J Athletic Train* 37(4):364–375, 2002.
8. Colloca CJ, Keller TS, Gunzburg R: Neuromechanical characterization of in vivo lumbar spinal manipulation. II Neurophysiological response, *J Manip Physiol Ther* 26:579–591, 2003.
9. Evans JM, Hill CR, Leach RA, Collins DL: The minimum energy hypothesis: a unified model of fixation resolution, *J Manip Physiol Ther* 25:105–109, 2002.
10. Ianuzzi A, Khalsa PS: Comparison of human lumbar facet joint capsule strains during simulated high-velocity, low-amplitude spinal manipulation versus physiological motions, *Spine* 5:277–290, 2005.
11. Pickar JG: Neurophysiological effects of spinal manipulation, *Spine* 2:357–371, 2002.
12. Pickar JG, McLain RF: Responses of mechanosensitive afferents to manipulation of the lumbar facet in the cat, *Spine* 20:2379–2385, 1995.
13. Pickar JG, Wheeler JD: Response of muscle proprioceptors to spinal manipulative-like loads in the anesthetized cat, *J Manip Physiol Ther* 24:2–11, 2001.
14. Vautravers P, Lecocq J: Common low back pain and vertebral manipulations: inventory, evaluation, presumptive mechanisms of action, problems, *Rev Rhum Ed Fr* 60:518–523, 1993.
15. Wright A: Hypoalgesia post-manipulative therapy: a review of a potential neurophysiological mechanism, *Man Ther* 5:11–16, 2000.
16. Maitland GD: *Vertebral manipulation*, London, 1986, Butterworth.
17. Soderberg GL: Muscle mechanics and pathomechanics: their clinical relevance, *Phys Ther* 63:216–220, 1983.
18. Bakewell S: Medical gymnastics and the Cyriax collection, *Med Hist* 41:487–495, 1997.
19. Cyriax J: *Textbook of orthopedic medicine, vol 1, Diagnosis of soft tissue lesions*, London, 1982, Ballière Tindall.
20. Cyriax J: Clinical rheumatology and orthopaedic medicine, *Br Med J* 1:1353, 1977.
21. Cyriax JH: Lesions of the lumbar disk: conservative treatment, *Acta Chir Orthop Traumatol Cech* 35:388–392, 1968.
22. Sheng B, Yi-Kai L, Wei-dong Z: Effect of simulating lumbar manipulations on lumbar nucleus pulposus pressures, *J Manip Physiol Ther* 25:333, 2002.
23. Ben Eliyahu DJ: Magnetic resonance imaging and clinical follow-up: study of 27 patients receiving chiropractic care for cervical and lumbar disc herniations, *J Manip Physiol Ther* 19:597–606, 1996.

24. Ye RB, Zhou JX, Gan MX: Clinical and CT analysis of 35 cases of lumbar disc herniation before and after non-operative treatment, *Zhong Xi Yi Jie He Za Zhi (Chinese Journal of Modern Developments in Traditional Medicine)* 10:667–668, 1990 645.
25. Ottenbacher K, Difabio RP: Efficacy of spinal manipulation/mobilization therapy: a meta analysis, *Spine* 10:833–837, 1985.
26. Bronfort G, Haas M, Evans RL, Bonter LM: Efficacy of spinal manipulation and mobilization for low back pain and neck pain: a systematic review and best evidence synthesis, *Spine J* 4:335–356, 2004.
27. Arnold JJ, Ehleringer SR: Is spinal manipulation an effective treatment for low back pain? Yes: evidence shows benefit in most patients, *Am Fam Physician* 85:756–758, 2012.
28. Bergmann TF, Jongeward BV: Manipulative therapy in lower back pain with leg pain and neurological deficit, *J Manip Physiol Ther* 21:288–294, 1998.
29. Crockard HA, Sen CN: The transoral approach for the management of intradural lesions at the craniovertebral junction: review of 7 cases, *Neurosurgery* 28:88–98, 1991.
30. Erhard RE, Welch WC, Liu B, et al: Far-lateral disk herniation: case report, review of the literature, and a description of nonsurgical management, *J Manip Physiol Ther* 27:123–128, 2004.
31. Browning JE: Chiropractic distractive decompression in the treatment of pelvic pain and organic dysfunction in patients with evidence of lower sacral nerve root compression, *J Manip Physiol Ther* 11:426–432, 1988.
32. Cassidy JD, Thiel HW, Kirkaldy-Willis WH: Side posture manipulation for lumbar intervertebral disk herniation, *J Manip Physiol Ther* 16:96–103, 1993.
33. Lisi AJ, Bhardwaj MK: Chiropractic high-velocity low-amplitude spinal manipulation in the treatment of a case of postsurgical chronic cauda equina syndrome, *J Manip Physiol Ther* 27:574–578, 2004.
34. Oliphant D: Safety of spinal manipulation in the treatment of lumbar disk herniations: a systematic review and risk assessment, *J Manip Physiol Ther* 27:197–210, 2004.
35. Assendelft WJ, Bouter LM, Knipschild PG: Complications of spinal manipulation: a comprehensive review of the literature, *J Fam Pract* 42:475–480, 1996.
36. Haldeman S, Rubinstein SM: Cauda equina syndrome in patients undergoing manipulation of the lumbar spine, *Spine* 17:1469–1473, 1992.
37. Balblanc JC, Pretot C, Ziegler F: Vascular complication involving the conus medullaris or cauda equina after vertebral manipulation for an L4-L5 disk herniation, *Rev Rhum Engl Ed* 65:279–282, 1998.
38. Li JS: Acute rupture of lumbar intervertebral disc caused by violent manipulation, *Zhonghua Wai Ke Za Zhi (Chinese Journal of Surgery)* 27:477–478, 1989.
39. Powell FC, Hanigan WC, Olivero WC, et al: A risk/benefit analysis of spinal manipulation therapy for relief of lumbar or cervical pain, *Neurosurgery* 33:73–79, 1993.
40. Stevinson C, Ernst E: Risks associated with spinal manipulation, *Am J Med* 112:566–571, 2002.
41. Saunders HD: Use of spinal traction in the treatment of neck and back conditions, *Clin Orthop Relat Res* 179:31–38, 1983.
42. Gose EE, Naguszewski WK, Naguszewski RK: Vertebral axial decompression therapy for pain associated with herniated or degenerated discs or facet syndrome: an outcome study, *Neurol Res* 203:186–190, 1998.
43. Ramos G, Martin W: Effects of vertebral axial decompression on intradiscal pressure, *J Neurosurg* 81:350–353, 1994.

44. Sherry E, Kitchener P, Smart R: A prospective randomized controlled study of VAX-D and TENS for the treatment of chronic low back pain, *Neurol Res* 23:780–784, 2001.
45. Medical Services Advisory Committee (MSAC): *Vertebral axial decompression (VAX-D) therapy for low back pain.* Available at http://www.health.gov.au/msac/pdf/msac1012.pdf. (Accessed 02.04.04.)
46. Washington State Department of Labor and Industries, Office of the Medical Director: *Vertebral axial decompression (Vax-D): technology assessment.* Available at http://www.lni.wa.gov/omd/TechAssessDocs. (Accessed 07.08.03.)
47. Deen HG, Rizzo TD, Fenton DS: Sudden progression of lumbar disc protrusion during vertebral axial decompression traction therapy, *Mayo Clin Proc* 78:1554–1556, 2003.
48. Wang G: *Powered traction devices for intervertebral decompression: health technology assessment update.* Available at www.lni.wa.gov/ClaimsIns/Files/OMD/TractionTechAssessJun142004.pdf. (Accessed 28.02.05.)
49. Fritz JM, Whitman JM, Flynn TW, et al: Factors related to the inability of an individual with a spinal manipulation, *Phys Ther* 84:173–190, 2004.
50. Cookson JC: Orthopedic manual therapy: an overview. II. The spine, *Phys Ther* 59:259–267, 1979.
51. Grieve GP: Lumbar instability, *Physiotherapy* 68:2–9, 1982.
52. Meadows J: *Orthopedic differential diagnosis in physical therapy: a case study approach*, New York, 1999, McGraw-Hill.
53. Schneider G: *Lumbar Instability*, ed 2, Edinburgh, 1994, Churchill Livingstone.
54. Flynn T, Fritz J, Whitman J, et al: A clinical prediction rule for classifying patients with low back pain who demonstrate short-term improvement with spinal manipulations, *Spine* 27:2835–2843, 2002.
55. Pearcy MJ, Tibrewal SB: Axial rotation and lateral bending in the normal lumbar spine measured by three-dimensional radiography, *Spine* 9:582–587, 1984.
56. Pearcy MJ, Whittle MW: Movements of the lumbar spine measured by three-dimensional x-ray analysis, *J Biomed Eng* 4:107–112, 1982.
57. Oxland TR, Crisco JJ, Panjabi MM, et al: The effect of injury on rotational coupling at the lumbosacral joint: a biomechanical investigation, *Spine* 17:74–80, 1992.
58. Jette DU, Jette AM: Physical therapy and health outcomes in patients with spinal impairments, *Phys Ther* 76:930–941, 1996.
59. Hancock MJ, Maher CG, Latimer J: Spinal manipulative therapy for acute low back pain: a clinical perspective, *J Man Manip Ther* 16:198–203, 2008.
60. Henschke N, Maher C, Ostelo R, et al: Red flags to screen for malignancy in patients with low-back pain, *Cochrane Database Syst Rev* 2:Feb 2013 CD008686.
61. Downie A, Williams C, Henschke N, et al: Red flags to screen for malignancy and fracture in patients with low back pain: systematic review, *BMJ* 347:f7095, 2013.
62. Greenhalgh S, Selfe J: A qualitative investigation of red flags for serious spinal pathology, *Physiother* 95:223–226, 2009.
63. Leerar PJ, Boissonnault W, Domholdt E, et al: Documentation of red flags by physical therapists for patients with low back pain, *J Man Manip Ther* 15:42–49, 2007.
64. Ferguson F, Holdsworth L, Rafferty D: Low back pain and physiotherapy use of red flags: the evidence from Scotland, *Physiother* 96:282–288, 2010.

CHAPTER 14

Lumbar Spine: Treatment of Motor Control Disorders

PAUL W. HODGES, PAULO H. FERREIRA, MANUELA L. FERREIRA

INTRODUCTION

Interventions that aim to modify the manner in which patients with low back pain (LBP) control their spine and pelvis have become popular over the past few decades. These interventions are based on the premise that a patient's pain is related to loading of spine and pelvis tissues and the potential role of suboptimal posture and postural alignment, muscle activation and movement in this loading. These motor control features may either be a precursor to the onset of pain or injury (e.g., repetitive suboptimal loading of tissues) or a consequence of pain or injury (e.g., adaptation of motor control to protect an injured structure or poor control linked to some "inhibitory" process). There is substantial evidence for the efficacy of these approaches,[1] but the application of each approach has important considerations. Although some approaches have advocated relatively straightforward application of exercise, the prevailing view is that exercise must be tailored to the individual patient.[2]

Although, historically, there had been an assumption that pain is related to "instability,"[3] it is increasingly clear that patients can present across a spectrum from too little to too much control, and the focus on "instability" is too narrow and poorly defined. Instead, the focus has shifted to dynamic control of the spine and pelvis.[4] With this in mind, it is clear that exercise interventions aimed at rehabilitation and prevention of low back and pelvic pain should not simply maximize stiffness but instead must optimize the balance between movement and stiffness as appropriate for specific functions. Many exercise interventions have been proposed to improve control of the spine and pelvis, and much has been written about the goals of training and how this can be achieved.[5] The approach outlined in this chapter assumes that features of the manner in which an individual controls his or her spine and pelvis may suboptimally load the tissues, and through careful consideration of muscle activation, posture and postural alignment, movement, sensation (both

proprioception and kinesthesia as well as other sensory inputs) and the multiple functions of the trunk muscles, within a biopsychosocial view of a patient, this approach aims to restore optimal loading. This may involve targets as diverse as increased or decreased muscle activation, modification of spinal alignment, optimized load sharing between adjacent body segments, coordination of postural and respiratory functions of the trunk, and exposure to threat. This diverse approach requires careful assessment and precise application of training strategies. The purpose of this chapter is to consider the requirements for optimal motor control of the spine and pelvis, review the changes in this system in the presence of low back and pelvic pain, provide an overview of clinical assessment of the patient with pain, introduce strategies to train or restore optimal motor control of the spine and pelvis, and review the evidence for the efficacy of interventions that aim to improve the motor control of the spine and pelvis.

DYNAMIC CONTROL OF THE LUMBAR SPINE AND PELVIS

Requirements for Dynamic Motor Control of the Lumbar Spine and Pelvis

For function the spine and pelvis must be controlled dynamically. The requirements for dynamic control can be described in terms of a range of interdependent goals that ultimately must be integrated to meet the objectives of stiffness and movement. The term *stability* is generally defined as the property of a structure that allows it to return to equilibrium if perturbed.[5] This applies to both a position and a trajectory of movement: to maintain or return to a specific alignment or to a path of movement. Thus, by definition, stability is achieved by a balance between movement and stiffness, depending on the task (e.g., high stiffness may be required when lifting a weight from the floor; whereas motion is required during walking to transfer and dampen forces, and minimize energy expenditure). This contrasts the simple assumption that is commonly applied in clinical interventions that implies the spine must be stiffened. Rather than describing poor spine control in terms of "more" or "less" stability (i.e., "instability"), it has been argued that control of the spine is best described in terms of "robustness."[6] A robust system is one in which control of position or movement can be maintained despite various challenges, whereas a system with low robustness fails even in the presence of minor challenges. This robust system is maintained by a combination of movement and stiffness, depending on the task. For instance, if the stiffness of the spine is high in quiet standing, balance is compromised even with minor disturbances,[7] yet if the spine moves and is controlled dynamically, the robustness of maintenance of spine control is enhanced and the body can respond effectively to more challenging disturbances.

Clinical Note

A robust spine is one in which control of a static position or a dynamic movement is maintained despite different challenges being applied to the spine.

Whether the objective is to move or stiffen the spine, the moving or stiffening depends on the contribution of muscles. In vitro experiments have shown that the lumbar spine without muscle buckles when loaded with as little as 9 kg (~90 N).[8] Buckling of the spine (i.e., lack of stability of individual segments) can involve any combination of the six degrees of freedom that must be controlled at each intervertebral segment (i.e., three rotations and three translations) and at the sacroiliac joints (Figure 14-1). It is the static control of rotation buckling that is the primary consideration in most contemporary models of spine stability.[5,8,9]

Stiffening the muscles and their tendons can stabilize the spine. In this sense, it may be assumed that the stiffer the spine, the better. If the spine is stiffened by muscle contraction, then greater force is required to perturb it. Stiffness control by co-contraction of the trunk muscles is one of the mechanisms used by the nervous system to meet the demands for stability and to control buckling of the spine. However, stiffening the spine is not the only option available, and many functions do not involve simple co-contraction but instead use carefully orchestrated patterns of muscle activity using movement to absorb and dissipate forces, transfer loads, minimize energy expenditure, and enable coordination of spine control demands with the other functions of the trunk muscles (e.g., breathing). Although co-contraction and stiffening are used in some functional situations, they are not the only solution, because many functions involve dynamic control of the movement.

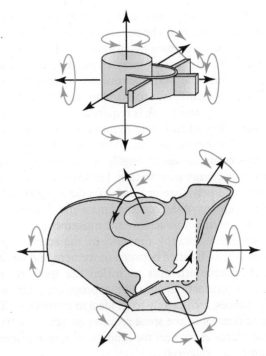

Figure 14-1 Six degrees of freedom, including rotation about and translation along each of the three orthogonal axes, must be controlled to maintain healthy spinal and pelvic function.

An illustration of the role of movement in the control of robust stability of the spine comes from the postural adjustment associated with arm movement. Studies of arm movement show that when a limb is moved, the nervous system does not simply stiffen the trunk to support the movement, but instead, the spine and pelvis are moved in the direction opposite to the perturbation in advance of the perturbation.[10,11] This is achieved by alternating activity of the trunk flexor and extensor muscles rather than co-contraction. Such movement will act to dampen the force impact on the spine, and limit the effect of the perturbation. People who stiffen their spines have an ability to allow greater perturbation to the spine[12] and to maintain balance.[13] Thus, although coordinated movement of the spine requires more complex control strategies than simple stiffening (and hence a more complicated controller), it is likely to be more ideal in the long term.

A final consideration is that, if one looks beyond the demand to control buckling of the spine and motion, it is obvious that the stability of other functions needs to be considered. For instance, the spine contributes to respiration. This is not only as a result of the direct contribution of spinal movement to expansion of the thorax during inspiration[14] but also because small-amplitude motions of the spine are required to compensate for the disturbance to balance caused by breathing.[15,16] If spine stability was maintained simply by stiffening, respiratory efficiency would be compromised because of the reduced contribution of spinal movement. Similarly, balance control requires a contribution from movement of the hips and trunk. Two basic balance strategies have been described:

the **"ankle" strategy** and the **"hip" strategy**.[17] Although postural equilibrium can be maintained in quiet stance and with minor perturbations by movements about the ankle with the body acting as an inverted pendulum (i.e., ankle strategy), when the perturbations are increased, torque at the ankle is insufficient to maintain balance and movement of the hip and trunk is required (i.e., hip strategy). Thus the ability of the spine to move in a manner that is essential to maintain balance. If movement is restricted, balance is compromised.[18] Finally, movement is required to minimize energy expenditure. For instance, rotation of the spine and pelvis around each axis during gait reduces the displacement of the center of mass and the associated energy requirement to achieve the movement.[19]

In summary, healthy function of the spine requires maintenance of balance between movement and stiffness. As such, simple attempts to stiffen the spine through muscle co-contraction, although appropriate under some circumstances, are unlikely to be ideal in many tasks. Thus dynamic control of the spine requires complex control of flexible strategies to meet the multiple demands placed on it to function effectively.

Guiding Principles for a Healthy Functioning Spine

- Static models are unlikely to be able to predict the ideal strategies for motor control.
- Optimal stability is not simply achieved by maximal stiffness.
- Spine requires movement for ideal function.

Guiding Principles: Requirements for Spinal Control

STATIC MAINTENANCE OF POSITION
- Control of postural alignment
- Control of segment translation/rotation

DYNAMIC CONTROL OF MOVEMENT
- Movement for function
- Movement for shock absorption and braking action
- Movement for force/load transfer
- Movement to minimize energy expenditure
- Movement for other functions, such as:
  - Respiration
  - Balance control

Neural Mechanisms for Dynamic Control of the Lumbar Spine and Pelvis

To meet the demands placed on the spine, Panjabi[1] recognized that lumbopelvic stability depends not only on the contribution of the passive elements (including the intervertebral discs, ligaments, joint capsules and facet joints) but also on the active elements (i.e., muscles) and

the controller (i.e., the nervous system). When the spine is considered in a static sense, only one muscle activation strategy is required to meet the demands of stability: co-contraction of the large superficial trunk muscles to increase spinal stiffness. Observations from a number of tasks such as lifting are consistent with this proposal.[20] Although control of buckling is critical for the maintenance of healthy spinal function, as mentioned in the previous section, this control fails to consider how *movement* of the spine is controlled or how *stability* of the movement trajectory is maintained. Furthermore, the contribution of trunk muscles to other homeostatic functions such as balance and breathing and continence further complicates the task for the nervous system in controlling the spine and pelvis. Strategies other than simple co-contraction are available and are necessary to control the spine and pelvis in a dynamic sense. It is unlikely one will be able to predict the ideal strategies for lumbopelvic control or the ideal exercise interventions for back pain from basic static models of stability.

The task for the nervous system to control the spine and pelvis is immense. It must detect the current status of the stability of the spine utilizing input from the range of mechanoreceptors in the muscles and passive structures of the spine/pelvis, in addition to input from the visual and vestibular systems regarding the status of the body with respect to the world. It must consider the demands of the intended action by consideration of the dynamics of the body using an internal model of body dynamics built up over a lifetime of movement experiences, and select an appropriate strategy of muscle activity to meet the demands of movement and stability to accomplish the desired task. It must initiate a muscle activation strategy, then determine the outcome, and make any appropriate adjustments to ensure success. The complexity of this control and the level of the nervous system involvement are primarily determined by temporal demands. When the nervous system responds to an unexpected disturbance such as a trip or a slip, the time delay must be short, the complexity is limited, and the strategy involves a combination of reflex and triggered (i.e., multisegmental responses that are faster than voluntary movement but more flexible than reflexes) components. This type of control is mediated by feedback (i.e., *feedback adjustment*). When the task is predictable (e.g., voluntarily initiated tasks such as lifting a mass or catching a ball), there can be sufficient time to plan and optimize the control. In this situation the postural adjustment precedes the movement and is referred to as a *feedforward or preparatory adjustment*.[11] Although the simplest strategy to meet the demands for control might appear to be stiffening the trunk by co-contraction, in view of the necessity to maintain mobility, more complex strategies are involved. A third type of control involves the *maintenance of low level tonic activation* of muscle.[21] The basis of this strategy is that, because reflexes involve a delay and not all challenges can be predicted, low-level tonic ongoing activity provides a first line of defense to control the segment in cases in which the spine is unexpectedly challenged. Feedforward and feedback strategies can add to this control as able or required. Trunk muscles are known to act in this manner. For example, gentle activity of a few percent of maximum voluntary contraction is maintained in quiet upright postures.[5]

Guiding Principles: Strategies Available for Optimal Spine Control

- *Reactive control*: feedback-mediated strategies in response to sensory input from unexpected challenges
- *Anticipatory control*: feedforward strategies initiated in advance of a predictable challenge
- *Ongoing tonic muscle activation*: first line of defense to provide control before reflexes can be initiated

---

A critical element in this system is accurate sensory information from the spine and pelvis. Afferent input from the mechanoreceptors in the intervertebral disc, joint capsules, ligaments, and muscles all contribute to the awareness of spinal position and movement. Muscle proprioceptors are particularly dense in the deep muscles,[22] providing the potential to detect small intervertebral motion. Furthermore, electrical stimulation of the mechanoreceptors in the intervertebral disc[23] and joint capsule of the sacroiliac joint[24] lead to short latency responses of the paraspinal and pelvic muscles. This provides evidence of basic spinal mechanisms to maintain spinal control. Of note, deficits in sensory function are commonly reported in LBP,[25,26] which may underlie changes in the accuracy of movement control.

One way to view movement control strategies is to consider a spectrum from static/stiffening control at one end and dynamic strategies involving movement at the other (Figure 14-2). Tasks that involve high load, poor predictability, and the necessity to maintain the alignment of the spine are likely to involve co-contraction strategies, as this is likely to provide the greatest amount of stiffness. In contrast, tasks that involve low load and greater predictability or tasks that require greater movement are likely to involve a more complex dynamic strategy. This simple conceptual model considers just a few of the large number of factors considered by the nervous system when selecting an appropriate response but can help us understand the decisions that are made and the muscle activation patterns that are initiated to meet the movement demands. The nervous system has a large number of muscles available to contribute to these control strategies. Although all muscles are likely to contribute to some extent, anatomical features are likely to influence the decision to recruit specific muscles for a particular function.

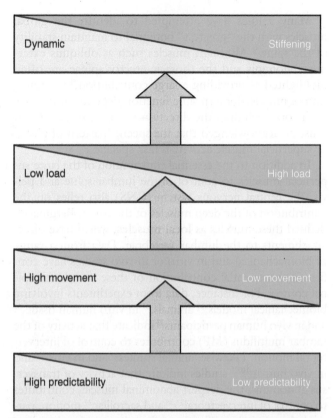

Figure 14-2 A spectrum of control strategies, ranging from dynamic control to static stiffening, is available to the nervous system, depending on task demands. The strategy used is influenced by a range of factors, including the load, movement requirement, and predictability.

Muscular Mechanisms for Control of the Spine and Pelvis

Large superficial muscles of the lumbar spine and pelvis are required for optimal control of the spine. Bergmark[27] defined the superficial muscles that cross from the pelvis to the rib cage as **global muscles**. Contraction of these muscles generates torque to oppose external forces and move the spine, pelvis, and whole body. Co-contraction of these muscles on either side of the trunk provide an ideal strategy to increase trunk stiffness and is common during tasks such as lifting.[20] However, during many functional activities, rather than simple co-contraction to increase trunk stiffness, activity of these muscles is carefully timed to perfectly match the movement and stability demands. For instance, the superficial trunk muscles such as obliquus externus abdominis and the lumbar erector spinae are active in alternating bursts in association with arm movements to oppose the reactive forces using a dynamic strategy of trunk movement rather than simple trunk stiffening.[10,12,28] Furthermore, during gait, global muscles co-contract at heel strike (the time of maximal impact to the spine) but have specific phasic bursts associated with forward propulsion of the body, displacement of the center of mass, and changes in direction of pelvic motion.[29]

Many studies have attempted to identify the global muscles with the "greatest" potential to maintain stability of the spine.[9] Although muscles such as obliquus externus abdominis and the thoracic erector spinae are often highlighted as providing a large contribution,[9] the selection of muscles for a specific function depends on a range of factors, including the direction of force. In general, it must be acknowledged that the specific pattern of global or superficial muscle activity is task specific.

In addition to the essential contribution of the large superficial muscles to control of the lumbar spine and pelvis, the central nervous system (CNS) also relies on the contribution of the deep muscles of the trunk. Bergmark[27] defined these muscles as **local muscles**, which have direct attachments to the lumbar vertebrae. Data from a range of biomechanical and in vitro or in vivo studies have confirmed the essential contribution of these muscles to spinal control. For instance, data from experiments involving biomechanical models,[30] animals,[31] in vitro human tissue,[32] and in vivo human participants[33] indicate that activity of the lumbar multifidus (MF) contributes to control of intervertebral motion. Likewise, animal studies[34] and in vitro[35] and in vivo human[10,11] studies indicate that activity of transversus abdominis, the deepest abdominal muscle, contributes to control of intervertebral[11,36] and sacroiliac[37] motion, particularly translation. These muscles, along with other deep muscles with segmental attachments (e.g., psoas major[38]), are often activated either early or tonically in a range of tasks and often in a manner that is not specific to the direction of forces acting on the spine.

If these muscles are inaccurately considered as flexors and extensors of the trunk (transversus abdominis has a minimal ability to act as a flexor as its fiber angle is only up to 12° from horizontal, and the short deep fibers of MF are close to the center of rotation of the lumbar joints with a trivial moment arm for extension), these muscles would be erroneously concluded to contribute little to spinal control. However, via contributions to intra-abdominal pressure, tensioning of the thoracolumbar fascia and the direct effects of contraction on the intervertebral segments, these muscles provide an additional contribution to intervertebral control.[34,35] In fact, as a result of the limited contribution to generation of torque at the trunk, these muscles provide a major advantage to the nervous system—the ability to influence intervertebral control during movement, without restricting range of motion[31] and without requiring control of other torques generated by muscle contraction. A major control issue for the more superficial global muscles is that these muscles also generate torque. This means that whenever they are recruited to provide control to the spine and pelvis, additional muscles must contract to control the complex torques generated by contraction of the superficial global muscles. Thus the deep muscles provide a possible solution to simplify control of the spine and, potentially, an ideal solution for maintenance of dynamic control by allowing control during movement, in conjunction with the activation of the global muscles to generate and control the torques. It is critical to note that most functional tasks require coordinated activity of both the deep and superficial muscles to meet the demands for control and movement. The balance between the deep and superficial muscles is likely to be guided by the principles outlined in Figure 14-2. In Figure 14-2 tasks that lie to the right involve greater co-contraction of the superficial muscles, with underlying activation of deep muscles. Tasks to the left are likely to have a greater contribution from deep muscles and the fine-tuned activation of the superficial muscles in a dynamic manner matched to the direction of force.

As intra-abdominal pressure and fascial tension are important for the control of intervertebral motion, other muscles that surround the abdominal cavity provide an additional contribution. This includes the diaphragm and pelvic floor muscles. Data from in vitro[39] and in vivo studies[40] confirm that activity of these muscles contributes to the control of the lumbar spine (Figure 14-3) and sacroiliac joints (Figure 14-4). Because of the dual role of these muscles in controlling stiffness and movement of the spine, as well as respiration and continence, additional complexity is introduced to the nervous system.

Guiding Principles: Selection of Muscle Activation Strategy

- Superficial global muscles co-contract to stiffen the trunk during tasks with high load, poor predictability
- Phasic bursts of superficial global muscles activity are matched to the demands of task to overcome external and internal forces
- Deep local muscles are generally active early and tonically, in a manner that is less dependent on the direction of force

---

The Challenge to Coordinate the Multiple Functions of the Trunk Muscles

In addition to the control of movement and stiffness of the spine and pelvis, trunk muscles also have important respiratory and continence functions. Breathing involves movement of the spine and pelvis. The diaphragm is the principal muscle of inspiration, depressing the central tendon and elevating the lower ribs to increase the vertical and lateral dimensions of the thorax. Other muscles, such as the erector spinae and latissimus dorsi, extend the spine to assist inspiration and oppose deflationary forces transmitted to the vertebral column by the rib cage articulations.[41] During strong expiratory efforts, activity of the paraspinal muscles is also likely to be required to counteract the flexion moment from activity of the expiratory abdominal muscles.

The abdominal muscles deflate the rib cage and elevate the diaphragm to assist expiration (Figure 14-5).[42] Although the abdominal muscles are active during quiet

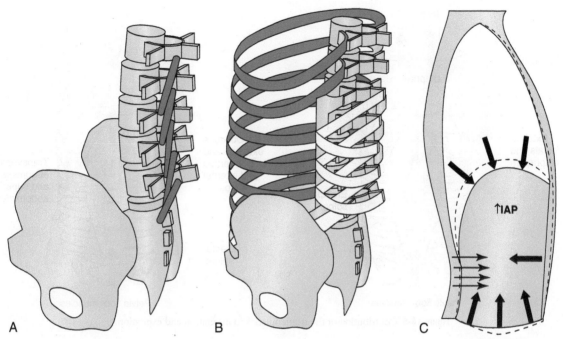

Figure 14-3 Deep muscles of the trunk contribute to control of the lumbar spine. **A,** Multifidus contributes to control of intervertebral motion by means of gentle compression between segments and control of posteroanterior translation. **B,** Transversus abdominis contributes to control of intervertebral motion by means of increased intra-abdominal pressure (IAP) and tension in the thoracolumbar fascia. **C,** These effects depend on co-contraction of the diaphragm and pelvic floor muscles.

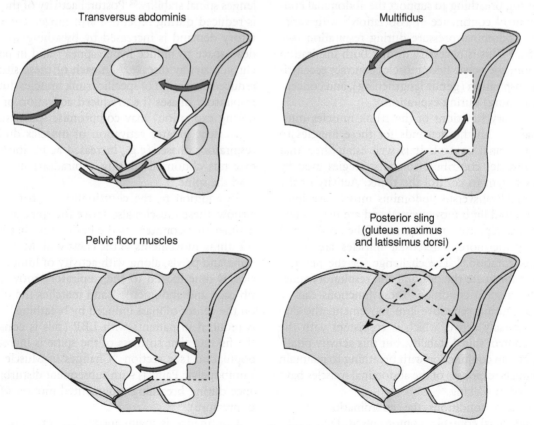

Figure 14-4 Deep muscles of the trunk contribute to the control of sacroiliac (SI) joint stability. Contraction of the transversus abdominis and the pelvic floor muscles provides compression to the SI joint. Although contraction of the pelvic floor muscles counternutates the sacrum (i.e., rotates the sacrum posteriorly relative to the ilia), which places the joint in a less stable position, this can be counteracted by activity of the multifidus and potentially the posterior sling muscles (i.e., gluteus maximus and latissimus dorsi) that attach to the thoracolumbar fascia.

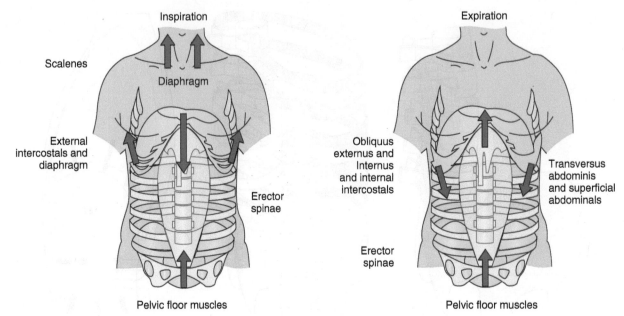

Figure 14-5 Contribution of the trunk muscles to inspiration and expiration.

breathing in supine with expiration produced by elastic recoil of the ribcage and lungs, when the trunk is upright, the abdominal muscles are recruited with quiet breathing. Furthermore, activity of the pelvic floor muscles is required during breathing to support the abdominal contents and control continence in association[43] with variation in intra-abdominal pressure during respiration (see Figure 14-5).[44] This is necessary during both inspiration and expiration; the pelvic floor muscles contract eccentrically during inspiration (gentle lengthening), and concentrically (shortening) during expiration.[43]

The respiratory functions of the trunk muscles must be coordinated with the demands for these muscles to contribute to spinal control. It is well established that respiratory muscles contribute to the strategies used by the nervous system to control the trunk. Activity of the diaphragm and transversus abdominis muscle are initiated prior to rapid limb movements[11] and are maintained tonically during repetitive movements of the arm[45,46] and walking.[47] Furthermore, intercostal muscles are active during trunk rotation.[48] The challenge for the nervous system is to coordinate the postural and respiratory functions. Under normal conditions these functions can be coordinated. During repetitive arm movement, the diaphragm is tonically active, which is consistent with the demand to control spinal stability, but this activity phasically modulates in conjunction with breathing to maintain airflow.[45] Similar responses of the abdominal muscles have been identified in walking.[47]

Under certain conditions the coordination of this breathing and spinal control is compromised. During lifting most individuals either hold their breath or expire.[49,50] Activity of the trunk muscles in association with spinal stability may be compromised when respiratory demand is increased. For instance, a potential conflict exists for contribution of abdominal muscles to spine control when ventilation is challenged during lifting[51] or other tasks such as repetitive arm movements, which repetitively challenges spinal stability.[52] Postural activity of the diaphragm is reduced during repetitive arm movement when respiratory demand is increased by breathing with increased dead-space to induce hypercapnea[52] and in patients with chronic airway disease.[53] In each of these situations, the reduced activation of specific trunk muscles during certain respiratory phases (i.e., reduced activation of diaphragm during expiration) may compromise spinal stability, and conversely, greater activation of muscles during certain respiratory phases (e.g., increased activation of obliquus externus abdominis during expiration) may excessively load the spine.[51]

In addition to the contribution of trunk muscles to airflow, these muscles also move the spine and pelvis in a manner that counteracts the body sway that is caused by breathing movements of the chest wall. Movement of the spine and pelvis, along with activity of lumbopelvic muscles, is time locked to the respiratory movement of the rib cage and abdomen[15,16] and matches the displacement on the center of mass induced by breathing. This motion is reduced in patients with LBP (this is consistent with the finding that stiffness of the spine is increased in this population [see section "Changes in Muscle Control in Lumbopelvic Pain"]) with subsequent disturbance to balance during breathing (augmented motion of the center of pressure).[54,55]

Continence is maintained when pressure in the urethra exceeds that in the bladder. Activity of the pelvic floor muscles contributes to the former, but abdominal and diaphragm muscle activation increases the latter.

For maintenance of lumbopelvic stability, activity of the pelvic floor muscles is necessary for elevation of intra-abdominal pressure, providing an indirect contribution to spinal control via the elevation of abdominal pressure and tension in the thoracolumbar fascia (which depends on pressure in the abdominal cavity to maintain geometry of the abdominal wall[56]).[40] In addition, tension in the pelvic floor muscles might also increase the stiffness of the sacroiliac joints in women.[39]

The demand for pelvic floor muscle activity to contribute to continence is generally consistent with the demands of lumbopelvic control, unless activation is excessive (as has been proposed in some conditions[57]). Consistent with this proposal, pelvic floor muscles contribute to the postural adjustment associated with perturbations to the spine from arm movement in women and men.[40,58] However, activity of the other muscles surrounding the abdominal cavity (e.g., diaphragm and abdominal muscles) to increased intra-abdominal pressure for spine control places additional demand on the pelvic floor muscles. In stress urinary incontinence, pelvic floor muscle activity may be compromised, and recent data suggest that women with this condition often have increased activity of the obliquus externus abdominis.[59,60] Together, these changes may be associated with a combination of incontinence and poor dynamic control of the spine and pelvis.

Static models of spinal control do not take into account the interaction between spinal control, breathing and continence. This is important because, although activation of a muscle such as obliquus externus abdominis may stiffen the spine when co-contracting with the paraspinal muscles, this may restrict the ability of the individual to expand the rib cage to breathe in. Static strategies for spinal stability that stiffen the spine and prevent spinal and rib cage movement are unlikely to be sustainable for anything other than brief efforts because of their effect on the essential demands of breathing. Without consideration of effects such as this, it is unlikely that static models will adequately explain the strategies used by the CNS to control spinal movement. From another perspective, it is important to consider that deficits in respiration and continence may lead to compromised spinal control. Epidemiological studies suggest that continence and respiration are associated with increased risk for LBP.[61,62]

Guiding Principles for a Dynamic Spine

- Trunk muscles contribute to a range of functions in addition to their role in controlling movement and stability of the spine
- Trunk muscles play major competing roles in breathing, continence, and balance
- Incontinence and breathing disorders are associated with an increased risk of developing low back pain

---

CHANGES IN DYNAMIC CONTROL WITH LUMBOPELVIC PAIN

Dynamic Control of the Spine in Low Back and Pelvic Pain

There is considerable variability regarding changes in control of the lumbopelvic stability in low back and pelvic pain. Increased,[63] decreased,[64] and no change[65,66] in muscle activity have been reported. Inconsistent and incomplete understanding of the motor adaptations in low back and pelvic pain has led to a major controversy in clinical practice. Although physiological/biomechanical studies suggest that spine stability is augmented in LBP as a result of adaptation in the activity of the trunk muscles,[67,68] paradoxically, much of the clinical literature argues that exercise should aim to increase stability to compensate for "spinal instability."[3] Variable trunk muscle activity in back pain and the narrow view that stability is synonymous with stiffness has led to confusion. Yet, there has been an explosion of exercise programs to enhance stability, despite lack of evidence that such programs reduce back pain. In contrast, strategies to restore muscle coordination improve outcomes.[69,70] Understanding the pathophysiology of trunk control changes in low back and pelvic pain is critical when considering the most effective preventative and rehabilitation strategies.

Changes in Posture and Postural Alignment in Lumbopelvic Pain

There is no definitive link between a single posture and pain. For every aspect of posture that is considered suboptimal, there will always be examples of individuals who frequently use the posture, without reporting symptoms. Although this has been used as evidence of lack of relevance of postural deviations to pain, it is important to consider that the relevance of a posture (i.e., a strategy for loading the spine) for development of pain depends not only on the amplitude of the load but also on the exposure (i.e., frequency with which the loading strategy is adopted)[71] and the tissue properties of the individual. Thus a specific posture (related to suboptimal loading strategy) may lead to pain only if there is sufficient exposure to exceed tolerance, and different patients will likely present with different postures. Recent work has indicated that patients with LBP commonly adopt postures that are more flexed or extended than pain-free individuals,[72] and this depends on their patient subgroup (see section "Patient Subgrouping"). Postural deviations may result from pain or be a precursor for future pain.

Changes in Muscle Control in Lumbopelvic Pain

Lumbopelvic pain is associated with vast array of changes in activity of the trunk muscles. Many of these changes are likely to affect the movement and stiffness of the spine and pelvis, but the nature of these changes is complicated; some changes suggest less stiffness whereas others suggest increased stiffness, both of which may underlie less robust stability. For instance, increased co-contraction of flexor and extensor muscles has been reported when a load is released from the trunk,[73] activity of erector spinae muscles is increased during gait[63] and during a sit-up,[74] and "bracing" of the abdominal muscles is increased during an active straight leg raise[75] in patients with chronic low back and/or pelvic pain. Furthermore, activity of the obliquus externus abdominis muscle is increased during shoulder movements during experimentally induced pain[76] or when pain is anticipated.[77] When healthy individuals are given experimental pain, most adapt muscle activity to increase stiffness and protection, but no two individuals achieve this with the same combination of muscle changes.[67] Consistent with this observation, inspection of the data presented by Radebold et al.[73] reveals increased activity of at least one superficial trunk muscle in all participants in a postural task but the specific muscles involved varied between individuals. Together these findings suggest that an increase in the protection of the spine and pelvis is common in LBP. This is supported by findings of reduced motion of the spine in patients with back pain; patients with LBP less commonly prepare the spine by movement in advance of rapid arm movements,[78] intervertebral motion is decreased during trunk flexion,[79] and counter-rotation of the shoulders and pelvis is reduced during locomotion.[80]

In contrast, other data tend to indicate that the control of the spine is compromised in the presence of pain. For instance, activity of transversus abdominis[81] and MF[82] muscles is delayed during arm movements, and tonic activity of transversus abdominis is reduced during walking[83] and with repetitive arm movements during experimentally induced back pain,[76] and amplitude of activity is reduced during leg movements.[84] There is also evidence for decreased cross-sectional area,[85] increased fatiguability,[86] and structural changes such as increased intramuscular fat [87,88] of the paraspinal muscles, particularly the lumbar MF. These measures, although not directly indicating changes in the ability to control movement, do suggest functional changes in specific trunk muscles. Findings of impaired structure and behavior of the deep trunk muscles have been interpreted to suggest that control of the spine and pelvis is impaired in many individuals with low back and pelvic pain. Although no studies have directly measured stability when activity of the deep muscles is removed, this hypothesis is based on the in vivo and in vitro evidence for a contribution of these muscles in spinal control.[31,34,36,89] Other data from specific back pain populations have provided direct evidence of impaired intervertebral control. For instance, intervertebral translation is abnormal in patients with spondylolisthesis,[90] and buckling has been observed with fluoroscopy in a single subject during a weight-lifting effort.[91]

In summary, patients can present with a complex mix of reduced and increased control. Although some may present at the extreme of a net excess or insufficiency of control, many will present with elements of both (e.g., excessive recruitment of long paraspinal muscles, with compromised control of MF). Identification of the relevance of individual variation in muscle activation can be simplified by consideration of patient subgroups (see section "Patient Subgrouping"). The substantial variability in the adaptation of the trunk muscles in patients with lumbopelvic pain is often interpreted to suggest that there is no consistent adaptation of muscle control during pain. But there may be a common goal that underpins the adaptation to pain in many patients. Despite the variability, the CNS may adapt to pain or injury by increasing spinal stiffness to increase the *safety margin*—that is, to protect the part from pain and/or (re)injury. In this case the nervous system may adopt a strategy to increase stiffness of the spine by increasing the co-contraction of trunk muscles. Thus, rather than selecting a strategy of coordination of deep and superficial muscle activation that is specific to a task, the nervous system may simplify control by stiffening the spine with reduced flexibility of movement choices. This may be specific to a direction of movement. With this strategy, the nervous system would decrease the potential for error, limit the impact of unanticipated disturbances to the spine, and limit the potential for further injury. In effect, rather than selecting a strategy from a spectrum of dynamic possibilities that are perfectly matched to the demands of the task, the nervous system may select a simple solution that provides reasonable (but perhaps not optimal) quality of movement control that satisfies the demands of a range of conditions. However, because many muscles can achieve the same goal (that is, the system is "redundant" as there are multiple solutions to the same problem), different individuals may select different combinations of muscle activity to achieve this goal and the strategy may differ between different tasks.

To test the idea that a range of different strategies of muscle activation achieve a similar outcome for the spine, van Dieen et al.[68] undertook a modeling experiment in which they simulated a range of strategies adopted by patients with back pain in a biomechanical model of stability. The outcome was that stability was increased by each alternative pattern of increased muscle activation, whether the strategy involved increased co-contraction of flexors and extensors, increased activity of the flexors alone or increased activity of the extensors alone. Consistent with this modeling study, recent data from a study of experimental pain suggest that, when pain is induced in healthy individuals, most subjects adopt a pattern of increased activity, but again the pattern varied between individuals.[67] Of note, these individuals also presented with impaired activity of the deep muscles. Thus an individual may present with changes in the deep muscles that would be consistent with compromised control, yet activity of the superficial muscles may be increased, which is consistent with increased stiffening of the spine. Despite the increased activity, the control of intervertebral motion may be compromised as a result of reduced or impaired activity of the deep muscles. Whether the poor control of the deep muscles leads to compensation by the more superficial muscles or whether overactivity of the superficial muscles supersedes the activity of the deep muscles is discussed in section "Mechanisms for Changes in Motor Control in Lumbopelvic Pain."

In summary, available data suggest that individuals with low back/pelvic pain present with a spectrum of changes that range from insufficient control to excessive control, and some present with elements of both underactivity and overactivity of muscles. Within this large variation, there is likely to be subgroups, which may be characterized by features of motor control that are provocative or relieving, and this may relate to specific patterns of muscle activation.

CHANGES IN MOVEMENT IN LUMBOPELVIC PAIN

As for the other dimensions of motor control, there is large diversity in the manner in which changes in movement present in patients with low back and pelvic pain. Movement may be considered as motion of the spine in space (e.g., flexion/extension of the entire spine), specific motion of a region of the spine (e.g., lordosis/kyphosis of the lumbar spine), relative motion of adjacent regions (e.g., lumbar spine relative to thoracolumbar junction, or hip relative to lumbar spine), or motion of intervertebral segments (e.g., translation at a segment or range of motion at a specific segment acting like a "hinge"). Evidence is variable. In general, studies that show modified motion has been derived from specific patient subgroups including modified control at a segmental level in patients with spondylolisthesis,[90] poor control of spine during hip movement in subgroups into an "extension-rotation" subgroup,[92-95] and reduced counter-rotation of the trunk in gait.[80] Thus modification to movement is common and may range from strategies that reduce motion to enhance protection to strategies that lead to excessive motion. That is, a spectrum of changes from too much to too little control. This underscores the necessity to consider patients individually to determine the relevance of motor control for their pain presentation.

Mechanisms for Changes in Motor Control in Lumbopelvic Pain

Why is control of the spine modified in patients with low back and pelvic pain? There are a number of questions to consider. One is whether the pain precedes the motor control changes or motor control changes precede pain (Figure 14-6). There is evidence for both. Several authors argue that changes in motor control can lead to the development of pain. Cholewicki et al.[96] reported an

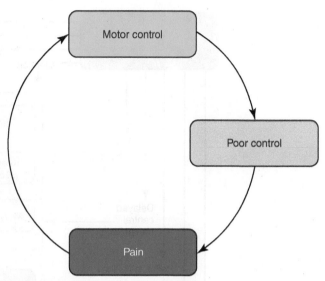

Figure 14-6 Vicious cycle of pain and motor control deficits. Although motor control deficits may lead to pain as a result of compromised control of the spine and pelvis, pain can also lead to changes in motor control. A patient who presents with pain has already entered the cycle; where the person entered it is less important.

association between delayed offset of activity of the superficial abdominal muscles and subsequent development of episodes of acute back pain in athletes. Early work by Janda[97] argued that children with "soft" neurological signs were at risk of developing back pain as adults. Sahrmann[92] argued that repeated movement with poor control (e.g., motion of the spine instead of the hip) was a precursor to pain. If true, there must be factors that "motivate" the adoption of the suboptimal control strategy prior to pain onset. Issues as diverse as habitual postures or movement patterns[92] and secondary consequence of breathing disorders or incontinence[61] have been implicated.

Conversely, it is also argued that pain and injury lead to changes in control and structure of the trunk muscles. For instance, experimental pain can cause changes in trunk muscle activity during gait[63] and other tasks such as arm movements[76]; experimental injury in animals leads to rapid muscle atrophy[98] and changes in muscle structure (i.e., muscle fiber types, connective tissue and fat[99]) in the MF muscle; and these changes are similar in many respects to those identified in patients with clinical pain.[81,85]

If pain and injury lead to changes in structure and behavior of the trunk muscles, what is the mechanism? Pain can affect control at multiple levels of the nervous system (Figure 14-7). In reality, when an individual presents with pain, whether the pain caused the changes or whether the changes caused the pain is to some extent irrelevant as the patient will already be in a cycle in which pain and injury have the potential to increase or perpetuate the changes in motor control. Motor control may be modified by mechanisms involving both the sensory and motor mechanisms at multiple levels of the nervous system. These mechanisms could be complementary, additive, or competitive.

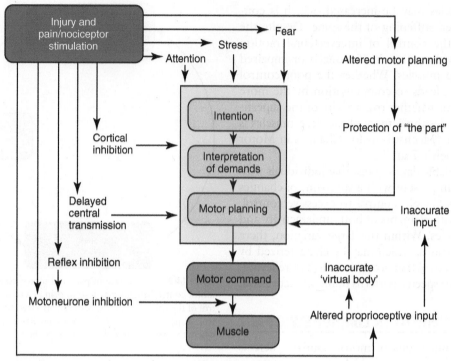

Figure 14-7 Possible mechanisms of pain that can affect the planning of movement and activation of trunk muscles.

Guiding Principles of Motor Control

- Changes in motor control may lead to pain and injury
- Pain and injury can change motor control
- Motor control may adapt by increasing the stability of the spine and pelvis
- There is substantial individual variation that must be considered when attempting to understand the relationship between pain and motor control

Sensory System Mechanisms

Deficits in the detection, transmission, integration, utilization, and perception of sensory information could modify motor control. Errors in the detection or interpretation of position or movement of the body would render optimal control of the lumbar spine and pelvis impossible. Proprioceptive deficits (e.g., detection or perception of position and movement) are commonly reported in LBP. These changes manifest as reduced ability to reposition the spine or pelvis to a target posture or alignment and decreasing sensitivity for detection movement.[25] Such changes will influence the quality of control of back motion and have several potential mechanisms:

1. Afferent input will be compromised by injury to mechanoreceptors (e.g. muscle spindles or mechanoreceptors in the intervertebral disc) or the tissues in which they reside.[100]
2. Processing of sensory information may be "ignored" by the nervous system, as a result of sensory "reweighting," which refers to the capacity of the nervous system to rely on information from multiple sources and reduce or increase reliance on a specific source. Despite the availability of afferent input from the injured part the nervous system may elect not to use it (e.g., decreased responsiveness to back muscle proprioception and increased responsiveness to ankle input,[101] or increased dependence on vision[102]).
3. The representation of the body region at the primary sensory cortex may be distorted[103] or the body schema altered.[104] Reorganization of the primary sensory cortex in chronic spinal pain involves enlargement and medial shift of the representation of the low back relative to that identified in pain-free individuals, and these changes are correlated with pain duration.[103] Sensory cortex activity measured from somatosensory evoked potentials indicate increased N80 component, which relates to the sensory-discriminative pain processing at the primary sensory cortex, and no change in the N150 component, which indicates processing in secondary sensory cortex.[105] Together, these data highlight the potential for reorganization (and possible sensitization) to the primary sensory cortex, which may contribute to modified motor control.[103]

Any of these changes in sensory function could underpin compromised control. Each would have different implications for management. For instance, injury to a mechanoreceptor may have limited potential for recovery, but reweighting and sensory cortex reorganization may be amenable to training.

Motor System Mechanisms

Many regions of the nervous system are involved in the planning and generation of movement, and changes at any site, including the motor cortex, subcortical, spinal, and peripheral sites, may contribute to motor control changes due to pain.

A key site of recent investigation has been the primary motor cortex. Studies in chronic LBP have revealed reorganization of the cortical territory with projections to trunk muscles. Similar to the changes in the primary sensory cortex,[103] recurrent nonspecific LBP involves more diffuse and posterolaterally shifted cortical representation of the deep trunk muscle, transversus abdominis, relative to pain-free individuals.[106] This change appears to have a behavioral relevance, as the cortical reorganization is correlated with changes in motor behavior (i.e., muscle activation during arm movements), which implies a potential role in the mechanism of the adapted behavior.[106] There is also reorganization of the representation of the paraspinal muscles. Transcranial magnetic stimulation and selective muscle recordings from deep fascicles of MF and the superficial longissimus with fine-wire electromyography demonstrate reduced excitability and a convergence (i.e., "smudging") of the cortical representations of each muscle group in chronic LBP.[107] Similar to other cortical changes, the magnitude of convergence of cortical areas appears related to the severity or location of pain and preliminary evidence implies convergence of discrete motor cortical representation is linked with the transition from acute to chronic back pain.[108]

The loss of discrete motor cortical representation for the paraspinal muscles helps explain features of motor dysfunction in chronic spinal pain. Evidence from other conditions implies that the presence of discrete cortical representation of individual muscles may have relevance for independent control of the different muscle layers. In another painful condition, focal hand dystonia, there is similar blurring and overlap of the cortical representation of individual fingers, which is associated with loss of independent finger movement and impaired hand function.[109] In a similar manner and unlike pain-free individuals who maintain separate control of individual back muscles, patients with LBP co-activate the deep and superficial back and abdominal muscles during arm movements[81,110] and with changes in sitting posture.[111] It is hypothesized that the reorganization of the motor cortex underpins adoption of new motor strategies that prioritizes protection of the spine with a simplified strategy of co-activation of the trunk muscles providing a greater safety margin, rather than the finely tuned coordination between multiple muscles, that although it may be more optimal, the finely tuned coordination has greater potential for error.[112] Indirect support of this hypothesis comes from other data, which show that when challenged by acute experimental pain, the excitability of the corticomotor pathway for the transversus abdominis muscle is reduced and that for obliquus externus abdominis muscle is increased,[107] again suggesting a shift in strategy from fine-tuned control to a simplified more protective solution. Several authors have argued that the CNS adopts this strategy to compensate for reduced osseoligamentous stability of the spine (Figure 14-8).[3,68] However, similar changes in motor control may be replicated when pain is induced experimentally by injection of hypertonic saline,[76] that is, when osseoligamentous stability has not changed. Furthermore, similar changes may occur even when pain is anticipated but not present.[77] For example, if painful electrical shocks to the back are provided every

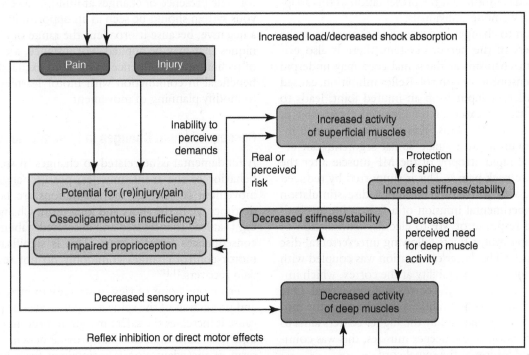

Figure 14-8 Possible factors that may explain the relationship between impaired activity of the deep muscles and increased activity of the superficial muscles. Pain and injury may lead to opposite changes in the deep and superficial muscles.

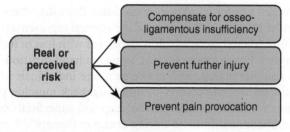

Figure 14-9 Motor control may change because of real or perceived risk to the spine as a result of instability and the risk of pain and injury or reinjury.

time an arm is moved, the response of the obliquus externus abdominis muscle is augmented and occurs earlier in association with arm movement, and this is maintained after the painful stimulation is no longer linked to the arm movement.[113] Thus adaptation may occur in a number of situations when the real or perceived control of the spine is decreased leading to a real or perceived risk of further injury or pain (Figure 14-9).

When dynamic control of the spine is considered, muscle activity is precisely matched to the demands to maintain stability of the trajectory and all other components of spinal control. However, this dynamic strategy has potential for error, if the timing or amplitude or muscle activation does not match the actual demand. In a healthy system, where there is tolerance for small errors, this is not problematic. However, if the tolerance for errors is reduced (e.g., as a result of osseoligamentous insufficiency, pain, or poor proprioception), the CNS may adopt a simplified more protective static strategy to increase spinal stiffness. Thus, rather than using a range of control alternatives, the preferred strategy adopted by the CNS may be a simplified solution, but the presentation of this adaptation will vary among individuals.

In addition to changes in descending control from the higher centers of the nervous system, there is also evidence that mechanisms at the spinal cord may underpin changes in sensorimotor control. Reflex inhibition, caused by altered afferent input from an injured joint, leads to reduced activity of extensor muscles and facilitation of flexors muscles in the limbs. This mechanism, which involves interneurons at a single spinal segment, can account for the rapid atrophy of the MF muscle after the onset of acute back pain.[85] This is supported by reduced responsiveness of MF to intervertebral disc stimulation following experimental infusion of a facet joint in pigs[23] and reduced response of MF to electrical stimulation of the descending motor tracts following intervertebral disc lesion in pigs.[114] This latter observation was coupled with evidence of increased excitability at the cortex, which implies competing effects at the cortex and spinal cord. One interpretation of this observation is that although the motor control strategy planned by the higher centers aims to augment activation of the deeper muscles, this was counteracted by inhibition at the spinal cord.

The ability to control posture/alignment and movement will be affected by changes in structural changes in muscles. These changes may include atrophy, muscle fiber changes, and fatty and connective tissue changes. LBP or injury are characterized by increased fatigability of back extensor muscles is increased,[86] atrophy of back muscles in the acute and chronic period (but not subacute period, thus highlighting the potential for different mechanisms at different time points),[85,98,115] fatty infiltration,[115] and transformation from type 1 (fatigue resistant) to type 2 (nonfatigue resistant) muscle fibers[99,116] of MF. Recent work suggests a role for pro-inflammatory cytokines in this structural remodeling of muscle,[112,117] which highlights the potential for complex neurobiological processes associated with injury and pain.

Changes in coordination of firing of motor units within muscles have been studied extensively for simple limb tasks. Voluntary contraction of limb muscles in pain involves redistribution of motor unit activity within and between muscles[118] rather than uniform inhibition of motoneuron discharge as was predicted by earlier theories.[119] Whether similar changes affect trunk muscles requires further investigation. As the motoneuron and muscle fibers are the final common pathways of the motor system, all these changes will have an impact on the output of the sensorimotor system.

Summary

In summary, multiple factors have the potential to change control of the muscle activity, posture/alignment, and movement before and after pain and injury. In most cases, it is likely that a range of factors is involved, and one issue for management is to consider the importance of each factor. The presence of changes at multiple levels of the nervous system should be seen as an opportunity rather than a negative, because it broadens the range of clinical techniques that may be applied. For instance, a combination of techniques to influence spinal cord excitability may be beneficial in conjunction with motor learning strategies to modify planning of movement.

Consequences of Changes in Dynamic Control

A fundamental issue related to changes in structure and behavior of the trunk muscles, posture/alignment and movement is whether the adaptations are beneficial or detrimental, in the short and long term. Changes in strategy that lead to increased and decreased stability may have consequences for the spine. This is significant because motor control changes commonly do not resolve when pain recovers.[81,120]

From one point of view, a strategy to increase stiffness and protection of the spine and pelvis may be positive because it increases the safety margin to prevent pain and reinjury.[3,121] Although this may provide benefit in the short term, if the adaptation is maintained for a long period, it is likely to have negative consequences for the spine and pelvis secondary to increased loading,[122,123] restriction of movement,[78] reduced variation, and inadequate fine-tuning of trunk movement (see Figure 14-8).

Loading on the spine is increased as a result of muscle co-contraction. This has been confirmed in studies of patients with back pain during lifting.[123] Although there is debate whether increased loading is detrimental to the spine, it is argued that high cumulative loads may lead to mechanical and physiological changes.[124,125] These changes may accelerate degeneration[126] and potentially increase the long-term risk of LBP recurrence.

A consequence of spinal stiffening and muscle co-contraction is the reduced availability of movement as a mechanism to absorb and dissipate force. As described earlier, movement presents a range of advantages to the control of forces at the spine. Some data show that patients with LBP are less likely to use movement as a component of the strategy to control the spine, which is associated with a greater perturbation to the trunk[78] and a greater time to recover balance after a perturbation.[13] Both of these issues are likely to have consequences in the long term. In addition, if spine movement is reduced, the contribution of spinal motion to respiration and balance control would be compromised. Consistent with this proposal, it has been reported that patients with LBP sway more with breathing[54,55] and have increased vertical motion of the rib cage with breathing.[127] This latter finding suggests restricted ability to use anteroposterior and lateral motion of the abdominal wall and rib cage secondary to increased activity of the superficial abdominal muscles. In terms of balance, increased spinal stiffness may limit the contribution of spinal movement to control postural equilibrium. Patients with LBP are less able to use a hip strategy to maintain balance when standing on a short support base,[18] and when lumbar motion is restricted by the application of a brace, balance quality is reduced.[7] Another important consideration is that if the nervous system adopts a control strategy that relies on spinal stiffening rather than movement, it may limit the ability of the CNS to perform some tasks. Although the stiffening strategy may be suitable for tasks where movement can be restricted (i.e., movement is not required, can be compensated elsewhere, or can be reduced without preventing the task from being completed), when movement is obligatory, an appropriate strategy may not be available. For instance, when standing on one leg, it is essential to shift the center of mass over the stance leg. Inappropriate control of the spine in this context through trunk stiffening makes the aforementioned task difficult to execute.[128]

Optimal control of any body segment depends on some variation. Although excessive variation is problematic, so is too little variation.[129] Variation is necessary to share the load around tissues such that no single muscle, ligament, or area of joint surface is loaded for every repetition of a task. Variation is also necessary for learning,

to be exposed to new movement solutions. One possible consequence of adaptation in motor control is reduced variation when patients adopt a more stereotypical movement pattern. This can be problematic in the long term. For instance, lower limb kinematics of runners with lower limb problems are characterized by less variation.[129]

Finally, impaired activity of the deep muscles, in conjunction with increased activity of the superficial muscles, is likely to have consequences for the control of movement and stability at the intervertebral level. As mentioned earlier, it is well accepted from a number of experimental models that deep muscle function is important for spinal control (see section "Muscular Mechanisms for Control of the Spine and Pelvis"). The contribution of the deep muscles in controlling the lumbar spine and pelvis is unlikely to be completely compensated for, or replicated by, activity of the larger, more superficial muscles, especially in dynamic situations. The models of Bergmark[27] and Crisco and Panjabi[130] predict that, without activity of the deeper muscles, the integrity of the spine cannot be maintained. Thus impaired function of these muscles is likely to render the entire spinal system, and its control, vulnerable, thus leading to compromised quality of control. Although this may not be a problem in the short term, as the increased activity of the superficial muscles is likely to stiffen and protect the spine, in the long term, this has the potential to be problematic.

For the reasons outlined above it could be argued that the muscle co-contraction strategy with its short-term benefit may lead to increased risk of back pain recurrence if the almost obligatory use of this strategy does not resolve after the resolution of pain. It is well accepted that previous back pain is a strong predictor of future back injury.[131] The failure of changes in trunk muscle control to resolve may be a mechanism underlying this finding. Data from numerous studies of individuals with a history of pain, but no pain at the time of testing, indicate that changes in motor control persist after the resolution of symptoms.[81,110] This implies that motor strategies do not resolve spontaneously after cessation of pain, at least in some individuals. The possibility that abnormal muscle activation leads to future LBP is supported by recent data that suggest delayed offset of activity of the abdominal muscles predicts LBP.[96] This feature of muscle activation was a predictor both for those with a history of LBP and for those with no history of pain. This indicates that factors other than pain could be responsible for the preexisting modifications in motor control. In another example, reduced cross-sectional area of the MF muscle that is not restored by specific training was associated with increased risk of back pain recurrence relative to individuals who did receive such training.[70] A key issue to consider is why some individuals go on to have back pain recurrence whereas others do not. Further work is required to determine possible factors that may contribute to back pain recurrence. Some data suggest that the failure of resolution of the motor adaptation may be linked to unhelpful attitudes and beliefs about pain.[132] As persistence or recurrence of LBP[133,134] and pain-related attitudes are associated with changes in motor strategy,[135] this may provide a link between physiological and psychological factors and back pain recurrence.

Guiding Principles: Adapted Motor Patterns in Low Back Pain May Have Negative Long-Term Consequences as a Result of:

- Increased loading as secondary to enhanced muscle co-contraction, or suboptimal movement and/or posture and postural alignment
- Increased stiffness and reduced shock absorption
- Decreased movement variation to share load and learn
- Decreased control quality of intervertebral motion

Interpretation of Motor Changes for Exercise Planning

The potential negative long-term effects of an adaptation that increases the stiffness of the spine challenges the view that exercise to enhance spinal stability is universally appropriate for management of LBP. In the management of a patient with low back and/or pelvic pain, an important consideration is whether the adaptation is beneficial or detrimental, that is, whether the adaptation should be encouraged or discouraged. On one hand, it may be necessary to maintain some element of adaptation to compensate for reduced osseoligamentous control (e.g., requirement for thigh muscle activation to compensate for reduced passive restraint of the knee in knee osteoarthritis), limited ability of the tissues to tolerate load and movement, poor awareness of position and/or movement, or sensitization of the tissues. This point of view has been argued by different authors[3,121] and forms the basis of a range of intervention strategies that aim to increase the stiffness and stability of the spine.[122]

The alternative point of view is that training a strategy that solely aims to increase stiffness of the spine may have negative consequences for the spine and contribute to maintenance or recurrence of back pain and injury for some individuals. The alternative view is that rehabilitation should aim to optimize control, and this involves training a balance between movement and stiffness, which involves training and refinement of the coordination between the deep and superficial muscles to restore an optimal dynamic strategy for control of the spine.[2] This highlights the need for comprehensive assessment of the patient to determine the relationship between motor control (i.e., posture and postural alignment, muscle activation and movement) and the presenting symptoms to identify which elements of the motor control system require enhancement and which elements should be reduced.

Guiding Principles of Motor Control Treatment

- Some elements of motor control require enhancement
- Some elements of motor control should be reduced
- Development of treatment goals can be achieved only through careful assessment and evaluation of the response to change

---

Summary

Optimal control of the spine and pelvis requires a carefully controlled dynamic system with a balance between movement and stiffness. Application of motor control principles to the management of low back and pelvic pain has evolved from a relatively straightforward approach that aimed to enhance stiffness, to an individualized approach where exercise is tailored to the individual to match the presentation in terms of the patient's unique presentation of posture and postural alignment, muscle activation and movement and their functional demands. Treatment planning relies on careful assessment and tailoring of exercises to meet the individual patient's needs. The following sections summarize key elements of this approach.

CLINICAL APPROACH TO MOTOR CONTROL TRAINING

Principles of Clinical Approach to Motor Control Training for Low Back and Pelvic Pain

Motor control training for low back and pelvic pain aims to restore optimal control of the spine and pelvis, with consideration of posture/postural alignment, muscle activation and movement. Sensation and the multiple functions of the trunk muscles (e.g., respiratory, continence, balance) are also key considerations. The objective of this approach is to optimize load on the structures of the spine and pelvis (that may be a source of ongoing nociceptor discharge), in a manner that is matched to the changes in motor control that are specific to the individual and matched to his or her functional demands. This requires consideration of the role of biology (e.g., role of ongoing nociceptor discharge in the maintenance of pain and/or the role of exposure to healthy movement to recovery) within the biopsychosocial presentation of the patient.

Although motor control training is unlikely to be appropriate for all patients with low back and pelvic pain, for those who retain a component of their condition related to loading of the spinal tissues, motor control training appears to be relevant. Motor control training requires careful assessment of each element of motor control, and the guiding principal is to use a clinical reasoning approach to apply specific tests to identify features of motor control that are relevant for the patient's symptoms. At the completion of the assessment, the clinician has a clear picture of whether or not motor control is altered in the patient, how it relates to pain provocation or relief and tissue loading, and a prioritized list of features of motor control to address with treatment. The intervention is specifically targeted to the presentation of the patient.

Motor Learning

Rehabilitation involves a motor learning approach.[2] Motor learning involves the acquisition and refinement of movement and coordination that leads to a permanent change in movement performance.[136] This can be achieved by drawing on the principles of motor training for skill learning. Different researchers have defined either two or three phases of motor learning. Fitts and Posner[137] proposed three phases. The **cognitive phase** focuses on cognitively based problems, and all components of the task are organized cognitively with attention to feedback, movement sequence, and quality of performance. The **associative phase** commences once the patient has acquired the fundamentals of the movement and the focus shifts to emphasize the consistency of performance and the cognitive demands are reduced. In the **automatic phase**, which is achieved after considerable practice, the demand for conscious intervention is reduced and the focus shift to transferring the task between environments. Gentile[138] proposes two phases, which parallel those of Fitts and Posner. In phase 1, the patient "gets the idea"; in phase 2, the emphasis is on fixation and diversification of the skill.

Motor learning principles provide guidance for a range of strategies for optimal training of motor function.

Motor learning of complex movements can be facilitated by *practice of parts* of the movement (i.e., segmentation) before practicing the whole movement. Learning can be facilitated by *simplification* of the task by modification of elements such as reducing the load, speed, or changing the body position to make it easier for the patient to correctly perform the task. Feedback is critical to ensure learning. Feedback of both the quality of performances and the results of the task can be provided.

Training of motor control of the trunk in the framework of motor learning involves training of the components of function that are found to be relevant for a patient's symptoms in the detailed assessment of posture and postural alignment, muscle activation and movement. The sequence of phases is outlined in Figure 14-10. The process involves progressive phases that increase the complexity of training to enable a patient to regain optimal motor control from the initial attempts to address the specific deficits in motor control through to high-level functional training. In addition to this basic sequence, there are other issues that may require consideration for specific individuals. For instance, it is critical to regain breathing during the early stages of training and throughout program progression, and this may be a specific problem for some individuals. The following sections outline the key aspects related to the methods used to guide the clinical reasoning approach based on subgrouping and important considerations for treatment planning based on the mechanisms of pain and the interaction between the biological, psychological, and social aspects of pain.

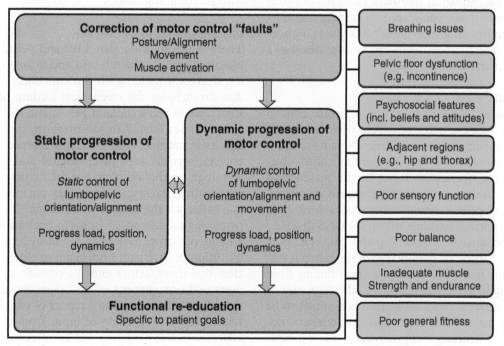

Figure 14-10 Progression of motor control training for dynamic control of the spine and pelvis. Items to the left-hand side indicate the basic progression of exercise from initial identification and retraining of specific features of sensorimotor control that are related to the patient's symptoms. Once skills are learned to correct motor control "faults," this is progressed through integration of control of these features in more demanding contexts via static and dynamic progressions. The final phase involves integration into functional tasks identified by the patient. Items to the right-hand side are features that may present as barriers to recovery of optimal motor control that should be screened for and included in the intervention as necessary for an individual patient.

Patient Subgrouping

Subgrouping of patients involves identification of features of a patient's presentation that can identify more homogeneous groups from within the heterogeneous population with low back and pelvic pain. Several approaches can be used, including those that allocate patients on the basis of their responsiveness to interventions (e.g., treatment based classification[139]), pathoanatomical diagnosis of the pain source,[140] a combination of both,[141] or on the basis of features of motor control that provide guidance for the prioritization of the features of posture or postural alignment, muscle activation, and movement that should be addressed with the treatment.[92,142] These latter approaches integrate well with the motor control approach outlined in this chapter. One of the features that characterize skilled clinical practice is recognition of patterns that can simplify and guide the selection of treatments. Subgrouping of a patient according to a cluster of features of pain provocation/relief (i.e., movements or positions that provoke or relieve pain) and motor control strategies (e.g., poor control of lumbar lordosis, relative flexibility of hip and spine) follows this philosophy and aims to facilitate the process for the clinician to identify the cluster of relevant features of the patients presentation and plan targeted treatment. The ultimate test of subgrouping will be to show, with clinical trials, that the outcomes are improved when intervention is based on the subgrouping. There is encouraging evidence from a recent study.[143] It is also necessary to consider the patient's pain presentation and the probable relevance of neurobiological processes and the psychological and social elements of a pain presentation, which are considered to varying amounts by different subgrouping strategies.[144] The following sections consider how these elements can be considered in a patient's presentation.

Neurobiology of Pain

A critical consideration for application of motor control training in low back and pelvic pain is the potential role of tissue loading in perpetuation of a patient's pain presentation. There is considerable debate regarding the involvement of ongoing nociceptive input in the presence of persistent pain. Although some ongoing pain states may be mediated by central sensitization mechanisms (i.e., amplification of neural signaling within the CNS that elicits pain hypersensitivity[145]) or neuropathic pain (i.e., pain attributable to a lesion or dysfunction in the nervous system[146]), patients may also maintain a contribution from nociceptive input from the periphery, although this is likely to be sensitized. Nociceptive pain is assumed to be predominantly maintained by activation of peripheral nociceptive sensory neurons.[147] Theoretically, it is individuals whose symptoms retain a contribution from activation of nociceptors who are likely to benefit from intervention that addresses suboptimal loading of tissues. Typical features of a nociceptive pain presentation are that the pain is localized to the area of injury or dysfunction; has a clear, proportionate mechanical or anatomical nature that responds predictably to aggravating and easing factors; is usually intermittent; may be manifested as sharp pain with movement or mechanical provocation; and may also present as a constant dull ache or throb at rest.[148] A recent study reported that, in a nonspecific LBP group, motor control training was more effective for individuals who scored higher on a questionnaire based on a consensus opinion of features that characterized lumbar "instability."[149] An issue for consideration is that the questionnaire is largely focused on features reflective of nociceptive type pain, and a plausible interpretation of the study was that the responsiveness of treatment was not based on the presence of "instability" but instead on the presence of nociceptive features to pain.

Pain related to central sensitization is characterized by a disproportionate, nonmechanical, and unpredictable pattern of pain in response to multiple or nonspecific aggravating or easing factors; an intensity that is disproportionate to the nature and extent of injury or pathology; a strong association with maladaptive psychosocial factors; and diffuse or nonanatomical areas of pain or tenderness on palpation.[150] Patients with this presentation may still benefit from exposure to "healthy" movement, but the attention to the detail of movement may be unnecessary or unhelpful if it focuses too much attention on protection of the tissues. Neuropathic pain, by definition, includes trauma to peripheral nerves and could benefit from modification of movement to alter the mechanical interface of the nerve with surrounding tissues.

Biopsychosocial Model of Pain

There is no question that LBP and pelvic pain include biological, psychological, and social aspects, with varying degrees depending on the individual. The biological domain includes the mechanical loading of the tissues/structures of the spine and pelvis, and the neurobiological processes related to sensitization, immune response and its interaction with nociceptive processing. This, of course, interacts with psychological and social features. Although psychological and social factors are unlikely to cause pain in the first instance, they can moderate the pain and influence the long-term outcome. The relevance of psychological and social issues in back pain is clear, and a range of factors have been found to be associated with transition of back pain from acute to chronic pain.[134] It is clear that these factors must be considered in the assessment and management of back pain. An important consideration is that a person's report of pain is not linearly related to the amplitude of input from the nociceptive afferents in the periphery but is influenced and molded by many issues including the individual's experience and other psychological and social issues.[151]

Pain catastrophizing, fear, and poor pain coping skills can influence neurobiology of pain, drive sensitization processes, and influence the manner in which the motor system adapts, often leading to motor adaptation that is *greater* than what is necessary, maintained *beyond* when it is necessary, or completely *inappropriate* for the health of the tissues.[112] It is increasingly recognized that motor control can be changed by psychological factors, which include, but are not limited to, stress and fear of pain and (re)injury. It has been reported that control of the trunk is changed during lifting under "stressful" conditions.[152] Furthermore, when a person anticipates back pain, changes in motor control are similar to those identified in clinical pain; for instance, the onset of activity in the deep abdominal muscles is delayed during arm movements[77] and activity of the superficial muscles occurs earlier.[113] Notably, these motor control features do not appear to recover rapidly in all individuals after the removal of the threat of pain. The failure of these changes to resolve on the resolution of symptoms has been linked with unhelpful attitudes about back pain.[132] In summary, biological (including features of motor control) and psychological changes are likely to be interdependent and require co-intervention in many cases. Effective management of the whole patient must include consideration of all aspects as each may present as a barrier to clinical improvement.

Summary

Optimal control of the spine and pelvis requires a carefully controlled dynamic system. In such a system, the nervous system matches the strategy of activation of the trunk muscles, control of posture and postural alignment, and movement to the multiple tasks that must be coordinated to achieve optimal control of the spine. On balance, data from patients with low back pain indicate that deficits are present in the ability of the nervous system to select the appropriate control strategy, and this may present across a spectrum from simple strategies that involve co-contraction to protect the spine and increase the safety margin to inadequate control of a movement/region/segment. Underlying these different movement presentations is a combination of suboptimal posture and postural alignment, muscle activation (i.e., variable presentation of decreased and increased activation of deep and superficial muscles), movement, sensory function, modification of control of the multiple functions of the trunk muscles and structural changes in muscle (i.e., atrophy, fatty infiltration, muscle stiffness/length changes). In view of the individual-specific nature of these changes, comprehensive rehabilitation will require comprehensive assessment (potentially guided by patient subgrouping), and a tailored motor learning approach to restore control. The following sections provide an overview of the assessment, training goals, and treatment options as well as guidelines for progression of exercise.

Practical Application of Clinical Approach to Motor Control Training

The purpose of the following sections is to provide an overview of the basis and application of motor control training to the management of patients with lumbopelvic pain and dysfunction. Optimization of motor control requires careful assessment and treatment planning. There is no single intervention that works for all patients, and a treatment can be planned only once the clinician has identified the features of control that require modification. This must be nested in a biopsychosocial framework to ensure that all aspects of the presentation and the interaction among them have been addressed. Many approaches to motor control training have been proposed, and the following information is an amalgamation of elements of many of these approaches. The combination of approaches enhances a clinician's toolbox from which to draw flexibility to match a package of intervention to the needs and preferences of the patient. Although clinical trials provide evidence of the efficacy of the approach, there are many elements that require further development. For instance, most assessments rely on the skilled observation of the clinician and have not been subjected to assessment of clinometric properties. Furthermore, the basis for the clinical decision making is based on clinical reasoning, rather than simplified algorithms because of the diversity of presentations. Although subgrouping can simplify the process of targeting treatment by aiding the identification of patterns, clinical skill is required to prioritize treatment targets and identify effective solutions.

Clinical Approach to Motor Control Training of Posture and Postural Alignment

Principles. At a basic level, the application of a motor control approach to posture and postural alignment aims to identify features of the manner in which the patient's posture deviates from "ideal" and how different postures either provoke or relieve pain. Although population studies generally indicate an unclear link between posture and pain,[153] major limitations of that work is the lack of recognition that there will not be a single posture related to pain, that the relationship between posture and pain will depend on exposure to the posture, and the failure to consider the unique manner in which a posture may relate to pain for an individual patient. A clear relationship is not always easily revealed, but for many patients, there are specific features that modify their pain in a predictable and repeatable manner. The challenge clinically is to identify the relevant features and find a strategy to induce a change in the postural behavior.

Assessment of posture and postural alignment of a patient with low back and pelvic pain involves identification of aspects that might be related to pain presentation. Three features can help determine potentially relevant features: (1) features that deviate from a predicted "ideal" posture, (2) elements of posture that provoke or relieve pain (e.g., curvature), and (3) muscle activation required to maintain the position (e.g., excessive activity [i.e., excessive loading of the posterior elements when sitting in excessive lumbar extension] or insufficient activity [i.e., excessive flexion loading of the spine in slump sitting]). What is *ideal* posture? A range of postures has been defined as "ideal" or "neutral" in the clinical literature (for review, see reference[154]). A postural alignment that is founded on several sources of evidence and appears clinically relevant is one that involves optimal sagittal balance (i.e., C7 over the sacrum), gentle curvature (i.e., cervical lordosis, thoracic kyphosis, a smooth transition to a gentle lumbar lordosis), and a pelvis that is level or slightly anteriorly tilted and symmetrical in the frontal and transverse planes. This posture is considered ideal because it (1) provides optimal sharing of loading between spinal structures[155]; (2) is midrange and thus avoids "creep" of viscoelastic tissues into flexion, extension, lateral flexion or rotation; (3) is associated with minimal activity of large, more superficial trunk muscles such as those required to overcome gravity if the center of mass of the trunk is biased anteriorly or posteriorly relative to the pelvis[156,157]; (4) is thought to encourage greater activity of the deeper muscles of the trunk,[156] including the pelvic floor muscles[158]; and (5) involves a more efficient breathing pattern.[159] Postural alignment is strongly associated with muscle activation; activation of the MF muscle and the lower regions of transversus abdominis and obliquus internus abdominis muscles is greatest when sitting with a lumbar lordosis associated with a smooth transition to kyphosis at the thoracolumbar junction, whereas thoracic erector spinae and obliquus externus abdominis muscle activity is greatest when the thoracolumbar region is extended; and activity of the extensor muscles is minimal in slumped sitting.[156,160] Swayback postures involve a tendency to "hang" on the obliquus externus abdominis muscle as a result of the more posterior alignment of the upper trunk relative to the pelvis.

Although this proposed "ideal" postural alignment is unlikely to be ideal for all individuals (for reasons such as pathology [e.g., spinal stenosis], spinal segmental mobility, function, habitual postures and movements, anthropometric features [e.g., lumbosacral angle], and other issues), it serves as a starting point for identification of features that can be evaluated for relevance to pain. In a way, it is the basic blueprint for postural alignment that acts as a starting point for assessment, but this needs to be molded by the specific presentation of the patient to identify the postural alignment that is ideal for their unique individual situation. If a feature of postural alignment is identified that deviates from ideal, it can be modified to assess the relationship to pain/muscle activation. If correction changes symptoms and/or reduces overactivity of muscle, then the feature is likely to be relevant to consider in planning of the motor control training program.

The key to application of motor control training for correction of posture or postural alignment is careful assessment to identify the features that are relevant to the patient's symptoms, and the evaluation of the outcome for his or her symptoms when specific features are modified. Clinicians have a host of techniques available to them to assist the patient in "correcting" the suboptimal

features of motor control and a trial and error approach to find the best solution is advocated.

Assessment and Treatment Goal Planning. Assessment of posture and postural alignment is undertaken in a range of positions. In addition to the specific posture that a patient indicates is problematic, it is common to assess posture in sitting and standing. There is a broad range of features that are considered (Table 14-1). The relevance of a specific feature of postural alignment for the patient's presentation can be supported if successful modification of the features makes a positive change in symptoms and/or reduces muscle overactivity/hyperactivity. In many patients, it will be possible to identify a predictable mechanical response to changes in posture and postural alignment, but this is not always the case. Considering the fact that pain has a nonlinear relationship to nociceptive input (see section "Neurobiology of Pain"), it is not surprising that for some patients there is no clear mechanical presentation to their symptoms, and a precise relationship between posture and pain may not be forthcoming. Furthermore, in some cases pain may be provoked only by prolonged posture. In these cases it may be more helpful to consider the optimization of muscle activity as an indicator of the target alignment.

At the conclusion of the assessment, the clinician records a list of key features that have been identified as having a relationship to the patient's symptoms. This list should be ranked in order of importance and highlighted for reference throughout the progression of rehabilitation of the patient. The optimization of posture and postural alignment can achieve a number of interconnected goals, which are outlined in Table 14-2.

Training. Training of posture and postural alignment involves identification of a strategy to modify the features that were identified to be relevant for the patient's presentation in the assessment and prioritized in treatment planning. Many possible training strategies are available, and once trialed, the strategy's outcome must be assessed. It is acceptable for the new posture to feel "odd" or "awkward," but it should not be painful or difficult to hold (i.e., it should not require substantial muscle activity to maintain the posture). This requires consideration of pathology if known (e.g., in advanced spinal stenosis, it is likely that pain will be provoked by trying to adopt a lordotic lumbar curve) and the individual patient's presentation. According to the principles of motor learning, the patient should be given a strategy to cognitively correct the posture with a feedback method to ensure he or she has performed the correct modification (e.g., feedback with mirror, manual cues). Once identified, training may commence with a few sessions throughout the day as a home program to learn to change posture. This should be progressed to frequent adoption of the posture at regular intervals throughout the day as required by the functions being performed. Table 14-3 presents a range of strategies that may be helpful to modify posture.

TABLE **14-1**

Assessment of Posture and Postural Alignment: Features Assessed for Deviation Relative to "Ideal" Posture and Relevance for Symptoms

Sagittal alignment/sagittal balance	• Alignment of C7 over sacrum; or manubriosternal junction over symphysis pubis o Sway (thorax posterior to pelvis), kyphotic/slump (thorax forward of the pelvis)

Spinal curves	• Start and finish of sagittal spinal curves, depth of curves
	  o Lumbar lordosis
	  o Thoracic kyphosis
	  o Transition from thoracic kyphosis and lumbar lordosis (i.e., flat, flexed, or extended at the thoracolumbar junction)
	  o Cervical lordosis and level head position
	• Segmental changes, such as segmental lordosis, segmental lumbar kyphosis (i.e., flexion at lumbosacral junction)
	• Pelvic position
	  o Anterior/posterior tilt; look at relation of anterior superior iliac spines to posterior superior iliac spines

Frontal plane (front/back)	• Lateral shift/list upper trunk • Pelvis lateral tilt/rotation • Right/left weight bearing • Scoliosis: structural versus functional • Infrasternal angle symmetry

Muscle activity	• Assessed with observation, palpation, electromyography, ultrasound imaging
	  o Hypertrophy/atrophy
	  o Hyperactivity/hypoactivity
	  o Asymmetry

Posture/postural alignment of adjacent segments	• Lower limb, including the feet
	  o Hip: flexed, neutral, extended, adducted, rotated
	  o Knee: flexed, neutral, (hyper)extended, medial (internal)/lateral (external) rotation of tibia and/or femur
	  o Foot/ankle: pronated/supinated
	• Shoulder girdle: scapular position and stability
	• Neck/thorax

TABLE **14-2**

Training Goals of Posture and Postural Alignment

Optimize lumbopelvic loading	• Avoid postures that do the following:
	  o Provoke pain
	  o Are difficult to maintain
	• Encourage postures that do the following:
	  o Relieve pain
	  o Correct asymmetry
	  o Minimize activity of hyperactive muscles (often superficial/global muscles)
	  o Enhance activity of hypoactive muscles (often deep/local muscles, but not limited to these muscles)
	• Avoid prolonged postures.
	• Encourage flexible use of posture/posture change.

Optimize respiratory pattern	• Change in posture will influence breathing pattern[159]
Optimize control of pelvic floor muscles	• Change in posture will influence pelvic floor muscle activity[158]

Clinical Approach to Motor Control Training of Muscle Activation

Principles. Activation of muscles of the lumbopelvic region influences the control of posture and postural alignment, and movement. Depending on the individual patient, modification of muscle activation may be the initial target for treatment. Alternatively, it may be easier to change muscle activation by modifying posture and postural alignment, or easier to modify posture and postural alignment, or movement by first changing muscle activation. Data from clinical trials highlight the value of detailed consideration of muscle activation. Motor control

TABLE **14-3**

Example Techniques for Correction of Posture and Postural Alignment

Instructions	• Verbal instructions are to guide the patient to modify the target feature of posture.
	• Examples:
	  ○ "Roll forward on your tailbone" to improve anterior tilt and lordosis of the lumbar spine; "breathe into base of ribs" to remove excessive extension of the thoracolumbar junction
	  ○ "Grow tall"
	  ○ "Position (or lift) ischial tuberosities while sitting, avoiding flexion at the lumbosacral junction"
	  ○ "Check that the shoulder girdle is relaxed"

Imagery (visual and proprioceptive)	• A "mental image" is selected that aids the patient to gain the understanding of the change that is required. • Example: ○ "Lengthening" of the spine may help reduce thoracic kyphosis

Manual guidance	• The clinician's or patient's hands may be placed on the patient's body to guide motion toward the corrected position.
	• Examples:
	  ○ Hand on sacrum to provide guidance of anterior rotation of the pelvis
	  ○ Hand on the thoracolumbar junction to provide guidance to relax into flattening in this region

Manual cues	• The patient places his or her hands on key landmarks of the body as a reference to monitor position/alignment. • Example: ○ Little finger and thumb of one hand on the xiphoid and navel to monitor the distance between these two landmarks as indirect feedback of changes in the angle of the thoracolumbar junction (i.e., distance reduces and increases with thoracolumbar flexion and extension)

"Dissociation" tasks	• Guidance is provided to change the relative motion of adjacent body regions.
	• Examples:
	  ○ "Waiter's bow" exercise to teach a patient to flex at the hips rather than flex the lumbar spine
	  ○ Attention to control of thoracolumbar junction curvature while rotating the pelvis and lower lumbar spine

Muscle activation	• Techniques are used to either increase or decrease activity of muscle(s) to aid movement to a specific posture.
	• Examples:
	  ○ Augmented feedback of muscle activity to aid in increasing or decreasing activity (by palpation, observation, electromyography, ultrasound imaging or biofeedback)
	  ○ Application of techniques to directly or indirectly change activity such as manual therapies (articular mobilization; connective tissue massage)
	  ○ Use of serratus anterior activation (reversed origin insertion) to facilitate a thoracic kyphosis

Cues/reminders	• Tape is applied to remind the patient to adjust posture if it is no longer maintained.
	• Examples:
	  ○ Application of therapeutic tape to the spine when positioned in lordosis to provide feedback by stretch sensation if curvature flattens; a software program that flashes a reminder on the computer screen at predetermined intervals
	  ○ Photos taken to show patient his or her posture in different positions; sticky dots placed over the tragus, middle of the shoulder (anteroposterior), middle of the hip, middle of the knee and anterior to the lateral malleolus to demonstrate the appropriate line of gravity

training approaches can successfully change muscle activation.[161,162] Furthermore, several studies have shown that a patient's ability to activate muscles at baseline predicts his or her response to motor control training,[163,164] and the degree of improvement of muscle activation is related to clinical improvement.[163–165] In a general sense, muscle activation may be either too much or too little, and these extremes of muscle activation may both present for different muscles in the same patient. Muscles may also present with inadequate strength and endurance. Furthermore, muscles may be atrophied or have undergone a process of structural remodeling with increased fat and connective tissue. There is considerable interindividual variation with respect to the muscles that are involved and the manner in which the muscle activation is changed. Clinical strategies to subgroup patients based on their motor control presentation can aid identification of common patterns of modified muscle activation, and can facilitate the clinical reasoning required for treatment selection. A rule of thumb is that a first step should be to correct the pattern of activation before adding a load to induce change in strength, endurance, and structure.[166]

There is no uniform strategy for training muscle activation and no single muscle that requires training in all patients. Instead, the strategy of motor control training depends on detailed assessment to identify suboptimal features of the muscle activation strategy. Ideally an assessment might involve detailed assessment of muscle activation used in multiple functions against known standards of muscle activation. Although clear in principle, this is difficult in reality because it would necessitate assessment of muscle activation with invasive procedures and detailed understanding of each task. In lieu of this complexity, specialized tests have been developed to provide insight into the features of the pattern of muscle activity that require training for an individual patient. The outcome of these tests is combined with insight gained from evaluation of the muscle activation patterns the patient uses in different postures and movements. Once the feature(s) of muscle activation that require attention have been identified, the challenge is then to find a technique that will encourage change in muscle recruitment and then transfer of the improved muscle activation pattern to function through progression of exercise.

Assessment and Treatment Goal Planning. Assessment of muscle activation strategy is complicated by difficulty associated with accurate assessment of muscle function in clinical practice in the absence of invasive recording methods. Although it may be relatively straightforward to assess the strength of a limb muscle by investigation of developed torque, when the target of assessment is to evaluate the quality of motor control, it is important to consider the subtle control of timing and amplitude of activity during the performance of a movement, and that requires consideration of muscles that are superficial and easily accessed plus deep muscles that cannot be easily assessed. Every time a patient moves and every posture he or she adopts will provide some information of muscle activation strategies, although methods to quantify activation are not readily available. As an alternative, assessments can be performed that evaluate a patient's ability to activate specific muscles. Table 14-4 presents details of the tests used to assess the potential impairment of activation of the deeper muscles of the trunk and any individual specific pattern of over activation of the more superficial muscles. The results of these tests have been shown to relate to the manner in which the muscles are functionally activated[167] and clinical rating scales (Table 14-5) are available to quantify the performance. These scales are repeatable and can discriminate between individuals with and without LBP.[168]

TABLE 14-4

Assessment of Muscle Activation: Test of Independent Activation of Deep Trunk Muscles to Determine the Ability of Patient to Activate the Deep Trunk Muscles and Any Strategy for Overactivity of the Superficial Trunk Muscles

Test principle	• Evaluate ability to activate short/deep muscles independently from long/superficial muscles; outcome is related to quality of control of the muscle during function.[167]
Task	• Ability to cognitively perform the motor skill of contraction of the transversus abdominis or multifidus muscle independently from the other superficial trunk muscles. Assessments have also been devised along similar principles for psoas and pelvic floor muscles, to name a few.
Measure	• Precision 　o Which muscles? 　　– By observation, palpation, electromyography, ultrasound imaging 　　– Aim for independent activation of deep muscle(s) without activation of the superficial muscles 　o What sequence? 　o What quality? 　　– Smooth, symmetrical, slow • Ideal response 　o Palpable slow gentle increase in tension of deep muscle 　o Co-contraction with other deep muscles 　o No or little activity of superficial muscles 　o Symmetrical contraction 　o Smooth and sustained (not jerky) contraction 　o Normal breathing 　o Repeat multiple contractions (up to 10×10 seconds)
Interpretation	• Ability to activate specific deep muscles equals well-controlled activation during function with relevance for predicting treatment efficacy.[163] • Strategy of hyperactivity of superficial trunk muscles. This generally forms the foundation (in addition to information gleaned from assessment of posture and movement) of identification of the muscles that may require reduction in activity to optimize load on the spine/pelvis.

TABLE 14-5

Clinical Rating Scale to Assess Quality of Muscle Contraction and Interaction between Deep and Superficial Muscles

Criteria	Score
Quality of Contraction	
No contraction	0
Rapid superficial contraction	1
Just perceptible contraction	2
Good quality gentle slow contraction	3
Substitution	
Resting substitution	0
Moderate to strong substitution	1
Subtle perceptible substitution	2
No substitution	3
Symmetry	
Unilateral contraction	0
Bilateral but asymmetrical contraction	1
Symmetrical contraction	2
Breathing	
Inability or difficulty with breathing during contraction	0
Able to hold contraction while maintaining breathing	1
Holding	
Hold <10 seconds	0
Hold ≥10 seconds	1

Training muscle activation aims to encourage a strategy of muscle activation that maintains optimal load on the spine and pelvis, by a combination of increasing and decreasing muscle activity as indicated by assessment of the individual patient. The outcome of the test will indicate whether deep muscles require training and, if so, which specific muscles are involved. The test will also identify which of the more superficial muscles is potentially overactive or hyperactive and require "downtraining." As with posture and postural alignment correction, training of muscle activation may achieve several goals (Table 14-6).

Training. Every attempt to modify motor control, including those that target posture and postural alignment, and movement will influence muscle activation. Although in some cases simply addressing posture and movement may be sufficient, for many, attention must also be placed on changing muscle activation patterns directly. Many techniques have been described in clinical practice to explicitly target changing muscle activation in order to modify the load on the tissues of the spine and pelvis; either by enhancing muscle activation to improve control of aberrant movement or reducing muscle activation to decrease overload. Some of these techniques are presented in Table 14-7.

As a basic principle it is necessary to identify (1) a strategy that works best for the patient to modify his or her pattern of muscle activation, which will generally include components that achieve the best contraction of underactive/hypoactive components and reduce overactive/hyperactive components; (2) a feedback technique so that the patient can be sure that he or she is practicing the correct exercise at home; and (3) the number of contractions and duration of holding that the patient can perform

TABLE 14-6

Training Goals of Muscle Activation

Optimize lumbopelvic loading	• Avoid muscle activity that does the following:
	  o Provokes pain by overloading tissues
	  o Prevents an ideal posture or motion path
	• Encourage muscle activity that does the following:
	  o Relieves pain
	  o Improves control by reducing aberrant motion or enables a more ideal loading strategy of posture or movement
	  o Corrects asymmetry
	  o Minimizes activity of overactive/hyperactive muscles (often superficial/global muscles)
	  o Enhances activity of underactive/hypoactive muscles (often deep/local muscles, but not limited to these muscles)
	• Avoid prolonged postures
	• Encourage variation in muscle activation strategy to "share the load"
	• Encourage functional use of improved muscle activation patterns in postures and movements

Optimize breathing pattern	
Optimize control of pelvic floor muscles	
Aim to increase endurance in muscles which control spinal posture	

TABLE **14-7**

Example Techniques to Train Muscle Activation

Techniques to reduce activity of overactive/hyperactive lumbopelvic muscles	• Whole body posture (in general, more activity requires more support to encourage reduction) • Spinal posture (in general, "neutral" spinal alignment involves less activity of superficial muscles) • Instruction • Breathing techniques • Feedback (e.g., electromyography, palpation) • Decreased effort • Connective tissue techniques, trigger point, dry needling • Inhibitory taping • Imagery
Techniques to increase activity of underactive/hypoactive lumbopelvic muscles	• Whole body posture (stretch on muscle) • Spinal posture (greater activity in neutral) • Instruction • Co-contraction with other muscles to facilitate contraction (e.g., pelvic floor muscles can be used to encourage improved contraction of transversus abdominis[169]) • Manual facilitation • Imagery • Feedback (i.e., observation, palpation, ultrasound imaging) • Taping

while maintaining the contraction quality. With this information, it is possible to design an effective home program for the patient to practice for two to three sessions per day initially. Progression involves increased hold time/repetition and decreased feedback. The aim is for a "confident" correction of the muscle activation strategy that can be performed independently, cognitively, with minimal feedback, minimal effort, held for at least 10 seconds, and all while the patient breathes normally.

Clinical Approach to Motor Control Training of Movement

Principles. As for the other components of the approach, motor control training that addresses movement aims to change features that are identified in the assessment as having relevance for a patient's symptoms. Features of movements may be relevant because they load the tissues through motion into a provocative position, they involve provocative muscle activation, or they may load the tissues inappropriately as a result of too much or too little control. There are many potential underlying mechanisms. For instance, movement may excessively load the spine secondary to poor interaction between adjacent body regions (e.g., movement of the spine instead of the hip), suboptimal postures, or suboptimal muscle activation. The principles for training are similar to those outlined for posture and postural alignment, with the exception that the goal of training is the control of a trajectory of dynamic movement rather than a specific position. As for the other elements of motor control, there is not a single feature that requires training in all individuals, and treatment must be targeted to the individual presentation after careful and detailed assessment. The clinician's goal is to find a clinical tool or technique to aid the patient to change his or her movement strategy. The key to

successful correction of movement is the accuracy of the assessment of the relevance of motor control for the patient's presentation (i.e., is the movement feature relevant to symptoms?) and the assessment of the outcome of the application of a treatment technique (has the technique made a difference to movement?). As outlined in section "Patient Subgrouping," a major focus in the recent clinical literature has been the identification of clinical subgroups; clusters of features that characterize a specific patient presentation. Subgrouping methods that include careful analysis of movement include those described by Sahrmann,[92] O'Sullivan,[142] and McKenzie.[141] The objective is to simplify the clinical reasoning approach by aiding the identification of patterns that can help the clinician select an appropriate course of treatment. Movement presentation forms a key element of many subgrouping approaches.[144] As always, careful assessment is critical.

Assessment and Treatment Goal Planning. For guidance of motor control training, movement assessment focuses on identification of features of movement that are related to symptoms and include feature(s) that suboptimally load the tissues in a manner that could be responsible for the development, provocation, or maintenance of symptoms. Identification of relevant features is guided by the pain response, comparison of the movement strategy against the expected optimal strategy for the task, and/or the muscle response. In addition to the observation of the movement, it is critical to consider the starting posture or position, as this will make an impact on the ensuing movement (e.g., motion of the lumbar spine during a function will differ depending on whether the lumbar region starts in a position of flexion or extension). Movement strategy can be assessed in several ways: (1) physiological movements (e.g., flexion in standing), (2) specific functional tasks (e.g., sit-to-stand),

(3) formal movement tests (e.g., assessment of dissociation of hip rotation from motion of the spine in prone), and (4) the functional task(s) that the patient indicates is problematic. In each case, the movement is observed in detail. Table 14-8 summarizes key principles of assessment of movement.

Similar to posture correction, strategies to change movement have many goals; these include, but are not limited to, changing movement to avoid provocative movements. Again, the key distinction is that, for movement correction, the objective is to change aspects that

TABLE **14-8**

Elements of Assessment of Movement Control Incorporating Tests from Multiple Subgrouping Paradigms

Features of Movement Evaluated	
Evaluation of changes in sagittal/frontal/transverse alignment during movement	• Timing • Amplitude • Sequence
Evaluation of muscle activity	• For example, palpation, observation, electromyography, ultrasound imaging
Evaluation of posture/ movement of adjacent segments and ability to dissociate movement of lumbopelvic region from adjacent segments	• Lumbar versus hip • Lumbar versus thoracolumbar junction • Lower limb and feet • Shoulder girdle • Neck/thorax

Specific Movement Tests	

Basic physiological movements	• Flexion in standing
	  o Observe for loss of motion, increased lumbar flexion/lateral shift, increased lumbar extension, increased thoracolumbar extension, increased posterior/anterior pelvic tilt, relationship between hip and lumbar motion
	• Return from flexion in standing
	  o Observe for relationship between hip and lumbar motion, increased thoracolumbar extension, anterior pelvic sway, increased or decreased extension, anterior pelvic rotation
	• Extension
	• Side bending (lateral flexion)
	• Side "glide"
	• Rotation
	• Response to axial loading

Standardized functional movement	• Sit-to-stand
	  o Stand after placing spine in neutral
	  o Observe ability to maintain lumbar lordosis; observe where the movement is initiated, increased lumbar flexion, decreased lumbar extension, increased thoracolumbar extension, increased posterior pelvic tilt, anterior pelvic sway, medial hip rotation, relationship between hip, and lumbar motion
	• Squat
	  o Observe ability to maintain lumbar lordosis; observe for increased lumbar flexion, decreased lumbar extension, increased thoracolumbar extension, increased posterior pelvic tilt, medial hip rotation, relationship between hip and lumbar motion
	  o Include single leg squat and minisquat
	• Single leg stance
	  o Observe ability to control pelvic/trunk movement during single leg stance; observe for Trendelenburg sign (i.e., drop of pelvis on side of lifted leg), lateral shift of thorax/ lateral flexion, medial hip rotation, pelvic sway
	  o Pelvic rotation
	  o Weight through heels not toes
	• Rolling
	  o Observe rotation of trunk and effect of control of rotation of trunk
	• Gait
	  o Observe for symmetry between sides, decreased motion, excessive pelvic rotation, relationship between hip and lumbar motion, increased lumbar flexion/lateral shift, increased thoracolumbar extension, increased anterior/posterior pelvic rotation, lack of thoracic rotation, limping

(Continued)

TABLE **14-8**

Elements of Assessment of Movement Control Incorporating Tests from Multiple Subgrouping Paradigms—cont'd

Specific Movement Tests

Specific movement tests	• Slump/rock backward in sitting
	• Sit upright/erect in sitting
	  o Observe for inability to move lumbar spine and pelvis independently from thoracolumbar regions
	• Neutral repositioning test in sitting
	  o Place in neutral, fully slump and return
	    – Observe for flexion at symptomatic segment
	  o Bend forward while maintaining neutral position
	    – Observe for flexion at symptomatic segment
	• Knee extension with ankle dorsiflexion
	  o Observe for inability to dissociate hip from spine
	• Hip abduction/lateral rotation with hips and knees flexed in supine
	  o Observe for ability to move hip independently of lumbar spine and pelvis, asymmetry
	• Knee flexion (active and passive) in prone
	  o Observe for pelvic rotation, anterior pelvic tilt
	• Hip rotation medial and lateral (active and passive) in prone
	  o Observe for pelvic rotation
	• Hip and knee extension in prone
	  o Observe for excessive lumbar extension or segmental extension, absence of gluteal muscle activation, excessive trunk rotation
	• Hip abduction/lateral rotation in side lying with heels together
	  o Observe for pelvic rotation
	• Hip and knee flexion in supine
	  o Observe for lumbar flexion, pelvic rotation with lumbar extension
	• Anterior pelvic rotation in supine
	  o Observe for ability to rotate pelvis and extend lumbar spine independent of thoracolumbar junction
	• Posterior pelvic rotation in supine
	  o Observe for ability to rotate pelvis and extend lumbar spine independent of hip
	• Lateral pelvic rotation in supine
	  o Observe for ability to rotate pelvis independent of thoracolumbar junction and hip
	• Four point kneeling
	  o Rock back and forward
	    – Observe for relative motion of hips and lumbar spine, hip motion independent of thoracolumbar junction, lateral deviation of pelvis, lumbar rotation
	  o Arm lift
	    – Observe for lumbar rotation
	  o Anterior and posterior pelvic tilt
	    – Observe for relative motion of lumbar spine and thoracolumbar junction, lateral deviation

Muscle length/stiffness tests	• Tensor fasciae latae, rectus femoris, psoas (Thomas test) • Hamstrings in supine • Paraspinal muscles • Tensor fasciae latae/iliotibial band in side-lying (Ober's test)

load the tissues suboptimally in a dynamic sense as the spine and pelvis move through a trajectory. Table 14-9 includes a summary of the multiple goals that may be targeted with correction of movement, each with varying relevance for individual patients.

Training. Training movement control aims to find a clinical technique to change movement such that it is performed in a manner that more optimally loads the tissues. A range of training techniques is available to encourage a change in movement strategy. After each technique is trialed, it is critical to identify whether the desired modification of movement has been achieved. It is acceptable for the new movement to feel "odd" or "unusual," but it should not be painful or difficult to maintain (i.e., muscle activity required to control the movement should not be excessive). As for posture or postural alignment correction, the target movement needs to be considered with respect to pathology (if it is known) and the individual patient's motor control presentation. The objective is to find an optimal method to modify the target feature(s) of

TABLE **14-9**

Training Goals for Movement Correction

Optimize lumbopelvic loading	• Avoid movements that do the following:
	○ Provoke pain
	○ Are difficult to maintain because of high muscular effort
	• Encourage movements that do the following:
	○ Relieve pain
	○ Correct asymmetry
	○ Correct specific movement faults
	– Dissociation between regions
	– Poor control at a specific segment/region
	– Maintain spinal alignment (e.g., lumbar lordosis, thoracic kyphosis and cervical lordosis)
	○ Minimize activity of overactive/hyperactive muscles (often superficial/global muscles)
	○ Enhance activity of underactive/hypoactive muscles (often deep/local muscles, but not limited to these muscles)
	• Avoid prolonged postures.
	• Encourage flexible use of posture and postural change
Optimize respiratory pattern	
Optimize control of pelvic floor muscles	

movement and identify a feedback technique (e.g., palpation, visual feedback with mirror) that the patient can use to confirm the correct performance. The home program commences with practice of the skill during a few sessions throughout the day and adoption of the corrected movement pattern as able during function.

Techniques to Correct Individual Specific Movement Faults

- Instructions (e.g., maintain lordosis when bending)
- Imagery (e.g., visual and proprioceptive)
- Manual guidance (e.g., hand on sacrum to facilitate anterior rotation of pelvis)
- Manual cues (e.g., finger on xiphoid and navel to control thoracolumbar junction)
- Dissociation tasks (e.g., separate lumbar from thoracolumbar junction motion, "waiter's bow")
- Muscle activation (e.g., palpation, observation, EMG biofeedback)
- Cues/reminders (e.g., taping)

Clinical Approach to Progression of Motor Control Training

Once a patient has mastered the skills to control posture and postural alignment, muscle activation, and movement, the next step is to challenge patients through a range of progressions to consolidate the improved motor control strategies and to challenge the patient for readiness for more challenging and more functional contexts. The program presented in Figure 14-10 shows a sequence through static and dynamic progressions, ultimately leading to function. The program also considers factors that may need to be included if they present as barriers for an individual patient. The following sections provide an overview of the principles applied in each progression.

Progression of Motor Control of the Spine and Pelvis with Static Training. Many clinical programs are available to progressively add load to progress training of control of static alignment of the spine and pelvis. In this phase, the patient is encouraged to maintain specific alignment of the spine and pelvis while load is applied to the trunk either directly or via limb movement or loading. Although many approaches begin training with this type of exercise from the outset, the alternative view promoted in this chapter is that the patient should first be trained to correct the relevant features of posture and postural alignment, muscle activation, and movement, and then train the control under load as a progression once he or she is confident with the correction. The basic sequence involves (1) correction of spine and pelvic alignment, (2) enhancement of contraction of the deep muscles, and (3) application of load or resistance to encourage activation of the more superficial muscles. The key feature that is monitored in the static phase of training is the ability to maintain the alignment of the spine and pelvis. If alignment cannot be maintained, then the load needs to be reduced to the point at which the control is challenged but not overcome. It is important to assess the threshold load that can be tolerated before control of alignment is lost; and any asymmetries in the control of alignment (such as lower threshold for loss of control of alignment in one direction when load is applied into rotation). The goals of static training are presented in Tables 14-10 and 14-11, which provide an overview of some common approaches to target this aspect of training.

Dynamic Control of the Spine and Pelvis and Motor Control Training. Training of dynamic control of the spine and pelvis follows the same overall principle as static progression (i.e., to monitor the patient's ability to control features of motor control while the spine is challenged). Although the goal in static progression is straightforward (i.e., to monitor and control of alignment of the spine and pelvis), the goal in dynamic progression is more complex. Every different movement has a different "ideal" against which the patient's performance is being judged. The clinician must have an understanding of the ideal performance of the task and a clear understanding of the patient's individual suboptimal features from the

TABLE **14-10**

Training Goals of Static Progression

Correct relevant features of motor control while the system is loaded	• Train integration of correct muscle activation • Train integration of correct posture and postural alignment • Train integration of correct movement (e.g., dissociation of hip from spine)

Focus on improving static control of lumbopelvic orientation/alignment	• Increase threshold load amplitude before loss of control of alignment
	• Target specific deficits in muscle system (e.g., asymmetries in load tolerance)
	• Target the functional needs of the patient
	• Train endurance
	• Progress by the following:
	  o Load
	    – ↑ Lever length
	    – ↑ Load/resistance
	  o Position
	    – Supported
	    – Unsupported
	  o Dynamic
	    – ↑ Speed of movement
	    – ↑ Instability

TABLE **14-11**

Example Clinical Options for Static Progression

Strategy	Principles	Example Exercises
Leg loading	In crook lying, load is applied in a progressive manner by moving the legs in different planes of motion. The patient is instructed to maintain the position of the spine and pelvis.	Bent knee fall-outs: leg is slowly lowered to the side while maintaining the position of the pelvis and spine. The position of the spine and pelvis can be monitored with a pressure biofeedback unit. Specific directions of greater and lesser control can be identified by directions of movement that are associated with loss of control of alignment.
Rhythmic stabilizations (proprioceptive neuromuscular facilitation)	The patient maintains a neutral position as force is applied to the body. Force is normally low (~30%), and the direction slowly alternates.	In sitting with neutral alignment, a rotary force can be applied to the shoulders in alternating directions. During the change in direction, the activation of the superficial muscles alternates over the top of the tonically maintained activation of the deeper muscles.
Limb loading	The neutral position of the spine is maintained in any body position as load is applied first through short levers (i.e., bent limbs) and then through longer levers with the limbs straight.	In a quadruped position, the position of the spine is maintained in neutral as either the arm or leg or both are moved to the side or in the sagittal plane. Postural preparations are required to ensure the center of mass is placed over the new base of support.
Pilates	Load is applied though the use of limb load, springs, and other equipment as the spine is maintained in a neutral position.	On a Pilates Reformer Bed® (sliding bed with springs adjusted to resist the motion of the bed), the patient precontracts the deep muscles and maintains the neutral position as the sliding surface is translated by extension and flexion of the bed. Although this technique often involves movement on expiration, it may be more ideal to train movement with both phases of breathing.
Large exercise balls	The neutral position of the spine is maintained while the body is partly or completely supported on a ball. Load can be added by addition of limb load.	Patients can sit in neutral on a large ball with the hips above 90°. Load can be applied by reduction of the base of support (e.g., lifting a leg) or by increasing the load (e.g., by movement of the arms or legs).

assessment of movement. Progression of training through dynamic control requires an individualized approach and requires greater skill of assessment and training to be able to ensure that the patient is successful and that he or she is sufficiently challenged.

The goals of dynamic training are presented in Table 14-12. Two common approaches to dynamic progression are (1) exercises that challenge control of the spine as it moves and (2) exercises that challenge control of the spine during dynamic balance control (e.g., unstable surfaces). In both of these situations the aim is to challenge the spine by increasing the requirement to move, and the patient aims to control the features of movement that were identified on the initial assessment to be problematic (e.g., feedback to maintain lumbar lordosis and not move into lumbar flexion while standing on a balance board). Care must be taken to ensure progression

occurs at a rate the patient can control, and not too fast. Table 14-13 presents common treatment approaches that may be applied in this phase of training.

Functional Retraining of Control of the Spine and Pelvis and Motor Control Training. A critical element of progression of exercise to function is that the best transfer to function is achieved the closer an exercise is to the function being targeted. The static and dynamic progressions discussed in preceding sections should ideally be linked to the functional needs of the patient, and the functional retraining phase of a motor control approach should be merely an extension of these earlier phases to ensure that the functional tasks that the patient highlighted in the initial assessment, or those that the patient continues to experience problems with are addressed.

The goal of functional retraining in the context of motor control training is to ensure that the correction

TABLE **14-12**

Training Goals of Dynamic Progression

Correct relevant features of motor control while the system is loaded dynamically	• Train integration of correct muscle activation • Train integration of correct posture and postural alignment • Train integration of correct movement (e.g., dissociation of hip from spine)

Focus on improved dynamic control of lumbopelvic movement	• Train control during changes in lumbopelvic position
	• Train incorporation of lumbopelvic movement into simple dynamic functions
	• Increase threshold load amplitude before loss of control of alignment
	• Target specific deficits in muscle system (e.g., asymmetries in load tolerance)
	• Target the functional needs of the patient
	• Train endurance
	• Progress by the following:
	  o Load
	    – ↑ Lever length
	    – ↑ Load/resistance
	  o Position
	    – Supported
	    – Unsupported
	  o Dynamic
	    – ↑ Speed of movement
	    – ↑ Instability

TABLE **14-13**

Example Clinical Options for Dynamic Progression

Strategy	Principles	Example Exercises
Unstable surfaces	The patient aims to maintain balance and alignment of the trunk when placed on an unstable surface. To maintain balance, movement of the spine is necessary, because it is impossible to maintain balance simply by control at the ankle. Careful attention is made to the features of muscle activity, alignment and/or movement that were identified to be poorly controlled in the assessment.	Balance boards Therapy balls
Function-specific tasks	Specific movements that are required for function are trained. The movement is segmented, simplified, and performed with reduced speed and reduced load.	Walking (progressing from side-side weight shift), trunk rotation

of motor control issues is integrated into function. Assessment of function relies on the principles described for dynamic and static progression and requires careful evaluation of the individual patient's key features of motor control (posture and postural alignment, muscle activation and movement) during the performance of the functional task. The target functions are assessed to determine which features are related to their symptoms. Those features are then modified using the skills the patients have learned in the early phase of correction and have reinforced through the phases of static and dynamic progression. It is necessary to draw on the principles of motor learning (i.e., segmentation, simplification and feedback) to optimize correction of performance of the function. Patients are challenged with increasing demand up to the intensity required for their natural performance. Clinical Application of Strategies to Manage Barriers to Recovery. In addition to attention to correction of the basic elements of motor control, comprehensive management of a patient's symptoms may require consideration of other issues that can commonly present as barriers to recovery for an individual patient. Although the effect of many of these issues may only be minor for many, in some patients, these

issues require careful attention in exercise prescription to achieve clinical change. The challenge for the clinician is to determine the importance of a potential barrier and to determine the amount of time and effort to devote to assessment and management. Table 14-14 presents a range of common barriers that may require consideration.

EVIDENCE FOR EFFICACY OF MOTOR CONTROL EXERCISES FOR SPINAL AND PELVIC PAIN

As described in the previous sections, rehabilitation of dynamic control of the spine and pelvis involves a motor learning approach targeted at all aspects of motor control. The intervention therefore involves more than a set of simple exercises targeted at specific muscles. Instead, the approach requires the clinician's attention to assessment of movement, posture and postural alignment, muscle activation (including detecting signs of overactivity and underactivity of specific muscle groups), in combination with consideration of other features including breathing, continence, balance, sensory function, and beliefs and attitudes about pain. Few clinical trials have investigated a comprehensive intervention. Most studies have been

TABLE **14-14**

Common Barriers to Training

Beliefs and attitudes	• Unhealthy attitudes and beliefs about back pain may compromise the attainment of motor control goals (e.g., fear of pain may encourage protective strategies). • Assessment and management of fear, catastrophizing, and pain coping skills may be required.
Breathing	• Because trunk muscles are involved in breathing and trunk control, modification of breathing pattern may challenge the control of the spine. • Careful assessment of the interaction of these functions and the effect of increased respiratory demand may be required.
Pelvic floor muscle function	• Issues of continence, pelvic organ support, and pelvic pain can all involve modified activation of the pelvic floor and abdominal muscles, which may interfere with progression of training for lumbopelvic control. • Specific assessment of the pelvic floor muscle dysfunction may be required.
Adjacent body regions	• Poor control of adjacent regions of the body will affect lumbopelvic control. • Biomechanical and neuromuscular interactions between the lower limbs and lumbopelvic region (e.g., pronation of the feet can lead to internal [medial] rotation of the femurs and anterior pelvic tilt), and between neck-thorax-shoulder require assessment and management if relevant.
Balance	• Patients with lumbopelvic pain often present with balance problems either secondary to reduced spinal motion (which is necessary for balance control) or poor sensory function of the spine.
Sensory function	• Training of posture and postural alignment, muscle activation, and movement includes a major sensory component associated with perception of incorrect and correct control of each element. • In some patients, additional attention to sensation may be required if it presents as a major factor.
Strength and endurance	• Although a major focus of motor control training is coordination of muscle activity, it is also necessary to address muscle strength and endurance if these features are compromised. • This may be particularly relevant in a more chronic context where structural remodeling of muscle (i.e., increased fat and connective tissue) is present. • Loading should not be commenced until muscle activity, alignment and/or movement can be controlled adequately.
Fitness	• Many patients with chronic pain are deconditioned and require general fitness training. • This should be commenced once the patient can control movement.

limited to investigation of the training of activation of the deep trunk muscles (i.e., transversus abdominis and MF) in isolation from the more superficial muscles. In some trials this is progressed to control of the muscles during static control of the trunk while adding load to the trunk via movement of the extremities. Furthermore, in most cases the intervention is applied in a generic manner, without individualization and to a participant group of nonspecific LBP. Unfortunately, most clinical studies include a limited description of the exercise intervention. If the description of the intervention is unclear, judging whether the study should be used to assess the efficacy of the intervention becomes difficult.

Several systematic reviews have been published that review the available literature and include meta-analysis of the outcomes.[1,170,171] These reviews conclude that motor control training is efficacious for reducing pain and/or disability in low back and pelvic pain. However, the comparison with other treatments remains unclear. A major limitation of the previous systematic reviews is the limited consideration of the content of the clinical program or the study population. This section provides an overview of evidence of efficacy of motor control training for spinal and pelvic pain with specific attention to these two aspects. The evidence discussed is restricted to studies that are conducted as randomized, controlled studies. A typical randomized, controlled study involves patients with a specific condition who are randomly allocated to a controlled group or to a group receiving the treatment of interest. To assess the efficacy of motor control exercises, only information provided by good quality studies is used. Good quality studies usually have a score of at least 3 on the 0-10 PEDro scale. The PEDro scale assesses the quality of randomized, controlled trials based on criteria such as allocation of patients and eligibility criteria.[172]

Randomized, controlled trials that included at least one exercise intervention that could be considered to involve elements of the motor control approach were identified. The comparison group could include no intervention, other exercise interventions, and other interventions, such as manual therapy techniques. Motor control training could be delivered in isolation or in combination with other treatments. Table 14-15 summarizes the study population, content of the motor control training program, comparison group, PEDro score, and outcome.

Can Motor Control Training Help in the Treatment of Acute Low Back Pain?

Can Motor Control Training Reduce Pain or Disability in Patients with Acute Low Back Pain?

One trial by Hides et al.[120] has addressed the issue of the efficacy of motor control exercises (involving training of MF in combination with transversus abdominis with a range of techniques and progressed into functional positions) in the treatment of pain and disability associated with acute first episode unilateral LBP. This trial

compared motor control training plus medical management to medical management alone for acute LBP. The majority of participants in both groups recovered, and the effect of motor control exercise on the short-term outcome of pain was small and not significant. Motor control training showed no effect on disability in the short term. However, the size of the MF was restored only in individuals who received the motor control intervention, and this was predicted to have a potential relevance for long-term outcome (see next section).

Can Motor Control Training Reduce Recurrence after an Acute Episode of Low Back Pain?

Hides et al. published a follow-up study examining the ability of motor control training to reduce the recurrence of episodes after acute unilateral LBP.[70] Motor control training plus medical management was substantially more effective than medical management alone for reducing recurrence at the 1- and 3-year follow-up. Individuals who did not receive the motor control intervention were 12.4 times more likely to suffer a subsequent episode of LBP.

Can Motor Control Training Help in the Treatment of

Clinical Point

Motor control training does not appear to offer substantial short-term benefit in reducing pain or disability in patients suffering from low back pain (LBP) of less than 3 months' duration. However, research has shown that acute LBP changes the pattern of muscle recruitment, possibly leading to further back pain; therefore this approach appears to be useful in reducing the number of future episodes of LBP. Patients should be advised that the *purpose of the intervention is to reduce the recurrence of back pain episodes* and that the intervention is unlikely to affect pain or disability dramatically in the short term.

Chronic Nonspecific Low Back Pain?

Is Motor Control Training More Helpful in Reducing Pain or Disability Than Usual Care, No/Minimal Interventions, or Placebo in Patients with Chronic Low Back Pain?

Six trials have examined the effects of motor control training compared with no treatment,[173] educational booklet,[174] placebo,[175] or usual care by a physical therapist[176] or general practitioner.[177,178] Most of these studies used an intervention limited to activation of the deep muscles with progression into functional postures. Only the study of Costa et al.[175] included consideration of posture and movement, and this was limited in scope. Three trials combined other treatments with the motor control interventions.[176–178] In general, the studies reported that motor control was efficacious for pain and/or disability in the short and long term, with better outcomes than the comparison group. However, this was not universal. Although motor control training was effective, one

TABLE 14-15

Randomized Clinical Trials of Motor Control Training

Author	Participants	Motor Control Program	Comparison	PEDro Score	Outcome
Acute LBP					
Hides et al.[120] Hides et al.[70]	Acute first episode unilateral LBP (<3 weeks)	Co-contraction of MF with TrA, feedback with ultrasound imaging, postural correction in standing + Medical management	Medical management (advice + medication)	7[120] 6[70]	Equal improvement in pain and disability at 4 weeks; symmetry of cross-sectional area of multifidus restored only for motor control group; decrease recurrence for motor control (1 year: 30% versus 84%, 3 years: 35% versus 75%)
Chronic Nonspecific LBP: Comparison with No/Minimal Intervention, Usual Care, or Placebo					
Costa et al.[175]	Chronic nonspecific LBP (>12 weeks)	Individualized exercise based on participant's presentation with aim to improve function of TrA and MF, progressed to basic correction of posture and movement	Placebo (detuned ultrasound therapy + detuned short-wave therapy)	9	Greater reduction in pain at 12 months, but not 2 or 6 months; significantly greater improvement in activity and global perceived effect for motor control at all time points
Niemisto et al.[178]	Chronic nonspecific LBP (>3 months)	Activation of TrA in prone, progressed to more functional positions and daily activities + Manual therapy and muscle energy	Usual general practitioner care (education booklet)	8	Greater improvement in pain and disability at 5 and 12 months
Cairns et al.[176]	Recurrent nonspecific LBP	Endurance training for TrA and MF muscles + Manual therapy	Conventional treatment	7	Equal improvement in pain and disability at treatment at 12 months
Moseley[177]	Chronic nonspecific LBP (>2 months)	Motor control exercises according to Richardson and Jull[179] (activation of TrA and MF in nonfunctional postures, progressed to static training with limb movements and muscle activation in functional positions) + manual therapy + education of neurophysiology of pain	Usual general practitioner care	6	Greater improvement in pain and disability for motor control at 1 and 12 months
Shaughnessy et al.[173]	Chronic nonspecific LBP (>12 weeks)	Activation of TrA and MF in nonfunctional postures, progressed to static training with limb movements	No intervention	5	Greater improvement in disability for motor control group
Goldby et al.[174]	Chronic nonspecific LBP (>12 weeks)	Training of co-contraction of TrA and MF, progressed to function	Education booklet	4	Equal improvement in pain and disability
Chronic Nonspecific LBP: Comparison with Manual Therapy					
Ferreira et al.[182]	Chronic nonspecific LBP (>3 months)	Training of co-contraction of TrA and MF with real-time ultrasound feedback Progressed to activation in functional positions and training the coordination of all trunk muscles during functional tasks	Spinal manipulative therapy	8	Equal improvements in pain and function at 8 weeks, 6 months, and 12 months

(Continued)

TABLE 14-15

Randomized Clinical Trials of Motor Control Training—cont'd

Author	Participants	Motor Control Program	Comparison	PEDro Score	Outcome
Critchley et al.[181]	Chronic non-specific LBP (>12 weeks)	Training of co-contraction of TrA and MF, progressed to group exercises that challenged stability	Manual therapy + home exercises pain management program	7	Equal improvements in pain and disability at 18 months
Rasmussen-Barr 2003[180]	Chronic nonspecific LBP (>12 weeks)	Training of co-contraction of TrA and MF, progressed to activation with limb loading, activation in functional task and in situations that provoke pain	Manual therapy	5	Greater reduction in disability after treatment and 12 months
Goldby et al.[174]	Chronic nonspecific LBP (>12 weeks)	Training of co-contraction of TrA and MF, progressed to function	Manual therapy	4	Greater reduction in pain and quality of life at 6 months

Chronic Nonspecific LBP: Comparison with Other Exercise

Author	Participants	Motor Control Program	Comparison	PEDro Score	Outcome
Macedo et al.[183,184]	Chronic nonspecific LBP (>12 weeks)	Individualized exercise based on participant's presentation with aim to improve function of TrA and MF, progressed to basic correction of posture and movement	Graded physical activity	8	Equal improvements in outcome at 2, 6, and 12 months; greater reduction in pain with motor for patients with high score on lumbar instability questionnaire
Ferreira et al.[182]	Chronic nonspecific LBP (>3 months)	Real-time ultrasound Progression by incorporating more functional positions and training the coordination of all trunk muscles during those functional tasks	General exercise (strengthening, stretching, and cardiovascular exercise)	8	Better function and global perceived effect for motor control at 8 weeks; outcome not different between groups at 6 and 12 months
França et al.[187]	Chronic nonspecific LBP (>3 months)	Exercises focused on the TrA and MF muscles progressed to upright postures	Muscle stretching exercise	8	Greater improvement in pain and disability with motor control at 6 weeks
Unsgaard-Tøndel[189]	Chronic nonspecific LBP	Training of co-contraction of TrA and MF with ultrasound imaging, progressed to activation in function	High load sling exercise or general exercise	7	Equal improvement in pain and disability at treatment conclusion and 1 year
França et al.[188]	Chronic nonspecific LBP (>3 months)	Training of co-contraction of TrA and MF progressed to upright postures	Strength training of global muscles	7	Greater improvement in pain and disability with motor control at 6 weeks
Koumantakis et al.[186]	Chronic nonspecific LBP (>6 months)	Training of co-contraction of TrA and MF in nonfunctional positions, progressed by incorporation into functional task and heavier load exercise tasks performed by comparison group	Higher load exercise for extensor and flexor muscles	7	Equal improvements in pain and disability at 2 and 5 months
Kladny et al.[190]	Chronic nonspecific LBP	Training of co-contraction of TrA and MF motor control exercises + General exercises	General exercises + manual therapy	5	Greater reduction in disability for motor control at end of treatment

Author	Participants	Motor Control Program	Comparison	PEDro Score	Outcome
Miller et al.[185]	Chronic nonspecific LBP (>7 weeks)	Activation of TrA (with MF), progressed to maintenance of activation while movement of extremities in multiple positions and functional tasks	McKenzie approach	5	Equal improvements in pain for both groups at 6 weeks
Stevens et al.[191]	Chronic nonspecific LBP	Training of co-contraction of TrA and MF progressed to contraction in different contexts + Manual therapy (10%)	General exercises of trunk muscle function and coordination	2	Greater improvement in pain for motor control in short term, then no difference

Chronic Nonspecific LBP: Comparison with Surgery

Author	Participants	Motor Control Program	Comparison	PEDro Score	Outcome
Brox et al.[193] Forholdt et al.[194]	Chronic LBP (>12 months) with spine degeneration or spondylosis	Training of co-contraction of TrA and MF + exercise for endurance and coordination + cognitive intervention	Lumbar fusion surgery	8	Equal improvement in disability at 1 and 9 years; greater improvement in fear avoidance for motor control group

Chronic LBP with Specific Diagnosis

Author	Participants	Motor Control Program	Comparison	PEDro Score	Outcome
Stuge et al.[195,196]	Pelvic girdle pain	Training of co-contraction of TrA and MF, progressed to global muscles with increased loading + manual therapy	Usual physical therapy	7	Greater improvement in pain and disability for motor control group at 20 weeks, 1 year, and 2 years
O'Sullivan et al.[69]	Chronic LBP with radiological diagnosis of spondylolysis or spondylolisthesis	Training of co-contraction of TrA and MF, progressed to activation with limb loading, activation in functional tasks and aggravating static postures	Usual general practitioner care	7	Greater reduction in pain and disability for motor control at 3, 6, and 30 months

MF, Multifidus; *TrA*, transversus abdominis; *LBP*, low back pain.

study showed that it was not more effective than a comprehensive physical therapy intervention for patients with recurrent LBP.[176] Notably, motor control training led to greater improvement in activity and had a greater global perceived effect than placebo at 12 months.

Is Motor Control Training More Helpful in Reducing Pain or Disability Than Manual Therapy in Patients with Chronic Low Back Pain?

Four trials have examined the effect of motor control training compared with manual therapy (i.e., spinal manipulative therapy).[174,180–182] In each trial, motor control training was limited to activation the deep trunk muscles with progression to functional positions and motor control training improved pain or disability. The effects were generally similar to those achieved with manual therapy in the short and long term, with the exception of outcomes favoring motor control training for reduction of disability at 12 months in one study[180] and pain and quality of life at 6 months in another.[174]

Clinical Point

Motor control training offers more benefits to patients with chronic LBP than does no provision of treatment or common traditional interventions such as educational booklets or treatment at the discretion of a medical practitioner. Patients with chronic LBP have altered patterns of muscle recruitment and a high level of disability. The effects of motor control training in reducing pain and disability appear to be similar to those seen with manual therapy treatment. Although some studies have attempted to identify subgroups of patients with LBP features that characterize patients who respond better to a particular intervention is still not known. Patients who benefit from motor control exercises show clinical patterns that have been suggested to indicate "spinal instability" (although the interpretation of this remains unclear as the scale used to assess "instability" may in fact provide information regarding pain characteristics [e.g., nociceptive versus central bias to symptoms] rather than "spinal instability"), probably more critically, signs of altered motor control. Although this issue has not been investigated extensively, *the authors recommend that clinicians assess patterns of movement and muscle recruitment to gain clinical insight into whether a patient would respond better to a motor control exercise approach or to treatment that focuses on mobilization of spinal joints.* Although the idea of treating patients with chronic LBP with a combination of motor control exercises and manual therapy seems appealing, this clinical question has not yet been investigated.

Is Motor Control Training More Helpful in Reducing Pain or Disability Than Other Forms of Exercises in Patients with Chronic Nonspecific Low Back Pain?

Nine trials have compared motor control exercises to other forms of exercises in nonspecific LBP.[182–191] The comparison exercise programs have included general exercises for muscle strength/endurance/flexibility,[182] graded physical activity using behavioral principles,[183,184] or other specific exercise approaches, including McKenzie exercises (i.e., end range repetitive spine motion)[185] and high load training for global trunk muscles.[186–189] Motor

control training has generally been limited to activation of deep muscles with progression to functional positions with or without static training with loading applied by movement of the extremities. One study involved some element of individualization of training with consideration of muscle activation and some consideration of posture and movement.[183,184] In general, for these studies of nonspecific LBP, motor control training targeted at activation of deep muscles was equally efficacious for improvements in either disability or pain at 12 months. Three studies found greater effect of motor control training than general exercises for pain and/or disability on short-term outcomes (3 months,[191] 6 weeks[187,188]) and another found greater global perceived effect at 8 weeks (the primary outcome measure of the study).[182] Macedo et al.[183,184] found that motor control training was more efficacious than a graded activity program for patients who had higher scores on a questionnaire based on the clinical consensus opinion of features that relate to lumbar spine instability.[192] This preliminary observation requires validation in a new study, and it remains to be determined whether these features are indicative of "instability" or simply reflect characteristics of nociceptive pain.

What Is the Efficacy of Motor Control Training Compared with Surgery for Patients with Chronic Low Back Pain?

One trial (quality score of 8[193] on the PEDro scale) examined the effect of motor control training and education compared to surgery and physical therapy treatment (advice and exercises). The two groups produced similar reductions in pain and disability at 12 months and 9 years.[194]

Clinical Point

Motor control training is effective when applied as part of a treatment package that usually includes sessions of manual therapy and education. Currently, it appears that when applied in a non-specific manner to patients with "non-specific" low back pain, motor control exercises offer similar effects in terms of pain and disability compared with other forms of exercises, although in the short term, motor control exercises appear to be more beneficial than general exercises, and there is preliminary evidence that baseline features of an individual's presentation may aid identification of patients who are likely to respond best to this treatment. Treatment packages that include motor control training produce reductions in pain and disability similar to those seen with surgical procedures, such as spinal fusion. Clinicians should keep this in mind when recommending exercises for chronic LBP, especially given the high cost and risks associated with surgical procedures.

Is Motor Control Training Helpful in the Treatment of Patients with Specific Back Pain Characteristics?

One study investigated the effect of motor control training for management of pelvic girdle pain.[195] In this trial, motor control training involved activation of deep muscles progressing to higher load exercises applied using a sling. The intervention included manual therapy and ergonomic advice and was compared to a conventional physical therapy program. When added to a conventional physical therapy program, motor control training was more effective than conventional physical therapy alone for all outcomes at 20 weeks and 1 year, and this was maintained at 2 years.[196]

One study investigated motor control training (i.e., co-contraction of transverse abdominus [TrA] and MF muscles, progressing to activation with limb loading and activation in functional tasks and aggravating static postures) for patients with chronic LBP associated with radiological diagnosis of spondylolysis or spondylolisthesis compared to usual care by a general practitioner.[69] Outcomes for pain and disability were superior for motor control training at all time points including 30-month follow-up.

An additional recent study (2013) evaluated a comprehensive motor control training program that addressed maladaptive movement/posture behaviors with integration into function (i.e., positive cognitive and lifestyle behaviors) for patients with chronic LBP that presented with a mechanical behavior (i.e., movement clearly associated with pain).[197] The treatment produced a greater improvement in pain and disability at 3 and 12 months than the comparison intervention. However, interpretation is complicated as both treatments addressed features of motor control; the comparison intervention combined manual therapy with simple nontargeted isolation of deep muscle activation, without consideration of progression or other elements of motor control.

Clinical Point

Approximately 50% of pregnant women experience lumbopelvic pain during pregnancy. It is known that specific deep abdominal and pelvic muscles maintain pelvic stability.[75] Pelvic pain has been associated with compromised control of the pelvic joints. The finding that motor control training is helpful in reducing pain and disability in patients with pregnancy-related pelvic pain[198] is important, both because of the prevalence of this condition and because of the lack of evidence of efficacy of other physical therapy interventions in its treatment.

Can Motor Control Training Change the Control of Muscle Activation, Posture, and Movement, and Is This Related to Outcome?

If motor control training is effective, it is important to consider whether the intervention can actually change the features of motor control it aims to address and, if so, whether improvements in motor control are associated with improvements in clinical outcomes. In terms of muscle activation, cognitive training of motor control of the deep muscles can change the timing of activation of the transversus abdominis muscle toward that identified for pain-free individuals,[199] the improvements in control persist when tested at 6 months after the intervention,[200] and the improvement in timing is related to restoration of the

organization of the representation of the muscle at the motor cortex.[201] Timing of activation of the transversus abdominis muscle was not restored by other exercise that activates TrA but without any cognitive attention to contraction of the muscle or modification of its activity (e.g., a sit-up[200] or during abdominal bracing maneuvers[202]). Other studies report greater thickening of the TrA on ultrasound imaging during leg movement (consistent with improved muscle activation) after a motor control intervention but not after a general exercise program or a course of manual therapy.[203] In terms of muscle structure, Hides et al.[120] reported that the cross-sectional area of the MF can be restored with low-intensity activation in patients with acute first-episode LBP. In contrast, Danneels et al.[115] reported that this approach could not restore MF cross-sectional area in chronic LBP and high-level training to overload the muscle was required.

In terms of correction of posture, one study of patients with neck pain has reported that a program of cognitive correction of spinal alignment can improve spontaneous posture.[204] Likewise, features of movement presentation can be corrected with cognitive training.[205] Further work is required to study the effect of training on transfer of modified strategies for control of movement and posture to functional activities.

The association between changes in motor control and clinical improvement has also been studied, but to date this has been limited to investigation of the relationship between changes in activation of transversus abdominis and clinical trial outcomes.[165,203] Two studies have investigated changes in recruitment of the TrA with ultrasound, after the application of motor control training. In one study, which compared motor control training to general exercise and manual therapy, a subset of 34 participants with chronic LBP were assessed for ability to recruit the TrA by means of ultrasound measurement during a leg movement task and this was compared with clinical outcomes of function, disability, and pain. Patients with chronic LBP who received motor control training showed greater increase in thickness of TrA than patients who received general and spinal manipulative therapy. A moderate but significant correlation was found between changes in recruitment of the TrA and changes in the clinical outcomes of global perceived effect and disability (Figure 14-11).[203] The other study showed a relationship between increased thickening of TrA on ultrasound imaging (and decreased thickening of obliquus internus abdominis on ultrasound imaging) during voluntary TrA activation and pain reduction after training. Of note, this relationship between improvement in activation of TrA was achieved with each of the exercise interventions included in the study and not limited to the group that received motor control training.

A final issue is whether activation of the deep muscles, before treatment, can be used to predict the potential effect of motor control training for the individual. Data from a study by Ferreira[203] suggest that patients with poorer activation of the TrA before treatment have a greater response.

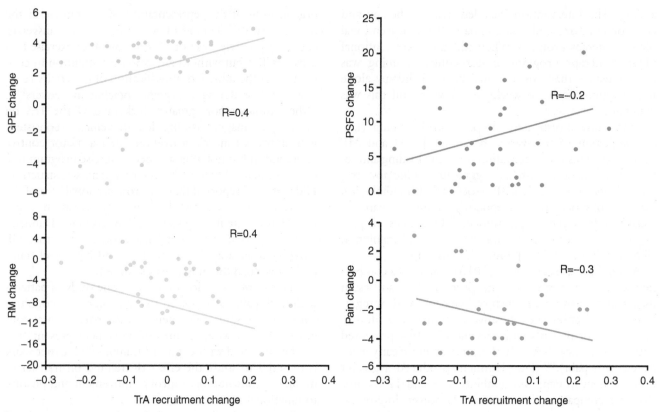

Figure 14-11 Correlation between changes in recruitment of the transversus abdominis measured with ultrasonography and changes in clinical outcomes. Lines represent R squared best of fit. *GPE*, Global perceived effect; *PSFS*, patient-specific functional scale; *RM*, Roland Morris.

In another study, individuals who improved the shortening/lateral slide of TrA observed on ultrasound imaging, after training, had higher odds for a clinically significant improvement at 12 months after an intervention.[164]

SUMMARY AND DIRECTIONS FOR THE FUTURE

Although existing studies are promising, further research is needed to further clarify the efficacy of motor control training in LBP. Critical issues that need to be addressed include the identification of subgroups that assist in the selection of the most appropriate treatment strategies and evaluation of the most appropriate clinical path for progression of exercise. Motor control training likely has a place in the management of many patients with low back and pelvic pain, but the relative contribution of the intervention to clinical outcomes will vary from individual to individual.

REFERENCES

1. Macedo LG, Maher CG, Latimer J, McAuley JH: Motor control exercise for persistent, nonspecific low back pain: a systematic review, *Phys Ther* 89:9–25, 2009.
2. Hodges PW, van Dillen L, McGill S, et al: Integrated clinical approach to motor control interventions in low back and pelvic pain. In Hodges PW, Cholewicki J, van Dieen J, editors: *Spinal control: the rehabilitation of back pain*, Edinburgh, 2013, Elsevier.
3. Panjabi MM: The stabilizing system of the spine. I. Function, dysfunction, adaptation, and enhancement, *J Spinal Dis* 5:383–389, 1992.
4. Hodges P, Cholewicki J: Functional control of the spine. In Vleeming A, Mooney V, Stoeckart R, editors: *Movement, stability and lumbopelvic pain*, Edinburgh, 2007, Elsevier.
5. Cholewicki J, Panjabi MM, Khachatryan A: Stabilizing function of trunk flexor-extensor muscles around a neutral spine posture, *Spine* 22:2207–2212, 1996.

6. Reeves NP, Narendra KS, Cholewicki J: Spine stability: lessons from balancing a stick, *Clin Biomech* 26:325–330, 2011.
7. Mok NW, Hodges PW: Movement of the lumbar spine is critical for maintenance of postural recovery following support surface perturbation, *Exp Brain Res* 231:305–313, 2013.
8. Crisco JJ, Panjabi MM, Yamamoto I, Oxland TR: Euler stability of the human ligamentous lumbar spine. II. Experiment, *Clin Biomech* 7:27–32, 1992.
9. McGill SM, Grenier S, Kavcic N, Cholewicki J: Coordination of muscle activity to assure stability of the lumbar spine, *J Electromyogr Kinesiol* 13:353–359, 2003.
10. Hodges PW, Cresswell AG, Thorstensson A: Preparatory trunk motion accompanies rapid upper limb movement, *Exp Brain Res* 124:69–79, 1999.
11. Hodges PW, Richardson CA: Feedforward contraction of transversus abdominis is not influenced by the di-

rection of arm movement, *Exp Brain Res* 114:362–370, 1997.
12. Mok NW, Brauer SG, Hodges PW: Failure to use movement in postural strategies leads to increased spinal displacement in low back pain, *Spine* 32:E537–E543, 2007.
13. Mok N, Brauer S, Hodges P: Changes in lumbar movement in people with low back pain are related to compromised balance, *Spine* 36:E45–E52, 2011.
14. DeTroyer A, Estenne M: Functional anatomy of the respiratory muscles. In Belman MJ, editor: *Respiratory muscles: function in health and disease*, Philadelphia, 1988, WB Saunders.
15. Gurfinkel VS, Kots YM, Paltsev EI, Feldman AG: The compensation of respiratory disturbances of erect posture of man as an example of the organisation of interarticular interaction. In Gelfard IM, Gurfinkel VS, Formin SV, Tsetlin ML, editors: *Models of the structural functional organisation of certain biological systems*, Cambridge, MA, 1971, MIT Press.

16. Hodges P, Gurfinkel VS, Brumagne S, et al: Coexistence of stability and mobility in postural control: evidence from postural compensation for respiration, *Exp Brain Res* 144:293–302, 2002.

17. Horak F, Nashner LM: Central programming of postural movements: adaptation to altered support-surface configurations, *J Neurophysiol* 55:1369–1381, 1986.

18. Mok N, Brauer S, Hodges P: Hip strategy for balance control in quiet standing is reduced in people with low back pain, *Spine* 29:E107–E112, 2004.

19. Perry J: *Gait analysis: normal and pathological function*, Thorofare, NJ, 1992, SLACK.

20. Cholewicki J, McGill SM, Norman RW: Lumbar spine loading during the lifting of extremely heavy weights, *Med Sci Sports Exerc* 23:1179–1186, 1991.

21. Johansson H, Sjolander P, Sojka P: A sensory role for the cruciate ligaments, *Clin Orthop Relat Res* 268:161–178, 1991.

22. Nitz AJ, Peck D: Comparison of muscle spindle concentrations in large and small human epaxial muscles acting in parallel combinations, *Am Surg* 52:273–277, 1986.

23. Indahl A, et al: Interaction between the porcine lumbar intervertebral disc, zygapophysial joints, and paraspinal muscles, *Spine* 22:2834–2840, 1997.

24. Indahl A, Kaigle A, Reikerås O, Holm S: Sacroiliac joint involvement in activation of the porcine spinal and gluteal musculature, *J Spinal Disord* 12:325–330, 1999.

25. Brumagne S, Cordo P, Lysens R: The role of paraspinal muscle spindles in lumbosacral position sense in individuals with and without low back pain, *Spine* 25:989–994, 2000.

26. Gill KP, Callaghan MJ: The measurement of lumbar proprioception in individuals with and without low back pain, *Spine* 23:371–377, 1998.

27. Bergmark A: Stability of the lumbar spine: a study in mechanical engineering, *Acta Orthop Scand* 60(Suppl 230):1–54, 1989.

28. Aruin AS, Latash ML: Directional specificity of postural muscles in feed-forward postural reactions during fast voluntary arm movements, *Exp Brain Res* 103:323–332, 1995.

29. Saunders SW, Schache A, Rath D, Hodges PW: Changes in three dimensional lumbo-pelvic kinematics and trunk muscle activity with speed and mode of locomotion, *Clin Biomech* 20:784–793, 2005.

30. Bogduk N: A reappraisal of the anatomy of the human lumbar erector spinae, *J Anat* 131:525–540, 1980.

31. Kaigle AM, Holm SH, Hansson TH: 1997 Volvo Award in biomechanical studies: kinematic behavior of the porcine lumbar spine—a chronic lesion model, *Spine* 22:2796–2806, 1997.

32. Wilke HJ, Wolf S, Claes LE, et al: Stability increase of the lumbar spine with different muscle groups: a biomechanical in vitro study, *Spine* 20:192–198, 1995.

33. Moseley GL, Hodges PW, Gandevia SC: Deep and superficial fibers of lumbar multifidus are differentially active during voluntary arm movements, *Spine* 27:E29–E36, 2002.

34. Hodges P, Kaigle Holm A, Holm S, et al: Intervertebral stiffness of the spine is increased by evoked contraction of the transversus abdominis and the diaphragm: in vivo porcine studies, *Spine* 28:2594–2601, 2003.

35. Barker P, Guggenheimer K, Grkovic I, et al: Effects of tensioning the lumbar fasciae on segmental stiffness during flexion and extension, *Spine* 31:397–405, 2005.

36. Hodges PW, Eriksson AE, Shirley D, Gandevia SC: Intra-abdominal pressure increases stiffness of the lumbar spine, *J Biomech* 38:1873–1880, 2005.

37. Richardson CA, Snijders CJ, Hides JA, et al: The relation between the transversus abdominis muscles, sacroiliac joint mechanics, and low back pain, *Spine* 27:399–405, 2002.

38. Park RJ, Tsao H, Cresswell AG, Hodges PW: Anticipatory postural activity of the deep trunk muscles differs between anatomical regions based on their mechanical advantage, *Neuroscience* 261:161–172, 2014.

39. Pool-Goudzwaard A, van Dijke GH, van Gurp M, et al: Contribution of pelvic floor muscles to stiffness of the pelvic ring, *Clin Biomech* 19:564–571, 2004.

40. Hodges PW, Sapsford RR, Pengel HM: *Feedforward activity of the pelvic floor muscles precedes rapid upper limb movements.* In VIIth international physiotherapy congress, Sydney, Australia, 2002.

41. Cala SJ, Edyvean J, Engel LA: Chest wall and trunk muscle activity during inspiratory loading, *J Appl Physiol* 73:2373–2381, 1992.

42. De Troyer A: Mechanics of the chest wall muscles. In Miller A, Bianchi A, Bishop B, editors: *Neural control of the respiratory muscles*, Boca Raton, FL, 1997, CRC Press.

43. Hodges PW, Pengel HM, Sapsford R: Postural and respiratory functions of the pelvic floor muscles, *Neurourol Urodyn* 26:362–371, 2007.

44. Campbell EJM, Green JH: The behaviour of the abdominal muscles and the intra-abdominal pressure during quiet breathing and increased pulmonary ventilation, *J Physiol* 127:423–426, 1955.

45. Hodges P, Gandevia S: Changes in intra-abdominal pressure during postural and respiratory activation of the human diaphragm, *J Appl Physiol* 89:967–976, 2000.

46. Hodges P, Gandevia S: Activation of the human diaphragm during a repetitive postural task, *J Physiol* 522:165–175, 2000.

47. Saunders S, Rath D, Hodges PW: Respiratory and postural activation of the trunk muscles changes with mode and speed of locomotion, *Gait Posture* 20:280–290, 2004.

48. Rimmer KP, Ford GT, Whitelaw WA: Interaction between postural and respiratory control of human intercostal muscles, *J Appl Physiol* 79:1556–1561, 1995.

49. Hagins M, Pietrek M, Sheikhzadeh A, et al: The effects of breath control on intra-abdominal pressure during lifting tasks, *Spine* 29:464–469, 2004.

50. Pietrek M, Sheikhzadeh A, Nordin M, Hagins M: Biomechanical modeling of intra-abdominal pressure generation should include the transversus abdominis, *J Biomech* 33:787–790, 2000.

51. McGill SM, Sharratt MT, Seguin JP: Loads on spinal tissues during simultaneous lifting and ventilatory challenge, *Ergonomics* 38:1772–1792, 1995.

52. Hodges PW, Heijnen I, Gandevia SC: Reduced postural activity of the diaphragm in humans when respiratory demand is increased, *J Physiol* 537:999–1008, 2001.

53. Hodges PW, McKenzie DK, Heijnen I, Gandevia SC: *Reduced contribution of the diaphragm to postural control in patients with severe chronic airflow limitation.* In Proceedings of the annual scientific meeting of the Thoracic Society of Australia and New Zealand, Melbourne, April 7–12 2000.

54. Grimstone SK, Hodges PW: Impaired postural compensation for respiration in people with recurrent low back pain, *Exp Brain Res* 151:218–224, 2003.

55. Gagey P: Postural disorders among workers on building sites. In Bles W, Brandt T, editors: *Disorders of posture and gait*, Amsterdam, 1986, Elsevier.

56. Tesh KM, Shaw Dunn J, Evans JH: The abdominal muscles and vertebral stability, *Spine* 12:501–508, 1987.

57. Pool-Goudzwaard AL, Slieker ten Hove MC, Vierhout ME, et al: Relations between pregnancy-related low back pain, pelvic floor activity and pelvic floor dysfunction, *Int Urogynecol J Pelvic Floor Dysfunct* 16:468–474, 2005.

58. Stafford RE, Ashton-Miller JA, Sapsford R, Hodges PW: Activation of the striated urethral sphincter to maintain continence during dynamic tasks in healthy men, *Neurourol Urodyn* 31:36–43, 2012.

59. Smith MD, Coppieters MW, Hodges P: *Effect of bladder fullness on postural control in women with and without incontinence.* In Musculoskeletal physiotherapy Australia, fourteenth biennial conference: positive precision performance, Brisbane, November 24–26, 2005.

60. Thompson JA, O'Sullivan PB, Briffa NK, Neumann P: Altered muscle activation patterns in symptomatic women during pelvic floor muscle contraction and Valsalva manouevre, *Neurourol Urodyn* 25:268–276, 2006.

61. Smith MD, Russell A, Hodges PW: The relationship between incontinence, breathing disorders, gastrointestinal symptoms and back pain in women: a longitudinal cohort study, *Clin J Pain* 30:162–167, 2013.

62. Smith MD, Russell A, Hodges PW: Do incontinence, breathing difficulties, and gastrointestinal symptoms increase the risk of future back pain? *J Pain* 10:876–886, 2009.

63. Arendt-Nielsen L, Graven-Nielsen T, Svarrer H, Svensson P: The influence of low back pain on muscle activity and coordination during gait: a clinical and experimental study, *Pain* 64:231–240, 1996.

64. Soderberg GL, Dostal WF: Electromyographic study of three parts of the gluteus medius muscle during functional activities, *Phys Ther* 58:691–696, 1978.

65. Alexiev AR: Some differences of the electromyographic erector spinae activity between normal subjects and low back pain patients during the generation of isometric trunk torque, *Electromyogr Clin Neurophysiol* 34:495–499, 1994.

66. Cohen MJ, Swanson GA, Naliboff BD, et al: Comparison of electromyographic response patterns during posture and stress tasks in chronic low back pain patterns and control, *J Psychosom Res* 30:135–141, 1986.

67. Hodges PW, Coppieters MW, MacDonald D, Cholewicki J: New insight into motor adaptation to pain revealed by a combination of modelling and empirical approaches, *Eur J Pain* 17:1138–1146, 2013.

68. van Dieen JH, Cholewicki J, Radebold A: Trunk muscle recruitment patterns in patients with low back pain enhance the stability of the lumbar spine, *Spine* 28:834–841, 2003.

69. O'Sullivan PB, Twomey LT, Allison GT: Evaluation of specific stabilizing exercise in the treatment of chronic low back pain with radiologic diagnosis of spondylolysis or spondylolisthesis, *Spine* 22:2959–2967, 1997.

70. Hides JA, Jull GA, Richardson CA: Long term effects of specific stabilizing exercises for first episode low back pain, *Spine* 26:243–248, 2001.

71. Dye SF: The knee as a biologic transmission with an envelope of function: a theory, *Clin Orthop Relat Res* 325:10–18, 1996.

72. Dankaerts W, O'Sullivan P, Burnett A, Straker L: Differences in sitting postures are associated with nonspecific chronic low back pain disorders when patients are subclassified, *Spine* 31:698–704, 2006.

73. Radebold A, Cholewicki J, Panjabi MM, Patel TC: Muscle response pattern to sudden trunk loading in healthy individuals and in patients with chronic low back pain, *Spine* 25:947–954, 2000.

74. Soderberg GL, Barr JO: Muscular function in chronic low-back dysfunction, *Spine* 8:79–85, 1983.

75. O'Sullivan PB, Beales DJ, Beetham JA, et al: Altered motor control strategies in subjects with sacroiliac joint pain during the active straight-leg-raise test, *Spine* 27:E1–E8, 2002.

76. Hodges PW, Moseley GL, Gabrielsson AH, Gandevia SC: Acute experimental pain changes postural recruitment of the trunk muscles in pain-free humans, *Exp Brain Res* 151:262–271, 2003.

77. Moseley GL, Nicholas MK, Hodges PW: Does anticipation of back pain predispose to back trouble? *Brain* 127(Part 10):2339–2347, 2004.

78. Hodges P, et al, editors: *Different range and temporal pattern of lumbopelvic motion accompanies rapid upper limb flexion in people with low back pain.* In Mok N, Brauer S, Fifteenth interdisciplinary world congress on low back and pelvic pain, Melbourne, November 10–13, 2004.

79. Kaigle AM, Wessberg P, Hansson TH: Muscular and kinematic behavior of the lumbar spine during flexion-extension, *J Spinal Disord* 11:163–174, 1998.

80. Lamoth CJ, Meijer OG, Wuisman PI, et al: Pelvis-thorax coordination in the transverse plane during walking in persons with nonspecific low back pain, *Spine* 27:E92–E99, 2002.

81. Hodges PW, Richardson CA: Inefficient muscular stabilisation of the lumbar spine associated with low back pain: a motor control evaluation of the transversus abdominis, *Spine* 21:2640–2650, 1996.

82. MacDonald D, Moseley GL, Hodges PW: *The function of the lumbar multifidus in unilateral low back pain.* In World congress of low back and pelvic pain, melbourne, November 10–13, 2004.

83. Saunders S, Coppieters M, Hodges P: *Reduced tonic activity of the deep trunk muscle during locomotion in people with low back pain.* In World congress of low back and pelvic pain, Melbourne, November 10–13, 2004.

84. Ferreira PH, Ferreira ML, Hodges PW: Changes in recruitment of the abdominal muscles in people with low back pain: ultrasound measurement of muscle activity, *Spine* 29:2560–2566, 2004.

85. Hides JA, Stokes MJ, Saide M, et al: Evidence of lumbar multifidus muscle wasting ipsilateral to symptoms in patients with acute/subacute low back pain, *Spine* 19:165–177, 1994.

86. Roy SH, DeLuca CJ, Casavant DA: Lumbar muscle fatigue and chronic low back pain, *Spine* 14:992–1001, 1989.

87. Alaranta H, Tallroth K, Soukka A, Heliaara M: Fat content of lumbar extensor muscles in low back disability: a radiographic and clinical comparison, *J Spinal Disord* 6:137–140, 1993.

88. Kjaer P, Bendix T, Sorensen JS, et al: Are MRI-defined fat infiltrations in the multifidus muscles associated with low back pain? *BMC Med* 5:2, 2007.

89. Barker PJ, Guggenheimer K, Grkovic I, et al: *Effects of tensioning the lumbar fasciae on segmental stiffness during flexion and extension.* In World congress of low back and pelvic pain, Melbourne, November 10–13, 2004.

90. Schneider G, Pearcy MJ, Bogduk N: Abnormal motion in spondylolytic spondylolisthesis, *Spine* 30:1159–1164, 2005.

91. Cholewicki J, McGill SM: Mechanical stability of the in vivo lumbar spine: implications for injury and chronic low back pain, *Clin Biomech* 11:1–15, 1996.

92. Sahrman S: *Diagnosis and treatment of movement impairment syndromes*, St Louis, 2002, Mosby.

93. Gombatto SP, Collins DR, Sahrmann SA, et al: Gender differences in pattern of hip and lumbopelvic rotation in people with low back pain, *Clin Biomech* 21:263–271, 2006.

94. Van Dillen LR, Gombatto SP, Collins DR, et al: Symmetry of timing of hip and lumbopelvic rotation motion in 2 different subgroups of people with low back pain, *Arch Phys Med Rehabil* 88:351–360, 2007.

95. Scholtes SA, Gombatto SP, Van Dillen LR: Differences in lumbopelvic motion between people with and

people without low back pain during two lower limb movement tests, *Clin Biomech* 24:7–12, 2009.

96. Cholewicki J, Silfies SP, Shah RA, et al: Delayed trunk muscle reflex responses increase the risk of low back injuries, *Spine* 30:2614–2620, 2005.

97. Janda V: Muscles, central nervous motor regulation and back problems. In Korr IM, editor: *The neurobiologic mechanisms in manipulative therapy*, New York, 1978, Plenum Press.

98. Hodges PW, Kaigle Holm A, Hansson T, Holm S: Rapid atrophy of the lumbar multifidus follows experimental disc or nerve root injury, *Spine* 31:2926–2933, 2006.

99. Hodges PW, James G, Blomster L, et al: Can pro-inflammatory cytokine gene expression explain multifidus muscle fiber changes after an intervertebral disc lesion? *Spine* 39:1010–1017, 2014.

100. Panjabi M: A hypothesis of chronic back pain: ligament subfailure injuries lead to muscle control dysfunction, *Eur Spine J* 15:668–676, 2006.

101. Brumagne S, Janssens L, Knapen S, et al: Persons with recurrent low back pain exhibit a rigid postural control strategy, *Eur Spine J* 17:1177–1184, 2008.

102. della Volpe R, Popa T, Ginanneschi F, et al: Changes in coordination of postural control during dynamic stance in chronic low back pain patients, *Gait Posture* 24:349–355, 2006.

103. Flor H, Braun C, Elbert T, Birbaumer N: Extensive reorganization of primary somatosensory cortex in chronic back pain patients, *Neurosci Lett* 224:5–8, 1997.

104. Moseley GL: I can't find it! Distorted body image and tactile dysfunction in patients with chronic back pain, *Pain* 140:239–243, 2008.

105. Schabrun SM, Jones E, Kloster J, Hodges PW: Temporal association between changes in primary sensory cortex and corticomotor output during muscle pain, *Neuroscience* 235:159–164, 2013.

106. Tsao H, Galea MP, Hodges PW: Reorganization of the motor cortex is associated with postural control deficits in recurrent low back pain, *Brain* 131(Pt 8):2161–2171, 2008.

107. Tsao H, Tucker KJ, Hodges PW: Changes in excitability of corticomotor inputs to the trunk muscles during experimentally induced acute low back pain, *Neuroscience* 181:127–133, 2011.

108. Schabrun S, Jones E, Elgueta-Cancino E, Hodges PW: *Understanding the transition from acute to chronic low back pain*, Melbourne, Australia, 2013, Australian Physiotherapy Association.

109. Schabrun SM, Stinear CM, Byblow WD, Ridding M: Normalizing motor cortex representations in focal hand dystonia, *Cereb Cortex* 19:1968–1977, 2009.

110. MacDonald D, Moseley GL, Hodges PW: Why do some patients keep hurting their back? Evidence of ongoing back muscle dysfunction during remission from recurrent back pain, *Pain* 142:183–188, 2009.

111. Claus AP, et al: *Spinal posture in sitting: how do we sit and how should we sit?* Bologna, Italy, 2009, International Society of Gait and Posture Research.

112. Hodges PW, Tucker K: Moving differently in pain: a new theory to explain the adaptation to pain, *Pain* 152(Suppl 3):S90–S98, 2011.

113. Moseley GL, Hodges PW: Are the changes in postural control associated with low back pain caused by pain interference? *Clin J Pain* 21:323–329, 2005.

114. Hodges PW, Galea MP, Holm S, Holm AK: Corticomotor excitability of back muscles is affected by intervertebral disc lesion in pigs, *Eur J Neurosci* 29:1490–1500, 2009.

115. Danneels LA, Vanderstraeten GG, Cambier DC, et al: Effects of three different training modalities on the cross sectional area of the lumbar multifidus muscle in patients with chronic low back pain, *Br J Sports Med* 35:186–191, 2001.

116. Mannion AF: Fibre type characteristics and function of the human paraspinal muscles: normal values and changes in association with low back pain, *J Electromyogr Kinesiol* 9:363–377, 1999.

117. Hodges PW, James G, Blomster L, et al: Multifidus muscle changes after back injury are characterized by structural remodeling of muscle, adipose and connective tissue, but not muscle atrophy: Molecular and morphological evidence, *Spine* 2015 (in press).

118. Tucker K, Butler J, Graven-Nielsen T, et al: Motor unit recruitment strategies are altered during deep-tissue pain, *J Neurosci* 29:10820–10826, 2009.

119. Lund JP, Donga R, Widmer CG, Stohler CS: The pain-adaptation model: a discussion of the relationship between chronic musculoskeletal pain and motor activity, *Can J Physiol Pharmacol* 69:683–694, 1991.

120. Hides JA, Richardson CA, Jull GA: Multifidus muscle recovery is not automatic after resolution of acute, first-episode low back pain, *Spine* 21:2763–2769, 1996.

121. Van Dieen JH, Selen LP, Cholewicki J: Trunk muscle activation in low-back pain patients: an analysis of the literature, *J Electromyogr Kinesiol* 13:333–351, 2003.

122. McGill S: *Low back disorders: evidence based prevention and rehabilitation*, Champaign, IL, 2002, Human Kinetics.

123. Marras WS, Ferguson SA, Burr D, et al: Spine loading in patients with low back pain during asymmetric lifting exertions, *Spine J* 4:64–75, 2004.

124. Kumar S: Cumulative load as a risk factor for back pain, *Spine* 15:1311–1316, 1990.

125. Norman R, Wells R, Neumann P, et al: A comparison of peak versus cumulative physical work exposure: risk factors for the reporting of low back pain in the automotive industry, *Clin Biomech* 13:561–573, 1998.

126. Ching CT, Chow DH, Yao FY, Holmes AD: The effect of cyclic compression on the mechanical properties of the inter-vertebral disc: an in vivo study in a rat tail model, *Clin Biomech* 18:182–189, 2003.

127. Hodges PW, Smith D, Chang A, Coppieters MW: *Breathing pattern changes and low back pain.* In Third world congress of international society for physical and rehabilitation medicine, São Paulo, April 10–14, 2005.

128. Hungerford B, Hodges P, Gilleard W: Evidence of altered lumbo-pelvic muscle recruitment in the presence of posterior pelvic pain and failed load transfer through the pelvis, *Spine* 28:1593–1600, 2003.

129. Hamill J, van Emmerik RE, Heiderscheit BC, Li L: A dynamical systems approach to lower extremity running injuries, *Clin Biomech* 14:297–308, 1999.

130. Crisco JJ, Panjabi MM: The intersegmental and multisegmental muscles of the lumbar spine: a biomechanical model comparing lateral stabilising potential, *Spine* 7:793–799, 1991.

131. Greene HS, Cholewicki J, Galloway MT, et al: A history of low back injury is a risk factor for recurrent back injuries in varsity athletes, *Am J Sports Med* 29:795–800, 2001.

132. Moseley GL, Hodges PW: Reduced variability of postural strategy prevents normalisation of motor changes induced by back pain: a risk factor for chronic trouble? *Behav Neurosci* 120:474–476, 2006.

133. Susan H, Picavet J, Vlaeyen J, Schouten J: Pain catastrophizing and kinesiophobia: predictors of chronic low back pain, *Am J Epidemiol* 156:1028–1034, 2003.

134. Burton A, Tillotson K, Main C, Hollis S: Psychosocial predictors of outcome in acute and subchronic low back trouble, *Spine* 20:722–728, 1995.

135. Watson PJ, Booker CK: Evidence for the role of psychological factors in abnormal paraspinal activity in patients with chronic low back pain, *J Musculoskelet Pain* 5:41–56, 1997.

136. Shumway-Cooke A, Woollacott MH: *Motor control*, Baltimore, 1995, Williams & Wilkins.

137. Fitts PM, Posner MI: *Human performance*, Belmont, CA, 1967, Brooks/Cole.

138. Gentile AM: Skill acquisition: action, movement and neuromuscular processes. In Carr JH, Shepherd RB, Gordon J, et al, editors: *Movement and science: foundations for physical therapy in rehabilitation*, Rockville, MD, 1987, Aspen.

139. Delitto A, Erhard RE, Bowling RW: A treatment-based classification approach to low back syndrome: identifying and staging patients for conservative treatment, *Phys Ther* 75:470–485, 1995. discussion 485–489.

140. Petersen T, Laslett M, Thorsen H, et al: Diagnostic classification of non-specific low back pain. A new system integrating patho-anatomic and clinical categories, *Physiother Theory Pract* 19:213–237, 2003.

141. McKenzie R, May S: *The lumbar spine, mechanical diagnosis and therapy*, ed 2, Waikanae, 2003, Spinal Publications New Zealand Ltd..

142. O'Sullivan P: Diagnosis and classification of chronic low back pain disorders: maladaptive movement and motor control impairments as underlying mechanism, *Man Ther* 10:242–255, 2005.

143. Vibe Fersum K, O'Sullivan P, Skouen JS, et al: Efficacy of classification-based cognitive functional therapy in patients with non-specific chronic low back pain: a randomized controlled trial, *Eur J Pain* 17:916–928, 2013.

144. Karayannis NV, Jull GA, Hodges PW: Physiotherapy movement based classification approaches to low back pain: comparison of subgroups through review and developer/expert survey, *BMC Musculoskelet Disord* 13:24, 2012.

145. Woolf CJ: Central sensitization: implications for the diagnosis and treatment of pain, *Pain* 152(Suppl 3):S2–S15, 2011.

146. Woolf CJ: Dissecting out mechanisms responsible for peripheral neuropathic pain: implications for diagnosis and therapy, *Life Sci* 74:2605–2610, 2004.

147. Scholz J, Woolf CJ: Can we conquer pain? *Nat Neurosci* (5 Suppl):1062–1067, 2002.

148. Smart KM, Blake C, Staines A, et al: Mechanisms-based classifications of musculoskeletal pain: part 3 of 3: symptoms and signs of nociceptive pain in patients with low back (± leg) pain, *Man Ther* 17: 352–357, 2012.

149. Macedo LG, Maher CG, Hancock MJ, et al: Predicting response to motor control exercises and graded activity for patients with low back pain: preplanned secondary analysis of a randomized controlled trial, *Phys Ther* 94:1543–1554, 2014.

150. Smart KM, Blake C, Staines A, et al: Mechanisms-based classifications of musculoskeletal pain: part 1 of 3: symptoms and signs of central sensitisation in patients with low back (± leg) pain, *Man Ther* 17:336–344, 2012.

151. Waddell G: *The back pain revolution*, Edinburgh, 1998, Churchill Livingstone.

152. Marras WS, Davis KG, Heaney CA, et al: The influence of psychosocial stress, gender, and personality on mechanical loading of the lumbar spine, *Spine* 25:3045–3054, 2000.

153. Griffith LE, Shannon HS, Wells RP, et al: Individual participant data meta-analysis of mechanical workplace risk factors and low back pain, *Am J Public Health* 102:309–318, 2012.

154. Claus AP, Hides JA, Moselely GL, Hodges PW: Is 'ideal' sitting posture real? Measurement of spinal curves in four sitting postures, *Man Ther* 14:404–408, 2009.

155. McGill SM: The influence of lordosis on axial trunk torque and trunk muscle myoelectric activity, *Spine* 17:1187–1193, 1992.

156. Claus AP, Hides JA, Moselely GL, Hodges PW: Different ways to balance the spine: subtle changes in sagittal spinal curves affect regional muscle activity, *Spine* 34:E208–E214, 2009.

157. Dankaerts W, O'Sullivan P, Burnett A, Straker L: Altered patterns of superficial trunk muscle activation during sitting in nonspecific chronic low back pain patients: importance of subclassification, *Spine* 31:2017–2023, 2006.

158. Sapsford RR, Richardson CA, Maher CF, Hodges PW: Pelvic floor muscle activity in different sitting postures in continent and incontinent women, *Arch Phys Med Rehabil* 89:1741–1747, 2008.

159. Lee LJ, Chang AT, Coppieters MW, Hodes PW: Changes in sitting posture induce multiplanar changes in chest wall shape and motion with breathing, *Respir Physiol Neurobiol* 170:236–245, 2010.

160. O'Sullivan P, Dankaerts W, Burnett A, et al: Evaluation of the flexion relaxation phenomenon of the trunk muscles in sitting, *Spine* 31:2009–2016, 2006.

161. Tsao H, Hodges PW: Immediate changes in feedforward postural adjustments following voluntary motor training, *Exp Brain Res* 181:537–546, 2007.

162. Tsao H, Hodges P: Persistence of improvements in postural strategies following motor control training in people with recurrent low back pain, *J Electromyogr Kinesiol* 18:559–567, 2008.

163. Ferreira PH, Ferreira ML, Maher CG, et al: Changes in recruitment of transversus abdominis correlate with disability in people with chronic low back pain, *Br J Sports Med* 44:1166–1172, 2010.

164. Unsgaard-Tøndel M, Lund Nilsen TI, Magnussen J, Vasseljen O: Is activation of transversus abdominis and obliquus internus abdominis associated with long-term changes in chronic low back pain? A prospective study with 1-year follow-up, *Br J Sports Med* 46:729–734, 2012.

165. Vasseljen O, Fladmark AM: Abdominal muscle contraction thickness and function after specific and general exercises: a randomized controlled trial in chronic low back pain patients, *Man Ther* 15:482–489, 2010.

166. Danneels L, Cools AM, Vanderstraeten GG, et al: The effect of 3 different training modalities on the cross sectional area of paravertebral muscles, *Scand J Med Sci Sports* 11:335–341, 2001.

167. Hodges PW, Richardson CA, Jull GA: Evaluation of the relationship between the findings of a laboratory and clinical test of transversus abdominis function, *Physiother Res Int* 1:30–40, 1996.

168. Pinto RZ, Franco HR, Ferreira PH, et al: Reliability and discriminatory capacity of a clinical scale for assessing abdominal muscle coordination, *J Manipulative Physiol Ther* 34:562–569, 2011.

169. Sapsford RR, Hodges PW, Richardson CA, et al: Co-activation of the abdominal and pelvic floor muscles during voluntary exercises, *Neurourol Urodyn* 20:31–42, 2001.

170. Ferreira PH, Ferreira ML, Maher CG, et al: Specific stabilisation exercise for spinal and pelvic pain: a systematic review, *Aust J Physiother* 52:79–88, 2006.

171. Hauggaard A, Persson AL: Specific spinal stabilisation exercises in patients with low back pain—a systematic review, *Phys Ther Rev* 12:233–248, 2007.

172. Maher C, Sherrington C, Herbert R: Reliability of the PEDro scale for rating quality of randomized controlled trials, *Phys Ther* 83:713–721, 2003.

173. Shaughnessy M, Caulfield B: A pilot study to investigate the effect of lumbar stabilization exercise training on functional ability and quality of life in patients with chronic low back pain, *Int J Rehabil Res* 27:297–301, 2004.

174. Goldby LJ, Moore AP, Doust J, Trew ME: A randomized controlled trial investigating the efficiency of musculoskeletal physiotherapy on chronic low back disorder, *Spine* 31:1083–1093, 2006.

175. Costa LO, Maher CG, Latimer J, et al: Motor control exercise for chronic LBP: a randomized placebo-controlled trial, *Phys Ther* 89:1275–1286, 2009.

176. Cairns MC, Foster NE, Wright C, et al: Randomized controlled trial of specific spinal stabilization exercises and conventional physiotherapy for recurrent LBP, *Spine* 31:E670–E681, 2006.

177. Moseley L: Combined physiotherapy and education is efficacious for chronic low back pain, *Aust J Physiother* 48:297–302, 2002.

178. Niemisto L, Lahtinen-Suopanki T, Rissanen P: A randomized trial of combined manipulation, stabilizing exercises, and physician consultation compared to physician consultation alone for chronic low back pain, *Spine* 28:2185–2191, 2003.

179. Richardson CA, Jull GA: Muscle control—pain control. What exercises would you prescribe? *Man Ther* 1:2–10, 1995.

180. Rasmussen-Barr E, Nilsson-Wikmar L, Arvidsson I: Stabilizing training compared with manual treatment in sub-acute and chronic low-back pain, *Man Ther* 8:233–241, 2003.

181. Critchley D, Ratcliffe J, Noonan S, et al: Effectiveness and cost-effectiveness of three types of physiotherapy used to reduce chronic low back pain disability: a pragmatic randomized trial with economic evaluation, *Spine* 32:1474–1481, 2007.

182. Ferreira M, Ferreira P, Latimer J, et al: Comparison of motor control exercise, general exercise and spinal manipulative therapy for chronic low back pain: a randomized trial, *Pain* 131:31–37, 2007.

183. Macedo LG, Latimer J, Maher CG, et al: Effect of motor control exercises versus graded activity in patients with chronic nonspecific LBP: a randomized controlled trial, *Phys Ther* 92:363–377, 2012.

184. Macedo LG, Maher CG, Hancock M, et al: Predicting response to motor control exercises and graded activity for LBP patients: preplanned secondary analysis of a randomized controlled trial, *Phys Ther* 94:1543–1554, 2014.

185. Miller E, Schenk R, Karnes J, et al: A comparison of the McKenzie approach to a specific spine stabilization program for chronic low back pain, *J Man Manip Ther* 13:103–112, 2005.

186. Koumantakis GA, Watson PJ, Oldham JA, et al: Supplementation of general endurance exercise with stabilisation training versus general exercise only: physiological and functional outcomes of a randomised controlled trial of patients with recurrent LBP, *Clin Biomech* 20:474–482, 2005.

187. França FR, Burke TN, Caffaro RR, et al: Effects of muscular stretching and segmental stabilization on functional disability and pain in patients with chronic LBP: a randomized, controlled trial, *J Manipulative Physiol Ther* 35:279–285, 2012.

188. França FR, Burke TN, Hanada ES, Marques AP: Segmental stabilization and muscular strengthening in chronic LBP: a comparative study, *Clinics (Sao Paulo)* 65:1013–1017, 2010.

189. Unsgaard-Tondel M, Fladmark AM, Salvesen O, Vasseljen O: Motor control exercises, sling exercises, and general exercises for patients with chronic LBP: a randomized controlled trial with 1-year follow-up, *Phys Ther* 90:1426–1440, 2010.

190. Kladny B, Fischer FC, Haase I, et al: Evaluation of specific stabilizing exercise in the treatment of LBP and lumbar disk disease in outpatient rehabilitation, *Z Orthop Ihre Grenzgeb* 141:401–405, 2003.

191. Stevens V, Crombez G, Parlevliet T: *The effectiveness of the specific exercise therapy versus device exercise therapy in the treatment of chronic low back*

pain patients. In Proceedings of the 6th interdisciplinary world congress of low back and pelvic pain, Spain, 2007, Barcelona.

192. Cook C, Brismee JM, Sizer PS Jr : Subjective and objective descriptors of clinical lumbar spine instability: a Delphi study, *Man Ther* 11:11–21, 2006.

193. Brox JI, Sorensen R, Friis A: Randomized clinical trial of lumbar instrumented fusion and cognitive intervention and exercises in patients with chronic low back pain and disc degeneration, *Spine* 28: 1913–1921, 2003.

194. Froholdt A, Reikeraas O, Holm I, et al: No difference in 9-year outcome in CLBP patients randomized to lumbar fusion versus cognitive intervention and exercises, *Eur Spine J* 21:2531–2538, 2012.

195. Stuge B, Laerum E, Kirkesola G, Vollestad N: The efficacy of a treatment program focusing on specific stabilizing exercises for pelvic girdle pain after pregnancy: a randomized controlled trial, *Spine* 29:351–359, 2004.

196. Stuge B, Veierod MB, Laerum E, et al: The efficacy of a treatment program focusing on specific stabilizing exercises for pelvic girdle pain after pregnancy: a two-year follow-up of a randomized clinical trial, *Spine* 29:E197–E203, 2004.

197. Vibe Fersum K, O'Sullivan P, Skouen JS, et al: Efficacy of classification-based cognitive functional therapy in patients with non-specific chronic LBP: a randomized controlled trial, *Eur J Pain* 17:916–928, 2013.

198. Kendall FP, McCreary EK: *Muscles: testing and function*, ed 3, Baltimore, 1983, Williams & Wilkins.

199. Tsao H, Hodges PW: Immediate changes in feedforward postural adjustments following voluntary motor training, *Exp Brain Res* 181:537–546, 2007.

200. Tsao H, Hodges PW: Persistence of improvements in postural strategies following motor control training in people with recurrent low back pain, *J Electromyogr Kinesiol* 18:559–567, 2008.

201. Tsao H, Galea MP, Hodges PW: Driving plasticity in the motor cortex in recurrent low back pain, *Eur J Pain* 14:832–839, 2010.

202. Hall L, Tsao H, MacDonald D, et al: Immediate effects of co-contraction training on motor control of the trunk muscles in people with recurrent low back pain, *J Electromyogr Kinesiol* 19:763–773, 2009.

203. Ferreira PH: *Effectiveness of specific stabilisation exercises for chronic low back pain*, PhD thesis; Sydney, 2005, University of Sydney.

204. Falla D, Jull G, Russell T, et al: Effect of neck exercise on sitting posture in patients with chronic neck pain, *Phys Ther* 87:408–417, 2007.

205. Hoffman SL, Johnson MB, Zou D, et al: Effect of classification-specific treatment on lumbopelvic motion during hip rotation in people with low back pain, *Man Ther* 16:344–350, 2011.

CHAPTER 15

Spinal Pathology
Nonsurgical Intervention

OMAR EL ABD, DANIEL CAMARGO PIMENTEL, JOAO EDUARDO DAUD AMADERA

INTRODUCTION

Painful spinal conditions are very common in the general population. The lifetime prevalence of back pain can be higher than 80%.[1] In 2011, episodes of back pain were responsible for more than 3.4 million visits to outpatients departments[2] and 3.9 million visits to emergency departments,[3] being the fourth leading symptom prompting patients to seek evaluation by a physician.[4] These conditions are responsible for much pain and physical suffering for patients and for social and financial pressures in the community. Interventional spinal techniques are a new and evolving field that combines different aspects of the medical field to manage patients with painful spinal conditions. These interventions combine various aspects of physical medicine and rehabilitation, orthopedics, pain management, radiology, rheumatology, neurology, and physical therapy. The objectives of these interventional techniques are to diagnose and efficiently treat painful spinal conditions and to minimize the persistence or recurrence of pain using minimally invasive procedures. These procedures are often faster, safer, and less costly than standard surgical techniques and produce successful outcomes when well indicated.

This chapter discusses painful spinal conditions and their management through interventional techniques. It provides an overview of the clinical presentations of different pathologies and, focusing on interventional spinal procedures, discusses appropriate imaging studies, indications, techniques, side effects, and complications.

EPIDEMIOLOGY

The incidence and prevalence of back pain have been the subjects of multiple epidemiological studies. The *incidence* is the rate at which healthy subjects report a new symptom or disease within a certain period. The *prevalence* is the number of subjects reporting certain symptoms or a certain disease at a particular period. Waterman et al.[5]

estimated a back pain incidence of 139/100,000 person-years with a bimodal distribution among age groups. Two peaks were found: between 25 and 29 years of age (258/100,000 person-years) and 95 and 99 years of age (147/100,000 person-years). Lawrence et al.[6] reported a prevalence of 59.1 million U.S. adults who have had back pain within the past 3 months. According to the American National Center for Health Statistics 2012 report,[7] 28.9% of all those living in the United States older than 18 years have had low back pain and 15.8% have had neck pain within the past 3 months. As reported by Balagué et al.,[1] the lifetime prevalence of back pain can be as high as 84%, and the prevalence of chronic back pain is approximately 23% with up to 12% of the population being disabled by this condition. Back pain also represents a heavy economic burden for industrialized countries. Annual direct costs related to back pain range from $22.7 to $82.6 billion, and the total cost can be as high as $238.1 billion a year.[8]

With regard to the location of pain, the prevalence of radiculopathy (9.9% to 25%)[9] is reported to be much lower than the prevalence of axial back pain (11% to 84%).[10] The percentage of patients who report an acute episode of back pain and later develop chronic pain (lasting 3 to 6 months or longer) is the subject of controversy. Several studies suggested that 75% to 90% of patients with an acute episode of back pain recover within 4 to 6 weeks.[11] However, studies have shown a higher incidence of recurrence and persistence of pain after the initial acute episode.[12] Although the findings of studies vary, clinicians encounter a number of patients who convert from acute to chronic pain.

ANATOMY AND PAIN-PRODUCING STRUCTURES

The human spine normally consists of 7 cervical, 12 thoracic, and 5 lumbar vertebral bodies, as well as 5 fused sacral vertebrae and 5 fused coccygeal vertebrae, although anomalies can sometimes occur. The spinal cord runs in the central canal and commonly ends at the L1-2 level.

Nerve roots emerge from the neural foramina. There are seven cervical intervertebral discs and eight cervical nerve roots. In the cervical region, the nerve roots emerge cephalad to their corresponding vertebral bodies except for the C8 nerve root, which emerges caudal to the C7 vertebral body. In the thoracic, lumbar, sacral, and coccygeal regions, nerve roots continue to emerge from the neural foramina just caudal to the corresponding vertebral bodies. The cauda equina develops at the L1-2 level; it is formed by an aggregation of lumbar, sacral, and coccygeal nerve roots. These nerve roots are present in the central canal and emerge at their corresponding neural foramina. Multiple ligaments and muscles support the spine. A spinal segment (Figure 15-1) consists of two vertebral bodies: an intervertebral disc and a set of two facets on each side (zygapophyseal joints). Pain can occur as a result of pathology involving a single element, multiple elements of a particular segment, or multiple segments.

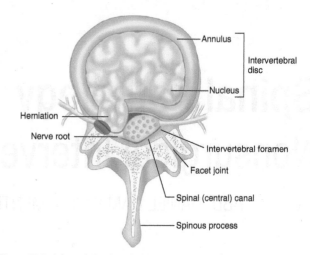

Figure 15-2 A lateral disc herniation compressing the exiting nerve root. (From Jandial R, Garfin SR: *Best evidence for spine surgery: 20 cardinal cases,* Philadelphia, 2012, Saunders.)

Radicular Pain

Involvement of nerve roots causes radicular pain. Nerve roots are affected secondary to mechanical pressure, inflammation, or both. Mechanical pressure usually occurs secondary to disc protrusion (herniation) or spinal stenosis. In the case of disc herniation, the nucleus pulposus protrudes through the annulus fibrosus and causes mechanical compression of the nerve root either in the central canal or in the intervertebral foramen (Figure 15-2). Acute disc herniations are accompanied by multiple inflammatory products (listed later in this chapter), which play an important role in the production of pain. Disc herniations occur in all age groups but are predominant in the young and middle aged. In contrast, spinal stenosis most often affects the elderly. This condition is a combination of disc degeneration, ligamentum hypertrophy and facet joint arthropathy, and/or spondylolisthesis, resulting in stenosis of the central spinal canal in the cervical and lumbar spine (Figure 15-3). Spinal stenosis causes pressure on and possibly dysfunction of the spinal cord (myelopathy) when it involves the central canal in the cervical and thoracic spine. In the lumbar spine, the cauda equina roots are involved, which causes neurogenic claudication.

With radiculopathy, symptoms are present along a nerve root distribution. This causes pain in the upper and lower extremities. It is worth mentioning that pain in the periscapular, pericostal, and buttock area can be radicular in origin. Sensory symptoms include pain, numbness, and

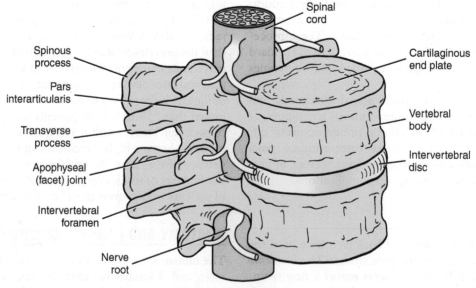

Figure 15-1 Spinal segment.

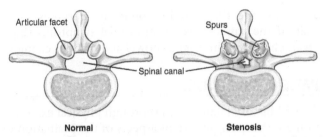

Figure 15-3 Axial cuts through vertebra showing a normal spinal canal (*left*), spinal stenosis (*right*). (From Lundy-Ekman L: *Neuroscience: Fundamentals for rehabilitation*, ed 3, St. Louis, 2007, Saunders.)

tingling that follow the distribution of a particular nerve root (see Figure 15-5 later in the chapter). The symptoms may be accompanied by motor weakness in a myotomal distribution.

Axial Pain

Axial pain occurs predominantly in the paraspinal areas and along the spinous processes. It also may be associated with pain in the extremities; however, by definition, paraspinal (axial) pain is more severe than the pain in the extremities.

Intervertebral Disc

Degenerative disc disease (spondylosis) is an important cause of axial pain. The pain from the intervertebral discs is located axially near the degenerated disc. The human disc is shaped like a donut and is formed of three distinct parts: the nucleus pulposus, the annulus fibrosus, and the cartilaginous end plates, which are adjacent to the vertebral bodies above and below. The nucleus pulposus is a semifluid mass of mucoid material composed of collagen fibers and proteoglycans. Water constitutes approximately 80% to 90% of the nucleus. As the disc ages, it loses its water content, which is replaced by fibrocartilage. The end plates function as the nutrient pathways for the disc. They are composed of hyaline cartilage, which is located toward the vertebral body surface, and fibrocartilage, which is concentrated toward the nucleus pulposus. Degeneration of the annulus predisposes the nucleus to herniation, which occurs most often at the annulus' weakest part, its posterolateral aspect. Good evidence indicates that, in addition to the pain caused by mechanical irritation of the sensory nociceptive fibers in the damaged intervertebral disc, discogenic pain occurs secondary to chemical irritation. Multiple inflammatory products are found in the painful disc tissue. These include phospholipase A2 (present in high levels), prostaglandin E, histamine-like substances, potassium ions, lactic acid, and substance P, as well as calcitonin gene-related peptide, vasoactive intestinal peptide, and other polypeptide amines, which can increase the excitability of the sensory neurons.[13,14]

The mechanism of pain referral is complex. Healthy lumbar intervertebral discs receive sensory supply into the annulus fibrosus, whereas diseased discs, according to one report, have an in-growth of nerve fibers that express substance P into their nuclei.[15] Two extensively interconnected nerve plexuses, the anterior and posterior plexuses, serve as the source of nerve endings within the lumbar intervertebral discs. The anterior plexus is formed from branches of both sympathetic trunks: the proximal ends of the gray ramii communicantes and the perivascular nerve plexuses of the segmental arteries. Therefore the anterior part of the disc is innervated solely by sympathetic fibers.[16,17]

The sinuvertebral nerves constitute the vast majority of the posterior plexus. Although some consider these nerves recurrent branches of the spinal nerves, others regard them as branches of spinal nerves with a sympathetic component. Luschka first described the sinuvertebral nerve as reentering the canal and providing innervation to the posterior longitudinal ligament and annulus fibrosus.[18] It now is widely accepted that the sinuvertebral nerve is the main nerve supply to all structures in the spinal canal. It enters the spinal canal through the intervertebral foramen. Once inside, it gives off multiple ascending and descending branches, which eventually combine to form a plexus along the posterior longitudinal ligament.[19,20] This plexus receives branches from the ipsilateral caudal and cephalic segments of the sinuvertebral nerve and as suggested the contralateral side as well.[21] Because of the interaction with the sympathetic system, as well as the segmental anastomosis, somatic pain referral is extremely common; that is, pain occurs in areas that commonly feel pain, such as the skin and underlying muscles.

Facet Joint

The facet (zygapophyseal) joints can be another source of axial pain. Pain is attributed to facet joint pathology in approximately 15% to 32% of patients who describe axial pain.[22] The facets are paired synovial joints located adjacent to the neural arches. They are formed by the superior articular process of the vertebra below and the inferior articular process of the vertebra above.

Pain is located predominantly in the paraspinal area. Pain originating from the facet joints can be either unilateral or bilateral. The results of multiple studies have led to the development of specific pain referral maps for the cervical facet joints. The facet joints receive their innervations from the medial branch of the dorsal ramii, with each medial branch innervating two joints.[23] Each joint is innervated by the medial branches rostral and caudal to that joint.[23] In the cervical spine, cervical facet pain can be accompanied by headaches in arthropathies of the atlantooccipital, atlantoaxial (C1-2 facet joint),

C2-3, and C3-4 facet joints. This is especially observed in patients with a history of whiplash events.[24,25] The third occipital nerve, which is the superficial medial branch of the C3 dorsal ramus, predominantly innervates the C2-3 joint, along with articular branches from the C2 dorsal ramus. At times, a small, inconsistent contribution arises from a communicating branch of the great occipital nerve.[26,27] The C1-2 lateral joints are innervated by the anterior ramii of C1 and C2.[28] Upon entering the spinal cord, the C1, C2, and C3 nerves converge with trigeminal nerve afferents on cells in the dorsal gray column of C1 to C3. This results in the communication between both afferents known as *trigeminal volleys*. The trigeminal nerve provides superficial sensations to most of the face and anterior scalp. Therefore pain is referred in the trigeminal nerve distribution.

Compression Fractures

Acute vertebral compression fractures are becoming an increasingly common cause of axial back pain. This increase in incidence is probably due to the aging population and the prevalence of osteoporosis. The pain usually is very severe and localized, and it usually occurs in the area overlying the involved vertebral body. Vertebral osteoporotic compression fractures most often occur in the thoracolumbar junction area. The occurrence of these fractures increases with age, and its prevalence is estimated to be 10% to 26% among women and men older than 50 years.[29] The pain usually is precipitated by trauma, although it has been reported to follow minor events, such as coughing. It also can occur spontaneously in patients with severe osteoporosis because osteoporotic vertebral bodies are unable to withstand stress. In addition, compression fractures may be caused by malignancies involving the spine.

Sacroiliac Joint

Sacroiliac (SI) joint arthropathy also can be a cause of axial back pain that affects 15% to 30% of individuals with chronic nonradicular pain.[30] The pain is located in the lumbosacral-buttock junction with referral to the lower extremities and to the groin area. Painful conditions of the SI joint can result from spondyloarthropathies, infection, malignancies, pregnancies, and trauma, or they can even occur spontaneously.

Referred Pain

Musculoskeletal structures and organs near the spine are potential sources of pain, from which the pain can be referred to the spine and the paraspinal area. A careful, detailed physical examination is needed to assess these conditions because various shoulder and hip conditions can mimic radiculopathies. Pelvic conditions and malignancies involving the supraclavicular area or the axilla should be considered if symptoms persist despite the absence of identifiable lesions on imaging studies, especially if the patient has constitutional symptoms (e.g., fever, chills, weight loss) or bowel and bladder changes.

PATIENT EVALUATION

Careful history taking and a thorough physical examination are the most important aspects of the evaluation of patients with a painful spinal condition. This process is necessary so that the clinician can interpret the imaging studies accurately in context and formulate the treatment plan.

History Taking

As in any clinical encounter, the clinician inquires about the history of the painful condition, including its location, onset, character, radiation, exacerbating and mitigating factors, and accompanying symptoms. It is crucial to establish which area is the most painful; this allows the clinician to formulate the preliminary differential diagnosis and to determine whether the pain is axial, radicular, or referred from other structures. Discogenic pain originating from painful disc conditions usually is difficult to localize. On questioning, patients frequently point to a general area of pain. This pain usually is exacerbated by sitting and mitigated by a change in position. Pain may be characterized but not limited to aching or a sharp sensation. In the cervical spine, upper cervical discs refer pain to the occipital area, causing headaches.[27] In the lumbar spine, pain may be referred to the abdominal and inguinal areas.[21]

Cervical facet joint pain is usually but not explicitly exacerbated by neck extension or lateral bending. In the lumbar region, pain from facet joints usually is exacerbated by standing and walking and mitigated by sitting; however, pain from lumbar facet joints can occur on forward flexion as well. Pain from facet joints usually overlies the facet joints in the paraspinal area and is more localized than discogenic pain. Pain can be referred ipsilaterally or bilaterally.

Specific diagrams are available that show the referral patterns for cervical facet joint pain (Figure 15-4). The referral pattern for cervical facet joint pain has been studied and established.[31] To map the pain referral patterns for the cervical facet joints, researchers stimulated the joints in healthy subjects and noted the painful locations.[26,32,33] Different studies produced essentially very similar pain referral maps in the cervical spine. However, the authors of the chapter are not aware of studies that consistently reproduced pain referral maps from the lumbar facet joints.

Patients with radicular symptoms usually describe pain predominantly in the extremities. The pain may start as axial pain (in the case of disc herniations), which is followed by the onset of limb pain as the axial pain improves. It is important to note that the buttocks and periscapular regions are considered part of the limbs. Pain predominantly in these locations is considered radicular pain rather than

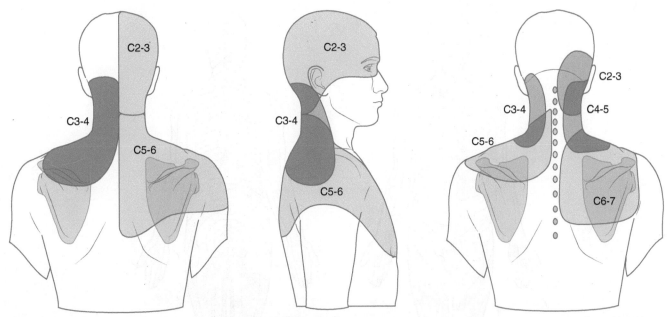

Figure 15-4 Referral patterns of cervical facet joint pain. *Dark brown* indicates overlap. In figure on the left, note that dermatomes overlap and different dermatomes are shown on each side. (From Slipman C, Derby R, Simeone F et al: *Interventional spine: an algorithmic approach*, p 614, Philadelphia, 2008, Saunders.)

axial pain. The pain often is described as shooting, stabbing, sharp, or burning, and patients often are able to localize the painful area accurately. The pain usually follows a specific nerve root distribution, with some variability.[34] Cervical radicular pain is exacerbated by cervical extension and lateral bending. The pain may be relieved by overhead elevation of the ipsilateral upper extremity because this maneuver reduces tension on the lower nerve roots (shoulder abduction relief sign).[35] Dermatome maps are available that outline the spinal nerve root distribution (Figure 15-5). It is important to note that these maps are not 100% accurate as nerve root distribution varies from individual to individual.

Clinical Note

Dermatome patterns can vary from individual to individual.

In cases of disc herniation and foraminal stenosis, lumbar radicular pain is often exacerbated by sitting and mitigated by walking. In cases of spinal stenosis, pain is generally exacerbated by walking (spinal extension) and mitigated by sitting (neurogenic claudication). Differentiating neurogenic claudication from vascular claudication, which occurs secondary to vascular insufficiency, is important because both conditions affect the same (elderly) population. Patients with vascular claudication feel relief from pain when they stop walking or when they stand rather than sit. Patients with neurogenic claudication have more pain when walking downhill (because of spinal extension) and less pain when walking with a walker or a shopping cart (because of spinal flexion). Pain

from neurogenic claudication follows a nerve root distribution, whereas pain from vascular claudication is present globally in the location supplied by specific arteries.

Pain referred from the SI joint should be suspected in patients who describe pain in the low back, predominantly in the sacral sulcus area, with or without radiation to the lower extremity and the groin area. Pain occurs secondary to systemic conditions (e.g., spondyloarthropathies, repetitive shear events) and after trauma, or it can occur spontaneously.[36]

Physical Examination

A focused physical examination based on the information acquired in the patient's history establishes a working differential diagnosis. Some elements of the general physical examination are essential in the evaluation of patients with painful spinal conditions. These elements are detailed in Table 15-1.

Spinal Physical Examination Maneuvers

Specific maneuvers are used to evaluate a variety of conditions and anatomical areas that may cause a patient pain. These maneuvers are outlined in Table 15-2. Discogenic provocative maneuvers provoke pain reproduction in patients with lumbar discogenic pain. Root tension signs in the upper and lower extremities reproduce radicular pain. SI provocative maneuvers are used to reproduce pain in patients with SI joint syndrome. These tests are neither specific nor sensitive. (More information on these tests and others can be found in Volume 1 of this series, *Orthopedic Physical Assessment*.)

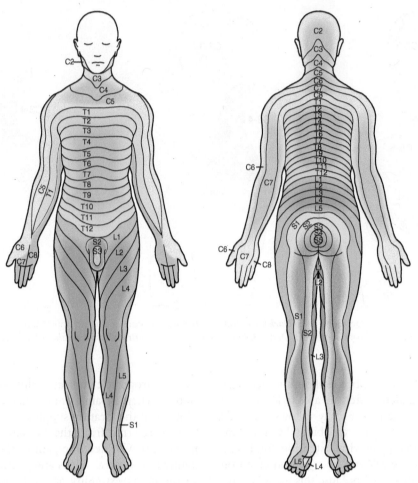

Figure 15-5 Dermatome maps. (From Marx J, Hockberger R, Walls, R: *Rosen's emergency medicine: concepts and clinical practice*, ed 8, Philadelphia, 2014, Saunders.)

TABLE **15-1**

General Physical Examination Elements that May Have Bearing on a Spinal Condition

Evaluation	Description	Rationale
Height and weight	Measurement	Height-weight ratio assessment, exercise and diet recommendations; unusual loss of weight requires medical workup
Deformity	Scoliosis, kyphosis, reduced lordosis (cervical or lumbar)	Sign of spinal pathology, postural changes, and possible causes of musculoskeletal imbalances
Muscle wasting	Inspection of the peripheral muscles	Sign of radiculopathy or other neurological disorder
Leg length discrepancy	Measurement	Postural changes and musculoskeletal imbalances
Examination of pulses	Arterial pulses in the upper and lower extremities	Peripheral vascular disease may result in painful conditions that mimic radiculopathy
Palpation of lymph nodes	Presence of lymph nodes in the neck, axilla, and inguinal area	Possible sign of occult malignancy resulting in metastasis to the spine
Palpation of tenderness	Over the spinous processes and facet and SI joints	Spine pathology, such as compression fractures and facet joint and SI joint arthropathy
Peripheral joint examination	Range of motion and specific joint maneuvers	Extraspinal source of pain with referral to the spine
Gait examination	Assessment of gait, heel walking, toe walking, and tandem walking	Good screening tool for evaluation of weakness and neurological disorders

SI, sacroiliac.

TABLE **15-2**

Spinal Physical Examination Maneuvers

Maneuver	Technique	Result
Pelvic rock	With the patient supine, flex the hips until the flexed knees approximate to the chest; then rotate the lower extremities from one side to the other	Provokes lumbar discogenic pain
Sustained hip flexion	With the patient supine, raise the extended lower extremities to approximately 60°. Ask the patient to hold the lower extremities in that position and release. The test result is positive with reproduction of low lumbar and/or buttock pain. Next, lower the extremities successively approximately 15° and at each point note the reproduction and intensity of pain	Provokes lumbar discogenic pain
Upper extremity: root tension signs	Perform contralateral neck lateral bending and abduction of the ipsilateral upper extremity	Reproduces cervical radicular pain in the periscapular area or in the upper extremity
Spurling's maneuver	Passively perform cervical extension, lateral bending toward the side of symptoms, and axial compression	Reproduces cervical radicular pain in the periscapular area or in the upper extremity
Straight leg raise	With the patient supine, the involved lower extremity is passively flexed to 30° with the knee in full extension	Reproduces pain in the buttock, posterior thigh, and posterior calf in conditions with S1 radicular pain
Reverse straight leg raise	With the patient prone, the involved lower extremity is passively extended, the knee flexed	Reproduces pain in the buttock and anterior thigh in conditions with high lumbar (e.g., L3 and L4) radicular pain
Crossed straight leg raise	With the patient supine, the contralateral lower extremity is passively flexed to 30° with the knee in full extension	Reproduces pain in the ipsilateral buttock, posterior thigh, and posterior calf in conditions with S1 radicular pain
Sitting root	With the patient sitting, the involved lower extremity is passively flexed with the knee extended	Reproduces pain in the buttock, posterior thigh, and posterior calf in conditions with S1 radicular pain
Lasegue's test	With the patient supine, the involved lower extremity is passively flexed to 90°	Reproduces pain in the buttock, posterior thigh, and posterior calf in conditions with S1 radicular pain
Bragard's maneuver	With the patient supine, the involved lower extremity is passively flexed to 30°, with dorsiflexion of the foot	Reproduces pain in the buttock, posterior thigh, and posterior calf in conditions with S1 radicular pain
Gaenslen's maneuver	Position the patient supine with the affected side flush with the edge of the examination table. The hip and knee on the unaffected side are flexed, and the patient clasps the flexed knee to the chest. The examiner then applies pressure against the clasped knee, extends the lower extremity on the ipsilateral side, and brings it under the surface of the examination table	Reproduces pain in patients with SI joint syndrome
SI joint compression	With the patient side lying, apply compression to the joint	Reproduces pain in patients with SI joint syndrome
Pressure at the sacral sulcus	With the patient in a prone position, apply pressure on the posterior superior iliac spine (PSIS) (dimple)	Reproduces pain in patients with SI joint syndrome
Patrick's test or FABER test	With the patient supine, the knee and hip are flexed. The hip is abducted and externally rotated	Reproduces pain in patients with SI joint syndrome, facet joint arthropathy (pain is reproduced in the low back), and degenerative joint disease of the hip (pain is reproduced in the groin)
Yeoman's test	With the patient prone, the hip is extended and the ilium is externally rotated	Reproduces pain in patients with SI joint syndrome
Iliac gapping test	Distraction to the anterior SI ligaments can be performed by applying pressure to the anterosuperior iliac spine	Reproduces pain in patients with SI joint syndrome

SI, sacroiliac.

The best diagnostic method for evaluating pain that emanates from the SI joint is a fluoroscopically guided, intra-articular diagnostic injection with a local anesthetic.[37]

Sensory Examination

Pinprick, light touch, position, and vibration sensation are examined, with particular emphasis on the limb with radicular pain. The sensations of vibration and position are diminished in severe spinal stenosis, especially in the cervical spine with central canal involvement. In radiculopathy, reduced pinprick and light touch sensations are noted in specific dermatomal distribution.

Spinal Sensory Changes with Pathology

- Spinal stenosis: sensations of vibration and position are affected
- Radiculopathy: sensations of pinprick and light touch are affected in specific dermatomes

Deep Tendon Reflexes

Examination of the deep tendon reflexes is helpful in the diagnosis of radiculopathies, especially if asymmetrical reflexes are present (Table 15-3). Deep tendon reflexes may be diminished secondary to multiple neurological conditions or as a result of age. In contrast, deep tendon reflexes may remain unaffected in radiculopathies or may even be hyperactive in radiculopathies accompanied by upper motor neuron lesions.

Manual Muscle Testing

Manual muscle testing is performed on the four extremities to determine whether a myotomic weakness is present. To detect myotomic weakness, two different muscles supplied by the same nerve root and two different peripheral nerves usually are tested. For example, to examine the L5 nerve root for muscle weakness, the extensor hallucis longus (L5, deep peroneal nerve) and gluteus medius and minimus (L5, superior gluteal nerve) are tested. This testing rules out different neurological conditions that cause weakness, such as myopathies, peripheral nerve injuries, and plexopathies.

TABLE 15-3

Deep Tendon Reflexes

Deep Tendon Reflex	Nerve Root Affected
Biceps	C6
Triceps	C7
Quadriceps	L4
Medial hamstring (not commonly elicited)	L5
Gastrocsoleus	S1

Spinal Range of Motion

Range of motion usually is restricted in patients with spinal pain because of degenerative spinal conditions and muscle guarding around the painful structure.

IMAGING STUDIES

Imaging studies are essential to confirm a suspected diagnosis. Furthermore, imaging must be done before spinal intervention procedures are performed. With the advances in imaging technology, a high number of false-positive findings may be encountered. Imaging of the spine solely identifies anatomical changes but not biochemical or physiological changes that cause pain. It is important to correlate the imaging findings with the clinical picture. For example, anatomical changes, which are visualized through various radiologic and imaging studies, can be attributable to the aging process. However, these changes may not cause symptoms. Ordering unnecessary imaging studies without a clear management plan is not beneficial. Sorting out the positive findings is really the clinician's task. When the imaging studies are properly correlated with the clinical picture and other investigations, the accuracy of the diagnosis, and therefore management, is optimized.

Clinical Note

The clinician must always correlate the findings from diagnostic imaging with the clinical findings for the diagnostic imaging findings to have clinical significance related to the patient's problems.

Radiographic Imaging

Traditionally, radiographic imaging is the first step in the evaluation of painful spinal disorders. Although x-ray films cannot be used to evaluate soft tissues, such as the intervertebral discs, nerves, ligaments, or spinal cord, they are useful for screening for fractures, bone changes, and anatomical deformities. Radiographic studies can be used to evaluate the alignment of the spine and the integrity and architecture of the radiopaque structures. Dynamic x-ray images, such as flexion and extension views, can be used to evaluate spinal instability.

Plain x-ray film anteroposterior, oblique, and lateral views constitute a routine examination. These views provide information about intervertebral disc heights, spondylotic changes, foraminal size variability, deformities, and bony alignment. X-ray films can be useful for identifying malignancy and destructive, metabolic, and rheumatological diseases. The usefulness of ordering x-ray films for acute low back pain is the subject of debate in the literature. Because the pain from this condition improves in a short time, radiographic results usually are not significant and do not affect management. X-ray films should be requested in atypical presentations. Deyo and Diehl[38] suggested criteria for ordering x-ray films to

TABLE **15-4**

Criteria for Use of X-Ray Imaging in Acute Low Back Pain

Criteria	Rationale
Age >50 years	Higher risk of osteoporotic fractures
Significant trauma	Risk of fractures
Neurological deficit	Sign of radiculopathy
Unexplained weight loss	Occult spinal lesion (e.g., malignancy)
Suspicion of ankylosing spondylitis	Spine and sacroiliac joint x-ray films are diagnostic for this condition
History of alcohol or drug abuse	Risk of infection (e.g., osteomyelitis)
History of cancer	Possible spinal metastasis
Corticosteroid use	Osteoporotic fractures
Fever	Possible osteomyelitis
Pain that persists longer than 1 month	Pain is becoming chronic, and further management is recommended
Litigation	To further establish the cause of pain

Data from Deyo RA, Diehl AK: Lumbar spine films in primary care: current use and effects of selective ordering criteria, *J Gen Intern Med* 1:20-25, 1986.

evaluate painful conditions of the lumbar spine. The purpose is mainly to exclude other significant conditions that can manifest as low back pain. These criteria and their rationales are summarized in Table 15-4.

Common Spinal Pathology X-ray Series

- Anteroposterior view
- Oblique view
- Lateral view

Computed Tomography

Computed tomography (CT) scans use two x-ray beams focused on a particular plane of an object. Multiple images are taken, and composite axial images are created using a computer and a rotating x-ray beam. With advances in digital reformatting of the axial images, coronal and sagittal images can be obtained as well as a digital three-dimensional image reconstruction.

A CT scan of the spine provides superior quality imaging of the bone structures. With a CT scan, the clinician can identify subtle fractures that are not identifiable on plain x-ray films. CT scans also provide information about destructive bone pathologies (e.g., infection and malignancy) and on bony union after surgery. Using myelography in conjunction with CT scans enhances imaging for painful spinal disorders. Myelography involves injection of a contrast material into the spinal canal, after

which the CT scan is performed. (Before the use of CT scans, myelography was performed with plain x-ray films.) CT scan myelography provides information about the status of the spinal canal in addition to the spinal bony elements. CT scans and CT myelograms are important in the postoperative workup of painful spinal conditions involving implanted ferromagnetic hardware and in patients unable to have magnetic resonance imaging (MRI) because of implanted devices.

Bone Scan

Bone scanning (also called *bone scintigraphy*) allows the clinician to assess both the anatomy and the physiological activity of tissues. It is an effective screening modality for evaluating systemic pathologies because it covers the whole body. Before and as part of the bone scan, the patient is given an intravenous injection of nuclear tracers that emit small amounts of γ-radiation proportional to the uptake from a specific tissue. Imaging of the radiation produced in tissues allows evaluation of the location of tissue metabolic pathologies. Technetium-99 m is used in the evaluation of bone pathologies, and gallium-67 is used in the evaluation of infections. Healthy bones are in a constant state of normal turnover of bone breakdown (osteoclast activity) and bone rebuilding (osteoblast activity). An increased concentration of the technetium-99 tracer suggests increased bone turnover, which can occur in pathologies such as osteoblastic malignant lesions and acute fractures. Lack of radioactive tracer activity indicates cessation of bone activity (cold defect), which can occur with osteonecrosis. Imaging of the radiotracer traditionally is performed in a uniplanar anteroposterior fashion. Single photon emission CT (SPECT) now allows tomographic images to be obtained, which improves the sensitivity and specificity of this modality.

Bone scanning is particularly useful for evaluating for occult lesions and suspected infections and as a screening tool for metastases. Because most metastatic spinal lesions are osteoblastic in origin, bone scans detect high bone turnover activity with these lesions. A minority of malignancies involving the spine (e.g., multiple myeloma) may involve osteoclastic activity; in these cases, a bone scan result is negative. If a bone scan result is positive, further imaging of the involved area(s) is performed using other modalities, such as CT scanning and MRI studies, which provide anatomical details.

Magnetic Resonance Imaging

MRI was first used in the late 1970s and had gained popularity by the mid-1980s. MRI has become the imaging modality of choice for evaluating painful spinal conditions. It provides a detailed anatomical picture that surpasses the results of other modalities, allowing the clinician to better visualize and evaluate structures, such as the nerve roots, spinal cord, paraspinal area, and soft tissues (e.g., intervertebral discs). MRI is sensitive to bone marrow abnormalities found in malignancy, infection, and disc degeneration. With the use of intravenous contrast (gadolinium), MRI provides optimum information on spinal cord lesions, demyelination, infections, fractures, and tumors. In the evaluation of postoperative spinal pain recurrence, comparison of the MRI images before and after intravenous administration of gadolinium contrast helps to differentiate new disc herniations, recurrence, and postoperative scarring.

MRI technology does not involve the use of ionizing radiation. Instead it uses magnetic fields and pulsed radiofrequency through which computer-generated sagittal, axial, and coronal images are produced. An external magnet polarizes the hydrogen protons in water molecules, and a specific radiofrequency is pulsed into the body. Images are generated according to the tissues' mobile intrinsic hydrogen ions.

Two frequency spin sequences are used for MRI imaging: T1-weighted imaging (the longitudinal relaxation time) and T2-weighted imaging (the transverse relaxation time). On T1-weighted images, fat-rich tissues have a bright signal. On T2-weighted images, extracellular free water has a bright signal.

The most common terminology used by clinicians to describe MRI spinal findings is presented in Table 15-5, and findings are shown in Figures 15-6 to 15-13.

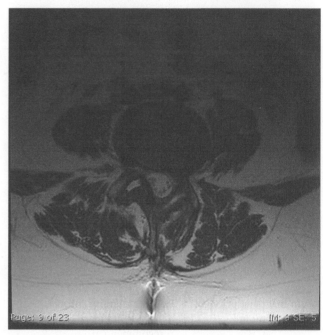

Figure 15-6 Axial T2-weighted image demonstrating fluid in the right L4-5 facet joint after left L4 laminectomy and facetectomy, indicating stress on the right L4-5 facet joint with possible pain.

TABLE **15-5**

Common Magnetic Resonance Imaging Terminology and Descriptions

Term	Description
Disc desiccation	Reduction of the bright nuclear signal on the sagittal T2-weighted images; this finding signifies disc degeneration and reduction of the water content of the nucleus
Disc bulge	Circumferential, broad-based extension of the annulus beyond the vertebral end plate
Disc herniation	General term used to describe the displacement of the nucleus pulposus beyond the disc itself
Focal disc protrusion	More specific term describing disc displacement. The nuclear material protrudes into the annulus without disrupting its outer wall; this results in a change in the contour of the annulus (see Figures 15-6 to 15-12)
Disc extrusion	Nuclear material protrudes through the outer wall of the annulus. The protruded material can remain contained by the posterior longitudinal ligament (subligamentous extrusion) or may extend beyond it (transligamentous extrusion)
Sequestered disc	Nuclear material is detached from the disc and migrates in the spinal canal cranially or caudally
High-intensity zone	An area of high intensity on T2-weighted images in the annulus;[39] it occurs secondary to an area of vascularized granulation tissue in the outer region of the annulus
Foraminal stenosis	Narrowing of the neural foramen; this commonly occurs secondary to a lateral disc herniation, bone spurs, or spondylolisthesis
Central stenosis	Narrowing of the central canal; this commonly occurs secondary to a combination of disc herniation and/or ligamentum hypertrophy, facet joint hypertrophy, and spondylolisthesis
Myelomalacia	T2-weighted signal changes in the spinal cord commonly present in severe central stenosis
End plate changes (Modic changes[40])	Changes in the end plates associated with degenerative disc disease at the level of involvement, first described by Modic et al.[40] Type 1 changes decrease signal intensity on T1-weighted images and increase signal intensity on T2-weighted images. Type 2 changes increase signal intensity on T1-weighted images and isointense or slightly increase signal intensity on T2-weighted images; type 3 changes show a decreased signal intensity on both T1- and T2-weighted images. These changes in signal intensity appear to reflect a spectrum of vertebral body marrow changes associated with degenerative disc disease

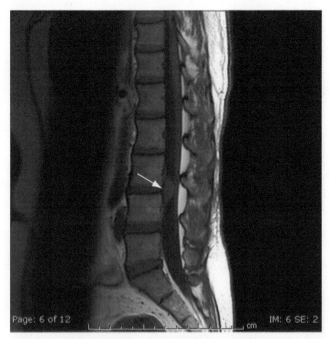

Figure 15-7 Sagittal T1-weighted image with a large focal protrusion at the L3-4 disc level.

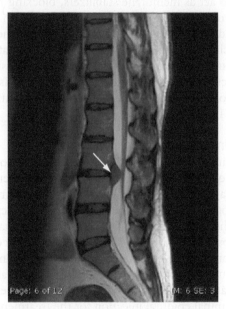

Figure 15-8 Sagittal T2-weighted image with a large focal protrusion at the L3-4 disc level.

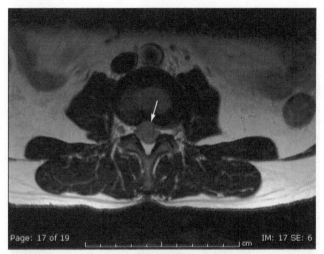

Figure 15-9 Axial T2-weighted image with a large focal protrusion at the L3-4 disc level.

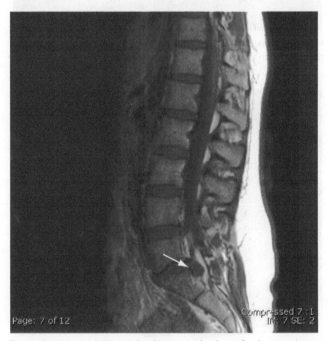

Figure 15-10 Sagittal T1-weighted image with a large focal protrusion at the L5-S1 disc level.

SPINAL INTERVENTION PROCEDURES

The two main types of spinal intervention procedures are diagnostic interventions and therapeutic interventions.

Diagnostic Intervention Procedures

The purpose of diagnostic spinal interventions is to establish and confirm a suspected diagnosis. In many cases the physical examination, imaging techniques, and electrodiagnostic studies fail to provide an accurate assessment of spinal pathologies. This often is due to multiple-level imaging findings or a lack of imaging or electrodiagnostic evidence of a painful spinal disorder. Through the use of local anesthetics, diagnostic interventions attempt either to "block" the painful structure and eliminate or reduce the pain or to provoke pain to allow an accurate assessment of the location of the pathology based on the patient's response.

Pharmacological Intervention Procedures

Local Steroid Injections

Therapeutic interventions are widely used to treat painful spinal conditions. These can include local steroid injections or other devices and procedures, such as

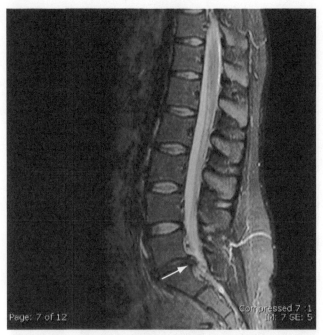

Page: 7 of 12   Compressed 7 :1   IM: 7 SE: 5

Figure 15-11 Sagittal T2-weighted image with a large focal protrusion at the L5-S1 disc level.

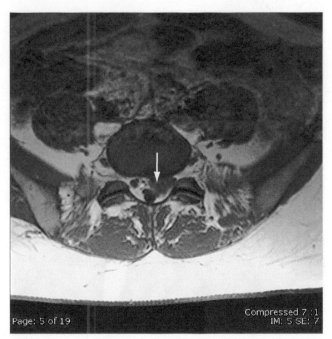

Page: 5 of 19   Compressed 7 :1   IM: 5 SE: 7

Figure 15-13 Axial T1-weighted image showing a large, left focal protrusion at the L5-S1 disc level compressing the left S1 nerve.

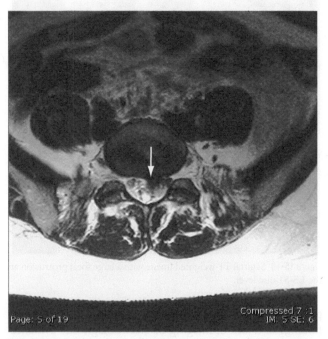

Page: 5 of 19   Compressed 7 :1   IM: 5 SE: 6

Figure 15-12 Axial T2-weighted image showing a large, left focal protrusion at the L5-S1 disc level compressing the left S1 nerve.

radiofrequency and percutaneous disc decompression. Administration of a local steroid injection in or around the painful structure is considered an efficient way to use steroids in small amounts without systemic side effects.

Steroids are a potent anti-inflammatory medication. They reduce inflammation around the intervertebral discs, spinal nerves, and facet joints. At the cellular level, steroids inhibit the action of phospholipase A2, preventing the formation of arachidonic acid and inflammatory mediators.

They also act as membrane stabilizers, blocking the conduction of nociceptive C fibers that carry pain signals. Steroids diminish the sensitization of the dorsal horn cells by reducing prostaglandins. After the inflammation has been reduced, edema around the nerve roots subsides and microcirculation is improved, reducing nerve ischemia. The steroids most often used in spinal interventions are listed in Table 15-6.

Interlaminar and Caudal Epidural Injections

Interlaminar epidural injections are the traditional and most frequently used spinal therapeutic intervention in the management of axial discogenic pain and radicular pain. Dogliotti[41] first introduced epidural injections in 1933. The injections were first used in the management of lumbosacral pain in 1952.[42] Currently the use of interlaminar and caudal epidural injections versus transforaminal epidural injections is the subject of debate, although the literature is increasingly showing more benefit of transforaminal epidural injection for the treatment of certain spine conditions as compared with other injections.[43] Interlaminar and caudal epidural injections are considered nontarget specific compared with transforaminal injections. Steroids are injected into the posterior epidural space but do not reach the anterior space because of the presence of ligaments. In a randomized, double-blind trial, Carette et al.[44] administered up to three interlaminar epidural injections of methylprednisolone acetate or isotonic saline to 158 patients with sciatica caused by a herniated nucleus pulposus (HNP). No significant differences in outcomes were seen in the short or long term (1 year). These researchers concluded that interlaminar epidural injections offered no significant functional

TABLE **15-6**

Common Medications Used for Spinal Intervention Procedures

	Hydrocortisone	Methylprednisolone (Depo-Medrol)	Triamcinolone Acetonide (Kenalog)	Betamethasone Sodium Phosphate and Acetate (Celestone, Soluspan)	Dexamethasone Sodium Phosphate (Decadron Phosphate)
Relative anti-inflammatory potency	1	5*	5*	25*	25*
pH	5-7	7-8	4.5-6.5	6.8-7.2	7-8.5
Onset	Fast	Slow	Moderate	Fast	Fast
Duration of action	Short	Intermediate	Intermediate	Long	Long
Concentration (mg/cc)	50	40-80	20	6	4 mg/cc
Relative mineralocorticoid activity	2+	0	0	0	0

*Relative to hydrocortisone as 1.

benefit, nor did they reduce the need for surgery. The major flaw in this study was that fluoroscopic guidance was not used. Needle positioning was not confirmed either with fluoroscopy or by adding local anesthetic, and transient sensory and motor deficits were not monitored after the epidural injection.

Koes et al.[45] reviewed data from 12 randomized studies and reported that the efficacy of interlaminar epidural steroid injections was not established. The benefits of epidural steroid injections, if any, were of short duration only. Watts and Silagy[46] reviewed 11 randomized studies involving a total of 907 patients and reported no long-term adverse outcomes. They also provided quantitative evidence from meta-analysis that epidural administration of corticosteroids is effective in the management of lumbosacral radicular pain. In a retrospective study of 75 patients, Manchikanti et al.[47] compared pain relief after blind interlaminar epidural injections, caudal epidural injections, and transforaminal epidural injections. The response was most favorable with transforaminal injections, followed by caudal injections, which surpassed the outcome for blind interlaminar injections.

Indications for Interlaminar and Caudal Epidural Injections

- Overall, studies have shown better outcomes for interlaminar and caudal epidural injections in acute rather than chronic pain, with a longer duration of improvement for radicular pain.
- Interlaminar epidural injections are declining in popularity among interventionalists, whereas transforaminal epidural injections are growing in popularity because of their better outcomes.

Interlaminar epidural injections are performed blindly or with fluoroscopic guidance. In a prospective study that included 316 patients undergoing blind epidural injections, needle positions were evaluated using fluoroscopy.[48]

Renfrew et al.[48] reported that, even in experienced hands, blind placement of the injection needle was optimal in only 60% of cases. They recommended fluoroscopic control and contrast administration to ensure correct needle placement and to prevent inadvertent vascular injections.

Technique for Interlaminar Epidural Injections. With fluoroscopic guidance, the level of the injection can be accurately assessed and the epidural location can be accurately confirmed using contrast. This reduces the patient's discomfort. Using contrast helps reduce the incidence of intravascular injections; such an injection can be readily identified because the contrast has a quick runoff (i.e., fast flow of contrast under fluoroscopy when the medium is injected into a blood vessel). The use of fluoroscopy and contrast is highly recommended in postoperative patients because it readily identifies the surgical level and confirms needle positioning.

The patient is placed in the prone position on the fluoroscopy table. A pillow is placed under the abdomen to open up the interlaminar space. Conscious sedation can be used but is not recommended; avoiding its use provides extra protection from accidental neural trauma. Light sedation is suggested if the patient is very anxious or has a history of vasovagal events. The blood pressure, pulse, and pulse oxymetry are monitored. The skin is prepped with iodine and draped with sterile drapes. The interlaminar space is properly identified under fluoroscopy by adjusting the end plates and aligning the spinous processes. A midline interspinous or slightly paraspinal entry point is identified. Using a 25-gauge, 4-cm (1.5-inch) needle, the clinician injects 0.5 cc of lidocaine 1% subcutaneously, forming a skin wheal. This injection is used to numb the skin, and it also provides the clinician with a needle introduction site.

For the intralaminar injection, 17- to 22-gauge Tuohy needles are used. These are special needles with curved tips designed to reduce the incidence of dural punctures. In most cases 9-cm (3.5-inch) needles are used, but 13-cm (5-inch) needles occasionally are needed for obese patients. Pencil point tip (Whitacre and Sprotte), sharp tip (Quincke), and blunt tip needles are also used.

The needle is introduced through the skin and advanced into the midline of the interlaminar space. The needle stylet is removed, and a loss of resistance syringe is applied. A "loss of resistance" syringe is a special syringe made of plastic or glass. The clinician introduces the needle, under fluoroscopic guidance, while applying continuous pressure on the syringe plunger. Once the needle passes through the thick ligamentum flavum, the clinician feels a sense of give and encounters a loss of resistance on the syringe plunger. Aspiration is performed to ensure that there is no leakage of cerebrospinal fluid. Contrast is injected to confirm the needle's position. When the epidural flow is confirmed, steroids and local anesthetics are injected. The needle is then removed. If the vital signs are stable, the patient is transferred by stretcher or wheelchair to the waiting area for monitoring for approximately 15 minutes. As soon as the lower extremities regain their full strength, the patient is discharged.

Evidence of Vasovagal Events (Vasovagal Attack)

- Lightheadedness (dizziness)
- Paleness
- Sweating
- Nausea
- Decreased blood pressure
- Decreased heart rate
- Loss of consciousness

The cervical spine is a narrower space; however, the same technique is used. Cervical interlaminar epidural injections are performed at the C6-7 or C7-T1 level because of the relative increase in spinal canal diameter at those levels. Performing the injections at these levels is relatively safer because the wider central canal reduces the chances of spinal cord injury and provides a better space for introducing catheters. A needle and catheter technique frequently is used to perform cervical interlaminar epidural injections. An epidural catheter is inserted through an epidural needle placed at the C6-7 or the C7-T1 level. The epidural needle is introduced with the loss of resistance technique. Once the positioning is confirmed with fluoroscopy, a 20-gauge catheter is introduced and driven cephalad in the epidural space near the level of the pathology. Contrast is used to confirm the catheter's presence in the epidural space before medications are injected. This technique has the advantage of introducing the medication near the pathology while accessing the epidural space in the lower cervical spine.

Lumbosacral or caudal epidural steroid injections are performed blindly or with fluoroscopic guidance.

In the blind technique, the patient is placed in the prone position, and the sacral hiatus is palpated. The skin is prepped and draped in the usual sterile manner. A spinal needle is introduced at 45°. A pop is felt as the needle passes through the sacrococcygeal ligament. The angle of the needle is reduced, and the needle is advanced superiorly. The "loss of resistance technique" is used to confirm the needle's position. Once the epidural positioning has been confirmed, a mixture of steroids and local anesthetics is injected. With the "fluoroscopically guided technique," the sacral hiatus is identified, the needle is inserted in a similar fashion to above but the needle is guided using a fluoroscope and its position is confirmed with contrast.

Transforaminal Epidural Injections

Transforaminal epidural injections are administered only under fluoroscopic guidance. This injection aims for the disc and spinal nerve interface. The needle is introduced into a triangular space within the anterosuperior third of the neural foramen; this space, known as the "safe triangle" (Figure 15-14), is bounded by the pedicle superiorly, exiting nerve inferomedially, and lateral margin of the neural foramen laterally. The needle is lodged at the 6 o'clock position, just inferior to the pedicle. If the needle is introduced farther medially, such that the safe triangle is violated, a dural puncture may result. Once the needle is in position, the medication can be efficiently injected into the lateral epidural space or around the emerging nerve root, depending on the needle position and the bevel (slanted) orientation.

This approach is commonly used in the treatment of radicular pain,[16] and it also is used in the management of axial discogenic pain. In experienced hands, the transforaminal technique is safe and produces a good outcome.

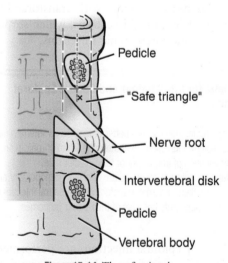

Figure 15-14 The safe triangle.

Transforaminal epidural steroid injection is gaining popularity over the interlaminar approach because it is more effective at administering the medication at the spinal nerve-disc interface in the lateral epidural space rather than in the dorsal epidural space, which is separated from the lateral epidural space by the ligamentum flavum. Fluoroscopic guidance is essential for this procedure, and administration of steroids at the level of the pathology is crucial to effectiveness.

Transforaminal epidural injections have both diagnostic and therapeutic value. If the pathology is unclear or if multiple pathologies are present, administration of local anesthetic (without a steroid) has diagnostic value if pain is relieved immediately after the injection is given. For therapeutic purposes, steroids are injected with the goal of pain relief 2 or 3 days after the injection. The effectiveness of therapeutic transforaminal epidural injections has been the subject of a number of studies. In a prospective study, Lutz and Wisneski[18] evaluated the outcomes of therapeutic transforaminal epidural steroid injections in 69 patients for a mean period of 80 weeks. They found that 75% of their patients reported improvement of pain intensity of at least 50% and near return to functional activities after 1.8 injections.

In a prospectively randomized study, Riew et al.[49] evaluated 55 patients with lumbar radicular pain with radiographic confirmation of nerve root compression. All of their patients had requested operative intervention and were considered surgical candidates. Instead the patients were randomized and underwent a selective nerve root injection with either bupivacaine alone or bupivacaine with betamethasone. The treating physicians and the patients were blinded to the medication. Twenty-nine patients did not have surgery during a follow-up period of 13 to 28 months. Of the 27 patients who had received bupivacaine alone, nine did not have surgery. Of the 28 patients who had received bupivacaine and betamethasone, 20 decided not to have surgery.

A study by Vad et al.[50] prospectively included 50 patients with lumbar radicular pain that had lasted longer than 6 weeks. All of the patients had MRI evidence of an HNP with less than 50% narrowing of the neural foramen, along with radicular pain corresponding to the MRI positive level of pathology. The patients were randomized into two groups. The treatment group received fluoroscopically guided transforaminal epidural injections, and the control group received trigger point injections. Forty-eight patients completed the study, and the average follow-up was 16 months. Outcome measures were the Roland Morris Questionnaire, a visual analogue scale, and the finger to floor test. An 84% improvement was seen in the study group, and only a 24% improvement in the control group.

In a prospective study, Botwin et al.[51] included 34 patients with unilateral radicular pain, caused by degenerative spinal stenosis, who were not responding to conservative management. Their patients received an average of 1.9 fluoroscopically guided transforaminal epidural injections on the symptomatic side. A visual analogue scale score, the Roland 5-point pain scale, standing and walking tolerance, and a patient satisfaction scale were assessed 2 and 12 months after the injections. The results showed that 75% of the patients reported a pain score reduction of greater than 50% after the injection therapy; in addition, 64% had improved walking tolerance and 57% had improved standing tolerance at 12 months.

Slipman et al.[16] retrospectively evaluated 20 patients who had had cervical radicular pain for longer than 5 months. Their patients received an average of 2.2 cervical transforaminal epidural injections in addition to physical therapy. The patients were followed for 21 months. Their pain scores, medication use, work status, and satisfaction were assessed. Sixty percent of the patients reported excellent or good outcomes, and 30% underwent surgery.

Huston et al.[17] prospectively studied the side effects and complications of transforaminal epidural injections. An analysis of 350 consecutive cervical and lumbar transforaminal injections identified no instance in which dural punctures occurred. Lutz and Wisneski[18] found no epidural punctures or other major complications in 50 patients who received lumbar transforaminal epidural injections. Botwin et al.[19] reviewed complications in 322 transforaminal lumbar epidural injections performed on 207 patients. They reported a complete absence of postdural puncture headache (PDHD). The most common complication found in their study was headache, which occurred in 3.1% of patients. These headaches were transient and resolved after 24 hours. These patients' epidurograms were reviewed, and no intrathecal pattern was noted.

Spinal cord injury has been reported after lumbosacral nerve root block with steroid injections.[52] This is postulated to occur secondary to an injury or to injection of particulate steroids in patients with an aberrant artery of Adamkiewicz. Another possibility is occlusion of the anterior spinal artery, with resultant spinal cord infarction, after inadvertent injection into a feeder artery in the neural foramen. A hypothesis for this occurrence is the use of Depo-Medrol and Kenalog preparations for the procedure; these preparations form large particulate granules, which can occlude the anterior spinal artery unless a meticulous technique is followed. El Abd et al.[53] demonstrated that the use of digital subtraction angiography (DSA) is capable of detecting intravascular needle placements that were missed by contrast injection under live fluoroscopy, thus adding a safety step before medication injection. In addition, the use of nonparticulate steroids, such as dexamethasone, is preferred as another safety measure to avoid vascular occlusion during transforaminal epidural injections.

Technique for Cervical Transforaminal Epidural Injections. The patient is placed in the supine position on the fluoroscopy table. A bolster is placed under the contralateral shoulder. The blood pressure, pulse, and pulse oxymetry are monitored. The fluoroscopy beam is rotated to visualize the neural foramen in a perpendicular plane to the radiographic imager. Once the neural foramen has been properly visualized, a 25-gauge needle is introduced through the skin. The needle is advanced until it abuts the superior articular process of the corresponding neural foramen. The needle then is slightly advanced into the foramen. Contrast (0.3 cc of Omnipaque 300) is used to confirm the needle's position. When contrast clearly outlines the exiting nerve root, 0.5 cc of lidocaine 1% is given and the patient is asked about unusual taste. This lidocaine test is performed as another safety measure to avoid vascular injection (intravascular lidocaine is known to produce a metallic taste). Then 1.5 cc of dexamethasone 10 mg/mL is administered (Figure 15-15). For diagnostic purposes only, 0.8 cc of lidocaine 2% is given without steroids (diagnostic injection).

Technique for Thoracic and Lumbar Transforaminal Epidural Injections. The patient is placed in the prone position on the fluoroscopy table. Blood pressure, pulse, and pulse oxymetry are monitored. The fluoroscopy beam is rotated to visualize the neural foramen in an oblique plane with the superior articular process dissecting the corresponding pedicle. Once the neural foramen has been properly visualized, a skin wheal is made with 0.5 cc of lidocaine 1%.

A 22-gauge needle is introduced through the skin and advanced to the 6 o'clock position under the pedicle (the safe triangle) under fluoroscopic guidance. Needle positioning is confirmed using the anteroposterior plane. The needle should not extend medial to the pedicle on the anteroposterior view. Contrast (0.3 cc of Omnipaque 300) is used to confirm the needle's position. When the contrast clearly outlines the exiting nerve root, the lidocaine test is performed with the injection of 1 cc of lidocaine 1%, followed by 2 cc of dexamethasone 10 mg/mL (Figures 15-16 and 15-17). For diagnostic purposes only, 0.8 cc of lidocaine 2% is given without steroids (diagnostic injection).

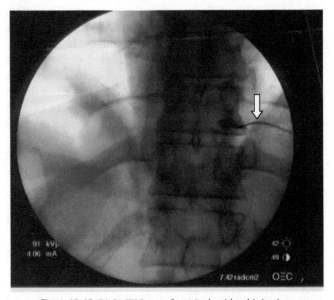

Figure 15-16 Right T10 transforaminal epidural injection.

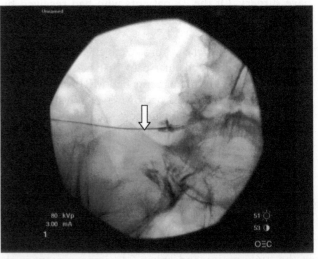

Figure 15-17 Left L5 transforaminal epidural injection. Note the presence of left S1 flow (an S1 transforaminal injection had been given just before the L5 injection).

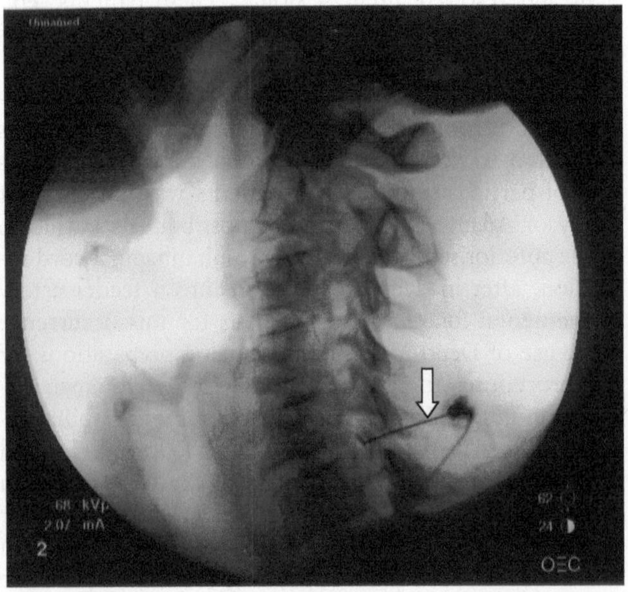

Figure 15-15 Left C6 transforaminal epidural injection.

Guiding Principles for Transforaminal Epidural Injections

- The needle must be carefully positioned in the safe triangle (see Figure 15-14).
- The needle's position must be confirmed radiographically in the anteroposterior plane.
- For a cervical transforaminal injection, oblique planes, rather than lateral planes, should be used to perform the injection. The depth of the needle cannot be noted if lateral planes are used.
- Live fluoroscopy should be used while contrast material is injected.
- If possible, dexamethasone should be used for cervical and thoracic injections. (Dexamethasone has less particulate substance than Depo-Medrol or Kenalog, which are suspected of causing vascular clogging.)
- Cervical and thoracic transforaminal injections should be administered only by a well-trained physician experienced in performing these procedures.
- With thoracic transforaminal injections, the risk of pneumothorax arises if the pleura is punctured. The interventionalist should always keep the needle medial to the costovertebral junction.

While performing the transforaminal epidural injections, the clinician must take special precautions to prevent vascular injections and spinal cord injuries.

Facet Joint Injections

Neither the clinical examination nor imaging studies can confirm a diagnosis of facet-mediated pain. The gold standard for this diagnosis is the use of a local anesthetic to block a particularly painful joint.[54] Barnsley et al.[55] evaluated the effect of intra-articular cervical facet joint steroid injections in 41 patients with chronic neck pain. The patients were carefully selected by means of differential diagnostic cervical facet joint block with a long-acting and a short-acting anesthetic. Under double-blind conditions, patients received intra-articular injections of either 1 cc of bupivacaine (20 patients) or 1 cc of betamethasone (21 patients). Patient follow-up was conducted either in the office or by telephone until the patient reported a return of 50% of the pain. The median time to a return of 50% of pain was 3 days in the steroid group and 3.5 days in the local anesthetic group. Only 20% of the patients had substantial relief after 1 month. The authors concluded that the improvement was due to either a placebo effect or secondary to facet joint distention. This study had some flaws; the sample number was small, and all the patients included had traumatic injury with whiplash.

Lilius et al.[56] evaluated 109 patients with chronic low back pain who did not respond to conservative management. Their patients were separated into three groups: the first received intra-articular steroid and a local anesthetic, the second received saline, and the third received pericapsular steroid and a local anesthetic. The authors reported improvement of pain in all three groups. The major flaw of this study was that the patients were selected without undergoing diagnostic injections to identify the level of therapeutic injections.

In a prospective study Carette et al.[57] compared the effect of intra-articular saline with that of intra-articular methylprednisolone in 101 patients after positive lidocaine joint injection. At 6 months 46% of the methylprednisolone group and 15% of the saline group reported marked pain relief.

In a prospective study Lynch and Taylor[58] evaluated 50 patients. Of these, 23 received extraarticular steroid injections and 27 received intra-articular steroid injections without a local anesthetic. Nine of the 27 patients who had received intra-articular injections had total improvement, whereas none of the control group (those who had received extraarticular injections) experienced total improvement. Only two members of the intra-articular group had no improvement.

Technique for Intra-articular Facet Joint Injections. These injections are performed only under live fluoroscopic visualization. For cervical facet joint injections, the patient is placed in the lateral position on the fluoroscopy table. A bolster is placed beneath the patient's head with the ipsilateral side bent 5° to 15° for better visualization of the upper joints. For C1-2 injections, the patient is positioned prone with the bolster placed beneath the forehead and the neck in slight extension of 5° to 10°. For lumbar facet joint injections, the patient is placed prone with or without a bolster under the ipsilateral side. The blood pressure, pulse, and pulse oxymetry are monitored. The skin is prepped and draped in the usual sterile manner. The target ipsilateral joint is properly identified in a plane perpendicular to the radiographic imager. A 25-gauge, 4-cm (1.5-inch) needle (for cervical injections) or a 22-gauge 9-cm (3.5-inch) spinal needle (for lumbar injections) is used. The needle is advanced to the midportion of the superior articular process (for level C1-2, the needle is introduced through the lateral third of the joint). After the depth has been checked, the needle is advanced to pierce the joint capsule (Figure 15-18). Approximately 0.15 cc of Omnipaque 300, a water-soluble contrast agent, is injected into the joint for proper identification. After a positive arthrogram has been identified, 0.8 cc of Xylocaine 2% is given as a diagnostic injection. A greater than 80% improvement in pain is considered a positive diagnostic injection. For therapeutic injections, 0.8 cc of Celestone (6 mg) (or another type of steroid) and 0.2 cc of lidocaine 1% are injected.

Medial branch blocks instead of intra-articular injections are primarily performed for the diagnosis of facet joint syndrome.[59] Technically, they are easier to perform than the intra-articular facet joint injections. The spinal needle is positioned at the junction of the superior articular process and the transverse process under fluoroscopic guidance (Figure 15-19).

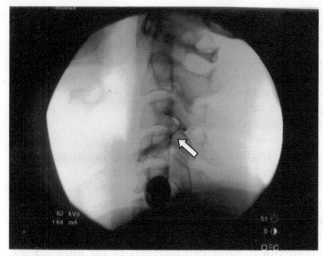

Figure 15-18 Left C3-4 intra-articular facet joint injection.

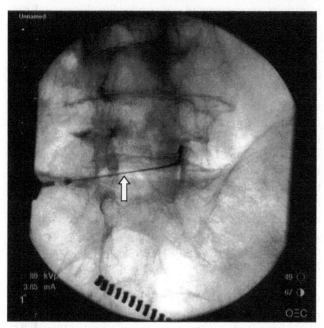

Figure 15-19 Right L5-S1 intra-articular facet joint injection.

Facet Joint Radiofrequency Ablation

From a spinal intervention perspective, radiofrequency ablation is considered the ultimate management of facet joint mediated pain. This procedure results in ablation of the medial branch nerves that provide sensory innervations to one or more facet joints. In a randomized, double-blind trial, Lord et al.[25] included 24 patients with chronic neck pain with a median duration of pain of 34 months. All the patients had developed pain after a motor vehicle accident. The radiofrequency procedure was compared with an identical procedure in which the machine was not turned on. The patients were split into two groups of 12 receiving each treatment. The radiofrequency level was selected using double-blind, placebo-controlled facet blocks. Follow-up consisted of clinic visits and phone interviews until the patient's pain

had returned to the 50% level. The median time for pain return was 263 days in the active treatment group and 8 days in the control group. At 27 weeks, seven patients in the active group and one patient in the control group were pain free. The study had a good design and good methodology; however, the sample size was small.

In a prospective study, Dreyfuss et al.[60] included 15 patients with chronic low back pain who reacted positively to a double local anesthetic comparative block (with lidocaine and bupivacaine). Patients underwent lumbar facet joint radiofrequency therapy and were followed for 12 months. To determine the outcome of the study, the investigators evaluated a number of factors: the patients' use of prescription analgesic medications; the results of the McGill Pain Questionnaire and Short Form SF-36; the North American Spine Society treatment expectations; the patient's ability to perform isometric push and pull, dynamic floor to waist lifts, and above the shoulder lifting tasks; and the results of needle electromyography of the L2 to L5 bands of the multifidus muscles performed before and 8 weeks after the procedure. Sixty percent of patients had at least a 90% pain reduction, and 87% of the patients had a 60% pain reduction for 12 months.

McDonald et al.[61] followed 28 patients for 5 years. All the patients underwent radiofrequency treatment of the cervical spine after undergoing placebo-controlled blocks. The median pain relief time after the first procedure was 219 days.

A systematic review of therapeutic lumbar facet joint interventions for the treatment of chronic low back pain conducted by Falco et al.[62] concluded that there was good evidence for the use of conventional radiofrequency neurotomy for the treatment of such conditions.

Technique for Radiofrequency Ablation of the Facet Joints. Radiofrequency ablation is performed only under live fluoroscopic visualization. Blood pressure, pulse, and pulse oxymetry are monitored. For cervical facet joint radiofrequency ablation, the patient is placed in the lateral position on the fluoroscopy table. A bolster is placed beneath the patient's head with the ipsilateral side bent 5° to 15° to allow better visualization of the upper joints. For treatment of a lumbar facet joint, the patient is placed in the prone position. The skin is prepped and draped in the usual sterile manner. A grounding pad is applied to the patient's shoulder (or any other area of dry skin) and connected to the radiofrequency generator.

For the cervical spine, the target facet joint is properly visualized in a plane perpendicular to the radiographic imager. A 22-gauge, 4-cm (1.5-inch), specially insulated needle is introduced and advanced under fluoroscopic guidance in a ventral and medial direction until it abuts the superior articular process, transverse process, and pedicle. The C3 medial branch (third occipital nerve) needs to be lesioned in two or three locations along the C2-3 facet because it is larger.

For the lumbar spine, the fluoroscopy beam is rotated 10° to 20° to visualize the ipsilateral superior articular process and the transverse process clearly. Then 0.5 cc of lidocaine 1% is injected subcutaneously. A 22-gauge, specially insulated spinal needle is introduced under direct fluoroscopic visualization. The needle is advanced until it abuts the junction of the base of the superior articular process, pedicle, and transverse process. The needle then is slightly "walked off" over the transverse process; this places the needle close to the medial branch at that level.

Once the needle is in the proper position, sensory testing is performed at 50 Hz with a voltage of 0 to 1 V. The patient is asked whether sensory symptoms ranging from pressure, tingling, burning, to pain are experienced. The symptoms must be localized in the paraspinal area and not in the extremities. If sensory symptoms are not elicited or are felt in the extremities, the needle's position is changed. Once sensory testing has been confirmed, motor testing is performed by switching the frequency to 2 Hz with a voltage of 1 to 10 V. The clinician's hand is placed over the immediate ipsilateral paraspinal area to check for rhythmic muscle contractions. When contractions are identified, the voltage is doubled and the clinician's hand is placed over the limb muscles supplied by the nerve root corresponding to the medial branch level. Neither the clinician nor the patient should feel any rhythmic contractions in the limb muscles. If contractions in the limb muscles are identified, the needle's position is changed. Sensory testing and motor testing confirm that the radiofrequency needle is positioned close to the medial branch and away from the corresponding nerve root.

Once correct positioning of the needle has been confirmed, 0.5 cc of lidocaine 2% is injected into the cervical levels and 3 cc of lidocaine 1% is injected into the lumbar spine. Radiofrequency lesioning is then performed at 80°C (176°F) for 90 seconds. The radiofrequency denervation of each facet joint implies lesioning of the medial branch at the joint level and the medial branch of the level cephalad to that joint.

Radiofrequency ablation is a safe procedure if performed according to the technique just described. The most common complication is the sensation of pain, which can last 7 to 10 days. Pain rarely lasts longer than 2 weeks[63] because of the denervation process of the ablated medial branches.

Sacroiliac Joint Injections

Injections into the SI joint are either diagnostic or therapeutic for SI joint syndrome. No physical examination test or imaging study can be used to confirm this diagnosis.[37,64] Diagnostic injections are used to further assess the pain emanating from the joint. If the patient has a positive response to the diagnostic injection, a therapeutic injection is administered.

Technique for Intra-articular SI Joint Injections. The patient is placed in the prone position on the fluoroscopy table. The skin is prepped and draped in the usual sterile manner. The blood pressure, pulse, and pulse oximetry are monitored. The fluoroscopy beam is slightly rotated

in an oblique position. The most caudal part of the joint is visualized with the ventral and the dorsal aspects superimposed. At the needle entry point, a skin wheal is made using 0.5 cc of lidocaine 1%. Under direct fluoroscopic visualization, a 22-gauge, 9-cm (3.5-inch) needle is introduced into the most caudal aspect of the SI joint. After the needle's positioning in the joint has been confirmed, 0.3 cc of contrast (Omnipaque 300) is injected. Intra-articular contrast should be properly visualized. For diagnostic injections, 1 cc of lidocaine 2% is used; for therapeutic injections, 0.8 cc of Celestone (6 mg) and 0.5 cc of lidocaine 2% are used.

DISCOGRAMS

Diagnostic Discograms

In 1970, Henry Crock first described **internal disc disruption syndrome (IDDS)** after conducting a retrospective analysis of patients who continued to experience leg and back pain despite multiple surgical procedures. He postulated that IDDS was caused by alterations in the internal structure and metabolic function of one or more discs, the alterations having developed after significant trauma.[65] Subsequent studies have established the morphology of the disrupted disc to be a degenerated nucleus pulposus with radial fissures extending to the periphery of the annulus fibrosus.[66] Patients with IDDS usually present with axial back pain that is dull or aching and difficult to localize and that often produces somatically referred symptoms.

Provocative discography is considered the best available test for diagnosing IDDS.[67] A discogram is considered only when the option of spinal fusion is entertained, whether for failure of conservative measures to control pain or for the management of spinal instability. A discogram confirms the disc level causing pain. However, discograms are plagued by a high false-positive rate of 5.6% for chronic pain, 15% for postdiscectomy, and 50% for patients with somatization disorder.[68] Because of that, even experienced physicians should perform the procedure meticulously. A patient undergoing a discogram should not be sedated and should be blinded to the disc level assessed. Sedation can cloud the patient's sensation of pain. It is important for the patient to be completely conscious so that the pain provoked during the test can be accurately described.

Technique for Diagnostic Lumbar Discogram

The patient starts the test in the side-lying position with a roll under the L4-5 area. Blood pressure, pulse, and pulse oximetry are monitored. The fluoroscopy beam is rotated to visualize the intervertebral discs with parallel end plates and dissected by the superior articular process. To visualize the L5-S1 disc, the fluoroscopy beam should be tilted caudally to avoid the ipsilateral iliac crest. Using a double-needle technique (an 18-gauge outer discography needle and a 22-gauge inner discography needle), the clinician places the needles into the disc using a posterolateral approach. After placement of the needles, the patient's position is changed to prone. Omnipaque 300 is used for disc injection, and needle placement is assessed using fluoroscopic imaging (Figure 15-20). The

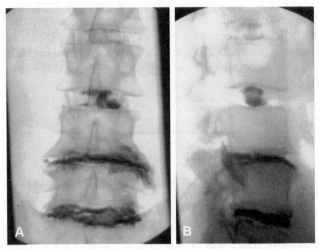

Figure 15-20 Fluoroscopic anteroposterior (**A**) and lateral (**B**) views of intradiscal contrast after a diagnostic lumbar discogram at L2-3, L3-4, L4-5, and L5-S1. The L4-5 and L5-S1 discs are degenerated, but only the L5-S1 level provoked concordant pain; therefore the L5-S1 level is the positive level.

patient is blinded to the intervertebral disc injected. The pain response and its distribution are recorded after each disc injection (P0, no pain on injection; P1, partial concordant pain; P2, discordant pain; and P3, concordant pain with same intensity and distribution). A discographic injection is considered positive if the pain response is P3 at the injected level. Negative levels are considered control levels in each discographic study. The pain response encompasses the skin, underlying soft tissue, and viscera located in these areas.

Immediately after discography, a CT scan is performed. Discs that appear lobular or cotton ball shaped (grade 0, 1, or 2 on the Modified Dallas Discogram Scale)[69] are classified as normal; discs that have an irregular discogram pattern with extravasation of dye to or through the outer annulus (grade 3, 4, or 5 on the Modified Dallas Discogram Scale) are classified as abnormal (Figure 15-21).

Percutaneous Discectomy

Patients who have radicular pain and fail to improve with conservative management, including spinal nerve root blocks, are candidates for percutaneous discectomy, an evolving spinal procedure. This procedure aims to achieve disc decompression without the side effects of conventional surgical procedures. Regardless of the technique used,

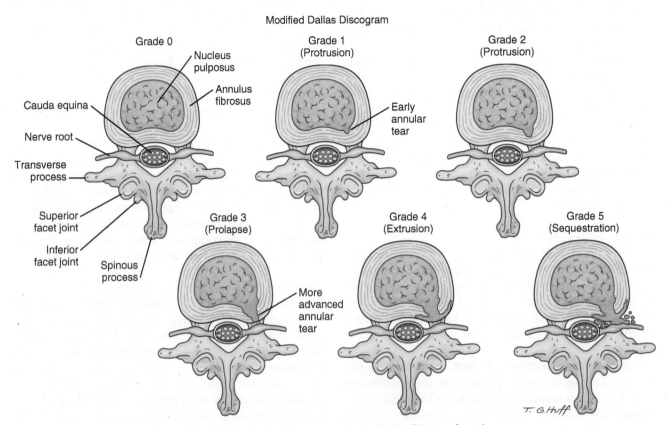

Figure 15-21 Modified Dallas Discogram Scale for CT classification of annular tears.

percutaneous disc decompression is based on the principle that a small reduction of volume in a closed hydraulic space, such as an intact disc, results in a disproportionately large drop in pressure. Once the intradiscal pressure declines, the disc is believed to downregulate inflammatory mediators and decrease in size, and a healing process is believed to commence, thereby alleviating the chemical, mechanical, and neural genesis of discogenic pain.[70]

Percutaneous discectomy was first introduced in 1964 with the use of intradiscal chymopapain injections (chemonucleolysis). However, chymopapain was reported to be associated with severe anaphylactic reactions and transverse myelitis, and its use has been discontinued.[71]

Hijikata[72] introduced instrumented percutaneous disc decompression in 1975. Although his procedure was reported to be effective, it did not become widely accepted. Among the reasons cited were the potential complications, including nerve root and/or vascular injury caused by the large canula (5 to 8 mm in diameter), repeated entrance into the disc space with an increased risk of infection, inability to relieve foraminal or lateral recess stenosis, lack of applicability among patients who had previously undergone surgery, difficulty performing the procedure on obese patients, and inaccessibility of the L5-S1 disc.

In 1985, Maroon and Onik introduced the automated lumbar discectomy device.[73] The device was criticized for its low success rate and for reports of major cauda equina injury. Laser discectomy became popular, but its use subsequently declined because of postprocedural complications, such as moderate-to-severe intraoperative pain secondary to the thermal effect of the laser, postoperative low back pain and spasm, bowel necrosis resulting from inadvertent perforation of the anterior annulus, nerve root injury, and inability to visualize the tip of the laser beam under fluoroscopy.[74] The technologically advanced devices nucleoplasty,[75] Dekompressor,[76] and hydrodiscectomy[77] were introduced most recently. Reports suggest that these devices are effective, especially in the management of small disc protrusions with radicular pain, and that they cause minimal and transient side effects and complications. Randomized studies to validate their use have yet to be performed to show supporting evidence, which up to now is limited.[78]

Technique for Lumbar Percutaneous Discectomy

The patient is placed in the side-lying position with a roll under the L4-5 area. The blood pressure, pulse, and pulse oxymetry are monitored. The fluoroscopy beam is rotated to visualize the intervertebral discs with parallel end plates and dissected by the superior articular process. To visualize the L5-S1 disc, the beam should be tilted caudally to avoid the ipsilateral iliac crest. Conscious sedation is used. A 17-gauge, 15-cm (6-inch) spinal needle is introduced into the disc using a posterolateral extrapedicular approach. The needle is positioned at the junction of the annulus and the nucleus. After the needle placement, the patient's position is changed to prone.

The discectomy device's catheter is placed into the spinal needle. Under real-time imaging, the tip of the catheter is withdrawn simultaneously with the introducer needle until it is positioned approximately 1 mm distal to the proximal annular-nuclear interface. The catheter then is advanced slowly until it reaches the distal nuclear-annular interface. The process of decompression involves advancing and withdrawing the catheter to form channels in the disc. A minimum of six channels is created, at the 12, 2, 4, 6, 8, and 10 o'clock positions. Additional channels, up to 12, are created if resistance to catheter advancement is perceived. Postoperatively, patients are allowed unlimited walking, standing, and sitting. They are instructed not to perform any lifting, bending, or stooping. Return to sedentary or light work is permitted at 3 to 4 days after the procedure. A lumbar stabilization program is started 2 weeks after the procedure.

Intradiscal Electrothermoplasty

Intradiscal electrothermoplasty (IDET) was introduced in 1997 for the management of discogenic axial pain. The procedure consists of the insertion of a flexible catheter in a circumferential manner into the annulus of a painful disc. Heating the annulus via the catheter is thought to coagulate the nerve fibers in the annulus and inflammatory products, stiffen the collagen fibers, and heal disc tears.[63,79] IDET gained popularity among clinicians shortly after its introduction. It is used in the management of discogenic pain proved by discography. IDET is seen as a last step before lumbar fusion surgery is considered. It is performed primarily in the lumbar spine and seldom in the thoracic spine.

Technique for Intradiscal Electrothermoplasty

The patient is placed in the side-lying position with a roll under the L4-5 area. Blood pressure, pulse, and pulse oxymetry are monitored. The fluoroscopy beam is rotated to visualize the intervertebral discs with parallel end plates and dissected by the superior articular process. To visualize the L5-S1 disc, the beam should be tilted caudally to avoid the ipsilateral iliac crest. Conscious sedation is used. A 17-gauge, 15-cm (6-inch) needle is introduced until it contacts the annulus fibrosis. After the needle placement, the patient's position is changed to prone. A flexible electrode is introduced through the needle and navigated through the posterior annulus. The catheter is heated for 16 minutes at 90°C (194°F). After the procedure, the patient wears a lumbar corset for 6 weeks.

Complications of Intradiscal Procedures

When good techniques are used, these interventional procedures are minimally invasive and have few complications or side effects. The side effects are transient and include temporary worsening of radicular or axial pain. Discitis is a possible complication, although the incidence is extremely low. Collis and Gardner[80] reported on 2187 disc injections and mentioned only one intervertebral disc infection. Wiley et al.[81] reported a review of the literature, which showed only 30 cases of discitis in approximately 5000 disc injections, an incidence of 0.6% per disc. Fraser et al.[82] reviewed 432 cases and found an overall infection rate of 2.3% of patients, or 1.3% per disc. The study breaks down the incidence of infection based on different techniques. The incidence of infection fell to 0.7% when a double-needle technique was used. Aprill[83] examined 2000 patients who had undergone discography involving a single-needle technique and reported only one case of acute discitis in that group.

PERCUTANEOUS VERTEBROPLASTY

Percutaneous vertebroplasty (PV) was first introduced in France in 1984 for the management of aggressive vertebral hemangiomas.[84] The procedure later was used in the management of painful vertebral compression fractures and painful vertebral malignancies. The procedure involves the injection of polymethylmethacrylate (PMMA; also called *bone cement*) into the vertebral body. PV is an outpatient procedure performed with the patient under conscious sedation. Sterile preparation is applied. The procedure is performed in the thoracic and lumbar spine using a transpedicular (posterior) approach. A 17-gauge needle is introduced into the vertebral body through the pedicles, and the needle is positioned in the junction between the posterior and middle thirds of the vertebral body. Once the needle's position has been confirmed, PMMA is injected. This process is performed either unilaterally or bilaterally.

Complications

Complications of PV are rare, and the use of good technique can obviate them. The most severe complication is injury to the spinal cord, nerve roots, or venous plexuses if the needle breaches the medial pedicle; this necessitates immediate surgical decompression. Pedicle fracture can occur, which is not destabilizing to the spine but may be painful for many weeks. Extravasation of bone cement into neural structures and blood vessels can occur, although the occurrence of this can be minimized by mixing the cement with the contrast and injecting them under live fluoroscopy.

KYPHOPLASTY

Kyphoplasty is a procedure for the management of compression fractures developed in the late 1990s.[85] A balloon is placed through a needle into the vertebral body. The balloon is inflated to reduce the fracture, and PMMA is injected under low pressure. The supporters of this procedure believe that the restoration of height of the vertebral body improves the biomechanics of the spine and may reduce kyphosis. The injection of PMMA under low pressure is also believed to reduce extravasation into surrounding structures.

SUMMARY

Nonsurgical interventional procedures for the spine are becoming a prominent management tool for painful spinal disorders. Physicians and surgeons currently consider using these procedures more frequently than recommending surgical interventions. These procedures, when performed by experienced physicians, have good outcomes and minimal complications. With advances in technology, improved techniques and the development of more effective equipment are expected. Interventions should always be followed up with an active spinal rehabilitation program after the patient's symptoms improve. Nonsurgical techniques, combined with a rehabilitation program, can restore function and minimize the recurrence of back pain.

REFERENCES

1. Balagué F, Mannion AF, Pellisé F, et al: Non-specific low back pain, *Lancet* 379:482–491, 2012.
2. Centers for Disease Control and Prevention, Available at: National hospital ambulatory medical care survey: factsheet outpatient department, 2011. http://www.cdc.gov/nchs/data/ahcd/NHAMCS_2011_opd_factsheet.pdf, Accessed May 12, 2015.
3. Centers for Disease Control and Prevention, Available at: National hospital ambulatory medical care survey: factsheet emergency department, 2011. http://www.cdc.gov/nchs/data/ahcd/NHAMCS_2011_ed_factsheet.pdf, Accessed May 12, 2015.
4. Centers for Disease Control and Prevention: Available at: National hospital ambulatory medical care survey: 2010 summary tables, 2010. http://www.cdc.gov/nchs/data/ahcd/namcs_summary/2010_namcs_web_tables.pdf, Accessed May 12, 2015.
5. Waterman BR, Belmont PJ Jr, Schoenfeld AJ: Low back pain in the United States: incidence and risk factors for presentation in the emergency setting, *Spine J* 12:63–70, 2012.
6. Lawrence RC, Felson DT, Helmick CG, et al: Estimates of the prevalence of arthritis and other rheumatic conditions in the United States. Part II, *Arthritis Rheum* 58:26–35, 2008.
7. National Center for Health Statistics, Available at: Health, United States, 2011: with special feature on socioeconomic status and health, 2012. http://www.cdc.gov/nchs/data/hus/hus11.pdf, Accessed May 12, 2015.
8. Ma VY, Chan L, Carruthers KJ: Incidence, prevalence, costs, and impact on disability of common conditions requiring rehabilitation in the United States: stroke, spinal cord injury, traumatic brain injury, multiple sclerosis, osteoarthritis, rheumatoid arthritis, limb loss, and back pain, *Arch Phys Med Rehabil* 95:986–995, 2014.
9. Van Boxem K, Cheng J, Patijn J, et al: Lumbosacral radicular pain, *Pain Pract* 10:339–358, 2010.
10. Kalichman L, Hunter DJ: Lumbar facet joint osteoarthritis: a review, *Semin Arthritis Rheum* 37:69–80, 2007.
11. Hallegraeff JM, Krijnen WP, van der Schans CP, et al: Expectations about recovery from acute non-specific low back pain predict absence from usual work due to chronic low back pain: a systematic review, *J Physiother* 58:165–172, 2012.
12. Waxman R, Tennant A, Helliwell P: A prospective follow up study of low back pain in the community, *Spine* 25:2085–2090, 2000.
13. Miyamoto H, Doita M, Nishida K, et al: Effects of cyclic mechanical stress on the production of inflammatory agents by nucleus pulposus and anulus fibrosus derived cells in vitro, *Spine* 31:4–9, 2006 (Phila PA 1976).
14. Schroeder M, Viezens L, Schaefer C, et al: Chemokine profile of disc degeneration with acute or chronic pain, *J Neurosurg Spine* 18:496–503, 2013.

15. Freemont AJ, Peacock TE, Goupille P, et al: Nerve ingrowth into diseased intervertebral disc in chronic back pain, *Lancet* 350:178–181, 1997.

16. Slipman C, Lipetz J, Jackson H, et al: Therapeutic selective nerve root blocks in the nonsurgical management of atraumatic cervical spondylotic radicular pain: a retrospective analysis with independent clinical review, *Arch Phys Med Rehabil* 81:741–746, 2000.

17. Huston C, Slipman C, Meyers J, et al: Side effects and complications of fluoroscopically guided nerve root injections, *Arch Phys Med Rehabil* 9:937, 1996.

18. Lutz G, Wisneski R: Fluoroscopic transforaminal lumbar epidural steroid injections: an outcome study, *Arch Phys Med Rehabil* 79:1362–1366, 1998.

19. Botwin K, Gruber R, Bouchlas C, et al: Complications of fluoroscopically guided transforaminal lumbar epidural injections, *Arch Phys Med Rehabil* 81:1045–1050, 2000.

20. Slipman CW, Plastaras C, Patel R, et al: Provocative cervical discography symptom mapping, *Spine J* 5:381–388, 2005.

21. El Abd O, Slipman CW, Brandys E, et al: The prevalence of abdominal and inguinal pain in patients with internal disc disruption syndrome, Chicago, October 9, 2003, PASSOR Annual Meeting Research Forum.

22. Laplante BL, DePalma MJ: Spine osteoarthritis, *PM&R* 4(5suppl):S28–S36, 2012.

23. Bogduk N: The clinical anatomy of the cervical dorsal rami, *Spine* 7:319–330, 1982.

24. Slipman CW, Lipetz JS, Plastaras CT, et al: Therapeutic zygapophyseal joint injections for headaches emanating from the C2-3 joint, *Am J Phys Med Rehabil* 80(3):182–188, 2001.

25. Lord S, Barnsley L, Wallis B, et al: Chronic cervical zygapophyseal joint pain after whiplash: a placebo-controlled prevalence study, *Spine* 21:1737–1745, 1996.

26. Fukui S, Ohseto K, Shiotani M, et al: Referred pain distribution of the cervical zygapophyseal joints and the cervical dorsal rami, *Pain* 68:79–83, 1996.

27. Gellhorn AC: Cervical facet-mediated pain, *Phys Med Rehabil Clin N Am* 22:447–458, 2011.

28. Bogduk N: The anatomy of occipital neuralgia, *Clin Exp Neurol* 17:167–184, 1980.

29. Rosen HN, Vokes TJ, Malabanan AO, et al: The official positions of the international society for clinical densitometry: vertebral fracture assessment, *J Clin Densitom* 16:482–488, 2013.

30. Cohen SP, Chen Y, Neufeld NJ: Sacroiliac joint pain: a comprehensive review of epidemiology, diagnosis and treatment, *Expert Rev Neurother* 13:99–116, 2013.

31. Gelhorn AC, Katz JN, Suri P: Osteoarthritis of the spine: the facet joints, *Nature Reviews Reumatology* 9:216–224, 2013.

32. Dwyer A, Aprill C, Bogduk N: Cervical zygapophyseal joint pain patterns. I. A study in normal volunteers, *Spine* 15:453–457, 1990.

33. Aprill C, Dwyer A, Bogduk N: Cervical zygapophyseal joint pain patterns. II. A clinical evaluation, *Spine* 6:458–461, 1990.

34. Slipman CW, Plastaras CT, Palmitier RA, et al: Symptom provocation of fluoroscopically guided cervical nerve root stimulation: are dynatomal maps identical to dermatomal maps? *Spine* 23:2235–2242, 1998.

35. Fast A, Parikh S, Marin EL: The shoulder abduction relief sign in cervical radiculopathy, *Arch Phys Med Rehabil* 70:402–403, 1989.

36. Chou L, Slipman CW, Bhagia S, et al: Inciting events initiating injection-proven sacroiliac joint syndrome, *Pain Med* 5:26–32, 2004.

37. Rupert MP, Lee M, Manchikanti L, et al: Evaluation of sacroiliac joint interventions: a systematic appraisal of the literature, *Pain Physician* 12:399–418, 2009.

38. Deyo RA, Diehl AK: Lumbar spine films in primary care: current use and effects of selective ordering criteria, *J Gen Intern Med* 1:20–25, 1986.

39. Aprill C, Bogduk N: High-intensity zone: a diagnostic sign of painful lumbar disc on magnetic resonance imaging, *Br J Radiol* 65:361–369, 1992.

40. Modic MT, Steinberg PM, Ross JS, et al: Degenerative disk disease: assessment of changes in vertebral body marrow with MR imaging, *Radiology* 166:193–199, 1988.

41. Dogliotti AM: Segmental peridural anesthesia, *Am J Surg* 20:107, 1933 (Abstract).

42. Robechhi A, Capra R: L'idrocortisone (composto F): rime esperinze cliniche in campo reumatologico, *Minerva Med* 98:1259–1263, 1952.

43. Rho ME, Tang CT: The efficacy of lumbar epidural steroid injections: transforaminal, interlaminar, and caudal approaches, *Phys Med Rehabil Clin N Am* 22:139–148, 2011.

44. Carette S, Leclaire R, Marcoux S, et al: Epidural corticosteroid injections for sciatica due to herniated nucleus pulposus, *N Engl J Med* 336:1634–1640, 1997.

45. Koes BW, Scholten RJ, Mens JM, et al: Efficacy of epidural steroid injections for low-back pain and sciatica: a systematic review of randomized clinical trials, *Pain* 63:279–288, 1995.

46. Watts RW, Silagy CA: A meta-analysis on the efficacy of epidural corticosteroids in the treatment of sciatica, *Anaesth Intensive Care* 23:564–569, 1995.

47. Manchikanti L, Pakanati RR, Pampati V: Comparison of three routes of epidural steroid injections in low back pain, *Pain Digest* 9:277–285, 1999.

48. Renfrew DL, Moore TE, Kathol MH, et al: Correct placement of epidural steroid injections: fluoroscopic guidance and contrast administration, *Am J Neuroradiol* 12:1003–1007, 1991.

49. Riew KD, Yin Y, Gilula L, et al: The effect of nerve-root injections on the need for operative treatment of lumbar radicular pain: a prospective, randomized, controlled, double-blind study, *J Bone Joint Surg Am* 82:1589–1593, 2000.

50. Vad V, Bhat A, Lutz G, et al: Transforaminal epidural steroid injections in lumbosacral radiculopathy: a prospective randomized study, *Spine* 27:11–16, 2002.

51. Botwin KP, Gruber RD, Bouchlas CG, et al: Fluoroscopically guided lumbar transforaminal epidural steroid injections in degenerative lumbar stenosis: an outcome study, *Am J Phys Med Rehabil* 81:898–905, 2002.

52. Houten JK, Errico TJ: Paraplegia after lumbosacral nerve root block: report of three cases, *Spine J* 2:70–75, 2002.

53. El Abd OH, Amadera JE, Pimentel DC, et al: Intravascular flow detection during transforaminal epidural injections: a prospective assessment, *Pain Physician* 17:21–27, 2014.

54. Falco FJ, Manchikanti L, Datta S, et al: An update of the systematic assessment of the diagnostic accuracy of lumbar facet joint nerve blocks, *Pain Physician* 15:E869–E907, 2012.

55. Barnsley L, Lord S, Wallis BJ, et al: Lack of effect of intraarticular corticosteroids for chronic pain in the cervical zygapophyseal joints, *N Engl J Med* 330:1047–1050, 1994.

56. Lilius G, Laasonen EM, Myllynen P, et al: Lumbar facet joint syndrome: a randomized clinical trial, *J Bone Joint Surg Br* 71:681–684, 1989.

57. Carette S, Marcoux S, Truchon R, et al: A controlled trial of corticosteroid injections into facet joints for chronic low back pain, *N Engl J Med* 325:1002–1007, 1991.

58. Lynch MC, Taylor JF: Facet joint injection for low back pain: a clinical study, *J Bone Joint Surg Br* 68:138–141, 1986.

59. Falco FJ, Erhart S, Wargo BW, et al: Systematic review of diagnostic utility and therapeutic effectiveness of cervical facet joint interventions, *Pain Physician* 12:323–344, 2009.

60. Dreyfuss P, Halbrook B, Pauza K: Efficacy and validity of radiofrequency neurotomy for chronic lumbar zygapophysial joint pain, *Spine* 25:1270–1277, 2000.

61. McDonald G, Lord S, Bogduk N: Long-term follow-up of patients treated with cervical radiofrequency neurotomy for chronic neck pain, *Neurosurgery* 45:61–66, 1999.

62. Falco FJ, Manchikanti L, Datta S, et al: An update of the effectiveness of therapeutic lumbar facet joint interventions, *Pain Physician* 15:E909–E953, 2012.

63. Saal JS, Saal JA: Management of chronic discogenic low back pain with a thermal intradiscal catheter. A preliminary report, *Spine* 25:382–388, 2000.

64. Slipman CW, Sterenfeld EB, Chou LH, et al: The value of radionuclide imaging in the diagnosis of sacroiliac joint syndrome, *Spine* 21:2251–2254, 1996.

65. Crock HV: A reappraisal of intervertebral disc lesions, *Med J Aust* 1:983–999, 1970.

66. Bogduk N: The lumbar disc and low back pain, *Neurosurg Clin North Am* 2:791–806, 1991.

67. Stout A: Discography, *Phys Med Rehabil Clin N Am* 21:859–867, 2010.

68. Provenzano DA: Diagnostic discography: what is the clinical utility? *Curr Pain Headache Rep* 16:26–34, 2012.

69. Sachs B, Vanharanta H, Spivey M, et al: Dallas discogram description: a new classification of CT discography in low back disorders, *Spine* 12:287–294, 1987.

70. Derby R, Kine G, Saal JA, et al: Response to steroid and duration of radicular pain as predictors of surgical outcome, *Spine* 17:S176–S183, 1992.

71. Javid MJ, Nordby EJ, Ford LT, et al: Safety and efficacy of chymopapain in herniated nucleus pulposus with sciatica, *JAMA* 249:2489–2494, 1983.

72. Hijikata S: Percutaneous nucleotomy: a new concept technique and 12 years' experience, *Clin Orthop* 238:9–23, 1989.

73. Maroon JC, Onik G: Percutaneous automated discectomy: a new method for lumbar disc removal, *J Neurosurgery* 66:143–146, 1987.

74. Hellinger J: Technical aspects of the percutaneous cervical and lumbar laser disc decompression and nucleotomy, *Neurol Res* 21:99–102, 1995.

75. Sharps L, Isaac Z: Percutaneous disc decompression using nucleoplasty, *Pain Physician* 5:121–126, 2002.

76. Alo KM, Wright RE, Sutcliffe J, et al: Percutaneous lumbar discectomy: one year follow-up in an initial cohort of fifty consecutive patients with chronic radicular pain, *Pain Pract* 5:116–124, 2005.

77. Hardenbrook M, Gannon D Jr, Younan E, et al: Clinical outcomes of patients treated with percutaneous hydrodiscectomy for radiculopathy secondary to lumbar herniated nucleus pulposus, *Internet J Spine Surg* 7:2013. Available at, http://ispub.com/IJSS/7/1/14479, Accessed, May 12, 2015.

78. Manchikanti L, Singh V, Falco FJ, et al: An updated review of automated percutaneous mechanical lumbar discectomy for the contained herniated lumbar disc, *Pain Physician* 16(suppl):SE151–SE184, 2013.

79. Karasek M, Bogduk N: Intradiscal electrothermal annuloplasty: percutaneous treatment of chronic discogenic low back pain, *Tech Reg Anesth Pain Manag* 5:130–135, 2001.

80. Collis JS Jr, Gardner WJ: Lumbar discography: an analysis of 1000 cases, *J Neurosurg* 19:452–461, 1962.

81. Wiley J, McNab I, Wortzman G: Lumbar discography and clinical applications, *Can J Surg* 11:280–289, 1968.

82. Fraser RD, Osti OL, Vernon-Roberts B: Discitis after discography, *J Bone Joint Surg Br* 69:26–35, 1987.

83. Aprill CN: Diagnostic lumbar injection. In Frymoyer JW, editor: *The adult spine*, ed 2, Philadelphia, 1997, Lippincott-Raven.

84. Galibert P, Deramond H, Rosat P, et al: Note preliminaire sur le traitement des angiomes vertebraux at des affections dolorigenes et fragilisantes du rachis, *Chirurgie* 116:326–335, 1990.

85. Peh WC, Munk PL, Rashid F, et al: Percutaneous vertebral augmentation: vertebroplasty, kyphoplasty and skyphoplasty, *Radiol Clin North Am* 46:611–635, 2008.

CHAPTER 16

Spinal Pathology, Conditions, and Deformities:
Surgical Intervention

ELIAS DAKWAR, ARMEN DEUKMEDJIAN, YOAV RITTER, C. DAIN ALLRED, GLENN R. RECHTINE II

INTRODUCTION

Successful surgical management of spinal pathology can be simplified into two basic concepts: decompression and stabilization. The neural elements, including the spinal cord and nerve roots, must be freed from impingement to halt the progression of neurological deficit and potentially to allow improvement in function. Segmental instability must also be addressed, because this leads to pain and deformity and may result in neurological impairment. This chapter focuses primarily on degenerative derangements of the spine; however, similar principles of decompression and stabilization hold true for spinal pathology caused by trauma, neoplasms, infection, and other etiologies.

Critical Questions Regarding Surgical Success

- Which neurological structure is compromised: spinal cord, nerve roots, or both?
- What is the source of compression (e.g., disc herniation, osteophyte, fracture fragment, tumor)?
- Does the compressive force arise from the anterior side, posterior side, or both?
- How many levels of the spine are involved?
- What is the spinal alignment?
- Are there different levels of segmental instability?
- What are the relevant medical co-morbidities?

Patient selection is perhaps more important than the technical aspects of surgery for achieving a successful surgical outcome in the treatment of spinal disorders. When surgery is indicated, careful planning of the operation is vital for success. This planning is based on a knowledge of the pathological process and its influence on local anatomy and neurological function. Armed with the answers to critical questions, the surgeon can select an operation that will adequately address the pathological condition, alleviate symptoms, and restore function.

CERVICAL DISC DISEASE

Degenerative cervical disc disease comprises a number of derangements of the cervical spine, ranging from isolated, single-level disc herniation to multilevel spondylosis with osteophyte formation. The clinical evaluation of patients with cervical disc disease requires interpretation of a detailed history, a meticulous examination, and appropriate diagnostic testing. Proper diagnosis and differentiation of patients with nerve root disorders (i.e., **radiculopathy**), spinal cord compression (i.e., **myelopathy**), cervical deformity, or axial neck pain give the clinician insight into the natural history of the process and direct the treatment plan.

Differential Diagnosis of Cervical Disc Disease

- Radiculopathy (nerve root)
- Myelopathy (spinal cord)
- Axial neck pain

Cervical spondylotic radiculopathy usually presents as upper extremity pain associated with dysesthesias or paresthesias in a dermatomal pattern. Symptoms stem from impingement of a single or multiple nerve roots as a result of the degenerative changes of the bony and soft tissue anatomy (e.g., intervertebral discs). The natural history of cervical radiculopathy is favorable. Radiculopathy appears to be a distinct disorder, because progression from radiculopathy to myelopathy is uncommon. Most patients' acute symptoms improve with nonoperative management as the inflammatory cycle initiated by nerve root compression resolves. The short-term success of medical management is generally accepted; however, over a longer period, radiculopathy commonly recurs. Gore et al.[1] reported that 50% of patients with cervical radiculopathy who were treated conservatively had persistent symptoms at 15-year follow-up. In their long-term observations, Lees and Turner[2] reported that 30% of patients complained of intermittent symptoms, whereas 25% experienced persistent radiculopathy. On plain x-ray films, separating normal, age-related degenerative changes from those causing symptoms often is difficult. In asymptomatic adults older than 50 years of age, the prevalence of significant radiographic degenerative changes mirrors age; that is, in a cohort of 60-year-olds, approximately 60% will have radiographic spondylosis, even with no symptoms.

Surgery for radiculopathy is indicated for patients who have demonstrated symptoms of sufficient duration and magnitude despite conservative management. Generally, patients considered for surgery are those with at least 3 months of persistent or recurrent arm pain or neurological deficits that interfere with personal or professional function and those for whom nonsurgical treatment has failed. Nonsurgical conservative treatments may include oral steroids, muscle relaxants, nonsteroidal anti-inflammatory drugs (NSAIDs), and physical therapy. A correlation of clinical findings with an identifiable lesion on neuroradiography also portends more consistent relief of symptoms after surgery.

Indications for Surgery for Radiculopathy

- Persistent or recurrent arm pain of more than 3 months' duration
- Neurological deficits that interfere with function
- Failure of conservative treatments

Upper motor neuron symptoms, including hyperreflexia, fine motor dysfunction, and gait disturbances, are the typical manifestations of cervical spondylotic myelopathy (CSM). The normal aging process of the spine starts with disc desiccation and loss of height. This leads to a degenerative cascade of events that includes osteophyte formation, ligament hypertrophy, and facet and uncovertebral joint (joints of Luschka) degeneration. When abnormal biomechanics of the spine are coupled with degenerative changes that narrow the spinal canal or compress the spinal cord, the result is a myelopathy. Spinal cord compression is dynamic and can change with flexion or extension of the neck. Flexion stretches the spinal cord, whereas extension causes buckling of ligaments and narrowing of the spinal canal.

The natural history of myelopathy is less favorable than that of radiculopathy, with a tendency for acute episodes of neurological decline separated by periods of relative stability of symptoms. Clarke and Robinson[3] first reported on the natural history of myelopathy. They reported that in more than 100 patients, motor symptoms worsened over time, and none of the patients returned to a normal neurological status. Lees and Turner[2] reported similar findings for long-term observations. Nurick[4] classified patients into six grades based on their disability with ambulation. His observations demonstrated long periods of no disease progression after early deterioration. Sumi et al.[5] reviewed 60 patients with mild cervical myelopathy and used magnetic resonance imaging (MRI) findings on a T1-weighted image (T1WI) to evaluate those patients who could tolerate having a cervical myelopathy without surgical treatment compared with those who could not tolerate the condition. They classified the spinal cord based on its presenting anatomical shape. If both sides were round and convex, they classified the cord as "ovoid deformity"; however, if a single side or both sides exhibited an acute angle to the lateral border, they defined the cord as "angular-edged deformity." In their review of a total of 55 cases with a mean of 94 months' follow-up, they noted global deterioration in 25% of myelopathies. There was a significant difference with respect to patients with "ovoid deformity," of whom 70% tolerated their mild myelopathy, compared with only 58% of those patients with "angular-edge deformity." Sumi et al.[5] concluded that surgery was a viable option for patients with mild cervical myelopathy and the "angular-edge deformity."

Surgical intervention can also be recommended when moderate to severe symptoms significantly affect a patient's quality of life or ability to work. Such symptoms include unsteady gait, hand dysfunction, or a neurogenic bowel or bladder. Surgery also is indicated when a patient has a clinical history of disease progression and, in milder cases, when significant stenosis is seen on imaging studies.

Indications for Surgery for Myelopathy

- Moderate to severe symptoms that affect the patient's quality of life or ability to work
- Unsteady gait
- Hand dysfunction
- Neurogenic bowel or bladder
- Spinal stenosis
- Progressive disease

Axial neck pain is pain that is localized to the cervical area and does not radiate into the upper extremities. It can manifest as unilateral or bilateral pain, headaches, or stiffness. The most common cause of axial neck pain is cervical strain, commonly referred to as whiplash or whiplash-associated disorders (WADs). Treatment for whiplash is universally nonoperative, and in most cases symptoms resolve within 6 to 8 weeks. Patients with cervical degenerative disease associated with axial pain are more challenging to manage. Surgical outcomes have been unpredictable, and success has been limited when the sole indication for operative intervention is neck pain.[6–8] However, more recent studies have reported that surgery has yielded beneficial results in patients with severe, persistent neck pain in whom the disease was limited to one or two levels while sparing the remaining discs. Garvey et al.[9] reported good or excellent results in 82% of their patients at follow-up beyond 4 years and concluded that single- or two-level cervical fusion could provide more reliable outcomes. Likewise, Palit et al.[10] demonstrated a 79% satisfaction rate among patients who underwent one-to three-level fusions. Despite these more promising reports, the surgeon should exercise considerable restraint in recommending operative care for axial neck pain, and the patient must understand the relative unpredictability of surgery in the relief of symptoms.

The main role of the cervical spine is twofold. First, the cervical spine is responsible for the head's location over the body. Second, horizontal gaze is very tightly controlled via the cervical spine. Scheer et al. and the International Spine Study Group[11] summarized some of the clinical correlations between cervical deformity, in particular, sagittal alignment and its relationship to axial neck pain and myelopathy. Evidence is mounting to support clinical correlation as it pertains to health-related quality of life with certain cervical spine radiographic parameters. Furthermore, sagittal alignment may play a leading role in adding to spinal cord compression, which in turn leads to cervical myelopathy.

Surgical Treatment of Cervical Radiculopathy

The surgical options for treating cervical radiculopathy include anterior cervical discectomy and fusion (ACDF), cervical disc arthroplasty, anterior corpectomy and fusion (ACF), posterior laminotomy with foraminotomy, and laminectomy or laminoplasty with or without fusion. The procedures most commonly performed for single-level cervical radiculopathy resulting from soft disc herniations are cervical arthroplasty, ACDF, and foraminotomy. The other procedures (ACF, laminectomy, and laminoplasty) are reserved for more advanced ankylosis and multilevel disease. (These are discussed in more detail in the section on the surgical management of myelopathy.) Robinson and Smith[12] first described a technique for ACDF in 1955. This procedure has the advantages of (1) halting further osteophyte formation, (2) leading to regression and remodeling of existing osteophytes after solid fusion, and (3) distracting the disc space, which reduces buckling of the ligamentum flavum and enlarges the neuroforamen.[13]

The Smith-Robinson technique uses a horseshoe-shaped, tricortical iliac crest bone graft (Figure 16-1). The graft height should be 2 mm more than the preexisting disc space, with a minimum height of 5 mm. Overdistraction can occur if an attempt is made to enlarge the disc space by more than 4 mm; this may result in overcompression, graft collapse, and pseudarthrosis. Various other graft configurations have been described, including the dowel-shaped Cloward graft, the iliac crest strut graft reported by Bailey and Badgley, and the keystone graft described by Simmons (Figure 16-2).[14–16] In addition to these techniques, which use autogenous bone graft, success has been reported with the use of allograft bone, carbon fiber composite cages, titanium-threaded cages, polymethylmethacrylate, coral, and ceramics. However, these have not been shown to be superior to autografting.[13] With respect to multilevel anterior cervical fusion procedures, Frenkel et al.[17] reported up to 20% pseudarthrosis. These authors used recombinant bone morphogenic proteins for multilevel ACDFs with good results. That being said, there have been multiple reports documenting worsening dysphagia and neck swelling

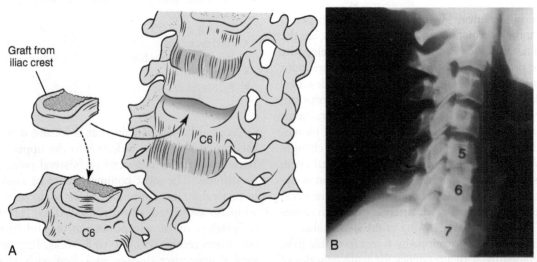

Figure 16-1 A, Illustration showing a Smith-Robinson graft (horseshoe-shaped tricortical iliac crest) placed in the disc space after excision of disc material. **B,** Lateral x-ray film showing ACDF at C5-C6 and C6-C7 using the Smith-Robinson technique. (**A** redrawn from Herkowitz HN, Garfin SR, Eismont FJ, et al, editors: *Rothman-Simeone: The spine,* ed 6, Philadelphia, 2011, Saunders; **B** from Herkowitz HN, Garfin SR, Balderson RA, et al, editors: *Rothman-Simeone: The spine,* ed 4, Philadelphia, 1999, Saunders.)

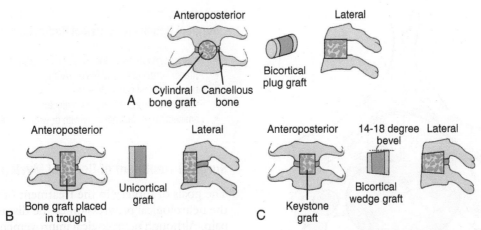

Figure 16-2 Schematic showing some of the various graft configurations for ACDF. **A,** Cloward dowel graft. **B,** Bailey and Badgley iliac strut. **C,** Simmons keystone graft. (Redrawn from Herkowitz HN, Garfin SR, Balderson RA et al, editors: *The spine,* ed 4, Philadelphia, 1999, Saunders.)

associated with the use of recombinant bone morphogenic proteins and overall their use should be considered only with strict caution.

The anterior cervical spine may be approached from the right or left side. After the skin and platysma have been incised, dissection is carried down to the spine, following the natural fascial planes. The sternocleidomastoid muscle and carotid sheath are retracted laterally, and the trachea, esophagus, and thyroid are moved medially. Along with the risk posed to these large structures, a risk of injury to the recurrent laryngeal nerve exists. The disc space is identified, and the annulus is incised. The disc contents and end plate cartilage are removed to the uncovertebral joints on either side and to the posterior longitudinal ligament (PLL) posteriorly. If sequestered disc material is behind the PLL or if a rent is noted in the PLL, the ligament is removed and the fragment is identified and excised; otherwise, the PLL may be left intact. The end plates are prepared to expose bleeding subchondral bone, and the contoured graft is placed into the disc space.

Controversy continues about the need for instrumentation in the surgical management of cervical disc disease. The purported advantages of internal fixation are to provide immediate stability, increase the fusion rate, prevent loss of graft fixation and position, improve postoperative rehabilitation, and reduce the requirement for a cervical orthosis.[18] Considerable debate exists about the efficacy of anterior cervical plating for single-level fusions. As the procedure is performed at an increasing number of levels, more compelling data support the use of rigid internal fixation because of the increased likelihood of bone graft nonunion (Figure 16-3).

Another option for the treatment of cervical radiculopathy at a single-level is disc arthroplasty. Upadhyaya et al.[19] reported on 1213 patients with symptomatic, single-level cervical disc disease who were randomly assigned to undergo either ACDF or disc arthroplasty (in three separate trials). A total of 621 patients received an artificial cervical disc, and 592 patients were treated with ACDF. Although both treatment arms yielded very good results, the arthroplasty was noted to yield a lower rate of

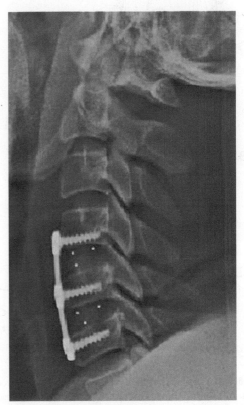

Figure 16-3 Lateral x-ray showing anterior discectomy and fusion (ACDF) of both C4/5 and C5/6 levels using cages and an anterior plate. As the number of fusion levels increases, internal fixation reduces the risk of pseudoarthrosis. (From Wang L, Hee HT, Wong HK: (iv) Cervical spondylotic myelopathy: a brief review of its pathophysiology, presentation, assessment, natural history and management, *Orthopaed Trauma* 25(3):181-189, 2011.)

secondary surgery and a higher rate of neurological success. It was also associated with a lower rate of adjacent-level disease at 2 years.

Posterior approaches can also be used effectively in the surgical treatment of cervical radiculopathy. Laminotomy with foraminotomy is used primarily for unilateral radiculopathy at one or more levels. This technique is particularly useful for disc herniations or osteophytes that occur in relatively lateral positions. An incision is made posteriorly

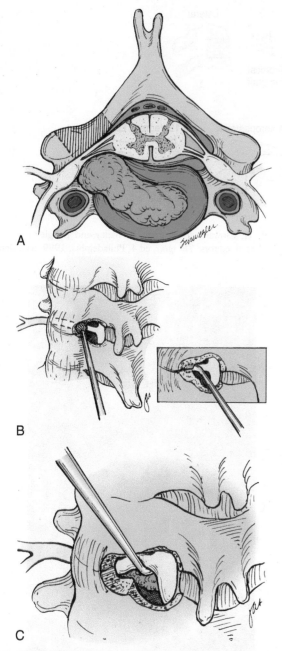

Figure 16-4 A, Posterolateral disc herniation causing nerve root compression. **B,** Laminotomy is performed; a portion of the laminae superiorly and inferiorly is removed, and the nerve root is identified. **C,** After foraminotomy, the nerve root is retracted, revealing the herniated disc, which is excised. (From Herkowitz HN, Garfin SR, Balderson RA et al, editors: *Rothman-Simeone: The spine,* ed 4, Philadelphia, 1999, Saunders.)

between the spinous processes at the affected level or levels, and dissection is carried down to expose the laminae on the symptomatic side. A keyhole-shaped laminotomy is performed using a combination of rongeurs, a high-speed burr, and angled curets (Figure 16-4). The nerve root can then be exposed, and a probe is used to ensure adequate decompression. If a soft disc herniation is present laterally, the nerve root can be retracted gently and the disc fragment excised. At least 50%, and preferably as much as 75%, of the facet joint surfaces should be preserved to prevent iatrogenic segmental instability.[20]

Surgical Options for Cervical Radiculopathy

- Anterior cervical discectomy and fusion (ACDF)
- Anterior corpectomy and fusion (ACF)
- Anterior cervical disc arthroplasty
- Posterior laminectomy with foraminotomy
- Laminectomy or laminoplasty with or without fusion

Surgical Treatment of Cervical Myelopathy

The goals of surgery in the treatment of CSM are to halt the neurological progression of the disease and to reduce pain. Although neurological improvement occurs in some cases, it cannot be reliably predicted, nor should it be the expected outcome for the patient or the clinician. Because neurological improvement cannot be ensured, when possible, surgical intervention should occur before the deficits progress to the level of disability. Patients who have had symptoms for more than 2 years show little or no improvement despite receiving treatment.[21] The choice of surgical technique and approach is based on the location of the neural compression, the number of involved levels, the presence of instability, the alignment in the sagittal plane, and the surgeon's familiarity and comfort level.

Surgical Considerations for Cervical Myelopathy

- Location of neural compression
- Number of levels involved
- Presence of instability
- Sagittal plane alignment
- Surgeon's experience

Because cervical spondylosis typically results in cord compression from anterior structures, the anterior approach allows for direct access to the pathological anatomy and decompression of the neural elements. Another advantage of the anterior approach is that it allows for better correction of sagittal plane deformity in patients with loss of normal cervical lordosis, a deformity that is more difficult to address with a posterior approach. Patients with compression of the cord primarily at the disc levels are candidates for ACDF using the techniques described previously. ACDF can be used successfully in single-level or multilevel disease; however, most surgeons do not advocate its use for more than three levels because of the increased risk of pseudarthrosis.[22] Posterior stabilization sometimes is added to improve rates of successful fusion when multiple levels are involved. As mentioned previously, iliac crest autograft is the gold standard, and the use of internal fixation becomes more important in two- and three-level procedures.

When myelopathy is caused by osteophytes, disc herniation, or ossification of the posterior longitudinal ligament (OPLL) that extends above or below the disc space (behind the vertebral bodies), corpectomy is indicated for satisfactory decompression of the spinal cord. The term *corpectomy* implies removal of the central portion of the vertebral body and the discs above and below, as well as decompression of the joints of Luschka. The anterior approach for ACF is the same as that for ACDF, that is, following the natural fascial planes between the trachea, esophagus, and thyroid medially and the sternocleidomastoid muscle and the carotid sheath laterally to expose the anterior cervical spine. The appropriate discs are incised and removed back to the PLL. A rongeur is used to remove the bulk of the central portion of the vertebral body (Figure 16-5). After this initial trough is made, a high-speed burr is used to remove the remaining vertebral body back to the posterior cortex. Small angled curets are then used to remove the posterior

cortex from the dura. The cervical spine is stabilized after corpectomy with strut grafts or cages made of titanium/PEEK.[23] The iliac crest or other interbody substitutes are used to promote structural support, to attempt to correct deformity, and to allow for fusion. Figure 16-6 shows the use of a fibular strut graft for a C3-C7 fusion after corpectomies. Internal fixation in the form of anterior cervical plating often is indicated to provide additional rigidity, reduce graft dislodgement, and possibly reduce the rate of pseudarthrosis (Figure 16-7). Postoperatively, a rigid cervical orthosis is often used. After prolonged surgery, the patient may remain intubated overnight to reduce the risk of respiratory complications.

Posterior surgery for the management of cervical myelopathy is indicated in patients with dorsal spinal cord compression, diffuse canal stenosis, multilevel spondylosis, and OPLL. Posterior surgery may be preferable to long anterior exposures for diffuse disease, because posterior approaches are less technically demanding and do not endanger structures such as the trachea, esophagus, and recurrent laryngeal nerve. For posterior decompression of the spinal cord to be effective, the cord must move posteriorly (dorsally) in the thecal sac. For this to occur, a lordotic alignment of the cervical spine is necessary; kyphosis in the sagittal plane is a relative contraindication to posterior surgery, because the spinal cord is less likely to move posteriorly when it is "draped over" the kyphotic vertebral bodies. Laminectomy (Figure 16-8) with or without fusion and laminoplasty are the principle posterior procedures used to treat myelopathy.

Isolated cervical laminectomy currently has narrow indications. Laminectomy alone can increase instability and lead to postoperative kyphosis, neurological deterioration,

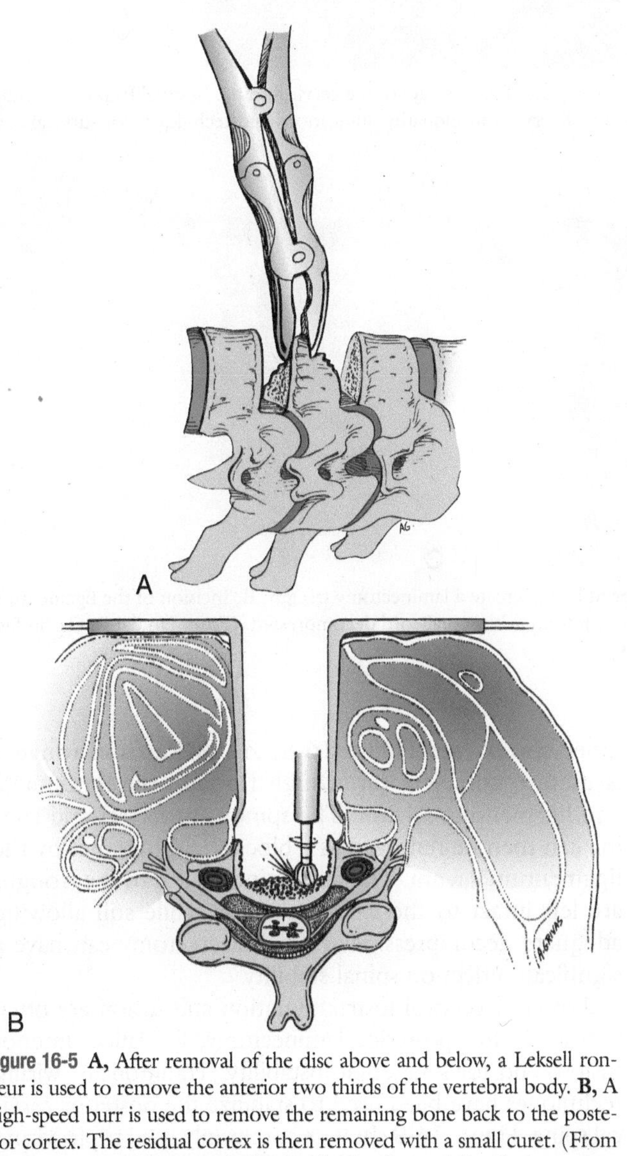

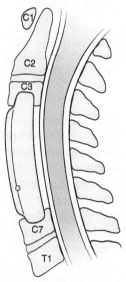

Figure 16-5 A, After removal of the disc above and below, a Leksell rongeur is used to remove the anterior two thirds of the vertebral body. **B,** A high-speed burr is used to remove the remaining bone back to the posterior cortex. The residual cortex is then removed with a small curet. (From Winter RB, Denis F, Lonstein JW, Smith M, editors: *Atlas of spine surgery,* Philadelphia, 1995, Saunders.)

Figure 16-6 Schematic showing corpectomies of C4-C6 with placement of a strut graft from C3 to C7. Note that the vertebral bodies have been notched to secure the graft in position. (Adapted from Smith MD: Cervical spondylosis. In Birdwell KH, DeWald RL, editors: *The textbook of spinal surgery,* ed 2, Philadelphia, 1997, Lippincott-Raven, p 1411.)

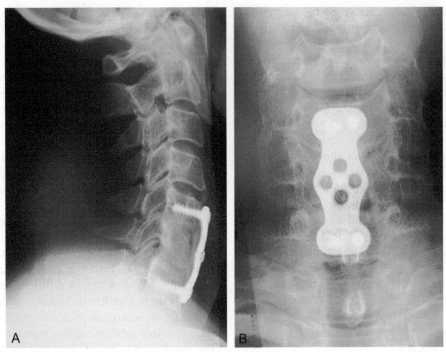

Figure 16-7 Lateral (**A**) and anterior posterior (**B**) postoperative cervical corpectomy and fusion x-rays of the cervical spine. Internal fixation provides additional stability. (From Medow JE, Trost G, Sandin J: Surgical management of cervical myelopathy: indications and techniques for surgical corpectomy, *Spine J*, 6(6):S233-S241, 2006.)

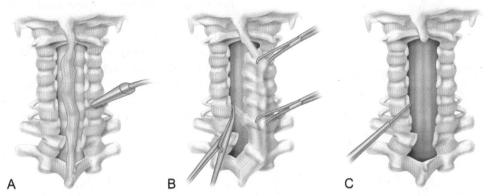

Figure 16-8 Posterior view of a cervical spine laminectomy. **A**, Use of high-speed bur to create a laminectomy trough. **B**, Incision of the ligamentum flavum and en bloc resection of the lamina from C3 to C7. **C**, Completed laminectomy with spinal cord decompressed. (From Jandial R, Garfin SR: *Best evidence for spine surgery: 20 cardinal cases*, Philadelphia, 2012, Saunders.)

and progression of OPLL. For these reasons, laminectomy without posterior stabilization probably should be reserved for patients with short segment posterior compressive lesions and a normal cervical lordosis. Kaptain et al.[24] reported that more than 20% of patients with no instrumented cervical laminectomy developed deformity progression. This percentile was significantly higher in patients who already had loss of cervical lordosis. With more diffuse disease, laminectomy should be combined with instrumentation and fusion. The procedure is performed through a posterior midline incision. The paraspinal muscles are dissected from the spinous processes and laminae bilaterally. A high-speed burr is then used to create two troughs at the lateral aspects of the laminae down to the

inner cortex (see Figure 16-8, *A*). A Kerrison rongeur is used to complete the trough through the inner table and ligamentum flavum. The spinous processes and lamina can then be removed as a block, held together by the ligamentum flavum. The facet joints lateral to the troughs are left intact to the extent possible while still allowing adequate decompression. Partial facetectomy can have a significant effect on spinal stability.

Posterior cervical instrumentation and fusion are often indicated after posterior laminectomy, for failed anterior fusion, and for segmental instability. Traditionally, wiring techniques have been used to stabilize the posterior cervical spine. Figure 16-9 shows a commonly used triple wiring technique, which also secures two corticocancellous strips

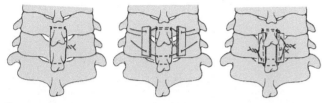

Figure 16-9 Triple wiring technique in the posterior cervical spine. This serves as a tension band as well as securing two corticocancellous strip grafts in position bilaterally. (From Benzel EC, editor: *Spine surgery: techniques, complication avoidance, and management,* ed 3, Philadelphia, 2012, Saunders.)

of bone graft. Most wiring techniques require the spinous processes as points of fixation; however, after laminectomy, these have been removed. Screw fixation is currently the mainstay for stabilization; this can be a plate and screw construct or a rod and screw construct (Figure 16-10).

Combined anterior and posterior approaches are necessary in some patients. This circumferential approach most often is indicated for patients with a combination of severe sagittal plane kyphosis and multilevel stenosis, postlaminectomy kyphosis, or severe osteoporosis. In these challenging cases, the anterior procedure (multilevel corpectomy with strut graft) is directed at restoring sagittal alignment and decompressing the spinal cord. The posterior procedure (using lateral mass screws with plate or rod fixation) typically is used to enhance stabilization, minimize anterior graft complications, and reduce pseudarthrosis rates. These can be done as one procedure or as staged procedures on different days.

Because of the high incidence of spinal cord compression secondary to OPLL in Japan, Japanese surgeons have been very innovative in developing decompressive procedures. Laminoplasty was designed to reduce postoperative instability while maintaining spinal motion. Although various laminoplasty techniques have been described, the common goal of each is to expand the area of the spinal canal (effecting decompression) while preserving the posterior bony and ligamentous structures. Retaining the posterior elements allows segmental muscle reattachment, promoting stability and allowing motion.

The two most common laminoplasty techniques are the open door technique, in which the posterior arch is opened on one side with the contralateral side acting as a hinge, and the French door technique, in which the lamina is opened in the midline with bilateral hinges.[25,26]

The exposure for laminoplasty is a posterior midline approach, dissecting the paraspinal musculature from the posterior elements. Care is taken to preserve the interspinous ligaments and facet joint capsules. A high-speed burr generally is used to create lateral troughs in the lamina bilaterally. The trough can then be completed and opened on one side and hinged on the other (open door technique) (Figure 16-11, *A*). A midline osteotomy can also be performed; the lamina is opened centrally, hinging on the bilateral troughs (French door technique) (Figure 16-11, *B*). Various methods of holding the laminoplasty open have also been detailed, including wiring, sutures, small plates, and interposition bone grafts.

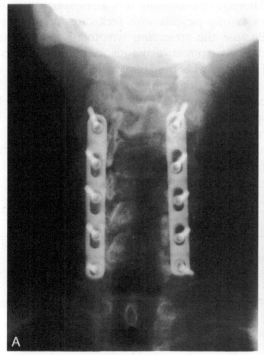
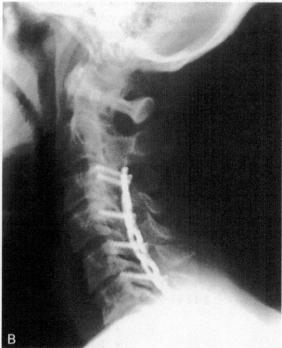

Figure 16-10 Anteroposterior (**A**) and lateral (**B**) x-ray films showing lateral mass plating and fusion from C3 to C7 after laminectomy for severe multilevel myelopathy. (Geck MJ, Eismont FJ: Surgical options for the treatment of cervical spondylotic myelopathy, *Orthop Clin North Am* 33(2):329-348, 2002.)

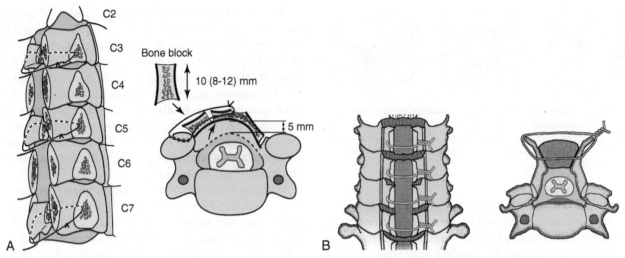

Figure 16-11 Two common techniques for vertebroplasty. **A,** Open door technique. **B,** French door technique. These procedures allow for preservation of motion and maintain the posterior ligamentous structures while decompressing the spinal canal. (**A** redrawn from Itoh T, Tsuji H: Technical improvements and results of laminoplasty for compressive myelopathy in the cervical spine, *Spine* 10:729-736, 1985; **B** from Herkowitz HN, Garfin SR, Balderson RA et al, editors: *The spine*, ed 4, Philadelphia, 1999, Saunders.)

Surgical Treatment of Axial Neck Pain

Operative treatment for axial neck pain has narrow indications and should be used when all nonoperative options have been exhausted. Surgery may be indicated for a patient who continues to have unrelenting neck pain despite conservative treatment and has one- or two-level cervical degenerative disease. ACDF and cervical disc arthroplasty are the primary procedures used to treat axial neck pain. Both procedures eliminate the diseased disc (thought to be the major pain generator). A posterior approach may also be helpful in patients with failed anterior surgery or when posterior decompression is indicated. The anterior approach generally is preferred, because it does not involve extensive paraspinal muscle stripping and the disc is removed in its entirety.

Rehabilitation Considerations

Data in the literature provide little evidence on ways to optimize postoperative rehabilitation. The surgeon's preference and local opinion generally influence the rehabilitation process, lending anecdotal guidance to such things as the use of bracing and activity limitations. With the improvement of spinal instrumentation through the use of more rigid constructs, the use of postoperative bracing has decreased. The authors' guidelines are outlined in Table 16-1; however, there is a wide range of variability among surgeons.

THORACIC DISC DISEASE

Thoracic disc herniation is a relatively unusual diagnosis among patients who seek care for spinal problems. Because the presenting symptoms can be quite varied, this uncommon diagnosis often goes unrecognized. However, with the improvement in MRI and other advanced imaging techniques, patients are being diagnosed earlier and with greater accuracy. Figure 16-12 shows spinal cord impingement caused by soft and hard disc herniations. Disc herniations in the thoracic spine mostly affect middle-aged individuals. Nearly 80% are seen in

TABLE **16-1**

Rehabilitation Considerations After Surgery on the Cervical Spine

Expected Hospital Course	Outpatient Course	Red Flags
• Length of stay: 0-2 days • Ambulation and upper extremity range of motion (ROM) • Bracing: may or may not be used (surgeon's preference, 2-12 weeks)	• Aerobic conditioning, upper extremity stretching/strengthening • Active cervical spine ROM when brace is removed • No passive ROM for 3 months (at affected levels) • May shower when wound is healed • For fusions: no heavy lifting/exercise for 3 months	• Change in neurological examination findings or symptoms • Worsening pain • Difficulty swallowing • Erythema/fever/wound drainage

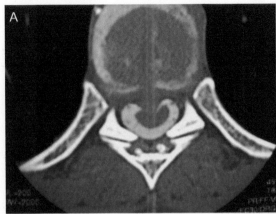 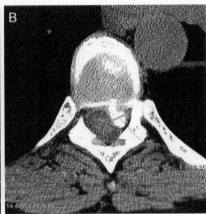

Figure 16-12 Thoracic disc herniations. **A,** Pre-operative computed tomography (CT)/myelogram showing central soft disc herniation at T6-T7. **B,** Pre-operative axial CT image showing a T8-T9 lateralized calcified thoracic disc herniation. (From Sheikh H, Samartzis D, Perez-Cruet MJ: Techniques for the operative management of thoracic disc herniation: minimally invasive thoracic microdiscectomy, *Orthop Clin North Am* 38(3):351-361, 2007.)

the fourth through sixth decades, with **33%** occurring in those in their forties.[27] Surgery for thoracic disc disease is estimated to account for **0.15%** to **1.8%** of all discectomies performed.[28,29] No clear-cut syndrome has been described for this condition, because the presentation varies considerably. The most common initial symptom is pain (in **57%** of patients), followed by sensory complaints and, least commonly, motor and bladder disturbances.[27] Three quarters of disc herniations in the thoracic spine occur between T8 and L1, with T11-T12 being the most affected level (**26%**).[27] This is thought to be related to the increased stress on the spine at the thoracolumbar junction.

Patients without myelopathy can be treated conservatively with narcotic pain medications, anti-inflammatory drugs, physical therapy, activity modification, and occasionally bracing. In general, surgery is regarded as the treatment of choice for symptomatic patients with myelopathy to prevent the sequelae of cord compression. Indications for operative intervention for herniated thoracic discs include progressive myelopathy, lower extremity weakness, and unremitting pain after conservative treatment.

Surgical Treatment

When surgery is indicated, the approach taken to remove the diseased disc is determined by its nature and location, the level of the pathology, and the surgeon's experience. Historically, thoracic myelopathy was treated with a direct posterior laminectomy and disc excision. This approach has been abandoned because of its unacceptably high rate of neurological deterioration, which results from manipulation of the spinal cord to access the disc for excision.[30] The widely accepted techniques for thoracic discectomy are the transthoracic approach, costotransversectomy, the transpedicular (posterolateral) approach, and video-assisted thoracoscopy (VATS).

With the evolvement of minimally invasive surgery, another technique being used is the minimally invasive lateral retropleural approach.[31]

The transthoracic approach gives the widest exposure to the disc space (especially for central and intradural herniations), accessibility of multiple levels, and the ability to place a bone graft. However, with these advantages comes the morbidity of a thoracotomy.[28] A left-sided approach usually is preferred to avoid the inferior vena cava and the liver in the lower thoracic spine. With the patient in the lateral decubitus position, a standard thoracotomy is performed, and the chest cavity is entered one or two levels above the level of interest. Mobilization of the parietal pleura and segmental vessels and nerves is then performed. Partial or complete discectomy can be undertaken anteriorly without manipulation of the spinal cord (Figure 16-13). Fusion is indicated when stability is compromised by the decompression, as in the case of complete discectomy with partial corpectomy. A chest tube is placed at the end of the surgery.

For posterolateral and lateral disc herniations, the costotransversectomy approach may be used. This approach has the advantages of avoiding entry into the pulmonary cavity and providing access to all thoracic levels, but it requires disruption of the paraspinal musculature and more extensive bone resection. The patient is positioned prone, and a paramedian incision is made. The paraspinal muscles are retracted medially or split transversely. The posterior medial portion of the rib is resected, and the pleura is mobilized and retracted anteriorly. The transverse process and pedicle on the affected side are excised, providing access to the lateral aspect of the disc. The disc fragment is removed, often along with a posterolateral portion of the adjacent vertebral bodies. Disc herniations that do not cross the midline can be effectively decompressed with this technique without manipulation of the spinal cord, minimizing neurological complications.

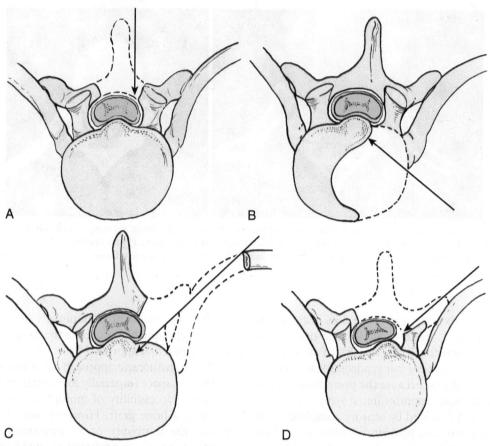

Figure 16-13 A, Decompression of thoracic disc herniations from a standard laminectomy approach requires manipulation of the spinal cord and results in a high rate of neurological injury. **B,** A transthoracic approach allows the most direct access to the disc without encountering the spinal cord. **C,** Decompression using a costotransversectomy approach allows safe excision of the disc posteriorly. **D,** For posterolateral and foraminal disc herniations, a transpedicular approach can give access to the lesion. (From Herkowitz HN, Garfin SR, Eismont FJ et al, editors: *Rothman-Simeone: The spine,* ed 6, Philadelphia, 2011, Saunders.)

A transpedicular (or posterolateral) approach to the thoracic spine is useful only for posterolateral or foraminal herniations. This approach gives only limited exposure of the disc, but it avoids thoracotomy, does not necessitate rib resection, and requires less extensive dissection. With the patient prone, a midline exposure is performed. The lamina, facet joint, and pedicle on the affected side are removed. The lateral portion of the involved disc can then be excised with small curets and pituitary rongeurs. Segmental stability may be compromised, depending on the amount of the facet and pedicle that are removed to facilitate visualization.

VATS may be able to provide the advantages of the anterior (or transthoracic) approach to thoracic disc pathology while minimizing the morbidity of thoracotomy (Figure 16-14). This approach is more technically demanding and has a steep learning curve for the surgeon and staff; incomplete decompression and failure to resolve symptoms can result from inadequate visualization or unreliable excision of disc material. Limited data are available on the effectiveness of VATS, because this technique is evolving; however, preliminary series in the literature appear promising.[32]

The operative technique for the minimally invasive surgery (MIS) lateral approach to the thoracic spine has previously been described.[33] After general endotracheal intubation, the patient is positioned in the true lateral decubitus position with the operative side up. Intraoperative fluoroscopy is used to ensure the patient is placed and secured in a true lateral orientation, with the working corridor to the disc space orthogonal to the floor (true 90° lateral trajectory).

For the retropleural approach, a 5- to 6-cm oblique incision is made directly over the rib that is overlying the targeted pathology on lateral fluoroscopy. Monopolar cautery is used to dissect through the subcutaneous tissue and muscle. The periosteum is elevated circumferentially off the rib, and approximately 6 cm of rib is resected. The plane between the parietal pleura and endothoracic fascia is developed in the cranial and caudal direction, as well as anteriorly, until the lateral surface of the vertebral bodies and disc spaces are visualized. A table-mounted retractor is then placed over the targeted level to maintain exposure. Once accurate placement of the retractor has been confirmed and adequate exposure

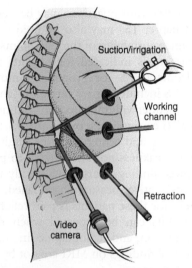

Figure 16-14 Diagram of the typical portals and instruments used in video-assisted thoracoscopy for decompression of a T8-T9 herniated disc. (From Herkowitz HN, Garfin SR, Eismont FJ et al, editors: *Rothman-Simeone: The spine*, ed 6, Philadelphia, 2011, Saunders.)

is achieved, the goals of surgery are accomplished in the traditional methods.

In a report from a multicenter study, Uribe et al.[31] described outcomes following MIS lateral approach for thoracic disc herniation in 60 consecutive patients treated at one of five international institutions with an average follow-up of 11 months. Myelopathy was improved in 83%; radiculopathy, in 87%; back pain, in 91%; and bladder and/or bowel dysfunction, in 88% of patients.

Rehabilitation Considerations

Little information is available in the literature about postoperative rehabilitation after surgery of the thoracic spine. Many surgeons routinely use rigid orthoses, whereas others believe that the inherent stability of the thoracic spine, combined with modern instrumentation (for more extensive procedures), is sufficient to forgo bracing. Table 16-2 presents the authors' preferred guidelines for rehabilitation.

LUMBAR DISC DISEASE

An estimated 80% of the population experiences low back pain at some time in their lives, resulting in one of the most common causes of disability among people living in industrialized nations.[34] In most patients, low back pain is self-limiting and requires no treatment; however, 7% to 14% of patients have symptoms that persist longer than 2 weeks, and 1% to 2% of patients eventually undergo surgery of the lumbar spine.[35] The most common disorders of lumbar discs can be divided into syndromes that cause predominantly back pain and those in which the primary complaint is leg pain (sciatica).

Statistics for Lumbar Disc Disease

- 80% of the population will experience low back pain
- 7%-14% will have symptoms longer than 2 weeks
- 1%-2% will undergo surgery

Discogenic pain syndromes of the lumbar spine present with low back pain as the chief symptom. Some associated buttock or sporadic leg pain also may be reported, but these are generally associated with irritation of the nerve root in the neural foramen. As the name implies, the lumbar intervertebral discs are thought to be the principal pain generators and are the focus of diagnosis and treatment. These syndromes can be classified into three categories: internal disc disruption (IDD), degenerative disc disease (DDD), and segmental instability. IDD usually follows trauma and is marked by damage to the internal structure and metabolic function of the intervertebral disc; imaging is generally normal. DDD, on the other hand, is atraumatic, with a gradual onset of symptoms that usually manifest in middle-aged individuals, and often involves anular tears, disc bulges, and disc herniation.[36] Radiographic findings include disc space narrowing, osteophyte formation, and end plate sclerosis. Segmental instability describes excessive motion, either

TABLE **16-2**

Rehabilitation Considerations After Surgery on the Thoracic Spine

Expected Hospital Course	Outpatient Course	Red Flags
• Length of stay: 3-7 days • Ambulation when able to be out of bed • Bracing: may or may not be used after chest tube is removed (surgeon's preference, 2-12 weeks)	• Aerobic conditioning, upper extremity/lower extremity stretching/strengthening • Active spinal range of motion (ROM) when brace is removed • No passive ROM for 3 months (at affected levels) • May shower when wound is healed • Brace off for shower, activities of daily living • No heavy lifting/exercise for 3 months	• Change in neurological examination findings or symptoms • Worsening pain • Shortness of breath • Erythema/fever/wound drainage

translational or rotational, of the spinal segments; this manifests as spondylolisthesis, lateral listhesis, rotatory subluxation, or scoliosis.

Disc Syndromes

- Internal disc disruption (IDD)
- Degenerative disc disease (DDD)
- Segmental instability

Lumbar disc herniation can cause impingement and inflammation of neural elements, most commonly the nerve roots. This leads to pain that radiates down the leg on the affected side, called *radiculopathy*. Irritation of the posterior primary ramus may result in localized back pain as well. In a healthy disc, the inner nucleus pulposus is contained by the annulus fibrosus. When fissuring or tearing of the inner annulus occurs but the outer portion remains intact, the nucleus can bulge or protrude posteriorly, causing nerve root impingement. As further fissuring occurs, the nucleus can push through and exit the annulus, causing extrusion of the disc material. When an extruded fragment becomes detached from the remaining nucleus pulposus, it is said to be sequestered (Figure 16-15). Nonoperative treatment of symptomatic lumbar disc disease often results in a return to normal activity. Conservative treatment plans commonly consist of several modalities, including drug therapies and the use of a wide variety of physical therapy interventions, such as exercise, traction, and counterirritation techniques to manage pain (e.g., electrical nerve stimulation, acupuncture, biofeedback), as well as bracing and manipulation. Epidural

and selective nerve root injections may be helpful. Facet blocks (see Chapter 15) may also be used to treat pain arising from microinstability of the facet joints.

Urgent surgery is indicated for patients with cauda equina syndrome (CES) or progressive motor deficit. Findings in CES include urinary retention (check a postvoid residual bladder volume), fecal incontinence, "saddle anesthesia" (i.e., numbness over buttocks, anus, lower genitals, perineum, and posterosuperior thighs), and significant motor weakness not attributable to pain. In the absence of these findings, surgery generally is indicated only after conservative measures have failed. The major goal of surgery for these patients is pain relief. The most predictable results can be expected when the history, physical examination, and radiographic findings are consistent. Abnormal findings on MRI are not by themselves an indication for surgery.

If surgery is indicated, the surgeon must determine whether decompression alone (i.e., discectomy) or decompression in conjunction with stabilization is the treatment of choice for the patient. Initially, discectomy alone is the treatment of choice for lumbar disc herniation with radiculopathy. In the event of multiple recurrent disc herniations, significant pain that has failed all conservative treatment, or evidence of instability, spinal fusion is recommended.

Surgical Procedures for Lumbar Disc Disease

- Discectomy
- Posterior lumbar interbody fusion (PLIF)
- Transforaminal lumbar interbody fusion (TLIF)
- Lateral lumbar interbody fusion (LLIF)
- Anterior lumbar interbody fusion (ALIF)
- Artificial disc replacement

Discectomy

Surgery is indicated for patients with unilateral radiculopathic leg pain for whom imaging studies confirm a correlating lumbar disc herniation, for patients in whom nonoperative management fails after a trial of 6 to 8 weeks, and for patients with severe or worsening motor deficit.[37,38] Conventional, or open, discectomy is performed with the patient positioned prone on a frame or in the kneeling position; this allows the patient's abdomen to hang free, preventing pressure on the vena cava, which reduces intraoperative bleeding. The proper spinal level is identified, and a small midline incision is made. Subperiosteal dissection is performed, exposing the spinous process and lamina. When proper exposure of the posterior elements is obtained, laminotomy (or laminectomy) of the affected side is carried out with the appropriate rongeurs and curets. Care must be taken not to cross the pars interarticularis and remove the entire facet,

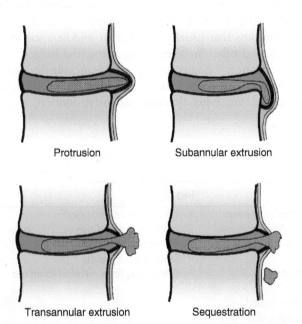

Protrusion   Subannular extrusion

Transannular extrusion   Sequestration

Figure 16-15 Classification of disc herniations. (Modified from Herkowitz HN, Garfin SR, Balderson RA et al, editors: *Rothman-Simeone: The spine,* ed 4, Philadelphia, 1999, Saunders.)

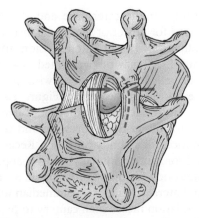

Figure 16-16 Technique for lumbar discectomy. Parts of the superior and inferior laminae and ligamentum flavum are removed to expose the nerve root and underlying disc herniation (*left arrow*). The disc fragment is excised, and a blunt probe is used to ensure adequate decompression. Excessive bone removal (past dotted line) can cause iatrogenic instability. (From Benzel EC, editor: *Spine surgery: techniques, complication avoidance, and management,* ed 3, Philadelphia, 2012, Saunders.)

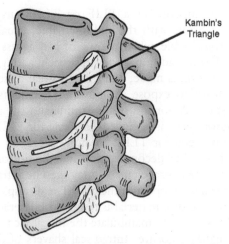

Figure 16-17 Drawing of lateral lumbar spine depicting Kambin's triangular safe working zone for percutaneous arthroscopic discectomy. This zone is a right triangle in which one arm is the thecal sac, the other arm is the end plate of the caudal body, and the hypotenuse is the exiting nerve root. (From Fessler RG, O'Toole JE, Eichholz KM, Perez-Cruet MJ: The development of minimally invasive spine surgery, *Neurosurg Clin North Am* 17:401-409, 2006.)

because this may result in iatrogenic instability. The ligamentum flavum is excised to expose the dura. The nerve root is inspected and retracted to reveal the underlying disc herniation (Figure 16-16). The PLL and posterior annulus are incised, and pituitary rongeurs are used to remove the herniation in a piecemeal fashion. A blunt probe can then be inserted to ensure that a sufficient amount of disc material has been removed for adequate decompression of the nerve root. After meticulous hemostasis is achieved, the wound is closed in layers.

Alternative forms of discectomy have been described, with the goal of reducing the size of the incision and limiting dissection, and thereby minimizing postoperative morbidity, reducing the potential for scar formation, and allowing for quicker mobilization and rehabilitation. Two of the more common alternative techniques are microdiscectomy and arthroscopically assisted microdiscectomy (AMD).

Using the operating microscope or loupes with a headlamp coaxial to the line of sight allows the surgeon to obtain illumination and visualization of deep spinal structures through a small incision. With this advantage, microdiscectomy can be performed through incisions 2 to 3 cm (1 to 1.2 inches) long. The surgical technique is similar to that for conventional discectomy, in which dissection of the paraspinals, laminotomy, and removal of the ligamentum flavum are required to allow visualization of the pathological disc and decompression of the nerve root. This operation can be safely performed as an outpatient procedure.[39] However, its role is somewhat controversial, because several reports show similar results for microdiscectomy and conventional open discectomy.[40,41]

AMD uses a percutaneous, posterolateral approach to the lumbar disc. The potential advantages of this technique are as follows: it does not require muscle stripping, bone resection, or retraction of inflamed nerve roots; it allows irrigation and dilution of inflammatory mediators;

and it minimizes epidural bleeding and subsequent scar formation.[42] For AMD, the patient is positioned prone on a radiolucent table, and standard sterile skin preparation and draping are followed. Under fluoroscopic guidance, a needle is inserted approximately 10 cm (4 inches) from the midline and directed toward the triangular working zone and into the disc (Figure 16-17).[42] A guidewire is placed through the needle, and the needle is removed. An obturator and canula are then advanced over the guidewire, providing access for the arthroscope and instruments. This approach allows for manual removal of the disc fragments causing nerve root compression, as well as annular fenestration, which reduces intradiscal pressure and creates a "path of least resistance" away from the nerve root for any future herniations. Success rates of 70% to 90% have been reported for AMD, with minimal complications.[43,44]

Posterior Lumbar Interbody Fusion/Transforaminal Lumbar Interbody Fusion

Numerous authors have reported on the success of posterior lumbar interbody fusion (PLIF) techniques in the treatment of lumbar degenerative disease, spondylolisthesis, and discogenic back pain. PLIF allows for *direct* decompression of the neural elements, distraction and realignment of the disc space, and stabilization of the painful motion segment. Some debate exists as to the surgical indications for PLIF (or a modification, transforaminal lumbar interbody fusion [TLIF]); however, most would agree that only patients who still have persistent, disabling pain after an aggressive, prolonged nonoperative therapy program should be recommended for the operation. Provocative discography has also been recommended as a diagnostic tool to confirm that a particular disc space is the focus of pain generation.[45]

Patients undergoing a PLIF or TLIF surgery are positioned prone with the abdomen free, usually on a Jackson spinal table, which allows for easy access of fluoroscopy. In the traditional open approach, a longitudinal midline incision is made, and subperiosteal dissection is carried down to expose the posterior elements of the lumbar spine. A portion of the lamina and the superior and inferior facets is removed (bilateral for PLIF; bilateral or unilateral for TLIF) to allow access to the spinal canal. Further decompression may be performed as necessary. The neural elements may then be retracted to expose the lateral aspect of the disc. The disc space is entered, and the disc material is removed bilaterally. Care must be taken not to manipulate the thecal sac too much to get medial exposure. Intradiscal shavers of different widths are used to excise the remaining disc material and prepare the end plates for fusion. Structural grafts are then placed in the interspace to restore alignment and allow for fusion (Figure 16-18). In a PLIF, two structural grafts are placed in the lateral disc space, whereas in a TLIF, one graft is placed anteromedially. Multiple techniques and graft choices have been described, including autograft bone, allograft bone, and metal and carbon fiber cages filled with cancellous bone, and all of these choices come in a number of shapes and configurations. Although most variations of the PLIF technique involve grafting of the interspace and the use of implants, the need for posterior segmental instrumentation and the addition of posterolateral fusion are the subject of debate. PLIF may be performed as a stand-alone procedure, or pedicle screw fixation with or without intertransverse fusion can be added (Figure 16-19). With a TLIF, one entire facet, or sometimes bilateral facets, are removed for direct decompression and thus require posterior fixation for stability purposes. Recent advances have allowed for more minimally invasive approaches to posterior interbody fusions. For example, an MIS TLIF involves a unilateral or bilateral paramedian incision and uses muscle dilation rather than cautery to prevent postoperative muscle atrophy.[46] All methods have been reported successful.[47-49]

Anterior Lumbar Interbody Fusion

Anterior lumbar interbody fusion (ALIF) has become an increasingly popular surgical option because it allows reconstruction of the anterior column, improves sagittal alignment (i.e., restores lumbar lordosis), stabilizes the painful motion segment, enlarges the neuroforamina through distraction of the disc space, and avoids paraspinal muscle damage and scarring. The primary indication for ALIF is chronic low back pain, generally caused by DDD,

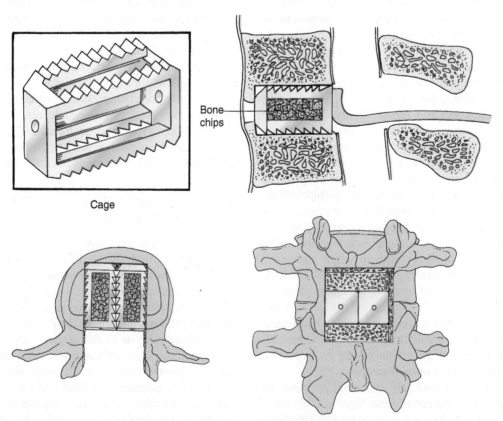

Figure 16-18 Posterior lumbar interbody fusion. The diagram shows the interbody positioning of two carbon fiber cages packed with cancellous bone graft. The cauda equina (not shown) is retracted to each side as the cage is impacted into the disc space. (From Benzel EC, editor: *Spine surgery: techniques, complication avoidance, and management,* ed 3, Philadelphia, 2012, Saunders.)

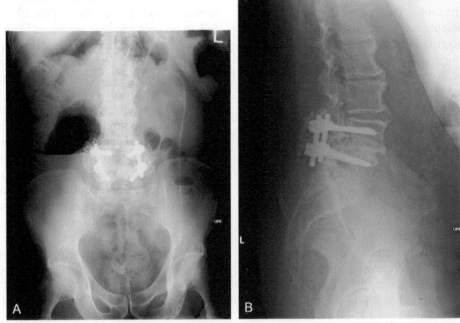

Figure 16-19 Anteroposterior (**A**) and lateral (**B**) x-ray films showing an instrumented PLIF of L4-L5. (From Benzel EC, editor: *Spine surgery: techniques, complication avoidance, and management,* ed 2, Philadelphia, 2005, Saunders.)

degenerative spondylolisthesis, or failed posterior surgery. As with other surgical techniques for the treatment of degenerative lumbar conditions, ALIF is indicated when disabling symptoms have persisted for a prolonged period and when conservative management options have been exhausted. It is used primarily in the treatment of L4-L5 and L5-S1, but it also may be used at more rostral levels. Neural compression is a relative contraindication for ALIF; decompression of the canal and neuroforamen is most safely and effectively carried out dorsally under direct vision. Indirect decompression of bilateral foramina may be accomplished with a large interbody graft using the lateral lumbar interbody fusion (LLIF), which is discussed in the following section.[50]

ALIF is performed with the patient supine on a radiolucent table. An anterior retroperitoneal approach is used, usually from the left side. An abdominal or vascular surgeon commonly performs the procedure in conjunction with the spinal surgeon. A paramedian incision is made low on the abdomen, the rectus sheath is incised, and the muscle is retracted. The retroperitoneal space is entered, and the peritoneum is mobilized and retracted to expose the lower lumbar spine. The iliac vessels are retracted to allow access to the disc space or spaces that are to be fused. The anterior longitudinal ligament and anterior annulus are excised, along with the remainder of the disc material. The subchondral bone of the end plates is prepared, and a graft slightly larger than the disc space is inserted to achieve the desired level of sagittal correction and distraction of the foramina. The choice of graft varies and, as with PLIF, successful outcomes and fusion have been achieved using tricortical autograft, shaped

allograft, and cages. Hemostasis is achieved, followed by a standard closure. A nasogastric tube is used postoperatively until bowel function returns. Retrograde ejaculation is a recognized complication that may develop after ALIF. It most often occurs after L5-S1 fusion and is a result of injury to the autonomic nerves overlying that interspace.

Lateral Lumbar Interbody Fusion

Recent advances in instruments, retractors, and techniques have tremendously propelled lumbar fusions, allowing near-total removal of discs and placement of large interbody grafts, thus increasing rates of fusion. With the LLIF technique, the disc space is accessed laterally, through the psoas muscle, allowing for minimal tissue disruption, decreased blood loss, reduced postoperative pain, and shorter recovery time.[51,52] Dural retraction is avoided, as well as destruction and denervation of the posterior musculature and removal of the posterior arch with its potential for instability. Compared with anterior approaches, there is reduced risk of vascular injury. The surgeon is maximizing the strongest areas of the end plate, with the implant placement spanning the ring apophysis.

The LLIF technique is indicated in many of the same cases as those where TLIF, PLIF, or ALIF is indicated. However, the main contraindication for LLIF at this point is at the L5-S1 level due to the iliac crest as a barrier, as well as the presence of the iliac vessels and lumbosacral plexus at that level. The lateral technique is also useful for adjacent segment disease, to avoid the prior scar, and to maximize fusion surface. Recently it has gained acceptance as an excellent tool in the treatment of spinal deformity, along with percutaneous pedicle screw fixation.

Preoperative imaging is essential, as it is with all spine surgery. If the majority of spinal stenosis or compression is dorsal in nature, a posterior approach may be more appropriate. However, the size of the neuroforamina is increased with placement of a large interbody graft, thus providing indirect decompression of the nerve roots. It is important also to recognize an extra lumbar segment (i.e., lumbarization of the sacrum) when it is present, because the lateral approach to the lower lumbar spine may not be feasible in these cases.[53] On MRI, the surgical level should have an adjacent healthy-appearing psoas muscle, and if it has moved anteriorly, then there is a likelihood of increased neural elements at the entrance to the disc space from the lateral side. Intraoperative neuromonitoring allows directional neuromonitoring with continuous electromyographic (EMG) monitoring of nearby nerves while traversing the psoas muscle. Fluoroscopy is essential during LLIF and will determine the outcome of each case.

The patient is placed in the lateral position and secured to the table using silk tape, with laterality determined preoperatively by the surgeon, taking into consideration MRI findings, elevation of iliac crest, symptomatology, and surgeon preference. The bed is then broken to open the disc space slightly and to allow improved access between the lowest rib and the iliac crest. Using fluoroscopy, the surgeon marks the skin with a target of the posterior third of the disc space. Using one or two incisions (the second used to guide the dilator), the surgeon uses blunt dissection to sweep the peritoneum anteriorly and feel for the transverse process and psoas muscle. The dilator is placed, and with constant checking of the neuromonitoring, sequential dilators are used until the retractor is placed. With the retractor anchored in place with a shim and articulating arm, a set of interbody instruments are used to prepare the interspace and place the graft. It is hypothesized that minimizing the time that the retractor is open will minimize risk of complications, including anterior thigh numbness or nerve injury.

Overall, LLIF is a powerful tool for lumbar interbody fusion, with short recovery times, relatively low complication risks, minimal blood loss, high fusion rates, and reduced overall health care costs compared with other maximally invasive procedures.[54]

Lumbar Artificial Disc Replacement

The U.S. Food and Drug Administration (FDA) has approved the use of lumbar artificial disc replacement for the treatment of symptomatic lumbar disc disease. The artificial disc is an alternative to fusion procedures. The proposed advantages of disc replacement are the ability to restore pain-free motion of the intervertebral segment and to protect adjacent segments from increased loading and failure. The current indications for disc replacement are quite limited; only about 5% of patients considered for surgical intervention meet the criteria.[55] Candidates for lumbar arthroplasty are patients 18 to 60 years old in whom nonoperative treatment for at least 6 months has failed, who have single-level DDD confirmed by MRI and discography, and who have no previous lumbar fusion, no instability, and no extruded disc material.[56] Proper patient selection has been advocated as the most important parameter for a successful clinical outcome.[57] There has been some difficulty in getting insurance reimbursement for these lumbar total disc replacements, which has stalled an otherwise potentially powerful tool.

The only implant currently approved in the United States is the SB-Charité disc prosthesis. Others currently in trials are the ProDisc-L (Depuy-Synthes), XL TDR (Nuvasive, Inc.), Maverick (Medtronic), and FlexiCore (Stryker Spine). The SB-Charité prosthesis consists of cast cobalt-chromium-molybdenum (Co-Cr-Mo) alloy end plates that engage the bone with small spikes and an ultra-high-molecular-weight polyethylene insert with a less constrained, mobile-bearing design (Figure 16-20). Short-term follow-up of these implants has demonstrated a relatively high success rate and has shown results equivalent to or slightly better than those in the ALIF control group (stand-alone BAK cages with autograft).[56] The approach for implantation is similar to that for ALIF, a left anterior retroperitoneal exposure of the lower lumbar spine. The disc is excised, and the end plates are prepared. The prosthetic end plates are sized and implanted, followed by a polyethylene spacer of the appropriate height to restore lordotic alignment of the segment. Long-term survival data are limited, as are reports of successful methods for revision or salvage when implant failure occurs.

Rehabilitation Considerations

Spinal surgeons vary widely in the use of postoperative bracing and activity restrictions after surgery to the lumbar spine, partly because of a lack of evidence-based literature. In a series of 50 open discectomies, Carragee et al.[58] urged patients to return to full activities as soon as possible, with no restrictions at all. They reported that this resulted in a quicker return to work and no increase in complications. This study is helpful for patients undergoing simple discectomy, but it should not be extrapolated to those undergoing fusion procedures. Patients who undergo arthroplasty do not require any postoperative orthosis. The authors' suggested guidelines for rehabilitation can be found in Table 16-3.

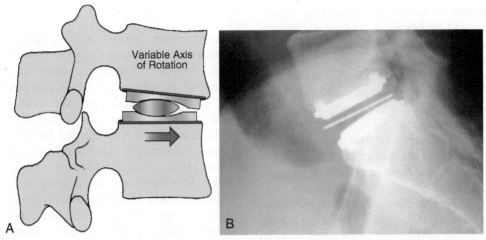

Figure 16-20 A, Schematic of SB-Charité artificial disc prosthesis. The mobile-bearing design of this device accommodates the dynamic changes in the spine's axis of rotation. **B,** Lateral x-ray film showing the SB-Charité device at the L5-S1 disc space of a 39-year-old woman. (From Benzel EC, editor: *Spine surgery: techniques, complication avoidance, and management,* ed 2, Philadelphia, 2005, Elsevier.)

TABLE **16-3**

Rehabilitation Considerations After Surgery on the Lumbar Spine

Expected Hospital Course	Outpatient Course	Red Flags
• Length of stay: 0-3 days for discectomy, laminectomy; 3-7 days for instrumented fusions • Nasogastric tube (for anterior approach) • Ambulation and upper extremity/lower extremity range of motion (ROM) • Bracing: may or may not be used (surgeon's preference, 2-12 weeks)	• Aerobic conditioning, upper extremity/lower extremity stretching/strengthening • Active spine ROM/strengthening • No passive ROM for 3 months (at affected levels) • May shower when wound is healed • Brace off for shower, activities of daily living • No heavy lifting/exercise for 3 months	• Change in neurological examination findings or symptoms • Worsening pain • Bowel/bladder changes • Erythema/fever/wound drainage

LUMBAR SPINAL STENOSIS AND SPONDYLOLISTHESIS

The term *lumbar spinal stenosis* describes a complex set of symptoms, physical findings, and radiographic abnormalities caused by narrowing of the spinal canal. The etiologies of spinal stenosis are degenerative, congenital, traumatic, and iatrogenic in nature, as well as a few others. The most common form of spinal stenosis is degenerative and usually occurs in the sixth and seventh decades.[59] The degenerative changes result in hypertrophy of the facet joints, capsule, and ligamentum flavum. In addition, disc degeneration leads to posterior bulging and loss of height, which add to both central and foraminal narrowing.

As would be expected in most degenerative disorders, the symptoms of lumbar stenosis can have an insidious onset. Initially they may include a low back ache that worsens with activity and is relieved by rest. As the stenosis progresses, symptoms of neurogenic claudication can begin to interfere with daily activities. These symptoms are classically described as vague cramping, aching, or burning pains in the back, buttocks, and legs that are exacerbated by standing or walking and relieved by sitting, squatting, or flexing the lumbar spine.[60] Spinal stenosis must be differentiated from vascular claudication, a somewhat similar but distinct symptom complex caused by peripheral vascular disease. With **vascular claudication**, symptoms generally cease when movement is halted, even while still standing. With **neurogenic claudication**, symptoms remain while still standing and generally improve with bending over and opening the neuroforamen. Lower extremity ultrasound can be used to rule out vascular claudication.

Lumbar spondylolisthesis can be classified into five groups according to the underlying abnormality[61]:

congenital (dysplastic), isthmic (spondylolytic), degenerative, traumatic, and pathological. The most common form is isthmic spondylolisthesis, which is associated with a defect in the pars interarticularis; this form can be found in 5% to 7% of adults in the United States.[62] Many of these individuals are asymptomatic. Back pain and hamstring tightness are the most common presenting complaints, and few progress to high-grade slips. The degenerative form, caused by intersegmental instability resulting from long-standing degenerative changes of the disc and facet joints (usually at L4-L5), can cause or contribute to spinal stenosis and symptoms of neurogenic claudication.

A commonly adopted method of grading spondylolisthesis is the Meyerding classification, based on the ratio of overhanging part of the superior vertebral body to anteroposterior length of the adjacent inferior vertebral body (Table 16-4).

Conservative management is the mainstay of treatment for most patients with spinal stenosis or degenerative spondylolisthesis. Pharmacological treatment (NSAIDs, antidepressants, pain relievers, and muscle relaxants), injections, manipulation, bracing, exercise, traction, and physical therapy all have been reported to be helpful. Because the natural history of this disorder suggests that few patients will have short-term deterioration, a thorough trial of these nonoperative measures is suggested before surgery is considered.[63] Patients with moderate symptoms may be treated conservatively for 2 to 3 years. Surgery is considered when the slippage is rapid or neurological signs start to become evident (Figure 16-21).

Surgical Procedures for Lumbar Spinal Stenosis and Spondylolisthesis

- Laminectomy
- Posterolateral fusion (no instrumentation)
- Posterior lumbar interbody fusion (PLIF)
- Transforaminal lumbar interbody fusion (TLIF)
- Lateral lumbar interbody fusion (LLIF)

TABLE **16-4**

Meyerding Classification for Spondylolisthesis

Grade	% Overhang/Slip
I	0%-25%
II	26%-50%
III	51%-75%
IV	76%-100%
V (spondyloptosis)	>100%

Lumbar Laminectomy

Decompressive laminectomy for spinal stenosis of the lumbar spine is indicated in patients with intractable pain recalcitrant to nonoperative treatment and those with neurological deficits that significantly impair their lifestyle and ability to function. Because of the potential destabilizing effects of lumbar decompression, laminectomy without stabilization is reserved for patients with no significant deformity or instability. Laminectomy is a safe, effective procedure; it may have a success rate in the range of 85% to 90% for eliminating neurogenic claudication.[64,65]

Laminectomy is performed with the patient positioned prone on a spine frame or in the kneeling position with the abdomen hanging free. A midline incision is made over the lumbar spine, and dissection proceeds down to expose the spinous processes and laminae bilaterally. The proper level or levels are identified radiographically, and the spinous processes are removed. The decompression is divided into three stages. In the first stage, the central canal is decompressed by means of removal of the laminae and ligamentum flavum (Figure 16-22). A number of methods can be used for this, including use of a high-speed burr, Kerrison rongeurs, or osteotomes, depending on the surgeon's familiarity and experience. In the second stage, hypertrophied tissue is removed from the lateral recesses. A Kerrison rongeur is used to excise the medial aspect of the inferior and superior facets, along with excess ligamentum flavum, out to the level of the pedicle. In the third stage, each individual neuroforamen is decompressed. The nerve roots are identified, and a blunt probe is used to palpate the foramen. The bone spurs and soft tissue are removed until the probe can be passed freely into the foramen. Care must be taken to preserve the integrity of the pars interarticularis as well as that of the facets. The wound is closed in layers, and a suction drain is commonly used.

Minimally invasive and microsurgical techniques have also been developed for lumbar decompression. Little difference is apparent in the long-term outcomes of these procedures compared with those achieved with the standard approach.[66,67] These techniques use the advantages of coaxial light and stereopsis, which the operating microscope provides, to perform the decompression through smaller incisions and with less morbid dissections. This may lead to less pain, shorter hospital stays, and quicker rehabilitation.[39] Preservation of the spinous processes, along with the interspinous and supraspinous ligaments, may also minimize the risk of iatrogenic instability and can be more easily performed with the advent of newer retraction systems.

Posterolateral Fusion

Dorsolateral arthrodesis of the lumbar spine may be used to treat many disorders that result in deformity

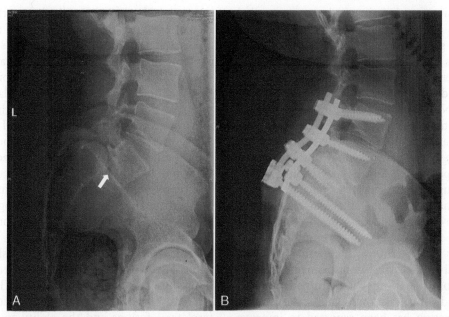

Figure 16-21 Lateral preoperative (**A**) and postoperative (**B**) radiographs of high-grade spondylolisthesis *(arrow)* demonstrating significant reduction after spinal instrumentation and fusion.

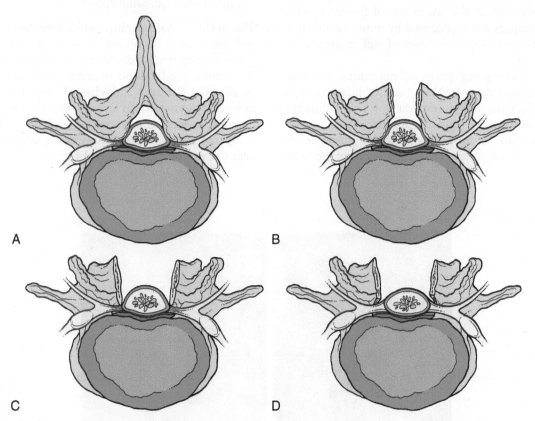

Figure 16-22 Lumbar laminectomy technique. **A,** Depiction of an axial view of the lumbar spine with typical hypertrophic degenerative changes. **B,** First stage: The spinous processes, midline laminae, and ligamentum flavum are removed to expose the dura. **C,** Second stage: Decompression of the lateral gutters is performed, with removal of the remaining laminae and the medial aspect of the superior facets. **D,** Third stage: Decompression of the neuroforamina is performed. (From Herkowitz HN, Garfin SR, Balderson RA et al, editors: *Rothman-Simeone: The spine,* ed 4, Philadelphia, 1999, Saunders.)

and instability. This procedure is widely recommended for many patients in whom trauma, tumor, or infection have rendered the spine unable to support physiological loading.[68] It also is indicated for instability secondary to previous surgery or isthmic spondylolisthesis. Its use in degenerative disorders, however, is the subject of considerable debate. No benefit has been shown to adding arthrodesis to routine discectomy or after laminectomy in the stable lumbar spine.[69] Controversy exists over the need for fusion in degenerative spondylolisthesis when decompression is performed for associated spinal stenosis. Recent data suggest that, when degenerative instability is present, more successful outcomes result when posterolateral arthrodesis is added to the decompressive operation.[70,71]

Indications for the addition of internal fixation, namely, segmental pedicle screw instrumentation, to posterolateral fusions are also debated. In patients with degenerative spondylolisthesis and spinal stenosis, segmental internal fixation has been reported to improve fusion rates, but this did not lead to improved clinical outcomes.[72] Instrumentation may help correct deformity, stabilize the spine, enhance arthrodesis rates, minimize the number of segments that need to be fused, and reduce rehabilitation time and brace wear. Instrumentation often is indicated in the treatment of fractures, when structural support is compromised by tumor or infection, for failed in situ fusion, or in cases of high-grade translational motion.

Patients undergoing posterolateral fusion are positioned kneeling on an Andrews table or prone on a radiolucent Jackson frame (especially for instrumented cases). Most often, a midline approach and subperiosteal dissection are done to expose the posterior elements. Exposure is continued out to the tips of the lateral processes. Decompression is then performed as needed. Decortication of the dorsal aspect of the transverse processes and the lateral aspect of the superior facets and pars interarticularis, as well as removal of the facet joint capsule and cartilage, prepares the spine bed for fusion. Instrumentation (if used) is then implanted, using screws that pass through the pedicles into the vertebral bodies interconnected with rods (Figures 16-23 and 16-24). The gutters overlying the lateral process are filled with bone graft, and the wound is closed in layers over a suction drain.

Complications of posterolateral fusion may include hemorrhage, infection, and neurological injury in the perioperative period. Later, pseudarthrosis, hardware failure, or recurrent symptoms may lead to failures of treatment. In cases of instability or risk of progression of deformity or spondylolisthesis, instrumented posterior spinal fusion is indicated (TLIF/PLIF) with or without interbody work. With improved fusion rates over posterolateral fusions and the ability to correct deformity, instrumented fusions are the treatment of choice when spinal fusion is required in patients with spinal stenosis or spondylolisthesis.

Rehabilitation Considerations

The authors' postoperative guidelines for laminectomy and dorsolateral fusion are the same as those for procedures treating lumbar disc disease (see Table 16-3). When the wound produces no drainage, early showering may be allowed. Carragee and Vittum[73] reported no increase in wound complications after posterior surgery when patients were allowed to shower 2 to 5 days after surgery, compared with a historic cohort by the same surgeon who kept the wound dry for 10 to 14 days.

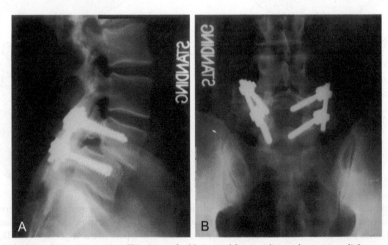

Figure 16-23 Postoperative lateral (**A**) and anteroposterior (**B**) views of a 31-year-old man who underwent pedicle screw instrumentation and posterolateral fusion for a grade II spondylolisthesis at L4-L5. (From Benzel EC, editor: *Spine surgery: techniques, complication avoidance, and management,* ed 2, Philadelphia, 2005, Elsevier.)

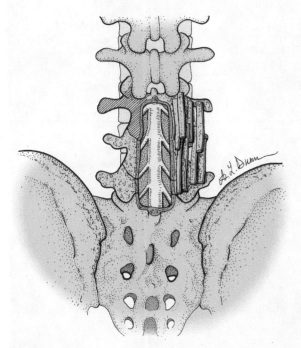

Figure 16-24 Diagram of a posterolateral fusion after lumbar laminectomy. Bone graft is shown in the lateral gutters; the fusion bed includes the transverse processes, the facet joints, and the pars interarticularis. (From Benzel EC, editor: *Spine surgery: techniques, complication avoidance, and management,* ed 2, Philadelphia, 2005, Elsevier.)

SPINAL DEFORMITIES

Spinal deformity generally is categorized as frontal plane deformity (scoliosis) or sagittal plane deformity (kyphosis). However, scoliosis most often includes a rotational or torsional malalignment and sagittal plane disturbance (Figure 16-25). In children and adolescents, scoliosis is broadly classified as idiopathic, congenital, neuromuscular, or syndrome related. Most cases of pediatric scoliosis are idiopathic (Figure 16-26). Kyphosis may be related to congenital abnormalities, neuromuscular disorders, trauma, infectious or neoplastic processes, or metabolic disorders, but Scheuermann's disease is the diagnosis in most cases. The magnitude and progression (or risk for progression) of the curve are the major indications for surgical treatment of scoliosis.

In adolescent idiopathic scoliosis (AIS), the risk for curve progression is largely a factor of growth remaining and the magnitude of the present curve. In a growing child, bracing usually is indicated when the curve reaches 25° to 30°, with an upper limit of approximately 45°, beyond which curves are less amenable to bracing. Most data have shown that bracing halts curve progression, but correction cannot be anticipated. Weinstein et al.[74] concluded that bracing significantly decreased the progression of high-risk curves to the threshold for surgery in patients with AIS. Longer hours of brace wear were associated with greater benefit. The indications for surgical correction in AIS are a growing child who presents with a curve of 40° to 45°, progression of a curve to 40° in

a child undergoing nonoperative treatment, and a curve greater than 50° to 60° in a skeletally mature adolescent.[75]

Scoliosis Treatment

- Bracing: Curve 25° to 45°
- Surgery: 1. Growing child with a curve of 40° to 45°
    2. Curve that progresses to 40° in a child undergoing bracing
    3. Curve greater than 50° to 60° in a skeletally mature adolescent

---

The normal range for thoracic kyphosis in the adolescent is generally considered to be 20° to 40°. Patients with Scheuermann's disease often have kyphosis greater than 45°, with associated end plate irregularities, Schmorl's nodes, and vertebral wedging on x-ray films. Deformity is the most common presenting complaint, and pain is another common symptom. Bracing for Scheuermann's disease has led to improvement in vertebral wedging and kyphotic angle but was less effective in patients with greater than 75° of initial kyphosis.[76] Surgical intervention may be indicated for rigid kyphosis greater than 75° and for those who have unrelenting pain despite conservative treatment.[77]

Deformity in adults presents a diagnostic as well as a therapeutic challenge for the clinician. Adult deformity most often can be divided into cases in which a curve was present before maturity, cases in which the curve developed de novo as a result of metabolic bone disease or degeneration, and cases in which degenerative changes are superimposed on pre-existing scoliosis. Nonoperative management is directed at treatment of symptoms, usually pain. Operative intervention is indicated to treat persistent, disabling pain that is refractory to conservative treatment; to correct and stabilize progressive deformity; to restore coronal and sagittal balance; and to decompress neural elements associated with spinal stenosis.[78]

Surgical Procedures for Spinal Deformities

- Posterior arthrodesis
- Anterior arthrodesis

Posterior Arthrodesis

Preoperative planning for surgical correction of thoracic and lumbar deformities is important. Standing posteroanterior (PA) and lateral x-ray films of the entire spine are used to gauge the magnitude of the deformity and spinal balance. Bending films are also commonly used to assess the flexibility of the curve. This information is used to determine which levels to include in the fusion and how much correction of deformity can be expected.

Posterior reconstructive surgery is performed with the patient prone on a radiolucent spine frame. A long midline incision is made, and subperiosteal dissection is carried deep to expose the spinous processes, laminae, and

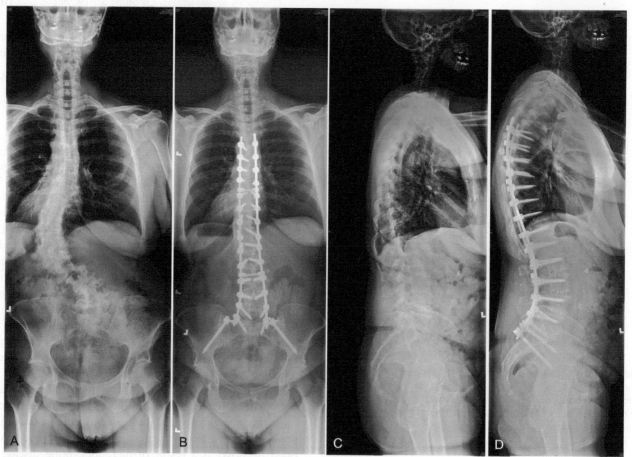

Figure 16-25 Preoperative (**A**) and postoperative (**B**) posteroanterior and preoperative (**C**) and postoperative (**D**) lateral radiographs of adult idiopathic scoliosis demonstrating significant correction of spinal deformity after spinal instrumentation and fusion.

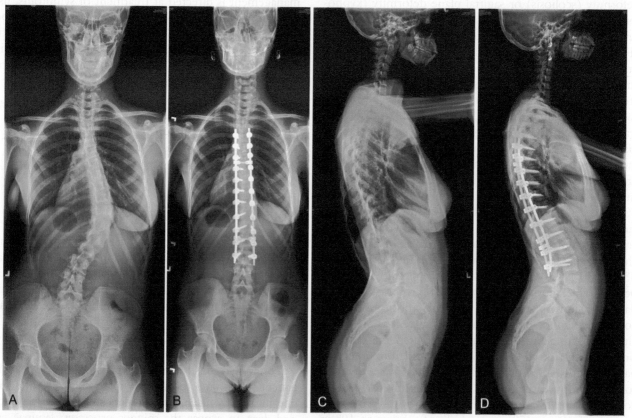

Figure 16-26 Preoperative (**A**) and postoperative (**B**) posteroanterior and preoperative (**C**) and postoperative (**D**) lateral radiographs of adolescent idiopathic scoliosis demonstrating significant correction of spinal deformity after spinal instrumentation and fusion.

lateral processes of the levels to be included in the fusion. Intraoperative x-ray film or fluoroscopy is used to positively identify the correct levels. The spinous processes generally are removed, the facet joint cartilage and capsule are excised, and decortication of the lateral processes and facet joints is performed to prepare the bed for later bone grafting.

Modern segmental instrumentation systems allow for multiple points of fixation along the spine. This enhances the procedure by adding stability to the construct, allow-ing for correction of deformity, improving fusion rates, and preserving normal sagittal plane alignment. Flat-back syndrome was common after nonsegmental Harrington rod fixation. Segmental fixation can be achieved using a number of techniques or combinations of techniques, including sublaminar wires or cables, hooks, and pedicle screws (Figures 16-27 to 16-29). These are affixed to rods, which are bent to accommodate the normal anat-omy while providing correction of the existing deformity.

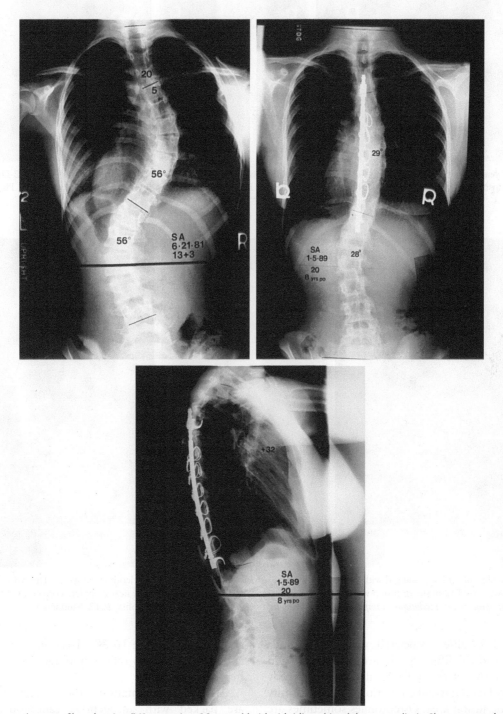

Figure 16-27 Preoperative x-ray films showing 56° curves in a 13-year-old girl with idiopathic adolescent scoliosis. She was treated with posterior fu-sion using the Harri-Luque technique (i.e., segmental fixation was obtained with sublaminar wires). The curves were corrected to 29° and 28°. (From Herkowitz HN, Garfin SR, Balderson RA et al, editors: *Rothman-Simeone: The spine*, ed 4, Philadelphia, 1999, WB Saunders, p 361.)

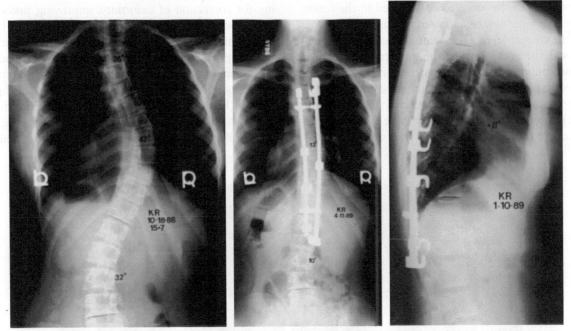

Figure 16-28 A 14-year-old with a 47° right thoracic curve. The condition was treated with posterior fusion from T4 to L1 using C-D instrumentation (hooks and rod construct). (From Herkowitz HN, Garfin SR, Balderson RA et al, editors: *Rothman-Simeone: The spine,* ed 4, Philadelphia, 1999, Saunders.)

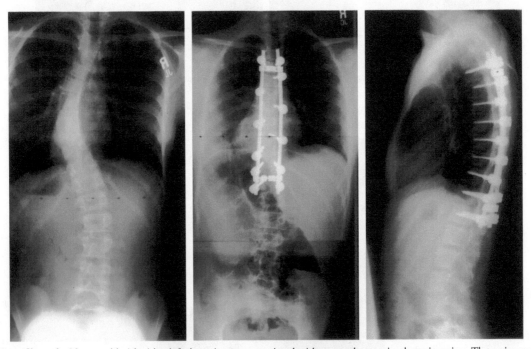

Figure 16-29 X-ray films of a 12-year-old girl with a left thoracic curve associated with a complex cervicothoracic syrinx. The syrinx was treated, and the patient underwent T4-T12 posterior fusion with pedicle screw fixation. Postoperative x-rays show near-complete correction of the curve. (From Benzel EC, editor: *Spine surgery: techniques, complication avoidance, and management,* ed 3, Philadelphia, 2012, Saunders.)

In adults, deformities associated with degenerative changes present added difficulty. These curves are stiff and cannot be passively corrected. Circumferential interbody techniques may be used to aid correction of the deformity and increase the fusion area. Osteotomies sometimes are needed in more severe cases to restore spinal alignment and balance (Figure 16-30). Decompressive surgery also is often required to relieve impingement of the cord or nerve roots.

After instrumentation, the posterolateral gutters are packed with autogenous cancellous bone graft. The wound is closed in layers. The rigidity of modern

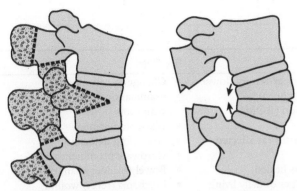

Figure 16-30 Schematic showing operative technique of lumbar pedicle subtraction osteotomy in the correction of lumbar kyphosis and sagittal imbalance (*stippled area removed*). (Modified from Benzel EC: *Spine surgery: techniques, complication avoidance and management*, ed 3, Philadelphia, 2012, Saunders.)

instrumentation reduces the need for postoperative bracing or casting. Patients may be mobilized early, and light activity advanced as pain permits.

Anterior Arthrodesis

For some thoracic and thoracolumbar curves, anterior instrumentation and fusion are preferred. The anterior approach has several potential advantages.[79] The crankshaft phenomenon, which may occur with continued growth after posterior arthrodesis, is essentially eliminated by anterior fusion. The hardware is anterior to the axis of rotation, making anterior fusion kyphogenic; this is helpful in AIS when hypokyphosis of the thoracic spine is present (although this can be a problem in the lumbar and thoracolumbar regions, where kyphosis is detrimental, or in the treatment of kyphotic deformities). In addition, anterior instrumentation in thoracolumbar curves allows correction while preserving additional lumbar motion segments.

The patient is placed in the lateral decubitus position, and the spine is approached from the side of the curve's convexity. Depending on the levels to be included, a thoracotomy, retroperitoneal approach, or combination of the two with detachment of the diaphragm is needed for adequate exposure. Thorascopic techniques have also been described, which have the potential to reduce the morbidity of the open exposures. The segmental vessels are ligated, and the psoas muscle is mobilized. The discs are excised, and the end plates are removed to expose bleeding surfaces for fusion. Screws are placed in the lateral aspect of the vertebral body and are measured to achieve bicortical fixation. A rod is placed into the screw heads, and correction is performed, converting scoliosis to lordosis (Figure 16-31). The disc spaces are packed with cancellous bone graft (usually from the rib, harvested during the exposure); vertebral compression and tightening of the screws follow, and the wound is closed. A chest tube and nasogastric tube are used postoperatively.

With adult deformity, an anterior approach often is combined with a posterior approach (described in the section on ALIF). This allows more complete excision of the disc, which improves the fusion area and allows oversized grafts to be placed to correct lumbar kyphosis.

Rehabilitation Considerations

Surgery to correct a spinal deformity often requires extensive exposures and operative times, with correspondingly longer periods of rehabilitation. It is important to begin

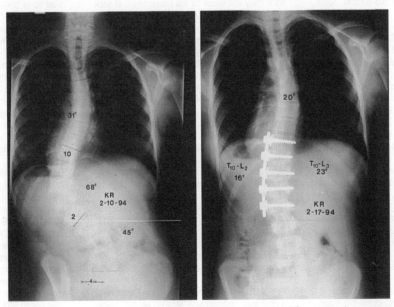

Figure 16-31 Adolescent girl with a progressive, 68° thoracolumbar curve that was treated with anterior instrumentation and fusion from T10 to L2. A standing postoperative x-ray film shows correction of the primary curve to 23°, with preservation of most of the lumbar segments. (From Herkowitz HN, Garfin SR, Balderson RA et al, editors: *Rothman-Simeone: The spine*, ed 4, Philadelphia, 1999, Saunders.)

TABLE **16-5**

Rehabilitation Considerations After Surgery for Spinal Deformity

Expected Hospital Course	Outpatient Course	Red Flags
• Length of stay: 4-7 days • Nasogastric tube (for anterior approach) • Ambulation when able to be out of bed • Bracing: may or may not be used after chest tube is removed (surgeon's preference, 2-12 weeks)	• Aerobic conditioning, upper extremity/lower extremity stretching/strengthening • Active spinal range of motion (ROM)/strengthening • No passive ROM for 3 months (at affected levels) • May shower when wound is healed • Brace off for shower, activities of daily living • No heavy lifting/exercise for 3 months	• Change in neurological examination findings or symptoms • Worsening pain • Worsening deformity • Hardware prominence • Bowel/bladder changes • Erythema/fever/wound drainage

ambulation as soon as it is medically tolerated to minimize deconditioning and complications from prolonged bed rest. Chest tubes, nasogastric tubes, Foley catheters, and central lines are removed as early as possible to facilitate this. Table 16-5 outlines the expected postoperative course, as well as red flags that may signal the development of complications.

SUMMARY

Spinal disorders result from a wide array of pathological processes, but symptoms and disability generally are consequences of impingement of the neural elements and/or instability of spinal segments. The primary goals of surgery are to decompress the neural elements and stabilize unstable segments. Debate remains in many cases with regard to the approach used, the use of autograft versus allograft, and the need for and type of hardware used. New techniques, including artificial disc replacement, focus on restoring functional motion and avoiding fusion, with hopes of preserving adjacent segments. Bone graft substitutes and osteoinductive agents may also improve fusion rates and limit morbidity. Current and future studies will help guide the use of these new technologies and improve the operative care of spinal disorders.

REFERENCES

1. Gore DR, Sepic SB, Gardner GM, Murray MP: Neck pain: a long-term follow-up of 205 patients, *Spine* 12:1–5, 1987.
2. Lees F, Turner JW: Natural history and prognosis of cervical spondylosis, *Br Med J* 5373:1607–1610, 1963.
3. Clarke E, Robinson PK: Cervical myelopathy: a complication of cervical spondylosis, *Brain* 79:483–510, 1956.
4. Nurick S: The natural history and the results of surgical treatment of the spinal cord disorder associated with cervical spondylosis, *Brain* 95:101–108, 1972.
5. Sumi M, Miyamoto H, Suzuki T, et al: Prospective cohort study of mild cervical spondylotic myelopathy without surgical treatment, *J Neurosurg Spine* 16:8–14, 2012.
6. Williams JL, Allen MB Jr, Harkess JW: Late results of cervical discectomy and interbody fusion: some factors influencing the results, *J Bone Joint Surg Am* 50:277–286, 1968.
7. White AA, Southwick WO, Deponte RJ, et al: Relief of pain by anterior cervical spine fusion for spondylosis: a report of sixty-five patients, *J Bone Joint Surg Am* 55:525–534, 1973.
8. Dohn DF: Anterior interbody fusion for treatment of cervical disk conditions, *JAMA* 197:897–900, 1966.
9. Garvey TA, Transfeldt EE, Malcolm JR, Kos P: Outcome of anterior cervical discectomy and fusion as perceived by patients treated for dominant axial-mechanical cervical spine pain, *Spine* 27:1887–1895, 2002, discussion, 1895.
10. Palit M, Schofferman J, Goldthwaite N, et al: Anterior discectomy and fusion for the management of neck pain, *Spine* 24:2224–2228, 1999.
11. Scheer JK, Tang JA, JS Smith, et al and the International Spine Study Group: Cervical spine alignment, sagittal deformity, and clinical implications, *J Neurosurg Spine* 19:141–159, 2013.
12. Robinson R, Smith G: Anterolateral cervical disc removal and interbody fusion for cervical disc syndrome, *Bull Johns Hopkins Hosp* 96:223–224, 1955.
13. Sidhu K, Herkowitz H: Surgical management of cervical disc disease. In Herkowitz H, Garfin S, Balderston R, et al, editors: *The spine, ed 4, vol I*, Philadelphia, 1999, WB Saunders.
14. Bailey RW, Badgley CE: Stabilization of the cervical spine by anterior fusion, *J Bone Joint Surg Am* 42:565–594, 1960.
15. Cloward RB: The anterior approach for removal of ruptured cervical disks, *J Neurosurg* 15:602–617, 1958.
16. Simmons EH, Bhalla SK: Anterior cervical discectomy and fusion: a clinical and biomechanical study with eight-year follow-up, *J Bone Joint Surg Br* 51:225–237, 1969.
17. Frenkel MB, Cahill KS, Javahary RJ, et al: Fusion rates in multilevel, instrumented anterior cervical fusion for degenerative disease with and without the use of bone morphogenetic protein, *J Neurosurg Spine* 18:269–273, 2013.
18. Herkowitz H: Internal fixation for degenerative cervical spine disorders. In Weisel S, editor: *Seminars in spine surgery: cervical disc disease*, Philadelphia, 1995, WB Saunders.
19. Upadhyaya CD, Wu J-C, Trost G, et al: Analysis of the three United States Food and Drug Administration investigational device exemption cervical arthroplasty trials, *J Neurosurg Spine* 16:216–228, 2012.
20. Zdeblick TA, Zou D, Warden KE, et al: Cervical stability after foraminotomy: a biomechanical in vitro analysis, *J Bone Joint Surg Am* 74:22–27, 1992.
21. Rao R: Neck pain, cervical radiculopathy, and cervical myelopathy: pathophysiology, natural history, and clinical evaluation, *Instr Course Lect* 52:479–488, 2003.
22. Emery SE, Bohlman HH, Bolesta MJ, Jones PK: Anterior cervical decompression and arthrodesis for the treatment of cervical spondylotic myelopathy: two to seventeen-year follow-up, *J Bone Joint Surg Am* 80:941–951, 1998.
23. Burkett CJ, Baaj AA, Dakwar E, Uribe JS: Use of titanium expandable vertebral cages in cervical corpectomy, *J Clin Neurosci* 19(3):402–405, 2012.
24. Kaptain GJ, Simmons NE, Replogle RE, Pobereskin L: Incidence and outcome of kyphotic deformity following laminectomy for cervical spondylotic myelopathy, *J Neurosurg* 93(2 Suppl):199–204, 2000.
25. Hirabayashi K, Satomi K: Operative procedure and results of expansive open door laminoplasty, *Spine* 13:870–876, 1988.

26. Tomita K, Nomura S, Umeda S, Baba H: Cervical laminoplasty to enlarge the spinal canal in multilevel ossification of the posterior longitudinal ligament with myelopathy, *Arch Orthop Trauma Surg* 107:148–153, 1988.

27. Arce CA, Dohrmann GJ: Herniated thoracic disks, *Neurol Clin* 3:383–392, 1985.

28. Bohlman HH, Zdeblick TA: Anterior excision of herniated thoracic disc, *J Bone Joint Surg Am* 70:1038–1047, 1988.

29. Otani K, Nakai S, Fujimura Y, et al: Surgical treatment of thoracic disc herniation using the anterior approach, *J Bone Joint Surg Br* 64:340–343, 1982.

30. Benjamin V: Diagnosis and management of thoracic disc disease, *Clin Neurosurg* 30:577–605, 1983.

31. Uribe JS, Smith WD, Pimenta L, et al: Minimally invasive lateral approach for symptomatic thoracic disc herniation: initial multicenter clinical experience, *J Neurosurg Spine* 16:264–279, 2012.

32. Anand N, Regan JJ: Video-assisted thoracoscopic surgery for thoracic disc disease: classification and outcome study of 100 consecutive cases with a 2-year minimum follow-up period, *Spine* 27:871–879, 2002.

33. Uribe JS, Dakwar E, Cardona RF, Vale FL: Minimally invasive lateral retropleural thoracolumbar approach: cadaveric feasibility study and report of 4 clinical cases, *Neurosurgery* 68(1 Suppl):32–39, 2011, discussion 9.

34. Quebec Task Force on Spinal Disorders: Scientific approach to the assessment and management of activity-related spinal disorders" a monograph for clinicians, *Spine* 12(7 Suppl):S1–S59, 1987.

35. Deyo RA, Loeser JD, Bigos SJ: Herniated lumbar intervertebral disk, *Ann Intern Med* 112:598–603, 1990.

36. Torgerson WR, Dotter WE: Comparative roentgenographic study of the asymptomatic and symptomatic lumbar spine, *J Bone Joint Surg Am* 58:850–853, 1976.

37. Errico TJ, Fardon DF, Lowell TD: Open discectomy as treatment for herniated nucleus pulposus of the lumbar spine, *Spine* 20:1829–1833, 1995.

38. Eysel P, Rompe JD, Hopf C: Prognostic criteria of discogenic paresis, *Eur Spine J* 3:214–218, 1994.

39. Bookwalter JW, Busch MD, Nicely D: Ambulatory surgery is safe and effective in radicular disc disease, *Spine* 19:526–530, 1994.

40. Daneyemez M, Sali A, Kahraman S, et al: Outcome analyses in 1072 surgically treated lumbar disc herniations, *Minim Invasive Neurosurg* 42:63–68, 1999.

41. Gibson JN, Grant IC, Waddell G: The Cochrane review of surgery for lumbar disc prolapse and degenerative lumbar spondylosis, *Spine* 24:1820–1832, 1999.

42. Kambin P: Arthroscopic microdiscectomy, *Arthroscopy* 8:287–295, 1992.

43. Hermantin FU, Peters T, Quartararo L, Kambin P: A prospective, randomized study comparing the results of open discectomy with those of video-assisted arthroscopic microdiscectomy, *J Bone Joint Surg Am* 81:958–965, 1999.

44. Schaffer JL, Kambin P: Percutaneous posterolateral lumbar discectomy and decompression with a 6.9-millimeter cannula: analysis of operative failures and complications, *J Bone Joint Surg Am* 73:822–831, 1991.

45. Schechter NA, France MP, Lee CK: Painful internal disc derangements of the lumbosacral spine: discographic diagnosis and treatment by posterior lumbar interbody fusion, *Orthopedics* 14:447–451, 1991.

46. Mummaneni PV, Rodts Jr. GE: The mini-open transforaminal lumbar interbody fusion, *Neurosurgery* 57(4 Suppl):256–261, 2005.

47. Cloward RB: Posterior lumbar interbody fusion updated, *Clin Orthop Relat Res* 193:16–19, 1985.

48. Gill K, Blumenthal SL: Posterior lumbar interbody fusion: a 2-year follow-up of 238 patients, *Acta Orthop Scand Suppl* 251:108–110, 1993.

49. Suk SI, Lee CK, Kim WJ, et al: Adding posterior lumbar interbody fusion to pedicle screw fixation and posterolateral fusion after decompression in spondylolytic spondylolisthesis, *Spine* 22:210–219, 1997, discussion, 219–220.

50. Castellvi AE, Nienke TW, Marulanda GA, et al: Indirect decompression of lumbar stenosis with transpsoas interbody cages and percutaneous posterior instrumentation, *Clin Orthop Relat Res* 472:1784–1791, 2014.

51. Spoor AB, Oner FC: Minimally invasive spine surgery in chronic low back pain patients, *J Neurosurg Sci* 57:203–218, 2013.

52. Ozgur BM, Aryan HE, Pimenta L, Taylor WR: Extreme Lateral Interbody Fusion (XLIF): a novel surgical technique for anterior lumbar interbody fusion, *Spine J* 6(4):435–443, 2006.

53. Smith WD, Youssef JA, Christian G, et al: Lumbarized sacrum as a relative contraindication for lateral transpsoas interbody fusion at L5-6, *J Spinal Disord Tech* 25:285–291, 2012.

54. McAfee PC, Phillips FM, Andersson G, et al: Minimally invasive spine surgery, *Spine* 35:S271–S273, 2010.

55. Huang RC, Lim MR, Girardi FP, Cammisa FP: The prevalence of contraindications to total disc replacement in a cohort of lumbar surgical patients, *Spine* 29:2538–2541, 2004.

56. German JW, Foley KT: Disc arthroplasty in the management of the painful lumbar motion segment, *Spine* 30(16 Suppl):S60–S67, 2005.

57. Zeegers WS, Bohnen LM, Laaper M, Verhaegen MJ: Artificial disc replacement with the modular type SB Charite III: 2-year results in 50 prospectively studied patients, *Eur Spine J* 8:210–217, 1999.

58. Carragee EJ, Helms E, O'Sullivan GS: Are postoperative activity restrictions necessary after posterior lumbar discectomy?: a prospective study of outcomes in 50 consecutive cases, *Spine* 21:1893–1897, 1996.

59. Johnsson KE, Rosen I, Uden A: The natural course of lumbar spinal stenosis, *Clin Orthop Relat Res* 279:82–86, 1992.

60. Hawkes CH, Roberts GM: Neurogenic and vascular claudication, *J Neurol Sci* 38:337–345, 1978.

61. Wiltse LL, Newman PH, Macnab I: Classification of spondylolysis and spondylolisthesis, *Clin Orthop Relat Res* 117:23–29, 1976.

62. Fredrickson BE, Baker D, McHolick WJ, et al: The natural history of spondylolysis and spondylolisthesis, *J Bone Joint Surg Am* 66:699–707, 1984.

63. Johnsson KE, Uden A, Rosen I: The effect of decompression on the natural course of spinal stenosis: a comparison of surgically treated and untreated patients, *Spine* 16:615–619, 1991.

64. Tile M, McNeil SR, Zarins RK, et al: Spinal stenosis: results of treatment, *Clin Orthop Relat Res* 115:104–108, 1976.

65. Yukawa Y, Lenke LG, Tenhula J, et al: A comprehensive study of patients with surgically treated lumbar spinal stenosis with neurogenic claudication, *J Bone Joint Surg Am* 84:1954–1959, 2002.

66. Postacchini F, Cinotti G, Perugia D, Gumina S: The surgical treatment of central lumbar stenosis: multiple laminotomy compared with total laminectomy, *J Bone Joint Surg Br* 75:386–392, 1993.

67. Weiner BK, Walker M, Brower RS, McCulloch JA: Microdecompression for lumbar spinal canal stenosis, *Spine* 24:2268–2272, 1999.

68. Zdeblick TA, Hanley EN, Sonntag VK, et al: Indications for lumbar spinal fusion. Introduction; 1995 Focus Issue Meeting on Fusion, *Spine* 20(24 Suppl):124S–125S, 1995.

69. Sonntag VK, Marciano FF: Is fusion indicated for lumbar spinal disorders? *Spine* 20(24 Suppl):138S–142S, 1995.

70. Herkowitz HN, Kurz LT: Degenerative lumbar spondylolisthesis with spinal stenosis: a prospective study comparing decompression with decompression and intertransverse process arthrodesis, *J Bone Joint Surg Am* 73:802–808, 1991.

71. Postacchini F: Management of lumbar spinal stenosis, *J Bone Joint Surg Br* 78:154–164, 1996.

72. Fischgrund JS, Mackay M, Herkowitz HN, et al: 1997 Volvo Award winner in clinical studies: degenerative lumbar spondylolisthesis with spinal stenosis—a prospective, randomized study comparing decompressive laminectomy and arthrodesis with and without spinal instrumentation, *Spine* 22:2807–2812, 1997.

73. Carragee EJ, Vittum DW: Wound care after posterior spinal surgery: does early bathing affect the rate of wound complications? *Spine* 21:2160–2162, 1996.

74. Weinstein SL, Dolan LA, Wright JG, Dobbs MB: Effects of bracing in adolescents with idiopathic scoliosis, *N Engl J Med* 369(16):1512–1521, 2013.

75. Winter RB, Lonstein JE: Juvenile and adolescent scoliosis. In Herkowitz HN, Garside SH, Balderston RA, et al, editors: *The spine*, ed 4, vol I, Philadelphia, 1999, WB Saunders.

76. Bradford DS, Moe JH, Montalvo FJ, Winter RB: Scheuermann's kyphosis and roundback deformity: results of Milwaukee brace treatment, *J Bone Joint Surg Am* 56:740–758, 1974.

77. An HS, Humphreys SC, Balderston RA: Juvenile kyphosis. In Herkowitz HN, Garfin SR, Balderston RA, et al, editors: *The spine*, ed 4, vol I, Philadelphia, 1999, WB Saunders.

78. Boachie-Adjei O, Gupta MC: Adult scoliosis and deformity. In Fardon DF, Garfin SR, editors: *Orthopaedic knowledge update: spine 2*, vol I, Rosemont, 2002, American Academy of Orthopedic Surgeons.

79. Lenke LG, Dobbs MB: Idiopathic scoliosis. In Frymoyer JW, Wiesel SW, editors: *The adult and pediatric spine*, ed 3, vol I, Philadelphia, 2004, Lippincott Williams & Wilkins.

CHAPTER 17

Highlights from an Integrated Approach to the Treatment of Pelvic Pain and Dysfunction

DIANE LEE*

INTRODUCTION

Optimal function of the pelvis is critical for the health of the musculoskeletal, urological, colorectal, sexual, and reproductive systems. Impaired pelvic function has been implicated in multiple conditions, including low back and pelvic pain, urinary impairments (retention, urgency incontinence), pelvic organ prolapse, constipation, fecal incontinence, and dyspareunia. Understanding the relationships between these systems and the consequences of impaired function of one on another is complex. Multiple health practitioners specialize in varying aspects of pelvic health, and treatment is often based on the practitioner's training and experience (e.g., manual therapy, core stability exercises, pelvic floor release and training, surgery, pessaries, injections, and/or medication). The best evidence-based treatment would consider all knowledge pertaining to pelvic health and thus require collaboration of multiple disciplines, a difficult task given the physical logistics of clinical practice. The organizers of the World Congress on Low Back and Pelvic Pain and the International Pelvic Pain Society have recognized the necessity of collaboration; both groups facilitate the exchange of knowledge between the multiple health disciplines involved in restoring pelvic health. To be fully evidence-based and informed practitioners, physical therapists can no longer work in isolation when treating patients with pelvic pain, incontinence, pelvic organ prolapse, and/or sexual dysfunction. In addition, conditions of the musculoskeletal pelvis (i.e., loss of mobility and/or control during functional tasks) should no longer be considered independent from those of the urological, reproductive, colorectal, and/or sexual systems. The

evidence, particularly from studies of women and their experiences with pregnancy, suggests these conditions coexist. The body of knowledge pertaining to pelvic health is extensive and cannot be contained in one chapter. The intent of this chapter is to present an overview of specific pathologies pertaining to the various systems of the pelvis and highlight how *"The Integrated Systems Model for Disability and Pain"* (ISM) can help clinicians organize their knowledge on these topics and facilitate evidence-based (or informed) management of the often complex patient with pelvic pain and dysfunction.

PREVALENCE AND POSSIBLE CAUSES OF PELVIC PAIN AND DYSFUNCTION

Pelvic pain and dysfunction are common, particularly for parous women. Twenty percent of women experience pelvic girdle pain (PGP) during or after their pregnancy,[1-3] and 8% of these go on to have severe disability.[4-6] Forty-eight percent of primiparous women experience urinary incontinence in the last trimester of their pregnancy, and this number increases to 85% with subsequent pregnancies.[7] Five to seven years after delivery, 44.6% of women continue to have some degree of incontinence,[8] and this number increases with age, with 55% of women over the age of 65 experiencing some form of urinary incontinence. Incontinence is the second most common reason for admission into assisted living.[9] Fifty percent of parous women have some degree of symptomatic or asymptomatic loss of pelvic organ support.[10] Fifty-two percent of women surveyed for low back pain or PGP also reported some form of pelvic floor dysfunction (e.g., incontinence, sexual dysfunction, and or constipation).[11] Sixty-six percent of women with a diastasis rectus abdominis (DRA)

*The author, editors, and publisher wish to acknowledge Linda-Joy Lee for her contributions on this topic in the previous edition.

have at least one support-related (e.g., stress urinary incontinence, fecal incontinence, pelvic organ prolapse) pelvic floor dysfunction.[12]

Clearly the conditions are related and common among parous women. Why? A shared feature of all pelvic conditions is the failure to regain optimal strategies for transferring loads through the pelvis and its organs. The possible causes are multiple and include impairments of the:

1. Articular system (e.g., injury to either the sacroiliac joints [SIJs] and/or pubic symphysis [PS])
2. Neural system (e.g., pudendal nerve damage, leading to pain and/or weakness of the pelvic floor muscles [PFMs], including altered timing and recruitment [e.g., delayed, absent, excessive, sustained, asymmetric] of the deep muscles of the trunk [transversus abdominis (TrA)], PFMs, deep multifidus [dMf]) and loss of neural or dural mobility
3. Myofascial system (e.g., tearing of parts of the levator ani from the arcus tendineus fascia pelvis [anterior or posterior] or arcus tendineus levator ani [ATLA], stretching of the linea alba [LA] and rectus abdominis [i.e., DRA])
4. Visceral system (e.g., lengthening of the uterosacral and cardinal ligaments supporting the superior aspect of the vagina, altered tension in the broad and round ligaments and/or pubovesical ligaments supporting the bladder)

Systemic physiological impairments persisting from pregnancy into postpartum (e.g., endocrine, vascular, respiratory changes) can also create nonoptimal strategies for pelvic health. This list is merely suggestive because any change in the structure or function of the trunk (and anything that influences that) can promote nonoptimal recruitment strategies and impact how loads are transferred. Further impact to the structure and function of the various support mechanisms over time can potentially lead to more dysfunction.

How can a clinician organize and translate the increasing body of knowledge for best treatment of the patient with poor pelvic health? Is there enough research evidence to guide clinical practice for the complex patient who has impairments in multiple systems? Even if we understood all the research evidence, is it accurately reflected in clinical practice? What is an evidence-based practitioner?

EVIDENCE-BASED PRACTICE—WHAT IS IT?

Evidence-based practice (EBP) embraces all disciplines of health care and has become synonymous with best practice, but what does the term really mean? To some, it appears that EBP means that a clinician should only use assessment tests and treatment techniques and protocols that have been validated through the scientific process with high-ranking studies as valued by the levels of evidence.[13] In 2010 at the World Congress on Low Back and Pelvic Pain, Maurice van Tulder stated: *"We should not start using interventions until there is sufficient evidence for them."*

This is difficult to adhere to for many reasons, one being that there is not enough evidence for the wide variety of complexities met in clinical practice. Furthermore, even highly ranked evidence can conflict. For example, in a randomized controlled trial (RCT), Stuge et al.[14] found a significant decrease in pain and a 50% reduction in disability (measured by the Oswestry Low Back Pain Questionnaire) when specific stabilization exercises were prescribed for women with PGP after pregnancy. Conversely, Gutke et al.[15] found no significant change in pain and no change in disability (measured by the Oswestry Low Back Pain Questionnaire) in their subjects with PGP who were prescribed specific stabilization exercises after pregnancy. On paper, the two RCTs appear similar, but the results are dramatically different. Which evidence is the clinician to believe?

Many studies have sought to classify, or subgroup, individuals with various pain disorders (e.g., chronic, acute, peripherally versus centrally mediated) or movement behaviors[16-18] in an attempt to provide more evidence for management; however, not every patient encountered in clinical practice fits into any of the classifications proposed. Classification systems that begin with pain, or restrict assessment to a certain movement analysis, do not appear to meet the needs of every patient. In fact, treatment that relieves pain does not guarantee restoration of function and performance.[19-21] In addition, what has meaning for the patient often goes beyond pain (e.g., my right side just doesn't feel right; my hip "jams" when I lunge; I leak urine when I jump or run; I don't trust my knee to hold me when I stand on one leg). Restoring optimal strategies for health requires more than removing pain; it requires an understanding of what is necessary for function and performance and knowledge of the multiple mechanisms that can drive the nonoptimal strategy. When faced with the task of helping individual, complex patients, the research rarely fits completely.

The original definition of EBP includes more than research; consideration is also given to clinical expertise and patient-centered values and goals (Figure 17-1).[22] Sackett et al.[22] define EBP as the integration of best research evidence with clinical expertise and patient values.

Clinical Note

"External clinical evidence can inform, but can never replace individual clinical expertise, and it is this expertise that decides whether the external evidence applies to the patient at all, and if so, how it should be integrated into a clinical decision."

(Sackett et al.[22])

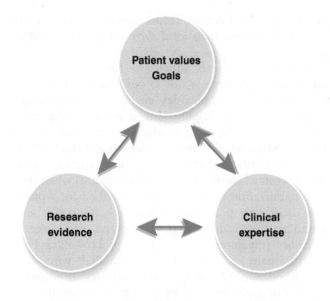

"External clinical evidence can inform, but can never replace individual clinical expertise, and it is this expertise that decides whether the external evidence applies to the patient at all, and if so, how it should be integrated into a clinical decision"
Sackett et al 2000

Figure 17-1 The three components of evidence-based practice as defined by Sackett et al.[22] (From Lee D: *The pelvic girdle*, ed 4, Edinburgh, 2011, Elsevier.)

What is clinical expertise? Clinical expertise comprises both propositional (i.e., declarative) and nonpropositional (i.e., procedural, craft, and personal) knowledge[23]; in other words, knowing how and what to do and when to do it so that the right thing is done at the right time. A clinical expert is able to "find a finding" (i.e., skill acquisition) and then interpret the finding relative to the patient's values and goals (i.e., clinical reasoning) to determine how the finding can direct treatment.

In the opening keynote address of the 2012 International Federation of Orthopaedic Manipulative Physical Therapists (IFOMPT) conference in Quebec, Professor Gwen Jull said, *"The future of physiotherapy continues with an informed clinically reasoned assessment approach to direct management of the individual patient."*

The goal of this chapter is to facilitate clinical reasoning for the treatment of pelvic pain and dysfunction by exploring some of the research evidence and clinical expertise pertaining to pelvic health. Being able to organize one's knowledge (i.e., research evidence and clinical expertise) for immediate use in the clinical setting is critical for best treatment. Clinical reasoning is known to suffer when there is a lack of knowledge organization.[24] Take a moment and imagine all your knowledge pertaining to pelvic health (i.e., the musculoskeletal, urological, colorectal, sexual, and reproductive systems) organized

within a framework similar to a closet for your clothing. Is your closet a disorganized collection of clothing, shoes, and accessories through which you have to dig to find the right shirt to go with the necessary shoes for the event planned? Are the right shoes missing? Or is your closet highly organized such that minimal time is spent putting together multiple options for a successful outfit? What would it take for your closet (and thus your treatment options) to be effective and efficient?

THE INTEGRATED SYSTEMS MODEL FOR DISABILITY AND PAIN (ISM): A FRAMEWORK TO ORGANIZE KNOWLEDGE

The ISM[25] is a framework (closet organizer), not a classification system, to help clinicians organize knowledge and develop clinical reasoning to facilitate wise decisions for treatment. Dr. Dan Siegel defines integration as "a process by which separate elements are linked together into a working whole. An integrated system is flexible, adaptive, coherent, energized and stable."[26] Doesn't this sound like what we are trying to achieve with our patients? What is a system? A body system, again defined by Siegel,[26] is a group of organs and/or structures with coordinated activities, achieving the same general function in the body. A system is composed of individual parts that interact with one another and share common characteristics, including structure, behavior, and interconnectivity. The Clinical Puzzle[27] (Figure 17-2) is a graphic conceptualization of the ISM and represents the person and his or her problem(s) (center of the puzzle) and the body systems that support optimal strategies for function and performance (i.e., articular, neural, myofascial, visceral [individual pieces], and physiological [center]). The outer circle of the Clinical Puzzle represents postures and movements that are essential for the patient to achieve their goals. The Clinical Puzzle is used to reflect on key findings from the assessment to clinically reason the best treatment plan.

The ISM approach is applicable to disability with or without pain (i.e., peripheral or centrally mediated) of any duration (i.e., acute or chronic) and is centered on the patient's values and goals, a key component of EBP. The assessment is meaningful to the patient's story and is not protocol-driven or based on clinical guidelines or prediction rules for regional pain. Every patient's experience and story is unique regardless of the location of his or her pain or impairment; thus no two assessments or treatment programs will be the same. This requires the clinician to have an inventory of assessment tests and to be able to clinically reason "on the fly" to choose subsequent tests that provide further information to support or negate an evolving hypothesis. For example, two women with a DRA can have a completely different exercise program yet a common goal of restoring optimal function of the abdominal wall. One may have a dominant internal

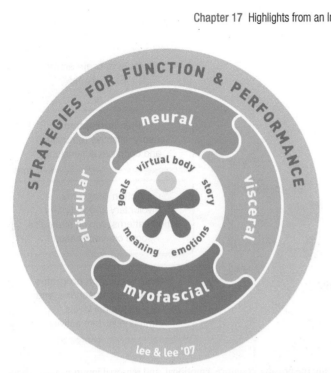

Figure 17-2 The Clinical Puzzle from The ISM.[25] The *Clinical Puzzle* conceptualizes *The ISM*. The outer circle of the puzzle represents the strategies for function and performance that the patient currently uses for meaningful tasks. The center circle of the puzzle represents several systems that relate to the person and the sensorial (i.e., sensations, perceptions), cognitive (i.e., beliefs, attitudes, motivations), and emotional (i.e., fears, anger, anxiety) dimensions of their current experience. It also includes systemic systems (such as endocrine balance, immune function) and genetic factors. It is the place where primary symptoms, goals, and barriers to recovery are noted. The four other pieces of the puzzle represent the various systems in which impairments are assessed and noted during the clinical examination. (From Lee DG, Lee LJ, McLaughlin L: Stability, continence and breathing: the role of fascia following pregnancy and delivery, *J Bodyw Mov Ther* 12:333-348, 2008.)

oblique (IO) strategy with delayed or absent activation of TrA, whereas another may have a dominant pelvic floor and external oblique (EO) strategy and asymmetric activation of TrA. Both strategies can result in separation of the recti (i.e., the impairment being diagnosed as a DRA); however, treatment of these two individuals is quite different. What is pulling excessively on the LA can be highly variable and requires individual assessment and treatment.

A key feature of this whole body and person approach is *Finding the Primary Driver*.[25] In short, this involves understanding the relationships between and within multiple regions of the whole body and how impairments in one region can impact the other. Specific tests are used to determine sites of nonoptimal alignment, biomechanics, and control (defined as failed load transfer [FLT]) during analysis of a task that is meaningful to the patient's story or complaint (meaningful task analysis). Subsequently the timing of FLT (which site fails first, second, third, etc.), as well as the impact of providing manual and/or verbal cues to correct one site on another, is noted. Clinical reasoning of the various results determines the site of the primary driver, or the primary region of the body, that if corrected

will have a significant impact on the function of the whole body/person. Sometimes two areas of the body require intervention (co-drivers), and sometimes one area requires most treatment (primary driver), whereas another requires some attention for the best outcome (secondary driver).

Further tests of specific systems (e.g., articular, neural, myofascial, visceral)[28] then determine the underlying impairment causing the nonoptimal alignment, biomechanics, and/or control of the driver(s) for the specific task being assessed. Once the impaired system has been determined, specific techniques and training for release, alignment, control, and integration into movement (including strength and conditioning) can be implemented to improve the function of the driver(s) and thus impact the function of the whole body and person.[29-31] Determining what has meaning is different for every patient. Strategies for function and performance for any task will not change unless one can help patients experience something different, hopefully better, in their bodies.

Clinical Note

Melzak[32,33] describes the gestalt of one's experience as follows:

"The body is felt as a unity, with different qualities at different times.... [Together all outputs] produce a continuous message that represents the whole body... felt as a whole body possessing a sense of self... as a flow of awareness."

Melzak's body-self neuromatrix (Figure 17-3) is useful for understanding how inputs to the matrix (i.e., the whole body nervous system) from:
1. cognitions (e.g., memories of past experiences, what we focus our attention on, what has meaning, beliefs),
2. sensations (e.g., cutaneous, nociceptive, visceral, musculoskeletal), and
3. emotions (e.g., fear, hyper vigilance, anger, sadness, grief) lead to outputs potentially producing:
1. pain,
2. involuntary and voluntary action patterns (i.e., increased neuromuscular tone in certain muscles, organs), and/or
3. activation of the stress-regulatory system (e.g., cortisol, norepinephrine and endorphin levels, dampening of the immune system).

These outputs are essentially related to the sympathetic nervous system's flight, fight, or freeze response to threat. No two individuals will have the same experience or behavior in response to threat (real or imagined) because how they manifest their pain or illness is shaped in part by who they are,[24] what they think, and how they feel. Understanding the person with poor pelvic health begins by hearing his or her story and experiences (in all three dimensions—cognitive, sensorial, emotional) and learning what has meaning for him or her. Table 17-1 outlines the three dimensions of the person's experience that should be determined from his or her story.

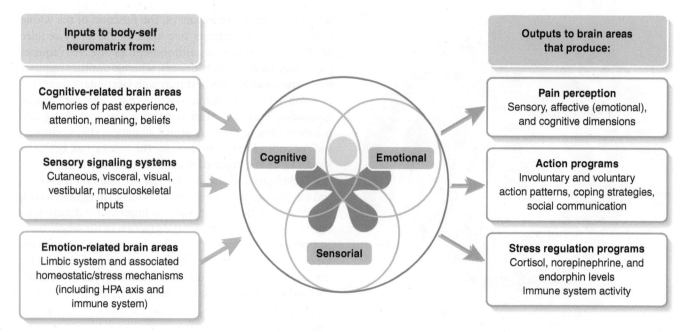

Figure 17-3 Melzak's body-self matrix[33] provides a framework for understanding the possible cognitive, emotional, and sensorial inputs to the embodied nervous system and how these inputs can collectively impact perceptions of pain, activate action programs (e.g., flight, flight, freeze), change social behavior, suppress the immune system, and stimulate stress responses. (From Lee D: *The pelvic girdle*, ed 4, Edinburgh, 2011, Elsevier.)

Key features from the patient's story are noted in the center of the Clinical Puzzle, including:

1. The patient's meaningful complaint—the primary symptom (i.e., thought, emotion, feeling) that has brought him or her for treatment.
2. The patient's meaningful task and goals—the aggravating posture or movement (e.g., "I have pelvic girdle pain when I run"), tasks which are difficult to perform (or avoided) and relate to their performance goals (e.g., "My hip 'jams' or 'doesn't feel right' when I do a lunge to the left and this is impacting many poses in my Yoga practice"), or tasks that create respiratory or urogynecological symptoms (e.g., "I get short of breath in spin class; I leak urine when I jump; I find sexual intercourse painful").
3. Any potential cognitive or emotional barriers to recovery or significant medical considerations.

Tasks for screening are then chosen based on the meaningful task and these are charted on the outer circle of the Clinical Puzzle. For example, if the meaningful complaint is PGP aggravated by sitting, then three useful screening tasks that are components of this meaningful task would be:

1. Standing posture (i.e., the position from which the task begins)
2. Squat
3. Sitting posture

Regional areas of the whole body are then assessed in each of the screening tasks to determine if the strategy is optimal or nonoptimal. An optimal strategy for any task will:

1. Have optimal alignment, biomechanics, and control
2. Distribute and balance pressure in all three canisters (cranium, thorax, abdomen)

3. Allow optimal respiration
4. Have sufficient mobility to accommodate perturbations to the system (breath, movement).

Optimal strategies look and feel good! Optimal strategies for the transference of load through the pelvis will support musculoskeletal, respiratory, urological, colorectal, sexual, and reproductive health. Nonoptimal strategies produce sites that fail to transfer load, and they often demonstrate poor alignment, biomechanics, and/or control or are associated with excessive increases in pressure, poor breathing patterns (e.g., breath holding), or rigidity inappropriate for the task. Nonoptimal strategies simply do not look good nor do they feel good.

If possible, the timing of FLT between the various sites is considered to determine which body region (e.g., foot, pelvis, thoracic ring, hip) fails first, second, or third (Figure 17-4). Then the clinician provides specific manual and verbal cues or corrections to one or more sites of FLT to determine which correction has the most positive impact (i.e., improvement in range of motion, decrease in effort, reduction in symptoms) on the screening task (#1, 2, 3 as previously indicated). The pelvis is corrected or controlled by manually restoring neutral alignment (if possible), centering the pelvic mass over the base of support (i.e., the feet), and then providing gentle compression. The patient then repeats the screening task to assess the impact of this correction on his or her ability to maintain optimal alignment of the thorax and move the hips. The thorax is corrected or controlled (being thoracic ring specific—see Chapter 11), and the task is repeated to assess any change in the patient's ability to stabilize the pelvic joints and move the hips. An enquiry is made as

TABLE **17-1**

Assessing the "Person"

Dimension	Description
Sensorial dimension of patient's experiences 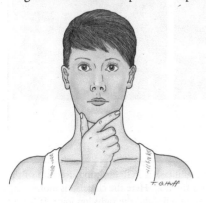 Front Back	Where is their meaningful complaint (e.g., pain, burning, tingling, numbness) located in their body and what is its behavior (i.e., aggravating and relieving features)? Try to determine the autobiographical details (i.e., what happened when) of the sensations and make a determination if the symptoms are now peripherally or centrally mediated.
Cognitive dimension of patient's experiences 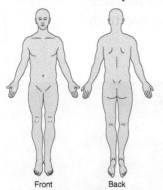	A simple question such as "What do you think is going on?" can provide much information as to the patient's cognitive beliefs pertaining to their experience. Listen carefully as this is often when "flags" appear in the story that can be the primary driver, or barrier, to physical interventions. Education plays a large role here to retrain negative thoughts (or inaccurate thoughts) that can contribute to nonoptimal movement and postural behavior.
Emotional dimension of patient's experiences 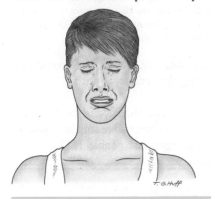	This is usually communicated both verbally and nonverbally. Watch for emotional posturing (defensive angry posturing is militant like whereas depressive giving-up posturing is collapsed) and behaviors that appear inconsistent with other features of the story. Not being able to answer the question asked, but only providing answers pertaining to how much pain he or she is in is another clue that the amygdala has this person "hi-jacked." Remember that individuals with poor pelvic health may have seen many professionals and be quite confused and frustrated. This is not an emotional barrier; this is the patient's reality.

Note: Understanding the person with poor pelvic health begins by hearing his or her story. The clinician needs to understand the "person behind the problem." This understanding can only be obtained by having time during the clinical sessions to truly hear the patient's story from his or her perspective.

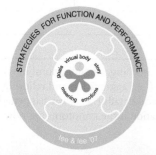

Finding the primary driver
when there are multiple sites of failed load transfer
(FLT) within and between regions of the whole body

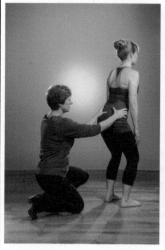
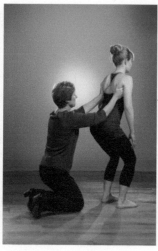
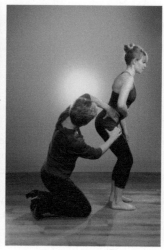
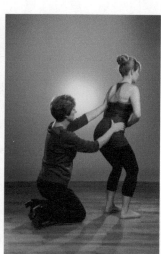

- *Which one shows FLT first?*
- *What is the impact of correcting one on the other?*

Figure 17-4 Determining the primary driver. Finding the primary driver for a squat task when the meaningful task is PGP in sitting. Regions of the body are assessed to determine if the alignment, biomechanics, and control are optimal or nonoptimal for the task. Here the clinician is monitoring from left to right the pelvis (in particular, the right SIJ), the mid thorax (in particular thoracic rings 3, 4, and 5), and the right hip joint. If two of more sites of FLT are identified, the clinician then must determine which one is the driver by noting the timing of the FLT and the impact of any correction. In the picture on the right, the clinician is assessing the timing of the FLT between an upper thoracic ring and the right SIJ. The site that fails first is often, but not always, the site of the primary impairment, the primary driver. To confirm this hypothesis, the clinician notes the impact of correcting the alignment, biomechanics, and control of the pelvis on the thorax and then the thorax on the pelvis. The site of correction that provides the best improvement in performance of the task determines the driver. (Copyright Diane G. Lee Physiotherapist Corp.)

to the difference in the "gestalt of the experience" when various body regions are corrected or controlled to not only confirm the hypothesis but also help the patient to become aware of the differing experiences of his or her body when sites distant from the pain are corrected or controlled. Collectively the timing and impact of various corrections on the screening determine the "driver" for that task. It is possible to have a pelvic-driven pelvis, thorax-driven pelvis, foot-driven pelvis, even a cranial-driven pelvis. Every pelvic pain patient is unique.

Once the driver is confirmed, the meaningful task is repeated to:

1. Confirm the hypothesis of the best place to begin treatment.
2. Create patient confidence and understanding as to how the regions of the body relate and why, sometimes, treatment has to begin distant from the site of their symptom(s).
3. Give the patient a different experience (gestalt) of his or her body and thus begin to change his or her "brain

map" or body schema because changing a motor output begins by changing the sensory input.

The next step is to determine the specific or combination of system impairment(s) responsible for the nonoptimal strategy for the meaningful task (Table 17-2).

Clinical Note

"The advantage of a clinical reasoning approach is that it is responsive to new knowledge and evidence, is flexible and allows for change and growth"
Professor Gwen Jull at the 2012 IFOMPT conference in Quebec.

The ISM[25] is such a clinical reasoning approach. It is a framework, not a classification, that considers all three dimensions of the patient's experience and the barriers that each may present to the recovery process for both acute and persistent conditions. Most tasks

TABLE **17-2**

Conditions Associated with the Various Systems of the Clinical Puzzle

System	Associated Condition

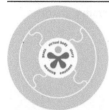	• Cognitive barriers (i.e., beliefs and memories from past experiences, thoughts "attended to")
	• Emotional barriers (i.e., anger, fear, depression)
	• Physiological and medical considerations
	   ○ Hormone health (neuroendocrine)
	   ○ Nutrition
	   ○ Hydration
	   ○ Disease (e.g., diabetes, cardiovascular)
	• Patient's values and goals (i.e., meaningful complaints and tasks)

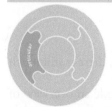	• Capsular sprain or tear • Ligament sprain or tear (grades I-III) • Labral or intra-articular meniscal tear • Intervertebral disc strain/tear/herniation/prolapse • Fracture • Joint fixation or dislocation • Periosteal contusion • Stress fracture • Osteitis, periostitis, apophysitis • Osteochondral and chondral fractures, minor osteochondral injury • Chondropathy (e.g., softening, fibrillation, fissuring, chondromalacia) • Synovitis • Apophysitis • Fibrosis/osteophytosis of the zygapophyseal and intervertebral joints, sacroiliac joint, hip joint

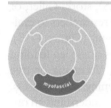	• Intramuscular strain/tear (grades I-III)
	• Muscle contusion
	• Musculotendinous strain/tear
	• Complete or partial tendon rupture or tear
	• Fascial strain/tear
	• Tendon pathology—tendon rupture, partial tendon tears, tendinopathy (acute or chronic), paratendinopathy, pantendinopathy
	• Skin lacerations/abrasions/puncture wounds
	• Bursa—bursitis
	• Muscular or fascial scarring or adhesions
	• Loss of fascial integrity of the anterior abdominal wall including
	   ○ Diastasis rectus abdominis
	   ○ Sports hernia (tear of transversalis fascia)
	   ○ Hockey hernia (tear of the external oblique)
	   ○ Inguinal hernia
	• Loss of fascial integrity of the endopelvic fascia leading to cystocoele, enterocoele, and/or rectocoele

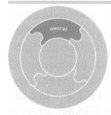	• Peripheral nerve trunk or nerve injury (i.e., neuropraxia, neurotmesis, axonotemesis)
	• Central nervous system injury
	• Altered motor control
	   ○ Absence of recruitment, inappropriate timing (early or late) of muscle recruitment,
	   ○ Inappropriate amount (increased of decreased) of muscle activity (all relative to demands of task)
	   ○ Overactivity or underactivity of muscles at rest
	• Altered neurodynamics
	• Sensitization of the peripheral or central nervous system
	• Altered central nervous system processing
	   ○ Altered body schema or virtual body

(*Continued*)

TABLE **17-2**

Conditions Associated with the Various Systems of the Clinical Puzzle—Cont'd

System	Associated Condition
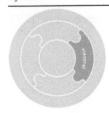	• Inflammatory organ disease or pathology (e.g., appendicitis cystitis, acute ulcerative gastritis, pleuritis, endometriosis) • Infective disorders of the pelvic organs • Organ disease • Lack of organ mobility/motility

Note: Conditions can be combined; for example, it is possible to have a stiff joint and an overactive muscle further compressing the joint. The articular system impairment is not identifiable until the compression from the neural system impairment has been released.

Adapted from Lee D: *The pelvic girdle,* ed 4, Table 7-4a, Edinburgh, 2011, Elsevier.

involve the whole body; thus assessment must include analysis of the relationship between the body regions and the impact and interplay of each. It is no longer acceptable to just assess the pelvic girdle and its contents when presented with a patient with pelvic pain; the source may reside far removed from the location of the symptoms.

THE STATE OF THE EVIDENCE ON PELVIC FUNCTION AND ASSESSMENT DURING A COMMON TEST—SINGLE LEG STANDING AND CONTRALATERAL HIP FLEXION

Increasing scientific evidence and clinical expertise confirm a key role for the pelvis in lumbopelvic health, and paradigms for assessment and treatment of pelvic pain have changed considerably since 1990.[34,35] It has been argued that optimal function of the pelvis is essential for musculoskeletal, urological, colorectal, sexual, and reproductive health, and yet agreement is lacking for what optimal function of the pelvis requires. The biomechanics of the SIJs and PS are poorly understood for many of the tasks that aggravate people with PGP. Agreement is still lacking for when the SIJ should move and when it should not.

Pathology and intervention in musculoskeletal rehabilitation assumes that as clinicians we are able to reach a functional diagnosis—for this chapter a diagnosis that pertains to pelvic health. Not only is there disagreement on the biomechanics of the pelvic joints, but agreement is also lacking for best ways to evaluate the functional status of the pelvis.[34,35] The form and force closure theories proposed by Snjiders et al.[36,37] and the motor control requirements for effective load transfer through the pelvis[38-52] are well accepted, and yet the best ways to translate this knowledge into clinical practice to determine if the patient's form closure, force closure, and/or motor control mechanisms are healthy are widely debated. In addition, the best ways to restore optimal function of the pelvis are unclear (i.e., when and how should the SIJ or PS be mobilized or stabilized?). Although much evidence

has been gained over the past 25 years, there is still much to do.

The intent of this chapter is to provide an overview of evidence-based (or informed) treatment for poor pelvic health and the clinical reasoning that supports treatment decisions. However, clinicians are a long way from agreeing on how to assess and determine the specific impairments of the pelvis, and this first needs to be acknowledged and discussed.

Standing on one leg and flexing the contralateral hip, a task known as the one leg standing (OLS), stork, Gillet, or kinetic test, is often used by clinicians and researchers to evaluate mobility and control of the pelvic joints (Figure 17-5). When a patient's meaningful task requires single leg loading (e.g., walking, running, climbing stairs, Vrksasana or tree pose in yoga), this is an appropriate screening task to assess. To interpret the findings, it is necessary to understand an optimal response—in other words, what should happen within the pelvis and between the pelvis and the hip, knee, and foot as well as between the pelvis and thorax, neck, and cranium when standing on one leg and flexing the contralateral hip. At this time, there are no studies that have considered the entire body when doing this task. A few studies have investigated the biomechanics of the pelvic girdle (mainly the osteokinematics) and the muscle recruitment strategies in subjects with and without pain during single leg standing with contralateral hip flexion.

Jacob and Kissling[53] determined that 0.4° to 4.3° of rotation (innominate relative to the sacrum) is possible in the non–weight-bearing SIJ in healthy, pain-free subjects between the ages of 20 and 50 years. Sturesson and coworkers[54-56] found no statistical differences in the available range of SIJ motion in subjects with PGP and impairment during single leg standing. These findings suggest that although mobility may vary between subjects, PGP is not predictive of more or less motion at the SIJ.

Hungerford et al.[57] found that the amplitude of SIJ motion was symmetric in healthy, pain-free subjects and asymmetric in those with PGP. However, Dreyfuss et al.[58] found that 20% of healthy, pain-free subjects had movement asymmetries of the SIJ, and again there appears to

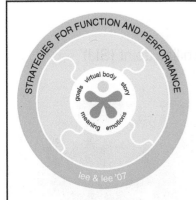

Active Mobility Test for the Sacroiliac Joint

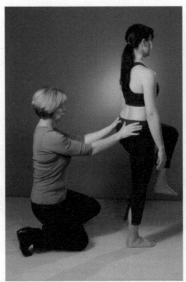
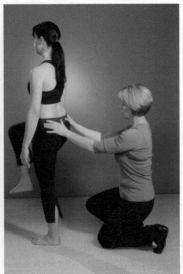

- *The innominate should posteriorly rotate relative to the ipsilateral sacrum during single leg standing with contralateral hip flexion*
- *The movement should be symmetric between sides*

Figure 17-5 Single leg standing with contralateral hip flexion. During this task, the non–weight-bearing innominate on the side of hip flexion should posteriorly rotate relative to the ipsilateral sacrum.[57] The amplitude of motion should be symmetric between the left and right sides. (From Lee D: *The pelvic girdle*, ed 4, Edinburgh, 2011, Elsevier.)

be no correlation between PGP and asymmetric SIJ motion. So the question remains as to when noted movement asymmetries of the SIJ are relevant to the clinical picture.

Asymmetric motion of the SIJs during single leg standing is a sign of FLT (i.e., nonoptimal alignment and biomechanics) and is a key feature of the ISM approach and requires that clinicians can reliably perceive these differences because one cannot interpret a finding one cannot find (Figure 17-6). Unfortunately, intertester reliability is lacking for SIJ mobility analysis during this test (Table 17-3).[58-62] Following a systematic review of commonly used mobility tests for the SIJ, Van der Wurff et al.[63] concluded: "*...at this time, it is questionable whether any SIJ tests are of any value for clinical [and that]... there are no indications that 'upgrading' of the methodological quality would have improved the final conclusions.*"

Sturesson et al. felt that their studies[55,56] supported their position that movement of the SIJ in weight bearing was too small for clinicians to feel. Vleeming et al.[34] go further and state, "*Assumed SIJ motion during this*

test does not occur. The authors conclude that movement of the external pelvis relative to the hips gives the (manual) illusion that the SIJ are repositioned." Vleeming believes clinicians were feeling an illusion of intrapelvic motion.[34,64] Most clinicians who use this test in clinical practice share the opinion that they can feel motion at the SIJ (i.e., intrapelvic motion differentiated from motion of the pelvic girdle on the femur at the hip joint) during single OLS on the non–weight-bearing side. Are clinicians being deluded by this illusion? Is the research evidence superior to clinical expertise with this test? Are clinicians being illuded by their senses and deluded by their beliefs? When the methods of the intertester reliability studies are considered, several questions arise. How did the testers perceive the information? Visually (i.e., watching the posterior superior iliac spine [PSIS] move relative to the sacrum), kinesthetically (i.e., feeling the PSIS move relative to the sacrum), or visually and kinesthetically or does this matter? Some clinicians appear to have better visual accuracy than kinesthetic, others have better

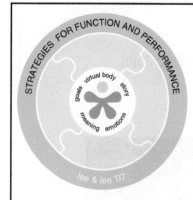

Active Mobility Test for the Sacroiliac Joint (SIJ)

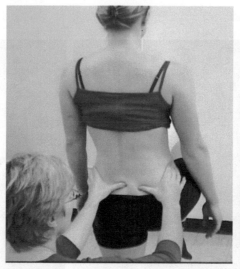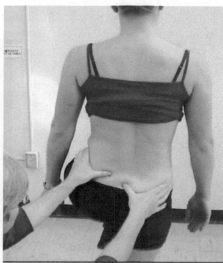

- *Note the obvious asymmetry of SIJ motion between the left and right sides*
- *Which side do you think looks like it is moving less?*

Figure 17-6 Single leg standing with contralateral hip flexion. When SIJ motion is reduced (for many different reasons) the amplitude of innominate motion relative to the sacrum is asymmetric and the pelvic girdle often compensates by tilting on the contralateral hip (i.e., extrinsic pelvic motion). This asymmetry can be seen and felt by trained clinicians. (Copyright Diane G. Lee Physiotherapist Corp.)

TABLE 17-3

Reliability of Commonly Used Tests for Mobility of the Sacroiliac Joint

Study	Palpation Points	Tactile versus Visual	Finding
Dreyfuss et al. 1994[58]	S2 and inferior PSIS	No comment on tactile vs. visual	Unreliable
Potter and Rothstein 1985[59]	S2 and inferior PSIS	No comment on tactile vs. visual	Unreliable
Carmichael 1987[60]	Several palpation points	Both visual and tactile	Unreliable
Herzog et al. 1989[61]	S2 and inferior PSIS	No comment on tactile vs. visual	Reliable
Meijne et al. 1999[62]	Several palpation points	Both visual and tactile	Unreliable
van der Wurff et al. 2000[63]			Systematic review of all mobility and pain provocation tests of the sacroiliac joint confirm lack of reliability and validity of all mobility tests

Note: On closer investigation of the methods, much information is missing that could directly influence the results of these trials.

PSIS, Posterior superior iliac spine.

kinesthetic sense, and a few are good at both. When the clinician is instructed to rely on their predetermined best sense (i.e., visual or kinesthetic), their intertester reliability appears to improve when tested informally during course instruction. Multiple mechanisms may drive this difference; however, those who are less reliable when using vision often have unilateral mobility restrictions of their upper neck. Were the testers in the reliability studies (see Table 17-3) screened for asymmetric mobility of their upper neck? How much compression was applied to the pelvis during the testing? The SIJ is easily influenced by the smallest amounts of compression,[65–69] which could be another confounding variable. There is no mention of compression control in any of the methods in the reliability studies reviewed.

> ### Clinical Note
>
> - Illusion: "A distortion of the senses, revealing how the brain normally organizes and interprets sensory stimulation. While illusions distort reality, they are generally shared by most people." (as defined by Wikipedia)
> - Delusion: "A belief held with strong conviction despite superior evidence to the contrary." (as defined by Wikipedia)

Hungerford et al.[57] also investigated control of SIJ motion on the weight-bearing side during single leg standing (Figure 17-7). The innominate remained posteriorly rotated relative to the sacrum in the pain-free subjects, whereas in the PGP population, the innominate rotated anteriorly relative to the sacrum—a movement that clinicians have found to be able to reliably palpate.[70] This research suggests that when assessing control of the SIJ, anterior rotation of the innominate relative to the sacrum should be noted because this is a sign of FLT when the pelvis is loaded.

Standing on one leg is a whole body task and a key component of many more complex functional tasks. Although the pelvis plays an essential role in standing on

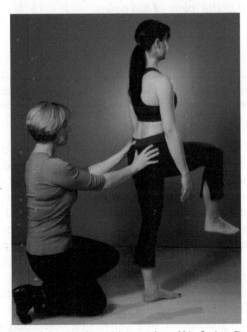

Figure 17-7 Single leg standing with contralateral hip flexion. During this task, the weight-bearing innominate should remain posteriorly rotated relative to the ipsilateral sacrum. This is the close-packed, self-braced position for the SIJ. (From Lee D: *The pelvic girdle*, ed 4, Edinburgh, 2011, Elsevier.)

one leg, the task requires more than optimal function of the pelvis. When the pelvis fails to transfer load optimally (i.e., loses control or fails to move when it should), it is important to consider the impact of the rest of the body on the pelvis and not just assume that the primary problem is within the pelvis (Figure 17-8).

Finding the Primary Driver for a Single Leg Standing Task with Contralateral Hip Flexion

Multiple studies on subjects with low back and pelvic pain suggest that motor control changes in the trunk are variable, individual, and task specific. Some muscles are compromised (i.e., timing of activation is delayed or absent), whereas others are augmented (i.e., early and increased activation). The common link between tasks and individuals is that the strategy chosen is nonoptimal and there are often multiple sites of FLT; so when are the asymmetries of active mobility of the SIJs noted during single leg standing and contralateral hip flexion relevant to the clinical picture? Loss of intrapelvic control during loading is always relevant and movement asymmetry is relevant when it presents during a task that requires movement, regardless of the location of symptoms.

The following two brief case reports demonstrate the relationship between the thorax and pelvis during single leg standing and contralateral hip flexion. They will highlight how the primary driver was determined to be the seventh thoracic ring in the first case and the pelvis in the second case, even though their meaningful complaint and task were similar in both cases (i.e., chronic right posterior PGP aggravated by running or walking).

Case Report 1—Thorax-Driven Pelvic Pain and Impairment

A female triathlete presented with a primary complaint of chronic right PGP (meaningful complaint), aggravated by running (meaningful task). The single leg standing task was used to screen intrapelvic mobility and control in that it pertained to her meaningful task. During left single leg standing with right hip flexion (Figure 17-9, *A*), her pelvis laterally tilted (abducted) at the left hip (extrinsic pelvic motion) and minimal motion of the right SIJ (intrapelvic motion) occurred compared with the left SIJ during right single leg standing with left hip flexion (Figure 17-9, *C*). In other words, there was an asymmetric intrapelvic motion noted on active mobility testing. The right SIJ was not moving when it should and therefore was noted as a site of FLT (first site of FLT noted). In addition, her seventh thoracic ring translated to the left and rotated to the right during the OLS test. Although these are optimal biomechanics for rotation of a thoracic ring,[75] rotation should not occur during this specific task, and therefore this is considered a second site of FLT in this case. Increased tone in a specific fascicle of the right iliocostalis extending

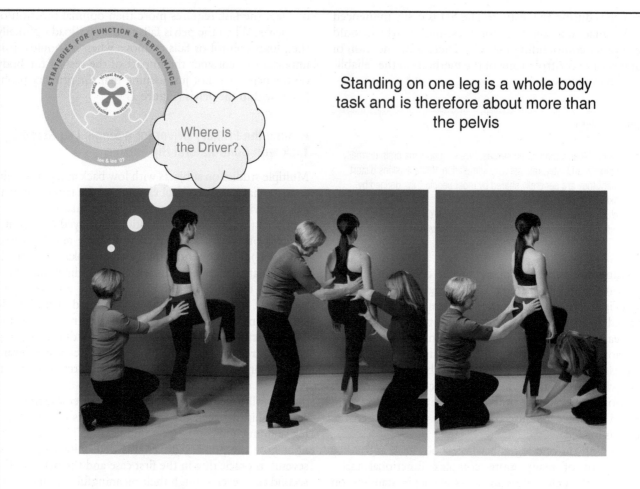

Figure 17-8 Standing on one leg and flexing the opposite hip is a whole body task and consideration must be given to how the rest of the body is influencing pelvic alignment, biomechanics, and control. The primary driver for this task can be anywhere from the cranium to the foot. (From Lee D: *The pelvic girdle*, ed 4, Edinburgh, 2011, Elsevier.)

from the iliac crest to the right seventh rib was palpable (Figure 17-9, *B*).

During right single leg standing, the right, weight-bearing SIJ lost control (i.e., loss of intrapelvic control with the right innominate anteriorly rotated relative to the sacrum) (Figure 17-10). The right SIJ had already been identified as a site of FLT (i.e., asymmetric intrapelvic motion); however, this additional finding (i.e., loss of control) ruled out a diagnosis of a stiff, fibrotic or fixated SIJ, which would not lose control. The patient's seventh thoracic ring continued to translate to the left and rotate to the right and persistent increased tone was noted again in the right iliocostalis.

There were two sites of FLT for both of these tasks, the seventh thoracic ring and right SIJ. To determine the primary driver (i.e., best region to begin to treat), the timing

of FLT was noted during both tasks. The seventh thoracic ring was translated laterally to the left and rotated to the right before initiation of weight transfer, and this translation and rotation increased before the right SIJ failed to move during left single leg standing and before the right SIJ lost control during right single leg standing. This suggests that the seventh thoracic ring was the primary driver, given that it failed before the SIJ during the task. Confirmation of this hypothesis required consideration of the impact of a correction of the pelvis on the seventh thoracic ring alignment, biomechanics, and control and then the impact of a pelvic ring correction on the seventh thoracic ring alignment, biomechanics, and control during both tasks. Correcting the seventh thoracic ring alignment and control[76] restored the mobility of the right SIJ during left single leg standing and control of

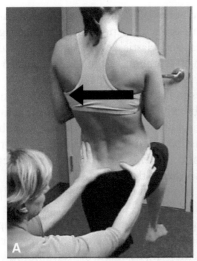
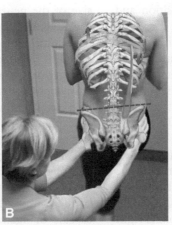
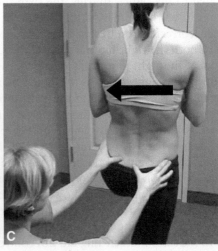

Figure 17-9 **A,** During this left single leg loading task, note that the pelvis has laterally tilted relative to the left femur (i.e., abducted at the left hip joint) and the thorax (in particular the seventh thoracic ring) has translated to the left and rotated to the right, both signs of FLT (i.e., nonoptimal alignment, biomechanics, and control) for this task. **B,** Increased activation of a specific fascicle of the right iliocostalis muscle (which arises from the right iliac crest and inserts into the posterior aspect of the right seventh rib) can create a vector of force that both destabilizes the right SIJ (causing the innominate to anteriorly rotate relative to the sacrum) and causes the seventh thoracic ring to translate to the left/rotate to the right. **C,** Note the difference in both the pelvic position relative to the femur and the position of the thorax relative to the pelvis in this right single leg standing task. Although not as easily seen, the seventh thoracic ring remained relatively left translated and right rotated during this task as well. (Copyright Diane G. Lee Physiotherapist Corp.)

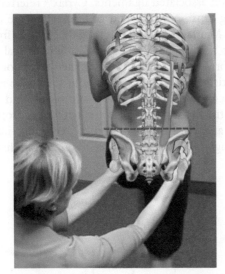

Figure 17-10 The right SIJ and the seventh thoracic ring also failed to transfer load effectively in the right single leg loading task. Which is the driver for this task—the seventh thoracic ring or the pelvis? What are the next tests the clinician would choose to determine treatment? (Copyright Diane G. Lee Physiotherapist Corp.)

the right SIJ during right single leg standing. Correcting the pelvis (i.e., alignment and control) had no impact on the seventh thoracic ring, which remained left translated and right rotated during the task. Therefore, the seventh thoracic ring was considered to be the driver as it gave the best overall body response when corrected for this task.

Specific system tests (articular, neural, myofascial, and visceral) pertaining to the seventh thoracic ring confirmed that the specific hypertonic fascicle noted in the right iliocostalis lumborum pars thoracic (ILPT) was,

in part, responsible for the nonoptimal alignment and biomechanics of both the seventh thoracic ring and the pelvic ring. This muscle was one of several trunk muscle dyssynergies. Because much of the neural drive for the abdominal wall and low back musculature comes from the lower thorax, it is plausible that low thoracic ring impairments could lead to some muscles being compromised and others augmented, as the evidence has clearly shown. However, what is not known from the research is the best way to restore synergy and optimal recruitment strategies. The patient's PGP was likely driven by nonoptimal function of thoracopelvic control mediated by an underlying neural system impairment (i.e., hypertonic fascicle of the right ILPT). Initial treatment focused on restoring optimal alignment, biomechanics, and control of the seventh thoracic ring (see Chapter 11), following which her PGP reduced and her pelvic alignment and control improved as well as her function and performance.

Case Report 2—A Thorax-Driven Pelvic Pain and Impairment Becomes a Pelvic-Driven Pelvic Pain and Impairment

This female patient presented with right-sided low back and PGP (meaningful complaint) aggravated by walking (meaningful task). The single leg standing task was chosen as an initial screening task to assess the patient's strategies for vertical loading through her low back and pelvis. She had three sites of FLT during right single leg standing: the right SIJ (i.e., the right innominate rotated anteriorly relative to the sacrum), right hip (i.e., the femur translated anterior when she shifted her weight to the right), and sixth thoracic ring (i.e., translated to the left and rotated to the right). Initially, the sixth thoracic ring was found to be the primary driver because it failed first and when corrected resulted in improved position and control of both the right hip and the right SIJ. Increased activation of the right iliocostalis combined with under-activation of the right TrA was the noted neural system impairment, causing the FLT of the sixth thoracic ring. Two years later, the patient's thoracopelvic function was reassessed. Both the intensity and frequency of her lum-bopelvic pain were less. However, there was still a control impairment of the right SIJ during right single leg stand-ing. Her sixth thoracic ring continued to translate left and rotate right during this task; however, controlling the right SIJ now restored the control of the sixth thoracic ring, whereas correcting the alignment and providing control to the sixth thoracic ring did not control the right SIJ during this task as it did 2 years ago. An evaluation of the patient's core muscles[28] (i.e., a neural system as-sessment) revealed delayed activation of the right TrA in response to a pelvic floor cue. This delay in activation was not improved by correcting the sixth thoracic ring. When the patient was given a cue to specifically recruit the right TrA (imagine a guy wire connecting the right anterior superior iliac spine (ASIS) to the midline), a symmetric coactivation response of the left and right TrA was felt. This strategy controlled the right SIJ during right single leg standing. Massed practice to improve the coactivation of the right and left TrA was now advised to build a new brain map for a better strategy for pelvic control.

In summary, although single leg standing with contra-lateral hip flexion is commonly used to identify nonopti-mal strategies for pelvic function, loss of intrapelvic control noted during this task does not necessarily mean the pelvis is the primary driver for the nonoptimal strategy noted.

SPECIFIC SYSTEMS TESTS TO DIRECT TREATMENT OF THE PRIMARY DRIVER

Once the primary driver for a specific task has been found, more tests can then be used to determine which impair-ments in which systems are responsible for the nonopti-mal strategy (i.e., articular, neural, myofascial, or visceral). The clinician's ability to do this relies entirely on his or her ability to accurately perceive visual and kinesthetic in-formation. Treatment will depend on the interpretation of this information through clinical reasoning and hy-pothesis development.

Joint Mobility Tests—What is Really Being Tested?

Passive physiological and passive accessory mobility tests provide information about more than just the joint, al-though historically the findings from these tests have been interpreted through the lens of the articular system. Overactive muscles can increase compression across a joint's surfaces, effectively reducing the size of both the

neutral and elastic zones of motion. Underactive muscles can reduce compression, thus potentially increasing the size of the neutral and elastic zones. Vectors of pull on the skeleton from attachments of the viscera can also pro-duce joint compression and alter passive and active joint mobility. Changes in fascial integrity and tension can also change joint mobility. Therefore, when testing active or passive physiological and passive accessory joint mobility, consideration must be given to more than just the ampli-tude of motion and the end feel to accurately interpret and clinically reason what the findings mean.

All joints have two zones of motion, a neutral and elas-tic zone (Figure 17-11).[50] The neutral zone is the part of the joint's range that is not influenced by the capsule or the capsular ligaments (i.e., there is no stress on the capsule or ligaments). In Maitland's[77] terminology, this range has been defined as 0 to R1 (first resistance). The amplitude of neutral zone motion varies between joints in the same body and between individuals (comparing the same joint). However, the amplitude of both zones should be similar between the left and right sides in the same individual. The elastic zone is the range that is influ-enced by increasing tension in various parts of the joint's capsule and associated ligaments. Cyriax[78] referred to the increasing tension at the end of a joint's range as "end feel" and Maitland[77] called this range R1 to R2 (from first resistance to the end of the joint's physiological range). It is important for clinicians to set their intention to feel the qualities of resistance throughout the entire range of motion (i.e., both neutral and elastic zones) and then to interpret the findings from this test with those from active mobility and control tests. Clinical reasoning involving the findings of all three tests generates a more likely and

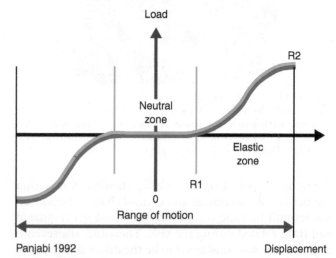

Figure 17-11 An adapted graphic representation of both Panjabi's[49,50] neutral and elastic zone representation of joint motion and Maitland's[77] joint movement diagram. Maitland's 0 to R1 is equivalent to Panjabi's neutral zone and R1 to R2 is equivalent to the elastic zone. Cyriax[78] described several different "qualities" of R1 to R2 which he called end-feel. (Copyright Diane G. Lee Physiotherapist Corp.)

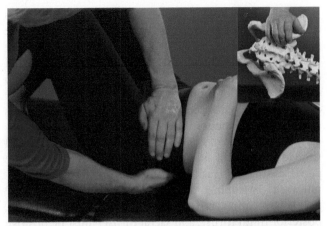

Figure 17-12 Passive accessory mobility testing of the SIJ. With the joint in its neutral, non–close-packed position (i.e., sacrum slightly counternutated), the innominate should be able to glide anteroposteriorly at all three parts of the SIJ: the superior, middle, and inferior parts. There should also be a very small craniocaudal glide. Interpretation of the joint glide findings requires clinical reasoning of multiple findings including those on active, passive accessory and control testing. The inset on the top right of this figure shows the specific finger placement of the right hand during this test; medial to the iliac crest and the PSIS of the innominate. (From Lee D: *The pelvic girdle*, ed 4, Edinburgh, 2011, Elsevier.)

probable hypothesis as to the specific impairment impacting the joint's neutral and elastic zones of motion.

Passive accessory, or arthrokinematic, mobility testing is initially performed with the joint in its neutral or loose-packed position (Figure 17-12). The amplitude of the neutral zone should be the greatest in this position because the capsule and ligaments are under the least amount of tension. For the SIJ, the loose-packed position is counternutation of the sacrum.[67,68] Providing there are no vectors from any system compressing the SIJ, the sacrum will be counternutated when the patient lies supine with his or her hips and knees flexed and supported over a bolster. Any activation of the deep abdominals, PFMs, gluteals, hamstrings, or adductors of the thigh has the potential to increase compression across the SIJ[40,66,79,80] and thus reduce the size of the neutral zone. This must be considered when comparing mobility between sides.

Passive tests for efficacy of the form closure mechanism (i.e., the ability of the passive components of the joint to resist shear forces) require that the joint be positioned in the close-packed position and then the passive accessory mobility of the neutral and elastic zones assessed. When the joint is close-packed, there should be maximum congruence of the articular surfaces and maximum tension in the major ligaments, and no motion should be possible in the neutral zone. For the SIJ, this position is nutation of the sacrum because nutation increases tension in the sacrotuberous, sacrospinous, and interosseus ligaments.[67,68] This is a simple test for addressing a cognitive belief (of either the patient or the clinician) that the SIJ is unstable. If the joint has a true articular system impairment that has rendered it unstable, motion will still be palpable

in the neutral zone even when the joint is close-packed. If neutral zone motion is well controlled in this close-packed position, the articular system can be ruled out as being the cause of the loss of joint control in loading tasks. If pain is provoked when the passive test moves beyond R1 (into the elastic zone), then one can conclude that there is nociceptive input arising from the ligaments of the SIJ.

Tests for efficacy of the force closure mechanism (i.e., the external forces necessary to control shear when a joint is in its neutral position) are inseparable from testing motor control strategies. When the recruitment strategy of the stabilizers of SIJ motion is optimal, there is no motion in the neutral zone even when the joint is positioned in neutral (i.e., the loose-packed position). The amount of activation necessary to control shear of a neutral joint varies according to the amplitude of the applied load.

Passive mobility testing remains essential in clinical practice, in spite of the difficulty to show intertester reliability for commonly used tests. How the results from these tests are interpreted has changed dramatically during three decades. It is now understood that joint mobility can be influenced by factors extrinsic to the joint and occasionally far removed. For example, impaired function at C3-4-5 can impact the range of motion at the hip through mechanisms mediated through changes in neural drive to the diaphragm through the phrenic nerve and thus distally to the hip via the psoas muscle. It is very common to find neuromuscular vectors responsible for nonoptimal alignment, biomechanics, and control of the mid-thorax impacting passive and active mobility as well as control of the SIJ. Vectors of pull from the visceral attachments to the skeleton can also compress and restrict SIJ motion, and it is manual testing that differentiates the underlying system impairments and thus directs specific treatment. In clinical practice, a diagnosis is not reached on one test alone. Restricted active and passive mobility of the SIJ does not always mean that the joint is stiff and requiring a mobilization technique or fixated and requiring a manipulation. Interpretive reasoning of the patient's story and all the clinical findings are necessary to reach a logical, sound hypothesis as to the primary driver and underlying system impairment(s). Once this is determined, pathology and intervention in musculoskeletal rehabilitation are clear. The reader is referred to other resources for further information on specific assessment techniques for the neural, myofascial, and visceral systems.[28]

THE PELVIC-DRIVEN PELVIS—PATHOLOGIES OR CONDITIONS

The next part of this chapter will focus on the management of the individual with pelvic-driven pelvic pain and impairment, whereby the best correction for the meaningful task is the pelvis. Clinical reasoning of the wide variety of possible findings from active, passive, and control tests for the SIJ will be discussed to facilitate an understanding of the specific pathologies so that the principles for evidence-informed and reasoned intervention can follow. It is not possible to cover every single condition responsible for poor pelvic health; common ones have been chosen for this chapter. Table 17-4 highlights key differential features between the specific system impairments described in the following.

The Painful Sacroiliac Joint—An Articular System Impairment

Pain that is nociceptive and arising from the SIJ (i.e., peripherally mediated) is located directly over the posterior aspect of the SIJ and can radiate to the groin and down the posterolateral thigh.[81,82] The SIJ alone does not cause low back pain; however, complex patients often present with both low back and PGP. When the painful SIJ is driving the movement behavior, the patient has difficulty weight bearing on the involved side and often uses a cane. There is either a history of trauma to the pelvis or an autoimmune disorder that is creating the intra-articular synovitis. When assessing the individual's strategies for function and performance, there is very early loss of control of the SIJ when the patient is asked to load the painful side in standing. Compression of the pelvis during this task increases the unilateral PGP significantly. In supine, three or four of the known PGP pain provocation tests (i.e., distraction, compression, posterior thigh thrust, and sacral thrust) must be positive

TABLE **17-4**

Differentiating Features of Common Clinical Conditions (Pathologies) Pertaining Specifically to the Sacroiliac Joint

Pathology	Story	Active Osteokinematic Mobility	Passive Arthrokinematic Mobility	Test for Weight-Bearing Control	Intervention
Articular system—painful SIJ	Trauma or autoimmune disorder	Too painful to test	Too painful to test	Early loss of SIJ control, worsens with any pelvic correction or compression	Refer to specialist for intra-articular injection
Articular system—stiff SIJ	Trauma, not recent	Reduced	Reduced—all 3 parts Position—intrapelvic torsion	No loss of control	Specific SIJ grade 4 mobilization
Articular system—fixated	Trauma recent or if in the past multiple episodes with intermittent relief with manipulation	Reduced	Reduced—all parts Position—apparent shear of either the innominate or the sacrum	No loss of control when the joint is fixated	Specific distraction manipulation focused to the subluxed part of the SIJ
Articular system—"loose"	Past history of trauma with or without episodic fixation	Variable, may be reduced or not	Excessive Form closure mechanism tests may be normal, i.e., neutral zone, motion controlled, or abnormal depending on resting tone of deep muscular stabilizers	Loss of control early in task	Depends on whether laxity is due to loss of capsular integrity or neuromuscular resting tone Options: Motor control training or prolotherapy
Neural system—excessive compression	Nothing that differentiates	Inconsistent, reduced, or normal and varies with task and repetition of task	Often reduced at one particular part of the joint	Loss of control at a variable time in the task, sometimes early, sometimes late	Release the overactive muscles, facilitate the underactive muscles, motor control training for optimal synchronicity and synergy (brain training)

(Continued)

TABLE **17-4**

Differentiating Features of Common Clinical Conditions (Pathologies) Pertaining Specifically to the Sacroiliac Joint—Cont'd

Pathology	Story	Active Osteokinematic Mobility	Passive Arthrokinematic Mobility	Test for Weight-Bearing Control	Intervention
Neural system—insufficient or inappropriate compression	PGP aggravated by vertical loading tasks of variable duration	Often normal mobility (symmetric)	Often normal mobility with no part of the SIJ compressed Symmetric	Inconsistent loss of control, varies with repetition and task dependent	Motor control training to restore optimal synchronicity and synergy (brain training) then strength and conditioning for tasks desired in life
Myofascial system—diastasis rectus abdominis—nonsurgical	Pregnancy-related, excessive IAP secondary to a fatty omentum Nonoptimal abdominal wall strategies	Variable depending on compensatory strategy used to transfer loads through the low thorax, lumbar spine, and pelvis	Variable	Loss of control with neural system deficits of insufficient force closure secondary to nonoptimal motor control strategies	Motor control training to restore optimal synchronicity and synergy (brain training) then strength and conditioning for tasks desired in life
Myofascial system—diastasis rectus adbdominis—surgical	Pregnancy-related or excessive IAP secondary to fatty omentum	Variable depending on compensatory strategy used to transfer loads through the low thorax, lumbar spine, and pelvis	Variable	Loss of control with optimal neural system and motor control that is unable to generate tension in the linea alba sufficient to force close and stabilize the joints of the low thorax, lumbar spine, and/or pelvis	Recti plication and abdominoplasty followed by motor control training
Visceral system—causing excessive compression of the SIJ	Low abdominal symptoms	Often reduced	Various parts of the SIJ are compressed and the vector of pull comes from inside the pelvis, i.e., from the visceral structures	Loss of control	Restore "alignment" position and mobility of pelvic organs in order to reduce compression of the SIJ

SIJ, Sacroiliac joint; *PGP,* pelvic girdle pain; *IAP,* intra-abdominal pressure.

for a definitive diagnosis of a painful SIJ.[83] This is not a common pathology, or condition, seen in outpatient orthopedic physical therapy practice. More often one of the four SIJ pain provocation tests is positive and more likely related to nociception arising from one or more of the SIJ ligaments. Vleeming et al.[84] found that 98% of patients with a positive Active Straight Leg Raise Test[65] had pain arising from the long dorsal sacroiliac ligament, a

ligament known to tense when the innominate anteriorly rotates or the sacrum counter-nutates.

Most modes of physical therapy (e.g., manual therapy, exercise, belts, taping) aggravate pain that is truly arising from the SIJ. In this author's experience, the best intervention for this pathology is an intra-articular injection of lidocaine and corticosteroid under fluoroscopic guidance. Once the joint pain subsides and pelvic correction and compression improve the ability to transfer loads through the pelvis, physical therapy can begin.

When the ligaments of the pelvis are the source of the patient's pain, treatment is indicated; however, the location of pain (and the specific structure) is often not helpful in patient management. Clinical reasoning of the multiple findings on movement analysis is necessary to generate a sound hypothesis as to why the ligament is generating pain. Then the appropriate intervention is clear.

The Stiff Sacroiliac Joint—An Articular System Impairment

Patients with a stiff SIJ present with a history of trauma that may not be recent. They often have a compensatory "irritated" contralateral SIJ and/or lumbosacral junction due to the altered biomechanics induced by the asymmetric intrapelvic mobility this impairment causes. Therefore the site of pain is often misleading. On active mobility testing (i.e., osteokinematics), the innominate will fail to posteriorly rotate relative to the ipsilateral sacrum and the pelvis may or may not laterally tilt on the contralateral hip joint. On passive mobility testing (i.e., arthrokinematics), the amplitude of motion in the neutral zone is reduced compared with the opposite side. This reduction in motion is apparent at all three parts of the joint (i.e., superior, middle, and inferior), and the end feel in the elastic zone is short, firm, and nonspringy. There is no loss of intrapelvic control during single leg standing. The pelvis is often twisted such that the innominate on the stiff side is anteriorly rotated relative to the contralateral innominate. This articular system impairment requires a specific mobilization technique and should be directed at all three parts of the SIJ (Figure 17-13).[29] Full range of motion of the stiff SIJ should be achieved in one or two treatment sessions.

The Fixated Sacroiliac Joint—An Articular System Impairment

There is some debate as to whether this condition truly exists or whether it is merely a severely compressed joint. Every time the author begins to be convinced that it does not exist, she sees a patient who convinces her that on the rare occasion, especially in a young individual with insufficient form closure, this can occur. The individual with a fixated SIJ presents with a history of trauma and can remember exactly when and what happened. Often the first thing noticed is the inability to weight bear on the affected side after the injury. Walking is difficult in the early stages of this impairment, and in all cases an obvious limp is present. If the patient has seen other practitioners, he or she may report intermittent relief of pain and restoration of partial function when the SIJ was manipulated. However, the reduction of pain and restoration of function often do not last. The findings vary and depend on whether or not the SIJ is fixated at the time of examination. The following describes the findings of a

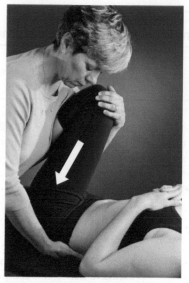

Figure 17-13 Passive mobilization technique for the stiff, "fibrotic" SIJ. After the SIJ is taken to the barrier for posterior rotation, the femur is slightly adducted and medially (internally) rotated. From here, the specific vector of resistance that is restricting motion of the SIJ is determined by applying a dorsolateral force (*arrow*) in a variety of directions. The clinician is looking for the vector of greatest resistance. Once this vector is found, a sustained grade 4 mobilization technique is used to release the joint. (From Lee D: *The pelvic girdle*, ed 4, Edinburgh, 2011, Elsevier.)

fixated SIJ. Of note is the immediate impression on palpating the pelvis that something is "not right" in that the shape of the pelvis is distorted. The shape of the pelvis with a fixated SIJ differs from the common intrapelvic torsion, in which one innominate is anteriorly rotated to the other and the sacrum is rotated in between. The fixated SIJ causes the pelvis to feel as though it has been sheared either in the craniocaudal plane (i.e., innominate upslip or downslip) or in the anteroposterior plane (i.e., sacral anterior-posterior shear lesion). Active SIJ mobility is not only reduced, but it feels like the joint is fused as well. There is no loss of control, and the ability to weight bear depends on the level of pain at the time of examination. Passively it is impossible to find the joint line to even test arthrokinematic mobility of the fixated SIJ. This system impairment requires a specific distraction manipulation focused on the most compressed part of the joint (Figure 17-14).[29] Immediately after the manipulation, many mobility findings change, including the SIJ's active mobility (restored), passive mobility (may be excessive), and control (usually there is now loss of control). To prevent refixation when the pelvis is next loaded, the joint should be well supported (compressed) with either tape or a sacroiliac belt (see *Role of Taping and Pelvic Belts* later).

The Loose Sacroiliac Joint—An Articular System Impairment

The individual with a loose SIJ may have true laxity of the passive restraints (i.e., capsule and ligaments) or more

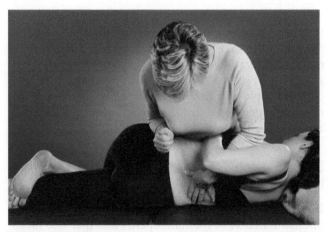

Figure 17-14 A high-velocity, low-amplitude thrust technique directed precisely at the fixated, or severely compressed, SIJ while stabilizing L5-S1 can have an immediate effect on improving the alignment and biomechanics of the SIJ. Subsequently, there is often loss of SIJ control, and the entire pelvic ring needs temporary support from an external force (e.g., taping or sacroiliac belt) until force closure and motor control strategies are restored. (From Lee D: *The pelvic girdle*, ed 4, Edinburgh, 2011, Elsevier.)

commonly a reduction in resting tone of the deep muscular stabilizers, giving a "false positive" for a loose joint. This patient may have been told that he or she has an "unstable SIJ," a cognitive belief with possible catastrophic results. A true loose SIJ is an articular instability and exists when the capsule and ligaments of the SIJ have been significantly stretched so that the force closure and motor control mechanisms cannot control shear between the innominate and the sacrum. This patient also reports pelvic trauma (with or without fixation of the SIJ), and when there is poor control, the ligaments of the joint are often nociceptive. Active mobility findings are variable and depend on the compensatory stabilization strategy chosen. Some strategies excessively compress the SIJ in an attempt to stabilize it and thus reduce mobility. Alternatively, the joint may appear to have symmetric, or excessive, mobility when compared with the noninjured side. Passively the amplitude of neutral zone motion is increased (R1 is much further from 0), and pain is readily provoked when the capsule and ligaments are stretched with motion testing in the elastic zone. The quality of the end feel in the elastic zone varies from "soft" to "empty" (i.e., no end feel). Tests for efficacy of the form closure mechanism are required to differentiate the true loose SIJ (i.e., an articular system impairment) from the loss of neuromuscular control (i.e., a neural system impairment). Integrity of the passive restraints is necessary for the SIJ to become close-packed.

If, on passive arthrokinematic mobility testing of the SIJ:
1. The innominate is mobile relative to the sacrum at all three parts of the joint, but
2. It is not possible to close-pack the SIJ, and
3. Motion is still palpable in the neutral zone when you attempt to tighten all the major ligaments of the SIJ, then the hypothesis (pathology) is an articular instability or true loose joint.

Treatment depends on whether the deep muscles can compensate and control shear or movement of the SIJ during specific loading tasks that are required in the individual's life. If yes, then the combination of motor control and movement training is the intervention.[30,31] If no, then prolotherapy for the posterior ligaments of the SIJ should be considered before training.

The Poorly Controlled, Excessively Compressed Sacroiliac Joint—A Neural System Impairment

Several muscles together with their fascial attachments can overly compress the SIJ and thus impact its function. The patterns are numerous; however, there are common features. First of all, nothing in the history clearly differentiates this system impairment. Symptom onset is often insidious and the patient may have difficulty identifying a precipitating event. Poor habitual postures or strategies for movement often underlie this impairment. Active mobility of the poorly controlled yet excessively compressed SIJ is variable and often inconsistent. At times, active mobility of the SIJ is reduced and at other times, normal. The amplitude of active mobility can vary between repetitions of the same task or between different tasks. Importantly, this individual would not be a good candidate for inclusion in an intratester reliability study for active mobility testing of the SIJ. Findings on passive mobility of the SIJ are also inconsistent with high variability in the amplitude of neutral zone motion between parts of the joint tested. Commonly, overactivation of the superficial fibers of the lumbar multifidus or the longissimus portion of the erector spinae compresses the superior part of the SIJ, reducing motion in the neutral zone but not in the middle or inferior parts of the joint. Piriformis can compress and reduce motion of the entire SIJ or just the middle part, whereas iliococcygeus and/or ischiococcygeus can compress the inferior part. Because of its fascial connections with iliococcygeus, obturator internus can also compress the inferior part of the SIJ when overactive. These are but a few of the common patterns of altered resting tone of muscles that can impact both active and passive mobility of the SIJ. The compressed SIJ secondary to a neural system impairment often loses control in weight bearing but not always and not consistently. Treatment requires restoring optimal alignment of the trunk and synergy of the deep segmental and superficial muscles, a complex topic that deserves a chapter of its own.[29–31] It is important to remember that the pelvis may not be the driver and treatment may begin elsewhere in the body.

The Poorly Controlled, Insufficiently Compressed Sacroiliac Joint—A Neural System Impairment

This neural system impairment is very common in both genders of all ages. It is a result of anything that disrupts optimal sequencing and timing of muscular activation. Dyssynergies of muscle activation (i.e., altered motor control[85–87]) can disturb the force closure mechanism and create excessive stress and strain on the tissues that eventually become symptomatic. Treatment is often sought once symptoms persist or there is a loss of function. Patients may remember an event or a point in their life when the symptoms or loss of function began. A motor vehicle-, work-, or sport-related accident, pregnancy and/or delivery, surgery, abdominal illness, or an emotional crisis (e.g., divorce, death, loss of a significant relationship or position) can precipitate this condition. Sometimes the patient cannot identify a triggering event and will often ask, "How or why did this happen?" The active and passive mobility of the SIJ on the side of the PGP is often unremarkable, yet patients demonstrate an inability to control loads through the pelvis on this side. This may be a consistent or inconsistent finding, and it can sometimes depend on repetition of the aggravating task and sometimes depends on the task itself. There is no loss of articular integrity of the SIJ, and the tests for the form closure mechanism are normal. Evaluation of the recruitment patterning of the muscles that provide control to the SIJ reveals a wide variety of dyssynergies, including:

1. Delayed or absent activation or overactivation of left and right TrA muscles
2. Delayed or absent activation or overactivation of the PFMs (i.e., all three layers' left and right sides in a variety of patterns)
3. Delayed or absent activation or overactivation of the deep lumbosacral multifidus muscle
4. Overactivation of the transverse, vertical, or oblique fibers of the left and right IO muscles
5. Overactivation of the superficial fibers of multifidus, iliocostalis, longissimus muscles
6. Delayed or absent activation or overactivation of the obturator internus or externus muscles
7. Delayed or absent activation or overactivation of the gluteals, tensor fascial lata, adductors (long and short), sartorius, and quadriceps muscles

Any pattern can be present. Assessment is essential to guide the appropriate intervention for this condition. Similar to the excessively compressed SIJ, this condition requires restoration of optimal alignment of the trunk and synergy of the deep segmental and superficial muscles, a complex topic that deserves a chapter of its own.[29-31] It must be remembered that the pelvis may not be the driver and treatment may begin elsewhere in the body.

Diastasis Rectus Abdominis—A Myofascial System Impairment

It has been well established that TrA plays a crucial role in optimal function of the lumbopelvis and that one mechanism by which this muscle contributes to intersegmental[39] and intrapelvic[88] control is through fascial tension. A DRA muscle has the potential to disrupt the force closure mechanism and is a common postpartum occurrence.[12,89] Universally the most obvious visible change during pregnancy is the expansion of the abdominal wall, and, although most abdomens accommodate this stretch very well, others are damaged extensively (Figure 17-15).

One structure particularly affected by the expansion of the abdomen is the LA, the complex connective tissue that connects the left and right rectus abdominis muscles.[90] The width of the LA is known as the inter-recti distance (IRD) and normally varies along its length from the xyphoid to the PS. Beer et al.[91] measured the width of the LA with ultrasound imaging in 150 nulliparous women aged 20 to 45 years and found the mean width to be highly variable, reporting 7±5 mm at the xyphoid, 13±7 mm 3 cm above the umbilicus, and 8±6 mm 2 cm below the umbilicus. Mendes et al.[92] showed that ultrasound imaging is an accurate method for measuring IRD, and others have used this tool to measure the behavior of the LA during a variety of tasks.[93,94] A DRA is commonly diagnosed when the IRD exceeds what is thought to be

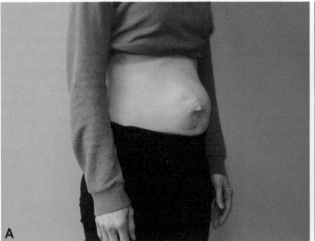
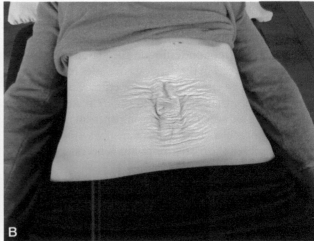

Figure 17-15 A, Standing relaxed abdominal profile of a woman with a DRA. **B,** When lying supine, the extensive damage to the midline abdominal skin is easily seen and this structural change extended through the layers of the superficial fascia to the LA. A comprehensive examination of the structure and behavior of the linea is necessary to determine whether trunk function can be restored with training or whether a surgical consultation should be considered. (Copyright Diane G. Lee Physiotherapist Corp.)

normal, although there is no standardized agreement as to what normal is.

There is little scientific literature on this condition. Boissonnault and Blaschak[95] found that 27% of women have a DRA in the second trimester and 66% in the third trimester of pregnancy. Fifty-three percent of these women continued to have a DRA immediately postpartum, and 36% remained abnormally wide at 5 to 7 weeks postpartum. Gilliard and Brown[89] reported that 100% of women had a DRA in their third trimester. Coldron et al.[93] measured the IRD from day 1 to 1 year postpartum and noted that the distance decreased markedly from day 1 to 8 weeks and that without any intervention there was no further reduction in the IRD at the end of the first year. In the urogynecological population, 52% of patients were found to have a DRA.[12] Sixty-six percent of these women had at least one support-related pelvic floor dysfunction (e.g., stress urinary incontinence, fecal incontinence, and/or pelvic organ prolapse). There are no studies to guide clinicians on what is the best treatment for postpartum women with DRA.

Clinically it appears that there are two subgroups of postpartum women with DRA:
1. Those who are able to restore optimal strategies for transferring loads through the trunk (including the pelvis) with or without achieving closure of the DRA through a multimodal treatment program, such as the ISM approach (Figure 17-16), and
2. Those who fail to achieve optimal strategies for transferring loads through the trunk, in spite of (a) having optimal function of the trunk musculature, (b) not having a loss of articular integrity of the SIJs or PS, and (c) in whom the IRD remains greater than normal (i.e., nonoptimal myofascial system).

In multiple vertical loading tasks (e.g., single leg standing, squatting, walking, moving from sit to stand, and climbing stairs), FLT through the joints of the lower thorax, lumbar spine, and/or pelvic girdle is consistently found.

The second subgroup of postpartum women with a DRA appear to have sustained significant damage to the midline fascial structures and can no longer generate sufficient tension through the abdominal wall for resolution of function (Figure 17-17). For this subgroup, a surgical plication of the recti along with an abdominoplasty to repair the midline abdominal fascia (i.e., the LA) and skin should be considered.[96]

The Poorly Controlled, Excessively Compressed Sacroiliac Joint—A Visceral System Impairment

The pelvic organs attach to the skeletal pelvis, and it is through these attachments that changes in pelvic alignment and excessive compression of the SIJ can be created. Assessment and specific treatment of the visceral system are outside the scope of this chapter except

to acknowledge the presence of these conditions and suggest how they can be differentiated from articular, neural, and myofascial system impairments. The key differentiating finding of this system impairment is the location of the vector of force creating compression of the SIJ noted during passive arthrokinematic mobility testing. The pull (vector) can clearly be felt and comes from inside the pelvis and not from the muscles on the outside of the skeleton or from the pelvic floor. If the pelvic organs (e.g., bladder, uterus, ovaries, fallopian tubes, sigmoid colon) are approximated toward the compressed SIJ and the passive mobility test is repeated and mobility is restored, then articular, neural, or myofascial system impairments can be ruled out. The reader is referred to the Barral Institute (www.barralinstitute.com) for more information, courses, and resources on visceral system impairments and their role in pelvic pain and impairments.

PRINCIPLES OF TREATMENT AND THE INTEGRATED SYSTEMS MODEL FOR DISABILITY AND PAIN

Restoring pelvic health requires a clinician to have both tools for releasing the nonoptimal strategies that perturb alignment, mobility, and control of the pelvic joints, myofascia, and organs, and tools for training new strategies for function and performance through a wide variety of tasks. In the ISM approach the first step is to determine the best place in the body to intervene—in other words, identifying the primary driver because loss of pelvic alignment, mobility, and control may be secondary to impairments elsewhere in the body (e.g., foot, thorax, neck, cranium). It is beyond the scope of this chapter to describe the necessary interventions for pelvic pain and impairment that is driven by body regions extrinsic to the pelvis. This chapter will focus on the principles of treatment interventions for pelvic pain and impairment that are driven by specific system impairments within the pelvis, in other words the pelvic-driven pelvis. There are four components to most treatment sessions, and they can be summarized by the acronym RACM: Release, Align, Connect (or control), and Move (Table 17-5). The first part of treatment is to release whatever is causing the nonoptimal strategy for alignment, biomechanics, and control of the primary driver (in this instance the pelvis) (Figure 17-18).[29]

Releasing the Pelvic-Driven Pelvis

Cognitions and Emotions
On occasion, thoughts and feelings (i.e., cognitions and emotions) are the primary driver of the patient's pelvic pain and impairment and require "release" and understanding before any physical intervention or movement training. Releasing cognitive and emotional barriers (i.e., psychosocial factors) requires patient education that includes:

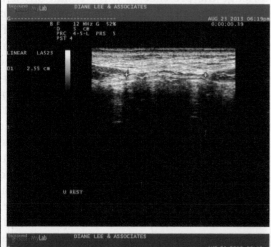

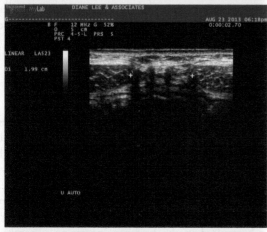

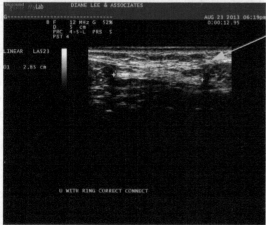

Note the difference in the inter-recti distance when two different abdominal strategies are used for the curl-up (CU) task

2.55 cm at rest

1.99 cm during CU with no transversus abdominis activation

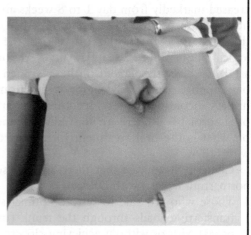

Note the shape and tension of the linea alba in this CU task

2.85 cm during CU with activation of transversus abdominis

Figure 17-16 This woman has a functional diastisis of the rectus abdominus muscles (DRA) that did not require a surgical intervention. Note the difference in the tension (echogenicity) and shape of the LA during the short head and neck curl up (CU) task with two different abdominal strategies. Also note how the IRD narrowed with the nonoptimal strategy that failed to generate tension in the LA (the gap closed from 2.55 cm at rest to 1.99 cm with the CU task), whereas when a coactivation of the deep and superficial abdominals occurred tension was generated in the LA and the IRD actually widened from 2.55 cm at rest to 2.85 cm. This finding was noted across multiple research subjects[96] and suggests that one should not be trying to narrow the IRD in patients with DRA. Focus should be on restoring optimal strategies of abdominal wall function that improve effective load transfer through the trunk. (From Jones MA, Rivett D: Jones MA, Rivett DA, eds: *Clinical reasoning for manual therapists*, ed 2, Edinburgh, 2017, Elsevier.)

1. Knowledge of the neuroscience of pain,[26,97,98] as well as
2. Provision of a logical hypothesis derived from the patient's history and clinical findings that explains both their experience (e.g., pain, numbness—the sensorial dimension) and their disability.

It is imperative that safe environments are created for this patient to explore his or her cognitive, emotional, and physical fears (i.e., fear-avoidance behavior) and to address comments such as "I'll never get better." Thoughts can become reality if the patient is convinced they are true.

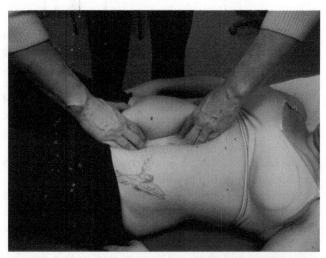

Figure 17-17 This woman's anterior abdominal wall required surgery to repair the midline LA. Despite having excellent motor control strategies, she was unable to stabilize the joints of her lower thorax, lumbar spine, or pelvic girdle due to the lack of force closure. Following surgery, specific motor control training restored function and reduced her multiple pain complaints. (Copyright Diane G. Lee Physiotherapist Corp.)

A significant part of treating a complex patient is to restore hope and have a treatment plan or intervention that resonates and seems reasonable. This is a starting point for facilitating change.[99] A primary goal of treatment is to "illuminate the path to change" and to empower the patient to take control of that path and be responsible for his or her pelvic health. For the patient with centrally sensitized pain, tools and techniques that reduce activity of the sympathetic nervous system and activate the parasympathetic nervous system can help to reduce the threat. These include various forms of meditation, Yoga Nidra, alternate nostril breathing (Nadi Shodhan or Anuloma Viloma Pranayama), and acupuncture, all helpful tools for empowering patients to take control of their nervous systems and change the input to their body–self neuromatrix. Change the sensory input, and the output will change. Helping the patient to create a cohesive story of their experience helps to integrate the amygdala (i.e., emotional memories of an experience) and hippocampus (i.e., autobiographical detail of that experience)[26] and again reduces the threat. Empower the patients with a sensitized nervous system such that they can take control and change their state of "flight, fright, or freeze" (i.e., states of threat) themselves.

Physical Impairments

Tools and techniques are also necessary to release the specific system impairments and change the sensory input to the neuromatrix from these sources. These include mobilization and manipulation techniques to release the stiff or fixated SIJ; release techniques for overactive muscles including release with awareness, muscle energy, and dry needling; fascial release techniques to restore inter- and intramuscular fascial mobility; techniques for restoring mobility of the dura and peripheral nerves (e.g., pudendal, sciatic, femoral, obturator, ilioinguinal, genitofemoral, lumbar plexus); and visceral release techniques. All of these release techniques are merely "clothes, shoes, and accessories in the closet," and the reader is encouraged to "shop" for lots of these tools. In my practice, the release with awareness technique combined with dry needling is highly useful for patients with pelvic pain.

Release with Awareness

This technique was first introduced in 2001[100] to treat "butt grippers"—individuals who habitually overactivate the ischiococcygeus muscles as part of their pelvic stabilization strategy. Release with awareness can be used on any muscle in the body that is facilitated due to increased neural drive—this is a neural system impairment. There is often a latent trigger point in the relevant muscle that the patient may not be aware of until the muscle is palpated. The trigger point is monitored with one hand with just enough pressure to increase the sensory awareness of the

---

TABLE **17-5**

Components of RACM—Release, Align, Connect and Control, and Move

Component	Description
Release	• Cognitive and emotional barriers are released with education as well as changing the "experience of the patient's body"—the clinical application of Melzak's body-self neuromatrix (see Figure 17-3) • Physical barriers require the clinician to have a wide variety of techniques to release articular, neural, myofascial, and visceral system impairments
Align	• Release cues and corrections are incorporated into movement practice to align the body both within and between regions
Connect and Control	• When necessary, specific connect cues are used to facilitate or "wake-up" more activation and coordination of the deep and superficial muscle systems of the trunk and also incorporated into the movement practice
Move	• The principles of neuroplasticity are used to rewire brain maps and create more efficient strategies for function and performance (put it all together to build a new brain map for the meaningful task) • Tissue healing and repair needs to be considered when adding loads to the movement program

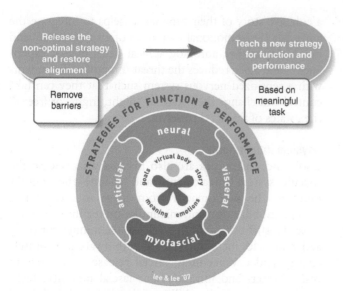

Figure 17-18 The two primary components of the treatment program according to *The ISM*. First, use techniques and movement training to release the barriers creating the nonoptimal strategy and then retrain (i.e., build) new strategies based on the meaningful task following neuroplastic and tissue repair principles. (From Lee D: *The pelvic girdle*, ed 4, Edinburgh, 2011, Elsevier.)

patient but not so much that it provokes pain. The joint or the muscle itself is moved so as to shorten the length of the muscle. This immediately reduces the afferent input to the spinal cord from the primary annulospiral ending in the intrafusal muscle fiber by reducing tension on the muscle spindle (Figure 17-19). Within 10 to 15 seconds a reduction in the tone of the muscle at the trigger point will be felt, if you wait for it. If you poke, prod, or provoke the muscle, it will defend against that sensory input and the reduction in tone will not occur.

The second part of the technique requires patients to be aware and engaged in what is happening in their body. They are asked to bring their attention to any sensation in the muscle being palpated while being given verbal cues by the clinician that facilitate relaxation or letting go. Clinicians provide cues that "stop the patients from doing something" as opposed to "patients doing something in addition to what they are already doing." For example, to release the ischiococcygeus the clinician can give cues such as "let my fingers sink into this muscle, let the sitting bones widen and your tailbone float" as opposed to "pull the sitting bones apart." The goal is to reduce activation. Therefore patients have to figure out how to stop doing something as opposed to adding on another layer of muscle activation that will further compress and restrict the joint. When the clinician feels the patient's nervous system respond to the manual and verbal cues, the patient is encouraged with positive reinforcement that the patient is on the right path. Patients will often say, "But I didn't do anything," to which the clinician can reply, "I don't want you to do something. I want you to stop doing something." Meanwhile the

clinician continues to move the joint in various combinations of movements that facilitate further relaxation of the muscle until no further release is obtained. If the clinician moves the joint from this point in any direction, another barrier will often be engaged. The osteopathic physicians call this a "still point." After a short period of time an "expansive release" occurs, following which the muscle(s) will relax further, allowing more lengthening and greater range of joint motion.

The last part of this *release with awareness* technique is to take both the muscle and joint through this new range (i.e., into stretch or elongation of the muscle and to the new end of joint range). More release techniques for specific muscles pertaining to the thorax, lumbar spine, and pelvis can be found in the 4th edition of *The Pelvic Girdle*.[29] If the technique is successful, there will be an immediate improvement in both the active and passive mobility of the joint.

Aligning the Pelvic-Driven Pelvis

Following release of the compressive vectors, alignment of the pelvis often improves; however, old habits are hard to break, and movement training is essential if the release obtained in the treatment session is to be maintained and transferred into functional tasks. When retraining a squat task for a patient who complains of pelvic pain with sitting, it can be helpful to incorporate the specific release cues used in the treatment session into their movement training to build a better strategy for this task.

Connecting and Controlling the Pelvic-Driven Pelvis

Releasing and aligning the primary driver (especially if the driver is outside the pelvis [e.g., thorax, neck, cranium, foot]) can result in a dramatic improvement in the recruitment strategy of the muscular stabilizers of the pelvis (see *Tiana's Story* later). When the pelvis is the driver of the pelvic pain/impairment, correcting the pelvic alignment often restores the activation and synergy of the deep muscles that stabilize the pelvis (i.e., TrA, the PFMs, and deep fibers of multifidus). On occasion, specific cueing is necessary to further augment or "wake-up" a muscle that has been inhibited for a prolonged period of time.[30] In the following are some "best cues" for activation of TrA, multifidus, and the various muscular layers of the pelvic floor.

Transversus Abdominis

Using MRI and ultrasound imaging, Hides et al.[101] investigated the response of the abdominal wall to the cue "draw in the abdominal wall without moving the spine," a cue often referred to as the drawing-in maneuver or the abdominal hollowing cue. Thickness of both the TrA and IO muscles increased significantly during this cue, suggesting that it results in coactivation rather than isolation of either abdominal muscle. There is ongoing debate in the literature as to the necessity of being able to isolate

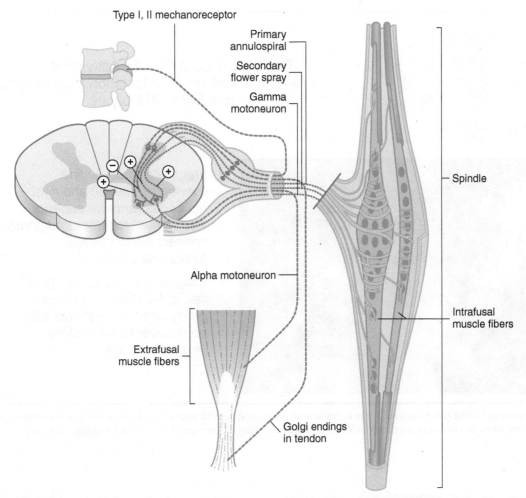

Figure 17-19 Activation of a muscle is influenced and controlled by many neural feedback loops involving the brain, spinal cord, and peripheral receptor systems. Changing the position of the joint and its associated muscles, tendons, and fascia can alter afferent input and thus efferent output to the related extrafusal muscle fiber. The result can be a decrease in activation of the targeted muscle at rest. This is called a *positional release*. Imagery and awareness can activate the higher centers that have a descending inhibitory influence on the efferent output to the extrafusal muscle fiber(s) and can further reduce a muscle's activation. (From Lee D: *The pelvic girdle*, ed 4, Edinburgh, 2011, Elsevier.)

TrA from IO, and clinically it appears more important that there is synergy of all muscles such that the strategy matches the demands of the task by providing mobility and control where needed. Strategies are highly individual and task specific. After the pelvis is released and neutral alignment restored, the following cues, asked of the patient, help to facilitate more activation of TrA:

1. Imagine a force, or line, connecting the left and right hip bones (ASISs) together and gently connect along this line (a bilateral cue) (Figure 17-20).
2. Imagine your hip bones (i.e., ASISs) are like an open book and gently close the right (or left) book cover to the midline (a unilateral cue).

Tactile cueing is given in conjunction with these verbal cues so that the brain receives consistent sensory input from several sources.

The Pelvic Floor Muscles

In a chapter pertaining to pelvic health, it is important to note the multiple functions of the PFMs, including but not limited to voiding, defecation, sexual arousal, pelvic organ support, breathing, and movement control of the joints of the pelvis, lumbar spine, and indirectly, the low thorax.

Optimal function of the pelvic floor requires not only that the anatomy and nerve supply be intact[102–104] but also that there be optimal coordination of contraction and relaxation (i.e., motor control of all three layers) as well as adequate strength and endurance for the specific task.

The pelvic floor is composed of three muscular layers, and each layer contains several muscles and related fascia (Figure 17-21). The most superficial layer (layer 1) contains the ischiocavernosus, bulbocavernosis (i.e., bulbo-spongiosus), superficial transverse perineal muscles, and the external anal sphincter. This layer has direct continuity with the short adductors of the thigh. The middle layer (layer 2) cannot be palpated, or assessed, externally and contains the compressor urethrae, external urethral sphincter, urethrovaginal sphincter, and deep transverse perineal muscles. The middle layer has direct continuity

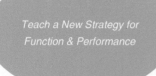

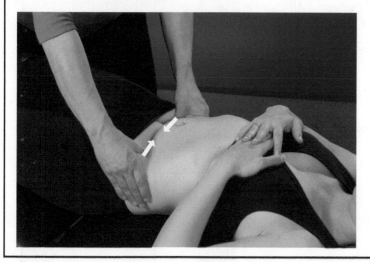

Finding the Best Cue for Activation of Transversus Abdominis in Isolation from Internal and External Oblique

- *Imagine a force, or line, connecting the left and right hip bones (anterior superior iliac spines) together and gently connect along this line (a bilateral cue)*

- *Imagine your hip bones (anterior superior iliac spines) are like an open book and gently close the right (or left) book cover to the midline (a unilateral cue)*

Figure 17-20 Manual and verbal cues to activate TrA in isolation from the more superficial internal and EO muscles. It is critical that the right layer is palpated, otherwise when TrA contracts, no tension will be felt in the fascial layer. (Copyright Diane G. Lee Physiotherapist Corp.)

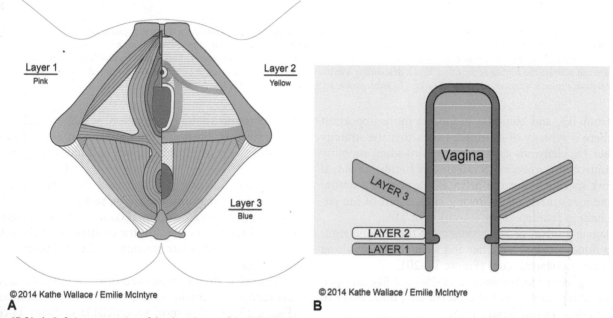

Figure 17-21 A, Inferior perspective of the three layers of the PFMs in the transverse plane. The first layer (*pink*) contains ischiocavernosus, bulbocavernosis, and the superficial transverse perineal muscles collectively known as the urogenital triangle and is easily palpated externally. The middle layer is not accessible to external palpation (*yellow*) and contains the perineal membrane (*yellow*), urethral sphincter (*circle* around the urethra), compressor urethra (extending from the pubic rami), urethrovaginalis (encompassing the urethra and the vagina), and deep transverse perineal muscles. The third and deepest layer is the levator ani (*blue*). The posterior part is accessible for external palpation and contains the puborectalis and iliococcygeus. The anterior and deeper parts of this layer (i.e., pubococcygeus, pubovisceralis, pubovaginalis) can only be palpated intravaginally. **B,** Coronal section through the three layers of the PFMs and illustrates the relationship and location of each layer to the vagina. Note that layer one is external to the vaginal entrance. (From Wallace K: *Reviving your sex life after childbirth, your guide to pain free and pleasurable sex after the baby*, pp 38, 115, Kathe Wallace, 2014. Copyright 2014 Kathe Wallace / Emilie McIntyre.)

with the fascia of TrA. The deepest layer of the pelvic floor (layer 3) is collectively called the levator ani, which is composed of the pubococcygeus (i.e., pubovisceralis, pubovaginalis), puborectalis, and iliococcygeus and has direct continuity through the arcus tendineus pelvis fascia and ATLA to the obturator internus and thus the hips. The posterior part of the levator ani can be palpated and assessed, externally.

In healthy individuals a gentle contraction of the pelvic floor results in an isolated contraction of TrA.[105] This does not occur in patients, especially those with pelvic pain, and this coactivation has not been found in those with urinary incontinence.[106] Assessment is always necessary to confirm the result of any given cue and many patterns will be found in clinical practice.

Many different dys-synergies exist in the three muscular layers of the pelvic floor, and it is common to need to release certain muscles and activate (i.e., wake-up) others. After the pelvis has been released and neutral alignment restored, the following cues can help to either facilitate more activation or release excessive activation of the various layers of the pelvic floor. These cues come from collaboration with Holly Herman and Kathe Wallace and their collective experience working with thousands of women with pelvic floor dysfunction and pelvic pain.

1. To activate the superficial layer: for women—nod the clitoris toward the vagina; for men—draw the glans of the penis in towards the body
2. To release the superficial layer: for women—imagine the clitoris lengthening away from the vagina; for men—think about lengthening the penis, widen the ischial rami (i.e., relax the superficial transverse perineal muscles)
3. To activate the middle layer—gently squeeze the muscles around the urethra as if to slow down the flow of urine
4. To release the middle layer—imagine the urethral tube expanding
5. To activate the deepest layer: levator ani—gently squeeze the anal sphincter and draw the anus up and forwards toward the back of the pubic bone
6. To release the deepest layer: levator ani—think about relaxing the anal sphincter to allow the passage of "wind" and let the distance between the tailbone and pubic bone lengthen

If the reflex connection between the PFMs and abdominal wall is impaired and coactivation does not occur, combining the abdominal and PFM cues may be useful.

The position of the lumbopelvis can influence activity of the PFMs.[107] In women with stress urinary incontinence, a reduced lumbar lordosis has been noted. An increased thoracic kyphosis and loss of lumbar lordosis is also associated with an increased incidence of vaginal prolapse.[108,109] PFM training is recommended as the first line of treatment for women with stress, urge, or mixed incontinence as well as pelvic organ prolapse.[110-112] However, debate continues as to the best way to train

the pelvic floor. Bump et al.[113] noted that 24% to 40% of women have decreased cortical awareness of their PFMs and will valsalva when attempting to do a PFM contraction. Alternatively, they may contract but not lift the levator plate. Others have good lift but are still incontinent.[114] When the PFMs are overactive, the lift of the levator plate may be restricted because this lift depends on the starting position of the PFMs.[115] Furthermore, the PFMs may be able to contract yet no tension is generated in the associated fascia due to loss of integrity.[103,104] Many individuals with pelvic pain and poor pelvic health present with asymmetry of resting tone, activation, and timing of contraction and relaxation of all, one, or a combination of the three layers of the pelvic floor. Asymmetric activation of the levator ani and ischiococcygeus has been found to displace the coccyx, innominate, and the femoral head,[116] providing evidence of the connectivity of this layer of the pelvic floor to the hip.

New perspectives from The ISM on how the PFMs function (e.g., activation, symmetry, relaxation) suggest that whenever the pelvis is twisted (i.e., intrapelvic torsion), there is a change in the neural drive to the PFMs and symmetry should not be expected. It is important to assess PFM function in both the habitual resting position of the pelvis and then with the pelvis manually corrected to neutral alignment to truly find the correlation between the activation pattern noted and the torsion. Then it is necessary to determine what is causing the torsion of the pelvis to direct treatment to the appropriate source of the problem (i.e., find the primary driver).

Multifidus

Multifidus is known to play a significant role in segmental control of the low back[117-119] and very likely the SIJ. Its deep segmental and superficial multisegmental fibers are differentially active during loading.[118] The central nervous system matches the activation of the deep and superficial multifidus to the demands of both the internal and external environments.[119] No studies have investigated whether this muscle coactivates with TrA or the PFMs, but clinically it appears to do so when strategies are optimal. Once again, the patterns of activation are highly variable in patients with PGP and/or poor pelvic health. It is known that within 48 hours of an acute low back injury, inhibition of the deepest fibers of multifidus occurs and recovery is not spontaneous.[120-122] No studies have specifically investigated whether the same inhibition occurs with an acute injury to the SIJ. Clinically, it appears that the deep fibers of the lumbosacral multifidus behave the same way such that both L5-S1 and the unilateral SIJ on the side of inhibition are affected.

The deep fibers of multifidus are contained in a fibroosseus compartment and act like a hydraulic amplifier[123] to stiffen the thoracolumbar fascia before loading. For this to occur, a certain size, or capacity, of the muscle is required in addition to an appropriate timing of activation.

In patients with unilateral PGP, it is common to find augmentation or increased resting tone of the superficial fibers of multifidus coexisting with inhibition of the deep fibers. This overactivation compresses the superior part of the SIJ, reducing both its active and passive mobility. It is also common in low back and pelvic pain patients to find augmentation of various parts of the erector spinae (i.e., iliocostalis or longissimus). MacIntosh and Bogduk[124] have identified the specific insertion point of each fascicle of iliocostalis and longissimus, which is interesting to consider clinically (Figure 17-22). Overactivation of longissimus from T6 to T12 will pull the sacrum cranially (i.e., increase nutation) and enhance stabilization of the SIJs because sacral nutation increases form closure of the SIJs. Conversely, overactivation of iliocostalis from T4 to T12 will pull the posterior aspect of the iliac crest cranially (i.e., increase anterior rotation of the innominate) and reduce stabilization of the SIJs (unless the circumferential deep muscles can compensate) because anterior rotation of the innominate decreases form closure of the SIJ. Both longissimus and iliocostalis can induce a "twist" or intrathoracic rotation of the specific thoracic ring to which they attach through an inferior pull on either the transverse process or the posterior aspect of the rib (see Figures 17-9 and 17-10). Thus it is important to understand the relationship between the alignment, biomechanics, and control of the thorax and that of the pelvis and to determine which region is primarily at fault—in other words, find the primary driver!

Often the superficial fibers of erector spinae require specific release[29] before training of the deeper muscles[30] can begin. Sometimes, releasing the superficial muscles results in an "automatic wake-up" of the deeper muscles and no specific "cueing" or augmentation is required, whereas at other times, specific deep muscle training is required. Again, assessment is essential; no assumptions can be made in clinical practice. The following cues, asked of the patient, help to facilitate greater activation of the deep fibers of multifidus (after releasing and aligning anything that is causing the pelvis, lumbar spine, and/or thorax to twist):

1. For the sacral fibers: imagine a force, or line, connecting the posterior aspect of your hip bones (PSISs) together and gently connect along this line (bilateral cue)
2. For the lumbosacral fibers: imagine a line running from your groin through your pelvis to the L5 vertebra and connect along this line and then gently suspend (or lift, create space) this vertebra 1 mm above the one below (Figure 17-23).

Tactile cueing is given in conjunction with these verbal cues so that the brain can receive the sensory input.

Functional Muscle Units Revisited

Recently, new anatomical studies[125,126] have suggested that the back and abdominal muscles should no longer be considered independently because their fascial connections and compartments suggest that they are truly one integrated myofascial system (Figure 17-24). For example, Scheunke et al.[125] noted that forces induced by activation of the abdominals (i.e., all three layers) are transmitted to the transverse and spinous processes only if there is sufficient stiffness in the middle and posterior laminar fibers of the thoracolumbar fascia. This stiffness is, in part, generated by activation of multifidus (both deep and superficial fibers), longissimus, and iliocostalis. Again, synergy and coactivation of muscles appear to be more important than training deep versus superficial or local versus global muscles. In addition, muscular capacity (i.e., size) is critical for the generation of sufficient fascial tension, thereby enabling the effective transference of load. A DRA has the potential to disrupt this force closure mechanism if the activation of the abdominal and back muscles cannot generate sufficient tension in the LA for the transference of loads.

The goal for this part of the treatment session (connect and control) is to create (or remember) new neural networks (i.e., brain maps) for more efficient strategies. The initial training for connecting and control follows the principles of neuroplasticity and because clinicians know that "neurons that wire together, fire together,"[98] it is important to train coactivation patterns. It is also important

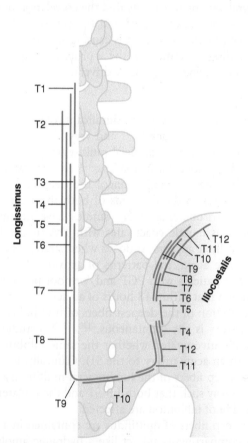

Figure 17-22 Note the specific point of insertion on the iliac crest of the fascicles of the iliocostalis muscle and on the lumbar and sacral spine of the longissimus muscle according to MacIntosh and Bogduk.[124] (Redrawn from MacIntosh JE, Bogduk N: The attachments of the lumbar erector spinae, *Spine* 16:783-792, 1991.)

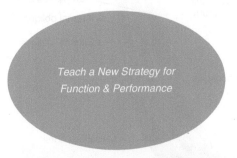

Finding the Best Cue for Activation of
Deep Multifidus in Isolation from
Superficial Multifidus and Erector Spinae

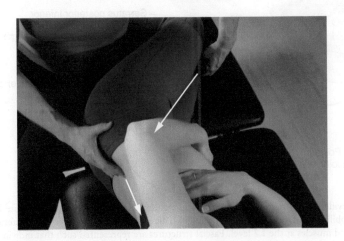

- Draw posterior superior iliac
  spines together

- "Guy wire" images combined
  with suspension cue

- Imagine a guy wire from:

  – Groin to segmental deep
    multifidus, then suspend
    this vertebra 1 mm above
    the one below

  – Leg to deep multifidus and
    then suspend the vertebra 1
    mm above the one below

Figure 17-23 Manual and verbal cueing for activating the deep fibers of lumbosacral multifidus in isolation from the superficial erector spine. (Copyright Diane G. Lee Physiotherapist Corp.)

to ensure that the patterns being trained are task specific and meet the functional requirements of the patient.

Movement Training for the Pelvic-Driven Pelvis

The principles of neuroplasticity[98,127,128] are used to create or rewire new brain maps for more efficient strategies for function and performance. Neuroplasticity has been defined as *"The ability of the nervous system to respond to intrinsic and extrinsic stimuli by reorganizing its structure, function and connections."*[127] The nervous system is embodied[26] and therefore influenced by our thoughts, feelings, and actions. Change is constantly occurring through our entire life.

Key Factors for Facilitating Neuroplastic Change

- Focused attention with awareness
- Train tasks that have meaning
- High-quality massed practice
- Normalize the sensory input
- Provide positive feedback of performance of task
- Train specificity of task
- Prescribe visualization

Clinical Note

"There is overwhelming evidence that the brain is continuously remodeled in response to new or novel experiences. Therefore, an appreciation of the influence of the central nervous system on all forms of movement as well as pain should underpin all forms of rehabilitation."

(Snodgrass et al.[127])

Re-wiring new brain maps is not easy and requires focused attention or awareness without distractions that take attention away from the body's experience when training. Learning and change can occur when there is awareness and is facilitated when tasks are trained that have meaning. Although correct instruction of supine bent knee fallout exercises can facilitate strength and endurance of the muscles that stabilize the pelvis and these exercises do play a role in rehabilitation,[30] the enhanced performance may not cross over into functional tasks, such as a squat or single leg stand (let alone exalted warrior in yoga).

Massed practice of high-quality strategies that normalize the sensory input to the neuromatrix will increase

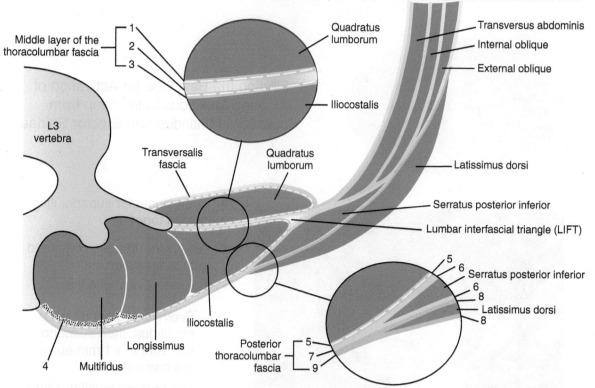

Figure 17-24 Anatomical and biomechanical studies provide evidence for training the deep and superficial systems synergistically because loads are distributed when there is appropriate coactivation such that mobility is not lost at the cost of stability. This is a transverse section of the posterior (PLF) and middle layer (MLF) of the thoracolumbar fascia and related muscles at the L3 level. Fascial structures are represented such that individual layers are visible, but not necessarily presented to scale. The serratus posterior inferior (SPI) often is not present caudal to the L3 level. The TrA muscle is covered with a dashed line on the peritoneal surface illustrating the transversalis fascia (TF). This fascia continues medially covering the anterior side of the investing fascia of the quadratus lumborum (QL). Anteriorly and medially, the TF also fuses with the psoas muscle fascia (not drawn). The IO and EO are seen external to TrA. SPI is highly variable in thickness and, more often than not, absent on the L4 level. Latissimus dorsi (LD) forms the superficial lamina of the PLF together with the SPI, when present. The three paraspinal muscles, multifidus, longissimus, and iliocostalis, are contained within the paraspinal retinacular sheath (PRS). The aponeurosis (tendon) of the paraspinal muscles (4) is indicated by stippling. The epimysium of the individual spinal muscles is very thin and follows the contours of each separate muscle within the PRS. The epimysium is not indicated in the present figure but lies anteriorly to the aponeurosis (4). The upper circle shows a magnified view of the different fascial layers contributing to the MLF. The picture shows that MLF is made up of three different structures: (1) this dashed line depicts the investing fascia of QL; (3) this dashed line represents the PRS, also termed the deep lamina of the PLF encapsulating the paraspinal muscles; (2) the thick dark line between the two dashed lines 1 and 3 represents the aponeurosis of the abdominal muscles especially deriving from TrA. Numbers 1, 2, and 3 form the MLF. The lower circle shows a magnified view of the different fascial layers constituting the PLF. The picture shows that on the L3 level, the PLF is also made up of three layers as the fascia of SPI is normally present on this level. (5) This dashed line depicts the PRS or deep lamina of the PLF encapsulating the paraspinal muscles; (6) the investing fascia of SPI is seen blending medially into the gray line marked (7) and representing the aponeurosis of SPI- posteriorly to the PRS; (8) this dark line represents the investing fascia of LD blending medially into the black line representing the LD aponeurosis (9) posteriorly to the SPI aponeurosis. Numbers 5, 7, and 9 form the PLF. Numbers 7 and 9 form the superficial lamina of the posterior layer (sPLF). (Redrawn from Schuenke MD, Vleeming A, Van Hoof T, Willard FH: A description of the lumbar interfascial triangle and its relation with the lateral raphe: anatomical constituents of load transfer through the lateral margin of the thoracolumbar fascia, *J Anat* 221:569, 2012.)

the speed of synaptic connectivity and thus the ease of use of the strategy. How much is enough? Research by Tsao and coworkers[129-131] suggested the following prescription for training new strategies for lumbopelvic control—the goal is to achieve three sets of 10, 10-second holds of the optimal strategy with a 2-minute rest in between sets and to perform this training at least twice, preferably 3 to 4 times per day. When compliant, the brain map will be consolidated and less conscious effort is required in as little as 2 weeks.[130] Patients need to have the awareness to know when they are using an optimal strategy for every training task and to only perform high-quality movement patterns. Attending to the effort

it takes to perform the task (e.g., single leg lift, bent knee fallout, clam shell, squat, single leg stance with weight shift, lunge, exalted warrior) will inform patients when the strategy is optimal or not because good strategies feel good (e.g., effortless, light, less symptomatic). The gestalt of their experience improves when patients train strategies that are better for their pelvic health. Imagery, or visualization, of what a good strategy "looks like" can also help.

When designing movement training for the restoration of pelvic health, consideration must be given to the entire body or whole kinetic chain because everything can have an impact on function and performance of the pelvis.[31]

At minimum, the following regions should be monitored during training:

1. Local control of:
   a. 3 pelvic joints
   b. 2 hip joints
   c. 15 lumbar joints
   d. 130 thoracic joints (10 complete thoracic rings), and
2. Interregional control between the:
   a. Thorax and pelvis
   b. Shoulder girdle and pelvis
   c. Feet-knees and pelvis
   d. Neck-cranium and pelvis, and
3. Postural and motion control between the body and the environment.

Role of Taping and Pelvic Belts

After the system impairments driving the nonoptimal strategy have been released, it is not uncommon to find poor control of the joints of the pelvis. Compression of the pelvis will now improve both the experience and performance of meaningful tasks. Neuromuscular retraining to create new motor strategies takes time, and the provision of temporary support via taping or belting the pelvis can be useful for mechanical and neuroplastic learning purposes.[69,132-134] Although general compression of the pelvis can help, more often, specific compression of the pelvis is necessary. The COM-PRESSOR SI belt and The Baby Belly Belt™ (Figure 17-25) are designed to apply pelvic compression specifically where it is needed and this can be highly individual. Both belts have an additional elastic strap that is versatile and can be applied to the underlying belt either anterior or posterior to the SIJ. The elastic straps are applied according to which compression location makes the meaningful task easier to perform. If the task does not improve with compression anywhere in the pelvis, belts or taping will not be helpful.

Getting to "WOW"!

Changing patients' experience of their body in tasks that have meaning for them often elicits comments such as "Wow! What did you do?" This is the first step to creating new, more efficient ways for them to live, move, and simply be in their bodies. Dan Siegel[26] calls this "SNAG the brain," his acronym for Stimulate Neuronal Activation and Growth and in the ISM is called "Getting to WOW!".

CLINICAL CASE

To pull this all together, a clinical case of a young woman who does not have a pelvic-driven pelvis but rather a thorax-driven pelvis and her meaningful complaint, stress urinary incontinence, will be shared. From her story, the reader will be able to appreciate that many clinicians would have treated her pelvis directly; however, The Integrated Systems Model directed the clinician elsewhere. It is reproduced here with permission.[135]

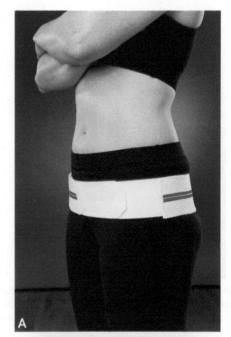

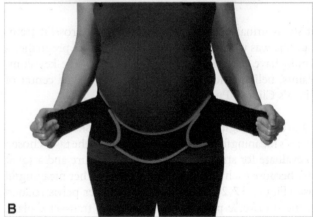

Figure 17-25 The COM-PRESSOR sacroiliac (SI) belt (**A**) and The Baby Belly Belt™ (**B**) are two SI belts designed by Diane Lee for the application of specific compression to the pelvis. Both belts are adaptable in that compression can be applied to the front or back (or to the front on one side and the back on the other) of the pelvis and specific assessment determines the best location. (**A**, From Lee D: *The pelvic girdle*, ed 4, Edinburgh, 2011, Elsevier; **B**, from Lee DG: New perspectives from the Integrated Systems Model for treating women with pelvic girdle pain, urinary incontinence, pelvic organ prolapse and/or diastasis rectus abdominis, *J Assoc Chartered Physiother Womens Health* 114:10-24, 2014.)

Tiana's Story

Tiana is a 25-year-old nurse who does CrossFit training five to six times per week and as a consequence of this high-intensity training has had multiple muscle strains and injuries. As her ability and training increased, she noticed increasing urinary frequency. Recently, she noticed that if she did not void often she experienced stress urinary incontinence especially with tasks that loaded the trunk or increased her intra-abdominal pressure (i.e., box jumps). Tiana is nulliparous.

Tiana's Meaningful Complaint

Primary concerns for Tiana included the increasing frequency of her need to void and the increasing incidence

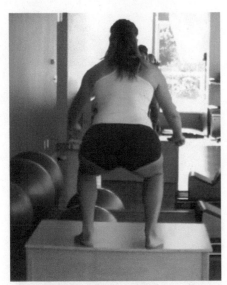

Figure 17-26 Tiana's meaningful task is a box jump. Note how in the landing phase of Tiana's box jump her weight is more to the right of her base of support. (Copyright Diane G. Lee Physiotherapist Corp.)

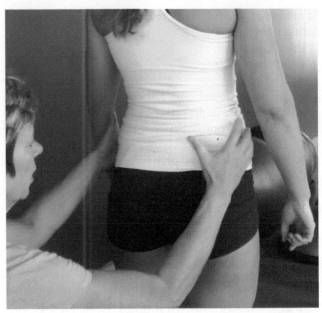

Figure 17-27 In standing, Tiana's pelvis was rotated to the right in the transverse plane (TPR right) and associated with a congruent right intrapelvic torsion (IPTR). (Copyright Diane G. Lee Physiotherapist Corp.)

of stress urinary incontinence during her CrossFit training. She was worried about the impact future pregnancies would have on her urinary continence. These key complaints, beliefs, and goals were entered into the center of Tiana's Clinical Puzzle.

Tiana's Meaningful Task and Screening Tasks

Tiana's meaningful task was a box jump and the tasks chosen to evaluate for strategy were standing posture and a squat task because each of these directly relate to her meaningful task (Figure 17-26). Tiana stood with her pelvis rotated in the transverse plane to the right (i.e., transverse plane to the right [TPR] right) and her pelvis in an intrapelvic torsion to the right (i.e., intrapelvic torsion to the right [IPTR] = left innominate anteriorly rotated relative to the right innominate, sacrum right rotated) (Figure 17-27). Her lower thorax (thoracic rings 8 to 10) was rotated to the left (i.e., TPR left lower), the seventh thoracic ring was shifted left and rotated right, and the sixth thoracic ring was shifted to the right and rotated to the left.

Correcting the alignment of the two thoracic rings (six and seven) improved the pelvic position, whereas correcting the alignment of the pelvis made the thorax posture and position worse. This suggested that the thorax was driving the pelvic position as opposed to the pelvis driving the thorax and that further investigation of what was causing the malalignment of the sixth and seventh thoracic rings was needed.

During a squat, the following sites of FLT (i.e., nonoptimal alignment, biomechanics, or control) were noted, including the timing of when they failed:

1. The seventh thoracic ring shifted further to the left and rotated to the right, and the sixth thoracic ring shifted further to the right and rotated to the left before
2. The left SIJ gave way (i.e., the left innominate anteriorly rotated relative to the sacrum)

When the alignment of the sixth and seventh thoracic rings was corrected, the left SIJ no longer failed. In comparison, when the left SIJ was controlled, the sixth and seventh thoracic rings continued to shift and rotate during the squat task, a sign of FLT. These findings suggested that the sixth and seventh thoracic rings were the primary driver and that further assessment should focus on determining what was causing the loss of alignment, biomechanics, and control of the sixth and seventh thoracic rings.

The supine bent leg raise task was not relative to her meaningful task of box jumping; however, for Tiana to know if she was correcting her thoracic rings properly, it was useful as part of her exercise training. Tiana found that more effort was required to lift her left leg (with the knee bent) than her right leg. No change in effort was noted when the twist was taken out of her pelvis (i.e., intrapelvic torsion right). However, the task was much easier to perform when the seventh thoracic ring was corrected (Figure 17-28). During this task, the sixth thoracic ring self-corrected when the seventh thoracic ring was corrected, so the focus of correction could be on just the seventh thoracic ring.

Hypothesis of Tiana's Primary Driver

Correction of the sixth and seventh thoracic rings improved the performance of Tiana's standing posture, squat task, and the ability to lift her left leg while supine. Thus these thoracic rings were hypothesized to be the primary driver. Further system analysis (i.e., neural, articular, myofascial, visceral [or combination]) was required to determine what was causing the nonoptimal alignment of the sixth and seventh thoracic rings across multiple tasks.

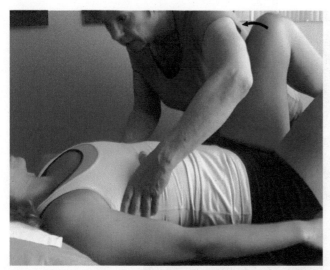

Figure 17-28 The active bent leg raise test was much easier for Tiana to perform on her left side when the seventh thoracic ring alignment was corrected, further supporting the hypothesis that the nonoptimal alignment and biomechanics of the seventh thoracic ring were impacting her ability to transfer loads effectively through her pelvic girdle in this task. (Copyright Diane G. Lee Physiotherapist Corp.)

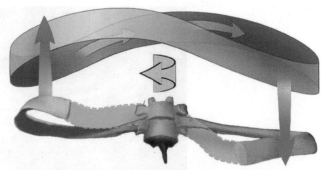

Figure 17-29 The left external oblique fascicle attaching directly to the left seventh rib can produce anterior rotation of this rib and thus right rotation of the entire seventh thoracic ring. (Copyright Diane G. Lee Physiotherapist Corp.)

Vector Analysis of Tiana's Primary Driver

When correcting the sixth and seventh thoracic rings, a resistant vector of force was felt from the left side of her upper abdominal wall. On palpation, increased tone was noted in the left EO muscle. The hypertonicity covered a number of thoracic rings and was regional, not fascicle specific. However, the primary impact was on the seventh thoracic ring. A specific fascicle of the EO muscle has the ability to anteriorly rotate one rib. However, this rib is part of an entire thoracic ring, such that when the rib anteriorly rotates on the left, it can potentially produce left translation and right rotation of the entire thoracic ring (Figure 17-29).[136] When the seventh thoracic ring was corrected, the sixth thoracic ring self-corrected, suggesting that the primary impaired thoracic ring was the seventh thoracic ring. The next question was, "What was the impact of this increased tone in the left external oblique muscle on the recruitment strategy of the entire abdominal wall?" This led to the next part of the examination, a neural system analysis of the abdominal wall.

Neural System Analysis of Tiana's Abdominal Wall

More palpable tension was noted superficially on the left side of Tiana's lower abdomen, likely due to the increased resting tone of the left EO muscle. When asked to gently contract her pelvic floor, increased activation of the left EO was palpable as an immediate first response. Ultrasound imaging revealed that the right TrA responded appropriately to this cue and the left TrA did not (Figure 17-30). When the seventh thoracic ring was corrected, there was less superficial abdominal tension and a symmetric activation of both the left and right TrA was felt and seen via ultrasound imaging (Figure 17-31).

Neural System Analysis of Tiana's Pelvic Floor

A transabdominal anteroposterior ultrasound evaluation of the pelvic organs and fascial support system revealed asymmetry of the bladder when the pelvis was resting in an IPTR (Figure 17-32, *A*). Contraction of the PFMs appeared to increase the asymmetry of her bladder. When the seventh thoracic ring was corrected (thus neutralizing the position of the pelvis), the shape of the bladder was more symmetric, as was the pelvic floor lift (Figure 17-32, *B*).

A transabdominal sagittal view of the pelvic floor contraction did not reveal any asymmetry because only the midline of the bladder and pelvic floor were imaged with this orientation. A good lift in an optimal location for urethral and bladder support was noted. A perineal real-time ultrasound view of Tiana's pelvic floor contraction when her pelvis was twisted (IPTR) revealed less lift (i.e., decreased amplitude) and less pelvic organ support during her cough (greater descent was seen) compared with when her pelvis was in a neutral position.

Intravaginal Examination of Tiana's Pelvic Floor

When Tiana's pelvis was in an IPTR, no activation of the left side of her levator ani was apparent on internal palpation (i.e., grade 0). The left side of the levator ani (i.e., iliococcygeus) was not hypertonic despite appearing to be elevated on the ultrasound examination. When her pelvic position was neutralized, better recruitment of the left side of her levator ani occurred immediately (i.e., grade 3); however, she could only hold this contraction for 5 seconds (i.e., an endurance deficit). Weakness and loss of endurance of the left side of the levator ani were still present in spite of removing the influence of the IPT on the recruitment strategy.

Hypothesis of Tiana's Story

The hypothesis was that Tiana had a muscle imbalance of abdominal wall (i.e., overactivation of the left EO muscle and underactivation of the left TrA muscle) creating a primary seventh thoracic ring shift to the left (i.e., seventh thoracic ring was right rotated). This thoracic ring shift appeared to be causing a compensatory rotation of the pelvis (i.e., TPR right and IPT right). There was insufficient activation of the deep muscle system (i.e., left TrA and PFM)

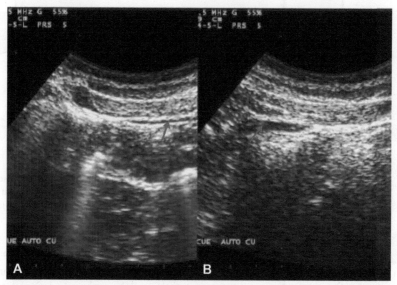

Figure 17-30 These are two ultrasound images captured from the video of the left (**A**) and right (**B**) sides of the abdominal wall in response to a verbal cue for Tiana to contract her pelvic floor muscles. Note the difference (*arrows*) in broadening and corseting of her transverse abdominis, in particular the lack of response on her left side. (Copyright Diane G. Lee Physiotherapist Corp.)

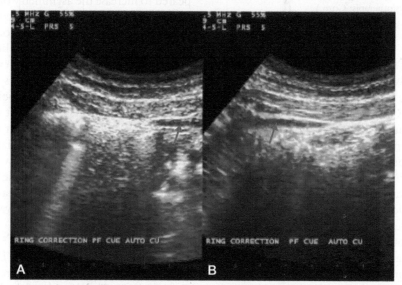

Figure 17-31 Note the increase (*arrow*) in the broadening of the left (**A**) transverse abdominis (TrA) (compared with Figure 17-30, *A*) with a verbal cue to contract the pelvic floor when the seventh thoracic ring is corrected. The broadening of the left (**A**) TrA is comparable with the right (**B**) TrA when the seventh thoracic ring is corrected (*arrows*). (Copyright Diane G. Lee Physiotherapist Corp.)

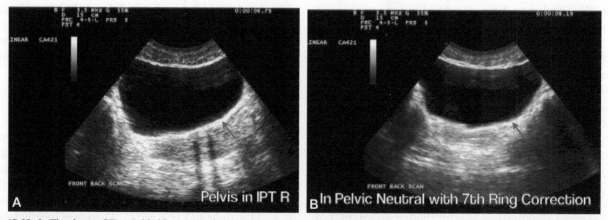

Figure 17-32 A, The shape of Tiana's bladder appeared asymmetric (imaged via ultrasound) when the pelvis was in a right intrapelvic torsion. **B,** Note the immediate change (*arrows*) in bladder shape when the pelvic alignment is corrected in response to the seventh thoracic ring correction. (Copyright Diane G. Lee Physiotherapist Corp.)

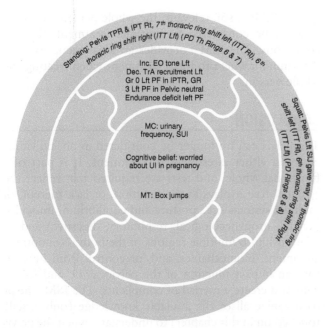

Figure 17-33 Tiana's completed Clinical Puzzle. *TPR*, Transverse plane to the right; *IPT*, intrapelvic torsion; *Rt*, right; *ITT*, intra-thoracic torsion; *Lft*, left; *PD*, primary driver; *Inc.*, increased; *EO*, external oblique; *Dec.*, decreased; *TrA*, tranversus abdominis; *PF*, pelvic floor; *IPTR*, intrapelvic torsion to the right; *MC*, meaningful complaint; *SUI*, stress urinary incontinence; *UI*, urinary incontinence; *MT*, meaningful task; *SIJ*, sacroiliac joint. (Copyright Diane G. Lee Physiotherapist Corp.)

and this was a likely cause for the loss of control of the left SIJ. The mechanism that changed the recruitment strategy of the left side of her pelvic floor was unclear. What was clear was that the left side of her levator ani was not recruited when her pelvis was twisted (IPTR). Although the activation improved when the twist of her pelvis was removed, there was an underlying strength and endurance deficit on this side of her pelvic floor. Collectively, all of this was creating poor urethral, bladder, pelvic, and sixth and seventh thoracic ring support during tasks which increased loading through the pelvis and its organs (i.e., the box jump). Her complete Clinical Puzzle is illustrated in Figure 17-33.

Treatment

According to the treatment principles of the Integrated Systems Model approach, the first step was to release the vectors that were creating nonoptimal alignment of the seventh thoracic ring and then restore optimal recruitment synergies of the abdominal wall.

Tiana's Treatment Program

STEP 1: Release the left external oblique (EO) muscle and align the sixth and seventh thoracic rings

STEP 2: Home exercise:

1. Supine: hook lying—ask patient to align the seventh thoracic ring and then breathe with a lateral costal expansion strategy for three to four breaths. Then, take the

patient's legs to the right on the inhale breath, hold and connect to TrA and the PFMs and then exhale to return the legs to neutral for three to four repetitions (Figure 17-34). Then, recheck the effort it takes to lift the left leg and it should be less.

2. Side-angle pose: position the left leg back and correct the seventh thoracic ring first. Next, unwind the right intrapelvic torsion, then rotate the thorax to the left to lengthen the left EO; hold this position for three breaths (Figure 17-35).

STEP 3: Connect and control and move

STEP 4: Home exercise:

1. Correct the alignment of the seventh thoracic ring, activate the pelvic floor (clinician feels for the contraction of the left side of the levator ani), and then perform three squats. (Note: The three home exercises should be performed before her CrossFit training workout.)

STEP 5: Strength and endurance training for the pelvic floor (home exercise)

1. Left side levator ani strength and endurance training: patient works up to 10 repetitions of 10-second holds in pelvic neutral, 3 times per day, at least 3 to 4 times per week. Clinician introduces both slow and fast contractions specific for CrossFit training after 4 to 6 weeks. Patient continues with intensive specific PFM training for at least 8 weeks.

FOLLOW-UP PLAN: Clinician reassesses symmetry of activation (i.e., motor control), strength, and endurance (i.e., performance) of the levator ani at 4 to 6 weeks, along with the ability to control the left SIJs, sixth and seventh thoracic rings, and maintain urethral closure during squats and box jumps. Pelvic floor muscle training can be progressed along with more advanced thoracopelvic alignment exercises as necessary at that time.

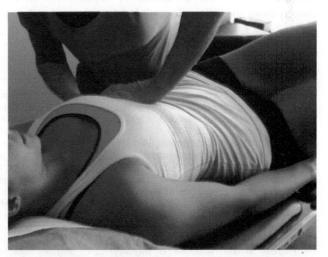

Figure 17-34 Release technique and home exercise practice for restoring adequate length and activation of the left external oblique (EO) muscle and thus the seventh thoracic ring. For the release technique, the therapist maintains the alignment of the seventh thoracic ring as the patient takes a deep lateral costal expansion breath and/or takes the knees to the right (thus, elongating the left EO). For the home exercise practice, the patient is taught to manually correct the seventh thoracic ring and to maintain the correction through the entire lateral costal expansion breath and while taking their knees to the right. (Copyright Diane G. Lee Physiotherapist Corp.)

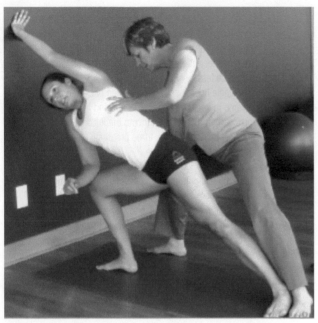

Figure 17-35 Modified extended side-angle pose (modified Parsvakonasana in yoga) is a useful exercise for releasing and aligning both the thorax (ring specific) and the pelvis to restore the relationship and between the multiple rings of the trunk. The focus in these tasks should always begin with correcting the primary driver. (Copyright Diane G. Lee Physiotherapist Corp.)

Summary

Tiana's story illustrates how nonoptimal strategies in the thorax can drive the loss of thoracic and pelvic ring control, as well as urinary frequency and incontinence. This is not uncommon yet is often missed when these patients are assessed "from the bottom up." Urinary frequency and incontinence can be caused by impairments far removed from the pelvic floor and although local training

of the PFMs is still relevant, the whole person and body need to be considered for optimal treatment of these conditions. The ISM[25] provides an ideal framework for determining where to focus treatment when treating the whole person.

CONCLUSION

The pelvis can no longer be considered as an individual entity in either assessment or treatment. It is part of a functional whole, and tests are required that reflect the essential role it plays in the function, or lack thereof, of multiple systems (i.e., posture and equilibrium, musculoskeletal, urogynecological, respiratory, digestive) and its relationship to multiple regions of the body. Nonoptimal alignment, biomechanics, and/or control from head to toe can impact function of the pelvic girdle and its organs and create a myriad of complaints. The ISM[25] helps to organize all of the available knowledge (only briefly touched on in this chapter) to understand when the pelvis is a victim (not the driver) and when it is the problem (the driver). Finding drivers requires the skill to not only interpret a finding but also find it reliably. For clinicians, visual and kinesthetic perceptions are foundational tools for assessing the human form in function. Understanding our individual strengths, weaknesses, accuracies, and misperceptions enhances our reliability and skills necessary to locate a finding. Clinical reasoning of the findings then determines its relevance to the clinical picture, which subsequently directs management of individual patients. Although clinical reasoning can be taught through texts and online media, there will always be a need for hands-on practical courses; this is the art and skill of physical therapy that is so difficult to measure with science.

REFERENCES

1. Larsen EC, Wilken-Jensen C, Hansen A, et al: Symptom-giving pelvic girdle relaxation in pregnancy. I: prevalence and risk factors, *Acta Obstet Gynecol Scand* 78:105–110, 1999.
2. Albert HB, Godskesen M, Westergaard JG: Incidence of four syndromes of pregnancy-related pelvic joint pain, *Spine* 27:28–31, 2002.
3. Östgaard HC, Andersson GJ, Karlsson K: Prevalence of back pain in pregnancy, *Spine* 16:549–552, 1991.
4. Östgaard HC, Zetherström G, Roos-Hansson E: Regression of back and posterior pelvic pain after pregnancy, *Spine* 21:2777-2780, 196.
5. Albert H, Godskesen M, Westergaard J: Prognosis in four syndromes of pregnancy-related pelvic pain, *Acta Obstet Gynecol Scand* 80:505–510, 2001.
6. Wu WH, Meijer OG, Uegaki K, et al: Pregnancy-related pelvic girdle pain (PPP), I: terminology, clinical presentation, and prevalence, *Eur Spine J* 13:575–579, 2004.
7. Morkved S, Bo K, Schei B, Salvesen KA: Pelvic floor muscle training during pregnancy to prevent urinary incontinence: a single blind randomized controlled trial, *Obstetr Gynecol* 101:313–319, 2003.
8. Wilson PD, Herbison P, Glazener C, et al: Obstetric practice and urinary incontinence 5-7 years after delivery, *ICS Proceedings Neurourology and Urodynamics* 21:284–300, 2002.
9. Mason DJ, Newman DK, Palmer MH: Changing urinary incontinence practice: this report challenges nurses to lead the way in managing incontinence, *Am J Nurs* 103(suppl):2–3, 2003.
10. Hagen S, Stark D: Conservative prevention and management of pelvic organ prolapse in women, *Cochrane Database Syst Rev* 12:2001, CD003882.
11. Pool-Goudzwaard A, Slieker ten Hove MC, Vierhout ME, et al: Relations between pregnancy-related low back pain, pelvic floor activity and pelvic floor dysfunction, *Int Urogynecol J Pelvic Floor Dysfunct* 16:468–474, 2005.
12. Spitznagle TM, Leong FC, Van Dillen LR: Prevalence of diastasis recti abdominis in a urogynecological patient population, *Int Urogynecol J Pelvic Floor Dysfunct* 18:321–328, 2007.
13. Cochrane AL: *Effectiveness and efficiency, random reflections on health services*, London, 1972, Nuffield Provincial Hospitals Trust, Reprinted in 1989 in association with the BMJ, Reprinted in 1999 for Nuffield Trust by the Royal Society of Medicine Press, London.
14. Stuge B, Lærum E, Kirkesola G, Vøllestad N: The efficacy of a treatment program focusing on specific stabilizing exercises for pelvic girdle pain after pregnancy, *Spine* 29:351–359, 2004.
15. Gutke A, Sjödahl J, Öberg B: Specific muscle stabilizing as home exercises for persistent pelvic girdle pain after pregnancy, a randomized, controlled clinical trial, *J Rehabil Med* 42:929–935, 2010.
16. McKenzie RA: *The lumbar spine: mechanical diagnosis and therapy*, Wellington, 1981, Spinal Publications.
17. Sahrmann S: *Diagnosis and treatment of movement impaired syndromes*, St. Louis, 2001, Mosby.
18. O'Sullivan P, Beales D: Diagnosis and classification of pelvic girdle pain disorders—Part 1: a mechanism based approach within a biopsychosocial framework, *Man Ther* 12:86–97, 2007.
19. Orchard J, Best TM: The management of muscle strain injuries: an early return versus the risk of recurrence, *Clin J Sport Med* 12:3–5, 2002.
20. Best TM, Garrett WE: Hamstring strains: expediting return to play, *Phys Sportsmed* 24:37–44, 1996.

21. Hoskins W, Pollard H: Hamstring injury management—Part 2: treatment, *Man Ther* 10:180–190, 2005.

22. Sackett DL, Straus S, Richardson WS, et al: *Evidence-based medicine. How to practice and teach EBM*, New York, 2000, Elsevier Science.

23. Jensen GM, Gwyer J, Hack LM, Shepard KF: *Expertise in physical therapy practice*, 2 ed, Philadelphia, 2007, Saunders.

24. Jones MA, Rivett D: Introduction to clinical reasoning. In Jones MA, Rivett DA, editors: *Clinical reasoning for manual therapists*, Edinburgh, 2004, Elsevier.

25. Lee L-J, Lee D: Clinical practice—the reality for clinicians. In Lee D, editor: *The pelvic girdle*, 4 ed, Edinburgh, 2011, Elsevier.

26. Siegel D: *Mindsight*, New York, 2010, Bantam Books.

27. Lee DG, Lee LJ, McLaughlin LM: Stability, continence and breathing: the role of fascia following pregnancy and delivery, *J Bodyw Mov Ther* 12:333–348, 2008.

28. Lee D, Lee L-J: Techniques and tools for assessing the lumbopelvic-hip complex. In Lee D, editor: *The pelvic girdle*, ed 4, Edinburgh, 2011, Elsevier.

29. Lee D, Lee L-J: Techniques and tools for addressing barriers in the lumbopelvic-hip complex. In Lee D, editor: *The pelvic girdle*, 4 ed, Edinburgh, 2011, Elsevier.

30. Lee L-J, Lee D: Tools and techniques for 'waking up' and coordinating the deep and superficial muscle systems. In Lee D, editor: *The pelvic girdle*, 4 ed, Edinburgh, 2011, Elsevier.

31. Lee L-J: Training new strategies for posture and movement. In Lee D, editor: *The pelvic girdle*, 4 ed, Edinburgh, 2011, Elsevier.

32. Melzack R: Pain and the neuromatrix in the brain, *J Dent Educ* 65:1378–1382, 2001.

33. Melzack R: Evolution of the neuromatrix theory of pain. The Prithvi Raj Lecture: Presented at the third World Congress of World Institute of Pain, Barcelona 2004, *Pain Pract* 5:85–94, 2005.

34. Vleeming A, Schuenke MD, Masi AT, et al: The sacroiliac joint: an overview of its anatomy, function and potential clinical implications, *J Anat* 221:537–567, 2012.

35. Lee D: *The pelvic girdle*, eds 1-4, Edinburgh, 1989–2011, Elsevier.

36. Snijders CJ, Vleeming A, Stoeckart R: Transfer of lumbosacral load to iliac bones and legs. 1: biomechanics of self-bracing of the sacroiliac joints and its significance for treatment and exercise, *Clin Biomech (Bristol, Avon)* 8:285–294, 1993.

37. Snijders CJ, Vleeming A, Stoeckart R: Transfer of lumbosacral load to iliac bones and legs. 2: loading of the sacroiliac joints when lifting in a stooped posture, *Clin Biomech (Bristol, Avon)* 8:295–301, 1993.

38. Hodges PW: Changes in motor planning of feedforward postural responses of the trunk muscles in low back pain, *Exp Brain Res* 141:261–266, 2001.

39. Hodges PW: *Neuromechanical control of the spine*, Stockholm, Sweden, 2003, Karolinska Institutet PhD thesis.

40. Hodges PW, Cholewicki JJ: Functional control of the spine. In Vleeming A, Mooney V, Stoeckart R, editors: *Movement, stability and lumbopelvic pain*, 2 ed, Edinburgh, 2007, Elsevier.

41. Hodges PW, Cresswell AG, Thorstensson A: Preparatory trunk motion accompanies rapid upper limb movement, *Exp Brain Res* 124:69–79, 1999.

42. Hodges PW, Kaigle Holm A, Holm S, et al: Intervertebral stiffness of the spine is increased by evoked contraction of transversus abdominis and the diaphragm: in vivo porcine studies, *Spine* 28:2594–2601, 2003.

43. Hodges PW, Moseley GL: Pain and motor control of the lumbopelvic region: effect and possible mechanisms, *J Electromyogr Kinesiol* 13:361–370, 2003.

44. Hungerford B, Gilleard W, Hodges P: Evidence of altered lumbopelvic muscle recruitment in the presence of sacroiliac joint pain, *Spine* 28(14):1593–1600, 2003.

45. Cresswell A: Responses of intra-abdominal pressure and abdominal muscle activity during dynamic loading in man, *Eur J Appl Physiol* 66:315–320, 1993.

46. Cresswell A, Grundstrom H, Thorstensson A: Observations on intra-abdominal pressure and patterns of abdominal intra-muscular activity in man, *Acta Physiol Scand* 144:409–418, 1992.

47. Cholewicki J, van Vliet JJ: Relative contribution of trunk muscles to the stability of the lumbar spine during isometric exertions, *Clin Biomech (Bristol, Avon)* 17:99–105, 2002.

48. Cholewicki J, Panjabi MM, Khachatryan A: Stabilizing function of trunk flexor-extensor muscles around a neutral spine posture, *Spine* 22:2207–2212, 1997.

49. Panjabi MM: The stabilizing system of the spine. Part I: function, dysfunction, adaptation, and enhancement, *J Spinal Disord* 5:383–389, 1992.

50. Panjabi MM: The stabilizing system of the spine. Part II. Neutral zone and instability hypothesis, *J Spinal Disord* 5:390–396, 1992.

51. Radebold A, Cholewicki J, Panjabi MM, et al: Muscle response pattern to sudden trunk loading in healthy individuals and in patients with chronic low back pain, *Spine* 25:947–954, 2000.

52. Radebold A, Cholewicki J, Polzhofer GK, et al: Impaired postural control of the lumbar spine is associated with delayed muscle response times in patients with chronic idiopathic low back pain, *Spine* 26:724–730, 2001.

53. Jacob HA, Kissling RO: The mobility of the sacroiliac joints in healthy volunteers between 20 and 50 years of age, *Clin Biomech (Bristol, Avon)* 10:352–361, 1995.

54. Sturesson B: *Load and movement of the sacroiliac joint*, Sweden, 1999, Lund University PhD thesis.

55. Sturesson B, Selvik G, Uden A: Movements of the sacroiliac joints: a Roentgen stereophotogrammetric analysis, *Spine* 14:162–165, 1989.

56. Sturesson B, Uden A, Vleeming A: A radiosteriometric analysis of movements of the sacroiliac joints during the standing hip flexion test, *Spine* 25:364–368, 2000.

57. Hungerford B, Gilleard W, Lee D: Alteration of pelvic bone motion determined in subjects with posterior pelvic pain using skin markers, *Clin Biomech (Bristol, Avon)* 19:456–464, 2004.

58. Dreyfuss P, Dryer S, Griffin J, et al: Positive sacroiliac screening tests in asymptomatic adults, *Spine* 19:1138–1143, 1994.

59. Potter NA, Rothstein J: Intertester reliability for selected clinical tests of the sacroiliac joint, *Phys Ther* 65:1671–1675, 1985.

60. Carmichael JP: Inter- and intra-examiner reliability of palpation for sacroiliac joint dysfunction, *J Manipulative Physiol Ther* 10:164–171, 1987.

61. Herzog W, Read L, Conway PJW, et al: Reliability of motion palpation procedures to detect sacroiliac joint fixations, *J Manipulative Physiol Ther* 12:86–92, 1989.

62. Meijne W, van Neerbos K, Aufdemkampe G, van der Wurff P: Intraexaminer and interexaminer reliability of the Gillet test, *J Manipulative Physiol Ther* 22:4–9, 1999.

63. van der Wurff P, Hagmeijer R, Meyne W: Clinical tests of the sacroiliac joint. A systematic methodological review: part 1: reliability, *Man Ther* 5:30–36, 2000.

64. Personal communication with Dr. Andry Vleeming.

65. Mens JMA, Vleeming A, Snijders CJ, et al: The active straight leg raising test and mobility of the pelvic joints, *Eur Spine* 8:468–473, 1999.

66. van Wingerden JP, Vleeming A, Buyruk HM, et al: Stabilization of the sacroiliac joint in vivo: verification of muscular contribution to force closure of the pelvis, *Eur Spine J* 13:199–205, 2004.

67. Vleeming A, Stoeckart R, Volkers AC, Snijders CJ: Relation between form and function in the sacroiliac joint. 1: clinical anatomical aspects, *Spine* 15:130–132, 1990.

68. Vleeming A, Volkers AC, Snijders CJ, Stoeckart R: Relation between form and function in the sacroiliac joint. 2: biomechanical aspects, *Spine* 15:133–136, 1990.

69. Vleeming A, Buyruk H, Stoechart R, et al: An integrated therapy for peripartum pelvic instability: a study of the biomechanical effects of pelvic belts, *Am J Obstetr Gynecol* 166:1243–1247, 1992.

70. Hungerford B, Gilleard W, Moran M, et al: Evaluation of the reliability of therapists to palpate intra-pelvic motion using the stork test on the support side, *Phys Ther* 87:879–887, 2007.

71. O'Sullivan PB, Beales DJ, Beetham JA, et al: Altered motor control strategies in subjects with sacroiliac joint pain during the active straight-leg-raise test, *Spine* 27:E1–E8, 2002.

72. Beales DJ, O'Sullivan PB, Briffa NK: Motor control patterns during active straight leg raise in pain-free subjects, *Spine* 34:E1–E8, 2009.

73. Reeves NP, Narendra KS, Cholewicki J: Spine stability: the six blind men and the elephant, *Clin Biomech (Bristol, Avon)* 22:266–274, 2007.

74. MacDonald DA, Moseley LG, Hodges PW: The lumbar multifidus: does the evidence support clinical beliefs? *Man Ther* 4:254–263, 2006.

75. Lee DG: Biomechanics of the thorax: a clinical model of in vivo function, *J Man Manipulative Ther* 1:13–21, 1993.

76. Lee L-J: Restoring force closure/motor control of the thorax. In Lee D, editor: *The thorax—an integrated approach*, White Rock, 2003, Diane G. Lee Physiotherapist Corp.

77. Maitland GD: *Vertebral manipulation*, ed 5, Oxford, England, 1986, Butterworth Heinemann.

78. Cyriax J: *Textbook of orthopaedic medicine*, London, 1954, Cassell.

79. Damen L, Stijnen T, Roebroeck ME, et al: Reliability of sacroiliac joint laxity measurement with Doppler imaging of vibrations, *Ultrasound Med Biol* 28:407–414, 2002.

80. Buyruk HM, Snijders CJ, Vleeming A, et al: The measurements of sacroiliac joint stiffness with colour Doppler imaging: a study on healthy subjects, *Eur J Radiol* 21:117–121, 1995.

81. Fortin JD, Dwyer A, Aprill C, et al: Sacroiliac joint pain referral patterns upon applying a new injection/arthrography technique. II: clinical evaluation, *Spine* 19:1483–1489, 1994.

82. Fortin JD, Dwyer A, West S, Pier J: Sacroiliac joint pain referral patterns upon application of a new injection/arthrography technique. I: asymptomatic volunteers, *Spine* 19:1475-1482.

83. Laslett M, Aprill CH, McDonald B, et al: Diagnosis of sacroiliac joint pain: validity of individual provocation tests and composites of tests, *Man Ther* 10:207–218, 2005.

84. Vleeming A, de Vries HJ, Mens JM, van Wingerden JP: Possible role of the long dorsal sacroiliac ligament in women with peripartum pelvic pain, *Acta Obstet Gynecol Scand* 81:430–436, 2002.

85. Van Dieen JH, Cholewicki J, Radebold A: Trunk muscle recruitment patterns in patients with low back pain enhance the stability of the lumbar spine, *Spine* 28:834–841, 2003.

86. Van Dieen JH, de Looze MP: Directionality of anticipatory activation of trunk muscles in a lifting task depends on load knowledge, *Exp Brain Res* 128:397–404, 1999.

87. Van Dieen JH, Selen LPJ, Cholewicki J: Trunk muscle activation in low-back pain patients, an analysis of the literature, *J Electromyogr Kinesiol* 13:333–351, 2003.

88. Richardson CA, Snijders CJ, Hides JA, et al: The relationship between the transversely oriented abdominal muscles, sacroiliac joint mechanics and low back pain, *Spine* 27:399–405, 2002.

89. Gilliard W, Brown CW: Structure and function of the abdominal muscles in primigravid subjects during pregnancy and the immediate postbirth period, *Phys Ther* 76:750–762, 1996.

90. Axer H, von Keyserlingk DG, Prescher A: Collagen fibers in linea alba and rectus sheaths. I. General scheme and morphological aspects, *J Surg Res* 96:127–134, 2001.

91. Beer GM, Schuster A, Seifert B, et al: The normal width of the linea alba in nulliparous women, *Clin Anat* 22:706–711, 2009.

92. Mendes D, Nahas FX, Veiga DF, et al: Ultrasonography for measuring rectus abdominis muscles diastasis, *Acta Cir Bras* 22:182–186, 2007.

93. Coldron Y, Stokes MJ, Newham DJ, et al: Postpartum characteristics of rectus abdominis on ultrasound imaging, *Man Ther* 13:112, 2008.

94. Lee D, Hodges PW: *Behaviour of the linea alba during a curl-up task in women with diastasis rectus abdominis*, *Man Ther*, 2015 (in press).

95. Boissonnault JS, Blaschak MJ: Incidence of diastasis recti abdominis during the childbearing year, *Phys Ther* 68:1082–1086, 1988.

96. Toranto IR: Resolution of back pain with the wide abdominal rectus plication abdominoplasty, *Plast Reconstr Surg* 81:777–779, 1988.

97. Butler DS, Moseley GL: *Explain pain*, Adelaide, Australia, 2003, NOI Group Publications.

98. Doidge N: *The brain that changes itself. Stories of personal triumph from the frontiers of brain science*, New York, 2007, Penguin Books.

99. Bialosky JE, Bishop MD, Cleland JA: Individual expectation: an overlooked, but pertinent, factor in the treatment of individuals experiencing musculoskeletal pain, *Phys Ther* 90:1345–1355, 2010.

100. Lee D: *Imagery for core stabilization*, 2001, VHS produced by Diane G. Lee Physiotherapist Corporation.

101. Hides J, Wilson S, Stanton W, et al: An MRI investigation into the function of the transversus abdominis muscle during "drawing-in" of the abdominal wall, *Spine* 31:E175–E178, 2006.

102. Ashton-Miller JA, Howard D, DeLancey JO: The functional anatomy of the female pelvic floor and stress continence control system, *Scand J Urol Nephrol Suppl* 207:1–7, 2001.

103. DeLancey JO, Kearney Q, Chou Q, et al: The appearance of levator ani muscle abnormalities in magnetic resonance images after vaginal delivery, *Obstet Gynecol* 101:46–53, 2003.

104. Dietz HP, Steensma AB: The prevalence of major abnormalities of the levator ani in urogynaecological patients, *Br J Obstet Gynecol* 113:225–230, 2006.

105. Sapsford RR, Hodges PW, Richardson CA, et al: Co-activation of the abdominal and pelvic floor muscles during voluntary exercises, *Neurourol Urodyn* 20:31–42, 2001.

106. Bo K, Morkved S, Frawley H: Evidence for benefit of transversus abdominis training alone or in combination with pelvic floor muscle training to treat female urinary incontinence: a systematic review, *Neurourol Urodyn* 28:368–373, 2009.

107. Sapsford RR, Richardson CA, Maher CF, Hodges PW: Pelvic floor muscle activity in different sitting postures in continent and incontinent women, *Arch Phys Med Rehabil* 89:1741–1747, 2008.

108. Mattox TF, Lucente V, McIntyre P, et al: Abnormal spinal curvature and its relationship to pelvic organ prolapse, *Am J Obstet Gynecol* 183:1381–1384, 2000.

109. Nguyen JK, Hall CD, Taber E, Bhatia NN: Sonographic diagnosis of paravaginal defects: a standardization of technique, *Int Urogynecol J Pelvic Floor Dysfunct* 11:341–345, 2000.

110. Bo K, Hilde G: Does it work in the long term? A systematic review on pelvic floor muscle training for female stress urinary incontinence, *Neurourol Urodyn* 32:215–223, 2013.

111. Dumoulin C, Hay-Smith J: Pelvic floor muscle training versus no treatment, or inactive control treatments for urinary incontinence in women, *Cochrane Database Syst Rev* 1:2010 Jan 20 CD005654.

112. Fritel X, Fauconnier A, Bader G, et al: Diagnosis and management of adult female stress urinary incontinence: guidelines for clinical practice from the French College of Gynaecologists and Obstetricians, *Eur J Obstet Gynecol Reprod Biol* 151:14–19, 2010.

113. Bump RC, Hurt GW, Fantl JA, et al: Assessment of Kegal pelvic muscle exercise performance after brief verbal instruction, *Am J Obstet Gynecol* 165:322–327, 1991.

114. Sherburn M, Murphy CA, Carroll S, et al: Investigation of transabdominal real-time ultrasound to visualise the muscles of the pelvic floor, *Austr J Physiother* 51:167–170, 2005.

115. Whittaker JL, Thompson JA, Teyhen DS, Hodges P: Rehabilitative ultrasound imaging of pelvic floor muscle function, *J Orthop Sports Phys Ther* 37:487–498, 2007.

116. Bendová P, Růzicka P, Peterová V, et al: MRI-based registration of pelvic alignment affected by altered pelvic floor muscle characteristics, *Clin Biomech (Bristol, Avon)* 22:980–987, 2007.

117. MacDonald D, Moseley GL, Hodges PW: Why do some patients keep hurting their back? Evidence of ongoing back muscle dysfunction during remission from recurrent back pain, *Pain* 142:183–188, 2009.

118. Moseley GL, Hodges PW, Gandevia SC: Deep and superficial fibers of the lumbar multifidus muscle are differentially active during voluntary arm movements, *Spine* 27:E29–E36, 2002.

119. Saunders S, Rath D, Hodges P: Postural and respiratory activation of the trunk muscles changes with mode and speed of locomotion, *Gait Posture* 20:280–290, 2004.

120. Hides JA, Richardson CA, Jull GA: Multifidus recovery is not automatic following resolution of acute first episode low back pain, *Spine* 21:2763–2769, 1996.

121. Hides JA, Stokes MJ, Saide M, et al: Evidence of lumbar multifidus muscles wasting ipsilateral to symptoms in patients with acute/subacute low back pain, *Spine* 19:165–172, 1994.

122. Hides J, Gilmore C, Stanton W, Bohlscheid E: Multifidus size and symmetry among chronic LBP and healthy asymptomatic subjects, *Man Ther* 13:43–49, 2008.

123. Gracovetsky S, Farfan H: The optimum spine, *Spine* 11:543–573, 1986.

124. MacIntosh JE, Bogduk N: The attachments of the lumbar erector spinae, *Spine* 16:783–792, 1991.

125. Schuenke MD, Vleeming A, Van Hoof T, Willard FH: A description of the lumbar interfascial triangle and its relation with the lateral raphe: anatomical constituents of load transfer through the lateral margin of the thoracolumbar fascia, *J Anat* 221:568–576, 2012.

126. Willard FH, Vleeming A, Schuenke MD, et al: The thoracolumbar fascia: anatomy, function and clinical considerations, *J Anat* 221:537–567, 2012.

127. Snodgrass SJ, Heneghan NR, Tsao H, et al: Recognising neuroplasticity in musculoskeletal rehabilitation: A basis for greater collaboration between musculoskeletal and neurological physiotherapists, *Man Ther* 19:614–617, 2014.

128. Boudreau SA, Farina D, Falla D: The role of motor learning and neuroplasticity in designing rehabilitation approaches for musculoskeletal pain disorders, *Man Ther* 15:410–414, 2010.

129. Tsao H, Hodges PW: Immediate changes in feedforward postural adjustments following voluntary motor training, *Exp Brain Res* 181:537–546, 2007.

130. Tsao H, Hodges PW: Persistence of improvements in postural strategies following motor control training in people with recurrent low back pain, *J Electromyogr Kinesiol* 18:559–567, 2007.

131. Tsao H, Druitt TR, Schollum TM, Hodges PW: Motor training of the lumbar paraspinal muscles induces immediate changes in motor coordination in patients with recurrent low back pain, *J Pain* 11:1120–1128, 2010.

132. Damen L, Mens JM, Snijders CJ: PhD thesis *The mechanical effects of a pelvic belt in patients with pregnancy-related pelvic pain*, Rotterdam, The Netherlands, 2002, Erasmus University.

133. Damen L, Spoor CW, Snijders CJ: Does a pelvic belt influence sacroiliac joint laxity? *Clin Biomech (Bristol, Avon)* 17:495–498, 2002.

134. Sichting F, Rossol J, Soisson O, et al: Pelvic belt effects on sacroiliac joint ligaments: A computational approach to understand therapeutic effects of pelvic belts, *Pain Physician* 17:43–51, 2014.

135. Lee DG: New perspectives from the Integrated Systems Model for treating women with pelvic girdle pain, urinary incontinence, pelvic organ prolapse and/or diastasis rectus abdominis, *J Assoc Chartered Physiother Womens Health* 114:10–24, 2014.

136. Lee D: *Manual therapy for the thorax*, Surrey, 1994, Diane Lee & Associates.

CHAPTER 18

Hip Pathologies: Diagnosis and Intervention

TIMOTHY L. FAGERSON, OLADAPO M. BABATUNDE, MARC R. SAFRAN

INTRODUCTION

This chapter explores adult hip pathologies, their diagnoses, and appropriate interventions. Most hip conditions are discussed, except for hip joint arthroplasty and pediatric conditions, which are covered elsewhere in this text (see Chapters 19 and 29). Clinicians require a good working knowledge of hip pathologies, which will enable them to select, perform, and interpret the appropriate tests for the diagnostic process and then decide what interventions need to be included to treat the patient's condition most effectively. Obviously, a good working knowledge of hip anatomy is also important; thus the "**4 layer concept**" and the "**3G approach**: groin, gluteal, and greater trochanter triangles" have been elucidated upon in this regard.[1,2]

Adult hip pathologies can be divided into six subcategories based on the type of disorder (Table 18-1). It also can be helpful to think of hip disorders in relation to age because their prevalence rate often is age dependent (Table 18-2).

Another useful approach is to classify a condition based on the need for diagnostic imaging or laboratory tests to confirm the diagnosis and initiate appropriate medical or surgical management. Clinicians commonly use the following diagnostic classification system in the absence of imaging or other diagnostic testing to not only classify the patient but also assist in determining when to refer to other colleagues for further diagnostic testing. These can be applied not only to hip pathologies but also to all clinical problems.[3]

1. Diagnoses that can be made on the basis of the history and physical examination alone (e.g., sprains, strains, muscles imbalances, nerve entrapments). Rehabilitation should be initiated as appropriate.
2. Diagnoses that tentatively can be made on the basis of the history and physical examination, but further diagnostic imaging and laboratory studies are necessary to confirm the diagnosis (e.g., osteoarthritis [OA], rheumatoid arthritis [RA], herniated disc). Rehabilitation can be initiated to assist symptom management and maintain maximum function while a definitive diagnosis is pursued.

3. Red flag diagnoses (e.g., fracture, dislocation, osteonecrosis, infection, metastatic disease). These conditions require definitive medical or surgical intervention. Rehabilitation should follow when appropriate.

When possible, a diagnosis should be the lowest common denominator driving a clinical presentation. Table 18-3 presents a summary of musculoskeletal diagnoses for rehabilitation management.[4]

When one of these lowest common denominators cannot be identified or associated with an anatomical structure and pathology (i.e., if a tissue level or pathoanatomical diagnosis cannot be made), one of the next levels of rehabilitation diagnosis should be used, for example, weak left gluteus medius (i.e., an **impairment-based diagnosis**) or difficulty walking (i.e., a **functional limitation–based diagnosis**).[5] Such impairment-based or functional limitation–based diagnosis can be helpful in the physical rehabilitation realm when a clear "**active pathology**"–**based diagnosis** cannot be definitively made or where multiple tissue level problems exist together and do not fit a unifying diagnostic entity (Figure 18-1).

Pain is the primary reason a patient seeks outpatient clinical care. The exact location of hip-mediated pain varies. Khan and Woolson[6] reported that, of patients presenting for total hip replacement, 73% had groin pain (Table 18-4). Other common locations were the lateral hip (trochanter) and buttocks (gluteals).[6] Hip pain from OA can also refer to the anterior knee and to the low back. Sometimes these are the only symptoms produced by hip OA. Although groin pain often is associated with hip pathology, the groin is not the only place that symptoms originating from the hip are felt, nor is the groin region immune to pain referral from sources other than the hip. In contrast with the findings of Khan and Woolson,[6] a study by Wroblewski[7] rated the groin area as the fourth most common site of pain in patients with OA of the hip, behind the greater trochanter, the anterior thigh, and the knee. Hip OA can also cause medial buttock, shin, and low back pain (LBP).[7] In addition to

TABLE 18-1

Types of Hip Disorders

Type of Disorder	Examples
Soft tissue disorders	• Bursitis • Tendonitis/tendinosis • Muscle strain • Osteitis pubis • Hip pointer • Snapping hip syndrome • Sports hernia • Contracture • Hip capsule contracture
Joint disorders	• Osteoarthritis • Femoroacetabular impingement • Labral tears • Loose bodies
Osseous disorders	• Osteonecrosis • Osteoporosis • Heterotopic ossification • Transient osteoporosis • Osteoid osteoma • Symptomatic herniation pit • Brodie's abscess
Fractures and dislocations	• Hip fracture • Femoral head fracture • Acetabular fracture • Stress fracture • Traumatic dislocation
Nerve entrapment syndromes (commonly described types)	• Piriformis syndrome • Meralgia paresthetica • Hamstring syndrome • Superior gluteal nerve entrapment
Pediatric disorders (not covered in this chapter)	• Developmental dysplasia of the hip (DDH) • Congenital coxa vara • Acute transient synovitis • Legg-Calvé-Perthes (LCP) disease • Slipped capital femoral epiphysis (SCFE) • Avulsion fracture

TABLE 18-2

Hip Disorders Related to Age

Disorder	Age
Developmental dysplasia of the hip	Newborn/infancy
Congenital coxa vara	1-3 years
Acute transient synovitis	2-10 years
Legg-Calvé-Perthes disease	2-10 years
Slipped femoral capital epiphysis	10-16 years
Avulsed ASIS, AIIS, lesser trochanter	12-16 years
Osteoid osteoma (femoral neck)	5-30 years
Malignancy	Any age
Rheumatoid arthritis	Any age (20-40 years)
Stress fractures	14-25 years
Avascular necrosis	20-40 years
Paget's disease	≥40 years
Osteoarthritis	≥45 years
Hip fracture	≥65 years

ASIS, Anterosuperior iliac spine; *AIIS,* anteroinferior iliac spine.
Modified from Fagerson TL, editor: *The hip handbook,* p 40, Boston, 1998, Butterworth-Heinemann.

TABLE 18-3

Manual Therapy Diagnoses

Principal Diagnosis	Type of Problem
Pain	• Mechanical • Chemical
Misalignment	• Structural • Functional
Hypomobility	• Contracture • Adhesion • Restriction
Hypermobility	• Instability • Tissue insufficiency
Weakness	• Motor control • Muscle imbalance • Tissue weakness

Modified from Dyrek DA: Assessment and treatment planning strategies for musculoskeletal deficits. In Sullivan SD, Schmitz TJ, editors: *Physical rehabilitation: assessment and treatment,* ed 3, pp. 61-82, Philadelphia, 1994, FA Davis.

pain referred from the hip, the buttock, lateral hip, and groin are common sites of pain referred from the lumbar spine and sacroiliac joints.[8,9]

DIFFERENTIATING HIP DISEASE FROM LUMBAR DISEASE BY PHYSICAL EXAMINATION

Because the lumbar spine can refer symptoms to the hip region (and to a lesser extent vice versa), the clinician should always rule out involvement of the lumbar spine when a hip problem is suspected. The examination therefore may be extensive, involving the hip, lumbar spine, and pelvis. The concept of **regional interdependence** is very applicable to the lumbopelvic–hip region.[10,11] Brown et al.[12] identified a limp, groin pain, and limited hip medial rotation as signs that significantly predicted a hip problem rather than a lumbar problem.[12] Clinically, Cyriax's screening tests for a noncapsular pattern of the hip and a positive "sign of the buttock" have been identified as predictors for further workup.[13] With a capsular pattern of the hip, the pattern of hypomobility is one in which medial rotation and abduction and flexion are the most limited motions.[14] Extension and lateral rotation may also be limited; adduction is the least limited in a

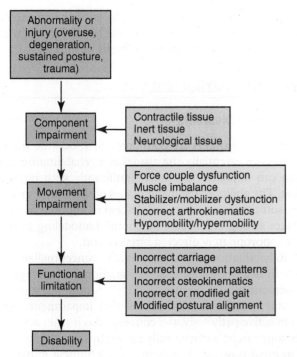

Figure 18-1 Diagnostic pathway for pathology. (Modified from Magee DJ, Zachazewski JE, Quillen WS, editors: *Scientific foundations and principles of practice in musculoskeletal rehabilitation*, p 403, St Louis, 2007 Saunders/Elsevier.)

Cyriax-described capsular pattern of the hip. It should be noted, however, that Klassbo et al.[15] warn against using hip capsular patterns as a diagnostic predictor of OA based on a study of passive range of motion (ROM) in subjects with and without hip OA.[15]

Cyriax[14] described the sign of the buttock as a means of differentiating a major lesion of the buttock (e.g., infection, tumor, fracture) from a minor lesion (e.g., bursitis, tendonitis, arthritis). Major lesions obviously are *red flags* indicating the need for further workup. For the sign of the buttock test, hip flexion is performed in the supine position, first with knee flexion and then with knee

extension. Normally, hip flexion combined with knee flexion results in a greater hip flexion ROM than does hip flexion with knee extension because hamstring muscle tension limits the motion when the knee is in extension. However, if the hip flexion ROM is the same with the knee extended and the knee flexed (i.e., an empty end feel is noted, usually the result of pain), this is a positive sign of the buttock (Figure 18-2).[13,14]

Signs Predicting a Hip Rather Than a Lumbar Problem[12]

- Limp
- Groin pain
- Limited hip medial rotation
- Capsular pattern of the hip (i.e., medial rotation, abduction, flexion)
- Positive "sign of the buttock"

The lumbar spine can refer symptoms into the hip region and lower extremity even when the lumbar spine itself is symptom free (Figure 18-3). The L1 dermatome covers the anterior and lateral hip. The L2 dermatome covers the iliac crest (buttock) and medial thigh. The L3 dermatome covers the iliac crest (buttock) and medial thigh and knee. The cluneal nerves, which supply the skin over the buttocks from the iliac crest to the greater trochanter, originate as the lateral branches of the dorsal primary divisions of the upper three lumbar nerves. A disc herniation at L4-L5 can cause groin pain via the sinuvertebral nerve.[8]

Restricted hip movement often can be an etiological factor in LBP. Greater limitation of medial than of lateral rotation of the hip is seen more frequently in patients

TABLE 18-4

Location and Frequency of Hip Pain in Patients with Intra-articular Hip Pathology

Location	Frequency (%)
Groin only	43
Trochanter only	18
Gluteal only	5
Groin/trochanter	12
Groin/gluteal	16
All locations	3
No hip pain	3
Groin only or groin with other locations	73

Modified from Khan NQ, Woolson ST: Referral patterns of hip pain in patients undergoing total hip replacement, *Orthopedics* 21:123-126, 1998.

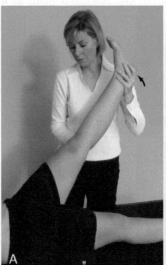
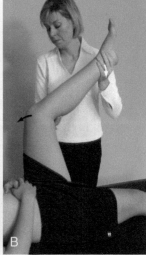

Figure 18-2 Sign of the buttock test. **A,** Hip is flexed with knee straight until resistance of pain is felt. **B,** The knee is then flexed to see whether further hip flexion can be achieved. If further hip flexion can be achieved, the test is negative. (From Magee DJ: *Orthopedic physical assessment*, ed 6, p 674, St. Louis, 2014, Saunders/Elsevier.)

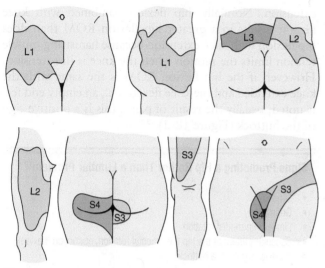

Figure 18-3 Dermatomes around the hip. Only one side is illustrated. (From Magee DJ: *Orthopedic physical assessment*, ed 6, p 731, St. Louis, 2014, Saunders/Elsevier.)

with LBP than in individuals without LBP.[16] Vad et al.[17,18] identified that professional golfers and professional tennis players with LBP had statistically significant limitations in lead hip rotation and lumbar extension.[17,18] Limited hip extension also has been correlated with an increased incidence of LBP.[19] Hip strength weakness and imbalance has also been correlated with LBP.[11]

During assessment, it should be also be noted that people with limited hip motion, as a result of OA or other hip pathology, will place more load on their lumbar spine during motion; that is, limited femoroacetabular motion will be compensated by increased lumbopelvic motion, much in the way people with frozen shoulder (i.e., limited glenohumeral motion) increase scapulothoracic motion to get their functional ROM. Also, hip pain, as in

OA, may result in compensation, favoring the affected extremity, resulting in weakness of the hip abductors, which results in trochanteric bursal/gluteus medius pain.

ADULT HIP PATHOLOGIES

Soft Tissue Disorders

Soft tissue disorders are considered first, because the soft tissues are essentially the tissues the rehabilitation clinician can influence the most significantly with intervention. The ability of the living tissues of the body, especially the soft tissues, to adapt and deform to imposed demands makes strong repair and functional remodeling possible with appropriately directed intervention.

Rehabilitation clinicians usually conceptualize their role in health care using some variation of the **Nagi disablement model** (Figure 18-4).[5,20-22] Although it is often assumed from the Nagi model that impairments result from active pathology, the converse also is true: active pathology can be partly or fully caused by impairments (e.g., abnormal postural alignment and/or muscle imbalances can lead to OA). Obviously, impairments and pathology can each affect the other. Sahrmann[23] defines these differing mechanisms as the **pathokinesiology model** (i.e., pathology causing impairments) and the **kinesiopathology model** (i.e., impairments causing pathology).

Greater Trochanteric Pain Syndrome

It can be difficult to distinguish bursitis from gluteal tendinitis and other lateral hip etiologies by signs and symptoms alone. For this reason, use of the term *lateral hip pain* or *greater trochanteric pain syndrome* (GTPS) has been suggested when an anatomical source cannot be specified by physical examination.[24] GTPS has ex-

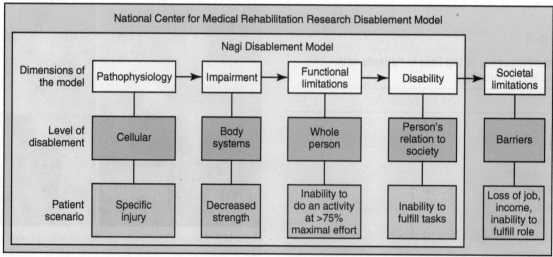

Figure 18-4 Modified disablement models: Nagi Disablement Model and National Centre for Medical Rehabilitation Research Disablement Model. (Modified from Synder AR, Parsons JT, Valovich McLeod TC et al: Using disablement models and clinical outcomes assessment to enable evidence-based athletic training practice. Part I: Disablement models, *J Athl Training* 43:428-436, 2008.)

panded as a clinical entity to cover several etiologies such as greater trochanteric bursitis (GTB), gluteus medius syndrome, gluteus medius and minimus tendinopathy, gluteus medius and minimus tears or strains, and lateral (external) snapping hip. The key to the best management relies on making an accurate diagnosis.

In these cases, imaging can be very helpful in identifying an etiology and to exclude any intra-articular causes of a patient's discomfort. Plain radiographs are initially obtained to investigate bony morphology and potential abnormalities, whereas diagnostic ultrasound can be used for soft tissue evaluation, particularly for fluid collections and tendinopathy. Magnetic resonance imaging (MRI) has become the mainstay for imaging because of the ability to comprehensively evaluate bone, chondral, and soft tissue causes for a patient's lateral hip pain. The following sections describe specific evaluation and management options for the most common anatomic causes of GTPS.

Greater Trochanteric Bursitis

In the region of the greater trochanter, three bursae are consistently present: two major bursae and one minor bursa (Figure 18-5).[25] The subgluteus maximus bursa lies between the greater trochanter and the fibers of the gluteus maximus and tensor fascia lata (TFL) muscles as they blend into the iliotibial band (ITB). The subgluteus medius bursa lies at the superoposterior tip of the greater trochanter and prevents friction between the gluteus medius muscle and the greater trochanter and also between the gluteus medius and gluteus minimus muscles. The subgluteus minimus bursa is a minor bursa lying between the gluteus minimus attachment and the superoanterior tip of the greater trochanter.

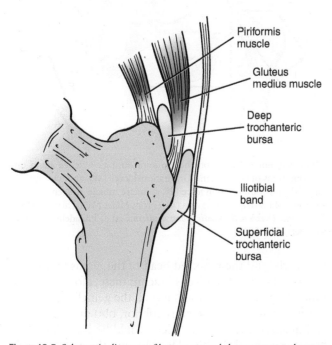

Figure 18-5 Schematic diagram of bursae around the greater trochanter.

Piriformis muscle

Gluteus medius muscle

Deep trochanteric bursa

Iliotibial band

Superficial trochanteric bursa

GTB is more common in arthritic conditions, with fibromyalgia, and with leg length discrepancies. It also is more common in females than in males (2-4:1 ratio), with a peak incidence occurring between 40 and 60 years of age.[25] GTB, especially in athletes, may result from a fall onto a hard surface (traumatic GTB) or friction of the ITB over the greater trochanter during repetitive flexion/extension motion of the hip, such as occurs in running (similar to ITB friction syndrome at the knee). Those with friction-related GTB often have tightness of the hip abductors/ITB or gluteus maximus or weakness of the ipsilateral hip abductors.

GTB is characterized by an aching pain over the lateral aspect of the hip accompanied by distinct tenderness on palpation around the greater trochanter. Patients may also report pain when lying on the affected hip. A widely accepted diagnostic classification for trochanteric bursitis includes both of these features and one of three other findings (see following textbox).[26] Symptom relief through peritrochanteric injection of a corticosteroid and an anesthetic is required for more definitive diagnosis of GTB. In a study by Shbeeb et al.,[27] 77% of patients treated for GTB with glucocorticosteroid injection had relief at 1 week after the injection, and 61% had lasting relief at 26 weeks.

Clinical Criteria for Diagnosis of Trochanteric Bursitis

1. *Both* of the following symptoms must be present:
   - Aching pain in the lateral aspect of the hip
   - Distinct tenderness around the greater trochanter
2. *One* of the following three symptoms must be present:
   - Pain at the extreme of rotation, abduction, or adduction, especially positive Patrick's (FABER) test
   - Pain on forced hip abduction
   - Pseudoradiculopathy (i.e., pain extending down the lateral aspect of the thigh)

Modified from Shbeeb MI, Matteson EL: Trochanteric bursitis (greater trochanter pain syndrome), *Mayo Clin Proc* 71:565-569, 1996; data from Ege Rassmusen KJ, Fano N: Trochanteric bursitis: treatment by corticosteroid injection, *Scand J Rheumatol* 14:417-420, 1985.

Rehabilitation intervention for GTB can include modalities such as therapeutic ultrasound/phonophoresis, iontophoresis, and nonsteroidal anti-inflammatory drugs (NSAIDs) to alleviate the inflammatory response; however, treatment also should include manual therapy/mobilization techniques and therapeutic exercises to address potential causative factors, such as ITB contracture; hip flexion contracture; abnormal lumbopelvic alignment, general lumbopelvic–hip mobility, and stability; and gluteus medius weakness. The patient should be advised to avoid aggravating activities or positions, such as lying on the painful side or engaging in excessive walking or running, until the inflammatory process abates. Use of a contralateral cane can prove useful in acute and irritable cases of GTB.

Typically, GTB responds well to nonoperative management that includes rest, NSAIDs, physical therapy focused on stretching, flexibility, and strengthening. In cases when symptoms are persistent despite the appropriate nonoperative management, a corticosteroid injection into the bursa has been shown to provide good pain relief, as stated earlier. Surgical treatment is reserved for refractory cases. Although originally performed as an open procedure, most surgeons currently prefer to treat GTB through endoscopy (i.e., hip arthroscopy). The most commonly cited technique is to access the lateral compartment for greater trochanter bursectomy and inspection of the ITB and gluteal insertions. A motorized shaver to debride the bone and a radiofrequency device to maintain hemostasis are typically used. For cases in which greater trochanter wear is observed, a partial release of the ITB has been shown to be beneficial.[28]

Gluteus Medius/Gluteus Minimus Tears and Tendinosis

The quadriceps muscle has been described as "the key to the knee"; similarly, the key muscle for hip joint function is the gluteus medius muscle.[5] The gluteus medius is critical for balancing the pelvis in the frontal plane during one-leg stance, which accounts for approximately 60% of the gait cycle.[5,29] Janda[30] has described the one-leg stance as the most common posture for humans because it is the lowest common denominator during locomotion, the primary functional task that humans perform. When the gluteus medius is weak, Trendelenburg's gait pattern or a compensated Trendelenburg's gait pattern is seen (Figure 18-6). During one-leg stance, approximately three times the body weight is transmitted through the hip joint, and two thirds of that is generated by the hip abductor mechanism (Figure 18-7). To reduce this load in cases of hip pain or dysfunction, the patient often shows a compensating Trendelenburg's lean over the affected hip; this reduces the lever arm for body weight and therefore the counterbalancing hip abductor contraction. This counterbalancing effect can stress the lumbar spine, and a cane in the opposite hand is an excellent alternative.[31] The contralateral cane can act as a gait assist to unload the abductors as the patient is progressively rehabilitated. Walking is an excellent endurance and strengthening activity for the hip abductors and is preferred over specific abductor strengthening exercises if the abductors are easily irritated. A cane in the contralateral hand (Figure 18-8) can help create the noncompensatory mechanical environment that assists a weak gluteus medius and gluteus minimus in regaining their strength.

The gluteus medius has been likened to the supraspinatus in the shoulder, and the hip can sustain rotator cuff–like injuries.[32,33] If the hip "complex" were compared to the glenohumeral "complex," the likenesses would be as follows: the gluteus medius would be comparable to the supraspinatus, the gluteus minimus to the infraspinatus, the piriformis to the teres minor, the iliopsoas to the sub-

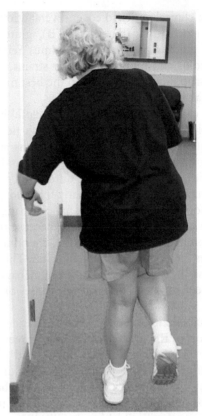

Figure 18-6 Compensated Trendelenburg's lurch over the left hip.

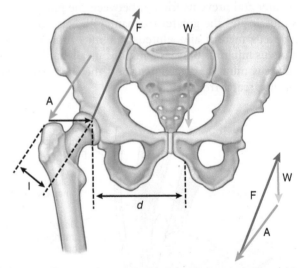

Figure 18-7 Forces acting on the hip joint during single-leg stand under conditions of equilibrium. Gravitational force (*W*), abductor muscle force (*A*), hip joint reaction force (*F*), abductor muscle moment arm (*I*), and force of gravity moment arm (*d*). (From Miller MD, Thompson SR: *DeLee and Drez's orthopaedic sports medicine*, ed 4, Philadelphia, 2013, Saunders/Elsevier.)

scapularis, and the reflected head of the rectus femoris to the long head of the biceps brachii; these, along with the other deep rotators of the hip (i.e., the gemellus superior, obturator externus, gemellus inferior, obturator internus, and quadratus femoris muscles) would be considered the "rotator cuff" of the hip. The TFL and the gluteus maxi-

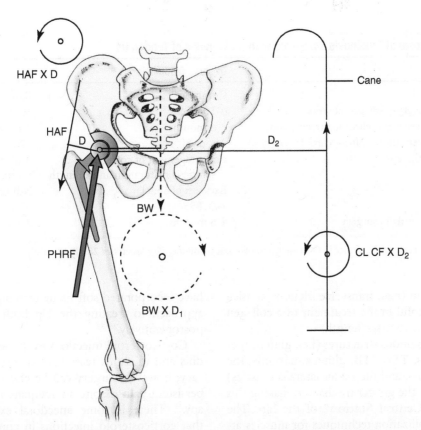

Figure 18-8 The balance of torques acting in the frontal plane about a right prosthetic hip while in single limb support. The diagram depicts a cane used contralateral to the prosthetic hip. Assuming static equilibrium, the sum of the clockwise torque produced by body weight (BW) (*dashed circle*) equals the combined counterclockwise torques produced by hip abductor force (HAF) and the contralateral cane force (CLCF) (*solid circles*). The prosthetic hip reaction force (PHRF) is shown directed toward the right prosthetic hip. The force vectors are not drawn to scale. *D,* Moment arm used by HAF; *D1,* moment arm used by BW; *D2,* moment arm used by CLCF. (Modified from Neumann DA: An electromyographic study of the hip abductor muscles as subjects with a hip prosthesis walked with different methods of using a cane and carrying a load, *Phys Ther* 79:1163-1173, 1999.)

mus, feeding into either side of the ITB proximally, act in a fashion similar to the deltoid in the shoulder; they provide a strong, superficial fascial umbrella around the hip. Sahrmann[23] emphasized the importance of enhancing motor control of the one-joint hip muscles (i.e., iliopsoas, gluteals, and deep lateral [external] rotator muscles), which control the position of the femoral head in the acetabulum, over the two-joint muscles (i.e., rectus femoris, hamstrings, TFL-ITB), which have distal attachments that are at a distance from the hip joint center.

"Rotator Cuff" Muscles of the Hip (with Shoulder Equivalents)

- Gluteus medius (supraspinatus)
- Gluteus minimus (infraspinatus)
- Piriformis (teres minor)
- Iliopsoas (subscapularis)
- Rectus femoris (long head of the biceps)
- Tensor fascia lata (deltoid)
- Gluteus maximus (deltoid)

Tendinosis and strains (tears) of the gluteus medius and gluteus minimus were a common finding in an MRI study of patients presenting with buttock, lateral hip, or groin pain.[34] Khan et al.[35] has reported that most cases of tendinopathy are, in fact, tendinosis, not tendinitis. The primary problem is collagen degeneration, not inflammation. Because differentiating tendinosis from tendinitis is difficult and because tendinosis is much more common than tendonitis, Khan et al.[35] suggested treating all cases initially as if the problem were collagen degeneration. The differences between overuse tendinosis and overuse tendonitis can be found in Table 18-5. Eccentric strengthening has been shown to be an effective method of treating tendinosis, probably because eccentric muscle action stimulates mechanoreceptors, which encourage tendon cells to produce collagen. Loading the tendon also improves collagen cross-linking and alignment, resulting in greater tensile strength.[35] As mentioned previously, walking is an excellent eccentric exercise for the gluteus medius, and it should be incorporated into any program. Other approaches (e.g., rest, ice, compression, ultrasound treatment, and anti-inflammatory medication) can and should be used when appropriate for acute injury.

TABLE **18-5**

Implications of a Diagnosis of Tendinosis Compared with a Diagnosis of Tendonitis

Trait	Overuse Tendinosis	Overuse Tendonitis
Prevalence	Common	Rare
Time required for recovery (early presentation)	6-10 weeks	Several days to 2 weeks
Time required for full recovery (chronic presentation)	3-6 months	4-6 weeks
Likelihood of full recovery to sport from chronic symptoms	About 80%	99%
Focus of conservative therapy	Encouragement of collagen-synthesis maturation and strength	Anti-inflammatory modalities and drugs
Role of surgery	Excision of abnormal tissue	Not known
Prognosis for surgery	70%-85%	95%
Time required to recover from surgery	4-6 months	3-4 weeks

From Khan KM, Cook JL, Taunton JE, Bonar F: Overuse tendinosis, not tendinitis, *Phys Sportsmed* 28:38-48, 2000.

Soft tissue mobilization (e.g., transverse frictions, passive stretching) can be helpful in the treatment of a collagen scar and can help improve tissue length.

Twelve musculotendinous structures (i.e., gluteus medius, gluteus minimus, TFL, ITB, gluteus maximus, the six short lateral rotators, and the vastus lateralis muscles) attach to or cross over the greater trochanter, making this region the **"Grand Central Station"** of the hip. The use of soft tissue mobilization techniques for muscles attaching to the greater trochanter is extremely beneficial for restoring optimal hip joint mechanics. Particularly beneficial is the application of sustained, deep pressure, load and release techniques to various points in the gluteus medius, gluteus minimus, and TFL muscles above the greater trochanter, combined with sustained ipsilateral passive hip abduction performed in the side-lying position (Figure 18-9). This technique helps release the abductor mechanism and thereby paradoxically improves hip abduction ROM by allowing the abductors to fold in on themselves. Loading the abductors just proximal to the greater trochanter with the hip in abduction also acts as a medioinferior mobilization of the hip capsule and pubofemoral ligament. Several case study–based reports

have incorporated soft tissue techniques in a multimodal approach to treating the hip both nonoperatively and postoperatively.[36–38]

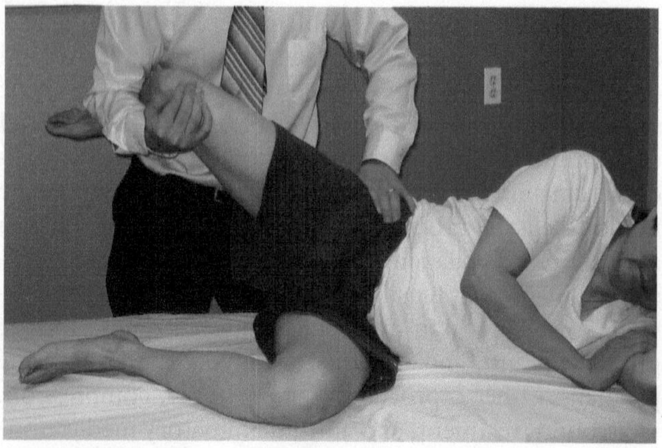

Corticosteroid injections in the setting of gluteus medius and minimus tears have demonstrated limited efficacy; however, surgery can be effective for patients with persistent pain despite an adequate trial of physical therapy.[39] There is some anecdotal experience suggesting that corticosteroid injections in conjunction with physical therapy may be beneficial for patients with gluteus medius and minimus tendinopathy and possibly smaller tears. Platelet-rich plasma (PRP) has also been found to be helpful anecdotally, although more research is needed in both of these areas.

Surgical treatment of persistent lateral hip pain from a gluteus medius/minimus tear is very similar to that of treating greater trochanter bursitis in that many surgeons prefer to use endoscopic techniques. Using a lateral entry point, the peritrochanteric compartment of the hip can be debrided. After inspection of the gluteal insertions, the decision can be made to debride or repair the tissues depending on the amount of tissue torn (Figure 18-10). Repair of the gluteal muscle can be achieved using suture anchors or transosseous tunnels.[40–42]

Proximal Iliotibial Band Syndrome

Proximal ITB tightness or contracture (whether that be true shortening, increased tone, tissue dehydration or a combination of these) can be a primary cause leading to a secondary effect such as GTB caused by compression and friction of the subgluteus maximus bursa between the tight ITB and the greater trochanter. Proximal ITB tightness may also be a secondary effect to a primary cause such as OA of the hip, labral tear, or gluteal tendinitis. The classic test for ITB contracture is **Ober's test**. For this test, the patient is in the side-lying position with the leg to be tested uppermost. In most cases the hip should be able to adduct so that the knee touches the table without the pelvis moving caudally. To prevent a

Figure 18-9 Hip abductor soft tissue release technique.

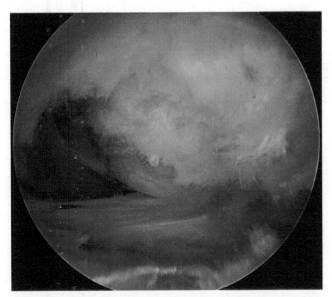

Figure 18-10 Arthroscopic picture of a medium full thickness avulsion tear of the gluteus medius.

false-negative result, the following are important: (1) the clinician should use one hand to firmly stabilize the patient's pelvis; (2) the hip should be extended to 0°, with the clinician using the other hand to engage the ITB over the greater trochanter; and, (3) the hip must not be allowed to flex or to rotate medially as the knee is lowered toward the table (Figure 18-11). To prevent a false-positive result, the clinician must ensure that the patient is fully relaxed and allows the leg to be lowered toward the table. Performing the test with the knee flexed 90° takes up slack in the rectus femoris and the anterior fascia lata and is more sensitive to change than performing the test with the knee extended. However, care must be taken to avoid excessive valgus stress to the medial knee when the knee is flexed for the test.

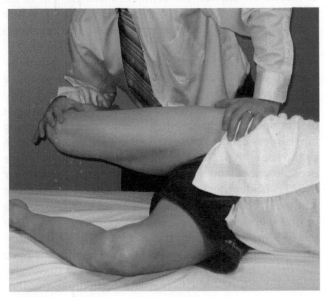

Figure 18-11 Ober's test.

ITB contracture is best treated using a combination of soft tissue mobilization and hold/relax-type stretching in the Ober's test stretch position. In addition, stretching of the rectus femoris and iliopsoas is important because these muscles are enveloped by the fascia lata. The patient should be taught self-stretching to maintain and improve what is achieved in manual therapy sessions (Figure 18-12). Foam rollers have become popular in the personal training arena as a means of self-mobilization of the ITB. Improving the strength and stability of the lumbopelvic region also is important to reduce tension in the ITB. The ITB and hip abductors can tighten in an ineffective attempt to compensate for lack of lumbar control and stability.

External and Internal Snapping Hip

Snapping hip is a phenomenon patients may experience in which there is an audible snap or pop as the hip moves through a ROM, usually when the flexed hip is extended.[43] It often is painless, but it can become symptomatic in athletic individuals. The syndrome is more common in young athletic females. The cause of the snapping or clicking can be intra-articular or extra-articular (Table 18-6).

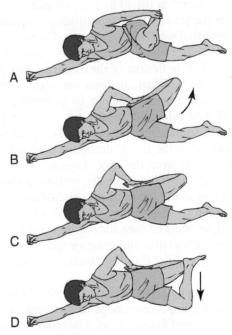

Figure 18-12 Iliotibial band stretch. The patient is in side lying with iliotibial band to be stretched uppermost. **A,** The patient flexes the upper hip and knee to grab dorsum of foot. **B,** While holding the foot, the patient extends and abducts the hip as far as possible. **C,** The patient holds the hip extended as far as possible with the knee flexed as far as possible (the heel should touch the patient's buttock on the same side) and adducts the hip. **D,** The patient lifts the opposite foot over the flexed knee and rests it on the outside of the opposite knee. The patient then uses the opposite foot (*right foot in this case*) to push the knee and thigh into further adduction. The patient should feel the stretch on the outside of the knee (*left knee in this case*) near the knee. (From Safran M, Zachazewski JE, Stone DA: *Instructions for sports medicine patients*, ed 2, p 338, Philadelphia, 2012, Saunders/Elsevier.)

TABLE **18-6**

Causes of Snapping Hip (Coxa Saltans)

INTRA-ARTICULAR	ANTERIOR		POSTERIOR
	Internal	External	
Loose bodies	Iliopsoas tendon snapping over pelvic brim	Iliotibial band snapping over greater trochanter	Long head of biceps femoris tendon sliding over ischial tuberosity
Synovial chondromatosis	Iliopsoas tendon snapping over femoral head	Gluteus maximus tendon snapping over greater trochanter	
Osteochondral injury	Iliopsoas tendon snapping over bony ridge on lesser trochanter		
Subluxation of the hip	Tendonitis of iliopsoas or rectus femoris		
Labral tears	Anterosuperior labrum most common site		

From Gruen GS, Scioscia TN, Lowenstein JE: The surgical treatment of internal snapping hip, *Am J Sports Med* 30:607-613, 2002.

External snapping hip can be caused by contracture or thickening of the ITB.[44] Often presenting as an audible or palpable sound as the ITB, TFL, or gluteus maximus slides over the greater trochanter during movement, this can be associated with or without pain. Diagnosis is made primarily by history and physical examination. A test for a snapping ITB is flexion of the adducted hip with the knee extended.[45] Often, patients can demonstrate the external snapping, while standing, by jutting their hip out to the affected side, and an obvious snap can be seen. Another test to demonstrate external snapping is having the patient lay in the lateral decubitus position with the affected hip away from the table. The patient then moves his or her hip, like riding a bicycle, with repetitive flexion and extension of the hip in neutral abduction. This often causes the hip to snap. Ober's test is also likely to show shortening of the ITB (see the section on ITB contracture). Plain radiographs and imaging such as MRI can be used to exclude other diagnoses such as a gluteus medius or minimus tear.[43]

Internal snapping hip is caused by the iliopsoas as it slides over the iliopectineal ridge or the anterior capsulolabral complex and femoral head. The classic test for snapping of the iliopsoas muscle over the anterior pelvic brim or hip is reproduction of the snap as the hip is extended from a position of flexion, abduction, and lateral rotation (the extension test). Although an audible clunk is often heard, it is helpful to identify the location of the snap or click by simultaneous palpation during the test. Often firm manual pressure during the extension test can reduce the snapping by preventing the lateral to medial subluxation of the tendon over the pelvic brim.[43] Other maneuvers that may reproduce internal snapping include lifting the leg of the supine patient about 46 cm (18 inches) from

the examination table and having the patient actively move his or her leg from abduction-lateral (external) rotation to adduction-medial (internal) rotation. A third test has the supine patient move his or her leg from flexion-abduction-lateral (external) rotation to extension-adduction-medial (internal) rotation. Commonly, shortening of the iliopsoas muscle and malalignment of the pelvis are associated with snapping of the iliopsoas muscle.

Treatment of both internal and external snapping hips with NSAIDs and ice can be helpful in the short term. For long-term benefit, the cause of the snapping must be resolved, or at least its frictional effect must be reduced. Treatment can involve soft tissue mobilization and stretching techniques for myotendinous contractures, correction of muscle imbalances, correction of malalignment of the pelvic girdle, movement pattern adjustments to minimize or abolish the click, and prescription orthotics for patients with pronating feet.

If conservative measures do not resolve symptoms associated with snapping hip syndrome, injections into the bursa can be utilized. Surgery is reserved for those who have recalcitrant symptoms despite an adequate attempt of nonoperative management. For external snapping hip, surgery can be performed via a small open approach to the lateral hip; however, endoscopic approaches have been described and are becoming more common. Once the ITB is identified, the surgeon can resect, release, or lengthen the ITB using techniques such as removing a central ellipse of ITB, cutting the posterior portion of the ITB, or Z-plasty lengthening.[43,45] Surgery for internal snapping hip can also be performed with an open approach; however, endoscopic approaches have also been recently described. In these procedures the iliopsoas can be released from either the lesser trochanter via a transcapsular technique at the level of the femoral neck of the hip in the peripheral compartment or off the anterior border of the acetabulum through a small capsulotomy.[46,47] All three techniques have promising results, and, in a study by Ilizaliturri et al.,[48] the transcapsular and resection off the lesser trochanter were found to have no differences in outcomes. A recent systematic review reported superior outcomes of endoscopic iliopsoas lengthening as compared with open iliopsoas lengthening.[49]

Flexion Contracture

Hip flexion contracture is common with hip dysfunction, probably as a result of protective guarding and the positioning of the hip into flexion (i.e., the resting position) in response to pain. The likely causes of hip flexion contracture can be one or more of the following: shortening of the iliopsoas muscle, shortening of the rectus femoris muscle, shortening of the TFL muscle, or contracture of the anterior hip capsule. Hip flexion contracture can occur in response to OA, after injury to the hip region, or as part of a repetitive, flexed posture or movement habit. As a consequence of hip flexion contracture, loading through the hip joint is shifted to a thinner region of hyaline cartilage in both the femur and the acetabulum, the pelvis is placed in anterior tilt with increased lumbar lordosis, and the hip extensors are placed in a state of constant, low-level muscle tension because the line of gravity shifts anterior to the center of mass.[50] Therefore it is important for the clinician to examine for flexion contracture and, if it is reversible, to intervene appropriately.

> ### Causes of Hip Flexion Contracture
>
> - Shortening of the iliopsoas
> - Shortening of the rectus femoris
> - Shortening of the tensor fascia lata
> - Shortening of the anterior hip capsule

The **Thomas test** assesses for contracture of the iliopsoas muscle. In this test the hip opposite the affected one is flexed to the point of flattening the lordosis in the lumbar spine, and the involved hip then is extended. If the involved hip stays flexed (i.e., is not able to extend to 0°), this is a positive test result for a flexion contracture (Figure 18-13). For an accurate test result, it is very important to negate the lumbar lordosis. For a more sensitive assessment when compared with the opposite side and certainly when the maneuver is used for treatment, the clinician should flex the opposite knee fully to the chest. During treatment, a rolled towel can be placed immediately distal to the ischial tuberosity to minimize anterior rotation torque of the innominate during hip extension. If the hip stays abducted during Thomas's test, it is indicative

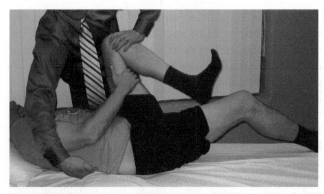

Figure 18-13 Thomas test. With the back flat to the table and the contralateral hip flexed, any flexion indicates a hip flexor contracture.

of a tight TFL; if the knee cannot be flexed beyond 90° in the stretch position, this is indicative of shortening of the rectus femoris.

In addition to testing the length of the iliopsoas muscle, it is important that the clinician palpate the iliacus muscle at its origin at the internal superior rim of the iliac crest and palpate the psoas major muscle down to the inguinal ligament to assess for increased density (Figure 18-14).

To ensure that palpation of the psoas major muscle occurs, and not loading of some other abdominal structure, the examiner resists active hip flexion by asking the patient to push up with his or her thigh against the examiner's caudal hand while simultaneously, with the cephalad hand, the examiner palpates the psoas major muscle in the abdomen a few inches lateral to the umbilicus.

> ### Clinical Note
>
> Because of the abdominal contents, *extreme caution* should be observed if this soft tissue technique is to be used; the aortic pulse should be identified and then avoided with the soft tissue load, and female patients of childbearing age should be queried about pregnancy.

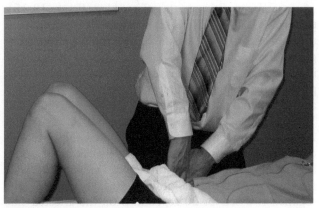

Figure 18-14 Iliacus soft tissue release.

Ely's test (i.e., prone knee flexion, then added hip extension) can be used to assess for contracture of the rectus femoris muscle; most athletes' knees can be flexed to touch the heel to the buttock in prone lying; however, the stretch should be stopped if pain is felt in the knee or lumbar spine. Hip joint capsuloligamentous contracture is distinguished from contracture of the rectus femoris by hip extension in the prone position with the knee extended and also by assessment of the end feel on a posteroanterior glide of the hip. Anterior hip capsule restriction can be treated with a combined hip extension and posteroanterior glide technique with the patient in the prone position.

Iliopsoas Syndrome (Iliopsoas Bursitis and Tendonitis)

Iliopsoas syndrome is defined as anterior hip pain associated with inflammation of the iliopsoas bursa or tendon. The condition often is the result of repetitive overuse of the bursa or tendon or sudden overload in sports. Iliopsoas bursitis or tendonitis can result from repetitive friction of the iliopsoas myotendon over the anterior femoral head or iliopectineal eminence. Signs and symptoms of this syndrome typically include tenderness in the femoral triangle over the iliopsoas myotendon, decreased hip extension ROM, hip flexion contracture, positive anterior snapping hip, and weakness of hip medial and lateral rotation at 90° hip flexion.[51] Additionally, pain with resisted hip flexion while seated may also be indicative of iliopsoas bursitis or tendinitis.

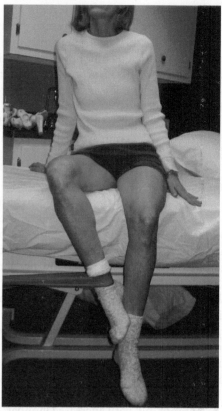

Figure 18-15 Sitting hip medial (internal) and lateral (external) rotation (illustrated) resistance.

Signs and Symptoms of Iliopsoas Syndrome

- Tenderness in the femoral triangle
- Decreased hip extension
- Hip flexion contracture
- Anterior snapping hip
- Medial and lateral rotation weakness at 90° hip flexion
- Pain with resisted hip flexion while seated

Johnston et al.[51] described a hip rotation strengthening program for treatment of iliopsoas syndrome. The program consists of medial and lateral rotation strengthening exercises in sitting to the affected leg (Figure 18-15), performed daily for 2 weeks, 3 sets of 20 repetitions on the weaker rotation, 2 sets of 20 repetitions on the stronger rotation. After 2 weeks the frequency of this exercise is reduced to two to three times a week. At the 2-week point, side-lying abduction/lateral (external) rotation against TheraBand resistance is introduced (Figure 18-16), with 3 sets of 20 repetitions on the affected side and 2 sets of 20 repetitions on the uninjured side, which is continued daily for 2 weeks. At the 4-week mark a one-leg standing minisquat is introduced, keeping the knee tracking over the outside of the foot (Figure 18-17); the regimen is 3 sets of 20 repetitions on the affected side and 2 sets of 20 repetitions on the uninjured side. At this

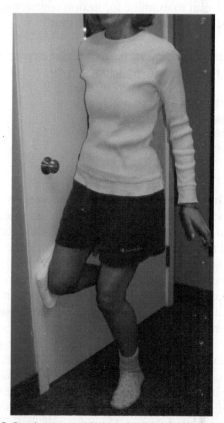

Figure 18-16 One-leg squat with contralateral abduction against a wall.

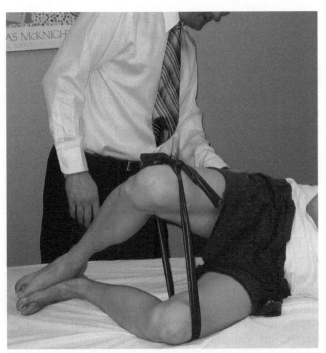

Figure 18-17 Side-lying hip abduction (clam) exercise with TheraBand. The focus should be on contraction of the posterior gluteus medius muscle and deep lateral (external) rotators.

point, all strength exercises were performed two to three times per week. The hip flexors, quadriceps, lateral hip/piriformis, and hamstrings are stretched daily. The patient is instructed to perform twice as many stretches on the affected side as the uninjured side and to repeat the stretches as often as possible during the day. The stretching program continues as long as the pain persists. Gluteal reeducation during gait is also incorporated with a conscious, voluntary contraction of the gluteal muscles of both the affected and the uninjured leg during the middle to late portion of the stance phase of the gait cycle. This is performed a maximum of 10 to 15 steps at a time, two or three times per day.[51] The advantages of this program are that it is cost-effective and practical for a patient to perform independently at home. Further research is necessary to corroborate the good results seen in the preliminary retrospective case series.[51]

Adhesive Capsulitis of the Hip

The capsule of the hip joint can develop a contracture similar to adhesive capsulitis in the shoulder (frozen shoulder). It can be primary or secondary and is most common in middle-aged women. Byrd and Jones[52] describe good response to manipulation under anesthetic followed by arthroscopy. The capsular pattern is the typical pattern of contracture of a joint capsule in cases of arthritis. At the hip joint, the most limited movements classically were described by Cyriax as "maximum loss of medial rotation, flexion, abduction and a minimal loss of extension."[14] Extension and lateral rotation can also be limited, and adduction is the least limited motion. In

fact, as abduction range decreases, adduction range can be seen to increase in patients with progressing OA of the hip. Kaltenborn[53] described the hip capsular pattern as an extension more limited than flexion, medial rotation more limited than lateral rotation, and abduction more limited than adduction. The only difference between the descriptions of Cyriax and Kaltenborn are the contributions of flexion and extension to a capsular pattern. These authors agree that abduction is more limited than adduction and medial rotation more limited than lateral rotation in a typical capsular pattern.

The arthrokinematic motions at the hip are anterior glide, posterior glide, medial glide, long axis distraction, lateral distraction, and short axis distraction. (Short axis distraction is a pull in line with the angle of the femoral neck, whereas lateral distraction is a direct lateral pull of the proximal end of the femur.) These accessory motions are used for joint mobilization purposes, primarily to treat a capsuloligamentous restriction. Mulligan[54] described a technique combining arthrokinematic with osteokinematic motions that he called *mobilization with movement* (MWM). Short axis distraction combined with medial or lateral rotation is particularly effective for improving rotation ROM (Figure 18-18).[54] Manual posterior mobilization can be useful for assessing and treating a posterior hip capsule contracture that would limit flexion and medial rotation ranges of motion (Figure 18-19). The literature has shown support for the use of manual mobilization techniques in conjunction with a home exercise program.[55]

End feel is an important component of joint mobility assessment, both in osteokinematic assessment of the quality of overpressure and in arthrokinematic assessment of the quality of end range tissue resistance.[5] Normal end feels at the hip are soft tissue approximation for flexion and a firm, capsuloligamentous end feel for extension, medial and lateral rotation, abduction, and adduction. Abnormal end feels common at the hip are a firm capsular

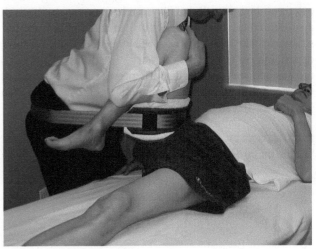

Figure 18-18 Mulligan's mobilization with movement (MWM) technique to increase range of motion of hip medial (internal) rotation.

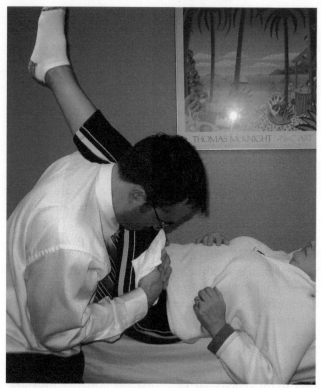

Figure 18-19 Posterior hip mobilization to stretch the posterior capsule of the hip.

end feel before the expected end range (e.g., from capsular contracture), an empty end feel from severe pain (e.g., very acute bursitis), and a bony block (e.g., from osteophytes in advanced OA).

General Muscle Strain Management

Management of muscle strains (tears) should follow a rational, evidence-based progression based on the extent, mechanism, symptoms, and healing stage of the injury. In the acute, or early, phase, the PRICEM regimen should be followed. Acute phase management should be used for the first 2 to 5 days and sometimes longer, depending on the extent of the injury. Rehabilitation then progresses through a subacute and late phase. Return to sport after a muscle strain may take anywhere from a few weeks to many months, depending on the extent of injury.[5] In addition to gluteus medius and minimus strains (see previous section), two of the more common muscle strain injuries in the hip region (i.e., hamstring strain and adductor strain) are reviewed.

Acute Injury Treatment Regimen

P	Protect injury, prevent further injury, promote healing
R	Relative rest
I	Ice/cryotherapy
C	Compression
E	Elevation
M	Modalities, medication, massage movement, mobilization

Proximal Hamstring Strains and Avulsions

Acute hamstring strains are common in sports involving high-speed movements (e.g., soccer, football, rugby) and also in dancers from prolonged end-range stretch positions.[56,57] Strains are often reported as the second and third most common injury (after knee and ankle sprains) in field sports, with it being most common in males and in positions involving explosive speed (e.g., running back, wide receivers in football).[58] Hamstring strains are, in fact, the most frequent injury in track and field and also the most common rugby training injury.[59,60] In a general sports medicine population, hamstring strains are the third most common hip or pelvic injury, after gluteus medius strain/tendonitis and GTB.[61]

Two types of hamstring injuries can occur: muscle strains/tears (grades I to III) and avulsions. Muscle strains tend to occur at the stress risers of the musculotendinous or tenoperiosteal junctions or at the site of scar tissue from a previous injury (i.e., an acquired form of stress riser). The most widely accepted theory about the hamstrings' vulnerability to injury is that they are a two-joint muscle functioning to eccentrically control knee extension and hip flexion at the same time. The biceps femoris muscle tends to be the most commonly injured component of the hamstrings, perhaps because the nerve supply to the short head of the biceps femoris is from the peroneal division of the sciatic nerve, whereas the long head of the biceps femoris and the other components of the hamstrings have their nerve supply from the tibial division of the sciatic nerve.[57,62] It is proposed that the differing nerve supplies to the biceps femoris may result in poor neuromuscular coordination between the two heads of the muscle and thus a greater susceptibility to injury.[63]

During walking and even jogging, the hamstrings are not fully recruited. It is with sprinting that high eccentric resistance from the hamstrings is required to decelerate the rapid leg swing (i.e., both knee extension and hip flexion); therefore, the hamstrings are most vulnerable to injury during sprinting. With running, the hamstrings have three primary functions: eccentric contraction to decelerate the leg swing that starts at approximately 30° flexion; eccentric contraction at foot strike to control and facilitate hip extension; and, eccentric contraction at push-off to assist the gastrocnemius in extending the knee.[62] If gluteus maximus recruitment for propulsive hip extension is insufficient at push-off, the hamstrings may have this additional role. Such hamstring dominance may be a factor predisposing the hamstring to injuries because inadequate recruitment from the gluteus maximus may result in overcompensation and strain of the proximal hamstrings.[64] Although the hamstrings are meant to assist the gluteus maximus in hip extension, they are not meant to be the primary or sole extensor.[65] For example, golfers can strain the proximal hamstring of the non–target-side leg from the propulsion required for the drive in the golf swing. The gluteus maximus should contract strongly on the non–target-side leg during the forward swing. Inadequate recruitment from the gluteus maximus may result in overcompensation and strain of the proximal hamstrings.[64]

A hamstring injury also can occur during eccentric control of hip flexion in sports (e.g., lunging for a ball in tennis). The injury may occur when a player has not sufficiently flexed the knee, causing the hamstrings to strongly contract and lengthen at the same time. An important component of rehabilitation of such hamstring strains is emphasizing to the player the importance of bending the knees for practically everything so that, even when a lunging, top-heavy movement occurs, it does not result in sudden or cumulative tissue overload. Another theory on rehabilitation of this mechanism is to strengthen the hamstrings for this type of function with activities such as single-leg stand windmill touches (Figure 18-20). In the controlled rehabilitation environment, this activity is appropriate for the few times this movement might occur in sport. However, during sport performance, such as tennis, bending the knees should be strongly encouraged for injury prevention of hamstring strains as well as being better for stroke mechanics than lunging for the ball over a straight knee.

Strain or overload of the hamstring tissues also may result from a pelvic alignment fault or malalignment that changes the length/tension relationship of the hamstrings. Athletes with hamstring strains often show an anterior innominate tilt or rotation on the affected side, and manipulation of the sacroiliac joint can enable these patients to regain muscle function and return to activity more quickly than those treated with more conservative measures.[66] This same response has been identified with runners experiencing anterior or lateral hip pain.[67]

Recurrence of hamstring injuries is a concern because levels of recurrence range from 12% to 62%.[56,68] This recurrence suggests that rehabilitation may have been inadequate or that the athlete has returned to play too soon. These questions have driven research into what optimal hamstring rehabilitation is. Progressive eccentric loading and neuromuscular control exercises have emerged as key variables to be included in a rehabilitation program.[69] Fredericson et al.[70] recommended incorporating eccentric hamstring strengthening based on the rationale that it is the only proven treatment for chronic tendinopathies.[70]

Clinical Note

Progressive eccentric strengthening/loading and neuromuscular control exercises are the key features in a hamstring rehabilitation program followed by a progressive running and agility program.

Rehabilitation of hamstring strains using progressive agility and trunk stabilization exercises (Box 18-1) was reported to be more effective than a program emphasizing isolated hamstring stretching and strengthening.[69] Sherry and Best[69] reported that only one of 13 subjects in the core stabilization group sustained a recurrent injury during the 1-year follow-up, whereas in the static hamstring stretch/progressive hamstring strengthening group, 7 of 10 subjects had recurrent hamstring strains. A subsequent study[56] reported that a progressive running and eccentric strengthening program had similar good results as a progressive agility and trunk stabilization program in recovery of hamstring function and return to sport. No doubt each of these four variables are important in a comprehensive hamstring strain rehabilitation. Brukner et al.[68] have proposed a seven-part management plan in applying the limited evidence on recurrent hamstring strains: (1) biomechanical assessment and correction, (2) neurodynamics, (3) core stability/neuromuscular control/lumbar spine strengthening, (4) increase strength in hamstrings using an eccentric-biased program, (5) overload running program, (6) injection therapies, and (7) stretching/yoga/relaxation. Silder et al.[56] identified that MRI, despite applying optimal rehabilitation principles and being cleared for return to sport clinically, was still not normal even at 12 months following hamstring strain. This finding echoes the advice of Orchard and Best,[71] who recommend that players, coaches, and clinicians embrace the notion of *"carrying an injury"* so that, even when cleared to return to sport, the risk of reinjury be appreciated and necessary preventive steps taken in the initial weeks to months after returning to sport.

Patients with hamstring injuries who do not respond to PRICEM regimen and rehabilitation may be candidates for PRP injections. The literature has reported mixed results on the efficacy of these injections. Hamid et al.[72] found that PRP combined with a rehabilitation program decreased

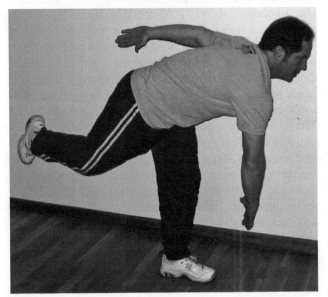

Figure 18-20 Windmill touches for eccentric hamstring contraction.

BOX **18-1**

Progressive Agility and Trunk Stabilization Approach for Treating Hamstring Strains

PHASE 1*

1. Low- to moderate-intensity† sidestepping: 3×1 minute
2. Low- to moderate-intensity grapevine stepping (lateral stepping with the trail leg going over the lead leg and then under the lead leg), both directions: 3×1 minute
3. Low- to moderate-intensity steps forward and backward over a tape line while moving sideways: 2×1 minute
4. Single-leg stand, progressing from eyes open to eye closed: 4×20 seconds
5. Prone abdominal body bridge (abdominal and hip muscles are used to hold the body in a face down, straight plank position with the elbows and feet as the only points of contact): 4×20 seconds
6. Supine extension bridge (abdominal and hip muscles are used to hold the body in a supine hook lying position with the head, upper back, arms, and feet as the points of contact): 4×20 seconds
7. Side bridge (i.e., side plank) each side: 4×20 seconds
8. Ice in long sitting: 20 minutes

PHASE 2

1. Moderate- to high-intensity sidestepping: 3×1 minute
2. Moderate- to high-intensity grapevine stepping: 3×1 minute
3. Moderate- to high-intensity steps forward and backward while moving sideways: 2×1 minute
4. Single-leg stand windmill touches: 4×20 seconds of repetitive alternate hand touches
5. Push-up stabilization with trunk rotation (starting at the top of a full push-up, the patient maintains this position with one hand while rotating the chest toward the side of the other hand as it is lifted to point toward the ceiling; the patient pauses and then returns to the starting position): 2×15 repetitions on each side
6. Fast feet in place (jogging in place with increasing velocity, picking up the feet only a few inches off the ground): 4×20 seconds
7. Proprioceptive neuromuscular facilitation trunk pull-downs using a TheraBand: 2×15 repetitions to the right and left
8. Symptom-free practice without high-speed maneuvers
9. Ice for 20 minutes if any symptoms of local fatigue or discomfort are present

Modified from Sherry M, Best T: A comparison of 2 rehabilitation programs in the treatment of acute hamstring strains, *J Orthop Sports Phys Ther* 34:116-125, 2004.
†*Low intensity* is a velocity of movement that is less than or near that of normal walking; *moderate intensity* is a velocity of movement greater than normal walking but not as great as sports activity; *high intensity* is a velocity of movement similar to sports activity.
* Progression criteria: The patient is progressed from exercises in phase 1 to exercises in phase 2 when the individual can walk with a normal gait pattern and do a high knee march in place without pain.

mean time to return to play compared with rehabilitation in a randomized controlled trial of 28 patients. However, Reurink et al.[73] reported no difference in return to play in a double-blind placebo-controlled trial of 80 patients. With research on both sides of the PRP debate, it is clear that, at this time, more research is needed to definitively include or exclude PRP in the management of muscle strains.

Intramuscular corticoid steroid injections have also been described as a treatment for hamstring injuries. A study by Levine et al.[74] reported on a retrospective review of 431 National Football League players who suffered hamstring injuries. Of these, 58 players (13%) with severe discrete injuries were treated with intramuscular injection of corticosteroid and anesthetic. No complications were reported, and only 9 of the 58 players (16%) missed a game as a result of their injury. Other studies have not reported consistent clinical efficacy of intramuscular corticosteroid injections. In fact, one in vitro study has shown cortisone injections to have negative long-term consequences on muscle injury repair.[75] Thus the use of intramuscular corticosteroid injections in acute hamstring injuries remains controversial.[76]

Sometimes the injury can be so severe as to cause an avulsion of the hamstring insertion into the ischial tuberosity of the pelvis (Figure 18-21). In these cases, a good physical examination may show tenderness at the insertion or origin of the hamstrings. Although in some situations, nonsurgical management may be appropriate, these patients should have a discussion with a surgeon to determine whether surgery is best for them. Currently, the literature suggests a controversy about whether to repair acute hamstring avulsions. A study by Hofmann et al.[77] reported that hamstring avulsions managed non-surgically yielded noticeable subjective strength deficits. Another study by Subbu et al.,[78] comparing those with acute repair versus those that are done in a delayed fashion, suggests that those with acute repairs do better. However, these studies are fraught with bias, as many patients do return to sports and do well with nonoperative treatment. Regardless, surgery is typically performed in hamstrings with a small open incision, although endoscopic techniques have also been described.[79] In both techniques, the avulsed hamstring tendon is identified and then secured to the insertion origin site using various methods such as suture anchors or interference screws.

Adductor Muscle Strains and Tendon Injuries

As in other regions of the body, contractile tissue injuries at the hip come in two forms: strain (a muscle tear) and tendonitis (acute inflammation) or tendinosis (chronic

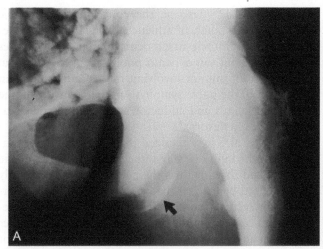
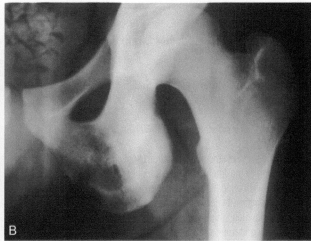

Figure 18-21 Ischial tuberosity avulsion fracture. **A,** Anteroposterior radiograph of the left hip demonstrates a crescentic hamstring avulsion fracture (*arrow*). Early callus formation is identified between the donor site and the fragment. **B,** Anteroposterior radiograph of the left hip in a different patient depicts abundant callus formation following avulsion fracture. The lesion was initially misinterpreted as tumor. (From Bencardino JT, Palmer WE: Imaging of hip disorders, *Radiol Clin North Am* 40:267-287, 2002.)

degeneration). Participants in sports such as soccer, hockey, and football are susceptible to adductor muscle pulls (i.e., a "groin" strain) because of the explosive lateral and rotatory hip movements involved, along with end range abduction stresses. Hyperabduction (overstretching) and forceful abduction of the thigh during adduction (e.g., during a soccer tackle) are the most common mechanisms of groin injury. Overuse adductor muscle injury also is common with repetitive, high-velocity limb movement that usually involves a change in direction (e.g., ice hockey or soccer). Adductor injuries usually are felt in the groin, and any of the adductor muscles can be affected, although the adductor longus is most commonly injured.[80]

Defects in the abdominal musculature (i.e., "sportsman hernia"), osteitis pubis, inguinal hernia, and referred pain from the hip joint or lumbar spine should be ruled out in any assessment of the hip. A general but useful test to differentiate abdominal injury from adductor injury is to have the patient perform a sit-up or a sit-up with trunk rotation; an abdominal injury is most likely to be painful with these maneuvers.

In a study comparing active and passive management of adductor strains, Holmich et al.[81] found the active treatment group (i.e., those who performed adductor strengthening, lumbopelvic strengthening and stabilization, and balance work) did much better than the passive treatment group (i.e., those who received transverse friction massage, transcutaneous electrical nerve stimulation, laser therapy, and adductor stretching). These findings support the notion that deficient collagen (i.e., quality and quantity) is part of the problem. An active loading program (that includes eccentric exercise) stimulates collagen synthesis and produces better long-term results than a passive loading program. Box 18-2 outlines an active loading program for adductor strain rehabilitation.

In addition to eccentric strengthening, prolotherapy (regeneration injection therapy) has demonstrated ef-

fectiveness at stimulating healing. Topol et al.[82] reported good results from dextrose prolotherapy injections in rugby and soccer players with groin pain. Schilders et al.[83] reported that pubic cleft injections gave relief for up to 1 year in competitive athletes with groin pain and normal MRI but recommended that injections be used diagnostically only if MRI demonstrated adductor enthesopathy (disorder of the tendon insertion). When conservative management has failed, selective adductor longus release has proven effective in professional athletes.[84]

Athletic Pubalgia ("Sports Hernia" or "Core Muscle Injury")

Athletic pubalgia is one cause of lower abdominal and/or groin pain that is often a **"diagnosis of exclusion"** in high-level athletes where other causes of groin pain have been ruled out.[85,86] Kachingwe and Greche[87] identified a cluster of five key findings in the clinical presentation of athletes with athletic pubalgia based on their research and a review of the literature.

This complex injury of the flexion/adduction apparatus of the hip occurs mostly in male elite athletes in ice hockey, soccer, and football who are involved in vigorous training and competition schedules and whose sport involves repetitive hyperextension of the hip along with

---

Key Findings for Diagnosing Athletic Pubalgia[87]

- Deep groin and/or lower abdominal pain
- Pain exacerbated by sport-specific activities (sprinting, cutting, kicking, shooting puck in hockey, hitting ball in golf) and/or sit-ups, and relieved by rest
- Tenderness on palpation of pubic ramus at insertion of rectus abdominus and/or conjoined tendon
- Pain with resisted hip adduction (at 0°, 45°, and/or 90° flexion)
- Pain with resisted abdominal curl-up

BOX **18-2**

Postinjury Program for Adductor Strain

PHASE I (ACUTE)

- Rest, ice, compression, and elevation (RICE)
- Nonsteroidal anti-inflammatory drugs (NSAIDs)
- Massage
- Transcutaneous electrical stimulation (TENS)
- Ultrasound
- Submaximum isometric adduction from knees bent to knees straight, progressing to maximum isometric adduction, pain free
- Non–weight-bearing hip progressive resistive exercise (PRE) with weight in antigravity position (all except abduction)
- Pain-free, low-load, high-repetition exercise
- Upper body and trunk strengthening
- Contralateral lower extremity (LE) strengthening
- Flexibility program for noninvolved muscles
- Bilateral balance board
  Clinical milestone: Concentric adduction against gravity without pain

PHASE II (SUBACUTE)

- Bicycling/swimming
- Sumo squats
- Single-limb stance
- Concentric adduction with weight against gravity
- Standing with involved foot on sliding board moving in frontal plane
- Adduction in standing position on cable column or with TheraBand
- Seated adduction machine
- Bilateral adduction on sliding board moving in frontal plane (i.e., bilateral adduction simultaneously)
- Unilateral lunges (sagittal) with reciprocal arm movements
- Multiplane trunk tilting
- Balance board squats with throwbacks
- General flexibility program
  Clinical milestone: Involved lower extremity passive range of motion (PROM) equal to that of the uninvolved side and involved adductor strength at least 75% that of the ipsilateral abductors

PHASE III (SPORT-SPECIFIC TRAINING)

- Phase II exercises with increase in load, intensity, speed, and volume
- Standing resisted stride lengths on cable column to simulate skating
- Sliding board
- On-ice kneeling adductor pull-togethers
- Lunges (in all planes)
- Correction or modification of ice skating technique
  Clinical milestone: Adduction strength 90% to 100% of abduction strength and involved muscle strength equal to that of the contralateral side

Modified from Tyler TF, Nicholas SJ, Campbell RJ, et al: The effectiveness of a preseason exercise program to prevent adductor muscle strain in professional ice hockey players. *Am J Sports Med* 30:680-683, 2002.

---

trunk rotation.[86] Abdominal hyperextension with thigh hyperabduction around the pivot of the "pubic joint" has also been reported as a mechanism.[85] Often patients report an initial incident of a hyperextension injury of the hip in which the anterior pelvis or pubic symphysis is the pivot. Both the rectus abdominis and adductor longus tendons insert at the pubic symphysis and are the most common sites of pain in athletic pubalgia along with tears of the abdominal fascia.[85]

Meyers et al.[88] describe the concept of the "pubic joint," because much of athletic pubalgia pathology relates to tears of muscle attachments injured by the stresses of rotation about this dynamic pubic complex. There can be a variety of injuries involving muscle attachments in the region of the pubic symphysis primarily involving the rectus abdominus and adductor attachments (and occasionally the hip flexors).[85,86,88]

Meyers et al.[85] hypothesized that the abdominal component of the injury usually is the initial injury in athletic pubalgia and that it allows the pelvis to rotate anteriorly (as evidenced by the fact that in the cadaver, when a portion of the rectus abdominis is cut, the pelvis rotates anteriorly with ease). The anterior tilt of the hemipelvis causes a compartment syndrome in the proximal adductor muscles because the adductor muscles are now relatively unopposed as a result of injury to the lower abdominals (creating an unbalanced force couple).[85,88]

Meyers et al.[85] described their pelvic floor (abdominal) repair as a broad surgical reattachment of the inferolateral edge of the rectus abdominis muscle and its fascia to the pubis and anterior ligaments. They also performed an adductor release that involved complete division of all the anterior epimysial fibers of the adductor longus 2 to 3 cm (1 to 1.2 inches) distal to the insertion on the pubis, as well as multiple longitudinal incisions at the tendinous attachment site on the pubis.[85] Surgical repair for athletic pubalgia boasts a 95% success rate.[85,86] A typical postoperative rehabilitating protocol is outlined in Box 18-3. Athletes usually are able to return to competitive sports by 12 weeks after surgery.

A course of conservative management should be attempted for sports pubalgia before surgery is considered. A key component of conservative rehabilitation is core

---

BOX **18-3**

Postoperative Protocol for Surgical Repair of a Sports Hernia

0-4 WEEKS

- Relative rest

4-6 WEEKS

- No resistive exercises
- Posterior pelvic tilt (5 to 6 second hold): sets of 10
- Gentle stretching (5 repetitions, hold 30 seconds each)
  - Side bending
  - Hip flexion
  - Quadriceps
  - Hamstrings
  - Adductors
- Pool exercises
  - Walking, forward and backward
  - Standing hip abduction/adduction/flexion/extension: 3×10 repetitions
  - Partial squats: 30 repetitions
  - Heel raises: 3×10 repetitions

6 WEEKS
- Progressive resistance exercises
  - Hip flexion/adduction/abduction/extension with body weight (add resistance in 1 pound [0.45 kg] increments as tolerated)
  - UE PREs: Light dumbbells
  - Cardiovascular exercises: 20 to 30 minutes in any combination of the following
    - Upper body ergometer (UBE)
    - Stairmaster
    - Stationary bike
    - Elliptical glider
- Pool exercises
  - Running, forward and backward
  - Side slides
  - Carioca
  - Jumping jacks
  - Swimming (flutter kick; *no butterfly*)

7 WEEKS
- Previous exercises, increase weights as tolerated
  - Strengthening
    - Abdominal crunches
    - Bridging
  - Jogging: 0.5 mile (0.8 km)
  - Backward jog: 100 yards (91.4 m) × 5 repetitions

8 WEEKS
- Previous PREs
- Trunk stabilization exercises
  - Lunges
  - Swiss ball
  - Crunches
  - Bridging
  - Obliques
  - Superman
  - Trunk extension
  - Reverse fly
- Jogging: mile (0.8-1.6 km)
- Backward jog: 100 yards (91.4 m) × 5 repetitions
- Agility drills
  - Sprinting: 50 yards (45.7 m); avoid sudden starts and stops
  - Figures-of-eight
  - Cariocas
- Plyometrics
  - Rope jumping
  - Side to side
  - Front to back

9 WEEKS
- Previous exercises
- LE PREs
- Sport-specific drills
  - Soccer—*No* shooting or long volleys

10-12 WEEKS
- Continued increase in exercise with the goal of return to play at 12 weeks after surgery

UE, Upper extremity; *PREs,* progressive resistance exercises; *LE,* lower extremity.
Modified from Meyers W, Ryan J: Drexel University College of Medicine, Department of Surgery, Hahnemann Sports Medicine Center.

strengthening, including emphasis on eccentric adductor and oblique abdominal strengthening.[89] A particularly effective form of core strengthening for athletic pubalgia uses diagonal elastic tubing resistance between the upper and lower extremities. Alex McKechnie[88] developed this approach and has had considerable success using it with professional athletes. A key component of this method is to have the patient simultaneously contract the pelvic floor and transversus abdominis and hold a low-level contraction while performing activities such as squats, lunges, and sport-specific moves repetitively, with additional core resistance coming from a TheraBand wrapped around each thigh and held in the contralateral hand (Figures 18-22 and 18-23) or by using the commercially available Core X System.

Joint Disorders

Osteoarthritis

OA is a complex disorder of synovial joints characterized by deterioration of articular cartilage and new bone formation, resulting in joint pain and dysfunction.[90] Radiographically, the deterioration of articular cartilage presents as joint space narrowing, and new bone formation presents as osteophytes. The hip is one of the more common sites of involvement, and OA of the hip affects approximately 1.5% of the adult population in the United

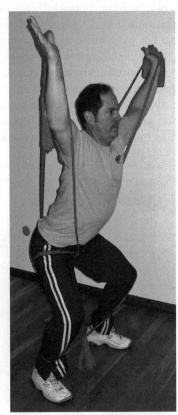

Figure 18-22 McKechnie squat with TheraBand. Note the TheraBand is wrapped around ankles, thighs, and hands so that when the TheraBand is stretched, it resists diagonal patterns of movement.

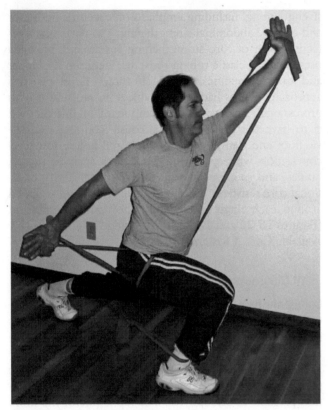

Figure 18-23 McKechnie lunge with TheraBand.

States.[91] Pain from OA of the hip usually is felt in the groin, lateral hip, and/or buttock.[6,7,91,92] Substantiated clinical presentation for hip OA is typically moderate anterior or lateral hip pain with weight bearing; age older than 50 years; morning stiffness for less than 1 hour; and limited hip medial (internal) rotation and flexion by 15° or more compared with the nonpainful side.[91,92]

OA can be divided into primary and secondary types. **Primary OA** occurs without some predisposing mechanical alignment factor. **Secondary OA** is the end result of

---

Clinical Presentation of Hip Osteoarthritis

- Pain in the lateral hip, groin, and/or buttock, especially on weight bearing
- Age older than 50 years
- Morning stiffness for less than an hour
- Medial rotation and flexion limited by 15° or more compared to unaffected side
- Joint space narrowing and osteophytes on x-ray

another disease process. Eighty percent of OA of the hip is secondary in nature.[93] Predisposing factors to secondary OA of the hip are disorders such as osteonecrosis, Legg-Calvé-Perthes disease, developmental dysplasia of the hip, slipped capital femoral epiphysis, congenital coxa vara or coxa valga, and hip fracture.

The primary signs and symptoms of OA are joint pain and stiffness. Radiographically, OA is characterized by joint space narrowing in the weight-bearing region and by osteophyte formation (Figure 18-24). RA, on the other hand, shows uniform joint space narrowing, which progresses to protrusio acetabuli (i.e., protrusion of the femoral head through the acetabulum) at the end stage. Routine radiographic views of the hip usually are sufficient to diagnose OA. Routine views for the hip are an anteroposterior (AP) pelvic view (which captures both proximal femurs, the pelvis, and the distal lumbar spine), AP hip view, and lateral hip view (either true lateral or frog lateral).

Routine X-Ray Views for the Hip

- Anteroposterior (AP) pelvis
- AP hip
- Lateral view (either true lateral or frog lateral)

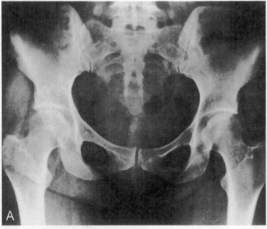
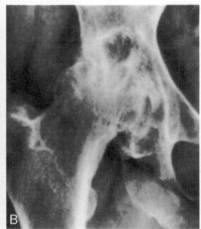

Figure 18-24 **A**, Normal hip joints on plain x-ray film, AP view. **B**, Osteoarthritis of the hip joint. Note the superior and lateral joint space narrowing, subchondral sclerosis, superior acetabular bone cyst, medial femoral neck, and lesser trochanteric sclerosis with buttressing. (From Frontera WR, Silver JK: *Essentials of physical medicine and rehabilitation*, Philadelphia, 2002, Hanley & Belfus.)

Advanced OA of the hip (i.e., radiographic evidence of OA with persistent severe symptoms or functional loss) can be effectively treated with total hip arthroplasty (THA), as discussed in Chapter 19. Because THA is not without risks and limitations, it is reserved for more advanced cases of OA that have not responded to medical management. A number of nonoperative (medical) approaches can be used to manage OA, including pharmacological and nonpharmacological measures. Nonpharmacological methods include patient education and physical and occupational therapy, which have been described as the foundation of treatment for patients with OA[94] and also help in postsurgical recovery should surgery become the treatment of choice.

Rehabilitation management of OA of the hip should be directed toward maintaining function, relieving symptoms, preventing deformity, and educating the patient in ways to protect the hip joint.[92] Function can be maintained by changing the person to fit the environment or by changing the environment to fit the person. Examples of factors that can be changed in the person are inflammation, joint alignment, ROM, and muscle length and strength. Changing the environment may involve activity modification, adaptive equipment, home modifications, and social services.

In published trials of nonmedicinal and noninvasive treatments for hip OA, aerobic-type exercise has been shown to have the greatest benefit.[95] Exercise therapy with the goals of improving muscle function (i.e., endurance, strength, and coordination), ROM, pain relief, and walking ability has been shown to be effective for OA of the hip.[96] However, in a study by Hoeksma et al.,[55] manual therapy for the hip was reported to be even more effective than exercise therapy in improving pain, stiffness, hip function, and ROM. The manual therapy these researchers used was stretching of the iliopsoas, quadriceps, TFL, sartorius, adductors, and gracilis with a hold time of 8 to 10 seconds for each muscle, repeated two times. The stretching was followed by a series of five traction manipulations (i.e., long axis traction), as described by Cyriax,[97] starting with the hip in the maximum loose-packed position; with each subsequent manipulation, the hip was placed in a position of more restriction.[55,97]

Combinations of manual soft tissue techniques, joint mobilization, and manual stretching are very effective in improving ROM and muscle length, reducing pain, and improving gait and other functions. A published case study[98] reported that ROM, strength, function, and gait can be improved and pain reduced in a person with hip OA who follows through with a rehabilitation program that includes manual therapy, therapeutic exercise, and education that addresses the presenting impairments. Patients with progressive OA may eventually need a hip replacement when walking becomes too painful, but the appropriate rehabilitation intervention can delay the operation and make for a better postoperative outcome. Delaying hip replacement too long, however, especially if function and exercise capability are significantly limited, is not wise, because it can result in worsening cardiovascular health in particular and prolonged or incomplete recovery.[99]

The decision to work on improving a joint's ROM depends on whether that joint's range can be expected to increase and whether the hip currently is functionally limited. The decision as to whether the joint's range can be increased depends primarily on the end feel. If the end feel is a bony block, the joint's range cannot be changed. If the end feel is not a bony block, the joint's range may be changeable. A balance between symptoms, range, and function must be found. Much of the pain from OA arises from the inflammatory process. In most cases, reducing inflammation produces concomitant symptom relief and functional improvements. A rationale for improving ROM is that restricted motion could be causing an inflammatory response as a result of abnormal joint surface arthrokinematics. If this hypothesis is not supported by treatment, the approach for improving ROM must be modified or discontinued.

It is important to teach the patient the principles of hip joint protection, especially considering that normal gait causes approximately three times the body's weight to load through the hip during walking (see Figure 18-7). These protection principles can be grouped into body weight reduction, load carrying modification, and assistive device use. For every pound of body weight lost, a 3-pound reduction in load through the hip occurs; therefore body weight reduction is an admirable goal. However, the weight-bearing exercise required to lose body weight can irritate the hip. Pool exercises, swimming, and upper body workouts can be used for weight reduction without exacerbating hip inflammation. Workouts on stationary bikes and rowing machines also are often well tolerated until OA is more advanced.

Hip Joint Protection Principles

- Weight reduction
- Exercise modification
- Load-carrying modification
- Use of assistive device

When the patient needs to carry something, it should be as light as possible and should be carried on the patient's back in a knapsack. If a unilateral load is carried, it should be carried on the side of the hip problem. A cane should be used on the side contralateral to the hip problem. Both the contralateral cane and ipsilateral load advice are based on the opposing torque forces.[100] For example, during one-leg stance on the right leg, the right hip has body weight creating a counterclockwise torque and the hip abductors creating a clockwise torque (see Figure 18-8).

Use of a cane in the contralateral (left) hand or holding a weight in the ipsilateral (right) hand also creates a clockwise torque about the right hip, thereby assisting the right hip abductors in clockwise torque generation.

Besides rehabilitation intervention, medication is an important component of nonoperative treatment for OA. The main indication for the use of medication in OA is pain relief.[94] Acetaminophen is recommended for mild to moderate pain because its efficacy is comparable with that of NSAIDs for this level of pain, and it has a more favorable side effect profile, provided the dosage does not exceed 4 g per day. NSAIDs are recommended for moderate to severe hip pain and in cases in which acetaminophen does not provide significant relief or the clinical presentation suggests significant inflammation.[94] Because of the cardiovascular risks associated with the cyclo-oxygenase-2 (COX-2) inhibitors, the nonselective traditional NSAIDs ibuprofen and naproxen are usually recommended as a first line of treatment. However, celecoxib (200 mg daily [qd]) and naproxen (500 mg twice per day [bid]) appear to be safer than other agents with regard to cardiovascular risk.[101] For long-term use of a nonselective NSAID, or in individuals with an increased risk of an upper gastrointestinal adverse event, a proton-pump inhibitor is recommended.[94]

Other pharmacological measures for hip OA are intra-articular injection of glucocorticosteroids, intra-articular injection of hyaluronan, and opioid analgesics (e.g., Tramadol).[94] Some patients find that glucosamine and/or chondroitin sulphate help take the edge off their symptoms.

Femoroacetabular Impingement

Although femoroacetabular impingement (FAI) was first recognized as a mechanism for early hip OA in 1965, it was not until recently that increased interest in this condition as a primary etiological factor behind labral tears and OA has been considered.[102,103] FAI has been identified as the most common cause of end-stage OA in young men and a common cause in young women.[104] Three mechanisms of impingement have been identified: **cam impingement**, caused by jamming of an abnormal femoral head (e.g., from pistol grip deformity) into the acetabulum with increasing hip flexion; **pincer impingement**, which occurs when the acetabular rim contacts the femoral head–neck junction at end range of flexion, causing a leverage of the opposite side of the femoral head up against the postero-inferior edge of the acetabulum; and the most common **mixed/combined type** that has components of both cam and pincer.[105]

Mechanism of Hip (Femoroacetabular) Impingement

- Cam
- Pincer
- Mixed/combined

Symptoms of FAI typically are seen in athletic, younger, and middle-aged individuals who experience groin pain with sports activity. The pain initially is intermittent and can be aggravated by increased athletic activity, especially in those involving end range hip movements, prolonged walking, and prolonged sitting.[105]

The **hip impingement test** is described as hip flexion to 90° and medial (internal) rotation of the adducted hip; this elicits groin pain with a positive test result.[105] Although this test is called the impingement test, it is not pathognomonic of FAI. The imaging workup should include an AP pelvis radiograph, along with a lateral view, which gives good visualization if either flattening of the normally concave femoral neck (i.e., a pistol grip deformity) and/or a nonspherical femoral head is present (Figure 18-25). The lateral view may either be a cross table lateral, a Dunn view, or modified Dunn view. Computed tomography (CT) scan can be a helpful adjunct in measuring acetabular version.

Conservative treatment involves activity modification to avoid the impingement positions and NSAIDs to reduce inflammation. To maintain a higher level of function and to manage pain, the surgeon and patient may opt for arthroscopic debridement/resection of the source of impingement through contouring of the femoral head and neck to a more normal anatomy (i.e., cheilectomy—surgery to remove bone spurs) or resecting part of the acetabulum that is overhanging. A periacetabular osteotomy may be needed if an acetabular torsion problem is present.[106] During surgery, debridement or repair of labral tears and debridement or microfracture may be indicated in the management of any chondral lesions that are present.[107] Further studies, including level I studies, are required to fully determine the cost benefit ratio and functional outcome of early operative intervention to prevent continued progression of OA of the hip.

Capsular Laxity and Microinstability

Capsular laxity and atraumatic hip instability can be a challenging diagnosis for the clinician and are less com-

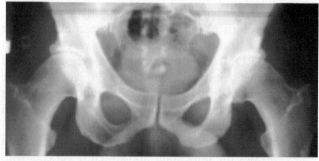

Figure 18-25 Plain x-ray film of the pelvis showing a "pistol grip" deformity of both proximal femora. This deformity is so named because the nonspherical femora resemble pistol grips. (From Shetty VD, Villar RN: Hip arthroscopy: current concepts and review of literature, *Br J Sports Med* 41:64-68, 2007.)

mon reasons for hip discomfort. However, instability, even microinstability, can be a cause of significant hip dysfunction and lead to labral tears and/or chondral damage. Capsular laxity and instability may be either a result of microtrauma and overuse or ligamentous laxity in conditions such as Marfan's syndrome or Ehlers-Danlos syndrome. In these patients, the history is very important because the patients can usually describe the motion that reproduces symptoms. Patients may also state that their leg "gives out" or they have a painful pop. On physical examination, increased passive ROM may be noted with soft endpoints, especially with lateral (external) rotation in extension. Hyperextension of the hip with lateral (external) rotation may also reproduce their symptoms. Radiographs will either be normal or may demonstrate some evidence of dysplasia such as a lower center-edge angle.[108,109]

Rehabilitation for hip microinstability is focused on strengthening of the muscle around the hip, proprioception training, core strengthening, optimization of muscular balance, and patient education about "at-risk" postures and movement habits. Often, patients with microinstability have an element of dysplasia (i.e., undercoverage of the femoral head) that enables them to achieve the extremes of ROM often required in their craft (e.g., dancers, gymnasts). The ability to control open-chain extreme range with one hip and closed-chain extreme range with the other hip is often an activity requirement (e.g., ballet). When an athlete is recovering from an injury that may involve hip microinstability, Pilates has been advocated as an effective non–weight-bearing strengthening and motor control environment before progressing to the demands of weight-bearing routines.[110]

If rehabilitation does not resolve the patient's symptoms, surgery may be warranted. Typically, an MRI is obtained before surgery to identify other pathological conditions that may be contributing and that may need to be addressed at the time of surgery. The preferred method for treating capsular laxity and microinstability in cases in which there are no large bony abnormalities is through an endoscopic technique. After routine portal placement, the hip is evaluated for any osseous, chondral, labral, and soft tissue or capsular defects. If identified, these are treated appropriately. With regard to capsular laxity, both thermocapsular shrinkage and capsular plication have been described. Thermal capsulorrhaphy is performed using a radiofrequency probe to heat the capsule and shrink it, thus reducing capsular volume.[108] There have been reports on the success of thermocapsular shrinkage; however, many surgeons are concerned with complications such as chondrolysis and nerve damage secondary to the elevation of joint temperature that have been seen in the shoulder.[110,111] Arthroscopic capsular plication of the hip performed by placing sutures in the medial and lateral limbs of the iliofemoral ligament and securing knots to tighten the capsule. This is repeated un-

til the desired effect is achieved. Short-term results have been promising.[111,112]

Postoperative management after capsular repair involves protecting the repair from elongation by restricting motions that would stress the repair until a sufficient cicatrix (i.e., scar) has formed. For example, after an anterior capsule repair (which is by far the most common), extension and lateral (external) rotation would be limited to neutral (0°) for the first 2 to 3 weeks followed by 3 weeks of gentle motion. A continuous passive motion (CPM) machine is often used for the first 2 to 4 weeks and weight bearing limited to 20 pounds foot flat for the first 2 to 4 weeks. It is important to encourage neutral rotation during gait and to prevent lateral (external) rotation when lying supine (CPM is useful for this and foot wraps are used when out of the CPM). Flexion may also be limited to 90° for the first 10 days and a hip brace worn to help with adherence to sagittal and transverse plane motion restrictions. A gradual progressive rehabilitation process is followed to obtain a good balance between hip stability and mobility with an approximate return to sport 4 to 6 months postoperatively.[113]

Labral Tears

With the advances in MRI imaging and the increasing use of arthroscopy at the hip, labral tears have been found to be more common than previously thought (Figure 18-26). Acetabular tears are one of the most common indications for hip arthroscopy. It is believed that labral tears may precipitate and/or accelerate the process of OA; however, recent studies have reported that up to 70% of asymptomatic individuals have labral tears.[114,115] Most labral tears (86%) are in the anterior quadrant of the labrum.[116] Chondral lesions double in the presence of a labral tear, and 40% of patients with a labral tear have severe chondral lesions.[116]

The mechanism for labral tears is often associated with either repetitive microtrauma associated with pivoting and twisting movements in sports or with a specific traumatic event. The specific traumatic event often involves extension and lateral (external) rotation, with the femoral head moving anteriorly and overstressing the anterior labrum.[116] However, atraumatic tears are also found, and recent research has indicated bony abnormalities such as FAI and dysplasia being present in a nearly 90% of patients who end up being treated with surgical arthroscopy.[117] Once the labrum has been torn, instability can occur in the joint and may lead to abnormal arthrokinematics and possibly further cartilage and labral damage. Less commonly, microinstability can be the primary cause of labral damage.[118]

The symptoms of a labral tear usually are mechanical in nature: buckling, catching, painful clicking, and restricted ROM. Several special tests have been described to assess for labral pathology; these tend to be variations of two primary tests[118-120]:

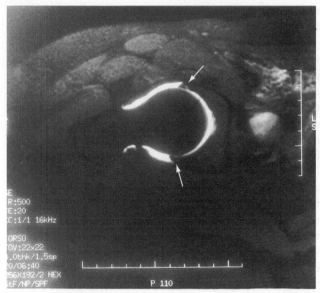

Figure 18-26 Magnetic resonance arthrogram showing an acetabular labral tear. (From DeLee J, Drez D, Miller M: *DeLee and Drez's orthopaedic sports medicine*, ed 2, Philadelphia, 2003, Saunders.)

1. The **hip impingement test** involves medial rotation of the flexed and adducted hip while it is held in at least 90° flexion and at least 15° adduction. If pain is not reproduced with the test performed slowly, a rapid application of the medial (internal) rotation at end range can reproduce symptoms. This test is suggestive of a wide range of anterior hip disorders, including anterior labral tear, anterosuperior impingement, and iliopsoas tendonitis.

2. The **hip apprehension test** consists of lateral (external) rotation of the extended hip. If symptoms are not reproduced, a rapid application of end range lateral (external) rotation can be performed. With a positive test result, this maneuver elicits apprehension or groin pain and suggests anterior hip instability, anterior labral tear, or posteroinferior impingement.

The **McCarthy hip extension sign** is a further test for labral pathology. In this test, both hips are flexed, and while the uninvolved hip is kept flexed, the involved hip is extended from the flexed position first in lateral (external) rotation and then in medial (internal) rotation. Reproduction of the patient's pain is a positive test result. McCarthy considered positive results on three different tests to be the key to predicting labral pathology: (1) pain with the McCarthy hip extension sign; (2) painful impingement with hip flexion, adduction, and lateral (external) rotation; and (3) inguinal pain on a resisted straight-leg raise.[121]

McCarthy's Signs Predicting Hip Labral Pathology

- Positive McCarthy hip extension sign
- Painful impingement on hip flexion, adduction, and lateral rotation
- Inguinal pain on resisted straight-leg raise (Stinchfield resisted hip flexion test)

The active and, if necessary, resisted straight-leg raise in the early range (test 3 in McCarthy's three-test battery) has been labeled the Stinchfield resisted hip flexion test, and the result is often positive with intra-articular disorders such as labral tears, arthritis, synovitis, occult femoral neck fractures, and prosthetic failure or loosening.[122] It also is positive with rectus femoris tendinitis and/or iliopsoas tendonitis/bursitis.

Fitzgerald[123] described the following variations to differentiate anterior from posterior labral tears. To test for *anterior* labral tears, the hip first is flexed with lateral (external) rotation and full abduction and then extended with adduction and medial (internal) rotation. A positive test result is hip pain with or without an associated click. To test for *posterior* labral tears, the hip is first fully flexed, adducted, and medially (internally) rotated. It then is extended with abduction and lateral (external) rotation. Again, a positive test result is pain with or without an associated click.[123]

Millis and Kim[120] found that MRI with gadolinium enhancement provides a more sensitive and specific diagnosis of labral tears than was previously possible (although it does not identify all tears present on arthroscopy), and arthroscopy provides a means to resect or stabilize the tear.[124]

Surgical treatment of labral tears is typically performed arthroscopically. Using portals in the hip, the surgeon can assess the joint and the degree of labral and or chondral involvement by doing a diagnostic arthroscopy (Figure 18-27). Next, the surgeon will proceed to either debride the unstable flap of labrum or repair it (often based on the location of the tear, as the labrum has limited blood supply, and thus, limited capacity to heal). For repairs, usually the substance of the labrum is intact, and the labrum injured at

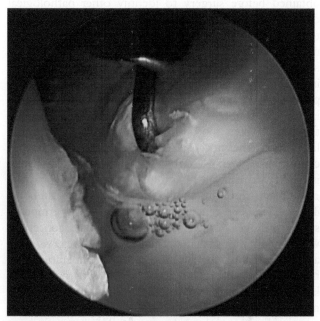

Figure 18-27 Labral tear seen arthroscopically.

the acetabular rim. The labrum is mobilized and a suture anchor is placed at the edge of the acetabulum. The sutures are then passed around or through the labrum and secured with knots or via a knotless technique.[125]

Focal Cartilage Injuries

Focal cartilage injuries can occur in association with FAI or in isolation. Focal cartilage injuries from FAI are typically the result of delamination from impingement and/or shearing from microinstability (Figure 18-28). Additionally, traumatic injuries can cause focal cartilage loss from axial loading or shear of the head within the socket (Figure 18-29). These types of injuries can often be difficult to diagnose and be an elusive source of hip pain. The pain typically occurs immediately after injury but may come and go. Persistent pain and symptoms of

catching or clicking should warrant advanced imaging such as an MRI to evaluate the joint. If cartilage injury is found, it often does not respond well to nonoperative treatment, and referral to an orthopedic surgeon is recommended. Recent advances in hip arthroscopy and surgical techniques have provided surgeons with several options to treat these types of injuries. Both open and hip arthroscopy techniques can be used to perform chondroplasties or stabilize loose cartilage flaps or even microfracture areas of exposed bone (Figure 18-30). There have been some reports of chondral repair, although the capacity of the cartilage to heal is limited, and the viability of the chondral flaps has been shown to be abnormal.[126,127] Another surgical option is to do a cartilage transplant procedure; however, there are limited reports on this technique.[128]

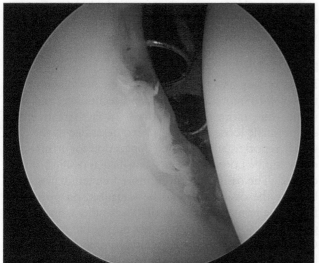

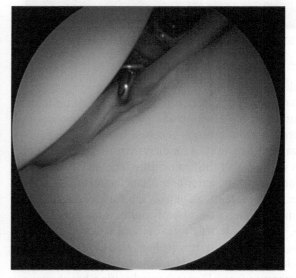

Figure 18-28 Labral chondral junction tear.

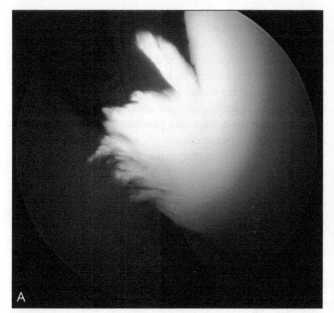

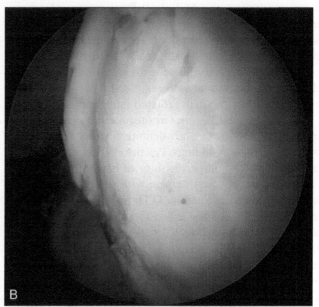

Figure 18-29 **A,** Hip chondral injury on femoral head before debridement. **B,** Exposed bone after cartilage debridement.

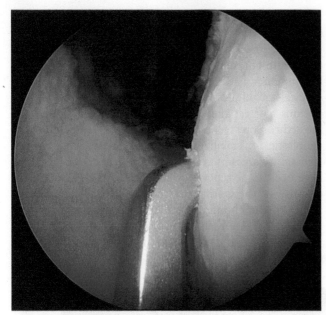

Figure 18-30 Microfracture of femoral head lesion.

Ligamentum Teres Injuries

There is no universal agreement on the ligamentum teres' contribution to hip function and pathology. Advances in hip arthroscopy has brought renewed interest in its function because it has allowed for direct visualization. Recent research suggests that the ligamentum teres may have analogous function to the anterior cruciate ligament (ACL) in the knee.[129] The ligament controls hip rotation in flexion. The ligamentum teres consistently tightens to limit hip abduction, medial (internal) rotation, and lateral (external) rotation, as shown by Martin et al.,[130] where they dissected eight cadavers and measured hip kinematics with regard to the ligamentum teres. Biomechanical testing has shown a similar load to failure, and anatomic studies have reported similar structure to the ACL.[131,132] Furthermore, the free nerve endings in the ligamentum teres suggest it may be involved in both proprioceptive and pain reception for the hip.[133] Another study by Martin et al.[134] reported increased hip excursion with a sectioned ligamentum teres particularly when the hip was laterally (externally) rotated in flexion and medially (internally) rotated in extension.

Diagnosis of ligamentum teres tears can be particularly challenging, as there are no definite history features or physical examination findings. Practitioners typically report that patients have nonspecific signs of hip irritability such as a positive log-roll test or pain with flexion, adduction and medial (internal) rotation. O'Donnell et al.[135] have recently reported a new test called the **ligament teres (LT) test.** The LT test is conducted with the hip flexed at 70° and 30° short of full abduction. The hip is then medially (internally) and laterally (externally) rotated to its limits of motion. Pain on either medial (internal) or lateral (external) rotation is consistent with a positive LT test result. O'Donnell et al.[135] found that this test was an effective way of assessing the presence of LT tears with moderate to high interobserver reliability. There is also a correlation with tears of the LT and symptoms of instability as reported by Martin et al.[130] who found that five of nine cases with arthroscopically proven ligamentum teres rupture had demonstrated symptoms of instability. Advanced imaging with MRIs has also proved to be challenging, because the findings are not always reliable. Byrd and Jones[136] were able to make the preoperative diagnosis of a ligamentum teres rupture in only 2 out of their 41 cases.

Surgical treatment has historically been focused on debriding the torn or injured ligamentum teres with a shaver or radiofrequency probe. If the cause of the ligament tear is present and identified, it should be addressed at the same time. There have also been reports of ligamentum teres reconstruction.[137,138] However, at this time, there is limited outcome data and reports have focused solely on techniques. More research is needed to determine not only whether this should be performed but also based on what indications.[139,140]

Loose Bodies

Loose bodies have been more frequently diagnosed in the hip with improved arthroscopic technology and technique—and more easily removed. In fact, treatment of symptomatic loose bodies has been described as the most widely reported and accepted application for arthroscopy of the hip.[141] Loose bodies are classified as ossified or nonossified. The ossified group is more frequently diagnosed because the ossification can be visualized on plain x-ray films. The primary symptom of loose bodies is anterior inguinal pain with locking episodes during hip movements. Other signs and symptoms include painful clicking, buckling, giving way, and persistent pain with activity.[141] Loose bodies can damage the articular cartilage of a joint, therefore prompt diagnosis and treatment are essential to prevent progression to OA.

Although arthroscopy has become the ideal method of addressing loose bodies definitively, Cyriax[14] described a technique for repositioning a loose body that may have some temporary benefit in lieu of arthroscopic removal. Cyriax[14] likened his technique for loose body treatment to repositioning a pebble in your shoe: you shake it around until it moves to a pain-free position. Cyriax[14] described loose bodies as presenting with sudden, sharp pain on weight bearing. The technique for "reducing" a loose body in the hip involves applying strong, long axis traction to the hip while it is in 80° flexion and then lowering the hip to 0° flexion while maintaining the traction and applying several small amplitude, high-velocity lateral (external) rotation maneuvers. If this method is unsuccessful, the procedure is performed again, but this time small thrusts into medial (internal) rotation are used. The effect on pain and function should be dramatic if indeed a mobile loose body is the culprit. The clinician should not persist if the treatment is not effective after several attempts, but if it works, it should be repeated as needed. It should be noted that there are no outcome reports on Cyriax loose body manipulation technique. If conservative treatment does not provide lasting relief, arthroscopy may be necessary to remove the loose bodies (Figure 18-31).

Hip Arthroscopic Technique Considerations

It is important for a rehabilitation specialist to understand the basics of hip arthroscopy. To start, the setup for hip arthroplasty is very different than other orthopedic procedures. The patient can be positioned either lateral or supine on a special table that helps distract the hip while the surgeon is able to work inside the joint (Figure 18-32). The hip needs to be distracted to allow the surgeon access to the central compartment—within the confines of the acetabulum. Because the hip is a deep structure surrounded by layers of soft tissue, fluoroscopy is necessary to provide guidance during the surgery. Portal placement is the most fundamental and often the most challenging for the surgeon and is extremely important to optimize maneuverability

and access around the hip joint. Additionally, poor placement can increase risk to important neurovascular structures around the hip (Figure 18-33). After successful establishment of both viewing and working portals, the surgeon then can use special hip arthroscopy tools to treat the pathology identified (Figure 18-34). The acetabular articular surface, the labrum, the ligamentum teres, and the femoral head articular surface are structures within the central compartment and can be seen and treated while the hip is distracted. With current techniques, traction is used to provide the distraction to the central compartment and is limited to 2 hours. Outside of the central compartment, cam deformities of FAI and usually loose bodies are seen along the femoral neck. These structures are within the joint capsule in an area called the peripheral compartment. An incision in the capsule in the peripheral compartment allows access to the iliopsoas for lengthening. Access to the

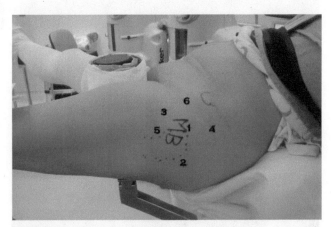

Figure 18-33 Hip arthroscopy portals. Dots represent the outline of the greater trochanter and the U outlines the anterior superior iliac spine (ASIS). (1) Position of the anterolateral portal. (2) Position of the posterolateral portal. (3) Position of the modified anterior portal about 5 to 7 cm distal and anterior to the anterior portal. (4) Proximal anterolateral portal. (5) Distal anterolateral portal. (6) Position of the anterior portal and the junction of the ASIS and greater trochanter.

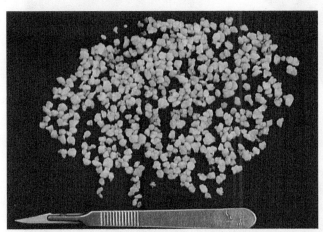

Figure 18-31 Loose bodies retrieved arthroscopically from the hip joint.

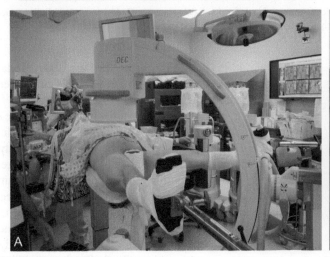

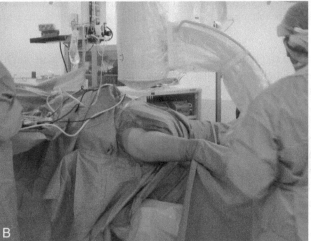

Figure 18-32 A, Room setup for supine patient positioning in hip arthroplasty. **B,** Intraoperative fluoroscopy used to help provide guidance during the surgery.

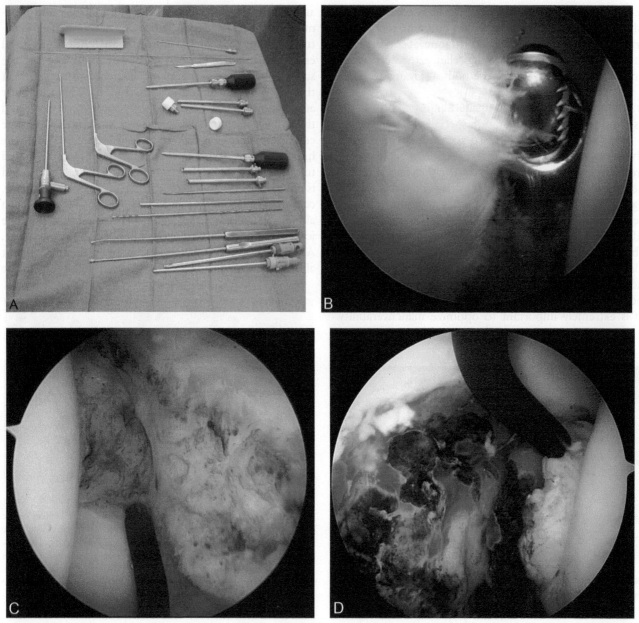

Figure 18-34 A, Commonly used tools in hip arthroplasty. **B,** Arthroscopic motorized shaver for tissue debridement. **C,** Arthroscopic radiofrequency device for ablating soft tissue. **D,** The radiofrequency probe can be actively bent by the surgeon to provide greater access around the hip.

lateral structures that cause greater trochanteric pain, such as trochanteric bursitis, external snapping hip, and gluteus medius tears are performed without traction.

Rehabilitation after Hip Arthroscopy

Numerous papers and also basic science research on rehabilitation of the hip following hip arthroscopy have been published over the last decade.[142–145] An example of one such protocol is provided in Figure 18-35. To optimize outcome and to reduce risk of complications, rehabilitation professionals treating postoperative hip arthroscopy patients should familiarize themselves with rehabilitation guidelines, in addition to the surgical and patient-related factors of the individual case.

Rehabilitation should progress through four fundamental stages: (1) protection and mobility, (2) controlled stability, (3) strengthening, and (4) return to activity.[142] Progression is based on both criteria and healing time/ experience. There are variations in rehabilitation guidelines based on whether surgery was a debridement only, involved a labral repair, involved cam or pincer impingement bone shaving/trimming, involved capsular repair, or involved chondroplasty with or without microfracture. The rehabilitation professional should make sure he or she knows the surgical details, postoperative orders, and rehabilitation progression guidelines of the surgeon and/ or surgery type for each patient. Typically, the rehabilitation process is 3 to 6 months after hip arthroscopy, which

Hip Arthroscopy for Labral Repair
Dr. Safran's Physical Therapy Protocol

Patient Checklist:

Weightbearing
FFWB x 2 weeks
(Flat Foot - 20 lb)

Continuous passive motion (CPM)
2 weeks
4-6 hrs/day

Lie on stomach:
1-2 hrs 2-3x/day

* *If Labral Repair:
* Rotational Boot:
* When laying on back
* and not in CPM
  18-21 days

* Brace:
* 0-90 x 10 days

* ROM Limits:
* Flexion: 90° x 10 days
* Extension: 0° x 3 wks
* Abduction: 25° x 3wks
* External (lateral) rotation: 0° x 3 wks
* Internal (medial) rotation: no limits

Modalities:
Active Release Technique
Ultrasound and electrical stimulation
as needed starting week 3.

Time Lines:
Week 1 (1-7 POD)
Week 2 (8-14 POD)
Week 3 (15-21 POD)
Week 4 (22-28 POD)

Phase I: Initial Exercises — Week:	1	2	3	4	5	6	7	9	13	17	21	25
Ankle pumps	■	■										
Gluteus slide	■	■										
→ do standing		■	■	■								
Isometrics	■	■										
Stationary bike with non resistance	■	■	■	■								
Passive Range of motion (ROM)/CIRCUMDUCTION	■	■	■	■	■	■						
→ add extension and external (lateral) rotation (FABER)				■	■	■						
Soft tissue massage and scar mobilization	■	■	■	■	■	■						
Passive stretching: quadriceps and piriformis	■	■	■	■	■	■						
→ add hip flexor stretching			■	■	■	■						
Deep water progression		■	■	■	■	■	■	■				
Quadruped rocking		■	■	■								
Standing hip internal rotation		■	■	■	■	■	■	■	■	■	■	■
Resisted prone internal/external rotation		■	■	■	■	■	■	■	■	■	■	■
Lower abdominal progression and transverse abdominals	■	■	■	■	■	■						
Gluteal progression	■	■	■	■	■	■						
Bridging progression			■	■	■	■						
Leg press (limited weight)					■	■						
Gait progression "crutch weaning"				■	■							
Short arc quadriceps and vastus medialis oblique strengthening	■	■										
Straight leg raises with transversus abduction		■	■									
Proprioception	■	■	■	■	■	■	■					
Phase II: Intermediate Exercises	1	2	3	4	5	6	7	9	13	17	21	25
Balance progression			■	■	■	■	■					
Stationary biking with resistance				■	■	■	■	■				
Double 1/3 knee bends				■	■	■	■	■				
Advanced core progression				■	■	■	■	■				
→ Pilates exercises (with instructor)						■	■	■	■			
Manual Mobilizations (with physical therapist)				■	■	■	■	■	■			
Side stepping						■	■	■	■			
Eliptical/stairclimber				■	■	■	■	■	■			
Single 1/3 knee bends (after OK double leg)							■	■	■	■		
→ Lateral step downs							■	■	■	■		
→ Balance squats							■	■	■	■		
Multidirectional lunges							■	■	■	■	■	
Phase III: Advanced Exercises	1	2	3	4	5	6	7	9	13	17	21	25
Plyometrics progression									■	■		
Side to side lateral movement										■		
Forward/backward running with cord									■	■		
Running/skating/golf/etc progression										■		
Agility drills - returning to sport										■		
Phase IV: High Level Activities	1	2	3	4	5	6	7	9	13	17	21	25
Functional sport testing										■		
Multi-plane agility										■	■	
Sport specific drills										■	■	■

Figure 18-35 Dr. Safran's physical therapy protocol following cheilectomy and/or labral repair. *FFWB*, Flatfoot weight bearing (sometimes called partial weight bearing [PWB]); *CPM*, continuous passive motion; *ROM*, range of motion; *Ext*, extension; *Abd*, abduction; *ER*, external (lateral) rotation; *IR*, internal (medial) rotation; *E-Stim*, electrical stimulation; *POD*, post operative day; *VMO*, vastus medialis obliquus; *OK*, okay. (Courtesy of Dr. Marc Safran, Department of Orthopedic Surgery, Stanford School of Medicine. Adapted from Stalzer S, Wahoff M, Scanlan M: Rehabilitation following hip arthroscopy, *Clin Sports Med* 25:337-357, 2006; and Wahoff M, Ryan M: Rehabilitation after femoroacetabular impingement arthroscopy, *Clin Sports Med* 30:463-482, 2011.)

may vary depending on the type of surgery and individual patient response.

The ideas of Sahrmann[23] are worth incorporating into both the nonoperative and postoperative rehabilitation of patients with labral pathology. Sahrmann emphasized the importance of keeping the femoral head well seated in the acetabulum. This requires accurate diagnosis of the movement impairment syndrome, followed by prescription of the appropriate stretches, motor control and strengthening exercises, and patient education. Sahrmann has identified 11 movement impairments at the hip, of which anterior femoral glide is the most common. **Anterior femoral glide syndrome** can result in injury to the anterior labrum of the hip through a directional susceptibility of the hip into extension (common in runners and dancers), which causes the femoral head to increase pressure against the anterior joint structures, causing irritation and injury. Anterior femoral glide syndrome can also cause impingement of anterior hip structures (e.g., the iliopsoas myotendon and anterior labrum) as a result of inadequate posterior glide of the femoral head during hip flexion. For treatment, the clinician should advise the patient to avoid activities and exercises that load the anterior labrum (e.g., into end range extension and/or lateral [external] rotation); prescribe exercises and activities that encourage posterior glide of the femoral head (e.g., rocking back and forward in the quadruped position while hinging at the hips with the back held flat in the neutral spine position); and emphasize control of one-joint hip stabilizers (e.g., iliacus, gluteus maximus, and posterior gluteus medius) and deemphasize two-joint stabilizers (e.g., hamstrings, rectus femoris).[23]

Sahrmann's Movement Impairments of the Hip

- Femoral anterior glide syndrome without medial rotation
- Femoral anterior glide syndrome with medial rotation
- Femoral anterior glide syndrome with lateral rotation
- Hip adduction syndrome without medial rotation
- Hip adduction syndrome with medial rotation
- Femoral lateral glide syndrome
- Hip extension with knee extension
- Hip extension with medial rotation
- Femoral hypomobility syndrome with superior glide
- Femoral accessory hypermobility syndrome
- Hip lateral rotation syndrome (shortened piriformis)

From Sahrmann SA: *Diagnosis and treatment of movement impairment syndromes,* pp 176-191, St Louis, 2002, Mosby.

Osseous Disorders

Osteonecrosis

Osteonecrosis is a multifactorial disease in which osteocyte death occurs in the femoral head via a variety of proposed pathogenic pathways. It has both clinically and radiographically recognizable patterns to aid diagnosis.

Osteonecrosis can occur anywhere in the body but is most common in the head of the femur.

The two general subtypes of osteonecrosis are traumatic osteonecrosis and nontraumatic osteonecrosis. The traumatic type often occurs secondary to a hip fracture or dislocation, and, for this reason, displaced femoral neck fractures are treated by surgically replacing the femoral head. With a hip dislocation, the risk for osteonecrosis is increased if hip reduction is not performed within 8 hours.[146]

Types of Osteonecrosis

- Traumatic
- Nontraumatic

In the nontraumatic type of osteonecrosis, the symptoms are hip pain (often a fairly abrupt onset of severe pain), decreased hip ROM, and stiffness. These symptoms are not specific to this condition, and no specific physical examination tests exist for osteonecrosis. The examiner therefore needs to rely on the history as the clue to pursue diagnostic imaging that would result in a definitive diagnosis. The male-to-female ratio for osteonecrosis is 4:1. The most common age range for onset is between the third and fifth decades. Bilateral involvement is seen in more than 50% of cases. *Red flags* for nontraumatic osteonecrosis include a history of corticosteroid use, alcohol abuse, or sickle cell disease. Clinicians should keep in mind that plain radiographs are not sensitive to osteonecrosis in the early stages; therefore being alert to any historical red flags is crucial. MRI is sensitive and specific for diagnosing osteonecrosis (Figure 18-36), and the classic MRI finding is the crescent sign. The crescent sign is seen early on MRI as decreased signal indicative of the necrotic bone; when the crescent sign is observed on plain films at a more advanced stage of the disease process it is from a subchondral fracture between necrotic bone and healthy bone.

Red Flags for Hip Osteonecrosis

- History of corticosteroid use
- Alcohol abuse
- Sickle cell disease
- Gaucher's disease (a genetic disease in which fatty deposits accumulate in cells and certain organs including bone)

Treatment for osteonecrosis covers the gamut of surgical options for treatment of the hip. Mild cases respond well to surgical core decompression, in which a hole is drilled up into the femoral head to release pressure and provide a pathway for new blood vessels to grow into

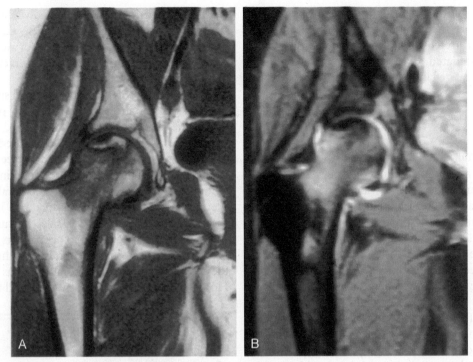

Figure 18-36 Osteonecrosis. Corresponding coronal T_1-weighted (TR/TE, 600/20) (**A**) and fat-suppressed fast T_2-weighted (TR/TE, 4000/70) (**B**) spin-echo magnetic resonance images reveal an area of osteonecrosis in the right femoral head, with associated articular collapse and joint effusion. Note the diffusely distributed abnormalities in the femoral head and neck compatible with marrow edema and the crescent sign on the superior femoral head. (From Resnick D, Kransdorf MJ: *Bone and joint imaging,* ed 3, p 1076, Philadelphia, 2005, Saunders.)

the area of necrotic bone. Moderately severe cases can be treated by osteotomy or vascularized fibular grafts. Severe or late stage cases require hemiarthroplasty or total hip replacement.[147]

It is important for clinicians to be aware of osteonecrosis because patients may be seen for hip pain that is mistakenly thought to be of soft tissue origin, when the real source of symptoms is osteonecrosis.[5] The prognosis is much better if the problem is diagnosed in the early stage, when core decompression can be performed.

Osteitis Pubis

Osteitis pubis is the most common inflammatory disorder affecting the pubic symphysis, which is part of the pelvis not of the hip.[148] It can, however, refer symptoms to the hip area. Generally, it is a self-limiting inflammation that occurs secondary to overuse, trauma, pelvic surgery, or childbirth. Although it can occur at any age, it is most common in males in their third or fourth decade. Those most at risk are athletes who participate in sports involving repetitive shearing forces at the pubic symphysis and multidirectional deceleration and acceleration forces (e.g., soccer, ice hockey). Long-distance runners are also prone to develop osteitis pubis. The gracilis muscle that attaches to the pubic symphysis has been implicated as a component in the etiology, and contracture or weakness (or both) of the gracilis often is seen with osteitis pubis.

A "groin burn" is a common complaint in patients with osteitis pubis. Depending on the irritability of the condition, the pain can be brought on by walking,

running, climbing stairs, one-leg stance, pivoting, kicking, and even coughing or sneezing. Rest usually relieves the pain. A prolonged, bilateral adductor muscle contraction with the patient squeezing the clinician's fist between the knees can elicit groin pain. Resisted rectus abdominis contraction (i.e., a sit-up) can also be painful. Tenderness is present at the superior or inferior pubic ramus (or both), and often both sides can be tender. Occasionally, pelvic compression may exacerbate symptoms of osteitis pubis. Other conditions to consider in the differential diagnosis are groin strain, pubic rami stress fracture, hernia, and infectious osteitis pubis (most often occurring after urological or gynecological surgery).[148]

The imaging studies of choice are plain radiographs and radionuclide bone scans. The radiographic findings, which may be negative in the early stage of osteitis pubis, usually include decreased definition of the cortical bone (i.e., irregular cortical margins and patchy sclerosis), and widening of the pubic symphysis may be seen. To assess for pubic symphysis widening, one-leg standing (flamingo) views are recommended. Bone scans usually show unilateral uptake at the pubic symphysis. Imaging helps differentiate osteitis pubis from other causes of groin pain, such as athletic pubalgia. MRI may also be used to diagnose osteitis pubis.

Treatment should begin with rest from the causative activity (e.g., soccer or running) and avoidance of aggravating activities. NSAIDs and ice can be helpful for the inflammation. If NSAIDs are not helpful, a corticosteroid injection into the site of maximum tenderness can be considered. Prolotherapy injections are also effective in some cases. Once the symptoms have abated, progressive rehabilitation stretching and strengthening of the hip musculature are initiated. Exercise in water can be particularly helpful. Heat-retaining compressive shorts can be helpful for dry land exercise and sport.[149]

Fractures and Dislocations

Hip (Proximal Femur) Fracture

Hip fractures are a common orthopedic injury with a high incidence, cost, and risk.[150] Worldwide, in the year 2000, there were estimated to be 1.6 million hip fractures, and, with the increasing elderly population, this is projected to increase to 6.26 million hip fractures worldwide by 2050.[151,152] More than 300,000 hip fractures occur each year in the United States, with a 1-year mortality rate of nearly 25%, a life expectancy reduction of 25%, and lifetime health care costs approaching $25 billion.[153] The morbidity rate after fracture is 32% to 80%.[153] One interpretation of this data is that a hip fracture is part of a downward spiral of health. Although partly true, this view ignores evidence that many older adults are able to tolerate and make improvements in physical attributes and function.[154-156]

Approximately 90% of elderly hip fractures result from a simple low-energy fall.[157] The most common risk factors for falls (and thus hip fractures) are age, gender, race, institutionalization/hospitalization, medical co-morbidities (e.g., cardiac disease, stroke, dementia, prior hip fracture, osteoporosis), hip geometry, medication, bone density and body habitus, diet, smoking, alcohol consumption, fluorinated water, urban versus rural residence, and climate.[158] Despite all these risk factors, a hip fracture occurs for many reasons that include, but are not limited to, poor balance reactions, decreased strength and weaker

(i.e., osteoporotic) bone. Older individuals tend to fall on the hip because of their slower gait speed (Figure 18-37), whereas younger elders often fall forward onto an outstretched arm, resulting in a Colles' fracture at the wrist (Figure 18-38).[159]

Most hip fractures need to be treated surgically to allow for pain control and early mobilization of the patient to reduce the risks associated with prolonged bed rest and immobilization. The type of fixation required depends on the age of the patient and location and degree of displacement of the fracture. Hip fractures are most simply categorized as intracapsular or extracapsular. A femoral neck fracture is the typical intracapsular fracture, and an intertrochanteric fracture is the typical extracapsular fracture. This distinction is important because, in older patients a displaced femoral neck fracture usually requires an arthroplasty because the blood supply to the femoral head has been disrupted. However, in young patients, surgeons will typically attempt

---

Risk Factors for Falls and Hip Fractures[158]

- Age: Incidence increases with age
- Gender: Increased incidence in females > males
- Race: Increased incidence in Caucasians
- Social living situation: Increased incidence with institutionalization
- Medical history: Increased incidence with multiple co-morbidities
- Falls risk: Increased incidence with poor balance
- Strength and endurance: Increased incidence with poor muscular strength and endurance
- Hip geometry: Increased with longer and/or narrower femoral neck
- Medication: Increased risk with multiple medications
- Bone density: Increased risk with low bone density
- Diet: Increased with low calcium and vitamin D
- Smoking: Increased with excessive use
- Alcohol consumption: Increased with excessive use
- Fluorinated water: Decreased with fluorinated water

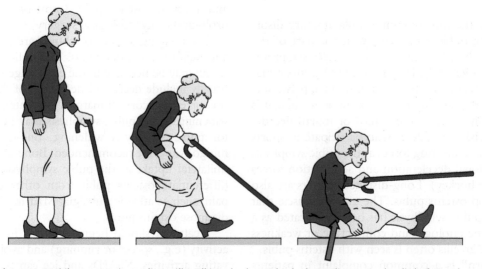

Figure 18-37 A fall that occurs while a person is standing still, walking slowly, or slowly descending a step has little forward momentum. With little forward momentum, the principal point of impact is near the hip. (Modified from Cummings SR, Nevitt MC: A hypothesis: the cause of hip fractures, *J Gerontol* 44: M107-M111, 1989.)

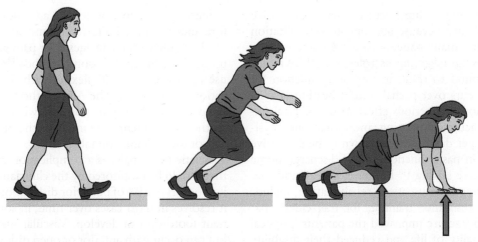

Figure 18-38 A fall that occurs while a person is walking rapidly has enough forward momentum to carry the individual onto the hands or knees instead of the hip. (Modified from Cummings SR, Nevitt MC: A hypothesis: the cause of hip fractures, *J Gerontol* 44: M107-M111, 1989.)

to do an urgent anatomic reduction to save the hip rather than perform a hip arthroplasty. The greater the displacement, the higher the risk of avascular necrosis of the femoral head. Thus, with a nondisplaced femoral neck fracture, a surgeon can often treat it with pins or screws.

Total hip arthroplasty (THA) has been advocated as the optimal treatment for displaced femoral neck fractures in the elderly because of the high rate of avascular necrosis as well as ease of mobilizing the patient earlier. THA is associated with more independent living, it is more cost-effective, and there is a longer interval to reoperation or death than with open reduction and internal fixation (ORIF) and unipolar or bipolar hemiarthroplasty.[160] A hemiarthroplasty replaces only the fractured ball side and does nothing to the acetabular side. There are two types of hemiarthroplasty: unipolar and bipolar. The bipolar implant has a pole of movement within the prosthesis that

is designed to reduce wear on the acetabular cartilage. The bipolar endoprosthesis is more expensive than the unipolar design and is used with younger patients (those younger than approximately 70 years of age) who might require revision to a total hip replacement during their lifetime usually because of acetabular cartilage degeneration. The original unipolar design (e.g., the Austin-Moore prosthesis) tends to be used on less active and older patients who are unlikely to outlive the hip implant.

For intertrochanteric fractures (stable or unstable), the sliding hip screw, which is available in a variety of designs, is the implant of choice.[157] Unstable intertrochanteric fractures sometimes are treated with an intramedullary device, but no difference in functional outcomes has been seen between it and the sliding hip screw when used for stable fractures.[157] Figure 18-39 shows some of the implants commonly used in hip surgery.

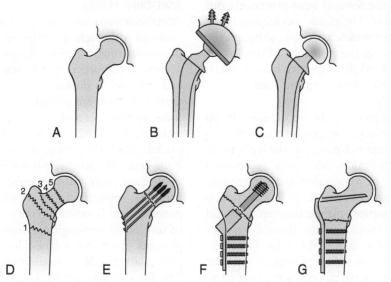

Figure 18-39 Various types of hip reconstructions and implants. **A,** Normal hip joint. **B,** Total hip arthroplasty (both femoral head and acetabulum replaced). **C,** Hemiarthroplasty (only femoral head and neck replaced). **D,** Levels of proximal femoral fractures: *1,* Subtrochanteric; *2,* intertrochanteric; *3,* basicervical; *4,* transcervical (femoral neck); *5,* subcapital. **E,** Multiple screw fixation of a femoral neck fracture. **F,** Screw and plate fixation of an intertrochanteric hip fracture. **G,** Blade plate fixation of a proximal femoral osteotomy. In this drawing, no rotation of the proximal fragment was performed (Modified from Shinar AA: Surgeries of the hip: the approaches and the basics. In Fagerson TL, editor: *The hip handbook,* p 239, Boston, 1998, Butterworth-Heinemann.)

Rehabilitation after a hip fracture must be intensive and multidisciplinary because appropriate rehabilitation efforts can restore many patients to a pre-fracture functional status.[5] Weight bearing as tolerated (WBAT) for gait has been found to result in improved function for hip fracture patients over partial weight-bearing (PWB) restriction, without deleterious effect to the surgical fixation.[161] In the acute care setting, more than one physical therapy visit per day has been shown to be predictive of achievement in basic function and of discharge home from the acute care setting.[150] Binder et al.[155] found that 6 months of extended outpatient rehabilitation, including progressive resistance training, for frail elderly patients with a hip fracture improved the patients' physical function and quality of life and reduced their disability compared with a low intensity "standard" home exercise program. Mangione et al.[156] found that a sample of frail elderly patients who had ORIF or hemiarthroplasty for a hip fracture could tolerate a moderate- to high-intensity home exercise program of either resistance training or aerobic exercise with appropriate supervision. A meta-analysis of 11 studies on extended rehabilitation after hip fracture, including those of Binder et al.[155] and Mangione et al.,[156] supports the findings that extended rehabilitation (often up to 12 months after surgery) is effective at improving functional abilities in this population.[162]

Traumatic Hip Dislocation

Dislocation of the hip in nonsurgical instances is rare. It usually occurs secondary to some form of trauma and often is associated with an acetabular and/or a femoral head fracture. Most traumatic hip dislocations are posterior (i.e., 85% to 90%), and this usually is related to a mechanism of injury in which the hip is flexed and in some degree of adduction and the knee is flexed while a dislocating force drives the femoral head posteriorly out of the acetabular socket.[163] The classic mechanism is the dashboard injury in motor vehicle accidents, although the use of seat belts is reducing the incidence of this injury. In contact sports (e.g., football, rugby, ice hockey, wrestling), a fall or tackle onto a flexed hip and knee can also drive the femur posteriorly.

Posterior hip dislocations can be recognized based on the mechanism of injury. The patient has considerable posterior thigh and buttock pain, and the leg appears shortened and is held in flexion, adduction, and medial (internal) rotation. Prompt recognition and early reduction are essential for a good outcome. Before reduction under anesthesia is attempted, plain radiographs should be taken to rule out a fracture of the femoral head or acetabulum. Reduction of a dislocated hip should be performed within 6 to 8 hours to reduce the risk of avascular necrosis of the femoral head, which occurs as a later complication in 10% to 15% of patients following posterior hip dislocation. For dislocated hips that are not reduced within 8 hours, the rate of femoral head osteonecrosis increases to 40%. Most traumatic dislocations of the hip are reduced using spinal or general anesthesia. However, before anesthesia is administered, one attempt at reduction can be made with an analgesic for pain and muscle spasm using the Allis or Stimson methods.[146] These methods use hip traction in 90° flexion with firm counterstabilization of the pelvis. The Allis method is performed with the patient in the supine position, whereas in the Stimson method the patient is prone with the hip flexed over the end of the examination table.[146]

Sciatic nerve palsy is a complication of hip dislocation that should be monitored by the clinician. Sciatic nerve injury occurs in 10% of posterior dislocations, and, although it resolves in most cases over time, in some cases, permanent footdrop can develop. Vascular insufficiency is rare but can occur with anterior or open dislocations. After hip reduction, radiographs should be obtained to make sure no loose bodies are preventing concentric reduction and that no fracture exists.

Once the dislocated hip has been reduced, management may require limited motion using a hip brace and patient education about risk positions. The risk position for posterior dislocation is combined flexion, adduction, and medial (internal) rotation. The risk position for anterior dislocation is combined extension and medial (internal) rotation. These movements, done rapidly, further increase the risk for re-dislocation.

Risk Positions for Hip Dislocation

- Posterior: Flexion, adduction, and medial rotation
- Anterior: Extension and lateral rotation

Acetabular Fracture

Acetabular fractures are socket-side hip fractures but are categorized with fractures of the pelvis, unlike fractures of the proximal femur, which are designated as hip fractures. Most acetabular fractures occur as a result of high-energy trauma, and they can be displaced or nondisplaced. Displaced acetabular fractures are treated with ORIF to allow earlier ambulatory function and to reduce the risk of posttraumatic arthritis. The ORIF hardware (i.e., screws and plates) is placed outside the joint to act as an "internal cast" until the bone heals. The hardware is not routinely removed.[164]

Perhaps more than in most other hip conditions or surgeries, application of a knowledge of in vivo force and pressure data is extremely important in the rehabilitation of surgical or nonsurgical acetabular fractures. Table 18-7 presents an evidence-based loading progression that is particularly useful for rehabilitation of acetabular fractures based on data from in vivo force and pressure measurements at the hip.[165] Most patients with an acetabular fracture begin with touch-down (i.e., feathering) weight bearing (TDWB), which, when performed correctly, results in less acetabular contact pressure than even non–weight bearing

TABLE **18-7**

Progression of Activities of Daily Living and Exercise Based on In Vivo Force and Pressure Data at the Hip

Low Load	Low-Moderate Load	Moderate Load	High-Moderate Load	High Load
TDWB gait performed correctly	PWB gait	FWB gait	AROM (standing) *no support*	Getting into and out of low chairs
NWB gait	Chair rise *with technique**	AROM (standing) *with support*	Maximum isometrics	Going up and down stairs
PROM	Stairs *with technique*	One-leg stance *(with support)*	One-leg stance *no support*	Accidental stumble
AAROM	AROM (supine and prone) *no resistance*	Hip abduction (side-lying) *no external resistance*	Slow jogging	Abductor resistance
Submaximum quad sets	Submaximum gluteal isometrics	Low-resistance exercise (supine and prone)		Jumping
Bridging	Bridging			Running
Double leg stance				
Bicycle (no resistance)				

With technique refers to the use of a load-modifying variable, which a physical therapist can teach a patient. For example, for a chair rise, this could involve use of the armrests, having the affected leg out in front, sitting in a higher chair, or a combination of these. For stairs, *with technique* could involve ascent and descent one leg at a time, use of a banister and a crutch, or both.

Modified from Fagerson TL: *Home study course: current concepts of orthopaedic physical therapy—hip*, La Crosse, WI, 2001, Orthopaedic Section, American Physical Therapy Association.

TDWB, Touch-down weight bearing; *NWB,* non–weight bearing; *PROM,* passive range of motion; *AAROM,* active-assisted range of motion; *PWB,* partial weight bearing; *AROM,* active range of motion; *FWB,* full weight bearing.

(NWB), which can cause joint loading from hip muscle co-contraction. The exercise program should also follow a graduated loading progression that mirrors the healing stages of the fracture and is in synchronization with the physician's prescribed weight-bearing status.

Femoral Head Fracture

Femoral head fractures are rare and are typically seen with traumatic posterior hip dislocations. The first step is to reduce the hip fracture then assess the fracture of the femoral head and its displacement. Nonsurgical management is only for nondisplaced Pipkin type 1 fractures, whereas most surgeons recommended surgical treatment for any other type (Figure 18-40). Many different surgical techniques and approaches have been described depending on the fracture size and amount of displacement. The core features of surgery are (1) a safe approach and (2) adequate fixation or excision of the fragment. If the fracture cannot be reduced and fixed, then arthroplasty is another treatment option but is not ideal for younger patients.[166]

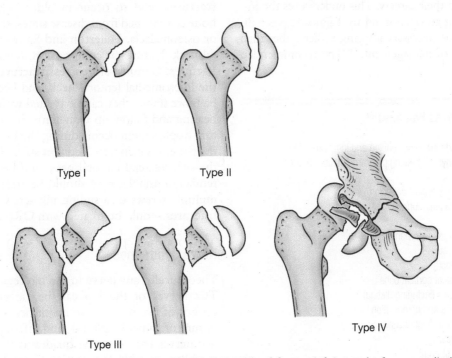

Figure 18-40 Pipkin classification for femoral head fractures. Type I: Femoral head fracture inferior to the fovea centralis. Type II: Femoral head fracture superior to the fovea centralis. Type III: Type I or II with an associated femoral neck fracture. Type IV: Type I, II, or III with an associated acetabular fracture.

There is very little in the literature about postoperative rehabilitation protocols for femoral head fractures. It is generally recommended to have a prolonged period of non–weight bearing for about 2 months followed by gradual progressive weight bearing for fractures that needed fixation. For excision cases, weight-bearing limitation may be very different depending on the surgeon. ROM and strengthening exercises can typically be started earlier, but this is also often decided on a case-by-case basis.

Stress Fracture

Stress fractures in the hip region usually are seen at the femoral neck, pubic rami, and proximal femoral shaft. Although most stress fractures occur in the lower leg and foot, 8.8% of lower extremity stress fractures are reported to occur in the hip and pelvic region.[167]

Stress fractures typically occur as a result of repetitive overuse that exceeds the intrinsic ability of bone to repair itself. Osteoclastic old bone resorption typically precedes osteoblastic new bone formation by 3 to 4 weeks, and increased stress to the bone during this time (e.g., an increase in running mileage) can result in microfractures, which result in a stress fracture if the increased stress to the bone is continued. Resting and unloading the bone can allow the osteoblastic new bone formation to catch up.[168]

Early detection and appropriate management of stress fractures of the proximal femur are very important because these fractures have a high rate of complication of nonunion, progression to complete fracture, and/or osteonecrosis.[169] A study of 23 athletes with femoral neck fractures found that the diagnosis was not confirmed, on average, until 14 weeks after the onset of symptoms, and this delay forced elite athletes to end their careers. This underscores the importance of keeping an open mind to diagnostic possibilities and ordering the necessary imaging earlier rather than later in the course of management.[170] The recommended imaging modalities for diagnosing stress fractures are bone scans or MRI because stress fractures often can be missed on plain x-ray films.[171] CT also can be used.

Safran et al.[172] identified that athletes diagnosed with femoral neck stress fractures have a higher incidence of pincer type FAI (particularly involving coxa profunda and acetabular retroversion). Patients with coxa profunda and acetabular retroversion are encouraged to improve their fracture risk factors such as maximizing bone density, core strengthening, and cross-training.[172]

The classic symptom of a lower extremity stress fracture is progressive, activity-related pain that is relieved by rest. Local tenderness often is present. A **single-leg hop test** usually reproduces symptoms, and percussion of bone distal to the fracture site may reproduce symptoms.[173] A femoral neck stress fracture causes anterior thigh or groin pain (often an ache) that is relieved by rest, although night pain may be present in chronic cases. An antalgic (painful) gait, pain at the extremes of hip rotations (especially medial [internal] rotation), and pain with axial compression are common findings.[174] Clinicians should consider referral for further workup for stress fractures if continuous therapeutic ultrasound increases the patient's pain, which has been reported for lower leg stress fractures, and although it is not a sensitive tool for this diagnosis, the occurrence of increased pain with ultrasound used in treatment of suspected soft tissue injury should be a prompt for further workup.[175]

Stress fractures can be defined as fatigue or insufficiency fractures. **Fatigue fractures** tend to occur in young and middle-aged individuals from repetitive mechanical stress (e.g., distance running or military training). **Insufficiency fractures** tend to occur in older individuals when the bone is weakened from disease states, such as osteoporosis or osteomalacia. Fullerton and Snowdy[176] defined femoral neck fractures as compression, tension, and displaced fractures. **Compression stress fractures** tend to occur in the inferomedial femoral neck, and because they tend to be more stable, they can be treated with protected weight bearing and follow-up x-ray films (to ensure that no fracture displacement occurs during the healing process) until the patient is pain free. **Tension stress fractures** occur on the superolateral femoral neck, and because they are potentially unstable, they should be treated surgically with multiple screws or a sliding hip screw. **Displaced stress fractures** should be treated with ORIF.[29]

Nerve Syndromes

Theoretically, any nerve in the hip region can be injured. The nerves of the hip can be categorized into three groups of five nerves: five major nerves (sciatic, femoral, obturator, superior gluteal, and inferior gluteal); five minor nerves (nerve to the quadratus femoris and inferior gemellus, pudendal, posterior femoral cutaneous, nerve to the obturator internus and superior gemellus, and lateral femoral cutaneous); and five "referring" nerves

---

Risk Factors for Stress Fractures[169]

- Participation in sports involving running and jumping
- Rapid increase in physical training program (intensity and/or duration)
- Poor preparticipation physical condition
- Recent change in training surface—harder
- Female gender
- Hormonal or menstrual disturbances
- Low bone turnover rate
- Decreased bone density
- Decreased thickness of cortical bone
- Nutritional deficiencies (including dieting)
- Extremes of body size and composition
- Running on irregular or angled surfaces
- Inappropriate footwear
- Inadequate muscle strength
- Poor flexibility
- "Type A" behavior

(iliohypogastric, ilioinguinal, genitofemoral, cluneal, and sinuvertebral). Irritation of nerve roots of the lumbar and sacral plexuses can also refer symptoms to the hip and buttock region.

Nerve injuries occur as a result of one of three mechanisms: compression, traction, or ischemia. The three types of nerve injury are neuropraxia, axonotmesis, and neurotmesis (described in more detail in Chapter 25). Most nerve injuries about the hip have been described as a complication of total hip replacement, in which injury to the sciatic nerve is by far the most common complication. Surgeons also are very aware that the incision must not be extended more than 6 cm (2.4 inches) directly proximal beyond the tip of the greater trochanter, to avoid causing denervation of a branch of the superior gluteal nerve.[177]

In the nonsurgical setting, most nerve injuries at the hip occur as the result of mechanical entrapment, which causes a neuropraxia. Neuropraxia is an intact neural structure with decreased function because of local pressure, which produces ischemia and contusion of the nerve. Usually full function is recovered after appropriate management. These nerve entrapments often are related to alignment, contractures, and repetitive or a single excessive overload or overstretch. The two most common nerve entrapments in relation to the hip are sciatic nerve entrapment by the piriformis muscle in the greater sciatic foramen and lateral femoral cutaneous nerve entrapment at the lateral edge of the inguinal ligament. Entrapments of other nerves in the hip region also have been reported in the literature, including the ilioinguinal nerve, femoral nerve, obturator nerve, genitofemoral nerve, lateral cutaneous branches of the subcostal and iliohypogastric nerves, and entrapment of the sciatic nerve at the level of the ischial tuberosity (sometimes called *hamstring syndrome*).[31]

Nerve entrapments or injuries are easiest to diagnose when the symptoms include specific neurological features (i.e., motor weakness, sensory changes [numbness or tingling], and reflex change). Nerve entrapments are most difficult to diagnose when the primary symptom is pain, especially buttock pain or groin pain that mimics a muscle strain or tendonitis. Causalgia-like pain or reflex sympathetic dystrophy occasionally complicates recovery after a nerve injury.[177]

Three nerve entrapments at the hip frequently described involve the sciatic nerve (i.e., piriformis syndrome), the pudendal nerve (i.e., pudendal neuralgia), and the lateral femoral cutaneous nerve (i.e., meralgia paresthetica).

Piriformis Syndrome

Piriformis syndrome is a confusing diagnosis because some practitioners believe that it is overdiagnosed, others that it is underdiagnosed, and some do not believe that it exists.[178] Often it is a **"diagnosis of exclusion"**, when no other reason for pain in the buttock can be determined. Piriformis syndrome may account for up to 5% of cases of low back, buttock, and leg pain. It most commonly is seen in the 30 to 40 age range, and it often is associated with some form of trauma to the buttock.[179] Buttock tenderness is present over the piriformis muscle (especially in the greater sciatic notch) and surrounding tissues, and referred leg symptoms can arise from sciatic nerve irritation or from trigger points in the muscle itself. Flexion, adduction, internal (medial) rotation (FLADIR) of the hip usually causes buttock pain with piriformis syndrome. Numerous tests for piriformis syndrome have been described in the literature. Basically, they involve either passive stretching or resisted contraction of the piriformis muscle, and a positive test result is reproduction of symptoms in or emanating from the buttock.[5]

The piriformis muscle is the only muscle that passes through the greater sciatic notch, along with six nerves (sciatic, superior gluteal, inferior gluteal, pudendal, posterior femoral cutaneous, and the nerve to the quadratus femoris) and three vessel sets (i.e., superior gluteal artery and vein, inferior gluteal artery and vein, and internal pudendal artery and vein). Therefore a problem with the piriformis logically would have magnified effects because of its close anatomical relationship to numerous other neurovascular structures. A change in sacral or innominate alignment can also change the position of or tension on the piriformis in relation to these structures and thus potentially cause buttock and/or referred pain.

Several definitions of piriformis syndrome have been presented in the literature.[179] These authors believe that treatment is best guided by an approach in which a diagnosis of piriformis syndrome is complemented by a statement of symptom mechanism and a statement of symptom distribution (e.g., "local buttock pain from fall onto buttock," or, "buttock and posterior leg pain to foot from sciatic irritation by piriformis muscle in greater sciatic notch"). Differentiating piriformis syndrome from other lumbopelvic causes of referred pain into the buttock and posterior leg is important.

Piriformis syndrome is characterized by symptoms in the sciatic nerve distribution. Pain in the buttock alone is not piriformis syndrome; the term *piriformis syndrome* is associated with sciatic nerve irritation by the piriformis muscle. As mentioned, the piriformis muscle is the only muscle that passes through the greater sciatic foramen, which makes it the most likely muscular source of sciatic entrapment.

Likely aggravating factors for piriformis syndrome are walking, stair-climbing, and activities involving trunk rotation. Less severe cases of piriformis syndrome can be exacerbated by repetitive or resistive lateral rotation (e.g., from kicking a soccer ball).[5] A positive piriformis test produces buttock pain with possible radiation into the leg. Travell and Simons[180] described the piriformis as "the double devil" because it can refer pain from irritation of the sciatic nerve or irritation of the piriformis trigger points.

Treatment can include gentle, static stretching; ice massage; a vapocoolant spray and stretch technique;

therapeutic ultrasound; and NSAIDs. Techniques to promote balanced and optimal alignment, mobility, and stability of the lumbopelvic region are also important. Gluteus maximus and gluteus medius strengthening with an emphasis of control of weight-bearing hip adduction and medial (internal) rotation has been demonstrated as an effective treatment for chronic piriformis syndrome.[181] A heel insert of up to 0.64 cm (0.25 inch) on the non-affected side may take some tension off the piriformis. Rest from sporting activity for several weeks often is necessary.[5]

Pudendal Neuralgia

Pudendal neuralgia is a rare pain syndrome involving the cutaneous distribution of the pudendal nerve and/or its three branches. Entrapment of the pudendal nerve was first described in 1988 in a group of competitive male cyclists and is sometimes called **cyclist's syndrome,** because compression and ischemic response of the pudendal nerve can result from a narrow bicycle seat.[182] Pudendal neuralgia can also be the cause of debilitating pelvic pain after trauma, after delivery, or after surgery, often from fibrotic scarring. It is a **"diagnosis of exclusion"** but should be considered in patients with chronic hip and pelvic region pain. The Nantes diagnostic criteria for pudendal neuralgia includes 5 criteria.[183]

Nantes Diagnostic Criteria for Pudendal Neuralgia[183]

1. Pain in anatomic distribution of pudendal nerve
2. Pain aggravated by sitting
3. Not awakened by pain at night
4. No objective sensory loss on clinical examination
5. Pain is improved with anesthetic pudendal nerve block

Physical therapy is considered an important component of the overall management of the patient with pudendal neuralgia advisably by a therapist trained in pelvic floor work.[182] Weiss and Prendergast[184] reported that patients with pudendal nerve entrapment often presented with some or all of these comorbidities, and the clinician should treat what he or she finds: connective tissue restrictions, adverse neural tension, intrapelvic and extrapelvic muscle hypertonicity and/or myofascial trigger points, biomechanical abnormalities (e.g., sacroiliac joint dysfunction), decreased core strength, or faulty neuromuscular recruitment patterns.

If the patient still has debilitating pain after a course of physical therapy and other conservative therapies (e.g., medication, counseling) a CT-guided pudendal nerve block can often be diagnostic and therapeutic. If CT-guided injections of the pudendal nerve give relief, albeit not lasting, then the patient may be a candidate for surgical decompression of the pudendal nerve.[182]

Meralgia Paresthetica

Entrapment of the lateral femoral cutaneous nerve of the thigh as it emerges from the pelvis adjacent to the anterior superior ischial spine (ASIS) can result in tingling, numbness, and pain in the nerve's sensory distribution on the anterolateral thigh. This condition is called **meralgia paresthetica.** It can present during pregnancy, in obese individuals, in laborers who carry heavy tool bags around their waist, and from direct trauma near the ASIS during sports. Sensory testing can confirm the diagnosis, and a positive Tinel's sign may be elicited by tapping adjacent to the ASIS and inguinal ligament. The diagnosis should not be made before other hip, lumbar, or intrapelvic pathology has been ruled out. Treatments that can be beneficial include correction of mechanical contributing factors as well as rest, ultrasound, and NSAIDs if needed. In some cases, injection of an analgesic and a corticosteroid is warranted. In rare cases, when conservative measures have failed, surgical release of the nerve can be performed.[185]

SUMMARY

Applying the information presented in this chapter to live clinical situations requires good clinical judgment. The most logical method for making clinical decisions is the risk–reward ratio: balancing cost (i.e., risk) against benefit (i.e., reward). The F balance (Figure 18-41) is an expansion of the risk–reward ratio that can be particularly helpful to the clinician in making decisions about a person presenting with hip pathology. In rehabilitation terms, clinicians balance achievement of best possible function against the risk of tissue failure (i.e., tissue breakdown or damage). Controlled forces (e.g., movement, mobilization, exercise) are used to improve form (e.g., strength, flexibility, endurance, balance), and both controlled forces and improved form are used to optimize function (e.g., transfers, walking, stairs, sports activity). The patient should always be the focus of the rehabilitation process—"feel" at the center of the F balance refers to the importance of asking "How does the patient feel?" and incorporating his or her goals into the treatment plan.

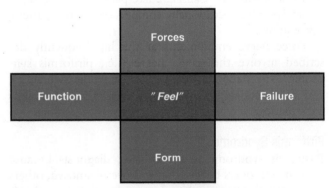

Figure 18-41 The F balance: A model for clinical decision making. (From Fagerson TL, editor: *The hip handbook,* p 248, Boston, 1998, Butterworth-Heinemann.)

REFERENCES

1. Edelstein J, Draovitch P, Kelly BT: The layer concept: utilization in determining the pain generators, pathology and how structure determines treatment, *Curr Rev Musculoskel Med* 5:1–8, 2012.

2. Franklyn-Miller A, Falvey E, McCrory P, Briggs C: Landmarks for the 3G approach: groin, gluteal and greater trochanter triangles—a patho-anatomical method in sports medicine, *Eur J Anat* 12:81–87, 2008.

3. Sahrmann SA: Diagnosis by the physical therapist: a prerequisite for treatment, *Phys Ther* 68:1703–1706, 1988.

4. Dyrek DA: Assessment and treatment planning strategies for musculoskeletal deficits. In Sullivan SD, Schmitz TJ, editors: *Physical rehabilitation: assessment and treatment*, 3 ed, Philadelphia, 1994, FA Davis.

5. Fagerson TL, editor: *The hip handbook*, Boston, 1998, Butterworth-Heinemann.

6. Khan NQ, Woolson ST: Referral patterns of hip pain in patients undergoing total hip replacement, *Orthopedics* 21:123–126, 1998.

7. Wroblewski BM: Pain in osteoarthrosis of the hip, *Practitioner* 1315:140–141, 1978.

8. Yukawa Y, Kato F, Kajino G, et al: Groin pain associated with lower lumbar disc herniation, *Spine* 22:1736–1740, 1997.

9. Kuslich SD, Ulstrom CL, Michael CJ: The tissue origin of low back pain and sciatica: a report of pain response to tissue stimulation during operations on the lumbar spine using local anesthesia, *Orthop Clin North Am* 22:181–187, 1991.

10. Wainner RS, Whitman JM, Cleland JA, Flynn TA: Regional interdependence: a musculoskeletal examination model whose time has come, *J Orthop Sports Phys Ther* 37:658–660, 2007.

11. Reiman MP, Weisbach PC, Glynn PE: The hip's influence on low back pain: a distal link to a proximal problem, *J Sport Rehabil* 18:1–10, 2009.

12. Brown MD, Gomez-Marin O, Brookfield KFW, Stokes Li P: Differential diagnosis of hip disease versus spine disease, *Clin Orthop* 419:280–284, 2004.

13. Greenwood MJ, Erhard RE, Jones DL: Differential diagnosis of the hip vs lumbar hip spine: five case reports, *J Orthop Sports Phys Ther* 27:308–315, 1998.

14. Cyriax J: *Textbook of orthopaedic medicine, vol 1, Diagnosis of soft tissue lesions*, ed 8, London, 1982, Baillière Tindall.

15. Klassbo M, Harms-Ringdahl K, Larrson G: Examination of passive ROM and capsular patterns in the hip, *Physiother Res Int* 8:1–12, 2003.

16. Ellison JB, Rose SJ, Sahrmann SA: Patterns of hip rotation range of motion: a comparison between healthy subjects and patients with low back pain, *Phys Ther* 70:537–541, 1990.

17. Vad VB, Bhat AL, Basrai D, et al: Low back pain in professional golfers: the role of associated hip and low back range-of-motion deficits, *Am J Sports Med* 32:494–497, 2004.

18. Vad VB, Gebeh A, Dines D, et al: Hip and shoulder internal rotation range of motion deficits in professional tennis players, *J Sci Med Sport* 6:71–75, 2003.

19. Mellin G: Correlations of hip mobility with the degree of back pain and lumbar spinal mobility, *Spine* 13:668–670, 1988.

20. Nagi SZ: An epidemiology of disability among adults in the United States, *Milbank Mem Fund Q Health Society* 54:439–467, 1976.

21. Synder AR, Parsons JT, Valovich McLeod TC, et al: Using disablement models and clinical outcomes assessment to enable evidence-based athletic training practice. Part I: disablement models, *J Athl Training* 43:428–436, 2008.

22. Eunice Kennedy Shriver National Institute of Child Health and Human Development: *Research plan for the national centre for medical rehabilitation research (NCMRR)*, NIH Publication No. 93-3509, Washington, DC, 1993, National Institute of Child Health and Human Development, National Institutes of Health, US Department of Health and Human Services.

23. Sahrmann SA: *Diagnosis and treatment of movement impairment syndromes*, St Louis, 2002, Mosby.

24. Del Buono A, Papalia R, Khanduja V, et al: Management of the greater trochanteric pain syndrome: a systematic review, *Br Med Bull* 102:115–131, 2012.

25. Shbeeb MI, Matteson EL: Trochanteric bursitis (greater trochanter pain syndrome), *Mayo Clin Proc* 71:565–569, 1996.

26. Ege Rassmusen KJ, Fano N: Trochanteric bursitis: treatment by corticosteroid injection, *Scand J Rheumatol* 14:417–420, 1985.

27. Shbeeb MI, O'Duffy JD, Michet CJ, et al: Evaluation of glucocorticosteroid injection for the treatment of trochanteric bursitis, *J Rheumatol* 23:2104–2106, 1996.

28. Craig RA, Gwynne Jones DP, Oakley AP, Dunbar JD: Iliotibial band Z-lengthening for refractory trochanteric bursitis (greater trochanteric pain syndrome), *ANZ J Surg* 77:996–998, 2007.

29. Egol KA, Koval KJ, Kummer F, Frankel VH: Stress fractures of the femoral neck, *Clin Orthop* 348:72–78, 1998.

30. Janda V: On the concept of postural muscles and posture in man, *Aust J Physiother* 29:83–84, 1983.

31. Fagerson TL: *Home study course: current concepts of orthopaedic physical therapy—hip*, La Crosse, WI, 2001, Orthopaedic Section, American Physical Therapy Association.

32. Bunker TD, Esler CAN, Leach WJ: Rotator-cuff tear of the hip, *J Bone Joint Surg Br* 79:618–620, 1997.

33. Domb BG, Nasser RM, Botser IB: Partial-thickness tears of the gluteus medius: rationale and technique for trans-tendinous endoscopic repair, *Arthroscopy* 26:1697–1705, 2010.

34. Kingzett-Taylor A, Tirman PF, Feller J, et al: Tendinosis and tears of gluteus medius and minimus muscles as a cause of hip pain: MR imaging findings, *Am J Roentgen* 173:1123–1126, 1999.

35. Khan KM, Cook JL, Taunton JE, Bonar F: Overuse tendinosis, not tendinitis, *Phys Sportsmed* 28:38–48, 2000.

36. Cashman GE, Mortenson WB, Gilbart MK: Myofascial treatment for patients with acetabular labral tears: a single-subject research design study, *J Orthop Sports Phys Ther* 44:604–614, 2014.

37. Lebeau RT, Nho SJ: The use of manual therapy post-hip arthroscopy when an exercise-based therapy approach has failed, *J Orthop Sports Phys Ther* 44:712–721, 2014.

38. Yazbek PW, Ovanessian V, Martin RL, Fukuda TY: Nonsurgical treatment of acetabular labrum tears: a case series, *J Orthop Sports Phys Ther* 41:346–353, 2011.

39. Labrosse JM, Cardinal E, Leduc BE, et al: Effectiveness of ultrasound-guided corticosteroid injection for the treatment of gluteus medius tendinopathy, *Am J Roentgenol* 194:202–206, 2010.

40. Byrd JW: Gluteus medius repair with double-row fixation, *Arthrosc Tech* 2:e247–e250, 2013.

41. Domb BG, Carreira DS: Endoscopic repair of full-thickness gluteus medius tears, *Arthrosc Tech* 2:77–81, 2013.

42. Voos JE, Shindle MK, Pruett A, et al: Endoscopic repair of gluteus medius tendon tears of the hip, *Am J Sports Med* 37:743–747, 2009.

43. Gruen GS, Scioscia TN, Lowenstein JE: The surgical treatment of internal snapping hip, *Am J Sports Med* 30:607–613, 2002.

44. Sher I, Umams H, Downie SA, et al: Proximal iliotibial band syndrome: what is it and where is it? *Skeletal Radiol* 40:1553–1556, 2011.

45. Brignall CG, Stainsby GD: The snapping hip: treatment by Z-plasty, *J Bone Joint Surg Br* 73:253–254, 1991.

46. Byrd JW: Hip arthroscopy, *J Am Acad Orthop Surg* 14:433–444, 2006.

47. Wettstein M, Jung J, Dienst M: Arthroscopic psoas tenotomy, *Arthroscopy* 22(907):e1–e4, 2006.

48. Ilizaliturri VM, Chaidez C, Villegas P, et al: Prospective randomized study of 2 different techniques for endoscopic iliopsoas tendon release in the treatment of internal snapping hip syndrome, *Arthroscopy* 25:159–163, 2009.

49. Khan M, Adamich J, Simunovic N, et al: Surgical Management of internal snapping hip syndrome: a systematic review evaluating open and arthroscopic approaches, *Arthroscopy* 29:942–948, 2013.

50. Neumann D: *Kinesiology of the musculoskeletal system: foundations for physical rehabilitation*, Philadelphia, 2002, Elsevier.

51. Johnston CAM, Lindsay DM, Wiley JP: Treatment of iliopsoas syndrome with a hip rotation strengthening program: a retrospective case series, *J Orthop Sports Phys Ther* 29:216–224, 1999.

52. Byrd JWT, Jones KS: Adhesive capsulitis of the hip, *Arthroscopy* 22:89–94, 2006.

53. Kaltenborn FM: *Manual mobilization of the extremity joints*, ed 4, Oslo, 1989, Olaf Norlis Bokhandel.

54. Mulligan BR: *Manual therapy: "NAGS", "SNAGS", "MWMS" etc*, ed 3, Wellington, 1995, Plane View Services.

55. Hoeksma HL, Dekker J, Ronday K, et al: Comparison of manual therapy and exercise therapy in osteoarthritis of the hip: a randomized clinical trial, *Arthritis Rheum* 51:722–729, 2004.

56. Silder A, Sherry MA, Sanfilippo J, et al: Clinical and morphological changes following 2 rehabilitation programs for acute hamstring strain injuries: a randomized clinical trial, *J Orthop Sports Phys Ther* 43:284–299, 2013.

57. Clanton TO, Coupe KJ: Hamstring strains in athletes: diagnosis and treatment, *J Am Acad Orthop Surg* 6:237–248, 1998.

58. Sherry MA, Best TM, Silder A, et al: Hamstring strains: basic science and clinical research applications for preventing the recurrent injury, *Strength Cond J* 33:56–71, 2011.

59. Malliaropoulos N, Mendiguchia J, Pehlivanidis H, et al: Hamstring exercises for track and field athletes: injury and exercise biomechanics, and possible implications for exercise selection and primary prevention, *Br J Sports Med* 46:846–851, 2012.

60. Brooks JHM, Fuller CW, Kemp SPT, Reddin DB: Epidemiology of injuries in English professional rugby union: part 2 training injuries, *Br J Sports Med* 39:767–775, 2005.

61. Lloyd-Smith R, Clement DB, McKenzie DC, Taunton JE: A survey of overuse and traumatic hip and pelvic injuries in athletes, *Phys Sportsmed* 13:131–141, 1986.

62. Agre JC: Hamstring injuries: proposed aetiologic factors, prevention, and treatment, *Sports Med* 2:21–33, 1985.

63. Opar DA, Williams MD, Shield AJ: Hamstring strain injuries: Factors that lead to injury and re-injury, *Sports Med* 42:209–226, 2012.

64. Belcher JR, Jobe FW, Pink M, et al: Electromyographic analysis of the hip and knee during the golf swing, *Clin J Sports Med* 3:162–166, 1995.

65. Goode AP, Reiman MP, Harris L, et al: Eccentric training for prevention of hamstring injuries may depend on intervention compliance: a systematic review and meta-analysis, *Br J Sports Med* Sep 16, 2014 (Epub ahead of print).

66. Cibulka MT, Rose SJ, Delitto A, Sinacore DR: Hamstring muscle strain treated by mobilizing the sacroiliac joint, *Phys Ther* 66:1220–1223, 1986.

67. Cibulka MT, Delitto A: A comparison of two different methods to treat hip pain in runners, *J Orthop Sports Phys Ther* 17:172–176, 1993.

68. Brukner P, Nealon A, Morgan C, et al: Recurrent hamstring muscle injury: applying the limited evidence in the professional football setting with a seven-point programme, *Br J Sports Med* 48:928–938, 2014.

69. Sherry MA, Best TM: A comparison of 2 rehabilitation programs in the treatment of acute hamstring strains, *J Orthop Sports Phys Ther* 34:116–125, 2004.

70. Fredericson M, Moore W, Guillet M, Beaulieu C: High hamstring tendinopathy in runners, *Phys Sportsmed* 33:32–43, 2005.

71. Orchard J, Best TM: The management of muscle strain injuries: an early return versus the risk of recurrence, *Clin J Sports Med* 12:3–5, 2002.

72. Hamid MS, Mohamed Ali MR, Yusof A, et al: Platelet-rich plasma injections for the treatment of hamstring injuries: a randomized controlled trial, *Am J Sports Med* 42:2410–2418, 2014.

73. Reurink G, Goudswaard GJ, Moen MH, et al: Platelet-rich plasma injections in acute muscle injury, *N Engl J Med* 370:2546–2547, 2014.

74. Levine WN, Bergfeld JA, Tessendorf W, Moorman CT: Intramuscular corticosteroid injection for hamstring injuries: a 13-year experience in the national football league, *Am J Sports Med* 28:297–300, 2000.

75. Beiner JM, Jokl P, Cholewicki J, Panjabi MM: The effect of anabolic steroids and corticosteroids on healing of muscle contusion injury, *Am J Sports Med* 27:2–9, 1999.

76. Hamilton B: Hamstring muscle strain injuries: what can we learn from history? *Br J Sports Med* 46:900–903, 2012.

77. Hoffman KJ, Paggi A, Connors D, Miller SL: Complete avulsion of the proximal hamstring insertion: functional outcomes after nonsurgical treatment, *J Bone Joint Surg Am* 96:1022–1025, 2014.

78. Subbu R, Benjamin-Laing H, Haddad F: Timing of surgery for complete proximal hamstring avulsion injuries: successful clinical outcomes at 6 weeks, 6 months, and after 6 months of injury, *Am J Sports Med*, Nov 17, 2014 (Epub ahead of print).

79. Dierckman BD, Guanche CA: Endoscopic proximal hamstring repair and ischial bursectomy, *Arthrosc Tech* 1:e201–e207, 2012.

80. Hasselman CT, Best TM, Garrett WE: When groin pain signals an adductor strain, *Phys Sportsmed* 23:53–60, 1995.

81. Holmich P, Uhrskou P, Ulnits L, et al: Effectiveness of active physical training as treatment for long-standing adductor-related groin pain in athletes: randomised trial, *Lancet* 353:439–443, 1999.

82. Topol GA, Reeves KD, Hassanien KM: Efficacy of dextrose prolotherapy in elite male kicking-sport athletes with chronic groin pain, *Arch Phys Med Rehabil* 86:697–702, 2005.

83. Schilders E, Bismil Q, Robinson P, O'Connor PJ, Gibbon WW, Talbot JC: Adductor-related groin pain in competitive athletes: role of adductor enthesis, magnetic resonance imaging, and entheseal pubic cleft injections, *J Bone Joint Surg Am* 89:2173–2178, 2007.

84. Schilders E, Dimitrakopoulou A, Cooke M, et al: Effectiveness of a selective partial adductor release for chronic adductor-related groin pain in professional athletes, *Am J Sports Med* 41:603–607, 2013.

85. Meyers WC, Foley DP, Garrett WE, et al: Management of severe lower abdominal or inguinal pain in high-performance athletes, *Am J Sports Med* 28:2–8, 2000.

86. Brannigan A, Kerin MJ, McEntee GP: Gilmore's groin repair in athletes, *J Orthop Sports Phys Ther* 30:329–332, 2000.

87. Kachingwe AF, Grech S: Proposed algorithm for the management of athletes with athletic pubalgia (sports hernia): a case series, *J Orthop Sports Phys Ther* 38:768–781, 2008.

88. Meyers WC, McKechnie A, Philippon MJ, et al: Experience with "sports hernia" spanning two decades, *Ann Surg* 248:656–665, 2008.

89. Johnson JD, Briner WW: Primary care of the sports hernia: recognizing an often overlooked cause of pain, *Phys Sportmed* 33:35–39, 2005.

90. Buckwalter JA, Saltzman C, Brown T: The impact of osteoarthritis: implications for research, *Clin Orthop Relat Res* 427S:S6–S15, 2004.

91. American Academy of Orthopaedic Surgeons: *Osteoarthritis of the hip: a compendium of evidence-based resources*, Rosemont, IL, 2004, American Academy of Orthopaedic Surgeons.

92. Cibulka MT, White DM, Whoerle J, et al: Hip pain and mobility deficits: hip osteoarthritis: clinical practice guidelines, *J Orthop Sports Phys Ther* 39:A1–A25, 2009.

93. Harris WH: Etiology of osteoarthritis of the hip, *Clin Orthop Relat Res* 213:20–33, 1986.

94. Hochberg MC, Altman RD, April KT, et al: American college of rheumatology 2012 recommendations for the use of nonpharmacologic and pharmacologic therapies in osteoarthritis of the hand, hip, and knee, *Arthritis Care Res* 64:465–474, 2012.

95. Puett DW, Griffin MR: Published trials of nonmedicinal and noninvasive therapies for hip and knee osteoarthritis, *Ann Intern Med* 121:133–140, 1994.

96. Van Baar ME, Assendelft WJ, Dekker J, et al: Effectiveness of exercise therapy in patients with osteoarthritis of the hip or knee: a systematic review of randomized clinical trials, *Arthritis Rheum* 25:1361–1369, 1999.

97. Cyriax JH: *Illustrated manual of orthopaedic medicine*, ed 2, London, 1996, Butterworth-Heinemann.

98. King L: Case study: physical therapy management of hip osteoarthritis prior to total hip arthroplasty, *J Orthop Sports Phys Ther* 26:35–38, 1997.

99. Fortin PR, Penrod JR, Clarke AE, et al: Timing of total joint replacement affects clinical outcomes among patients with osteoarthritis of the hip or knee, *Arthritis Rheum* 46:3327–3330, 2002.

100. Neumann DA: Biomechanical analysis of selected principles of hip joint protection, *Arthritis Care Res* 2:146–155, 1989.

101. The safety of COX-2 inhibitors: deliberations from the February 16-18, 2005, FDA meeting. American College of Rheumatology Hotline. Available at www.rheumatology.org.

102. Murray RO: The aetiology of primary osteoarthritis of the hip, *Br J Radiol* 38:810–824, 1965.

103. Wenger DE, Kendell KR, Miner MR, Trousdale RT: Acetabular labral tears rarely occur in the absence of bony abnormalities, *Clin Orthop Relat Res* 426:145–150, 2004.

104. Murphy S, Tannast M, Kim Y-J, et al: Debridement of the adult hip for femoroacetabular impingement: indications and preliminary clinical results, *Clin Orthop Relat Res* 429:178–181, 2004.

105. Ganz R, Parvizi J, Beck M, et al: Femoroacetabular impingement: a cause for osteoarthritis of the hip, *Clin Orthop Relat Res* 417:112–120, 2003.

106. Mardones RM, Gonzalez C, Chen Q, et al: Surgical treatment of femoroacetabular impingement: evaluation of the effect of the size of the resection, *J Bone Joint Surg Am* 87:273–279, 2005.

107. Bare AA, Guanche CA: Hip impingement: the role of arthroscopy, *Orthopedics* 28:266–273, 2005.

108. Philippon MJ, Schenker ML: Athletic hip injuries and capsular laxity, *Oper Tech Orthop* 15:261–266, 2005.

109. Shu B, Safran MR: Hip instability: anatomic and clinical considerations of traumatic and atraumatic instability, *Clin Sports Med* 30:349–367, 2011.

110. Turner R, O'Sullivan E, Edelstein J: Hip dysplasia and the performing arts: is there a correlation? *Curr Rev Musculoskel Med* 5:39–45, 2012.

111. Bayer JL, Sekiya JK: Hip instability and capsular laxity, *Oper Tech Orthop* 20:237–241, 2010.

112. Safran M, Kalisvaart MR: *Hip microinstability treated with arthroscopic capsular plication*. In Presented at the International Society for Hip Arthroplasty, Rio de Janeiro, Brazil. October 9-11, 2014.

113. Stalzer S, Wahoff M, Scanlan M: Rehabilitation following hip arthroscopy, *Clin Sports Med* 25:337–357, 2006.

114. Register B, Pennock AT, Ho CP, et al: Prevalence of abnormal hip findings in asymptomatic participants: a prospective, blinded study, *Am J Sports Med* 40:2720–2724, 2012.

115. Yuan BJ, Bartelt RB, Levy BA, et al: Decreased range of motion is associated with structural hip deformity in asymptomatic adolescent athletes, *Am J Sports Med* 41:1519–1525, 2013.

116. McCarthy JC, Noble PC, Schuck MR, et al: The role of labral lesions to development of early degenerative hip disease, *Clin Orthop Relat Res* 393:25–37, 2001.

117. Wegner DE, Kendell KR, Miner MR, Trousdale RT: Acetabular labral tears rarely occur in the absence of bony abnormalities, *Clin Orthop Relat Res* 426:145–150, 2004.

118. Safran MR: The acetabular labrum: anatomic and functional characteristics and rationale for surgical intervention, *J Am Acad Orthop Surg* 18:338–345, 2010.

119. Garbuz DS, Masri BA, Haddad F, Duncan CP: Clinical and radiographic assessment of the young adult with symptomatic hip dysplasia, *Clin Orthop Relat Res* 418:18–22, 2004.

120. Millis MB, Kim Y-J: Rationale of osteotomy and related procedures for hip preservation: a review, *Clin Orthop Relat Res* 405:108–121, 2002.

121. McCarthy JC, Lee J: Hip arthroscopy: indications, outcomes, and complications, *J Bone Joint Surg Am* 87:1138–1145, 2005.

122. McGrory BJ: Stinchfield resisted hip flexion test, *Hosp Physician* 9:41–42, 1999.

123. Fitzgerald RH: Acetabular labral tears: diagnosis and treatment, *Clin Orthop* 311:60–68, 1995.

124. McCarthy JC, Lee J: Arthroscopic intervention in early hip disease, *Clin Orthop* 429:157–162, 2004.

125. Kelly BT, Weiland DE, Schenker ML, Philippon MJ: Arthroscopic labral repair in the hip: surgical technique and review of the literature, *Arthroscopy* 21:1496–1504, 2005.

126. Stafford GH, Bunn JR, Villar RN: Arthroscopic repair of delaminated acetabular articular cartilage using fibrin adhesive. Results at one to three years, *Hip Int* 21:744–750, 2011.

127. Starman JS, Griffin JW, Kandil A, et al: What's new in sports medicine, *J Bone Joint Surg Am* 96:695–702, 2014.

128. Nam D, Shindle MK, Buly RL, et al: Traumatic osteochondral injury of the femoral head treated by mosaicplasty: a report of two cases, *HSS J* 6:228–234, 2010.

129. Kivlan BR, Richard Clemente F, Martin RRL, Martin HD: Function of the ligamentum teres during multi-planar movement of the hip joint, *Knee Surg Sports Traumatol Arthrosc* 21:1664–1668, 2013.

130. Martin RRL, Kivlan BR, Clemente FR: A cadaveric model for ligamentum teres function: a pilot study, *Knee Surg Sports Traumatol Arthrosc* 21:1689–1693, 2013.

131. Wenger D, Miyanji F, Mahar A, Oka R: The mechanical properties of the ligamentum teres: a pilot study to assess its potential for improving stability in children's hip surgery, *J Pediatr Orthop* 27:408–410, 2007.

132. Demange MK, Kakuda CMS, Pereira CAM, et al: Influence of the femoral head ligament on hip mechanical function. [Influência do ligamento da cabeça do fêmur na mecânica do quadril], *Acta Ortopedica Brasileira* 15:187–190, 2007.

133. Leunig M, Beck M, Stauffer E, et al: Free nerve endings in the ligamentum capitis femoris, *Acta Orthop Scand* 71:452–454, 2000.

134. Martin RL, Palmer I, Martin HD: Ligamentum teres: a functional description and potential clinical relevance, *Knee Surg Sports Traumatol Arthrosc* 20:1209–1214, 2012.

135. O'Donnell J, Economopoulos K, Singh P, et al: The ligamentum teres test: a novel and effective test in diagnosing tears of the ligamentum teres, *Am J Sports Med* 42:138–143, 2014.

136. Byrd JWT, Jones KS: Traumatic rupture of the ligamentum teres as a source of hip pain, *Arthroscopy* 20:385–391, 2004.

137. de Sa D, Phillips M, Philippon MJ, et al: Ligamentum teres injuries of the hip: a systematic review examining surgical indications, treatment options, and outcomes, *Arthroscopy* 30:1634–1641, 2014.

138. Mei-Dan O, McConkey MO: A novel technique for ligamentum teres reconstruction with "all-suture" anchors in the medial acetabular wall, *Arthrosc Techn* 3:e217–e221, 2014.

139. Simpson JM, Field RE, Villar RN: Arthroscopic reconstruction of the ligamentum teres, *Arthroscopy* 27, 2011. 436-441+e54.

140. Philippon MJ, Pennock A, Gaskill TR: Arthroscopic reconstruction of the ligamentum teres: technique and early outcomes, *J Bone Joint Surg Br* 94:1494–1498, 2012.

141. Krebs V: Loose bodies. In McCarthy JC, editor: *Early hip disorders*, New York, 2003, Springer-Verlag.

142. Wahoff M, Ryan M: Rehabilitation after femoroacetabular impingement arthroscopy, *Clin Sports Med* 30:463–482, 2011.

143. Dirocco S, McCarthy JC, Busconi BD, et al: Rehabilitation after hip arthroscopy. In McCarthy JC, editor: *Early hip disorders: advances in detection and minimally invasive treatment*, New York, 2003, Springer-Verlag.

144. Edelstein J, Ranawat A, Enseki KR, et al: Postoperative guidelines following hip arthroscopy, *Curr Rev Musculoskel Med* 5:15–23, 2012.

145. Wahoff M, Dischiavi S, Hodge J, Pharez JD: Rehabilitation after labral repair and femoroacetabular decompression: criteria-based progression through return to sport phase, *Int J Sports Phys Ther* 9:813–826, 2014.

146. Parris HG, Sallis RE, Anderson DV: Traumatic hip dislocation: reducing complications, *Phys Sportmed* 21:67–74, 1993.

147. Plancher K, Razi A: Management of osteonecrosis of the femoral head, *Orthop Clin North Am* 28:461–477, 1997.

148. Andrews SK, Carek PJ: Osteitis pubis: a diagnosis for the family physician, *J Am Board Fam Pract* 11:291–295, 1998.

149. Sing R, Cordes R, Siberski D: Osteitis pubis in the active patient, *Phys Sportsmed* 23:67–73, 1995.

150. Guccione AA, Fagerson TL, Anderson JJ: Regaining functional independence in the acute care setting following hip fracture, *Phys Ther* 76:818–826, 1996.

151. Johnell O, Kanis JA: An estimate of the worldwide prevalence and disability associated with osteoporotic fractures, *Osteoporos Int* 17:1726–1733, 2006.

152. Pitzul KB, Munce SEP, Perrier L, et al: Quality indicators for hip fracture patients: a scoping review protocol, *BMJ Open* 4:e006543, 2014.

153. Braithwaite RS, Col NF, Wong JB: Estimating hip fracture morbidity, mortality and costs, *J Am Geriatr Soc* 51:364–370, 2003.

154. Fiatarone MA, O'Neill EF, Ryan ND, et al: Exercise training and nutritional supplementation for physical frailty in very elderly people, *N Engl J Med* 330:1769–1775, 1994.

155. Binder EF, Brown M, Sinacore DR, et al: Effects of extended outpatient rehabilitation after hip fracture: a randomized controlled trial, *JAMA* 292:837–846, 2004.

156. Mangione KK, Craik RL, Tomlinson SS, Palombaro KM: Can elderly patients who have had a hip fracture perform moderate- to high-intensity exercise at home? *Phys Ther* 85:727–739, 2005.

157. Liporace FA, Egol KA, Tejwani N, et al: What's new in hip fractures?: current concepts, *Am J Orthop* 34:66–74, 2005.

158. Koval KJ, Zuckerman JD: *Hip fractures: a practical guide to management*, New York, 2000, Springer-Verlag.

159. Cummings SR, Nevitt MC: A hypothesis: the cause of hip fractures, *J Gerontol* 44:M107–M111, 1989.

160. Healey WL, Iorio R: Total hip arthroplasty: optimal treatment for displaced femoral neck fractures in elderly patients, *Clin Orthop Relat Res* 429:43–48, 2004.

161. Koval KJ, Sala DA, Kummer FJ, Zuckerman JD: Postoperative weight-bearing after a fracture of the femoral neck or an intertrochanteric fracture, *J Bone Joint Surg Am* 80:352–356, 1998.

162. Auais MA, Eilayyan O, Mayo NE: Extended exercise rehabilitation after hip fracture improves patients physical function: a systematic review and meta-analysis, *Phys Ther* 92:1437–1451, 2012.

163. Paterno SA, Lachiewicz PF, Kelley SS: The influence of patient-related factors and the position of the acetabular component on the rate of dislocation after total hip replacement, *J Bone Joint Surg Am* 79:1202–1210, 1997.

164. McGrory BJ, Evans PJ: Fractures of the pelvis and acetabulum, *Hosp Physician* 4:44–50, 2003.

165. Fagerson TL: Postoperative hip rehabilitation based on *in vivo* force and pressure data, *Topics Geriatr Rehabil* 29:268–271, 2013.

166. Droll KP, Broekhuyse H, O'Brien P: Fracture of the femoral head, *J Am Acad Orthop Surg* 15:716–727, 2007.

167. Matheson GO, Clement DB, McKenzie DC, et al: Stress fractures in athletes: a study of 320 cases, *Am J Sports Med* 15:46–58, 1987.

168. Perron AD, Brady WJ, Keats TA: Principles of stress fracture management, *Postgrad Med* 110:115–124, 2001.

169. Sanderlin BW, Raspa RF: Common stress fractures, *Am Fam Physician* 68:1527–1532, 2003.

170. Johansson C, Ekenman I, Tornkvist H, Eriksson E: Stress fractures of the femoral neck in athletes: the consequence of a delay in diagnosis, *Am J Sports Med* 18:524–528, 1990.

171. Rizzo PF, Gould ES, Lyden JP, Asnis SE: Diagnosis of occult fractures about the hip: magnetic resonance imaging compared with bone scanning, *J Bone Joint Surg Am* 75:395–401, 1993.

172. Safran MR, Goldin M, Anderson C, et al: The association of femoral neck stress fractures with femoral acetabular impingement, *Orthop J Sports Med* 1(suppl 1), 2013.

173. Browning KH: Hip and pelvis injuries in runners: careful evaluation and tailored management, *Phys Sportmed* 29:23–34, 2001.

174. Lacroix VJ: A complete approach to groin pain, *Phys Sportmed* 28:66–86, 2000.

175. Romani WA, Perin DH, Dussault RG, et al: Identification of tibial stress fractures using therapeutic continuous ultrasound, *J Orthop Sports Phys Ther* 30:444–452, 2000.

176. Fullerton LR, Snowdy HA: Femoral neck stress fractures, *Am J Sports Med* 16:365–377, 1988.

177. Lewallen DG: Neurovascular injury associated with hip arthroplasty, *J Bone Joint Surg Am* 79:1870–1880, 1997.

178. Silver JK, Leadbetter WB: Piriformis syndrome: assessment of current practice and literature review, *Orthopedics* 21:1133–1135, 1998.

179. Papadopoulis EC, Khan SN: Piriformis syndrome and low back pain: a new classification and review of the literature, *Orthop Clin North Am* 35:65–71, 2004.

180. Travell JG, Simons DG: *Myofascial pain and dysfunction: the trigger point manual, vol 2, the lower extremities*, Baltimore, 1992, Williams & Wilkins.

181. Tonley JC, Yun SM, Kochevar RJ, et al: Treatment of an individual with piriformis syndrome focusing on hip muscle strengthening and movement reeducation: a case report, *J Orthop Sports Phys Ther* 40:103–111, 2010.

182. Hibner M, Desai N, Robertson LJ, Nour M: Pudendal neuralgia, *J Minim Invasive Gynecol* 17:148–153, 2010.

183. Labat J-J, Riant T, Robert R, et al: Diagnostic criteria for pudendal neuralgia by pudendal nerve entrapment (Nantes criteria), *Neurourol Urodyn* 27:306–310, 2008.

184. Weiss JM, Prendergast SA: Pitfalls in the effective diagnosis and treatment of pudendal nerve entrapment, *Vision—Newsletter of the International Pelvic Pain Society* 13:1–3, 2006.

185. Grossman MG, Ducey SA, Nadler SS, Levy AS: Meralgia paresthetica: diagnosis and treatment, *J Am Acad Orthop Surg* 9:336–344, 2001.

CHAPTER 19

Physical Rehabilitation after Total Hip Arthroplasty

JEANNA ALLEGRONE, JAMES GREEN II, DAVID NICOLORO, DIANE M. HEISLEIN, ERIC O. EISEMON, EDGAR T. SAVIDGE, SANAZ HARIRI, HARRY E. RUBASH

INTRODUCTION

Indications for Total Hip Arthroplasty

The most common indication for primary total hip arthroplasty (THA) is osteoarthritis (OA). Clinically, symptomatic OA is defined as pain occurring on most days during the past month in addition to radiographic changes (i.e., osteophytes, subchondral sclerosis, and joint space narrowing). Approximately 10% to 12% of adults have symptomatic OA. Conversely, approximately 50% of people with radiographic evidence of OA are asymptomatic.[1]

Other indications for THA include rheumatoid arthritis, avascular necrosis, traumatic arthritis, certain hip fractures, benign and malignant bone tumors, arthritis associated with Paget's disease, ankylosing spondylitis, and juvenile rheumatoid arthritis (Table 19-1). Contraindications to THA include active local or systemic infections and medical conditions that significantly increase the risk of serious perioperative morbidity and mortality (see Table 19-1).[2]

Prevalence of Total Hip Arthroplasty

Rates of THA have increased worldwide, with more than 1 million procedures being performed annually.[3] Projections expect this trend to increase exponentially during the next 15 years.[4] The reasons for the increase are multifactorial, including a higher incidence of OA secondary to an aging population and a worldwide obesity epidemic. Furthermore, younger patients are now considered candidates for THA due to increased survivorship of the prosthesis (>80% at 25-year follow-up), along with evidence that early intervention for OA may provide better functional outcomes. By 2030, patients <65 years old are projected to represent 50% of the hip arthroplasty population.[3,5]

Hip Osteoarthritis Patient Management and Surgical Decision Making

Diagnosis and management of hip OA can be delayed because of patient and clinician difficulty in identifying that the hip is the source of pain and the functional limitations. Compared with painful conditions in other joints, such as the knee, hip pain is particularly difficult to define for three reasons: (1) the joint is deep, therefore pain arising from it can be felt across a broader region; (2) pain from structures outside the hip (e.g., the lower back, groin, and urinary and genital tracts) can cause referred pain in the hip region; and (3) delineating a specific topographical area that can be defined as "the hip" is difficult.[7]

Nonsurgical treatment for OA is often recommended before THA. A systematic review identified several nonsurgical alternatives that could be effective in the management of hip OA pain before surgery, including self-management, education, exercise, weight reduction, acupuncture, and medical pharmaceutical management (e.g., acetaminophen, nonsteroidal anti-inflammatory drugs [NSAIDs], opioids, corticosteroids, glucosamine sulfate, diacerein, hyaluronic acid, and homeopathic remedies). This same systematic review identified THA as effective in improving the quality of life of hip OA patients who did not respond to nonsurgical treatments.[8]

TABLE **19-1**

Indications and Contraindications for Total Hip Arthroplasty

Indications	• Osteoarthritis • Rheumatoid arthritis and juvenile rheumatoid arthritis • Avascular necrosis • Traumatic arthritis • Certain hip fractures (e.g., femoral neck fracture in an older, active adult) • Benign and malignant bone tumors • Arthritis associated with Paget's disease • Ankylosing spondylitis
Relative contraindications	• Age under 60 years • Obesity • Neurological disease (increases the risk of postoperative dislocation)
Absolute contraindications	• Active local or systemic infections • Unstable medical conditions that significantly increase the risk of serious perioperative morbidity and mortality (e.g., cardiac conditions, such as a recent myocardial infarction [MI]; also pulmonary, liver, genitourinary, or metabolic disease)

As of 2015, there are no international consensus guidelines to assist orthopedic surgeons as to when to perform THA.[3] In addition to symptomatic OA, functional limitations and physical examination findings can factor into the decision to operate, as well as other patient- and physician-related factors (see Table 19-1). A 2006 study identified differences between referring physicians' and orthopedic surgeons' opinion on the effect of disease severity and quality of life in the decision to pursue THA. They concluded that referring physicians were more likely to think that patients had to have a higher disease severity to warrant operation and were more apt to consider social factors and quality of life issues versus orthopedic surgeons.[9]

Appropriate patient selection is an important consideration for THA. Obesity, advanced age, and medical comorbidities may make a surgical candidate less optimal; however, these are not absolute contraindications for surgery (see Table 19-1). There is a 40% increased risk of complications for each decade above 65 years old. For younger patients, particularly those <50 years old, survivorship of the prosthesis needs to be considered, given the higher activity level of this patient population.[3] The timing of THA from onset of symptomatic OA is also an important consideration. Studies have shown that patients who wait less than 3 months for surgery have better functional improvement postoperatively than patients who wait 6 months or more.[3]

TOTAL HIP ARTHROPLASTY

Surgical Approaches

There are several different surgical approaches, as well as modifications to these approaches, to perform a THA. The three most common approaches are the anterior, anterolateral, and posterior approach. Each approach has specific advantages and disadvantages, and if done correctly, there is no significant difference in outcomes between the approaches.

The choice of approach is primarily based on the surgeon's experience and the ability to achieve a reproducible result. Occasionally, a patient-specific factor (e.g., neuromuscular disease, anatomical abnormality, or flexion contracture) will lead surgeons to vary their standard approach. Each approach has specific rehabilitation guidelines with respect to dislocation precautions, movement restrictions, and weight-bearing restrictions, and therefore it is important to be familiar with the major approaches and the rationale behind their associated precautions.

The anterior approach has increased in popularity in the United States as of 2015.[10,11] Patients are positioned supine on either a special traction table or regular operating room table. The skin incision starts approximately 3 cm distal and lateral from the anterior superior iliac spine (ASIS) and goes in a distal and lateral direction. The deep dissection goes through an intranervous plane between the sartorius muscle (supplied by the femoral nerve) and tensor fascia lata (supplied by the superior gluteal nerve). This approach is considered "muscle sparing" because it maintains the muscle attachments. Other than the reflected head of the rectus femoris muscle, which is directly over the anterior capsule, no muscles are incised or removed from their attachment to bone.[12] The hip is dislocated anteriorly during the procedure. The advantages of this approach are thought to be a low dislocation rate, decreased damage to the musculature, a faster rehabilitation rate, and potentially no need for dislocation precautions.[13–16] The disadvantages of this approach include the difficulty with exposure affecting implant positioning and risk of iatrogenic fracture, significant surgeon learning curve for performing the procedure, and anterior dislocations.[17]

The anterolateral approach is performed either supine or in a lateral decubitus position. The skin incision is started at the greater trochanter with the proximal portion angled toward the ASIS and the distal incision following along the shaft of the femur. After the iliotibial band and tensor fascia lata are incised, a common modification of this approach is performed with the anterior one third of the abductor muscles released directly off the greater trochanter. The abductor muscles are repaired during the closure. Similar to the anterior approach, the hip is dislocated anteriorly. The anterolateral approach is very versatile, allowing excellent exposure of the acetabulum and the femur and has a low dislocation rate. This approach is usually chosen for patients who are at high risk for dislocation (i.e., patients with hip fractures, dementia, large range of motion [ROM], abductor muscle tears, or neuromuscular disease).[18] Due to the abductor muscles repair, active abduction is not immediately recommended to protect the repair for a period of approximately 6 weeks.

The posterior approach is the most common approach used for hip replacement. Patients are placed in a lateral decubitus position for surgery. The skin incision is centered on the greater trochanter, similar to the anterolateral approach. The proximal incision is in line with the posterior superior iliac spine, then follows the mid shaft of the femur from the tip of the greater trochanter distally. The abductor muscles are protected and the lateral (external) rotator muscles and capsule are taken off the back of the femur to allow the hip to be dislocated posteriorly. In addition to being a very familiar approach for most orthopedic surgeons, this approach has excellent exposure to the acetabulum and femur. It can be extended proximally to gain additional exposure to the posterior column of the acetabulum or distally to expose the femur.

Types of Fixation

The type of implant fixation can affect a patient's weight-bearing activities postoperatively. Fixation of the femoral or acetabular components can be achieved with or without the use of cement. Methyl methacrylate is used as cement to hold either the acetabular or most commonly the femoral components in place. A technique including a cemented femoral component and cementless acetabular component is called hybrid fixation. Fixation using cement is achieved at the time of surgery because it interdigitates with the host bone and forms a secure housing for the implant's smooth surface. Cementless implants obtain their initial hold in bone during surgery as they are impacted into either the prepared acetabulum or femur. The roughened stems allow for the host bone to grow around or into the actual implant on its roughened surface, which holds the implant in place. This process of ingrowth takes approximately 6 weeks.

Nontraditional Hip Arthroplasty Options

Surgical implant types for hip arthroplasty have evolved, resulting in more options for both surgeons and patients. In part, this evolution has been driven by the need for arthroplasty options for patients who, beyond the desire of restoring basic functional activity (e.g., walking and performing activities of daily living [ADLs]), have the additional goal of returning to recreational and sport-type activities. The desire to promote early return of function and minimize surgical trauma (and resulting pain and edema) has also prompted the development of alternative

surgical approaches (such as the direct anterior and 2-incision minimally invasive THA).

Minimally invasive surgery (MIS) is a term used to describe either a smaller incision (typically half of the length of the traditional incision) or an approach that does not involve cutting tendons or splitting muscles. There has been considerable debate as to the possible benefits of MIS, including decreased blood loss and pain and earlier functional recovery. Disadvantages of MIS are primarily considered to be an increased prevalence of complications, such as fracture, infection, component malposition, undesired muscle damage, and heterotopic ossification.[19-21]

In the mid-1990s the renewed development of metal-on-metal (MOM) hip prostheses in England resulted in a prosthesis called the hip resurfacing arthroplasty (HRA).[22-24] This approach offers an alternative for younger patients, allowing return to high-level recreational and sport activities. Advantages of MOM are the theoretical long-term high tolerance to stress and load bearing that a traditional, non-MOM prosthesis does not allow without early implant failure.[22-24] Returning to all or near-all recreational activities has been observed in the HRA population.[25]

Despite successful outcomes, MOM implants have also revealed their own challenges. In HRA, many potential outcomes were theorized, such as avascular necrosis of the femoral head, femoral neck thinning (and possibly fracture), and edge wear of the metal implants, resulting in the release of metal ions into the surrounding tissues and blood stream.[26-28] Many, if not all, of these instances, require removal of the prosthesis and conversion to a traditional THA prosthesis.[27,28] At the time of this writing, multiple prosthetic developers have issued recalls on their MOM implants as a result of the wear and cobalt and chromium metal ion release. The impact of these ion releases is not fully understood, although local tissue destruction and formation of pseudo-tumors have been observed in these cases and attributed to the metal debris.[27-29]

Total Hip Arthroplasty Revision

Revision THA has a variety of indications. Patients typically present with a new onset of disabling pain, stiffness, and functional impairment after their primary THA, unrelieved by appropriate medical management and lifestyle modifications. A U.S. study using the Healthcare Cost and Utilization Project Nationwide Inpatient Sample database identified the primary indications for THA revision surgery as instability or dislocation (22.5%), mechanical loosening (19.7%), and infection (14.8%).[2,30] The most common types of revision are all component (41.1%), followed by femoral component only (13.2%), acetabular component only (13.2%), and isolated femoral head and acetabular liner exchange.[30]

Indications for Revision THA Surgery

- Disabling pain
- Stiffness
- Functional impairment
- Bone loss (on radiographs)
- Implant loosening (on radiographs)
- Malpositioned components (on radiographs)
- Fracture
- Recurrent dislocation
- Infection

In situations in which infection of the joint space has been identified before revision THA, patients often require removal of the prosthesis, with implantation of a temporary antibiotic-infused "spacer," followed by a period of intravenous antibiotic treatment (typically 6 to 8 weeks), and then reimplantation of a new THA prosthesis after resolution of the infection.

COMPLICATIONS OF TOTAL HIP ARTHROPLASTY

Hip dislocation is one of the most common complications following THA. Rates vary widely in the literature, between 0.3% and 10% incidence after primary THA, and up to 28% incidence after revision THA.[31,32]

Data from a study of U.S. Medicare recipients quantified the risk of the other most common short-term postoperative complications of primary elective THA and revision THA (Table 19-2).[33] During the 17-year time frame (1991 to 2008) in which these data were collected, the authors noted that overall medical and surgical complexity for elective primary THA and revision THA had increased in this elderly population. There was a trend toward higher rates of diabetes, congestive heart failure (CHF), obesity, and renal failure in this population, and the overall number of significant co-morbidities had increased. Despite this, complications of primary THA dramatically decreased over this time frame before stabilizing or slightly worsening in 2008, whereas the revision THA complications have increased.

In addition to the above-mentioned complications, postoperative limp is another issue that can impact the outcome of THA. The most common causes of a postoperative limp are a leg length discrepancy (LLD) and abductor muscle disruption during surgery. LLD can occur in up to 3% of THA cases; however, it is generally accepted that discrepancies of <1 cm are well tolerated by patients.[31] Beyond the limp, significant LLD can lead to low back pain and functional impairments and can lead to litigation[31] and revision THA. Although the surgeon aims to keep the limb lengths equal, hip stability is a higher priority. An interplay exists between leg length and hip stability—that is, the longer the operative leg length, the tighter the soft tissue and therefore the more stable the hip. Conversely, the shorter the operative limb, the more lax the soft tissue around the hip and therefore, the greater the risk of dislocation.

The surgical approach can have an effect on limb length and postoperative limp. The anterior approach provides opportunity for direct measurement of leg length and thus has less than average LLD and preserves the major abductor muscle attachment.[10,31] The anterolateral approach has been associated with an elevated risk of a postoperative limp as high as 10% 2 years postoperatively and a 2.8% incidence of severe heterotopic ossification.[34] However, other studies have not shown a clinically significant difference in gait between the approaches (i.e., anterolateral, direct lateral, and posterior) at 1 year postoperatively.[35] The direct lateral approach can have variable effects on LLD but does disrupt the abductor muscle mechanism, which can be associated with postoperative limp.[10,31] Positioning for the posterolateral approach makes it difficult to accurately measure leg length, and overlengthening can more commonly occur.[31] However, with a strict posterior approach, the abductor musculature is spared, and thus, this approach is associated with a lower incidence of postoperative limp.[10]

Preoperative and postoperative patient education is essential with respect to actual or perceived LLD. Patients should understand the possibility that their limb might be lengthened during surgery to increase stability. Patients should be informed that the perception that the operative leg feels longer is a normal physiological reaction to THA. Patients who have a perceived LLD preoperatively have a higher likelihood of a perceived LLD postoperatively.[31] Less common causes of a limp are loose implants, biological problems (e.g., sepsis, neuromuscular imbalance, contractures), and extrapelvic causes (e.g., degenerative spine, knee, and ankle pathology).[36]

TABLE **19-2**

Ninety-Day Complications of Primary Elective Total Hip Arthroplasty (THA) and Revision of Primary Elective Total Hip Arthroplasty

Complication	THA (%)	Revision THA (%)
Mortality	0.8	3.0
Deep vein thrombosis	0.6	0.7
Pulmonary embolism	0.4	0.3
Wound Infection	0.6	2.5
Hemorrhage	0.7	1.4
Myocardial infarction	0.7	1.0
Sepsis	0.4	1.1
All-Causes Hospital Readmission	10.9	17.6

Data from Wolf BR, Lu X, Li Y et al: Adverse outcomes in hip arthroplasty: long-term trends, *J Bone Joint Surg Am* 94:8, 2012.

REHABILITATION FOLLOWING TOTAL HIP ARTHROPLASTY

Rehabilitation following THA is a multidisciplinary effort that requires effective and timely communication and coordination. Decisions about the rehabilitation plan of care and discharge are based on patient and surgical considerations but may be influenced by the different members of the health care team.

Patient function varies greatly for THA candidates. For example, for very sedentary individuals, the maximum functional requirement may be to ambulate short household distances; in contrast, high functioning individuals want to return to sports and recreational activities, such as tennis, golf, and hiking. Therefore, it is important that the patient remains the center of the decision-making process throughout the course of treatment, from the choice of prosthetic device and surgical technique to the rehabilitation plan of care.

The patient and family remain at the center of the team, which includes the orthopedic surgeon, primary care physician, physical and occupational therapists, nurse, case manager, and other specialists as needed. A patient may be discharged from the acute care hospital to a rehabilitation facility or home, based on the rehabilitation clinicians' input about function, the nurse's and physician's (or physician's assistant's) input about medical status, and the patient's and family's input about social supports and environmental constraints. Case managers coordinate with insurance companies to facilitate the appropriate resources and a timely transition to a rehabilitation facility or home with nursing and rehabilitation services.

Multidisciplinary Decision Making for Hospital Discharge

Hospital discharge requires input from:
- The rehabilitation clinicians, about function
- The nurse and physician or physician assistant, about the patient's medical status
- The patient and family, about special supports and environmental constraints
- Case managers, about available resources

A multidisciplinary, organized team approach including participation by the patient, surgeons, anesthesiologists, physical therapists, and occupational therapists is essential for improving patient outcomes. The literature shows that preoperative patient education is associated with reduced hospital length of stay (LOS) and improved patient reported outcome measures. MIS has been associated with better pain control, shorter LOS, and less use of assistive devices postoperatively. Aggressive pain management via use of regional and local analgesia may improve postoperative pain, reduce the use of narcotics, and therefore increase patient participation in physical therapy (PT) and ultimately reduce LOS. There is also evidence that

early rehabilitation (including same day mobilization) decreases postoperative pain and reduces LOS.[37,38]

Patient-Related Factors

Throughout the episode of care, a variety of patient-related factors influence rehabilitation decision making, including the patient's previous level of function, social support, environment, co-morbidities, and age. Care should be taken to individualize the examination and evaluation of patients after THA because many individual patient-related factors will influence the patient's progression.

Factors Impacting Rehabilitation Decision Making

- Surgical approach used and any modifications
- Surgical complications
- Medication
- Limitations or restrictions imposed by the surgeon or the surgery
- Age
- Prior level of function
- Medical status and medical history
- Social supports
- Environmental constraints

Preoperative Level of Function

Patients functioning at a high activity level (e.g., recreational activities and sports) may have better strength, cardiovascular endurance, and flexibility than those with low activity tolerance and should be expected to return to a higher level of activity after surgery.[39] The previous level of function influences decisions about exercise prescription, the timing of intervention, and activity restrictions. Patients with low activity levels before surgery may have secondary impairments, such as diminished strength and ROM, as well as greater functional limitations, which may need to be addressed with basic exercise and early intervention. A healthy, highly functioning individual may not require as much skilled intervention until healing has occurred, at which point, functionally based high-level exercise may be prescribed that would be inappropriate for a sedentary patient.

Social Support and Home Environment

The availability of social support influences discharge decision making because patients who live alone may be unable to care for themselves at home and therefore may require a short inpatient rehabilitation stay before returning home.[40-44] Social support and home environment also play a large part in determining a patient's early rehabilitative plan of care because the presence of stairs or other fixed environmental barriers may necessitate the use of assistive devices and specific training in their use. It is important to identify any potential barriers early, to develop an appropriate plan of care to address each patient's individual needs.

Medical Co-morbidities

Trends have shown that patients undergoing THA have a greater number of medical co-morbidities and that an increased number of obese patients are undergoing the procedure.[45] The patient's medical history and co-morbidities must be factored into the decision-making process because these may affect healing time, postoperative complications, and overall functional mobility. It will also factor into the patient's specific functional needs and potential. However, obese patients (with high body mass index [BMI]) are shown to have greater improvement in function and greater satisfaction post-THA than normal-weight patients, potentially due to lower baseline function.[46] Furthermore, patients with serious co-morbidities may require a longer hospital stay and are more likely to require inpatient rehabilitation before returning home.[43,44,47] Diabetes has been shown as one of the strongest predictors of postoperative complications.[48] Specific medical co-morbidities need to be considered when developing an appropriate plan of care because certain interventions may be contraindicated given their co-morbid condition.

Age

Age has been shown to influence postoperative function, mortality, and risk of revision. Older patients undergoing THA are at higher risk of postoperative mortality and experience less improvement in function. However, younger patients are at higher risk of requiring revision surgery.[49] In addition, age can affect the postacute care discharge destination. Patients more than 70 years old are more likely to be discharged to an inpatient rehabilitation facility because of the increased incidence of co-morbidities, reduced mobility, and a greater likelihood of living alone.[*]

Postoperative Considerations

It is essential that the surgeon inform the rehabilitation clinician of the approach used, whether the approach was modified in any way (e.g., trochanteric osteotomy), and whether there were any intraoperative complications (e.g., femoral fracture). All these factors can affect the patient's postoperative weight-bearing status, ROM limitations, and exercise prescription.

Weight-Bearing Restrictions

The patient's weight-bearing status ultimately depends on the surgeon's preference and patient-specific intraoperative findings. Historically, surgeons allowed full weight bearing or weight bearing as tolerated (WBAT) only after cemented THA, based on the principle that adequate fixation is achieved only with cement. Uncemented THA has been associated with micro motion at the bone-prosthetic interface, causing concern for compromised stability and ingrowth of the prosthesis. Thus patients with uncemented THA have traditionally had reduced weight bearing orders for 4 to 12 weeks postoperatively.[51,52]

More recently, many surgeons allow WBAT for uncemented THAs. In uncemented THAs, press-fit stems often are strong enough to withstand the effects of early weight bearing while awaiting bony ingrowth. In fact, some prosthetic designs have been designed to withstand loads of 300% body weight.[52] In a long-term study of more than 300 patients who were allowed WBAT after cementless THA, 99.5% of patients had successful osteointegration of the femoral THA component by 3 months postoperatively, as confirmed by imaging.[51] A 2-year follow-up randomized controlled trial (RCT) comparing partial weight bearing (PWB) to WBAT after cementless THA demonstrated no significant difference in ROM, functional outcome scores, and pain at 3 and 24 months postoperatively. In this study, more patients who were allowed WBAT were able to wean from a cane versus the PWB group (74% to 67%) at 3 months, without compromised fixation at 2 years by imaging.[52]

If the optimum press fit is not possible in an uncemented THA, the patient is made PWB or touch-down weight bearing (TDWB) (i.e., the foot is allowed to touch the ground for balance and stability, without any weight acceptance) for 4 to 12 weeks to allow bone ingrowth into the porous component. Caution should be used with rehabilitation even after cemented THA because it is sometimes used when bone quality is questionable. Careful consideration should be given to exercise or functional movements that may impose an increased load across the femur or pelvis.

If an intraoperative complication arose, such as a crack in the proximal femur (often cerclage wires around the proximal femur indicate such a complication), the patient's weight-bearing status may be downgraded to TDWB. If an osteotomy of the greater trochanter was performed, the patient typically is restricted to TDWB or PWB for up to 12 weeks to allow the osteotomy to heal. It may seem intuitive that keeping a patient non-weight bearing on the affected extremity, rather than TDWB, would better protect the hip; however, keeping a patient non-weight bearing actually places more stress across the hip joint because patients must use their hip musculature to keep the leg lifted off the ground.

Dislocation Precautions

Although a variety of surgical procedures can be used for THA, the common approaches are posterior, posterolateral, anterior, anterolateral, and direct lateral. As detailed previously, they differ in the location where the primary incision is made through the integument, fascia, muscle, and joint capsule to gain access to the hip. Soft tissues that have been transected and then repaired are weaker and present a risk for hip dislocation. Consequently, it is important that the clinician understand the surgical approach and recognize the precautions that must be taken

---

*References 40, 41, 43, 44, 47, 50.

to prevent hip dislocation. A combination of certain movements poses the greatest risk for dislocation. A large part of the rehabilitation clinician's role is to instruct the patient in how to prevent a hip dislocation, which includes education and reinforcement throughout functional movements. For example, a patient who had a posterior approach THA should not bend forward to put on or take off shoes, and compensatory strategies using an assistive device are required for independence in this activity. Dislocation precautions also affect therapeutic exercise interventions. End-range exercise for strengthening, flexibility, and ROM should be avoided until the soft tissues have healed adequately and the surgeon has discontinued hip dislocation precautions.

After surgery, the surgeon wants the patient to avoid the very maneuver that was used intraoperatively to dislocate the hip. For example, to dislocate a hip during a posterior or posterolateral approach, the hip must be flexed, adducted, and medially (internally) rotated. It follows logically that precautions against posterior hip dislocation consist of no hip flexion past 90° in conjunction with hip adduction past midline and hip medial rotation past neutral (Table 19-3). Figure 19-1 depicts an example of modifying ADLs to maintain the hip flexion precaution for the posterior approach THA. A pillow may be positioned between the patient's legs in supine to prevent adduction. Abduction braces are sometimes used to keep the hip in slight lateral (external) rotation and abduction for a patient with a high risk of dislocation after a posterior approach THA. However, there is little evidence in the literature to support use of the brace.[53] Studies looking at bracing after closed reduction of a dislocation[54] and bracing after all-cause revision THA[55] concluded that there is no benefit to bracing versus no brace to prevent short-[55] or long-term[54] dislocation.

Precautions against anterior dislocation include avoiding hip extension and lateral rotation beyond neutral (as detailed in Table 19-3). To help reinforce these precautions, the patient can be positioned in bed with a trochanteric roll at the lateral hip to prevent lateral rotation

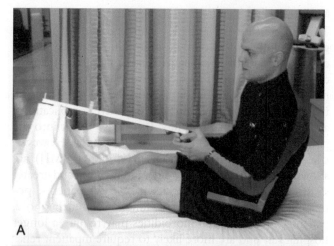
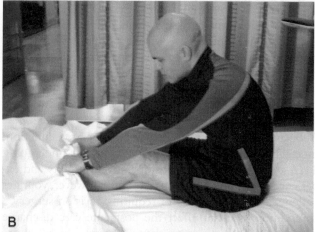

Figure 19-1 Maintaining ≤90° hip flexion after a posterior approach THA. **A,** Correct method using tool. **B,** Incorrect method.

(Figure 19-2). Patients can be educated to avoid bridging past neutral hip extension in hook lying and to avoid pivoting or lunging away from the operated side while standing to avoid the combination of hip extension and lateral rotation.

When a transtrochanteric approach is used, "trochanter off" precautions are prescribed. This is not a dislocation precaution but a restriction of active contraction of the musculature attached to the trochanter to allow the bone to heal. This approach involves bony repair of the greater trochanteric osteotomy; therefore the repair must be protected to minimize the risk of nonunion. Because the abductor muscles (e.g., gluteus medius and minimus) insert into the greater trochanter, no active abduction is allowed for at least 6 weeks after surgery (see Table 19-3). Patients sometimes have active abduction restriction after a lateral approach, to protect the reattachment of the abductor muscles to the trochanter after surgery.

Studies have differed in their assessment of risks for hip dislocation by surgical approach. The literature demonstrates that 75% to 90% of dislocations happen posteriorly.[32,56,57] Historically, higher rates of dislocation have been observed for the posterior or posterolateral versus

TABLE **19-3**

Treatment Precautions to Prevent Hip Dislocation or Delay Muscle or Bone Healing

Type of Procedure	Precautions
Posterior or posterolateral approach	No hip flexion past 90° in conjunction with hip adduction past midline and hip medial rotation past neutral
Anterior or anterolateral approach	No hip extension or lateral rotation beyond neutral
Transtrochanteric or lateral approach	No active abduction

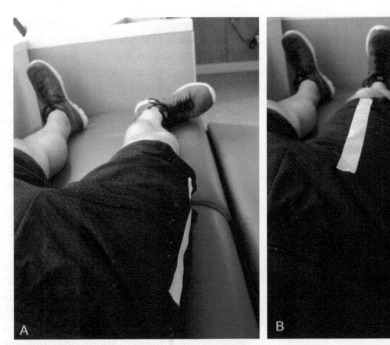

Figure 19-2 A, Improper positioning of the lower extremity with hip lateral rotation. **B,** Corrected by positioning with a trochanteric roll to maintain neutral position after an anterior approach THA.

anterolateral approach.[32,53,58-60] More recently, a comprehensive meta-analysis found that the combined dislocation rate was 1.27% for the transtrochanteric approach, 3.23% for the posterior approach (3.95% without a posterior capsular repair and 2.03% with the repair), 2.18% for the anterolateral approach, and 0.55% for the direct lateral approach.[61] A 2006 systematic review reported no significant difference between the dislocation rate for the posterior approach versus the direct lateral approach (1.3% versus 4.2%, respectively) but reports that the evidence is not strong enough to be conclusive about this complication risk.[62] A subsequent RCT[63] documented a 3% dislocation rate for the lateral approach compared with zero dislocations for the posterior approach over an average 38-month follow-up. In contrast, a study based on the Swedish Hip Arthroplasty Register found the posterior approach had an increased risk of dislocation (relative risk [RR] 1.3, confidence interval [CI] 1.1-1.7) compared to the direct lateral approach.[64] In a community-based population, Khatod et al.[65] did not find a correlation between the surgical approach and the rate of dislocation.

A larger femoral head diameter is associated with a lower long-term cumulative risk of dislocation in all operative approaches, but especially with the posterolateral approach.[59] Soft tissue repair when the posterior approach is used has been shown to reduce the dislocation rate from 4.46% to 0.49%. Most surgeons currently repair the posterior capsule[32,53,61,66-68] and short lateral (external) rotators[31] to achieve these improved results. In a systematic review of the literature, when the soft tissue was repaired in the posterior approach, the dislocation rate was comparable for the anterolateral, direct lateral, and posterior approaches (0.7%, 0.43%, and 1.01%, respectively).[69]

Several patient-related factors are associated with increased risk of hip dislocation. Historically, women were thought to be twice as likely as men to dislocate, but recent studies have challenged this finding.[53] Patients with neuromuscular and cognitive disorders, such as cerebral palsy, muscular dystrophies, psychoses, dementia, and alcoholism, have been associated with higher dislocation rates.[32,53] Weakness, noncompliance with hip precautions, and balance issues are underlying causes for this finding.[32] Other risk factors include prior hip surgery, history of fracture, developmental dysplasia, osteonecrosis, or inflammatory arthropathy.[53] In fact, prior open hip surgery is likely to double the risk of instability due to scarring, laxity, and soft tissue compromise.[32]

The need for patient dislocation restrictions after an anterolateral approach THA has been called into question. A prospective, randomized study evaluated the effect of postoperative functional restrictions on the prevalence of dislocation after an uncemented, anterolateral approach THA.[70] The study participants were divided into a "restricted" group and an "unrestricted" group. Both groups were asked to limit the ROM of the hip to less than 90° flexion and 45° lateral and medial rotation and to avoid adduction for the first 6 weeks after surgery. In addition to these baseline restrictions, during the first 6 weeks after surgery, patients in the restricted group (1) had an abduction pillow placed between their legs in the operating room before bed transfer and used pillows to maintain abduction while in bed; (2) used elevated toilet seats and elevated chairs in the hospital, in the rehabilitation facility, and at home; and (3) were prevented from sleeping on their side, driving, and being a passenger in an automobile. Of the 303 THAs studied, the only dislocation was in the restricted group, and it occurred as the patient was transferred from the operating table to a bed with an abduction pillow in place. Patients in the unrestricted group returned to side sleeping sooner, rode and drove in automobiles more often, returned to work sooner, and had a higher level of satisfaction with the pace of their recovery than those in the restricted group. An additional expenditure of approximately U.S. $655 per patient was made in the restricted group for additional adaptive equipment.

A small, 2009 randomized prospective study also studied patients who had an anterolateral approach[71] and restricted versus unrestricted activities. The restricted group was instructed to avoid hip flexion greater than 90°, crossing legs at the thighs, and riding in a car for 1 month postoperatively versus the "early" group who were advised only to avoid crossing their thighs. There were no dislocations in either group, but significant differences were found in functional progression. The unrestricted group progressed earlier to use of a cane, weaning off all assistive devices, walking without a limp, and driving compared with the restricted group.

In a study of 6623 consecutive cemented primary Charnley THAs (90% via transtrochanteric approach, 9% via anterolateral, and 1% posterolateral), the cumulative risk of a first-time dislocation was 1% at 1 month and 1.9% at 1 year; it then rose at a constant rate of approximately 1% every 5 years to 7% at 25 years for patients who had not had a revision by that time.[72] This study is one of the few that have studied the long-term risk of dislocation; however, surgical techniques have improved since this study which likely has decreased the long-term risk of dislocation. More research on this topic should shed additional light on whether all THA patients need to adhere to dislocation precautions postoperatively, possibly depending on their surgical approach.

Little consensus is found among surgeons on the length of time the patient should follow these dislocation precautions. The duration ranges from a few weeks to lifelong, depending on the surgeon's preference. The capsule and connective tissues should heal by 6 to 12 weeks; therefore patients are advised to follow the hip dislocation precautions for at least this duration of time.

STAGES OF REHABILITATION MANAGEMENT

Rehabilitation from THA requires a multidisciplinary approach and often begins before surgery. Patients may have preoperative education followed by inpatient rehabilitation while in the acute care hospital. Postacute care rehabilitation may occur in an inpatient rehabilitation, home care, or outpatient setting. Patients will often receive care in more than one setting to achieve full return to their desired function, ranging from short-distance ambulation to sports-level activity. Transition from one stage to the next is dictated by the patient's functional abilities within the constraints of the person's individual environment, available supports, and co-morbidities. For multiple rea-

sons, the length of the acute care stay has been declining from the early 1990s to the time of this publication, with earlier transition to the next postacute care phase of rehabilitation (inpatient rehabilitation, home care, and/or outpatient), depending on the needs of the patient.

Like primary THA, rehabilitation following a revision THA needs to be individualized to the patients based on the same inherent preoperative, perioperative, and postoperative considerations, challenges, and surgeon orders. Similar short- and long-term outcomes that have been observed following primary THA have been observed in revision THA.

Preoperative Rehabilitation

Before undergoing surgery, many patients attend a THA education class (if offered by the facility in which they are having surgery), which may include a physician and/or surgeon, nurse, rehabilitation clinicians, and a case worker, discharge planning nurse, or social worker. Patients are educated about preparing for surgery, the surgical procedure, the postoperative course, applicable precautions, early postoperative exercise, functional mobility with a walker and/or crutches, and discharge planning from hospital to home or to inpatient rehabilitation or extended care facility (ECF).[73,74]

One of the primary roles of preoperative education is the influence it can have on patient expectations regarding long-term outcome after surgery, course of hospitalization, and transition from the hospital into the postacute care phase.[74,75] Evidence has shown that patients who receive preoperative education demonstrate improved achievement of preoperative expectations (such as symptom relief and improved function), significantly less preoperative anxiety, and decreased incidence of postoperative complications (such as hip dislocation).[74–77] Education about hip dislocation precautions, the proper use of assistive devices, early postoperative exercise, and mobility may be more effective before surgery, when pain, the effects of anesthesia, and postoperative anxiety do not interfere with the patient's ability to concentrate and process information. The textbox on the following page outlines a sample syllabus for a preoperative education class.

The literature is conflicting on the effect of preoperative educational sessions on short- and long-term THA outcomes. In one study, patients who received preoperative education and therapy to increase strength and ROM performed transfer activities sooner postoperatively than those who did not receive preoperative training; however, no significant difference was seen in pain or in the **Harris Hip Score (HHS)**.[78] In another randomized, controlled prospective study, Giraudet-Le Quintrec et al.[76] compared patients who had received a preoperative information leaflet (control group) with patients who had attended a collective, multidisciplinary information session 2 to 6 weeks before surgery. The patients who had attended

---

Sample Syllabus for Preoperative Education on Total Hip Replacement

- Definition of items used during your hospital stay
- Preparing your home before surgery and items to bring with you
- Planning your discharge
- Admission to the hospital
- Operating room
- Recovery room
- What to expect each day in the hospital
- Total hip replacement dislocation precautions
- Prevention of dislocation after total hip replacement
- Instructions for sitting and rising from a chair
- Walker, crutches, and cane use
- Gait training
- How to climb stairs
- How to get into and out of a car
- How to get into and out of a stall shower or tub shower
- Rehabilitation
- Exercises
- Sexual activity after hip replacement
- Skin care
- Wound care, signs of infection, signs of a blood clot
- When to call your doctor and what to do in an emergency
- How to contact your surgeon
- How to contact the orthopedic nurse education coordinator
- When to return for follow-up appointments
- Antibiotic prophylaxis after a total hip replacement
- Venous thromboembolism prophylaxis

---

the information session were significantly less anxious just before surgery than the patients in the control group. They also had less pain before surgery, and they were able to stand sooner; however, the trend toward lower anxiety scores was not statistically significant after surgery.[75,76]

Discussions and decisions about discharge planning and destination (i.e., home or rehabilitation facility) should begin preoperatively via formalized screening. Studies have shown that factors available to providers before surgery, such as age, gender, presence of co-morbidities, living situation, and presurgical function, are all factors in the recommendation for discharge destination.[79,80] Since 1999, use of formalized preoperative screening tools has also assisted in anticipating likely discharge destination after the hospital stay. Oldmeadow et al. developed the **Risk Assessment and Prediction Tool (RAPT)** for total joint arthroplasty patients (Figure 19-3).[81] Information such as age, gender, preoperative walking ability, preoperative use of assistive walking aids, and available social supports are collected by the multidisciplinary team. This information is entered into a formula that generates a prediction score for likely discharge destination (i.e., home versus inpatient rehabilitation). This tool has been validated in multiple studies to aid early discharge planning.[82,83] Early planning to arrange alternative short-term living arrangements or support may allow patients who live alone to avoid discharge to an inpatient rehabilitation setting.[81]

Acute Care Rehabilitation

Over time, the LOS in hospital after THA has decreased dramatically, due to the rising costs of THA and increased volume of patients. Among Medicare recipients in the United States, LOS after primary THA has decreased from 8 to 3 days between 1991 and 2008. A similar decrease has been observed for revision THA over the same time frame, from 9 to 4 days.[33] Currently, there are fast-track and enhanced recovery programs (ERPs) that target an even shorter LOS (≤2 days). Hospitals are tasked with minimizing hospital stay to reduce costs. Rehabilitation professionals are, therefore, tasked with optimizing patient outcomes in a shorter perioperative period of time.[37]

In the acute care setting, the primary role of physical and occupational therapists with patients who are post THA is to promote mobility and functional independence.[84-87] For many patients, demonstrating independence with functional activities, such as bed mobility, transfers, ambulation, stair walking, and self-care activities, is achievable during the acute care stay (which can be as short as 2 to 3 days).[85-88]

Rehabilitation after THA is usually started within the first 24 hours following surgery and continues throughout the acute care stay until the patient meets goals for discharge home or is transferred to an inpatient rehabilitation facility.[85,86,88] With changes in the demographics of patients, surgical techniques, surgical blood loss mitigation, anesthetic techniques, and optimized pain control, rehabilitation clinicians should anticipate being able to successfully mobilize patients within hours of the completion of surgery.[85,86,88,89] As part of preparing for patient care in the acute care phase, rehabilitation clinicians must take into account medical aspects of patients after THA that are often unique to the acute care environment, including pain management, hemodynamic issues, and medical complications.

Pain Management

Optimizing pain management in the acute care phase is essential to promote both early mobility and achievement of patient and clinician goals.[90-92] Given that rehabilitation is going to be occurring within the time frame of the normal physiological inflammatory response to soft tissue and bone trauma (i.e., the first 48 to 72 hours), pain perceived and reported by patients after THA is anticipated to be at its peak.[93,94] Both multimodal pharmaceutical and nonpharmaceutical pain management approaches have proven successful in the acute care environment.[90-92] Multimodal pharmaceutical management typically consists of narcotic and nonnarcotic and nonsteroidal anti-inflammatory medications.[90-92] Nonpharmaceutical pain management may consist of ice, compression (via abdominal binders deliberately placed lower around the hips), and promotion of early ROM and movement (as promotion of exercise and ROM before THA has been shown to decrease pain).[86,93,95]

The Risk Assessment and Prediction Tool (RAPT) for Hip or Knee Arthroplasty

This Risk Assessment and Prediction Tool (RAPT) is a very useful tool developed independently by the American Congress of Rehabilitation Medicine and the American Academy of Physical Medicine and Rehabilitation.

The RAPT approach is recommended for use in helping general practitioners (GPs) assess their patients.

With support from this simple guideline, GPs are able to assess whether a patient is a suitable candidate for an integrated surgery and prehabilitation and rehabilitation program as part of their treatment program.

To be completed by the patients undergoing elective Hip or Knee replacement surgery prior to discussion with your orthopedic surgeon or attending pre-admission clinic.
Name _____
DOB _____
Address _____
Surgeon _____

Study	Value	Score
1. What is your age group?	50-65y 66-75y >75y	=2 =1 =0
2. Gender?	Male Female	=2 =1
3. How far, on average, can you walk? (a block is 200m)	Two blocks or more (± rests) 1-2 blocks (the shopping centre) Housebound (most of time)	=2 =1 =0
4. Which gait aid do you use? (more often than not)	None Single-point stick Crutches/frame	=2 =1 =0
5. Do you use community supports? (home help, meals-on-wheels, district nurse)	None or 1 per week Two or more per week	=1 =0
6. Will you live with someone who can care for you after your operation?	Yes No	=3 =0
	Your score (out of 12)	

KEY: Destination at discharge from acute care predicted by score:

Scores <6   extended inpatient rehabilitation

Scores 6-9   directly home after additional acute intervention

Scores >9   directly home

Patient's expectation of discharge destination is also a determinant. The prediction indicated by the score is discussed with the patient and the destination agreed to.

Patient's preference	Prediction	Agreed destination

Figure 19-3 The Risk Assessment and Prediction Tool (RAPT) for Hip or Knee Arthroplasty. (Modified from 2004 American Congress of Rehabilitation Medicine and the American Academy of Physical Medicine and Rehabilitation.)

For rehabilitation clinicians, coordinating administration of pain medications by nursing staff before therapy sessions is essential (especially given that different medications have their own frequency and timing of administration). With this approach, the patient is best able to tolerate the rehabilitation activities and interventions from a pain perspective.

> **Clinical Note**
>
> Ideally, rehabilitation clinicians should coordinate their patient treatment times with the administration of pain medications given by the nursing staff.

Hemodynamic Issues

As a result of blood lost from the surgery, patients who are post THA often have decreases in hematocrit (HCT) and hemoglobin (Hgb) within 24 hours following surgery.[96-98] Despite decreased HCT/Hgb, literature has demonstrated that safe mobilization of patients is possible as long as hemodynamic stability is maintained and symptoms of hemodynamic intolerance are monitored.[99,100] If a patient demonstrates repeated hemodynamic instability with position change or activity in the presence of a low HCT, the decision for blood transfusion may be made to prevent continued hemodynamic instability.[101] Although not contraindicated, clinical treatments during a blood transfusion should be performed cautiously, with a focus on a patient's hemodynamic tolerance to activity and care to maintain the integrity of the intravenous line providing the transfusion.

Assessment of the patient's hemodynamic status before initiating and during clinical sessions is essential. Although there is a plethora of evidence supporting successful mobilization out of bed in the very early postoperative period, rehabilitation clinicians do need to be aware of possible adverse hemodynamic responses to activity and position changes that may compromise a patient's safety. As a result of acute changes in blood and fluid volumes, the side effects of pain medicines and anesthesia, cardiac medicines taken by patient for co-morbidities, and in some cases, prolonged horizontal body positioning in bed, patients in the first 24 hours following surgery may demonstrate activity-induced hypotension (or bradycardia) with movement into sitting or standing or walking positions.[102,103] This is typically accompanied by subjective reports of lightheadedness, nausea, and/or fatigue. Acute hypotension can lead to syncope along with potential hypoxia and injury to key vital organ systems.[102,104-106] In addition, if a patient were to have a syncopal episode while standing or walking, this could result in additional injury to the patient and potentially the health care provider due to an uncontrolled or controlled fall to the ground.[104]

> **Clinical Note**
>
> It is essential that rehabilitation clinicians monitor the patient's vital signs prior to and during changes in patient position, especially during the early postoperative period.

To prepare for this possible adverse reaction, rehabilitation clinicians should take baseline resting vital signs on all patients during all treatment sessions during this early postoperative period and continue to check the vital signs with all changes in patient body position. Prior studies have defined a systolic blood pressure (SBP) decrease of >10 mm Hg during exercise as "exercise-induced hypotension."[107] However, the change in SBP should be considered in relation to the patient's baseline blood pressure (BP). Clinicians should mobilize patients with caution if decreasing BPs are observed with activity. It is strongly recommended that if the decreasing BP is accompanied by associated symptoms, activity should cease and patients should be returned to a supine position. Once supine, it is expected that SBP will return to baseline level and resolution of adverse signs and symptoms will occur. If a patient does not demonstrate improved hemodynamics and resolution of symptoms in supine, placing the patient in a **Trendelenberg position** (supine with head 15° to 30° lower than feet) may assist with stabilization of cardiovascular symptoms. If the patient's symptoms do not resolve or worsen, the patient should be evaluated by the medical team.

Medical Considerations

Clinicians also must be aware of other, infrequent contraindications to rehabilitation intervention, including new-onset arrhythmia, active work-up for acute cardiac event or pulmonary embolus (PE), or acute change in mental status that prevents the patient from following commands and participating in physical therapy treatment.

> **Contraindications to Rehabilitation**
>
> - New onset arrhythmia
> - Acute cardiac event
> - Pulmonary embolism
> - Acute change in mental status

Deep vein thrombosis (DVT) prophylaxis has progressed significantly between 2006 and 2014, resulting in significant decreases in the occurrence of DVT postoperatively. Literature has reported DVT occurrence after THA to be between 1.3% and 10.0%.[108] DVT prophylaxis is achieved through a multimodal approach, including medication, mechanical compression devices, compression hosiery, and early mobilization of the patient. Medication options and standards for DVT prophylaxis have evolved, with the American College of Chest Surgeons stating that aspirin use for DVT prophylaxis is acceptable in patients with low risk for DVT and is compliant with the Joint Commission's "Surgical Care Improvement Project" (SCIP).[109] Oral medicines such as Coumadin and injectable medicines such as Lovenox are also used routinely for DVT prophylaxis.[109-111] Rehabilitation clinicians should be aware of signs and symptoms that may indicate presence of DVT and warrant consultation with the patient's clinical care team for further evaluation and diagnostic workup. Physiological signs, although relevant, have been shown to be poor predictors of the presence or absence of DVT.[112] Therefore Homan's sign has been shown to be largely unhelpful in identifying DVT in patients.[113] However, the Wells Criteria[114] have been well validated for clinical probability in the assessment of DVT. Clinical signs of DVT alone are not diagnostic but warrant referral for further evaluation.[115]

Wells Clinical Prediction Rules for Likelihood of Deep Vein Thrombosis (DVT)

- Active cancer
- Paralysis, paresis, or recent plaster immobilization of lower extremities
- Recently bedridden for >3 days or major surgery within 4 weeks
- Localized tenderness along distribution of deep venous system
- Entire leg swollen
- Calf swelling >3 cm when compared with asymptomatic leg
- Pitting edema
- Collateral superficial veins (non-varicose)
- Previously documented DVT
- Alternative diagnosis as likely or greater than that of DVT

Scoring: +1 for each factor above except −2 for last criterion (alternative diagnosis likely). A cumulative score of ≥2 is likely DVT, whereas <2 means DVT is unlikely.

Modified from Wells PS, Anderson DR, Rodger M et al: Evaluation of D-dimer in the diagnosis of suspected deep-vein thrombosis, *New Engl J Med* 349:1228, 2003.

Interventions

In the acute care setting, physical therapists focus their postoperative care in three areas: functional mobility training, therapeutic exercise, and patient education.

Functional Mobility Training. The mainstay of rehabilitation in the inpatient setting is functional mobility training, which is progressed or limited according to patient tolerance and surgical and weight-bearing precautions.[84-88] Typical activities for functional mobility training include bed mobility (e.g., supine to sit, sit to supine, rolling), sit to stand, bed to chair transfers, ambulation with assistive devices, and stair training.[84-88] The most current evidence recommends patients be progressed as tolerated with functional activities, irrespective of the postoperative day from surgery.[85] When determining "tolerance," the clinician should consider the patient's overall fitness level/cardiovascular conditioning, pain levels with activity, and hemodynamic response to activity.

Functional mobility training should emphasize safe, efficient mobility that complies with any applicable ROM and weight-bearing precautions and minimizes pain. Further consideration is given to assistive devices, and starting ambulation with a walker will allow patients to maximize their ability to maintain balance while initiating early weight bearing on the operated limb. Progression to other assistive devices (such as crutches or a cane) is dependent on both patient factors and postoperative activity limitations, and may take place at different points in the overall recovery process.

As a patient progresses to walking activities, instruction on gait pattern and correction of modifiable gait deviations also becomes a focus of treatment. Patients may demonstrate gait deviations that are related to compensations made presurgery or postsurgery as a result of pain or discomfort, weakness, joint and soft tissue restrictions, or edema or swelling. Patients should be given verbal, visual, and manual cues to correct any modifiable gait deviations as soon as possible without compromising the patient's safety, activity tolerance, or ability to meet any goals for discharge.

Therapeutic Exercise. Exercise prescription is important in the early postoperative phase to address impairments of pain, edema, ROM, strength, and motor control, and to prevent secondary complications.[84-86]

Supine exercises performed in bed include active-assisted ROM (AAROM) and active ROM (AROM) at the hip, knee, and ankle and isometric exercise of the quadriceps and gluteals.[84-86,116] As functional mobility progresses to sitting, standing, and ambulation, the therapeutic regimen should include sitting and standing AROM exercises. Typical exercises prescribed during the acute care stay are listed in Table 19-4.[84-86]

Patient Education. In the acute care phase, patient education focuses on multiple topics.[84,86,117] Instruction in activity modification in the setting of any applicable postoperative surgeon-specific limitations (such as weight-bearing status and hip dislocation precautions) and surgical side effects (i.e., pain and edema) is often led by rehabilitation clinicians.[84,86] This includes potential modifications for moving from supine to sit and vice versa; standing from and sitting onto beds, chairs, toilets; self-care management for ADLs; gait sequencing on level surfaces and stairs; and use of assistive devices for walking and ADLs. These instructions and recommendations

---

TABLE **19-4**

Postoperative Exercises

Supine	• Ankle pumps
	• Heel slides
	• AROM and AAROM hip abduction and adduction to neutral
	• AROM hip lateral rotation and internal rotation to neutral
	• Quadriceps and gluteal isometrics
Sitting	• AROM knee flexion and extension
	• AROM hip external rotation
Standing	• AROM hip abduction
	• AROM hip extension
	• AROM hip flexion (marching)
	• Heel raises

AROM, active range of motion; *AAROM,* active-assisted range of motion

are to maximize independence and safety of patients after THA and limit preventable adverse events (such as hip dislocation).

Edema and nonpharmaceutical pain management are also key areas of education that rehabilitation clinicians provide. These include the use of cryotherapy at and around the surgical site to assist in edema and pain reduction.[86] Ice has long been shown to assist with management of edema and pain, and as a result contributes to improved outcomes.[117] Limb and joint positioning is also important to assist patients in maximizing comfort and preventing passive migration of the surgical hip into undesired positions (that may increase either the patient's pain or risk of dislocation).

Discharge Planning. Rehabilitation clinicians play a primary role in providing recommendations for an appropriate discharge plan from the acute care setting following THA (including destination, and frequency and intensity of rehabilitation services).[81,82,118] An appropriate discharge plan for patients following THA is essential to both achieve a safe level of function and promote the patients' achievement of their individual long-term goals. The two primary postacute care discharge destinations are "home" or an extended care facility (ECF).[79,81,82,118]

Home represents the patient's own home or that of a care plan partner. ECF represents a health care facility, such as acute rehabilitation hospital or skilled nursing facility.[79] When considering home as a destination, rehabilitation clinicians must also consider whether the patient will receive care in the patient's home (i.e., home care) or in an outpatient setting. Frequency and intensity of services are based on the scope of the patient's health care needs (i.e., physical and/or occupational therapy [OT], along with other skilled health care needs) and the anticipated duration of need for rehabilitation services to meet the patient's goals for recovery.

The rationale for a given discharge recommendation depends on a number of individual patient factors including those discussed previously as well as the patient's medical and functional ability status during and at the time of discharge from acute care.[47,118,119] Once a patient's discharge recommendation is agreed upon by the patient and members of the health care team, the patient's plan of care will be progressed accordingly by PT and/or OT.

Although there are no absolute guidelines, the consensus in the literature is that a patient is appropriate for a home discharge plan when he or she demonstrates:[85,118,120]

- Independence with supine to sit and sit to supine movements (typically from a flat position to simulate a patient's bed at home)
- Independence with sit to stand and stand to sit movements from bed, chair, and toilet (with any needed modification to elevate toilet height if patient has posterior hip precautions)
- Independence with ambulation with needed assistive device of 100 to 150 feet (30.5 to 45.7 m)
- Supervised or independent ambulation on stairs

These guidelines are not all encompassing, and a small percentage of patient situations may allow for a patient to safely transition home without having achieved all of the above-listed functional tasks.

For all other patients who have not yet achieved these goals, discharge to an ECF is typically recommended. For these patients, an ECF allows for the continued opportunity to work with rehabilitation clinicians on a frequent basis and provides a longer time period to achieve these goals. In addition, the ECF may allow for more consistent continued management of co-morbidities and/or postsurgical conditions (e.g., pain control, wound care) that is not possible with home care services.

Inpatient Rehabilitation in the Extended Care Facility

For patients following THA who have transitioned to an ECF, rehabilitation clinicians must consider the patient's physiological state of recovery as well as the resources of the ECF when establishing plan of care. Physiologically, assuming the patient has transitioned to an ECF 72 hours or more following his or her procedure, the patient should be beyond the peak inflammatory response to the surgical trauma.[93,121] Acute pain levels should be well controlled by this point; blood and fluid levels have also likely stabilized.[121] However, individual patient factors may prolong the time frame for healing and pain resolution, and the ECF setting allows for further management of these issues over a broader time frame, which can lead to more rapid and meaningful progress toward functional and discharge goals.

The ECF setting also provides greater access to rehabilitation services compared with home care. Whether it is in the skilled nursing facility setting or acute inpatient rehabilitation setting, clinicians are typically able to provide 2 to 3 hours of therapy per day versus a similar number of hours per week in home care.[121,122] For patients with certain co-morbidities or limited social support upon discharge, this higher frequency of therapy can be of great benefit by allowing these patients to overcome impairments (such as diminished endurance and activity tolerance) or provide greater opportunities to practice key functional tasks independently.

Interventions

In the inpatient rehabilitation setting, the focus of rehabilitation is very similar to the acute care setting. That focus is a continuation of functional mobility training, therapeutic exercise, patient education, as well as ADL training that was initiated in the immediate postoperative period.[121,122] Similar to the acute care setting, patients work toward demonstrating independence with bed mobility, transfers, ambulation with appropriate assistive device, and stair negotiation.[121,122] Therapeutic exercise for patients in this setting may expand to include sitting, standing, and possibly resisted exercises, given that pain tolerance has likely improved. Patient education continues to focus on activity modification in the setting of applicable postoperative precautions or guidelines, assistive device use, and ADLs.[121,122]

Home Care Rehabilitation

Rehabilitation in the home care setting is parallel to care in the ECF. Goals of treatment are a continuation of care initiated in the acute care setting. Typically, a home care clinician visits patients during the first several weeks after surgery, when tissue healing and pain limit the intensity and type of treatment. Home safety should be at the forefront of a clinician's mind, and recommendations should be made for environmental modifications because many patients may not receive home OT following discharge from the hospital.

As in the acute care setting, the home care therapist must screen for DVT and infection, to reduce risk of significant postoperative complications. Because the physical therapist may be the only provider consistently seeing the patient in the home setting, he or she should also routinely inspect the surgical incision for any erythema or drainage indicative of potential wound infection.

Functional milestones for discharge from home care services have not been defined in the literature, but Medicare provides a guideline to assist in this decision process. A patient is eligible for home care services if leaving the home requires a "considerable and taxing effort."[123] Home care clinicians prescribe exercise, balance training, and functional training to enable mobility outside the home. Generally, patients at some point should be able to ambulate out of the home with close to normal gait speed and negotiate curbs and stairs. Once no longer homebound, the patient may continue with the exercise program independently and may transition to outpatient rehabilitation when recommended by the surgeon and physical therapist.

Home Safety

Safety is always a priority when discharging a patient home because balance and stability are limited as a result of pain, decreased motor control, decreased ROM, and narcotic use. A fall may increase the risk of dislocation, fracture, and other trauma that would negatively affect recovery and outcome. Loose area rugs and throw rugs should be removed, exposed wiring and cords should be protected, and hallways and common walkways (e.g., the path to the bathroom) should be lit at night. Grab bars and railings may be recommended for safe mobility in the home.

Home Safety Tips for Total Hip Arthroplasty Patients

- Loose area rugs or throw rugs should be removed
- Electrical cords should be protected
- Hallways and walkways should be lighted
- Grab bars and railings should be installed where appropriate
- Raised and firm seating surfaces should be used (if posterior precautions)
- Shower and tub chairs and raised toilet seat should be used if needed

---

Interventions

Taking into account the patient's particular home environment, functional training teaches safe function within the home. Emphasis is on safe negotiation of the home environment, including stairways, landings, bathrooms (including toilet and shower and bath transfers), and other common areas. Outdoor mobility on curbs and inclines may also be incorporated into treatment as needed. As function and stability improve and pain diminishes, patients may begin using a unilateral assistive device, such as a cane, instead of crutches or a walker. A cane or single crutch in the contralateral hand reduces the hip abduction moment and hip joint reaction forces in the involved hip,[124] allowing a normalized gait despite hip abduction weakness while providing support during bony and soft tissue healing.[125]

Cryotherapy and analgesic interventions should be continued as needed to adequately control pain and allow patients to fully participate in their rehabilitation sessions. Both narcotic and nonnarcotic pain management strategies should be timed to provide optimum pain control before the therapy visits. The use of ice should be continued as well at the surgical site for edema and pain reduction.[86,117]

Therapeutic Exercise

Evidence exists for the use of early resistance training of the quadriceps muscle for increasing muscular strength as well as functional performance, specifically in sit-to-stand performance. As function improves, exercise should incorporate functional weight bearing and eccentric exercise in addition to "open chain" exercise (i.e., non–weight-bearing movement of the lower extremity). Sashika et al.[126] demonstrated improved gait speed and hip abduction strength after THA with a 6-week home program that emphasized weight-bearing eccentric exercise compared with isometrics and open chain exercise alone. Eccentric hip abduction strengthening using low, nonprogressive resistance continues to show an increase in hip abduction strength even within 2 or more months after surgery.[127]

Outpatient Rehabilitation

Referral to outpatient rehabilitation is based on the surgeon's recommendation and the patient's continued functional limitations. Outpatient rehabilitation may begin as soon as a patient is capable of arranging for and attending clinic visits. Consideration must be given to the time frame for bony and soft tissue healing, as well as any relevant precautions or contraindications when selecting examination and intervention techniques. Intervention is driven by the patient's functional abilities and examination findings, as well as surgical precautions (see Table 19-3). Strength, stability, and gait deviations can continue to limit functional mobility, ambulation, and return to the desired activity level 6 months to 1 year after surgery.[128–134]

Therapeutic Exercise

As bony and soft tissue healing progress, patients are able to tolerate increasingly higher intensity exercise. Many patients show decreased hip strength months after THA[128,133,134] compared with healthy individuals because of pain and immobility that were present before surgery, surgical disruption of nerves and muscles,[135] and decreased activity and weight bearing after surgery. Hip abductor muscle weakness may contribute to a limp during gait (Trendelenburg gait as depicted in Figure 19-4) and decreased function. Maximal strength training, specifically open chain hip abduction and leg presses, has been shown to be safe and effective following hip arthroplasty,[136] but it may not be tolerated by or appropriate for all patients.

Progressive resistive exercise individualized for the patient's age and ability has been shown to increase hip strength after THA, as well as gait speed and distance.[128,130,137] Common strengthening exercises at this stage may include bridging, side-lying hip abduction, and lateral (external) rotation with resistance. In addition, intervention that includes weight bearing and postural stability training improves strength, stability, and function up to 12 months compared with AROM and isometrics alone.[130] Wall slides, mini-squats, and weight-shifting exercise help promote strength, postural stability, and balance and proprioception. Table 19-5 details common exercises for the outpatient phase of THA rehabilitation.

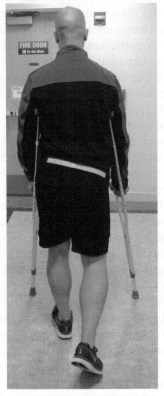

Figure 19-4 Trendelenburg's sign, seen with hip abduction weakness on the right.

TABLE 19-5

Common Exercises for the Outpatient Phase of Rehabilitation

Range of motion	• Hip flexor stretching (modified Thomas test, rectus femoris stretch) • Hamstring stretch • Gastrocnemius stretch • Passive range of motion (PROM) hip flexion and lateral rotation
Strengthening	• Side-lying hip abduction and lateral rotation with resistance • Bridging • Wall slides • Mini squats • Calf raises • Step up and downs
Balance and proprioception	• Tandem stance and single-leg stance (stable and unstable surfaces) • Balance boards

ROM exercises (see Table 19-5) continue to address motion restrictions that are functionally relevant, particularly hip extension and flexion, which may affect terminal stance in gait and lower body dressing, respectively. Consideration of the surgical approach and hip dislocation precautions is crucial with all ROM and strengthening exercises. Communication with the patient's surgeon will help to clarify how long the patient must adhere to the surgeon's hip dislocation precautions. Further consideration is important with uncemented THAs because twisting closed chain exercises may cause loosening of the femoral stem in the medullary canal. Cardiovascular conditioning should be incorporated into the patient's overall treatment program. The use of a stationary bike[138] is ideal because this will cause less wear on the hip joint than other high-impact weight-bearing exercises.[39] The patient's functional goals are central in prescribing therapeutic exercise. The ROM, strength, and balance requirements for a particular task must all be considered when an exercise program is devised.

Caution: Exercises and Uncemented Total Hip Arthroplasty

• Twisting closed chain exercise may place undue stress on the hip and lead to loosening of the femoral stem

---

Manual Therapy Treatment

Soft tissue mobilization may improve scar mobility, restore muscle length, and improve hip ROM. Joint mobilization to the affected hip generally is considered a contraindication because of the time frame for healing, especially with revision and uncemented surgeries, as well as the altered mechanics of the implant itself.

Aquatic Therapy

Aquatic therapy is an increasingly used tool for postoperative rehabilitation. Although aquatic therapy has been studied in the immediate postoperative phase,[139,140] it is common to wait for wound healing to occur to minimize the risk of both wound infection and contamination of the aquatic environment.[140] Advantages of aquatic therapy include decreased loading due to buoyancy in the water and hydrostatic forces creating varying resistance as velocity of movement changes. Aquatic therapy has been shown to increase hip strength and function while decreasing pain and stiffness when compared to land-based therapy.[139,141]

Functional Milestones and Return to Recreation or Sports

Function typically progresses from ambulation with a walker or crutches to a cane and finally to ambulation without an assistive device, depending on the patient's previous level of function and co-morbidities. The final functional milestones to be reached typically are high-level activities for recreation and sports, such as golf, tennis, biking, and hiking. The time frames and guidelines for return to sports and recreational activities depend on the surgeon's preference, surgical procedure (i.e., approach and fixation), and patient's previous and current functional abilities.[39]

In 2007, Klein et al. surveyed a total of 549 surgeons from the Hip Society and American Association of Hip and Knee Surgeons regarding their recommendations for activity following a "standard" primary THA.[142] Surgeons were asked to categorize their recommendations into one of four categories (allowed, allowed with experience, not allowed, or undecided). This survey also showed that 32% of surgeons allowed return to activity at 1 to 3 months postoperatively, whereas 59% waited until 3 to 6 months

---

Surgeon Consensus Guidelines for Return to Sport Following Total Hip Arthroplasty: Activities Allowed[142]

- Bowling
- Dancing (ballroom, jazz, square)
- Doubles tennis
- Elliptical
- Golf
- Hiking
- Low-impact aerobics
- Road cycling
- Rowing
- Speed walking
- Stairclimber
- Stationary cycling
- Stationary skiing
- Swimming
- Treadmill
- Walking
- Weight machines

Surgeon Consensus Guidelines for Return to Sport Following Total Hip Arthroplasty: Activities Allowed with Experience[142]

- Cross-country skiing
- Downhill skiing
- Ice skating and roller blading
- Pilates
- Weight lifting

Surgeon Consensus Guidelines for Return to Sport Following Total Hip Arthroplasty: Activities Not Allowed[142]

- Baseball and softball
- Contact sports (football, basketball, soccer)
- High-impact aerobics
- Jogging
- Racquetball and squash
- Snowboarding

Surgeon Consensus Guidelines for Return to Sport Following Total Hip Arthroplasty: Undecided if Activities Allowed[142]

- Martial arts
- Singles tennis

---

before allowing activity. The textboxes outline the consensus guidelines on which sports are or are not allowed and which ones surgeons were undecided about.

Patients who participate in athletic activities that are too strenuous after joint replacement put themselves at greater risk for traumatic complications (e.g., dislocation, periprosthetic fracture, and implant breakage) compared with sedentary patients who have joint replacements. Another major consideration for return to recreation and sports is the wear placed on prosthetic-bearing surfaces. Body weight and the number of steps affect component wear; therefore activities that require more weight-bearing steps cause greater wear on the prosthesis. Activities such as jogging, hiking, and power walking impose up to 5 times body weight across the joint, whereas cycling imposes less than 1.5 times body weight. Despite prosthetic wear, these activities are beneficial from a strength, flexibility, and cardiovascular standpoint. Therefore, a balance is required between the health benefits of exercise and some increased risk of prosthetic wear. If an activity is to be performed with high frequency and long duration, as is required in sports, then low-impact activities, such as swimming, cycling, golf, and doubles tennis, should be recommended. If only occasional recreational activity is desired, higher-impact activities, such as hiking, power walking, and singles tennis, may be safe because of the low frequency and short duration of the activity.[39]

OUTCOMES AND ASSESSMENT TOOLS

Interest in assessing the outcome of hip arthroplasty has grown significantly in an effort to inform best practice and to provide patients with objective information regarding the expected outcomes of the procedure specific to their clinical presentation. The HHS is perhaps the most commonly used system for assessing patients who have undergone THA. This instrument is used by the clinician to rate the patient's pain, function, and joint mobility. Scores range from 0 to 100 with higher scores indicating better outcomes. The **36-item Medical Outcomes Study Short-Form Health Survey (SF-36)** supplements the HHS well by also capturing quality of life domains that are influenced by THA.[143] The SF-36 is often considered the "gold standard" of health outcome assessment tools. This self-reported outcome tool examines eight dimensions, including physical function, social function, physical and emotional role, pain, mental health, vitality, and general health. Scores range from 0 to 100 with higher scores indicating better health status. Due to the broad nature of the areas examined, it is less sensitive to changes in functional ability following THA and typically is used in conjunction with instruments that are more specific to THA.

The **Western Ontario and McMaster Universities Arthritis Index (WOMAC)** is an arthritis-specific evaluation tool that also is frequently used to assess patients who have had THA.[144] Pain, stiffness, and function are self-rated on a Likert scale with an ordinal scale of 0 to 4. A maximum score of 20, 8, and 68, respectively, can be reported for each subcategory as well as a global score by summing the three subscale scores. Lower scores indicate lower levels of symptoms or physical disability. A study of the SF-36, WOMAC, and HHS has shown them all to have high validity and reliability in assessing the outcome of THA.[145,146]

The **Hip Disability and Osteoarthritis Outcome Score (HOOS)** examines five domains of pain, symptoms, ADLs, sport and recreation, and hip-related quality of life by self-report. It has been validated for use in patients with hip arthroplasty and has been found to be more responsive than the WOMAC.[147] The **Lower Extremity Functional Scale (LEFS)** is a common tool used to assess a broad range of lower extremity disorders and is more sensitive to change in function than the SF-36. This scale rates the patient's ability to perform 20 physical tasks on a Likert scale of 0 to 4 with higher scores indicating better function and a maximum score of 80. It has excellent psychometric properties and is easy to administer and score.[148] The **University of California–Los Angeles activity scale** has been found to be a valuable tool for assessing patients' overall activity level postoperatively.[149] This scale provides a simple rating from 1 to 10 to describe the patient's activity level from no physical activity to regular participation in impact sports, similar to the **Tegner Activity Level Scale**.[150]

Despite the number of self-reported assessment tools available for use in patients following THA, there is a known discord between self-report and performance-based measures of function following hip arthroplasty.[151] Self-reported measures tend to show the most significant improvements in the early phases of rehabilitation, whereas performance-based measures may take a longer time into recovery to demonstrate change. In addition to the use of the above-described self-reported scales of function, common performance-based assessments for patients following THA include the **6-Minute Walk Test (6MWT)**, the **Timed Up and Go Test**, and other time-based measures, such as gait speed, timed sit to stand, and timed stair climbing. The 6MWT is a reliable performance-based test examining the maximum distance hip arthroplasty patients can ambulate in 6 minutes over a 50-m walkway at a self-selected speed. Patients can use assistive devices as needed and results can be compared over time to measure improvement.[152] The Timed Up and Go assessment examines the time it takes the patient to stand from a chair, walk 3 m, and return to the chair. This test was designed to assess mobility, balance, walking ability, and fall risk in the older adults and has been used in the OA population as a predictor of function post arthroplasty.[153]

SUMMARY

The prevalence of both primary and revision THAs has increased dramatically from 1993 to 2005, and this trend is expected to continue between 2005 and 2030. This is partially due to an aging population, obesity epidemic, and improved prosthetic survivorship (which expands THA appropriateness to a younger population). OA continues to be the most common indication for primary THA. Anterolateral and posterior surgical techniques are most commonly used for THA, but the direct anterior approach is becoming more common, particularly in the United States. Each surgical approach has its advantages, disadvantages, and implications for rehabilitation, which specifically affect postoperative weight-bearing status, dislocation precautions, and rehabilitation progression. Typically, an uncomplicated THA patient is allowed WBAT. Although most THA patients have hip dislocation precautions, outcome data have fueled debate regarding the need for dislocation precautions, particularly for the anterolateral or anterior approaches, and some surgeons do not require hip dislocation precautions for certain patients.

Successful rehabilitation after THA requires effective communication and coordination among all members of the health care team, the patient, and the patient's family. Decision making on the plan of care, intervention, and discharge destination is influenced by surgical factors, patient characteristics, the stage of tissue healing, and the PT examination. It is vital that the rehabilitation clinician consider all factors to ensure the optimum surgical outcome and to allow the patient to be progressed appropriately throughout the episode of care. In the current era of decreased hospital LOS, early and accelerated rehabilitation programs have become more common.

Revision THAs and minimally invasive THAs are addressed with decelerated and accelerated rehabilitation plans of care, respectively. The most commonly used THA outcome tools are the HHS, SF-36, and WOMAC. Research examining THA outcomes has become increasingly available, due to the interest in promoting evidence-based practice among surgeons and rehabilitation clinicians.

REFERENCES

1. Hunter DJ, Guermazi A, Roemer F, et al: Structural correlates of pain in joints with osteoarthritis, *Osteoarthritis Cartilage* 21:1170–1178, 2013.
2. National Institutes of Health: *Total hip replacement: consensus development conference statement*, Accessed April 26, 2014. Available at http://consensus.nih.gov/1994/1994HipReplacement098html.htm.
3. Pivec R, Johnson AJ, Mears SC, Mont MA: Hip arthroplasty, *Lancet* 380:1768–1777, 2012.
4. Kurtz S, Ong K, Lau E, et al: Projections of primary and revision hip and knee arthroplasty in the United States from 2005 to 2030, *J Bone Joint Surg Am* 89:780–785, 2007.
5. Maillefert JF, Roy C, Cadet C, et al: Factors influencing surgeons' decisions in the indication for total joint replacement in hip osteoarthritis in real life, *Arthritis Rheum* 59:255–262, 2008.
6. Mota REM, Tarricone R, Ciani O, et al: Determinants of demand for total hip and knee arthroplasty: a systematic literature review, *BMC Health Serv Res* 12:225, http://dx.doi.org/10.1186/1472-6963-12-2252012.
7. Birrell F, Lunt M, Macfarlane GJ, Silman AJ: Defining hip pain for population studies, *Ann Rheum Dis* 64:95–98, 2005.
8. Zhang W, Nuki G, Moskowitz RW, et al: OARSI recommendations for the management of hip and knee osteoarthritis part III: changes in evidence following systematic cumulative update of research published through January 2009, *Osteoarthritis Cartilage* 18:476–499, 2010.
9. Dreinhofer KE, Dieppe P, Sturmer T, et al: Indications for total hip replacement: comparison of assessments of orthopaedic surgeons and referring physicians, *Ann Rheum Dis* 65:1346–1350, 2006.
10. Queen RM, Schaeffer JF, Butler RJ, et al: Does surgical approach during total hip arthroplasty alter gait recovery during the first year following surgery? *J Arthroplasty* 28:1639–1643, 2013.
11. Bal BS: Clinical faceoff: anterior total hip versus mini-posterior which one is better? *Clin Orthop Relat Res* 473:1192–1196, 2015.
12. Matta JM, Shahrdar C, Ferguson T: Single-incision anterior approach for total hip arthroplasty on an orthopaedic table, *Clin Orthop Relat Res* 441:115–124, 2005.
13. Meneghini RM, Pagnano MW, Trousdale RT, Hozack WJ: Muscle damage during MIS total hip arthroplasty: Smith-Petersen versus posterior approach, *Clin Orthop Relat Res* 453:293–298, 2006.
14. Nakata K, Nishikawa M, Yamamoto K, et al: A clinical comparative study of the direct anterior with mini-posterior approach: two consecutive series, *J Arthroplasty* 24:698–704, 2009.
15. Rodriguez JA, Deshmukh AJ, Rathod PA, et al: Does the direct anterior approach in THA offer faster rehabilitation and comparable safety to the posterior approach? *J Arthroplasty* 472:455–463, 2014.
16. Alecci V, Valente M, Crucil M, et al: Comparison of primary total hip replacements performed with a direct anterior approach versus the standard lateral approach: perioperative findings, *J Orthop Traumatol* 12:123–129, 2011.
17. Hallert O, Li Y, Brismar H, Lindgren U: The direct anterior approach: initial experience of a minimally invasive technique for total hip arthroplasty, *J Orthop Surg Res* 7:17, 2012.
18. Berend M: Anterolateral approach for primary total hip replacement. In Berry DM, Lieberman J, editors: *Surgery of the hip*, Philadelphia, 2012, Elsevier.
19. Pagano MW, Leone JM, Lewallen DG, et al: Two-incision total hip arthroplasties had modest outcomes and some substantial complications, *J Arthroplasty* 21:305, 2006.
20. Feinblatt JS, Berend KR, Lombardi AV: Severe symptomatic heterotopic ossification and dislocation: a complication after two-incision minimally invasive total hip arthroplasty, *J Arthroplasty* 20:802–806, 2005.
21. Parratte S, Pagnano MW: Mayo experience with two-incision total hip arthroplasty: the added technical difficulty has not been rewarded, *Sem Arthroplasty* 19:170–174, 2008.
22. Newman MA, Barker KL, Pandit H, et al: Outcomes after metal-on-metal hip resurfacing: could we achieve better function, *Arch Phys Med Rehabil* 89:660–666, 2008.
23. Muirhead-Allwood S, Sandiford M, Kabir C: Total hip resurfacing as an alternative to total hip arthroplasty: indications and precautions, *Sem Arthroplasty* 19:274–282, 2008.
24. The Alberta Hip Improvement Project, Mackenzie JR, O'Connor GJ, et al: Functional outcomes for 2 years comparing hip resurfacing and total hip arthroplasty, *J Arthroplasty* 27:750–757, 2012.
25. Le Duf MJ, Amstutz HC: Sporting activity after hip resurfacing: changes over time, *Orthop Clin North Am* 42:161–167, 2011.
26. Kohan L, Field CJ, Keer DR: Early complications of hip resurfacing, *J Arthroplasty* 27:997–1002, 2012.
27. Weegen WVD, Sijbesma T, Hoekstra HJ, et al: Treatment of pseudotumors after metal-on-metal hip resurfacing based on magnetic resonance imaging, metal ion levels, and symptoms, *J Arthroplasty* 29:416–421, 2014.
28. Gross TP, Liu F: Outcomes after revision of metal-on-metal hip resurfacing arthroplasty, *J Arthroplasty* 29(9 suppl):219–223, 2014.
29. Memon AR, Galbraith JG, Hart JA, et al: Inflammatory pseudotumor causing deep vein thrombosis after metal-on-metal hip resurfacing arthroplasty, *J Arthroplasty* 28:197, 2013 e9-12.
30. Bozic KJ, Kurtz SM, Lau E, et al: The epidemiology of revision total hip arthroplasty in the United States, *J Bone Joint Surg Am* 91:128–133, 2009.
31. Berend KR, Sporer SM, Sierra RJ, et al: Achieving stability and lower-limb length in total hip arthroplasty, *J Bone Joint Surg Am* 92:2737–2752, 2010.
32. Werner BC, Brown TE: Instability after total hip arthroplasty, *World J Orthop* 3:122–130, 2012.
33. Wolf BR, Lu X, Li Y, et al: Adverse outcomes in hip arthroplasty: long-term trends, *J Bone Joint Surg Am* 94:8, 2012.
34. Mulliken BD, Rorabeck CH, Bourne RB, Nayak N: A modified direct lateral approach in total hip arthroplasty: a comprehensive review, *J Arthroplasty* 13:737–747, 1998.
35. Queen RM, Appleton S, Butler RJ, et al: Total hip arthroplasty surgical approach does not alter postoperative gait mechanics one year after surgery, *Phys Med Rehabil* 6:221–226, 2013.
36. Austin MS, Hozack WJ, Sharkey PF, Rothman RH: Stability and leg length equality in total hip arthroplasty, *J Arthroplasty* 18(3 suppl 1):88–90, 2003.
37. Ibrahim MS, Twaij H, Giebaly DE, et al: Enhanced recovery in total hip replacement: a clinical review, *Bone Joint J* 95-B:1587–1594, 2013.
38. Sharma V, Morgan PM, Cheng EY: Factors influencing early rehabilitation after THA, *Clin Orthop Relat Res* 467:1400–1411, 2009.
39. Kuster MS: Exercise recommendations after total joint replacement: a review of the current literature and proposal of scientifically based guidelines, *Sports Med* 32:433–445, 2002.
40. Jones CA, Voaklander DC, Johnston DW, Suarez-Almazor ME: The effect of age on pain, function, and quality of life after total hip and knee arthroplasty, *Arch Intern Med* 161:454–460, 2001.
41. Mahomed NN, Liang MH, Cook EF, et al: The importance of patient expectations in predicting functional outcomes after total joint arthroplasty, *J Rheumatol* 29:1273–1279, 2002.
42. Munin MC, Rudy TE, Glynn NW, et al: Early inpatient rehabilitation after elective hip and knee arthroplasty, *JAMA* 279:847–852, 1998.
43. Epps CD: Length of stay, discharge disposition, and hospital discharge predictors, *AORN J* 79:975–976, 2004 979-981, 984-988.
44. Forrest GP, Roque JM, Dawodu ST: Decreasing length of stay after total joint arthroplasty: effect on referrals to rehabilitation units, *Arch Phys Med Rehabil* 80:192–194, 1999.
45. Cram P, Lu X, Kaboli PJ, et al: Clinical characteristics and outcomes of Medicare patients undergoing total hip arthroplasty, 1991-2008, *JAMA* 305:1560–1567, 2011.
46. Villalobos PA, Navarro-Espigares JL, Hernandez-Torres E, et al: Body mass index as predictor of health-related quality-of-life changes after total hip arthroplasty: a cross-over study, *J Arthroplasty* 28:666–670, 2013.
47. Munin MC, Kwoh CK, Glynn N, et al: Predicting discharge outcome after elective hip and knee arthroplasty, *Am J Phys Med Rehabil* 74:294–301, 1995.
48. Soohoo NF, Farng E, Lieberman JR, et al: Factors that predict short-term complication rates after total hip arthroplasty, *Clin Orthop Relat Res* 468:2363–2371, 2010.
49. Santaguida PL, Hawker GA, Hudak PL, et al: Patient characteristics affecting the prognosis of total hip and knee joint arthroplasty: a systematic review, *J Can Chiro* 51:428–436, 2008.
50. Freburger JK: An analysis of the relationship between the utilization of physical therapy services and outcomes of care for patients after total hip arthroplasty, *Phys Ther* 80:448–458, 2000.

51. Taunt CJ, Finn H, Baumann P: Immediate weight bearing after cementless total hip arthroplasty, *Orthopedics* 31:223, 2008.

52. Markmiller M, Weib T, Kreuz P, et al: Partial weight-bearing is not necessary after cementless total hip arthroplasty, *Int Orthop* 35:1139–1143, 2011.

53. Patel PD, Potts A, Froimson MI: The dislocating hip arthroplasty: prevention and treatment, *J Arthroplasty* 22:86–90, 2007.

54. DeWal H, Maurer SL, Tsai P, et al: Efficacy of abduction bracing in the management of total hip arthroplasty dislocation, *J Arthroplasty* 19:733–738, 2004.

55. Murray TG, Wetters NG, Moric M, et al: The use of abduction bracing for the prevention of early postoperative dislocation after revision total hip arthroplasty, *J Arthroplasty* 27(suppl 1):126–129, 2012.

56. Morrey BF: Instability after total hip arthroplasty, *Orthop Clin North Am* 23:237–248, 1992.

57. Soong M, Rubash HE, Macaulay W: Dislocation after total hip arthroplasty, *J Am Acad Orthop Surg* 12:314–321, 2004.

58. Woo RY, Morrey BF: Dislocations after total hip arthroplasty, *J Bone Joint Surg Am* 64:1295–1306, 1982.

59. Berry DJ, von Knoch M, Schleck CD, Harmsen WS: Effect of femoral head diameter and operative approach on risk of dislocation after primary total hip arthroplasty, *J Bone Joint Surg Am* 87:2456–2463, 2005.

60. Ritter MA, Harty LD, Keating ME, et al: A clinical comparison of the anterolateral and posterolateral approaches to the hip, *Clin Orthop Relat Res* 385:95–99, 2001.

61. Masonis JL, Bourne RB: Surgical approach, abductor function, and total hip arthroplasty dislocation, *Clin Orthop Relat Res* 405:46–53, 2002.

62. Jolles BM, Bogoch ER: Posterior versus lateral surgical approach for total hip arthroplasty in adults with osteoarthritis, *Cochrane Database Syst Rev* 3:2006 CD003828.

63. Ji HM, Kim KC, Lee YK, et al: Dislocation after total hip arthroplasty: a randomized clinical trial of a posterior approach and a modified lateral approach, *J Arthroplasty* 27:378–385, 2012.

64. Hailer NP, Weiss RJ, Stark A, Karrholm J: The risk of revision due to dislocation after total hip arthroplasty depends on surgical approach, femoral head size, sex, and primary diagnosis, an analysis of 78,098 operations in the Swedish hip arthroplasty register, *Acta Orthop* 83:442–448, 2012.

65. Khatod M, Barber T, Paxton E, et al: An analysis of the risk of hip dislocation with a contemporary total joint registry, *Clin Orthop Relat Res* 447:19–23, 2006.

66. White RE, Forness TJ, Allman JK, Junick DW: Effect of posterior capsular repair on early dislocation in primary total hip replacement, *Clin Orthop Relat Res* 393:163–167, 2001.

67. Goldstein WM, Gleason TF, Kopplin M, Branson JJ: Prevalence of dislocation after total hip arthroplasty through a posterolateral approach with partial capsulotomy and capsulorrhaphy, *J Bone Joint Surg Am* 83(suppl 2):2–7, 2001.

68. Pellicci PM, Bostrom M, Poss R: Posterior approach to total hip replacement using enhanced posterior soft tissue repair, *Clin Orthop Relat Res* 355:224–228, 1998.

69. Kwon MS, Kuskowski M, Mulhall KJ, et al: Does surgical approach affect total hip arthroplasty dislocation rates? *Clin Orthop Relat Res* 447:34–38, 2006.

70. Peak EL, Parvizi J, Ciminiello M, et al: The role of patient restrictions in reducing the prevalence of early dislocation following total hip arthroplasty: a randomized, prospective study, *J Bone Joint Surg Am* 87:247–253, 2005.

71. Ververeli PA, Lebby EB, Tyler C, Fouad C: Evaluation of reducing postoperative hip precautions in total hip replacement: a randomized prospective study, *Orthopedics* 32:889, 2009.

72. Berry DJ, von Knoch M, Schleck CD, Harmsen WS: The cumulative long-term risk of dislocation after primary Charnley total hip arthroplasty, *J Bone Joint Surg Am* 86:9–14, 2004.

73. Yoon RS, Nellans KW, Geller JA, et al: Patient education before hip or knee arthroplasty lowers length of stay, *J Arthroplasty* 25:547–551, 2010.

74. Mancuso CA, Graziano S, Briskie LM, et al: Randomized trials to modify patients' preoperative expectation of hip and knee arthroplasties, *Clin Orthop Relat Res* 466:424–431, 2008.

75. McDonald S, Hetrick SE, Green S: Pre-operative education for hip or knee replacement, *Cochrane Database Syst Rev* 1:2004 CD003526.

76. Giraudet-Le Quintrec J, Coste J, Vastel L, et al: Positive effect of patient education for hip surgery: a randomized trial, *Clin Orthop Relat Res* 414:112–120, 2003.

77. Lubbeke A, Suva D, Perneger T, et al: Influence of preoperative education on the risk of dislocation after primary total hip arthroplasty, *Arthritis Care Res* 61:552–558, 2009.

78. Gocen Z, Sen A, Unver B, et al: The effect of preoperative physiotherapy and education on the outcome of total hip replacement: a prospective randomized controlled trial, *Clin Rehabil* 18:353–358, 2004.

79. Bozic KJ, Wagie A, Naessens JM, et al: Predictors of discharge to an inpatient extended care facility after total hip or knee arthroplasty, *J Arthroplasty* 21:151–156, 2006.

80. Barsoum WK, Murray TG, Klika AK, et al: Predicting patient discharge disposition after total joint arthroplasty in the United States, *J Arthroplasty* 25:885–892, 2010.

81. Oldmeadow LB, McBurney H, Robertson VJ: Predicting risk of extended inpatient rehabilitation after hip or knee arthroplasty, *J Arthroplasty* 18:775–779, 2003.

82. Dauty M, Schmitt X, Menu P, et al: Using the Risk Assessment and Predictor Tool (RAPT) for patients after total knee replacement surgery, *Ann Phys Rehabil Med* 55:4–15, 2012.

83. Ariza G, Badia M, Cuixart A, et al: Quality of life after knee arthroplasty: utility of the RAPT scale, *Rehabilitacion* 46:147–156, 2012.

84. Brander V, Stulberg SD: Rehabilitation after hip and knee joint replacement. An experience- and evidence-based approach to care, *Am J Phys Med Rehabil* 85(11 suppl):S98–S118, 2006.

85. Chen AF, Stewart MK, Heyl AE, et al: Effect of immediate postoperative physical therapy on length of stay for total joint arthroplasty patients, *J Arthroplasty* 27:851–856, 2012.

86. Wainwright T, Middleton R: An orthopaedic enhanced recovery pathway, *Curr Anaesth Crit Care* 21:114–120, 2010.

87. Kimmel LA, Oldmeadow LB, Sage C, et al: A designated three day elective orthopaedic surgery unit: first year's results for hip and knee replacement patients, *Int J Orthop Trauma Nursing* 15:29–34, 2011.

88. Smith TO, McCabe C, Lister S, et al: Rehabilitation implications during the development of the Norwich Enhanced Recovery Programme (NERP) for patients following total knee and total hip arthroplasty, *Orthop Traumatol Surg Res* 98:499–505, 2012.

89. Robbins CE, Bierbaum BE, Ward DM: Total hip arthroplasty: day of surgery physical therapy intervention, *Curr Orthop Pract* 20:157–160, 2009.

90. Goyal N, Parikh A, Austin M: Pain management after total joint arthroplasty, *Sem Arthroplasy* 19:226–230, 2008.

91. Pasero C, McCaffrey M: Orthopaedic postoperative pain management, *J Perinesth Nurs* 22:160–174, 2007.

92. Hebl JR, Dilger JA, Byer DE, et al: A pre-emptive multimodal pathway featuring peripheral nerve block improves perioperative outcomes after major orthopedic surgery, *Reg Anesth Pain Med* 33:510–517, 2008.

93. Kellet J: Acute soft tissue injuries-a review of the literature, *Med Sci Sports Exerc* 18:489–500, 1986.

94. Zhang J, Pan T, Wang JHC: Cryotherapy suppresses tendon inflammation in an animal model, *J Orthop Translation* 2:75–81, 2014.

95. Gill SD, McBurney H: Does exercise reduce pain and improve physical function before hip or knee replacement surgery? A systematic review and meta-analysis of randomized controlled trials, *Arch Phys Med Rehabil* 94:164–176, 2013.

96. Liu X, Zhang X, Chen Y, et al: Hidden blood loss after total hip arthroplasty, *J Arthroplasty* 26:1100–1106, 2011.

97. Yoshihara H, Yoneoka D: Predictors of allogenic blood transfusion in total hip and knee arthroplasty in the United States, 2000-2009, *J Arthroplasty* 29:1736–1740, 2014.

98. Fan YX, Liu FF, Jia M, et al: Comparison of restrictive and liberal transfusion strategy on post-operative delirium in aged patients following total hip replacement: a preliminary study, *Arch Gerontol Geriatr* 59:181–185, 2014.

99. Foss NB, Kristensen MT, Kehlet H: Anaemia impedes functional mobility after hip fracture, *Age Aging* 37:173–178, 2008.

100. Ranucci M, La Rovere M, Castelvecchio S, et al: Postoperative anemia and exercise tolerance after cardiac operations in patients without transfusion: what hemoglobin level is acceptable? *Ann Thorac Surg* 92:25–31, 2011.

101. Hardy JF: Current status of transfusion triggers for red blood cell concentrates, *Transfusion Apheresis Sci* 31:55–66, 2004.

102. Wilkins I, Wheeler D: Recognizing and treating postoperative complications, *The Foundation Years* 2:244–250, 2006.

103. Rockwood MRH, Howleet SE, Rockwood K: Orthostatic hypotension and mortality in relation to age, blood pressure, and frailty, *Arch Gerontol Geriatr* 54:e255–e260, 2012.

104. Irvin DJ, White M: The importance of accurately assessing orthostatic hypotension, *Geriatr Nurs* 25:99–101, 2004.

105. Shibao C, Grijalva CG, Lipsitz LA: Early discontinuation of treatment in patients with orthostatic hypotension, *Auton Neurosci* 177:291–296, 2013.

106. Shibao C, Lipsitz L, Biaggioni I: Evaluation and treatment of orthostatic hypotension, *J Am Society Hypertension* 7:317–324, 2013.

107. Low DA, Nobrega ACL, Mathias CJ: Exercise-induced hypotension in autonomic disorders, *Auton Neurosci* 171:66–78, 2012.

108. Shimoyama Y, Sawai T, Tatsumi S, et al: Perioperative risk factors for deep vein thrombosis after total hip arthroplasty or total knee arthroplasty, *J Clin Anesthesia* 24:531–536, 2012.

109. Mont MA, Hozack WJ, Callaghan JJ: Venous thromboemboli following total joint arthroplasty: SCIP measures moves us closer to an agreement, *J Arthroplasty* 29:651–652, 2014.

110. Xing KH, Morrison G, Lim W, et al: Has the incidence of deep vein thrombosis in patients undergoing total hip/knee arthroplasty changed over time? A systematic review of randomized controlled trials, *Thrombosis Res* 123:24–34, 2008.

111. Hamilton SC, Whang WW, Anderson BJ, et al: Inpatient enoxaparin and outpatient aspirin chemoprophylaxis regimen after primary hip and knee arthroplasty: a preliminary study, *J Arthroplasty* 27:1594–1598, 2012.

112. Merli GJ: Pathophysiology of venous thrombosis, thrombophilia, and the diagnosis of deep vein thrombosis-pulmonary embolism in the elderly, *Clin Geriatr Med* 22:75–92, 2006.

113. Urbano FL: Homans' sign in the diagnosis of deep vein thrombosis, *Hosp Physician* 37:22–24, 2001.

114. Wells PS, Anderson DR, Rodger M, et al: Evaluation of d-dimer in the diagnosis of suspected deep-vein thrombosis, *New Engl J Med* 349:1227–1235, 2003.

115. Bounameaux H, Perrier A, Righini M: Diagnosis of venous thromboembolism: an update, *Vasc Med* 15:399–406, 2010.

116. Suetta C, Magnusson SPD, Rosted A, et al: Resistance training in the early postoperative phase reduces hospitalization and leads to muscle hypertrophy in elderly hip surgery patients: a controlled, randomized study, *J Am Geriatr Soc* 52:2016–2022, 2004.

117. Cabrera Martimbianco AL, Gomes da Silva BN, Viegas de Carvalho AP, et al: Effectiveness and safety of cryotherapy after arthroscopic anterior cruciate ligament reconstruction. A systematic review of the literature, *Phys Ther Sport* 15:261–268, 2014.

118. Oldmeadow LB, McBurney H, Robertson VJ, et al: Targeted postoperative care improves discharge outcome after hip or knee arthroplasty, *Arch Phys Med Rehabil* 86:1424–1427, 2004.

119. O'Brien S, Ogonda L, Dennison J, et al: Day two post operative 'fast track' discharge following primary total hip replacement, *J Orthop Nurs* 9:140–145, 2005.

120. Husted H, Holm G: Fast track in total hip and knee arthroplasty-experiences from Hvidore University Hospital, Denmark, *Injury* 37:S31–S35, 2006.

121. Vincent HK, Vincent KR: Influence of admission hematocrit on inpatient rehabilitation outcomes after total knee and hip arthroplasty, *Am J Phys Med Rehabil* 86:806–817, 2007.

122. Vincent KR, Vincent HK, Lee LW, et al: Outcomes after inpatient rehabilitation of primary and revision total hip arthroplasty, *Arch Phys Med Rehabil* 87:1026–1032, 2006.

123. Archer D, Lin F, Etiebet M: Medicare home health eligibility. Accessed August 28, 2006. Available at http://www.medicarerights.org/maincontenthomehealtheligibility.html; also Medicare Rights Center, http://www.medicarerights.org.

124. Bateni H, Maki BE: Assistive devices for balance and mobility: benefits, demands, and adverse consequences, *Arch Phys Med Rehabil* 86:134–145, 2005.

125. Ajemian S, Thon D, Clare P, et al: Cane-assisted gait biomechanics and electromyography after total hip arthroplasty, *Arch Phys Med Rehabil* 85:1966–1971, 2004.

126. Sashika H, Matsuba Y, Watanabe Y: Home program of physical therapy: effect on disabilities of patients with total hip arthroplasty, *Arch Phys Med Rehabil* 77:273–277, 1996.

127. Di Monaco M, Vallero F, Tappero R, Cavanna A: Rehabilitation after total hip arthroplasty: a systematic review of controlled trials on physical exercise programs, *Eur J Phys Rehabil Med* 45:303–317, 2009.

128. Shih CH, Du YK, Lin YH, Wu CC: Muscular recovery around the hip joint after total hip arthroplasty, *Clin Orthop Relat Res* 302:115–120, 1994.

129. Tanaka Y: Gait analysis of patients with osteoarthritis of the hip and those with total hip arthroplasty, *Biomed Mater Eng* 8:187–196, 1998.

130. Trudelle-Jackson E, Smith SS: Effects of a late-phase exercise program after total hip arthroplasty: a randomized controlled trial, *Arch Phys Med Rehabil* 85:1056–1062, 2004.

131. Madsen MS, Ritter MA, Morris HH: The effect of total hip arthroplasty surgical approach on gait, *J Orthop Res* 22:44–50, 2004.

132. Loizeau J, Allard P, Duhaime M, Landjerit B: Bilateral gait patterns in subjects fitted with a total hip prosthesis, *Arch Phys Med Rehabil* 76:552–557, 1995.

133. Downing ND, Clark DI, Hutchinson JW, et al: Hip abductor strength following total hip arthroplasty: a prospective comparison of the posterior and lateral approach in 100 patients, *Acta Orthop Scand* 72:215–220, 2001.

134. Bertocci GE, Munin MC, Frost KL, et al: Isokinetic performance after total hip replacement, *Am J Phys Med Rehabil* 83:1–9, 2004.

135. Baker AS, Bitounis VC: Abductor function after total hip replacement: an electromyographic and clinical review, *J Bone Joint Surg Br* 71:47–50, 1989.

136. Husby VS, Helgrud J, Bjorgen S, et al: Early maximal strength training is an efficient treatment for patients operated with total hip arthroplasty, *Arch Phy Med Rehabil* 90:1658–1667, 2009.

137. Wang AW, Gilbey HJ, Ackland TR: Perioperative exercise programs improve early return of ambulatory function after total hip arthroplasty: a randomized, controlled trial, *Am J Phys Med Rehabil* 81:801–806, 2002.

138. Gilbey HJ, Ackland TR, Wang AW, et al: Exercise improves early functional recovery after total hip arthroplasty, *Clin Orthop Relat Res* 408:193–200, 2003.

139. Rahmann AE, Brauer SG, Nitz JC: A specific inpatient aquatic physiotherapy program improves strength after total hip or knee replacement surgery: a randomized controlled trial, *Arch Phys Med Rehabil* 90:745–755, 2009.

140. Liebs TR, Herzberg W, Ruther W, et al: Multicenter randomized controlled trial comparing early versus late aquatic therapy after total hip or knee arthroplasty, *Arch Phys Med Rehabil* 93:192–199, 2012.

141. Giaquinto S, Ciotola E, Dall'Armi V, Margutti F: Hydrotherapy after total hip arthroplasty: a follow up study, *Arch Gerontol Geriatr* 50:92–95, 2010.

142. Klein GR, Levine BR, Hozack WJ, et al: Return to athletic activity after total hip arthroplasty, *J Arthroplasty* 22:171–175, 2007.

143. Lieberman JR, Dorey F, Shekelle P, et al: Outcome after total hip arthroplasty: comparison of a traditional disease-specific and a quality-of-life measurement of outcome, *J Arthroplasty* 12:639–645, 1997.

144. Ethgen O, Bruyere O, Richy F, et al: Health-related quality of life in total hip and total knee arthroplasty: a qualitative and systematic review of the literature, *J Bone Joint Surg Am* 86:963–974, 2004.

145. Soderman P, Malchau H: Is the Harris Hip Score system useful to study the outcome of total hip replacement? *Clin Orthop Relat Res* 384:189–197, 2001.

146. Soderman P, Malchau H, Herberts P: Outcome of total hip replacement: a comparison of different measurement methods, *Clin Orthop Relat Res* 390:163–172, 2001.

147. Nilsdotter AK, Lohmander LS, Klässbo M, Roos EM: Hip disability and osteoarthritis outcome score (HOOS)—validity and responsiveness in total hip replacement, *BMC Musculoskelet Disord* 4:10, 2003.

148. Binkley JM, Stratford PW, Lott SA, Riddle DL: The lower extremity functional scale (LEFS): scale development, measurement properties, and clinical application, *Phys Ther* 79:371–383, 1999.

149. Beaule PE, Dorey FJ, Hoke R, et al: The value of patient activity level in the outcome of total hip arthroplasty, *J Arthroplasty* 21:547–552, 2006.

150. Tegner Y, Lysholm J: Rating systems in the evaluation of knee ligament injuries, *Clin Orthop Relat Res* 198:43–49, 1985.

151. Stratford PW, Kennedy DM, Maly MR, MacIntyre NJ: Quantifying self-report measures' overestimation of mobility scores postarthroplasty, *Phys Ther* 90:1288–1296, 2010.

152. Kennedy DM, Stratford PW, Wessel J, et al: Assessing stability and change of four performance measures: a longitudinal study evaluating outcome following total hip and knee arthroplasty, *BMC Musculoskelet Disord* 6:3, 2005.

153. Nankaku M, Tsuboyama T, Akiyama H, et al: Preoperative predication of ambulatory status at 6 months after total hip arthroplasty, *Phys Ther* 93:88–93, 2013.

CHAPTER 20

Knee: Ligamentous and Patellar Tendon Injuries

ERIC M. BERKSON, DAVID NOLAN, KRISTINA FLEMING, ROBERT SPANG, JEFF WONG, PETER ASNIS, JAESON KAWADLER*

INTRODUCTION

Successful nonsurgical and surgical management of knee ligament and patellar tendon injuries requires knowledge of the functional anatomy and biomechanics of the knee. This understanding forms the basis for the physical examination of the knee and foundation for treatment options. When a patient sustains a knee ligament injury or patellar tendon injury, the clinician must be able to integrate this information to evaluate the knee and to develop an appropriate treatment regimen.

This chapter presents the scientific background of the principles of treatment of knee ligament and patellar tendon injuries. The functional anatomy and biomechanics of the knee are presented as a foundation for clinical decision making. Specific ligamentous injuries are then discussed in terms of epidemiology, operative and nonoperative approaches to treatment, and rehabilitation.

FOUNDATION FOR SURGICAL AND NONSURGICAL MANAGEMENT OF LIGAMENT AND PATELLAR TENDON INJURIES OF THE KNEE

Functional Anatomy and Biomechanics of the Knee

The knee joint consists of articulations among the femur, tibia, and patella. The distal end of the femur and the proximal end of the tibia form the tibiofemoral joint, whereas the distal end of the femur and the

articular side of the patella form the patellofemoral articulations, which participate in the flexion-extension movement of the knee. The proximal tibiofibular joint assists in lateral stability of the knee.[1] The femoral condyles are convex in the anterior and posterior and the medial and lateral directions. They are separated by the trochlear groove, which guides the patella during flexion and extension. The intercondylar notch serves as the site of attachment for the anterior and posterior cruciate ligaments. The width of the intercondylar notch may be an important consideration for the risk of injury to the cruciate ligaments and for the development of loss of extension after reconstruction of the anterior cruciate ligament (ACL). The transverse anterior to posterior dimension of the lateral femoral condyle is greater than that of the medial femoral condyle (Figure 20-1).[2] As a result, the lateral femoral condyle projects farther anteriorly than the medial femoral condyle, providing a bony buttress to minimize lateral displacement of the patella. The radius of curvature of the femoral condyles decreases from anterior to posterior and is shorter on the medial side than on the lateral side.[3] The anterior to posterior length of the articular surface of the medial femoral condyle is longer than that of the lateral femoral condyle.[2] The longer articular surface of the medial femoral condyle facilitates lateral (external) rotation of the tibia as the knee approaches terminal extension.

The medial tibial plateau is concave from anterior to posterior and from medial to lateral, whereas the lateral tibial plateau is convex from anterior to posterior

*The authors, editors, and publisher wish to acknowledge Michael M. Reinold, James J. Irrgang, Marc R. Safran, and Freddie H. Fu for their contributions on this topic in the previous edition.

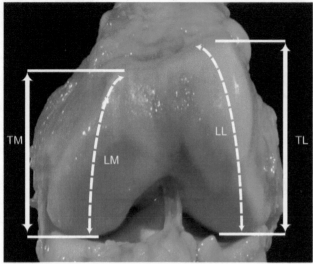

Figure 20-1 Cadaveric specimen of the distal femur. The transverse anterior-posterior dimension of the lateral femoral condyle *(TL)* is greater than that of the medial femoral condyle *(TM)*. The anterior to posterior length of the articular surface of the medial femoral condyle *(LM)* is longer than the anterior to posterior length of the articular surface of the lateral femoral condyle *(LL)*. (TL>TM; LM>LL.)

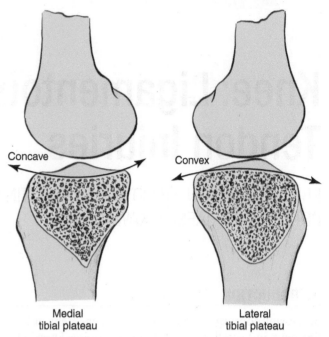

Figure 20-2 The medial tibial plateau is concave anterior to posterior, whereas the lateral tibial plateau is convex anterior to posterior. (From Kapandji IA: *The physiology of the joints: annotated diagrams of the mechanics of the human joints,* Edinburgh, 1970, Churchill Livingstone.)

Static (Passive) Restraints of the Knee

- Ligaments, primarily:
  - Medial collateral ligament
  - Lateral collateral ligament
  - Anterior cruciate ligament
  - Posterior cruciate ligament
  - Posterior oblique ligament
  - Posterolateral corner
- Joint capsule
- Menisci (2)
- Iliotibial band

Dynamic (Active) Restraints of the Knee

- Quadriceps
- Hamstrings
- Gastrocnemius
- Gracilis
- Sartorius
- Popliteus

(Figure 20-2). The concavity of the tibial plateaus is increased by the presence of the menisci. The bony configuration of the knee lends little inherent stability. Stability of the knee depends on static and dynamic restraints. The static restraints include the joint capsule, ligaments, and menisci. Dynamic stability is provided by muscles that cross the knee, including the quadriceps, hamstrings, popliteus, and gastrocnemius.

The ligamentous restraints of the knee include the collateral, cruciate, and capsular ligaments. The medial collateral ligament (MCL) is a broad band that runs from the medial epicondyle of the femur to insert on the tibia approximately 10 cm below the medial joint line (Figure 20-3). The MCL, which has been described as a thickening of the medial capsule, is divided into deep and superficial layers. The deep MCL is intimately attached to the medial meniscus and consists of the tibiomeniscal and femoromeniscal ligaments. The superficial band of the MCL runs from the medial epicondyle to insert distal to the tibial plateau. The ligament joins the posterior joint capsule where it forms the posterior oblique ligament.[4,5] Because the superficial band of the MCL is farther from the center of the knee, it is the first ligament injured when a valgus stress is applied. The MCL courses anteriorly as it runs from the femur to the tibia.

The lateral (fibular) collateral ligament (LCL) is a cordlike structure that runs from the lateral epicondyle of the femur to the fibular head (Figure 20-4). The LCL courses somewhat posteriorly as it passes from the femur to the fibular head. It is separated from the lateral meniscus by the popliteus tendon, which partly explains the increased mobility of the lateral meniscus.

The ACL arises from the tibial plateau just anterior and medial to the tibial eminence. From the tibia, the ACL courses superiorly, laterally, and posteriorly to insert on the posterior margin of the medial wall of the lateral femoral condyle (Figure 20-5). The ACL is composed of two distinct bundles: the anteromedial bundle, which is taut in 60° or more of flexion, and the posterolateral bundle, which is

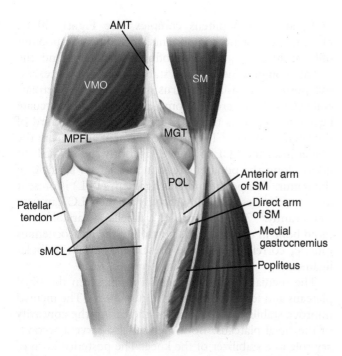

Figure 20-3 Structures of the medial side of the knee. *VMO*, Vastus medialis obliquus muscle; *MPFL*, medial patellofemoral ligament; *POL*, posterior oblique ligament; *sMCL*, superficial medial collateral ligament; *SM*, semimembranosus muscle; *MGT*, medial gastrocnemius tendon; *AMT*, adductor magnus tendon. (From LaPrade RF, Engebretsen AH, Ly TV et al: The anatomy of the medial part of the knee, *J Bone Joint Surg Am* 89:2003, 2007.)

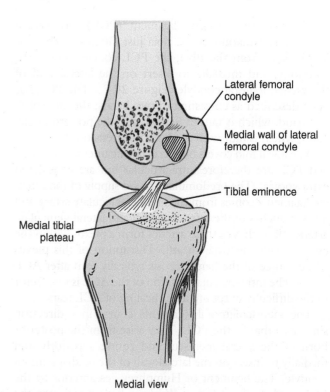

Medial view

Figure 20-5 The anterior cruciate ligament arises from the tibial plateau anterior and medial to the tibial eminence and courses superiorly, laterally, and posteriorly to insert on the medial wall of the lateral femoral condyle. (From Zachazewski JE, Magee DJ, Quillen WS, editors: *Athletic injuries and rehabilitation*, p 625, Philadelphia, 1996, WB Saunders.)

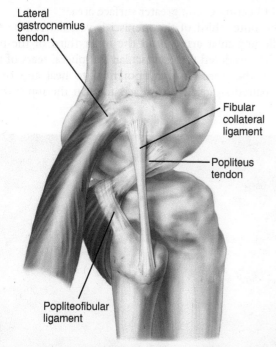

Figure 20-4 Structures of the lateral side of the knee. Illustration demonstrates the isolated fibular collateral ligament, popliteus tendon, popliteofibular ligament, and lateral gastrocnemius tendon (lateral view, right knee). (From LaPrade RF, Ly TV, Wentorf FA, Engebretsen L: The posterolateral attachments of the knee: a qualitative and quantitative morphologic analysis of the fibular collateral ligament, popliteus tendon, popliteofibular ligament, and lateral gastrocnemius tendon, *Am J Sports Med* 31:856, 2003.)

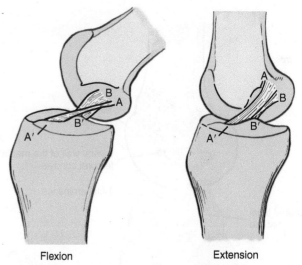

Flexion   Extension

Figure 20-6 The anterior cruciate ligament is composed of two bundles. The anteromedial bundle (A-A′) is taut in flexion. The posterolateral bundle (B-B′) is taut in extension. (From Zachazewski JE, Magee DJ, Quillen WS, editors: *Athletic injuries and rehabilitation*, p 625, Philadelphia, 1996, WB Saunders.)

taut in extension and medial (internal) and lateral (external) rotation (Figure 20-6). The anteromedial and posterolateral bundles both provide anteroposterior (AP) stability to the knee, whereas the posterolateral bundle has been shown to also provide rotational stability to the knee.[6-8]

The posterior cruciate ligament (PCL) arises from the posterior margin of the tibia just inferior to the tibial plateau. From the tibia, the PCL courses superiorly, anteriorly, and medially to insert on the lateral wall of the medial femoral condyle (Figure 20-7). The PCL has been described as consisting of two bands: the anterolateral band, which is taut in flexion, and the posteromedial band, which is taut with the knee in extension.

A synovial fold covers both cruciate ligaments. The ACL and PCL are therefore intra-articular but are considered extrasynovial. The predominant blood supply of the cruciate ligaments comes from the middle geniculate artery and a few branches of the inferior medial and lateral geniculate arteries. Branches of these arteries form a plexus within the encompassing synovial sheath.[9] Disruption of this plexus is the source of the hemarthrosis typically seen after ACL injury. The intra-articular position of the ACL is one factor in the difficulty in spontaneous healing of ACL tears.

The meniscofemoral ligaments course in a direction similar to that of the PCL. They arise from the posterior horn of the lateral meniscus and course superiorly and medially to insert on the lateral wall of the medial femoral condyle. The ligament of Humphrey lies anterior to the PCL, and the ligament of Wrisberg lies posterior to the PCL. The meniscofemoral ligaments become taut with internal rotation of the tibia.

The posterolateral corner (PLC) of the knee has a complex anatomy consisting of the biceps femoris, the LCL, and the popliteus complex (see Figure 20-4). Dynamic and static components, including the popliteofibular ligament, the fabellofibular ligament, and the arcuate complex, add to this stability and prevent excessive posterior translation, varus rotation, and posterolateral rotation. The arcuate complex consists of the arcuate ligament, popliteus tendon, LCL, and posterior third of the lateral capsule.[10] The arcuate ligament arises from the fibular head and LCL to course superiorly and medially to insert along the popliteus tendon and lateral condyle of the femur. The popliteofibular ligament (PFL) is present in 98% of knees, but the anatomy of the PLC can vary significantly.[11] The presence of a fabella, a variable sesamoid bone in the tendinous portion of the gastrocnemius muscle, correlates with the presence of a fabellofibular ligament.

The medial and lateral menisci lie between the tibial plateaus and femoral condyles (Figure 20-8). The menisci improve stability of the knee by increasing the concavity of the tibial plateaus. Both menisci also serve a secondary role as a stabilizer of the knee. The posterior horn of the medial meniscus serves a secondary stabilizing effect resisting anterior tibial translation.[12,13] Levi et al.[14] documented a 58% increase in anterior tibial translation with a medial meniscectomy in the flexed ACL-deficient knee. The lateral meniscus also serves as a stabilizer, which is particularly important in axial and rotatory loading of the knee.[15] The menisci also absorb shock and distribute weight bearing over a greater surface area.

The outer third of the menisci is vascularized by the middle genicular artery, and the inner third of the menisci is considered to be avascular. Peripheral tears of the menisci therefore have the potential to heal and often are repaired surgically; however, tears in the inner third

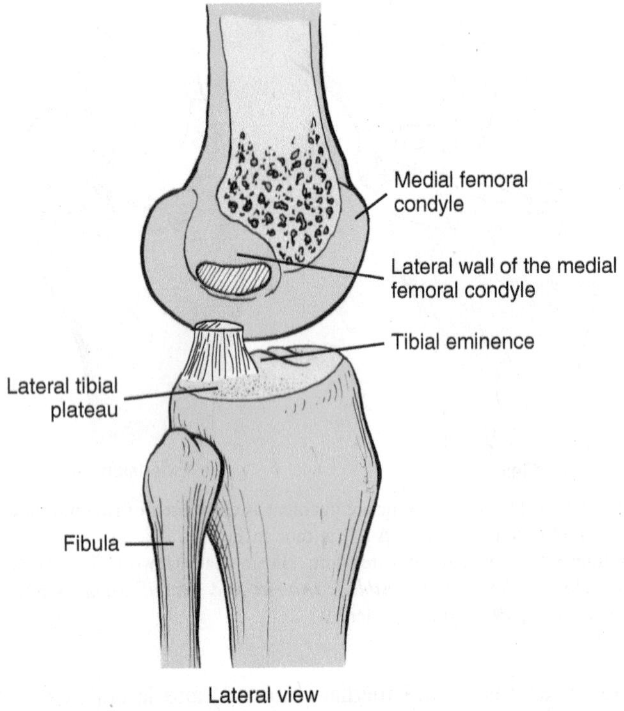

Figure 20-7 The posterior cruciate ligament arises from the posterior margin of the tibial plateau and courses superiorly, medially, and anteriorly to insert on the lateral wall of the medial femoral condyle. (From Zachazewski JE, Magee DJ, Quillen WS, editors: *Athletic injuries and rehabilitation,* p 625, Philadelphia, 1996, WB Saunders.)

Medial femoral condyle

Lateral wall of the medial femoral condyle

Tibial eminence

Lateral tibial plateau

Fibula

Lateral view

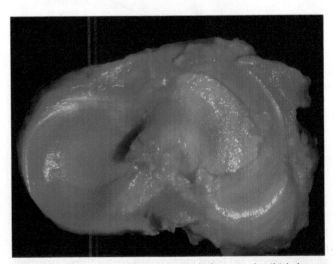

Figure 20-8 The medial and lateral menisci lie between the tibial plateaus and femoral condyles and have different shapes because of the structure of the tibial plateau. The medial meniscus is longer in the anteroposterior direction with a smaller anterior horn than its posterior. The lateral meniscus is more symmetrical but has fewer capsular and ligamentous attachments and is thus more mobile.

(the avascular "white–white" zone) do not heal, and partial meniscectomy often is required. Baratz et al.[16] reported the effects of a partial or total meniscectomy on the articular contact area and stress in the human knee. Total meniscectomy resulted in a concentration of high contact forces on a small area of the tibial plateau. Partial meniscectomy resulted in a smaller increase in contact stress. With a total meniscectomy, the increased tibiofemoral contact forces that result may predispose the patient to long-term degenerative changes. Therefore, partial meniscectomy is preferred to minimize this risk. Because of the convex articulation of the tibia on the lateral side, partial meniscectomy of the lateral meniscus results in greater contact stresses and increased risk for progression of osteoarthritis than the medial side.[17]

During flexion and extension of the knee, the menisci move posteriorly and anteriorly, respectively (Figure 20-9). This movement is a result of the bony geometry of the tibiofemoral joint. Posterior movement of the medial meniscus during flexion also is partly because of the insertion of a portion of the semimembranosus into the posterior horn of the medial meniscus. Similarly, fibers from the popliteus tendon inserting on the posterior horn of the lateral meniscus pull the lateral meniscus posteriorly during flexion. AP movement of the lateral meniscus is greater than that of the medial meniscus, which reduces the susceptibility of the lateral meniscus to injury. During rotation of the knee, the menisci move relative to the tibial plateaus. During lateral (external) rotation of the tibia, the medial meniscus moves posteriorly relative to the medial tibial plateau, whereas the lateral meniscus moves anteriorly relative to the lateral tibial plateau. During medial (internal) rotation of the tibia, movement of the menisci relative to the tibial plateaus is reversed.[3]

Flexion and extension of the knee combine rolling and gliding of the joint surfaces to maintain congruency of these surfaces. During flexion of the knee, the femur rolls posteriorly and glides anteriorly. During extension, the femur rolls anteriorly and glides posteriorly. The combined rolling and gliding of the joint surfaces maintains the femoral condyles on the tibial plateaus. Disruption of the normal arthrokinematics of the knee results in increased translation of the joint surfaces, which can lead to progressive degenerative changes of the articular surfaces.

Muller[18] described the ACL and PCL as a four-bar linkage system that maintains the normal arthrokinematics of the knee (Figure 20-10, *A*). Two of the four bars are the ACL and PCL. The remaining two bars are the line connecting the femoral attachments of the ACL and PCL and the line connecting the tibial attachments of the ACL and PCL. The ACL and PCL are inelastic and maintain a constant length as the knee flexes and extends. As a result, the four-bar linkage system controls rolling and gliding of the joint surfaces as the knee moves. During flexion, the femur rolls posteriorly. This increases the distance between the tibial and femoral insertions of the ACL. Because the ACL cannot lengthen, it guides the femoral condyles anteriorly (Figure 20-10, *B*). Conversely, during extension of the knee, the femoral condyles roll anteriorly and the distance between the femoral and tibial insertions of the PCL increases. Because the PCL cannot lengthen, it pulls the femoral condyles posteriorly as the knee extends (Figure 20-10, *C*). Disruption of the ACL or PCL disrupts the four-bar linkage system and results in abnormal translation of the femoral condyles. Disruption of the normal arthrokinematics of the knee may lead to repetitive injury of the menisci and joint surfaces and to the development of progressive degenerative changes over time.

Ligamentous Restraints of the Knee

The primary restraint to anterior translation of the tibia is the ACL, which provides approximately 85% of the total restraining force to anterior translation of the tibia.[19,20]

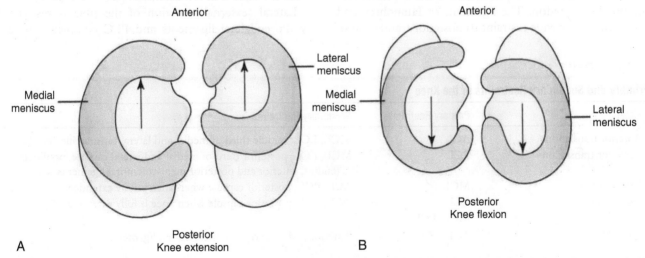

Figure 20-9 The menisci move anteriorly with extension (**A**) and posteriorly with flexion (**B**). The right knee is shown. (Redrawn from Kapandji IA: *The physiology of the joints: annotated diagrams of the mechanics of the human joints,* Edinburgh, 1970, Churchill Livingstone.)

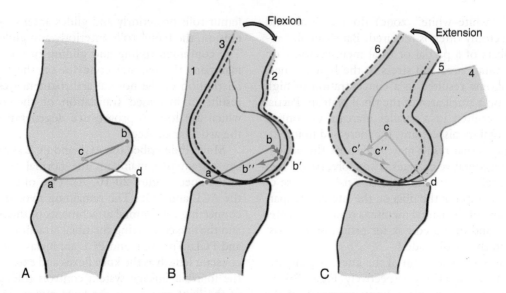

Figure 20-10 Four-bar linkage system. **A,** The four bars consist of the anterior cruciate ligament (ACL) *(line ab);* the posterior cruciate ligament (PCL) *(line cd);* the line connecting the femoral attachments of the ACL and PCL *(line cb);* and the line connecting the tibial attachments of the ACL and PCL *(line ad).* **B,** During flexion, the femur rolls posteriorly; this increases the distance between the tibial and femoral insertions of the ACL. Because the ACL cannot lengthen, it guides the femoral condyles anteriorly. *1,* The position of the femur in extension; *2,* position of the knee if anterior sliding of the femur did not occur with rolling during flexion; *3,* actual position of the femur with flexion because of the pull of the anterior cruciate ligament causing the femur to slide forward during the roll. **C,** During extension of the knee, the femoral condyles roll anteriorly, and the distance between the femoral and tibial insertions of the PCL increases. Because the PCL cannot lengthen, it pulls the femoral condyles posteriorly as the knee extends. *4,* The position of the femur in flexion; *5,* position of the knee if posterior sliding of the femur did not occur with rolling during extension; *6,* actual position of the femur with extension because of the pull of the posterior cruciate ligament causing the femur to slide backward during the roll. (Modified from Kapandji LA: *The physiology of the joints: annotated diagrams of the mechanics of the human joints,* Edinburgh, 1970, Churchill Livingstone.)

The remaining 15% of the restraining ligamentous force to anterior displacement of the tibia is provided by the collateral ligaments, the middle portion of the medial and lateral capsules, and the iliotibial band (Table 20-1).

The primary restraint to posterior displacement of the tibia is the PCL. The PCL provides approximately 85% to 95% of the total restraining force to posterior translation of the tibia.[19] The remaining 5% to 15% of the total ligamentous restraining force to posterior displacement of the tibia is provided by the collateral ligaments, the posterior portion of the medial and lateral capsules, and the popliteus tendon. The ligaments of Humphrey and Wrisberg also provide restraint to posterior translation of

the tibia, and their ability to do so increases with medial (internal) rotation of the tibia (see Table 20-1).

The primary restraint to valgus rotation is the MCL. The ACL and PCL serve as secondary restraints to valgus rotation. When the knee is in full extension, the posterior capsule becomes a significant restraint to valgus rotation (see Table 20-1). For varus rotation, the primary restraint is the LCL, and the ACL and PCL serve as secondary ligamentous restraints. The restraining force provided by the ACL and PCL, as well as the posterior capsule, increases when the knee is in full extension (see Table 20-1).

Lateral (external) rotation of the tibia is restrained by the collateral ligaments and PLC complex, whereas

TABLE 20-1

Primary and Secondary Restraints of the Knee

Tibial Motion	Primary Restraint	Secondary Restraints
Anterior translation	ACL	MCL, LCL; middle third of medial and lateral capsule; iliotibial band
Posterior translation	PCL	MCL, LCL; posterior third of medial and lateral capsule; popliteus tendon; anterior and posterior meniscofemoral ligaments
Valgus rotation	MCL	ACL, PCL; posterior capsule when knee is fully extended
Varus rotation	LCL	ACL, PCL; posterior capsule when knee is fully extended
Lateral (external) rotation	MCL, LCL	
Medial (internal) rotation	ACL, PCL	Anterior and posterior meniscofemoral ligaments

ACL, Anterior cruciate ligament; *MCL,* medial collateral ligament; *LCL,* lateral collateral ligament; *PCL,* posterior collateral ligament.
From Zachazewski JE, Magee DJ, Quillen WS, editors: *Athletic injuries and rehabilitation,* p 627, Philadelphia, 1996, WB Saunders.

medial (internal) rotation is restrained by the cruciate ligaments, the posteromedial capsule, and the ligaments of Humphrey and Wrisberg (see Table 20-1).

The quadriceps and hamstrings serve as dynamic stabilizers of the knee. In doing so, they assist the passive restraints in controlling kinematics of the knee. These muscles work synergistically with the cruciate ligaments to dynamically control motion of the knee. Unopposed contraction of the quadriceps is synergistic to the PCL and antagonistic to the ACL. Conversely, isolated contraction of the hamstrings is synergistic to the ACL and antagonistic to the PCL. It is theorized that activities that promote co-contraction of the hamstrings and quadriceps minimize tibial translation, and activities of this type have been advocated for rehabilitation of knee ligament injuries.[21] Dynamic stabilization of the knee to control abnormal motion depends on muscular strength and endurance, as well as on the development of appropriate neuromuscular control.

Role of Proprioception

Researchers have shown increased interest in the role of proprioception in the prevention and progression of knee injuries.[22-25] A systematic review by Cooper et al.[26] detailed decreased proprioception in populations with ACL deficiency as well as the postoperative ACL reconstruction population. Proprioception has been described as a variation in the sense of touch. It includes the senses of joint motion (i.e., kinesthesia) and joint position. Proprioception is mediated by mechanoreceptors in the skin, the musculotendinous units, ligaments, and the joint capsule. These sensory receptors transduce mechanical deformation to a neural signal, which modulates conscious and unconscious responses. Although local receptors are disrupted in ligamentous rupture, it is theorized that other knee joint receptors may play a compensatory role in aiding in the stability of the knee, via increased muscle spindle sensitivity and protective muscle activation.[26] The role of proprioception in providing smooth, coordinated movement and dynamic stabilization has been well documented.[24,27-29]

Proprioceptive reflexes originating from the joint capsule or musculotendinous units likely also play a role in knee stability, although they have been reported to have relatively long latency in humans.[30] This was demonstrated by Solomonow et al.,[24] who reported increased hamstring electromyographic (EMG) activity in a patient with an ACL-deficient knee during maximum slow-speed isokinetic testing of the quadriceps. The increased hamstring EMG activity occurred simultaneously with anterior subluxation of the tibia at approximately 40° knee flexion and was associated with a sharp decrease in quadriceps torque and inhibition of quadriceps EMG activity. Because the ACL was ruptured, reflex contraction of the hamstrings could not have been mediated by receptors originating in the ACL. They proposed that this reflex contraction is mediated by receptors in the joint capsule or hamstring muscles.

Several clinical studies have evaluated proprioception in terms of threshold to detection of passive motion and reproduction of passive joint position. Barrack et al.[22] reported deficits in threshold to detection of passive motion in subjects with a unilateral ACL-deficient knee. Barrett[28] reported high correlations between measurements of proprioception and function ($r=0.84$) and patient satisfaction ($r=0.90$) in 45 patients who had undergone ACL reconstruction. Standard knee scores and clinical examination results correlated poorly with the patient's own opinion and the results of functional tests. Lephart et al.[25] studied the threshold to detection of passive movement in patients who had undergone ACL reconstruction. Testing was performed at 15° and 45° flexion. Three trials were performed, moving into flexion and extension. The results indicated that the threshold to detection of passive movement was less sensitive in the reconstructed knee than the noninvolved knee. Also, the threshold to detection of passive motion was more sensitive in both the reconstructed knee and the normal knee at 15° flexion than at 45° flexion. Sensitivity to detection of passive motion was enhanced by the use of a neoprene sleeve, which has implications for bracing after ACL injury and/or reconstruction. Use of a sleeve or compressive wrap or garment may help the patient develop a greater sense of perception of the knee during rehabilitation and progressive activity.

Several studies have also examined the relationship between neuromuscular/proprioceptive training and single-leg hop test scores in a population of patients with ACL deficiency.[31-33] Groups who engaged in neuromuscular training as part of their rehabilitation program displayed significantly improved single-leg hop test scores compared with those of a standard training group. Liu-Ambrose et al.[34] failed to note similar results in patients after surgical ACL reconstruction. It was hypothesized that patients with ACL deficiency may rely more heavily on compensatory muscle activation than patients who undergo ACL reconstruction because of the lack of integrity of the static stabilizing structures of the knee.[34]

Furthermore, Liu-Ambrose et al.[34] examined the effect of proprioceptive training on concentric and eccentric quadriceps and hamstring strength. The proprioceptive training group demonstrated significantly greater improvement in concentric quadriceps strength and eccentric hamstring strength over a 12-week period, compared with a standard strength-training group.

Beard et al.[35] and Fitzgerald et al.[32] examined passive laxity using a KT1000 and KT2000 after a proprioceptive training program. Neither study reported an increase in sagittal plane motion after rehabilitation programs in either the treatment or the control groups. Therefore, it can be concluded that neuromuscular training programs involve minimal risk and can provide improvements in strength, proprioception, and functional outcome testing (i.e., hop testing).

Injury to the knee may result in abnormal sensory feedback and altered neuromuscular control, which may lead to recurrent injury. Proprioceptive training after knee injury and/or surgery should attempt to maximize the use of sensory information mediated by the ligaments, joint capsule, and/or musculotendinous unit to stabilize the joint dynamically. Proprioceptive training requires repetition to develop motor control of abnormal joint motion and may be enhanced with the use of EMG biofeedback. Initially, control of abnormal joint motion requires conscious effort. Through repetitive training, motor control of abnormal movement becomes automatic and occurs subconsciously. It should be noted, however, that the extent to which an individual can develop neuromuscular control of abnormal joint motion to stabilize the knee dynamically is currently unknown.

Biomechanics of Exercise

Open kinetic chain (OKC) exercise is exercise in which the distal segment is free to move, resulting in isolated movement at a given joint. At the knee, OKC exercise results in isolated flexion and extension. OKC knee extension is a result of isolated contraction of the quadriceps, and OKC knee flexion occurs as a result of isolated contraction of the hamstrings. Baratta et al.[29] and Draganich et al.[36] reported low levels of co-activation of the quadriceps and hamstrings during OKC knee extension. It is hypothesized that the hamstrings become active during the terminal range of extension to decelerate the knee and act as a synergist to the ACL to minimize anterior tibial translation produced by contraction of the quadriceps. During OKC knee extension, the flexion moment arm increases as the knee is extended from 90° flexion to full extension (0°). This requires increasing quadriceps and patellar tendon tension, which can increase the load on the patellofemoral and tibiofemoral joints.

During closed kinetic chain (CKC) exercises, the distal segment is relatively fixed; therefore movement at one joint results in simultaneous movement of all other joints in the kinetic chain in a predictable manner. The lower extremity functions as a CKC when a person squats over the fixed foot, resulting in simultaneous movement of the ankle, knee, and hip. CKC exercises for the lower extremity result in contraction of muscles throughout the lower extremity. During CKC exercises for the lower extremity, the flexion moment arms at the knee and hip increase as the squat is performed, and increased force of contraction of the quadriceps and hamstrings is required to control the knee and hip, respectively.

OKC and CKC exercises have different effects on tibial translation and ligamentous strain and load. During active OKC knee extension, the shear component produced by unopposed contraction of the quadriceps depends on the angle of knee flexion (Figure 20-11). Sawhney et al.[37]

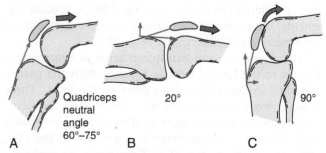

Figure 20-11 During open-chain knee extension, tibial translation is a function of the shear force produced by the patellar tendon. **A,** Quadriceps neutral position. The patellar tendon force is perpendicular to the tibial plateaus and results in compression of the joint surfaces without shear. **B,** At flexion angles less than the angle of the quadriceps neutral position, orientation of the patellar tendon produces anterior shear of the tibia. **C,** At angles greater than the angle of the quadriceps neutral position, patellar tendon force causes a posterior shear of the tibia. (From Daniel DM, Stone ML, Barnett P, Sachs R: Use of the quadriceps active test to diagnose posterior cruciate ligament disruption and measure posterior laxity of the knee, *J Bone Joint Surg Am* 70:386-391, 1988.)

investigated the effects of isometric quadriceps contraction on tibial translation in subjects with an intact knee. Tibial translation was measured with the KT1000 Ligament Arthrometer (MEDmetric, San Diego, CA) at 30°, 45°, 60°, and 75° flexion. OKC isometric quadriceps contraction against 10 pounds (4.5 kg) of resistance applied to the distal aspect of the leg resulted in anterior tibial translation at 30° and 45° flexion. No significant tibial translation occurred at 60° or 75° flexion. It was determined that the quadriceps-neutral Q angle (i.e., the angle at which quadriceps contraction produces no anterior or posterior tibial translation) occurs at 60° to 75° flexion (see Figure 20-11, *A*). OKC knee extension at angles less than the quadriceps-neutral position results in anterior translation of the tibia. This was reported by Grood et al.[20] in intact cadaveric knees. Anterior translation of the tibia during OKC knee extension increased with loading of the quadriceps at angles less than 60° flexion. Sectioning of the ACL increased anterior translation during loaded and unloaded OKC knee extension. Anterior tibial translation produced by the quadriceps at knee flexion angles less than the quadriceps-neutral angle is a result of the anteriorly directed shear component of the patellar tendon force (see Figure 20-11, *B*). OKC knee extension at knee flexion angles greater than the quadriceps-neutral position results in posterior tibial translation. This is the result of a posteriorly directed shear component of the patellar tendon force at these angles of knee flexion (see Figure 20-11, *C*).

OKC knee flexion is produced by isolated contraction of the hamstrings. This has been shown to result in posterior translation of the tibia and was reported by Lutz et al.,[38] who found posterior tibial shear forces during isometric OKC knee flexion at 30°, 60°, and 90° knee flexion. The posterior shear force increased as flexion progressed from 30° to 90° flexion.

Several methods of biomechanical analysis have been used to study rehabilitation of the knee, including cadaveric, EMG, kinematic, kinetic, mathematical modeling, and in vivo strain gauge measurements. These studies are best evaluated by delineating the findings according to the tissue or structure examined, such as the ACL, the PCL, and the patellofemoral joint.

Anterior Cruciate Ligament

Most biomechanical research on rehabilitation of the knee has focused on the ACL. After years of theoretical and anecdotal assumptions, researchers now are better able to scrutinize more closely the efficacy of OKC and CKC exercises. Markolf et al.[39] examined the effect of compressive loads on cadaveric knees to simulate body weight. These authors reported that compressive forces reduce strain on the ACL, compared with OKC exercises, thus providing a protective mechanism. Fleming et al.[40] investigated this theory using in vivo strain gauge measurements in the ACL. This method allows direct measurement of ACL strain during activity. The authors noted that strain on the ACL increased from −2% during non–weight bearing to 2.1% in a weight-bearing position. Although an increase in ACL strain was observed in a weight-bearing position, it still is unclear whether a 2% strain is detrimental to a healing ACL graft. Clinical experience has demonstrated that early weight bearing does not result in poor functional outcomes in postoperative ACL reconstructions.

CKC exercises have also been theorized to reduce ACL strain by providing co-contraction of the hamstrings and quadriceps. Wilk et al.[41] examined the EMG activity of the quadriceps and hamstrings during the CKC squat and leg press and the OKC knee extension. These authors noted that co-contraction occurred from 30° to 0°, during the ascent phase of the squat, when the body is positioned directly over the knees and feet, but it did not occur at other ranges of motion or during the CKC leg press or OKC knee extension. Therefore not all CKC exercises produce a co-contraction of the quadriceps and hamstrings. Rather, several factors appear to affect muscle activation during CKC exercises, including the knee flexion angle, body position relative to the knee, and the direction of movement (i.e., ascending or descending). Clinically, exercises performed in an upright and weight-bearing position with the knee flexed to approximately 30° (e.g., squats and lateral lunges) may be used during knee rehabilitation to promote co-contraction of the quadriceps and hamstrings.

Wilk et al.[41] also used mathematical modeling to estimate the shear forces at the tibiofemoral joint during the squat, leg press, and knee extension exercise (Figure 20-12). The authors reported that a posterior tibiofemoral shear force was observed during the entire range of motion (ROM) during both the CKC squat and leg press (peak, 1500 Newtons [N]), and during deep angles of OKC

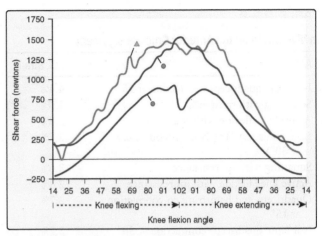

Figure 20-12 Tibiofemoral shear forces observed throughout the range of motion during closed kinetic chair squat (*green triangle*) and leg press (*blue circle*) exercises and open kinetic chain knee extension exercises (*red circle*). (Redrawn from Wilk KE, Escamilla RF, Fleisig GS et al: A comparison of tibiofemoral joint forces and electromyographic activity during open and closed kinetic chain exercises, *Am J Sports Med* 24:522, 1996.)

knee extension from 100° to 40° (peak, 900 N). Anterior tibiofemoral shear force (peak, 250 N) and, theoretically, ACL strain were observed during the OKC knee extension exercise from 40° to 10°.

Similar to the results of Wilk et al.,[41] Beynnon et al.,[42] using in vivo strain gauge measurements, found that the greatest amount of ACL strain (2.8%) occurred during 40° to 0° OKC knee extension. This strain was found to increase significantly in a linear fashion with the application of an external 45 Newton boot (3.8%). However, the authors also reported an ACL strain of 3.6% during the CKC squat exercise. In contrast, application of external loading did not significantly increase the amount of strain on the ACL (4%).

Based on the findings of Fleming et al.,[40] Wilk et al.,[41] and Beynnon et al.,[42] both OKC and CKC exercises should be performed during rehabilitation of a reconstructed ACL, although the patient often is limited to 90° to 40° during the OKC knee extension when heavy resistance is applied.

The bicycle and stair climbers also are commonly used during ACL rehabilitation. Fleming et al.[43] analyzed six different bicycle riding conditions, manipulating speed and power. These authors found no significant differences among these conditions (minimal mean ACL strain of 1.7%). The greatest amount of strain was observed when the knee reached the greatest amount of extension. Similarly, Fleming et al.[44] analyzed two cadences of stair climbing (80 and 112 steps per minute) and noted a similar 2.7% strain on the ACL. Again, the greatest strain was observed during terminal knee extension. Therefore both bicycling and stair climbing are two safe exercises that put low strain on the ACL compared with other rehabilitation exercises (Table 20-2). Furthermore, the finding that the greatest

TABLE 20-2

In Vivo Strain on the Anterior Cruciate Ligament

Activity	ACL Strain
Isometric quadriceps contraction at 15°	4.4%
Squatting with resistance	4.0%
Active knee flexion with resistance	3.8%
Lachman's test (150 N of anterior shear at 30°)	3.7%
Squatting without resistance	3.6%
Active knee flexion without resistance	2.8%
Quadriceps and hamstring co-contraction at 15°	2.7%
Isometric quadriceps contraction at 30°	2.7%
Stair climbing	2.7%
Anterior drawer test (150 N anterior shear at 90°)	1.8%
Stationary bicycle	1.7%
Quadriceps and hamstrings co-contraction at 30°	0.4%
Passive knee range of motion	0.1%
Isometric quadriceps contraction at 60° and 90°	0.0%
Quadriceps and hamstrings co-contraction at 60° and 90°	0.0%
Isometric hamstring contraction at 30°, 60°, and 90°	0.0%

Modified from Fleming BC, Beynnon BD, Renstrom PA et al: The strain behavior of the anterior cruciate ligament during stair climbing: an in vivo study, *Arthroscopy* 15:185-191, 1999.

TABLE 20-3

Posterior Tibiofemoral Shear Forces

Source	Activity	Knee Angle (Degrees)	Force (× Body Weight)
Kaufman[47]	60°/sec flexion isokinetic	75	1.7
	180°/sec flexion isokinetic	75	1.4
Morrison[45,46]	Level walking	5	0.4
	Descending stairs	5	0.6
	Ascending stairs	45	1.7
Smidt[48]	Isometric flexion	45	1.1

amount of strain occurred as the knee moved into terminal knee extension was similar to the results seen by Wilk et al.[41] and Beynnon et al.[42] during OKC and CKC exercises.

Posterior Cruciate Ligament

Historically, rehabilitation after injury to the PCL has had mixed results. Poor functional outcomes have often been attributed to residual laxity after surgical reconstruction. The biomechanics of the tibiofemoral joint during exercise must be understood so that the rehabilitative process does not have deleterious effects on the PCL.

Posterior tibiofemoral shear forces that occur during specific activities, such as level walking,[45] ascent up and descent down stairs,[46] and resisted knee flexion exercises,[47,48] have been documented.[49] Level walking and descent down stairs have a relatively low posterior tibiofemoral shear force, 0.4×body weight (BW) and 0.6×BW, respectively (Table 20-3). However, high posterior shear force has been noted during several commonly performed activities of daily living (ADLs), such as climbing stairs (1.7×BW at 45° knee flexion)[46,50] and squatting (3.6×BW at 140° knee flexion), which may have an effect on residual laxity after surgery. Further studies have reported that isometric knee flexion at 45° places a posterior shear force of 1.1×BW on the tibiofemoral joint.[48]

Tremendous shear forces on the PCL and the tibiofemoral joint occur during OKC resisted knee flexion. Posterior tibial displacement is attributed to the high EMG activity of the hamstring muscles during resistive knee flexion. Lutz et al.[38] reported a maximum shear force of 1780 N at 90°, 1526 N at 60°, and 939 N at 30° during isometric knee flexion. Kaufman et al.[47] also noted a PCL load of 1.7×BW at 75° during isokinetic knee flexion exercise. Because PCL stress increases with the knee flexion angle, isolated OKC knee flexion exercises should be avoided for at least 8 weeks after surgery or in patients who did not undergo surgery, until symptoms subside.

Excessive stress on the PCL has also been observed during deeper angles of OKC knee extension. Several studies have proven that resisted knee extension at 90° flexion causes a posterior tibiofemoral shear and potential stress on the PCL.[24,37,38,41,51] Wilk et al.[41] documented a posterior shear force from 100° to 40° with resisted OKC knee extension. The greatest amount of stress on the PCL was seen at angles of 85° to 95° during active resisted knee flexion. Conversely, the lowest amount of posterior shear force occurred from 60° to 0° of resisted knee extension.[41] Kaufman et al.[47] also reported that posterior shear forces were exerted until 50° to 55° knee flexion. Jurist and Otis[51] documented stress on the PCL at 60° flexion during an isometric knee extension exercise when resistance was applied at the proximal tibia. To reduce the excessive posterior shear force on the PCL, OKC resisted knee extension should be performed from 60° to 0°.[49]

The stress applied to the PCL during CKC exercises depends on the knee flexion angle produced during the exercise. Wilk et al.[41,52] reported an increase in posterior shear force as the knee flexion angle increased during CKC exercise. Stuart et al.[53] also documented a linear increase in posterior shear force from 40° to 100° knee flexion during the front squat maneuver. Therefore, to reduce PCL stress during CKC exercises, leg presses and squats should be performed from 0° to 60° knee flexion.[49]

Patellofemoral Joint

The effects of OKC versus CKC exercises on the patellofemoral joint must be considered in a rehabilitation regimen after knee ligament injury and/or surgery. The patellofemoral joint consists of the articulation between the patella and the distal end of the femur. The patella is embedded in the knee extensor mechanism and is the largest sesamoid bone in the body. Proximally, the quadriceps inserts into the patella through the quadriceps tendon. Distally, the patella is connected to the tibia through the patellar tendon. The patella protects the anterior aspect of the knee, increases the effective moment arm of the knee extensor mechanism, and centralizes the divergent forces produced by the quadriceps. The tendency of the patella to sublux laterally (i.e., produced by the Q [quadriceps] angle, the vastus lateralis, and the lateral retinacular structures) must be counterbalanced by the oblique fibers of the vastus medialis. Maintaining this balance is crucial to normal function of the knee extensor mechanism.

The patella is a triangular bone with the base directed superiorly and the apex directed inferiorly. The patella is described as having three facets on its posterior aspect. A central ridge that runs from superior to inferior divides the patella into medial and lateral facets. The odd facet lies on the medial border of the patella and engages the femur only during the extreme range of flexion. The posterior margin of the patella is covered by a thick layer of articular cartilage, which is thicker centrally than peripherally. This layer of articular cartilage is thicker than at any other joint in the body, perhaps up to 5 mm thick.[54] It is important for reducing friction and aiding lubrication of the patellofemoral joint.

The stability of the patellofemoral joint depends on static and dynamic restraints. Static restraints consist of the shape of the patellofemoral joint and the medial and lateral patellofemoral ligaments. The lateral femoral condyle projects farther anteriorly than the medial femoral condyle and serves as a buttress to minimize lateral displacement of the patella. Dynamic stability of the patellofemoral joint is provided by the quadriceps. The vastus medialis oblique (VMO) and medial retinaculum provide medial stabilization of the patella. The vastus lateralis, lateral retinaculum, and iliotibial band pull the patella laterally. The Q angle is the angle formed by lines that connect the anterior superior iliac spine to the midpatella and the midpatella to the tibial tubercle. The Q angle results in lateral displacement of the patella when the quadriceps contracts. Lateral displacement of the patella is dynamically resisted by the VMO and medial retinaculum. Weakness of the VMO allows the patella to track laterally. In addition, tightness of the lateral retinaculum and overpull from the vastus lateralis and iliotibial band can result in lateral displacement of the patella.

Prevention and/or treatment of patellofemoral symptoms after knee ligament injury or surgery should seek to maintain or restore the balance of the medial and lateral stabilizers of the patellofemoral joint.

Hungerford and Barry[55] described the patellofemoral contact pattern as the knee moves through a full ROM (Figure 20-13). The patella initially makes contact with the femur in the trochlear groove at approximately 20° flexion. Initial contact is between the trochlear groove and the inferior pole of the patella. As flexion progresses, the contact area on the patella progresses superiorly, so that by 90° flexion, the entire articular surface of the patella, except for the odd medial facet, has articulated with the femur. As flexion continues beyond 90°, the quadriceps tendon articulates with the trochlear groove and the patella moves into the intercondylar notch area of the femur. At full flexion, the odd medial facet and lateral facet of the patella articulate with the intercondylar notch. The odd medial facet articulates with the femur only at the end range of flexion.

Knowledge of the patellofemoral contact pattern is useful for determining the limits of motion when patients with patellofemoral symptoms perform OKC and CKC exercises. It should also be noted that the patellofemoral contact area increases from 20° to 90° flexion. This increase helps distribute patellofemoral joint reaction forces over a larger area to reduce patellofemoral contact stress per unit of area. (Chapter 22 presents a more detailed discussion of the impact of patellofemoral forces and mechanics during rehabilitation and activity.)

Clinical Note

Generally, exercises for the patellofemoral joint should be performed in the pain-free and crepitus-free ROM.

Alterations in the Q angle often are associated with patellofemoral disorders. They may alter the contact areas and thus the amount of joint reaction forces of the

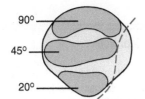
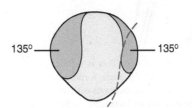

Figure 20-13 Areas of contact of the patella during different degrees of flexion. (From Magee DJ: *Orthopedic physical assessment*, ed 6, p 767, St. Louis, 2014, Saunders/Elsevier.)

patellofemoral joint. Huberti and Hayes[56] examined the in vitro patellofemoral contact pressures at various degrees of knee flexion from 20° to 120°. The maximum contact area occurred at 90° knee flexion, where contact pressure was estimated to be 6.5×BW. An increase or decrease in the Q angle of 10° resulted in increased maximum contact pressure and a smaller total area of contact throughout the ROM.

Patellofemoral joint reaction force is a function of quadriceps and patellar tendon tension and of the angle formed between the quadriceps and patellar tendons (Figure 20-14). This force compresses the patellofemoral joint, with increasing patellar and quadriceps tendon tension and an increasing angle of knee flexion. Patellofemoral joint reaction forces during functional CKC activities were calculated by Reilly and Martens[57] and were found to be 0.5×BW during level walking, 3.3×BW on stairs, and 7.8×BW during a full squat. These results are consistent with activities that increase patellofemoral symptoms.

OKC and CKC exercises produce different effects on patellofemoral joint reaction force and contact stress per unit area. During OKC knee extension, the flexion moment arm for the knee increases as the knee is extended

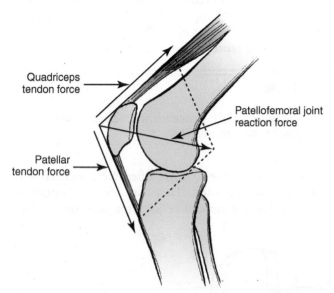

Figure 20-14 Patellofemoral joint reaction force. This is a function of patellar and quadriceps tendon tension and the angle formed between the quadriceps and patellar tendons. This force increases with increasing patellar and quadriceps tendon tension and an increasing angle of knee flexion. (From Zachazewski JE, Magee DJ, Quillen WS, editors: *Athletic injuries and rehabilitation*, p 633, Philadelphia, 1996, WB Saunders.)

from 90° flexion to full extension (0°), which results in increased quadriceps and patellar tendon tension and increasing patellofemoral joint reaction forces. For CKC exercises, the flexion moment arm of the knee increases as the angle of knee flexion increases. In the case of OKC exercises, the patellofemoral joint reaction forces may be concentrated in a relatively small contact area, resulting in larger contact stresses per unit area; this can create forces that ultimately result in symptoms such as pain and possibly degenerative change. Conversely, for CKC exercises, the flexion moment arm of the knee increases as the knee flexion angle increases. Greater quadriceps and patellar tendon tension is required to counteract the increasing flexion moment arm. By controlling the position of the foot, ankle, knee, and hip in this weight-bearing position, it may be possible to influence the position and "tracking" of the patella, which results in increasing patellofemoral joint reaction force as the knee flexes. This force is distributed over a larger patellofemoral contact area, minimizing the increase in contact stress per unit area.

Steinkamp et al.[59] analyzed patellofemoral joint biomechanics during the leg press and extension exercises in 20 normal subjects. Patellofemoral joint reaction force, stress, and moments were calculated during both exercises. At 0° to 46° knee flexion, the patellofemoral joint reaction force was less during the CKC leg press. Conversely, at 50° to 90° knee flexion, joint reaction forces were lower during the OKC knee extension exercise. Joint reaction forces were minimal at 90° knee flexion during the knee extension exercise. Similar findings have been reported by Escamilla et al.,[60] who studied patellofemoral compressive forces during the OKC knee extension and the CKC leg press and vertical squat. OKC knee extension produced significantly greater forces at angles less than 57° knee flexion, whereas both CKC activities produced significantly greater forces at knee angles more than 85°.

In analyzing the biomechanics of the OKC knee extension, Grood et al.[20] reported that quadriceps force was greatest near full knee extension and increased with the addition of external loading. The small patellofemoral contact area observed near full extension, as previously discussed, and the increased amount of quadriceps force generated at these angles may make the patellofemoral joint more susceptible to injury. At lower angles of extension (i.e., closer to full extension, or 0°), a greater magnitude of quadriceps force is focused onto a more condensed location on the patella. Therefore, if the results of Steinkamp et al.,[59] Escamilla et al.,[60] and Grood et al.[20] are applied, it appears that during OKC knee extension, as the contact area of the patellofemoral joint decreases, the force of quadriceps pull subsequently increases; as a result, a large magnitude of patellofemoral contact stress is applied to a focal point on the patella while it is seated in the trochlear groove in a position to articulate with the femur. In contrast, during CKC exercises, the quadriceps force increases as the knee continues into flexion. However, the area of patellofemoral contact also increases as the knee flexes, leading to a wider dissipation of contact stress over a larger surface area.

In 1999, Witvrouw et al.[61] prospectively studied the efficacy of OKC and CKC exercises during nonoperative patellofemoral rehabilitation. Sixty patients participated in a 5-week exercise program consisting of either OKC or CKC exercises. Subjective pain scores, functional ability, quadriceps and hamstring peak torque, and hamstring, quadriceps, and gastrocnemius flexibility were all recorded before and after rehabilitation and at 3 months after the program ended. Both treatment groups reported a significant decrease in pain, increase in muscle strength, and increase in functional performance at 3 months after intervention.

The studies seem to show that both OKC and CKC exercises can be used to maximize the outcomes for patellofemoral patients if they are performed within a safe ROM. Exercises prescribed by the clinician should be individualized according to the patient's needs and the clinician's assessment. If CKC exercises are less painful than OKC exercises, then that form of muscular training is encouraged. In addition, for postoperative patients, regions of articular cartilage wear must be considered carefully before an exercise program is designed. Clinicians most often allow OKC exercises, such as knee extension at 90° to 40° knee flexion. This ROM provides the lowest patellofemoral joint reaction forces while providing the greatest amount of patellofemoral contact area. CKC exercises, such as the leg press, vertical squats, lateral step-ups, and wall squats (i.e., wall slides), are performed initially at 0° to 16° and then progressed to 0° to 30°, where patellofemoral joint reaction forces are lower. As the patient's symptoms subside, the ranges of motion performed are progressed to allow greater muscle strengthening in larger ranges. Exercises are progressed

based on the patient's subjective reports of symptoms and the clinical assessment of swelling, ROM, and painful crepitus.

EVALUATION OF KNEE INJURIES

Subjective Assessment and History

A thorough history and physical examination are essential for making the correct diagnosis and determining appropriate treatment. Most injuries about the knee can be diagnosed with a thorough clinical evaluation, which often can eliminate the need for advanced imaging. (A full discussion of the history and physical examination can be found in *Orthopedic Physical Assessment*, Chapter 12, volume I of this series.)

The history can help determine the patient's activity level before injury and expectations after recovery. This can help in the planning and timing of treatment and in ensuring that patients have a realistic expectation of the outcome after the injury. For athletes, understanding current and past level of play, hours played per week, skill level, potential, and athletic goals is important because these factors play a role in surgical decision making.[62]

The clinician first must determine whether the injury is of traumatic origin. With traumatic injuries, the patient should be asked about the mechanism of injury and the location of the pain. This information provides a clue as to which anatomic structures are at risk. The examiner should determine whether the foot was planted, whether the injury was a twisting injury, whether the injury resulted from direct contact, and the direction of the forces involved. It is important to determine whether the patient had injured the same knee before and, if so, how it was treated. Was the patient able to leave the scene unassisted or was assistance required? This may indicate the severity of the injury. The patient may be able to relate hearing or feeling a pop at the time of injury, which may indicate a cruciate ligament tear or osteochondral fracture. Determining whether any deformity was present that may have been reduced before the patient was evaluated is helpful in diagnosing a patellar or tibiofemoral dislocation or periarticular fracture. Determining the time course of swelling of the knee after injury also is helpful because an acute effusion or hemarthrosis may differentiate an intra-articular fracture or torn cruciate ligament from a peripheral meniscal tear or patellar dislocation.

The same history is required for a subacute or chronically dysfunctional knee because the injury may have been initiated by a traumatic event but never treated. The examiner must determine when the symptoms began in relation to a traumatic event. The patient must relate whether the primary complaint is popping or clicking, giving way (instability), locking, pain, or swelling. The relationship between activity and the patient's symptoms can also be helpful in determining the cause of the problem. Pain on takeoff (and, to a lesser extent, landing) when jumping often is because of extensor mechanism problems (i.e., patella, patellar tendon, quadriceps tendon), whereas instability on landing suggests ACL insufficiency or quadriceps weakness. A history of popping or clicking frequently is elicited, and these sounds can be caused by a variety of conditions, both pathological and normal.

Instability often is described as giving way, sliding, slipping out of socket, buckling, or having a sensation that the knee may give out. Giving way usually indicates intra-articular pathology, including a displaced meniscal tear or cruciate ligament injury, resulting in a loose body or rotary instability. Impending giving way may be due to patellar subluxation or weakness of the extensor mechanism. Most patients with chronic rotatory instability can ambulate and perform ADLs without pain or instability. These patients complain of buckling during activities such as running, jumping, pivoting, or cutting. True locking is a mechanical block to full extension with uninhibited flexion, and it usually indicates a displaced meniscal tear. Other causes of locking include loose bodies, joint effusion, hamstring spasm, posterior capsulitis, and sometimes disruption of the quadriceps mechanism.

A history of swelling commonly is obtained after an injury; however, the time from injury to the onset of swelling and the location and amount of swelling should be determined, as well as its response to rest, activity, and medications. The development of a large, acute hemarthrosis within 2 to 6 hours after injury occurs secondary to an ACL rupture approximately 70% of the time,[63] although it also may be due to an intra-articular or osteochondral fracture. Alternatively, an acute hemarthrosis may be due to patellar dislocation; however, because the capsule is torn, the swelling usually is not as large as with a cruciate ligament disruption or fracture. An effusion that develops 1 day or more after injury usually is a hydrarthrosis, which occurs secondary to a meniscal tear, synovitis, or sympathetic effusion. Chronic synovitis and its attendant effusion indicate intra-articular inflammation. It usually is caused by a meniscal tear, advanced chondromalacia patella (e.g., patellar dysfunction, or excessive lateral patellar compression syndrome), rotatory instability, or loose bodies. The differential diagnosis must also include pigmented villonodular synovitis, osteochondritis dissecans, inflammatory and/or rheumatological arthritis, and other causes of synovitis.

Physical Examination

A thorough physical examination complements a good history. We recommend that the reader review *Orthopedic Physical Assessment*, Chapter 12, volume I of this series for a detailed explanation of how to complete various physical examination techniques associated with examination of the knee. An understanding of the rationale for using specific examination techniques is required to diagnose ligamentous instability. The physical examination entails multiple steps, including inspection, ROM and strength testing, more specific tests, and palpation.

The motion resulting from a clinical test in a relaxed patient depends on the position of the limb at the start of the test, the point of application and direction of the force, and the examiner's ability to detect displacement. Manual examination of the knee compares the two sides to differentiate normal laxity from pathological instability. In a normal patient, left-to-right and side-to-side differences usually are negligible; therefore an internal control often exists for most patients. Most knee ligament tests assess for pathological motion by stressing a specific ligament or ligament complex. The motion detected during this examination depends on whether the primary or the secondary restraints have been disrupted (see Table 20-1). When a primary restraint is disrupted, pathological motion occurs, but its extent is limited by the remaining structures, called *secondary restraints*. Disruption of a secondary restraint does not result in pathological motion if the primary restraint is intact; however, disruption of the secondary restraint when the primary restraint is disrupted enhances pathological motion. For all clinical laxity tests, the femur is held steady and the tibial translation or rotation (i.e., joint space opening) is measured. A summary of the examination of the knee is presented in Box 20-1.

Specific Tests

Please see *Orthopedic Physical Assessment* for detailed explanations about properly performing each test.

Medial Collateral Ligament

Testing begins by palpation at the proximal or distal end of the ligament. This is important prognostically because proximal MCL injuries may have a slower recovery of full ROM compared with distal injuries.[64] The **abduction (valgus stress) test** assesses the integrity of the MCL and medial instability (Figure 20-15). This should be performed first in full extension and again in 20° to 30° knee flexion, which relaxes secondary restraints. It is imperative to examine both knees because some ligamentous laxity may be normal in some individuals. The severity of injury to the MCL and associated structures can be determined by the amount of medial joint line opening. If increased medial joint line opening is seen in the affected knee at 20° to 30° flexion, the posterior oblique ligament and posteromedial capsule may be injured.

If excessive medial joint opening is seen in full extension, a more severe injury to the secondary structures must be assumed. Medial joint line opening with the knee in full extension indicates injury to the MCL (superficial and deep fibers), posterior oblique ligament, ACL,

Physical Examination of the Knee

STANDING POSITION
- Mechanical alignment and symmetry of the lower extremity
- Foot type
- Gait
- Heel-and-toe walking
- "Duck" walk

SITTING POSITION
- Palpation:
  - Medial joint line
  - Lateral joint line
  - Patellar tendon
  - Tibial tubercle
  - Proximal tibia (pes anserine bursa, Gerdy's tubercle)
- Sulcus–tubercle angle (Q angle at 90°)

SUPINE POSITION WITH KNEES EXTENDED
- Palpation:
  - Warmth
  - Swelling
  - Patellar facets
  - Quadriceps tendon
  - Lateral collateral ligament in figure-of-four position
- Active and passive flexion and extension
- Patellofemoral and tibiofemoral crepitus
- Sag sign
- Godfrey's sign
- Quadriceps active test
- Anterior and posterior drawer tests
- Lachman's test
- Varus–valgus stress test
- O'Donoghue-McMurray test
- Dial test
- Reverse pivot shift test
- External rotation recurvatum test
- Quadriceps atrophy
- Hamstring and calf tightness

SIDE-LYING POSITION
- Ober's test

PRONE POSITION
- Heel height difference (flexion contracture)
- Apley's compression/distraction test
- External rotation of the tibia at 30° and 90° flexion
- Reverse Lachman's test
- Quadriceps flexibility

From Zachazewski JE, Magee DJ, Quillen WS, editors: *Athletic injuries and rehabilitation*, p 639, Philadelphia, 1996, WB Saunders.

PCL, posteromedial capsule, medial quadriceps expansion and retinaculum, and semimembranosus. With this more severe injury, the results of one or more rotatory instability tests are also positive. Where complete injury to medial structures is present, a positive dial test may result (Figure 20-16).[65]

Lateral Collateral Ligament

Adduction (Varus Stress) Test. The varus stress test assesses the integrity of the LCL and, thus, lateral instability (Figure 20-17). Both knees are tested first in full extension and again in 30° knee flexion.

The severity of injury to the LCL and associated structures can be determined by the amount of lateral joint line opening in extension and slight flexion. With the knee in full extension, capsular and other secondary restraints (e.g., the biceps femoris and popliteus) resist varus stress, even when the LCL is disrupted. Flexion helps relax the secondary restraints for primary testing of the LCL.[66]

If excessive lateral joint line opening is seen in full extension, a more severe injury to the secondary structures must be assumed. Lateral joint space opening with the knee in full extension indicates some degree of injury to the LCL, posterolateral capsule, arcuate–popliteus complex, iliotibial band, biceps femoris tendon, ACL, PCL, and lateral head of the gastrocnemius. With this more severe injury, the results of one or more rotatory instability tests are also positive.

Anterior Cruciate Ligament

Lachman's Test. Outside of the operating room, Lachman's test is the most sensitive clinical test for determining disruption of the ACL, particularly the anteromedial band.[67-69] Lachman's test isolates the ACL, which acts as the primary restraining force preventing anterior translation of the tibia relative to the femur (Figure 20-18, *A*). Similar to testing of the MCL and LCL, the leg is held in approximately 20° to 30° of flexion to relax secondary stabilizers. The amount of anterior translation and the quality of the end point indicate potential injury to the ACL. The grade of laxity is measured in comparison to the normal contralateral knee, not as the degree of absolute translation. Greater laxity of the uninjured knee may be associated with poorer outcomes after reconstruction.[70] The degrees of anterior translation can be affected by several other factors. A large effusion or displaced meniscal tear can diminish the degree of translation. Muscular guarding and the position of the foot can also affect the side-to-side difference. With an incompetent PCL, the tibia sags posteriorly at rest, giving a false sense of increased anterior translation. Also, a false-negative result on Lachman's test can occur if the ACL scars to the PCL to the roof of the intercondylar notch. A pseudo-end point is detected in these cases. A meta-analysis of 20 studies showed the overall sensitivity of Lachman's test was 81% and specificity 81%; with anesthesia, the sensitivity was 91% and specificity was 78%.[71]

Anterior Drawer Test. The anterior drawer test is the oldest test but has been shown to be the least sensitive for detecting ACL injuries because it is generally positive only with loss of both ACL and the secondary restraints such as the posterior horn of the medial meniscus. False-negative results also can occur with a displaced ("bucket handle")

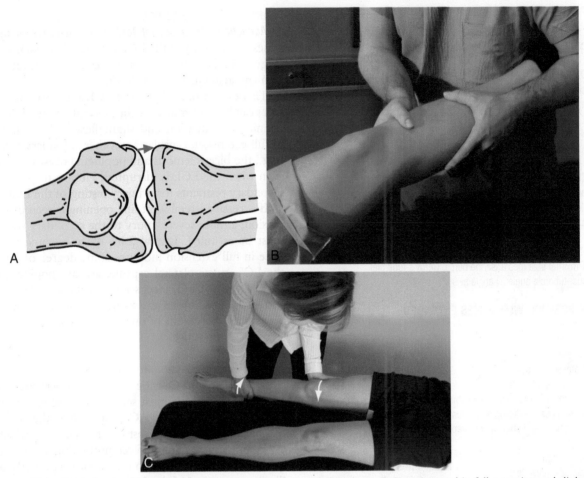

Figure 20-15 Abduction (valgus) stress test. **A,** Gapping of the medial aspect of the knee. **B,** Knee is tested in full extension and slightly flexed (20° to 30°). **C,** Valgus stress applied with thigh supported on examination table. (**A** and **C,** From Magee DJ: *Orthopedic physical assessment*, ed 6, p 812, St. Louis, 2014, Saunders/Elsevier.)

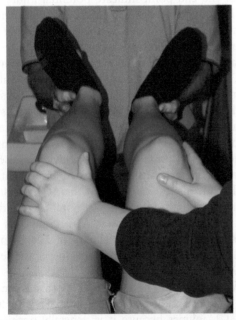

Figure 20-16 Tibial lateral (external) rotation (dial) test. Side-to-side differences in tibial external (lateral) rotation are compared at 90° of knee flexion. A side-to-side difference of more than 15° suggests posterolateral corner involvement.

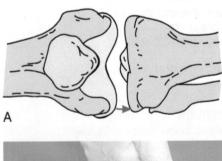

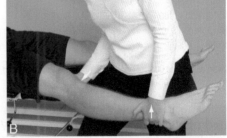

Figure 20-17 Adduction (varus stress) test. **A,** One-plane lateral instability "gapping" on the lateral aspect. **B,** Positioning for testing lateral collateral ligament in extension. (From Magee DJ: *Orthopedic physical assessment*, ed 6, p 814, St. Louis, 2014, Saunders/Elsevier.)

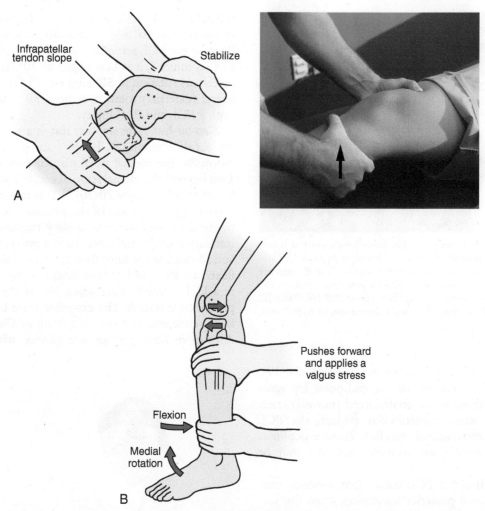

Figure 20-18 Physical examination of the ACL. **A,** Lachman's test is performed with the knee in about 30° of flexion and provides the most sensitive and specific test for the ACL in the office setting. **B,** The pivot shift test. This test is performed with the patient supine. The examiner places the heel of one hand behind the head of the fibula and the other hand on the foot. With the knee in full extension and hip in slight flexion and abduction, lateral (external) rotation of the tibia is combined with an axial load and valgus force to the knee. A positive pivot results at about 20° of flexion as the lateral tibial plateau reduces back into position. This test is very specific but often requires muscle relaxation in the operating room to increase sensitivity. (**A** [*line art only*] and **B,** From Magee DJ: *Orthopedic physical assessment*, ed 6, pp 817, 824, St. Louis, 2014, Saunders/Elsevier.)

meniscal tear, hamstring spasm, and hemarthrosis. For the anterior drawer test, the sensitivity has been reported to be 38% and specificity was 81%.[71]

Pivot Shift Test. The pivot shift test is used to test for injury to the ACL and to assess anterolateral rotatory instability of the knee.[72-74] During this test, the tibia subluxes anterolaterally on the femur (Figure 20-18, *B*).[74] This recreates the anterior subluxation-reduction phenomenon that occurs during functional activities when the ACL is torn. A positive pivot shift test is pathognomonic for ACL deficiency. Unfortunately, the sensitivity of the test is affected by guarding and muscular splinting. The sensitivity improves dramatically if the test is done with the patient under anesthesia.[75] Varying the position of the hip (i.e., into abduction and slight flexion) and lateral (external) rotation of the tibia can enhance the pivot shift.[72] Many other modifications have been proposed to improve the

accuracy of the pivot shift test.[76] This test can differentiate partial tears of the ACL from complete injuries. A tear is considered complete if rotational instability is demonstrated by a positive pivot shift test result. Meta-analysis showed the pivot shift test to have sensitivity of 28% and specificity of 81%, which improved with anesthesia to 73% sensitivity and 98% specificity.[71] Because of its specificity, the pivot shift test, particularly under anesthesia, can be considered the most important assessment in the evaluation of an ACL injury.

Posterior Cruciate Ligament and Posterolateral Corner

Posterior Drawer Test. An isolated tear of the PCL leads to increased posterior translation of the tibia that increases with knee flexion. The most accurate means of diagnosing this injury is the posterior drawer test with the knee flexed at 90°.[77,78] The test is performed as described

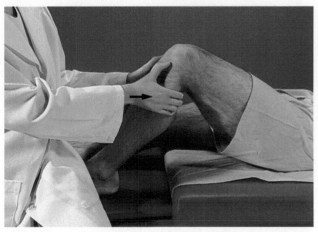

Figure 20-19 Posterior drawer test. The posterior drawer test is performed with the knee in 90° flexion. The examiner palpates the hamstrings posteriorly to make sure they are relaxed. The thumbs are placed in the anterior joint line to palpate posterior translation of the tibia when a posterior force is applied. (From Ball JW, Dains JE, Flynn JA, et al: *Seidel's guide to physical examination*, ed 8, St. Louis, Mosby, 2015.)

in *Orthopedic Physical Assessment* (Figure 20-19). The amount of translation and the end point are again compared with those in the contralateral (normal) knee. If excessive posterior translation is evident, the PCL (primarily the anterolateral bundle), arcuate–popliteus complex, posterior oblique ligament, and ACL may be injured.

Truly isolated acute PCL tears often produce only minimally increased posterior translation when the secondary restraints of the knee are intact, particularly the posterior capsule and posteromedial and posterolateral structures. Some studies have suggested that the meniscofemoral ligaments are strong and may act as secondary stabilizers to PCL function. A posterior drawer test with the leg in medial (internal) rotation is reduced if the posterolateral structures or, as some investigators have suggested, the meniscofemoral ligaments are intact.[79] Some investigators believe that a posterior drawer cannot occur with an intact arcuate–popliteus complex, although laboratory studies have revealed that a posterior drawer of no more than 10 mm (0.5 inch), as compared with the contralateral side, can occur with an isolated PCL injury. False-negative results can occur with a displaced bucket handle meniscal tear, hamstring or quadriceps spasm, and hemarthrosis. In combination, tests for PCL injury have an accuracy of 96%, sensitivity of 90%, and specificity of 99%.[80] Although it is important also to assess the end point of the posterior drawer test, the end point may return to a normal, firm feel in chronically PCL-deficient knees. Thus the quality of the end point is not as sensitive as with Lachman's test.

Tibial External Rotation (Dial Test) (see Figure 20-16). Because isolated PCL injury does not increase tibial rotation, a PLC injury should be suspected if there is any increased lateral (external) rotation. The dial test examines the side-to-side difference in lateral (external) rotation of the tibia at 90° and then at 30° of knee flexion.[66,81,82] Because the PCL serves as a secondary restraint when the PLC is injured, it is best tested at 90°. Increased lateral (external) rotation at 30° suggests PLC injury. Increased lateral (external) rotation at both 30° and 90° suggests both a PCL and PLC injury.

Step-off Test. The step-off test is a sensitive uniplanar test for determining PCL injury and posterior instability. Normally, the medial tibial plateau protrudes anteriorly 1 cm beyond the medial femoral condyle when the knee is flexed to 90° (Figure 20-20).[83] This step-off is lost when there is a posterior sag of the tibia associated with injury to the PCL and other secondary restraints to posterior translation of the tibia. Similarly, a **posterior sag test** involved viewing the knee from the lateral side with the hip flexed to 45° and the knee flexed to 90° and is positive in a PCL-deficient knee when loss of the tibial tubercle prominence is seen. The examiner must be aware of tibial tubercle enlargement (as a result of Osgood-Schlatter disease) or tibial plateau osteophytes, which can give a

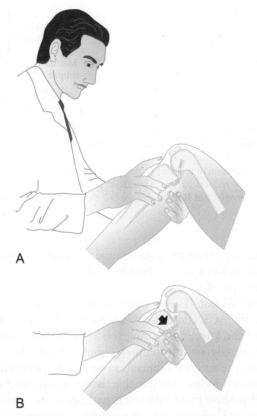

Figure 20-20 Step-off test. **A,** Normal relationship of the tibiofemoral joint. The medial tibial plateau protrudes anteriorly approximately 1 cm (0.5 inch) beyond the medial femoral condyle. **B,** With injury to the posterior cruciate ligament, the step-off is lost. The medial tibial plateau now lies either in line with or posterior to the medial femoral condyle. (Adapted from Miller MD, Harner CD, Koshiwaguchi S: Acute posterior cruciate ligament injuries. In Fu FH, Harner CD, Vince KG, editors: *Knee surgery*, vol 1, Baltimore, 1994, Williams & Wilkins.)

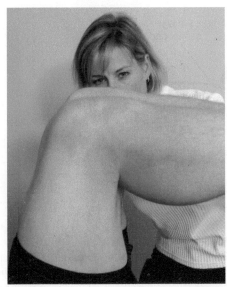

Figure 20-21 Godfrey's test. This posterior sag test is performed with the patient's hips and knees flexed to 90°. Examiner watches for posterior shift, which is not evident in this case. (From Magee DJ: *Orthopedic physical assessment*, ed 6, p 820, St. Louis, 2014, Saunders/Elsevier.)

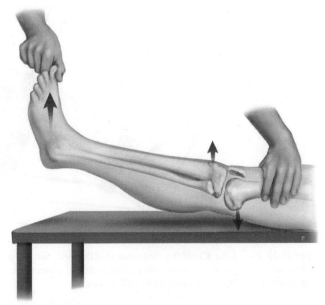

Figure 20-22 External rotation recurvatum test. To perform this test, the examiner grasps the individual's big toes and lifts the leg, allowing both knees to go into passive hyperextension. The test result is positive if the affected knee hyperextends to a greater degree than the noninvolved knee and appears to be in valgus alignment. Also, the tibial tuberosity is displaced laterally as the lateral tibial plateau subluxes posteriorly. (Redrawn from LaPrade RF, Ly TV, Griffith C: The external rotation recurvatum test revisited, *Am J Sports Med* 36:709–771, 2008.)

false-negative result. Different degrees of posterior sag represent varying degrees of injury to the PCL, arcuate–popliteus complex, posterior oblique ligament, and ACL. The quadriceps active drawer test[84] and Godfrey's sign (Figure 20-21) also can be used to test the PCL.

Hughston's Posteromedial and Posterolateral Drawer Signs. Although an isolated injury to the PCL has little effect on tibial rotational laxity or varus or valgus angulation, concomitant injury to the secondary extra-articular restraints results in some aspects of rotatory instability. Posteromedial and posterolateral drawer tests assess rotatory instability combined with PCL injury and are analogous to the Slocum test for rotatory instability associated with ACL injury.[85] With the patient positioned as for the posterior drawer test, the foot is medially (internally) rotated 30°. Posteromedial rotatory instability is present if most of the posterior translation occurs on the medial side of the knee and/or if the amount of posterior translation increases or does not change. Posteromedial rotatory instability is a result of varying degrees of injury to the PCL, posterior oblique ligament, MCL (deep and superficial), semimembranosus muscle, posteromedial capsule, and ACL (posteromedial corner).

Next, the patient's foot is placed in 15° lateral (external) rotation as the examiner sits on the patient's forefoot. If most of the posterior translation occurs on the lateral side of the knee and/or if the amount of posterior translation increases or does not change, posterolateral rotatory instability is present, indicating an injury to the PCL, arcuate–popliteus complex, LCL, biceps femoris tendon, posterolateral capsule, and ACL (i.e., posterolateral corner). Over-rotating the foot can lead to a false-negative test because this can tighten other secondary and tertiary restraints.

External Rotation Recurvatum Test (Figure 20-22). In some cases of posterolateral rotatory instability, lifting the big toe of the individual causes a hyperextended knee, which rotates into valgus to a greater extent than the uninvolved side.[85]

Reverse (Jakob) Pivot Shift Test. The reverse (Jakob) pivot test is the most sensitive test for posterolateral rotatory instability and is analogous to the pivot shift for ACL deficiency.[86,87] Unfortunately, the test is not pathognomonic for PCL injury because up to 35% of normal knees may have a positive reverse pivot test result.[88]

Instrumented Testing of the Knee

Evaluation of the ligamentous instability of the knee has been classically defined by its associated physical examination findings. Lachman's test is a sensitive indicator of ACL injury, and the pivot shift is highly specific. These tests, however, suffer from different interobserver and intraobserver variability. Several knee ligament arthrometers have been developed as a means to standardize and quantify ligamentous examinations. Several ligament testing devices are commercially available for clinical use to quantify laxity of the knee. These include the KT1000 Knee Ligament Arthrometer, the Acufex Knee Signature System (Acufex Microsurgical, Norwood, MA), the Genucom Knee Analysis System (FaroMedical, Toronto, Canada), the Rolimeter (Aircast, Boca Raton, FL), and the Stryker Knee Laxity Tester (Stryker Corp., Kalamazoo, MI). Of these, the KT1000 arthrometer has been most widely used (Figure 20-23).

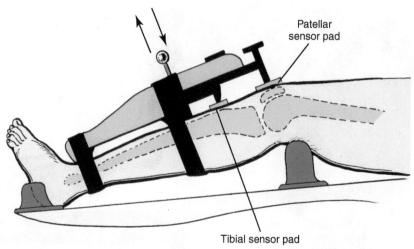

Figure 20-23 Use of the KT1000 arthrometer (MEDmetric, San Diego, CA) to quantify tibial translation. Relative movement of the tibiofemoral joint is measured as motion between the patellar and tibial sensor pads. (From Zachazewski JE, Magee DJ, Quillen WS, editors: *Athletic injuries and rehabilitation*, p 650, Philadelphia, 1996, WB Saunders.)

The reliability and validity of these devices have been widely studied.[89-101] The Acufex and Genucom arthrometers appear to be less reliable than the KT1000 with higher standard deviation (SD) of measurements.[95,96] Intratester reliability and intertester reliability for the KT1000 have been reported to be high, both within and between days.[100] Wroble et al.[96] indicated that the 90% confidence limit for right-left difference with the KT1000 was ±1.6 mm when measured at 89 N and ±1.5 mm when measured at 134 N. A confidence interval of this magnitude is within acceptable limits for the clinical diagnosis of ACL injuries. In vitro and in vivo studies have shown the KT1000 to be a valid measure for the detection of ACL injury. The correlation between measurements made with the KT1000 and those made with direct transducer readings in cadaveric knees was 0.97.[89] The mean anterior displacement in ACL-intact cadaveric knees was found to be 5.8 mm, which increased to 12.1 mm when the ACL was sectioned. In vivo studies reported that 92% of normal subjects had a side-to-side difference in anterior displacement of less than 2 mm, whereas 96% with confirmed unilateral disruption of the ACL had a side-to-side difference in anterior displacement more than 2 mm.[89] Based on this research, the KT1000 appears to be a clinically applicable instrument that can be used to assess anterior laxity in patients with an ACL-deficient knee.

Importantly, before using the KT1000 to assess AP laxity of the knee, the clinician must screen for PCL injury. This is done by observing for lack of a step-off between the medial femoral condyle and the medial tibial plateau. The posterior sag test or the active quadriceps drawer test (or both) also can be done to rule out injury to the PCL. Failure to detect a PCL-deficient knee before testing with the KT1000 may result in a false-positive result for anterior laxity, so the test procedure must be modified. Please refer to *Orthopedic Physical Assessment* for more specifics regarding KT1000 testing.

Clinical Note

Before doing instrumented testing of the knee for ACL injury, the knee must be cleared for PCL deficiency.

The major criticism of instrumented testing of the knee, including use of the KT1000, has been that it does not quantify rotation. A clinical failure with a positive pivot shift, could have a normal Lachman's test result and normal KT1000 parameters. For this reason, various techniques[102] have been developed to assess rotation stability of the knee via MRI,[103] inertial and gyroscopic sensors,[104,105] and optical tracking systems.[106]

Special Diagnostic Studies

Radiography

Radiographs of the knee should be obtained after any acute trauma. If the trauma was severe and the patient reports pain when the knee is moved, radiographs should be obtained before the physical examination is started. Fractures must be ruled out before the knee is moved through any ROM or manipulated because displacement of the fracture may damage other structures, including neurovascular structures.

Our standard radiographic series for the knee includes a 45° flexion weight-bearing posteroanterior (PA), AP, lateral, and merchant views. Because ligaments and menisci are radiolucent, radiography is used for the most part to exclude other causes of knee pain, swelling, deformity, and/or loss of function. Other radiographs obtained in special circumstances that may be beneficial include a long cassette AP weight-bearing view to assess alignment; stress radiographs in cases of suspected rotational injury; a cross-table lateral view to look for hemarthrosis with a fat-fluid level, an indication of a fracture; and lateral (external) and medial (internal) rotation views to look for loose bodies or oblique fracture lines.

Standard Radiographic Series for the Knee

- 45° flexion weight-bearing posteroanterior view
- Anteroposterior view
- Lateral view
- Merchant view

When viewing standard radiographs of the knee, the examiner should look for any obvious intra-articular or osteochondral fractures, calcifications, joint space narrowing, epiphyseal damage, osteophytes or lipping, loose bodies, tumors, accessory ossification centers, alignment deformity (varus–valgus), patellar alta or baja, asymmetry of the femoral condyles, and dislocations. Secondary signs can be seen on plain radiographs to help diagnose ligamentous or meniscal injury.

Soft tissue swelling as seen on radiographs is helpful when the injured structures are surrounded by fat. An MCL injury may reveal only soft tissue swelling on the medial aspect of the knee. A bloody effusion, often associated with intra-articular ligament damage, is detected as a soft tissue density in the suprapatellar pouch on the lateral view. Fat in the effusion, or lipohemarthrosis, suggests a fracture (e.g., osteochondral or intra-articular) and is identified as a fat-fluid level on a cross-table lateral projection. Although fat globules occasionally are seen in many other types of effusions, the accumulation of fat is much greater in cases of trauma.[107] Meniscal tears, although often associated with effusions, do not produce as large an effusion as a cruciate ligament disruption or intra-articular fracture. Furthermore, the timing of the radiograph in relation to the time of injury is important because cruciate ligament injuries are associated with acute effusions, but meniscal tears usually do not produce a significant effusion for at least 12 hours.

Although extensive fractures about the knee are readily identified by standard radiographs, careful evaluation of the films may be required to detect avulsion injuries at the attachment sites of ligaments. This is particularly true in children, in whom cruciate ligament injuries frequently involve avulsion fractures. An avulsion of the ACL insertion may be seen on the flexion AP radiograph or on the lateral view by identifying the displaced fragment superior and anterior to the tibial spine.[108] **Segond's fracture**, also known as the **lateral capsular sign**, is an avulsion fracture of the lateral capsule posterior to Gerdy's tubercle on the proximal lateral tibia.[109] This fracture, seen on AP radiographs, is an indirect sign of ACL injury. The thin fragment of bone is vertically oriented and located proximal and anterior to the

fibular head and should not be confused with a lateral ligamentous injury. Avulsion of the tibial insertion of the PCL may be seen on lateral radiographs in the posterior intercondylar area. A PCL avulsion may be a small flake of bone or a large bony fragment. Lateral ligamentous injury may be identified on an AP or external rotation view as an avulsion of the biceps femoris or LCL insertion from the fibular head, or the **"arcuate sign."**[110] Uncommonly, the MCL or LCL may avulse from the femoral condyle with a bony fragment. These injuries can be identified on AP radiographs.

A lateral radiograph can be used to identify a **lateral femoral notch sign**, a deepening of the terminal sulcus and a sign of an ACL-deficient knee.[111,112] Located on the lateral femoral condyle at the junction between the weight-bearing tibial articular surface and the patellar articular surface, the terminal sulcus is the usual location of the impaction injury caused by collision of the femoral condyle with the posterior tibial plateau. Depressions more than 2 mm in this area may represent osteochondral fractures and are often correlated with higher energy pivoting injuries and lateral meniscal tears.[113]

Chronic knee injuries may also produce abnormal findings on radiographic studies. A chronic MCL injury may result in calcification at the site of injury. When this occurs at the femoral origin of the MCL, it is called **Pellegrini-Stieda disease**. Although the natural history of isolated cruciate ligament injuries is debated, most authors agree that if left untreated, the unstable knee develops degenerative osteoarthritic changes. Osteoarthritic change in the cruciate-deficient knee tends to occur first in the medial compartment, but the compartment with meniscal pathology often develops degenerative changes.[114] This is best seen on 45° flexion, weight-bearing PA radiographs.[115] Degenerative changes identified on radiographs in a patient with a history of trivial trauma with signs of possible meniscal pathology may suggest a degenerative meniscal tear.

Stress radiography has been advocated for knee ligament injuries, but it is difficult to carry out after acute trauma.[111] In a chronic injury or in the anesthetized patient, these radiographs are more easily obtained and can be valuable. Stress radiography is particularly popular in Europe to document knee instability in the sagittal and frontal planes[116–120]; however, it is not used as often in the United States. For MCL injury, manual stress radiographs show significant medial joint gapping.[121] Recently, the importance of stress radiography in evaluating PLC and other rotational stabilities of the knee has been advocated (Figure 20-24).[122]

Arthrography

Traditionally, single-contrast and double-contrast arthrography served as the gold standard for evaluating the menisci and plica and, to a lesser extent, the cruciate

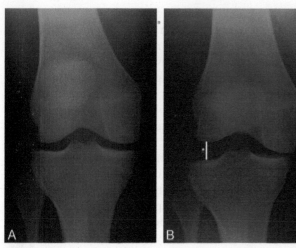

Figure 20-24 Stress radiographs of the knee. **A,** Non–weight-bearing AP radiograph in a suspected posterolateral corner injury. **B,** Varus stress radiograph in the same knee. The degree of opening of the lateral compartment (*) has correlated with posterolateral corner injury and can aid in decision making regarding surgical intervention. (From Gwathmey FW Jr, Tompkins MA, Gaskin CM, Miller MD: Can stress radiography of the knee help characterize posterolateral corner injury? *Clin Orthop Relat Res* 470:770, 2012.)

ligaments and articular surfaces.[123-129] However, this method is limited in that it is an uncomfortable, invasive procedure that requires a great deal of expertise to perform and interpret, and it exposes the patient to irradiation. It was more widely used before the advent of arthroscopy and magnetic resonance imaging (MRI). Arthrography has been largely replaced by those two modalities in most centers, but it still may be used in specialized situations to resolve a specific question or when the availability or quality of MRI is limited.

Radionuclide Scintigraphy

Radionuclide scintigraphy uses technetium-99 methylene diphosphonate (MDP) to screen for a variety of abnormalities. In general, the scintigram reflects the relative blood flow to an area and the degree of bone turnover (i.e., osteogenesis and osteolysis). The test is sensitive but nonspecific. It provides more information about osseous physiology than structural characteristics. The technique traditionally has been used to evaluate arthritic joints, stress fractures, tumors, osteonecrosis, infection, osteolysis, metabolic or metastatic bone disease, and reflex sympathetic dystrophy. Increased osseous metabolic activity, as determined by scintigraphy, has also been seen with knee disorders previously considered to involve only soft tissue failure, including symptomatic tears of the ACL.[130-136]

Diagnostic Ultrasonography

Ultrasonography has been used to evaluate various structures of the knee, including the menisci and ligaments.[137] It is most useful in the evaluation of patellar tendonitis

and partial patellar tendon tears. This technique is technician dependent, and although it is inexpensive, it has not been popularized for routine use in the evaluation of ligamentous and meniscal injuries. It is used in the United States primarily for evaluating patellar tendonitis and masses about the knee.

Computed Tomography

Ever since the early application of computed tomography (CT) to the musculoskeletal system, this technique has been used to evaluate many disorders of the knee.[138-140] However, CT scanning is best used for bony detail because soft tissue detail is better seen with MRI or arthroscopy. Many conflicting descriptions have been reported with respect to the need for and type of intraarticular contrast material and patient positioning in the CT scanner. Therefore, clinical use of CT scanning after meniscal and ligamentous injury currently is not widely accepted.

Magnetic Resonance Imaging

MRI is a sensitive, noninvasive, nonionizing radiation means of evaluating the structural integrity of the knee. It is particularly helpful for visualizing soft tissue structures. At first, MRI met some resistance because initial studies were less accurate than double contrast arthrography, and the procedure was time-consuming and expensive.[141-144] Improvements in hardware and software, as well as increasing expertise in the interpretation of these studies, have overcome these problems, and MRI has become the procedure of choice for evaluating acute knee injuries.[145-150] Partial and complete tears of ligaments and menisci, as well as other pathological changes, such as bone bruises and effusions, can be identified with MRI. Evaluation of the knee by MRI is reader dependent, but its accuracy approaches 100% in diagnosing lesions of the PCL, ACL, medial meniscus, and lateral meniscus (diagnosis is least accurate with the lateral meniscus).[145,148,150-153] Some clinicians believe this technique is overused,[154] and in the future its use may be limited by the expense. Nonetheless, MRI can help diagnose injuries when the patient cannot relax for an adequate examination and can provide additional information about concomitant intra-articular knee injuries.

Increased signal intensity in the subchondral bone (i.e., bone bruises) has been found in specific patterns. Up to 80% of patients with an ACL injury show increased subchondral signal in the posterior aspect of the lateral tibial plateau and the anterior aspect of the lateral femoral condyle as a result of abnormal impaction of these surfaces secondary to the transient subluxation of the lateral compartment after an ACL injury (Figure 20-25).[155-157] This pattern is distinctly different from bone bruises seen after patellar dislocation and PCL injury. Bone bruises are less common after isolated PCL injuries.

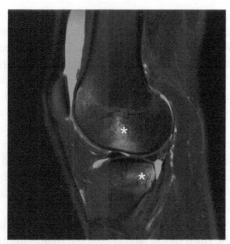

Figure 20-25 MRI of a knee demonstrating bone bruises (*) on the posterolateral tibia and at the anterior lateral femoral condyle characteristic of the knee subluxation seen with ACL injury.

Indications for an MRI

- An acutely injured knee in which an ACL tear is likely but it is unclear whether the patient has associated meniscal or chondral pathology
- Complete evaluation for preoperative planning for a knee with multiple-ligament injuries
- Unclear diagnosis based on the history, physical examination, and standard radiographs
- A patient who cannot relax or cooperate during the physical examination
- Clinical course not commensurate with the clinical diagnosis
- A high-level athlete with an acute injury who needs an immediate, thorough evaluation to determine the extent of injury and the need for surgical or nonoperative treatment
- Evaluation of an occult fracture or to assess physeal injury
- Investigation of the cause of poor ROM after ligament reconstruction surgery

Other uses of MRI include evaluation for soft tissue masses, tumors, osteonecrosis, osteochondritis dissecans, and extensor mechanism injuries, including tendonitis.

Arthroscopy

Arthroscopy currently is the most commonly performed orthopedic procedure in the United States. It allows for direct visualization of all intra-articular structures, and it can be used to diagnose and surgically treat lesions of the knee. For many acute knee injuries, the best opportunity for complete recovery is with prompt, appropriate surgical treatment. The benefit of arthroscopy, therefore, is that all pathology can be correctly identified and treated as needed. Arthroscopy uses smaller incisions than open surgery, allows better visualization with less morbidity, and can be performed without the use of a tourniquet. Partial tears of the ACL sometimes cannot be differentiated from complete tears, even with an examination

under anesthesia. Using arthroscopy, the surgeon can determine whether the ACL is partially or completely torn. Furthermore, if the ligament is partially torn, the extent of injury can be ascertained to guide treatment. Arthroscopy can also be used to evaluate meniscal pathology and determine whether the lesion should be left alone, repaired, or excised. It also has been shown that complete, isolated PCL disruptions may yield a negative posterior drawer sign, even under anesthesia, but these can be diagnosed with arthroscopy.[158]

Although invasive, arthroscopy is a relatively low-risk procedure; it has a complication rate of less than 1% and an infection rate of approximately 0.1%.[159-161] Although the risk of anesthesia exists, some authors have reported local anesthesia to be effective and safe.[162-166] This is important because several investigators are evaluating the efficacy of diagnostic and therapeutic office arthroscopy.[167-170] Nonetheless, diagnostic arthroscopy has been largely replaced by MRI.

EPIDEMIOLOGY, BIOMECHANICS, AND CLASSIFICATION OF KNEE LIGAMENT INJURIES

Straight Plane versus Rotatory Instabilities

The terminology used to classify knee ligament injuries is the source of much confusion. This partly arises from the use of inappropriate terminology to describe and classify movement of the knee. Noyes et al.[171,172] defined terms that should be used to describe the motion and position of the knee. Motion of the knee is accompanied by rotation and translation of the joint surfaces. *Translation* refers to movement that results when all points of an object move along paths parallel to each other. A fixed point on one surface engages successive points on the opposing surface, much like a tire sliding on an ice patch when the brakes are locked. In the knee, translation of the tibia has three independent components, known as *translational degrees of freedom:* medial-lateral translation, anterior-posterior translation, and proximal-distal translation. Translation of the tibia is commonly reported in millimeters of motion.

Rotation occurs when successive points on a given surface meet successive points on an adjacent surface. The surface appears to be going in circles about an axis of rotation. Rotation of the joint is similar to a tire rolling down a road. In the knee, rotation has three independent degrees of freedom. Flexion and extension rotation occurs in the sagittal plane about an axis located through the femur, which lies in the coronal plane. Abduction and adduction rotation occurs in the coronal plane through an axis in the sagittal plane. Internal (medial) and external (lateral) rotation occurs in the transverse plane around a vertical axis, which is located near the PCL. Rotation of the knee is measured in degrees of motion.

Motion of the knee involves a complex combination of rotation and translation of the joint surfaces. Based on the convex–concave rule, flexion of the knee is associated with posterior translation and rotation of the tibia. When the tibia is fixed, flexion of the knee occurs as posterior rotation and anterior translation of the femur. Extension of the knee involves anterior rotation and translation of the tibia. When the tibia is fixed, extension of the knee involves anterior rotation and posterior translation of the femur. This combination of rotation and translation is necessary to keep the femur centered over the tibial plateau throughout the ROM. As described earlier, rotation and translation of the joint surfaces during movement of the knee are controlled by the geometry of the joint surfaces, tension in the ligamentous structures, and muscular contraction. Disruption of ligamentous or musculotendinous structures alters the normal arthrokinematics of the knee and may lead to progressive degeneration of the joint surfaces.

The terms *laxity* and *instability* often are used interchangeably. The meaning of these terms must be clarified to improve communication among health care professionals in the evaluation and treatment of knee ligament injuries. The term *laxity* can be used to indicate slackness or lack of tension in a ligament or to describe looseness of a joint. *Laxity* also is used to indicate the amount of joint motion or play that results with the application of forces and moments. Laxity of a joint can be normal or abnormal; therefore the adjective *abnormal* should be used to indicate laxity that is pathological. In addition, *laxity* can refer to either translation or rotation, and this should be clearly specified. For example, *anterior laxity* of the knee can refer either to anterior translation or to rotation of the tibia. If *anterior laxity* is used to describe translation of the tibia, the more precise (and preferable) term is *anterior translation*. The amount of laxity often is recorded as the difference between the involved and noninvolved knees, and this should be clearly indicated. Owing to the ambiguity in the use of the term *laxity,* Noyes et al.[173] recommended that it not be used to describe joint motion or displacement. They recommended that the term be used in a more general sense to indicate slackness or lack of tension in a ligament. When referring to motion of the knee, it is preferable to describe the specific motion as *translation* or *rotation.*

According to Noyes et al.,[171] the term *instability* can be used to describe the symptom of giving way or the physical sign of increased mobility of the joint. To avoid ambiguity, they recommend avoiding use of the term *instability* to indicate an episode of giving way. They prefer to use it to indicate a physical sign that is characterized by an increased or excessive displacement of the tibia resulting from traumatic injury to the stabilizing structures.

Ligamentous injury to the knee results in varying degrees of abnormal laxity or instability, as just described. Hughston et al.[174] classified instability that arises as a result of a knee ligament injury as straight plane or rotatory instability, with straight plane implying equal translation of the medial and lateral tibial plateaus. Rotatory instabilities involve unequal movement of the medial and lateral tibial plateaus and can include anteromedial, anterolateral, and posterolateral instabilities. Anteromedial rotatory instability occurs when the medial compartment ligaments, including the posterior oblique ligament, are torn. Anteromedial rotatory instability may be accentuated by a tear of the ACL. With anteromedial rotatory instability, a valgus stress test at 30° flexion is positive. In addition, increased anterior translation of the medial tibial plateau is seen when an anterior drawer test is performed with the tibia laterally (externally) rotated, and the medial pivot shift test may be positive.

Anterolateral rotatory instability occurs with injury to the middle third of the lateral capsular ligaments and is accentuated by a tear of the ACL. With anterolateral instability, an anterior drawer test results in increased anterior translation of the lateral tibial plateau. The lateral pivot shift test also is positive.

Posterolateral rotatory instability implies greater posterior translation of the lateral tibial plateau compared with the medial tibial plateau when a posterior drawer force is applied. Posterolateral instability occurs with a tear of the arcuate complex, which results in a positive varus stress test at 30° flexion. The external (lateral) rotation recurvatum test also is positive.

Combined rotatory instabilities, such as anteromedial and anterolateral rotatory instability, also can occur.

Butler et al.[19] developed the concept of primary and secondary ligamentous restraints. For each plane of motion of the knee, one ligamentous structure serves as the primary restraint. This structure is responsible for restraining most of the motion in a given direction. For example, the ACL is the primary restraint for anterior translation of the tibia, providing approximately 85% of the restraining force.[19] As the name implies, secondary restraints are structures that take on a secondary role in restraining motion in a particular direction. For example, the secondary restraints for anterior tibial translation are the collateral ligaments, the middle portion of the medial and lateral capsule, and the iliotibial band. These structures are responsible for providing approximately 15% of the total restraining force to anterior translation of the tibia.[19]

Care must be taken to avoid thinking solely in terms of straight plane stability versus rotatory instabilities and primary versus secondary restraints. There are many components to stability including bony, capsular, ligamentous, and musculotendinous structures that contribute to a functionally stable knee. As such, it is vitally important to accurately diagnose instability and, in particular, to look for concomitant injuries because missed instability components negatively impact outcomes. For example, knees with untreated combined ACL–MCL injuries showed increased valgus laxity and a reduction in tissue quality of the healed MCL.[175] Early ACL reconstruction in combined ACL and MCL injuries may provide a more stable environment for MCL healing.[176] In combined ACL and PLC injuries, failure to address the PLC injury will lead to failure of the ACL reconstruction. Thus, one must consider that rotatory instabilities and combined injuries exist, and that missed injuries lead to poor results.

The amount of ligament laxity or instability after injury to the ligamentous structures of the knee depends on the extent of injury and the amount of force applied. Injury to the primary restraint that leaves the secondary restraints intact may result in a minimal increase in laxity during manual examination of the knee. However, if both the primary and secondary restraints are injured or stretched, clinical tests for laxity may demonstrate a large increase in motion compared with the noninvolved side. For example, isolated injury to the ACL may result in only a slight increase in anterior tibial translation if the secondary restraints are intact. Over time, with repeated episodes of giving way, the secondary restraints may stretch out, resulting in increased anterior tibial translation. Similarly, when posterior drawer testing shows more than 10 mm posterior tibial translation, associated ACL and/or PLC injury should be suspected in addition to PCL injury. It is important to note that the secondary stabilizers are not as effective as the primary stabilizers in restraining motion in a particular direction. Therefore, over time, the secondary restraints tend to stretch out gradually when the primary restraint has been lost.

Another important consideration for clinicians in performing and interpreting a clinical laxity test is the amount of force applied to the knee. Forces applied during a clinical laxity test are small, ranging from 9.1 to 18.1 kg (20 to 40 pounds). This is much less than the forces involved in in vivo activities, which may exceed 45.4 kg (100 pounds) with strenuous exercise.[19] As a result, clinical laxity tests may not accurately describe the stability of the knee in performing strenuous physical activities. The clinical laxity test may demonstrate only a slight degree of increased laxity. When more strenuous activities are performed, higher loads are placed on the knee, which may result in greater laxity and in complaints of giving way.

Anterior Cruciate Ligament

The ACL is one of the most commonly injured ligaments in the knee. The ACL is the primary stabilizer for resisting anterior translation of the tibia on the femur and serves to control hyperextension of the knee. The ACL also serves as a secondary stabilizer to resist internal (medial) and external (lateral) rotation, as well as varus and valgus stress. The ACL can be injured by contact or noncontact mechanisms of injury. Pathomechanics include a valgus force applied to a flexed, laterally (externally) rotated knee with the foot planted, or hyperextension, often combined with medial (internal) rotation. Less common mechanisms of injury include hyperflexion or a direct valgus force.

Mechanisms of Injury to the Anterior Cruciate Ligament

- Valgus force applied to a flexed, laterally rotated knee with the foot planted
- Hyperextension (often combined with medial rotation)
- Hyperflexion
- Direct valgus force

Daniel et al.[62] reported that the incidence of acute ACL injury among members of a managed health care plan was 31 per 100,000 members annually. Ninety percent of ACL injuries occurred in patients 15 to 45 years of age. Most ACL injuries occur as a result of sports activities, particularly those that place high demands on the knee (e.g., those involving jumping and hard cutting).[177] Skiing may be a particularly high-risk activity; the incidence of ACL injury among adult skiers is 1 in 2000.[178]

A narrow intercondylar notch or the notch geometry itself may place a patient at greater risk of injury.[179] LaPrade and Burnett[180] reported a higher incidence of acute ACL injuries in individuals with a narrow notch width index. The notch width index is the ratio of the width of the anterior outlet of the intercondylar notch divided by the total condylar width at the level of the popliteal groove. These researchers' prospective study involved 213 athletes at a Division I university, representing 415 ACL-intact knees. Intercondylar notch stenosis was found in 40 knees (i.e., a notch width index less than 0.2), and 375 individuals had a normal notch width index. During the 2-year follow-up period, seven ACL injuries occurred, six in knees with a narrow notch, and one in a knee with a normal notch width. Souryal and Freeman[181] reported similar results in 902 high school athletes followed prospectively. The overall rate of ACL injury during the 2-year follow-up was 3%. Athletes who sustained noncontact ACL tears had a statistically smaller notch width index. Of the 14 athletes with noncontact ACL injuries, 10 had a notch width index at least 1 SD below the mean. Notch geometry has been proposed as one anatomic factor leading to an increased risk of ACL injury in women.

Female athletes have a four to eight times the risk for ACL injury over their male counterparts. Malone[182] reported that women participating in National Collegiate Athletic Association (NCAA) Division I basketball were eight times more likely than their male counterparts to sustain an ACL injury. Females appear to have some unique characteristics that may predispose them to ACL injury, including a wider pelvis, increased genu valgum, altered muscular recruitment patterns, increased ligament laxity, and different biomechanical movement patterns during athletic participation.[182–185] Females have increased quadriceps to hamstring strength ratios and land in a more erect posture, which may place greater strain on the ACL.[172,186] Altered valgus knee torques and neuromuscular control of the trunk predict ACL injury risk in female athletes and have been the subject of neuromuscular training interventions designed to prevent ACL injury.[187,188]

Of ACL ruptures, 75% occur in the midsubstance, 20% involve the femoral attachment, and 5% involve the tibial attachment.[189] Associated injuries include meniscal tears in 50% to 70% of acutely injured knees and in up to 90% of chronic, ACL-deficient knees,[63,158,190] chondral injuries in 6% to 20% of ACL-injured knees,[63,158] collateral ligament injuries in 40% to 75% of ACL-injured knees,[190,191] and occasionally capsular injuries and knee dislocations.

Up to 80% of patients have reported hearing or feeling an audible crack or pop at the time of initial injury.[63] The acute hemiarthrosis from the ACL tear produces knee swelling within the first 2 to 6 hours after injury. A slower appearance of knee swelling, however, can be indicative of capsular injury, or even an acute on chronic ACL injury.

Classification of ACL injuries is based on the extent of the tear and the resulting instability and is largely a clinical diagnosis. Patients with partial tears have increased anterior translation, as documented by the Lachman's test or instrumented laxity testing, but they have a negative pivot shift test under anesthesia. If loss of ligament function and rotational instability are demonstrated by a positive pivot shift test, the ACL tear is considered complete. Although this determination can often be made in the clinic, an examination under anesthesia may be required to establish a definitive diagnosis.

The natural history of an ACL-deficient knee is still unclear. A torn ACL does not heal, although research investigating the use of bioenhanced ACL repair with a bioactive scaffold has reported some promise.[192–194] ACL deficiency leads to rotatory instability in many patients and results in functional disability. This instability can occur with ADLs in some, with sports activities such as running and stopping (i.e., deceleration), cutting, and jumping in others, and with no functional instability in still another undetermined group. Repetitive episodes of instability may result in meniscal tears, which can result in arthritis. Debate exists as to whether isolated ACL tears, without meniscal pathology, result in degenerative changes within the knee joint.[62,73,190,192,195–197] ACL-deficient patients who undergo meniscectomy without ACL reconstruction develop degenerative changes more quickly; this is more apparent in patients having higher activity levels.[198] A direct relationship exists between giving way (i.e., instability) and the activity level, but many patients with an ACL-deficient knee can return to sports at a less stressful level of activity. Furthermore, functional instability may also be related to meniscal pathology. As is discussed later in this chapter, meniscal injury directly relates to the level of disability, pain, and swelling and the frequency of reinjury.

Posterior Cruciate Ligament

Although the true incidence of PCL injuries is unknown, they are thought to account for 3% to 40% of all knee injuries.[199–202] PCL injury may be more common than realized. PCL injuries are easily missed because clinicians are less familiar with the clinical examination findings.

The PCL is the strongest ligament in the knee,[203] and a significant force is required to rupture it. Most PCL injuries occur as a result of athletic, motor vehicle, or industrial accidents. The mechanism of most athletic PCL injuries is a fall on the flexed knee with the foot and ankle plantar-flexed.[79,204] This imparts a posteriorly directed force on the proximal tibia, which ruptures the taut ligament that is parallel to the force vector, usually resulting in an isolated PCL injury.[205] Similarly, in a motor vehicle accident, the knee is flexed and the tibia is forced posteriorly on impact with the dashboard. Another mechanism of injury to the PCL is a downwardly directed force applied to the thigh while the knee is hyperflexed, such as when landing from a jump.[75] Hyperflexion of the knee without a direct blow to the tibia can also result in an isolated PCL injury.[206]

Mechanisms of Injury to the Posterior Cruciate Ligament

- Fall on a flexed knee with the ankle plantar flexed
- Dashboard injury
- Downward force to the thigh while the knee is hyperflexed
- Hyperflexion

Other mechanisms can result in injury to the PCL, but these usually also involve injury to other ligaments. Forced hyperextension does not commonly result in injury to the PCL.[207] Rather, hyperextension is more likely to lead to injury to the posterior knee capsule, popliteal vessel, and/or ACL.[200] A posteriorly directed force applied to the anteromedial tibia with the knee in hyperextension may also cause injury to the posterolateral corner[200] and results in lateral and posterolateral instability. Significant varus or valgus stress injures the PCL only after rupture of the appropriate collateral ligament. Therefore, when the PCL is torn, the integrity of the rest of the knee must be carefully evaluated.

Clinical Note

If the posterior cruciate has been torn, the integrity of the other ligaments, posterior corners, capsule, and menisci must be carefully examined.

Seventy percent of PCL disruptions occur on the tibial side, with or without an associated bony fragment; 15% occur on the femoral side, and 15% involve midsubstance tears.[189] Associated injuries with acute "isolated" PCL tears include chondral defects in 12% and meniscal tears in 27%, which occur more commonly in the lateral compartment.[208] As with chronic ACL tears, the incidence of meniscal and chondral lesions is higher in chronic PCL-deficient knees,[208] although in contrast with acute injuries, these more commonly involve the medial compartment.

The patient often reports an audible crack or pop at the time of the initial injury. The patient also notes mild to moderate swelling within the first 2 to 6 hours; however, unlike with ACL injuries, these individuals may return to activity, and the injury often is thought to be a minor event. Patients frequently complain of an unstable gait, but pain with weight bearing or anterior knee pain is common. Pain in patients with a chronic PCL-deficient knee also may be partly due to degeneration of the medial or patellofemoral compartments.[207] Walking down stairs loads the patellofemoral compartment and will often exacerbate the pain.

As with the classification of ACL injuries, grading of PCL injuries depends on the extent of the tear and the degree of resulting laxity. A grade I PCL sprain involves microscopic partial tearing of the ligament, which overall remains intact. The ligament fibers are stretched, causing hemorrhage and microscopic disruption of the ligament. Examination of a grade I PCL injury reveals no increased laxity compared with the contralateral knee, and the end point is firm. A grade II sprain is also a partial tear, although the injury results in partial loss of function, as determined by a slight increase in posterior translation during a posterior drawer test; however, a definite end point is noted, and the reverse pivot shift test is negative. This may be a macroscopic or microscopic tear that results in hemorrhage and stretching of the ligament, but the ligament is still in continuity and functions to some degree. A grade III sprain of the PCL is a complete tear of the ligament. Loss of both ligament function and joint stability are seen; the posterior drawer test result is 2+ to 3+; and the posterior sag test, Godfrey's sign, the quadriceps active drawer test, and the reverse pivot shift test are positive. Posterior tibial translation is excessive, and the end point is soft.

The natural history of the PCL-deficient knee remains controversial, and experience with treatment of PCL ruptures is not as advanced as with ACL injuries because PCL injuries are less common and more difficult to treat surgically. Some of these patients experience almost no functional limitation and compete in high-level athletics, whereas others are severely limited during ADLs.[204,206,209,210] Parolie and Bergfeld[204] suggested that, if adequate quadriceps strength can be obtained, most patients do well with nonoperative treatment. Dejour et al.[211] suggested that patients are symptomatic for the first 12 months, during which time they learn to adapt to the PCL injury. After this time, patients do well, and a high percentage returning to sports. They also reported the development of degenerative changes involving the medial and anterior compartment in chronic PCL-deficient knees,[211] but this finding has not been reported by others.[79,204,209]

Not all authors agree on the success of nonoperative treatment. Clancy et al.[79] reported degenerative changes in the medial compartment in 90% of patients at a 4-year follow-up. Dandy and Pusey[212] followed patients for an average of 7.2 years. Of these patients, 70% had pain while walking, and 55% had patellofemoral symptoms. No correlation was seen between ligament laxity and functional results in the group. Keller et al.[210] reported on a series of 40 patients at the 6-year follow-up. They found the longer the interval between injury and follow-up, the lower the knee score. The presence of radiographic degenerative changes directly correlated with lower knee scores despite excellent muscular strength. In PCL-deficient knees, altered kinematics result in a shift in the tibiofemoral contact location and increased medial compartment cartilage deformation beyond 75° of knee flexion.[213] Similarly, with long-term follow-up (15 years), Dejour et al.[211] found progressive deterioration of outcomes. Eighty-nine percent of patients with isolated PCL injuries had pain, and 79% of knees had degenerative changes. These researchers described the natural history of PCL deficiency as having three phases: functional adaptation, functional tolerance, and osteoarthritic deterioration.

A recent larger study by Shelbourne,[214] however, prospectively evaluated a series of 68 patients with isolated PCL injuries treated nonoperatively for an average of 17.6 years. Subjective clinical scores were good and patients remained active.[214] Surprisingly, moderate to severe arthritis was noted in only 11% of patients.

Whether surgical reconstruction for PCL tears can alter the development of long-term degenerative changes is unclear. Furthermore, in some patients the PCL apparently may heal although in a lengthened position.[215] This may explain the variable results of long-term studies of the PCL-deficient knee.

Medial Collateral Ligament

The MCL is the most commonly injured ligament in the knee.[199] However, the incidence of grade III injuries to the MCL may be lower than the incidence of high-grade ACL tears.[199] The MCL is injured by a valgus stress to the knee that exceeds the strength of the MCL. This most commonly occurs from a blow to the lateral aspect of the knee during a sports event. Uncommonly, a noncontact valgus injury to the knee, such as occurs in skiing, can produce an isolated tear of the MCL. Approximately 60% of skiing knee injuries affect the MCL.[216] The most injurious sports for MCL injury include wrestling, hockey, judo, and rugby.[217] Males are at greater risk than female athletes, and the average amount of time lost per injury has been reported as 23 days.[217]

Mechanism of Injury to the Medial Collateral Ligament

- Valgus stress to a weight-bearing knee

MCL injuries most commonly involve the femoral insertion site, which accounts for approximately 65% of all MCL sprains. Approximately 25% of MCL sprains involve the tibial insertion. The remaining 10% of MCL injuries involve a deep portion of the MCL at the level of the joint line.[189] Associated tears of the medial meniscus occur in 2% to 4% of grade I and grade II MCL sprains, but medial meniscal tears generally do not occur with grade III MCL sprains.[218-220] This is most likely because compression of the medial compartment is required to tear the medial meniscus, whereas injury to the MCL requires tension that unloads the medial compartment.

The diagnosis of an MCL injury can be made from the history and physical examination alone and usually does not require MRI or arthroscopy. However, if the physical examination is difficult to perform because of pain or muscle spasm or if damage to other intra-articular structures is suspected, an MRI can be helpful for determining the full extent of the injury. The patient often recalls being hit by another athlete while the foot was planted, feeling the impact on the lateral aspect of the knee and pain on the medial aspect of the knee. In rare cases, patients may note a pop at the time of injury, but they more commonly state that they felt a tearing or pulling on the medial aspect of the knee. Swelling occurs quickly at the site of injury, and ecchymosis may develop 1 to 3 days after injury. With a grade I or II sprain, the patient may be able to continue to play, but with a grade III sprain, the patient usually cannot continue to participate in sports. These patients usually walk with a limp and with the knee partially flexed because extension stretches the ligament and causes further pain. The patient may not have an effusion if the injury is isolated to the MCL.

Classification of MCL sprains depends on the extent of the tear and the degree of laxity that results. A grade I sprain involves microscopic tearing of the ligament, which overall remains intact. The ligament fibers are stretched, causing hemorrhage and microscopic disruption of the ligament. Examination of the MCL by the aforementioned tests reveals no increase in laxity compared with the contralateral knee, and the end point is firm. However, tenderness is present along the ligament. A grade II sprain of the MCL is also a partial tear, but the injury results in partial loss of function, as determined by a slight degree of increased joint opening (i.e., 3 to 5 mm) on a valgus stress test with the knee in 30° flexion and a definite end point is noted. In full extension, the knee joint opens less than 2 mm more than the contralateral knee. A grade II sprain may represent macroscopic or microscopic tearing, resulting in hemorrhage and stretching of the ligament,

but the ligament is still in continuity and functions to some degree. An acute grade II MCL injury is tender to palpation, and the patient notes pain with stress testing. A grade III sprain is a complete tear (i.e., both superficial and deep fibers) of the ligament. Loss of ligament function occurs, and a joint space opening of more than 5 mm compared with the noninvolved knee is seen on a valgus stress test at 30° flexion while an opening of more than 3 mm compared with the noninvolved knee occurs in full extension. Also, no definite end point is noted with stress testing. Significant joint opening in full extension indicates medial capsular injury and possibly injury to the cruciate ligaments.

Transection of the MCL results in 2° to 5° of laxity or 3 to 5 mm of joint opening when a valgus stress is applied, whereas transection of both the MCL and the posteromedial capsule results in 7° to 10° of laxity, indicating that both MCL and capsule play an important role in resisting valgus stress.[221] The severity of tenderness does not correlate with the extent of injury. A grade III sprain usually hurts less than a grade II or grade I injury because complete tearing eliminates stress to ligament fibers.

Use of MRI has allowed for accurate diagnoses of MCL sprains. Ligament tears can be classified by their involvement of the deep and superficial portions of the MCL. This is important, as a "complete" tear of the deep MCL is a very different clinical entity than a "complete" tear of the superficial MCL.

The natural history of isolated MCL tears is a process of healing after the injury, regardless of the degree of injury.[219,220,222-226] Patients with proximal injuries involving the femoral insertion tend to have a higher incidence of stiffness. Also, proximal MCL injuries heal with less residual laxity compared with injuries involving the tibial (distal) end. Partial and complete MCL tears significantly increase the load on the ACL, an important factor to consider in patients with multiligamentous injuries.[227]

Posteromedial Corner of the Knee

In addition to MCL injury, it is important to consider and assess for injury to the posterior oblique ligament (POL) and posterior capsule, which have been shown to be important valgus and rotational stabilizers of the knee.[228,229] In one series of surgically treated isolated and combined medial-sided knee injuries, 99% of the knees were found to have an injury to the POL, 70% had injury of the semimembranosus capsular attachment, and 30% were found to have complete peripheral detachment of the meniscus.[230]

In addition to valgus stress testing in flexion, the clinician must assess for opening of the medial joint space with the knee in full extension. The POL, posteromedial capsule, MCL, and cruciates all contribute to knee stability in full extension. Asymmetrical joint opening in full extension makes an isolated MCL injury unlikely, and one should suspect concomitant injury to the posteromedial capsule and POL, and possibly the ACL in addition to the MCL injury. An anterior drawer test in lateral (external) rotation may provide additional information regarding medial-sided injuries. With POL and capsular injury leading to grade III laxity in full extension, patients may have an avulsion of the posterior horn of the medial meniscus root that may require surgical intervention. The POL has also been shown to have an important role in preventing additional posterior tibial translation in the knee with PCL injury.[231]

Investigating the extent of injury to the POL and posterior capsule is important in decision making because nonoperative treatment of these injuries may be more likely to lead to unsatisfactory results. The resulting rotational instability, in addition to valgus laxity, may not be tolerated by athletes participating in pivoting sports.

Lateral Collateral Ligament

Isolated injuries to the LCL of the knee are uncommon. In fact, they tend to be the least common injury to the knee, causing only 2% of all knee injuries that result in pathological motion (i.e., grade III injuries).[199] The injury usually is the result of a direct varus stress to the knee, generally with the foot planted and the knee in extension.[159] Injury to the LCL tends to occur as a result of nonsport, high-energy activities[159,199] because a direct blow to the medial aspect of the knee is an unusual occurrence in sports. Varus stress to the knee may also occur during the stance phase of gait, with sudden imbalance and a shift of the center of gravity away from the side of injury resulting in tension on the lateral structures. This mechanism does not require an external force to the knee. Another cause of a varus stress to the knee is a sideswipe injury, in which one knee has a valgus stress and the other a varus stress. The varus injury often has a rotational component.

Mechanism of Injury to the Lateral Collateral Ligament

- Varus stress to a weight-bearing, extended knee

Straight varus injuries can result in LCL disruptions. These injuries tend to be tears from the fibular head, with or without avulsion in 75% of cases, from the femoral side in 20%, and midsubstance tears in 5%.[189] Associated peroneal nerve injuries are common (up to 24%) because the nerve is tethered as it courses around the fibular head.[159] These nerve palsies have a poor prognosis for complete recovery.[232]

Patients with injury to the LCL may hear or feel a pop in the knee and have lateral knee pain. An intra-articular effusion may represent a capsular injury or an associated meniscal or chondral lesion. Because the LCL is extra-articular, isolated LCL lesions do not commonly result in an effusion of the knee.

Often, LCL injuries occur in association with injury to other ligaments in the knee. A severe varus stress results in an LCL disruption, followed by disruption of the posterolateral capsule and PCL. The PLC should be assessed with stress tests for increased varus rotation and lateral (external) rotation at 30° and 90° and compared with the opposite knee (Dial test).[81,82]

Classification of LCL sprains depends on the extent of the tear and the resulting degree of laxity. A grade I sprain involves microscopic partial tearing of the ligament, but the ligament overall remains intact. The ligament fibers are stretched, causing hemorrhage and microscopic disruption within the ligament. Varus stress testing reveals no increase in laxity compared with the contralateral knee, and the end point is firm; however, tenderness is present along the ligament. A grade II sprain is also a partial tear, but the injury results in partial loss of function, as determined by a slight increase in joint opening with varus stress testing (i.e., 3 to 5 mm) compared with the noninvolved knee with the knee in 30° flexion and a definite end point is noted. In full extension, the knee joint opens less than 2 mm more than the contralateral knee. A grade II LCL sprain may represent macroscopic or microscopic tearing, resulting in hemorrhage and stretching of the ligament, but the ligament is still in continuity and functions to some degree. A grade II acutely injured LCL is tender to palpation, and the patient notes pain with stress testing. A grade III sprain is a complete tear of the ligament. Loss of ligament function occurs, and a joint space opening of more than 5 mm compared with the noninvolved knee is seen with varus stress testing in 30° flexion. An opening of 3 mm or more than the noninvolved knee is seen in full extension. In addition, no definite end point is noted with varus stress testing. Palpation of the ligament in the figure-of-four position reveals absence of tension in the ligament proximal to the fibular head.

The natural history of the untreated, complete LCL disruption has yet to be determined. Only a few studies with a limited number of subjects have involved isolated LCL injuries. DeLee et al.[159] suggested that severe, straight lateral instability with more than 10 mm of joint opening compared with the contralateral knee usually implies that the ACL or the PCL (or both) has been injured. From the few studies that have been reported, truly isolated LCL injuries appear to do well with nonoperative treatment.[159,223,226]

Posterolateral Corner of the Knee

Most PLC injuries occur during athletics, motor vehicle accidents, and falls.[233–236] A typical mechanism involves a posterolaterally directed force to the anteromedial tibia, leading to hyperextension and a varus force being applied to the knee. Other mechanisms include knee hyperextension or severe tibial lateral (external) rotation in a partially flexed knee.[237] A study investigating ultra-low-velocity knee dislocations in obese patients found 50% had injury to the lateral-sided structures.[238] The PLC (Figure 20-26) is the primary stabilizer of lateral (external) tibial rotation at all knee flexion angles.

Isolated PLC injuries are rare, because they are more commonly associated with concomitant ligamentous injuries such as ACL and PCL tears or with tibial plateau fractures. Approximately 9% of patients presenting with a knee hemarthrosis had a PLC injury in one study.[239] Recognizing vascular injury is of crucial importance, particularly in the dislocated or multiligamentous injured knee. Most patients have swelling diffusely over the posterolateral joint, and all have tenderness.[240] Varus stress examination is important, with both knees in full extension as well as at 30° of flexion. Tests directed at the PLC can be performed.

PLC injuries are most commonly classified based on varus instability. Grade I injuries are sprains, without significant varus instability. Grade II injuries are partial, with minimal laxity (i.e., approximately 6 to 10 mm). Grade III injuries are complete disruptions with more than 10 mm of laxity. Rotational stability should also be assessed, for example, via the Dial test. Varus-stress radiographs

showing increased lateral joint space widening of 4.0 mm suggests an isolated grade III PLC injury; widening of 6.6 mm suggests a combined posterolateral corner and ACL tear, while widening of 7.8 mm suggests posterolateral corner, ACL, and PCL injuries.[241]

An alternative classification system attempts to incorporate lateral (external) rotation instability in addition to varus instability. This divides injuries into type A or isolated rotational injury to the PFL and popliteus tendon complex. Type B is a rotational injury with mild varus component, indicating injury to PFL and popliteus tendon as well as LCL attenuation. Type C posterolateral instability has significant rotational and varus components due to complete disruption of the PFL, popliteus tendon complex, LCL, lateral capsule, and cruciate ligament(s).[242]

Correctly recognizing and treating PLC injuries and resultant rotatory instability is of critical importance because failure to address such injuries has a negative impact on outcomes. Concomitant cruciate ligament reconstructions have inferior outcomes when combined with grade II posterolateral injuries treated conservatively.[243-245] Thus posterolateral injuries and rotatory instabilities must be recognized and addressed so as to not jeopardize outcomes.

DISLOCATIONS AND MULTIPLE-LIGAMENT KNEE INJURIES

Knee dislocations and other, less severe multiple-ligament injuries account for approximately 20% of all grade III ligament injuries of the knee.[199] This diverse group of injuries has a variable severity and co-morbidity. Other than combined ACL–MCL injuries, combined ligament injuries account for fewer than 2% of all knee ligament injuries.[199] Frequent combinations of two-ligament injuries include the ACL–MCL (most common), PCL–MCL, PCL–LCL, ACL–LCL, and ACL–PCL.

To dislocate the knee, at least three ligaments must be torn.[246] In most knee dislocations, both cruciate ligaments and one collateral ligament are torn. Fractures occasionally are associated with knee dislocations, but these fracture-dislocations are considered a different entity from a dislocated knee and involve injury only to the ligaments.

A person may dislocate the knee by simply stepping in a hole and hyperextending the knee (low energy) or from a high-energy blow to the knee, such as can occur in a motor vehicle accident. Athletes have sustained low energy knee dislocations during collisions in baseball, rugby, football, and soccer.

Neurovascular injury is uncommon with knee injuries that involve only two ligaments. However, an LCL injury combined with a cruciate ligament injury can result in enough lateral joint opening to produce injury to the peroneal nerve.

Although the knee can dislocate in any direction, the most common directions are anterior and posterior.[247,248]

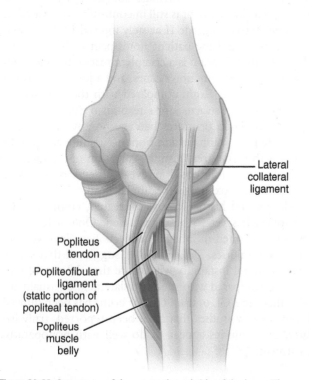

Lateral collateral ligament

Popliteus tendon

Popliteofibular ligament (static portion of popliteal tendon)

Popliteus muscle belly

Figure 20-26 Structures of the posterolateral side of the knee. The popliteofibular ligament or static portion of the popliteus tendon arises from the posterior aspect of the fibular head then travels with the main popliteus tendon to its insertion site on the lateral femur. This static portion of the popliteus tendon is nearly isometric and is positioned to resist posterolateral tibial rotations. (From Canale ST, Beaty JH: *Campbell's operative orthopaedics,* ed 12, Philadelphia, 2013, Elsevier.)

Knee dislocations may involve damage to multiple structures within the knee, including the cruciate and collateral ligaments, capsular structures, menisci, articular surface, tendons, and neurovascular structures. The nerves and blood vessels in the popliteal space of the knee are easily stretched and torn during dislocation of the knee, and neurovascular injury must be ruled out in all cases. Associated injuries include vascular damage in 20% to 40% of knee dislocations and nerve damage in 20% to 30%. Some knee dislocation case series reports have an amputation rate of the involved extremity of up to 49%.[247,249,250] Posterior knee dislocations are associated with the highest incidence of popliteal artery injury,[247] and posterolateral rotatory dislocations have the highest incidence of nerve injury.[251] Some evidence suggests that low-velocity knee dislocations may uncommonly result in neurovascular injury.[252] On the other hand, ultra-low-velocity knee dislocations in morbidly obese individuals have a very high rate of vascular injury.[253] The likelihood of combined neurovascular injury tends to increase as body mass index (BMI) increases.[238] These individuals may also have a greater incidence of postoperative complications.[254]

Evaluation of vascular status should include palpation of pulses and comparison of the ankle-brachial index (ABI). This test involves taking the blood pressure at the ankle and on the arm at rest and is repeated at both sites after 5 minutes of treadmill walking. It is used to predict the severity of peripheral arterial disease (PAD). If pulses are asymmetrical or if an abnormal ABI is obtained, an arteriogram is required. Recent evidence suggests that serial vascular examinations may replace the arteriogram if ABIs are normal.[255]

Osteochondral and meniscal injuries are rare, particularly with low-velocity knee dislocations. This is most likely due to a distraction force being required to dislocate the knee, whereas osteochondral and meniscal injuries are caused by compressive forces.[251]

The patient with a multiple-ligament injury frequently gives a history of severe injury to the knee, although, as noted earlier, the mechanism may be trivial. The patient often hears a pop. Swelling occurs within the first few hours, but it is not always large because of the associated capsular injury and extravasation of the hemarthrosis into the surrounding tissue. The patient may note deformity of the knee if the knee dislocated and remains unreduced. The patient complains of instability and inability to continue with sports and ADLs.

Tibiofemoral dislocations are classified by the direction in which the tibia translates in relation to the femur. As mentioned, the knee can dislocate in any direction. For example, if the tibia lies anterior to the femur, the injury is an anterior dislocation. Posterior, medial, and lateral dislocations of the knee also can occur. Rotatory dislocations occur when the knee dislocates in more than one direction; these include anteromedial, anterolateral, posteromedial, and posterolateral dislocations. Unfortunately, knee dislocations can reduce spontaneously; therefore this classification

scheme is not useful. Furthermore, the amount of tibial displacement that occurs at the time of injury cannot be estimated from physical or radiographic findings. It therefore is helpful to describe the dislocated knee by the ligamentous structures that have been disrupted.

The natural history of knee dislocations and multiple-ligament injuries is unknown. This is because of the uncommon nature of these injuries and the many types of dislocations and mechanisms of injury (e.g., low velocity versus high velocity) that can occur. However, vascular injury associated with a knee dislocation, if left untreated or if not repaired within 8 hours of the time of injury, results in an 86% amputation rate. If surgery to correct vascular injury is completed within 6 to 8 hours, the amputation rate is only 11%.[252] Associated nerve injuries have a poor prognosis for recovery, regardless of the treatment.[256,257]

The development of instability, loss of motion, and arthritis at the knee is unclear with nonoperative treatment. The level of function of patients with multiple-ligament injuries is worse than those with an isolated knee ligament injury. Knee dislocations treated with immobilization and aggressive rehabilitation have surprisingly good results with regard to stability, absence of pain, and the range of knee flexion up to 90°.[258] The incidence of arthritis after multiple-ligament injuries has yet to be determined, but increased instability would be expected to result in a greater degree of arthritic change. Controversies exist regarding the treatment of knee dislocations and multiligament reconstruction, particularly with regard to role of arteriography, acute surgical treatment, role of joint-spanning external fixation, and approach to ligamentous repair or reconstruction.[259]

TREATMENT OF KNEE LIGAMENT INJURIES

Guidelines for Progression of Rehabilitation

Progression of the rehabilitation program after knee ligament injury and/or surgery should proceed in a logical sequence. Generally, the phases of this progression overlap. For example, muscle function may be addressed before full ROM and flexibility has been restored. Progression of the patient through the sequence must be individualized and depends on the nature of the injury and/or surgery, principles of tissue healing, individual signs and symptoms, and the response to treatment. Adequate time must be allowed for tissue healing and remodeling. During rehabilitation, care must be taken to avoid overaggressive treatment, which is indicated by a prolonged increase in pain after treatment and/or regression in the patient's progress.

Clinical Note

Overaggressive treatment may lead to increased pain after treatment or regression of the patient's progress.

Determinants of Rehabilitation Progression

- Nature of injury
- Nature of surgery
- Tissue healing principles
- Tissue healing timelines
- Patient's signs and symptoms
- Patient's response to treatment

The initial phase of the rehabilitation program should promote tissue healing and reduce pain and swelling. During this period, treatments such as cryotherapy and compression may be beneficial for decreasing pain and swelling. A balance must be achieved between mobility and immobility. The healing tissues must not be overloaded; however, some amount of stress is believed to be necessary for proper tissue strength and alignment, as discussed later in the chapter. Overaggressive treatment during this period can disrupt the healing process, but prolonged immobilization also can have adverse effects. Prolonged immobilization is associated with decreased bone mass, changes in the articular cartilage, synovial adhesions, and decreased muscle strength and increased stiffness of ligaments and the joint capsule, which lead to joint contracture and loss of motion. Disuse results in atrophy and diminished oxidative capacity of muscle. Immobilization appears to affect slow muscle fibers more than fast muscle fibers.[260,261]

The time required for soft tissue healing varies. The response of soft tissue to injury is acute inflammation, which typically lasts several days or until the noxious stimulus has been neutralized. During this period, applications of cold and compression may be used to limit and control acute inflammation. Inflammation is followed by fibroplasia, which involves the proliferation of fibroblasts and the formation of collagen fibers and ground substance. Fibroplasia usually lasts for several weeks and results in the formation of granulation tissue, which is fragile, vascularized connective tissue. During this period, protected motion is encouraged because it stimulates collagen formation and alignment. Excessive loading of the healing tissue should be avoided because it may disrupt the healing tissue and reinitiate the inflammatory process. Over time, granulation tissue matures and remodels and can withstand greater loads. This process is gradual and depends on the stresses imposed on the tissue; stresses should be gradually and progressively increased to allow the tissues to adapt to the functional demands placed on them.

Rehabilitation of the knee should ensure that full symmetrical motion to the involved knee is restored. Loss of motion after knee ligament injury and/or surgery adversely affects function. Loss of extension affects gait and results in patellofemoral symptoms. Loss of flexion interferes with activities such as stair climbing, squatting, and running. In the early phases of rehabilitation, passive, active-assisted, and active ROM exercises can be used to increase and/or maintain motion of the knee. In the latter stages of rehabilitation, active and passive stretching can be used to restore motion. Stretching should be sustained (e.g., L3D technique—low load, long duration) and should use low force to maximize creep and relaxation of connective tissue to produce permanent elongation. Application of heat before and during the stretch and maintaining the stretch during cooling may also help produce permanent elongation.[262] Neurophysiological stretching techniques, such as contract/relax or contract/relax/contract, can help restore motion if the limitation is caused by muscular tightness.

Mobilization of the patella also may be helpful in restoring motion. Inferior glide of the patella is necessary for flexion, and superior glide is necessary for normal functioning of the extensor mechanism. Decreased superior mobility of the patella interferes with the ability of the quadriceps to pull through the knee extensor mechanism and results in the development of a knee extensor lag. Medial glide and lateral tilt of the patella are necessary to stretch the lateral retinacular structures. The force used during patellar mobilization must be appropriate for the degree of inflammation present. Overly aggressive patellar mobilization aggravates pain and swelling, which can contribute to loss of motion. Mobilization of the tibiofemoral joint is rarely necessary but can help restore motion if the limitation of motion is due to hypomobility of the tibiofemoral joint.

Rehabilitation after knee ligament injury and/or surgery must restore function of the muscles that cross the knee as well as the muscles that influence segments proximal and distal to the knee. After acute knee injury or in the immediate postoperative period, the emphasis should be on regaining motor control. Often acute pain and swelling result in inhibition of the quadriceps muscles, and a knee extensor lag develops. During this period, quadriceps sets, straight-leg raises (SLRs), co-contraction in weight bearing (i.e., CKC), and isometric hamstring exercises can be performed. Facilitation techniques such as vibration and tapping, as well as biofeedback and electrical stimulation, may be helpful in regaining motor control. Generally, gaining quadriceps control is more difficult than gaining control of the hamstring muscles.

Resistive exercises are initiated when the individual has regained full active motion of the knee. Initially, resistive exercises should be performed with light resistance and high repetitions to improve muscle endurance. This minimizes stress on healing structures about the knee and improves the aerobic capacity of slow twitch muscle fibers. OKC exercises can be used to provide isolated exercise for the hamstring and quadriceps muscles. Precautions must be taken to avoid overloading healing tissues and to prevent the development of patellofemoral symptoms. CKC exercises can be used to improve muscle function in functional patterns while minimizing patellofemoral stress. CKC exercises are progressed as tolerated and may include wall slides, minisquats, step-ups, and leg presses. Cycling is an excellent exercise for developing endurance of the lower extremity musculature while minimizing stress on the patellofemoral and tibiofemoral joints. Other forms of endurance exercise for the lower extremities include step machines, cross-country ski machines, and swimming.

In the later phases of rehabilitation, resistive exercises can be progressed to high-resistance, low-repetition exercises to develop muscle strength and power. High-resistance, low-repetition OKC exercises are used to improve isolated muscle strength, but care must be taken to avoid overloading the patellofemoral joint, as described earlier in this chapter. High-resistance, low-repetition CKC exercises can be used to improve strength in functional patterns with less risk of patellofemoral symptoms; however, patellofemoral mechanisms should always be considered with the rehabilitation of any knee injury.

Exercises should incorporate the concentric and eccentric phases of contraction. Concentric muscle function is necessary to accelerate the body, whereas eccentric muscle function is necessary to decelerate the body and to act as a shock absorber. During a concentric contraction, the muscle shortens as it contracts, whereas during an eccentric contraction, the muscle elongates as it contracts. The force–velocity relationship is different for concentric and eccentric contractions. During a concentric contraction, muscle force decreases as the speed of shortening increases. During an eccentric contraction, muscle force increases as the speed of lengthening increases. Eccentric contractions produce higher levels of force as a result of lengthening of the series elastic component and facilitation of the stretch reflex. Failure to incorporate eccentric exercise into the rehabilitation program results in the development of muscle soreness and an increased risk of reinjury with return to activity. Econcentric (i.e., pseudoisometric) exercises should also be included in the middle and late stages for two joint muscles (i.e., quadriceps, hamstrings, and gastrocnemius) because this action is how these muscles act functionally (e.g., flexing hip and knee at same time, as in running, causes the rectus femoris to shorten at the hip and lengthen at the knee while the hamstrings lengthen at the hip and shorten at the knee).

For athletes who require power to perform their sport, plyometric exercises should be incorporated into the final stages of the rehabilitation program. Plyometric exercises develop power and speed and incorporate lengthening of the muscle immediately before a powerful concentric contraction. These exercises include depth drops and jumps from heights of 15 to 46 cm (6 to 18 inches), bounding, hopping, and ricochets. The plyometric program must be carefully planned and implemented to avoid injury.

Once the strength and endurance of the lower extremity musculature have been established, neuromuscular control must be developed to enhance dynamic stability of the knee. This requires learning how to recruit muscles with the proper force, timing, and sequence to prevent abnormal joint motion. Initially, it requires conscious effort, often with the help of biofeedback. Through practice and repetition, control of abnormal joint motion becomes automatic and occurs subconsciously.

Proprioceptive neuromuscular facilitation techniques, such as rhythmic stabilization and timing for emphasis, may be helpful for developing dynamic stability. A variety of functional activities also can be used to develop dynamic control of abnormal joint motion. These activities generally are progressed from slow to fast speed, from low to high force, and from controlled to uncontrolled activities. The emphasis should be on establishing proper movement patterns to enhance dynamic stability of the joint. EMG biofeedback may be used to ensure that muscles are being recruited in the proper sequence to maintain joint stability. Activities for enhancing dynamic stability progress from walking, jogging/running, acceleration/deceleration, sprinting, jumping, cutting, pivoting, and twisting.

Anterior Cruciate Ligament Injuries

Treatment of ACL injuries must be individualized and depends on the extent of pathology and the level of disability experienced by the patient during sports and ADLs. Therefore decisions regarding the treatment of the ACL-deficient knee must be made in collaboration with the patient, physician, physical therapist, and athletic trainer. The type of treatment depends on many factors, including age, activity level, occupation, desire to continue sports, amount of functional instability, presence of associated injuries and arthritic changes, and amount of laxity. The patient's willingness to modify activity to a level compatible with functional stability is the most important factor governing treatment options.

Most studies of the natural history of conservative treatment of ACL injuries have shown poor results in young patients. Persistent instability is common. Noyes et al.[263] reported a 65% incidence of giving way during activity, which was associated with persistent pain and disability for several days thereafter. Hawkins et al.[264] reported that 86% of patients in his case series had similar findings. Furthermore, the ability to return to strenuous activity is limited without reconstruction; only 14% to 22% of patients in this younger age group return to the same level as their previous activity.[264-266]

In older patients, who accept limitations on their activities, results generally are better. Ciccotti et al.[267] evaluated a series of 40- to 60-year-old patients who were treated conservatively for ACL tears. Ninety-seven percent had a grade 2 or grade 3 on Lachman's test, and 83% had a positive result on the pivot shift test; the overall satisfaction rate was 83%.

Even so, without treatment, ACL insufficiency predisposes the patient to injury of other knee structures. The risk for additional lesions of the menisci and cartilage increases with time, potentially as a result of decreased rotational stability.[192,266,268-272] Progressive degeneration of the knee has been cited, especially when associated with meniscal tears.[266,273] At 20-year follow-up, osteoarthritic changes have been noted to occur with ACL insufficiency in 21% to 100% of patients and in 14% to 37% of patients after ACL reconstruction.[274]

A systematic review of outcomes after ACL injury evaluated 27 cohorts containing 1585 patients who had undergone reconstruction and compared 13 cohorts containing 685 patients treated nonoperatively.[275] Results at a mean of 14 years demonstrated patients who underwent ACL reconstruction had fewer subsequent meniscal injuries, less need for further surgery, and better improvement in activity level. Both groups had similar rates of development of radiographically evident osteoarthritis.

Researchers have attempted to classify patients by defining risk for instability. Factors associated with a good outcome for nonoperative treatment include intact collateral ligaments, absence of meniscal injury and/or arthritis, and participation in low-demand sports that do not require running, jumping, or cutting. At the same time, side-to-side laxity alone has not been shown to predict the need for surgery, and classification algorithms to date have not been successful in defining operative or nonoperative patients.[276-278]

Surgical reconstruction of the ACL-deficient knee should be considered if instability of a knee prevents the patient from participating in sports and other activities. It also should be considered if associated collateral ligament damage or meniscal injury is present or if a large increase in anterior tibial translation is seen with laxity testing. Surgery should be considered in most patients who have high expectations and plan to compete in sports that place high demands on the knee.

Partial tears of the ACL involving more than 50% of the ligament are more likely to progress to complete tears if treated nonsurgically.[173] In general, however, there is little correlation between the percentage of the tear and the clinical outcome.[173] Also, the extent of tearing may be difficult to quantify accurately. For this reason, the distinction between a partially torn ACL and a complete tear usually is a clinical one. A positive result on the pivot shift test, regardless of whether the patient is awake or under anesthesia, defines functional instability and an incompetent ACL.

ACL tears in skeletally immature individuals have been increasing in incidence. Although nonoperative management, including delayed reconstruction in this population, is appealing, clinical results of nonoperative management of complete tears of the ACL generally have not been favorable.[279-281] Up to 50% of children in this setting do not return to athletic activity.[282] Partial tears in this population

can also be difficult. Kocher studied a population of 45 skeletally immature patients with partial tears of the ACL and found that 31% required surgical reconstruction.[283] Partial tears that were more than 50% or involved the posterolateral bundle of the ACL were more likely to require further intervention. Surgical reconstruction techniques remain controversial, but physeal (i.e., growth plate) sparing techniques allow near-anatomic reconstructions with far less risk for growth disturbance.[284]

Nonoperative Treatment

Nonoperative treatment after injury to the ACL generally has fallen out of favor because advances in surgical and rehabilitative techniques have improved outcomes and reduced morbidity. Nonetheless, conservative treatment of ACL injuries may be indicated for more sedentary individuals who have an isolated injury without damage to other structures and who are willing to modify their lifestyle to avoid activities that cause pain, swelling, and/or episodes of instability. Nonoperative treatment of ACL injuries does not mean that the injury is ignored. Treatment should actively involve the patient and includes exercise, functional training, bracing, and patient education.

Treatment after acute injury to the ACL should focus on resolving inflammation, restoring ROM, regaining muscle control, and protecting the knee from further injury. Cryotherapy and compression can be used to decrease pain and swelling. ROM exercises should be performed to restore motion, which should improve as pain and swelling subside. Failure to regain motion, particularly extension, may indicate a torn meniscus, and further diagnostic studies and/or surgery may be indicated. Isometric exercises for the quadriceps and hamstring muscles should be initiated to regain motor control and minimize atrophy. Assistive devices should be used for ambulation while the knee is still actively inflamed. The use of assistive devices can be discontinued once the patient has regained full extension without a quadriceps lag and can walk normally, without gait deviations.

More aggressive rehabilitation can begin once inflammation has resolved and full ROM has been restored. The emphasis at this time should be on improving the strength and endurance of the muscles that cross the knee. Particular emphasis should be placed on the muscles that pull the tibia posteriorly (i.e., the hamstrings and gastrocnemius). The normal quadriceps to hamstring ratio at a slow contractile velocity is approximately 3:2. It has been suggested that rehabilitation of an ACL-deficient knee should strive to develop a hamstring-dominant knee so that the quadriceps to hamstring ratio approaches 1:1. This seems to be a logical goal for rehabilitation of ACL injuries, but it should not be achieved at the expense of quadriceps weakness.

OKC and CKC exercises can be used to improve strength and endurance. OKC exercises can be used to provide isolated exercise for the hamstring and quadriceps muscles. Precautions must be taken to prevent the development of patellofemoral symptoms with OKC knee extension. Standing and seated calf raises can be used to develop the gastrocnemius and soleus, respectively. CKC exercises can be used to develop strength and endurance of the muscles of the lower extremity in functional patterns while minimizing patellofemoral stress. CKC exercises are progressed as tolerated.

Once the strength and endurance of the lower extremity muscles have been established, neuromuscular control must be developed to enhance dynamic stability of the knee. Emphasis should be placed on learning to recruit the posterior muscles to minimize anterior translation of the tibia.

Sherrington[285] proposed co-activation of the antagonist during contraction of the agonist. Baratta et al.[29] and Draganich et al.[36] demonstrated co-activation of the hamstrings during resisted OKC knee extension. Antagonist–agonist co-activation probably originates from the motor cortex in the phenomenon known as *direct common drive*.[286] Activation of the muscle spindle can also facilitate contraction of the antagonist.[24] As the knee extends, muscle spindles lying within the hamstrings are activated and facilitate contraction. By training the hamstrings to stabilize the knee dynamically, the clinician can capitalize on the phenomenon of co-activation.

A functional brace may be helpful as the patient returns to activity but does not fully stabilize an ACL-deficient knee. Exactly how knee braces work is unclear, but many patients report improved function with the use of a knee brace. Whether functional braces provide a physical restraint to abnormal joint motion is doubtful. Several studies[287–289] have indicated that knee braces may restrain tibial translation at low-force levels but are ineffective at controlling abnormal joint motion at functional force levels. It has been proposed that knee braces function by improving proprioception. Lephart et al.[25] reported enhanced awareness of joint movement sense with the application of a neoprene sleeve. Application of a knee brace may stimulate cutaneous receptors and enhance proprioception. In addition, knee braces may enhance conscious or subconscious awareness of the injury, helping the individual to protect oneself from further injury. Studies of bracing in ACL-deficient knees have not offered a definitive answer. One prospective randomized study of ACL-deficient knees with functional bracing demonstrated no difference in functional outcome measures or peak torque of the hamstrings or the quadriceps muscles, although subjective stability is increased.[290] A study of ACL-deficient skiers, however, demonstrated a statistically decreased risk of subsequent knee injury.[291]

Another important component of nonoperative management of ACL injuries is modification of the patient's lifestyle to avoid activities associated with pain, swelling, and episodes of instability. Repeated episodes of instability cause further injury to the joint, including stretching of secondary restraints and injury to the menisci and joint surfaces. Recurrent pain and swelling with activity indicate additional damage to the joint. Activities that are not tolerated by the joint should be eliminated to prevent irreversible degenerative changes. Activities that place high stress on the ACL-deficient knee include those that involve jumping, landing, cutting, pivoting, and rapid acceleration or deceleration on the involved extremity. Nonoperative management is likely to fail in patients who are unwilling or unable to modify their lifestyle to avoid activities associated with increased pain, swelling, and instability. These individuals should consider surgical reconstruction.

Clinical Note

Activities that place high stress on the knee ligaments and in the ACL-deficient knee include jumping and landing, cutting, pivoting, and acceleration and deceleration.

Surgical Treatment

Because the ACL tends to stretch before it tears, surgical treatment of ACL injuries usually requires reconstruction with an autograft or allograft. From a historical perspective, results of direct repair have been poor,[191,292,293] and reconstructions using synthetic ligaments have led to early failure and the development of wear particle debris that leads to reactive synovitis.[294–296]

Although ACL reconstruction has been performed since the beginning of the twentieth century and is one of the most common orthopedic procedures, there is still debate in orthopedic literature about the optimal technique. Timing, graft choice, number of tunnels, tunnel location, fixation techniques, and rehabilitation protocols still continue to be refined.

The timing of surgery after acute injury is an important consideration in minimizing the risk of postoperative loss of motion. A decreased incidence of loss of motion and a faster return of quadriceps strength were noted when surgery was delayed 3 to 4 weeks after acute ACL injury.[252,297,298] Other studies have demonstrated excellent results with early reconstruction and a postoperative rehabilitation protocol emphasizing terminal extension and early ROM. A meta-analysis, performed in 2010, demonstrated no clinical difference between early reconstruction (i.e., within 3 weeks of injury) and late reconstruction (i.e., after 6 weeks of injury).[299] Even so, most authors recommend delaying surgery until inflammation has subsided (about 2 to 3 weeks) and ROM and muscle function have been restored, and the only strong indication for immediate surgery is avulsive ligamentous injuries and reparable meniscal injuries.[300–302]

Currently, ACL reconstruction is most commonly performed using an arthroscopically assisted technique with the goal of recreating the normal anatomy of the ACL.

An arthroscope is inserted into the knee through two or three small portals. A tibial tunnel is drilled with an intra-articular exit point at the posterior half of the native ACL insertion. A second tunnel is drilled in the femur at the origin of the native ACL. Different options exist for drilling the femoral tunnel arthroscopically, including through the tibial tunnel (trans-tibial), via a separate anteromedial portal, or use of an inside-out technique drilling through the femur itself. Regardless of technique, tunnels are precisely positioned to recreate the native footprints of the ACL on the tibia and femur.

Multiple surgical variables contribute to the success of the operation. Tunnel placement, graft type, graft fixation, tension, rotation, and notch preparation affect the biomechanics of the reconstruction. Graft fixation can be performed by multiple techniques. If a patellar tendon graft is used, fixation usually is achieved with interference screws (Figure 20-27). Soft tissue grafts (e.g., hamstring) can be fixed with an EndoButton, spiked washers, or a special interference screw. Enlarging the intercondylar notch with a "notchplasty" should be considered if the graft impinges in this area. This is especially important in female patients where a narrowed notch is one factor leading to increased prevalence of ACL injury. Excessive

notchplasty, though, may have biomechanical implications on tunnel placement and anterior laxity and is avoided when not necessary.[303]

ACL reconstruction techniques have evolved with advances in the biomechanical evaluation of the knee. Computer-assisted surgery, high-resolution MRI, evaluation of in vivo three-dimensional kinematics, as well as a better understanding of the ligamentous anatomy, recently provided new insights into functional performance of ACL reconstructions. These analyses have led to an increased emphasis on optimization of graft placement and an anatomic reconstruction technique. Too vertical of a placement of the femoral tunnel of the ACL preferentially reconstructs the anteromedial bundle at the expense of the posterolateral bundle and leads to persistent rotational instability of the knee. Attempts at addressing this problem with double-bundle,[304] anteromedial tunnel drilling,[305,306] or even two-incision approaches[307,308] have shown equivalent positive clinical outcomes. Current reconstructive techniques focus on positioning the femoral and tibial tunnels in optimal anatomic positions to recreate both the anteromedial and posterolateral bundles and thus simulating the biomechanics of the ACL better than previous techniques.

Multiple types of grafts are available to reconstruct the ACL. Autograft reconstructions, including bone–patellar tendon–bone (BPTB),[79,309,310] hamstring tendons,[311-313] and quadriceps tendon,[314] have the advantage of ease of availability, earlier incorporation into bone, and avoidance of possible disease transmission. The use of allograft tissue (i.e., tissue from another human being) for reconstruction has the advantage of avoidance of donor morbidity and a shorter surgical time.[315-317] Meta-analyses of BPTB autografts versus allografts have shown equivalent clinical outcomes once irradiated, and chemically processed allografts were excluded.[318,319] Allografts may have a higher failure rate in young active patients. A retrospective cohort study found that patients 25 and younger had a 29.2% failure rate with allograft tissue compared with an 11.8% failure rate with BPTB autografts.[320] At the same time, better results were seen in allografts in older individuals.

Comparison of BPTB and hamstring autografts showed lower rates of graft failure (4.9% versus 1.9%) and less anterior laxity in the BPTB group. The BPTB group, however, had higher reported percentage of anterior knee pain and increased risk for lysis (i.e., loosening) of adhesions.[321] Hamstring autografts may be associated with hamstring weakness and an increased risk of infection. A Cochrane Review demonstrated no significant clinical difference between hamstring and BPTB autografts.[322] In fact, no single graft source has been found to be clearly superior to others.[323] Ultimate decision for graft choice is an individual one commonly guided by physician experience and recommendations.[324]

Differences in graft tissue strength, stiffness, and graft fixation strength lead to differences in surgical technique

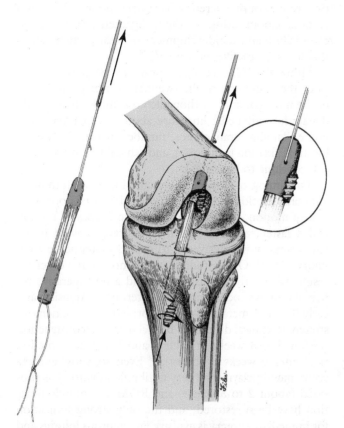

Figure 20-27 Anterior cruciate ligament reconstruction using a bone–patellar tendon–bone graft. Interference screw fixation is used to fix the graft within the tunnels. (From Zachazewski JE, Magee DJ, Quillen WS, editors: *Athletic injuries and rehabilitation,* p 665, Philadelphia, 1996, WB Saunders.)

TABLE 20-4

Ultimate Load to Failure and Stiffness of Various Graft Selections

Graft Selection	Ultimate Strength to Failure (Newtons)	Stiffness (Newton-Meters)
Native anterior cruciate ligament (Woo et al.[327])	2160	240
Patellar tendon (Race and Amis[328])	2977	455
Quadrupled hamstring (Hamner et al.[326])	4140	807
Quadriceps tendon (Staubli et al.[329])	2353	326

and postoperative rehabilitation. Although the quadrupled hamstring tendon graft is approximately 91% stronger than the native ACL and 39% stronger than the patellar tendon, all autografts and patellar tendon allografts have greater tensile strength and stiffness than the native ACL (Table 20-4).[325,326] Because of this, graft fixation strength must be factored into the equation when a rehabilitation program is developed.

Brand et al.[330] reported biomechanical data on various graft fixation techniques for ACL reconstruction. These authors reported that the tibial fixation strength for a patellar BPTB graft had a load to failure of 678 to 758 N[331] while femoral fixation with an interference screw was 640 N.[332,333] Soft tissue fixation strength for an EndoButton with no. 5 suture on the femoral side was 800 N.[334,335] Noyes et al.[336] have estimated the strength required for ADLs to be 454 N.

The authors' clinical approach to designing a rehabilitation program based on ACL graft selection is to be less aggressive initially with soft tissue grafts, such as the quadrupled hamstring grafts. This approach is based on the premise that soft tissue to bone healing takes approximately 12 weeks, whereas bone to bone healing occurs in approximately 8 weeks in most cases. With our current operative technique, patients generally return to sports within 6 to 9 months.

Postoperative Management for Reconstruction of the Anterior Cruciate Ligament

Rehabilitation after ACL reconstruction must consider graft type, initial graft strength, fixation, and healing and maturation of the graft. Initial graft strength depends on the type, quantity, and quality of the material used and is described earlier in detail.

Graft strength is strongest at the time of reconstruction. Over time, the graft undergoes necrosis and remodeling. Healing and maturation of autogenous BPTB grafts in the animal model[337-340] and in humans[337,341] have been described, as have healing and maturation of allograft BPTB

grafts in animal models[341-345] and humans.[342] Initially, the graft is avascular. By 6 weeks, the graft is enveloped in a synovial sheath. Revascularization begins 8 to 10 weeks after surgery and is nearly complete by 16 weeks. Histologically, the graft shows signs of avascular necrosis 6 weeks after reconstruction. The graft is invaded by mesenchymal cells 8 to 10 weeks after reconstruction. These cells proliferate and form collagen by postoperative week 16. One year after reconstruction, the graft takes on the appearance of a ligament, with dense, oriented collagen bundles. Graft strength decreases during the period of necrosis and then increases as the graft remodels and matures.

Although the graft takes on the appearance of a normal ligament, it does not function the same as the native ACL. Evidence suggests that, at 6 months after surgery, allografts demonstrate a greater decrease in their structural properties from the time of implantation, a slower rate of biological incorporation, and prolonged presence of an inflammatory response compared with autografts.[345] Although long-term clinical results have not demonstrated a significant difference between allograft and autograft reconstruction, rehabilitation after allograft reconstruction may need to be less aggressive than that after autograft reconstruction. Despite the research, little is known about the graft's ability to withstand loads and strain during healing and maturation. Therefore, it is difficult to base rehabilitation after ACL reconstruction strictly on the time required for healing and maturation of the graft. Recent research favors the use of criterion- and milestone-based rehabilitation progressions.

Clinical Note

Rehabilitation should be less aggressive after allograft reconstruction than autograft reconstruction.

Interest has developed in accelerated rehabilitation after ACL reconstruction, which initially was popularized by Shelbourne and Nitz in 1990.[346] These researchers discovered that an early accelerated rehabilitation program resulted in an earlier and more complete return of full extension and an earlier return to final flexion without any adverse effect on the stability of the knee, as indicated by side-to-side differences in knee laxity scores.[346] In addition, isokinetic testing of the quadriceps revealed a higher mean percentage of involved to noninvolved scores from 4 to 10 months postoperatively. However, these differences in isokinetic scores were eliminated 1 year after surgery. No differences were seen in the patients' subjective assessment of their knee function. A second surgical procedure to recover loss of extension was required less often in patients who underwent the accelerated program. Based on these results, the use of an accelerated rehabilitation program after ACL reconstruction was recommended because it resulted in earlier restoration of motion, strength, and function without compromising stability of the knee.

Loss of motion, especially in extension, has been described as a common complication after ACL reconstruction.[301,347–351] Sachs et al.[350] reported a 24% incidence of a knee flexion contraction more than 5° after ACL reconstruction. This was positively correlated with quadriceps weakness and patellofemoral pain. Harner et al.[301] reported an 11% incidence of loss of motion, which they defined as a knee flexion contracture of 10° or more and/or knee flexion less than 125°. All patients with loss of motion experienced loss of extension, and two thirds also had loss of flexion. Factors significantly related to the development of loss of motion included reconstruction within 4 weeks of the initial injury, concomitant knee ligament surgery involving the medial capsule, and gender (i.e., male). Patients with loss of motion tended to have had an autograft rather than an allograft and to be older, but these trends did not reach statistical significance. Also, patients who developed loss of motion used a postoperative brace that limited full extension more often than did patients who had normal motion after surgery. Loss of extension after ACL reconstruction leads to an abnormal gait, altered joint arthrokinematics, increase patellofemoral and tibiofemoral contact pressures, and even quadriceps weakness.

The goal for postoperative management after ACL reconstruction is to provide a stable knee that allows return to the highest level of function while minimizing the risk for loss of motion. To reduce the risk of loss of motion, postoperative management after ACL reconstruction should emphasize control of inflammation, restoration of full extension symmetrical to the noninvolved knee, early ROM and quadriceps exercises, and restoration of normal gait.

Clinical Note

To reduce risk of loss of ROM, rehabilitation should emphasize the following:

- Inflammation control
- Early ROM
- Restoration of full extension (actively and passively)
- Quadriceps exercises
- Restoration of normal gait

Adams et al.[352] outlined an excellent multiphased criterion-based rehabilitation approach that encompassed all aspects of the rehabilitation until return-to-sport. The phases include the presurgical phase, the immediate postoperative phase, the early postoperative phase, the intermediate postoperative phase, the late postoperative phase, and the transitional phase. Each phase with the appropriate milestones are outlined in Table 20-5.

TABLE 20-5

Criterion-Based Milestones for Treatment Progression

Phase	Milestones
Immediate postoperative	• Knee ROM 0°-90° • Active quadriceps contraction with superior patellar glide
Early postoperative	• Knee flexion >110° • Pain-free ambulation without crutches • Stationary bicycle without difficulty • Full knee extension during gait • Reciprocal stair-climbing • Straight-leg raise without extension lag • Knee Outcome Survey ADL subscale >65%
Intermediate postoperative	• Knee flexion within 10° of contralateral side • Quadriceps index >60% of contralateral side
Late postoperative	• Normal gait pattern • Quadriceps index >80% of contralateral side • Symmetrical ROM (compared with contralateral side) • Knee effusion of trace or less
Transitional postoperative	• Maintenance of quadriceps index >80% • Hop tests >80% of contralateral side at 12 wk • Knee Outcome Survey Sports subscale >70%

ROM, Range of motion.
Modified from Adams D, Logerstedt DS, Hunter-Giordano A et al: Current concepts for anterior cruciate ligament reconstruction: a criterion-based rehabilitation progression, *J Orthop Sports Phys Ther* 42:601-614, 2012.

In the **preoperative phase**, an emphasis is placed on regaining full ROM, decreasing joint effusion, and normalizing quadriceps strength. Patients who achieve minimal to no joint effusion, full return of ROM, and the ability to perform an SLR without an extensor lag have been shown to experience better postoperative outcomes.[300]

Preoperative Phase Goals

- Regain full ROM
- Decrease joint effusion
- Normalize quadriceps muscle strength

The **immediate postoperative phase** encompasses the first week and focuses on early ROM and reactivating the quadriceps muscles. Neuromuscular electrical stimulation (NMES) has been found to be an effective way to facilitate quadriceps activation and has been shown to improve postoperative outcomes.[353] This improves the patient's ability to generate a quadriceps contraction, as effusion and subsequent arthrogenic inhibition generally result in decreased volitional quadriceps activation after surgery. OKC exercises initiated at this time include hip abduction and adduction and knee extension in a restricted ROM (90° to 40°). This restricted range has been shown to reduce strain on the healing ACL graft.[41] The milestones to progress to the early postoperative phase of the rehabilitation progression are 0° to 90° ROM and the ability to actively perform a quadriceps contraction with a superior (i.e., upward) patellar glide.

Goals of Immediate Postoperative Phase (Week 1)

- Reduce pain
- Reduce swelling
- Establish ROM 0° to 90°
- Reactivate quadriceps muscles
- Initiate OKC exercises (90° to 40°)

The **early postoperative phase** generally occurs during the second postoperative week and is marked by the introduction of CKC and terminal knee extension strengthening. Weight-bearing exercise can include wall slides, minisquats, leg press, weight-shifting, and forward/lateral step-ups, all within a pain-free ROM. The patient also can begin riding a stationary bicycle during this phase, once 100° of knee flexion has been achieved. Milestones to progress to the intermediate phase of the rehabilitation program are knee flexion more than 110°, full active knee extension during gait, ambulation without an assistive device, use of a bicycle without difficulty, reciprocal stair climbing, SLR without an extensor lag, and a knee outcome survey ADL subscale score more than 65%.

Goals of Early Postoperative Phase (Week 2)

- Achieve terminal knee extension
- Introduce CKC exercises
- Begin stationary bike
- Improve pain-free ROM

The **intermediate postoperative phase** incorporates neuromuscular training, balance, and proprioceptive exercises, as well as continued quadriceps strengthening. Proprioceptive exercises can be utilized to improve outcomes without increased risk of injury. The milestones to progress to the late phase of the rehabilitation program are knee flexion ROM within 10° of the contralateral side and a quadriceps index score of more than 60%. The quadriceps index is defined as the ratio of uninvolved to involved quadriceps strength and can be measured isometrically with a dynamometer at 60° of knee flexion.

Goals of Intermediate Postoperative Phase

- Reestablish neuromuscular control
- Establish normal ROM
- Improve proprioception
- Improve strength

Once the incision has fully healed, an aquatic therapy program can be initiated, which will allow the patient to begin early running and agility drills in the pool. The buoyancy of the water assists the patient by reducing the percentage of BW and the loads applied to the lower extremity.

In the **late postoperative phase**, intensity of strengthening continues to increase to include low work to rest ratios. That is, high intensity, near-maximal bouts of exercise allowing for appropriate recovery time. Balance and proprioception exercises are progressed to include perturbations and distractions (e.g., a ball toss). To advance to the transitional postoperative phase, the patient must achieve a quadriceps index of more than 80%, a normal gait pattern, full ROM, and knee effusion of trace or less (as graded by a stroke test) (Table 20-6). Once a patient demonstrates understanding of normal and abnormal soreness patterns and the previously listed criteria have been met, a jogging progression may also be initiated within the late postoperative phase. It is outside the scope of this text to discuss a detailed jogging progression; however, the patient should remain pain free during all activities; the program should be reviewed and activities decreased if lasting soreness is experienced after any training session.

TABLE **20-6**

Grading Knee Effusion Using the Stroke Test

Grade	Presentation
0	No wave produced on downstroke
Trace	Small wave on medial side with downstroke
1+	Larger bulge on medial side with downstroke
2+	Effusion spontaneously returns to medial side after upstroke
3+	It is not possible to displace the fluid from the medial side of the knee

From Sturgill LP, Snyder-Mackler L, Manal TJ, Axe MJ: Interrater reliability of a clinical scale to assess knee joint effusion, *J Orthop Sports Phys Ther* 39:845-849, 2009.

Goals of Late Postoperative Phase

- Continue strengthening
- Establish neuromuscular control drills
- Achieve quadriceps index of more than 80% along with a normal gait pattern

The **transitional postoperative phase** includes plyometrics and sport-specific training and can begin as early as 8 weeks postoperatively, as long as the patient has met the previously listed criteria. Early plyometrics begin with double leg box jumps (i.e., jumping up to small step) and then are progressed to flat ground jumping and eventually double leg drop jumps. Emphasis is placed throughout the plyometric progression on proper jumping and landing techniques. Once the patient is able to consistently demonstrate proper hip and knee alignment with double-leg jumping in all directions, a similar single-leg jumping program can commence.

Goals of Transitional Postoperative Phase

- Continue sport-specific training
- Initiate early plyometric activity
- Ensure normal functional movement patterns
- Emphasize normal functional gait during activity

Functional testing before return to sport is essential to determine the athlete's strength, neuromuscular control, confidence in the limb, and ability to tolerate loads related to sport-specific activities.[354] A series of 4 single-leg hop tests have been studied and proved to be valid and reliable performance-based outcome measures.[355] The hop tests described include single hop for distance, 6-meter timed hop, triple hop for distance, and crossover hop for distance. Variation exists in exact passing return-to-sport criteria, but greater than or equal to 90% of the contralateral side in hop testing and the quadriceps index is suggested prior to clearing an athlete for return to participation.[353]

Another critical consideration in the rehabilitation of a patient after ACL reconstruction, in addition to physical and surgical factors, is the *patient's psychological readiness to return to sport*. Research has supported the use of the **ACL–return to sports after injury (ACL–RSI) scale** as a measure of an athlete's fear of psychological readiness, and includes questions such as "Are you fearful of reinjuring your knee by playing sports?" and "Are you confident you can perform at your previous level of sports participation?" Athletes who returned to sport at 12 months postoperatively scored higher on the ACL–RSI both in a preoperative assessment, as well as at 4 months postoperatively, compared with athletes who did not return to sport.[356] Furthermore, Ardern et al.[356] revealed a relationship between psychological readiness to return to

sport, the patient's estimated number of months it would take to return to sport, locus of control, and return to sport by 12 months postoperatively. An ACL–RSI score of less than 56 points has been found to indicate an increased risk of failing to return to preinjury level of participation. In these populations, health coaching, patient education, and change in locus of control can all be effective techniques to improve the likelihood of successful rehabilitation and return to sport.

Clinical Note

Patients must be physiologically and psychologically ready to progress through the different levels of rehabilitation and especially before return to the activity that caused the physical injury.

Posterior Cruciate Ligament Injuries

Although similar in presentation, PCL injuries differ from ACL injuries due to their potential for intrinsic healing. Isolated injury to the PCL does not produce the same degree of functional instability and disability seen with injury to the ACL. Many patients with an isolated PCL injury can return to their previous level of function with minimal symptoms. The level of function and patient satisfaction appear to be related to the ability of the quadriceps to stabilize the knee dynamically. Parolie and Bergfeld[204] reported the long-term results of 25 patients with PCL injuries who were managed without surgery. All patients who returned to their previous level of function and were satisfied with their results had isokinetic quadriceps torque values on the involved side more than 100% of those on the noninvolved side. Conversely, patients who were not satisfied with their knees had isokinetic torque values on the involved side that were less than 100% of those on the noninvolved side. Shelbourne and Muthukaruppan[357] prospectively evaluated 215 patients treated nonoperatively for an isolated PCL injury grade II or less and found subjective scores did not correlate with degree of laxity. Others have noted that the level of function after PCL injury did not appear to be related to the degree of instability.[204,212]

Although clinical outcomes have been found to be good in the short term, concern over long-term degenerative changes from the altered arthrokinematics of the PCL-deficient knee have been proposed. PCL-deficient knees experience increased contact pressures in the patellofemoral and medial compartments.[358] Long-term evaluations of patients treated nonoperatively have demonstrated some risk of this increased degenerative disease.[211,359] In contrast, Shelbourne et al.[214] prospectively evaluated a series of 68 patients with isolated PCL injuries treated nonoperatively for an average of 17.6 years. Subjective clinical scores were good and patients were able to remain active. Moderate to severe arthritis was noted in only 11% of patients.[214]

As PCL reconstruction has not demonstrated successful restoration of normal knee kinematics,[360] treatment for isolated grade II or less PCL injuries has generally been nonoperative, with surgery reserved for those patients failing a conservative treatment protocol. There is less controversy regarding multiple ligament injuries, grade III PCL injuries, or avulsive ligamentous injuries for which operative reconstruction of the PCL is recommended.

Nonoperative Management

Even though PCL injures may have an inherent ability to heal themselves, gravitational forces and hamstring muscle tension can often cause the tibia to be positioned posteriorly relative to the femur. Healing of the PCL in this elongated position can cause an increase in chronic instability and disability.[361] Some authors have gone so far as to advocate use of a cylindrical cast to avoid this laxity.[362] Use of a dynamic anterior drawer brace or hinged knee brace[363] may provide some support to prevent posterior translation of the tibia.

Treatment after acute injury to the PCL is similar to the management of acute ACL injuries. Nonsurgical treatment approaches rely on physical therapy and temporary bracing or immobilization to restore normal tibiofemoral positioning.[364] Rehabilitation should focus on resolving inflammation, restoring ROM, and regaining motor control of the knee. PRICE (i.e., protect, rest, ice, compression, and elevation) is used to reduce pain and swelling, while active assistive and passive motion exercises are performed to restore full ROM. ROM should be performed in the prone position to prevent hamstring activation and posterior sag of the tibia due to gravity, which would place increased stress on the healing ligament.[364] As the least amount of stress placed on the PCL occurs between 40° and 90°,[365,366] ROM exercises should be limited to 90° for the first 2 weeks. Isometric exercises for the quadriceps, such as prone quadriceps sets are used to minimize quadriceps atrophy. Hamstring exercises are avoided at this time and can be delayed up to 12 weeks after injury[364] because they contribute to increased posterior laxity. Also, the hamstring muscles do not appear to be as susceptible as the quadriceps muscles to disuse atrophy. Assistive devices are used for ambulation while the knee is still actively inflamed and are discontinued when the patient has regained full extension without a quadriceps lag and can walk normally, without gait deviations.

OKC knee flexion exercises should be avoided because they contribute to increased posterior tibial translation by incorporating hamstring activation. For patients with a PCL-deficient knee, hamstring strengthening is performed using OKC and CKC hip extension with the knee near terminal extension, which minimizes posterior tibial translation. During CKC exercises, the hamstrings function to counteract the flexion moment arm at the hip. Their effect (i.e., producing posterior tibial translation of the knee) is offset by simultaneous activation of the quadriceps muscles. Proprioceptive training for the PCL-deficient knee should emphasize recruitment of the quadriceps muscles to control posterior translation of the tibia dynamically.

More aggressive rehabilitation can begin once inflammation has resolved and full ROM has been restored. The emphasis at this time is on improving the endurance and strength of the quadriceps muscles. OKC knee extension exercises should be modified if the patient complains of pain or crepitus. CKC exercises are initiated and progressed as tolerated to improve the endurance and strength of the muscles of the lower extremity in functional patterns. Patients may begin a jogging progression once they demonstrate full ROM, 85% limb symmetry index, and trace or less effusion at rest and after activity. Sport-specific drills may commence once the patient performs a jogging progression pain free and exhibits 85% limb symmetry on dynamic stability testing (i.e., hop testing). Sport-specific drills may include changes in speed and direction and progress from proactive to reactive drills (i.e., reacting to an opponent).

Generally, patients with a PCL-deficient knee do not complain of instability during physical activity, and a functional brace is not necessary. If a patient does complain of instability, a functional brace specifically designed for a PCL-deficient knee and specifically limiting posterior tibial translation is recommended. This is a critical distinction, as most functional knee braces are designed for ACL-deficient knees and will not assist in the control of posterior tibial translation. Many patients with a PCL-deficient knee complain of patellofemoral symptoms, and may benefit from the use of a neoprene patellar sleeve.

Because of the tendency for progressive deterioration of the anterior and medial compartments of the knee, patients with a PCL-deficient knee should be educated to avoid activities that cause pain and swelling. Repetitive activities that involve high loading of the patellofemoral and tibiofemoral joints may accelerate this degenerative process and should be avoided.

Return to sport generally is delayed for several months, but the time frame in elite athletes can be as little as 6 to 8 weeks with the expected risk of increased residual joint laxity.[364] Patients who fail conservative treatment should be reassessed and considered for surgical repair or reconstruction. Chronic isolated PCL injuries may require serial PCL stress radiographs to objectively gauge injury progression and dictate treatment modifications.[364]

Surgical Treatment

Clinicians must take into account a number of important variables when deciding how best to manage a PCL injury. These include the type of injury; whether associated structures have been damaged; the patient's symptoms, activity level, goals, and expectations; and the acuity or chronicity of the injury. The goal of treatment is to restore the stability and normal kinematics of the knee and to allow the patient to return to the preinjury level of activity. The best way to achieve this is still the subject of debate.

For interstitial tears of the PCL, the decision to perform surgery is based on the degree of resulting functional instability and injuries to associated ligamentous structures. Surgical reconstruction is recommended for isolated PCL disruptions that result in more than 10 mm of increased posterior tibial translation compared with the noninvolved side or when injury to the PCL is accompanied by injury to other ligamentous structures. Acute repair of a PCL avulsed from the bone or avulsed with bone may be possible with a single screw or suture technique. Most series have shown that reconstructions do better in chronic cases, because the potential for stretching out of secondary restraints increases with time.

It is important to note that a posterior drawer of more than 15 mm can indicate a combined injury to the PCL and posterolateral structures.[66] An occult injury to the PLC shoulder be evaluated and concomitantly treated.

PCL tears can be reconstructed using an open or an arthroscopic technique. We prefer performing PCL reconstruction using an arthroscopically assisted technique. Although it is technically more demanding, it is believed to reduce operative morbidity and to hold promise for improved clinical results. As with reconstruction of the ACL, PCL reconstruction has been performed using a variety of graft materials, including patellar and Achilles tendon allografts, patellar tendon, fascia lata, medial head of the gastrocnemius, semitendinosus–gracilis, and meniscus autografts, and synthetic replacements. Procedures in which the medial head of the gastrocnemius,[83,367–371] the semitendinosus–gracilis,[368,369] the iliotibial band,[370] the meniscus,[371,372] Gore-Tex synthetic ligament,[373] and primary unaugmented repair[374–376] have all failed to produce consistent, objective results.

Techniques for PCL reconstruction can be divided into transtibial and tibial inlay. Transtibial techniques utilize a tunnel in the tibia exiting posteriorly. The graft makes an acute turn as it exits the tibia toward the femur. This "killer turn" has been implicated as a cause of graft failure. To address this potential problem, a tibial inlay technique has been advocated where the PCL graft is affixed to the posterior tibia directly.[377] Biomechanical studies of these techniques suggest that posterior laxity may increase to a greater degree with cyclic loading in the transtibial technique compared with the tibial inlay.[378] Clinical studies, however, have reported no meaningful difference between the two techniques. Attempts have been made to reduce the effects of the "killer turn" by smoothing the tunnel,[379] approaching from the anterolateral tibia,[380] and using an aperture fixation at the posterior portion of the tunnel.[381]

Single- versus double-bundle reconstruction of the PCL is also controversial. Single-bundle PCL reconstruction consists of reproducing the anterolateral bundle of the ligament because this is the largest and strongest band, and it functions primarily with the knee in flexion. The procedure is performed by drilling the tibial tunnel (so that it reproduces the distolateral portion of the tibial insertion site) and drilling the femoral tunnel (so that it reproduces the anterior portion of the femoral insertion site). An Achilles tendon allograft is passed through the femoral and tibial tunnels. The authors prefer to use an Achilles tendon allograft because of its length and strength, availability, lack of morbidity to the patient, and ease of passage; one end of the graft is without a bony block and can easily be passed through the acute angle required to go from the femoral to the tibial tunnel. The femoral side, which includes the Achilles bone plug, is fixed with an interference screw, and the tibial side is fixed to the tibia with a screw and soft tissue spiked washer (Figure 20-28).

Although a single-bundle reconstruction may reduce posterior tibial translation at the time of surgery, anatomical and biomechanical studies have shown that the two bundles of the PCL have different roles in the normal arthrokinematics of the knee. The anterolateral bundle becomes taut in flexion, and the posteromedial bundle becomes taut in extension. For this reason, a double-bundle technique has been advocated for reconstruction of the PCL. This procedure, which uses two separate grafts to restore both the anterolateral and posteromedial bundles of the PCL, requires two femoral tunnels and one common tibial tunnel. During reconstruction, the anterolateral

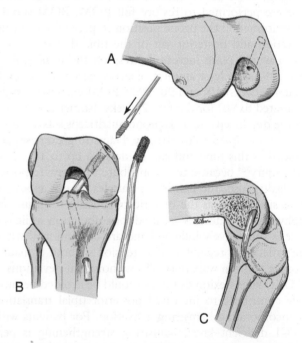

Figure 20-28 Posterior cruciate ligament (PCL) reconstruction. **A,** PCL reconstruction is performed with an Achilles tendon allograft passed through the femoral and tibial tunnels. **B,** The femoral side is fixed with an interference screw. **C,** The tibial side is fixed with a soft tissue spiked washer and screw. (From Zachazewski JE, Magee DJ, Quillen WS, editors: *Athletic injuries and rehabilitation,* p 670, Philadelphia, 1996, WB Saunders.)

bundle is tensioned in flexion, and the posteromedial bundle is tensioned in extension. Harner et al.[382] reported that double-bundle reconstruction more closely restores the normal tibial translation and biomechanics of the knee than the single-bundle technique. Several authors have described the double-bundle procedure in detail.[50,383,384] Nonetheless, the advantages of the double-bundle technique have not been confirmed in the literature, and much debate still exists over the best technique for PCL reconstruction.

Postoperative Management for Reconstruction of the Posterior Cruciate Ligament

Little is known about the healing and maturation of PCL grafts. Bosch et al.[385] studied PCL graft fixation in sheep using a free patellar tendon graft and demonstrated good bone to bone incorporation at 6 weeks. In their study, postoperative management consisted of immediate partial weight bearing and ROM beginning 2 weeks after surgery. Clancy et al.[339] demonstrated revascularization of free patellar tendon grafts 8 weeks after surgery in rhesus monkeys. As yet, no studies on graft fixation and incorporation after PCL reconstruction have been performed in humans.

The rehabilitation program after PCL reconstruction has evolved dramatically over the past several years as a result of advances in researchers' understanding of the anatomy and biomechanics of the knee and improved surgical techniques.

The goals of rehabilitation include restoring full range of knee motion, preventing wear of the articular cartilage, gradually increasing the stress applied to the healing PCL graft, and improving dynamic stabilization of the knee joint. Rehabilitation of PCL injuries focuses on regaining quadriceps strength and control. In fact, earlier quadriceps contraction in the gait cycle can increase dynamic stability in the knee enough to overcome the instability from an incompetent PCL.[386] Rehabilitation therefore focuses on regaining or exceeding normal quadriceps strength.[387]

Overall Goals in PCL Rehabilitation

- Restore full ROM
- Prevent excess articular cartilage wear
- Gradually increase stress to PCL
- Improve dynamic stabilization
- Regain quadriceps strength
- Minimize posterior tibial translation

It is important to minimize posterior tibial translation during rehabilitation.[38] This is accomplished by protecting against gravity-induced posterior sag and by avoiding OKC hamstring exercises. CKC exercises, such as the squat, produce less tibiofemoral shear force and increase overall dynamic stability about the knee joint. OKC quadriceps extension exercises should begin in the prone position to prevent posterior sag of the tibia. SLRs may be introduced once the quadriceps is able to lock the joint in terminal knee extension and no lag is present. The patient can then progress knee extension exercises in the sitting and supine positions.

Clinical Note

After PCL surgery, posterior translation of the tibia must be minimized during active and passive ROM and exercise training, and functional activities.

Several early progressive rehabilitation protocols after PCL reconstruction have been proposed and evaluated.[364,388] Our current milestone-based program consists of five phases designed to progress the patient gradually to full, unrestricted activities by 6 to 9 months after surgery, although individualized for each patient (Table 20-7). The protocol focuses on quadriceps strengthening and restoration of ROM while avoiding stress on the graft. The protocol has been developed based on the findings from the Pierce, O'Brien, Wohlt, and LaPrade review.[364]

Immediately after surgery, the knee is wrapped with a compression dressing and continuous cryotherapy is applied. The patient is educated on how to reduce swelling and pain using the PRICE method. The patient's knee

TABLE 20-7

Criterion-Based Progression of Postoperative Isolated PCL Reconstruction

Phase	Treatment Goals
Phase I (0-6 wk)	Protect reconstruction Reactivate quadriceps Decrease effusion
Phase II (6-12 wk)	Normalize gait Restore ROM Improve quadriceps strength Improve balance
Phase III (13-18 wk)	Improve neuromuscular control Continue quadriceps strengthening Progress hamstring strengthening
Phase IV (19-24 wk)	Continue quadriceps strengthening Continue neuromuscular control Improve muscular and cardiovascular endurance
Phase V (25-36 wk)	Initiate jogging progressions Initiate plyometric progression Initiate sport-specific/agility drills as indicated

ROM, Range of motion.

Modified from Pierce CM, O'Brien L, Griffin LW, Laprade RF: Posterior cruciate ligament tears: functional and postoperative rehabilitation, *Knee Surg Sports Traumatol Arthrosc* 21:1071-1084, 2013.

remains locked in full extension in a knee immobilizer throughout the first day and the patient is taught to ambulate with bilateral axillary crutches, bearing weight as tolerated. A dynamic anterior drawer brace, or other PCL brace, is used with therapy when prescribed by the surgeon.

Phase I (0 to 6 weeks) focuses on protecting the reconstruction, reducing knee effusion, regaining quadriceps control. Passive knee flexion is performed in the prone position and is limited to 90° for the first 2 weeks, then progressed as tolerated. Hyperextension is to be avoided until 12 weeks postoperatively. Isolated hamstring exercises are contraindicated for the first 4 months because of the large posterior shear force generated with hamstring contraction. ROM and patellar mobilizations, particularly superior patellar glides, are performed four to five times throughout the day to help restore motion. NMES is applied in conjunction with these exercises to facilitate a quadriceps contraction.[389–391] Cryotherapy is commonly used for 15 minutes after treatment to control pain and effusion.

Goals of Phase I PCL Rehabilitation (0 to 6 Weeks)

- Protect the repair
- Reduce swelling
- Restore quadriceps control
- Restore ROM
- Mobilize patella
- Avoid hyperextension
- Avoid isolated hamstring exercises for 16 weeks

Precautions after Isolated PCL Reconstruction

Timeframe	Precautions
0-2 weeks	ROM 0°-90°; then gradual progression to full ROM
0-6 weeks	Weight bearing as tolerated (WBAT) with bilateral crutches; then discharge when patient exhibits normal gait
0-6 weeks	Locked in full extension in knee immobilizer, except during ROM and quadriceps strengthening
0-4 months	No open-chain or isolated hamstring strengthening

At 6 weeks, the patient may begin to ambulate with one crutch. Once the patient demonstrates a normal, pain-free gait pattern, he or she may completely discontinue crutch use. The knee immobilizer may be discontinued after 6 weeks, once the patient is able to perform an SLR without an extension lag.

Phase II (generally 6 to 12 weeks) focuses on normalization of gait, restoration of full ROM, continued quadriceps strengthening, and balance/proprioception exercises. Minisquats are performed from 0° to 45°. Because the loss of proprioception after PCL injury is well documented,[392] the authors begin proprioceptive

drills, such as weight shifting on a stable platform. Neuromuscular control drills that train muscular co-activation for dynamic stabilization are also incorporated at this time. The stationary bicycle may be used for quadriceps strengthening, motion stimulation, and cardiovascular training when ROM permits and is not to exceed 115° knee flexion. Also at this time, an aquatic therapy program consisting of pool walking, light kicking, and other land exercises that are permitted via protocol is added. CKC exercises are progressed through the squat progression, which entails squat to squat with calf raise to squat with weight shift.[364] Lateral step-downs are also incorporated to encourage single-leg strengthening and motor control. Hamstring bridges are performed on a ball with the knees extended and double leg press can begin. The patient may progress to phase III of the rehabilitation program once he or she demonstrates normal, pain-free gait, full knee ROM, good control with single-leg step-down, and single-leg balance for more than 15 seconds.

Goals of Phase II PCL Rehabilitation (6 to 12 Weeks)

- Normalize gait
- Restore full ROM
- Improve quadriceps strength
- Improve proprioception/balance

Phase III generally spans about 13 to 18 weeks postoperatively and emphasizes continued quadriceps strengthening and neuromuscular control. Balance exercises are performed on variable surfaces and perturbations are added. Progressive hamstring strengthening with a bent knee is also implemented in this phase, with single-leg bridges and *isolated* hamstring strengthening delayed until week 16.

Goals of Phase III PCL Rehabilitation (13 to 18 Weeks)

- Quadriceps strengthening
- Neuromuscular control
- Progressive hamstring exercises

Phase IV (generally 19 to 24 weeks) emphasizes single-leg strength and endurance with an increasing emphasis on power and the initiation of sport-specific drills near the end of the phase. The patient may also increase duration and resistance on the stationary bicycle to address muscular and cardiovascular endurance.

Goals of Phase IV PCL Rehabilitation (19 to 24 Weeks)

- Emphasize single-leg strength and endurance
- Begin activity-specific drills

During **phase V** (generally 25+ weeks), plyometric exercises are used to enhance dynamic joint stabilization and neuromuscular control. The rapid dynamic loading of the musculature during plyometric drills helps train the stretch–shortening cycle of the musculature. Plyometric drills are progressed from the leg press machine to box jumps, then flat-ground jumps, drop jumps, and single-leg jumps. A jogging progression is initiated once the patient demonstrates full ROM, no effusion at rest or after activity, and more than 85% quadriceps strength index. Agility drills and sport- or activity-specific training drills may be incorporated at this time if the patient demonstrates more than 85% limb symmetry in hop testing and has performed a jogging progression without incident. If satisfactory results are seen on the clinical examination, the return to sport phase is initiated and gradually progressed in intensity over the course of 4 to 6 weeks.

Goals of Phase V PCL Rehabilitation (25+ Weeks)

- Dynamic joint stabilization
- Neuromuscular control
- Plyometric exercises
- Activity-specific drills

The authors periodically assess the knee laxity of patients with a reconstructed PCL throughout the program. A KT2000 arthrometer (MEDmetric, San Diego, CA) is used to assess the AP laxity of the knee joint at 2, 4, 6, 8, and 12 weeks and at 4, 6, 12, and 24 months after surgery. The test is performed at the quadriceps-neutral angle to ensure that AP laxity is measured accurately. Serial assessment of knee laxity is useful to the rehabilitation specialist for evaluating the integrity of the graft. Some physicians have utilized a PCL stress radiograph to objectively assess the healing of the PCL.[364] The rehabilitation program is assessed on the basis of the results of the arthrometric testing and is adjusted accordingly.

In the authors' experience, patients typically can return to noncontact sports at 6 months after surgery and to contact sports at 7 to 9 months. The authors tend to be more cautious with skiers because of the highly dynamic nature of the sport; we generally permit skiing at 8 to 9 months after surgery.

Medial Collateral Ligament Injuries

The MCL possesses the greatest capacity to heal of any of the four major knee ligaments and a conservative nonsurgical approach to isolated injuries of the MCL has demonstrated good results in up to 90% of cases.[99,196,219,220,222–226,393,394] Even so, in those cases that fail conservative management, or are associated with other ligamentous injuries, surgical repair and/or reconstruction may be necessary.

Acute treatment of isolated MCL injuries depends on the stability of the joint, the grade of injury, and the location of the tear. Grade I and grade II MCL sprains that are stable when valgus stress tested are treated with a brief period of immobilization and protected weight bearing with crutches. Controlled knee flexion and extension begins as soon as symptoms allow and sometimes necessitate the use of a hinged knee brace.

Grade III MCL injuries are more complex. Indelicato[220] classically prospectively evaluated 36 patients with grade III MCL complex injuries to compare operative versus nonoperative treatment. Although patients in the operative group had better stability (94% versus 85% good to excellent results), no functional difference was noted between groups. For this reason, most isolated grade III MCL injuries are also initially treated nonoperatively.[395]

Results of nonoperative treatment programs have indicated some residual instability with greater knee laxity noted in higher grade injuries. Up to 70% of patients had residual knee laxity in a study of football players with an early aggressive rehabilitation program.[396] Even in Indelicato's original study, notable laxity was seen in both operative and nonoperative groups.[220] Due to the generally excellent clinical results in these studies, it is thought that this residual valgus laxity has little effect on knee function. Even so, it can often be difficult to determine which medial injuries are indeed isolated compared with those involving more of the posteromedial capsule and posterior oblique ligament. Nonoperative management can lead to residual instability in this setting, especially in pivoting activities. Posteromedial corner injuries have been increasingly recognized and may serve as a separate indication for surgical intervention.[229,397,398]

Patients with combined ACL–MCL injuries may also require specific attention to the MCL during treatment. There is notable load sharing of the ACL and MCL. Increased forces on a reconstructed ACL are seen with MCL deficiency.[227,399,400] A goat model has supported the concept that ACL reconstruction can reduce forces on the MCL.[401] Knees with untreated combined ACL–MCL injuries have shown increased valgus laxity and a reduction in tissue quality of the healed MCL.[175] Early ACL reconstruction in combined ACL and MCL injuries may provide a more stable environment for MCL healing.[176] Because of this, the authors' preferred treatment approach utilizes a 4- to 6-week preoperative rehabilitation program that allows for MCL complex healing. This also decreases preoperative swelling and allows the patient to regain normal ROM and strength, maximizing the postoperative outcome. An intraoperative assessment of the MCL is made after ACL reconstruction, and a repair or reconstruction of the MCL is performed if necessary.

Combined PCL and medial-sided injuries also represent an indication for surgical reconstruction of both ligaments for similar reasons.[402,403]

For acute injuries requiring surgical intervention, repair is attempted at the site of injury. This repair is usually at the distal MCL on the tibia because femoral-sided injuries may heal more reliably. Tightening of the posterior capsule and posterior oblique ligament is performed based on clinical assessment and with an understanding of risk of postoperative stiffness. Several anatomic techniques have been described for this repair.[404,405]

Surgical reconstruction is performed using an allograft or autograft. Anatomic reconstructions have been advocated by several authors and focus on recreation of both the superficial and deep portions of the MCL.[229,405] For those knees requiring reconstruction of the posteromedial knee, improved mechanics and stability has been seen in additional reconstruction of the posterior oblique ligament.[406,407]

Nonoperative/Postoperative Management of Medial Collateral Ligament Injuries

Acute nonoperative treatment of isolated MCL injuries depends on the stability of the joint. Grades I and II MCL sprains that are stable with valgus stress testing are treated symptomatically without the use of a rehabilitation brace. Patients with isolated grade III MCL injuries who are unstable with valgus stress testing and who have a soft end point are treated with a hinged rehabilitation brace for 4 to 6 weeks. The brace typically is set to permit 0° to 90° of motion. The brace controls valgus stresses, allowing the ligament to heal while permitting limited motion of the knee.

Nonoperative treatment of acute grade III MCL injuries initially focuses on edema control and quadriceps reactivation, with the focus then shifting to restoration of full ROM. Valgus stress testing and side-to-side movements are discouraged in the first 3 to 4 weeks to ensure proper healing of the ligament. Once the clinical examination reveals improved stability to valgus stress, balance and proprioceptive exercises can begin. Assistive devices are used for ambulation until the patient demonstrates full extension of the knee without an extensor lag and can walk normally, without gait deviations. Healing is generally complete by 5 to 7 weeks, at which point an ACL reconstruction can be performed, if indicated. As soon as appropriate return of strength, ROM, and balance has been achieved, progression to sport-specific exercises can also be initiated.[398]

In the postoperative management of isolated MCL reconstruction patients, communication between each member of the rehabilitation team is essential. In general, 0° to 90° of motion should be achieved by the second postoperative week and full ROM by the sixth week. Additional immediate emphasis is placed on edema management, patellofemoral mobilizations, and quadriceps reactivation. SLRs and hip strengthening are encouraged early, with careful avoidance of valgus stresses at the knee. CKC strengthening can begin as soon as the patient is cleared for full weight bearing, generally by 6 weeks after surgery. With appropriate return of strength, ROM, and balance, plyometric progressions can begin at approximately 16 weeks. It is important to recognize that concurrent anterior or posterior ligament reconstruction will dramatically alter the postoperative course, and communication with the surgeon is essential to ensure appropriate management.

Criteria for Return to Sport after Isolated MCL Reconstruction

- Full, symmetrical ROM
- No knee effusion during or after activity
- Pain-free jogging progression
- Pain-free multidirectional plyometrics/speed/agility training
- 85% limb symmetry index (hop testing, isokinetic strength, functional testing)
- Ability to avoid valgus stresses with all activities listed here

Adapted from Laprade RF, Wijdicks CA: The management of injuries to the medial side of the knee, *J Orthop Sports Phys Ther* 42:221-233, 2012.

Lateral and Posterolateral Corner Injuries of the Knee

Treatment decisions regarding the PLC are based on the extent of injury and functional instability. Isolated grade I LCL sprains that are stable with varus stress testing are treated symptomatically and produce consistently good results. Physical therapy is directed at quadriceps strengthening and ROM. Grade II injuries also do well with a nonoperative approach but can be associated with residual functional instability.[409] Surgical intervention is considered for residual functional instability or with concomitant ACL or PCL injuries where reconstruction of the PLC may also provide protection for the reconstructed cruciate ligaments.[245] Grade III LCL injuries have inferior outcomes compared with those treated surgically, and surgery is generally recommended in this setting.[409,410]

Nonoperative Management of Posterolateral Corner Injuries

Isolated grade I and II PLC injuries may be treated conservatively, as long as the patient does not present with concomitant ligamentous injury for which surgery would be indicated. Nonoperative rehabilitation is similar to the

---

Typical Nonoperative Time Frames for Return to Sport after Isolated MCL Injury

Grade	Timeframe
I	1-2 wk[218,408]
II	3-6 wk[218,408]
III	8-12 wk[225]

postoperative protocol described in detail later in this chapter; however, more accelerated progressions are typically tolerated, because treatment is not dependent on graft healing times. Lunden et al.[235] outlined a comprehensive, multiphased nonoperative rehabilitation progression (Table 20-8).

The focus of **phase I** is edema management, restoration of ROM, and reactivation of the quadriceps. Once the patient achieves full knee extension, has 120° of knee flexion, and is able to perform an SLR without an extensor lag, he or she can be progressed to phase II.

Phase II emphasizes normalization of gait and continued quadriceps strengthening. Gastrocnemius, hamstring, and lumbopelvic muscle strengthening are also initiated in this phase, with careful avoidance of varus stresses at the knee (i.e., antigravity hip abduction). The patient may progress to phase III when he or she demonstrates a normal gait pattern.

Phase III is marked by the initiation of neuromuscular training, including balance and proprioception exercises. Functional strength is emphasized in this phase, with cueing for the patient to avoid tibial lateral (external) rotation and knee varus. Hop testing, timed balance, and squat depth testing are also performed late in this phase. The patient may begin sport-specific drills (**phase IV**) when he or she achieves 85% limb symmetry index on all functional testing. A medial compartment unloader brace may be indicated for high-level activities in patients with continued lateral knee instability.

TABLE 20-8

Criterion-Based Progression of Nonoperative Posterolateral Corner Injuries

Phase	Treatment Focuses	Milestones
Phase I	Edema management Restoration of ROM Reactivation of quadriceps	Full extension ROM >120° knee flexion Straight-leg raise without lag
Phase II	Normalization of gait Continued quadriceps strengthening Lumbopelvic strengthening	Normal, pain-free gait
Phase III	Neuromuscular control Functional strengthening	>85% limb symmetry index (hop testing, squat depth, timed balance)
Phase IV	Sport-specific drills	Return to sport

ROM, Range of motion.

Modified from Lunden JB, Bzdusek PJ, Monson JK et al: Current concepts in the recognition and treatment of posterolateral corner injuries of the knee, *J Orthop Sports Phys Ther* 40:502-516, 2010.

Surgical Management of Posterolateral Corner Injuries

Surgical management of posterolateral corner injuries involves decisions regarding repair or reconstruction of the involved structures. Historically, standard of care called for primary repair of PLC structures within a 3-week time span following injury. Recent studies have called this into question. LaPrade[410] noted poor healing potential of the LCL and popliteus tendon. Levy et al.[259] reported a 40% failure rate of repair compared with 6% failures for reconstruction in patients with multiligamentous injuries. Stannard reported similar rates of failure.[411] Geeslin and LaPrade[412] found better results with combined repair and reconstruction. Because of this, primary repair alone has been limited to the acute setting where structures are in good condition and have been avulsed off their attachments, and surgical reconstruction of the PLC is more common. The authors' preferred technique is to repair avulsions of the LCL when it avulses off the fibular head with the biceps tendon as soon as possible after injury. The repairs are then frequently reinforced with a staged reconstructive procedure at a later date. Timing for surgical intervention has become less important given that reconstruction can be performed in the acute and chronic setting.

Several techniques for surgical reconstruction exist. A biceps tenodesis uses a portion of the biceps and or a strip of the biceps tendon to reinforce the LCL and popliteofibular ligament.[413,414] Assessing alignment of the knee may improve outcomes, especially in the setting of multiple ligament injuries. A high tibial osteotomy can be used to correct coronal alignment while a change in slope may decrease force on the posterolateral corner.[415]

Reconstruction of the lateral collateral ligament, popliteus tendon, or PFL can be performed via LaPrade's anatomic technique or an anatomic repair that is fibula based. In LaPrade's technique, grafts are fixed to the fibular head, and as a final step, the graft is brought through from the posterior to the anterior tibia.[416-418] A fibula-based reconstruction avoids fixation within the fibular head and does not utilize the transtibial tunnel (Figure 20-29).[419-421]

In all reconstructions of the LCL and posterolateral corner, the common peroneal nerve must be identified and protected. The LCL remnants are sutured to the graft to provide added healing potential and possibly proprioceptive function.[422]

Postoperative Management of Posterolateral Corner Injuries

The variability in surgical techniques is described in detail earlier in this chapter; therefore the clinician must have an understanding of the technique used and the structures involved before beginning a rehabilitation program. The following information describes a rehabilitation progression that has been modeled for LaPrade's anatomic

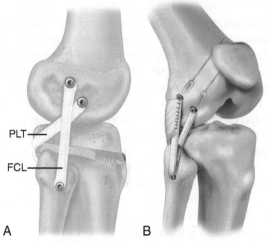

Figure 20-29 Anatomic posterolateral corner reconstructions. **A,** Diagrammatic representation of LaPrade's reconstructive technique. *PLT,* Popliteus tendon; *FCL,* fibular collateral ligament. **B,** Posterolateral capsular shift with a fibular sling. The capsular shift attempts to increase rotational stability by attaching the posterolateral capsule to the fibular collateral ligament (FCL) graft. (**A,** Redrawn from LaPrade RF, Johansen S, Wentorf FA et al: An analysis of an anatomical posterolateral knee reconstruction: an in vitro biomechanical study and development of a surgical technique, *Am J Sports Med* 32:1410, 2004. **B,** From Moulton SG, Geeslin AG, LaPrade RF: A systematic review of the outcomes of posterolateral corner knee injuries, Part 2: Surgical treatment of chronic injuries, *Am J Sports Med,* Aug 2015 [Epub ahead of print]).

technique explained earlier, involving the popliteus tendon, popliteofibular ligament, and LCL.

After PLC reconstruction, the patient is instructed to remain in a knee immobilizer locked in full extension at all times for the first 6 weeks, except when performing ROM and quadriceps strengthening exercises. The patient will also remain non–weight bearing for 6 weeks. For the first 4 months postoperatively, the patient will be instructed to avoid tibial lateral (external) rotation, especially in sitting. This can occur with movements such as sitting cross-legged, standing and pivoting, and engaging/disengaging cycling cleats. OKC hamstring strengthening is also avoided for 4 months and CKC squatting exercises are limited to 70° flexion.

Precautions after Isolated Posterolateral Corner Reconstruction

Timeframe	Precautions
6 wk	Non–weight bearing
6 wk	Locked in knee immobilizer in full extension, except during ROM and quadriceps strengthening
4 mo	No tibial external (lateral) rotation, especially in sitting
4 mo	No open-chain hamstring strengthening
4 mo	No CKC squats beyond 70° knee flexion

Adapted from Lunden JB, Bzdusek PJ, Monson JK et al: Current concepts in the recognition and treatment of posterolateral corner injuries of the knee, *J Orthop Sports Phys Ther* 40:502-516, 2010.

Phase I of postoperative rehabilitation generally encompasses the first 6 weeks. The immediate focus of rehabilitation is edema management, gentle ROM, and quadriceps reactivation. The patient remains in the knee immobilizer in full extension for the first 1 to 2 weeks to allow for the proliferation of fibroblasts and the formation of collagen. Excessive hyperextension is avoided.[235] Gentle ROM is then progressed to achieve 90° by the end of week 2 and full ROM by week 6. Once 100° of knee flexion has been reached, the patient can begin riding the stationary bicycle, with careful avoidance of tibial lateral (external) rotation. Isometric quadriceps strengthening is performed with quadriceps sets and SLR with NMES, and the patient is encouraged to perform up to 30 repetitions, five to six times per day.[235] The patient remains in the immobilizer when ambulating until able to perform an SLR without an extension lag. Lumbopelvic strengthening is also prescribed in this phase, but it is critical that the clinician be mindful of avoiding varus stresses at the knee, such as those incurred during antigravity hip abduction. To progress to phase II of the rehabilitation program, the patient must demonstrate no signs of knee effusion, an ability to perform an SLR without extension lag (i.e., 0° of knee extension) in supine, and more than 120° of knee flexion.

Phase II is marked by progression to full weight bearing. The patient is gradually weaned off crutches until the patient demonstrates a normal gait pattern, which generally takes about 2 weeks. If a **varus thrust** (a lateral bowing of the knee while weight bearing) was observed preoperatively, careful attention is directed at avoiding this motion during gait. Hamstring strengthening is performed with the knee extended (e.g., bridges with the feet on a ball or chair, progressing to standing single/double leg deadlifts) to avoid posteriorly directed forces at the knee. Balance and proprioception are a critical focus of the second postoperative phase, allowing the patient to regain neuromuscular control and confidence in the limb. CKC strengthening is initiated with partial BW leg press, then progressed to standing double-limb squats, without exceeding 70° of knee flexion. Perturbations can be applied in a static squat or lunged position to improve dynamic stability. Swimming with a flutter kick can begin at 8 weeks postoperatively, but the patient should be instructed to avoid flip turns and strokes that involve whip-kicks. To progress to phase III of the rehabilitation progression, the patient must demonstrate: no evidence of joint effusion at rest or with activity, normal pain-free gait pattern, and maintenance of full knee ROM.

Phase III continues with core and lower extremity strengthening, and a brisk walking progression may commence once the aforementioned criteria have been met. The patient is instructed to begin walking for 20 minutes and increase by 5 minutes per week. In order to begin a jogging progression, the patient must be able to ambulate pain free 3 to 5 km with brisk bouts on variable terrain.

Additionally, Lunden et al.[235] recommend that the patient be able to perform 20 repetitions of single-limb squatting with good neuromuscular control prior to beginning a jogging program. Once jogging has begun, step-ups and squatting may be performed at depths of more than 70°, and lateral and rotational components are added. A forward lunge can be utilized with the affected limb leading, with a medicine ball chop toward the medial side to promote varus control.[235] Proprioception exercises are advanced to include perturbations on unstable surfaces and distractions (e.g., ball tosses) to simulate sports activities.

Clinical Note

It has been recommended that a patient be able to do 20 single-leg squats with good control before beginning a jogging program.

Functional testing is similar in this population, as with many other knee injury populations, and can include hop testing, isokinetic or isometric strength testing, squat depth, and single-leg balance testing.[235] Furthermore, a truncated version of the star excursion balance test has been found to be reliable and is used to measure dynamic balance and limb confidence.[423] Like many of the other rehabilitation programs discussed in this chapter, once the patient achieves 85% limb symmetry index on the measures described earlier, he or she may begin sport-specific activities. It is also critical to qualitatively evaluate the patient's performance during functional tests to ensure proper jumping and landing techniques and dynamic avoidance of varus stress. Following this rehabilitation program, a patient can generally expect to return to activity and sports participation in 6 to 9 months, without the presence of concomitant ligamentous injury.

Multiple-Ligament Knee Injuries

Treatment of multiple-ligament injuries of the knee includes a wide spectrum of pathology and requires evaluation of many factors. A knee dislocation can be limb threatening because it is associated with a high incidence of neurological and vascular injuries. Immediate surgical intervention is necessary if the multiple-ligament injured knee is associated with a vascular injury or compartment syndrome. A grossly unstable knee can be stabilized initially with an external fixator. Delayed ligament reconstruction can be completed at a later time after all acute issues have been addressed.

Many knee dislocations reduce spontaneously. If three or more ligaments of the knee are injured, a knee dislocation should be suspected, and appropriate neurovascular examinations should be performed. Initial clinical assessment of a patient with a suspected knee dislocation should include a physical examination and measurement of an

ABI. An arteriogram should be obtained in patients with an abnormal physical examination.

Knee dislocations can result from low- or high-energy injuries. Low-energy injuries often are athletic injuries and have a better prognosis because fewer associated injuries are involved. High-energy injuries have a higher incidence of other organ system injuries and neurovascular compromise. However, ultra-low-velocity injuries in patients with a BMI of 40 or higher may have a very high rate of neurovascular injuries, and a significantly increased incidence of postoperative complications.[253,254,424]

Based on the work of Taylor et al.[258] on nonoperative versus operative treatment of knee dislocations, it is reasonable to conclude that nonoperative management could result in a functional knee, depending on the patient's age and functional demands. However, most authors support surgical reconstruction in an attempt to restore stability and improve functional outcomes.[248,300,425–428] Surgical management of a knee with a multiple-ligament injury may also prevent or delay the onset of arthritis by improving joint stability. Functional deficiency that results from a multiple-ligament knee injury must be evaluated relative to the patient's age, occupation, and recreational interests and the neurovascular status of the affected extremity before a decision is made to treat the condition surgically. Absolute indications for surgery include irreducible dislocations, dysvascular (i.e., defective blood supply) limbs, and open injuries.

When the authors opt for surgical management of this injury, reconstruction usually is delayed for 3 weeks after injury to allow soft tissue swelling to decrease. "Sealing" of the capsular injury occurs within a week, which permits the use of arthroscopically assisted techniques. Delayed reconstruction can also prevent the risk of arthrofibrosis by allowing time to regain motion after injury.[251,429] Even so, early repair of the PLC can be considered before 3 weeks to allow for the possibility of a primary repair of these structures. In this case, the PLC is repaired in this initial stage, and cruciate ligament reconstruction is performed several weeks later, after ROM has been regained. A few studies have suggested that acute ligament reconstruction (i.e., less than 2 to 3 weeks after injury) results in better functional outcome scores.[301,430] However, multiple confounding factors make the results difficult to interpret because surgery in patients with severe soft tissue trauma or other concomitant injuries often mandates delayed definitive reconstruction. These patients often have worse outcomes given the delayed timing of surgery and other injuries sustained from their initial trauma. Thus, prospective trials with closely matched groups are necessary to clearly delineate the benefits of early versus late ligamentous reconstruction after a knee dislocation.

In general, the treatment of each individual ligament injury is similar to that for an isolated injury of that ligament. Knees with an MCL injury are braced for the first 4 to 6 weeks to allow healing preoperatively. Reconstruction of the cruciate ligaments is then performed concomitantly. The authors prefer reconstruction using allograft tissue to reduce surgical time and patient morbidity. Use of allograft tissue also ensures the availability of graft tissue and minimizes difficulty with graft passage. The procedure is performed arthroscopically for reconstruction of the ACL and PCL. Open reconstruction is used for LCL/PLC and/or MCL/posteromedial corner injuries.

Postoperative rehabilitation for acute ligament reconstructions depends largely on the procedure performed and requires communication between the surgeon and therapist. ROM limits, time immobilized in extension, weight-bearing status, and brace use will depend on the extent of surgical reconstruction, the quality of the repair, and surgeon preferences. Return to functional activities also varies but is typically longer than that of individual ligaments.

TREATMENT OF PATELLAR TENDON INJURIES

Patellar Tendinopathy

Patellar tendinopathy is one of the most common causes of anterior knee pain in the athletic population. Activities that involve repetitive jumping, such as basketball and volleyball, have a high rate of patellar tendon pathology because of the repetitive eccentric contractions of the quadriceps muscles. Theories about the etiology of these injuries vary and include both intrinsic factors (e.g., muscle tightness, strength imbalances) and extrinsic factors (e.g., sport, training frequency), and both likely contribute to the pathological process.

The progression of symptoms has been described by Blazina et al.[431] and can be classified into four stages. Stage I tendinopathy typically occurs after a recent change in sports activity or a change in the intensity of the current sports activity. This stage is characterized by pain that is experienced after activity. Symptoms do not typically limit participation at this stage of the pathology. Stage II is characterized by pain at the start of activities that subsides, only to return as the patient begins to fatigue toward the end of participation. Stage III involves constant symptoms that limit the activity. Stage IV is defined as tendon rupture.

The stages of pathology defined by Blazina et al.[431] correspond well with the stages of tendinopathy defined by Nirschl.[432] He described an acute period of inflammation of the tendon and paratenon sheath surrounding the tendon (**stage I**). As the chronicity of symptoms continues, the underlying tendon tissue begins to develop tendinosis, whereas the paratenon continues to show an inflammatory response (**stage II**). Eventually the pathology becomes chronic enough that inflammation subsides and tendinosis of the tendon continues (**stage III**). To develop an appropriate treatment program for patellar

tendinopathy, it is imperative that the clinician differentially diagnose the appropriate stage of pathology and treat the patient accordingly.

On clinical examination, the patient often is point tender to palpation at the inferior patellar pole at the site of origin of the patellar tendon. The patient also may have symptoms in the midportion or distal attachment of the tendon, although these findings are less common. Resisted quadriceps contraction may elicit symptoms, and the patient often has tightness of the quadriceps musculature. The patient will likely complain of difficulty descending stairs, jumping/hopping, and squatting. Witvrouw et al.[61] prospectively evaluated predictive factors in the development of patellar tendinopathy and reported that the most common factor was the loss of quadriceps soft tissue flexibility. Decreased ankle dorsiflexion ROM has also been strongly correlated with an increased risk of patellar tendinopathy.[433] MRI studies show abnormal signals in the tendon but are often time-consuming and expensive. Ultrasound has become the method of choice for evaluation of tendons because it is inexpensive, noninvasive, repeatable, and allows for dynamic examination and administration of ultrasound-guided injections.[434,435] Hypoechoic regions can be visualized in symptomatic patellar tendons; furthermore, asymptomatic patellar tendons with areas of hypoechoicity are at an increased risk of developing patellar tendinopathy.[435]

Nonoperative Treatment

Conservative treatment for patellar tendinopathy must be appropriate for the stage and progression of pathology. The primary goals of rehabilitation are to control the applied loads and create an environment for proper healing. For patients in stage I and early stage II tendinopathy with an acute onset of symptoms and pain after activity, treatment aims at reducing the inflammatory response and balancing the strength and flexibility of the lower extremity. Traditional anti-inflammatory treatments are used, including cryotherapy and nonsteroidal anti-inflammatory medications. The use of modalities, including iontophoresis, ultrasound, and electrical stimulation, has not been supported for the treatment of tendinopathy in recent research.[436] Patients should attempt to minimize activities that irritate the tendon, and the concept of "relative rest" should be encouraged. The patient should continue to work on enhancing quadriceps strength, lower extremity muscle balance, and soft tissue flexibility. Abstaining from all activities and relying on rest and ice often cause further loss of strength and flexibility, which can result in a recurrence of symptoms when activities are resumed.

The treatment of more chronic stage II and stage III tendinopathies varies greatly from that used for the acute condition. As the chronicity of the pathology progresses, inflammation subsides and tissue degeneration occurs, creating a tendinosis rather than tendonitis. Thus, anti-inflammatory treatments are avoided, and a healing environment is encouraged by attempting to stimulate blood flow to the area. Several authors have encouraged the use of eccentric exercise for patellar tendinopathy to increase the amount of force applied to the tendon.[437-439] Furthermore, eccentric decline squats have been identified as an excellent exercise to increase and isolate the load through the patellar tendon, showing 25% to 30% higher loads as opposed to flat-ground squats.[436,440] Young et al.[441] demonstrated that decline squats are more effective than a traditional eccentric training program at reducing pain and improving physical function in a group of elite volleyball players. In addition to decline squats, deep transverse friction massage is recommended to encourage a healing environment and promote normalized collagen alignment.[436] Drop squats are added late in the eccentric training program to replicate high-speed eccentric loads. A gradual progression through plyometric and running activities precedes the return to full activity participation, which can generally be achieved within 2 to 3 months.[436]

In the treatment of patients with chronic patellar tendinopathy, the authors recommend a decline squat program including 2 sets of 15 decline squats, twice daily. Exercising into slight pain (up to 5 out of 10 on the VAS) is encouraged, without exceeding a 70° squat depth, to minimize patellofemoral joint loads. Furthermore, the clinician or the patient should perform deep transverse friction massage to the patellar tendon for 5 to 10 minutes per day.

As noted earlier, intrinsic factors are often the primary cause of this condition; therefore an evaluation of the entire kinetic chain is essential to neutralize potential risk factors. A comprehensive program will often include posterolateral hip strengthening and/or foot mobilizations, as indicated.

Platelet-rich plasma (PRP) is a recent nonoperative treatment modality that has been gaining interest. PRP is a sample of autologous blood with concentrations of platelets above baseline values. It is created through a two-phase centrifugation process where the liquid and solid components of anticoagulated blood are separated. The platelet-rich preparation can then be isolated and injected locally into an affected area in the body. In addition to platelets, PRP contains cells such as monocytes and neutrophils that can potentially create beneficial effects in tissue healing by causing a localized inflammatory effect. The inclusion of white blood cells in PRP can vary. Proteins such as platelet-derived growth factor, vascular endothelial growth factor, endothelial cell growth factor and basic fibroblast growth factor can be detected at high concentrations in PRP. Currently, more than 40 commercial systems are available, which can result in variable contents and concentrations of growth factors and cells in the PRP preparation.[442] A recent randomized trial comparing PRP injection to dry needling for patellar tendinopathy showed that a regimen of eccentric exercises and leukocyte rich PRP injection

with dry needling accelerates recovery relative to exercise and dry needling alone at 12 weeks. However, functional outcome scores between the two groups showed no difference at 26 weeks.[443] Another study has evaluated outcomes after three consecutive PRP injections delivered 1 week apart for patients with chronic patellar tendinopathy refractory to conservative treatment. Charousset et al.[444] reported that functional scores all significantly improved at the 2-year follow-up, and 75% of patients returned to their presymptom sporting level at 3 months after the procedure. Follow-up MRI also showed improved structural integrity of the tendon at a 3-month follow-up.[444] The cost-effectiveness and clinical evidence of PRP injections remains somewhat unclear in the setting of patellar tendinopathy, and more research is required to clearly delineate if there is a true clinical benefit with this technique.

Surgical Treatment

Surgery generally is performed for chronic tendinosis that has not responded to conservative treatment after 3 to 6 months. The surgery typically involves debridement of degenerative tissue, which creates an inflammatory response and facilitates a healing response. An anterior incision is made directly over the area of tendinosis, and dissection is carried down to the underlying tendon. The paratenon is preserved, and the patellar tendon is divided longitudinally. Degenerative patellar tendon tissue is debrided, and the patellar tendon is reapproximated with a high-tensile-strength suture. Several surgeons advocate additional stimulation of a healing response by drilling adjacent bone with a Kirschner wire (K-wire).

Postoperative rehabilitation focuses on minimizing pain and swelling and gradually restoring strength and ROM in the knee. ROM is initiated immediately to stimulate healing and collagen tissue organization. The patient typically achieves full knee extension immediately, and full knee flexion is restored gradually over the first 4 to 6 weeks. Bahr et al.[438] have outlined a comprehensive rehabilitation program. In the first week postoperatively, the patient performs quadriceps sets and pain-free ROM exercises, as well as standing weight-shifting. In the second postoperative week, the patient may begin weaning from crutches, and he or she may ambulate without an assistive device once he or she has a pain-free, nonantalgic gait. Stationary cycling may begin in the third week, in addition to minisquats with arm support. By weeks 4 and 5, the patient may begin step-ups and step-downs using a 2-inch step, respectively. Eccentric strengthening is initiated in the sixth postoperative week, but unlike nonoperative patellar tendinopathy, the patient is discouraged from exercising into pain. Return to jogging can generally begin at 3 to 4 months. In contrast, Shelbourne et al.[445] outlined an aggressive rehabilitation program that involved active and passive full flexion and extension ROM on the same day as the patient's surgery as well as unrestricted full weight bearing.[445] Patients in their study performed supervised resisted concentric and eccentric leg press using a portable, low-resistance leg press machine, once they arrived to their inpatient hospital room and twice per day for the first week. At that point, patients were allowed to begin step-up exercises and step height was progressively increased as pain allowed. Sport-specific drills were allowed once the patient achieved 85% isokinetic quadriceps strength, typically at about 2 months postoperatively. In this study, 14 of 16 patients were able to resume sports participation at their presymptom level in an average of 8.1 months. It is important to note that all of the patients in this study were elite-level athletes, including NCAA Division I and professional football, volleyball, basketball, and track athletes.[445]

Patellar Tendon Rupture

Patellar tendon rupture is a disabling injury that results in complete disruption of the extensor mechanism and the inability to actively obtain and maintain knee extension. Ruptures (grade III strains) often occur in sports as a result of a violent contraction of the quadriceps muscle as the foot is planted and the knee moves into flexion, producing an eccentric contraction of the quadriceps muscles. Forces causing rupture of the patellar tendon typically are more than $17 \times BW$.[446] In patients younger than 40 years of age, these forces are highest at the insertion of the tendon and therefore commonly produce tears at the inferior pole of the patella. Ruptures of the patellar tendon may be more prominent with systemic inflammatory disease, diabetes mellitus, or chronic renal failure. In these patients, rupture of the patellar tendon may more likely occur midsubstance than at the tendo-osseous junction.

One of the most commonly observed causative factors in patellar tendon rupture is chronic patient complaints of patellar tendinopathy. Kelly et al.[447] reported a correlation between preexisting patellar tendinosis and patellar tendon rupture. The relatively poor vascularity and chronic degeneration of tissue associated with patellar tendinosis, combined with repetitive microtrauma, eventually may result in complete rupture of the tendon.

Patients almost always report an acute incident and present with pain, swelling, and the inability to actively extend the knee. They may, however, be able to hold the knee in extension using the iliotibial band especially if gravity is eliminated. A palpable defect often is noted upon examination. The patient also has a visible antalgic and quadriceps avoidance gait pattern as the hip musculature and iliotibial band attempts to substitute for the lack of quadriceps control. Plain film radiographs are commonly taken as part of the evaluation. A superiorly oriented patella, or patella alta, on the lateral view may indicate rupture of the tendon. A MRI can confirm the diagnosis of a ruptured tendon and can aid the assessment for concomitant pathology.

Surgical Management

The treatment of an acute tear of the patellar tendon depends on the extent of the tear. If the patient is able to perform an SLR without a quadriceps lag (i.e., inability to fully extend the knee), nonoperative treatment can be considered. However, in most cases, patellar tendon rupture results in a disruption of the extensor mechanism and should be repaired surgically.

An anterior longitudinal incision over the knee permits exposure of both the patellar tendon and the patella. Because most ruptures occur at the tendo-osseous junction at the inferior pole of the patella, the patellar tendon cannot usually be simply reapproximated. Instead, three longitudinal drill holes spaced slightly apart are made in the patella. A running locking stitch is placed in the patellar tendon, and sutures are passed from the tendon through the drill holes in the patella and tied over a bony bridge at the proximal aspect of the patella. The paratenon of the patella is repaired, and the patient is placed in a knee immobilizer or cast.

Postoperative Treatment for Patellar Tendon Repair

The rehabilitation program following a patellar tendon repair is critical to the long-term success of the procedure. Rehabilitation must protect the healing tendon while gradually returning the patient to functional activities. Traditional rehabilitation programs involve approximately 6 to 8 weeks of immobilization and unloading of the lower extremity after surgery. Although this may be appropriate for patients with poor tissue status, a very active person or competitive athlete who wants to return to vigorous activities may risk the development of joint stiffness and arthrofibrosis if this pathway is followed. We prefer a program that gradually progresses ROM and weight bearing but does not overload the healing tissue; this is believed to minimize the risk of complications such as knee flexion limitations, patella immobility, and patella baja.[448] The specific pace of the rehabilitation program is based on the quality of surrounding tissue and the fixation strength of the repair. Communication with the surgeon is vital to develop an appropriate postoperative program.

The immediate postoperative goals include reducing pain and swelling, restoring patellar mobility, initiating early, controlled quadriceps muscle contraction, and gradually restoring ROM. The patient is instructed to use a brace locked in extension for ambulation. Immediate toe touch weight bearing is initiated, progressing to about 25% of BW by week 2 and 50% of BW by week 3. The patient typically progresses to weight bearing as tolerated without crutches by 6 weeks. At this time, the patient may unlock the brace during ambulation but is advised to continue wearing the brace for approximately 8 weeks.

The restoration of passive ROM is one of the most difficult goals to achieve. Full knee extension is encouraged immediately after surgery, although flexion is limited to 30° for the first 5 days and to 45° by the end of week 1. Motion is gradually progressed to 60° by week 2, 75° by week 4, and 90° by week 6. The rate of progression should be carefully monitored, and a continuous passive motion (CPM) machine may be useful at home. ROM is gradually progressed to 105° by week 8, 115° by week 10, and at least 125° by week 12.

Restoring Flexion after Patellar Tendon Repair

First 5 days	30°
Week 1	45°
Week 2	60°
Week 4	75°
Week 6	90°
Week 8	105°
Week 10	115°
Week 12	125°

Initial isometric exercises for the quadriceps and other lower extremity muscles are encouraged. These exercises include quadriceps setting and multiangle SLRs by the end of week 2. Use of the pool and gentle cycling may also be beneficial for the patient when ROM and incision healing permits, typically by 4 to 6 weeks. Gentle CKC exercises, such as weight shifting and minisquats to 30°, are initiated during week 4 and progressed to include the leg press, wall squats, front lunges, and other lower extremity exercises by weeks 10 to 12. Active OKC knee extension is avoided for the first 8 to 12 weeks. Patients who want to begin a running program are allowed to do so after a satisfactory clinical examination and appropriate functional goals have been met. Running typically begins around 5 to 6 months after surgery, with a gradual return to sports activity at 7 to 9 months.

ASSESSMENT OF FUNCTIONAL OUTCOME

Historically, outcome studies related to treatment of knee ligament injuries have focused on reporting physical impairment of the knee, including limitations in ROM, strength, and stability. Functional performance tests may be better predictors of functional limitations and disability than measurements of physical impairment after knee ligament injury. Deficits in functional performance tests probably would result in functional limitations and disability for a patient. Functional performance tests that reproduce the stresses and strains on the knee that occur during activities may be more likely to demonstrate functional limitations and disability. For example, carioca that involves a cross-cutting maneuver reproduces the pivot shift associated with anterolateral instability. This maneuver would be expected to be more stressful than a one-legged hop for distance in an individual with an ACL-deficient knee. Additional research is needed to identify functional performance tests that can accurately predict functional limitations and disability after a knee ligament injury.

Functional limitations and disability experienced by a patient after a knee ligament injury may have multiple causes. Disability may be related to a combination of factors, such as the type and extent of injury, symptoms, and physical impairment and to psychological factors, such as apprehension, lack of confidence, and fear of reinjury. This diversity has led researchers to use a combination of quality of life and disease-specific evaluation tools.

Multiple measures of patient outcomes have been used to measure clinical success. Questionnaires can be used to measure general health status, pain, functional status, or patient satisfaction. Physiological outcomes, utilization measures, or cost measures can also be defined as end points. Assessment tools can be driven by the health care provider or by patients themselves. Objective measures used by the health care provider can include ROM, strength, endurance, structural measures (radiographs), proprioception, and joint laxity. Subjective measures, derived from patient-driven data, include general health, pain perception, psychometric evaluations, disability predictions, and overall patient satisfaction. Subjective measurements have been found to be valid measurements of outcome and, in many cases, were more reliable than the "objective" tests health care providers have relied on for years. The most appropriate set of tools depends on the question to be evaluated and the patient population; usually a combination of these techniques is required.

Some common knee outcome measures include the Short-Form 36 (SF-36), the Modified Lysholm Scale, the Cincinnati Knee Rating Score, the Activities of Daily Living Scale, the Knee Injury and OA Outcomes Score, the Quality of Life Outcome Measure for Chronic ACL Deficiency (ACL-QoL), and the International Knee Documentation Committee (IKDC). Test-test reliability (reproducibility), responsiveness (i.e., the ability to detect clinically important change), and construct validity are usually defined for each outcome tool. Successful application of these tools to assess functional outcome requires an understanding of the patient population and the research question at hand.[449] An instrument validated for one population may not be the correct tool to measure a different population. The Western Ontario and McMaster Universities (WOMAC) Osteoarthritis Index, for example, was developed and validated to assess osteoarthritis outcomes in a relatively older population.[450] The usefulness of its comparisons in a population of younger patients with knee instability is uncertain. See *Orthopedic*

Physical Assessment for more information about the functional assessment of the knee.

SUMMARY

Successful treatment and rehabilitation of ligamentous and patellar tendon injuries of the knee requires a full understanding of the anatomy and biomechanics of the knee. Although imaging techniques continue to advance technologically, the physical examination remains the most important diagnostic tool. Each knee injury must be treated as an individual and unique case; however, application of the principles outlined in this chapter can lead to improved outcomes over time.

REFERENCES

1. Sanchez AR, Sugalski MT, LaPrade RF: Anatomy and biomechanics of the lateral side of the knee, *Sports Med Arthrosc* 14:2–11, 2006.
2. Calliet R: *Knee pain and disability*, Philadelphia, 1978, FA Davis.
3. Kapandji IA: *The physiology of the joints, vol 2, Lower limb*, London, 1970, Churchill Livingstone.
4. Hughston JC, Eilers AF: The role of the posterior oblique ligament in repairs of acute medial (collateral) ligament tears of the knee, *J Bone Joint Surg Am* 55:923–940, 1973.
5. LaPrade RF, Morgan PM, Wentorf FA, et al: The anatomy of the posterior aspect of the knee. An anatomic study, *J Bone Joint Surg Am* 89:758–764, 2007.
6. Fu FH, Shen W, Starman JS, et al: Primary anatomic double-bundle anterior cruciate ligament reconstruction: a preliminary 2-year prospective study, *Am J Sports Med* 36:1263–1274, 2008.
7. Scopp JM, Jasper LE, Belkoff SM, Moorman CT: The effect of oblique femoral tunnel placement on rotational constraint of the knee reconstructed using patellar tendon autografts, *Arthroscopy* 20:294–299, 2004.
8. Zantop T, Herbort M, Raschke MJ, et al: The role of the anteromedial and posterolateral bundles of the anterior cruciate ligament in anterior tibial translation and internal rotation, *Am J Sports Med* 35:223–227, 2007.
9. Arnoczky SP: Blood supply to the anterior cruciate ligament and supporting structures, *Orthop Clin North Am* 16:15–28, 1985.
10. Blackburn TA, Craig E: Knee anatomy: a brief review, *Phys Ther* 60:1556–1560, 1980.
11. Seebacher JR, Inglis AE, Marshall JL, Warren RF: The structure of the posterolateral aspect of the knee, *J Bone Joint Surg Am* 64:536–541, 1982.
12. Bedi A, Maak T, Musahl V, et al: Effect of tibial tunnel position on stability of the knee after anterior cruciate ligament reconstruction: is the tibial tunnel position most important? *Am J Sports Med* 39:366–373, 2011.
13. Shoemaker SC, Markolf KL: The role of the meniscus in the anterior-posterior stability of the loaded anterior cruciate-deficient knee. Effects of partial versus total excision, *J Bone Joint Surg Am* 68:71–79, 1986.
14. Levy IM, Torzilli PA, Warren RF: The effect of medial meniscectomy on anterior-posterior motion of the knee, *J Bone Joint Surg Am* 64:883–888, 1982.
15. Musahl V, Citak M, O'Loughlin PF, et al: The effect of medial versus lateral meniscectomy on the stability of the anterior cruciate ligament-deficient knee, *Am J Sports Med* 38:1591–1597, 2010.
16. Baratz ME, Fu FH, Mengato R: Meniscal tears: the effect of meniscectomy and of repair on intraarticular contact areas and stress in the human knee. A preliminary report, *Am J Sports Med* 14:270–275, 1986.
17. Alford JW, Lewis P, Kang RW, Cole BJ: Rapid progression of chondral disease in the lateral compartment of the knee following meniscectomy, *Arthroscopy* 21:1505–1509, 2005.
18. Muller M: The angles of femoral and tibial axes with respect to the cruciate ligament four-bar system in the knee joint, *J Theor Biol* 161:221–230, 1993.
19. Butler DL, Noyes FR, Grood ES: Ligamentous restraints to anterior-posterior drawer in the human knee: a biomechanical study, *J Bone Joint Surg Am* 62:259–270, 1980.
20. Grood ES, Suntay WJ, Noyes FR, Butler DL: Biomechanics of the knee-extension exercise: effect of cutting the anterior cruciate ligament, *J Bone Joint Surg Am* 66:725–734, 1984.
21. Palmitier RA, An KN, Scott SG, Chao EY: Kinetic chain exercise in knee rehabilitation, *Sports Med* 11:402–413, 1991.
22. Barrack RL, Skinner HB, Buckley SL: Proprioception in the anterior cruciate deficient knee, *Am J Sports Med* 17:1–6, 1989.
23. Kennedy JC, Weinberg HW, Wilson AS: The anatomy and function of the anterior cruciate ligament as determined by clinical and morphological studies, *J Bone Joint Surg Am* 56:223–235, 1974.
24. Solomonow M, Baratta R, Zhou BH, et al: The synergistic action of the anterior cruciate ligament and thigh muscles in maintaining joint stability, *Am J Sports Med* 15:207–213, 1987.
25. Lephart SM, Kocher MS, Fu FH, et al: Proprioception following anterior cruciate ligament reconstruction, *J Sport Rehabil* 1:188–196, 1992.
26. Cooper RL, Taylor NF, Feller JA: A systematic review of the effect of proprioceptive and balance exercises on people with an injured or reconstructed anterior cruciate ligament, *Res Sports Med* 13:163–178, 2005.
27. Walla DJ, Albright JP, McAuley E, et al: Hamstring control and the unstable anterior cruciate ligament-deficient knee, *Am J Sports Med* 13:34–39, 1985.
28. Barrett DS: Proprioception and function after anterior cruciate reconstruction, *J Bone Joint Surg Br* 73:833–837, 1991.
29. Baratta R, Solomonow M, Zhou BH, et al: Muscular coactivation : the role of the antagonist musculature in maintaining knee stability, *Am J Sports Med* 16:113–122, 1988.
30. Krogsgaard MR, Dyhre-Poulsen P, Fischer-Rasmussen T: Cruciate ligament reflexes, *J Electromyogr Kinesiol* 12:177–182, 2002.
31. Ageberg E, Zätterström R, Moritz U, Fridén T: Influence of supervised and nonsupervised training on postural control after an acute anterior cruciate ligament rupture: a three-year longitudinal prospective study, *J Orthop Sports Phys Ther* 31:632–644, 2001.
32. Fitzgerald GK, Axe MJ, Snyder-Mackler L: The efficacy of perturbation training in nonoperative anterior cruciate ligament rehabilitation programs for physically active individuals, *Phys Ther* 80:128–140, 2000.
33. Zätterström R, Fridén T, Lindstrand A, Moritz U: Rehabilitation following acute anterior cruciate ligament injuries – a 12-month follow-up of a randomized clinical trial, *Scand J Med Sci Sports* 10:156–163, 2000.
34. Liu-Ambrose T, Taunton JE, MacIntyre D, et al: The effects of proprioceptive or strength training on the neuromuscular function of the ACL reconstructed knee: a randomized clinical trial, *Scand J Med Sci Sports* 13:115–123, 2003.
35. Beard DJ, Dodd CA, Trundle HR, Simpson AH: Proprioception enhancement for anterior cruciate ligament deficiency. A prospective randomised trial of two physiotherapy regimes, *J Bone Joint Surg Br* 76:654–659, 1994.
36. Draganich LF, Jaeger RJ, Kralj AR: Coactivation of the hamstrings and quadriceps during extension of the knee, *J Bone Joint Surg Am* 71:1075–1081, 1989.
37. Sawhney R, Dearwater S, Irrgang JJ, Fu FH: *Quadriceps exercise following anterior cruciate ligament reconstruction without anterior tibial displacement*. In Presented at the Annual Conference of the American Physical Therapy Association, Anaheim, CA, June 24-28, 1990.
38. Lutz GE, Palmitier RA, An KN, Chao EY: Comparison of tibiofemoral joint forces during open-kinetic-chain and closed-kinetic-chain exercises, *J Bone Joint Surg Am* 75:732–739, 1993.
39. Markolf KL, Gorek JF, Kabo JM, Shapiro MS: Direct measurement of resultant forces in the anterior cruciate ligament: an in vitro study performed with a new experimental technique, *J Bone Joint Surg Am* 72:557–567, 1990.
40. Fleming BC, Renstrom PA, Beynnon BD, et al: The effect of weight bearing and external loading on anterior cruciate ligament strain, *J Biomech* 34:163–170, 2001.
41. Wilk KE, Escamilla RF, Fleisig GS, et al: A comparison of tibiofemoral joint forces and electromyographic activity during open and closed kinetic chain exercises, *Am J Sports Med* 24:518–527, 1996.
42. Beynnon BD, Johnson RJ, Fleming BC, et al: The strain behavior of the anterior cruciate ligament during squatting and active flexion-extension: a comparison of an open and a closed kinetic chain exercise, *Am J Sports Med* 25:823–829, 1997.
43. Fleming BC, Beynnon BD, Renstrom PA, et al: The strain behavior of the anterior cruciate ligament during bicycling: an in vivo study, *Am J Sports Med* 26:109–118, 1998.
44. Fleming BC, Beynnon BD, Renstrom PA, et al: The strain behavior of the anterior cruciate ligament during stair climbing: an in vivo study, *Arthroscopy* 15:185–191, 1999.
45. Morrison JB: The mechanics of the knee joint in relation to normal walking, *J Biomech* 3:51–61, 1970.
46. Morrison JB: Function of the knee joint in various activities, *Biomed Eng* 4:573–580, 1969.
47. Kaufman KR, An KN, Litchy WJ, et al: Dynamic joint forces during knee isokinetic exercise, *Am J Sports Med* 19:305–316, 1991.
48. Smidt GL: Biomechanical analysis of knee flexion and extension, *J Biomech* 6:79–92, 1973.

49. Wilk KE: Rehabilitation of isolated and combined posterior cruciate ligament injuries, *Clin Sports Med* 13:649–677, 1994.

50. Clancy WG: Repair and reconstruction of the posterior cruciate ligament. In Chapman MW, editor: *Operative orthopaedics*, Philadelphia, 1988, JB Lippincott.

51. Jurist KA, Otis JC: Anteroposterior tibiofemoral displacements during isometric extension efforts: the roles of external load and knee flexion angle, *Am J Sports Med* 13:254–258, 1985.

52. Wilk KE, Zheng N, Fleisig GS, et al: Kinetic chain exercise: implication for the ACL patient, *J Sport Rehabil* 6:125–143, 1997.

53. Stuart MJ, Meglan DA, Lutz GE, et al: Comparison of intersegmental tibiofemoral joint forces and muscle activity during various closed kinetic chain exercises, *Am J Sports Med* 24:792–799, 1996.

54. Williams PL, Warwick R: *Functional neuroanatomy of man*, Edinburgh, 1975, Churchill Livingstone.

55. Hungerford DS, Barry M: Biomechanics of the patellofemoral joint, *Clin Orthop Relat Res* 144:9–15, 1979.

56. Huberti HH, Hayes WC: Patellofemoral contact pressures: the influence of Q-angle and tendofemoral contact, *J Bone Joint Surg Am* 66:715–724, 1984.

57. Reilly DT, Martens M: Experimental analysis of the quadriceps muscle force and patello-femoral joint reaction force for various activities, *Acta Orthop Scand* 43:126–137, 1972.

58. Wilk KE, Reinold MM: Closed kinetic chain exercises and plyometric activities. In Bandy WD, Sanders B, editors: *Therapeutic exercise: techniques for intervention*, Baltimore, 2001, Lippincott Williams & Wilkins.

59. Steinkamp LA, Dillingham MF, Markel MD, et al: Biomechanical considerations in patellofemoral joint rehabilitation, *Am J Sports Med* 21:438–444, 1993.

60. Escamilla RF, Fleisig GS, Zheng N, et al: Biomechanics of the knee during closed kinetic chain and open kinetic chain exercises, *Med Sci Sports Exerc* 30:556–569, 1998.

61. Witvrouw E, Bellemans J, Lysens R, et al: Intrinsic risk factors for the development of patellar tendinitis in an athletic population: a two-year prospective study, *Am J Sports Med* 29:190–195, 2001.

62. Daniel DM, Stone ML, Dobson BE, et al: Fate of the ACL-injured patient. A prospective outcome study, *Am J Sports Med* 22:632–644, 1994.

63. Noyes FR, Bassett RW, Grood ES, Butler DL: Arthroscopy in acute traumatic hemarthrosis of the knee: incidence of anterior cruciate tears and other injuries, *J Bone Joint Surg Am* 62:687–695, 757 1980.

64. Robins AJ, Newman AP, Burks RT: Postoperative return of motion in anterior cruciate ligament and medial collateral ligament injuries. The effect of medial collateral ligament rupture location, *Am J Sports Med* 21:20–25, 1993.

65. Griffith CJ, LaPrade RF, Johansen S, et al: Medial knee injury: Part 1, static function of the individual components of the main medial knee structures, *Am J Sports Med* 37:1762–1770, 2009.

66. Gollehon DL, Torzilli PA, Warren RF: The role of the posterolateral and cruciate ligaments in the stability of the human knee: a biomechanical study, *J Bone Joint Surg Am* 69:233–242, 1987.

67. Torg JS, Conrad W, Kalen V: Clinical diagnosis of anterior cruciate ligament instability in the athlete, *Am J Sports Med* 4:84–93, 1976.

68. Jonsson T, Althoff B, Peterson L, Renstrom P: Clinical diagnosis of ruptures of the anterior cruciate ligament: a comparative study of the Lachman test and the anterior drawer sign, *Am J Sports Med* 10:100–102, 1982.

69. Katz JW, Fingeroth RJ: The diagnostic accuracy of ruptures of the anterior cruciate ligament comparing the Lachman test, the anterior drawer sign, and the pivot shift test in acute and chronic knee injuries, *Am J Sports Med* 14:88–91, 1986.

70. Kim SJ, Lee SK, Kim SH, et al: Does anterior laxity of the uninjured knee influence clinical outcomes of ACL reconstruction? *J Bone Joint Surg Am* 96:543–548, 2014.

71. van Eck CF, van den Bekerom MP, Fu FH, et al: Methods to diagnose acute anterior cruciate ligament rupture: a meta-analysis of physical examinations with and without anaesthesia, *Knee Surg Sports Traumatol Arthrosc* 21:1895–1903, 2013.

72. Bach BR, Warren RF, Wickiewicz TL: The pivot shift phenomenon: results and description of a modified clinical test for anterior cruciate ligament insufficiency, *Am J Sports Med* 16:571–576, 1988.

73. Fetto JF, Marshall JL: Injury to the anterior cruciate ligament producing the pivot-shift sign, *J Bone Joint Surg Am* 61:710–714, 1979.

74. Galway HR, MacIntosh DL: The lateral pivot shift: a symptom and sign of anterior cruciate ligament insufficiency, *Clin Orthop Relat Res* 147:45–50, 1980.

75. Nogalski MP, Bach BR: Acute anterior cruciate ligament injuries. In Fu F, Harner CD, Vince KG, editors: *Knee surgery*. Baltimore, 1994, Williams and Wilkins.

76. Lane CG, Warren R, Pearle AD: The pivot shift, *J Am Acad Orthop Surg* 16:679–688, 2008.

77. Covey CD, Sapega AA: Injuries of the posterior cruciate ligament, *J Bone Joint Surg Am* 75:1376–1386, 1993.

78. Markolf KL, Slauterbeck JR, Armstrong KL, et al: A biomechanical study of replacement of the posterior cruciate ligament with a graft. I. Isometry, pretension of the graft, and anterior-posterior laxity, *J Bone Joint Surg Am* 79:375–380, 1997.

79. Clancy WG, Shelbourne KD, Zoellner GB, et al: Treatment of knee joint instability secondary to rupture of the posterior cruciate ligament: report of a new procedure, *J Bone Joint Surg Am* 65:310–322, 1983.

80. Harner CD, Hoher J: Evaluation and treatment of posterior cruciate ligament injuries, *Am J Sports Med* 26:471–482, 1998.

81. Bae JH, Choi IC, Suh SW, et al: Evaluation of the reliability of the dial test for posterolateral rotatory instability: a cadaveric study using an isotonic rotation machine, *Arthroscopy* 24:593–598, 2008.

82. Jung YB, Lee YS, Jung HJ, Nam CH: Evaluation of posterolateral rotatory knee instability using the dial test according to tibial positioning, *Arthroscopy* 25:257–261, 2009.

83. Insall JN: Bone-block transfer of the medial head of the gastrocnemius for posterior cruciate insufficiency, *J Bone Joint Surg Am* 65:691–699, 1982.

84. Daniel DM, Stone ML, Barnett P, Sachs R: Use of the quadriceps active test to diagnose posterior cruciate ligament disruption and measure posterior laxity of the knee, *J Bone Joint Surg Am* 70:386–391, 1988.

85. Hughston JC, Norwood LA: The posterolateral drawer test and external rotational recurvatum test for posterolateral rotatory instability of the knee, *Clin Orthop Relat Res* 147:82–87, 1980.

86. Jakob RP, Staubli HU, Deland JT: Grading the pivot shift. Objective tests with implications for treatment, *J Bone Joint Surg Br* 69:294–299, 1987.

87. Jakob RP, Hassler H, Staeubli HU: Observations on rotatory instability of the lateral compartment of the knee: experimental studies on the functional anatomy and the pathomechanism of the true and the reversed pivot shift sign, *Acta Orthop Scand Suppl* 191:1–32, 1981.

88. Cooper DE: Tests for posterolateral instability of the knee in normal subjects: results of examination under anesthesia, *J Bone Joint Surg Am* 73:30–36, 1991.

89. Daniel DM, Stone ML, Sachs R, Malcom L: Instrumented measurement of anterior knee laxity in patients with acute anterior cruciate ligament disruption, *Am J Sports Med* 13:401–407, 1985.

90. Stratford PW, Miseferi D, Ogilvie R: Assessing the responsiveness of five KT1000 knee arthrometer measures used to evaluate anterior laxity at the knee joint, *Clin J Sport Med* 1:225–228, 1991.

91. Highgenboten CL, Jackson AW, Jansson KA, Meske NB: KT1000 arthrometer: conscious and unconscious test results using 15, 20, and 30 pounds of force, *Am J Sports Med* 20:450–454, 1992.

92. Wroble RR, Grood ES, Noyes FR, Schmitt DJ: Reproducibility of Genucom knee analysis system testing, *Am J Sports Med* 18:387–395, 1990.

93. Boniface RJ, Fu FH, Ilkhanipour K: Objective anterior cruciate ligament testing, *Orthopedics* 9:391–393, 1986.

94. King JB, Kumar SJ: The Stryker knee arthrometer in clinical practice, *Am J Sports Med* 17:649–650, 1989.

95. Riederman R, Wroble RR, Grood ES, et al: Reproducibility of the knee signature system, *Am J Sports Med* 19:660–664, 1991.

96. Wroble RR, Van Ginkel LA, Grood ES, et al: Repeatability of the KT1000 arthrometer in a normal population, *Am J Sports Med* 18:396–399, 1990.

97. Highgenboten CL, Jackson A, Meske NB: Genucom, KT1000, and Stryker knee laxity measuring device comparisons: device reproducibility and interdevice comparison in asymptomatic subjects, *Am J Sports Med* 17:743–746, 1989.

98. Steiner ME, Brown C, Zarins B, et al: Measurement of anterior-posterior displacement of the knee: a comparison of the results with instrumented devices and with clinical examination, *J Bone Joint Surg Am* 72:1307–1315, 1990.

99. Anderson AF, Snyder RB, Federspiel CF, Lipscomb AB: Instrumented evaluation of knee laxity: a comparison of five arthrometers, *Am J Sports Med* 20:135–140, 1992.

100. Hanten WP, Pace MB: Reliability of measuring anterior laxity of the knee joint using a knee ligament arthrometer, *Phys Ther* 67:357–359, 1987.

101. Muellner T, Bugge W, Johansen S, et al: Inter- and intratester comparison of the Rolimeter knee tester: effect of tester's experience and the examination technique, *Knee Surg Sports Traumatol Arthrosc* 9:302–306, 2001.

102. Lam MH, Fong DT, Yung PS, Chan KM: Biomechanical techniques to evaluate tibial rotation. A systematic review, *Knee Surg Sports Traumatol Arthrosc* 20:1720–1729, 2012.

103. Haughom BD, Souza R, Schairer WW, et al: Evaluating rotational kinematics of the knee in ACL-ruptured and healthy patients using 3.0 Tesla magnetic resonance imaging, *Knee Surg Sports Traumatol Arthrosc* 20:663–670, 2012.

104. Petrigliano FA, Borgstrom PH, Kaiser WJ, et al: Measurements of tibial rotation during a simulated pivot shift manoeuvre using a gyroscopic sensor, *Knee Surg Sports Traumatol Arthrosc*, 2014 [Epub ahead of print].

105. Kopf S, Kauert R, Halfpaap J, et al: A new quantitative method for pivot shift grading, *Knee Surg Sports Traumatol Arthrosc* 20:718–723, 2012.

106. Pearle AD, Solomon DJ, Wanich T, et al: Reliability of navigated knee stability examination: a cadaveric evaluation, *Am J Sports Med* 35:1315–1320, 2007.

107. Resnick D, Goergen TG, Niwayama G: Physical injury. In Resnick D, Niwayama G, editors: *Diagnosis of bone and joint disorders*, 2 ed Philadelphia, 1988, WB Saunders.

108. Pavlov H: The radiographic diagnosis of the anterior cruciate ligament deficient knee, *Clin Orthop Relat Res* 172:57–64, 1983.

109. Dietz GW, Wilcox DM, Montgomery JB: Segond tibial condyle fracture: lateral capsular ligament avulsion, *Radiology* 159:467–469, 1986.

110. Lee J, Papakonstantinou O, Brookenthal KR, et al: Arcuate sign of posterolateral knee injuries: anatomic, radiographic, and MR imaging data related to patterns of injury, *Skeletal Radiol* 32:619–627, 2003.

111. Warren RF, Kaplan N, Bach BR: The lateral notch sign of anterior cruciate ligament insufficiency, *Am J Knee Surg* 1:119–124, 1988.

112. Cobby MJ, Schweitzer ME, Resnick D: The deep lateral femoral notch: an indirect sign of a torn anterior cruciate ligament, *Radiology* 184:855–858, 1992.

113. Herbst E, Hoser C, Tecklenburg K, et al: The lateral femoral notch sign following ACL injury: frequency, morphology and relation to meniscal injury and sports activity, *Knee Surg Sports Traumatol Arthrosc*, 2014 [Epub ahead of print].

114. Jacobsen K: Osteoarthrosis following insufficiency of the cruciate ligaments in man: a clinical study, *Acta Orthop Scand* 48:520–526, 1977.

115. Rosenberg TD, Paulos LE, Parker RD, et al: The forty-five–degree posteroanterior flexion weight-bearing radiograph of the knee, *J Bone Joint Surg Am* 70:1479–1483, 1988.

116. Jacobsen K: Stress radiographical measurement of the anteroposterior, medial and lateral stability of the knee joint, *Acta Orthop Scand* 47:335–344, 1976.

117. Jacobsen K: Gonylaxometry: stress radiographic measurement of passive stability in the knee joints of normal subjects and patients with ligament injuries—accuracy and range of application, *Acta Orthop Scand Suppl* 194:1–263, 1981.

118. Kennedy JC, Fowler PJ: Medial and anterior instability of the knee: an anatomical and clinical study using stress machines, *J Bone Joint Surg Am* 53:1257–1270, 1971.

119. Franklin JL, Rosenberg TD, Paulos LE, France EP: Radiographic assessment of instability of the knee due to rupture of the anterior cruciate ligament: a quadriceps contraction technique, *J Bone Joint Surg Am* 73:365–372, 1991.

120. Torzilli PA, Greenberg RL, Insall J: An in vivo biomechanical evaluation of anterior-posterior motion of the knee: roentgenographic measurement technique, stress machine, and stable population, *J Bone Joint Surg Am* 63:960–968, 1981.

121. Laprade RF, Bernhardson AS, Griffith CJ, et al: Correlation of valgus stress radiographs with medial knee ligament injuries: an in vitro biomechanical study, *Am J Sports Med* 38:330–338, 2010.

122. Gwathmey Jr. FW, Tompkins MA, Gaskin CM, Miller MD: Can stress radiography of the knee help characterize posterolateral corner injury? *Clin Orthop Relat Res* 470:768–773, 2012.

123. Gillies H, Seligson D: Precision in the diagnosis of meniscal lesions: a comparison of clinical evaluation, arthrography, and arthroscopy, *J Bone Joint Surg Am* 61:343–346, 1979.

124. Brown DW, Allman FL, Eaton SB: Knee arthrography: a comparison of radiographic and surgical findings in 295 cases, *Am J Sports Med* 6:165–172, 1978.

125. Crabtree SD, Bedford AF, Edgar MA: The value of arthrography and arthroscopy in association with a sports injuries clinic: a prospective and comparative study of 182 patients, *Injury* 13:220–226, 1981.

126. Daniel D, Daniels E, Aronson D: The diagnosis of meniscus pathology, *Clin Orthop Relat Res* 163:218–224, 1982.

127. Dumas JM, Edde DJ: Meniscal abnormalities: prospective correlation of double-contrast arthrography and arthroscopy, *Radiology* 160:453–456, 1986.

128. Nicholas JA, Freiberger RH, Killoran PJ: Double-contrast arthrography of the knee: its value in the management of two hundred and twenty-five knee derangements, *J Bone Joint Surg Am* 52:203–220, 1970.

129. Thijn CJ: Accuracy of double-contrast arthrography and arthroscopy of the knee joint, *Skeletal Radiol* 8:187–192, 1982.

130. Dye SF, Andersen CT, Stowell MT: Unrecognized abnormal osseous metabolic activity about the knee of patients with symptomatic anterior cruciate ligament deficiency, *Orthop Trans* 11:492, 1987.

131. Marks PH, Goldenberg JA, Vezina WC, et al: Subchondral bone infractions in acute ligamentous knee injuries demonstrated on bone scintigraphy and magnetic resonance imaging, *J Nucl Med* 33:516–520, 1992.

132. Bauer HCF, Persson PE, Nilsson OS: Tears of the medial meniscus associated with increased radionuclide activity of the proximal tibia, *Int Orthop* 13:153–155, 1989.

133. Dye SF, Chew MH, McBride JT, Sostre G: Restoration of osseous of the knee following meniscal surgery, *Orthop Trans* 16:725, 1992.

134. Lohmann M, Kanstrup IL, Gergvary I, Tollund C: Bone scintigraphy in patients suspected of having meniscus tears, *Scand J Med Sci Sports* 1:123–127, 1991.

135. Marymont JV, Lynch MA, Henning CE: Evaluation of meniscus tears of the knee by radionuclide imaging, *Am J Sports Med* 11:432–435, 1983.

136. Mooar P, Gregg J, Jacobstein J: Radionuclide imaging in internal derangements of the knee, *Am J Sports Med* 15:132–137, 1987.

137. Teitz CC: Ultrasonography in the knee: clinical aspects, *Radiol Clin North Am* 26:55–62, 1988.

138. Passariello R, Trecco F, De Paulis F, et al: Computed tomography of the knee joint: technique of study and normal anatomy, *J Comput Assist Tomogr* 7:1035–1042, 1983.

139. Passariello R, Trecco F, De Paulis F, et al: Computed tomography of the knee joint: clinical results, *J Comput Assist Tomogr* 7:1043–1049, 1983.

140. Pavlov H: Computed tomography of the cruciate ligaments, *Radiology* 132:389–393, 1979.

141. Reicher MA: Meniscal injuries: detection using MR imaging, *Radiology* 159:753–757, 1986.

142. Reicher MA, Bassett LW, Gold RH: High-resolution magnetic resonance imaging of the knee joint: pathologic correlations, *Am J Roentgenol* 145:903–909, 1985.

143. Reicher MA, Rauschning W, Gold RH, et al: High-resolution magnetic resonance imaging of the knee joint: normal anatomy, *Am J Roentgenol* 145:895–902, 1985.

144. Silva I, Silver DM: Tears of the meniscus as revealed by magnetic resonance imaging, *J Bone Joint Surg Am* 70:199–202, 1988.

145. Jackson DW, Jennings LD, Maywood RM, Berger PE: Magnetic resonance imaging of the knee, *Am J Sports Med* 16:29–38, 1988.

146. Polly DW, Callaghan JJ, Sikes RA, et al: The accuracy of selective magnetic resonance imaging compared with the findings of arthroscopy of the knee, *J Bone Joint Surg Am* 70:192–198, 1988.

147. Crues JV, Mink J, Levy TL, et al: Meniscal tears of the knee: accuracy of MR imaging, *Radiology* 164:445–448, 1987.

148. Fischer SP, Fox JM, Del Pizzo W, et al: Accuracy of diagnoses from magnetic resonance imaging of the knee: a multi-center analysis of one thousand and fourteen patients, *J Bone Joint Surg Am* 73:2–10, 1991.

149. Raunest J, Oberle K, Loehnert J, Hoetzinger H: The clinical value of magnetic resonance imaging in the evaluation of meniscal disorders, *J Bone Joint Surg Am* 73:11–16, 1991.

150. Gross ML, Grover JS, Bassett LW, et al: Magnetic resonance imaging of the posterior cruciate ligament: clinical use to improve diagnostic accuracy, *Am J Sports Med* 20:732–737, 1992.

151. Mandelbaum BR, Finerman GA, Reicher MA, et al: Magnetic resonance imaging as a tool for evaluation of traumatic knee injuries: anatomical and pathoanatomical correlations, *Am J Sports Med* 14:361–370, 1986.

152. Mink JH, Levy T, Crues JV: Tears of the anterior cruciate ligament and menisci of the knee: MR imaging evaluation, *Radiology* 167:769–774, 1988.

153. Vellet AD, Marks P, Fowler P, Munro T: Accuracy of nonorthogonal magnetic resonance imaging in acute disruption of the anterior cruciate ligament, *Arthroscopy* 5:287–293, 1989.

154. Oberlander MA, Shalvoy RM, Hughston JC: The accuracy of the clinical knee examination documented by arthroscopy: a prospective study, *Am J Sports Med* 21:773–778, 1993.

155. Rosen MA, Jackson DW, Berger PE: Occult osseous lesions documented by magnetic resonance imaging associated with anterior cruciate ligament ruptures, *Arthroscopy* 7:45–51, 1991.

156. Speer KP, Spritzer CE, Bassett FH, et al: Osseous injury associated with acute tears of the anterior cruciate ligament, *Am J Sports Med* 20:382–389, 1992.

157. Johnson DL, Bealle DP, Brand JC, et al: The effect of a geographic lateral bone bruise on knee inflammation after acute anterior cruciate ligament rupture, *Am J Sports Med* 28:152–155, 2000.

158. DeHaven KE: Diagnosis of acute knee injuries with hemarthrosis, *Am J Sports Med* 8:9–14, 1980.

159. DeLee JC, Riley MB, Rockwood CA: Acute straight lateral instability of the knee, *Am J Sports Med* 11:404–411, 1983.

160. McGinty JB: Complications of arthroscopy and arthroscopic surgery. In McGinty JB, Caspari RB, Jackson RW, Poehling GG, editors: *Operative arthroscopy*, ed 2 Philadelphia, 1996, Lippincott-Raven.

161. Jameson SS, Dowen D, James P, et al: The burden of arthroscopy of the knee: a contemporary analysis of data from the English NHS, *J Bone Joint Surg Br* 93:1327–1333, 2011.

162. Wertheim SB, Klaus RM: Arthroscopic surgery of the knee using local anesthesia with minimal intravenous sedation, *Am J Arthrosc* 1:7–10, 1991.

163. Shapiro MS, Safran MR, Crockett H, Finerman GA: Local anesthesia for knee arthroscopy: efficacy and cost benefits, *Am J Sports Med* 23:50–53, 1995.

164. Besser MI, Stahl S: Arthroscopic surgery performed under local anesthesia as an outpatient procedure, *Arch Orthop Trauma Surg* 105:296–297, 1986.

165. McGinty JB, Matza RA: Arthroscopy of the knee: evaluation of an out-patient procedure under local anesthesia, *J Bone Joint Surg Am* 60:787–789, 1978.

166. Minkoff J, Putterman E: The unheralded value of arthroscopy using local anesthesia for diagnostic specificity and intraoperative corroboration of therapeutic achievement, *Clin Sports Med* 6:471–490, 1987.

167. Baeten D, Van den Bosch F, Elewaut D, et al: Needle arthroscopy of the knee with synovial biopsy sampling: technical experience in 150 patients, *Clin Rheumatol* 18:434–441, 1999.

168. Meister K, Harris NL, Indelicato PA, Miller G: Comparison of an optical catheter office arthroscope with a standard rigid rodlens arthroscope in the evaluation of the knee, *Am J Sports Med* 24:819–823, 1996.

169. Halbrecht JL, Jackson DW: Office arthroscopy: a diagnostic alternative, *Arthroscopy* 8:320–326, 1992.

170. Voigt JD, Mosier M, Huber B: In-office diagnostic arthroscopy for knee and shoulder intra-articular

injuries its potential impact on cost savings in the United States, *BMC Health Serv Res* 14:203, 2014.

171. Noyes FR, Mooar LA, Moorman CT, McGinniss GH: Partial tears of the anterior cruciate ligament: progression to complete ligament deficiency, *J Bone Joint Surg Br* 71:825–833, 1989.

172. Sell TC, Ferris CM, Abt JP, et al: The effect of direction and reaction on the neuromuscular and biomechanical characteristics of the knee during tasks that simulate the noncontact anterior cruciate ligament injury mechanism, *Am J Sports Med* 34:43–54, 2006.

173. Noyes FR, Grood ES, Suntay WJ: Three-dimensional motion analysis of clinical stress tests for anterior knee subluxations, *Acta Orthop Scand* 60:308–318, 1989.

174. Hughston JC, Andrews JR, Cross MJ, Moschi A: Classification of knee ligament instabilities. Part II. The lateral compartment, *J Bone Joint Surg Am* 58:173–179, 1976.

175. Woo SL, Young EP, Ohland KJ, et al: The effects of transection of the anterior cruciate ligament on healing of the medial collateral ligament. A biomechanical study of the knee in dogs, *J Bone Joint Surg Am* 72:382–392, 1990.

176. Millett PJ, Pennock AT, Sterett WI, Steadman JR: Early ACL reconstruction in combined ACL-MCL injuries, *J Knee Surg* 17:94–98, 2004.

177. Hirshman HP, Daniel DM, Miyasaka K: The fate of unoperated knee ligament injuries. In Daniel DM, Akeson WH, O'Connor JJ, editors: *Knee ligaments: structure, function, injury, and repair*, New York, 1990, Raven.

178. Deibert MC, Aronsson DD, Johnson RJ, et al: Skiing injuries in children, adolescents, and adults, *J Bone Joint Surg Am* 80:25–32, 1998.

179. Whitney DC, Sturnick DR, Vacek PM, et al: Relationship between the risk of suffering a first-time noncontact ACL injury and geometry of the femoral notch and ACL: a prospective cohort study with a nested case-control analysis, *Am J Sports Med* 42:1796–1805, 2014.

180. LaPrade RF, Burnett QM: Femoral intercondylar notch stenosis and correlation to anterior cruciate ligament injuries: a prospective study, *Am J Sports Med* 22:198–202, 1994.

181. Souryal TO, Freeman TR: Intercondylar notch size and anterior cruciate ligament injuries in athletes: a prospective study, *Am J Sports Med* 21:535–539, 1993.

182. Malone TR: *Relationship of gender in anterior cruciate ligament (ACL) injuries of NCAA Division I basketball players.* In Paper presented at Specialty Day Meeting of the American Orthopedic Society for Sports Medicine, Washington, DC, February 23, 1992.

183. Barrett GR, Noojin FK, Hartzog CW, Nash CR: Reconstruction of the anterior cruciate ligament in females: a comparison of hamstring versus patellar tendon autograft, *Arthroscopy* 18:46–54, 2002.

184. Ferrari JD, Bach BR, Bush-Joseph CA, et al: Anterior cruciate ligament reconstruction in men and women: an outcome analysis comparing gender, *Arthroscopy* 17:588–596, 2001.

185. Wilk KE, Arrigo C, Andrews JR, Clancy WG: Rehabilitation after anterior cruciate ligament reconstruction in the female athlete, *J Athl Train* 34:177–193, 1999.

186. Barber-Westin SD, Noyes FR, Smith ST, Campbell TM: Reducing the risk of noncontact anterior cruciate ligament injuries in the female athlete, *Phys Sportsmed* 37:49–61, 2009.

187. Hewett TE, Myer GD, Ford KR, et al: Biomechanical measures of neuromuscular control and valgus loading of the knee predict anterior cruciate ligament injury risk in female athletes: a prospective study, *Am J Sports Med* 33:492–501, 2005.

188. Hewett TE, Ford KR, Myer GD: Anterior cruciate ligament injuries in female athletes: part 2, a meta-analysis of neuromuscular interventions aimed at injury prevention, *Am J Sports Med* 34:490–498, 2006.

189. Tria AJ, Klein KS: *An illustrated guide to the knee*, New York, 1992, Churchill Livingstone.

190. Andersson C, Odensten M, Good L: Surgical or nonsurgical treatment of acute rupture of the anterior cruciate ligament: a randomized study with long-term follow-up, *J Bone Joint Surg Am* 71:965–974, 1989.

191. Sommerlath K, Lysholm J, Gillquist J: The long-term course after treatment of acute anterior cruciate ligament ruptures: a 9 to 16 year followup, *Am J Sports Med* 19:156–162, 1991.

192. McDaniel WJ, Dameron TB: Untreated ruptures of the anterior cruciate ligament: a follow-up study, *J Bone Joint Surg Am* 62:696–705, 1980.

193. Warren RF, Marshall JL: Injuries of the anterior cruciate and medial collateral ligaments of the knee: a long-term follow-up of 86 cases. Part II, *Clin Orthop* 136:198–211, 1978.

194. Murray MM, Fleming BC: Use of a bioactive scaffold to stimulate anterior cruciate ligament healing also minimizes posttraumatic osteoarthritis after surgery, *Am J Sports Med* 41:1762–1770, 2013.

195. Johnson RJ: The anterior cruciate ligament problem, *Clin Orthop* 172:14–18, 1983.

196. Sandberg R, Balkfors B, Nilsson B, Westlin N: Operative versus non-operative treatment of recent injuries to the ligaments of the knee: a prospective randomized study, *J Bone Joint Surg Am* 69:1120–1126, 1987.

197. Wroble R, Brand R: Paradoxes in the history of the anterior cruciate ligament, *Clin Orthop Relat Res* 259:183–191, 1990.

198. Nebelung W, Wuschech H: Thirty-five years of follow-up of anterior cruciate ligament–deficient knees in high-level athletes, *Arthroscopy* 21:696–702, 2005.

199. Miyasaka KC, Daniel DM, Stone ML, Hirschman P: The incidence of knee ligament injuries in the general population, *Am J Knee Surg* 4:43–48, 1991.

200. Cooper DE, Warren RF, Warner JJP: The posterior cruciate ligament and posterolateral structures of the knee: anatomy, function, and patterns of injury, *Instr Course Lect* 40:249–270, 1991.

201. L'Insalata JC, Harner CD: Treatment of acute and chronic posterior cruciate ligament deficiency: new approaches, *Am J Knee Surg* 9:185–193, 1996.

202. Clendenin MB, DeLee JC, Heckman JD: Interstitial tears of the posterior cruciate ligament of the knee, *Orthopedics* 3:764–772, 1980.

203. Kennedy JC, Hawkins RJ, Willis RB, Danylchuck KD: Tension studies of human knee ligaments: yield point, ultimate failure, and disruption of the cruciate and tibial collateral ligaments, *J Bone Joint Surg Am* 58:350–355, 1976.

204. Parolie JM, Bergfeld JA: Long-term results of non-operative treatment of isolated posterior cruciate ligament injuries in the athlete, *Am J Sports Med* 14:35–38, 1986.

205. Trickey EL: Injuries to the posterior cruciate ligament: diagnosis and treatment of early injuries and reconstruction of late instability, *Clin Orthop Relat Res* 147:76–81, 1980.

206. Fowler PJ, Messieh SS: Isolated posterior cruciate ligament injuries in athletes, *Am J Sports Med* 15:553–557, 1987.

207. Duri ZA, Aichroth PM, Zorrilla P: The posterior cruciate ligament: a review, *Am J Knee Surg* 10:149–164, 1997.

208. Geissler WB, Whipple TL: Intraarticular abnormalities in association with posterior cruciate ligament injuries, *Am J Sports Med* 21:846–849, 1993.

209. Torg J, Barton T, Pavlov HMD, Stine R: Natural history of the posterior cruciate ligament–deficient knee, *Clin Orthop Relat Res* 246:208–216, 1989.

210. Keller PM, Shelbourne KD, McCarroll JR, Rettig AC: Nonoperatively treated isolated posterior cruciate ligament injuries, *Am J Sports Med* 21:132–136, 1993.

211. Dejour H, Walch G, Peyrot J, Eberhard P: The natural history of rupture of the posterior cruciate ligament, *Rev Chir Orthop Reparatrice Appar Mot* 74:35–43, 1988.

212. Dandy DJ, Pusey RJ: The long-term results of unrepaired tears of the posterior cruciate ligament, *J Bone Joint Surg Br* 64:92–94, 1982.

213. Van de Velde SK, Bingham JT, Gill TJ, Li G: Analysis of tibiofemoral cartilage deformation in the posterior cruciate ligament-deficient knee, *J Bone Joint Surg Am* 91:167–175, 2009.

214. Shelbourne KD, Clark M, Gray T: Minimum 10-year follow-up of patients after an acute, isolated posterior cruciate ligament injury treated nonoperatively, *Am J Sports Med* 41:1526–1533, 2013.

215. Tewes DP, Fields MD, Fritts HM: *Longitudinal comparison of MRI findings in knees with posterior cruciate ligament injuries.* In Paper presented at the Specialty Day Meeting of the American Orthopaedic Society for Sports Medicine, February 17, 1994.

216. Pressman A, Johnson DH: A review of ski injuries resulting in combined injury to the anterior cruciate ligament and medial collateral ligaments, *Arthroscopy* 19:194–202, 2003.

217. Roach CJ, Haley CA, Cameron KL, et al: The epidemiology of medial collateral ligament sprains in young athletes, *Am J Sports Med* 42:1103–1109, 2014.

218. Derscheid GL, Garrick JG: Medial collateral ligament injuries in football: nonoperative management of grade I and grade II sprains, *Am J Sports Med* 9:365–368, 1981.

219. Holden DL, Eggert AW, Butler JE: The nonoperative treatment of grade I and II medial collateral ligament injuries to the knee, *Am J Sports Med* 11:340–344, 1983.

220. Indelicato PA: Non-operative treatment of complete tears of the medial collateral ligament of the knee, *J Bone Joint Surg Am* 65:323–329, 1983.

221. Wymenga AB, Kats JJ, Kooloos J, Hillen B: Surgical anatomy of the medial collateral ligament and the posteromedial capsule of the knee, *Knee Surg Sports Traumatol Arthrosc* 14:229–234, 2006.

222. Ballmer PM, Jakob RP: The nonoperative treatment of isolated complete tears of the medial collateral ligament of the knee, *Arch Orthop Trauma Surg* 107:273–276, 1988.

223. Ellsasser JC, Reynolds FC, Omohundro JR: The non-operative treatment of collateral ligament injuries of the knee in professional football players: an analysis of seventy-four injuries treated non-operatively and twenty-four injuries treated surgically, *J Bone Joint Surg Am* 56:1185–1190, 1974.

224. Fetto JF, Marshall JL: Medial collateral ligament injuries of the knee: a rationale for treatment, *Clin Orthop Relat Res* 132:206–218, 1978.

225. Indelicato PA, Hermansdorfer J, Huegel M: Nonoperative management of complete tears of the medial collateral ligament of the knee in intercollegiate football players, *Clin Orthop Relat Res* 256:174–177, 1990.

226. Jones R, Henley M, Francis P: Nonoperative management of isolated grade III collateral ligament injury in high school football players, *Clin Orthop Relat Res* 213:137–140, 1986.

227. Battaglia MJ, Lenhoff MW, Ehteshami JR, et al: Medial collateral ligament injuries and subsequent load on the anterior cruciate ligament: a biomechanical

evaluation in a cadaveric model, *Am J Sports Med* 37:305–311, 2009.

228. Wijdicks CA, Ewart DT, Nuckley DJ, et al: Structural properties of the primary medial knee ligaments, *Am J Sports Med* 38:1638–1646, 2010.

229. Laprade RF, Wijdicks CA: Surgical technique: development of an anatomic medial knee reconstruction, *Clin Orthop Relat Res* 470:806–814, 2012.

230. Sims WF, Jacobson KE: The posteromedial corner of the knee: medial-sided injury patterns revisited, *Am J Sports Med* 32:337–345, 2004.

231. Petersen W, Loerch S, Schanz, et al: The role of the posterior oblique ligament in controlling posterior tibial translation in the posterior cruciate ligament-deficient knee, *Am J Sports Med* 36:495–501, 2008.

232. Terranova WA, McLaughlin RE, Morgan RF: An algorithm for the management of ligamentous injuries of the knee associated with common peroneal nerve palsy, *Orthopedics* 9:1135–1140, 1986.

233. Covey DC: Injuries of the posterolateral corner of the knee, *J Bone Joint Surg Am* 83:106–118, 2001.

234. Chen FS, Rokito AS, Pitman MI: Acute and chronic posterolateral rotatory instability of the knee, *J Am Acad Orthop Surg* 8:97–110, 2000.

235. Lunden JB, Bzdusek PJ, Monson JK, et al: Current concepts in the recognition and treatment of posterolateral corner injuries of the knee, *J Orthop Sports Phys Ther* 40:502–516, 2010.

236. Ranawat A, Baker CL, Henry S, Harner CD: Posterolateral corner injury of the knee: evaluation and management, *J Am Acad Orthop Surg* 16:506–518, 2008.

237. Ricchetti ET, Sennett BJ, Huffman GR: Acute and chronic management of posterolateral corner injuries of the knee, *Orthopedics* 31:479, 2008.

238. Azar FM, Brandt JC, Miller RH, Phillips BB: Ultra-low-velocity knee dislocations, *Am J Sports Med* 39:2170–2174, 2011.

239. LaPrade RF, Wentorf FA, Fritts H, et al: A prospective magnetic resonance imaging study of the incidence of posterolateral and multiple ligament injuries in acute knee injuries presenting with a hemarthrosis, *Arthroscopy* 23:1341–1347, 2007.

240. DeLee JC, Riley MB, Rockwood CA: Acute posterolateral rotatory instability of the knee, *Am J Sports Med* 11:199–207, 1983.

241. LaPrade RF, Heikes C, Bakker AJ, Jakobsen RB: The reproducibility and repeatability of varus stress radiographs in the assessment of isolated fibular collateral ligament and grade-III posterolateral knee injuries. An in vitro biomechanical study, *J Bone Joint Surg Am* 90:2069–2076, 2008.

242. Fanelli GC, Larson RV: Practical management of posterolateral instability of the knee, *Arthroscopy* 18:1–8, 2002.

243. LaPrade RF, Resig S, Wentorf F, Lewis JL: The effects of grade III posterolateral knee complex injuries on anterior cruciate ligament graft force. A biomechanical analysis, *Am J Sports Med* 27:469–475, 1999.

244. Dhillon M, Akkina N, Prabhakar S, Bali K: Evaluation of outcomes in conservatively managed concomitant Type A and B posterolateral corner injuries in ACL deficient patients undergoing ACL reconstruction, *Knee* 19:769–772, 2012.

245. Kim SJ, Choi DH, Hwang BYL: The influence of posterolateral rotatory instability on ACL reconstruction: comparison between isolated ACL reconstruction and ACL reconstruction combined with posterolateral corner reconstruction, *J Bone Joint Surg Am* 94:253–259, 2012.

246. Cooper D, Speer K, Wickiewicz T, Warren R: Complete knee dislocation without posterior cruciate ligament disruption: a report of four cases

and review of the literature, *Clin Orthop Relat Res* 284:228–233, 1992.

247. Green NE, Allen BL: Vascular injuries associated with dislocation of the knee, *J Bone Joint Surg Am* 59:236–239, 1977.

248. Roman PD, Hopson CN, Zenni EJ: Traumatic dislocation of the knee: a report of 30 cases and literature review, *Orthop Rev* 16:917–924, 1987.

249. DeBakey M, Simeone F: Battle injuries in World War II: an analysis of 2,471 cases, *Ann Surg* 123:534–579, 1946.

250. Phifer T, Gerlock A, Vekovius W, McDonald J: Amputation risk factors in concomitant superficial femoral artery and vein injuries, *Ann Surg* 199:241–243, 1984.

251. Shelbourne KD, Pritchard J, Rettig AC: Knee dislocations with intact posterior cruciate ligament, *Orthop Rev* 21:607–611, 1992.

252. Shelbourne KD, Porter DA, Clingman JA, et al: Low-velocity knee dislocation, *Orthop Rev* 20:995–1004, 1991.

253. Hagino RT, DeCaprio JD, Valentine RJ, Clagett GP: Spontaneous popliteal vascular injury in the morbidly obese, *J Vasc Surg* 28:458–462, 1998.

254. Werner BC, Gwathmey FW, Higgins ST, et al: Ultra-low velocity knee dislocations: patient characteristics, complications, and outcomes, *Am J Sports Med* 42:358–363, 2014.

255. Miranda FE, Dennis JW, Veldenz HC, et al: Confirmation of the safety and accuracy of physical examination in the evaluation of knee dislocation for injury of the popliteal artery: a prospective study, *J Trauma* 52:247–252, 2002.

256. White J: The results of traction injury to the common peroneal nerve, *J Bone Joint Surg Br* 50:346–350, 1968.

257. Towne LC, Blazina ME, Marmor L: Lateral compartment syndrome of the knee, *Clin Orthop Relat Res* 76:160–168, 1971.

258. Taylor AR, Arden GP, Rainey HA: Traumatic dislocation of the knee: a report of 43 cases with special reference to conservative treatment, *J Bone Joint Surg Br* 54:96–102, 1972.

259. Levy BA, Fanelli GC, Whelan DB, et al: Controversies in the treatment of knee dislocations and multi-ligament reconstruction, *J Am Acad Orthop Surg* 17:197–206, 2009.

260. Sargeant AJ, Davies CT, Edwards RH, et al: Functional and structural changes after disuse of human muscle, *Clin Sci Mol Med* 52:337–342, 1977.

261. Haggmark T, Jansson E, Eriksson E: Fiber type area and metabolic potential of the thigh muscle in man after knee surgery and immobilization, *Int J Sports Med* 2:12–17, 1981.

262. Lehmann JF, Masock AJ, Warren CG, Koblanski JN: Effect of therapeutic temperatures on tendon extensibility, *Arch Phys Med Rehabil* 51:481–487, 1970.

263. Noyes FR, Matthews DS, Mooar PA, Grood ES: The symptomatic anterior cruciate-deficient knee. Part II: the results of rehabilitation, activity modification, and counseling on functional disability, *J Bone Joint Surg Am* 65:163–174, 1983.

264. Hawkins RJ, Misamore GW, Merritt TR: Follow-up of the acute nonoperated isolated anterior cruciate ligament tear, *Am J Sports Med* 14:205–210, 1986.

265. Noyes FR, Mooar PA, Matthews DS, Butler DL: The symptomatic anterior cruciate-deficient knee. I. The long-term functional disability in athletically active individuals, *J Bone Joint Surg Am* 65:154–162, 1983.

266. Seitz H, Schlenz I, Mueller E, Vécsei V: Anterior instability of the knee despite an intensive rehabilitation program, *Clin Orthop Relat Res* 328:159–164, 1996.

267. Ciccotti MG, Lombardo SJ, Nonweiler B, Pink M: Non-operative treatment of ruptures of the anterior cruciate ligament in middle-aged patients: results after long-term follow-up, *J Bone Joint Surg Am* 76:1315–1321, 1994.

268. O'Connor DP, Laughlin MS, Woods GW: Factors related to additional knee injuries after anterior cruciate ligament injury, *Arthroscopy* 21:431–438, 2005.

269. Giove TP, Miller SJI, Kent BE, et al: Non-operative treatment of the torn anterior cruciate ligament, *J Bone Joint Surg Am* 65:184–192, 1983.

270. McDaniel WJ, Dameron TB: The untreated anterior cruciate ligament rupture, *Clin Orthop Relat Res* 172:158–163, 1983.

271. Odensten M, Hamberg P, Nordin M, et al: Surgical or conservative treatment of the acutely torn anterior cruciate ligament: a randomized study with short-term follow-up observations, *Clin Orthop Relat Res* 198:87–93, 1985.

272. Bray RC, Dandy DJ: Meniscal lesions and chronic anterior cruciate ligament deficiency. Meniscal tears occurring before and after reconstruction, *J Bone Joint Surg Br* 71:128–130, 1989.

273. Sherman M, Warren R, Marshall JMD, Savatsky G: A clinical and radiographical analysis of 127 anterior cruciate insufficient knees, *Clin Orthop Relat Res* 227:229–237, 1988.

274. Louboutin H, Debarge R, Richou J, et al: Osteoarthritis in patients with anterior cruciate ligament rupture: a review of risk factors, *Knee* 16:239–244, 2009.

275. Chalmers PN, Mall NA, Moric M, et al: Does ACL reconstruction alter natural history? A systematic literature review of long-term outcomes, *J Bone Joint Surg Am* 96:292–300, 2014.

276. Eastlack ME, Axe MJ, Snyder-Mackler L: Laxity, instability, and functional outcome after ACL injury: copers versus noncopers, *Med Sci Sports Exerc* 31:210–215, 1999.

277. Hurd WJ, Axe MJ, Snyder-Mackler: A 10-year prospective trial of a patient management algorithm and screening examination for highly active individuals with anterior cruciate ligament injury: part 1, outcomes, *Am J Sports Med* 36:40–47, 2008.

278. Clancy WG, Ray JM, Zoltan DJ: Acute tears of the anterior cruciate ligament. Surgical versus conservative treatment, *J Bone Joint Surg Am* 70:1483–1488, 1988.

279. Lawrence JT, Argawal N, Ganley TJ: Degeneration of the knee joint in skeletally immature patients with a diagnosis of an anterior cruciate ligament tear: is there harm in delay of treatment? *Am J Sports Med* 39:2582–2587, 2011.

280. Millett PJ, Willis AA, Warren RF: Associated injuries in pediatric and adolescent anterior cruciate ligament tears: does a delay in treatment increase the risk of meniscal tear? *Arthroscopy* 18:955–959, 2002.

281. Henry J, Chotel F, Chouteau J, et al: Rupture of the anterior cruciate ligament in children: early reconstruction with open physes or delayed reconstruction to skeletal maturity? *Knee Surg Sports Traumatol Arthrosc* 17:748–755, 2009.

282. Mizuta H, Kubota K, Shiraishi M, et al: The conservative treatment of complete tears of the anterior cruciate ligament in skeletally immature patients, *J Bone Joint Surg Br* 77:890–894, 1995.

283. Kocher MS, Micheli LJ, Zurakowski D, Luke A: Partial tears of the anterior cruciate ligament in children and adolescents, *Am J Sports Med* 30:697–703, 2002.

284. Fabricant PD, Jones KJ, Delos D, et al: Reconstruction of the anterior cruciate ligament in the skeletally immature athlete: a review of current concepts: AAOS exhibit selection, *J Bone Joint Surg Am* 95:e28, 2013.

285. Sherrington C: Reciprocal innervation of antagonist muscles: fourteenth note on double reciprocal innervation, *Proc R Soc (London)* B91:244–268, 1909.

286. Basmajian J, Deluca C: *Muscles alive*, ed 5, Baltimore, 1985, Williams & Wilkins.

287. Bassett GS, Fleming BW: The Lenox Hill brace in anterolateral rotatory instability, *Am J Sports Med* 11:345–348, 1983.

288. Beck C, Drez D, Young J, et al: Instrumented testing of functional knee braces, *Am J Sports Med* 14:253–256, 1986.

289. Colville MR, Lee CL, Ciullo JV: The Lenox Hill brace: an evaluation of effectiveness in treating knee instability, *Am J Sports Med* 14:257–261, 1986.

290. Swirtun LR, Jansson A, Renstrom P: The effects of a functional knee brace during early treatment of patients with a nonoperated acute anterior cruciate ligament tear: a prospective randomized study, *Clin J Sport Med* 15:299–304, 2005.

291. Kocher MS, Sterett WI, Briggs KK, et al: Effect of functional bracing on subsequent knee injury in ACL-deficient professional skiers, *J Knee Surg* 16:87–92, 2003.

292. Kaplan N, Wickiewicz TL, Warren RF: Primary surgical treatment of anterior cruciate ligament ruptures: a long-term follow-up study, *Am J Sports Med* 18:354–358, 1990.

293. Andersson C, Gillquist J: Treatment of acute isolated and combined ruptures of the anterior cruciate ligament: a long-term follow-up study, *Am J Sports Med* 20:7–12, 1992.

294. Shelbourne KD, Whitaker HJ, McCarroll JR, et al: Anterior cruciate ligament injury: evaluation of intraarticular reconstruction of acute tears without repair—two to seven year followup of 155 athletes, *Am J Sports Med* 18:484–488, 1990.

295. O'Brien SJ, Warren RF, Pavlov H, et al: Reconstruction of the chronically insufficient anterior cruciate ligament with the central third of the patellar ligament, *J Bone Joint Surg Am* 73:278–286, 1991.

296. Buss DD, Warren RF, Wickiewicz TL, et al: Arthroscopically assisted reconstruction of the anterior cruciate ligament with use of autogenous patellar ligament grafts: results after twenty-four to forty-two months, *J Bone Joint Surg Am* 75:1346–1355, 1993.

297. Cosgarea AJ, Sebastianelli WJ, DeHaven KE: Prevention of arthrofibrosis after anterior cruciate ligament reconstruction using the central third patellar tendon autograft, *Am J Sports Med* 23:87–92, 1995.

298. Shelbourne KD, Foulk DA: Timing of surgery in acute anterior cruciate ligament tears on the return of quadriceps muscle strength after reconstruction using an autogenous patellar tendon graft, *Am J Sports Med* 23:686–689, 1995.

299. Smith TO, Davies L, Hing CB: Early versus delayed surgery for anterior cruciate ligament reconstruction: a systematic review and meta-analysis, *Knee Surg Sports Traumatol Arthrosc* 18:304–311, 2010.

300. Shelbourne KD, Wilckens JH, Mollabashy A, DeCarlo M: Arthrofibrosis in acute anterior cruciate ligament reconstruction. The effect of timing of reconstruction and rehabilitation, *Am J Sports Med* 19:332–336, 1991.

301. Harner CD, Irrgang JJ, Paul J, et al: Loss of motion after anterior cruciate ligament reconstruction, *Am J Sports Med* 20:499–506, 1992.

302. Niska J, Petrigliano F, McAllister DR: Anterior cruciate ligament injuries (including revision). In Miller MD, Thompson S, editors: *DeLee & Drez's orthopaedic sports medicine: principles and practice*, Philadelphia, 2015, Saunders/Elsevier.

303. Keklikci K, Yapici C, Kim D, et al: The effect of notchplasty in anterior cruciate ligament reconstruction: a biomechanical study in the porcine knee, *Knee Surg Sports Traumatol Arthrosc* 21:1915–1921, 2013.

304. Meredick RB, Vance KJ, Appleby D, Lubowit JH: Outcome of single-bundle versus double-bundle reconstruction of the anterior cruciate ligament: a meta-analysis, *Am J Sports Med* 36:1414–1421, 2008.

305. Riboh JC, Hasselblad V, Godin JA, Mather RC: Transtibial versus independent drilling techniques for anterior cruciate ligament reconstruction: a systematic review, meta-analysis, and meta-regression, *Am J Sports Med* 41:2693–2702, 2013.

306. Tompkins M, Milewski D, Brockmeier SF, et al: Anatomic femoral tunnel drilling in anterior cruciate ligament reconstruction: use of an accessory medial portal versus traditional transtibial drilling, *Am J Sports Med* 40:1313–1321, 2012.

307. Smith PA, Schwartzberg RS, Lubowitz JH: No tunnel 2-socket technique: all-inside anterior cruciate ligament double-bundle retroconstruction, *Arthroscopy* 24:1184–1189, 2008.

308. Sgaglione NA, Schwartz RE: Arthroscopically assisted reconstruction of the anterior cruciate ligament: initial clinical experience and minimal 2-year follow-up comparing endoscopic transtibial and two-incision techniques, *Arthroscopy* 13:156–165, 1997.

309. Shelbourne KD, Gray T: Anterior cruciate ligament reconstruction with autogenous patellar tendon graft followed by accelerated rehabilitation. a two- to nine-year follow-up, *Am J Sports Med* 25:786–795, 1997.

310. Bach BR, Jones GT, Sweet FA, Hager CA: Arthroscopy-assisted anterior cruciate ligament reconstruction using patellar tendon substitution: two- to four-year follow-up results, *Am J Sports Med* 22:758–767, 1994.

311. Aglietti P, Buzzi R, Menchetti PM, Giron F: Arthroscopically assisted semitendinosus and gracilis tendon graft in reconstruction for acute anterior cruciate ligament injuries in athletes, *Am J Sports Med* 24:726–731, 1996.

312. MacDonald PB, Hedden D, Pacin O, Huebert D: Effects of an accelerated rehabilitation program after anterior cruciate ligament reconstruction with combined semitendinosus-gracilis autograft and a ligament augmentation device, *Am J Sports Med* 23:588–592, 1995.

313. Yasuda K, Tsujino J, Ohkoshi Y, et al: Graft site morbidity with autogenous semitendinosus and gracilis tendons, *Am J Sports Med* 23:706–714, 1995.

314. Rabuck SJ, Musahl V, Fu FH, West RV: Anatomic anterior cruciate ligament reconstruction with quadriceps tendon autograft, *Clin Sports Med* 32:155–164, 2013.

315. Bach BR, Aadalen KJ, Dennis MG, et al: Primary anterior cruciate ligament reconstruction using fresh-frozen, nonirradiated patellar tendon allograft: minimum 2-year follow-up, *Am J Sports Med* 33:284–292, 2005.

316. Andrews M, Noyes FR, Barber-Westin SD: Anterior cruciate ligament allograft reconstruction in the skeletally immature athlete, *Am J Sports Med* 22:48–54, 1994.

317. Shino K, Inoue M, Horibe S, et al: Maturation of allograft tendons transplanted into the knee: an arthroscopic and histological study, *J Bone Joint Surg Br* 70:556–560, 1988.

318. Krych AJ, Jackson JD, Hoskin TL, Dahm DL: A meta-analysis of patellar tendon autograft versus patellar tendon allograft in anterior cruciate ligament reconstruction, *Arthroscopy* 24:292–298, 2008.

319. Mariscalco MW, Magnussen RA, Mehta D, et al: Autograft versus nonirradiated allograft tissue for anterior cruciate ligament reconstruction: a systematic review, *Am J Sports Med* 42:492–499, 2014.

320. Barrett AM, Craft JA, Replogle WH, et al: Anterior cruciate ligament graft failure: a comparison of graft type based on age and Tegner activity level, *Am J Sports Med* 39:2194–2198, 2011.

321. Freedman KB, D'Amato MJ, Nedeff DD, et al: Arthroscopic anterior cruciate ligament reconstruction: a metaanalysis comparing patellar tendon and hamstring tendon autografts, *Am J Sports Med* 31:2–11, 2003.

322. Mohtadi NG, Chan DS, Dainty KN, Whelan DB: Patellar tendon versus hamstring tendon autograft for anterior cruciate ligament rupture in adults, *Cochrane Database Syst Rev* 9:2011 CD005960.

323. Carey JL, Dunn WR, Dahm DL, et al: A systematic review of anterior cruciate ligament reconstruction with autograft compared with allograft, *J Bone Joint Surg Am* 91:2242–2250, 2009.

324. Rice RS, Waterman BR, Lubowitz JH: Allograft versus autograft decision for anterior cruciate ligament reconstruction: an expected-value decision analysis evaluating hypothetical patients, *Arthroscopy* 28:539–547, 2012.

325. Stäubli HU, Schatzmann L, Brunner P, et al: Mechanical tensile properties of the quadriceps tendon and patellar ligament in young adults, *Am J Sports Med* 27:27–34, 1999.

326. Hamner DL, Brown CH, Steiner ME, et al: Hamstring tendon grafts for reconstruction of the anterior cruciate ligament: biomechanical evaluation of the use of multiple strands and tensioning techniques, *J Bone Joint Surg Am* 81:549–557, 1999.

327. Woo SL, Hollis JM, Adams DJ, et al: Tensile properties of the human femur-anterior cruciate ligament-tibia complex. The effects of specimen age and orientation, *Am J Sports Med* 19:217–225, 1991.

328. Race A, Amis AA: The mechanical properties of the two bundles of the human posterior cruciate ligament, *J Biomech* 27:13–24, 1994.

329. Stäubli HU, Schatzmann L, Brunner P, et al: Quadriceps tendon and patellar ligament: cryosectional anatomy and structural properties in young adults, *Knee Surg Sports Traumatol Arthrosc* 4:100–110, 1996.

330. Brand J, Weiler A, Caborn DN, et al: Graft fixation in cruciate ligament reconstruction, *Am J Sports Med* 28:761–774, 2000.

331. Kohn D, Rose C: Primary stability of interference screw fixation: influence of screw diameter and insertion torque, *Am J Sports Med* 22:334–338, 1994.

332. Pena F, Grontvedt T, Brown GA, et al: Comparison of failure strength between metallic and absorbable interference screws: influence of insertion torque, tunnel-bone block gap, bone mineral density, and interference, *Am J Sports Med* 24:329–334, 1996.

333. Steiner ME, Hecker AT, Brown CH, Hayes WC: Anterior cruciate ligament graft fixation. Comparison of hamstring and patellar tendon grafts, *Am J Sports Med* 22:240–246, 1994.

334. Milano G, Mulas PD, Ziranu F, et al: Comparison between different femoral fixation devices for ACL reconstruction with doubled hamstring tendon graft: a biomechanical analysis, *Arthroscopy* 22:660–668, 2006.

335. Fabbriciani C, Mulas PD, Ziranu F, et al: Mechanical analysis of fixation methods for anterior cruciate ligament reconstruction with hamstring tendon graft: an experimental study in sheep knees, *Knee* 12:135–138, 2005.

336. Noyes FR, Butler DL, Grood E: Biomechanical analysis of human ligament grafts used in knee-ligament repairs and reconstructions, *J Bone Joint Surg Am* 66:344–352, 1984.

337. Alm A, Gillquist J, Stromberg B: The medial third of the patellar ligament in reconstruction of the anterior cruciate ligament: a clinical and histologic study by means of arthroscopy or arthrotomy, *Acta Chir Scand Suppl* 445:5–14, 1974.

338. Arnoczky SP, Warren RF, Ashlock MA: Replacement of the anterior cruciate ligament using a patellar tendon allograft: an experimental study, *J Bone Joint Surg Am* 68:376–385, 1986.

339. Clancy WG, Narechania AG, Rosenberg TD: Anterior and posterior cruciate ligament reconstruction in rhesus monkeys, *J Bone Joint Surg Am* 63:1270–1284, 1981.

340. Shino K, Inoue M, Horibe S, et al: Surface blood flow and histology of human anterior cruciate ligament allografts, *Arthroscopy* 7:171–176, 1991.

341. Yasuda K, Tomiyama Y, Ohkoshi Y, Kaneda K: Arthroscopic observations of autogeneic quadriceps and patellar tendon grafts after anterior cruciate ligament reconstruction of the knee, *Clin Orthop Relat Res* 246:217–224, 1989.

342. Shino K, Kawasaki T, Hirose H, et al: Replacement of the anterior cruciate ligament by an allogeneic tendon graft: an experimental study in the dog, *J Bone Joint Surg Br* 66:672–681, 1984.

343. Arnoczky SP: Anterior cruciate ligament replacement using patellar tendon: an evaluation of graft revascularization in the dog, *J Bone Joint Surg Am* 64:217–224, 1982.

344. Drez DJ, DeLee J, Holden JP, et al: Anterior cruciate ligament reconstruction using bone–patellar tendon–bone allografts: a biological and biomechanical evaluation in goats, *Am J Sports Med* 19:256–263, 1991.

345. Jackson DW, Grood ES, Goldstein JD, et al: A comparison of patellar tendon autograft and allograft used for anterior cruciate ligament reconstruction in the goat model, *Am J Sports Med* 21:176–185, 1993.

346. Shelbourne KD, Nitz P: Accelerated rehabilitation after anterior cruciate ligament reconstruction, *Am J Sports Med* 18:292–299, 1990.

347. Mohtadi NG, Webster-Bogaert S, Fowler PJ: Limitation of motion following anterior cruciate ligament reconstruction: a case-control study, *Am J Sports Med* 19:620–624, 1991.

348. Noyes F, Wojtys E, Marshall M: The early diagnosis and treatment of developmental patella infera syndrome, *Clin Orthop Relat Res* 265:241–252, 1991.

349. Paulos LE, Rosenberg TD, Drawbert J, et al: Infrapatellar contracture syndrome: an unrecognized cause of knee stiffness with patella entrapment and patella infera, *Am J Sports Med* 15:331–341, 1987.

350. Sachs RA, Daniel DM, Stone ML, Garfein RF: Patellofemoral problems after anterior cruciate ligament reconstruction, *Am J Sports Med* 17:760–765, 1989.

351. Strum G, Friedman M, Fox J, et al: Acute anterior cruciate ligament reconstruction: analysis of complications, *Clin Orthop Relat Res* 253:184–189, 1990.

352. Adams D, Logerstedt DS, Hunter-Giordano A, et al: Current concepts for anterior cruciate ligament reconstruction: a criterion-based rehabilitation progression, *J Orthop Sports Phys Ther* 42:601–614, 2012.

353. Kim KM, Croy T, Hertel J, Saliba S: Effects of neuromuscular electrical stimulation after anterior cruciate ligament reconstruction on quadriceps strength, function, and patient-oriented outcomes: a systematic review, *J Orthop Sports Phys Ther* 40:383–391, 2010.

354. Logerstedt D, Grindem H, Lynch A, et al: Single-legged hop tests as predictors of self-reported knee function after anterior cruciate ligament reconstruction: the Delaware-Oslo ACL cohort study, *Am J Sports Med* 40:2348–2356, 2012.

355. Reid A, Birmingham TB, Stratford PW, et al: Hop testing provides a reliable and valid outcome measure during rehabilitation after anterior cruciate ligament reconstruction, *Phys Ther* 87:337–349, 2007.

356. Ardern CL, Taylor NF, Feller JA, et al: Psychological responses matter in returning to preinjury level of sport after anterior cruciate ligament reconstruction surgery, *Am J Sports Med* 41:1549–1558, 2013.

357. Shelbourne KD, Muthukaruppan Y: Subjective results of nonoperatively treated, acute, isolated posterior cruciate ligament injuries, *Arthroscopy* 21:457–461, 2005.

358. Van de Velde SK, Gill TJ, Li G: Dual fluoroscopic analysis of the posterior cruciate ligament-deficient patellofemoral joint during lunge, *Med Sci Sports Exerc* 41:1198–1205, 2009.

359. Boynton MD, Tietjens BR: Long-term followup of the untreated isolated posterior cruciate ligament-deficient knee, *Am J Sports Med* 24:306–310, 1996.

360. Gill TJ, Van de Velde SK, Wing DW, et al: Tibiofemoral and patellofemoral kinematics after reconstruction of an isolated posterior cruciate ligament injury: in vivo analysis during lunge, *Am J Sports Med* 37:2377–2385, 2009.

361. Shelbourne KD, Jennings RW, Vahey TN: Magnetic resonance imaging of posterior cruciate ligament injuries: assessment of healing, *Am J Knee Surg* 12:209–213, 1999.

362. Jung YB, Tae SK, Lee YS, et al: Active non-operative treatment of acute isolated posterior cruciate ligament injury with cylinder cast immobilization, *Knee Surg Sports Traumatol Arthrosc* 16:729–733, 2008.

363. Jacobi M, Reischl N, Wahl P, et al: Acute isolated injury of the posterior cruciate ligament treated by a dynamic anterior drawer brace: a preliminary report, *J Bone Joint Surg Br* 92:1381–1384, 2010.

364. Pierce CM, O'Brien L, Griffin LW, Laprade RF: Posterior cruciate ligament tears: functional and postoperative rehabilitation, *Knee Surg Sports Traumatol Arthrosc* 21:1071–1084, 2013.

365. Fox RJ, Harner CD, Sakane M, et al: Determination of the in situ forces in the human posterior cruciate ligament using robotic technology. A cadaveric study, *Am J Sports Med* 26:395–401, 1998.

366. Pandy MG, Shelburne KB: Dependence of cruciate-ligament loading on muscle forces and external load, *J Biomech* 30:1015–1024, 1997.

367. Roth JH, Bray RC, Best TM, et al: Posterior cruciate ligament reconstruction by transfer of the medial gastrocnemius tendon, *Am J Sports Med* 16:21–28, 1988.

368. Wirth CJ, Jager M: Dynamic double tendon replacement of the posterior cruciate ligament, *Am J Sports Med* 12:39–43, 1984.

369. Lipscomb AB, Anderson AF, Norwig ED, et al: Isolated posterior cruciate ligament reconstruction: long-term results, *Am J Sports Med* 21:490–496, 1993.

370. Ogata K: Posterior cruciate ligament reconstruction: a comparative study of two different methods, *Bull Hosp Joint Dis Orthop Inst* 51:186–198, 1991.

371. Tillberg B: The late repair of torn cruciate ligaments using menisci, *J Bone Joint Surg Br* 59:15–19, 1977.

372. Lindstrom N: Cruciate ligament plastics with meniscus, *Acta Orthop Scand* 29:150–152, 1959.

373. Jones RC, Ab R: GORE-TEX posterior cruciate ligament replacement: preliminary clinical results, *Orthop Trans* 14:123–124, 1990.

374. Shirakura K, Kato K, Udagawa E: Characteristics of the isokinetic performance of patients with injured cruciate ligaments, *Am J Sports Med* 20:754–760, 1992.

375. Pournaras J, Symeonides PAN: The results of surgical repair of acute tears of the posterior cruciate ligament, *Clin Orthop Related Res* 267:103–107, 1991.

376. Bianchi M: Acute tears of the posterior cruciate ligament: clinical study and results of operative treatment in 27 cases, *Am J Sports Med* 11:308–314, 1983.

377. Papalia R, Osti L, Del Buono A, et al: Tibial inlay for posterior cruciate ligament reconstruction: a systematic review, *Knee* 17:264–269, 2010.

378. McAllister DR, Markolf KL, Oakes DA, et al: A biomechanical comparison of tibial inlay and tibial tunnel posterior cruciate ligament reconstruction techniques: graft pretension and knee laxity, *Am J Sports Med* 30:312–317, 2002.

379. Weimann A, Wolfert A, Zantop T, et al: Reducing the "killer turn" in posterior cruciate ligament reconstruction by fixation level and smoothing the tibial aperture, *Arthroscopy* 23:1104–1111, 2007.

380. Huang TW, Wang CJ, Weng LH, Chan YS: Reducing the "killer turn" in posterior cruciate ligament reconstruction, *Arthroscopy* 19:712–716, 2003.

381. Gill TJ, Van de Velde SK, Carroll KM, et al: Surgical technique: aperture fixation in PCL reconstruction: applying biomechanics to surgery, *Clin Orthop Relat Res* 470:853–860, 2012.

382. Harner CD, Janaushek MA, Kanamori A, et al: Biomechanical analysis of a double-bundle posterior cruciate ligament reconstruction, *Am J Sports Med* 28:144–151, 2000.

383. Race A, Amis AA: PCL reconstruction. In vitro biomechanical comparison of 'isometric' versus single and double-bundled 'anatomic' grafts, *J Bone Joint Surg Br* 80:173–179, 1998.

384. Wilk KE, Andrews JR, Clancy WG, et al: Rehabilitation programs for the PCL-injured and reconstructed knee, *J Sport Rehabil* 8:333–361, 1999.

385. Bosch U, Kasperczyk W, Marx M, et al: Healing at graft fixation site under functional conditions in posterior cruciate ligament reconstruction, *Arch Orthop Trauma Surg* 108:154–158, 1989.

386. Cain TE, Schwab GH: Performance of an athlete with straight posterior knee instability, *Am J Sports Med* 9:203–208, 1981.

387. Moyer RA, Marchetto PA: Injuries of the posterior cruciate ligament, *Clin Sports Med* 12:307–315, 1993.

388. Nyland J, Hester P, Caborn DN: Double-bundle posterior cruciate ligament reconstruction with allograft tissue: 2-year postoperative outcomes, *Knee Surg Sports Traumatol Arthrosc* 10:274–279, 2002.

389. Snyder-Mackler L, Delitto A, Bailey SL, Stralka SW: Strength of the quadriceps femoris muscle and functional recovery after reconstruction of the anterior cruciate ligament: a prospective, randomized clinical trial of electrical stimulation, *J Bone Joint Surg Am* 77:1166–1173, 1995.

390. Eriksson E, Haggmark T: Comparison of isometric muscle training and electrical stimulation supplementing isometric muscle training in the recovery after major knee ligament surgery: a preliminary report, *Am J Sports Med* 7:169–171, 1979.

391. Morrissey MC, Brewster CE, Shields CL, Brown M: The effects of electrical stimulation on the quadriceps during postoperative knee immobilization, *Am J Sports Med* 13:40–45, 1985.

392. Safran MR, Harner C, Giraldo JL, et al: Effects of injury and reconstruction of the posterior cruciate ligament on proprioception and neuromuscular control, *J Sport Rehabil* 8:304–321, 1999.

393. Weiss JA, Woo SLY, Ohland KJ, et al: Evaluation of a new injury model to study medial collateral ligament healing: primary repair versus nonoperative treatment, *J Orthop Res* 9:516–528, 1991.

394. Hastings DE: The non-operative management of collateral ligament injuries of the knee joint, *Clin Orthop Relat Res* 147:22–28, 1980.

395. Wijdicks CA, Griffith CJ, Johansen S, et al: Injuries to the medial collateral ligament and associated medial structures of the knee, *J Bone Joint Surg Am* 92:1266–1280, 2010.

396. Reider B, Sathy MR, Talkington J, et al: Treatment of isolated medial collateral ligament injuries in athletes with early functional rehabilitation. A five-year follow-up study, *Am J Sports Med* 22:470–477, 1994.

397. Tibor LM, Marchant MH, Taylor DC, et al: Management of medial-sided knee injuries, part 2: posteromedial corner, *Am J Sports Med* 39:1332–1340, 2011.

398. Laprade RF, Wijdicks CA: The management of injuries to the medial side of the knee, *J Orthop Sports Phys Ther* 42:221–233, 2012.

399. Matsumoto H, Suda Y, Otani T, et al: Roles of the anterior cruciate ligament and the medial collateral ligament in preventing valgus instability, *J Orthop Sci* 6:28–32, 2001.

400. Ichiba A, Nakajima M, Fujita A, Abe M: The effect of medial collateral ligament insufficiency on the reconstructed anterior cruciate ligament: a study in the rabbit, *Acta Orthop Scand* 74:196–200, 2003.

401. Ma CB, Papageogiou CD, Debski RE, Woo SL: Interaction between the ACL graft and MCL in a combined ACL+MCL knee injury using a goat model, *Acta Orthop Scand* 71:387–393, 2000.

402. Noyes FR, Barber-Westin SD: Posterior cruciate ligament revision reconstruction, part 1: causes of surgical failure in 52 consecutive operations, *Am J Sports Med* 33:646–654, 2005.

403. Iwata S, Sua Y, Nagura T, et al: Posterior instability near extension is related to clinical disability in isolated posterior cruciate ligament deficient patients, *Knee Surg Sports Traumatol Arthrosc* 15:343–349, 2007.

404. Canata GL, Chiey A, Leoni T: Surgical technique: does mini-invasive medial collateral ligament and posterior oblique ligament repair restore knee stability in combined chronic medial and ACL injuries? *Clin Orthop Relat Res* 470:791–797, 2012.

405. Lind M, Jakobsen BW, Lund B, et al: Anatomical reconstruction of the medial collateral ligament and posteromedial corner of the knee in patients with chronic medial collateral ligament instability, *Am J Sports Med* 37:1116–1122, 2009.

406. Coobs BR, Wijdicks CA, Armitage BM, et al: An in vitro analysis of an anatomical medial knee reconstruction, *Am J Sports Med* 38:339–347, 2010.

407. Griffith CJ, Wijdicks CA, LaPrade RF, et al: Force measurements on the posterior oblique ligament and superficial medial collateral ligament proximal and distal divisions to applied loads, *Am J Sports Med* 37:140–148, 2009.

408. Wilson B, Johnson D: Medial Collateral ligament and posterior medial corner injuries. In Miller MD, Thompson S, editors: *DeLee & Drez's orthopaedic sports medicine: principles and practice*, Philadelphia, 2015, Saunders/Elsevier.

409. Kannus P: Nonoperative treatment of grade II and III sprains of the lateral ligament compartment of the knee, *Am J Sports Med* 17:83–88, 1989.

410. LaPrade RF, Wentorf FA, Crum JA: Assessment of healing of grade III posterolateral corner injuries: an in vivo model, *J Orthop Res* 22:970–975, 2004.

411. Stannard JP, Brown SL, Farris RC, et al: The posterolateral corner of the knee: repair versus reconstruction, *Am J Sports Med* 33:881–888, 2005.

412. Geeslin AG, LaPrade RF: Outcomes of treatment of acute grade-III isolated and combined posterolateral knee injuries: a prospective case series and surgical technique, *J Bone Joint Surg Am* 93:1672–1683, 2011.

413. Kim SJ, Shin SJ, Choi CH, Kim HC: Reconstruction by biceps tendon rerouting for posterolateral rotatory instability of the knee: modification of the Clancy technique, *Arthroscopy* 17:664–667, 2001.

414. Kim SJ, Shin SJ, Jeong JH: Posterolateral rotatory instability treated by a modified biceps rerouting technique: technical considerations and results in cases with and without posterior cruciate ligament insufficiency, *Arthroscopy* 19:493–499, 2003.

415. Savarese E, Bisicchia S, Romeo R, Amendola A: Role of high tibial osteotomy in chronic injuries of posterior cruciate ligament and posterolateral corner, *J Orthop Traumatol* 12:1–17, 2011.

416. LaPrade RF, Johansen S, Wentorf FA, et al: An analysis of an anatomical posterolateral knee reconstruction: an in vitro biomechanical study and development of a surgical technique, *Am J Sports Med* 32:1405–1414, 2004.

417. LaPrade RF: Anatomic reconstruction of the posterolateral aspect of the knee, *J Knee Surg* 18:167–1871, 2005.

418. Laprade RF, Griffith CJ, Coobs BR, et al: Improving outcomes for posterolateral knee injuries, *J Orthop Res* 32:485–491, 2014.

419. Verma NN, Mithöfer K, Battaglia M, MacGillivray J: The docking technique for posterolateral corner reconstruction, *Arthroscopy* 21:238–242, 2005.

420. Bicos J, Arciero RA: Novel approach for reconstruction of the posterolateral corner using a free tendon graft technique, *Sports Med Arthrosc* 14:28–36, 2006.

421. Rios CG, Leger RR, Cote MP, et al: Posterolateral corner reconstruction of the knee: evaluation of a technique with clinical outcomes and stress radiography, *Am J Sports Med* 38:1564–1574, 2010.

422. Safran MR, Johnston-Jones K, Kabo JM, Meals RA: The effect of experimental hemarthrosis on joint stiffness and synovial histology in a rabbit model, *Clin Orthop Relat Res* 303:280–288, 1994.

423. Plisky PJ, Gorman PP, Butler RJ, et al: The reliability of an instrumented device for measuring components of the star excursion balance test, *N Am J Sports Phys Ther* 4:92–99, 2009.

424. Ridley TJ, Cook S, Bollier M, et al: Effect of body mass index on patients with multiligamentous knee injuries, *Arthroscopy* 30:1447–1452, 2014.

425. Meyers MH, Harvey JP: Traumatic dislocation of the knee joint, *J Bone Joint Surg Am* 53:16–29, 1971.

426. Meyers MH, Moore TM, Harvey JP: Traumatic dislocation of the knee joint [Follow-up notes on article previously published in the Journal], *J Bone Joint Surg Am* 57:430–433, 1975.

427. Sisto D, Warren R: Complete knee dislocation: a follow-up study of operative treatment, *Clin Orthop Relat Res* 198:94–101, 1985.

428. Dedmond BT, Almekinders LC: Operative versus nonoperative treatment of knee dislocations: a meta-analysis, *Am J Knee Surg* 14:33–38, 2001.

429. Fanelli GC, Edson CJ: Arthroscopically assisted combined anterior and posterior cruciate ligament reconstruction in the multiple ligament injured knee: 2- to 10-year follow-up, *Arthroscopy* 18:703–714, 2002.

430. Liow RY, McNicholas MJ, Keating JF, Nutton RW: Ligament repair and reconstruction in traumatic dislocation of the knee, *J Bone Joint Surg Br* 85:845–851, 2003.

431. Blazina ME, Kerlan RK, Jobe F: Jumper's knee, *Orthop Clin North Am* 4:665–678, 1973.

432. Nirschl RP: Elbow tendinosis/tennis elbow, *Clin Sports Med* 11:851–870, 1992.

433. Malliaras P, Cook JL, Kent P: Reduced ankle dorsiflexion range may increase the risk of patellar tendon injury among volleyball players, *J Sci Med Sport* 9:304–309, 2006.

434. Cook JL, Khan KM, Kiss ZS, Griffiths L: Patellar tendinopathy in junior basketball players: a controlled clinical and ultrasonographic study of 268 patellar tendons in players aged 14-18 years, *Scand J Med Sci Sports* 10:216–220, 2000.

435. Fredberg U, Bolvig L: Significance of ultrasonographically detected asymptomatic tendinosis in the patellar and achilles tendons of elite soccer players: a longitudinal study, *Am J Sports Med* 30:488–491, 2002.

436. Rutland M, O'Connell D, Brismée JM, et al: Evidence-supported rehabilitation of patellar tendinopathy, *N Am J Sports Phys Ther* 5:166–178, 2010.

437. Warden SJ, Brukner P: Patellar tendinopathy, *Clin Sports Med* 22:743–759, 2003.

438. Bahr R, Fossan B, Løken S, Engebretsen L: Surgical treatment compared with eccentric training for patellar tendinopathy (jumper's knee). A randomized, controlled trial, *J Bone Joint Surg* 88:1689, 2006.

439. Panni AS, Tartarone M, Maffulli N: Patellar tendinopathy in athletes: outcome of nonoperative and operative management, *Am J Sports Med* 28:392–397, 2000.

440. Frohm A, Halvorsen K, Thorstensson A: Patellar tendon load in different types of eccentric squats, *Clin Biomech (Bristol, Avon)* 22:704–711, 2007.

441. Young MA, Cook JL, Purdam CR, et al: Eccentric decline squat protocol offers superior results at 12 months compared with traditional eccentric protocol for patellar tendinopathy in volleyball players, *Br J Sports Med* 39:102–105, 2005.

442. Hsu WK, Mishra A, Rodeo SR, et al: Platelet-rich plasma in orthopaedic applications: evidence-based recommendations for treatment, *J Am Acad Orthop Surg* 21:739–748, 2013.

443. Dragoo JL, Wasterlain AS, Braun HJ, Nead KT: Platelet-rich plasma as a treatment for patellar tendinopathy: a double-blind, randomized controlled trial, *Am J Sports Med* 42:610–618, 2014.

444. Charousset C, Zaoui A, Bellaiche L, Bouyer B: Are multiple platelet-rich plasma injections useful for treatment of chronic patellar tendinopathy in athletes? a prospective study, *Am J Sports Med* 42:906–911, 2014.

445. Shelbourne KD, Henne TD, Gray T: Recalcitrant patellar tendinosis in elite athletes: surgical treatment in conjunction with aggressive postoperative rehabilitation, *Am J Sports Med* 34:1141–1146, 2006.

446. Zernicke RF, Garhammer J, Jobe FW: Human patellar tendon rupture, *J Bone Joint Surg Am* 59:179–183, 1977.

447. Kelly DW, Carter VS, Jobe FW, Kerlan RK: Patellar and quadriceps tendon ruptures: jumper's knee, *Am J Sports Med* 12:375–380, 1984.

448. Marder RA, Timmerman LA: Primary repair of patellar tendon rupture without augmentation, *Am J Sports Med* 27:304–307, 1999.

449. Zarins B: Are validated questionnaires valid? *J Bone Joint Surg Am* 87:1671–1672, 2005.

450. Roos EM, Klassbo M, Lohmander LS: WOMAC osteoarthritis index: reliability, validity, and responsiveness in patients with arthroscopically assessed osteoarthritis—Western Ontario and MacMaster universities, *Scand J Rheumatol* 28:210–215, 1999.

CHAPTER 21

Injuries to the Meniscus and Articular Cartilage

THOMAS J. GILL IV, OWEN P. MCGONIGLE, ALEX PETRUSKA, DAVID J. MAYMAN

INTRODUCTION

Injuries to the articular cartilage and meniscus of the knee are common. They can be caused by work activities and athletic injuries as well as activities of daily living and degeneration. They can occur as isolated injuries or in combination with injury to ligaments and other knee structures. Meniscal tears and chondral injuries can cause significant clinical symptoms of pain, swelling, loss of motion, and locking, often requiring surgical intervention. Arthroscopic treatment of meniscal tears has become one of the most common procedures in the United States.[1]

To evaluate and treat these injuries, the clinician must have an understanding of the anatomy, histology, and function of the meniscus and articular cartilage. This chapter reviews the anatomy and histology of both the articular and meniscal cartilage and the signs and symptoms of injuries to these structures; diagnostic studies and treatment alternatives are then discussed.

MENISCUS

Anatomy

The meniscus was first described by Bland-Sutton[2] in 1897 as "the functionless remnants of intra-articular leg muscles." Since that time the meniscal anatomy has been studied extensively. From a gross anatomical perspective, the menisci are two fibrocartilaginous structures that have strong bony attachments to the anterior and posterior tibial plateau.

In the C-shaped medial meniscus, the anteroposterior (AP) dimension of the posterior horn is larger than the AP dimension of the anterior horn. Some variation is seen in the bony attachments of the medial meniscus. Berlet and Fowler[3] have described four types of anterior horn meniscal attachments, three of which attached to bone. The type four variant had no firm bony attachment, but this type was found in only one of 34 specimens. A similar attachment was described by Nelson and LaPrade[4]; 14% of their specimens had no direct bony attachment of the anterior horn. The remainder of the medial meniscus is attached to the knee joint capsule. The capsular attachment of the meniscus to the tibia is called the **coronary ligament.** The posterior bony attachment consistently lies anterior to the tibial insertion of the posterior cruciate ligament. Johnson et al.[5] studied the surface area of the meniscal bony attachments and found that the anterior horn of the medial meniscus has the largest footprint (61.4 mm²) and that the posterior horn of the lateral meniscus has the smallest (28.5 mm²) (Figure 21-1).

The lateral meniscus, which is more semicircular in shape, also has anterior and posterior bony attachments. The lateral meniscus covers a larger area of the tibial articular surface than the medial meniscus. A lateral disc-shaped or discoid meniscus that covers the entire tibial articular surface has been reported in 3.5% to 5% of cases.[6] Discoid menisci are the result of a developmental anomaly and may have a familial pattern; they are rarely found medially, are generally thicker than normal, and lack normal posterior attachments. The bony attachment sites of the normally shaped lateral meniscus, the anterior and posterior horns, are much closer together in the lateral meniscus than in the medial meniscus. The anterior horn attaches just adjacent to the anterior cruciate ligament (ACL). The bony attachment site of the posterior horn is located behind the tibial spines and anterior to the insertion site of the medial meniscus. The Wrisberg variant of the discoid meniscus lacks a posterior bony attachment, which leaves the posterior meniscofemoral ligament of Wrisberg as the only posterior stabilizing structure; this often allows excess motion and posterior horn instability. The anterior meniscofemoral ligament of Humphrey runs from the posterior horn of the lateral meniscus to the posterior cruciate ligament and femur. In the posterolateral corner of the knee, the popliteus tendon lies between the knee joint capsule and the lateral meniscus. This region is

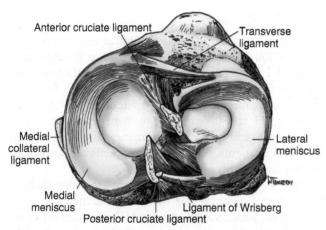

Figure 21-1 Anatomy of the menisci. (From Warren R, Arnoczky SP, Wickiewicz TL: Anatomy of the knee. In Nicholas JA, Hershamn EB, editors: *The lower extremity and spine in sports medicine*, p 687, St. Louis, 1986, Mosby.)

called the **popliteal hiatus.** Attachments also are found between the tibia and meniscus through the capsule, but these are not as well developed as on the medial side. Because of the differences in the attachment to the tibia,

the lateral meniscus has more mobility through knee joint motion (Figure 21-2). Thompson et al.[7] have demonstrated 11.2 mm of posterior excursion of the lateral meniscus during knee joint flexion, compared with 5.2 mm of excursion of the medial meniscus.

Blood Supply

The entire meniscus is vascular at the time of birth. By 9 months of age, the inner one third has become avascular. The vascularity of the meniscus decreases until approximately age 10, at which time it reaches its adult condition. Ten percent to 25% of the lateral meniscus is vascular, and 10% to 30% of the medial meniscus is vascular (Figure 21-3).[8]

The vascular supply of the menisci is the superior and inferior branches of the medial and lateral genicular arteries. These vessels form a perimeniscal capillary plexus. The region of the popliteal hiatus is a relatively avascular zone of the lateral meniscus. Cell nutrition to the inner 70% to 90% of the menisci comes from diffusion or mechanical pumping.[9]

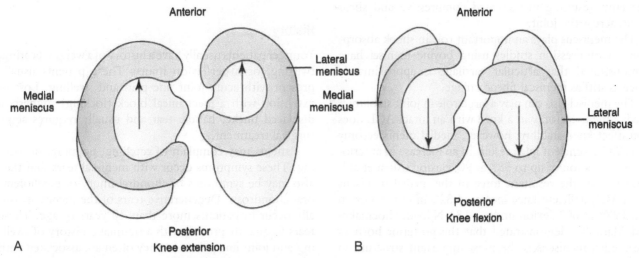

Figure 21-2 Menisci move anteriorly with extension (**A**) and posteriorly with flexion (**B**). The right knee is shown. (Redrawn from Kapandji IA: *The physiology of the joints: annotated diagrams of the mechanics of the human joints,* Edinburgh, 1970, Churchill Livingstone.)

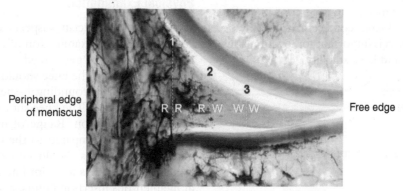

Figure 21-3 Blood supply to meniscus. A 5-mm-thick frontal section of the medial compartment of a human knee (Spalteholz preparation). Branching radial vessels from the perimeniscal capillary plexus penetrate the peripheral border of the medial meniscus. Vascularity and potential for healing: *RR,* Red-red zone (excellent); *RW,* red-white zone (variable); *WW,* white-white zone (poor). (Modified from Arnoczky SP, Warren RF: Microvasculature of the human meniscus, *Am J Sports Med* 10:90-95, 1982.)

Innervation

The menisci are innervated by myelinated and unmyelinated nerve fibers. Neural elements are most abundant in the outer portion of the meniscus. The anterior and posterior horns of the meniscus are innervated with mechanoreceptors that may play a role in proprioceptive feedback in the knee.[10]

Function

The menisci are critical structures in the knee. They take load from the femur and distribute it over the entire articular surface of the tibial plateau. The menisci transmit at least 50% to 70% of the load when the knee is in extension. Load transmission increases to 85% at 90° flexion.[11] Radin et al.[12] showed that removal of the medial meniscus resulted in a 50% to 70% decrease in femoral condyle surface contact area and an increase in joint reactive forces of 100%. Total lateral meniscectomy led to a 40% to 50% decrease in contact area and an increase in contact stresses of 200% to 300%.[12-14] In addition to being increased, stresses within the joint are distributed unevenly, resulting in increased compressive and shear forces across the joint.

The meniscus plays an important role in shock absorption.[15] Compression studies using bovine menisci have demonstrated that articular cartilage is approximately twice as stiff as meniscal fibrocartilage.

The menisci also can play a large role in joint stability.[16] Medial meniscectomy in a knee with an intact ACL does not affect knee stability; however, medial meniscectomy in an ACL-deficient knee results in an increase in anterior tibial translation of up to 58% at 90° flexion. Allen et al.[17] showed that the resultant force in the medial meniscus of an ACL-deficient knee increased 52% in full extension and 197% at 60° flexion under a 134-N load. Shoemaker and Markolf[18] demonstrated that the posterior horn of the medial meniscus is the most important structure in the knee for resisting an anterior tibial force applied to an ACL-deficient knee.

The inner two thirds of the menisci are important for shock absorption and for increasing joint contact surface area and therefore for reducing contact stresses. The peripheral ring of the menisci is important for load transmission, shock absorption, and knee stability.

Functions of the Menisci

- Load sharing
- Reducing joint contact stresses (by increasing contact surface area)
- Shock absorption
- Passive joint stabilization
- Limiting extremes of flexion and extension
- Proprioception

Epidemiology

The mean annual incidence of meniscal tears is 60 to 70 per 100,000,[19,20] and the ratio of males to females varies from 2.5:1 to 4:1. Approximately one third of all meniscal tears are associated with a tear in the ACL.[21] The peak incidence of meniscal tears associated with ACL injury occurs at 21 to 30 years of age in males and at 11 to 20 years of age in females. A traumatic cause is more likely in younger patients, whereas older patients are more likely to have degenerative meniscal tears.

Patients with an acute ACL injury are more likely to have a lateral meniscal tear than a medial meniscal tear.[22] In contrast, patients with chronic ACL-deficient knees are more likely to develop a medial meniscal tear; the role of the medial meniscus as an AP joint stabilizer in ACL-deficient knees is thought to be the reason for this phenomenon.

DIAGNOSIS OF MENISCAL TEARS

Meniscal tears can be diagnosed through a combination of a careful history, a thorough physical examination, and the appropriate diagnostic tests.

History

Younger patients usually have a history of a weight-bearing, twisting, or hyperflexion injury. These patients usually present with acute joint line pain and swelling. Loss of extension with a mechanical block (locking) suggests a displaced bucket handle tear and usually requires acute surgical treatment.

Patients may complain of catching, popping, or locking. These symptoms occur with meniscal tears, but they also may be symptoms of chondral injury or patellofemoral chondrosis. Degenerative tears of the meniscus usually occur in patients more than 40 years of age. These tears frequently present with a traumatic history of swelling and joint line pain, and they often are associated with some degree of chondral damage.

Physical Examination

Whenever the clinician suspects meniscal pathology, a complete physical examination of the low back and lower extremities must be performed.

Examination of the knee should begin with inspection of the skin and surrounding tissues. Quadriceps atrophy should be assessed. The knee should be examined for evidence of an effusion. Range of motion (ROM) should be assessed and compared to the opposite side. The ligamentous structures should be tested. The joint should be palpated to assess for joint line tenderness, tenderness at ligamentous insertion points, and tenderness in the region of the pes anserine bursa. The patellofemoral region also should be palpated.

Numerous special tests have been used to assess for meniscal pathology. Taken in isolation, the various physical examination tests for meniscal tears do not have high sensitivities, specificities, or positive predictive values. These tests include joint line palpation, the flexion McMurray test, and Apley's grind test. These tests have been shown to have mixed results. Evans et al.[23] looked at the flexion McMurray test to determine intraobserver reliability and accuracy. They found that a medially based "thud" with rotation and flexion was the only McMurray sign to correlate with meniscal pathology. This finding had 98% specificity but only 15% sensitivity for medial meniscal tears.[23] Weinstabl et al.[24] found that joint line tenderness was the best clinical sign of a meniscal tear, with a sensitivity of 74% and a 50% positive predictive value. The presence of an ACL injury makes joint line tenderness less helpful. Shelbourne et al.[25] showed an accuracy of 54.9% for medial meniscal tears and 53.2% for lateral meniscal tears. Terry et al.[26] examined the accuracy of a thorough history, physical examination, and plain radiographs to predict meniscal pathology preoperatively. The overall clinical evaluation had a sensitivity of 95%, specificity of 72%, and positive predictive value of 85% for tears of the medial meniscus; it had a sensitivity of 88%, specificity of 92%, and positive predictive value of 58% for tears of the lateral meniscus. All tears were confirmed arthroscopically.[26]

Diagnosis of Meniscal Pathology

- History of twisting while weight bearing
- History of hyperflexion of the knee
- Joint line tenderness
- Minimal to moderate synovial swelling
- Pain or forced flexion
- Limited extension with spring block end feel
- Magnetic resonance imaging
- High level of suspicion

Diagnostic Studies

Several types of imaging studies can be used as an adjunct to the history and physical examination. Radiographs, arthrography, magnetic resonance imaging (MRI), and arthroscopy have all been used to help define meniscal pathology.

Radiography

Plain radiographic films should be obtained in the evaluation of all knee pathology. A standard knee series should include a posteroanterior/anteroposterior (PA/AP) weight-bearing view in 30° flexion (Rosenberg view), a true lateral view, and a tangential image, such as a Merchant or skyline view (Figure 21-4). These images will not confirm the diagnosis of a meniscal tear, but they are still important.

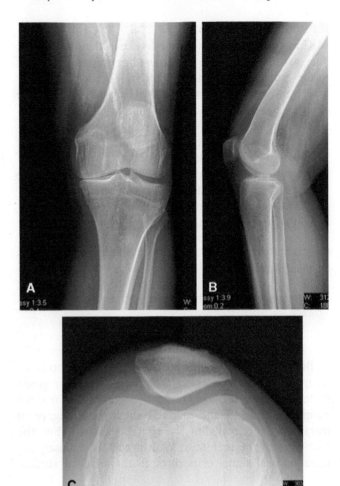

Figure 21-4 Standard radiographic views. **A,** AP weight-bearing view of the knee showing medial joint space loss. **B,** Lateral radiograph of the knee. **C,** Tangential view of the patellofemoral joint.

Plain radiographic films can be used to assess the knee for joint space narrowing, osteophyte formation, subchondral cysts, and subchondral sclerosis, all findings of osteoarthritis of the knee. Early degenerative changes are better seen on PA/AP views in 30° flexion because degenerative changes usually are more severe on the posterior femoral condyles than on the distal femur.[27,28] Non–weight-bearing radiographic films are not useful for determining joint space narrowing. The tangential view is best for assessing the patellofemoral joint, which can be a cause of medial or lateral knee pain. Plain radiographic films can also help determine whether any other bony pathology is present. If any question arises about lower limb alignment, 3-foot (1.0 m) standing films should be obtained to determine the anatomical and mechanical axis of the lower extremity.

Standard Knee Radiographic Films

- PA/AP weight-bearing view in 30° flexion (Rosenberg view)
- Lateral view
- Merchant or skyline view

Magnetic Resonance Imaging

MRI has proven to be a great advance in the diagnosis of knee pathology, but the scans must be read in the context of the patient's history and the physical examination findings. Some of the advantages of MRI are: (1) it allows the clinician to see the ligamentous and cartilaginous structures in the knee, (2) it does not require the use of ionizing radiation, and (3) it is noninvasive. Disadvantages of MRI include: (1) a relatively high cost, (2) the amount of time required to obtain the scan, and (3) the tight space in which the patient must lie unless an open magnet machine is used. Normal menisci appear as low signal intensity on all image sequences.

Clinical Note

MRI scans must be read in the context of the patient's history and the physical examination findings.

Based on its MRI appearance, the meniscus tear or injury can be categorized according to a four-grade system (Figure 21-5). Grade 0 represents a normal meniscus. Grade I and grade II show some degree of intrameniscal signal, but the signal does not abut the free edge of the meniscus. With grade III menisci, the intrameniscal signal exits through the articular surface of the meniscus. The grade III pattern is consistent with a meniscal tear.[29]

MRI is a powerful tool in the diagnosis of meniscal pathology. Several studies have shown meniscal tears on MRI scans of asymptomatic patients. Boden et al.[30] studied 74 asymptomatic patients. Sixty-three were under age 45, and eight of these (13%) were found to have meniscal tears. Eleven patients were over age 45, and four (36%) had positive findings on MRI.[30] LaPrade et al.[31] found MRI scans to be positive in 5.6% of knees in asymptomatic patients 18 to 39 years of age who had normal physical examination findings.[31]

Arthroscopy

Arthroscopy is the gold standard for the diagnosis of meniscal tears. Arthroscopic examination allows direct visualization of the tibial and femoral articular surfaces of the meniscus and the meniscocapsular junction. It also allows visualization of the lateral meniscus at the popliteal hiatus and probing to determine whether hypermobility is present.

Classification of Meniscal Tears

Meniscal tears can be classified as oblique, vertical longitudinal, radial (or transverse), horizontal cleavage, or complex (Figure 21-6). Several authors have evaluated the incidence of these tear patterns. Metcalf et al.[32]

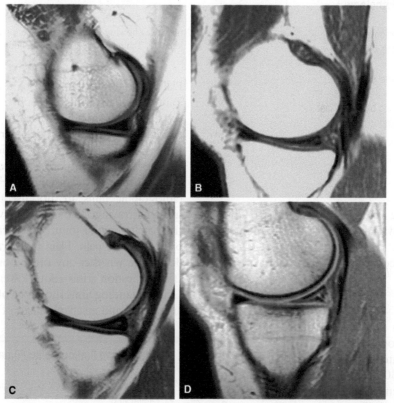

Figure 21-5 Categorization of menisci according to MRI results. **A,** Grade 0: normal meniscus. **B,** Grade I: mild intrameniscal signal. **C,** Grade II: intrameniscal signal. **D,** Grade III: complex tear of the medial meniscus.

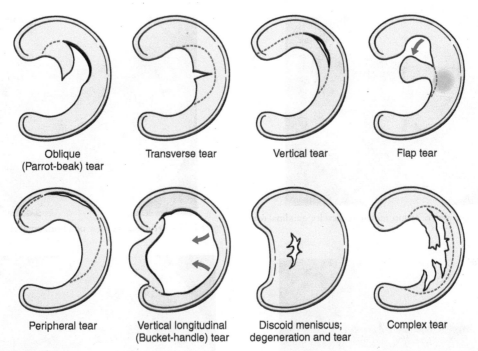

Figure 21-6 Types of meniscal tears.

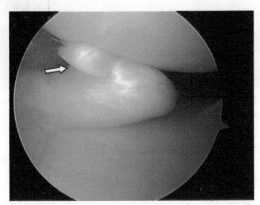

Figure 21-7 Arthroscopic view of an oblique (parrot beak) tear of the meniscus. Symptoms likely result from the flap getting caught in the joint and pulling on the meniscocapsular junction. This also could lead to propagation of the tear.

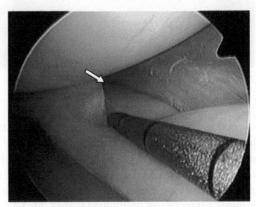

Figure 21-8 Arthroscopic view of a bucket handle tear of the meniscus.

determined that 81% of tears were oblique or vertical longitudinal. As patients get older, the incidence of complex tears increases. Most meniscal pathology is found in the posterior horns.

Oblique tears are most commonly found at the junction of the posterior and middle thirds of the meniscus. These tears are commonly called "flap" or "parrot beak" tears (Figure 21-7).

Vertical longitudinal tears, also called "bucket handle" tears, occur most often in young patients. These tears are commonly associated with ACL tears. Binfield et al.[33] showed a 9% incidence of bucket handle tears of the medial meniscus in ACL-deficient knees. Bucket handle tears occur more often in the medial meniscus, probably because of its more rigid attachments and susceptibility to

shear forces. A study by Binfield et al.[33] evaluated knees that on average had suffered an ACL injury 23.3 months earlier. This interval is sufficient from the time of original injury for knee instability to generate medial meniscal tears. Vertical longitudinal tears occur most often in the posterior horn of the meniscus and can involve the entire meniscus (Figure 21-8).

Bucket handle tears are unstable and, if large enough, can dislocate into the intracondylar region, causing a mechanical block to extension (locking). Incomplete vertical longitudinal tears can occur on the femoral or tibial surface of the meniscus (Figure 21-9).

The clinical significance of incomplete bucket handle tears is questionable. Fitzgibbons and Shelbourne[34] found that incomplete vertical longitudinal tears of the lateral meniscus that had been found at the time of ACL

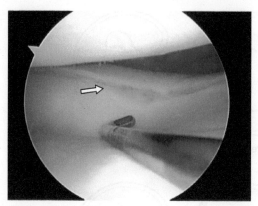

Figure 21-9 Arthroscopic view of an incomplete vertical longitudinal tear of the meniscus.

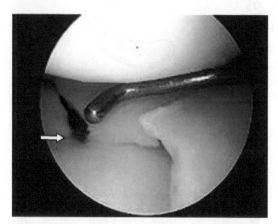

Figure 21-10 Arthroscopic view of a radial meniscal tear.

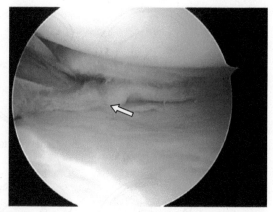

Figure 21-11 Arthroscopic view of a horizontal cleavage tear.

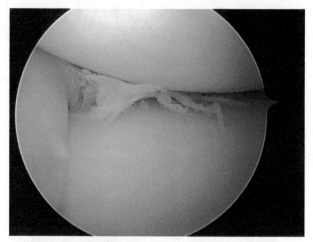

Figure 21-12 Arthroscopic view of a complex meniscal tear. Note the shredding of the meniscus.

reconstruction remained asymptomatic after ACL reconstruction if they were stable at the time of surgery.

Radial, or transverse, tears of the meniscus usually are located at the junction of the posterior and middle thirds of the meniscus. Complete radial tears disrupt the circumferential fibers of the meniscus (Figure 21-10). Jones et al.[35] showed that a complete radial tear completely disrupts the function of the meniscus, leading to significantly increased joint contact stresses.

Horizontal cleavage tears start near the inner margin of the meniscus and extend toward the capsule. Shear forces within the meniscus during load transmission likely cause a separation of the horizontally oriented collagen fiber bundles. The incidence of horizontal cleavage tears increases with age (Figure 21-11). Parameniscal cysts are most often associated with these tears. These cysts often form when horizontal cleavage tears reach the parameniscal region.[36]

Complex tears of the meniscus, often called **degenerative tears,** occur in multiple planes (Figure 21-12). Most patients with complex tears are more than 40 years of age. These tears most often occur at the posterior horn of the medial or lateral meniscus and are commonly associated with degenerative changes in the articular cartilage of the knee.

TREATMENT OF MENISCAL TEARS

Indications for Surgical Treatment

Not all meniscal tears require surgical intervention. Before deciding on surgery for meniscal pathology, the clinician must exclude other causes of knee pain, such as degenerative chondral changes. For surgery to be considered, symptoms of meniscal injury should limit activities of daily living, work, or sports. Some meniscal tears heal spontaneously; therefore a trial of conservative management with activity modification and rehabilitation should be attempted before surgical intervention. Henning et al.[37] showed that some tears heal spontaneously or remain asymptomatic, including short vertical tears (less than 10 mm), stable vertical longitudinal tears, partial-thickness tears (less than 50% of meniscal depth) on the tibial or femoral surfaces, and small radial tears (less than 3 mm).

In patients with evidence of knee osteoarthritis and an atraumatic degenerative meniscal tear, a prolonged trial of conservative treatment may be warranted. Nonoperative management has been shown to provide equivalent outcomes to partial meniscectomy at 6 and 12 months, after presentation with symptoms.[38] However, greater than 30% of patients who are treated nonoperatively will ultimately elect to undergo a partial meniscectomy due to persistence of symptoms.

Evidence has also questioned the utility of arthroscopic debridement of degenerative meniscal tears in middle-aged patients with little to no concomitant osteoarthritis.[39,40] These studies have been criticized for a very narrow patient inclusion criteria, and many have cautioned against the application of their findings to all patients with degenerative meniscal tears. Until further evidence is available, surgical decision making must be individualized and rely on mechanical symptoms, degenerative versus traumatic onset of symptoms, other possible pain generators (arthritis, plica, synovitis), and effect of previous nonoperative treatments.

Indications for Meniscal Surgery

- Symptoms limit activities of daily living, work, or sports
- Conservative treatment has not improved symptoms

If the meniscal injury is associated with an ACL injury, the timing of surgery usually is dictated by the acute rehabilitation after the ACL injury. Factors such as swelling and ROM dictate the timing of ACL reconstruction. Meniscal pathology usually can be addressed at the time of ACL reconstruction. If a displaced bucket handle meniscal tear is limiting recovery of extension after an ACL injury, the meniscal tear should be dealt with on an urgent basis to allow the patient to regain full extension before proceeding with ACL reconstruction.

Surgical Intervention

Surgeons should develop a standard approach to knee arthroscopy. A diagnostic arthroscopy of the entire knee should be performed as the initial portion of all knee arthroscopies. This diagnostic arthroscopy can be performed in a number of ways, but each surgeon should choose one routine and stick to it to avoid missing pathology. The final decision as to whether the meniscal tear should be repaired or excised should be made after the diagnostic arthroscopy. Most meniscal tears are not amenable to repair. These tears usually require partial meniscectomy to relieve the patient's pain and mechanical symptoms. When a partial meniscectomy is performed, as much of the functioning meniscus as possible is left to maximize the function of the remaining meniscus and minimize the effect on joint biomechanics.

Indications for meniscal repair can be divided into patient factors and meniscal factors. Patient factors include the chronicity of symptoms, patient's ability to tolerate the longer rehabilitation required after repair, and risk of failure of the repair. The patient's age also should be factored into the equation because younger patients are likely to have a greater chance of progression to arthritis after meniscectomy. Meniscal factors that are favorable for repair include a complete vertical tear longer than 10 mm, a tear within the peripheral 10% to 30% or within 3 to 4 mm of the meniscocapsular junction (red-red zone), an unstable tear that can be displaced by probing, a tear without secondary degeneration or deformity, and tears in stable knees or associated with concomitant ligamentous reconstruction.[30] If both patient and meniscal factors indicate that the tear is amenable to surgical repair, then repair should be performed.

As previously mentioned, some meniscal tears heal spontaneously or remain asymptomatic. If one of these tears is seen at the time of diagnostic arthroscopy and the knee is stable or is undergoing ACL reconstruction, the meniscus can be left alone, or **trephination (i.e., surgical excision of a circular piece of tissue)** and rasping can be performed without surgical stabilization.[37] Weiss et al.[41] reviewed 52 patients with stable vertical longitudinal meniscal tears (i.e., tears with less than 3 mm of displacement with probing) and performed repeat arthroscopy. Complete healing was noted in 65% of these patients. Only six patients required further treatment, and four of those had suffered a new traumatic event.[41]

Meniscal Resection

Total meniscectomy used to be a very common procedure. Fairbank[42] first described the damaging effects of total meniscectomy in 1948. As long-term results became available, the progression to osteoarthritis was noted; consequently, total meniscectomy has become a very uncommon procedure.[43,44] With arthroscopic techniques, partial meniscectomy has become feasible (Figure 21-13).

When meniscal repair is not indicated, surgeons now perform a partial meniscectomy. Metcalf et al.[32] established guidelines for meniscal resection. All mobile fragments of the meniscus that can be pulled past the inner margin of the meniscus into the center of the joint should

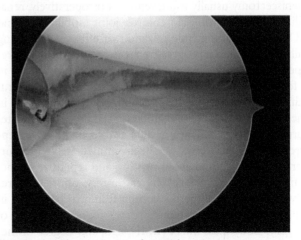

Figure 21-13 Arthroscopic view of a partial meniscectomy.

be resected. The remaining meniscal rim should be smoothed to remove any sudden changes in contour that may lead to further tearing. A perfectly smooth rim is not necessary. A probe should be used to gain information about the stability or mobility of the remaining meniscus. The meniscocapsular junction and the meniscal rim should be retained, if at all possible, to preserve the load transmission properties of the meniscus. Motorized and manual instruments should be used. Manual instruments are more accurate, and motorized shavers can remove loose debris and smooth frayed edges.

Partial Meniscectomy

Studies on the short-term outcome of partial meniscectomy have shown 80% to 90% good results at less than 2-year follow-up.[45] A number of long-term follow-up studies have shown progression of arthritis radiographically after partial meniscectomy. Fauno and Nielsen[46] found that with 8 years of follow-up, radiographic changes occurred in 53% of knees that had undergone partial meniscectomy, compared with 27% of untreated, contralateral knees. Schimmer et al.[47] found good or excellent results in 91.7% of partial meniscectomies at 4 years, but this dropped to 78.1% at 12 years. Articular cartilage damage associated with the meniscal tear had the greatest impact on the long-term outcome. Sixty-two percent of patients who had articular cartilage damage at the time of the index operation had a good or excellent result at final follow-up. In patients with no articular cartilage damage, 94.8% had good or excellent results.[47] In a review of the literature, Fabricant and Jokl[48] found age and sex had no association with clinical or radiographic outcomes up to 15 years postoperatively. Patients with flap tears had slower return to sports and more revision surgery than those with bucket handle tears. They found no difference in outcomes between medial and lateral meniscectomies. Patients with less than 50% of their meniscal rim remaining after partial meniscectomy had worse radiographic outcomes at 12 years than those with greater than 50% remaining.[48]

Postoperative Rehabilitation. Rehabilitation after partial meniscectomy usually is uneventful. Postoperatively, rehabilitation focuses on pain control, joint mobilization and ROM, gait training, minimization of effusion, regaining full strength, and a progressive return to preinjury or preoperative activity. These goals can be achieved either in a formal rehabilitation setting or with home treatment. Icing and elevation can help minimize pain and effusion in the knee. ROM exercises can be started immediately after surgery. Patients may bear weight as tolerated. Quadriceps strengthening exercises can begin immediately after surgery. Patients should avoid twisting and repetitive impact activities for 4 to 6 weeks after surgery. Short-term recovery following surgery has been found to be slower in women and those with worse arthritis found at the time of surgery. Body mass index (BMI), age, and degree of meniscal resection were not found to have an effect.[49]

Meniscal Cysts

As mentioned, meniscal cysts occur most often with horizontal cleavage tears. A retrospective review of 167 knee MRIs with findings of either intrameniscal (38%) or parameniscal (62%) cysts showed 59% of cysts were located in the medial meniscus and 41% in the lateral meniscus. Fifty-eight percent of these cysts were associated with a meniscal tear found on MRI.[50] These cysts usually can be decompressed at the time of partial meniscectomy from within the joint. Metcalf et al.[32] showed that meniscal cysts rarely recur if the meniscal pathology is dealt with appropriately. The results of arthroscopic decompression of cysts range from 90% to 100% without recurrence. If the cyst is not easily identified from within the joint, a needle can be passed percutaneously through the cyst into the joint and the location of the cyst identified arthroscopically. The cyst then can usually be decompressed by probing or shaving from within the joint.[51,52] If the cyst cannot be decompressed arthroscopically, an open cyst excision should be performed.

Meniscal Repair

Some meniscal tears can heal without fixation. As previously mentioned, meniscal tears that can be left to heal without fixation include vertical longitudinal tears less than 10 mm long, incomplete tears, and stable tears that move less than 3 mm with probing.[34] In such cases, the surgeon can attempt to enhance the healing response with abrasion of the synovial surfaces and meniscal trephination.[53] Synovial abrasion causes a vascular pannus that migrates into the tear and helps to produce a healing response. Meniscal trephination is a variation of creating vascular access channels. Horizontally oriented holes are made using a spinal needle through the peripheral vascularized region of the meniscus. Fox et al.[54] showed a 90% success rate in healing incomplete tears with trephination.

When a meniscal tear is found to be amenable to repair and the patient understands the risks of meniscal repair and the rehabilitation required (described later in this chapter), a series of steps must be taken to maximize the chances of success of the repair. First, the meniscal bed must be prepared. Loose edges of the tear should be debrided. The torn meniscal edges should be abraded with a rasp or shaver. Rasping of the synovial fringe is also helpful in creating a synovial pannus that can creep into the tear and aid the healing response. Tears that extend into the avascular zone have a lower healing rate. Some think that this can be improved somewhat with trephination.

Open Repair Techniques. Open meniscal repair was first reported by Annandale[55] in 1885. Meniscal repair did not become widely used until it was popularized by DeHaven[56] and Wirth.[57] Open meniscal repair currently is most useful with multiple-ligament injuries, in which the collateral ligament injuries may require open repair, or tibial plateau fractures that require open reduction and internal fixation. With open repair, the meniscus can be sutured directly. The success rate for open meniscal repair is high in multiple-ligament injuries likely because of the peripheral nature of the tears and the acuteness of the injury and the ensuing hemarthrosis. Rockborn and Gillquist[58] reported a 71% success rate in a 13-year follow-up of patients with open meniscal repairs. Brucker et al. reported on average 20.6-year follow-up of open meniscal repair in 26 patients. Eight patients (30%) were noted to have rerupture of the meniscus. Of the 18 remaining, 72% reported excellent results and on average there was no significant increase in arthritis development or progression compared with the contralateral knee.[59] Some surgeons still advocate open meniscal repair, suggesting that meniscal preparation and suturing are more readily achieved with an open approach and that the incisions do not need to be much larger than with inside-out arthroscopic repairs.

Arthroscopic Repair. Arthroscopy allows evaluation and treatment of meniscal tears that are not possible with open techniques. Three basic suturing techniques have been used with arthroscopic procedures: the inside-out technique, outside-in technique, and all-inside technique. Arthroscopic repairs also can be performed using bioabsorbable implants and suture anchors.

Inside-Out Technique. The inside-out technique was first popularized by Henning et al.[37] in the early 1980s. This technique uses double-armed sutures with long needles, which are positioned through arthroscopically directed cannulas. Skin incisions are then made between the two needles. Soft tissues are dissected down to the capsule, with care taken that no neurovascular structures are trapped between the sutures, and the sutures are then tied, reducing the meniscus. A significant advantage of this technique is that it allows accurate suture placement in the meniscus. The main disadvantage of this technique is the risk to neurovascular structures and the need for incisions between the sutures.

When this technique is performed on the medial side of the knee, branches of the saphenous nerve are most commonly injured.[60] Injuries to the saphenous nerve can cause localized numbness or a painful neuroma. The standard medial incision is a vertical incision approximately 3 cm (1.2 inches) long that starts just above the joint line and runs distally. The incision is made with the knee in 90° flexion. The infrapatellar branch of the saphenous nerve runs approximately 1 cm (0.5 inch) proximal to the joint line. The saphenous nerve usually lies below the subcutaneous fat on the deep fascia covering the sartorius muscle. Keeping the knee in 90° flexion allows the sartorius and saphenous nerve to fall posteriorly. Once the subcutaneous tissue has been bluntly dissected down to the sartorius fascia, the fascia is opened in the direction of its fibers and a plane is dissected down to the knee joint capsule. A retractor can then be placed in this plane, protecting the saphenous nerve. The needles can be visualized as they pass through the capsule.

On the lateral side of the knee, the peroneal nerve is most at risk. The popliteal artery and tibial nerve are at risk as the sutures move more posteriorly. The lateral capsule should be exposed before needles are inserted from within the knee joint. An incision is made on the lateral side of the knee just posterior to the fibular collateral ligament. Dissection is again performed with the knee in 90° flexion. The peroneal nerve is protected by finding the interval between the biceps femoris and iliotibial band and retracting the biceps and peroneal nerve posteriorly. The lateral gastrocnemius muscle is found and its fascia is divided in the direction of its fibers. Fibers of the lateral head of the gastrocnemius are dissected off of the posterior capsule. A retractor then can be placed posteriorly in the knee to protect the neurovascular structures. Once this dissection has been performed, needles can be safely passed from inside the knee and retrieved as they exit the capsule, without risk of neurovascular injury.

After the appropriate exposure and neurovascular protection have been obtained, attention can be returned to the meniscal pathology. The meniscal bed is prepared (Figure 21-14), and sutures then can be passed through the meniscus, exiting the knee joint capsule. The sutures should be passed in a vertical mattress pattern for maximum strength; ideally, they should be placed at 2- to 3-mm intervals (Figure 21-15).[61]

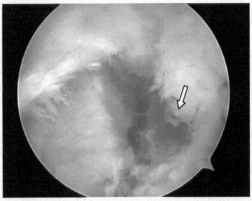

Figure 21-14 Arthroscopic view of a bleeding edge in the red zone of the meniscus.

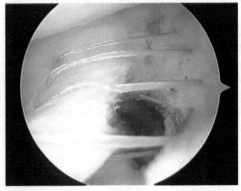

Figure 21-15 Arthroscopic view of vertical mattress sutures in place, ready to be tightened and tied.

Outside-In Technique. The outside-in technique was developed as an attempt to avoid the neurovascular complications that can occur with the inside-out technique. The outside-in technique uses a spinal needle passed percutaneously through the subcutaneous tissue, through the meniscal tear, into the knee joint. A suture then is passed into the joint through the needle and brought out through the anterior portal. A knot is tied in the free end of the suture, and the suture is pulled back into the joint, reducing the meniscal tear. Adjacent sutures are tied to each other outside the capsule.[62] A small incision is made between the two sutures, the soft tissues are cleared between the sutures down to the capsule (with care taken that no neurovascular structures are caught between the sutures), and the sutures are then tied as in the inside-out technique.

Modifications of the original outside-in technique have emerged. In one such modification, a needle is placed percutaneously as previously described to pass the first suture into the knee, followed by a parallel needle with a wire suture retrieval loop. The first suture is passed through the loop and pulled out of the knee joint through the second needle, leaving one intact suture that can be tied outside the capsule. This essentially leaves the patient with the same final configuration of sutures as an inside-out technique.

The outside-in technique is most useful for tears in the anterior or middle third of the meniscus. To perform this technique for posterior tears, the surgeon must use an open approach to allow safe passage of the needles into the knee joint.

All-Inside Technique. The all-inside suture repair is useful for tears of the posterior portion of the medial or lateral meniscus. The all-inside technique is advantageous in that it does not require any accessory incisions and therefore has a decreased risk to neurovascular structures, making it faster and easier than traditional repair techniques. The newest generation all-inside devices are passed through an anterior arthroscopic portal. The insertion device is passed through the meniscus tear in the desired location and an anchor is deployed extraarticularly behind the peripheral meniscus on the capsular surface. The insertion device is withdrawn into the joint and the process is repeated to place the second anchor in its desired location. A nonabsorbable suture attached to both anchors forms a suture bridge over the meniscal tear. The suture has a pretied, sliding, self-locking knot which is tensioned to close the gap in the meniscus and compress the meniscal repair site. Both horizontal and vertical suture orientation is possible.

Meniscal Repair Devices. A number of devices have been developed to allow meniscal repair without the risk of neurovascular injury or the need for secondary incisions (Figure 21-16). These devices have progressed through several "generations" with increasing strength of repair while decreasing complications from their use.

First-generation devices, described by Morgan[63] in 1991, used curved suture hooks through accessory posterior portals to pass sutures across the tear. Sutures were

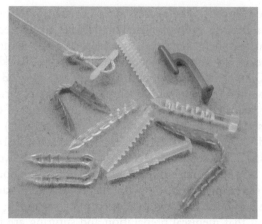

Figure 21-16 Examples of meniscal repair implant devices that vary in design and permit an all-inside meniscal repair without the need for accessory portals or incisions. (From Miller MD, Cole BJ: *Textbook of arthroscopy,* Philadelphia, 2004, Saunders/Elsevier.)

then retrieved and tied arthroscopically. The technique was technically demanding, and it continued to place the neurovascular structures at risk.

The second generation of all-inside meniscal repairs introduced the concept of devices placed across the tear and anchored peripherally. These generally consisted of a polyethylene bar with an attached suture, deployed through a sharp needle or cannula to capture the peripheral meniscus or capsule. Adjacent sutures were then secured with arthroscopic knots pushed onto the meniscal surface. The complications associated with these devices came from the arthroscopic knots leading to chondral abrasion and the inability to tension the knots after placement.

The third generation consisted of a similar design as the second generation but with bioabsorbable fixation devices, including arrows, screws, darts, and staples. Initial repair results were quite good with some studies showing a 91% healing rate.[64,65] These results were noted to significantly deteriorate with longer term follow-up. Kurzweil et al.[66] reported an overall failure rate of 28% with the meniscus arrow, at average follow-up of 54 months. Numerous device-specific complications have also been reported, including transient synovitis, inflammatory reaction, cyst formation, device failure, device migration, and chondral damage.

The fourth generation as described earlier in the technique section was developed to address concerns with the previous generations of fixation devices. These devices are flexible, and suture based, have a lower profile, and allow for variable compression and retensioning across the meniscal tear.

Studies comparing early generations of all-inside repair devices to inside-out repair techniques showed the all-inside techniques to have higher failure rates. With the newer-generation implants, biomechanical studies have demonstrated strength and load-to-failure characteristics comparable to mattress suture constructs and significantly better than earlier-generation devices.[67] Rosso et al.[68]

compared repair strengths between all-inside devices and inside-out suture repair and found no difference in biomechanical properties and failure rates between techniques after 100,000 loading cycles.

Results of Meniscal Repair. Meniscal repairs have been evaluated using second-look arthroscopy, double-contrast arthrography, MRI, and clinical examination with the absence of symptoms referable to meniscal pathology. To evaluate the success rates for meniscal repair found in the literature, readers must take into account the definition of successful repair. Success rates are higher for patients who undergo ACL reconstruction at the time of meniscal repair than for patients who have isolated meniscal repairs. Cannon and Vittori[69] looked at stable knees and knees that underwent ACL reconstruction at the time of meniscal repair. Of the stable knees, 50% healed, whereas 90% of the knees that underwent concomitant ACL reconstruction healed. The location of the tear within the meniscus must also be considered. Buseck and Noyes[70] reviewed 66 repairs associated with ACL reconstruction. All patients underwent second-look arthroscopy. Eighty percent were completely healed, 14% were partially healed, and 6% failed. Ninety-eight percent of tears in the outer one third healed. Finally, the length of follow-up must be evaluated. Many studies have been published on the short-term results of meniscal repair, but success rates decline if patients are followed for longer than 2 years.[71]

Numerous studies have presented outcomes on specific all-inside implant systems with success rates ranging from 63% to 96% excellent-to-good clinical results.[72-77] Many of these studies are limited by short-term follow-up periods

as discussed previously. Short-term outcomes with new fixation devices have been particularly promising; however, long-term outcomes are still needed to proclaim their equivalence or superiority to older treatment strategies. Grant et al.[78] performed a systematic review comparing all-inside (with devices from all generations) to inside-out techniques in patients with isolated meniscal tears. They found the failure rate for inside-out technique was 17% and all-inside was 19%. Functional outcomes were also reviewed and found to be no different between the two groups. Given the diverse and evolving evidence on meniscal repair technique, the surgeon should ultimately be guided by the clinical scenario surrounding the tear: concomitant injuries, tear chronicity, tear location, tear pattern, and surgeon comfort with available fixation techniques.

Indicators of Successful Meniscal Repairs

- Repairs are performed at the same time as ACL reconstruction
- Lateral meniscal repairs are more successful than medial meniscal repairs
- Tear is in the peripheral one third of the meniscus
- A functioning meniscus is present

Postoperative Rehabilitation. Rehabilitation after meniscal repair depends on whether ACL reconstruction was performed at the same time. Although many protocols exist, the principles of rehabilitation include an initial period of non-weight bearing and limitation of flexion. Standard meniscal repair guidelines are presented in Table 21-1.

TABLE 21-1

Rehabilitation Protocol after Meniscal Repair

	Weeks 1-2	Weeks 3-4	Weeks 5-6	Weeks 7-8	Weeks 9-16	Weeks 17-20	Weeks 21-24
Brace	Immobilized	Immobilized	No brace	No brace	No brace	No brace	No brace
WB	NWB	PWB	WB as tolerated	WB as tolerated	WB as tolerated	WB as tolerated	WB as tolerated
ROM	0°-90°	0°-90°	0°-120°	Full ROM	Full ROM	Full ROM	Full ROM
Exercises	Isometric Quad Exercises • Quad sets • SLR	Isometric Quad Exercises • Quad sets • SLR	Begin closed-chain exercises	Closed-chain exercises Hamstrings Stationary bike	Closed-chain exercises Hamstrings Stationary bike Stair climber	Running, straight	Cutting
Manual therapy	Patellar mobilization	Patellar and joint mobilization Passive ROM to 90°	Patellar and joint mobilization Passive ROM to 120°	Patellar and joint mobilization			

NWB, Non–weight-bearing; *PWB*, partial weight bearing; *ROM*, range of motion; *WB*, weight bearing; *Quad*, quadriceps; *SLR*, straight leg raise.

If ACL reconstruction is performed concomitantly with the meniscal repair, more aggressive ROM exercises should be performed. Flexion should be limited to 90° for the first 4 to 6 weeks. Arnoczky et al.[79] showed that the meniscus is subject only to small amounts of motion and stress between 15° and 60° flexion. After 6 weeks, more aggressive closed kinetic chain activities can be started. Return to pivoting sports should not be allowed before 6 months.

Complications of Meniscal Repair. The most common complication of meniscal repair is failure of healing and the need for subsequent partial meniscectomy. Other complications specifically associated with meniscal repair include injury to the saphenous nerve or vein, peroneal or tibial nerve, and popliteal artery or vein. Loss of motion after repair also can be associated with meniscal repairs.[62,80,81] Deep vein thrombosis, pain, infection, and hemarthrosis can occur but are not seen at a higher rate than with partial meniscectomy. Shelbourne and Johnson[82] reported a 25% incidence of stiffness when ACL reconstruction was performed at the same time as repair of a locked bucket handle meniscal tear. Meniscal repair performed at the same time as ACL reconstruction does appear to be a risk factor for postoperative stiffness; however, meniscal healing rates are higher when meniscal repair and ACL reconstruction are performed at the same time.

Complications of Meniscal Surgery

- Nerve injury (saphenous, peroneal, tibial)
- Vascular injury (saphenous, popliteal)
- Loss of range of motion (stiffness)
- Deep vein thrombosis
- Pain
- Infection
- Hemarthrosis

Meniscal Transplantation

Transplantation of the meniscus was first described by Milachowski et al.[83] in 1989. The experience with human meniscal transplantation was preceded by clinical studies in animals and cadavers. Cadaveric models have shown decreased contact pressures and increased contact surface areas after meniscal transplantation. Both the anterior and posterior horns of the meniscus must be securely attached in their anatomical positions to gain these biomechanical advantages. When both anterior and posterior attachments are released, the decrease in contact stresses is completely lost. If one attachment site is lost, some biomechanical benefit is obtained, but it is significantly reduced.[84]

Arnoczky et al.[85] transplanted cryopreserved medial meniscal allografts in 14 dogs. These menisci healed to the capsule by fibrovascular scar. At 3 months they

maintained a normal gross appearance. Histological studies showed that the transplanted menisci maintained a normal cellular distribution. Jackson et al.[86] used a goat model to compare autograft to fresh allograft and cryopreserved allograft. At 6 months the implanted menisci appeared very similar histologically to the controls. A slight decrease was seen in the cellularity in the central portions of the menisci. Peripheral vascularity was almost normal. The water content of the meniscus was increased and the proteoglycan content was decreased compared with controls. In another study, Fabriciani et al.[87] demonstrated little difference between cryopreserved and deep-frozen meniscal transplants. Their study showed nearly complete remodeling at 6 and 12 months. Debeer et al.[88] showed that 95% of the deoxyribonucleic acid (DNA) in a human transplanted meniscus was identical to that of the recipient at 1 year, which indicated that the host had repopulated the meniscal cells.

Indications for Meniscal Transplantation. The ideal patient for meniscal transplantation is one who previously has undergone complete or near-complete meniscectomy and has joint line pain, early chondral damage, a stable knee, and normal lower limb alignment. Meniscal transplantation can be considered at the same time as ACL reconstruction in an ACL-deficient knee. If axial malalignment is present, tibial or femoral osteotomy should be considered to correct it. Meniscal transplantation is contraindicated in patients with advanced chondral changes.[89] At this point, no evidence supports meniscal transplantation in asymptomatic patients who have undergone complete or near-complete meniscectomy. As longer-term results become available, the indications may expand to cover asymptomatic young patients with complete meniscectomies.

Indications for Meniscal Transplantation

- Previous complete or near-complete meniscectomy
- Joint line pain
- Early chondral damage
- Stable knee
- Normal lower limb alignment

Graft Sizing. Graft sizing is extremely important. To obtain the beneficial biomechanical effects of meniscal transplantation, the transplanted meniscus should vary less than 5% from the original meniscus. Various studies have used computed tomography (CT) scans, MRI, and plain radiography for meniscal allograft sizing. A study by Shaffer et al.[89] showed that MRI was accurate to within 5 mm of width and length measurements in 84% of cases, compared with 79% of cases measured with plain radiographs. Most tissue banks use plain radiographs for allograft sizing.[90]

Surgical Technique. The insertion of meniscal allografts has been described using an open technique with collateral ligament detachment, an open technique without collateral ligament detachment, an arthroscopically assisted technique, and an all-arthroscopic technique. The results of meniscal transplantation seem to depend on patient selection, graft sizing, and secure graft fixation more than surgical technique. As described previously, to increase the contact surface area and reduce contact stresses, the surgeon must securely fix the anterior and posterior horns. Soft tissue fixation, fixation with bone plugs, and fixation with a bony bridge inserted into a trough in the tibial plateau have been described as techniques for secure anterior and posterior horn fixation (Figure 21-17).

Results. The results of meniscal transplantation vary significantly with patient selection. Hommen et al.[91] showed that patients with lower preoperative Lysholm scores also had inferior postoperative results. Stollsteimer et al.[92] reported better results with weight <225 lb and Outerbridge grade of <2 in all compartments. Noyes[93] reported on a series of 96 meniscal allografts. MRI and arthroscopic evaluations were used in this study to determine graft success rates. Twenty-two percent healed, 34% partially healed, and 44% failed. When these results were broken down, normal knees had a 70% healing rate, with the other 30% partially healed, whereas knees with severe arthrosis had a 50% failure rate and 50% partial healing. Cameron and Saha[94] reported on 67 meniscal allografts with 87% good or excellent results using a modified Lysholm rating score. These authors performed 34 tibial osteotomies and suggested in their conclusions that limb alignment was important to their success rates. Other studies have shown that meniscal transplantation performed with appropriately sized grafts with secure fixation in patients with normal alignment and only early chondral changes can predictably reduce pain and in-crease knee function.[90] A systematic review by Hergan et al.[28] found 68% to 89% of patients rated their postoperative activity level as normal to nearly normal. As with meniscal repair, a longer-term follow-up of clinical outcomes seems to show deterioration of clinical results over time.[95] Overall failure of the meniscal transplant varies in studies between 0% and 37.5%[96] with early failure (<2 years) of approximately 10%. However, these results are somewhat ambiguous because the definition of failure was not universally defined among studies.

The theoretical chondroprotective effect of meniscal transplant has yet to be definitively shown in the literature. Studies evaluating this have produced different outcomes. Homen et al.[25] found compartment degeneration in 10 of 15 patients, whereas Roumazeille et al.[97] reported no average change in 22 patients. The variation in findings may be partially due to lack of standardized evaluation methods, with multiple different grading scores used to evaluate joint changes across multiple studies.

Postoperative Rehabilitation. Rehabilitation protocols vary among surgeons who perform meniscal allograft transplantation but these protocols are generally similar to those for meniscal repair. Patients are kept non-weight or partial weight bearing for the first 4 to 6 weeks. ROM is allowed but is limited to 90° flexion for the first 4 to 6 weeks. Muscle strengthening is progressed gradually with closed-chain quadriceps and hamstring exercises. Pivoting activities are restricted for the first 6 months. Return to sports participation should be guarded given a high meniscal tear rate. In particular, restriction of high-impact activities with cutting and pivoting is warranted.

Summary

The treatment of meniscal pathology is a continually changing field. The art and science of meniscal repairs have advanced tremendously. The future holds potential for meniscal allograft transplantation and for the development of meniscal replacements.

ARTICULAR CARTILAGE LESIONS

The treatment of full-thickness articular cartilage lesions in the knee is a field that is quickly evolving. Untreated articular cartilage lesions have little or no potential to heal. However, some studies show that a large number of patients will have isolated chondral defects and remain asymptomatic without treatment. Messner and Maletius[98] reviewed a series of 28 patients with isolated chondral lesions; 22 had either good or excellent clinical results without treatment 14 years after diagnosis. Most of these 22 patients had abnormal radiographic findings suggesting progressive degenerative changes. Although these data suggest that isolated chondral defects may predispose patients to the development of further degenerative changes in the knee, long-term prospective data

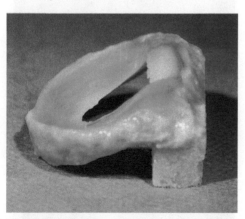

Figure 21-17 Meniscal allograft with bony attachments. (From Insall JN, Scott WN: *Surgery of the knee*, ed 3, p 552, New York, 2001, Churchill Livingstone.)

have not been obtained that link isolated chondral defects to progressive degenerative arthritis of the knee that compromises a patient's level of function.

History

The clinical presentation of a full-thickness chondral defect can vary. Some patients complain of loose body–type symptoms with locking, catching, and clicking. Other patients complain of crepitus with intermittent mechanical symptoms, and a third group presents with pain as the only symptom. The clinician should obtain a careful history to determine whether the symptoms are indeed coming from within the knee joint and, if so, whether they are coming from the medial, lateral, or patellofemoral compartment.

Physical Examination

A thorough physical examination should be performed for all patients suspected of having chondral defects of the knee. The clinician should begin the examination by watching the patient stand and walk, noting limb length and alignment and observing any gait abnormalities, such as valgus or varus thrust during the stance phase of gait. A low back examination and a complete distal neurological and vascular examination should also be performed. Examination of the hip is critical in any patient presenting with knee symptoms. A systematic examination of both knees should be performed. Thigh circumference and ROM should be compared between the two sides. Pain experienced by the patient during ROM should be noted. The knee should be examined for an effusion.

Knee stability should be examined, including testing of the anterior and posterior cruciate ligaments, the tibial (medial) collateral ligament, the fibular (lateral) collateral ligament, and the posterolateral (popliteus) corner. The knee should be palpated for any local tenderness. The extensor mechanism should be examined for continuity, and the alignment of the extensor mechanism (Q angle) should be measured. The mechanics of the patellofemoral articulation should be examined, and the clinician should observe for a **patellar "J" sign** (i.e., deviation of the patella cephalically and laterally in the pattern of an upside-down J), lateral tilt of the patella, lateral retinacular tightness, and patellofemoral crepitation.

Diagnostic Imaging

Diagnostic imaging should begin with plain radiographic films. A standing PA flexion view should be included in the standard knee series. A tangential view of the patellofemoral joint (e.g., Merchant view) should also be included. These plain radiographic films can show joint space narrowing, osteochondral defects, and patellofemoral tilt or subluxation. However, isolated chondral defects often cannot be seen on plain radiographic films.

The imaging study of choice for chondral defects is MRI because of its excellent sensitivity and specificity for this type of lesion. Bredella et al.[99] reported on 130 patients undergoing knee arthroscopy for suspected internal derangement. Of 86 arthroscopically proven abnormalities, 81 were detected with MRI. MRI performed with a T2-weighted, fast spin-echo sequence with fat saturation had a sensitivity of 94% and a specificity of 99% compared with arthroscopy (Figures 21-18 and 21-19).

Nonoperative Management

The goal of nonoperative management of chondral lesions is to minimize symptoms and allow maximum activity. Maintenance of ROM, muscle strengthening, and a variety of therapeutic modalities to reduce pain and inflammation all can minimize symptoms. Orthotics, bracing, and gait

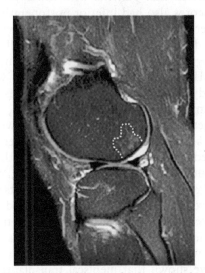

Figure 21-18 T2-weighted MRI scan of a chondral defect (outlined by *white dotted line*) of the posterior condyle.

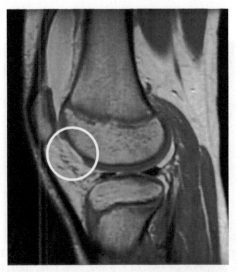

Figure 21-19 T1-weighted MRI scan of a trochlear chondral defect (*circled*).

training can minimize the stresses on the affected region of the joint. Weight loss in overweight patients can dramatically improve symptoms by reducing patellofemoral and tibiofemoral contact stresses.

Surgical Management

The ultimate goal of surgical treatment is restoration of the microarchitecture of the articular cartilage, which allows complete restoration of the biomechanical and physiological function of the knee. A number of techniques for cartilage repair and regeneration have been developed. The following sections present a detailed look at each of these modalities and review the basic science, surgical techniques, and rehabilitation principles and results.

Abrasion Arthroplasty

The idea of doing something to eburnated bone to cause a reparative tissue response was first proposed by Pridie[100] in 1959. He recommended joint debridement, removal of osteophytes, retention of the patella, shaving of fissured articular cartilage, and drilling of eburnated bone. He described fibrous, reparative-type tissue filling and covering 0.5 cm (0.25 inch) cortical drill holes through the femoral condyle. Most of his poor results involved patients in whom he also performed a patellectomy. Akeson et al.[101] attempted to confirm Pridie's findings in laboratory animals. They removed the articular cartilage and subchondral bone of dog femoral heads. At 1-year follow-up, they concluded that excessive loading destroyed the initial reparative tissue. These results also showed that the proteoglycan concentrations in the reparative tissue were less than half that of normal articular cartilage. Mitchell and Shepard[102] studied rabbit knee joints. They found that after multiple small holes were drilled into the subchondral bone, reparative tissue was stimulated to cover large areas of articular surfaces. The reparative tissue grew out from the drill holes and then spread over the exposed bone. This tissue began to fibrillate and break down within 1 year.[102] These two studies were the first to demonstrate that a fibrocartilaginous repair tissue could be stimulated to form on large areas of articular surface. However, these studies also showed that this reparative tissue did not have the proteoglycan concentration of articular cartilage and that it started to break down quickly with excessive loading.

Abrasion arthroplasty using motorized instrumentation was introduced by Johnson[103] in 1981. Whether the abrasion should be intracortical or cancellous bone should be exposed is the subject of debate. Hjertquist and Lemperg[104] reported that cartilage tissue of mature appearance forms only if the debridement is superficial enough to maintain a cortex.

Surgical Technique. The procedure introduced by Johnson in 1981 is essentially an extension of that described by Pridie. Along with debridement of the joint, a superficial layer of subchondral bone (1 to 3 mm deep)

is removed to expose interosseous vessels. This theoretically results in a hemorrhagic exudate that forms a fibrin clot and allows fibrous repair tissue to form over the area of exposed bone. Minimizing excessive subchondral bone destruction is an important and challenging part of the procedure. With increasing debridement and destruction of the subchondral bone, the risk of thermal necrosis to the surrounding area increases.

Rehabilitation. Regeneration of articular cartilage benefits from motion and from limiting the compressive force on the articular cartilage from weight bearing. Patient adherence to a program of motion with limited or no weight bearing is critical. To assist with this, the use of continuous passive motion (CPM) often is considered. Weight bearing often is restricted for up to 12 weeks, with daily CPM, especially in the early postoperative period. Active and passive ROM are encouraged throughout the postoperative course until weight bearing and strength training can begin.

Results. Eight knees were biopsied in Johnson's original series.[103] Of those eight biopsy specimens, only one showed any type II collagen typical of hyaline cartilage. All other biopsy specimens showed a combination of type I and type III collagen. Bert and Maschka[105] reviewed a series of 59 patients who underwent abrasion arthroplasty with a minimum 5-year follow-up. Of the 59 patients, 15 had conversion to total knee arthroplasty. Biopsies were performed on any remaining fibrous tissue. The fibrous tissue was stained with safranin O to look for proteoglycan. The fibrous surface did not stain, indicating the lack of proteoglycan.

Microfracture

Microfracture is a surgical option used to treat small areas of damaged cartilage (<2 cm). A small sharp pick (awl) is used to create small holes (microfractures) in the bone to stimulate circulation and the growth of fibrocartilage. Microfracture can be performed on the patellar, tibial, or femoral articular surface. The general indication for microfracture is a full-thickness chondral defect in either a weight-bearing region or a region of contact between the femur and patella. Microfracture can also be performed after debridement of unstable chondral flaps. Contraindications to microfracture include axial malalignment, partial-thickness chondral defects, and a patient who is unable or unwilling to comply with a strict postoperative rehabilitation protocol, including minimal weight bearing. Joint space narrowing, bipolar lesions, subchondral bone loss, chronic lesions, and inability to use a CPM machine may affect the outcome but are not strict contraindications.

Surgical Technique. Microfracture can be performed arthroscopically with a combination of shavers, curettes, and picks. The technique has been described by Steadman et al.[106] Three portals are made, allowing use of an inflow canula, the arthroscope, and the working instruments.

A diagnostic arthroscopy is performed, and the full-thickness chondral defect is identified. Any other work that needs to be performed in the knee is completed before the microfracture procedure is begun. The chondral defect is then inspected, and all cartilage remnants are debrided (Figure 21-20).

The articular cartilage surrounding the defect is inspected and any loose, delaminated cartilage is removed. A perpendicular edge of healthy cartilage is obtained circumferentially around the lesion. The calcified cartilage layer is removed, while care is taken not to debride through the subchondral plate.

An arthroscopic awl with the appropriate angle then is used to create perforations in the subchondral plate that are perpendicular to the surface. The awl allows the surgeon to make holes (microfractures) in the subchondral bone with control and without any worry of heat necrosis (Figure 21-21). Attention first is given to the periphery of the lesion. Holes are made at 3- to 4-mm intervals around the periphery and are approximately 3 to 4 mm deep. Once the holes have been made around the periphery, the remaining surface of the lesion is addressed. Holes should be spaced as close together as possible without fracturing

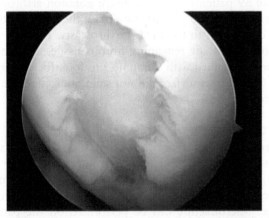

Figure 21-20 Arthroscopic view of a chondral defect debrided to subchondral bone. The calcified cartilage layer has been removed.

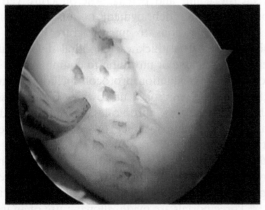

Figure 21-21 Arthroscopic view of a microfracture technique. Multiple pick holes are spaced 3 to 4 mm apart.

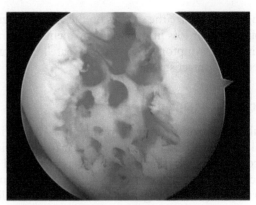

Figure 21-22 Arthroscopic view of a microfracture after reduction of pump pressure shows bleeding from all holes.

the subchondral bone between two holes (approximately 3 to 4 mm). After the holes have been made, a shaver is used to remove all bony debris. The pump pressure then is turned down to enable the surgeon to visualize fat droplets and blood exiting from all holes (Figure 21-22).

Any holes that do not show bleeding should be checked and possibly made deeper to allow bleeding. After the surgeon has made sure that all holes have been made appropriately, the knee is irrigated, instruments are removed, and the joint is evacuated of fluid. Incisions are closed, and a sterile dressing is applied. The key to this procedure is to establish a clot of pluripotent marrow cells that can then differentiate into stable cartilage under the right conditions.

Clinical Point

A strict rehabilitation program is essential after microfracture treatment of chondral lesions of the knee.

Rehabilitation. Microfracture creates an environment in which pluripotent marrow cells can be stimulated to produce cartilage. However, the rehabilitation program ultimately determines the success of the procedure. To design an appropriate rehabilitation program after microfracture, the clinician must think about the region that was affected and the kinematics of the knee. The ideal rehabilitation program encourages motion but limits weight bearing and shear stresses on the affected region. For these reasons, the rehabilitation protocol is very different for weight-bearing femoral condyle lesions than it is for patellar or trochlear lesions. All patients are put in a CPM machine postoperatively, and the patient is asked to use the CPM machine up to 10 hours/day.[107] The rate of motion usually is 1 cycle per minute. The CPM is started in a comfortable range and increased as tolerated. Patients with femoral condyle lesions are kept on toe-touch weight bearing with crutches for 6 to 8 weeks. At 8 weeks, the patient can progress to weight bearing as tolerated and can begin a more vigorous program of active motion. Strength training with weights or machines should be avoided for 16 weeks. Return to sports that involve cutting, pivoting, and jumping can be allowed at 4 to 6 months.

Patients who have patellar or trochlear lesions are allowed to bear weight as tolerated immediately after surgery; however, the knee must be protected from loaded motion where the defect is engaged. At the time of arthroscopy, the knee joint can be taken through a ROM to see specifically where the lesion is in contact with the opposing articular surface. In general, a patient with a trochlear or patellar microfracture can be put in a hinged knee brace with the brace set to move from full extension to 20° flexion. The knee should be taken out of the brace for CPM but should be braced at all other times to avoid shear forces across the lesion. The brace can be discontinued at 8 weeks. A study by Gill et al.[108] suggested that the period of restricted weight bearing should be increased to 12 weeks. This study evaluated the healing process in cynomolgus macaques. Histological analysis was performed 6 and 12 weeks after microfracture. At 6 weeks, limited chondral repair and ongoing resorption of subchondral bone were seen. By 12 weeks, the cartilage defects were completely filled and showed more mature cartilage and bone repair. Further studies in humans are needed to determine whether this additional length of time makes a clinically significant difference in the long-term outcome.

Results. Steadman et al.[109] looked at a series of 75 knees in 72 patients who underwent microfracture for full-thickness traumatic chondral defects. Follow-up was 7 to 17 years. Their three inclusion criteria were: (1) a traumatic full-thickness chondral defect, (2) no meniscal or ligamentous injury, and (3) patient age less than 45 years. Significant improvements were found according to the Lysholm and Tegner knee rating scales. At 7 years after surgery, 80% of patients stated that they were better than before surgery. Some patients took up to 2 years to obtain maximum improvement. Mithoefer et al.[110] performed an evidenced-based systematic analysis of the efficacy of the microfracture technique for articular cartilage repair in the knee. Twenty-eight studies and 3122 patients were included. The study found that microfracture effectively improved knee function during the first 24 months after surgery, but results were conflicting with longer-term follow-up, and there was insufficient evidence to suggest improved function beyond that point. Other factors they found to positively affect outcome were age less than 40 years, duration of symptoms less than 12 months, lesion less than 4 cm², BMI less than 30 kg/m², and higher preoperative activity level.

Mosaicplasty

Autologous osteochondral grafting has shown great promise in that it is a means to transplant bone and hyaline cartilage to a region of a chondral or osteochondral defect. Lane et al.[111] showed that the hyaline cartilage remains viable 12 weeks after transfer. However, two problems were encountered with single plug osteochondral transfers: donor-site morbidity and surface incongruity at the recipient site. Mosaicplasty was developed in an attempt to minimize these problems. Mosaicplasty involves the transfer of multiple small osteochondral plugs to a region of chondral or osteochondral defects. The use of multiple small grafts allows for maintenance of donor-site integrity and contouring of the new surface.

Surgical Technique. Autologous osteochondral mosaicplasty involves harvesting and transferring small, cylindrical osteochondral grafts (2.7 to 8.5 mm in diameter) from non–weight-bearing areas of the femur and transplanting them to prepared recipient sites in the region of the chondral or osteochondral defect.

Combination of different graft sizes allows for coverage of approximately 80% of the lesion. The areas between the osteochondral cylinders will fill with fibrocartilage. At the time of the procedure, a diagnostic arthroscopy is performed. The chondral or osteochondral defect is identified and inspected. All loose cartilage fragments are debrided back to stable, normal articular cartilage. The defect then is sized to determine the number and sizes of grafts needed. If the defect can be accessed adequately arthroscopically, the procedure can be performed arthroscopically. A mini-arthrotomy may be required. The grafts can be obtained from either the medial or lateral peripheral margins of the femoral condyles at the level of the patellofemoral joint (Figure 21-23), distal medial trochlea, or intercondylar notch.[112] The appropriate-sized tube chisel is introduced perpendicular to the donor site, and the harvester is driven into the donor site. For chondral defects, a 15-mm graft is taken. For osteochondral defects, a 25-mm graft is obtained. The chisel is twisted to break the cancellous bone, and the graft is removed. All grafts are harvested with a similar technique (Figure 21-24).

Attention is then turned to the recipient site. Recipient tunnels are created with drill bits and then an appropriately sized dilator. The grafts are inserted with an adjustable plunger device. It is extremely important to ensure that a smooth surface is created, without prominent or sunken grafts (Figure 21-25).

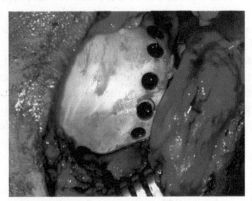

Figure 21-23 View of a graft donor site on the periphery of the lateral femoral condyle.

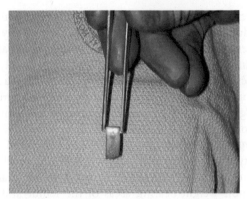

Figure 21-24 Single osteochondral plug.

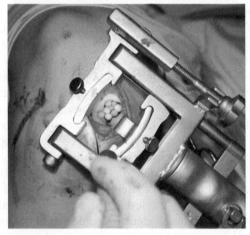

Figure 21-25 Defect filled with multiple osteochondral plugs. (From Insall JN, Scott WN: *Surgery of the knee,* ed 3, p 358, New York, 2001, Churchill Livingstone.)

After all grafts have been put in place, the knee is irrigated and all wounds are closed. Some surgeons place a drain in the knee to try to prevent large postoperative hematomas.

Rehabilitation. Rehabilitation after osteochondral autograft transplantation focuses on early return of ROM and protected weight bearing. ROM exercises can be initiated immediately after surgery. Patients are kept to toe-touch weight bearing for 6 weeks to allow healing of the bony portion of the graft. Patients are allowed to progress to weight bearing as tolerated after 6 weeks and can return to sports activity as soon as they have regained adequate ROM and strength.

Results. The results of multiple osteochondral autograft transplantation have been promising. Chow et al.[113] reported on 33 patients with 2- to 5-year follow-up. Eighty-seven percent of patients reported their knee as being normal or nearly normal using the International Knee Documentation Committee (IKDC) assessment. Jakob et al.[114] reported on 52 patients with 2- to 5-year follow-up. Ninety-two percent of patients had improvement in knee function at the final follow-up. Hangody et al.[115] reviewed 831 patients undergoing mosaicplasty. Good-to-excellent results were obtained in 92% of pa-

tients with femoral condylar defects, 87% of patients with tibial defects, and 79% of patients with patellar or trochlear defects. Three percent of patients reported donor-site morbidity, and 4% reported painful postoperative hemarthroses. Erdil et al.[116] presented mid-term follow-up of 65 knees after mosaicplasty with an average follow-up of 82 months. They reported improved outcomes using the Tenger activity scale, Lysholm scale, and the IKDC subjective knee evaluation form. They found no correlation between functional results and age, defect location, or additional knee pathology. They reported that only four patients required repeat arthroscopy for continued subjective complaints. In these patients, the resurfaced area showed intact cartilage. In contrast to the findings of these studies, Bentley et al.[117] reported that only 69% of patients had good or excellent clinical results as assessed by the modified Cincinnati and Stanmore scores. Painful postoperative hemarthroses continue to be a significant complication after mosaicplasty. Feczko et al.[118] used a German Shepherd model and tested donor-site plugs. They found that compressed collagen minimized blood loss from the donor sites while still allowing gradual substitution with bone and formation of a fibrocartilage cap at the articular surface.

Gudas et al.[119] conducted a prospective randomized trial comparing mosaicplasty (28 patients) to microfracture (29 patients) in athletes (mean age 24.3 years). They found both groups to have significant clinical improvement; however, mosaicplasty had 96% good-to-excellent results compared with 52% in microfracture at an average of 37 months follow-up. They concluded that in young athletic patients, mosaicplasty was superior to microfracture.

Autologous Chondrocyte Transplantation

Chesterman and Smith[120] first successfully isolated and grew chondrocytes in culture in 1965. They took epiphyseal chondrocytes from rabbits, grew them in culture, and then implanted them into articular defects in the tibia. They did not show any significant repair. In 1982, Grande et al.[121] began growing articular chondrocytes in culture and then transplanting them into a patellar defect covered with a periosteal flap. These initial results were presented in 1984 and showed 80% filling of the defect with hyaline-like cartilage. In 1987, the first autologous chondrocyte transplantation was performed in the human knee in Sweden. Brittberg et al.[122] reported on the results of the first 23 procedures. Fourteen of 16 patients with femoral lesions had good or excellent results, whereas only two of seven patients with patellar lesions had good or excellent results.

Surgical Technique. Autologous chondrocyte transplantation requires two operative procedures. The first procedure is a diagnostic arthroscopy and harvesting of chondrocytes. The cultured chondrocytes are implanted during the second procedure. A diagnostic arthroscopy is performed, and the chondral defect is assessed. The defect is not debrided. Any meniscal lesions should be dealt with during the first procedure. Once it has been decided that the patient could benefit from autologous chondrocyte transplantation, cartilage is harvested, typically from the upper medial or upper lateral condyle of the femur. Cartilage most often is taken from the upper medial condyle of the femur at the level of the patellofemoral joint. Three to four slices of cartilage, 3 to 4 mm by 10 mm, should be harvested down to subchondral bone. Two hundred to 300 mg of articular cartilage is required for enzymatic digestion and cell culturing. After harvesting of the cartilage, the knee is irrigated, all arthroscopic instruments are removed, and wounds are closed. The cartilage tissue is sent to a commercial laboratory where it is enzymatically degraded to isolate the chondrocytes. The chondrocytes are cultured over 4 to 6 weeks and sent back for reimplantation during the second procedure.

The second procedure involves implantation of the cultured chondrocytes into the articular defect under a periosteal or collagen membrane patch. A small peripatellar incision is performed to expose the chondral defect. The area of the defect is debrided, with cut vertical edges creating an abrupt transition from healthy cartilage to defect. The excised area is debrided down to subchondral bone without causing bleeding. If bleeding occurs from the subchondral bone, it must be stopped before implantation of the chondrocytes. Depending on the desired patch material, a separate incision can be made to harvest a periosteal flap, which usually is obtained from the upper medial tibia. The desired flap is sutured into the healthy cartilage surrounding the defect. In a periosteal flap the cambium layer of the flap must face the subchondral bone of the defect. Sutures are placed at 5- to 6-mm intervals, and intervals between the sutures are sealed off with fibrin glue. An opening is left in the periosteal patch for injection of the chondrocytes. After injection of the cells, closure of the periosteal patch is completed with sutures and fibrin glue (Figures 21-26 to 21-28).

Collagen patches, although not currently Food and Drug Administration (FDA)-approved for use in autologous chondrocyte implants (ACIs), are becoming increasingly common in use. A collagen patch offers a couple of advantages over the periosteal patch. First, there is decreased patient morbidity by avoiding periosteal harvesting. Second, there is decreased graft hypertrophy (25% with periosteal sleeve versus 5% collagen patch),[123] a complication which can be a significant source of postoperative symptoms (i.e., popping or catching) and lead to reoperation for debridement. The use of a collagen matrix does add significant cost to the initial surgery; however, Samuelson et al.[124] found them to be more cost effective than periosteal patches due to the high rate of complications associated with periosteal patches.

Rehabilitation. Rehabilitation after autologous chondrocyte transplantation can be broken down into ROM,

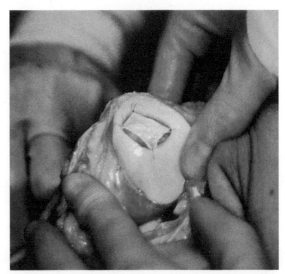

Figure 21-26 Periosteal patch being sewn into place. (From Insall JN, Scott WN: *Surgery of the knee,* ed 3, p 349, New York, 2001, Churchill Livingstone.)

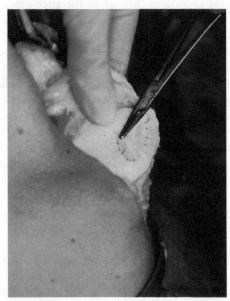

Figure 21-27 Completion of the periosteal patch. (From Insall JN, Scott WN: *Surgery of the knee,* ed 3, p 349, New York, 2001, Churchill Livingstone.)

CPM, weight bearing, strengthening, and functional training. Patients can begin working on ROM immediately after surgery. Trochlear groove patients should not work on active extension for the first 4 weeks because active extension increases patellofemoral contact stresses. CPM should be used as much as possible for the first 6 weeks. Most patients should be non–weight bearing for at least the first 2 weeks. Patients then can progress to partial weight bearing. All patients should be in a hinged knee brace that is locked in extension for ambulation. Femoral condyle patients can progress to weight bearing as tolerated at 6 weeks. Trochlear patients can progress to weight bearing as tolerated as soon as they are

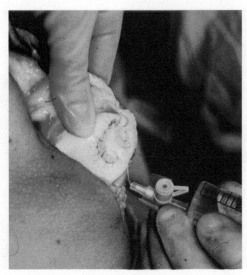

Figure 21-28 Injection of chondrocytes beneath the periosteal patch. (From Insall JN, Scott WN: *Surgery of the knee,* ed 3, p 349, New York, 2001, Churchill Livingstone.)

comfortable as long as they are in the knee brace locked in extension. This keeps the patella out of the trochlear groove and protects the repair. Strengthening can begin in the first 2 weeks with isometric quadriceps sets and straight leg raises. Closed-chain activities can be started at 6 weeks. Positions that stress the region of chondrocyte implantation should be avoided. For anterior femoral condyle lesions, loading in full extension should be avoided. For posterior femoral condyle lesions, loading in flexion should be avoided. For trochlear lesions, deep squats should be avoided. Functional training can begin between weeks 8 and 12.

Clinical Point

It is imperative that the surgeon inform the rehabilitation team of the range of motion allowed to prevent loading, as determined from intraoperative viewing of the lesion during knee range of motion. This allows optimum rehabilitation and protection of the repair.

Positions to Avoid with Autologous Chondrocyte Transplantation

- Anterior femoral condyle lesions—avoid loading in full extension
- Posterior femoral condyle lesions—avoid loaded flexion
- Trochlear lesions—avoid deep squats

Low-impact activities, such as cycling, rollerblading, and skating, can be started 9 to 12 months after surgery. Repetitive impact loading, such as jogging and aerobics, can be started at 13 to 15 months, and high-level sporting activities can be started 16 to 18 months after surgery.

Results. Peterson et al.[125] reported on 101 patients treated with ACIs with 2- to 9-year follow-up. Ninety-two percent of patients with isolated femoral lesions had good or excellent results. Sixty-five percent of patients with patellar defects had good-to-excellent results. Second-look arthroscopy was performed in 53 patients. Of these, 26 had a hypertrophic response of the periosteum or graft. Seven of these 26 were symptomatic. The incidence of graft failure was 7%. Peterson et al.[126] followed a group of 61 patients treated for isolated femoral or patellar defects for 5 to 11 years to determine the durability of the repair tissue. At 2 years, 50 of 61 patients had good-to-excellent results. At 5- to 11-year follow-up, 51 of 61 patients had good-to-excellent results.

Several studies have been performed to evaluate the outcome of ACIs compared with the outcomes with microfracture and mosaicplasty. Knutsen et al.[127,128] performed a randomized clinical trial comparing microfracture and ACI for isolated chondral defects. Eighty patients were enrolled in the study. Microfracture was performed on 40 patients, and ACI was performed on the other 40. An independent observer performed the follow-up data collection at 12 and 24 months and the lead author for the 5-year follow-up. Both groups showed improvement at all follow-up time points. According to the Short Form-36 (SF-36) outcome measurement tool, the microfracture group had a significantly greater improvement in the physical component at 24 months, but this did not persist at the 5-year follow-up. No difference in improvement was seen between the treatment arms based on the International Cartilage Repair Society (ICRS), Tegner, Lysholm, and SF-36 mental component scores. Biopsy specimens were obtained from 84% of patients at 2 years. Histological evaluation of repair tissues showed no significant differences between the two groups. Interestingly, no association was found between the histological specimens and the clinical outcome; however, none of the patients with the highest quality appearing cartilage failed. Horas et al.[129] compared ACI with osteochondral cylinder transplantation. Forty patients with isolated femoral defects were randomized to ACI or osteochondral cylinder transplantation. Using Lysholm scores, recovery from ACI was slower than recovery from osteochondral cylinder transplantation. After 2 years, clinical results were equal between the two groups. Histomorphological examination of the ACI patients showed a stable resurfacing of the defect in all patients. The tissue consisted mainly of fibrocartilage, with localized areas of hyaline-like regenerative cartilage close to the subchondral bone. Examination of biopsies from the osteochondral cylinder transplantation showed remaining gaps between the graft and intact articular cartilage, but no histological difference was seen between the osteochondral transplants and the surrounding original cartilage. Bentley et al.[117] compared ACI to mosaicplasty in a prospective, randomized controlled trial (RCT). Fifty-eight patients underwent ACI, and 42 underwent mosaicplasty. The average size defect was $4.66\,cm^2$. At 1 year, good-to-excellent results were seen in 88% of the ACI patients versus 69% in the mosaicplasty patients. This difference did not reach statistical significance. Second-look arthroscopy at 1 year demonstrated excellent or good repairs in 82% after ACI and 34% after mosaicplasty. The authors concluded superiority of ACI over mosaicplasty despite limited follow-up time. Vanlauwe et al.[130] evaluated microfracture versus ACI in another RCT. Outcome scores showed no difference at 6, 12, 18, and 60 months. Biopsy at 18 months showed improved structural regeneration in ACI compared with microfracture patients. The authors also noted that in a subgroup analysis of outcomes after 60 months, ACI resulted in better outcomes in patients who had their procedure less than 3 years after onset of symptoms.

SUMMARY

The treatment of chondral injuries has become an increasingly popular field. As outlined in this chapter, a number of different options are available to today's orthopedic surgeon. The different techniques have varying advantages and disadvantages, which must be considered when deciding on a treatment plan. Many of the studies evaluating these modalities report only short- to intermediate-term outcomes, and perhaps as long-term outcomes become available ideal usage for each of these options will become better defined. The rehabilitation team needs to understand the biology of the repair technique, the biomechanics of the knee, and how the location of the chondral defect affects the biomechanics to develop the best rehabilitation program and offer the best rehabilitation advice to each patient.

REFERENCES

1. Renstrom P, Johnson RJ: Anatomy and biomechanics of the menisci, *Clin Sports Med* 9:523–538, 1990.
2. Bland-Sutton J, editor: *Ligaments: their nature and morphology*, ed 2, London, 1897, JK Lewis.
3. Berlet GC, Fowler PJ: The anterior horn of the medial meniscus: an anatomic study of its insertion, *Am J Sports Med* 26:540–543, 1998.
4. Nelson EW, LaPrade RF: The anterior intermeniscal ligament of the knee: an anatomic study, *Am J Sports Med* 28:74–76, 2000.
5. Johnson DL, Swenson TM, Livesay GA, et al: Insertion-site anatomy of the human menisci: gross, arthroscopic, and topographical anatomy as a basis for meniscal transplantation, *Arthroscopy* 11:386–394, 1995.
6. Vandermeer RD, Cunningham FK: Arthroscopic treatment of the discoid lateral meniscus: results of long-term follow-up, *Arthroscopy* 5:101–109, 1989.
7. Thompson WO, Thaete FL, Fu FH, Dye SF: Tibial meniscal dynamics using three-dimensional reconstruction of magnetic resonance images, *Am J Sports Med* 19:210–216, 1991.
8. Arnoczky SP, Warren RF: Microvasculature of the human meniscus, *Am J Sports Med* 10:90–95, 1982.
9. Mow VC, Fithian DC, Kelly MA: Fundamentals of articular cartilage and meniscus biomechanics. In Ewing JW, editor: *Articular cartilage and knee joint function: basic science and arthroscopy*, New York, 1990, Raven.
10. Dye SF, Vaupel GL, Dye CC: Conscious neurosensory mapping of the internal structures of the human knee without intraarticular anesthesia, *Am J Sports Med* 26:773–777, 1998.
11. Ahmed AM, Burke DL: In-vitro measurement of static pressure distribution in synovial joints. I. Tibial surface of the knee, *J Biomech Eng* 105:216–225, 1983.
12. Radin EL, de Lamotte F, Maquet P: Role of the menisci in the distribution of stress in the knee, *Clin Orthop* 185:290–294, 1984.
13. Kettelkamp DB, Jacobs AW: Tibiofemoral contact area: determination and implications, *J Bone Joint Surg Am* 54:349–356, 1972.
14. Fukubayashi T, Kurosawa H: The contact area and pressure distribution pattern of the knee: a study of normal and osteoarthrotic knee joints, *Acta Orthop Scand* 51:871–879, 1980.
15. Voloshin AS, Wosk J: Shock absorption of meniscectomized and painful knees: a comparative in-vivo study, *J Biomed Eng* 5:157–161, 1983.
16. Levy IM, Torzilli PA, Warren RF: The effect of medial meniscectomy on anterior-posterior motion of the knee, *J Bone Joint Surg Am* 64:883–888, 1982.
17. Allen CR, Wong EK, Livesay GA, et al: Importance of the medial meniscus in the anterior cruciate ligament–deficient knee, *J Orthop Res* 18:109–115, 2000.
18. Shoemaker SC, Markolf KL: The role of the meniscus in the anterior-posterior stability of the loaded anterior cruciate–deficient knee: effects of partial versus total excision, *J Bone Joint Surg Am* 68:71–79, 1986.
19. Hede A, Jensen DB, Blyme P, et al: Epidemiology of meniscal lesions in the knee: 1,215 open operations in Copenhagen, 1982-84, *Acta Orthop Scand* 61:435–437, 1990.
20. Nielsen AB, Yde J: Epidemiology of acute knee injuries: a prospective hospital investigation, *J Trauma* 31:1644–1648, 1991.
21. Poehling GG, Ruch DS, Chabon SJ: The landscape of meniscal injuries, *Clin Sports Med* 9:539–549, 1990.
22. Duncan JB, Hunter R, Purnell M, et al: Meniscal injuries associated with acute anterior cruciate ligament tears in Alpine skiers, *Am J Sports Med* 23:170–172, 1995.
23. Evans PJ, Bell GD, Frank C: Prospective evaluation of the McMurray test, *Am J Sports Med* 21:604–608, 1993.
24. Weinstabl R, Muellner T, Vecsei V, et al: Economic considerations for the diagnosis and therapy of meniscal lesions: can magnetic resonance imaging help reduce the expense? *World J Surg* 21:363–368, 1997.
25. Shelbourne KD, Martini DJ, McCarroll JR, et al: Correlation of joint line tenderness and meniscal lesions in patients with acute anterior cruciate ligament tears, *Am J Sports Med* 23:166–169, 1995.
26. Terry GC, Tagert BE, Young MJ: Reliability of the clinical assessment in predicting the cause of internal derangements of the knee, *Arthroscopy* 11:568–576, 1995.
27. Rosenberg TD, Paulos LE, Parker RD, et al: The forty-five degree posteroanterior flexion weight-bearing radiograph of the knee, *J Bone Joint Surg Am* 70:1479–1483, 1988.
28. Muellner T, Weinstabl R, Schabus R, et al: The diagnosis of meniscal tears in athletes: a comparison of clinical and magnetic resonance imaging investigations, *Am J Sports Med* 25:7–12, 1997.
29. Fu FH, Harner CD, Vince KG, et al, editors: *Knee surgery*, vol 1, Philadelphia, 1994, Williams & Wilkins.
30. Boden SD, Davis DO, Dina TS, et al: A prospective and blinded investigation of magnetic resonance imaging of the knee: abnormal findings in asymptomatic subjects, *Clin Orthop* 282:177–185, 1992.
31. LaPrade RF, Burnett II QM, Veenstra MA, et al: The prevalence of abnormal magnetic resonance imaging findings in asymptomatic knees with correlation of magnetic resonance imaging to arthroscopic findings in symptomatic knees, *Am J Sport Med* 22:739–745, 1994.
32. Metcalf RW, Burks RT, Metcalf MS, et al: Arthroscopic meniscectomy. In McGinty JB, Caspari RB, Jackson RW, et al, editors: *Operative arthroscopy*, ed 2, Philadelphia, 1996, Lippincott-Raven.
33. Binfield PM, Maffulli N, King JB: Patterns of meniscal tears associated with anterior cruciate ligament lesions in athletes, *Injury* 4:557–561, 1993.
34. Fitzgibbons RE, Shelbourne KD: "Aggressive" nontreatment of lateral meniscal tears seen during anterior cruciate ligament reconstruction, *Am J Sports Med* 23:156–159, 1995.
35. Jones RS, Keene GC, Learmonth DJ, et al: Direct measurement of hoop strains in the intact and torn human medial meniscus, *Clin Biomech* 11:295–300, 1996.
36. Ferrer-Roca O, Vilalta C: Lesions of the meniscus. II. Horizontal cleavages and lateral cysts, *Clin Orthop Relat Res* 146:301–307, 1980.
37. Henning CE, Clark JR, Lynch MA, et al: Arthroscopic meniscus repair with a posterior incision, *Instr Course Lect* 37:209–221, 1988.
38. Katz JN, Brophy RH, Chaisson CE, et al: Surgery versus physical therapy for a meniscal tear and osteoarthritis, *New Engl J Med* 368:1675–1684, 2013.
39. Sihvonen R, Paavola M, Malmivaara A, et al: Arthroscopic partial meniscectomy versus sham surgery for a degenerative meniscal tear, *New Engl J Med* 369:2515–2524, 2013.
40. Khan M, Evaniew N, Bedi A, et al: Arthroscopic surgery for degenerative tears of the meniscus: a systematic review and meta-analysis, *Can Med Assoc J* 186:1057–1064, 2014.
41. Weiss CB, Lundberg M, Hamberg P, et al: Nonoperative treatment of meniscal tears, *J Bone Joint Surg Am* 71:811–822, 1989.

42. Fairbank TJ: Knee joint changes after meniscectomy, *J Bone Joint Surg Br* 30:664–670, 1948.

43. Wroble RR, Henderson RC, Campion ER, et al: Meniscectomy in children and adolescents: a long-term follow-up study, *Clin Orthop* 279:180–189, 1992.

44. Jørgensen U, Sonne-Holm S, Lauridsen F, et al: Long-term follow-up of meniscectomy in athletes: a prospective longitudinal study, *J Bone Joint Surg Br* 69:80–83, 1987.

45. Northmore-Ball MD, Dandy DJ, Jackson RW: Arthroscopic, open partial, and total meniscectomy: a comparative study, *J Bone Joint Surg Br* 65:400–404, 1983.

46. Fauno P, Nielsen AB: Arthroscopic partial meniscectomy: a long-term follow-up, *Arthroscopy* 8:345–349, 1992.

47. Schimmer RC, Brulhart KB, Duff C, et al: Arthroscopic partial meniscectomy: a 12-year follow-up and two-step evaluation of the long term course, *Arthroscopy* 14:136–142, 1998.

48. Fabricant PD, Jokl P: Surgical outcomes after arthroscopic partial meniscectomy, *J Am Acad Orthop Surg* 15:647–653, 2007.

49. Fabricant PD, Rosenberger PH, Jokl P, et al: Predictors of short-term recovery differ from those of long-term outcome after arthroscopic partial meniscectomy, *Arthroscopy* 24:769–778, 2008.

50. Anderson JJ, Connor GF, Helms CA: New observations on meniscal cysts, *Skeletal Radiol* 39:1187–1191, 2010.

51. Glasgow MM, Allen PW, Blakeway C: Arthroscopic treatment of cysts of the lateral meniscus, *J Bone Joint Surg Br* 75:299–302, 1993.

52. Ryu RK, Ting AJ: Arthroscopic treatment of meniscal cysts, *Arthroscopy* 9:591–595, 1993.

53. DeHaven KE: Meniscus repair, *Am J Sports Med* 27:242–250, 1999.

54. Fox JM, Rintz KG, Ferkel RD: Trephination of incomplete meniscal tears, *Arthroscopy* 9:451–455, 1993.

55. Annandale T: Excision of the internal semilunar cartilage, resulting in perfect restoration of the joint movements, *Br Med J* 1:291–292, 1889.

56. DeHaven KE: Peripheral meniscus repair: an alternative to meniscectomy, *Orthop Trans* 5:399–400, 1981 [Abstract].

57. Wirth CR: Meniscus repair, *Clin Orthop* 157:153–160, 1981.

58. Rockborn P, Gillquist J: Results of open meniscus repair: long-term follow-up study with a matched uninjured control group, *J Bone Joint Surg Br* 82:494–498, 2000.

59. Brucker PU, von Campe A, Meyer DC, et al: Clinical and radiological results 21 years following successful, isolated, open meniscal repair in stable knee joints, *Knee* 18:396–401, 2011.

60. Small NC: Complications in arthroscopic meniscal surgery, *Clin Sports Med* 9:609–617, 1990.

61. Post WR, Akers SR, Kish V: Load to failure of common meniscal repair techniques: effects of suture technique and suture material, *Arthroscopy* 13:731–736, 1997.

62. Rodeo SA: Arthroscopic meniscal repair with use of the outside-in technique, *J Bone Joint Surg Am* 82:127–141, 2000.

63. Morgan CD: The "all-inside" meniscus repair, *Arthroscopy* 7:120–125, 1991.

64. Albrecht-Olsen P, Kristensen G, Burgaard P, et al: The arrow versus horizontal suture in arthroscopic meniscus repair. A prospective randomized study with arthroscopic evaluation, *Knee Surg Sports Traumatol Arthrosc* 7:268–273, 1999.

65. Gill SS, Diduch DR: Outcomes after meniscal repair using the meniscus arrow in knees undergoing concurrent anterior cruciate ligament reconstruction, *Arthroscopy* 18:569–577, 2002.

66. Kurzweil PR, Tifford CD, Ignacio EM: Unsatisfactory clinical results of meniscal repair using the meniscus arrow, *Arthroscopy* 21:905, 2005.

67. Borden P, Nyland J, Caborn DN, Pienkowski D: Biomechanical comparison of the FasT-Fix meniscal repair suture system with vertical mattress sutures and meniscus arrows, *Am J Sports Med* 31:374–378, 2003.

68. Rosso C, Müller S, Buckland DM, et al: All-inside meniscal repair devices compared with their matched inside-out vertical mattress suture repair introducing 10,000 and 100,000 loading cycles, *Am J Sports Med* 42:2226–2233, 2014.

69. Cannon Jr. WD, Vittori JM: The incidence of healing in arthroscopic meniscal repairs in anterior cruciate ligament–reconstructed knees versus stable knees, *Am J Sports Med* 20:176–181, 1992.

70. Buseck MS, Noyes FR: Arthroscopic evaluation of meniscal repairs after anterior cruciate ligament reconstruction and immediate motion, *Am J Sports Med* 19:489–494, 1991.

71. Lee GP, Diduch DR: Deteriorating outcomes after meniscal repair using the meniscus arrow in knees undergoing concurrent anterior cruciate ligament reconstruction increased failure rate with long-term follow-up, *Am J Sports Med* 33:1138–1141, 2005.

72. Hantes ME, Zachos VC, Varitimidis SE, et al: Arthroscopic meniscal repair: a comparative study between three different surgical techniques, *Knee Surg Sports Traumatol Arthrosc* 14:1232–1237, 2006.

73. Asik M, Sen C, Erginsu M: Arthroscopic meniscal repair using T-fix, *Knee Surg Sports Traumatol Arthrosc* 10:284–288, 2002.

74. Haas AL, Schepsis AA, Hornstein J, Edgar CM: Meniscal repair using the FasT-Fix all-inside meniscal repair device, *Arthroscopy* 21:167–175, 2005.

75. Kocabey Y, Nyland J, Isbell WM, Caborn DN: Patient outcomes following T-Fix meniscal repair and a modifiable, progressive rehabilitation program, a retrospective study, *Arch Orthop Trauma Surg* 124:592–596, 2004.

76. Kotsovolos ES, Hantes ME, Mastrokalos DS, et al: Results of all-inside meniscal repair with the FasT-Fix meniscal repair system, *Arthroscopy* 22:3–9, 2006.

77. Quinby JS, Golish SR, Hart JA, Diduch DR: All-inside meniscal repair using a new flexible, tensionable device, *Am J Sports Med* 34:1281–1286, 2006.

78. Grant JA, Wilde J, Miller BS, Bedi A: Comparison of inside-out and all-inside techniques for the repair of isolated meniscal tears a systematic review, *Am J Sports Med* 40:459–468, 2012.

79. Arnoczky SP, Warren RF, Spivak JM: Meniscal repair using an exogenous fibrin clot: an experimental study in dogs, *J Bone Joint Surg Am* 70:1209–1217, 1998.

80. Small NC: Complications in arthroscopic surgery performed by experienced arthroscopists, *Arthroscopy* 4:215–221, 1988.

81. Austin KS, Sherman OH: Complications of arthroscopic meniscal repair, *Am J Sports Med* 21:864–869, 1993.

82. Shelbourne KD, Johnson GE: Locked bucket-handle meniscal tears in knees with chronic anterior cruciate ligament deficiency, *Am J Sports Med* 21:779–782, 1993.

83. Milachowski KA, Weismeier K, Wirth CJ: Homologous meniscus transplantation: experimental and clinical results, *Int Orthop* 13:1–11, 1989.

84. Paletta Jr. GA, Manning T, Snell E, et al: The effect of allograft meniscal replacement on intraarticular contact area and pressures in the human knee: a biomechanical study, *Am J Sports Med* 25:692–698, 1997.

85. Arnoczky SP, Warren RF, McDevitt CA: Meniscal replacement using a cryopreserved allograft: an experimental study in the dog, *Clin Orthop* 252:121–128, 1990.

86. Jackson DW, McDevitt CA, Simon TM, et al: Meniscal transplantation using fresh and cryopreserved allografts: an experimental study in goats, *Am J Sports Med* 20:644–656, 1992.

87. Fabbriciani C, Lucania L, Milano G, et al: Meniscal allografts: cryopreservation versus deep-frozen techniques—an experimental study in goats, *Knee Surg Sports Traumatol Arthrosc* 5:124–134, 1997.

88. Debeer P, Decorte R, Delvaux S, Bellemans J: DNA analysis of a transplanted cryopreserved meniscal allograft, *Arthroscopy* 16:71–75, 2000.

89. Shaffer B, Kennedy S, Klimkiewicz J, Yao L: Preoperative sizing of meniscal allografts in meniscus transplantation, *Am J Sports Med* 28:524–533, 2000.

90. Rodeo SA: Meniscal allografts: where do we stand? *Am J Sports Med* 28:524–533, 2001.

91. Hommen JP, Applegate GR, Del Pizzo W: Meniscus allograft transplantation: ten-year results of cryopreserved allografts, *Arthroscopy* 23:388–393, 2007.

92. Stollsteimer GT, Shelton WR, Dukes A, Bomboy AL: Meniscal allograft transplantation: a 1-to 5-year follow-up of 22 patients, *Arthroscopy* 16:343–347, 2000.

93. Noyes FR: Irradiated meniscus allografts in the human knee: a two to five year follow-up study, *Orthop Trans* 20:513, 1996 (abstract).

94. Cameron JC, Saha S: Meniscal allograft transplantation for unicompartmental arthritis of the knee, *Clin Orthop* 337:164–171, 1997.

95. Rosso F, Bisicchia S, Bonasia DE, Amendola A: Meniscal allograft transplantation: a systematic review, *Am J Sports Med* June 2014 [Epub ahead of print].

96. Hergan D, Thut D, Sherman O, Day MS: Meniscal allograft transplantation, *Arthroscopy* 27:101–112, 2011.

97. Roumazeille T, Klouche S, Rousselin B, et al: Arthroscopic meniscal allograft transplantation with two tibia tunnels without bone plugs: evaluation of healing on MR arthrography and functional outcomes, *Knee Surg Sports Traumatol Arthrosc* 23:264–269, 2015.

98. Messner K, Maletius W: The long-term prognosis for severe damage to weight-bearing cartilage in the knee: a 14-year clinical and radiographic follow-up in 28 young athletes, *Acta Orthop Scand* 67:165–168, 1996.

99. Bredella MA, Tirman PF, Peterfy CG, et al: Accuracy of T2-weighted fast spin-echo MR imaging with fat saturation in detecting cartilage defects in the knee: comparison with arthroscopy in 130 patients, *Am J Roentgenol* 172:1073–1080, 1999.

100. Pridie AH: The method of resurfacing osteoarthritic knee joints, *J Bone Joint Surg Br* 41:618–619, 1959.

101. Akeson WH, Miyashita C, Taylor TK, et al: Experimental arthroplasty of the canine hip: extracellular matrix composition in cup arthroplasty, *J Bone Joint Surg Am* 51:149–164, 1969.

102. Mitchell N, Shepard N: The resurfacing of adult rabbit articular cartilage by multiple perforation of the subchondral bone, *J Bone Joint Surg Am* 58:230–233, 1976.

103. Johnson LL: Arthroscopic abrasion arthroplasty: historical and pathological perspective—present status, *Arthroscopy* 2:54–69, 1986.

104. Hjertquist SO, Lemperg R: Histological, autoradiographic and microchemical studies of spontaneously healing osteochondral articular defects in adult rabbits, *Calcif Tissue Res* 8:54–72, 1971.

105. Bert JM, Maschka K: The arthroscopic treatment of unicompartmental gonarthrosis: a five-year follow-up study of abrasion arthroplasty plus ar-

throscopic debridement and arthroscopic debridement alone, *Arthroscopy* 5:25–32, 1989.

106. Steadman JR, Rodkey WG, Singleton SB, Briggs KK: Microfracture technique for full-thickness chondral defects: technique and clinical results, *Op Tech Orthop* 7:300–304, 1997.

107. Rodrigo JJ, Steadman JR, Silliman JF, Fulstone HA: Improvement of full-thickness chondral defect healing in the human knee after debridement and microfracture using continuous passive motion, *Am J Knee Surg* 7:109–116, 1994.

108. Gill TJ, McCulloch PC, Glasson SS, et al: Chondral defect repair after the microfracture procedure: a nonhuman primate model, *Am J Sports Med* 33:680–685, 2005.

109. Steadman JR, Briggs KK, Rodrigo JJ, et al: Outcomes of microfracture for traumatic chondral defects of the knee: average 11-year follow-up, *Arthroscopy* 19:477–484, 2003.

110. Mithoefer K, McAdams T, Williams RJ, et al: Clinical efficacy of the microfracture technique for articular cartilage repair in the knee: an evidence-based systematic analysis, *Am J Sports Med* 37:2053–2063, 2009.

111. Lane JG, Tontz Jr. WL, Ball ST, et al: A morphologic, biochemical, and biomechanical assessment of short-term effects of osteochondral autograft plug transfer in an animal model, *Arthroscopy* 17:856–863, 2001.

112. Ahmad CS, Cohen ZA, Levine WN, et al: Biomechanical and topographic considerations for autologous osteochondral grafting in the knee, *Am J Sports Med* 29:201–206, 2001.

113. Chow JC, Hantes ME, Houle JB, Zalavras CG: Arthroscopic autogenous osteochondral transplantation for treating knee cartilage defects: a 2 to 5 year follow-up study, *Arthroscopy* 20:681–690, 2004.

114. Jakob RP, Franz T, Gautier E, Mainil-Varlet P: Autologous osteochondral grafting in the knee: indication, results, and reflections, *Clin Orthop Relat Res* 401:170–184, 2002.

115. Hangody L, Rathonyi GK, Duska Z, et al: Autologous osteochondral mosaicplasty: surgical technique, *J Bone Joint Surg Am* 86(suppl 1):65–72, 2004.

116. Erdil M, Bilsel K, Taser OF, et al: Osteochondral autologous graft transfer system in the knee; mid-term results, *Knee* 20:2–8, 2013.

117. Bentley G, Biant LC, Carrington RW, et al: A prospective, randomised comparison of autologous chondrocyte implantation versus mosaicplasty for osteochondral defects in the knee, *J Bone Joint Surg Br* 85:223–230, 2003.

118. Feczko P, Hangody L, Varga J, et al: Experimental results of donor site filling for autologous osteochondral mosaicplasty, *Arthroscopy* 19:755–761, 2003.

119. Gudas R, Kalesinskas RJ, Kimtys V, et al: A prospective randomized clinical study of mosaic osteochondral autologous transplantation versus microfracture for the treatment of osteochondral defects in the knee joint in young athletes, *Arthroscopy* 21:1066–1075, 2005.

120. Chesterman PJ, Smith AU: Homotransplantation of articular cartilage and isolated chondrocytes: an experimental study in rabbits, *J Bone Joint Surg Br* 50:184–197, 1968.

121. Grande DA, Pitman MI, Peterson L, et al: The repair of experimentally produced defects in rabbit articular cartilage by autologous chondrocyte transplantation, *J Orthop Res* 7:208–218, 1989.

122. Brittberg M, Lindahl A, Nilsson A, et al: Treatment of deep cartilage defects in the knee with autologous chondrocyte transplantation, *N Engl J Med* 331:889–895, 1994.

123. Gomoll AH, Probst C, Farr J, et al: Use of a type I/III bilayer collagen membrane decreases reoperation rates for symptomatic hypertrophy after autologous chondrocyte implantation, *Am J Sports Med* 37(1 suppl):20S–23S, 2009.

124. Samuelson EM, Brown DE: Cost-effectiveness analysis of autologous chondrocyte implantation a comparison of periosteal patch versus type i/iii collagen membrane, *Am J Sports Med* 40:1252–1258, 2012.

125. Peterson L, Minas T, Brittberg M, et al: Two- to 9-year outcome after autologous chondrocyte transplantation of the knee, *Clin Orthop* 374:212–234, 2000.

126. Peterson L, Brittberg M, Kiviranta I, et al: Autologous chondrocyte transplantation: biomechanics and long-term durability, *Am J Sports Med* 30:2–12, 2002.

127. Knutsen G, Engebretsen L, Ludvigsen TC, et al: Autologous chondrocyte implantation compared with microfracture in the knee: a randomized trial, *J Bone Joint Surg Am* 86:455–464, 2004.

128. Knutsen G, Drogset JO, Engebretsen L, et al: A randomized trial comparing autologous chondrocyte implantation with microfracture. Findings at five years, *J Bone Joint Surg Am* 89:2105–2112, 2007.

129. Horas U, Pelinkovic D, Herr G, et al: Autologous chondrocyte implantation and osteochondral cylinder transplantation in cartilage repair of the knee joint: a prospective, comparative trial, *J Bone Joint Surg Am* 85:185–192, 2003.

130. Vanlauwe J, Saris DB, Victor J, et al: Five-year outcome of characterized chondrocyte implantation versus microfracture for symptomatic cartilage defects of the knee early treatment matters, *Am J Sports Med* 39:2566–2574, 2011.

CHAPTER 22

Patellofemoral Joint

CHRISTOPHER M. POWERS, RICHARD B. SOUZA, JOHN P. FULKERSON

INTRODUCTION

Patellofemoral pain (PFP) is one of the most common disorders of the knee.[1] Patellofemoral-related problems are prevalent in a wide range of individuals, but the highest incidence is seen in physically active people, such as runners, tennis players, and military recruits.[2-4] In general, the incidence of patellofemoral-related problems is higher in females than in males.[5]

Despite the high incidence of PFP in the general population, the pathophysiology of this disorder is sometimes elusive. This is supported by the fact that no clear consensus exists on how PFP should be treated. For example, a myriad of conservative procedures have been advocated (e.g., bracing, taping, foot orthotics, strengthening, stretching), and numerous surgical techniques have been described. Initially, nonoperative care is preferred, but surgical intervention is considered if conservative care fails.

The problem of PFP is highlighted by the fact that 70% to 90% of individuals with this condition have recurrent or chronic pain.[6] Although interventions for PFP have resulted in positive short-term outcomes, long-term clinical outcomes are less compelling. This is illustrated by the fact that 80% of individuals who completed a rehabilitation program for PFP still reported pain, and 74% had reduced their physical activity at a 5-year follow-up.[7] The apparent lack of long-term success in treating this condition may be because the underlying factors that contribute to the development of PFP are not being addressed. Although it is generally agreed that the etiology of PFP is multifactorial in nature, it is generally accepted that the root cause or causes of this condition are not well understood.[8-10]

The difficulty involved in treating PFP reflects the complexity of the patellofemoral joint and the multifactorial nature of the disorder. To treat this condition effectively, the clinician must clearly identify the primary cause or causes of the pain. The purpose of this chapter is to provide the reader with an understanding of the relevant anatomy, kinesiology, and biomechanics of the patellofemoral joint and to review current theories related to the etiology of PFP, evaluation methods, and treatment strategies.

FUNCTIONAL ANATOMY

The patellofemoral joint consists of the articulation of the patella and the trochlear surface of the femur. The patella is an integral part of the knee extensor mechanism and plays a key role in normal knee function and lower extremity biomechanics. The ability of the patellofemoral joint to improve the mechanical efficiency of the extensor mechanism and to accept and redirect forces depends on a host of factors, including the joint's osseous structure and contributions from various soft tissues, such as the quadriceps musculature, quadriceps tendon, patella tendon, and retinaculum. Clinicians must have an understanding of the anatomical structure of this joint to appreciate both normal and pathological function.

Osseous Structure

Patella

Contained within the quadriceps tendon, the patella has the distinction of being the largest sesamoid bone in the body. The patella consists primarily of cancellous bone covered by thin, compact lamina; its axial length is approximately 4 to 4.5 cm (1.6-1.8 inches), and it is approximately 5 to 5.5 cm (2-2.2 inches) wide. The thickness of the patella varies considerably, attaining a maximum height of 2 to 2.5 cm (0.77-1 inch) at its central portion.[11]

The articular surface of the patella is divided into the medial and lateral facets by a vertical ridge (median ridge) that roughly bisects the patella (Figure 22-1).[12] The lateral facet often is slightly larger than the medial facet.[13] The medial facet is subdivided by a less prominent vertical ridge that separates the medial facet proper and the smaller, odd facet (see Figure 22-1). The articulating surfaces of the patella are covered with aneural hyaline cartilage, the thickest cartilage in the body.[14] Maximum cartilage thickness is found at the central portion of the patella (approximately 4-5 mm) and decreases from the median ridge to the medial and lateral borders.

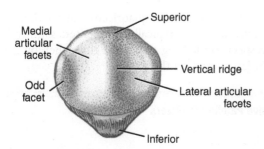

Figure 22-1 Articular side of the patella. (From Neumann DA: *Kinesiology of the musculoskeletal system: foundations for rehabilitation,* ed 2, St. Louis, 2010, Mosby.)

Trochlear Surface of the Femur

The femoral condyles form the trochlear groove that provides the articulating surface of the femur. Similar to the articular surface of the patella, the trochlear surface is divided into medial and lateral facets, the lateral facet being larger and extending more proximally and anteriorly than its medial counterpart (Figure 22-2). The larger lateral femoral condyle provides a bony buttress that helps provide lateral patellar stability.[15] The trochlear groove is shallower proximally than distally, indicating that bony stability is compromised as the patella moves superiorly during terminal knee extension. The cartilage covering the trochlear surface of the femur is much thinner than that covering the patella (i.e., 2-3 mm).[14]

Soft Tissue Structures

Synovium

The synovial lining of the patellofemoral joint, which is essentially the synovium of the anterior portion of the knee, has three components: the suprapatellar synovium, the peripatellar synovium, and the infrapatellar synovium. These three portions blend imperceptibly with each other, allowing free communication with the knee joint proper.[16] The peripatellar synovium creates a small synovial fold or fringe less than 1 cm (0.5 inch) wide that surrounds the patella; this generally is regarded as the true synovium of the patellofemoral joint.[14] Inflammation or scarring of this synovial fold (i.e., plica) can produce symptoms similar to those of cartilage degeneration.[17]

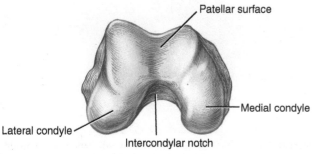

Figure 22-2 Inferior aspect of the distal end of the femur. (From Neumann DA: *Kinesiology of the musculoskeletal system: foundations for rehabilitation,* ed 2, St. Louis, 2010, Mosby.)

> **Portions of the Synovial Lining of the Patellofemoral Joint**
>
> - Suprapatellar synovium (pouch)
> - Peripatellar synovium (plica)
> - Infrapatellar synovium

Fat Pads

Three fat pads occupy the anterior knee: the quadriceps fat pad, the prefemoral fat pad, and the infrapatellar fat pad (Figure 22-3).[18] The infrapatellar fat pad, or Hoffa's fat pad, is the largest fat pad in the region and has been studied extensively because of its proposed role in various pathologies.[18-22] It is a voluminous structure located just inferior to the infrapatellar pole.[19] It extends inferiorly to the deep infrapatellar bursa at the insertion of the patellar ligament into the tibial tuberosity. Hoffa's fat pad attaches to several structures, including the intercondylar notch via the ligamentum mucosum, the patella tendon, the inferior pole of the patella, and the anterior horns of the menisci.[18]

The quadriceps fat pad, also known as the *anterior suprapatellar fat pad,* lies superior to the suprapatellar pole between the distal quadriceps tendon anteriorly and the suprapatellar recess posteriorly.[23] Just deep (posterior) to the suprapatellar recess and the suprapatellar bursa is the prefemoral fat pad, which is anterior to the femoral shaft and superior trochlear groove.[16]

> **Fat Pads of the Patellofemoral Joint**
>
> - Infrapatellar (Hoffa's) fat pad
> - Quadriceps (anterior suprapatella) fat pad
> - Prefemoral fat pad

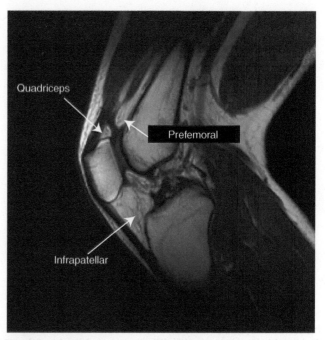

Figure 22-3 Sagittal magnetic resonance imaging (MRI) scan of the knee showing the fat pads that occupy the anterior aspect of the knee.

The fat pads of the knee house neurovascular projections. The infrapatellar fat pad is highly vascularized and highly innervated. Terminal extensions of the inferior genicular arteries anastomose in the infrapatellar fat pad, richly supplying it and its synovial coverings.[21] Substance P immunoreactive pain fibers are widespread and equally distributed throughout the fat pad, retinaculum, and synovium.[22]

Several functions have been proposed for the fat pads, including secretion of synovial fluid, occupation of dead space, and joint stability. Current research concludes that the infrapatellar fat pad appears to play a role in biomechanical support and neurovascular supply to the adjacent structures.[18]

Proposed Functions of Fat Pads

- Synovial fluid secretion
- Occupiers of dead space
- Joint stability
- Neurovascular supply

Soft Tissue Stabilizers

Because the patellofemoral joint lacks a tightly closed capsule, external assistance is required to achieve patellar stability within the trochlear groove; this assistance is provided by soft tissue stabilizers. In general, the soft tissue stabilizers of the patellofemoral joint can be described as passive stabilizers or active stabilizers.

Passive Stabilizers

Passive stabilizing structures include the patella tendon inferiorly and the medial and lateral retinaculum (Figure 22-4). The patella tendon functions to transmit the forces generated by quadriceps contraction to the tibia. This structure typically is oriented slightly lateral with respect to the long axis of the tibia, thereby creating a slight lateral pull on the patella.[14]

Passive Patella Stabilizers

- Patella tendon
- Medial retinaculum
- Lateral retinaculum

The normal patella retinaculum consists of layered, fibrous connective tissue that traverses the medial and lateral margins of the patella with attachments to the femur, tibia, patella, and patellar ligament.[24] The superficial fibers of the retinaculum originate from the vastus lateralis (VL) and vastus medialis (VM) fascia, linking the quadriceps muscles to the patella (Figure 22-5).[25] This linkage is responsible for the dynamic influence of the quadriceps muscles on the patellofemoral joint during active knee motion.

The lateral retinaculum is composed of two distinct portions: a thinner superficial layer and a thicker deep layer. The deep layer is further divided into three fibrous components: the epicondylopatellar band (or lateral patellofemoral ligament), the deep transverse retinaculum, and the patellotibial band (Figures 22-6 and 22-7). These

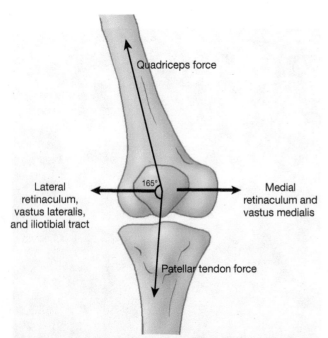

Figure 22-4 Active and passive soft tissue stabilizers of the patella. (From Andrews JR, Harrelson GL, Wilk KE: *Physical rehabilitation of the injured athlete,* ed 4, Philadelphia, 2012, Saunders.)

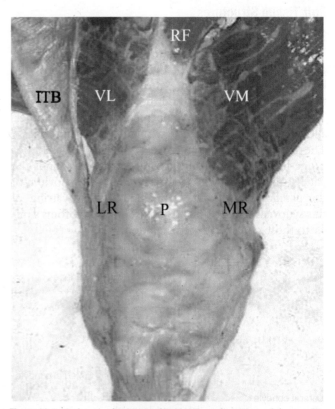

Figure 22-5 Cadaveric dissection showing interdigitation of the quadriceps musculature and iliotibial band with the peripatellar retinaculum. *VM,* Vastus medialis; *RF,* rectus femoris; *P,* patella; *VL,* vastus lateralis; *ITB,* iliotibial band; *LR,* lateral retinaculum; *MR,* medial retinaculum.

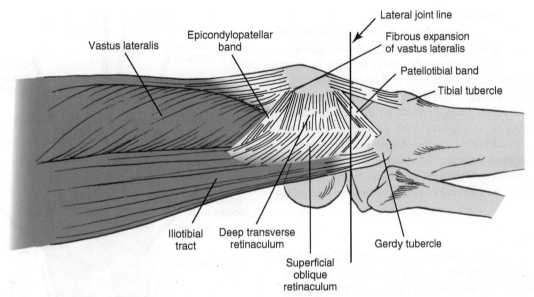

Figure 22-6 Anatomy of the lateral extensor mechanism and retinaculum showing the orientation of the elements that make up the superficial and deep layers. (Redrawn from Fulkerson JP, Gossling HR: Anatomy of the knee joint lateral retinaculum, *Clin Orthop* 153:183-188, 1990.)

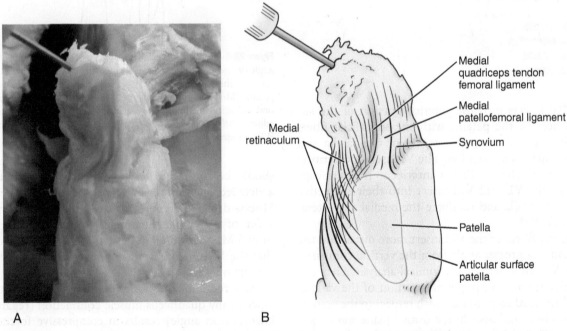

Figure 22-7 A, Transverse section of patella and medial retinaculum. **B,** Illustration to show how medial retinacular and medial patellofemoral ligament (MPFL) and medial quadriceps tendon-femoral ligament (MQTFL) blend in with extensor expansion over patella.

structures connect the patella to the iliotibial band (ITB) and help prevent medial patella excursion.[25] Because most of the lateral retinaculum originates from the ITB, this structure is drawn posteriorly with knee flexion, placing a lateral force on the patella.[26]

The medial retinaculum includes the medial patellofemoral and medial quadriceps ligaments. This complex forms a tough, fibrous layer that helps limit

lateral patellar excursion. The components of the medial retinacular complex are sometimes surgically imbricated or replicated in the interest of restoring medial support for the patella after a lateral dislocation.[27]

The specific role of the peripatellar retinaculum as a frontal plane stabilizer of the patellofemoral joint has been well established.[28,29] However, because of its unique orientation, the peripatellar retinaculum plays a complementary load-sharing role with respect to the patellar ligament by resisting tensile forces created by the extensor mechanism.[30] Similar to the patellar ligament, the patellar retinaculum provides distal inferior support for the patella through the medial and lateral meniscopatellar ligaments, which connect the patella to the tibia.[28]

The lateral retinaculum contains small nerve endings, which suggests that this structure can be a source of symptoms.[14] In addition, Sanchis-Alfonso et al.[31] reported on the widespread presence of substance P in this area. Fulkerson et al.[32] reported that nerve injury in the lateral retinaculum can be a source of pain and may be related to chronic tension.

Active Stabilizers

Active stabilizers of the patella consist of the four heads of the quadriceps femoris muscle (the VL, VM, vastus intermedius [VI], and rectus femoris [RF]), which fuse distally to form the quadriceps tendon. These muscles, which can be identified at their insertion into the patella, provide dynamic control of the patellofemoral joint.

Active Patella Stabilizers

- Vastus lateralis
- Vastus intermedius
- Vastus medialis
- Rectus femoris

The RF inserts into the anterior portion of the superior aspect of the patella, with the superficial fibers continuing over the superior aspect of the patella and ending in the patellar tendon. The VI inserts posteriorly into the base of the patella but anterior to the joint capsule. Both the VL and VM insert into their respective sides of the patella and reinforce the medial and lateral retinaculum.[33,34]

The lower fibers of the VM insert more distally on the patella and at a greater angle from the vertical compared with the VL. In a detailed anatomical analysis, Lieb and Perry[35] determined the angle of insertion of the various heads of the quadriceps muscle with respect to the vertical axis. The fiber alignment in the frontal plane was as follows: VL, 12° to 15° laterally; RF, 7° to 10° medially; and VM, upper fibers, 15° to 18° medially, lower fibers, 50° to 55° medially (Figure 22-8).[35] The fibers of the VI were found to lie parallel to the shaft of the femur.

The distinct and abrupt change in the fiber orientation between the superior and inferior portions of the VM led Lieb and Perry[35] to designate the inferior portion the **vastus medialis oblique (VMO)** and the superior portion the **vastus medialis longus (VML).** Although the fiber orientation of the VMO makes this structure particularly effective in providing medial patella stability,[35] there is debate as to whether the VMO and VML

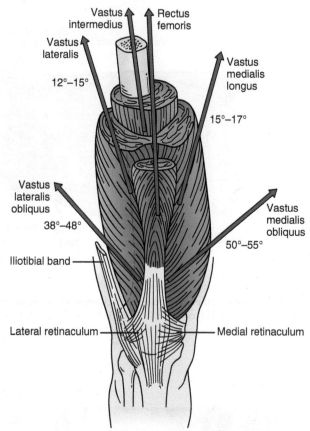

Figure 22-8 Components of the quadriceps–femoris complex. Note the angle of insertion of the various components of the complex. The orientation of the muscle fibers dictates the line of action and the pull on the patella. (Modified from McConnell J, Fulkerson J: The knee: patellofemoral and soft tissue injuries. In Zachazewski JE, Magee DJ, Quillen WS, editors: *Athletic injuries and rehabilitation,* p 697, Philadelphia, 1996, WB Saunders.)

should be considered separate anatomical structures. In a detailed anatomical study of 324 cadaver specimens, Hubbard et al.[36] reported that there is no aponeurotic sheet of epimysium anatomically separating the VMO from VML. This finding has led the authors to conclude that the VMO should not be considered a separate and distinct muscle.

As a result of the posterior origin of the vasti (linea aspera), any quadriceps muscle contraction (regardless of knee flexion angle) results in compressive forces acting on the patellofemoral joint (Figure 22-9). Even when the knee is fully extended, substantial joint compression can occur. The posterior angulation of the VM and VL fibers has been reported as approximately 55° from the vertical.[37]

In summary, the bony confines of the trochlea combined with the passive and active soft tissue stabilizers define the limit of patellar excursion and contribute significantly to stability of the patellofemoral joint. The balance between medial and lateral stability is essential for maintaining appropriate alignment of the extensor mechanism and normal biomechanics of the patellofemoral joint.

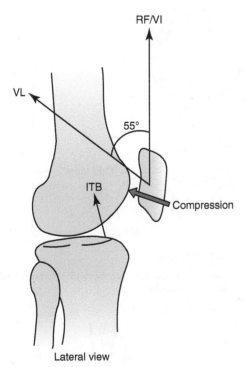

RF/VI

VL

55°

ITB

Compression

Lateral view

Figure 22-9 The posterior angulation of the vasti with respect to the femur results in compression of the patella with quadriceps contraction, regardless of the knee flexion angle. *VL,* vastus lateralis; *RF,* rectus femoris; *VI,* vastus intermedius; *ITB,* iliotibial band. (Modified from Powers CM, Lilley JC, Lee TQ: The effects of axial and multi-plane loading of the extensor mechanism on the patellofemoral joint, *Clin Biomech* 13:616-624, 1998.)

KINESIOLOGY

Normal Patellar Kinematics

The inability to visualize the relationship between the patella and the trochlear groove makes clinical assessment of patella tracking an imprecise task. Also, identifying abnormal patella motion is difficult if "normal" patella tracking has not been clearly defined. Kinematic magnetic resonance imaging (KMRI) has been used to quantify patellar movement during resisted knee extension from 45° flexion to full knee extension (0°).[38,39] Assessment of patella kinematics in this arc of knee motion is clinically relevant, because this is the range in which tracking abnormalities occur. KMRI has a distinct advantage over static imaging procedures in that the contribution of the extensor mechanism to patellofemoral joint kinematics can be assessed.[39]

Frontal Plane Movements

The normal position of the patella is slight lateral displacement throughout knee flexion and extension. The normal pattern of patellar motion in the frontal plane is characterized by slight medial displacement from 45° to 15° knee flexion, followed by slight lateral displacement at the end range of extension (15° to 0°).[40] This motion has been described previously as the C-curve pattern.[41] The estimated

amount of medial and lateral movement is about 3 mm in each direction based on quantitative analysis.[40]

The tendency of the patella to displace medially during knee extension is related to the geometry of the femoral trochlear groove. Because the lateral femoral condyle typically is larger and projects farther anteriorly than the medial condyle, the trochlear surface is angled slightly medially when viewed from distal to proximal positions (Figure 22-10).[42] In addition, the shift from medial to lateral patellar translation during terminal knee extension can be explained, in part, by the screw home mechanism of the knee. During terminal extension of the non–weight-bearing knee, the tibia rotates laterally as a result of the unequal curvature between the femoral condyles.[43] As was demonstrated by van Kampen and Huiskes,[42] patellar motion is highly influenced by rotation of the tibia, and lateral rotation induces a lateral patella displacement.

Transverse Plane Movements

During knee extension from 45° to 0°, the patella tilts medially (5° to 7°) from a laterally tilted position of 10°.[40] As with medial and lateral patella displacement, this motion pattern appears to be related to the geometry of the femoral trochlear groove.[40] The fact that the patella typically is laterally tilted throughout knee extension suggests that patella malalignment is more an issue of degree rather than position.

Sagittal Plane Movements

The motions of the patella in the sagittal plane consist of flexion and extension. *Flexion* is defined as the motion in which the inferior pole of the patella moves posteriorly, whereas *extension* is defined as the motion in which the

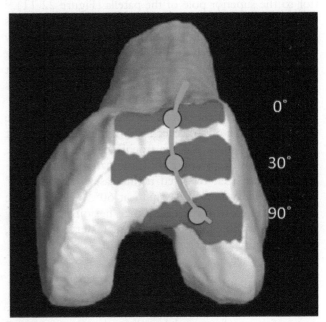

0°

30°

90°

Figure 22-10 Patellar motion in the frontal plane is dictated by the shape and orientation of the trochlear groove as the knee flexes and extends.

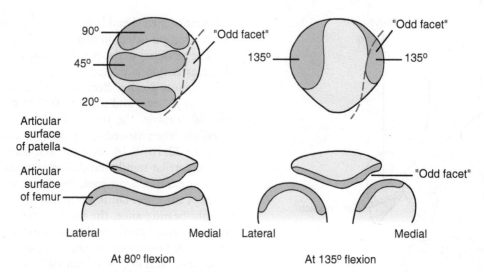

Figure 22-11 Contact area patterns on the patella as a function of the knee flexion angle. In general, contact area increases with increasing knee flexion. (Modified from Magee DJ: *Orthopedic physical assessment*, ed 6, p 767, St. Louis, 2014, Saunders/Elsevier.)

inferior pole moves anteriorly. Flexion of the patella occurs in conjunction with knee flexion; however, the magnitude of patellar flexion is about 20° less than that of knee flexion.[42] For example, when the knee is flexed to 60°, the patella typically is flexed to 40°. Similarly, as the knee extends, the patella also extends from the flexed position.[42]

Patellofemoral Joint Contact Area

During knee flexion, the patella moves from the superior (shallower) portion of the trochlear groove to the inferior (deeper) portion.[40] As such, the articulating surface of the patella on the femur varies throughout the range of knee motion. Movement from full extension to 90° flexion results in a band of contact that moves from the inferior to the superior pole of the patella (Figure 22-11).[44] Normally, the odd facet makes no contact during this range. Between 90° and 135°, the patella rotates laterally with the ridge between the medial and odd facets, making contact with the medial condyle. At 135°, the odd facet and the lateral portion of the lateral facet make contact, as does the quadriceps tendon (see Figure 22-11).[44]

Because the patella enters the deeper portion of the trochlear groove during knee flexion, the area of contact between the patella and the trochlear groove increases. With the quadriceps contracted, the patellofemoral contact area has been reported to increase from 146 mm² at 0° to a maximum of 345 mm² at 60°.[45] This increase in contact area with increased knee flexion functionally serves to distribute joint forces over a greater surface area, thereby minimizing joint stress.

Frontal Plane Influences

Fulkerson and Hungerford[14] described the natural tendency of the patella to track laterally as the "law of valgus." This tendency is a result of the valgus orientation of the

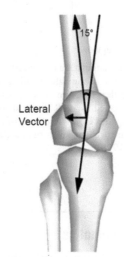

Figure 22-12 The orientation of the quadriceps force vector and patella ligament force vectors creates a lateral force acting on the patella. (From Powers CM: The influence of altered lower-extremity kinematics on patellofemoral joint dysfunction: a theoretical perspective, *J Orthop Sports Phys Ther* 33:639-646, 2003.)

lower extremity. As the quadriceps muscle follows the longitudinal axis of the femur, the quadriceps angle (Q angle) is formed, creating a lateral force vector that acts on the patella (Figure 22-12). This predisposes the patella to lateral tracking forces with quadriceps muscle tension.[46]

Clinically, the Q angle is measured as the angle formed by the intersection of a line drawn from the anterosuperior iliac spine (ASIS) to the midpoint of the patella and a proximal extension of a line drawn from the tibial tubercle to the midpoint of the patella.[47] The Q angle is greater in women than in men because women have a wider pelvis; the average Q angle is 15° to 18° in women and approximately 12° in men.[15] This variation between the genders may partly explain the higher incidence of PFP in females, because a larger Q angle creates a larger valgus vector and therefore a potentially greater predisposition to lateral tracking.[48]

JOINT BIOMECHANICS

The patellofemoral joint is susceptible to the largest loads in the body.[49] Because abnormal forces and stresses are thought to be a primary factor in the origin of PFP, it is important that clinicians understand the normal biomechanics of this joint.

Function of the Patella

The primary function of the patella is to facilitate knee extension.[50] This mechanical attribute has been described in detail and has been shown to increase the functional lever arm of the extensor mechanism.[50] Documentation of strength losses in subjects who have undergone patellectomy supports this concept. Fletcher et al.[51] reported a 49% reduction in the torque output of the extensor mechanism after patellectomy.

The quadriceps muscle lever arm varies throughout the knee range of motion, with reported maximum values ranging from 4.9 cm (1.9 inches) at 30° flexion[52] to 7.8 cm (3.1 inches) at 15° flexion.[53] The effectiveness of the patella diminishes with full flexion because the patella sinks into the trochlear groove, reducing the anterior displacement of the quadriceps tendon. The extensor lever arm is only slightly reduced with full extension (4.4 cm [1.7 inches]).[52]

Apart from improving the moment arm of the quadriceps muscle, the patella provides protection for the articular cartilage of the trochlea and prevents excessive friction between the quadriceps tendon and the femoral condyles, permitting the patellofemoral joint to tolerate high compressive loads. The patella also acts as a guide for the converging heads of the quadriceps muscle, facilitating transmission of the muscular forces to the patella tendon.[50]

Patellofemoral Joint Reaction Force

Because the quadriceps is the only muscle to cross the patellofemoral joint, the patellofemoral joint reaction force (PFJRF) is determined by the force and moment balance of the quadriceps force vector and the patella ligament force vector.[54] Early biomechanical descriptions of the patellofemoral joint characterized this articulation as a frictionless pulley where the patellar ligament force (F_{PL}) was assumed to be equal to the force applied by the quadriceps tendon (F_Q).[55,56] However, subsequent experimental studies and mathematical representations of the patellofemoral joint suggested that the patella also acted as a lever, thereby creating a force differential between the quadriceps tendon and the patella ligament.[54] This force differential is thought to occur as a result of the varying geometry and shape of the distal femur and patella, as well as the changing point of contact between the patella and femur as the knee flexes and extends.

The PFJRF is the measurement of compression of the patella against the femur and is dependent on the angle of knee flexion, as well as the degree of muscle tension.[57]

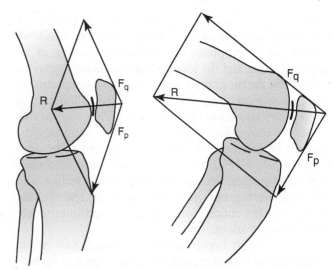

Figure 22-13 The patellofemoral joint reaction force increases as a function of quadriceps force and knee angle. F_q, Force of the quadriceps tendon; F_p, force of the patella tendon; R, patellofemoral joint reaction force. (From McConnell J, Fulkerson J: The knee: patellofemoral and soft tissue injuries. In Zachazewski JE, Magee DJ, Quillen WS, editors: *Athletic injuries and rehabilitation*, p 700, Philadelphia, 1996, WB Saunders.)

The resultant value of the quadriceps muscle force vector and the patella tendon force vector is equal and opposite to the PFJRF, which evokes compressive stresses on the patellofemoral articular cartilage (Figure 22-13).[58] Previous investigations have indicated that the PFJRF for level walking is approximately 1 times body weight; it is 3.8 times body weight during stair ascent and descent[59-61] and can be as high as 7 to 11 times body weight during running.[62]

Patellofemoral Joint Stress

From a mechanical standpoint, patellofemoral joint stress (or pressure) is defined as the PFJRF divided by the patellofemoral joint contact area. A high PFJRF is not necessarily harmful to the patellofemoral joint, because this force can be offset by a large contact area. However, a high joint reaction force combined with a small contact area may be detrimental.

Numerous studies have been undertaken to measure stresses directly from cadaveric knees using pressure-sensitive film. In addition, patellofemoral joint stress has been estimated in vivo by dividing the estimated PFJRF by the patellofemoral joint contact area obtained from the literature or MRI. It has been reported that peak patellofemoral joint stress can vary from 2 megapascals (MPa) for level walking to 6 MPa for stair ambulation.[59,60]

PATHOMECHANICS

As mentioned earlier, the cause of PFP can be elusive, and it may have multiple origins. For example, tissues such as the subchondral bone, synovium, retinaculum, and fat pad have been implicated as potential sources of patellofemoral joint symptoms.[63] Excessive mechanical stresses in these tissues are believed to stimulate pain receptors. Dye[63] proposed that differential loading of innervated tissue and the loss of tissue homeostasis may be responsible for the genesis of patellofemoral symptoms. In turn, restoration of tissue homeostasis (i.e., alleviation of stress in irritated tissue) is thought to reduce symptoms.

Several studies have provided evidence supporting the concept of differential loading as a factor in the development of pain.[60,64,65] Because the primary goal of conservative and surgical management of PFP is to reduce pain and improve function, it is important that the clinician understand the mechanisms that may contribute to abnormal joint loading.

As outlined by Fredericson and Powers,[66] factors that contribute to excessive patellofemoral stress can be broken down into three categories: local factors (abnormal patellofemoral joint mechanics), biomechanical factors (abnormal lower extremity kinematics), and overuse.

Local Factors: Abnormal Patellofemoral Joint Mechanics

When the patella is not properly situated within the trochlear groove owing to improper alignment or maltracking, contact between the patella and trochlear surfaces is diminished and stress is increased. Two of the more common examples of abnormal patella alignment and maltracking are excessive lateral patellar tilt and lateral patellar subluxation.

Excessive Lateral Pressure Syndrome

Ficat et al.[67] first proposed excessive lateral pressure as a causative factor in patellofemoral articular cartilage pathology. These authors proposed that the laterally tilted patella increased the compression between the lateral facet and the lateral femoral condyle (Figure 22-14). This patellar posture also unloads the medial facet.

Tilting of the patella can be isolated, or it can be associated with lateral patellar subluxation.[68-70] Chronic lateral tilt is determined radiologically and has been reported to have a deleterious effect on the articular cartilage. Lateral facet overload and deficient medial facet contact can lead to articular cartilage degeneration at both sites. Abnormal articular cartilage loading of the lateral facet may cross the threshold of cartilage resistance, leading to failure.[14] The primary area of lateral facet degeneration corresponds to the areas of contact in the 40° to 80° knee flexion range.[71]

The mechanism of medial facet articular cartilage damage in excessive lateral pressure syndrome (ELPS) appears to be different from that of lateral facet degeneration, because this area is susceptible to deficient contact. This form of degeneration likely can be attributed to impaired nutrition to the cartilage, because diminished joint compression results in decreased flow of synovial fluid.[72] Seedholm et al.[71] have stated that areas of relative contact deficiency develop mild degenerative changes and are most probably

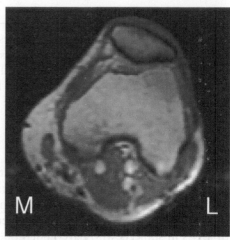

Figure 22-14 Axial MRI of the patellofemoral joint showing excessive lateral tilting of the patella, resulting in increased pressure between the lateral facet and the lateral femoral condyle. *M*, medial; *L*, lateral.

asymptomatic. When combined with the shearing of the medial facet associated with lateral patellar subluxation, more extensive medial facet degeneration may occur.[14]

Etiology of Excessive Lateral Patella Syndrome. The natural history of ELPS has been described as being congenital followed by adaptive shortening of the lateral retinaculum.[14] The significance of a tight lateral retinaculum is the increased posterolateral pull on this structure with knee flexion. This, in turn, accentuates lateral facet compression. Insall[73] stated that adaptive shortening of the lateral retinaculum was more likely the result of habitual lateral patella tracking.

Disruption of the medial stabilizers (the VM and the medial patellofemoral ligament) also has been implicated as a possible cause of excessive lateral patella tilt. Ahmed et al.[74] conducted a mechanical study to measure the static pressure distribution on the retropatellar surface. The results from 24 cadaveric specimens showed that a release of VMO tension created a pressure shift that was transferred almost entirely to the lateral facet of the patella. In addition, the change in the orientation of the pressure zone suggested a considerable frontal plane rotation of the patella relative to the femur.

Evidence exists that the shortened retinaculum and/or insufficient dynamic medial stabilizers contribute to lateral patellar tilt. Fulkerson et al.[75] demonstrated the effectiveness of surgical release of the lateral retinaculum in reducing lateral patella tilt. Based on preoperative and postoperative computed tomography (CT) evaluation, these authors reported a mean tilt improvement of 6° at 10° knee flexion and 15° at 20° knee flexion. These improvements brought the tilt angles of these subjects well within the normal range, as demonstrated in the control group. Douchette and Goble[76] demonstrated the importance of quadriceps muscle weakness and tightness of the lateral structures as contributors to ELPS. These authors found a significant decrease in patella tilt in patients who participated in an

8-week program of quadriceps muscle strengthening and ITB stretching. In addition, 84% of the previously symptomatic patients were pain free after this program.

Lateral Patellar Subluxation

Patella subluxation is abnormal medial or lateral movement of the patella. Abnormal patellar tracking, such that transient medial or lateral displacement occurs during flexion and extension, has been documented as a cause of articular cartilage damage and pain.[77,78] Subluxation of the patella is differentiated from patella instability or dislocation in that the patella stays in the trochlear groove rather than leaving it (i.e., dislocating).

In general, subluxation typically involves increased lateral displacement of the patella[14]; however, medial displacement also can occur.[79] Fulkerson and Hungerford[14] described three types of subluxation: minor recurrent subluxation, major recurrent subluxation, and permanent lateral subluxation. In minor recurrent subluxation, the patella deviates little from its normal course; this type of subluxation is not associated with clinically apparent relocation. In major recurrent subluxation, the patella comes across the lateral trochlear facet and returns to the trochlear groove with an audible snap. Permanent lateral subluxation is a stable lateral displacement in which there was no centering of the patella.

Etiology of Lateral Patella Subluxation. As mentioned previously, both static and dynamic structures provide resistance to the natural lateral forces acting on the patella. Disruption of the normal equilibrium of forces may lead to patella malalignment and associated pathology. To understand the etiology of a patient's symptoms and to formulate an effective treatment program, the clinician must understand the specific mechanisms involved.

Bony Abnormalities. Anatomical variations of the patella or distal femur (or both) can contribute to recurrent lateral patellar subluxation. Patellar or trochlear dysplasia compromises the inherent stability afforded by the bony structure, making the patella more susceptible to laterally directed forces. Wiberg[13] proposed a system for classifying patella shapes based on axial view radiographs:

- *Type I:* Both facets are slightly concave and symmetrical, and the medial and lateral facets are equal in size (Figure 22-15).

- *Type II:* The medial facet is distinctly smaller than the lateral facet. The lateral facet is concave, whereas the medial facet is more flat (see Figure 22-15). Wiberg found this to be the most common shape of the patella.

- *Type III:* The medial facet is slightly convex and considerably smaller, with marked lateral facet predominance (see Figure 22-15). Wiberg considered this shape a frank dysplastic form.

Apart from the shape of the patella, its position with respect to the trochlear groove can be a potential causative factor in lateral subluxation. **Patella alta,** as described by Insall,[46] is evident when the resting position of the patella is above the femoral groove (Figure 22-16). The high-riding patella does not sink adequately into the trochlear groove with knee flexion and therefore is prone to lateral displacement. In addition, individuals with patella alta are predisposed to elevated joint stresses, because the contact area is minimal, particularly when the knee is extended.[80] Patella alta is detected with lateral radiographs, and a positive sign is a patella tendon that is 20% longer than the patella. The excessive length of the patella tendon is thought to be the primary cause of this condition.[81]

Another bony etiological factor related to lateral patella subluxation is **trochlear dysplasia.** The trochlear groove of the femur, especially the larger anterior protrusion of the lateral femoral condyle, provides significant bony stability for the patella.[82] The normal trochlear facet (sulcus) angle was established by Brattstrom[82] using radiological techniques. Evaluation of 100 normal knees showed that the values for sexes were similar, with a mean angle of 143° for males and 142° for females. Higher sulcus angles represented a shallower trochlear groove and were associated with recurrent patella subluxation (Figure 22-17).[82,83] According to Hvid et al.,[84] a sulcus angle greater than 150° indicates trochlear dysplasia.

Studies by Powers[69] and Varadarajan et al.[85] have reported that the sulcus angle is significantly correlated with mediolateral patellar displacement and tilt. In contrast, Harbaugh et al.,[86] as well as Teng et al.,[87] reported that the inclination of the lateral anterior femoral condyle, as opposed to the sulcus angle, was more important in determining lateral tracking of the patella. In addition, the angle of inclination of the lateral trochlea has been reported to be associated with cartilage and bone marrow lesions on the lateral aspect of the patellofemoral joint.[88]

Abnormal Skeletal Alignment. Abnormal skeletal alignment has been reported to have a profound effect on the magnitude of the Q angle and the subsequent laterally directed component of the quadriceps muscle force.[78,89] Huberti and Hayes[89] documented the deleterious effects of an increased Q angle by measuring patellofemoral contact pressures in 12 fresh cadaver specimens. These authors found that a 10° increase in the Q angle resulted in a 45% increase in peak contact pressure at 20° of knee flexion. In half of these specimens, the area of patella

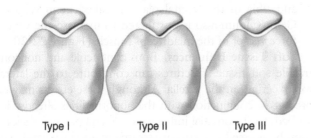

Figure 22-15 Classification of patella shapes based on axial view radiographs. (From Hunter RE, Sgaglione NA: *AANA advanced arthroscopy: the knee,* Philadelphia, 2010, Saunders.)

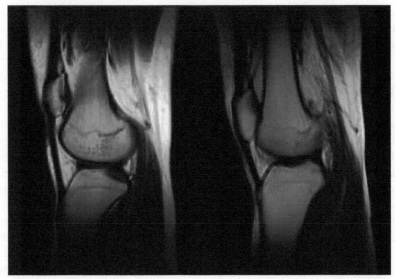

Figure 22-16 Sagittal MRI of the knee obtained at 0° showing patella alta *(left)* and the normal vertical position of the patella *(right)*.

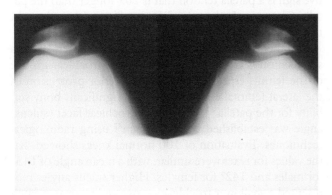

Figure 22-17 Skyline (sunrise) view of patellofemoral joints. Note the lateral displacement of both patellae and shallow trochlea (trochlear dysplasia), especially the one on the right. Note also the alpine hunter's cap shape of the patella. (From Magee DJ: *Orthopedic physical assessment,* ed 6, p 867, St. Louis, 2014, Saunders/Elsevier.)

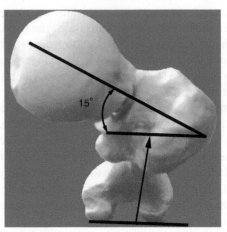

Figure 22-18 Femoral anteversion is measured by comparing the femoral neck and posterior condylar axes in the transverse plane. Normal anteversion is approximately 15°.

contact shifted laterally and the peak pressures were evident on the medial portion of the lateral facet.

An increased Q angle often is present with rotational malalignments of the femur and tibia. Such abnormalities include excessive femoral anteversion, lateral tibial torsion and/or lateral displacement of the tibial tubercle, and genu valgum.

- *Excessive femoral anteversion:* In the transverse plane, the neck of the femur forms an angle of about 15° with the transverse axis of the femoral condyles (Figure 22-18). This places the femoral head anterior to the femoral condyles. An increase in this angle, or *excessive femoral anteversion,* is associated with medial femoral rotation (Figure 22-19).[90-93] Excessive femoral anteversion and subsequent medial femoral rotation cause the trochlear surface of the femur to be placed medially with respect to the tibial tubercle, functionally increasing the Q angle.[94] Clinically, this is manifested by a toed-in gait and the appearance of "squinting patellae."[90]

- *Lateral tibial torsion and/or lateral displacement of the tibial tubercle:* A laterally displaced tibial tuberosity with respect to the midline of the tibia and the anterior superior iliac spine (ASIS) acts to increase the Q angle.[14] This anatomical variation typically is the result of increased lateral tibial torsion.

- *Genu valgum:* Increased valgus angulation of the femur and tibia in the frontal plane is called genu valgum. Genu valgum also is postulated to increase the valgus force vector of the quadriceps muscle (Figure 22-20).[94]

Soft Tissue Influences. Both contractile and noncontractile soft tissue structures can contribute to the lateral forces acting on the patella. Although these effects may be present in conjunction with the abnormalities already described, their potential influence on lateral patellar tracking must be assessed if an effective treatment is to be formulated.

Passive Structures. As mentioned previously, the lateral retinaculum has been implicated as a cause of

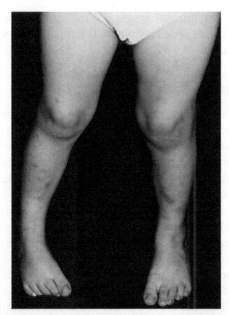

Figure 22-19 Excessive femoral anteversion is associated with increased femoral medial (internal) rotation. Note that this posture increases the quadriceps angle (Q angle). (Courtesy Michael Sherlock, M.D., Lutherville, MD. In Zitelli BJ, McIntire SC, Nowalk AJ: *Zitelli and Davis' atlas of pediatric physical diagnosis*, ed 6, Philadelphia, 2012, Saunders.)

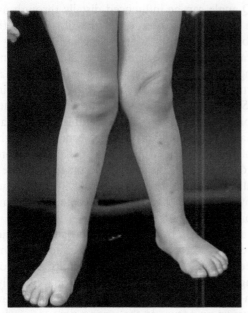

Figure 22-20 Increased angulation of the femur and tibia in the frontal plane is described as genu valgum. Note that this posture increases the Q angle. (From Zitelli BJ, McIntire SC, Nowalk AJ: *Zitelli and Davis' atlas of pediatric physical diagnosis*, ed 6, Philadelphia, 2012, Saunders.)

excessive lateral patellar tilt and is capable of exerting a lateral force on the patella, potentially contributing to subluxation. Because the lateral retinaculum has an extensive attachment to the ITB, contraction of the tensor fascia lata muscle may exert a dynamic lateral force through this connection.[95] In some cases this attachment may be

excessive, causing recurrent dislocation of the patella. Puniello[26] demonstrated a strong relationship between ITB tightness and decreased passive medial patella glide in a group of 17 subjects with patellofemoral dysfunction. Hughston and Deese[96] reported a high incidence (50%) of medial patella subluxation after lateral retinacular release, which indicates that this structure also plays a role in pulling the patella laterally.

Dynamic Structures. Historically, a force imbalance between the VM and the VL has been accepted as a principal cause of patella subluxation.[97-99] As such, clinical emphasis has been placed on the dynamic factors associated with patellar instability (i.e., VM weakness). The VM has been identified as the primary structure capable of counteracting the VL in maintaining patellar alignment. VM insufficiency has been associated with muscle atrophy,[97,100] hypoplasia,[97] inhibition caused by pain and effusion,[101,102] and impaired motor control.[103]

According to Fox,[97] hypoplasia of the extensor mechanism is found to a varying degree in 40% of the population. This hypoplasia manifests as incomplete development of the VM, because it is the last of the quadriceps muscle to develop phylogenetically.[97] The effect of an underdeveloped VM is a patellar alignment that is influenced by an overpowering VL; more specifically, the patella is situated more laterally and proximally. The more hypoplastic the VM, the more lateral the position of the patella. In addition, the superior and lateral pull of the patella can cause the development of patella alta. This hypoplasia also has been theorized to influence the development of the tibia, because the unchecked pull of the VL can result in lateral tibial rotation, lateral placement of the tibial tubercle, and genu recurvatum.[97]

Fox[97] theorized that the VM was the weakest muscle phylogenetically and therefore the first component of the quadriceps muscle to atrophy after injury or disuse. Fox considered the potential muscular imbalance between the medial and lateral dynamic stabilizers as a result of this atrophy or weakness to be the major predisposing factor for "hypermobile patella syndromes." Atrophy of the VM was observed by Smillie,[104] who stated that the apparent wasting of the VM was associated with the inability to complete terminal knee extension. To the contrary, Lieb and Perry[35] stated that apparent atrophy of the VM was the result of a thinner fascial covering (i.e., half the thickness) compared with the VL, which made atrophy of the VL less perceptible.

Atrophy of the quadriceps muscle group is thought to be caused by reflex inhibition,[101] with the stimulus being pain[105] or effusion.[106] Inhibition is the result of afferent stimuli from receptors in or around the injured knee that prevent activation of the α-motor neurons in the anterior horn of the spinal cord.[107] Spencer et al.[101] reported that infusion of only 20 to 30 mL of saline into the knee joint exceeded the threshold for quadriceps muscle inhibition, in contrast to other authors, who have proposed much larger volumes (e.g., 100 mL).[101] In an attempt to determine whether selective inhibition of the different heads of the quadriceps muscle was possible, Spencer et al.[101] examined Hoffman's reflex in the individual muscles after intra-articular infusion of saline into the knee. Although the VM appeared to be affected more by small amounts of induced effusion, no statistically significant differences were seen. This finding supported previous work that showed that reflex inhibition caused by effusion affects the entire extensor mechanism and does not predispose the patellofemoral joint to an imbalance of dynamic forces.

Documenting imbalances between the VM and the VL in patients with PFP has been of primary interest to the practicing clinician, because conservative treatment of this disorder typically focuses on restoring normal function of the dynamic stabilizers. Despite the interest in the function of the quadriceps femoris in patients with PFP, evidence supporting the concept of vasti muscle imbalance as a cause of lateral patella subluxation is limited.

Because in vivo strength assessment of the individual vastus muscle is not possible, electromyography (EMG) has been used to compare the relative recruitment of these muscles, under the rationale that decreased activity or impaired timing of the VM relative to the VL may indicate compromised medial patellar stability. Many investigators have studied the EMG activity of the dynamic patellar stabilizers in individuals with PFP; however, the results of these studies are equivocal. Some studies have found significant differences in VM and VL activity in patients with PFP,[108–110] whereas others have not.[111–114] Similarly, some authors have reported that the onset of VL activity precedes that of VM activity in persons with PFP[115,116]; however, vasti timing differences have not been reported in all studies.[117] Direct comparisons of these studies are difficult because of differences in experimental technique, methods of quantifying EMG, and the inherent variability associated with such data.

Another reason for the inconsistent results in these investigations may be the inherent variability among patients with PFP. Because the etiology of PFP has been considered a dynamic entity, a deficiency of the medial stabilizers logically should result in lateral displacement of the patella. However, radiological examinations have documented that fewer than 50% of patients with PFP show isolated lateral subluxation.[118] This suggests that lateral patellar tracking is not a universal finding in this disorder, and therefore such an inference cannot be generalized to all patients.

Etiology of Medial Patella Subluxation. Medial subluxation of the patella is less commonly seen than lateral patellar subluxation. The causes of lateral patellar subluxation are related more to anatomical and soft tissue abnormalities, whereas the etiology of medial subluxation is almost always iatrogenic.[79,96] This condition most commonly is caused by excessive medialization of the extensor mech-anism in realignment surgery or by lateral retinacular release in which little or no patella lateralization was done preoperatively.[96]

Abnormal Lower Extremity Kinematics

Researchers recently have recognized that the patellofemoral joint can be influenced by the segmental interactions of the lower extremity.[94,119] Abnormal motions of the tibia and femur in the transverse and frontal planes can have a substantial effect on patellofemoral joint mechanics and therefore PFP. An understanding of how the lower kinetic chain can influence the patellofemoral joint is important, because interventions to control abnormal lower extremity mechanics are not focused on the area of pain but rather on the joints proximal and distal to the patellofemoral joint (i.e., the hip and/or foot and ankle). As noted previously, structural deformities can lead to an increase in the Q angle and the lateral forces acting on the patella; however, abnormal motions of the lower extremity also can be contributing factors.[94,119] Three principal lower limb motions can influence the *dynamic* Q angle: tibial rotation, femoral rotation, and knee valgus.

Tibial Rotation

The Q angle can be influenced distally through motions of the tibia. Lateral rotation of the tibia moves the tibial tuberosity laterally, thereby increasing the Q angle, whereas tibial medial rotation decreases the Q angle by moving the tibial tuberosity medially (Figure 22-21, *A*). In turn, tibial rotation is influenced by subtalar joint motion. Subtalar joint pronation causes medial rotation of the tibia, and supination causes the tibia to rotate laterally. Normal subtalar joint pronation occurs during the first 30% of the gait cycle, during which the tibia rotates medially 6° to 10°.[120] This motion occurs in response to the medial rotation of the talus as it falls into the space created by the inferior and lateral movement of the anterior portion of the calcaneus.

As a result of this close biomechanical relationship between the rearfoot and the tibia, abnormal pronation has been linked to several lower extremity conditions, including patellofemoral joint dysfunction. Typically, pronation is considered abnormal if the amount of motion is excessive or occurs at the wrong time (i.e., when the foot should be supinating). When excessive pronation is related to various clinical entities, an assumption is made that abnormal pronation results in excessive tibial medial rotation and that this motion places a rotatory strain on soft tissues of the lower extremity. Although this may be the case with respect to the tibiofemoral joint, the same assumption does not hold true for the vertically aligned patellofemoral joint. In fact, excessive tibial medial rotation caused by subtalar joint pronation would actually *decrease* the Q angle and the lateral forces acting on the patella (see Figure 22-21, *A*).

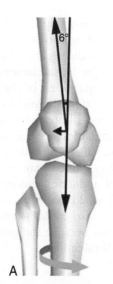 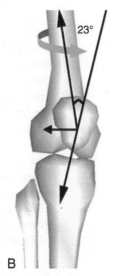 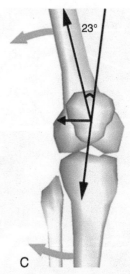

Figure 22-21 Schematic of the influence of femoral and tibial motion on the Q angle. **A,** Tibial medial (internal) rotation results in a decrease in the dynamic Q angle. **B,** Femoral medial (internal) rotation increases the dynamic Q angle. **C,** Femoral adduction or tibial abduction results in knee valgus and an increase in the dynamic Q angle. (From Powers CM: The influence of altered lower-extremity kinematics on patellofemoral joint dysfunction: a theoretical perspective, *J Orthop Sports Phys Ther* 33:639-646, 2003.)

This discrepancy was discussed by Tiberio,[121] who described a scenario in which excessive pronation could affect normal patellofemoral joint function. Tiberio postulated that to achieve knee extension in midstance, the tibia must rotate laterally relative to the femur to ensure adequate motion for the screw home mechanism. To compensate for this lack of tibial lateral rotation because of the failure of the foot to resupinate, the femur would have to rotate medially on the tibia such that the tibia was in relative lateral rotation. This compensatory medial rotation of the femur would permit the necessary screw home mechanics to allow for knee extension. However, excessive medial rotation of the femur would move the patella medially with respect to the ASIS, thereby increasing the Q angle and the lateral component of the quadriceps muscle vector (Figure 22-21, *B*). This would appear to be a plausible biomechanical means by which pronation could influence the patellofemoral joint; however, to do so, such motion ultimately would have to influence the femur.

An assumption made in the scenario just described is that if excessive pronation is evident in midstance, then excessive medial rotation of the tibia also should be evident. However, Reischl et al.[120] reported that the magnitude of foot pronation did not predict the magnitude of tibial or femoral rotation. Also, the magnitude of tibial rotation did not predict the magnitude of femoral rotation, which indicates that excessive rotation of the tibia did not translate into excessive femoral rotation. This is not surprising, considering that the knee has the potential to absorb rotatory forces through its transverse plane motion. It should be noted that all subjects in this study demonstrated pronation and tibial medial rotation during early stance. However, this motion was not a 1:1 ratio. Individual factors, such as the orientation of the subtalar joint axis and the amount of transverse plane motion between the rearfoot and the lower leg, likely influence the degree to which pronation can influence the magnitude of tibial rotation.

Femoral Rotation

The Q angle can be influenced proximally through motions of the femur. As described previously, increased femoral medial rotation results in a larger Q angle, because the patella is moved medially with respect to the ASIS and tibial tuberosity (see Figure 22-21, *B*). Consequently, femoral lateral rotation minimizes the Q angle, because the resultant line of action of the extensor mechanism is more in line with the ASIS.

Apart from increasing the Q angle and the laterally directed forces on the patella, femoral medial rotation can influence patella alignment and tracking. Because the patella is tethered in the quadriceps tendon, it is not obligated to follow the motions of the femur (i.e., trochlear groove), especially when the quadriceps muscles are contracted. In fact, during weight-bearing activities, medial rotation of the femur can occur independent of patella motion, thereby bringing the lateral anterior femoral condyle in close approximation to the lateral facet of the patella. Using dynamic MRI methods under weight-bearing conditions (i.e., a single-leg partial squat), Powers et al.[122] demonstrated that the primary contributor to lateral patella tilt in a group of individuals with patella instability was femoral motion (medial rotation), not patella motion (Figure 22-22). This finding was confirmed in a follow-up study a few years later.[123] The findings of these studies call into question the long-held assumption that lateral patella subluxation is the result of the patella moving on the femur. Although this may be the case during non–weight-bearing activities in which the femur is fixed (i.e., during knee extension in sitting), these studies provide evidence that lateral subluxation of the patella during

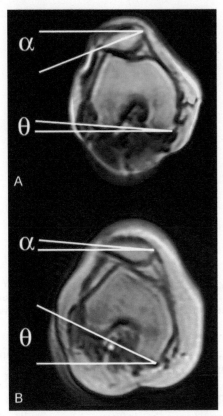

Figure 22-22 Influence of femoral rotation on lateral patella tilt at 0° knee flexion. During the non–weight-bearing condition (**A**), lateral patella tilt was the result of patella rotation (α) on a relatively horizontal femur (θ). During the weight-bearing condition (**B**), lateral patella tilt was a result of medial (internal) rotation of the femur (θ) under a relatively horizontal patella (α). (From Powers CM, Ward SR, Fredericson M et al: Patellofemoral kinematics during weight-bearing and non-weight-bearing knee extension in persons with lateral subluxation of the patella: a preliminary study, *J Orthop Sports Phys Ther* 33:677-685, 2003.)

weight-bearing activities may be the result of the femur rotating underneath the patella.

A biomechanical study by Souza and Powers[124] reported that females with PFP exhibited significantly greater peak hip medial (internal) rotation than did a control group (7.6° versus 1.2°), when averaged across three different tasks (running, step-down, and landing from a jump). Clinically, weakness of the hip lateral (external) rotators (i.e., gluteus maximus and deep rotators) may underlie the tendency of the hip to "rotate the thigh inward" during weight-bearing tasks. This concept is supported by several studies that have reported hip strength deficits in this population.[124-126]

Knee Valgus

Apart from abnormal motions in the transverse plane, excessive frontal plane motions can influence the patellofemoral joint. Most notably, valgus at the knee increases the Q angle, because the patella is displaced medially with respect to the ASIS (Figure 22-21, *C*). In comparison, a varus position of the knee decreases the Q angle, because the patella is brought more in line with the ASIS.

Knee valgus can be the result of thigh adduction, tibial abduction, or a combination of these two (see Figure 22-21, *C*). Excessive femoral adduction during dynamic tasks can be the result of weakness of the hip adductors, particularly the gluteus medius. The upper fibers of the gluteus maximus and the tensor fascia lata also assist in abduction at the hip and, if weak, may contribute to excessive thigh adduction. Structural abnormalities of the femur (i.e., excessive anteversion and coxa valga) can reduce the moment arm of the gluteus medius, which may result in a functional weakness.[127] Tibial abduction can be the result of excessive pronation or frontal plane motion at the ankle. However, tibial abduction also could be an accommodation to femoral adduction, because the proximal tibia is obligated to follow the distal femur.

Overuse

Because only 50% of patients with PFP have tracking abnormalities, other factors must be involved. If patellofemoral joint function and gait mechanics are normal, patellofemoral joint pathology may be related to excessive activity levels or overuse. For example, the peak PFJRF during weight acceptance has been calculated as 7 to 11 times body weight for healthy runners, a value estimated to be near the physiological limit of the involved tissues.[62] Therefore, for a given knee flexion angle, high forces result in elevated patellofemoral joint stress and may be problematic because of the repetitive nature of such activity. This concept is supported by the work of Thomee et al.,[128] who studied 40 women with PFP and concluded that chronic overloading and temporary overuse were the primary causes of symptoms.

Overuse injuries are a function of the magnitude of the applied force and the number of cycles the load is applied. For example, as the load increases, the number of repetitions necessary to cause injury decreases. Conversely, as the load decreases, the number of repetitions necessary to cause injury increases. Activities commonly associated with overuse histories include long-distance running and cycling.

Summary

Figure 22-23 summarizes the potential factors that may lead to patellofemoral joint dysfunction and pain. To treat PFP effectively, the clinician must address the root causes of the pain and dysfunction. Therefore the goal of the examination is to identify the likely cause or causes of symptoms so that the most effective interventions can be applied.

Clinical Note

To treat patellofemoral pain effectively, the clinician must determine the root causes of the pain and dysfunction, of which there are many.

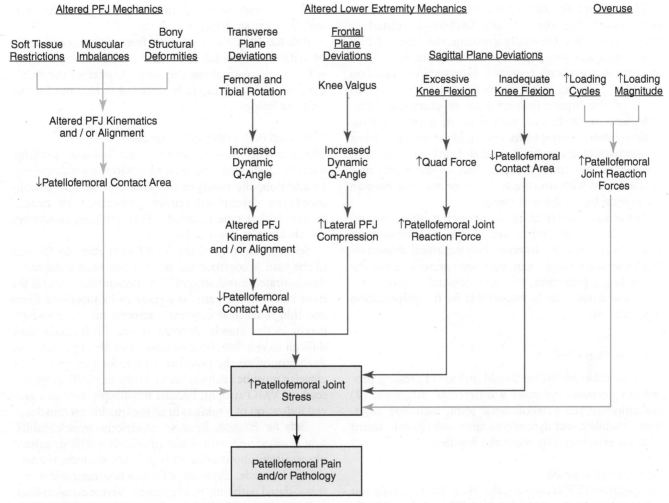

Figure 22-23 Flow diagram of potential mechanisms of patellofemoral pain and/or pathology. *PFJ*, Patellofemoral joint; *Quad*, quadriceps.

EXAMINATION

The goal of the examination is to obtain pertinent data to allow the formulation of a hypothesis about the cause of the symptoms. The examination should include both subjective and objective physical components.

Subjective Examination

The subjective examination is essential for making an accurate diagnosis. When taking a patient's history, the clinician should determine what problems are important and what types of examinations may be useful. Key information to obtain includes the patient's current complaints, symptoms, and the mechanism of injury.

Patients typically report pain as diffuse and arising from the anterior aspect of the knee.[128] However, sharp, "stabbing" symptoms can be elicited with provocative testing. Pain often is induced by activity and aggravated by functions that increase patellofemoral compressive forces, such as ascending and descending stairs, inclined walking, squatting, and prolonged sitting. The sensation of

"giving way" also may be reported and should be differentiated from tibiofemoral joint instability (i.e., ligament tear) or quadriceps muscle inhibition.

Pain along the medial and lateral borders of the patella is a common complaint, and retropatellar and inferior pain often is reported. Patients frequently report crepitus during knee flexion, but this should not by itself cause concern, because asymptomatic patellofemoral crepitus is very common.[129] Painful crepitus may be related to tightness of the deep retinacular tissues, plicae, or patellofemoral joint instability; it is not necessarily suggestive of arthritic changes.

According to Grelsamer and McConnell,[130] the location of symptoms may indicate the specific structures involved and provide direction with respect to a differential diagnosis:
- *Lateral:* Small nerve injury in the lateral retinaculum
- *Medial:* Recurrent stretching of the medial retinaculum/medial patellofemoral ligament
- *Retropatellar:* Articular cartilage damage; stress borne on subchondral bone
- *Superior:* Quadriceps tendonitis/tendinosis
- *Inferior:* Patella tendonitis/tendinosis; fat pad irritation

Throughout the history process, it is important to ascertain whether the patient's disability is related to pain or instability. Generally speaking, the onset of PFP is insidious and progression is slow. A specific episode or event is not always reported. However, the clinician should pay careful attention to the patient's perceived cause of the injury, making note of changes in lifestyle, activity levels and, with athletes, training habits. A slow onset of symptoms may indicate an underlying biomechanical error or structural faults that manifest themselves over time. A rapid onset of symptoms may be associated with overuse and may or may not have an underlying biomechanical cause.

Histories related to traumatic injury (i.e., direct falls on the patella) or instability related to pain are fairly obvious and self-explanatory. However, biomechanical abnormalities or structural faults may have been present before the injury (e.g., pronation, excessive femoral anteversion), and these factors may be responsible for the perpetuation of symptoms.

Physical Examination

The physical examination should include (1) testing procedures necessary to make a differential diagnosis; (2) evaluation of the patellofemoral joint, including alignment, mobility, and dynamic motion; and (3) assessment of lower extremity alignment and function.

Differential Diagnosis

To diagnose PFP accurately, the clinician must rule out other structures as potential sources of anterior knee pain symptoms.

Patella Tendonitis/Tendinosis. The symptoms of patella tendonitis/tendinosis can be very similar to those of PFP, because pain is often induced by activity, especially during high-speed eccentric contractions of the quadriceps muscles. A clear distinction can be made between tendonitis/tendinosis and PFP through careful palpation. Local tenderness to the quadriceps tendon (i.e., superior to the patella) and patella tendon (i.e., inferior to the patella) indicates tendonitis/tendinosis and should not be confused with retropatellar pain or medial or lateral patella pain.

Iliotibial Band Friction Syndrome. ITB friction syndrome is characterized by localized pain in the lateral aspect of the knee (i.e., lateral epicondyle of the femur). Occasionally crepitus or "snapping" can be palpated as the ITB crosses the lateral femoral condyle (approximately 30° flexion). Occasionally, this is mistaken for patellofemoral joint crepitus.

Meniscal and Ligamentous Structures. Structures of the tibiofemoral joint should be ruled out as possible causes of symptoms. Meniscal tests, such as joint line tenderness, McMurray's test, Apley's compression test, and the bounce home test, should be performed to rule out meniscus injury.[131] Likewise, ligamentous tests (e.g., Lachman's test, varus and valgus stress tests) should be performed, especially in patients with traumatic histories and/or acute swelling.

Referred Pain. Referred pain from compression and/or irritation of the L3 or L4 nerve roots can manifest itself as vague pain along the lateral border of the thigh. Patients should be carefully screened to rule out lumbar spine pathology.

Evaluation of the Patellofemoral Joint

The examiner should observe any redness, swelling, warmth, dystrophic changes, or obvious joint deformity. In addition, the presence of quadriceps muscle atrophy should be determined (either qualitatively or quantitatively with a tape measure). With athletes, quadriceps muscle atrophy may not be present.

Selective atrophy of the VMO in relation to the rest of the vasti is controversial and has not been consistently demonstrated across studies.[132,133] Because the VMO is the most visible of the vasti (as a result of its superficial fibers and thin retinacular covering), atrophy may be more apparent in this muscle. Atrophy of the VL is much more difficult to visualize, because most of its fibers are deep and wrap around to the posterior femur; for this reason, the clinician must be cautious about attributing PFP symptoms solely to VMO atrophy, because this atrophy may be a general indication of weakness in all the quadriceps muscles.

Tests for Effusion. Because quadriceps muscle inhibition is associated with slight (minimal) swelling, general observations about effusion (e.g., joint warmth, redness) should be made. Typically, PFP of a nontraumatic nature is associated with only mild effusion. Severe effusion likely indicates a more serious ligamentous injury. Major effusion can be assessed by compressing the patella into the trochlea. A positive ballotable or "floating" patella sign is seen when the patella quickly "rebounds" or "floats" when compressed into the trochlea.[131]

Minimal joint effusion can be assessed with the knee extended by "milking" fluid from the suprapatellar pouch and the lateral side of the knee into the medial side of the knee. A small bulge medially is a positive sign of mild swelling.[131]

Patellar Alignment. The patella should be assessed for gross alignment abnormalities. Typically this is done with the patient in supine, the knee extended, and the quadriceps muscle relaxed. According to McConnell[134] the most commonly observed abnormalities in individuals with PFP are as follows:

- *Lateral glide (i.e., lateral displacement):* The distance from the medial epicondyle of the femur to the center of the patella is greater than the distance from the lateral epicondyle of the femur to the center of the patella (Figure 22-24, *B*). Normally, the two distances are equal (Figure 22-24, *A*).
- *Lateral tilt:* The lateral border of the patella is lower than the medial border (as viewed in the transverse plane; Figure 22-24, *C*).

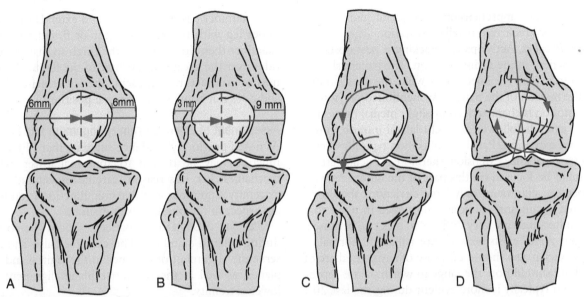

Figure 22-24 Assessment of the patellar glide component. Ideally, the patella should be centered on the superior portion of the femoral articular surface at 20° flexion. **A,** Ideal alignment. **B,** Lateral glide of the patella. **C,** Lateral tilt of the patella. **D,** Lateral rotation ("spin") of inferior pole of patella. (Modified from McConnell J, Fulkerson J: The knee: patellofemoral and soft tissue injuries. In Zachazewski JE, Magee DJ, Quillen WS, editors: *Athletic injuries and rehabilitation,* pp 711-712, Philadelphia, 1996, WB Saunders.)

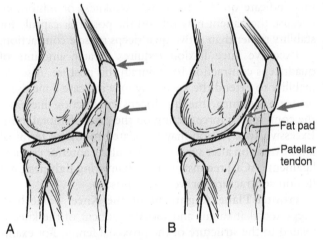

Figure 22-25 Assessment of the anteroposterior component of the patella. Ideally, the superior and inferior poles of the patella should be in line with the long axis of the femur. Excessive inferior tilt of the patella may irritate the infrapatellar fat pad. **A,** Ideal alignment. **B,** Posterior tilt of the inferior pole. (Modified from McConnell J, Fulkerson J: The knee: patellofemoral and soft tissue injuries. In Zachazewski JE, Magee DJ, Quillen WS, editors: *Athletic injuries and rehabilitation,* p 712, Philadelphia, 1996, WB Saunders.)

- *Lateral rotation:* The inferior pole of the patella is rotated externally with respect to the midline of the thigh (as viewed in the frontal plane; Figure 22-24, *D*).
- *Inferior tilt:* The inferior pole of the patella is tilted posteriorly compared with the superior pole (sagittal plane; Figure 22-25).

Although this classification system is widely used, both the validity and reliability of these techniques in assessing patella alignment have been challenged.[135,136] Care must

be taken in the interpretation of the results of patellar alignment testing, especially because the resting position of the patella tends to be one of slight lateral displacement and lateral tilt. Only obvious abnormalities should be considered relevant.

McConnell's Assessment Criteria for Patella Alignment

- Lateral glide (displacement)
- Lateral tilt
- Lateral rotation
- Inferior tilt

Passive Patella Mobility. In addition to static alignment, passive patella mobility should be evaluated. Because motion of the patella is necessary for normal joint function, assessment of patella mobility is an important component of the examination. The patella should be able to freely glide superiorly and inferiorly, as well as medially and laterally. Also, the clinician should be able to tilt the patella medially to raise the lateral border. Quite often patella mobility is restricted after prolonged immobilization or surgery. Tightness of the lateral retinaculum is the most common limiting factor and manifests as decreased medial patella glide and inability to tilt the patella medially. As the patella moves inferiorly and superiorly and the knee flexes and extends, adequate motion is essential to ensure normal knee motion.

When assessing passive patellar mobility, the clinician also should note excessive translations and/or apprehension to such movements. Excessive lateral translation of the patella may indicate tearing of the medial patellofemoral ligament. Patient apprehension to a lateral glide of the patella suggests recurrent patella dislocation

Patella Tracking. Active patella tracking is best observed with the patient in the sitting position. The patient should be asked to extend the knee slowly while the clinician observes the motion of the patella. As mentioned previously, normal motion is characterized by slight medial motion as the knee extends followed by slight lateral motion in terminal knee extension. Patellar subluxation typically occurs during terminal knee extension; therefore particular attention should be focused on this part of the range. As with static patellar alignment, only large deviations should be considered significant. Clinicians must keep in mind that subtle subluxations are very difficult to pick up, because a large "gray zone" exists between normal and abnormal.

The clinician also should be aware of any painful arc of motion and should note the range in which pain is reproduced. Pain typically is more evident during the last 20°, because greater quadriceps muscle forces are necessary to complete terminal knee extension, and the patellofemoral joint contact area decreases (resulting in elevated patellofemoral joint stress).

As the knee is extending, the examiner should make a qualitative assessment of the state of quadriceps muscle contraction. Does the knee appear to have difficulty completing terminal extension (suggestive of quadriceps muscle weakness), or is muscle "quivering" present (suggestive of reflex inhibition)?

Quadriceps Muscle Weakness. General quadriceps muscle weakness or atrophy (or both) is a hallmark of PFP. However, ascertaining whether true weakness is present is difficult, because pain commonly is reproduced with quadriceps muscle contraction and the patient may be hesitant to give maximal effort, thereby invalidating results.

Tests for Soft Tissue and Muscle Tightness. Tightness of various soft tissues and muscles that cross the knee can have an adverse effect on patellofemoral joint function. In particular, tightness of the RF muscle and tensor fascia lata–ITB complex should be evaluated.

Tightness of the RF muscle can result in excessive patellofemoral joint compression, especially when the knee is flexed and the hip is extended. This posture is particularly evident during the swing phase of the running cycle or with the trail limb during lunging tasks. The length of the RF muscle is best assessed using Thomas's test.[137] With the patient supine, both knees are brought to the chest to flatten the lumbar lordosis. The leg being tested then is allowed to extend such that it comes to rest on the table in a neutral position. If the knee cannot flex to 90° with the hip in a neutral position, the RF muscle is considered to be tight.

As noted previously, the interdigitation of the ITB and the lateral retinaculum suggests that tightness of this structure may produce a lateral force on the patella, potentially contributing to lateral subluxation and ELPS. Ober's test assesses for tightness of the ITB and tensor fascia lata. For this test, the patient is placed in the side-lying position.

The examiner passively abducts and extends the patient's upper leg with the knee straight or flexed to 90°. The examiner then slowly lowers the thigh so that the tendon rides over the greater trochanter of the femur.[137] If tightness or contracture is present, the leg remains abducted and does not come to the neutral position.

Assessment of Lower Extremity Alignment and Function

As noted previously, evidence suggests that PFP and dysfunction may be related to abnormal lower extremity mechanics. For this reason, careful assessment of lower extremity alignment and dynamic function is an important aspect of the physical examination.

Standing Posture. The patient should be observed during relaxed standing. The examiner also should observe the alignment of the knee in the sagittal and frontal planes, as well as the transverse plane alignment of the lower extremity.

Sagittal Plane Alignment of the Knee. The knee should be evaluated for hyperextension or excessive knee flexion. Knee hyperextension (i.e., genu recurvatum) may result in compression of the inferior pole of the patella into the infrapatellar fat pad. A hyperextended knee also may indicate quadriceps muscle weakness or inhibition, because the patient may rely on the posterior capsule for stability rather than active quadriceps muscle contraction.

Excessive knee flexion requires greater amounts of quadriceps contraction to maintain this posture. Also, an inability to extend the knee fully may indicate a meniscus problem. In turn, the quadriceps contraction increases the compressive forces acting on the patellofemoral joint. Excessive knee flexion may be related to loss of terminal knee extension after surgery (particularly anterior cruciate ligament [ACL] reconstruction), hamstring tightness, hip flexion contracture, or weak calf muscles.

Frontal Plane Alignment of the Knee. Some have suggested that valgus and varus alignment of the knee is related to the structure of the proximal femur. For example, the normal inclination between the femoral neck and the femoral shaft is 125°.[138] A reduction of this angle (i.e., coxa vara) results in a valgus orientation of the knee. An increase in the angle of inclination results in a varus orientation of the knee. Knee valgus tends to increase the Q angle and the lateral forces acting on the patella, whereas knee varus has the opposite effect. However, coxa valga reduces the lever arm of the gluteus medius muscle, thereby reducing the torque-producing capacity of this muscle.[139]

Transverse Plane Alignment of the Lower Extremity. Medial rotation of the femur (i.e., medial femoral torsion) results in "squinting patellae," whereas lateral rotation of the femur (i.e., lateral femoral torsion) results in the patella pointing outward (i.e., "grasshopper eyes"). (Note: Torsion implies actual anatomical rotation of the femur, not the physiological movement of the femur.) Femoral medial rotation may indicate excessive femoral anteversion or femoral torsion, whereas femoral lateral rotation may suggest femoral retroversion or lateral femoral torsion. Careful attention must be paid to whether foot pronation is evident and whether the entire lower extremity is in a posture of medial rotation or whether the medially rotated position of the femur appears to be an isolated entity.

Dynamic Function. Perhaps one of the most important aspects of the examination is observation of dynamic movement. This observation should include analysis of level walking, as well as higher demand activities, such as running, ascending and descending stairs, squatting, and jumping, especially if assessing active people. Careful attention should be paid so as to identify movement patterns that increase quadriceps demand and/or increase the dynamic Q angle. Observations also should be made with respect to the speed of ambulation, the force of impact during loading response, and any reproduction of symptoms. Components of the dynamic evaluation should be used to confirm or refute suspected abnormalities based on static testing procedures. Movements should be observed from both the frontal and sagittal views.

Sagittal View. The primary deviations for which the examiner should watch in the sagittal plane are inadequate knee flexion or hyperextension during weight acceptance and excessive knee flexion during stance. Decreased knee flexion during weight acceptance and knee hyperextension during the stance phase may indicate a **quadriceps avoidance gait pattern** caused by weakness or pain. The functional significance of inadequate knee flexion during weight acceptance is that shock absorption is impaired, and the tibiofemoral joint may be susceptible to excessive impulse loading. In addition, decreased knee flexion reduces the contact area between the patella and femur and therefore may contribute to elevated joint stress.

Excessive knee flexion during stance increases PFJRFs, because the quadriceps muscles are overly active supporting the flexed knee posture. Causes of excessive knee flexion include knee flexion contracture, hamstring tightness or spasticity, hip flexion contracture, meniscus pathology, and weak calf muscles.[140]

Frontal View. In the frontal view, rotation and valgus of the lower extremity are particularly important. An attempt should be made to evaluate for the following abnormalities:
1. Does the patient pronate the foot excessively? If so, does this result in excessive medial rotation of the tibia and femur?
2. Does the patient exhibit excessive medial rotation of the femur? If so, does this medial rotation tend to be present throughout the gait cycle (suggesting a fixed, bony deformity, such as excessive femoral anteversion), or does the patient "collapse" into medial rotation during weight acceptance? The latter is more indicative of poor muscular control or weakness of the hip lateral rotator muscles (Figure 22-26).
3. Does the patient exhibit excessive adduction of the femur and/or a contralateral pelvic drop? This indicates poor muscular control of the hip abductor muscles.

In many instances, frontal and transverse plane abnormalities are not readily evident during walking; therefore higher demand or functional activities specific to the patient need to be assessed. The **repetitive step-down test** is useful in this respect. The patient stands on a 0.2-m (8-inch) step and then lowers himself or herself with the painful leg and touches the heel to the floor (Figure 22-27). This is repeated 10 times without stopping unless the movement becomes too painful for the patient.

In general, an attempt should be made to determine whether frontal and transverse plane deviations

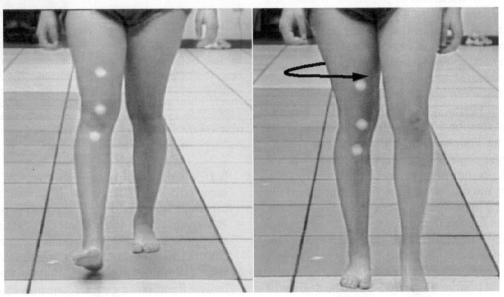

Figure 22-26 Frontal plane observational gait analysis of an individual with patellofemoral pain. Note the collapse into femoral internal rotation in midstance. Markers placed on the distal thigh, patella, and tibial tuberosity aid visualization of segment motions.

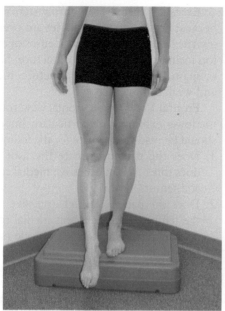
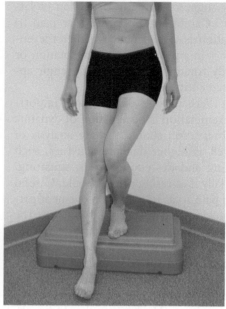

Figure 22-27 Assessment of lower extremity dynamic control. The patient slowly lowers herself with the extremity of interest and touches the heel to the floor without transferring weight to the descending limb. This patient shows medial collapse of the knee (excessive femoral adduction and medial [internal] rotation).

are occurring from the foot upward or from the pelvis downward. If the primary cause of the abnormality is identified, the correct treatment can be applied (i.e., proximal control through the hip versus distal control through the foot).

Additional Tests. Depending on the findings of the assessment of lower extremity alignment and dynamic function, the clinician may require additional information to formulate a hypothesis about the cause of the posture or motion abnormalities. The following tests may be useful:

- *Muscle testing of the hip lateral (external) rotators, abductors, and hip extensors:* If excessive dynamic medial rotation and/or adduction of the femur is observed during the dynamic assessment and muscle weakness is suspected, muscle performance testing of the hip abductors, lateral rotators, and extensors is warranted.
- *Assessment of hip range of motion:* Hip range of motion should be evaluated because restricted lateral rotation range of motion can bias a patient into a medial rotation position. Tightness of the hip flexors also can create a medial rotation bias. Hip flexor tightness can be assessed using Thomas's test, as described previously.
- *Craig's test of femoral anteversion:* Excessive femoral anteversion can contribute to medial (internal) rotation of the femur and can have a significant influence on the patellofemoral joint. Craig's test is performed with the patient prone and the knee flexed to 90°. The examiner palpates the posterior aspect of the greater trochanter of the femur, and the hip then is passively rotated medially and laterally until the greater trochanter reaches its most lateral position (Figure 22-28). The degrees of anteversion can be estimated based on the angle of the lower leg with the vertical. Normal femoral anteversion

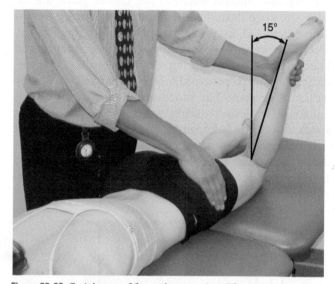

Figure 22-28 Craig's test of femoral anteversion. The examiner palpates the greater trochanter of the femur and rotates the femur internally and externally until the greater trochanter is at its most laterally prominent position. The angle of anteversion is estimated by measuring the angle created by the tibial shaft and a vertical line. Normal femoral anteversion is approximately 15°.

is 15°. It should be noted, however, that the measurement error with Craig's test is approximately 12°, so care must be made in the interpretation of findings.[141]

- *Foot evaluation:* If subtalar joint pronation is identified as a potential contributor to faulty lower extremity mechanics, the foot should be examined closely for fixed, bony deformities (e.g., rearfoot varus, forefoot varus), muscle tightness (e.g., gastrocnemius and soleus), and weakness of dynamic stabilizers (e.g., tibialis posterior and peroneal muscles).

DIAGNOSTIC IMAGING

Basic Radiographic Methods

The anteroposterior (AP) view is used to evaluate the patella for any fracture or bipartite configuration and for gross positional changes, such as dislocation or abnormalities of patella height. Asymmetry of the femoral condyles may indicate abnormal femoral torsion or femoral neck anteversion. A 30° knee flexion, weightbearing, posteroanterior (PA) view is most important for evaluating joint space and assessing for evidence of osteoarthritis.

Radiographs for Patellofemoral Pain

- Anteroposterior view in extension
- Anteroposterior view in 30° flexion
- Lateral view in full extension
- Lateral view in 30° flexion
- Axial view in 45° flexion
- Tangential view

The lateral view in full extension and at 30° knee flexion is used to determine patellar height and the patella's relationship to the trochlea. At full extension, the lateral view should show the distal articular surface of the patella just at the center of the trochlea. Other authors have proposed reliable methods for assessment of patella alta and patella baja.[81,142]

The patellofemoral joint also is visualized on an axial or tangential view. The axial view describes the parallel relationship of the x-ray beam with respect to the axis of the anterior tibia, whereas the tangential view describes the perpendicular relationship of the x-ray beam to the joint surfaces.[143] Both of these methods provide cross-sectional information about the relationship of the patella to the trochlear groove.[141] Overall, the most useful axial radiograph is the simple 30° or 45° knee flexion axial view. It is most important to ensure an accurate, reproducible 30° or 45° flexion view. A wooden leg holder with pins at the desired flexion angle is helpful.

For reproducible tangential views, certain requirements must be met. The x-ray beam and x-ray plate must be perpendicular to prevent distortion.[143,144] Views with the knee flexed more than 45° may be used[141,143,145] but are much less helpful. The position of potential maximum instability is 0° to 30°, but this position is technically difficult to capture on an axial radiograph.[146,147] For the most reliable and reproducible results, 45° seems to be the preferred position.[148] Some authors contend that tangential projections throughout the range (i.e., 30°, 60°, and 90°) are vital to the assessment of dynamic tracking of the patella.[146,147]

Computed Tomography

CT offers the advantage of a specific, definable plane. In general, CT is best performed using a midpatella transverse image, including the posterior condyles of the femur. This view enables the clinician to understand the relationship of the articulating midportion of the patella with its reciprocal portion of the trochlea at any degree of knee flexion. Midpatella transverse images through the posterior condyles with the knee flexed at 0°, 15°, 30°, and 45° provide an excellent depiction of how the patella enters the trochlea during flexion (Figure 22-29). The images may be taken with the quadriceps contracted or relaxed.

Magnetic Resonance Imaging

Early MRI had limited value in the evaluation of patients with PFP. The use of MRI was prohibitive, based on time and expense and on the quality and usefulness of the information obtained about patella position and tracking. More recently, however, CT and MRI have been used to image the patellofemoral joint during active or dynamic flexion and extension activities.[39,118,149,150] Kinematic and conventional modes of MRI of the patellofemoral joint offer advantages over CT in that they do not require radiation, and they allow depiction of important passive and active soft tissue stabilizers of the patellofemoral joint.[39,118,149] It has been suggested that dynamic or kinematic MRI, which allows assessment of the contribution of activated muscles and other soft tissue structures, is more sensitive than static imaging for demonstrating patellofemoral alignment and tracking abnormalities.[39] Statistically significant differences in patella tracking patterns and imaging parameters (e.g., patella tilt angle, bisect offset, lateral patella displacement) between active

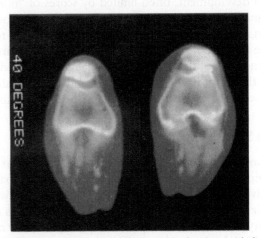

Figure 22-29 CT scan of lateral patella tilt and displacement with the knee in 40° flexion. Precise midpatella transverse CT images at 0°, 15°, 30°, and 45° knee flexion give an accurate impression of patella alignment. (From McConnell J, Fulkerson J: The knee: patellofemoral and soft tissue injuries. In Zachazewski JE, Magee DJ, Quillen WS, editors: *Athletic injuries and rehabilitation*, p 709, Philadelphia, 1996, WB Saunders.)

and passive knee extension have been demonstrated by Brossmann et al.[149] To date, constraints have been encountered in the form of image acquisition time (i.e., 0.5-1 images/sec).[39,118,149] The use of echoplanar MRI in the future may dramatically reduce image acquisition time and greatly improve resolution, allowing images of moving or changing structures to be acquired at near-real-time rates of 10 to 16 frames/sec.[151]

The use of quantitative and semiquantitative scoring of cartilage using MRI has grown in recent years. Several investigators have explored patellar cartilage compositional properties in vivo, quantified through T1rho or T2 relaxation time mapping, delayed gadolinium-enhanced MRI of cartilage (i.e., dGEMRIC), or sodium imaging.[152–156] These studies have generally found evidence of disruption of the normal biochemical composition of the articular cartilage in persons with PFP and patellofemoral joint osteoarthritis. Cartilage T1rho and T2 relaxation mapping allows for identification of prearthritic changes and has been shown effective at predicting future development of cartilage lesions.[152] However, challenges with high cost, long MRI scan times, and postprocessing time burdens have remained as critical barriers to widespread clinical adoption of these methods.

Semiquantitative scoring systems also have been described for morphological features of patellar cartilage and surrounding tissues. Specialized scoring systems designed expressly for patients following ACL injury or cartilage repair interventions, as well as those with primary knee osteoarthritis, have been described.[157–161] These scoring systems generally include categorical variables for various morphological features (e.g., cartilage lesions, meniscal tears, bone marrow edema) and are scored in several anatomical subcompartments (including patella and trochlea). It should be noted that these scoring systems are insensitive to incremental worsening of cartilage before lesion development, often limited by scores of "normal" or "increased signal inhomogeneity." However, once a lesion is present, there are several categorical levels to describe the lesion. Although these scoring systems are not designed for subtle compositional changes associated with PFP, they have been widely studied and provide valuable disease severity metrics for patients with advanced disease.

Bone Scan

A bone scan can reveal whether true intraosseous dysfunction is present and may localize the source of pain. A positive bone scan result after knee trauma objectifies the problem. It may even demonstrate whether there is more activity proximally or distally in the patella and may reveal a problem in the trochlea or elsewhere. Dye et al.[162] have been particularly influential in emphasizing the dynamic function of bone in PFP and the usefulness of following this with bone (radionuclide) scans.

CONSERVATIVE (NONOPERATIVE) TREATMENT

The treatment of PFP should be dictated by objective data obtained through a thorough examination. Treatment decisions also should be based on a solid scientific and biomechanical rationale. Once the examination has been completed, data should be compiled and a hypothesis formulated regarding the cause of the pain. The clinician should attempt to classify patients based on whether the suspected mechanism is a result of local patellofemoral joint dysfunction, lower quarter dysfunction, or overuse. Treatment decisions should focus on the identified impairments.

Treatment Classification for Patellofemoral Pain Based on Mechanism

- Local patellofemoral joint dysfunction
- Lower quarter dysfunction
- Overuse

Patellofemoral Joint Dysfunction

Specific treatment strategies for patellar malalignment and/or altered patellofemoral joint mechanics should be based on identified causes. As mentioned previously, possible contributing factors are bony and structural abnormalities, tightness of lateral structures, decreased patella mobility, and quadriceps muscle weakness. From a rehabilitation standpoint, little can be done to correct bony deformities. Although the influence of the Q angle can be minimized through the interventions described later in this chapter, conditions such as patella alta, trochlear dysplasia, femoral anteversion, and a laterally displaced tibial tuberosity are likely to require surgical intervention.

Tightness of Lateral Structures

If tightness of the lateral retinaculum is found to be contributing to ELPS or lateralization of the patella, treatment interventions should include soft tissue mobilization techniques (e.g., passive stretch, transverse frictions, deep tissue massage) to increase extensibility of the retinaculum. Soft tissue techniques in the area of the ITB and its interdigitation with the lateral retinaculum may prove useful (Figure 22-30). Because the ITB is a very dense, fibrous tissue, some clinicians question whether this structure can be stretched; however, longitudinal deep tissue massage may facilitate the breaking up of adhesions between the ITB and the overlying fascia.

Stretching of the tensor fascia lata also should be considered, because this muscle can influence the tension in the ITB (Figure 22-31). Also, patellar mobilization and patellar taping techniques (discussed in a later section) can be used for passive stretching of the lateral

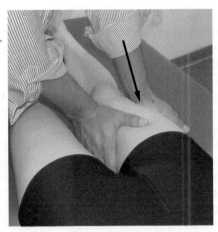

Figure 22-30 Soft tissue techniques in the area of the iliotibial band and its interdigitation with the lateral retinaculum may prove useful for increasing patella mobility. The arrow indicates the line of force application.

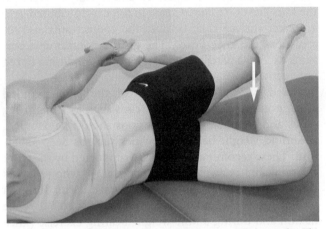

Figure 22-31 Self-stretch of the tensor fascia lata (TFL) muscle. This muscle can influence the patellofemoral joint through its insertion into the iliotibial band. The arrow indicates the line of force application by the contralateral heel.

structures. Low-load, prolonged passive stretching (L3D technique) is preferred so as to take advantage of the creep effect of soft tissue.

Decreased Patellar Mobility

Patellar oscillatory mobilization techniques combined with passive stretching should be performed to improve patellar mobility superiorly and inferiorly, as well as medially and laterally (see Figure 22-31). If the patella lacks normal mobility, forces may be concentrated in localized areas. The most common reasons for reduced patella mobility are prolonged immobilization, postoperative scarring, and quadriceps tightness.

When oscillatory mobilization techniques are performed, care should be taken to prevent excessive patellofemoral joint compression. To facilitate mobilization of the patella, the knee should be in extension or only slightly flexed (Figure 22-32). If the knee is flexed beyond 20°, the patella becomes seated within the trochlear groove which limits mobility of the patella.

Clinical Note

Generally speaking, an inferior glide of the patella facilitates knee flexion, whereas a superior glide of the patella facilitates knee extension. Mediolateral patellar mobilization restores the normal patella translations that occur during knee flexion and extension.

Quadriceps Muscle Weakness or Inhibition

Rehabilitation of the extensor mechanism continues to play a significant role in the treatment of PFP. With quadriceps muscle inhibition, pain and swelling must be controlled before a quadriceps exercise program is initiated. Pain modalities (e.g., transcutaneous electronic stimulation [TENS]), as well as methods to minimize effusion (e.g., ice, electrical stimulation), should be used as necessary.

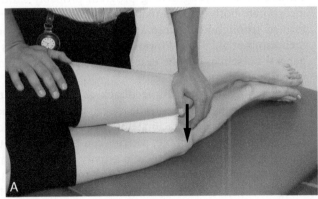
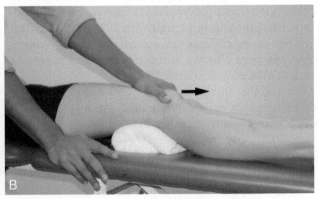

Figure 22-32 Patellofemoral joint mobilization techniques. Examples of medial glide (**A**) and inferior glide (**B**). Care should be taken to prevent direct joint compression. The arrows indicate the lines of force application.

As mentioned previously, the treatment of PFP using therapeutic exercise traditionally has focused on restoring dynamic patella stability through strengthening of the VMO. Such clinical practice is based on the assumption that the VMO is disproportionately weak relative to the VL, even though the strength of the VMO cannot be quantified in vivo.

Theories on VMO Strengthening. The concept of VMO strengthening is based on the belief that the VMO can be selectively recruited, independent of the VL, through various exercises.[98,134,163] The most common activities that have been postulated to facilitate VMO strengthening are various quadriceps muscle exercises (e.g., straight leg raises, isometric quadriceps sets, terminal knee extension), hip adduction, and medial tibial rotation.

A review of 20 existing EMG studies revealed that altering lower limb alignment or adding co-contraction through hip adduction does not preferentially enhance VMO activation relative to the VL.[164] This finding suggests that *isolated* recruitment of the VMO does not occur with exercises that are commonly prescribed for the treatment of PFP and that selective strengthening is unlikely. Even if greater EMG activity could be elicited in the VMO relative to the VL, the magnitude of VMO contraction would have to be at least 60% of maximum to stimulate hypertrophy.[165] As such, it appears that isolated recruitment or strengthening of the VMO through selected exercises may not be a realistic goal and that any emphasis on selective strengthening of the VMO most likely translates into a general quadriceps muscle strengthening effect.[166]

General Quadriceps Muscle Strengthening. Convincing evidence indicates that improving quadriceps muscle strength is an important aspect of treatment for PFP. For example, a study by Natri et al.[167] revealed that restoration of quadriceps muscle strength was a significant predictor of improved long-term outcomes (i.e., 7-year follow-up). Furthermore, work by Powers et al.[168] suggests that enhanced locomotor function in individuals with PFP is associated with increased torque of the quadriceps femoris muscle, which lends support to the concept of strengthening as a useful treatment option. A systematic review of the literature related to quadriceps strengthening in persons with PFP concluded that there was strong evidence that isolated quadriceps strengthening was more effective in reducing pain and improving function than education alone.[169]

Despite the apparent benefits of quadriceps muscle rehabilitation in patients with PFP, the mechanism by which strengthening improves PFP symptoms and functional ability has not been fully established. However, data provided by Chiu et al.[170] suggest that quadriceps strengthening increased patellofemoral joint contact area. An increase in contact area could reduce patellofemoral stress and therefore pain.

The goal of the therapeutic exercise program should be to facilitate quadriceps muscle strength while minimizing patellofemoral joint stress. Clinicians can benefit from an understanding of the biomechanics of weight-bearing and non–weight-bearing exercises, two methods commonly used to strengthen the knee extensor mechanism.

Weight-Bearing versus Non–Weight-Bearing Exercises. During non–weight-bearing knee extension (i.e., resistance applied at the ankle), the amount of quadriceps muscle force required to extend the knee steadily increases as the knee moves from 90° to full knee extension.[166] This increase in force is attributed to a decrease in mechanical advantage of the knee extensor mechanism.[171] In addition to the increase in quadriceps muscle force as the knee extends, the patellofemoral contact area steadily decreases. This combination of increased quadriceps muscle force and decreased contact area during terminal knee extension results in greater patellofemoral joint stress and pressure than what is seen with greater knee flexion angles in which the quadriceps muscle force is not as great and the contact area is larger.[166]

Conversely, during weight-bearing exercises (e.g., squatting), the quadriceps muscle force is relatively minimal when the knee is extended and steadily increases as the knee flexes.[166] The increase in force is distributed over a greater surface area, because the contact area also increases as the knee flexes. The greater contact area prevents excessive patellofemoral joint pressure during flexed knee activities.[166]

Based on the biomechanics of the patellofemoral joint, non–weight-bearing exercises such as straight leg raises and terminal knee extensions should be avoided, as should weight-bearing activities such as deep squatting. These recommendations are supported by the work of Steinkamp et al.[172] and Powers et al.,[173] who reported that greater patellofemoral stress was evident during a weight-bearing exercise (leg press) at 48° to 90° knee flexion and during a non–weight-bearing exercise (knee extension) at 48° to 0° knee flexion (Figure 22-33).

Quadriceps muscle strengthening apparently can be performed safely throughout the 0° to 90° knee flexion range by varying the mode of exercise. Both weight-bearing and non–weight-bearing exercises can be used to promote quadriceps muscle hypertrophy; therefore a comprehensive strengthening program probably should incorporate both types so that strengthening can be performed throughout a large arc of motion. The data of Steinkamp et al.[172] and Powers et al.[173] can be used as a general guideline, but the exact exercise prescription will vary from patient to patient.

Electromyographic Biofeedback as an Adjunct to Strengthening. EMG biofeedback can be a valuable tool for helping the patient facilitate contraction of the quadriceps muscle. For example, patients can be instructed to monitor their quadriceps muscle activity while performing functional tasks such as step-downs and partial squats. The goal is to provide patients with immediate feedback to increase general quadriceps muscle recruitment, especially during eccentric contractions (Figure 22-34). Although comparison of raw EMG signals between muscles (i.e., to document "muscle imbalance") is not appropriate,[166]

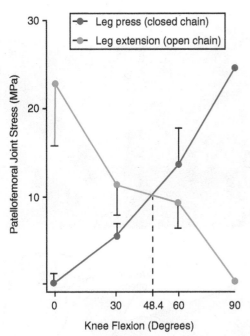

Figure 22-33 Patellofemoral joint stress as a function of knee angle during open- and closed-chain activities. The greatest stresses occur at high knee flexion angles during closed-chain activities and at low knee flexion angles during open-chain activities. (From Steinkamp LA, Dillingham, Markel MD et al: Biomechanical considerations in patellofemoral joint rehabilitation, *Am J Sports Med* 21:438-444, 1993.)

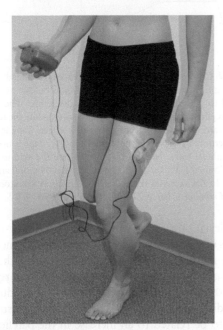

Figure 22-34 Electromyographic biofeedback can be used to facilitate quadriceps recruitment during functional tasks.

EMG biofeedback can be a useful tool for assessing general quadriceps muscle activation.

Taping and Bracing as an Adjunct to Strengthening. External patellar supports are commonly used in the management of PFP, typically as an adjunct to other treatment methods (e.g., strengthening). The primary goal of patellofemoral joint bracing and taping is to centralize the patella within the trochlear groove, thus improving patellar tracking.[174] The various patellofemoral braces on the market have used a number of methods to improve patellar tracking, including neoprene sleeves with patellar cutouts, lateral buttresses, air bladders, and various Velcro straps (Figure 22-35). However, the clinical effectiveness of patella stabilizing braces is questionable.[175,176] In contrast, the patellar taping technique described by McConnell[130,134] has been shown to be an effective option to reduce pain (Figures 22-36 and 22-37). In this protocol, rigid strapping tape is applied to the patella to correct malalignment (as determined by clinical evaluation). Various clinical studies support the therapeutic success of use of patellar taping to reduce pain in conjunction with other treatment methods.[177-179]

The fact that the various forms of external patellar supports have proved to be effective in reducing symptoms immediately after application[180-182] indicates that such orthoses have a mechanical effect on the patellofemoral joint. Although the literature supports the premise that bracing and/or taping reduces pain, the mechanism underlying this pain reduction does not appear to be related to changes in patellar tracking. For example, kinematic MRI studies have shown that patellar bracing has little effect on patellar tracking.[183,184] However, alternative mechanisms have been proposed. Using high-resolution MRI, Powers et al.[185] reported that patellar bracing had only a small influence on patellar alignment (i.e., lateral tilt and displacement); however, large increases in contact area between the patella and the trochlear groove were observed (Figure 22-38).

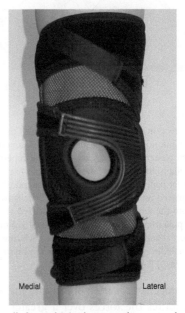

Figure 22-35 Patellofemoral joint brace used to control excessive lateral patella tracking (True-Pull, DJO Global, Inc., Vista, CA). The proximal and inferior straps attached to the lateral buttress are designed to limit lateral patella displacement.

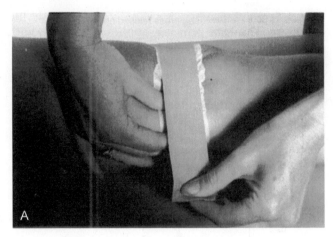

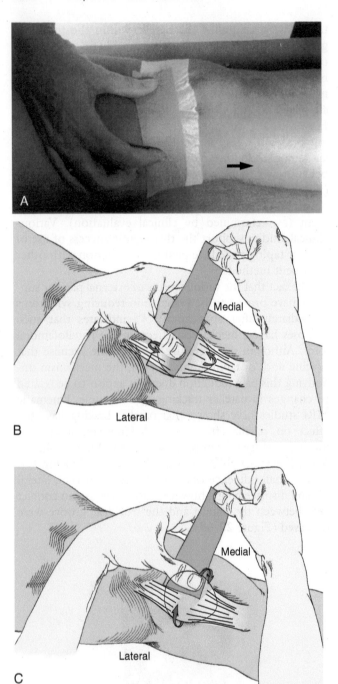

Figure 22-36 Correction of posterior and lateral tilt of the patella. **A** and **B,** To correct an inferior tilt, tape is placed on the superior half of the patella. An anteroposterior force is exerted on the superior aspect (the base) of the patella to lift the inferior pole (the apex) up and away from the infrapatellar fat pad. **A** and **C,** To correct a lateral tilt, anteroposterior pressure is placed on the medial half of the patella to lift the lateral border away from the femur while the tape is started at the midline of the patella and pulled medially. (From McConnell J, Fulkerson J: The knee: patellofemoral and soft tissue injuries. In Zachazewski JE, Magee DJ, Quillen WS, editors: *Athletic injuries and rehabilitation,* p 715, Philadelphia, 1996, WB Saunders.)

From a biomechanical standpoint, any increase in contact area distributes the forces over a greater surface area, thereby reducing joint stress (i.e., force per unit area). The results of the study by Powers et al.[185] suggest that changes in patellar alignment, by themselves, may not be responsible

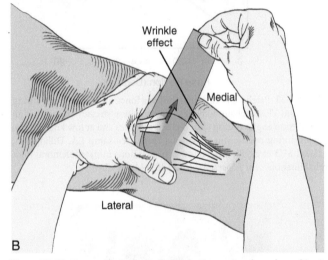

Figure 22-37 Correction of patella glide (excessive lateral tracking). **A** and **B,** Tape is placed just lateral to the lateral border of the patella and is used to glide the patella medially in the femur. The clinician's thumb helps glide the patella medially, if necessary, while the fingers pull the skin toward the patella, creating a wrinkle effect. Tape is anchored on the posteromedial aspect of the medial condyle. Tape is not brought into the popliteal fossa, because this may irritate the skin in this area. (From McConnell J, Fulkerson J: The knee: patellofemoral and soft tissue injuries. In Zachazewski JE, Magee DJ, Quillen WS, editors: *Athletic injuries and rehabilitation,* p 715, Philadelphia, 1996, WB Saunders.)

for the alleviation of pain with bracing. A follow-up study by Powers et al.[186] confirmed this hypothesis. Biomechanical modeling methods were used to demonstrate that application of a patellofemoral brace resulted in a reduction in both pain and patellofemoral stress in individuals with long-standing symptoms.[186] The reduction in stress was reported to be related to an increase in the patellofemoral joint contact area (as determined with MRI).

The literature makes it clear that external patellar supports can offer pain relief. This is significant from a clinical standpoint, because pain may influence quadriceps muscle inhibition. If the goal of conservative treatment of PFP is to strengthen the extensor mechanism, pain reduction is likely to facilitate recruitment of the quadriceps muscle. Such a reduction in pain allows for adequate exercise progression and subsequent muscle hypertrophy.

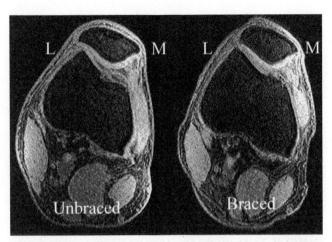

Figure 22-38 Axial MRI scans of the patellofemoral joint showing increased patellofemoral joint contact area after bracing. Note the increase in cartilage on cartilage contact (i.e., white on white) in the braced condition. *M,* medial; *L,* lateral.

Lower Extremity Dysfunction

In considering a treatment approach for abnormal lower extremity motions, it is important that the clinician keep in mind that altered mechanics can be driven from the foot upward or from the hips and pelvis downward. The ultimate goal in treatment of the lower extremity is to restore normal dynamic alignment and function. In many cases, interventions should be applied to both ends of the kinetic chain for maximum benefit.

Clinical Note

Treatment of patellofemoral pain syndrome involves not only treating the knee but also addressing leg and foot problems and especially balanced strength and endurance of the muscles of the hip.

Abnormal Foot Pronation

The decision of whether to use foot orthotics to control abnormal foot pronation should be based on a careful examination of the patient's gait or running pattern (or both). Patients who exhibit abnormal pronation and corresponding medial rotation of the tibia and femur are candidates for orthotics. If the patient shows excessive pronation but that motion does not appear to be transferred proximally (i.e., it is absorbed at the talocrural joint), orthotics may not be indicated. The clinician may want to consider a temporary orthotic to evaluate whether this approach is effective.

There is mixed evidence regarding the use of orthoses either in isolation or in combination with an exercise-based program for patients with PFP. However, at least one randomized, controlled trial[187] supported the short-term use of orthoses over placebo. The orthoses evaluated in this study were prefabricated, commercially available products and were noted to result in significant improved pain and function at 6 weeks. However, no differences were noted

between the group receiving orthoses and the placebo group at 12 weeks or 1 year. These data are consistent with the findings of Eng and Pierrynowski,[188] who found that both an orthotic group and a control group had significant reductions in pain after 8 weeks but that the orthotic group had significantly greater pain reduction than the control group. A series of studies have evaluated the predictors of success for orthoses in persons with PFP with varying results.[189-192] A systematic review on this topic concluded that foot orthoses for the treatment of PFP was most effective in older patients and those with greater forefoot valgus and rearfoot eversion, whereas exercise was more effective for younger patients.[193]

Abnormal Hip Medial Rotation and Adduction

If the femur is seen to "collapse" into medial rotation and/or adduction during the dynamic examination and this motion appears to originate from the hip or pelvis (as opposed to being influenced by tibial rotation), strengthening of the lateral rotators and abductors of the hip may be indicated. With excessive medial rotation, the emphasis should be on the gluteus maximus, because this muscle is optimally suited to control medial rotation of the femur. The posterior fibers of the gluteus medius and the deep rotators also contribute to dynamic stability of the femur; however, their lateral rotation torque capability at the femur is small in comparison. With excessive abduction, the focus should be on the gluteus medius. The upper fibers of the gluteus maximus also have an abduction component and should be addressed if excessive adduction is observed.

There is growing evidence that hip muscle strengthening is an important component of the rehabilitation plan for patients with PFP.[194-199] Two studies reported that isolated hip muscle and core strengthening resulted in superior pain relief in the short term and earlier pain relief in comparison to an exercise program focused on isolated knee muscle strengthening.[195,197] A separate randomized, controlled trial demonstrated that combining hip muscle strengthening along with knee muscle strengthening resulted in longer term reductions in pain and improved function at 1 year in comparison to a program focused solely on knee muscle strengthening.[194] Furthermore, Khayambashi et al.[199] reported that hip strengthening was superior to quadriceps strengthening in females with PFP, although it should be noted that both groups improved with respect to pain and function compared with baseline.

If hip weakness and altered hip motion are observed during the examination, patients should be placed on an exercise program that focuses on hip and pelvis stability during the performance of active lower extremity movements. According to Nadler et al.,[200] it is important to establish satisfactory lumbopelvic control to ensure that the proximal attachment sites for the hip abductors and lateral rotators are stable. Mascal et al.[201] outlined a three-phase treatment progression to enhance proximal control:

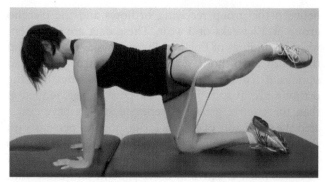

Figure 22-39 Non–weight-bearing exercise with band resistance to isolate the gluteus maximus. The hip should be extended, abducted, and laterally (externally) rotated.

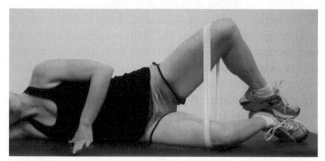

Figure 22-40 Side-lying (clam) exercise to strengthen the gluteus medius. Note that the hip rotates laterally (externally) during abduction.

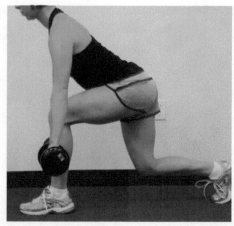

Figure 22-41 To increase the demand on the hip extensors, the forward lunge exercise should be performed with the trunk in a forward position.

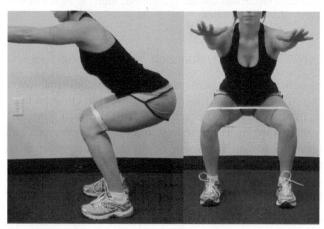

Figure 22-42 A TheraBand can be used to facilitate hip abductor and external rotator muscle action during the squat exercise. To increase hip extensor demand, the trunk should be in the forward position.

Treatment to Enhance Hip Control (Phase 1: Non–Weight-Bearing Hip Activation). Before dynamic weight-bearing strengthening of the hip musculature is started, patients should perform non–weight-bearing exercises with band resistance to isolate the gluteus maximus (Figure 22-39) and gluteus medius (Figure 22-40). When performing activation exercises for the gluteus medius, the patient must take care to minimize the contribution of the tensor fascia lata, because contraction of this muscle contributes to medial rotation of the lower extremity. Once the patient can isolate the muscles of interest while doing non–weight-bearing exercises and maintaining a stable pelvis, progression to weight-bearing strengthening can begin.

Treatment to Enhance Hip Control (Phase 2: Weight-Bearing Hip Strengthening). Weight-bearing exercises should include exercises performed in bilateral and single-limb stance. At this time, the patient should be introduced to the concept of a *hip strategy*. This involves doing exercises with increased hip flexion and a forward trunk lean. During a lunging exercise for example, increasing the forward trunk lean has been reported to increase the hip extensor torque along with activation of the gluteus maximus (Figure 22-41).[202] In addition, squat exercises should be performed with forward trunk posture. A band placed above the knees during squatting will facilitate the action of the gluteal muscles by adding concurrent resistance to hip abduction and lateral (external) rotation (Figure 22-42). With all exercises, care must be taken to ensure that the knee does not move forward or medial to the toes.

If the patient has a difficult time maintaining proper lower extremity alignment during the initiation of weight-bearing exercises, femoral strapping can be used to provide kinesthetic feedback and to augment muscular control and proprioception (Figure 22-43). Having patients perform weight-bearing exercises in front of a mirror can be useful. Also, taping or bracing of the patellofemoral joint may be used if pain is limiting the patient's ability to engage in a meaningful weight-bearing exercise program.

Treatment to Enhance Hip Control (Phase 3: Functional Movement Training). Once the patient can perform weight-bearing strengthening exercises without pain, exercises can be progressed to become more dynamic and functional. Patients should be encouraged to return to their sport or activity gradually once they can achieve satisfactory dynamic control. With competitive or recreational athletes who will be returning to full participation, plyometric training (i.e., jump training) should be considered as part of this transition period.

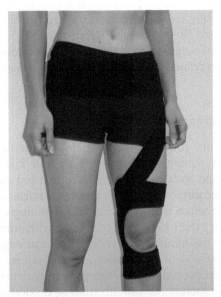

Figure 22-43 Femoral strapping (SERF Strap, DJO Global, Inc., Vista, CA) can be used to improve lower extremity control and kinematics during the rehabilitation program and functional activities.

Abnormal Gait Deviations

Facilitation of normal gait function is an essential component of the overall treatment plan. This is particularly important for the athlete (especially runners), in whom even a slight gait deviation can be exaggerated and can lead to injury at other joints. Clinicians should pay particular attention to reversal of the **quadriceps avoidance gait pattern** (i.e., walking with the knee extended or hyperextended). Because knee flexion during weight acceptance is critical for shock absorption, this key function must be restored to prevent the deleterious effects of high-impact loading.

As noted previously, the primary causes of quadriceps avoidance are pain, effusion, and quadriceps muscle weakness. As these components are addressed in other aspects of treatment, the clinician should keep in mind that resolution of symptoms may not readily translate into a more "normal" gait pattern. This is particularly evident in a patient with long-term pain and dysfunction. Movement patterns can be "learned," and the patient may need to be "reeducated" with respect to key gait deficiencies. EMG biofeedback can be an effective tool for this purpose, because visualization of quadriceps muscle activity can augment the reversal of the quadriceps avoidance gait pattern.

Overuse

A lack of significant findings on the physical examination (e.g., normal patella mechanics, normal lower extremity function) suggests that the source of symptoms may be related to overuse. This is typically the case in athletes. The treatment of choice for these individuals is control of symptoms and/or effusion, combined with rest and

activity modification. Muscle stretching and bracing of the patella also can be used if indicated. Reducing the repetitive forces applied through the joint allows healing of involved structures. Return to activity should be gradual and closely monitored. The training regimen should be evaluated for obvious errors, such as increasing exercise intensity too quickly and not allowing adequate time for recovery. When extended time-off is required, quadriceps and hip muscle strength should be maintained through careful application of resistive exercises (see the previous discussion).

SURGICAL CONSIDERATIONS

Conservative treatment for PFP may fail, even with the best therapy, medical management, bracing, and modification of activity. Some mechanical disorders of the knee extensor mechanism are too severe to respond fully to nonoperative treatment. Conditions that may resist nonoperative treatment include persistent patellar tilt, with or without chondrosis (i.e., cartilage deterioration) or subluxation; pathological plica; infrapatellar contracture; severe posttraumatic chondrosis-arthrosis (cartilage and joint deterioration); postoperative neuroma or scar pain; and recurrent dislocation. A tendency has arisen to use lateral release to treat any persistent anterior knee pain problem, rather than identifying a specific procedure to correct the underlying abnormality. This approach is not acceptable. For example, lateral release is appropriate only to relieve objectifiable tilt of the patella when nonoperative measures have failed.

Patellofemoral Joint Problems Requiring Surgery

- Persistent patella tilt
- Pathological plica
- Infrapatellar plica
- Severe posttraumatic chondrosis/arthrosis
- Postoperative neuroma
- Scar pain
- Recurrent dislocation

Obtaining a complete history before surgery is imperative. The clinician should determine what caused the onset of pain or instability. Was there a history of trauma, and is there any suggestion of generalized arthritis, referred pain, underlying structural deformity, or secondary pain? The clinician also should gain a feeling for the patient's personality (patients with dependent personalities are less likely to improve). If the onset of pain is spontaneous, the patient is more likely to have an underlying structural malalignment. The clinician should establish whether the primary problem is instability of the patella (i.e., subluxation or dislocation) or pain. If the problem is primarily pain, the clinician should determine whether it is more intra-articular or periarticular.

The physical examination is similar to that for a patient being evaluated for nonoperative treatment; however, greater emphasis is placed on identifying the specific sources and mechanical origins of pain, impairment, and dysfunction that require surgical intervention and that have not responded to conservative management.[203,204]

The knee should be evaluated for evidence of patella tilt, skin change, surgical scars, excessive varus or valgus, and contracture. The peripatellar retinaculum, patellar tendon, distal quadriceps, and infrapatellar area must be examined closely for evidence of neuroma, pain, and contracture. All surgical scars, including arthroscopy portals, should be palpated for induration and tenderness. Running a thumbnail along the scar easily determines pain (which, if present, suggests a scar neuroma). If the patient has had previous surgery, direct palpation should be performed to determine whether a tender residual band of the lateral retinaculum is present. Patellar alignment should be evaluated actively and passively. The examiner should note if the patella tracks laterally and if the patella appears to be above the level of the trochlea (i.e., patella alta) with the knee extended. Hypermobility, as well as abnormalities of medial and lateral displacement, should be noted. In particular, the examiner should note apprehension upon medial or lateral displacement of the patella as indicators of pathological instability. The examiner should firmly press on the patella to determine whether pain occurs on compression that reproduces the patient's complaints of discomfort. Pain reproduced by compression suggests articular cartilage breakdown (i.e., chondrosis).

The examiner also should note the degree of knee flexion pain or crepitation, because this helps localize a painful articular lesion (proximal lesions are painful in flexion past 75° to 80°, whereas distal lesions are painful close to full extension). This distal lesion, sometimes only softening of the distal pole patella, is common in young women with chronic lateral patellar tracking in early knee flexion. This is a source of unrelenting pain in some and commonly is missed, because alignment of the patella further into flexion as the trochlea deepens is often normal.

Any evidence of tilt or subluxation should be noted. In particular, the clinician must attempt to elevate the lateral patella away from the lateral trochlea to determine whether tethering of the patella laterally is present. Any alteration of normal skin temperature should be noted, such as might occur with reflex sympathetic dystrophy. The surgeon must take into consideration all diagnostic imaging studies in determining the significance of tilt or subluxation.

At the conclusion of the preoperative evaluation, the clinician should decide whether surgical treatment offers the patient a reasonable hope of improvement. A specific, correctable problem that can be defined must be identified. Is it tilt? Is arthrosis or chondrosis present, and if so, where is the lesion located? Is there a specific tender band of retinaculum or patella tendon? Does the patella track laterally so that the extensor mechanism needs to be realigned (in addition to lateral release)? Is there any evidence of neuroma or scar pain from previous surgery? Is the pain related to malalignment, or is it posttraumatic pain?

Lateral Release

Specific indications exist for lateral retinacular release, and many patients with resistant anterior knee pain do not respond to lateral retinacular release but can benefit from other surgical procedures. Surgical release of the lateral retinaculum is used to reduce a pathological patellar tilt (greater than 12°) in an individual with anterior knee pain who has minimal evidence of articular degeneration (e.g., arthrosis) or subluxation. Lateral release is not an appropriate procedure for treating many patients with significant instability (i.e., subluxation or dislocation) of the patella–extensor mechanism. Lateral release has been (and occasionally still is) recommended to treat patellar subluxations; however, axial radiography, CT, and laboratory studies using a cadaver knee model have clearly shown that lateral release does not consistently relieve signs and symptoms of patellar subluxation.[14,205]

Lateral release is not generally effective in relieving pain related to articular degeneration of the patella.[206] Once the lateral facet of the patella has collapsed and degeneration is evident,[67] releasing the lateral retinaculum does about as much to relieve contact stress on the degenerated cartilage as releasing the medial collateral ligament of a patient with medial compartment knee arthritis.

The clinician must also recognize that a lateral release is unlikely to lead to any meaningful change in a normally aligned patella that has been severely traumatized (e.g., fracture, dashboard injury) unless the patient has some secondary retinacular contracture and resulting patella tilt that needs to be released. Finally, lateral release, when done for the wrong reason, can leave a patient with a debilitating medial patella subluxation.[207]

Persistent Patella Tilt

Some patients with pathological patella tilt, with or without chondrosis or subluxation, do not respond to nonoperative treatment. In these patients the appropriate surgical procedure is best determined after the extent and location of articular lesions have been considered and the knee has been evaluated for evidence of subluxation associated with the tilt. In short, tilt with minimal evidence of articular degeneration or subluxation usually responds well to lateral release alone.[14] A possible exception is a patient with chondral softening on the medial facet, because these patients may have greater contact pressure on soft cartilage after lateral release.

Postoperative rehabilitation is aimed at maintaining the mobility of the lateral structures by taping the patella as soon as the sutures from the arthroscopy site have been removed and keeping the patella in the trochlea. Emphasis also must be placed on training of the gluteal muscles of the hip to minimize any increase in tension in an overactive tensor fascia lata and a tight ITB.

If grade 3 or grade 4 articular breakdown[208] is present on the lateral or distal medial facet in association with patellar tilt, an anteromedial tibial tubercle transfer (Trillat's procedure) is more effective than a lateral release,[209,210] particularly with any associated lateral patellar subluxation (Figure 22-44). If articular disease is not present but symptomatic subluxation is associated with patellar tilt, Trillat's procedure may be most appropriate when all nonoperative measures to control the instability have failed to provide adequate relief.[211]

Pathological Plica

Nonoperative treatment fails in some patients because of a persistent pathological plica. Most significant pathological plicae occur in the medial infrapatellar region and can be readily identified on clinical examination. To make this diagnosis, the clinician should be able to reproduce the patient's pain by palpating the plica. In most cases the plica is a prominent, palpable band. In our experience, arthroscopic excision of a pathological plica results in relief of pain in most patients. However, Broom and

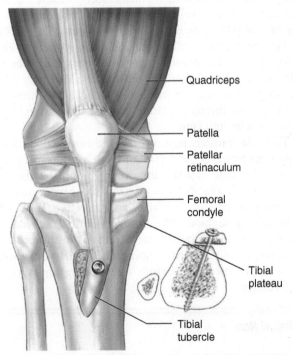

Figure 22-44 Medial tibial tubercle transfer. A distal bone–periosteum hinge is left, and one screw is used to fixate the osteotomy. The transfer reduces contact stress on the patella while the extensor mechanism has a more medial orientation, thus reducing the likelihood of lateral patellar dislocation of subluxation. (From Scott WN: *Insall and Scott surgery of the knee*, ed 5, Philadelphia, 2012, Churchill Livingstone.)

Labels in figure: Quadriceps; Patella; Patellar retinaculum; Femoral condyle; Tibial plateau; Tibial tubercle

Fulkerson[212] noted that pathological plicae sometimes may be associated with patellar malalignment. In patients with plicae, therefore, the examiner should be careful not to overlook other sources of pain related specifically to malalignment.

Infrapatellar Contracture

Infrapatellar contracture may occur after trauma or surgery involving the anterior knee. Although classic patella baja may occur, some patients with more subtle infrapatellar contractures may have persistent pain with relatively little evidence of contracture. Only a careful, pointed physical examination can detect this. Such patients usually have rather diffuse retropatellar tendon pain that often can be aggravated by squeezing or palpating the infrapatellar tendon area. An associated tightness of the medial and lateral retinaculum usually is noted.

In the authors' experience, once conservative rehabilitation fails, this condition must be evaluated arthroscopically, and open release of the contracture then is performed, usually through a short lateral incision. In most cases, lateral release is necessary, which often reveals a dense, tight infrapatellar fat pad. Release of the fat pad allows the surgeon to tilt the patella gradually up onto its medial edge, perpendicular to the trochlea. Complete release of infrapatellar scars, meticulous hemostasis, and immediate postoperative knee mobilization to full flexion are imperative in these patients. The results generally are excellent in properly selected patients when adequate release and debridement are performed.

Posttraumatic Chondrosis or Arthrosis

Time is particularly important in the treatment of patients who have sustained trauma to the anterior knee. The clinician should remember that intraosseous homeostasis can take 18 months or longer after injury.[213] The clinician must carefully assess the degree of pain and whether the patient can reasonably tolerate a prolonged period of activity modification and supportive management to allow spontaneous homeostasis. However, it is impossible to know whether pain relief will be obtained after such a long period, and patients with more severe pain cannot always tolerate this much time without treatment. Supportive measures include repeated ice applications, nonsteroidal anti-inflammatory medications, bracing, taping, and reassurance. Exercising, particularly resisted knee extension, is counterproductive in some of these patients.

Once the decision has been made to operate, the problem is whether the patella can be salvaged. Arthroscopic examination and debridement allow the surgeon to evaluate the extent of chondral injury once all soft tissue and retinacular problems have been addressed. At the time of an initial arthroscopic procedure, any posttraumatic neuroma, indurate (painful) retinaculum or tendon, and thickened plica or fibrillated articular cartilage should be excised. In most patients the lateral retinaculum need not be released unless a significant tilt aggravates the problem. Patellectomy is not commonly performed as the initial procedure, because many patients may benefit from soft tissue (i.e., retinacular) and articular (i.e., chondroplasty) debridement or patella realignment. If articular debridement has been performed, the clinician initially must avoid compression on the newly debrided area and must communicate with the surgeon to determine the site of the chondroplasty. Resurfacing of a severely damaged patella, sometimes in combination with an unloading tibial tubercle osteotomy, may be helpful in attempts to salvage the joint.[203]

If arthroscopic treatment fails, a decision should be made as to whether the articular cartilage is sufficient to allow transposition of the tibial tubercle (usually either medially, anteriorly, or both) to shift contact stress from damaged to healthy cartilage. In patients with extensive articular damage and intractable pain, patellectomy and patellofemoral resurfacing may be the only viable options. Resurfacing possibilities include autologous cartilage transplantation, allograft osteochondral transplantation, patellofemoral arthroplasty, and total knee replacement.

If healthy cartilage is present proximally on the patella, the tibial tubercle may be moved anteriorly. If the best remaining cartilage is proximal and medial, the patella should be moved anteromedially. Long-term results with this procedure have been favorable.[214] If the proximal patellar cartilage is severely damaged (as it often is after a dashboard injury), tibial tubercle anteriorization is less likely to be successful. In this case patellectomy or resurfacing may need to be considered.

Postoperative Neuroma or Scar Pain

A patient who has already had surgery and who complains of persistent pain that is different from the original pain may have a postoperative neuroma or painful scar. This is a clinical diagnosis, and it usually is not difficult to determine as long as the examiner is looking for it. The thumbnail test (running the dorsum of the thumbnail over each scar) elicits the sharp pain of a neuroma in most cases. The clinician must make sure that this is not a diffuse sensitivity, suggesting reflex sympathetic dystrophy. Patients with reflex sympathetic dystrophy are not surgical candidates and may require pain management programs, sympathetic blocks, or surgical sympathectomy.

Sensitive scar or neuroma can be relieved transiently in the office by injection of a local anesthetic (this confirms the diagnosis). Administration of corticosteroids in conjunction with the local anesthetic does not usually provide lasting benefit to patients with a neuroma. In general, if nonoperative management has failed and the patient demonstrates a localized focus of pain in a scar, excision of this painful segment of tissue may be curative.

Recurrent Patellar Dislocation

Recurrent patellar dislocation can be devastating to the patellar articular cartilage, and this condition generally warrants early surgery if nonoperative treatment fails to restore stable tracking of the patella. Each patellar dislocation may result in a shearing off of articular cartilage from the medial patella facet or lateral femoral trochlea. The cartilage may be stripped from the bone so that it cannot be replaced. Consequently, restoration of stable patella tracking is important, preferably before serious cartilage damage occurs.

After an acute patellar dislocation, any fragment of articular cartilage with bone attached should be replaced anatomically, generally using an open lateral release incision and eversion of the patella to expose its medial facet for reconstruction. Very fine absorbable sutures (8-0 or smaller) may help approximate the cartilage edges.

In the authors' experience, patellar stability is best restored using a lateral release and tibial tubercle transfer as described by Trillat et al.[215] and reviewed by Cox[211] when the patella is tracking laterally with an elevated Q angle or tibial tubercle–trochlear groove (TT-TG) measurement. Overzealous medial imbrication (i.e., overlapping of free edges) poses a substantial risk of increasing contact pressure on the medial patella facet (because the medial retinaculum is oriented so that its imbrication pulls the medial patella facet posteriorly as well as medially). If damage to the medial patella already is present after dislocation, anteromedial transfer of the tibial tubercle minimizes the load increase on the medial patella while reorienting the extensor mechanism medially to minimize and eliminate the risk of lateral patellar dislocation in patients with maltracking.

Tubercle transfer, however, should not be considered in patients with trochlear dysplasia who have normal tracking of the patella. It is also important to note whether the patient has patella alta, because this too predisposes the individual to patellar instability and therefore, should be corrected by slight distalization of the tibial tubercle at the time of tibial tubercle transfer. It is most important, however, to reiterate the importance of first exhausting conservative measures before undertaking any surgical intervention.

Clinical Note

Conservative treatment measures for patellofemoral problems should be exhausted before surgical intervention is contemplated.

In cases of involving minimum degrees of subluxation and minimal trochlear dysplasia, stability usually can be

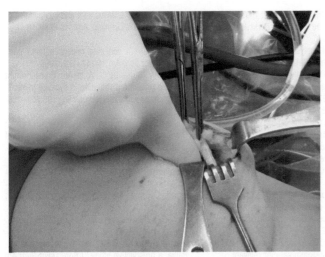

Figure 22-45 Palpation of the medial quadriceps tendon–femoral ligament (MQTFL).

restored through specific advancement of the medial retinaculum, including the medial quadriceps tendon–femoral ligament (MQTFL) (see Figure 22-7), which interdigitates with the VMO. The MQTFL remnant can be easily palpated through a small incision after the VMO has been lifted off the patella (Figure 22-45).[216,217] In our experience, after dislocation, the MQTFL remnant usually heals and provides a satisfactory structure for advancement,

such that formal tendon transfer reconstruction of the MQTFL is rarely indicated. Nonetheless, full MQTFL reconstruction sometimes is needed. This procedure is technically demanding; small errors in graft placement can lead to overload and even late destruction of the patellofemoral joint.[218] Tibial tubercle transfer should not be performed in a skeletally immature patient. Lateral release and careful MQTFL advancement, properly performed, should provide adequate stability in most cases.

SUMMARY

Surgical treatment can be extremely helpful in the management of patients with anterior knee pain resistant to nonoperative treatment. It is most important to direct surgical treatment specifically to the precise cause of the knee pain. Painful articular lesions should be debrided and unloaded, painful segments of the retinaculum or scar excised, alignment corrected, tilt relieved by lateral release, pathological plicae excised, and contractures released. Surgery should not be undertaken until the clinician has a clear concept of what needs to be corrected and the patient understands the risks involved and the potential benefits. The chosen surgical procedure requires appropriate postoperative management to optimize outcomes.

REFERENCES

1. Wood L, Muller S, Peat G: The epidemiology of patellofemoral disorders in adulthood: a review of routine general practice morbidity recording, *Prim Health Care Res Dev* 12:157–164, 2011.
2. Boling MC, Padua DA, Marshall SW, et al: A prospective investigation of biomechanical risk factors for patellofemoral pain syndrome: the Joint Undertaking to Monitor and Prevent ACL Injury (JUMP-ACL) cohort, *Am J Sports Med* 37:2108–2116, 2009.
3. Renstrom AF: Knee pain in tennis players, *Clin Sports Med* 14:163–175, 1995.
4. Taunton JE, Ryan MB, Clement DB, et al: A retrospective case-control analysis of 2002 running injuries, *Br J Sports Med* 36:95–101, 2002.
5. Boling M, Padua D, Marshall S, et al: Gender differences in the incidence and prevalence of patellofemoral pain syndrome, *Scand J Med Sci Sports* 20:725–730, 2010.
6. Stathopulu E, Baildam E: Anterior knee pain: a long-term follow-up, *Rheumatology* 42:380–382, 2003.
7. Blond L, Hansen L: Patellofemoral pain syndrome in athletes: a 5.7-year retrospective follow-up study of 250 athletes, *Acta Orthop Belgica* 64:393–400, 1998.
8. Davis IS, Powers CM: Patellofemoral pain syndrome: proximal, distal and local factors an international retreat, *J Orthop Sports Phys Ther* 40:A1–A16, 2010.
9. Powers CM, Bolgla LA, Callaghan M, et al: Patellofemoral pain: proximal, distal and local factors, 2nd International Research Retreat, *J Orthop Sports Phys Ther* 42:A1–A54, 2012.
10. Witrouw E, Callaghan MJ, Stefanik JJ, et al: Patellofemoral pain: consensus statement from the 3rd International Patellofemoral Pain Research Retreat held in Vancouver, September 2013, *Br J Sports Med* 48:411–414, 2014.
11. Reider B, Marshall JL, Koslin B, et al: The anterior aspect of the knee joint, *J Bone Joint Surg Am* 63:351–356, 1981.
12. Calliet R: *Knee pain and disability*, ed 2, Philadelphia, 1990, FA Davis.
13. Wiberg G: Roentgenographic and anatomic studies on the femoro-patellar joint, *Acta Orthop Scand* 12:319–410, 1941.
14. Fulkerson JP, Hungerford DS: *Disorders of the patellofemoral joint*, ed 2, Baltimore, 1990, Williams & Wilkins.
15. Hertling D, Kessler RM: *Management of common musculoskeletal disorders: physical therapy principles and methods*, ed 2, Philadelphia, 1990, JB Lippincott.
16. Romanes GJ: *Cunningham's textbook of anatomy*, ed 12, New York, 1981, Oxford University Press.
17. Hughston J, Andrews J: The suprapatella plica and internal derangement, *J Bone Joint Surg Am* 55:1318–1319, 1973.
18. Gallagher J, Tierney P, Murray P, et al: The infrapatellar fat pad: anatomy and clinical correlations, *Knee Surg Sports Traumatol Arthrosc* 13:268–272, 2005.
19. Aydingoz U, Oguz B, Aydingoz O, et al: Recesses along the posterior margin of the infrapatellar (Hoffa's) fat pad: prevalence and morphology on routine MR imaging of the knee, *Eur Radiol* 15:988–994, 2005.
20. Bohnsack M, Meier F, Walter GF, et al: Distribution of substance-P nerves inside the infrapatellar fat pad and the adjacent synovial tissue: a neurohistological approach to anterior knee pain syndrome, *Arch Orthop Trauma Surg* 125:592–597, 2005.
21. Scapinelli R: Vascular anatomy of the human cruciate ligaments and surrounding structures, *Clin Anat* 10:151–162, 1997.
22. Witonski D, Wagrowska-Danilewicz M: Distribution of substance-P nerve fibers in intact and ruptured human anterior cruciate ligament: a semi-quantitative immunohistochemical assessment, *Knee Surg Sports Traumatol Arthrosc* 12:497–502, 2004.
23. Roth C, Jacobson J: Jamadar et al: Quadriceps fat pad signal intensity and enlargement on MRI: prevalence and associated findings, *Am J Roentgenol* 182:1383–1387, 2004.
24. Starok M, Lenchik L, Trudell D, et al: Normal patellar retinaculum: MR and sonographic imaging with cadaveric correlation, *Am J Roentgenol* 168:1493–1499, 1997.
25. Fulkerson JP, Gossling HR: Anatomy of the knee joint lateral retinaculum, *Clin Orthop* 153:183–185, 1993.
26. Puniello MS: Iliotibial band tightness and medial patellar glide in patients with patellofemoral dysfunction, *J Orthop Sports Phys Ther* 17:144–148, 1993.
27. Fulkerson JP, Edgar C: Medial quadriceps tendon-femoral ligament: surgical anatomy and reconstruction technique to prevent patella instability, *Arthrosc Tech* 2:125–128, 2013.
28. Farahmand F, Naghi Tahmasbi M, Amis A: The contribution of the medial retinaculum and quadriceps muscles to patellar lateral stability: an in vitro study, *Knee* 11:89–94, 2004.

29. Ishibashi Y, Okamura Y, Otsuka H, et al: Lateral patellar retinaculum tension in patellar instability, *Clin Orthop Rel Res* 397:362–369, 2002.

30. Powers CM, Chen YJ, Farrokhi S, et al: The role of the peripatellar retinaculum in the transmission of forces within the extensor mechanism, *J Bone Joint Surg Am* 88:2042–2048, 2006.

31. Sanchis-Alfonso V, Rosello-Sastre E, Revert F: Immunohistochemical analysis for neural markers of the lateral retinaculum in patients with isolated symptomatic patellofemoral malalignment: a neuroanatomic basis for anterior knee pain in the active young patient, *Am J Sports Med* 28:725–731, 2000.

32. Fulkerson J, Tennant R, Jaivin J, et al: Histologic evidence of retinacular nerve injury associated with patellofemoral malalignment, *Clin Orthop* 197:196–205, 1985.

33. Dye SF: Patellofemoral anatomy. In Fox JM, Del Pizzo W, editors: *The patellofemoral joint*, New York, 1993, McGraw-Hill.

34. Terry GC: The anatomy of the extensor mechanism, *Clin Sports Med* 8:163–177, 1989.

35. Lieb FJ, Perry J: Quadriceps function: an anatomical and mechanical study using amputated limbs, *J Bone Joint Surg Am* 50:1535–1548, 1968.

36. Hubbard JK, Sampson HW, Elledge JR: Prevalence and morphology of the vastus medialis oblique in human cadavers, *Anat Rec* 249:135–142, 1997.

37. Powers CM, Lilly JC, Lee TQ: The effects of anatomically based multi-planar loading of the extensor mechanism on patellofemoral joint mechanics, *Clin Biomech* 13:608–615, 1998.

38. Shellock FG, Mink JH, Deutsch A, et al: Kinematic MRI of the joints: techniques and clinical applications, *Magn Reson Q* 7:104–135, 1991.

39. Shellock FG, Mink JH, Deutsch AL, et al: Patellofemoral joint: identification of abnormalities using active movement, "unloaded" versus "loaded" kinematic MR imaging techniques, *Radiology* 188:575–578, 1993.

40. Powers CM, Shellock FG, Pfaff M: Quantification of patellar tracking using MRI, *J Magn Reson Imaging* 8:724–732, 1998.

41. Hungerford DS, Barry M: Biomechanics of the patellofemoral joint, *Clin Orthop Relat Res* 144:9–15, 1979.

42. Van Kampen A, Huiskes R: The three-dimensional tracking pattern of the human patella, *J Orthop Res* 8:372–382, 1990.

43. Soderberg GL: *Kinesiology: application to pathological motion*, Baltimore, 1986, Williams & Wilkins.

44. Goodfellow J, Hungerford DS, Zindel M: Patellofemoral joint mechanics and pathology: functional anatomy of the patello-femoral joint, *J Bone Joint Surg Br* 58:287–290, 1976.

45. Salsich GB, Ward SR, Ter MR, et al: In vivo assessment of patellofemoral joint contact area in individuals who are pain free, *Clin Orthop Rel Res* 414:277–284, 2003.

46. Insall J: Patellar malalignment syndrome, *Orthop Clin North Am* 10:117–122, 1979.

47. Smith LK, Weiss W, Lehmkuhl LD: *Brunnstrom's clinical kinesiology*, ed 5, Philadelphia, 1996, FA Davis.

48. Schulthies SS, Francis RS, Fisher AG, et al: Does the Q angle reflect the force on the patella in the frontal plane? *Phys Ther* 75:24–30, 1995.

49. Dye SF: Functional anatomy and biomechanics of the patellofemoral joint. In Scott WN, editor: *The knee*, St Louis, 1994, Mosby.

50. Kaufer H: Mechanical function of the patella, *J Bone Joint Surg Am* 53:1551–1560, 1971.

51. Fletcher SS, Thompson CH, Lipke J, et al: The effect of patellectomy on knee function, *J Bone Joint Surg Am* 58:537–540, 1976.

52. Smidt GL: Biomechanical analysis of knee flexion and extension, *J Biomech* 6:79–92, 1973.

53. Perry J, Antonelli D, Ford W: Analysis of knee joint forces during flexed-knee stance, *J Bone Joint Surg Am* 57:961–967, 1975.

54. Yamaguchi GT, Zajac FE: A planar model of the knee joint to characterize the knee extensor mechanism, *J Biomech* 22:1–10, 1989.

55. Maquet PG: *Biomechanics of the knee: with application to the pathogenesis and the surgical treatment of osteoarthritis*, ed 2, Berlin, 1984, Springer-Verlag.

56. Reilly DT, Martens M: Experimental analysis of the quadriceps muscle force and patello-femoral joint reaction force for various activities, *Acta Orthop Scand* 43:126–137, 1972.

57. Hungerford DS, Lennox DW: Rehabilitation of the knee in disorders of the patellofemoral joint: relevant biomechanics, *Orthop Clin North Am* 14:397–402, 1983.

58. Buff HU, Jones LC, Hungerford DS: Experimental determination of forces transmitted through the patellofemoral joint, *J Biomech* 21:17–23, 1988.

59. Brechter JH, Powers CM: Patellofemoral joint stress during stair ascent and descent in persons with and without patellofemoral pain, *Gait Posture* 16:115–123, 2002.

60. Heino-Brechter JG, Powers CM: Patellofemoral joint stress during level walking in subjects with and without patellofemoral joint pain, *Med Sci Sports Exerc* 32:1582–1593, 2000.

61. Salsich GB, Brechter JH, Powers CM: Lower extremity kinetics during stair ambulation in patients with and without patellofemoral pain, *Clin Biomech* 16:906–912, 2001.

62. Scott S, Winter DA: Internal forces at chronic running injury sites, *Med Sci Sports Exerc* 22:357–369, 1990.

63. Dye SF: Therapeutic implications of a tissue homeostasis approach to patellofemoral pain, *Sports Med Arthrosc Rev* 9:306–311, 2001.

64. Farrokhi S, Keyak JH, Powers CM: Individuals with patellofemoral pain exhibit greater patellofemoral joint stress: a finite element analysis study, *Osteoarthritis Cartilage* 19:287–294, 2011.

65. Ho KY, Keyak JH, Powers CM: Comparison of patella bone strain between females with and without patellofemoral pain: a finite element analysis study, *J Biomech* 47:230–236, 2014.

66. Fredericson M, Powers CM: Practical management of patellofemoral pain, *Clin J Sport Med* 12:36–38, 2002.

67. Ficat P, Ficat C, Bailleux A: Syndrome d'hyperpression externe de la rotule, *Rev Chir Orthop* 61:39–59, 1975.

68. Powers CM: Patellar kinematics. I. The influence of vastus muscle activity in subjects with and without patellofemoral pain, *Phys Ther* 80:956–964, 2000.

69. Powers CM: Patellar kinematics. II. The influence of the depth of the trochlear groove in subjects with and without patellofemoral pain, *Phys Ther* 80:965–978, 2000.

70. Schutzer SF, Ramsby GR, Fulkerson JP: The evaluation of patellofemoral pain using computerized tomography: a preliminary study, *Clin Orthop* 204:286–293, 1986.

71. Seedholm BB, Takeda T, Tsubuku M, et al: Mechanical factors and patellofemoral osteoarthritis, *Ann Rheum Dis* 38:307–316, 1979.

72. Linn FC, Sokoloff L: Movement and composition of interstitial fluid of cartilage, *Arthritis Rheum* 8:481–494, 1965.

73. Insall J: Current concepts review: patellar pain, *J Bone Joint Surg Am* 64:147–152, 1982.

74. Ahmed AM, Burke DL, Yu A: In-vitro measurement of static pressure distribution in synovial joints. II. Retropatellar surface, *J Biomed Eng* 105:231–236, 1983.

75. Fulkerson JP, Schutzer SF, Ramsby GR, et al: Computerized tomography of the patellofemoral joint before and after lateral release or realignment, *Arthroscopy* 3:19–24, 1987.

76. Douchette SA, Goble EM: The effects of exercise on patellar tracking in lateral patellar compression syndrome, *Am J Sports Med* 20:434–440, 1992.

77. Heywood WB: Recurrent dislocation of the patella, *J Bone Joint Surg Br* 43:508–517, 1961.

78. Insall J, Falvo KA, Wise DW: Chondromalacia patellae: a prospective study, *J Bone Joint Surg Am* 58:1–8, 1976.

79. Shellock FG, Mink JH, Deutsch A, et al: Evaluation of patients with persistent symptoms after lateral retinacular release by kinematic magnetic resonance imaging of the patellofemoral joint, *Arthroscopy* 6:226–234, 1990.

80. Ward SR, Powers CM: The influence of patella alta on patellofemoral joint stress during normal and fast walking, *Clin Biomech* 19:1040–1047, 2004.

81. Insall J, Salvati E: Patellar position in the normal knee joint, *Radiology* 101:101–109, 1971.

82. Brattstrom H: Shape of the intercondylar groove normally and in recurrent dislocation of the patella, *Acta Orthop Scand* 68:85–138, 1964.

83. Vainionpaa S, Laasonen E, Patiala H, et al: Acute dislocation of the patella: clinical, radiographic and operative findings in 64 consecutive cases, *Acta Orthop Scand* 57:331–333, 1986.

84. Hvid I, Lars LI, Schmidt H: Patellar height and femoral trochlear development, *Acta Orthop Scand* 54:91–93, 1983.

85. Varadarajan KM, Freiberg AA, Gill TJ, et al: Relationship between three dimensional geometry of the trochlear groove and in vivo patellar tracking during weight-bearing knee flexion, *J Biomech Eng* 132:061008, 2010.

86. Harbaugh CM, Wilson NA, Sheehan FT: Correlating femoral shape with patellar kinematics in patients with patellofemoral pain, *J Orthop Res* 28:865–872, 2010.

87. Teng HL, Chen YJ, Powers CM: Predictors of patella alignment: an examination of patella height and trochlea geometry, *Knee* 21:142–146, 2014.

88. Stefanik JJ, Roemer FW, Zumwalt AC, et al: Association between measures of trochlear morphology and structural features of patellofemoral joint osteoarthritis on MRI: the MOST study, *J Orthop Res* 30:1–8, 2012.

89. Huberti HH, Hayes WC: Patellofemoral contact pressures: the influence of Q angle and tendofemoral contact, *J Bone Joint Surg Am* 66:715–724, 1984.

90. Crane LC: Femoral torsion and its relation to toeing-in and toeing-out, *J Bone Joint Surg Am* 41:421–428, 1959.

91. Kozic S, Gulan G, Matovinovic D, et al: Femoral anteversion related to side difference in hip rotation, *Acta Orthop Scand* 68:533–536, 1997.

92. Staheli LT: Medial femoral torsion, *Orthop Clin North Am* 11:39–49, 1980.

93. Svenningsen S, Terjesen T, Auflem M, et al: Hip rotation and in-toeing gait: a study of normal subjects from four years until adult age, *Clin Orthop Rel Res* 251:177–182, 1990.

94. Powers CM: The influence of altered lower-extremity kinematics on patellofemoral joint dysfunction: a theoretical perspective, *J Orthop Sports Phys Ther* 33:639–646, 2003.

95. Jeffreys TE: Recurrent dislocation of the patella due to abnormal attachment of the ilio-tibial tract, *J Bone Joint Surg Br* 45:740–743, 1963.

96. Hughston JC, Deese M: Medial subluxation of the patella as a complication of lateral release, *Am J Sports Med* 16:383–388, 1988.

97. Fox TA: Dysplasia of the quadriceps mechanism: hypoplasia of the vastus medialis muscle as related to the hypermobile patella syndrome, *Surg Clin North Am* 55:199–226, 1975.

98. Hanten WP, Schulthies SS: Exercise effect on electromyographic activity of the vastus medialis oblique and the vastus lateralis muscles, *Phys Ther* 70:561–565, 1990.

99. Reynolds L, Levin TA, Medeiros JM, et al: EMG activity of the vastus medialis oblique and the vastus lateralis in their role in patellar alignment, *Am J Phys Med* 62:61–70, 1983.

100. Basmajian JV, Harden TP, Regenos EM: Integrated actions of the four heads of quadriceps femoris: an electromyographic study, *Anat Rec* 172:15–20, 1972.

101. Spencer JD, Hayes KC, Alexander IJ: Knee joint effusion and quadriceps reflex inhibition in man, *Arch Phys Med Rehabil* 65:171–177, 1984.

102. Stratford P: Electromyography of the quadriceps femoris muscles in subjects with normal knees and acutely effused knees, *Phys Ther* 62:279–283, 1981.

103. Bennett JG, Stauber WT: Evaluation and treatment of anterior knee pain using eccentric exercise, *Med Sci Sports Exerc* 18:526–530, 1986.

104. Smillie IS: *Injuries of the knee joint*, ed 3, Baltimore, 1962, Williams & Wilkins.

105. Stener B: Reflex inhibition of quadriceps elicited from subperiosteal tumour of the femur, *Acta Orthop Scand* 40:86–91, 1969.

106. DeAndrade JR, Grant C, Dixon A: Joint distension and reflex muscle inhibition in the knee, *J Bone Joint Surg Am* 47:313–322, 1965.

107. Stokes M, Young A: Investigations of quadriceps inhibition: implications for clinical practice, *Physiotherapy* 70:425–428, 1984.

108. Mariani PP, Caruso I: An electromyographic investigation of subluxation of the patella, *J Bone Joint Surg Br* 61-B:169–171, 1979.

109. Souza DR, Gross MT: Comparison of vastus medialis obliquus: vastus lateralis muscle integrated electromyographic ratios between healthy subjects and patients with patellofemoral pain, *Phys Ther* 71:310–316, 1991.

110. Wise HH, Fiebert IM, Kates JL: EMG biofeedback as treatment for patellofemoral pain syndrome, *J Orthop Sports Phys Ther* 6:95–103, 1984.

111. Boucher JP, King MA, Lefebvre R, et al: Quadriceps femoris muscle activity in patellofemoral pain syndrome, *Am J Sports Med* 20:527–532, 1992.

112. MacIntyre DL, Robertson GE: Quadriceps muscle activity in women runners with and without patellofemoral pain syndrome, *Arch Phys Med Rehabil* 73:10–14, 1992.

113. Moller BN, Krebs B, Tidemand-Dal C, et al: Isometric contractions in the patellofemoral pain syndrome: an electromyographic study, *Arch Orthop Trauma Surg* 105:24–27, 1986.

114. Wild JJ, Franklin TD, Woods GW: Patellar pain and quadriceps rehabilitation: an EMG study, *Am J Sports Med* 10:12–15, 1982.

115. Cowan SM, Bennell KL, Hodges PW, et al: Delayed onset of electromyographic activity of vastus me-

116. Cowan SM, Hodges PW, Bennell KL, et al: Altered vastii recruitment when people with patellofemoral pain syndrome complete a postural task, *Arch Phys Med Rehabil* 83:989–995, 2002.

117. Powers CM, Landel R, Perry J: Timing and intensity of vastus muscle activity during functional activities in subjects with and without patellofemoral pain, *Phys Ther* 76:946–955, 1996.

118. Shellock FG, Mink JH, Deutsch AL, et al: Kinematic MR imaging of the patellofemoral joint: comparison of passive positioning and active movement techniques, *Radiology* 184:574–577, 1992.

119. Powers CM: The influence of abnormal hip mechanics on knee injury: a biomechanical perspective, *J Orthop Sports Phys Ther* 40:42–51, 2010.

120. Reischl SF, Powers CM, Rao S, et al: The relationship between foot pronation and rotation of the tibia and femur during walking, *Foot Ankle Int* 20:513–520, 1999.

121. Tiberio D: The effect of excessive subtalar joint pronation on patellofemoral joint mechanics: a theoretical model, *J Orthop Sports Phys Ther* 9:160–169, 1987.

122. Powers CM, Ward SR, Fredericson M, et al: Patellofemoral kinematics during weight-bearing and non-weight-bearing knee extension in persons with lateral subluxation of the patella: a preliminary study, *J Orthop Sports Phys Ther* 33:677–685, 2003.

123. Souza RB, Draper CE, Fredericson M, et al: Femur rotation and patellofemoral joint kinematics: a weight-bearing MRI analysis, *J Orthop Sports Phys Ther* 40:277–285, 2010.

124. Souza RB, Powers CM: Differences in hip kinematics, muscle strength and muscle activation between subjects with and without patellofemoral pain, *J Orthop Sports Phys Ther* 39:12–19, 2009.

125. Ireland ML, Willson JD, Ballantyne BT, et al: Hip strength in females with and without patellofemoral pain, *J Orthop Sports Phys Ther* 33:671–676, 2003.

126. Bolgla LA, Malone TR, Umberger BR, et al: Hip strength and hip and knee kinematics during stair descent in females with and without patellofemoral pain syndrome, *J Orthop Sports Phys Ther* 38:12–18, 2008.

127. Souza RB, Powers CM: Predictors of hip rotation during running: an evaluation of hip strength and femoral structure in women with and without patellofemoral pain, *Am J Sports Med* 37:579–587, 2009.

128. Thomee R, Tenstrom P, Karlsson J, et al: Patellofemoral pain syndrome in young women: a critical analysis of alignment, pain parameters, common symptoms and functional activity level, *Scand J Med Sci Sports* 5:237–244, 1995.

129. Abernathy PJ, Townsend P, Rose R, et al: Is chondromalacia a separate clinical entity? *J Bone Joint Surg Br* 60-B:205–210, 1978.

130. Grelsamer RP, McConnell J: *The patella: a team approach*, Gaithersburg, MD, 1998, Aspen.

131. Hoppenfeld S: *Physical examination of the spine and extremities*, Norwalk, CT, 1976, Appleton-Century-Crofts.

132. Pattyn E, Verdonk P, Steyaert A, et al: Vatus medialis obliquus atrophy: does it exist in patellofemoral pain syndrome? *Am J Sports Med* 39:1450–1455, 2011.

133. Balcarek P, Oberthür S, Frosch S, et al: Vastus medialis obliquus muscle morphology in primary and

recurrent lateral patellar instability, *Biomed Res Int* 2014:326586, 2014. Epub 2014 Apr 29.

134. McConnell J: The management of chondromalacia patellae: a long term solution, *Aust J Physiother* 32:215–223, 1986.

135. Powers CM, Mortenson S, Nishimoto D, et al: Concurrent criterion-related validity of a clinical measurement used for determining the medial/lateral component of patellar orientation, *J Orthop Sports Phys Ther* 29:372–377, 1999.

136. Watson CJ, Propps M, Galt W, et al: Reliability of McConnell's classification of patellar orientation in symptomatic and asymptomatic subjects, *J Orthop Sports Phys Ther* 29:378–385, 1999.

137. Konin JG, Wiksten DL, Isear JA: *Special tests for orthopedic examination*, Thorofare, NJ, 1997, Slack.

138. Neumann DA: *Kinesiology of the musculoskeletal system: foundations for physical rehabilitation*, St Louis, 2002, Mosby.

139. Arnold AS, Komattu AV, Delp SL: Internal rotation gait: a compensatory mechanism to restore abduction capacity decreased by bone deformity, *Dev Med Child Neurol* 39:40–44, 1997.

140. Perry J: *Gait analysis: normal and pathological function*, ed 2, Thorofare, NJ, 2010, Slack.

141. Souza RB, Powers CM: Concurrent criterion-related validity and reliability of a clinical test to measure femoral anteversion, *J Orthop Sports Phys Ther* 39:586–592, 2009.

142. Insall J, Goldberg V, Salvati E: Recurrent dislocation and the high riding patella, *Clin Orthop* 88:67–69, 1972.

143. Laurin C, Levesque H, Dussault S, et al: The abnormal lateral patellofemoral angle, *J Bone Joint Surg Am* 60:55–60, 1978.

144. Laurin CA: Patellar position, patellar osteotomy: their relationship to chondromalacia—x-ray diagnosis of chondromalacia. In Pickett J.C., Radin E.L., editors: Chondromalacia of the patella, vol 2, Baltimore, 1983, Williams & Wilkins.

145. Bradley W, Ominsky S: Mountain view of the patella, *Am J Radiology* 136:53–57, 1981.

146. Imai N, Tomatsu T, Nakaseko J, Terada H: Clinical and roentgenological studies on malalignment of the patellofemoral joint. II. Relationship between predisposing factors and malalignment of the patellofemoral joint, *J Jpn Orthop Assoc* 61:1191–1202, 1987.

147. Newberg AH, Seligson D: The patellofemoral joint: 30 degrees, 60 degrees, and 90 degrees, *Radiology* 137:57–61, 1980.

148. Merchant AC, Mercer RL, Jacobsen RH, et al: Roentgenographic analysis of patellofemoral congruence, *J Bone Joint Surg Am* 56:1391–1396, 1974.

149. Brossmann J, Muhle C, Schorder C, et al: Patellar tracking patterns during active and passive knee extension: evaluation with motion triggered cine MR imaging, *Radiology* 187:207–212, 1993.

150. Stanford W, Phelan J, Kathol MH, et al: Patellofemoral joint motion: evaluation by ultrafast computed tomography, *Skel Radiol* 17:487–492, 1988.

151. Cohen MS: Rapid MR imaging: techniques and performance characteristics. In In Taveras J.T., Ferrucci J.T., editors: Radiology: diagnosis/imaging/intervention, vol 1, Philadelphia, 1992, JB Lippincott.

152. Liebl H, Joseph G, Nevitt MC, et al: Early T2 changes predict onset of radiographic knee osteoarthritis: data from the osteoarthritis initiative, *Ann Rheum Dis* 74:1353–1359, 2015. 2014 Mar 10. Epub ahead of print.

153. Farrokhi S, Colletti PM, Powers CM: Differences in patellar cartilage thickness, transverse relaxation time, and deformational behavior: a comparison of young women with and without patellofemoral pain, *Am J Sports Med* 39:384–391, 2011.

154. Thuillier DU, Souza RB, Wu S, et al: T1ρ imaging demonstrates early changes in the lateral patella in patients with patellofemoral pain and maltracking, *Am J Sports Med* 41:1813–1818, 2013.

155. Nojiri T, Watanabe N, Namura T, et al: Utility of delayed gadolinium-enhanced MRI (dGEMRIC) for qualitative evaluation of articular cartilage of patellofemoral joint, *Knee Surg Sports Traumatol Arthrosc* 14:718–723, 2006.

156. Staroswiecki E, Bangerter NK, Gurney PT, et al: In vivo sodium imaging of human patellar cartilage with a 3D cones sequence at 3T and 7T, *J Magn Reson Imaging* 32:446–451, 2010.

157. Peterfy CG, Guermazi A, Zaim S, et al: Whole-Organ Magnetic Resonance Imaging Score (WORMS) of the knee in osteoarthritis, *Osteoarthritis Cartilage* 12:177–190, 2012.

158. Hunter DJ, Guermazi A, Lo GH, et al: Evolution of semi-quantitative whole joint assessment of knee OA: MOAKS (MRI Osteoarthritis Knee Score), *Osteoarthritis Cartilage* 19:990–1002, 2011.

159. Hunter DJ, Lo GH, Gale D, et al: The reliability of a new scoring system for knee osteoarthritis MRI and the validity of bone marrow lesion assessment: BLOKS (Boston Leeds Osteoarthritis Knee Score), *Ann Rheum Dis* 67:206–211, 2008.

160. Roemer FW, Guermazi A, Trattnig S, et al: Whole joint MRI assessment of surgical cartilage repair of the knee: cartilage repair osteoarthritis knee score (CROAKS), *Osteoarthritis Cartilage* 22:779–799, 2014.

161. Roemer FW, Frobell R, Lohmander LS, et al: Anterior Cruciate Ligament OsteoArthritis Score (ACLOAS): Longitudinal MRI-based whole joint assessment of anterior cruciate ligament injury, *Osteoarthritis Cartilage* 22:668–682, 2014.

162. Dye S, Staubli H-U, Biedert R: The mosaic of pathophysiology causing patellofemoral pain, *Op Tech Sports Med* 7:46–54, 1999.

163. Hodges PW, Richardson CA: The influence of isometric hip adduction on quadriceps femoris activity, *Scand J Rehab Med* 25:57–62, 1993.

164. Smith TO, Bowyer D, Dixon J, et al: Can vastus medialis oblique be preferentially activated? A systematic review of electromyographic studies, *Physiother Theory Pract* 25:69–98, 2009.

165. MacDougall JD: Morphological changes in human skeletal muscle following strength training and immobilization. In Jones NL, McCartney N, McComas AJ, editors: *Human muscle power*, Champaign, IL, 1986, Human Kinetics.

166. Powers CM: Rehabilitation of patellofemoral joint disorders: a critical review, *J Orthop Sport Phys Ther* 28:345–354, 1998.

167. Natri A, Kannus P, Jarvinen M: Which factors predict the long-term outcome in chronic patellofemoral pain syndrome? A 7-year prospective follow-up study, *Med Sci Sports Exerc* 30:1572–1577, 1998.

168. Powers CM, Perry J, Hsu A, et al: Are patellofemoral pain and quadriceps strength associated with locomotor function? *Phys Ther* 77:1063–1074, 1997.

169. Kooiker L, Van De Port IG, Weir A, et al: Effects of physical therapist-guided quadriceps-strengthening exercises for the treatment of patellofemoral pain syndrome: a systematic review, *J Orthop Sports Phys Ther* 44:391–401, 2014.

170. Chiu JK, Wong YM, Yung PS, et al: The effects of quadriceps strengthening on pain, function, and patellofemoral joint contact area in persons with patellofemoral pain, *Am J Phys Med Rehabil* 91:98–106, 2012.

171. Lieb FJ, Perry J: Quadriceps function: an electromyographic study under isometric conditions, *J Bone Joint Surg Am* 53:749–758, 1971.

172. Steinkamp LA, Dillingham MF, Markel MD, et al: Biomechanical considerations in patellofemoral joint rehabilitation, *Am J Sports Med* 21:438–444, 1993.

173. Powers CM, Ho KY, Chen YJ, et al: Patellofemoral joint stress during weightbearing and non-weightbearing quadriceps exercises, *J Orthop Sport Phys Ther* 44:320–327, 2014.

174. Hunter LY: Braces and taping, *Clin Sports Med* 4:439–454, 1985.

175. Lun VM, Wiley JP, Meeuwisse WH, et al: Effectiveness of patellar bracing for treatment of patellofemoral pain syndrome, *Clin J Sport Med* 15:235–240, 2005.

176. Finestone A, Radin EL, Lev B, et al: Treatment of overuse patellofemoral pain: prospective randomized controlled clinical trial in a military setting, *Clin Orthop* 293:208–210, 1993.

177. Crossley KM, Bennell KL, Green S, et al: Physical therapy for patellofemoral pain. A randomized, double-blinded, placebo-controlled trial, *Am J Sports Med* 30:857–865, 2002.

178. Whittingham M, Palmer S, Macmillan F: Effects of taping on pain and function in patellofemoral pain syndrome: a randomized controlled trial, *J Orthop Sports Phys Ther* 34:504–510, 2004.

179. Mason M, Keays SL, Newcombe PA: The effect of taping, quadriceps strengthening and stretching prescribed separately or combined on patellofemoral pain, *Physiother Res Int* 16:109–119, 2011.

180. Powers CM, Landel R, Sosnick T, et al: The effects of patellar taping on stride characteristics and joint motion in subjects with patellofemoral pain, *J Orthop Sports Phys Ther* 26:286–291, 1997.

181. Salsich GB, Brechter JH, Farwell D, et al: The effects of patellar taping on knee kinetics, kinematics and vastus lateralis muscle activity during stair ambulation in individuals with patellofemoral pain, *J Orthop Sport Phys Ther* 32:3–10, 2002.

182. Powers CM, Doubleday KL, Escudero C: The influence of patellofemoral bracing on pain, knee extensor torque and gait function in females with patellofemoral pain, *Physiother Theory Pract* 24:1–9, 2008.

183. Koskinen SK, Kujala UM: Effect of patellar brace on patellofemoral relationships, *Scand J Med Sci Sports* 1:119–122, 1991.

184. Shellock FG, Mink JH, Deutsch AL, et al: Effect of a patellar realignment brace on patellofemoral relationships: evaluation with kinematic MR imaging, *J Magn Reson Imaging* 4:590–594, 1994.

185. Powers CM, Shellock FG, Beering TV, et al: The effect of bracing on patellar kinematics in patients with patellofemoral pain, *Med Sci Sports Exerc* 31:1714–1720, 1999.

186. Powers CM, Ward SR, Chen YJ, et al: The effect of bracing on patellofemoral joint stress during free and fast walking, *Am J Sports Med* 32:224–231, 2004.

187. Collins N, Crossley K, Beller E, et al: Foot orthoses and physiotherapy in the treatment of patellofemoral pain syndrome: randomised clinical trial, *BMJ* 24:337, 2008.

188. Eng JJ, Pierrynowski MR: The effects of foot orthotic on three-dimensional lower-limb kinematics during walking and running, *Phys Ther* 74:836–844, 1994.

189. Vicenzino B, Collins N, Cleland J, et al: A clinical prediction rule for identifying patients with patellofemoral pain who are likely to benefit from foot orthoses: a preliminary determination, *Br J Sports Med* 44:862–866, 2010.

190. Barton CJ, Munteanu SE, Menz HB, et al: The efficacy of foot orthoses in the treatment of individuals with patellofemoral pain syndrome: a systematic review, *Sports Med* 40:377–395, 2010.

191. Sutlive TG, Mitchell SD, Maxfield SN, et al: Identification of individuals with patellofemoral pain whose symptoms improved after a combined program of foot orthosis use and modified activity: a preliminary investigation, *Phys Ther* 84:49–61, 2004.

192. Barton CJ, Menz HB, Levinger P, et al: Greater peak rearfoot eversion predicts foot orthoses efficacy in individuals with patellofemoral pain syndrome, *Br J Sports Med* 45:697–701, 2011.

193. Lack S, Barton C, Vicenzino B, et al: Outcome predictors for conservative patellofemoral pain management: a systematic review and meta-analysis, *Sports Med* 44:1703–1716, 2014.

194. Fukuda TY, Melo WP, Zaffalon BM, et al: Hip posterolateral musculature strengthening in sedentary women with patellofemoral pain syndrome: a randomized controlled clinical trial with 1-year follow-up, *J Orthop Sports Phys Ther* 42:823–830, 2012.

195. Dolak KL, Silkman C, Medina McKeon J, et al: Hip strengthening prior to functional exercises reduces pain sooner than quadriceps strengthening in females with patellofemoral pain syndrome: a randomized clinical trial, *J Orthop Sports Phys Ther* 41:560–570, 2011.

196. Ferber R, Bolgla L, Earl-Boehm JE, et al: Strengthening of the hip and core versus knee muscles for the treatment of patellofemoral pain: a multicenter, randomized controlled trial, *J Athl Train* 50:366–377, 2015. 2014 Nov 3. Epub ahead of print.

197. Ismail MM, Gamaleldein MH, Hassa KA: Closed kinetic chain exercises with or without additional hip strengthening exercises in management of patellofemoral pain syndrome: a randomized controlled trial, *Eur J Phys Rehabil Med* 49:687–698, 2013.

198. Khayambashi K, Mohammadkhani Z, Ghaznavi K, et al: The effects of isolated hip abductor and external rotator muscle strengthening on pain, health status, and hip strength in females with patellofemoral pain, *J Orthop Sports Phys Ther* 42:22–29, 2012.

199. Khayambashi K, Fallah A, Movahedi A, et al: Posterolateral hip muscle strengthening versus quadriceps strengthening for patellofemoral pain: a comparative control trial, *Arch Phys Med Rehabil* 95:900–907, 2014.

200. Nadler SF, Malanga GA, Feinberg JH, et al: Relationship between hip muscle imbalance and occurrence of low back pain in collegiate athletes: a prospective study, *Am J Phys Med Rehabil* 80:572–577, 2001.

201. Mascal CL, Landel R, Powers C: Management of patellofemoral pain targeting hip, pelvis, and trunk muscle function: 2 case reports, *J Orthop Sports Phys Ther* 33:647–660, 2003.

202. Farrokhi S, Pollard CD, Souza R, et al: Trunk position influences lower extremity demands during the forward lunge exercise, *J Orthop Sports Phys Ther* 38:403–409, 2008.

203. Fulkerson J: Awareness of the retinaculum in evaluating patellofemoral pain, *Am J Sports Med* 10:147–151, 1982.

204. Fulkerson J: Evaluation of the peripatellar soft tissues and retinaculum in patients with patellofemoral pain, *Clin Sports Med* 8:197–202, 1989.

205. Post W, Fulkerson J: Distal realignment of the patellofemoral joint, *Orthop Clin North Am* 23:6–11, 1992.
206. Shea K, Fulkerson J: Pre-operative computed tomography scanning and arthroscopy in predicting outcome after lateral release, *Arthroscopy* 8:327–334, 1992.
207. Fulkerson J: A clinical test for medial patella tracking, *Tech Orthop* 12:144, 1997.
208. Outerbridge R: Further studies on the etiology of chondromalacia patella, *J Bone Joint Surg Br* 46:179–190, 1964.
209. Fulkerson J: Anteromedialization of the tibial tuberosity for patellofemoral malalignment, *Clin Orthop Rel Res* 177:176–181, 1983.

210. Fulkerson J, Schutzer S: After failure of conservative treatment for painful patellofemoral malalignment: lateral release or realignment? *Orthop Clin North Am* 17:283–288, 1986.
211. Cox JS: Evaluation of the Roux-Elmslie-Trillat procedure for knee extensor realignment, *Am J Sports Med* 10:300–310, 1983.
212. Broom JM, Fulkerson JP: The plica syndrome: a new perspective, *Orthop Clin North Am* 17:279–281, 1986.
213. Minas T, Peterson L: Autologous chondrocyte transplantation, *Op Tech Sports Med* 8:144–157, 2000.
214. Buuck D, Fulkerson J: Anteromedialization of the tibial tubercle: 4-12 year follow up, *Op Tech Sports Med* 8:131–137, 2000.

215. Trillat A, Dejour HL, Coutette A: Diagnostic et traitement des subluxations recidivantes de la rotule, *Rev Chir Orthop* 50:813–824, 1964.
216. Fulkerson J, editor: *Common patellofemoral disorders (monograph series)*, Rosemont, IL, 2005, American Academy of Orthopedic Surgeons.
217. Nam E, Karzel R: Mini open medial reefing and arthroscopic lateral release for treatment of recurrent patellar dislocation, *Am J Sports Med* 33:220–230, 2005.
218. Elias JJ, Cech JA, Weinstein DM, et al: Reducing the lateral force acting on the patella does not consistently decrease patellofemoral pressures, *Am J Sports Med* 32:1202–1208, 2004.

CHAPTER 23

Physical Rehabilitation after Total Knee Arthroplasty

DIANE M. HEISLEIN, ERIC O. EISEMON*

INTRODUCTION

The primary indication for total knee arthroplasty (TKA) is to relieve pain caused by severe arthritis.[1,2] Osteoarthritis (OA) of the knee is prevalent, with radiographic evidence of degenerative joint disease in approximately 50% of patients age 75 years or older.[3] Furthermore, symptomatic OA develops at a rate of 1% per year in patients with a mean age of 70 years. Risk factors associated with the development of knee OA include obesity, female gender, previous knee trauma, presence of hand OA, and older age.[4] TKA is an elective procedure that is indicated when the joint no longer functions satisfactorily because of advanced disease. Because of the aging of the U.S. population and the prevalence of OA, the demand for primary total knee replacements continues to rise each year.[5-11]

Rates of Total Knee Arthroplasty in the United States[5-11]

- In 2004, approximately 267,000 primary total knee replacements were performed.
- By 2010, this number had increased significantly to more than 600,000 primary total knee replacements.
- Demand for total knee replacements is expected to exceed 3 million by 2030.

Three key elements must be considered in the decision to proceed with TKA: (1) whether the patient has debilitating pain, (2) whether less invasive treatments have failed to reduce pain and maintain the patient's desired level of activity, and (3) whether the patient is medically suited to respond to surgery. Therefore, TKA is appropriately reserved for patients with disease and symptoms that are unremitting despite judicious medical management, including anti-inflammatory medications, activity modification, weight loss, physical therapy, bracing and other biomechanical modifications, and use of a cane for ambulation. Moreover, the expected survival of the arthroplasty implant at 15 years is projected to be between 81% and 92%.[12] Actual implant survival on a per patient basis is hard to predict because it is dependent on surgical considerations, activity levels, and co-morbidities.

Indications for Knee Arthroplasty

- Debilitating pain
- Failure of conservative treatment
- Patient medically suitable for surgery

TKA has been shown to be an effective treatment for patients more than 60 years of age with end-stage OA of one or more compartments of the knee. In these patients with symptomatic OA, outcomes are excellent in part because the patient's overall activity level has diminished and their expectations after TKA (i.e., the level of physical activity possible) are reasonable. In addition, because of the activity level and age of these patients, the revision rate is minimal. In contrast, in patients younger than 60 years of age, activity levels remain high, and the higher rates of aseptic failure may be related to the unique demands that they place on the implant.[13] Therefore, revision rates remain relatively high in this group of patients, and the timing of surgical intervention must be chosen carefully. Conservative management of OA should be maximized before any decision is made to proceed with surgical intervention for this age group.

Rehabilitation after TKA is described according to the typical stages through which a patient proceeds after the surgery, including preoperative considerations, acute care, post-acute care, outpatient, and return to sports, vocation, and leisure activities. Variations in surgical procedures are discussed, including any modifications that need to be considered in the rehabilitation process; however,

---

*The authors, editors, and publisher acknowledge Drs. Nina Shervin and Harry Rubash for their contributions on this topic in the previous edition.

the chapter focuses on primary TKA performed for a patient with underlying severe OA because this scenario accounts for most of the TKAs currently performed.

PREOPERATIVE REHABILITATION

The impetus for preoperative rehabilitation has been prompted by evidence that the best predictors of the outcome of arthroplasty are the patient's preoperative status, including the knee range of motion (ROM), distance walked, and Western Ontario and McMasters Universities (WOMAC) OA Index scores.[14-16] Patients with advanced OA have a variety of options available, both surgical and nonsurgical. From a rehabilitation perspective, the programs established for patients in an effort to delay surgical intervention also offer the opportunity to address many impairments and functional limitations that can impede a patient's progress after surgery; therefore continuation of these programs is recommended right up to the time of surgery. Most rehabilitation programs aimed at preoperative TKA patients have attempted to address impairments in ROM, strength, and limited aerobic capacity or endurance, as well as functional limitations in ambulation, stair climbing, and performing activities of daily living (ADLs), such as dressing and bathing (Table 23-1).

Advanced OA results in an overall decrease in functional mobility as pain and deformity worsen. This gradual decline in functional status ultimately contributes to the patient's loss of strength in the involved limb and overall endurance and strength. Programs designed to address these deficits include a variety of exercise interventions, such as functional training activities, aquatic programs, and strength training programs.

Functional training activities incorporate functional movements, such as sit to stand, squatting, and step ups, as a way to improve strength and function. Targeted areas of weakness most commonly involve the quadriceps and the gluteal musculature. All of these tasks can address strength deficits; however, pain usually is a limiting factor in the patient's ability to tolerate these activities because of the high loads they create in the knee joint. Strategies to unload body weight (e.g., upper extremity support) may allow the patient to continue with these exercises without exacerbation of pain symptoms.

If patients are unable or unwilling to use functional movements for strengthening, more traditional exercises can be incorporated into the patient's program, such as straight leg raises, cycling, seated knee extension exercises, and supine or side-lying hip abduction exercises. Resistance from the weight of the limb often is sufficient early on, and as the patient progresses, low-load cuff weights or resistance equipment can be used to maximize the patient's strength.

Aquatic programs designed for patients with OA are commonly offered in community and rehabilitation settings. These programs use the buoyancy of water to facilitate movement in very weak limbs. Patients perform slow movements that require initiation of movement through the patient's musculature; however, the patient does not have to move the entire weight of the limb against gravity. As the patient progresses in these programs, increased speed of movement creates additional resistance, so that patients are always challenged to increase their strength. Aquatic programs typically are held in heated pools that induce relaxation and help reduce the joint stiffness commonly associated with OA. In addition to strengthening exercises, the pool can be used to address aerobic capacity and endurance limitations through swimming, jogging, or walking in the water. Again, slow movements are facilitated by the buoyancy of the water, and faster movement creates additional resistance to these activities.

Even though the preoperative level of physical function (ROM, strength, and the distance the patient can walk) are predictors of the success of TKA,[8,9,17] intervention studies that have examined the effect of preoperative rehabilitation on outcomes currently do not support the use of preoperative physical therapy for patients undergoing TKA.[18-23] However, the literature on preoperative rehabilitation is limited, and factors such as the specific impairments measured, measurement tools used, timing of outcome measurements, and intensity of the exercise programs may all contribute to this lack of evidence.

Patient education has been an additional focus of preoperative arthroplasty programs. Patients who fully understand the postoperative expectations and clinical care protocol have demonstrated better coping strategies postoperatively.[20,24,25] Clinically this is quite evident in patients who undergo a second arthroplasty because they are familiar with the expected daily progression of the rehabilitation program and the effort required of them for a successful outcome. Many hospitals have reduced the length of stay (LOS) after arthroplasty to reduce the overall costs associated with this procedure. Currently the acute care stay can range from 1 to 3 days after TKA.[26] Given this much shorter LOS, the effect of preoperative education should be examined more closely with regard to patient anxiety, coping strategies, and achievement of functional milestones after surgery.

TABLE 23-1

Preoperative Goals and Intervention Techniques

Goals	Types of Interventions
Maintain or maximize knee range of motion (ROM)	ROM exercises Stretching Joint mobilization
Maintain or maximize strength of lower extremity muscles, especially the quadriceps and hip musculature	Strengthening exercises Functional training activities
Maintain or improve aerobic capacity	Aerobic activities: • Walking • Stationary biking • Swimming

SURGICAL TECHNIQUE

The aim of TKA is to resurface the deficient and damaged tibiofemoral and patellofemoral joint surfaces with metal components and provide a low-friction articulation with a polyethylene bearing. The mechanical alignment and soft tissue balance around the knee should be anatomically restored for optimum function and longevity of the knee replacement.

The selection of regional or general anesthesia is made after a preoperative discussion between the anesthesiologist and the patient with input from the surgical team. This decision is affected by the patient's medical condition, although the cardiovascular outcomes, cognitive function, and mortality rates of regional and general anesthesia have not been proven to be significantly different.

The knee joint is accessed anteriorly through a medial parapatellar approach (although some surgeons use a lateral or subvastus approach). Osteophytes and intraarticular soft tissues are cleared. Bone cuts in the distal femur are made perpendicular to the mechanical axis, usually using an intramedullary alignment system. The proximal tibia is cut perpendicular to the mechanical axis of the tibia using either intramedullary or extramedullary alignment rods. Restoration of mechanical alignment is important to allow optimum load sharing and prevent eccentric loading through the prosthesis. Sufficient bone is removed so that the prosthesis will recreate the level of the joint line (Figure 23-1). This allows ligaments around the knee to be balanced accurately and prevents alteration of the height of the patella, which can have deleterious effects on patellofemoral mechanics. It is important to note that some extra-articular ligaments may be contracted secondary to preoperative deformity. These ligaments need to be carefully released in a stepwise fashion to balance the soft tissues around the knee and allow optimum knee kinematics.

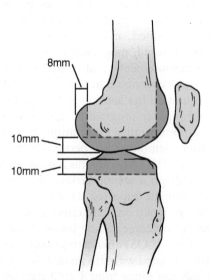

Figure 23-1 In the measured resection technique, as much bone and/or cartilage is removed as will be replaced by the thickness of the arthroplasty components. This method attempts to restore the anatomical joint line level.

If the patellofemoral joint is significantly diseased, the patella is resurfaced with a polyethylene button. Patellofemoral tracking is assessed with trial components in place. The definitive components usually are cemented into place with polymethylmethacrylate cement. In younger patients, some surgeons are using cementless implants; however, this does not change the postoperative rehabilitation program. The wound then is copiously irrigated, the tourniquet is deflated, hemostasis is achieved, a Hemovac drain is placed in some cases to prevent hematoma formation, and an occlusive dressing is applied.

Many implant options are available to the orthopedic surgeon for primary TKA. Most surgeons select a specific implant with which they are most familiar and that has worked well in their practice. The two main types of implant designs are described by whether or not the posterior cruciate ligament (PCL) is retained or removed. With the cruciate retaining (CR) design, the anterior cruciate ligament (ACL) is removed and the PCL is retained to provide anterior-posterior stability to the knee joint. The cruciate-sacrificing, posterior stabilized (PS) design involves removal of both the ACL and PCL, and the role of the PCL in knee motion is replaced by a post within the implant. There is great debate as to which is the better design; however, there is no conclusive evidence to point to one system being superior.[27]

The term *minimally invasive surgery* (MIS) has been used to describe operations that involve smaller skin incisions and therefore less soft tissue dissection. Typically, MIS TKA techniques involve smaller incisions, a proximal incision that goes through the vastus medialis oblique (VMO) rather than along the quadriceps tendon, and the patella is subluxed laterally rather than everted. The theoretical advantage of this approach is less pain and improved postoperative quadriceps strength.

Computer-navigated or -assisted surgery is employed in some centers. The role of this technique is to improve implant position with respect to the mechanical alignment of the limb. This is accomplished by placing several markers on the leg and using a computer to determine the femoral and tibial cuts. Although this has been shown to decrease outliers, there is no consensus on whether this improves patient outcomes.[28]

POSTOPERATIVE ACUTE CARE REHABILITATION

Clinical pathways have been developed as a standardized way to organize patient management after common surgical procedures, including TKA. The driving force behind the use of clinical pathways is the fact that early identification of deviations from optimum care can be identified and addressed, which streamlines the overall care of the patient and should reduce the overall cost of care. These pathways outline all aspects of care provided for the patient from all disciplines involved in the individual's care. The literature supports the use of clinical pathways for postoperative care of patients who have undergone TKA. Quality of care improves and LOS can be reduced without any increase in complications, readmissions, or changes in the patient's overall function.[29-34] Further studies are warranted to examine the cost effectiveness of clinical pathways for TKA.

Considerations for rehabilitation begin once the patient leaves the operating room. A major goal after TKA is to restore knee ROM as quickly as possible because this has been linked to improved functional mobility. Early restoration of ROM prevents the development of postoperative fibrosis, which may require manipulation or additional surgical intervention.

Use of continuous passive motion (CPM) was considered standard care for patients during the acute care stay in previous decades. Research examining the effect of CPM on outcomes is not conclusive; however, most research fails to find a significant long-term benefit of CPM use after TKA in terms of ROM results, pain, LOS, cost, and complications.[35-47] CPM has been shown to improve ROM in the early phases of rehabilitation,[36,48,49] but no long-term carryover has been seen 1 year after TKA.

Protocols for the use of CPM have not been studied. Reports on the initial ROM settings, amount of progression per day, and amount of time spent in the CPM are limited in the literature.[50] CPM may be used to augment the patient's rehabilitative care starting with a setting of 0° to ≥30° of knee flexion on postoperative day 1 (POD 1). Progression of the range is determined by the patient's tolerance. The duration of daily CPM use has not been studied specifically in patients who have had TKA. Most surgeons prefer their patients to use the CPM for several hours a day, but continuous use is discouraged because it limits the patient's ability to practice functional mobility training, as well as the amount of time out of bed. The overall use of CPM has declined, given the limited research supporting its use, the expense, and constraints on functional activities while in the device.

Rehabilitation interventions are developed based on a comprehensive examination of the patient, and goals are tailored to the specific needs of the individual patient (Table 23-2). Intervention on POD 1 focuses primarily on initiating ROM exercises to the involved knee and initiating therapeutic exercises for the lower extremities. Isometric contractions that target the quadriceps and gluteal muscles, as well as active exercises for ankle plantar flexion and dorsiflexion, are commonly prescribed. Prevention of thromboses is addressed by means of active ankle exercises and mobilizing the patient out of bed in addition to pharmacological and mechanical measures. The pulmonary system also is addressed because the patient is at risk for developing secondary complications as a result of the effects of anesthesia and from being in a supine position for prolonged periods. Instruction in deep

TABLE 23-2

Goals for Acute Rehabilitation and Types of Intervention

Goals	Types of Interventions
Maximize knee range of motion (ROM): 0° to 120° flexion	ROM exercises
Prevent secondary complications	Pulmonary toilet Breathing exercises Active exercise of the lower extremities Functional training
Improve strength and motor control	Therapeutic exercise focusing on strength
Achieve independent transfers	Transfer training
Achieve independent ambulation	Gait training with assistive device
Achieve independent basic self-care, activities of daily living	Assistive devices and training

breathing exercises, effective airway clearance strategies, and manual techniques as needed are of paramount importance in the days immediately after surgery.

Pain control is another factor that must be considered because pain greatly affects the patient's ability to participate in exercise and functional training. Various methods of pain control have been described for patients who have undergone TKA, and a number of factors must be considered for each individual patient to achieve adequate pain control while avoiding significant side effects of altered mental state, nausea, or vomiting. Finding the right balance for each patient is the goal of the health care team; the patient's pain complaints must be addressed, yet the person must be able to participate fully in the rehabilitation process. TKA procedures can be very painful for patients, especially in the first 24 to 48 hours after surgery. However, patients usually report progressive improvement in their pain levels over the course of their acute care stay and are able to be discharged on oral analgesics. Administering a patient's pain medication before rehabilitation is important because functional mobilization, especially ROM, can escalate pain significantly. Reports on the options available for pain control show that the use of multimodal pain management strategies is the most effective way to manage post TKA pain immediately after surgery. These pain management strategies may include the use of "preemptive" medications (including acetaminophen or selective nonsteroidal anti-inflammatory drugs [NSAIDs], antineuropathic and antinausea agents), femoral nerve blocks or periarticular injections, and scheduled dosing with oral opioid analgesics.[51-54] Despite improvements in pain control, further research is needed to determine the optimum dosing, timing, and anesthetic agents to provide the most pain relief with minimal side effects.

Rehabilitation Goals following Knee Arthroplasty

- Increase or restore ROM
- Prevent thrombosis
- Prevent secondary pulmonary complications
- Control pain
- Provide functional training (transfers, gait training)
- Improve strength
- Improve aerobic capacity

With the patient premedicated, the clinician can address ROM and strength issues through exercise. The other focus of treatment on POD 1 is functional training, which includes teaching the patient how to transfer into and out of bed and to begin pregait training activities in the standing position. Progression to gait training on POD 1 depends on the patient's pain level, tolerance of change in position, and overall well-being. In addition to pain, common problems that limit the patient are lightheadedness, nausea, and/or vomiting, often associated with orthostatic hypotension (low blood pressure when standing up), or side effects from narcotic medication. If abnormal, vital sign responses occur with changes in position or increased activity, the clinician must determine whether the intervention should be discontinued. Patients with underlying co-morbidities in the cardiovascular and/or pulmonary systems need to be monitored carefully for adverse responses in the first days after surgery. A full discussion of these responses is beyond the scope of this chapter; however, any indications of cardiac arrhythmia, ischemia, or oxygen desaturation should warrant careful progression with functional training.

Functional Training

Functional training includes teaching the patient how to transfer effectively from a supine to a sitting position. Some institutions use a knee immobilizer or brace that limits any knee flexion during the initial days of functional training. If this is available, it can be helpful to patients while the quadriceps are inhibited by pain, swelling, or residual effects from a femoral nerve block because it allows the patient to control the leg independently during transfers; otherwise the patient will require assistance to move the limb. Patients can use a direct supine to sit or a supine to side-lying to sit transfer, depending on their ability and preference. Sit to stand transfers can be facilitated early on by elevating the bed and/or chair to minimize the workload on the uninvolved limb in attaining full upright standing.

Patients require an assistive device to begin ambulation training. Most often, they will use a walker, although crutches can be used; this also depends on the patient's skill and agility. Weight bearing as tolerated (WBAT) usually is allowed immediately after surgery; therefore an assistive device is required primarily because of motor control problems in the limb. Patients can be advanced to less restrictive devices (one crutch or cane) as strength and motor control return. Most patients are allowed to discontinue the use of any assistive device at 6 weeks after surgery if the patient can demonstrate adequate motor control and at least 4 out of 5 strength of the involved limb on manual muscle testing of the quadriceps that allows for safe, stable ambulation. Before discharge and depending on the patient's home environment, instruction on stair ascent and descent may be required. Even if the patient does not have any stairs outside or in the home, instruction and practice are important for community ambulation and street curb negotiation.

Therapeutic Exercise

For most patients, the area of focus for strengthening immediately after surgery is the quadriceps muscle to allow the individual to gain motor control of the leg and knee during functional transfers. Isometric quadriceps setting exercises are initiated on POD 1. Often, facilitation techniques, such as tactile cueing, overflow feedback from the uninvolved leg, biofeedback, or even electrical stimulation, may be required to overcome the reflexive inhibition of the quadriceps that commonly occurs because of swelling in the knee joint.[55] Once the patient is able to actively contract the quadriceps, exercises can be advanced to include terminal knee extension or short arc quadriceps exercises consisting of knee extension from a slightly flexed position over a bolster or towel or pillow roll (Figure 23-2). Additional progressions using the weight of the limb for resistance can include eccentric lowering of the leg from a fully extended position in sitting and concentric knee extension in sitting. For the more advanced patient, manual resistance, cuff weights, or resistive bands can add additional resistance. However, most patients are not ready

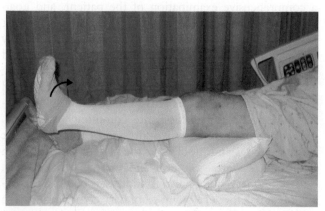

Figure 23-2 Quadriceps strengthening using terminal knee extension exercise.

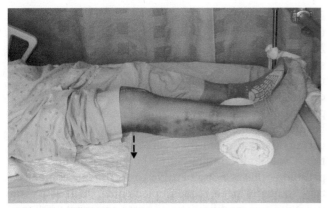

Figure 23-3 Positioning for passive knee extension ROM.

for any additional resistance beyond the effect of gravity on the lower leg during the first few days after surgery.

ROM exercises are initiated passively and progressed to active-assisted exercises. Emphasis on knee extension is more easily accomplished with the limb fully supported on the bed and with additional towel rolls or bolsters under the heel to passively stretch the knee into extension (**L3D technique - low load, long duration**) (Figure 23-3). For patients who have difficulty gaining knee extension, sleeping with the knee in an immobilizer can be effective for prolonged low load stretching. When working on knee flexion ROM, patients should be in the sitting position to allow gravity to assist with the motion. Once patients can place the foot on the floor, they can use a variety of techniques to enhance their own knee flexion, including sliding the foot under the chair, pushing the leg into more knee flexion with the opposite leg, or planting the foot firmly on the ground and scooting forward in the chair to flex the knee. Providing various methods for patients to gain ROM independently allows the knee to be ranged multiple times per day because most patients, while in the hospital, work with a physical therapist only once or twice a day at most.

Aerobic Capacity and Endurance Training

Early focus on aerobic capacity training often is accomplished merely by the effort required of patients for basic functional mobility. For the more advanced patient, increasing the distance ambulated in the hospital and the frequency of ambulation taxes the cardiopulmonary system adequately for a training effect. For patients with underlying co-morbidities in these areas, specific training parameters should be set, and the patient should use either heart rate or the **Rating of Perceived Exertion (RPE)** scale as a guide to the amount of activity that is appropriate for aerobic capacity training.

Discharge Planning

Because the LOS after TKA has declined significantly since the late 1990s, patients routinely are discharged

from the acute care setting in 1 to 3 days.[26] Many patients return directly home, whereas others need additional care in a post-acute care setting. The clinician is responsible for providing input on discharge planning, and this begins on the initial day of intervention. Interdisciplinary collaboration among the patient's health care providers is important for determining the best discharge plan for the patient's unique needs. Factors that are important to consider include the presence and extent of any co-morbidities that will influence the expected rate of recovery; the amount of support the patient will have at home from family or friends to assist in ADLs, basic household management, meal preparation, and food shopping; and the physical environment to which the patient is returning. Patients who live alone, have multiple co-morbidities, or have an environmentally challenging home situation may need to be discharged to an inpatient facility for ongoing rehabilitation until the patient has achieved a level of function sufficient to return to their home setting.[56-58] In contrast, patients with minimal medical issues, available social support, and a home setting that has minimal environmental and structural obstacles should be able to go directly home from the acute care facility and continue their rehabilitation either through home care services or in an outpatient setting.

Oldmeadow et al.[59] have developed a preoperative screening tool to assist in determining the likely discharge destination after the acute care stay. The **Risk Assessment and Prediction Tool (RAPT)** (see Figure 19-3) for total joint arthroplasty patients generates a score and the likelihood of discharge directly home or to an inpatient rehabilitation setting based on information, such as age, gender, preoperative walking ability, preoperative use of assistive walking aides, and available social supports. The use of this tool has been validated in several studies to aid in early discharge planning.[60-62]

Factors to Consider in Discharge Planning

- Presence and extent of co-morbidities
- Social support for the patient at home
- Physical environment to which the patient is returning
- Patient's level of function (physical capacity)
- Patient's ability to use or need for assistive devices

Regardless of the discharge destination after the acute care stay, patients need some training and support with assistive devices for basic ADLs before they are discharged home. For some, this training occurs in the acute care facility; patients transferred to a post-acute facility receive their training and equipment there. The most common items issued for patients include long-handled implements, such as a bathing sponge, dressing aid, and reacher to assist the patient in gaining complete independence in bathing and dressing activities. Additional items may include elastic shoelaces, depending on the type of footwear the patient owns and wears. For a taller patient who may have difficulty with sit to stand transfers, a raised toilet seat may help the patient gain complete independence in toileting, and a tub bench is recommended to allow the patient to remain seated during showering for safety reasons. Additional modifications to the home may include grab bars in the bathroom for safety and ramps for home entrances if the patient has difficulty on stairs.

POST-ACUTE CARE INPATIENT REHABILITATION

The post-acute care level of rehabilitation may be provided in an inpatient facility, such as a rehabilitation hospital, a transitional care unit, or skilled nursing facility. Regardless of the setting, the goal of rehabilitation is an extension of the care initiated in the acute care setting (Table 23-3). Patients typically remain at this level of care after discharge from the acute care setting, often on POD 2 to 4, and continue care for 9 days on average.[63] Predictors of increased LOS for inpatient rehabilitation include age more than 80 years, revision surgery, and multiple co-morbidities or illnesses.[64]

One of the main goals during inpatient rehabilitation is to progress the patient's mobility and safety to a level sufficient to allow the patient to return home. As with discharge from the acute care setting, social supports, environmental constraints, and the patient's overall physical capacity affect how quickly the individual returns home. Many patients discharged from a post-acute care inpatient facility continue their rehabilitation through home care services until they are ready for an outpatient setting.

Interventions in the post-acute care inpatient setting primarily continue with the treatments established in the acute care setting. Attention to maximizing ROM of the

knee and quadriceps strength to allow independence in transfer and ambulation is the prime focus of treatment. Many of these patients have additional co-morbidities that slow their progress in achieving independence in functional milestones. Frequently co-morbidities in the cardiovascular and/or pulmonary systems require a slower pace in this rehabilitative setting. These patients tend to be more deconditioned going into surgery and require pacing strategies until their aerobic capacity increases. If they have significant limitations because of an underlying pathology that is not amenable to treatment, compensatory strategies need to be implemented, such as pacing strategies and modifications of home environmental constraints to allow the patient to achieve safe and effective functional mobility.

Strength training and aerobic conditioning are additional components of the rehabilitation program that can be implemented in the post-acute care setting because patients typically have less pain that limits their tolerance of treatment. Exercises such as upper body ergometry and progression to stationary biking can be initiated once the patient has sufficient ROM to allow full cycling with the pedals. Discharge from the post-acute care inpatient setting to home occurs when the patient can demonstrate the ability to achieve independence in transfers, ambulation, ADLs, and instrumental activities of daily living (IADLs), including household management for patients returning to home alone (see volume 1 of this series, *Orthopedic Physical Assessment,* Chapter 1).

HOME CARE REHABILITATION

Once the patient has arrived home after discharge from either the acute care or post-acute inpatient setting, home care services can provide ongoing rehabilitation services if deemed necessary. Home care rehabilitation services often are provided to evaluate the patient's ability to negotiate the home environment safely and to provide ongoing interventions for functional training and therapeutic exercise. The primary reason patients continue with home care services after a post-acute care inpatient stay is inadequate knee ROM (<90° flexion) for functional activities. Patients can follow independent exercise programs to maintain and gain ROM independently, but the shift in home exercise programs now focuses more on strength gains and endurance training (see Table 23-3). Patients can use walking, swimming, or stationary biking for endurance and aerobic capacity training in addition to strengthening exercises that emphasize the quadriceps and hip musculature.

OUTPATIENT REHABILITATION

When the patient is able to get out into the community and has transportation to an outpatient rehabilitation facility, care is transitioned from the home care setting

TABLE **23-3**

Goals of Post-acute Care and Home Rehabilitation and Types of Interventions

Goals	Types of Interventions
Maximize knee range of motion (ROM): 0° to 120° flexion	ROM exercises Prolonged stretching
Improve strength and motor control	Therapeutic exercise focusing on strength
Achieve independent transfers	Transfer training
Achieve independent ambulation	Gait training with assistive device
Achieve independent basic self-care, activities of daily living	Assistive devices and training
Maximize aerobic capacity and endurance	Aerobic capacity training

to the outpatient setting. At this point the patient is not considered homebound and in the United States does not qualify for ongoing home care services under Medicare rules.[65] In addition, the outpatient clinic offers a variety of options in equipment to supplement the rehabilitation process.

The primary focus of treatment in the outpatient setting is strengthening, to facilitate the patient's return to full function. Residual deficits in ROM also are addressed through passive stretching and exercises that can be augmented with modalities as indicated (e.g., superficial heat, ultrasound). For patients with residual strength deficits, electrical stimulation can be used to enhance strength training regimens.[66,67] Quadriceps weakness, due in part to muscle activation deficits, often contributes to long-term limitations in functional ability. Emerging trends in high-intensity strengthening programs[68] and the use of neuromuscular electrical stimulation (NMES) as early as 2 days postoperatively are showing promise in reversing this pervasive impairment associated with TKA.[69] The continuum of rehabilitation in the outpatient setting takes the patient to the end point in functional rehabilitation after TKA and should include return to sport-specific activities if the patient so desires. Additional exercise equipment, such as isokinetic devices, pulley systems, and stair climbers, can be used for strengthening purposes of the lower extremities. Aerobic conditioning can be performed with walking, stationary bicycles, upper body ergometers, elliptical and standard treadmills, or cross-country ski machines, depending on the patient's overall endurance, balance, agility, and preferred mode of exercise.

Rehabilitation programs continue to be supplemented by progressive home exercise programs that focus on the goals of the rehabilitation program (Table 23-4). These most often include resistive exercises with cuff weights, resistance bands (Figure 23-4), or body weight in closed chain exercises, as well as ROM exercises with an emphasis on prolonged stretches to regain end range flexion or extension, depending on the patient's presentation. Gait training often continues in the outpatient setting; initially the patient is weaned off any assistive devices, and then the gait is fine-tuned as ROM and strength improve to restore a normal gait pattern and minimize any excessive loading on the joints from abnormal gait patterns. The frequency and duration of treatment are based on

TABLE **23-4**

Goals of Outpatient Rehabilitation and Types of Interventions

Goals	Types of Interventions
Maximize knee range of motion (ROM)	ROM exercises Prolonged stretching Manual techniques
Maximize strength	Aggressive strength training
Achieve normal gait without assistive device	Gait training Balance training
Achieve independence in self-selected activities (sports, leisure)	ROM Strengthening exercises Balance exercises Endurance training as required for activity

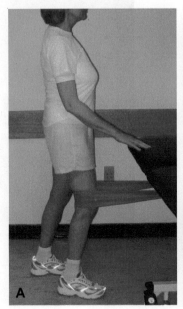 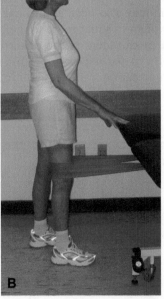

Figure 23-4 Quadriceps strengthening in closed chain using resistive elastic bands. **A,** Starting position (knee flexed). **B,** Finishing position (knee extended).

the patient's presentation and goals; however, a greater number of visits may be required if the patient needs manual techniques and stretching to improve ROM or if a treatment requires specific equipment (e.g., electrical stimulation). Outpatient rehabilitation often lasts at least 6 to 8 weeks because of the time needed to achieve true strength gains.

Regrettably, many presurgical patients have stopped participating in sports-related activities because of the pain associated with increased activity and advanced arthritis. For an increasing number of patients, TKA offers the hope of returning to meaningful activities, including a variety of sports and leisure activities. Sport-specific training often is included at the end of the rehabilitation process. A number of high-loading, repetitive sports activities, such as running, basketball, soccer, high-impact aerobics, singles tennis, squash, racquetball, and Alpine skiing, are not recommended after TKA because these types of activities have been associated with early arthroplasty failure.[70] Lower-load activities, such as walking, biking, golfing, swimming, tai chi, and bowling are encouraged because these activities help maintain strength gained in rehabilitation and provide the overall health benefits derived from regular physical activity.

When patients have completed rehabilitation after TKA, they may choose to seek out additional assistance in returning to a specific leisure activity. Their sport or activity of choice may have specific ROM, strength, or endurance requirements that call for additional training to allow the patient to participate fully at peak performance. Patients who want to return to cycling may need adjustments to their bicycles and additional work on ROM to maximize their tolerance of this activity. Golfers may need to address balance issues for the uneven terrain of the golf course to function confidently in this sport and may also need additional knee flexion ROM to allow them to squat to view lines for putting. Often the patient can identify the obstacles that impede their ability to participate fully in a sports activity, and this information can help guide both the examination and treatment focus of sport-specific rehabilitation.

Caution: High-Load Activities Not Recommended after Total Knee Arthroplasty

- Running
- Basketball
- Soccer
- High-impact aerobics
- Singles tennis
- Squash
- Racquetball
- Alpine skiing

ADDITIONAL SURGICAL CONSIDERATIONS FOR KNEE ARTHROPLASTY PATIENTS

Unicompartmental knee arthroplasties (UKAs) increasingly are performed for patients with advanced arthritic changes in one compartment of the knee, most often the medial compartment. These patients undergo a similar surgical event except that the prosthesis implanted resurfaces only one compartment (medial or lateral) of the tibiofemoral joint (Figure 23-5). After surgery, these patients follow a rehabilitation protocol that parallels that of patients who have had a TKA. The primary difference in patients with a UKA is that they undergo a less invasive surgical procedure that preserves more of the joint anatomy. Therefore they often have less blood loss at surgery, a shorter duration of anesthesia, and often less postoperative pain.[71,72] All these factors result in a faster recovery. Most of these patients are discharged directly home after the acute care stay, and they often are discharged home on POD 2.[73] They may require some rehabilitation services in the home initially but are moved into the outpatient setting more quickly and follow an outpatient rehabilitation process similar to that for primary TKA.

The other surgical arthroplasty consideration involves patients with bilateral knee OA. Because of the pathophysiology of OA, more than 80% of patients presenting with debilitating knee pain for evaluation have bilateral symptoms. In fact, in a study by Mont et al.,[74] 43% of

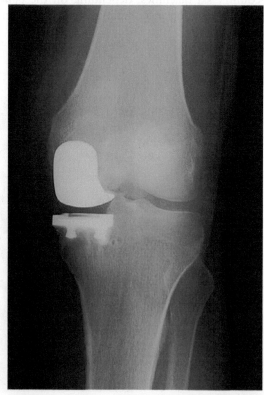

Figure 23-5 Anteroposterior radiograph of unicompartmental knee arthroplasty.

those presenting for unilateral TKA eventually had the other knee replaced as well; other researchers have had similar findings.[75-77] Patients who need bilateral knee replacements have a choice regarding the timing of the two procedures. A one-stage bilateral TKA may be performed, in which one TKA is performed, the tourniquet is deflated, and the contralateral tourniquet is inflated and the second TKA is performed, or both knees are done simultaneously by two teams at the same time. As an alternative, the patient may opt for two separate procedures done days, weeks, or months apart (two-stage TKA).

The overall complication rates in patients undergoing bilateral rather than unilateral TKA are similar, which suggests that for the average patient, the larger bilateral surgery appears to pose no increased risk.[78-80] However, it is clearly evident that the operative insult of bilateral one-stage procedures is greater, involving increased blood loss, greater hemodynamic effects, an increased risk of anesthetic complications from longer operative times, and a greater risk of embolization of fat and marrow contents. For these reasons, patients older than 75 years and those with significant cardiovascular co-morbidities are at increased risk of fatal complications and therefore should undergo a two-stage procedure.[79,81-83]

Patients who undergo a two-stage TKA follow the rehabilitation course outlined previously. Depending on the surgeon's and patient's preferences, the second TKA may be performed as early as 10 days after the first, or the two stages may be performed 3 or more months apart. For patients with a short interval between the two surgeries, the primary focus after the first procedure is to gain sufficient ROM and strength in the quadriceps muscle to allow this leg to act as the "strong" leg after the second procedure. These patients then follow a rehabilitation process similar to that outlined in the next paragraph for patients who undergo a one-stage bilateral TKA. Patients who have several months between procedures focus on fully rehabilitating the first knee before the second surgical procedure is performed.

One-stage bilateral TKAs present a unique challenge to the patient and rehabilitation professional. These patients need intensive rehabilitation services because both knees require treatment to address ROM and strength issues as outlined for single TKAs. Early postoperative functional training poses additional challenges because the patient often does not have sufficient knee ROM or strength to succeed in sit to stand transfers. Compensatory strategies, such as elevating the bed (Figure 23-6) and using knee immobilizers, may help the patient succeed with transfers the first few days after surgery. If CPM is used, it is alternated between the knees because the size of the CPM machine makes it difficult to position the patient on two at one time. CPM use should be considered judiciously as the increased time in the device for each knee will limit the patient's ability to be out of bed and working on

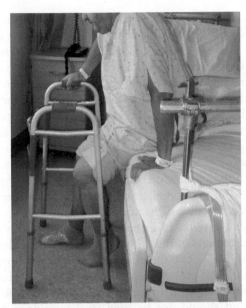

Figure 23-6 Assisted sit-to-stand transfers using elevation of the bed.

functional activities. Sufficient pain management is paramount in these patients because pain often impairs motor control. These patients usually require discharge to an inpatient rehabilitation facility for ongoing rehabilitation because most patients who have simultaneous bilateral TKAs do not achieve independence in functional mobility until 10 to 14 days after surgery. These patients' overall condition is also influenced by longer anesthetic times and increased blood loss and their associated side effects, which hamper progress in rehabilitation. The advantage of this procedure is that once patients have progressed through the initial phases of rehabilitation, they do not have a knee with advanced OA impeding their progress in rehabilitation, as is often seen in patients with bilateral knee OA who opt for two procedures many months apart.

COMPLICATIONS AFTER TOTAL KNEE ARTHROPLASTY

Common complications immediately after surgery include pulmonary complications, such as postoperative atelectasis and pneumonia, vascular complications (including deep vein thrombosis [DVT] and pulmonary embolus [PE]), and local wound problems or infection. For the clinician, a knowledge of the complications that may arise after TKA is important for early detection and referral to appropriate providers for management. Careful monitoring of the patient's heart rate, respiratory rate, oxygen (O_2) saturation levels, and body temperature can aid early detection of pulmonary complications. Interventions such as instruction in deep breathing exercises and manual techniques can help prevent and/or treat these pulmonary complications, which can be life threatening in older patients.

The frequency of thromboembolic disease in individuals who do not receive prophylactic therapy can be higher than 50%.[84] The risk of DVT is highest in the early postoperative period. Warfarin and low molecular weight heparins (blood-thinning drugs) reduce the risk of postoperative DVT in patients with TKA. Physical methods, including compression stockings, pneumatic compression devices, and early mobilization are useful adjuncts for preventing DVT but have not been proven to substitute for pharmacological prophylaxis. Although the overall incidence of symptomatic DVT after TKA is low,[85,86] the seriousness of this complication warrants close observation and prophylactic anticoagulation.

Patient reports of increased pain, swelling, warmth, and/or redness in the leg may accompany the development of DVT, but these clinical findings are poor predictors of the presence or absence of DVT.[87] Homan's sign is neither sensitive nor specific for the presence of DVT and should not be used to determine if a DVT is present.[88,89] Wells developed a clinical prediction rule (Table 23-5) to provide guidance on the probability of DVT. **Wells Clinical Prediction Rules for DVT** has been well validated for clinical probability assessment of DVT. A total score of <1 indicates low probability, 1 or 2 moderate, and >2 high probability that a DVT is present.[90,91]

Complications of Total Knee Arthroplasty

- Atelectasis (collapse of alveoli)
- Pneumonia
- Deep vein thrombosis (DVT)
- Pulmonary embolism (PE)
- Wound problems
- Infection
- Medial collateral ligament injury
- Extensor mechanism failure (patellar tendon rupture)
- Arthrofibrosis (stiff knee)
- Periprosthetic fracture
- Unstable or loosened prosthesis
- Heterotopic ossification

Immunosuppression, diabetes, smoking, previous knee surgery, and obesity are known risk factors for postoperative knee infection, which can be a devastating complication requiring emergent irrigation and debridement and long-term intravenous (IV) antibiotics. Infection can be prevented by perioperative use of IV antibiotics and attention to careful surgical technique and soft tissue handling, which have been shown to minimize wound healing problems. In addition, laminar airflow and having a dedicated surgical team and reduced surgical time have been shown to reduce the risk of infection in patients with TKA.[92,93] Early signs and symptoms of infection, which present primarily in the area of the

TABLE 23-5

Clinical Model for Predicting Pretest Probability of Deep Vein Thrombosis (DVT)* (Wells Clinical Prediction Rules for DVT)

Clinical Finding	Score
Active cancer (treatment ongoing, within previous 6 months, or palliative)	1
Paralysis, paresis, or recent plaster immobilization of lower extremities	1
Recently bedridden for 3 days or more, or major surgery within the previous 12 weeks requiring general or regional anesthesia	1
Localized tenderness along the distribution of the deep venous system	1
Entire leg swelling/calf swelling at least 3 cm larger than that on the asymptomatic leg (measured 10 cm below the tibial tuberosity)	1
Pitting edema confined to the symptomatic leg	1
Collateral superficial veins (nonvaricose)	1
Previously documented DVT	1
Alternative diagnosis that is at least as likely as DVT (e.g., cellulitis, calf strain, postoperative swelling)	−2

*In patients with symptoms in both legs, the more symptomatic leg is used. A cumulative score of >2 is likely DVT, whereas <2 means DVT is unlikely.

Modified from Wells PS: Advances in the diagnosis of venous thromboembolism, *J Thromb Thrombolysis* 21:32, 2006.

incision, include increased redness, warmth, edema, and possibly drainage from the surgical wound. Infection after wound closure can be either superficial (e.g., a cellulitis) or a deep infection in the joint or bone. Symptoms of progressively worsening pain accompanied by cardinal signs of systemic infection (e.g., fever, rigors [shivering]) should prompt the clinician to notify the surgeon because early management of infection is critical for a successful outcome.

Additional mechanical complications in TKA can include medial collateral ligament (MCL) injury, extensor mechanism failure, arthrofibrosis, and/or periprosthetic fracture. Iatrogenic intraoperative disruption of the MCL during TKA typically has been treated with implantation of a more constrained prosthesis that provides varus-valgus restraint. In addition, repair and/or reattachment of the ligament has proven successful, with postoperative knee scores and ROM equivalent to those in knees without this complication. Rehabilitation for these patients must be modified slightly because they wear a brace for 6 weeks after surgery and follow an MCL injury protocol to allow healing of the ligament.

Rupture of the patellar tendon is another rare but devastating complication of knee arthroplasty. Nonsurgical treatment and primary repair have not proven successful. Reconstruction with fresh-frozen extensor mechanism allograft is preferred because of the improved ability of both bone and tendon to incorporate. Nonabsorbable suture fixation of the allograft tendon onto a broad base of healthy quadriceps musculature allows reliable incorporation. Furthermore, fracture of the patella may also occur. Three aspects of the extensor mechanism must be assessed: whether the patellar component is loose, whether the extensor mechanism is partly or completely disrupted, and the extent of the remaining patellar bone. Nonsurgical treatment is successful if the extensor mechanism remains functional and the patellar component remains well fixed. Surgery is indicated in patients showing marked disruption of the extensor mechanism.[94,95] Postoperative management must initially allow for healing of the tendon repair, which will significantly impact the rate of progress in gaining ROM, strength, and functional mobility.

Postoperative stiff knee is a sign of failure of TKA and remains an unsolved problem. The best predictor of postoperative ROM is preoperative motion. When arthrofibrosis is diagnosed early, it can be managed successfully with manipulation under anesthesia. Late treatment of stiffness is less likely to respond to manipulation.[96]

Although the prevalence of postoperative periprosthetic fracture is fairly low (less than 2% of cases), treatment remains a challenge to all orthopedic surgeons, and the complication rates remain high. The main goal of treatment is to maintain alignment and fracture stability, and early ROM is essential to prevent stiffness. Surgery is indicated when the fracture is significantly displaced, stability of the prosthesis is compromised, and quality of bone is suboptimal. Failed prosthesis, demonstrated by a loose implant, requires revision arthroplasty. Displaced fractures associated with well-fixed implants are best treated with reduction and rigid fixation to allow early ROM.

Heterotopic ossification, another potential complication, results in calcium deposition within soft tissues around the joint. Although uncommon, this complication may directly impede progress with ROM and possibly strengthening exercises. Management may involve medication, radiation therapy, and possibly surgical excision, which will clearly alter the goals and rehabilitation treatment program.

The survival rate for primary TKA implants is >90% 10 years after the surgery.[97] Late complications after TKA primarily include prosthetic loosening.[98] A new onset of pain in either the distal thigh or leg may indicate loosening of the prosthesis, and these symptoms typically worsen with weight-bearing activities and progressively worsen over time. Again, early referral to the surgeon is indicated because appropriate surgical intervention is required. A painful TKA requires a broad systemic workup that includes both intrinsic (knee-related) and extrinsic sources of pain. It is important to note that despite the widely taught precept that knee pain can originate outside the

knee, patients continue to present to referral centers with pain in a replaced knee following an extensive and inconclusive workup of the knee joint when the origin of their pain is from an arthritic hip or lumbar spine.[8] Therefore protocols for evaluating a painful TKA begin with clinical and radiographic examination of extraarticular sites. Routine aspiration should be performed for a replaced knee suspicious for infection. White blood cell counts of $25,000/mm^3$ or higher provide a strong suspicion for an infected TKA that needs to be surgically debrided.[92,93,99]

Failure of a replaced knee results in rapid acceleration of pain symptoms, functional decline, and the need for revision arthroplasty. Revision surgery is indicated for gross loosening of the implants, instability, infection, malalignment, wear, osteolysis, or disruption of the extensor mechanism. Gross loosening of the implants may occur secondary to wear and osteolysis, malalignment, or infection. Therefore routine knee aspiration is indicated.[100] A midline incision is made, but when multiple incisions are present, it is important to use the most lateral incision because of the soft tissue blood supply. It also is important to assess the bone integrity, remaining bone stock, and the extensor mechanism and collateral ligament integrity. Furthermore, it is important to restore the anatomical joint line, which generally is 1.5 cm (0.6 inch) proximal to the tip of the fibula. Elevation of the joint line results in patellar impingement and reduced quadriceps strength. The complication rate for revision TKA is much higher than for primary TKA, approaching 25%. Infection, dysfunction of the extensor mechanism, instability, fixation failure, and periprosthetic fracture all can compromise the outcome of revision surgery. Although most of these complications require intervention from providers other than the physical therapist, early recognition of complications and appropriate referral are important.

OUTCOMES OF TOTAL KNEE ARTHROPLASTY

Outcomes after TKA have been reported in the literature for decades, and the majority of studies have focused on the technical aspects of prosthetic implant survivability and design. More recent research has embraced the need also to address the impact of this procedure on quality-of-life issues important to the patient. More standardized outcome tools are being used to assess patient outcomes, with the most common ones being the WOMAC, Oxford-12, and Short Form 12 (SF-12); however, a single ideal outcome tool to assess patients after TKA does not exist.

Overall, TKA for patients with end-stage OA is considered a successful surgical intervention, with implant survivability reported to be greater than 81% to 92% 15 years after surgery.[12] The primary factor that influences ROM outcome is preoperative ROM. Despite the intent of PCL-sparing or substitution (high flexion) prosthetic designs, studies have failed to find a significant difference in ROM outcomes using these implants compared with standard posterior constrained devices.[101-104] It is important for the clinician to have an understanding of the type of implant used and the expected ROM that can be achieved to establish realistic ROM goals for the patient. Constrained and rotating hinge devices, which are inherently more stable by design, may limit flexion ROM and have the potential to transfer more shear and rotatory forces to the bone-prosthesis interface, potentially contributing to early loosening of the prosthesis.[98]

UKA has a reported greater than 80% survival at 10 years. These devices tend to be used in younger patients who have a higher preoperative level of function, but also have higher expectations of functional performance post surgery. The most common reason for early failure of UKA is a lack of symptomatic improvement resulting in conversion to a TKA. Appropriate patient selection is the key to preventing early conversion to TKA.[105-108]

Additional considerations on prosthetic design have focused on the effect of preserving the PCL as a soft tissue structure that can contribute proprioceptive and kinesthetic input to the knee. The rationale for leaving the PCL intact is to enhance joint position sense and provide important feedback for balance mechanisms. Studies have shown that proprioception and kinesthesia improve after TKA, most likely because of the reduction in pain and inflammation and postoperative changes to the capsuloligamentous structures, not necessarily because of preservation of the PCL.[109] Further studies that specifically address balance and proprioceptive training after TKA with both PCL-sparing and PCL-substituting devices may shed more light on this design feature.

The strongest predictors of outcomes following knee arthroplasty surgery include preoperative pain, function, and WOMAC scores.[14-16,110] Patients with anxiety or depression, pain in the operative or contralateral knee, or preoperative knee weakness have poorer outcomes and residual participation restrictions.[108,111,112]

The timing of measurement and the tools used to measure function vary in the literature. The **WOMAC OA Index** and the **6-Minute Walk Test (6MWT)** have been reported to be most responsive when patients are examined 0 to 4 months after surgery.[113] Performance-based testing after TKA needs to consider the recovery time frame. Early postoperative assessments should include the 6MWT as the most responsive test. The timed stair ascent is not responsive early on because many patients are unable to complete this task in the first 4 months after surgery.[113] The 6MWT has also been shown to be predictive of functional ambulation and correlates well with longer walk tests in individuals 12 to 18 months post TKA.[114]

The **Knee Society Clinical Rating Scale** and the WOMAC are the most responsive outcome measures for TKA.[115] Both are disease-specific scales that rate function, pain, and stiffness—the primary symptoms associated with OA. Patient perception of functional recovery has multiple interactions, including psychological issues, which may influence the patient's report of function.[116-118] Comprehensive management, which includes psychological aspects, should be considered in the overall patient care plan.

A major focus in recent outcomes studies on patients who underwent TKA has been the correlation between strength and function. Many studies have reported residual weakness in patients who have completed rehabilitation,[116,118-121] which affects the patients' gait speed[122,123] and stair ascent strategy.[124] Experimental designs that focus specifically on additional interventions to address strength deficits have shown promise in improving strength and related functional activities.[67-69,122,125-127] Further research into interventions is important to determine the optimum treatment for developing postoperative protocols that will rehabilitate patients to their fullest potential and restore their functional ability to that of age- and gender-matched controls. As patients' expectations for postoperative function change, rehabilitation programs must evolve to meet these needs fully.

SUMMARY

TKA is a successful intervention for patients with end-stage arthritis of the knee. Rehabilitation is an essential component of the overall management of these patients. Coordinated, individualized care from all health care providers, from the preoperative phase through the continuum of postoperative rehabilitation, maximizes the patient's functional level and ability to resume meaningful activities. Ongoing advancements in surgical instrumentation and techniques, coupled with progressive rehabilitation programs, will continue to improve the long-term results and expectations for TKA.

REFERENCES

1. Vaccaro AR: *Orthopaedic knowledge update 8*, Rosemont, 2005, American Academy of Orthopaedic Surgeons.
2. Ranawat CS, Flynn WF, Saddler S, et al: Long-term results of the total condylar knee arthroplasty: a 15 year survivorship study, *Clin Orthop Relat Res* 286:94–102, 1993.
3. Suri P, Morgenroth DC, Hunter DJ: Epidemiology of osteoarthritis and associated comorbidities, *Phys Med Rehabil* 4(5 suppl):S10–S19, 2012.
4. Blagojevic M, Jinks C, Jeffery A, Jordan KP: Risk factors for onset of osteoarthritis of the knee in older adults: a systematic review and meta-analysis, *Osteoarthritis Cartilage* 18:24–33, 2010.
5. Feng EL, Stulberg SD, Wixson RL: Progressive subluxation and polyethylene wear in total knee replacements with flat articular surfaces, *Clin Orthop Relat Res* 299:60–71, 1994.
6. Kleinbart FA, Bryk E, Evangelista J, et al: Histologic comparison of posterior cruciate ligaments from arthritic and aged-matched knee specimens, *J Arthroplasty* 11:726–731, 1996.
7. Haverbush TH: *Online orthopedics 2000-2006.* (Accessed 12.07.06). Available at www.orthopodsurgeon.com.
8. Callaghan JJ, Rosenberg AG, Rubash HE, et al, editors: *The adult knee*, Philadelphia, 2003, Lippincott Williams & Wilkins.
9. Cram P, Lu X, Kates SL, et al: Total knee arthroplasty volume, utilization, and outcomes among medicare beneficiaries 1991-2010, *JAMA* 308:1227–1236, 2012.

10. Kurtz SM, Lau E, Ong K, et al: Future young patient demand for primary and revision joint replacement: national projections from 2010 to 2030, *Clin Orthop Relat Res* 467:2606–2612, 2009.

11. Kurtz S, Ong K, Lau E, et al: Projections of primary and revision hip and knee arthroplasty in the United States from 2005 to 2030, *J Bone Joint Surg Am* 89:780–785, 2007.

12. Roberts VI, Esler CNA, Harper WM: A 15-year follow-up study of 4606 primary total knee replacements, *J Bone Joint Surg Br* 89:1452–1456, 2007.

13. Aggarwal VK, Goyal N, Deirmengian G, et al: Revision total knee arthroplasty in the young patient: is there trouble on the horizon? *J Bone Joint Surg Am* 96:536–542, 2014.

14. Jones CA, Voaklander DC, Suarez-Almazor ME: Determinants of function after total knee arthroplasty, *Phys Ther* 83:696–706, 2003.

15. Parent E, Moffet H: Preoperative predictors of loomotor ability two months after total knee arthroplasty for severe osteoarthritis, *Arthritis Rheum* 49:36–50, 2003.

16. Kahn TL, Soheili A, Schwarzkopf R: Outcomes of total knee arthroplasty in relation to preoperative patient-reported and radiographic measures: data from the osteoarthritis initiative, *Geriatr Orthop Surg Rehabil* 4:117–126, 2013.

17. Topp R, Swank AM, Quesada PM, et al: The effect of prehabilitation exercise on strength and functioning after total knee arthroplasty, *Phys Med Rehabil* 1:729–735, 2009.

18. D'Lima DD, Colwell CW, Morris BA, et al: The effect of preoperative exercise on total knee replacement outcomes, *Clin Orthop Relat Res* 326:174–182, 1996.

19. Weidenhielm L, Mattson E, Brostrom L, Wersall-Robertsson E: Effect of preoperative physiotherapy in unicompartmental prosthetic knee replacement, *Scand J Rehab Med* 25:33, 1993.

20. Rodgers JA, Garvin KL, Walker CW, et al: Preoperative physical therapy in primary total knee arthroplasty, *J Arthroplasty* 13:414–421, 1998.

21. Beaupre LA, Lier D, Davies DM, Johnston DBC: The effect of a preoperative exercise and education program on functional recovery, health related quality of life, and health service utilization following primary total knee arthroplasty, *J Rheumatol* 31:1166–1173, 2004.

22. Baker CS, McKeon JM: Does preoperative rehabilitation improve patient-based outcomes in persons who have undergone total knee arthroplasty? A systematic review, *Phys Med Rehabil* 4:756–767, 2012.

23. Jordan RW, Smith NA, Chahal GS, et al: Enhanced education and physiotherapy before knee replacement; is it worth it? A systematic review, *Physiotherapy* 100:305–312, 2014. http://dx.doi.org/10.1016/j.physio.2014.03.003.

24. Lin PC, Lin LC, Lin JJ: Comparing the effectiveness of different educational programs in patients with total knee arthroplasty, *Orthop Nurs* 6:43–49, 1997.

25. Daltroy LH, Morlino CI, Eaton HM, et al: Preoperative education for total hip and knee replacement patients, *Arthritis Care Res* 11:469–478, 1998.

26. Healthcare Cost and Utilization Project (HCUP). (Accessed 28.07.14). Available at http://hcup-us.ahrq.gov/reports/projections/2012-03.pdf.

27. Ritter MA, Herbert SA, Keating EM, et al: Long-term survival analysis of a posterior cruciate–retaining total condylar total knee replacement, *Clin Orthop Relat Res* 309:136–145, 1994.

28. Spencer JM, Chauhan SK, Sloan K, et al: Computer navigation versus conventional total knee replacement no difference in functional results at two years, *J Bone Joint Surg Br* 89:477–480, 2007.

29. Kim S, Losina E, Solomon DH, et al: Effectiveness of clinical pathways for total knee and total hip arthroplasty, *J Arthroplasty* 18:69–74, 2003.

30. Pennington JM, Jones DPG, McIntyre S: Clinical pathways in total knee arthroplasty: a New Zealand experience, *J Orthop Surg* 11:166–173, 2003.

31. Healy WL, Iorio R, Ko J, et al: Impact of cost reduction programs on short-term patient outcome and hospital cost of total knee arthroplasty, *J Bone Joint Surg Am* 84:348–353, 2002.

32. Isaac D, Falode T, Liu P, et al: Accelerated rehabilitation after total knee replacement, *Knee* 12:346–350, 2005.

33. Teeny SM, York SC, Benson C, Perdue ST: Does shortened length of hospital stay affect total knee arthroplasty rehabilitation outcomes? *J Arthroplasty* 20:39–45, 2005.

34. Barbieri A, Vanhaecht K, Van Herck P, et al: Effects of clinical pathways in the joint replacement: a meta-analysis, *BMC Med* 7:32, 2009.

35. Denis M, Moffet H, Caron F, et al: Effectiveness of continuous passive motion and conventional physical therapy after total knee arthroplasty: a randomized clinical trial, *Phys Ther* 86:174–185, 2006.

36. Bennett LA, Brearley SC, Hart JAL, Bailey MJ: A comparison of two continuous passive motion protocols after total knee arthroplasty: a controlled and randomized study, *J Arthroplasty* 20:225–233, 2005.

37. Davies DM, Johnston DWC, Beaupre LA, Lier DA: Effect of adjunctive range-of-motion therapy after primary total knee arthroplasty on the use of health services after hospital discharge, *Can J Surg* 46:30–36, 2003.

38. Lenssen AF, de Bie RA, Bulstra SK, van Steyn MJA: Continuous passive motion (CPM) in rehabilitation following total knee arthroplasty: a randomized controlled trial, *Phys Ther Rev* 8:123–129, 2003.

39. Chen B, Zimmerman JR, Soulen L, et al: Continuous passive motion machine after total knee arthroplasty: a prospective study, *Am J Phys Med Rehabil* 79:421–426, 2000.

40. Worland RL, Arrendondo J, Angles F, et al: Home continuous passive motion machine versus professional physical therapy following total knee replacement, *J Arthroplasty* 13:784–787, 1998.

41. Ververeli PA, Sutton DC, Hearn SL, et al: Continuous passive motion after total knee arthroplasty: analysis of cost and benefits, *Clin Orthop Relat Res* 321:208–215, 1995.

42. Pope RO, Corcoran S, McCaul K, et al: Continuous passive motion after primary total knee arthroplasty: does it offer any benefits? *J Bone Joint Surg Br* 79:914–917, 1997.

43. Lachiewicz PF: The role of continuous passive motion after total knee arthroplasty, *Clin Orthop Relat Res* 380:144–150, 2000.

44. Kumar PJ, McPherson EJ, Dorr LD, et al: Rehabilitation after total knee arthroplasty: a comparison of two rehabilitation techniques, *Clin Orthop Relat Res* 331:93–101, 1996.

45. Herbold JA, Bonistall K, Blackburn M, et al: Randomized controlled trial of the effectiveness of continuous passive motion after total knee replacement, *Arch Phys Med Rehabil* 95:1240–1245, 2014.

46. Maniar RN, Baviskar JV, Singhi T, Rathi SS: To use or not to use continuous passive motion post–total knee arthroplasty: presenting functional assessment results in early recovery, *J Arthroplasty* 27:193–200, 2012.

47. Harvey LA, Brosseau L, Herbert RD: Continuous passive motion following total knee arthroplasty in people with arthritis, Feb 6, *Cochrane Database Syst Rev* 2,2014, CD004260.

48. Brosseau L, Milne S, Wells G, et al: Efficacy of continuous passive motion following total knee arthroplasty: a meta-analysis, *J Rheumatol* 31:2251–2264, 2004.

49. Milne S, Brosseau L, Robinson V, et al: Continuous passive motion following total knee arthroplasty, *Cochrane Database Syst Rev*, 2003, CD004260.

50. Chiarello CM, Gundersen L, O'Halloran T: The effect of continuous passive motion duration and incremental range of motion in total knee arthroplasty patients, *J Orthop Sports Phys Ther* 25:119–127, 1997.

51. Seet E, Leong WL, Yeo AS, Fook-Chong S: Effectiveness of 3-in-1 continuous femoral block of differing concentrations compared to patient controlled intravenous morphine for post total knee arthroplasty analgesia and knee rehabilitation, *Anaesth Intensive Care* 34:25–30, 2006.

52. YaDeau JT, Cahill JB, Zaqwadsky MW, et al: The effects of femoral nerve blockade in conjunction with epidural analgesia after total knee arthroplasty, *Anesth Analg* 101:891–895, 2005.

53. Venditoli PA, Makinen P, Drolet P, et al: A multimodal analgesia protocol for total knee arthroplasty, *J Bone Joint Surg Am* 88:282–289, 2006.

54. Baratta JL, Gandhi K, Viscusi ER: Perioperative pain management for total knee arthroplasty, *J Surg Orthop Adv* 23:22–36, 2014.

55. McNair PJ, Marshall RN, Maguire K: Swelling of the knee joint: effect of exercise on quadriceps muscle strength, *Arch Phys Med Rehab* 77:896–899, 1996.

56. Munin MC, Kwoh CK, Glynn N, et al: Predicting discharge outcomes after elective hip and knee arthroplasty, *Am J Phys Med Rehab* 74:294–301, 1995.

57. Bozic KJ, Wagie A, Naessens JM, et al: Predictors of discharge to an inpatient extended care facility after total hip or knee arthroplasty, *J Arthroplasty* 21:151–156, 2006.

58. Barsoum WK, Murray TG, Klika AK, et al: Predicting patient discharge disposition after total joint arthroplasty in the United States, *J Arthroplasty* 25:885–892, 2010.

59. Oldmeadow LB, McBurney H, Robertson VJ: Predicting risk of extended inpatient rehabilitation after hip or knee arthroplasty, *J Arthroplasty* 18:775–779, 2003.

60. Dauty M, Schmitt X, Menu P, et al: Using the Risk Assessment and Predictor Tool (RAPT) for patients after total knee replacement surgery, *Ann Phys Rehabil Med* 55:4–15, 2012.

61. Ariza G, Badia M, Cuixart A, et al: Quality of life after knee arthroplasty: utility of the RAPT scale, *Rehabilitation* 46:147–156, 2012.

62. Hansen VJ, Gromov K, Lebrun LM, et al: Does the risk assessment and prediction tool predict discharge disposition after joint replacement? *Clin Orthop Relat Res* 473:597–601, 2015.

63. Graham JE, Deutsch A, O'Connell AA, et al: Inpatient rehabilitation volume and functional outcomes in stroke, lower extremity fracture, and lower extremity joint replacement, *Med Care* 51:404–412, 2013.

64. Lin JJ, Kaplan RJ: Multivariate analysis of the factors affecting duration of acute inpatient rehabilitation after hip and knee arthroplasty, *Am J Phys Med Rehab* 83:344–352, 2004.

65. *Medicare and home health care.* (Accessed 13.08.14.) Available at www.medicare.gov.

66. Stevens JE, Mizner RL, Snyder-Mackler L: Quadriceps strength and volitional activation before and after total knee arthroplasty for osteoarthritis, *J Orthop Res* 21:775–779, 2003.

67. Stevens JE, Mizner RL, Snyder-Mackler L: Neuromuscular electrical stimulation for quadriceps muscle strengthening after bilateral total knee arthroplasty: a case series, *J Orthop Sports Phys Ther* 34:21–29, 2004.

68. Bade MJ, Stevens-Lapsley JE: Early high-intensity rehabilitation following total knee arthroplasty improves outcomes, *J Orthop Sports Phys Ther* 41:932–941, 2011.

69. Stevens-Lapsley JE, Balter JE, Wolfe P, et al: Early neuromuscular electrical stimulation to improve quadriceps muscle strength after total knee arthroplasty: a randomized controlled trial, *Phys Ther* 92:210–226, 2012.

70. Youm T, Mauer SG, Stuchin SA: Postoperative management after total hip and knee arthroplasty, *J Arthroplasty* 20:322–324, 2005.

71. Hall VL, Hardwick M, Reden L, et al: Unicompartmental knee arthroplasty (alias uni-knee): an overview with nursing implications, *Orthop Nurs* 23:163–171, 2004.

72. Bonutti PM, Mont MA, McMahon M, et al: Minimally invasive total knee arthroplasty, *J Bone Joint Surg Am* 86(suppl 2):26–32, 2004.

73. Bolognesi MP, Greiner MA, Attarian DE, et al: Unicompartmental knee arthroplasty and total knee arthroplasty among medicare beneficiaries, 2000 to 2009, *J Bone Joint Surg Am* 95:2013, e174.

74. Mont MA, Mitzner DL, Jones LC, et al: History of the contralateral knee after primary knee arthroplasty for osteoarthritis, *Clin Orthop Relat Res* 321:145–150, 1995.

75. Jankiewicz JJ, Sculco TP, Ranawat CS, et al: One stage versus two stage bilateral total knee arthroplasty, *Clin Orthop Relat Res* 309:94–101, 1994.

76. Liu TK, Chen SH: Simultaneous bilateral total knee arthroplasty in a single procedure, *Int Orthop* 22:390–393, 1998.

77. McMahon M, Block JA: The risk of contralateral total knee arthroplasty after knee replacement for osteoarthritis, *J Rheumatol* 30:1822–1824, 2003.

78. Ritter M, Mamlin LA, Melfi CA, et al: Outcome implications for the timing of bilateral total knee arthroplasties, *Clin Orthop Relat Res* 345:99–105, 1997.

79. Morrey BF, Adams RA, Ilstrup DM, et al: Complications and mortality associated with bilateral or unilateral total knee arthroplasty, *J Bone Joint Surg Am* 69:484–488, 1987.

80. Poultsides L, Memtsoudis S, Della Valle AG, et al: Perioperative morbidity and mortality of same-day bilateral TKAs, *Clin Orthop Relat Res* 472:111–120, 2014.

81. Kolettis GT, Wixson RL, Peruzzi WT, et al: Safety of one stage bilateral total knee arthroplasty, *Clin Orthop Relat Res* 309:102–109, 1994.

82. Memtsoudis SG, Hargett M, Russell LA, et al: Consensus statement from the consensus conference on bilateral total knee arthroplasty group, *Clin Orthop Relat Res* 471:2649–2657, 2013.

83. Poultsides LA, Rasouli MR, Maltenfort MG, et al: Trends in same-day bilateral total knee arthroplasty, *J Arthroplasty* 29:1713–1716, 2014. http://dx.doi.org/10.1016/j.arth.2014.04.021.

84. Geerts WH, Pineo GF, Heit JA, et al: Prevention of venous thromboembolism: the seventh ACCP conference on antithrombotic and thrombolytic therapy, *Chest* 126:338S–400S, 2004.

85. Callahan CM, Drake BG, Heck DA, Dittus RS: Patient outcomes following tricompartmental total knee replacement: a meta-analysis, *JAMA* 271:1349–1357, 1994.

86. Xing KE, Morrison G, Lim W, et al: Has the incidence of deep vein thrombosis in patients undergoing total hip/knee arthroplasty changed over time? A systematic review of randomized controlled trials, *Thrombosis Res* 123:24–34, 2008.

87. Merli GJ: Pathophysiology of venous thrombosis, thrombophilia, and the diagnosis of deep vein thrombosis-pulmonary embolism in the elderly, *Clin Geriatric Med* 22:75–92, 2006.

88. Urbano FL: Homans' sign in the diagnosis of deep vein thrombosis, *Hosp Physician* 37:22–24, 2001.

89. Bounameaux H, Perrier A, Righini M: Diagnosis of venous thromboembolism: an update, *Vasc Med* 15:399–406, 2010.

90. Wells PS, Hirsh J, Anderson DR, et al: Accuracy of clinical assessment of deep vein thrombosis, *Lancet* 345:1326–1330, 1995.

91. Wells PS: Advances in the diagnosis of venous thromboembolism, *J Thromb Thrombolysis* 21:31–40, 2006.

92. Duff GP, Lachiewicz PF, Kelley SS: Aspiration of the knee joint before revision arthroplasty, *Clin Orthop Relat Res* 331:132–139, 1996.

93. Install JN, Thompson FM, Brause BD: Two-stage reimplantation for the salvage of infected total knee arthroplasty, *J Bone Joint Surg Am* 84:490, 2002.

94. Mahoney OM, McClung CD, dela Rosa MA, Schmalzried TP: The effect of total knee arthroplasty design on extensor mechanism function, *J Arthroplasty* 17:416–421, 2002.

95. Silva M, Shepard E, Jackson W, et al: Knee strength after total knee arthroplasty, *J Arthroplasty* 18:605–611, 2003.

96. Seyler TM, Marker DR, Bhave A, et al: Functional problems and arthrofibrosis following total knee arthroplasty, *J Bone Joint Surg Am* 89:59–69, 2007.

97. Pabinger C, Berghold A, Boehler N, Labek G: Revision rates after knee replacement. Cumulative results from worldwide clinical studies versus joint registers, *Osteoarthritis Cartilage* 21:263–268, 2013.

98. Martin SD, Scott RD, Thornhill TS: Current concepts of total knee arthroplasty, *J Orthop Sports Phys Ther* 28:252–261, 1998.

99. Coyte PC, Hawker G, Croxford R, Wright JG: Rates of revision knee replacement in Ontario, Canada, *J Bone Joint Surg Am* 81:773–782, 1999.

100. Partington PF, Sawhney J, Rorabeck CH, et al: Joint line restoration after revision total knee arthroplasty, *Clin Orthop Relat Res* 367:165–171, 1999.

101. Chiu KY, Ng TP, Tang WM, Yau WP: Review article: knee flexion after total knee arthroplasty, *J Orthop Surg* 10:194–202, 2002.

102. Guild GN, Labib SA: Clinical outcomes in high flexion total knee arthroplasty were not superior to standard posterior stabilized total knee arthroplasty. A multicenter, prospective, randomized study, *J Arthroplasty* 29:530–534, 2014.

103. Lützner J, Hartmann A, Lützner C, Kirschner S: Is range of motion after cruciate-retaining total knee arthroplasty influenced by prosthesis design? A prospective randomized trial, *J Arthroplasty* 29:961–965, 2014.

104. Verra WC, van den Boom LG, Jacobs W, et al: *Retention versus sacrifice of the posterior cruciate ligament in total knee arthroplasty for treating osteoarthritis (Review), Cochrane Database Syst Rev* Oct 11;10:CD004803, 2013.

105. Iorio R, Healy WL: Current concepts review unicompartmental arthritis of the knee, *J Bone Joint Surg Am* 85:1351–1364, 2003.

106. Newman JH, Ackroyd CE, Shah NA: Unicompartmental or total knee replacement? Five-year results in a prospective, randomized trial of 102 osteoarthritic knees with unicompartmental arthritis, *J Bone Joint Surg Br* 80:862–865, 1998.

107. Lyons MC, MacDonald SJ, Somerville LE, et al: Unicompartmental versus total knee arthroplasty database analysis. Is there a winner? *Clin Orthop Relat Res* 470:84–90, 2012.

108. Niinimaki T, Eskelinen A, Makela K, et al: Unicompartmental knee arthroplasty survivorship is lower than TKA survivorship: a 27-year Finnish registry study, *Clin Orthop Relat Res* 472:1496–1501, 2014.

109. Swanki CB, Lephart SM, Rubash HE: Proprioception, kinesthesia, and balance after total knee arthroplasty with cruciate-retaining and posterior stabilized prostheses, *J Bone Joint Surg Am* 86:328–334, 2004.

110. Judge A, Arden NK, Cooper C, et al: Predictors of outcomes of total knee replacement surgery, *Rheumatology* 51:1804–1813, 2012.

111. Maxwell JL, Keysor JJ, Niu J, et al: Participation following knee replacement: The MOST cohort study, *Phys Ther* 93:1467–1474, 2013.

112. Mizner RL, Petterson SC, Stevens JE, et al: Preoperative quadriceps strength predicts functional ability one year after total knee arthroplasty, *J Rheumatol* 32:1533–1539, 2005.

113. Parent E, Moffet H: Comparative responsiveness of locomotor tests and questionnaires used to follow early recovery after total knee arthroplasty, *Arch Phys Med Rehab* 83:70–80, 2002.

114. Ko V, Naylor JM, Harris IA, et al: The six-minute walk test is an excellent predictor of functional ambulation after total knee arthroplasty, *BMC Musculoskelet Disord* 14:145, 2013.

115. Kreibich DN, Bourne RB, Rorabeck CH, et al: What is the best way of assessing outcome after total knee replacement? *Clin Orthop Relat Res* 331:221–225, 1996.

116. Finch E, Walsh M, Thomas SG, Woodhouse LJ: Functional ability perceived by individuals following total knee arthroplasty compared to age-matched individuals without knee disability, *J Orthop Sports Phys Ther* 27:255–263, 1998.

117. McGuigan FX, Hozack WJ, Moriarty L, et al: Predicting quality-of-life outcomes following total joint arthroplasty, *J Arthroplasty* 10:742–747, 1995.

118. Caracciolo B, Giaquinto S: Self-perceived distress and self-perceived functional recovery after recent total hip and knee arthroplasty, *Arch Gerontol Geriatr* 41:177–181, 2005.

119. Silva M, Shephard EF, Jackson WO, et al: Knee strength after total knee arthroplasty, *J Arthroplasty* 18:605–611, 2003.

120. Mizner RL, Stevens JE, Snyder-Mackler L: Voluntary activation and decreased force production of the quadriceps femoris muscle after total knee arthroplasty, *Phys Ther* 83:359–365, 2003.

121. Rossi MD, Hasson S: Lower-limb force production in individuals after unilateral total knee arthroplasty, *Arch Phys Med Rehab* 85:1279–1284, 2004.

122. Walsh M, Woodhouse LJ, Thomas SG, Finch E: Physical limitations and functional limitations: a comparison of individuals 1 year after total knee arthroplasty with control subjects, *Phys Ther* 78:248–258, 1998.

123. Oullet D, Moffet H: Locomotor deficits before and two months after knee arthroplasty, *Arthritis Rheum* 47:484–493, 2002.

124. Bryne JM, Gage W, Prentice SD: Bilateral lower limb strategies used during a step-up task in individuals who have undergone unilateral total knee arthroplasty, *Clin Biomech* 17:580–585, 2002.

125. Avramidis K, Strike PW, Taylor PN, Swain ID: Effectiveness of electrical stimulation of the vastus medialis muscle in the rehabilitation of patients after total knee arthroplasty, *Arch Phys Med Rehab* 84:1850–1853, 2003.

126. Mizner RL, Petterson SC, Snyder-Mackler L: Quadriceps strength and the time course of functional recovery after total knee arthroplasty, *J Orthop Sports Phys Ther* 35:424–436, 2005.

127. Moffet H, Collet JP, Shapiro SH, et al: Effectiveness of intensive rehabilitation on functional ability and quality of life after first total knee arthroplasty: a single-blind randomized controlled trial, *Arch Phys Med Rehab* 85:546–556, 2004.

CHAPTER 24

Rehabilitation of Leg, Ankle, and Foot Injuries

D.S. BLAISE WILLIAMS III, JAY HERTEL, CHRISTOPHER D. INGERSOLL, DAVID P. NEWMAN

INTRODUCTION

Injuries to the lower leg, ankle, and foot often result in disability because of the loss of the ability of the foot and ankle complex to support and drive the gait cycle. Rehabilitation for injuries to this region requires restoration of mobility as early as possible. It is imperative that the clinician balance the focus on early mobility with protection of injured tissues in order to allow for optimal healing and restoration of normal neuromuscular recruitment strategies for movement execution. Overuse injuries are common at the foot and ankle complex and even more so in the lower leg as a result of the need to eccentrically control motion during landing activities. Because the foot and lower leg motion are tightly coupled during walking and running, forces are transferred up the kinetic chain. This places an even greater importance on the evaluation and treatment of foot and ankle morphology and mechanics during weight bearing. A quick return to activity after an acute injury without proper assessment of lower leg and foot structure and mechanics to guide rehabilitation may predispose the patient to a subsequent injury. For these reasons, clinicians must exercise sound clinical judgment in assessing patient function and structure when designing and implementing rehabilitation programs for injuries to the lower leg, ankle, and foot.

PRINCIPLES OF REHABILITATION PROGRESSION FOR LOWER LEG, ANKLE, AND FOOT INJURIES

When treating injuries to the lower leg, ankle, and foot, the clinician must consider functional limitations in the entire lower extremity. Such limitations typically fall into the categories of restricted range of motion (ROM), reduced muscular strength and endurance, and impaired proprioception and neuromuscular control. A paradigm such as the rehabilitation pyramid[1] (Figure 24-1) is useful for designing treatment and rehabilitation programs.

The base of the rehabilitation pyramid emphasizes control of pain and inflammation and provision of a treatment environment that allows injured tissues to heal. Each of these components will vary greatly, depending on the patient's specific pathology. Initial treatment should be focused on the promotion of healing tissue and reduction of inflammation. Rest, ice compression, and elevation (RICE) are the accepted protocol for acute injuries. Pain and inflammation can be controlled further with physical agents such as compression cryotherapy and electrical stimulation, as well as with analgesic and anti-inflammatory medication. Provision of an environment that allows tissues to heal often is accomplished with some type of immobilization device, such as a cast, brace, or walking boot (Figures 24-2 to 24-4). Devices that assist ambulation, such as crutches and canes, also are often critical elements in creating an environment conducive to protection, tissue healing, and mobilization.

Progression through the rehabilitation pyramid centers on issues of neuromuscular control. The left side of the pyramid comprises three levels of neuromuscular control: control of volitional contractions, control of reflex reactions, and control of functional movement patterns. When neuromuscular control is established at multiple levels of rehabilitation progression, patients may be less likely to develop inefficient and potentially deleterious movement strategies that may slow their recovery or predispose them to subsequent injuries. Although neuromuscular control training has been shown to be of great importance in rehabilitation of particular injuries,[2] other functional limitations, such as restricted ROM and reduced muscular strength and endurance, must be addressed simultaneously.

Levels of Neuromuscular Control

- Control of voluntary movements
- Control of reflex reactions
- Control of functional movement patterns

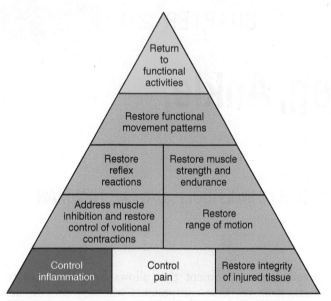

Figure 24-1 Rehabilitation pyramid. (Modified from Hertel J, Deneger CR: A rehabilitation paradigm for restoring neuromuscular control following injury, *Athl Ther Today* 3:12-16, 1998.)

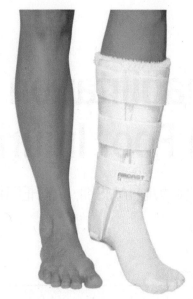

Figure 24-3 Aircast leg brace. (Courtesy of Donjoy, Vista, CA.)

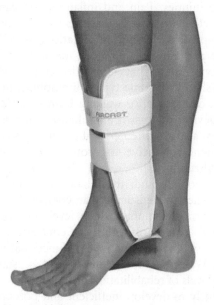

Figure 24-2 Aircast ankle brace. (Courtesy of Donjoy, Vista, CA.)

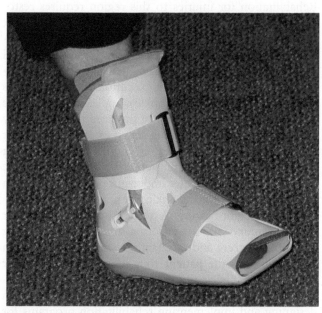

Figure 24-4 Walking boot (cam walker).

The cause of reduced ROM must be considered before efforts are initiated to restore this motion. After long periods of immobilization, ROM in the joints of the ankle and foot often is reduced, and tissue adaptations have occurred in the musculotendinous and collagenous structures, such as the joint capsule. Early emphasis on joint mobilizations often is helpful for alleviating capsular adhesions and reducing joint stiffness.[3] Before these treatments are started, it is important for the clinician to make sure that no contraindications exist to joint mobilizations, such as the use of surgical intra-articular fixations to stabilize fractures. Active and passive ROM exercises may also yield increases in joint ROM soon after immobilization

has ended. Specifically, if musculotendinous structures are tight, exercises and muscle-specific mobilization techniques targeted directly at improving flexibility in these structures may be initiated (Figure 24-5).

Muscle strengthening of foot and ankle muscles, as well as muscles surrounding the hips and knees, must also be addressed. Muscle strength is easily compromised after injury and immobilization. It is important to emphasize adequate neuromuscular control over volitional isometric contractions before advancing to isotonic contractions. Inability to initiate strong isotonic muscle contractions may be the result of **arthrogenic muscle inhibition (AMI)**. AMI is a reflex inhibition of the musculature surrounding

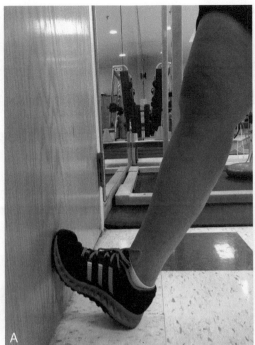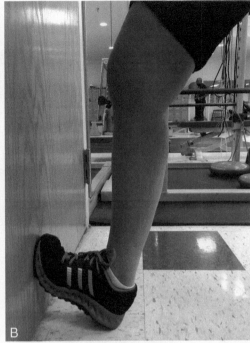

Figure 24-5 Stretching. **A,** Gastrocnemius (knee straight). **B,** Soleus (knee bent).

a joint after distension caused by swelling or damage to the joint structures.[4] As a result of AMI, fewer recruitable motor units are available during a voluntary contraction, which may lead to decreased force production. Attempting to progress exercise intensity or complexity while a muscle is in an inhibited state may cause a patient to develop compensatory motor unit recruitment patterns. With continued muscle inhibition, clinicians may observe severe muscle weakness, pain, and muscle atrophy that can prolong the rehabilitation period.

Strategies to reduce AMI, including cryotherapy and transcutaneous electrical nerve stimulation (TENS), should be used before the patient is progressed through a rehabilitation program. Cryotherapy may decrease the firing of the inhibitory interneuron involved in the reflex, thus reducing the inhibition of the voluntary muscle contraction. TENS, on the other hand, stimulates cutaneous type I nerve endings, which may disrupt the flow of information from joint receptors in the injured area to the spinal cord through competition with the same type I afferent fibers. Cryotherapy and TENS have been reported to diminish AMI and, if incorporated, should be applied before therapeutic exercise.[5] Cryotherapy before exercise or TENS before and during exercise creates a more normal muscle state, allowing the muscle to contract with increased and therefore more normal, motor unit activity.

Once volitional control has been established, isotonic, single-joint resistance exercises performed in an **open kinetic chain (OKC)** can begin. OKC exercises can be used to isolate specific joints or muscles to improve ROM, strength, and movement patterns while controlling compensatory movement patterns or forces that may occur during weight-bearing exercises. Similarly, the acuity of the injury or postoperative restrictions may require limited weight bearing. Therefore, OKC exercises may be an option for early strengthening. Resistive exercises performed with resistive bands or tubing are particularly useful for strengthening the muscles about the ankle, provided the movement is performed in a controlled fashion (Figure 24-6).[6] Both concentric and eccentric contractions should be performed.

After adequate neuromuscular control and strength have been restored in isolated open-chain activities, **closed kinetic chain (CKC)** exercises can be initiated. CKC exercises are more consistent with functional activities (e.g., walking, squatting, stair climbing) and involve all the joints of the lower extremity.[7] Most CKC exercises are multijoint in nature, although activities such as heel raises, emphasize primarily one joint. As the patient improves, both OKC and CKC activities can be advanced. However, advancing exercises must progress slowly and carefully in an attempt to maintain protection of injured structures and decrease the risk of reinjury.

Returning to athletic or recreational activities requires the development and maintenance of muscular endurance. Muscle endurance is the ability or capacity of a muscle group to perform repeated contractions against a load.[8] **Muscle endurance** usually takes much longer to return than strength, and many patients may not regain normal muscle endurance until they reverse the muscle atrophy that accompanies musculoskeletal injuries.[9] It is crucial to include muscle endurance activities later in rehabilitation programs so that patients are able to return to full activity.

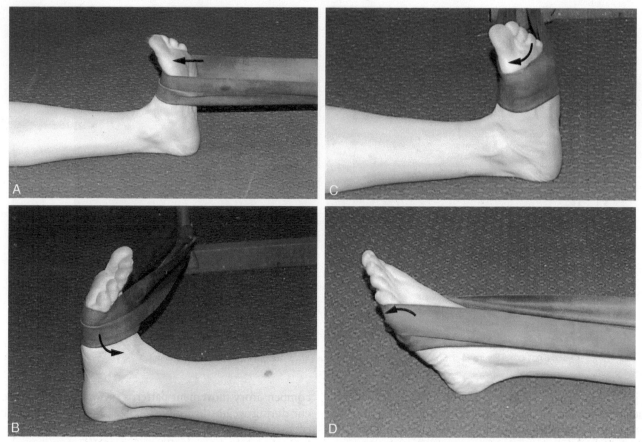

Figure 24-6 Four-way tubing exercises. **A,** Dorsiflexion. **B,** Eversion. **C,** Inversion. **D,** Plantar flexion.

Muscular endurance is trained with high repetitions at lower loads. It is important to have the patient perform exercises at speeds that simulate the speed of the functional activity or athletic performance. Power training during rehabilitation is important for strength at various speeds.[10] Most sport activities, even endurance activities, include components that require powerful muscle activation. **Power training** is the inclusion of exercises at low repetition under load and increasing velocities. This is important because it is a necessary component in the complete rehabilitation of the patient and for full, unrestricted return to play.

Exercises to address impairments in neuromuscular control and proprioception should be used throughout the rehabilitation process. Specifically, activities that challenge balance and postural control can aid in the restoration of normal proprioception, kinesthesia, and neuromuscular control. Exercises such as squatting, performing a plié in dancing, and bridging can be used effectively for balance training.[11] Progressions for balance training are presented in Table 24-1 and Figure 24-7.

In the final stages of rehabilitation, eccentric exercises and controlled plyometrics play an important role in ensuring the patient can return to normal activity. The eccentric exercises help train the muscles controlling the leg and foot to act as shock absorbers during motion and also to function as "dynamic brakes" to slow motion down.

Because prolonged limping may reinforce faulty neuromuscular recruitment and movement patterns, gait training should be incorporated in the rehabilitation process as early as possible for any lower extremity injury. An asymmetrical gait pattern (i.e., limping) at any point during rehabilitation is cause for concern because it may result in prolonged compensatory movement patterns. Assistive devices such as axillary crutches or a cane can be used initially to reduce weight bearing through the injured extremity. These can be discontinued when the patient can execute a symmetrical gait pattern. In addition, these devices can be used during rehabilitation sessions to help train the symmetrical pattern. When using axillary crutches, the patient should use a heel–toe gait pattern and bear weight as tolerated (or as allowed per postsurgical protocol). Before full weight bearing, gait training activities such as weight shifts forward and backward or sidestepping can be performed in the parallel bars or in a pool. To further challenge the patient, treadmill ambulation while changing the incline or speed can be incorporated.

TABLE **24-1**

Variables That Can Be Manipulated during Balance Training*

Stance	Visual Input	Surface	Arm Position	Patient Attention
Double limb	Eyes open	Firm	Outstretched	Concentrate only on balancing
Single limb	Eyes closed	Foam or Airex pad	At side	Recite by rote memory (ABCs), closed eyes
		Unstable (wobble board, trampoline)	Across chest	Perform simple computations (serial 7 s—counting in increments of 7; e.g., 7, 14, 21, and so on)
		Balance beam		External stimuli (ball toss, ball throw, rhythmic stabilization)

*Conditions are listed from easiest to hardest in each column.

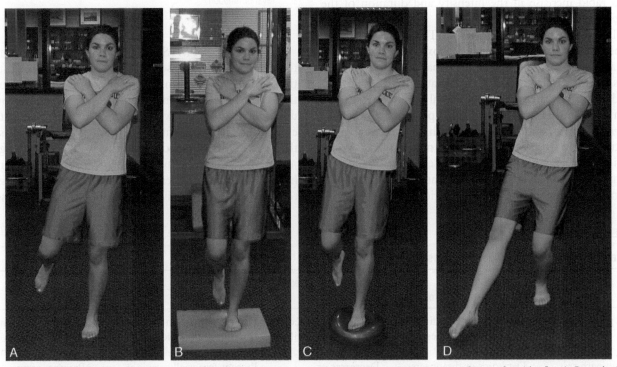

Figure 24-7 Balancing on different surfaces and the Star Excursion Balance Test (SEBT). **A,** Balancing on a firm surface (the floor). Perturbations can be added to increase the difficulty. **B,** Balancing on foam. **C,** Balancing on an air disc. **D,** Star Excursion Balance Test; point toes in different directions around the body.

Clinical Point

During the rehabilitation process, if a patient can only walk with a limp, assistive devices such as crutches and canes should be used.

The clinician must identify and address specific limitations that lead to gait abnormalities (e.g., inadequate dorsiflexion ROM). These limitations should be addressed with specific interventions aimed at improving ROM or strength *and* during gait retraining activities, such as heel walking, toe walking, and backward walking (retro-walking). Performing these activities in front of a mirror can provide the patient with feedback and can be particularly effective.[12]

EXERCISE-RELATED LEG PAIN

Exercise-related leg pain (ERLP) encompasses several disorders characterized by diffuse pain along the tibia caused by exertional or overuse activities.[13] Tissues and structures in the lower limb often are unable to withstand repetitive bouts of mechanical loading, which may result in tissue fatigue and eventual tissue failure. This is true for passive strain placed on the tissues and active strain from muscle activation. In general, these pathologies may progress from acute tendonitis to periostitis (commonly called *stress reaction*). If left untreated, tibial periostitis is likely to progress to a stress fracture or, possibly, to a complete fracture (see Chapter 26 for more detailed information on stress reactions and fractures of the lower leg).

Medial Tibial Stress Syndrome

Medial tibial stress syndrome (MTSS), a common overuse syndrome, is a periostitis or stress reaction characterized by diffuse pain along the posteromedial border of the tibia and associated with the tendon of the soleus.[14] The term *shin splints* traditionally has been used synonymously with MTSS. However, this term is ill defined and can encompass multiple causes of leg pain. Pain associated with MTSS typically is exacerbated by weight-bearing activities, such as walking, running, jumping, or standing for prolonged periods. MTSS often is linked to faulty lower extremity mechanics related to hyperpronation, as well as to a rapid increase in the intensity and duration of the aggravating activity.[15]

The actual pain generator for MTSS is the subject of debate. Suggestions include the proximal tendon of the tibialis posterior tendon, the proximal tendon of the soleus, and the tibial periosteum.[16] Anatomically, the origin of the tibialis posterior is more lateral than the typical origin of MTSS. However, the tibialis posterior, flexor digitorum longus, and soleus all attach to the distal tibial fascia placing stress on the posterior medial tibia.[17] When designing a rehabilitation plan, the clinician should recognize what MTSS is not. MTSS clearly is not a compartment syndrome of the deep posterior compartment of the leg, nor is it a tibial stress fracture. Differentiation of MTSS from a stress fracture is best confirmed by a bone scan (Table 24-2).[18,19]

General Treatment Considerations of Exercise-Related Leg Pain

- Treat the symptoms
- Eliminate or modify the cause
- Maintain or restore fitness
- Design rehabilitation programs to return the person to the previous level of function

Management of MTSS involves eliminating the potential biomechanical causes of the pathology and treating the patient's symptoms. Addressing abnormal pronation is an issue clinicians often face when treating overuse injuries of the lower extremity. It is important to emphasize that abnormal pronation is a dynamic issue that occurs during landing during walking, running or jumping. Many static malalignments, such as pes planus, hypermobile first ray, excessive forefoot varus, excessive rearfoot valgus, excessive lateral tibial torsion, excessive

TABLE **24-2**

Differential Diagnosis of Repetitive Stress Shin Pain

	Chronic Exertional Compartment Syndrome	Shin Splints* (Stress Reaction)	Stress Fracture	Tumor
Type of pain	Severe cramping, diffuse pain, and tightness	Diffuse along medial two thirds of tibial border	Deep, nagging, and localized with minimal radiation	Deep and nagging (bone) with some radiation
Pain with rest	Decreases or disappears	Decreases or disappears	Present, especially at night	Present, often night pain
Pain with activity	Increases	Increases	Present (may increase)	Present
Pain with warm-up	May increase or may manifest eventually	May disappear	Unilateral	Unilateral
Range of motion	Limited in the acute phase	Limited	Normal	Normal
Onset	Gradual to sudden	Gradual	Gradual	?
Altered sensation	Sometimes	No	No	Sometimes
Muscle weakness or paralysis	Maybe	No	No	Not usually
Stretching	Increases pain	Increases pain	Minimal pain alteration	No increase in pain
Radiography	Normal	Normal	Early, negative; late, positive (?)	Usually positive
Bone scan	Negative	Periosteal uptake	Positive	Positive
Pulse	Affected sometimes	Normal	Normal	Normal
Palpation	Tender, tight compartment	Diffuse tenderness	Point tenderness	Point or diffuse tenderness
Cause	Muscle expansion	Overuse	Overuse	?
Duration and recovery	None without surgery	None without rest	Up to 3 months	None with treatment

*Shin splints and stress fractures are different stages of tibial stress syndrome.

From Magee DJ: *Sports physiotherapy manual,* Edmonton, AB, Canada, 1988, University of Alberta Bookstore.

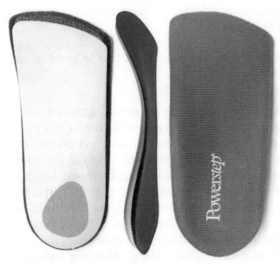

Figure 24-8 Foot orthotics. (Courtesy Powerstep.)

genu valgum, and excessive femoral anteversion, have been associated with abnormal pronation during gait. If these structural abnormalities are present in patients who exhibit abnormal pronation, foot orthotic devices may be used to reduce the magnitude or velocity of pronation during gait (Figure 24-8). Patients with MTSS who demonstrate abnormal pronation have benefited from intervention with foot orthotic devices.[20]

The symptoms associated with MTSS are often self-limiting. The intensity and duration of irritating activities must be modified to allow tissues to heal. Anti-inflammatory and analgesic medications and some therapeutic modalities may also be used initially to treat the symptoms, with limited success.[21] There is some evidence to suggest that mobilization of trigger points in the posterolateral leg results in positive outcomes for performance and pain (Figure 24-9).[22] Once symptoms begin to reduce, treatment of MTSS should include strengthening exercises focused on the muscles of that

dynamically control pronation (i.e., tibialis posterior tibialis anterior and peroneus longus) and the soleus. Also, the flexibility of the lower leg musculature should be addressed for the gastrocnemius, soleus, and anterior lower leg muscles.

Once symptoms resolve, return to full activity must proceed gradually and cautiously. Non–weight-bearing or reduced weight-bearing activities, such as cycling or underwater running, should be mixed with weight-bearing activities. As long as symptoms continue to improve, non–weight-bearing activities gradually can be reduced while weight-bearing activities, such as light plyometrics and gait activities, can be initiated. If faulty biomechanical parameters are present, they must be addressed with gait training or foot orthotic devices. In addition, the patient must maintain adequate muscular strength, endurance, and flexibility once he or she returns to full activity.

Tibial Stress Fractures

The tibia is the most common site for a stress fracture in the lower extremity. Matheson et al.[23] reported that more than 50% of stress fractures in athletes are in the leg, and they usually are seen in running and jumping athletes. Furthermore, females appear to be more susceptible than men with prevalence in runners as high as 28%.[24] Stress fractures are a result of overuse that result in failure of the bone along a continuum of failed adaptation from accelerated osteoclastic remodeling to a complete fracture. With stress fracture, bone attempts to remodel in response to repetitive subthreshold stress. Particularly with muscle fatigue, there is a reduction in the dampening or shock absorbing effect of normal muscle activity in response to repetitive ground reactive forces present in walking, running, or jumping. Constraint overload leads to a stress reaction and potentially a stress fracture.

Stress fractures also can occur at sites of repetitive muscle tension on bone, such as at the insertion of the soleus to the medial border of the tibia. Stress fractures can also occur in individuals with weakened bones. Female runners who may develop disordered eating, secondary amenorrhea, and resultant osteopenia (female athlete triad) are particularly at risk.[25] Complaints of night pain or a focal area that is acutely sensitive to ultrasound as the sound head is passed over it are indicative of stress fractures.

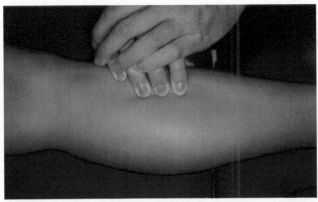

Figure 24-9 Trigger point therapy to the anteromedial leg for medial tibial stress syndrome.

Red Flags for Tibial Stress Fracture

- Night pain
- Focal pain (not diffuse pain)
- Tender area that is acutely sensitive to ultrasound

The treatment of uncomplicated stress fractures involves modified rest with non–weight bearing, pool running, swimming, or cycling until the patient can perform pain-free hopping. Modified rest should last at least 3 weeks from the confirmation of the stress fracture, and all symptoms must subside before a graduated return to activity program can be initiated (Table 24-3).[26] Patients with tibial stress injuries may be fitted with an Aircast brace with anterior compression during the period of modified rest, although improved results with the Aircast are questionable.[27] As weight-bearing activity is gradually increased, emphasis must be placed on *pain-free* activity. If any symptoms recur during or after activity during rehabilitation, the intensity of the activity should be reduced to ensure optimal healing conditions for the fracture. The entire lower extremity will require functional strengthening and retraining because of likely disuse atrophy resulting from the extended period of modified rest. The average tibial stress fracture completely resolves over 8 to 12 weeks after the offending stress has been removed.[23]

> **Clinical Note**
>
> With tibial stress fractures, emphasis must be placed on pain-free activities.

Rehabilitation efforts for stress fractures focus on determining the cause and alleviating the factors that led to the problem. Appropriate footwear and orthotics should be considered for patients who may require control of pronation or shock absorption. Increased loading rates after initial contact is a common occurrence in individuals with stress fractures, and reductions have been realized through feedback.[28] Tibial stress fractures also are seen commonly in individuals with excessive pronation and resultant medial tibial rotation. Most are training errors such as overtraining, inadequate rest, or rapid increases in activity duration and intensity. These training errors must be avoided in an attempt to prevent recurrence (Table 24-4).

TABLE **24-3**

Sample Walk–Run Program for Return to Activity after Gastrocnemius–Soleus Strain and Stress Fracture*

Week	Monday	Wednesday	Friday
1	10-min walk	20-min walk	30-min walk
2	6×(4.5-min walk+0.5-min run)	6×(4-min walk+1-min run)	6×(3.5-min walk+1.5-min run)
3	6×(3-min walk+2-min run)	6×(2.5-min walk+2.5-min run)	6×(2-min walk+3-min run)
4	6×(1.5-min walk+3.5-min run)	6×(1-min walk+4-min run)	6×(0.5-min walk+4.5-min run)
5	30-min run	30-min run	30-min run

*The walk–run program is started after a patient has demonstrated the ability to walk 30 minutes consecutively, without injury, three times per week on alternate days. The goal is to run pain free for 30 minutes three times per week. The program involves a total activity period of 30 minutes, which is structured into six sets of 5 minutes on alternate days. Each set involves a combination of running and walking, and the running component is increased after each session by 30 seconds.

From Kolt SK, Snyder-Mackler L, editors: *Physical therapies in sport and exercise*, p 434, Edinburgh, 2003, Churchill Livingstone.

TABLE **24-4**

Common Exercise Training Errors That May Lead to Overuse Injuries in the Lower Extremity

Mode	Error
Duration	• Increasing total time of exercise bouts too quickly
Frequency	• Increasing number of weekly exercise bouts too quickly
Intensity	• Increasing the physiological demands of exercise bouts too quickly
Environment	• Sudden change of surface (especially softer surfaces to hard surfaces) • Not alternating sides when running on crowned roads or sidewalks • Not alternating directions when running on oval tracks (especially indoors)
Equipment	• Poorly fitting or worn down shoes

CHRONIC EXERTIONAL COMPARTMENT SYNDROME

Chronic exertional compartment syndrome (CECS) must be considered as a cause of lower leg pain in athletes, especially those in endurance sports. The lower leg usually is divided into four discrete compartments (anterior, lateral, superficial posterior, and deep posterior; Figure 24-10), and CECS may occur in any of them. Some authors add a fifth compartment containing the tibialis posterior muscle as an occasional separate unit within the deep posterior compartment.[29,30] Each compartment encompasses muscles and the associated neurovascular bundle. Rarely, compartment syndromes can occur in the foot and can have causes similar to those in the leg of active individuals.[31]

CECS presents with transient symptoms that usually present during exercise or activity. The volume of exercising muscle may increase by as much as 20%, a result of an increase in blood volume and transcapillary filtration of intravascular fluid.[32] Venous and lymphatic return are limited by the increased volume within the compartment. Because the fascial sheath cannot significantly stretch to accommodate the abnormally increased volume, CECS occurs during exercise (see Table 24-2). CECS is characterized by severe cramping, diffuse pain, and tightness in one or more of the leg compartments. The patient will report compartment tightness that occurs during and/or after exercise, which is often more intense the next day. Associated swelling of the affected compartment occurs, although it may be difficult to visualize. This swelling is often palpable through increased turgor (i.e., rigidity) over the muscle. In some cases the patient may have a sensation of fatigue, weakness, or heaviness of the compartment muscles.

CECS may be difficult to diagnose because the symptoms present during exercise and begin to subside with rest. However, the signs and symptoms are fairly consistent in that they will occur at the same time, distance, and intensity of exercise and are consistent with deep aching pain, nerve pain (i.e., stinging, burning, numbness), and decreased function of the ankle dorsiflexors (i.e., foot slap or drop). A treadmill stress test with measurement of intracompartmental pressures may be necessary for a definitive diagnosis of CECS because this is considered the gold standard.[33] However, there has been some question as to the validity and necessity of such testing.[34]

Treatment of CECS may involve both conservative and surgical measures. Conservative measures have been questioned in terms of their effectiveness.[35] Fasciotomy is the definitive treatment, but in some cases, the condition resolves with activity modifications such as reduction in training volume or intensity. Other conservative treatment involves icing, stretching, muscle strengthening, proper footwear, and orthotic intervention, when appropriate. Recently evidence from a case series of two runners suggests that modifications in heel strike pattern may be successful in reducing symptoms.[36] If these measures are successful, a gradual return to activity and loading can be initiated. If these conservative measures fail, fasciotomy is commonly recommended. After surgery, the patient may be able to return to running in approximately 3 weeks.[37] The results are usually good, unless the area of fascia cut was not sufficient or ischemic changes and morphological muscle damage have occurred as a result of intense training in the presence of CECS.

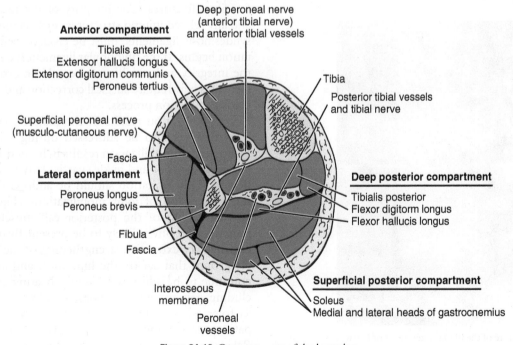

Figure 24-10 Compartments of the lower leg.

FRACTURES OF THE TIBIA AND FIBULA

Many different types of fractures can occur to the tibia and fibula (Figures 24-11 to 24-13). Complete fractures of the tibia and fibula may occur during sport activities that involve high torques and compression loads commonly placed on the lower leg. Fractures of the tibia may require internal fixation for stabilization and long periods

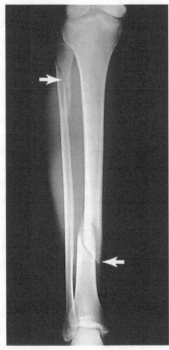

Figure 24-11 Fracture of tibia and fibula. (From Frank ED, Long BW, Smith BJ: *Merrill's atlas of radiographic positioning and procedures*, ed 11, St. Louis, 2007, Mosby.)

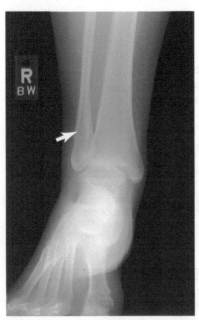

Figure 24-12 Fracture of the fibula, anteroposterior view (demonstrating subtle compaction fracture of distal fibula). (From Swain J, Bush KW, Brosing J: *Diagnostic imaging for physical therapists*, St. Louis, 2009, Saunders.)

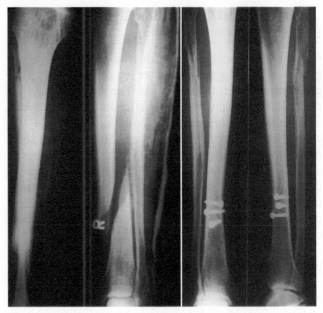

Figure 24-13 Displaced long spiral fracture of tibia fixed internally with interfragmentary screws. (From Canale ST, editor: *Campbell's operative orthopaedics*, ed 10, Philadelphia, 2003, Mosby.)

of immobilization because the tibia is the primary weight-bearing bone in the lower leg. Prolonged immobilization can lead to severe disuse atrophy of the entire lower extremity if not properly managed during the immobilization phase. It is crucial to maintain strength and mobility of the muscles surrounding the more proximal knee and hip joints as well as the joints of the foot. Some fractures of the fibula may require internal fixation, but immobilization time is shorter compared with the time required for tibial fractures. The integrity of the healed fracture and any related injured structures, such as the tibiofibular syndesmosis ligaments, must be ensured before rehabilitation begins. If the tibiofibular ligament is compromised, the integrity and stability of the ankle mortise has been lost. This may require surgical correction and will prolong the rehabilitation process.

Immobilization results in the majority of the problems that need to be addressed during rehabilitation. Prolonged immobilization results in limited ROM of the joints of the foot and ankle, particularly of ankle dorsiflexion. This limitation should be addressed with careful progression of joint mobilizations (Figure 24-14) and stretching of the posterior calf muscles. Because muscular atrophy is likely to be present throughout the entire lower extremity, strengthening of the major muscle groups that act on the hip, knee, and ankle should continue to be addressed. Weight-bearing exercises, including gait training activities, should be incorporated as tolerated throughout the rehabilitation process for patients recovering from tibial and/or fibular fractures. Balance and proprioceptive intervention will also be compromised and should be addressed as early in the rehabilitation process as possible.

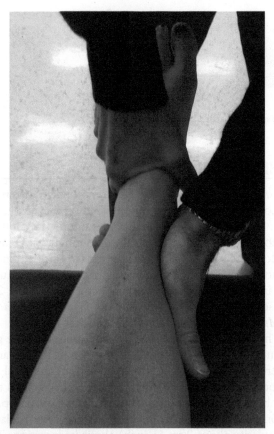

Figure 24-14 Posterior talar mobilization.

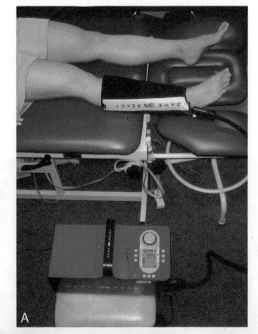

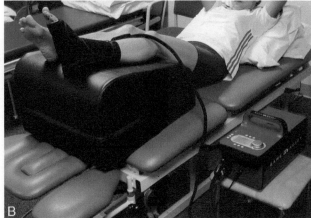

Figure 24-15 Game Ready® apparatus (CoolSystems, Inc., Concord, CA) used to apply compression and cold to the leg (**A**) and to the ankle (**B**).

GASTROCNEMIUS STRAINS

Gastrocnemius strains, sometimes referred to as "tennis leg," are frequently seen in explosive sports that require quick movements in multiple directions. Sports such as tennis require the athlete to bear weight on the forefoot (i.e., balls of the feet) and make powerful movements in different directions. The common mechanism for this injury is forced dorsiflexion while the knee is extended or forced knee extension while the foot is dorsiflexed. Both of these movements cause passive stress or stretch to the gastrocnemius muscle, which crosses the posterior portion of the knee and ankle. This, in combination with active contraction of the muscles, places the muscle in a poor length–tension relationship. This injury occurs primarily in the medial head of the gastrocnemius muscle and differs distinctly from partial tears or ruptures of the Achilles tendon.

For acute strains, treatment should follow the RICE protocol; weight bearing to tolerance is allowed in the first weeks after injury. A compression wrap (Figure 24-15, A) applied from the foot to a point just distal to the knee can be used to provide external pressure to the injured limb. A normal gait pattern is encouraged, with use of an assistive device for partial weight-bearing gait if the patient cannot ambulate without a limp. In all probability, the patient will have difficulty with push-off during gait, and bilateral heel lifts may be temporarily helpful

in reducing pain and activation of the gastrocnemius muscle.[38] Heel lifts (Figure 24-16) place the ankle in a plantar-flexed position during weight bearing and reduce the active and passive tension applied to the injured muscle. As dorsiflexion ROM returns, heel lift height can be reduced to allow normal active movement during weight bearing.

In the days after injury, active ROM exercises of the foot and ankle can be performed within the pain-free range. Cryotherapy may be used before and after exercise to control pain and localized inflammation in the early stages of recovery. Aggressive stretching of the gastrocnemius muscle must be avoided throughout the treatment process. Manual resistance exercises for the ankle muscles other than the plantar flexors may also be performed. Low-resistance plantar flexion exercises against elastic tubing are started when the patient is pain free (Figure 24-17). As the patient progresses, standing closed-chain exercises, including partial weight-bearing heel raises, squats, and

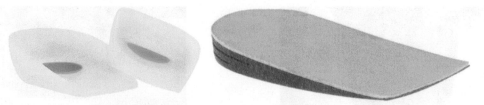

Figure 24-16 Heel lift examples. (Courtesy Breg, Carlsbad, CA.)

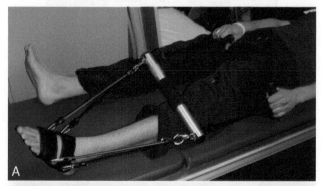

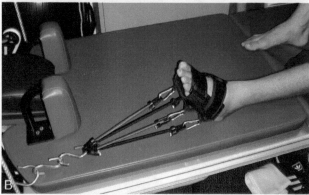

Figure 24-17 Ankle-Foot Maximizer® (AFX) (Progressive Health Innovations Inc., Port Moody, BC Canada) used to provide ankle exercises. **A,** Plantar flexion. **B,** Dorsiflexion.

lunges, may be initiated. To promote muscle tissue healing and fiber reorganization, low-intensity pulsed ultrasound may be used.[39] Soft tissue mobilization may also be beneficial in promoting healing and decreasing abnormal activation of surrounding muscle fibers.[40]

As ankle ROM returns, strengthening exercises using elastic resistance for all ranges are instituted (see Figure 24-6). The elastic resistance provides easy control over the variables of ROM, load, contraction type (concentric or eccentric), sets, and repetitions and allows control of speed and change of direction, which are difficult to duplicate using other exercise modalities. The intensity of closed-chain exercises should be increased gradually and may be advanced through a progression of leg press, hopping, and jumping activities. Prolonged walking, jogging, or running must be implemented in a pain-free manner. If the patient cannot perform these activities without limping or if the injured area swells with activity or pain is increased, progression is proceeding too quickly.

ACHILLES TENDINOPATHY

The Achilles tendon is the most common site of tendon pathology (i.e., tendinopathy) in the lower leg, ankle, and foot. Injuries can range from peritendinitis (i.e., inflammation of the peritendon sheath surrounding the Achilles tendon), tendinosis (i.e., degeneration of the tendon without inflammation), partial and complete ruptures, and insertional lesions, such as bursitis (see volume 2 of this series, *Scientific Foundations and Principles of Practice in Musculoskeletal Rehabilitation,* Chapter 3).

The Achilles tendon, the common tendon of the gastrocnemius and soleus muscles, inserts into the calcaneal tuberosity. The tendon is enveloped by the superficial and retrocalcaneal bursae near its insertion. The Achilles tendon has a peritendon sheath rather than a synovial (paratenon) sheath. The tendon itself has an area of relative avascularity about 2 cm (1 inch) above its insertion. This is the area where partial tears with secondary nodule formation and degenerative cysts are seen in tendinosis.

Common symptoms of Achilles tendinopathy are stiffness, pain with elongation or stretching, pain under load (e.g., going up onto the toes), and pain with running. The clinical examination may reveal signs of local tenderness, crepitus, palpable nodules in the tendon or peritendon, and limited dorsiflexion ROM. Limited power at push-off is commonly noted as a result of pain and subsequent disuse atrophy. If the condition is chronic, atrophy of the calf muscles may be observed.

Treatment for acute tendinopathy, associated bursitis, and insertional tendinopathy or enthesopathy is conservative in most cases. A careful history and full lower extremity examination (including gait assessment) is important to determine whether the pathological condition is related to overuse, mechanical problem, or possible compensation for other muscle weakness. If overuse is identified as a contributing factor, alterations in training that allow for rest and recovery will be necessary. If mechanical problems are a factor, they must be corrected before recovery can occur. Impairments at both proximal[41] and distal[42] parts of the tendon have been associated with the presence of Achilles pathology. Although there are suggestions that abnormal pronation and associated movements may be related to Achilles tendinopathy,[42,43] the relationships are unclear. Hyperpronation can cause the Achilles tendon to whip or twist when the foot bears weight during running, which can cause increased torque to the tendon.[44]

Early in the treatment process, emphasis should be placed on symptom management. This should include the use of analgesic and anti-inflammatory medications and modalities, as well as rest from aggravating activities. Pain-free ROM and low-intensity strengthening exercises may be implemented early in the treatment process. Temporary heel lifts (see Figure 24-16) made from high-density foam or orthopedic felt may be used in both shoes to reduce stress on the tendon. The height of the lifts can be reduced as pain-free ROM improves.

Once symptoms are under control, progressive stretching and strengthening of the gastrocnemius and soleus muscles may be undertaken. Thermal modalities such as continuous therapeutic ultrasound can be paired with cross-friction massage to help break up tendinous nodules, which are common in patients with Achilles tendinosis. These treatments should be followed by stretching of the Achilles tendon, either in a long sitting using a towel or rope to stretch the Achilles tendon or in the standing position with the patient pushing against a wall or table (see Figure 24-5). Stretching should be done with the knee straight for the gastrocnemius muscle and then in a bent knee position to isolate the soleus muscle. Elastic bands or tubing can be used to perform resistive exercises of the muscles acting on the ankle (see Figure 24-6). Plantar flexion exercises should include open- and closed-chain exercises. Progressions should follow principles described previously for gastrocnemius strains or those outlined by Curwin (see volume 2 of this series, *Scientific Foundations and Principles of Practice in Musculoskeletal Rehabilitation*, Chapter 3). Emphasis should be placed on eccentric training of the plantar flexors.[45]

Clinicians must be alert to the possibility of **Sever's disease** in physically active children and adolescents who present with insertional heel pain. Sever's disease (Figure 24-18) is an apophysitis at the insertion of the Achilles tendon. It is most common in boys ages 10 to 12 and girls ages 8 to 10. Children with Sever's disease must stop physical activity for at least 2 weeks to allow the symptoms to resolve. Upon resolution of symptoms, emphasis must be placed on increasing the flexibility of the gastrocnemius–soleus complex and a gradual return to activity. Typically, these patients have generalized lower extremity tightness, especially in the hamstrings and hip flexors that also require stretching. Footwear considerations should be made because many of these patients participate in sports with restrictive footwear (e.g., soccer).

ACHILLES TENDON RUPTURE (THIRD-DEGREE STRAIN)

Achilles tendon ruptures can be treated either surgically or conservatively. Conservative treatment typically is more successful for sedentary individuals. Nonoperative treatment is seldom used for physically active people, because once the tendon heals after immobilization, tensile

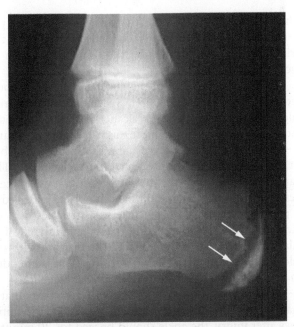

Figure 24-18 Radiograph reveals fragmentation of calcaneal apophysis in a child diagnosed with Sever's disease. (From Cuppett M, Walsh KM: *General medical conditions in the athlete*, ed 2, St. Louis, 2012, Mosby.)

strength is reduced to about 30% of normal, and the chance of rerupturing the tendon is greater.[46] In the rehabilitation program for a conservatively treated patient, more caution must be exercised not to aggravate the healing tissue.

Surgical repair of the Achilles tendon may be an open or a closed procedure, although open repair tends to have the best outcome.[47] After surgery, the patient is immobilized for 6 to 8 weeks. After complete immobilization, patients are placed in a cam walker (see Figure 24-4) with heel lifts. Over the next 4 to 6 weeks, weight bearing is progressively increased and the heel lifts are progressively reduced to neutral. The rehabilitation process follows a course similar to that for gastrocnemius strains but at a much slower pace. Special care must be taken not to stress the repaired tissue too soon. Any stretching that is done should be gentle. The foot should be kept in a neutral position (i.e., no inversion or eversion) during stretching, because this position reduces abnormal stresses on the medial or lateral sides of the tendon.

ANKLE SPRAINS

Ankle sprains are one of the most common athletic injuries and are often underestimated by both clinicians and patients. In fact, lateral ligament injuries account for 15% to 25% of all sports injuries.[48] The most common predisposition to an ankle sprain is a previous ankle sprain on the same side. For example, basketball players demonstrate recurrence rates as high as 80%.[49] Overall, up to 30% of individuals who suffer an initial ankle sprain eventually develop chronic ankle instability, which is characterized by long-standing symptoms of pain and instability.[50]

These findings indicate that the treatment of many patients with ankle sprains has been inadequate. One of the primary goals of rehabilitation should be prevention of recurrent injuries.

The lateral ligaments of the ankle are the most commonly injured (Figure 24-19). Specifically, the anterior talofibular ligament and the calcaneofibular ligament are most often affected. The mechanism of injury is plantar flexion and inversion, stressing first the anterior talofibular ligament and then the calcaneofibular ligament. The patient initially presents with pain, swelling, muscle weakness, difficulty with gait, and in some cases, joint laxity. A positive anterior drawer or inversion stress test will indicate that the lateral structures have been injured. The talar tilt is performed by inverting the rearfoot with the talocrural joint in a dorsiflexed position. This is intended to be a specific test for the calcaneofibular ligament.

Initial management should focus on decreasing inflammation and protecting the injured tissues. In the initial days after injury, the ankle should be iced for 20 minutes at least once a day (Figure 24-15, *B*). The ankle should be elevated whenever possible during the acute phase. In addition, a felt horseshoe pad should be held snugly around the lateral malleolus with a compression wrap. Alternatively, an Aircast brace (see Figure 24-2) can be used. Patients who are unable to ambulate without a limp should use crutches or a cane. The ankle should be placed in neutral dorsiflexion to keep the joint stable and decrease capsular distension. During the first 1 to 3 weeks (depending on severity), the ankle should be protected from inversion to prevent formation of type III collagen, which leads to elongation of the ligament.[51] Exercises

should be focused in the sagittal plane. Early mobility is important to stimulate collagen type I formation as it responds best to tension.[52]

ROM exercises may begin within a few days of injury in even the most severe cases. Gentle active range of motion (AROM) exercises in a pain-free ROM may be performed to improve ankle mobility and also to help reduce local swelling and edema (Figure 24-20). Pain-free movement of the ankle (i.e., ankle pumps: plantar flexion–dorsiflexion) and intrinsic foot crunches (Figure 24-21) can aid venous and lymphatic fluid return via a pump mechanism of alternating voluntary contraction and relaxation of the muscles around the lower leg. Ankle pumps may be performed in a cold whirlpool to decrease pain and metabolic function in the early stages of the injury. Light isometric resistance exercises can begin in the days after injury. As pain allows, partial weight-bearing activities may be

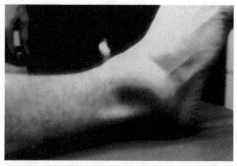

Figure 24-20 Swelling within the talocrural and subtalar joint capsule. (From Magee DJ: *Orthopedic physical assessment*, ed 6, p 897, St. Louis, 2014, Saunders.)

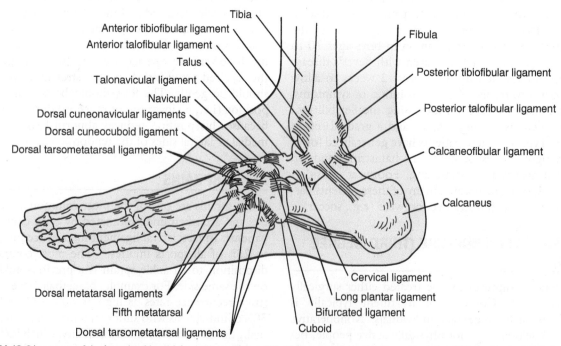

Figure 24-19 Ligaments of the lateral ankle and foot. (From Magee DJ: *Orthopedic physical assessment*, ed 6, p 889, St. Louis, 2014, Saunders.)

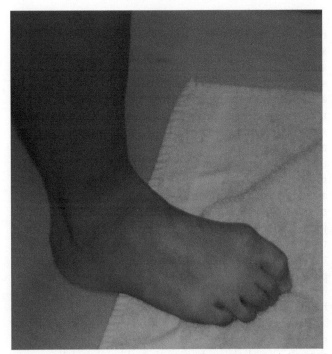

Figure 24-21 Intrinsic foot exercises: toe curls using towel.

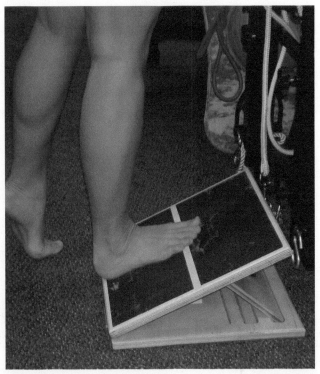

Figure 24-22 Slant board stretching.

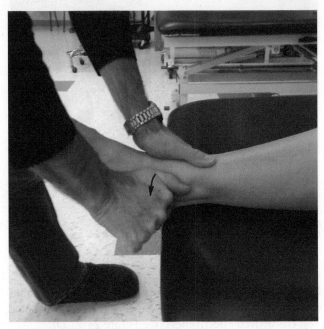

Figure 24-23 Distal fibular mobilization.

initiated in an effort to restore function. Wobble board exercises with the patient in the sitting position can be initiated and they can be progressed as pain allows.

Limited ankle dorsiflexion is a common occurrence after ankle sprains. Loss of dorsiflexion results in changes in functional activities such as walking and running. At least 10° of dorsiflexion is necessary for normal walking, and running requires 20° to 30° of dorsiflexion.[53,54] Traditional rehabilitation programs have emphasized stretching of the Achilles tendon on slant boards (Figure 24-22). However, talocrural joint mobilizations are also an important intervention,[55] especially if improved ROM is delayed or restrictions in capsular mobility are noted upon assessment. Mobility of the subtalar and calcaneocuboid joints should also be assessed, and joint mobilization of these joints should be used if restrictions are present (Figures 24-23 to 24-25). Posterior mobilizations of the talus on the tibia (talocrural joint) help increase dorsiflexion ROM and result in quicker return to symmetrical gait patterns than traditional treatments.[55] Posterior mobilization of the distal fibula on the tibia have also demonstrated positive results in dorsiflexion ROM.[56]

Strengthening exercises should advance from isometric contractions to isotonic exercises using elastic bands or tubing. Emphasis should be placed on eccentric training of the peroneal muscles and ankle dorsiflexors. Closed-chain strengthening exercises, including heel raises, squats, and lunges, also can be performed as tolerated. Strengthening should not be limited to the ankle, as weakness of proximal muscles has been reported.[57]

Balance exercises are a critical component in the rehabilitation for ankle sprains, particularly because they are effective in preventing the recurrence of ankle sprains (Figure 24-26).[55-60] Single-leg exercises can be started as soon as the patient can perform weight-bearing activities without pain. Progressions can be made by altering the visual input (eyes open, then closed), surface (firm surface, then foam, then balance disc; see Figures 24-7, *A-C*), and arm position (arms abducted to 90°, then at the sides, then folded across chest, then catching and throwing balls).

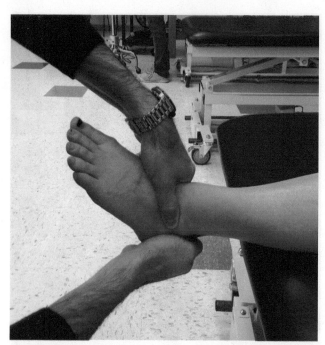

Figure 24-24 Subtalar mobilization.

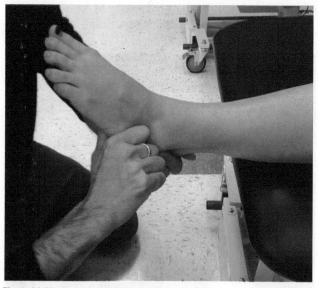

Figure 24-25 Calcaneocuboid mobilization.

Lunging and squatting exercises can be performed to train dynamic balance. In particular, the Star Excursion Balance Test has proved effectiveness (see Figure 24-7, D).

Shoe wear, bracing, and taping may also be important adjuncts to treatment of the lateral ankle sprain. Braces have been reported to reduce inversion velocity, and taping and high-top shoes have been reported to decrease the inversion moment when the ankle is placed in varying degrees of plantar flexion.[61-63] Everter strength has been shown to be important in the decrease of the inversion moment during weight-bearing activities.[64]

Gait training should be incorporated throughout the rehabilitation program. Emphasis should be placed on symmetrical, pain-free gait. For physically active patients, straight ahead jogging followed by running activities should be performed without pain. Once the physically active patient can run straight ahead without pain, movements requiring changes in direction should be emphasized. These may include side-to-side changes in direction and cutting maneuvers (Figure 24-27). Hopping activities also should be performed to prepare the ankle for a return to high-level functional activities. Hopping is characterized by low-amplitude quick landings on the balls of the feet, where most of force is absorbed by the ankle joint. Hopping should be performed in multiple directions in an effort to stress the joint in different planes of motion (Figure 24-28). Once hopping activities can be performed safely and without pain, more ballistic activities can be added, such as jumping and landing from a height.

Patients who suffer mild or moderate ankle sprains often return to activity within a few weeks of injury, even though the clinician knows that the injured ligaments have not had adequate time to heal. This may be the reason recurrence rates are so high. However, conclusive evidence shows that supervised rehabilitation, carried out for at least 4 weeks after an ankle sprain, can reduce the risk of recurrence by more than 50%.[65]

If an ankle sprain does not appear to be improving within the normal time frame, consideration should be given to other pathological conditions, which may require orthopedic referral. Such complications may include syndesmosis involvement (high ankle sprain), sinus tarsi syndrome, osteochondral fractures of the talus, and peroneal nerve palsy (Figure 24-29).

Ankle sprains that include damage to the tibiofibular syndesmosis and/or anterior inferior tibiofibular ligament are referred to as **high ankle sprains**. This injury is less common than lateral ankle sprains but may be seen in conjunction with lateral ankle ligament injuries. The mechanism of injury at this joint is usually one of lateral (external) rotation of the foot and medial (internal) rotation of the tibia (Figure 24-30). These high ankle sprains must be treated more conservatively than lateral ankle sprains so that the ligaments stabilizing the syndesmosis can heal. Therefore, the time frame for return to normal activities is longer for high ankle sprains than for lateral ankle sprains. These injuries should be immobilized for a minimum of 7 days after injury. If the ankle is not immobilized, the healing ligaments will be stressed repeatedly, because the wide anterior portion of the talus will spread the syndesmosis apart each time the ankle is dorsiflexed. Commonly, the average time of return to high-level functional activity after syndesmosis sprain is 6 weeks.[66]

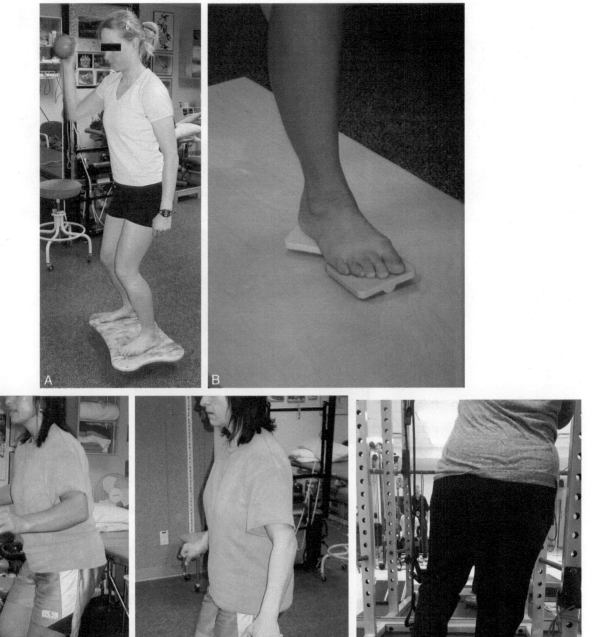

Figure 24-26 Balancing exercise examples. **A,** Balance board while throwing weighted ball. **B,** Propriofoot® (Össur hf., Reykjavik, Iceland). **C,** Bosu® balance (BOSU, Ashland, OH). **D,** Brazilian balance apparatus. **E,** Airex® pad.

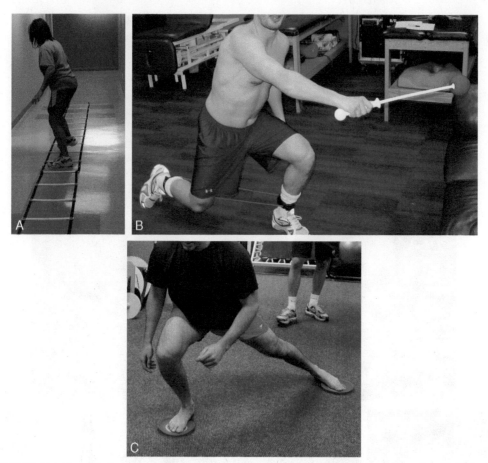

Figure 24-27 Activities with change in direction. **A,** With ladder. **B,** Mimicking activity with ankle tubes. **C,** Slider discs.

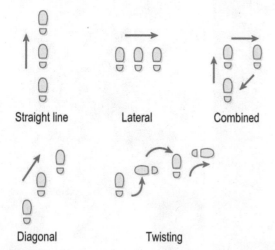

Figure 24-28 One-leg hopping patterns. (From Norris CM: *Managing sports injuries,* ed 4, London, Churchill Livingston, 2011.)

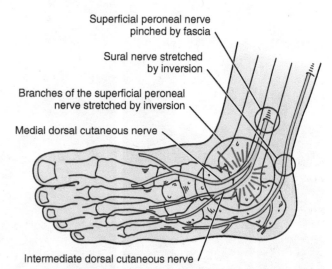

Figure 24-29 Stretching of the superficial peroneal nerve as a result of inversion of the ankle. (From Magee DJ: *Orthopedic physical assessment,* ed 6, p 945, St. Louis, 2014, Saunders/Elsevier.)

TARSAL TUNNEL SYNDROME

Tarsal tunnel syndrome is a neuropathy of the tibial nerve where it passes posterior to the medial malleolus from the leg to the foot (Figure 24-31). The nerve may be injured acutely in conjunction with a fracture foot the medial malleolus, or the condition may be an overuse injury.

In the latter case, excessive pronation may contribute to traction on or compression of the tibial nerve. Symptoms typically include paresthesia on the medial aspect of the ankle extending into the plantar aspect of the foot and, in severe cases, atrophy of the intrinsic muscles of the

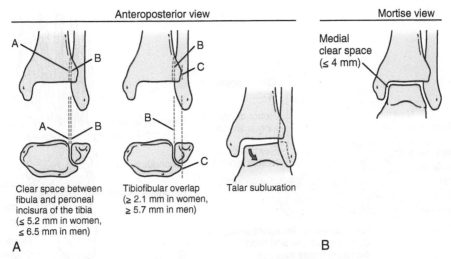

Figure 24-30 Syndesmotic radiographic criteria. A finding outside any of these criteria indicates a syndesmosis injury. **A**, Anteroposterior view. **B**, Mortise view. *A*, Lateral border of posterior tibial malleolus; *B*, medial border of fibula; *C*, lateral border of anterior tibial tubercle. (From Magee DJ: *Orthopedic physical assessment*, ed 6, p 957, St. Louis, 2014, Saunders/Elsevier.)

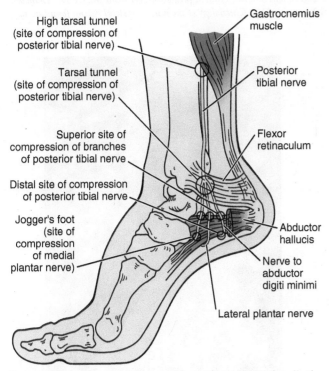

Figure 24-31 Tarsal tunnel syndrome. (From Magee DJ: *Orthopedic physical assessment*, ed 6, p 947, St. Louis, 2014, Saunders/Elsevier.)

foot. Changes in muscle function may be associated with cramping or clawing of the lesser toes. Some cases of tarsal tunnel syndrome, including those in conjunction with tibial fractures, must be treated surgically.

Conservative management of tarsal tunnel syndrome consists of anti-inflammatory medications, rest, ice, and correction of faulty foot mechanics. When excessive pronation is a contributing factor, the patient should be carefully evaluated for orthotic intervention. Strengthening may be necessary for the intrinsic muscles if muscle dysfunction is present. These exercises should include short

foot exercises, barefoot single-leg balance on soft surfaces, towel curls (see Figure 24-21), marble pickups, or walking in sand. The short foot exercise[67] is performed by keeping the heel and the metatarsal heads on the floor while contracting the muscles of the longitudinal arch in an effort to lift the arch off the floor. This exercise initially can be performed in a bilateral stance and progressed to a single-leg stance for increased balance demands.

TIBIALIS (POSTERIOR) TENDINOPATHY

Posterior tibialis tendinopathy can be the result of overuse usually related to an inability to adequately control some aspect of pronation. Acute posterior tibialis tendinopathy (i.e., tendonitis) is the injury that is sometimes referred to as shin splints. This injury is seen in runners or in athletes whose sport requires a great deal of running. This is because of the role of the posterior tibialis muscle in controlling pronation eccentrically during the loading phase of gait. The demand on this muscle (and others) becomes increased during running because the joint excursions, velocities, and forces are significantly increased.[68] Posterior tibialis tendinopathy may also result after the tendon has remained in a shortened position for a period of time. This can be the result of immobilization after fracture, a plantar-flexed posture of the rearfoot, or a cavus medial longitudinal arch.

In patients with posterior tibial pathology, there is usually tenderness just posterior to the medial malleolus and perhaps proximally along the posteromedial portion of the tendon on the tibia (Figure 24-32). If pain is significant along the tibia, the pathology should be differentially diagnosed from MTSS, which is more likely referred to as shin splints.[69] Additionally, the presence of paresthesia or radicular pain in the foot may indicate the presence of a tarsal tunnel syndrome. The patient with posterior tibialis

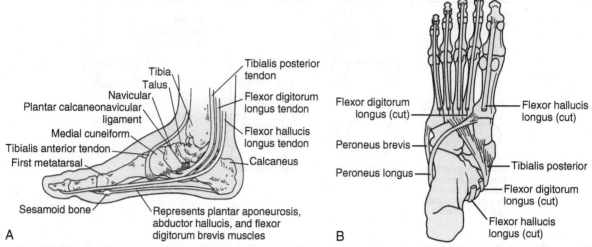

Figure 24-32 Posterior tibialis tendinopathy. **A,** Pathway of tibialis posterior. **B,** Plantar view of the right foot shows the distal course of the tendons of the peroneus longus, peroneus brevis, and tibialis posterior. The tendons of the flexor digitorum longus and flexor hallucis longus are cut. Note the force couple relationship between the two peroneal muscles and tibialis posterior to control inversion and eversion along with the long flexors and extensors. In both **A** and **B,** note how insertion of the tibialis posterior and tibialis anterior control pronation. (**A** from Magee DJ: *Orthopedic physical assessment*, ed 6, p 904, St. Louis, 2014, Saunders. **B** redrawn from Neumann DA: *Kinesiology of the musculoskeletal system: foundations for physical rehabilitation*, St. Louis, 2010, Mosby.)

tendinopathy may also report pain with palpation over the navicular, pain with resisted plantar flexion and inversion, and pain with passive eversion and dorsiflexion. Passive dorsiflexion and eversion can be accomplished functionally with relaxed single-leg stance.

Management of posterior tibialis tendonitis can be challenging because the foot must pronate (and supinate) even during normal ambulation. Therefore, completely decreasing stress on the tendon may be impossible without immobilization or casting. However, this is usually not a necessary nor desired treatment management strategy. The acute phase of rehabilitation should include management of pain and any swelling. Rest or complete cessation of activity appears to be the best for the patient in the acute stage. The patient may still remain active during this stage through cross-training as long as the activity does not increase the symptoms at the posterior tibialis tendon. Nonsteroidal anti-inflammatory drugs, ice, and other inflammation-reducing modalities are also beneficial during this stage.

Passive ROM for eversion and dorsiflexion should be the focus of the next stage of treatment. However, care should be exercised because excessive passive loading of the tendon can result in prolonged healing of the tissue. Regaining a normal resting length of the tendon is imperative in restoring the patient to normal function. Although deterioration of pain and other symptoms should guide treatment, increasing passive ROM is important, because decreased tendon length will likely be a main limiting factor to progress if not regained early. If increased pronation is a major mechanical problem leading to symptoms, this is a good time in the treatment to introduce some support to the medial longitudinal arch. Arch taping (Figure 24-33) or over-the-counter foot orthotic devices

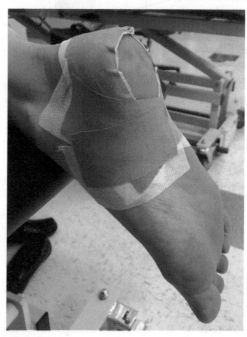

Figure 24-33 Arch taping.

may help temporarily while custom-molded orthoses are being fabricated. Because posterior tibialis pathology is so often associated with *excessive* pronation, external devices such as custom-molded orthoses may be necessary to control excess motion in the midfoot and rearfoot.

CKC activities and eccentric strengthening are the goals of the final stage of rehabilitation. Single-leg standing eccentric controlled heel drops loads the posterior tibialis tendon in a functional situation (Figure 24-34). Wobble boards in both a clockwise and counterclockwise

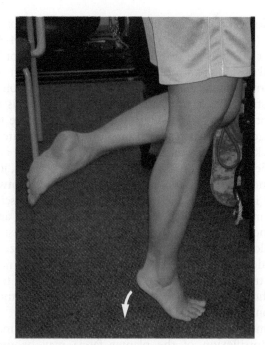

Figure 24-34 Eccentrically controlled heel drops.

direction provide training of multidirectional control of pronation and supination. Sidestepping and cariocas away from the affected side place increased eccentric demand on the tibialis posterior tendon. Finally, controlled landing activities from progressively increasing step heights train the patient to control pronation during running, and landing from a jump.

PERONEAL TENDINOPATHY

Peroneal tendinopathy is a result of overuse of either the peroneus longus or peroneus brevis tendons (Figure 24-35).

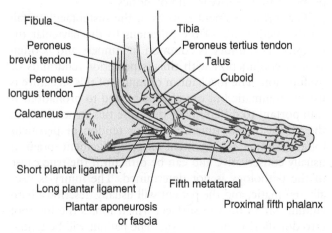

Fibula

Peroneus
brevis tendon

Peroneus
longus tendon

Calcaneus

Tibia

Peroneus tertius tendon

Talus

Cuboid

Short plantar ligament

Long plantar ligament

Plantar aponeurosis
or fascia

Fifth metatarsal

Proximal fifth phalanx

Figure 24-35 Supports of the lateral longitudinal arch of the foot, including peroneal tendons: plantar aponeurosis (including the abductor digiti minimi and the flexor digitorum brevis IV and V); long plantar ligament; short plantar ligament. (From Magee DJ: *Orthopedic physical assessment*, ed 6, p 904, St. Louis, 2014, Saunders.)

This injury is most often seen in conjunction with lateral ankle sprains and may be the cause or the result of lateral ankle instability. However, isolated peroneal tendinopathies are somewhat rare. Peroneal tendinopathy differs in its mechanism of injury depending on whether the longus or the brevis is involved. Peroneus brevis involvement is more commonly associated with supination overuse as it is stressed in the inverted position of the foot and ankle. A slightly different mechanism is usually attributed to peroneus longus tendinopathy. Like the brevis, the peroneus longus plantar flexes and everts the foot running beneath the plantar surface of the foot to attach to the first metatarsal (see Figure 24-32, *B*). Hypermobility of the first ray allows for excessive dorsiflexion, which forces the forefoot into pronation during weight-bearing activities. Therefore, the inability to control pronation by the peroneus longus may result in overuse.

Tenderness to palpation distal and posterior to the lateral malleolus is most common in peroneal tendinopathy.[70] The patient may also be tender proximal to the malleolus and, depending on the structure involved, at the base of the first or fifth metatarsal. Regardless of the specific structure, the patient will experience pain with resisted plantar flexion and eversion. Passive inversion and dorsiflexion may be painful for the peroneus brevis and likely the peroneus longus. Passive first metatarsal dorsiflexion also may be painful if the peroneus longus is involved.

The acute phase of rehabilitation should include management of any swelling and pain. Taping or bracing may help prevent the tendon from further tension injury, especially if any instability or weakness is present. After the acute phase, passive ROM and concentric resistive exercises should begin. Often, a muscle imbalance has developed, so stretching and strengthening antagonists such as the tibialis anterior and posterior muscles may be necessary, especially in the patient with a cavus foot. Eccentric and concentric training of first ray plantar flexion may also be beneficial. However, it is likely that the patient with a hypermobile first ray will not be able to gain enough dynamic strength to control forefoot pronation, and an orthosis or metatarsal support may be necessary.

Functional activities should complete the rehabilitation of the patient with peroneal tendinopathy. Single-leg standing exercises advancing to transverse plane rotations should be included, because patients must regain eccentric control during functional activities. This is especially important in athletes with associated lateral ankle sprains, because they will have decreased proprioceptive ability.[71] Wobble boards and minitramp standing with a ball toss will help control eccentric supination or pronation (see Figure 24-26, *A*). If instability or decreased proprioception remains toward the end of rehabilitation, taping or orthoses may be necessary in order for the athlete to return to play safely.

PLANTAR FASCIITIS

Plantar fasciitis is the result of stress injury to the plantar fascia and typically causes symptoms near its calcaneal origin. The plantar fascia normally stabilizes and locks the foot in supination before push-off. The plantar fascia is put under strain by the "windlass mechanism," which occurs during push-off when the metatarsophalangeal joints are hyperextended. It also is stressed by hyperpronation of the foot, as the medial longitudinal arch collapses. The condition is found in both rigid and hypermobile feet. Decreased flexibility in the gastrocnemius–soleus complex is commonly found, especially if the condition is seen in the cavus foot. A periosteal reaction at its origin can result in hemorrhage and, ultimately, a heel spur. In many cases, heel spurs (Figure 24-36) are asymptomatic, but if present, they are a sign of stress overload to the plantar fascia.

Biomechanical abnormalities of the foot may be significant contributing factors in the development of plantar fasciitis. Excessive pronation and the resulting stretch and wringing of the plantar fascia during the stance phase can lead to straining of these tissues. If tight posterior muscles limit dorsiflexion, they may force the rearfoot into pronation or the midfoot into dorsiflexion about the oblique midtarsal joint axis. These pathomechanics result in excessive stress on and subsequent injury to the plantar fascia.

Treatment of plantar fasciitis is aimed at reducing the inflammation and the tension on the plantar fascia, restoring tissue strength and mobility, and controlling any biomechanical abnormality. Inflammation can be controlled with ice, anti-inflammatory medication, and in recalcitrant

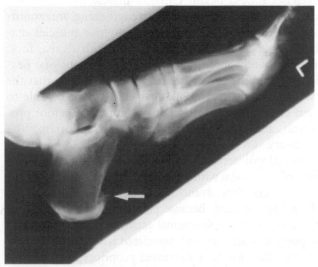

Figure 24-36 Heel spur. (From Magee DJ: *Orthopedic physical assessment*, ed 6, p 959, St. Louis, 2014, Saunders.)

cases, local corticosteroid injection.[72] A combination of arch taping (see Figure 24-33), low-dye taping (Figure 24-37), and/or off-the-shelf orthotics can help hold the foot in a neutral position and protect the plantar tissues from constant irritation during the early stages of rehabilitation.

Gastrocnemius and soleus muscle stretching is important to increase dorsiflexion and to prevent the foot from going into increased pronation to compensate for the lack of dorsiflexion in the ankle. Heel lifts, heel cups, modified arch taping, massage of the plantar fascia, joint play mobilizations, and assessment for proper footwear all are important in the management of plantar fasciitis. Assessment and mobilization of the joints of the ankle and foot also are important. Of particular interest are the talocalcaneal joint, which often needs mobilization into adduction, and the talonavicular joint, which needs good translation of the navicular inferiorly on the talus. All other joints of the foot should be assessed, and mobilization should be performed as needed.

If morning stiffness persists, a night splint to maintain dorsiflexion of the plantar fascia may be useful (Figure 24-38). With the rare persistent case, surgical consultation is required. Surgery involves release of the plantar fascia at its origin, removal of heel spurs, and exploration for nerve entrapment in scar tissue.

In some instances, an acute sprain of the medial longitudinal arch (plantar calcaneonavicular or "spring" ligament) may occur distal to the origin of the plantar fascia (Figure 24-39). The medial longitudinal arch is maintained by its bony arrangement, ligaments, and muscles and by the plantar fascia. The soft tissue may become overloaded during weight bearing, resulting in a sprain, often leading to the navicular bone being forced downward as a result of the weight of the body on the foot. This injury may lead to hyperpronation and lower extremity dysfunction. Clinicians should treat the symptoms and restore proper foot mechanics, which may involve intrinsic foot exercises (including the adductor hallucis muscle), proper-fitting footwear, and orthotics.

The spring ligament runs from the sustentaculum tali on the medial side of the calcaneus to the navicular tuberosity. This injury is common in runners and is often seen in conjunction with tibialis posterior tendonitis or dysfunction. The mechanism of injury of this structure is usually traumatic but can also be related to pronation. It is important to differentially diagnose this structure from the plantar fascia, tibialis posterior tendon or peroneus longus tendon. Management of spring ligament sprains is usually conservative and can be difficult if the true cause of the pathology is not determined. The injury is usually traumatic, and the patient will usually describe a hard landing on an uneven surface, which forces the forefoot into dorsiflexion or pronation. The patient will be tender

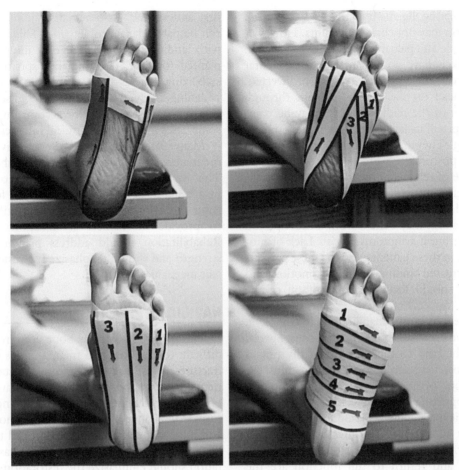

Figure 24-37 Low-dye taping. (From Nawoczenski DA, Epler ME: *Orthotics in functional rehabilitation of the lower limb*, Philadelphia, 1997, Saunders.)

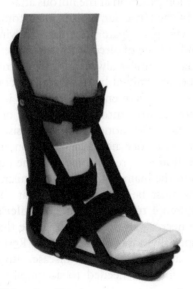

Figure 24-38 Night splint. Note how toes are in extension. (Courtesy of The Brace Shop, Boca Raton, FL.)

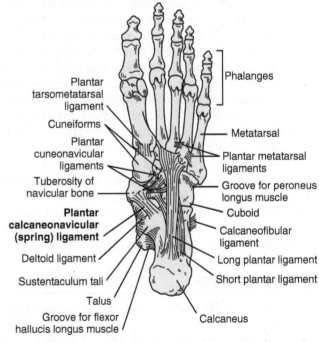

Figure 24-39 Ligaments on plantar aspect of foot. Note plantar calcaneonavicular (spring) ligament. (From Magee DJ: *Orthopedic physical assessment*, ed 6, p 891, St. Louis, 2014, Saunders/Elsevier.)

directly over the spring ligament with deep palpation. Superficial palpation may not elicit complaints. However, there may be a visible and palpable swelling over the area. The patient will likely have no pain with resisted plantar flexion when the rearfoot is neutral, everted, or inverted. Direct tension placed on the spring ligament through passive dorsiflexion of the midtarsal joints may be painful. Finally, patients will usually report discomfort during single-leg standing. They may also often present with a pronated midfoot posture.

The acute phase of rehabilitation should include management of any effusion and pain. Any painful activity should be avoided, and weight-bearing status should be monitored. The patient may benefit from a short period of non–weight bearing if symptoms persist. Lack of motion is not an issue in these patients. In fact, these patients usually have an increased amount of midfoot motion, and further treatment should focus on stabilization of the midfoot.

Once the acute phase of rehabilitation is complete, progressive resistive exercises should be the focus. Special attention should be paid to the strength of the tibialis anterior, tibialis posterior, and peroneus longus muscles. Arch taping or foot orthoses may decrease tension to the structures supporting the medial longitudinal arch. Taping and orthotic management should focus on placing the forefoot in an adducted and plantar flexed position relative to the rearfoot.

CKC activities and return to full function are the goals of the final stage of rehabilitation. Activities that focus on the functional strength of the tibialis posterior and peroneus longus muscles should be included. Single-leg standing on uneven surfaces or on the minitramp will aid in training these muscles. Balance beam activities focusing on eccentric control of pronation may also be beneficial. Long term, patients should be aware of any dorsal foot pain that occurs, because this can be a result of midfoot hypermobility and early dorsal compression syndrome.[73] As the midfoot deforms under load, it is capable of moving in three planes. A mobile midfoot would have a low (medial-lateral) oblique axis and therefore, would have a greater component of dorsiflexion available. Because the bony architecture of the midfoot does not allow for sagittal plane motion, the dorsal surfaces of the cuboid, navicular, and cuneiforms are likely to abut and result in potential chondral or arthritic changes.

MIDFOOT SPRAINS

Sprains to any of the numerous joints between the distal tarsal bones and the bases of the metatarsal heads can lead to considerable instability and disability. Injuries to the first and second tarsometatarsal joints (Lisfranc's joint) can be particularly problematic. This injury often occurs with landing from a height or a jump or rotating on a planted forefoot, resulting in a sprain of the ligaments stabilizing the tarsometatarsal joints and a diastasis, or widening, of the bases of the first and second metatarsals. In severe cases there may be accompanying fractures, and some cases may require surgical intervention.

Many cases are treated conservatively. Initial treatment must emphasize protection of the healing tissues. This early treatment often consists of immobilization in a walking boot (see Figure 24-4) for several weeks. After the boot is removed, an orthotic should be used to provide mechanical stabilization to the midfoot. Rehabilitation should address plantar intrinsic muscle strength and should emphasize the restoration of normal gait mechanics.

NAVICULAR FRACTURES

Fractures of the navicular bone are rare but can be very difficult to diagnose and treat. Injuries include complete fractures, stress fractures, and in skeletally immature patients, traction apophysitis. Fractures and stress fractures of the navicular are notorious for being nonunion fractures.[74] Prolonged immobilization (not modified rest) and bone stimulators are often needed to aid the healing of these fractures. Once the fracture has healed, rehabilitation should emphasize the restoration of ankle and foot ROM, strength, and endurance, as well as normal gait mechanics.

Physically active adolescents, particularly those with excessive foot pronation, can develop traction stress at the insertion of the tibialis posterior into the navicular. Many, in fact, have an accessory navicular bone that develops a traction irritation at the fibrous attachment to the main body of the navicular. This is most commonly seen in patients who participate in sports involving running, jumping, and change of direction (e.g., dancers). The differential diagnosis must always include a stress fracture, which can be determined by bone scan or computed tomography scan. Treatment is directed at inflammation and pronation control through the use of orthotics and appropriate shoes for motion control. Resistant cases of symptomatic accessory navicular irritation may require surgical resection with reattachment of the tibialis posterior tendon to the main body of the navicular.

Clinicians must be cautious of pain at the navicular bone in children 4 to 9 years of age. **Kohler's disease** is an avascular necrosis of the navicular bone that occurs in children, especially boys (Figure 24-40). Rest is the most important treatment for Kohler's disease, although a long leg cast sometimes is needed to accomplish this in an

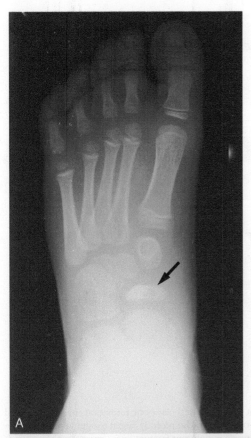

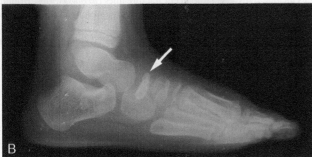

Figure 24-40 Kohler's disease showing affected navicular (*arrow*). **A**, Anteroposterior view. **B**, Lateral view. (From Chambers HG, Haggerty CJ: The foot and ankle in children and adolescents, *Op Tech Sports Med* 14:173-187, 2006.)

active child. This condition typically resolves on its own, with no lasting effects.

METATARSAL FRACTURES

The most common fractures of the metatarsals involve the second or third metatarsal (**march fracture**) (Figure 24-41) and the shaft of the fifth metatarsal just proximal to the styloid process (**Jones fracture**) (Figure 24-42).[75] Metatarsal stress fractures occur most often in the second and third metatarsals and are common in those who engage in running and jumping sports. Common causative factors, as initially proposed by James et al.,[76] include training errors, changes in exposure to different surfaces, strength/flexibility dysfunction, poor shoes, and biomechanical variants, such as excessive rearfoot and forefoot varus. Crichton et al.[77] noted that the second metatarsal is the most prone to stress fracture because the base of the second metatarsal extends proximally into the distal row of tarsal bones and is held rigid and stable by the bony architecture and ligament support. In addition, if the second metatarsal is longer than the first, as is seen with the Morton-type foot, it theoretically is subject to greater bone stress. Also, in a hypermobile forefoot, the second and third metatarsals are subjected to more rotational stress associated with excessive foot pronation.

These stress fractures heal well when treated for 4 to 6 weeks with modified rest and non–weight-bearing exercise (e.g., cycling, swimming, running in water), which maintain the patient's cardiovascular fitness. A gradual return to running and jumping activities with supportive footwear and orthotics is important in the postimmobilization stage in an attempt to reduce risk of reinjury.

A Jones fracture may be an acute fracture that occurs during sudden changes in direction, or it may be an overuse injury. Overuse injuries are especially common in individuals with rigid, cavus feet. Like navicular fractures, Jones fractures often result in nonunion and must be treated surgically.[78] As with other overuse foot injuries, appropriate shoes with adequate stability and shock absorption are essential for returning the individual to high-level functional activity. Attention must also be given to foot control, if necessary, through the use of orthotics. Rehabilitation should emphasize restoration of ankle and foot ROM, strength, and endurance, as well as normal gait mechanics.

METATARSALGIA

Metatarsalgia is a general term for forefoot pain in the area of the lesser metatarsal heads. However, this common term is nondescript and does not identify the specific source of pathology. Two common causes of metatarsalgia are transverse metatarsal arch sprains and Freiberg's infarction.

Transverse Metatarsal Arch Sprain

Transverse metatarsal arch sprains may be caused by an acute or chronic mechanism of injury. The plantar ligaments supporting the arch are injured, allowing the adjacent metatarsal heads to excessively plantar flex or drop and can lead to clawing of the toes. This can irritate the

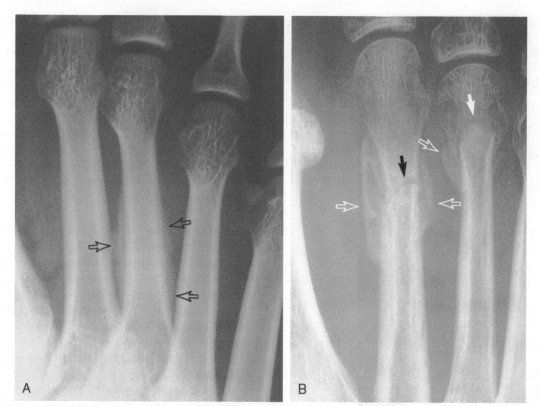

Figure 24-41 March stress fracture. **A,** Early findings. In this patient with exercise-induced foot pain, periosteal new bone formation envelops the third metatarsal diaphysis (*open arrows*). No fracture line is seen. **B,** Later findings. In this 34-year-old woman who recently began a jogging program, observe the fatigue fractures of the second and third metatarsal shafts. The findings include transverse radiolucent fracture lines (*arrows*) with surrounding periostitis (*open arrows*). Stress fractures commonly affect the metatarsal bones and accompany marching, ballet dancing, prolonged standing, foot deformities, and foot surgery. The middle and distal portions of the second and third metatarsals are most commonly affected. Such fractures, referred to as march fractures, may be imperceptible radiographically in the early stages. Bone scans, magnetic resonance images, or serial radiographs are often necessary to confirm the diagnosis. Stress fractures of the metatarsal heads are less common than those of the shaft and neck and are more frequently overlooked. (From Taylor JAM, Hughes TH, Resnick D: *Skeletal imaging: atlas of the spine and extremities,* ed 2, St. Louis, 2010, Saunders.)

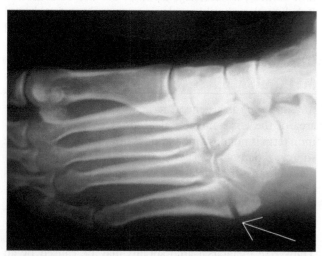

Figure 24-42 Jones fracture. (From Porter DA, Schon LC: *Baxter's the foot and ankle in sport,* ed 2, Philadelphia, 2008, Mosby.)

metatarsal heads and the subcutaneous tissues on the plantar aspect of the foot. A metatarsal felt pad placed just over the second to fourth metatarsal heads can be used to support the injured structures. If metatarsophalangeal extension is present, suggesting intrinsic weakness, exercises emphasizing strength of the plantar intrinsic muscles should be performed as well.

Freiberg's Infarction

Freiberg's infarction is a painful avascular necrosis of the second or, rarely, the third metatarsal head (Figure 24-43). It typically is seen in adolescents or young adults, who often are involved in running and jumping activities. Early radiographs may be normal, with later development of flattening of the involved metatarsal head. If the condition is caught early, deformity of the metatarsal head, which leads to early degenerative changes, can be prevented. Early treatment consists of exercise modification to eliminate excessive running and jumping plus orthotic foot support with a metatarsal pad or bar to unload the involved metatarsal head. A rocker bar on the shoe may also be required. If pain persists and deformity develops with degenerative osteophytes, surgical consultation is appropriate. Surgical management involves either a cheilectomy (cutting away of bony irregularities on the rim of the affected joint and capsular release) or, with more extensive damage, resection arthroplasty.

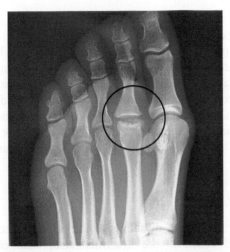

Figure 24-43 Radiographic appearance of Freiberg infarction (*circled area*). (From Miller MD: *Review of orthopeadics,* ed 6, Philadelphia, 2012, Saunders.)

MORTON'S NEUROMA

Morton's neuroma, or **interdigital neuritis**, is an injury to one of the common digital nerves as it passes between the metatarsal heads. The classic location is between the third and fourth metatarsal heads, where the nerve is thickest, receiving both branches from the medial and lateral plantar nerves. The digital nerves enter the forefoot between the superficial and deep transverse metatarsal ligaments in the interdigital space. Nerve irritation can then occur, with compression between the metatarsal heads. Narrow shoe width is often cited as a predisposing factor, because women are diagnosed with this pathology more often than men. A flat transverse metatarsal arch and/or excessive foot pronation can also be predisposing factors, with more metatarsal shearing forces occurring with the prolonged forefoot abduction.[79]

Morton's neuroma must be differentially diagnosed from a march stress fracture. Symptoms include a burning paresthesia in the forefoot, often localized to the third web space and radiating to the toes. The symptoms are increased with hyperextension of the toes on weight bearing, as in squatting, stair-climbing, or running. Additionally, the symptoms may be worse in shoes with a narrow toe box and higher heels. With ongoing nerve irritation and surrounding fibrous reaction or neuroma formation, the pain can become constant. Treatment is aimed at reducing inflammation and unloading the interspace between the bones. Anti-inflammatory medications and modalities may be used in an attempt to provide a local reduction in inflammation. Local corticosteroid injections may be helpful, along with an orthotic to prevent excessive pronation and a metatarsal pad to restore the transverse arch and separate the metatarsal heads.[80] Shoes with low heels and a wide toe box are essential. Failure of conservative management requires surgical excision of the neuroma, which is best done with a dorsal incision.

FIRST RAY INJURIES

Injuries to the first ray (big toe) are particularly problematic because the center of force distribution goes through the first ray during the terminal parts of stance and push-off in the gait cycle. Specific injuries include sesamoiditis, hallux valgus, hallux rigidus, and turf toe.

Sesamoiditis

Sesamoiditis involves trauma to the sesamoid bones in the tendons of the flexor hallucis brevis at its attachments to the base of the proximal phalanx of the hallux on the plantar aspect of the foot. This trauma can include a stress fracture, contusion, osteonecrosis, chondromalacia, or osteoarthritis of the sesamoid bones as they slide over and articulate with the head of the first metatarsal. Weight bearing on the toes increases the stress across the sesamoid bones. The patient reports localized tenderness to the medial (tibial) or lateral (fibular) sesamoid, with localized swelling and pain on weight bearing that increases when on the toes. The diagnosis typically is confirmed with a bone scan.

The sesamoid bones are imbedded within the tendon of the flexor hallucis brevis. Sesamoiditis does not refer to the direct inflammation of the bones themselves but rather the soft tissue surrounding the bones. Most individuals with sesamoid pain are those with a cavus foot. These individuals usually present with a rigid midfoot and forefoot and a plantar-flexed first ray.[81] However, individuals who pronate and place excess force on the medial side of the first metatarsophalangeal joint during push-off are also susceptible to sesamoiditis. The pathology can result from repetitive trauma as described earlier or an acute incident of high impact (i.e., landing from a jump).

Because the medial sesamoid is most often involved, radiographs may be inconclusive as to whether a fracture is present and contributing to symptoms. Tenderness to palpation over the involved sesamoid is most often present and may also present with a thickening or swelling of the tendinous sheath. The patient will be painful upon weight bearing, especially with the shoes off. Passive or active dorsiflexion of the first metatarsophalangeal joint will be painful. In addition, rising onto the toes may be painful or difficult for this patient.

The acute phase of rehabilitation should include controlling pain and decreasing first metatarsophalangeal dorsiflexion ROM. Taping the joint in neutral or slight plantar flexion decreases the stress on the flexor tendons and weight bearing on the sesamoids. Additionally, plantar flexion of the first ray should be minimized because this imparts a relative dorsiflexion at the first metatarsophalangeal joint.[70] Therefore, a metatarsal pad placed just proximal to the first metatarsal head will limit plantar flexion of the first ray. Decreasing heel height, especially in women's shoes, will also decrease the amount of first metatarsophalangeal dorsiflexion.

Management of sesamoiditis is usually handled with orthoses or shoe inserts. Because the symptoms are often a result of a structural deviation, support of the first ray in either a supinated or pronated foot is important. A metatarsal pad under the first ray may be enough to support the medial column. However, in more severe cases, a full custom-molded orthotic device with significant medial midfoot support may be necessary. Cutouts in the orthosis under the first metatarsal head may also decrease pressure on the sesamoids.[82]

Hallux Valgus

Hallux valgus is a condition that has a hereditary factor and is often familial. It is usually seen in patients with excessive foot pronation who use narrow footwear. Hallux valgus may occur with widening of the forefoot on weight bearing, resulting in increased laxity of the ligaments of the forefoot, particularly of the first and fifth metatarsal heads.[83] The metatarsal angle increases with hallux valgus from 1° to 2° to approximately 12°, resulting in increased valgus deviation of the great toe toward the second toe. With this altered

position, and with pronation and/or compression by footwear, the clinician can see the development of a callus, an exostosis, and a bursa thickening (all three make up a bunion) on the lateral side of the first metatarsal head. Treatment is directed at controlled foot pronation using an orthotic and motion control footwear with adequate forefoot width. The callus can be trimmed, and icing and other modalities (e.g., ultrasound) can be used to treat the bursitis. If not treated adequately, hallux valgus will continue to progress and often is treated surgically if severe and painful.

Hallux Rigidus

Hallux rigidus is a disabling condition associated with decreased ROM at the first metatarsophalangeal joint accompanied by degenerative changes in the joint. Extension usually is reduced more than flexion, which makes climbing stairs extremely painful. Hallux rigidus is most frequently the result of repeated trauma, but it also can be seen after joint immobilization for a single traumatic episode or infection. The condition progresses, with increasing restriction of joint motion. Radiographic films confirm the hypertrophic degenerative features, such as joint space narrowing, often dorsal osteophytes,

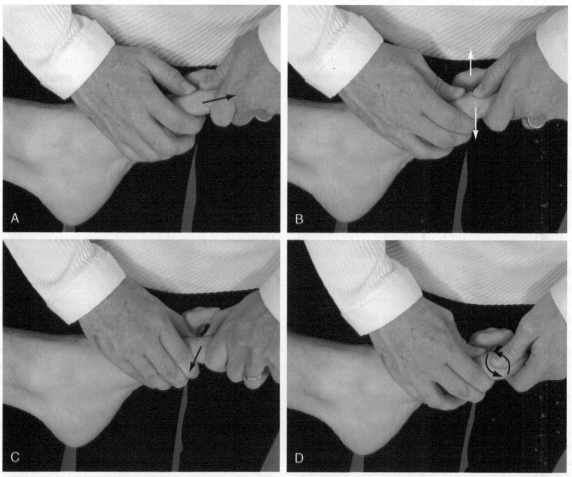

Figure 24-44 Joint play movements at the metatarsophalangeal and interphalangeal joints. **A,** Long-axis extension. **B,** Anteroposterior glide. **C,** Side glide. **D,** Rotation. (From Magee DJ: *Orthopedic physical assessment*, ed 6, p 951, St. Louis, 2014, Saunders.)

TABLE **24-5**

Non–Weight-Bearing and Partial Weight-Bearing Exercises That May be Initiated When Patients with First Ray Injuries are Unable to Bear Full Weight

Body Position	Exercise
Long sitting	• Open-chain toe extension active range of motion (AROM) • Open-chain toe flexion AROM
Seated with foot flat on floor	• Open-chain toe extension AROM (lift toes off floor while keeping heel on floor) • Closed-chain toe extension AROM (lift heel off ground while keeping toes on floor) • Closed-chain toe flexion AROM (clawing) • Closed-chain circumduction (lift heel off ground and put weight on lateral forefoot; roll from lateral to medial and then lateral again, making a complete circle around the ball of the foot)

Modified from Sammarco JG: How I manage turf toe, *Phys Sports Med* 16:113-118, 1988.

transverse joint space widening, and subchondral bone sclerosis. In late stages, as the metatarsophalangeal joint stiffens, hyperextension may be noted at the interphalangeal joint. Treatment is similar to that for turf toe.

Turf Toe

"Turf toe" is a sprain of the first metatarsophalangeal joint that typically occurs when the great toe is forced into hyperextension. It is often associated with sports played on artificial turf when a player catches the toe in a seam, but the condition also is common in those in the performing arts, such as ballet. Treatment is aimed at reducing the inflammation, protection, and restoration of normal ROM. Anti-inflammatory and analgesic medications and modalities (e.g., ice, iontophoresis) can be used in the early stages after injury. ROM exercises are used early on, with at least 10° of extension required for walking and stair-climbing. ROM exercises can be performed in a cold whirlpool, or contrast baths may be used during the inflammatory stage.

Passive joint mobilizing techniques can be effective for pain relief, starting with accessory (joint play) movements and moving into physiological movement patterns when accessory movements are pain free (Figure 24-44).[84] Sammarco[85] outlined a non–weight-bearing exercise program for rehabilitation of turf toe that involves stretching and strengthening

(Table 24-5); this program is also useful for hallux rigidus. The program is combined with taping of the big toe to prevent hyperextension. If normal ROM cannot be achieved, an orthotic with a rocker bar or a stiff-soled shoe with a rocker bar may be used to allow a pain-free gait. When the individual returns to activity, a properly fitted shoe with a stiffer sole should be used. The shoe can be combined with taping or a stiff insert to prevent hyperextension at the metatarsophalangeal joint. If an orthotic or shoe modification fails to provide relief, surgical consultation is needed. Cheilectomy is the usual procedure because it improves ROM without sacrificing joint stability.

SUMMARY

The rehabilitation of patients with foot, ankle, and lower leg injuries should emphasize a return to functional mobility with early attention to healing tissue. Because the foot is the contact point with the ground, changes here often result in changes further up the kinematic chain. Understanding injuries and rehabilitation at the foot and ankle can help understand injuries throughout the entire lower extremity. Rehabilitation of foot, ankle, and lower extremity injuries is challenging and requires attention to ROM, strength, balance, and functional activities. Finally, attention to sport-specific activities is crucial for full, safe return to play.

REFERENCES

1. Hertel J, Denegar CR: A rehabilitation paradigm for restoring neuromuscular control following athletic injury, *Athl Ther Today* 3:12–16, 1998.
2. Wortmann MA, Docherty CL: Effect of balance training on postural stability in subjects with chronic ankle instability, *J Sport Rehabil* 22:143–149, 2013.
3. Loudin JK, Bell SA: The foot and ankle: an overview of selected joint techniques, *J Athl Train* 31:173–178, 1996.
4. Hopkins JT, Ingersoll CD: Arthrogenic muscle inhibition: a limiting factor in joint rehabilitation, *J Sport Rehabil* 9:253–262, 2000.
5. Hopkins JT, Ingersoll CD, Edwards J, et al: Cryotherapy and transcutaneous electric neuromuscular stimulation decrease arthrogenic muscle inhibition of the vastus medialis after knee joint effusion, *J Athl Train* 37:25–31, 2002.
6. Docherty CL, Moore JH, Arnold BL: Effects of strength training on strength development and joint position sense in functionally unstable ankles, *J Athl Train* 33:310–314, 1998.
7. Snyder-Mackler L: Scientific rationale and physiological basis for the use of closed kinetic chain exercises in the lower extremity, *J Sport Rehabil* 5:2–12, 1996.
8. Bergfield JA, Anderson TE: Achieving mobility, strength, and function of the injured knee. In Hunter LY, Funk FJ, editors: *Rehabilitation of the injured knee*, St Louis, 1984, Mosby.
9. Leach RE: Overall view of rehabilitation of the leg for running. In Mack RP, editor: *AAOS symposium on the foot and leg in running sports*, St Louis, 1982, Mosby.
10. Lorenz DS: Variable resistance training using elastic bands to enhance lower extremity strengthening, *Int J Sports Phys Ther* 9:410–414, 2014.
11. Ferrell WR, Tennant N, Sturrock RD, et al: Amelioration of symptoms by enhancement of proprioception in patients with joint hypermobility syndrome, *Arthritis Rheum* 50:3323–3328, 2004.
12. Willy RW, Davis IS: Varied response to mirror gait retraining of gluteus medius control, hip kinematics, pain, and function in 2 female runners with patellofemoral pain, *J Orthop Sports Phys Ther* 43:864–874, 2013.
13. Reinking MF: Exercise-related leg pain in female collegiate athletes: the influence of intrinsic and extrinsic factors, *Am J Sports Med* 34:1500–1507, 2006.

14. Holder LE, Michael RH: The specific scintigraphic pattern of "shin splints in the lower leg": concise communication, *J Nucl Med* 25:865–869, 1984.

15. Viitasalo JT, Kvist M: Some biomechanical aspects of the foot and ankle in athletes with and without shin splints, *Am J Sports Med* 11:125–130, 1983.

16. Detmer DE: Chronic shin splints: classification and management of medial tibial stress syndrome, *Sports Med* 3:436–446, 1986.

17. Bouché RT, Johnson CH: Medial tibial stress syndrome (tibial fasciitis): a proposed pathomechanical model involving fascial traction, *J Am Podiatr Med Assoc* 97:31–36, 2007.

18. Matire JR: Differentiating stress fracture from periostitis: the finer points of bone scans, *Phys Sportsmed* 22:71–81, 1994.

19. Magee DJ: *Sports physiotherapy*, Edmonton, AB, Canada, 1988, University of Alberta.

20. Gross ML, Davlin LB, Evanski PB: Effectiveness of orthotic shoe inserts in the long-distance runner, *Am J Sports Med* 19:409–412, 1991.

21. Winters M, Eskes M, Weir A, et al: Treatment of medial tibial stress syndrome: a systematic review, *Sports Med* 43:1315–1333, 2013.

22. Grieve R, Barnett S, Coghill N, et al: Myofascial trigger point therapy for triceps surae dysfunction: a case series, *Man Ther* 18:519–525, 2013.

23. Matheson GO, Clement DB, McKenzie DC, et al: Stress fractures in athletes: a study of 320 cases, *Am J Sports Med* 15:46–58, 1987.

24. Rauh MJ, Koepsell TD, Rivara FP, et al: Epidemiology of musculoskeletal injuries among high school cross-country runners, *Am J Epidemiol* 163:151–159, 2006.

25. Barrack MT, Gibbs JC, De Souza MJ, et al: Higher incidence of bone stress injuries with increasing female athlete triad-related risk factors: a prospective multisite study of exercising girls and women, *Am J Sports Med* 42:949–958, 2014.

26. Romani WA, Gieck JH, Perrin DH, et al: Mechanisms and management of stress fractures in physically active persons, *J Athl Train* 37:306–314, 2002.

27. Allen CS, Flynn TW, Kardouni JR, et al: The use of a pneumatic leg brace in soldiers with tibial stress fractures—a randomized clinical trial, *Mil Med* 169:880–884, 2004.

28. Clansey AC, Hanlon M, Wallace ES, et al: Influence of tibial shock feedback training on impact loading and running economy, *Med Sci Sports Exerc* 46:973–981, 2014.

29. Davey JR, Rorabeck CH, Fowler PJ: The tibialis posterior muscle compartment: an unrecognized cause of exertional compartment syndrome, *Am J Sports Med* 12:391–397, 1984.

30. Ruland RT, April EW, Meinhard BP: Tibialis posterior muscle: the fifth compartment? *J Orthop Trauma* 6:347–351, 1992.

31. Lokiec F, Siev-Ner I, Pritsch M: Chronic compartment syndrome of both feet, *J Bone Joint Surg Br* 73:178–179, 1991.

32. Bong MR, Polatsch DB, Jazrawi LM, et al: Chronic exertional compartment syndrome: diagnosis and management, *Bull Hosp Joint Dis* 62:77–84, 2005.

33. Tucker AK: Chronic exertional compartment syndrome of the leg, *Curr Rev Musculoskelet Med* 2(3):32–37, 2010.

34. Tiidus PM: Is intramuscular pressure a valid diagnostic criterion for chronic exertional compartment syndrome? *Clin J Sport Med* 24:87–88, 2014.

35. Brennan FH Jr., Kane SF: Diagnosis, treatment options, and rehabilitation of chronic lower leg exertional compartment syndrome, *Curr Sports Med Rep* 2:247–250, 2003.

36. Diebal AR, Gregory R, Alitz C, et al: Effects of forefoot running on chronic exertional compartment syndrome: a case series, *Int J Sports Phys Ther* 6:312–321, 2011.

37. Detmer DE, Sharpe K, Sufit RL, et al: Chronic compartment syndrome: diagnosis, management, and outcomes, *Am J Sports Med* 13:162–170, 1985.

38. Akizuki KH, Gartman EJ, Nisonson B, et al: The relative stress on the Achilles tendon during ambulation in an ankle immobiliser: implications for rehabilitation after Achilles tendon repair, *Br J Sports Med* 35:329–333, 2001.

39. Montalti CS, Souza NV, Rodrigues NC, et al: Effects of low-intensity pulsed ultrasound on injured skeletal muscle, *Braz J Phys Ther* 17:343–350, 2013.

40. Best TM, Gharaibeh B, Huard J: Stem cells, angiogenesis and muscle healing: a potential role in massage therapies? *Br J Sports Med* 47:556–560, 2013.

41. Chuter VH, Janse de Jonge XA: Proximal and distal contributions to lower extremity injury: a review of the literature, *Gait Posture* 36:7–15, 2012.

42. Williams DS, Zambardino JA, Banning VA: Transverse-plane mechanics at the knee and tibia in runners with and without a history of achilles tendonopathy, *J Orthop Sports Phys Ther* 38:761–767, 2008.

43. Ryan M, Grau S, Krauss I, et al: Kinematic analysis of runners with achilles mid-portion tendinopathy, *Foot Ankle Int* 30:1190–1195, 2009.

44. Clement DB, Taunton JE, Smart GW: Achilles tendonitis and peritendinitis: etiology and treatment, *Am J Sports Med* 12:179–184, 1984.

45. Rees JD, Wilson AM, Wolman RL: Current concepts in the management of tendon disorders, *Rheumatology* 45:508–521, 2006.

46. Jones DC: Tendon disorders of the foot and ankle, *J Am Acad Orthop Surg* 1:87–94, 1993.

47. Bhandare N, Guyatt GH, Siddgui F, et al: Treatment of acute Achilles tendon ruptures: a systematic overview and metaanalysis, *Clin Orthop Relat Res* 400:190–200, 2002.

48. Adamson C, Cymet T: Ankle sprains: evaluation, treatment, rehabilitation, *Md Med* J 46:530–537, 1997.

49. Yeung MS, Chan K, So CH, et al: An epidemiological survey on ankle sprain, *Br J Sports Med* 28:112–116, 1994.

50. Itay SA, Ganel H, Horoszowski H, et al: Clinical and functional status following lateral ankle sprains, *Orthop Rev* 11:73–76, 1982.

51. Lynch SA, Renström PA: Treatment of acute lateral ankle ligament rupture in the athlete. Conservative versus surgical treatment, *Sports Med* 27:61–71, 1999.

52. Buckwalter JA, Cooper RR: Bone structure and function, *Instr Course Lect* 36:27–48, 1987.

53. Inman VT: *The joint of the ankle*, Baltimore, 1976, Williams & Wilkins.

54. Lindsjo U, Danckwardt-Lilliestrom G, Sahlstedt B: Measurement of the motion range in the loaded ankle, *Clin Orthop Relat Res* 199:68–71, 1985.

55. Green T, Refshauge K, Crosbie J, et al: A randomized controlled trial of a passive accessory joint mobilization on acute ankle inversion sprains, *Phys Ther* 81:984–994, 2001.

56. Collins N, Teys P, Vicenzino B: The initial effects of a Mulligan's mobilization with movement technique on dorsiflexion and pain in subacute ankle sprains, *Man Ther* 9:77–82, 2004.

57. Bullock-Saxton JE: Local sensation changes and altered hip muscle function following severe ankle sprain, *Phys Ther* 74:17–28, 1994.

58. Verhagen E, van der Beek A, Twisk J, et al: The effect of a proprioceptive balance board training program for the prevention of ankle sprains: a prospective controlled trial, *Am J Sports Med* 32:1385–1395, 2004.

59. Mohammadi F: Comparison of 3 preventive methods to reduce the recurrence of ankle inversion sprains in male soccer players, *Am J Sports Med* 35:922–926, 2007.

60. Tropp H, Askling C, Gillquist J: Prevention of ankle sprains, *Am J Sports Med* 13:259–262, 1985.

61. Ottaviani RA, Ashton-Miller JA, Kothari SU, et al: Basketball shoe height and the maximal muscular resistance to applied ankle inversion and eversion moments, *Am J Sports Med* 23:418–423, 1995.

62. Shapiro MS, Kabo JM, Mitchell PW, et al: Ankle sprain prophylaxis: an analysis of the stabilizing effects of braces and tape, *Am J Sports Med* 22:78–82, 1994.

63. Vaes PH, Duquet W, Casteleyn PP, et al: Static and dynamic roentgenographic analysis of ankle stability in braced and nonbraced stable and functionally unstable ankles, *Am J Sports Med* 26:692–702, 1998.

64. Ashton-Miller JA, Ottaviani RA, Hutchinson C, et al: What best protects the inverted weightbearing ankle against further inversion? Evertor muscle strength compares favorably with shoe height, athletic tape, and three orthoses, *Am J Sports Med* 24:800–809, 1996.

65. Holme E, Magnusson SP, Becher K, et al: The effect of supervised rehabilitation on strength, postural sway, position sense and re-injury risk after acute ankle ligament sprain, *Scand J Med Sci Sport* 9:104–109, 1999.

66. Wright RW, Barile RJ, Surprenant DA, et al: Ankle syndesmosis sprains in National Hockey League players, *Am J Sports Med* 32:1941–1945, 2004.

67. Greenman PE: *Principles of manual therapy*, ed 3, Philadelphia, 2003, Lippincott Williams & Wilkins.

68. Mann RA, Hagy J: Biomechanics of walking, running, and sprinting, *Am J Sports Med* 8:345–350, 1980.

69. Mubarak SJ, Gould RN, Lee YF, et al: The medial tibial stress syndrome. A cause of shin splints, *Am J Sports Med* 10:201–205, 1982.

70. Mann RA, Coughlin MJ: *Surgery of the foot and ankle*, ed 6, St. Louis, 1993, Mosby-Yearbook.

71. Beckman SM, Buchanan TS: Ankle inversion injury and hypermobility: effect on hip and ankle muscle electromyography onset latency, *Arch Phys Med Rehabil* 76:1138–1143, 1995.

72. Kosmahl EM, Kosmahl HE: *Painful plantar heel, plantar fasciitis, and calcaneal spur: etiology and treatment*, *J Orthop Sports Phys Ther* 9:17–24, 1988.

73. Kirby KA: *Foot and lower extremity biomechanics: a ten year collection of precision intricast newsletters*, Payson, AZ, 1997, Precision Intricast, Inc.

74. Torg JS, Pavlov H, Cooley LH, et al: Stress fractures of the tarsal navicular: a retrospective review of twenty-one cases, *J Bone Joint Surg* 64:700–712, 1982.

75. Eisele SA, Sammarco GJ: Fatigue fractures of the foot and ankle in the athlete, *J Bone Joint Surg Am* 75:290–298, 1993.

76. James SL, Bates BT, Ostering LR: Injuries to runners, *Am J Sports Med* 6:40–50, 1978.

77. Crichton PA, Fricker PA, Purdam CR, et al: Injuries to the pelvis and lower limb. In Bloomfield J, Fricker PA, Fitch KD, editors: *Textbook of science and medicine in sport*, Oxford, 1992, Blackwell Scientific.

78. Quill GE: Fractures of the proximal fifth metatarsal, *Orthop Clin North Am* 26:353–361, 1995.

79. Schamberger W: Nerve injuries around the foot and ankle, *Med Sport Sci* 23:105–120, 1987.

80. Saygi B, Yildirim Y, Saygi EK, et al: Morton neuroma: comparative results of two conservative methods, *Foot Ankle Int* 26:556–559, 2005.

81. Axe MJ, Ray RL: Orthotic treatment of sesamoid pain, *Am J Sports Med* 16:411–416, 1988.

82. Sammarco VJ, Nichols R: Orthotic management for disorders of the hallux, *Foot Ankle Clin* 10:191–209, 2005.

83. Gould N: Splayfoot, hallux valgus and hallux rigidus, *Med Sport Sci* 23:121–127, 1987.

84. Maitland GD: *Peripheral manipulation*, ed 2, London, 1977, Butterworth.

85. Sammarco JG: How I manage turf toe, *Phys Sports Med* 16:113–118, 1988.

CHAPTER 25

Peripheral Nerve Injuries

CAROLINE DRYE TAYLOR, RAFAEL ESCAMILLA, JAMES E. ZACHAZEWSKI*

INTRODUCTION

Peripheral nerve injuries occur infrequently compared with the multitude of other injuries with which the physician, physical therapist, or athletic trainer must contend. Because they are infrequent, they may be overlooked in the process of differential diagnosis. The authors' purpose in writing this chapter is to alert clinicians to a class of injuries that, although infrequent, can have potentially devastating functional implications.

There is increased documentation in the literature regarding the incidence of peripheral nerve injuries, particularly in literature related to surgery, athletic injuries, and trauma. Krivickas and Wilbourn[1] reviewed more than 200 cases and reported that 86% of peripheral nerve injuries in athletics occurred in the upper extremity. More than one third of those injuries were sustained by individuals playing American football, and the most common injury was to the brachial plexus. Takazawa et al.[2] reviewed 9550 injuries treated over a span of 95 years at the clinic of the Japanese Athletic Association. During that period, only 28 cases of peripheral nerve injury were documented. This contrast may be due to the different type of sports or athletic activities in each study and within different cultures. Hirasawa and Sakakida[3] reviewed 18 years of experience with peripheral nerve injuries and reported that only 5.7% (66 of 1167 cases) were associated with athletes. The brachial plexus was involved most often, accounting for 24.2% of injuries (16 of 66). However, this study did not include high-contact sports, such as American football.

Noble et al.[4] reported a prevalence of peripheral nerve injuries of 2.8% in a trauma population of 5777. In this study 83% of the patients were male, and a motor vehicle accident (MVA) was the most common cause of injury (46%). The most frequently injured nerves were the radial nerve in the upper extremity and the common fibular (peroneal) nerve in the lower extremity. A study of war wounds sustained by British soldiers in Iraq and Afghanistan reported that of 261 peripheral nerve injuries sustained by 100 consecutively injured men and women,

63% were caused by explosions. The main nerves injured were the ulnar, common fibular (peroneal), and tibial nerves. Nerve injuries were highly associated (82%) with open wounds.[5]

Peripheral nerves may be vulnerable during surgery as a result of prolonged pressure from patient positioning or retraction of surrounding tissues. A study in 1999 by the American Society of Anesthesiologists evaluated more than 4000 adverse anesthetic outcomes from the files of professional liability insurance companies, and nerve damage was the second most common cause of claims, accounting for 16% of cases.[6,7] Injury to the ulnar nerve occurs in as many as 1 in 200 adult surgical cases and is more common in men than in women.[7] Injury is caused by direct trauma when surgery is performed near the cubital tunnel (e.g., during ulnar collateral ligament reconstruction surgery) or the wrist or from compression of the nerve as a result of poor upper extremity positioning. The likelihood of sciatic nerve injury during total hip arthroplasty (1.3%) increases if there is a preexisting congenital hip dysplasia or dislocation (5.2%) or in cases of revision of prior hip arthroplasties (3.6%).[8]

During normal joint and body movements, the normal nervous system adapts to tensile, shear, and compressive loads. This requires gliding (i.e., excursion) relative to adjacent structures, stretching (by increasing strain), and a capacity to tolerate compression from adjacent or external structures, all the while maintaining its ability to transmit neural impulses.[9] However, when these loads become excessive, axonal transport and intraneural blood supply may decrease, producing peripheral nerve injuries and concomitant signs and symptoms. These are discussed in detail later in this chapter. Various nervous system mobilization techniques have been developed and are also described; and these can be used for both diagnostic purposes and conservative treatment to restore the normal biomechanical function of the nervous system.[10] Mobilizing the nervous system may reduce edema and central sensitization, and the mechanical effects of nerve excursion (i.e., gliding) may gradually result in a normally functioning nervous system.[11]

---

*The authors, editors, and publisher wish to acknowledge Robert J. Nee for his contributions on this topic in the previous edition.

ETIOLOGY

Injury to a peripheral nerve can occur by means of several mechanisms: stretching, compression (i.e., sustained compression or blunt trauma), friction, inflammation, or laceration. The clinical results of stretching or compression of the nerve vary depending on whether the insult has a rapid onset or is the result of a gradual change. A sudden insult does not allow for any adaptive change in the connective tissue of the nerve and is more likely to cause acute disruption of the nerve's blood supply or connective tissue. Conversely, the nerve can adapt amazingly well to a slow increase in tensile or compressive forces, such as that brought on by a growing osteophyte.[12] A classification of peripheral nerve injuries is presented in Table 25-1.[13-16]

Mechanisms of Peripheral Nerve Injury

- Stretching
- Compression
- Friction
- Inflammation
- Laceration

Compression of the nerve can be caused by external sources or by swelling (e.g., inflammation) with a concomitant increase in pressure in a rigid compartment (e.g., carpal tunnel syndrome [CTS] compressing the median nerve at the wrist or anterior compartment [exertional] syndrome of the leg compressing the deep fibular [peroneal] nerve).[17] A nerve can be directly compressed,

TABLE **25-1**

Classification of Nerve Injuries[13-16]

TYPE	FUNCTION			
Seddon's Classification	Sunderland's Classification	Pathological Basis	Possible Causes	Prognosis
Neurapraxia	**Type 1:** • Focal conduction block • Primarily motor function and proprioception are affected • Some sensation and sympathetic function possibly present	• Local myelin injury, primarily larger fibers • Axonal continuity • No Wallerian degeneration	• Electrolyte imbalances • Deformation of myelin sheaths • Ischemia caused by compression or traction	• Recovery within minutes, hours, or days if lesion was caused by anoxia or ionic imbalances • Mechanical compression or stretch may recover in weeks to months
Axonotmesis	**Type 2:** • Loss of nerve conduction at injury site and distally	• Disruption of axonal continuity with Wallerian degeneration • Connective tissue elements of the nerve remain intact	• Compression	• Axonal regeneration required for recovery • The length of time for regeneration will depend on the distance of the injury from the end of the nerve • Good prognosis
	Type 3: • Loss of nerve conduction at injury site and distally	• Loss of axonal continuity and endoneurial tubes • Perineurium and epineurium preserved	• Compression	• Disruption of endoneurial tubes, hemorrhage, and edema, producing scarring • Axonal misdirection possible • Poor prognosis • Surgery possibly required
	Type 4: • Loss of nerve conduction at injury site and distally	• Damage to endoneurium and perineurium • Epineurium remains intact	• Compression	• Intraneural scarring and axonal misdirection • Poor prognosis • Surgery required
Neurotmesis	**Type 5:** • Loss of nerve conduction at injury site and distally	• Severance of entire nerve	• Compression • Traction • Laceration	• Surgical resection and repair only means of recovery; full recovery unlikely • Factors that affect extent of recovery: nerve injured, level at which nerve is damaged, extent of injury, time elapsed since injury, patient's age

Modified from Dumitru D: *Electrodiagnostic medicine,* Philadelphia, 1995, Hanley & Belfus.

such as when the tibial nerve is entrapped and compressed within the tarsal tunnel during running.

In 1973 Upton and McComas[18] theorized that compression at one point along the nerve trunk increased the vulnerability of distal points along the nerve as a result of the effects of the compression. They hypothesized that the proximal compression disrupted axonal transport of vital nutrients and possibly the blood supply to the nerve, and they called this type of lesion a *double crush lesion*. They also noted that nerves with some other type of preexisting physiological disturbance (e.g., diabetic peripheral neuropathy) are more vulnerable to compressive lesions.

Friction over a nerve trunk can cause inflammation and fibrosis of the nerve's connective tissue elements. Fibrosis of the nerve trunk reduces its extensibility. Loss of extensibility at one site along the nerve trunk may cause other portions of the nerve to bear increasing tensile loads when the nerve bed is elongated,[19] leading to a mechanical form of a double crush syndrome.[12]

Injury to tissues adjacent to nerve trunks can cause extensive scarring around the nerve trunk, which may impair the nerve's ability to move relative to its interfacing tissue or may compress the nerve if it is enclosed in a rigid space.[12] This may be one mechanism for nerve injury following radiotherapy in addition to fibrosis of the nerves and adjacent blood vessels. Laceration injuries from trauma and surgery can sever the nerve.

Detailed information on the pathology of nerve injuries can be found in volume 2 of this series, *Scientific Foundations and Principles of Practice in Musculoskeletal Rehabilitation*, Chapter 8.

INJURIES TO THE CERVICAL NERVE ROOTS AND BRACHIAL PLEXUS

Etiology

Brachial plexus injuries are becoming more common as patients are surviving more severe trauma to the head, chest, spine, and shoulder.[20] The peak incidences of brachial plexus injuries are at birth, from obstetrical trauma, and at 20 to 40 years of age, as a result of MVAs or knife or bullet wounds. Up to 10% of all injuries to the peripheral nervous system involve the brachial plexus.[21]

The brachial plexus is vulnerable to injury during surgical procedures, such as scoliosis repair involving the upper ribs,[22] median sternotomy for open heart surgery,[16,23] or shoulder reconstruction. It also may be compromised by positioning during surgical procedures or during procedures such as axillary arteriography, venous cannulation, and administration of regional anesthetic blocks.[7,16] Damage to the brachial plexus is estimated to occur in between 0.2% and 0.6% of all surgeries.[8]

Neoplastic disease also can affect the brachial plexus. Primary brachial plexus tumors are rare; these include schwannomas, neurilemmomas, neurinomas, and

neurofibromas. Secondary neoplastic disease of the upper lobe of the lung (Pancoast's or superior sulcus tumors) and breast tissue are the more common causes of brachial plexus lesions. Radiation treatment to the breast and lung may further damage the brachial plexus either by direct fibrosis of the nerves or by damage to the vascular tissue and Schwann cells.[16] Radiation-induced peripheral neuropathy may not be clinically evident for several years.[24]

Brachial plexus injuries are the most common nerve injuries in athletics, although they occur infrequently except in American football; the reported incidence in college football players ranges from 52% to 70%.[25] To obtain a thorough understanding of the epidemiological factors associated with brachial plexus injuries in football, the clinician must consider the mechanism of injury and the player's position, along with other biomechanical and physical factors.

Classically, the following three distinct mechanisms of injury to the brachial plexus and cervical nerve roots have been described in the literature:

- Head and neck lateral flexion with shoulder depression, causing an ipsilateral traction injury to the brachial plexus (a contralateral compression injury to the brachial plexus may also occur) (Figure 25-1).[26-33]
- A direct blow to the supraclavicular region in the area of **Erb's point** (union of C5 and C6 nerve roots located 2 to 3 cm above the clavicle in the posterior triangle of the neck), causing direct compression of the brachial plexus at its most superficial point (Figure 25-2).[26,27,30,34]
- Cervical hyperextension and lateral (side) flexion, causing ipsilateral compression of the nerve roots within the

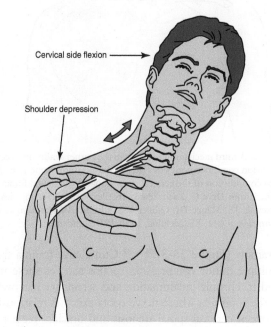

Cervical side flexion

Shoulder depression

Figure 25-1 The combination of shoulder depression and contralateral cervical side (lateral) flexion can lead to a traction injury to the brachial plexus; this is commonly referred to as a *burner*. (Modified from Drye C, Zachazewski JE: Peripheral nerve injuries. In Zachazewski JE, Magee DJ, Quillen WS, editors: *Athletic injuries and rehabilitation*, p 442, Philadelphia, 1996, WB Saunders.)

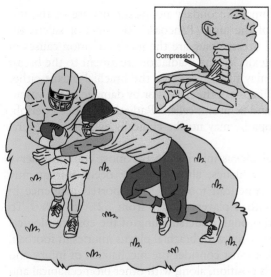

Figure 25-2 A second mechanism for a burner is a direct blow to the base of the neck (Erb's point). This leads to a compression injury to the trunks of the brachial plexus. (Modified from Drye C, Zachazewski JE: Peripheral nerve injuries. In Zachazewski JE, Magee DJ, Quillen WS, editors: *Athletic injuries and rehabilitation,* p 443, Philadelphia, 1996, WB Saunders.)

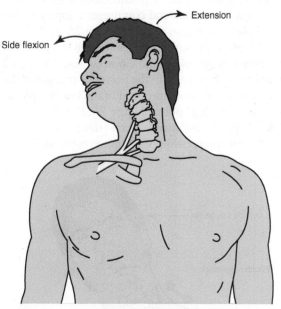

Figure 25-3 A third mechanism of injury in the burner syndrome is cervical extension combined with side (lateral) flexion to the same side. This leads to compression of the cervical nerve roots in the neural foramina. (Modified from Drye C, Zachazewski JE: Peripheral nerve injuries. In Zachazewski JE, Magee DJ, Quillen WS, editors: *Athletic injuries and rehabilitation,* p 444, Philadelphia, 1996, WB Saunders.)

foramina (Figure 25-3).[28,34–37] Cumulative trauma from multiple minor compression sprains such as these may lead to chronic inflammation and secondary narrowing of the foramina where nerve roots exit.[35] A relationship between cervical spinal stenosis and brachial plexus injuries has been demonstrated, with injuries caused by the extension and compression mechanism described earlier.[35]

CLINICAL PRESENTATION

Brachial plexus injuries in American football usually are the result of tackling or blocking. Therefore the incidence is highest among defensive players, such as linemen, linebackers, and defensive backs.[38,39] This injury is commonly referred to as a *burner* or *stinger.* The athlete experiences transient weakness of the shoulder musculature accompanied by upper extremity paresthesia. In the acute syndrome, symptoms usually last several seconds to a few minutes and are followed by complete recovery. Neck pain may or may not be present.[32,40]

The injury usually affects the upper trunk of the brachial plexus (i.e., C5-C6 nerve roots).[27–29,41] Immediately after injury, weakness can be found in the biceps, deltoid, supraspinatus, and infraspinatus muscles, which are all muscles that have their innervation by C5-C6 nerve roots. Deep tendon reflexes of the biceps may also be diminished. Symptoms often can be reproduced by cervical extension and lateral (side) flexion toward the involved extremity (compression on the brachial plexus) or lateral (side) flexion away from the involved extremity (tension on the brachial plexus).[33,40] Any restriction of cervical movement or spinal pain should alert the examiner to the possibility of cervical spine injury. True burners rarely involve restricted cervical mobility.[38] Restriction of shoulder range of motion should alert the clinician to the possibility of a clavicular fracture or acromioclavicular separation.

The injury to the nerve usually is considered a neurapraxic lesion, because it recovers almost immediately.[32,40] A thorough neurological examination can help differentiate spinal cord trauma from injury to the nerve root or brachial plexus (Table 25-2). The patient's neurological status should be monitored closely for several days after the injury to determine the level of recovery accurately. Patients with persistent weakness or sensory loss should be referred to a physician for follow-up evaluation for possible axonotmesis or neurotmesis, which are more severe nerve lesions compared with neurapraxia.

Electromyographic (EMG) studies do not differentiate denervation from Wallerian degeneration for 10 to 20 days after injury[33]. Garrick and Webb[31] suggested that EMG studies be performed 6 weeks after injury. Clinically, Speer and Bassett[30] reported that strength deficits at 72 hours after injury equaled those at 4 weeks after injury.

Clinical Note

EMG studies generally are not performed until a minimum of 2 to 3 weeks after injury to allow time for Wallerian degeneration to occur.

Acute management mainly involves resting the extremity. If strength and function return completely in 1 to 2 minutes, returning the athlete to play could be considered.[40] If any neurological deficits persist after this time, the athlete should not be allowed to continue

TABLE **25-2**

Neurological Evaluation of Brachial Plexus Injury

Lesion (Root Level)	Motor Findings (Resisted Tests)	Sensory Findings (Light Touch or Pinprick)
C4	Upper trapezius: shoulder elevation	Top of shoulders (acromioclavicular joint)
C5	Supraspinatus and deltoid: shoulder abduction	Lateral upper arm (lower deltoid) and lateral cubital fossa
C6	Biceps: elbow flexion	Lateral forearm, thumb
C7	Triceps: elbow extension	Index and middle fingertips
C8	Extensor pollicis longus: extension of distal phalanx of thumb	Fourth and fifth fingers and hypothenar eminence; medial forearm; medial cubital fossa
T1	Intrinsics of the hand: abduction/adduction of fingers	Medial arm
Suspected spinal cord lesions	Diffuse motor loss, bilateral weakness, lower extremity motor loss	Diffuse paresthesia and numbness, bilateral sensory loss (nondermatomal)

Modified from Drye C, Zachazewski JE: Peripheral nerve injuries. In Zachazewski JE, Magee DJ, Quillen WS, editors: *Athletic injuries and rehabilitation*, p 444, Philadelphia, 1996, WB Saunders.

participation until full strength, range of motion, and sensation are restored in the cervical spine and extremity. However, the athlete could be susceptible to further injury with a subsequent similar mechanism of injury of a smaller magnitude as a result of enhanced tissue sensitivity. Caution should be exercised in this decision, because athletes may often mask their symptoms because of their desire to play. Historically, Wroble et al.[38] have advocated for the use of ice and various modalities for subjective symptom management (transcutaneous electrical nerve stimulation [TENS], ultrasound), as well as anti-inflammatory medications if pain and tenderness of the cervical spine and shoulder persist. Neck and shoulder strengthening exercises are prescribed to address any residual weakness.[42]

Postural changes (e.g., a depressed shoulder), atrophy of the shoulder muscles, or both may occur.[34] Clearly, more severe neurological losses and the need for longer periods of recuperation indicate that it is less advisable for the athlete to return to play.[38]

Padded neck rolls and shock-absorbing shoulder pads may be of some assistance in preventing recurrent burner injuries in American football players.[20,23] However, they have been evaluated carefully only in controlled laboratory testing and not on the field. Gorden et al.[43] tested a variety of collars and did not find any collars that limited lateral flexion, only hyperextension. An appropriately fitted collar should be worn close to the neck and should restrict cervical extension and lateral flexion (Figure 25-4). Fitted properly, the collar does not restrict cervical

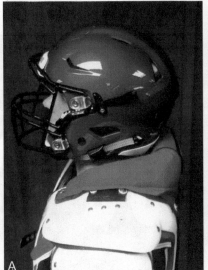
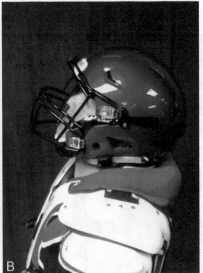

Figure 25-4 Neck rolls often are used to prevent excessive lateral (side) flexion of the cervical spine during tackling in American football. **A,** Properly fit collar and shoulder pads. **B,** Proper fit will assist in preventing excessive lateral flexion and extension of the cervical spine during tackling in American football.

rotation. Often the athlete wears the neck roll too low on the shoulder pads in an effort to be able to move the head and neck and see the football more easily; this renders the neck roll ineffective (Figure 25-5). At no time should straps running from the shoulder pads to the helmet be used to prevent head and neck movement. Use of straps may predispose the cervical spine to excessive axial loading and resultant fracture or fracture-dislocation by preventing movement of the cervical spine. In 1993 the U.S. Military Academy designed augmented shoulder pads that

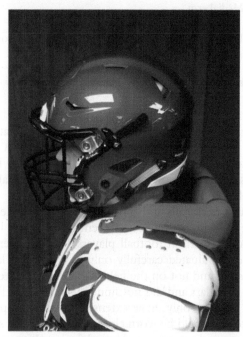

Figure 25-5 Position of collar and shoulder pad determine effective protection of cervical spine from injury. Placement too far posterior, either by collar position or shoulder pad fit, will allow too much extension and side (lateral) bending during tackling, which may cause injury.

added buffer padding to the neck in an effort to prevent compressive injuries to the brachial plexus.[34] These concepts have now been incorporated into commercially available shoulder pads, resulting in collars and shoulder pad combinations that vary based on the size of the player and position played (Figure 25-6).

Cervical nerve root avulsion injuries can occur with more severe injuries. Frequently, more than one nerve root level avulses at the time of injury, with the most common pattern in one study involved the C5-T1 nerve roots.[41] Adjacent roots are always involved if more than one level is avulsed, and associated vascular damage may occur.[20] The patient has complete motor loss in muscles innervated by the affected nerve root levels, and spontaneous recovery does not occur because of a neurotmesis nerve injury. Diagnostic findings may include fractures of the transverse processes on cervical radiographs.[42] Rehabilitation consists of maintaining range of motion in the involved upper extremity and reconstructive surgery to restore as much function as possible.

Acute Brachial Neuropathy

Acute brachial neuropathy is a rare syndrome characterized by acute or subacute intense shoulder pain, accompanied by weakness and wasting of various muscles of the shoulder and proximal arm. It should be considered a possible diagnosis if the patient has no clear trauma or history of overuse. The incidence is higher in males than in females, and patients in their 30s or 70s are affected more frequently.[44] The disorder has no clear pattern of motor nerve or brachial plexus involvement. Denervation may be limited to only one muscle supplied by a peripheral nerve (e.g., a normally innervated infraspinatus muscle with denervation of the supraspinatus muscle). Sensory loss usually is limited. Most reported cases occur in the

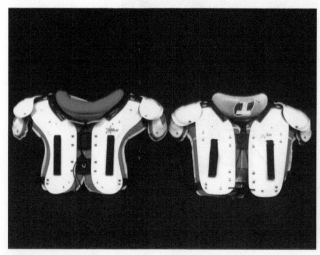
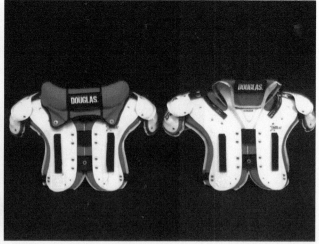

Figure 25-6 Shoulder pads and collar combinations used to assist in prevention of injury come in various sizes, shapes, and configurations depending on player position. Smaller pads and collars are used for position players such as defensive backs and receivers, whereas larger pads and collars are used for linemen.

dominant upper extremity.[40,45] The cause of acute brachial neuropathy is unknown.

Management in the acute phase includes rest and analgesics. The patient begins rehabilitation as soon as the pain subsides.[38] The prognosis generally is good, but residual weakness is common for several months or even years after diagnosis.

PERIPHERAL NERVE INJURIES IN THE UPPER QUARTER

Nerve Injuries of the Neck and Upper Limb

- Thoracic outlet syndrome
- Spinal accessory nerve
- Long thoracic nerve
- Axillary nerve
- Suprascapular nerve
- Musculocutaneous nerve
- Radial nerve
- Ulnar nerve
- Median nerve
- Combined lesions

Thoracic Outlet Syndrome

Thoracic outlet syndrome (TOS) is a controversial diagnosis consisting of neural and/or vascular compression in the thoracic outlet. TOS has a variety of clinical manifestations, depending on the site of compression and the neurovascular structures involved, as shown in Figure 25-7. Vascular symptoms are less common than neurogenic symptoms, but underlying vascular insufficiency must be considered. Molina and D'Cunha[46] have documented that, using Doppler ultrasound, 51% of the patients in their study ($n=148$) with neurogenic TOS were found to have arterial occlusion during TOS testing maneuvers and 8% had compression of the subclavian vein.

Subclavian-axillary vein effort thrombosis (i.e., Paget-Schroetter syndrome), although relatively uncommon, remains the most frequently encountered vascular disorder in young competitive athletes.[46] This condition was previously thought to be from an acute subclavian vein injury with superimposed thrombosis. However, it is now believed to be an acute clinical presentation secondary to a chronic condition characterized by a repetitive mechanical venous injury with exertional activity during arm elevation. The elevated arm increases the likelihood of subclavian vein compression in the costoclavicular space, because this space narrows with arm elevation. Thus, athletes or others involved in overhead activities may have a higher likelihood of subclavian-axillary vein effort thrombosis. Repetitive compression may injure the vein, stimulating localized tissue repair with fibrosis within and around the vein wall. With chronic and repetitive injury, scar tissues ensues. The formation of venous collaterals may limit symptoms for months or years after the original injury. Eventually, turbulent blood flow within the narrowed vein leads to thrombosis formation in the subclavian vein and may also lead to occlusion of the distal axillary vein. When symptoms are finally manifested, they may include arm swelling, cyanotic discoloration, heaviness, pain, and fatigue during or after exertional efforts such as what occurs in sport and exercise.

The most common neurogenic signs of TOS arise from compression of the lower trunk (i.e., C8-T1 nerve roots) of the brachial plexus; these include symptoms such as pain and paresthesias of the medial arm and hand, upper extremity fatigue, and weakness and atrophy of muscles innervated by C8-T1, such as the intrinsic hand muscles.[46]

TOS may occur in patients with excessive shoulder girdle (i.e., scapula and clavicle) depression[47] or overly developed trapezius and neck musculature (e.g., hypertrophy of scalenus anterior and medius) and in those whose work requires repetitive overhead use of the upper extremity or prolonged wear of heavy body armor, such as for combat soldiers. Violinists and violists can develop symptoms from an overly depressed position of the shoulder girdle as they support their instrument on their shoulder. Swimmers may develop symptoms as a result of hypertrophy of the pectoralis minor muscle and thus a decreased coracopectoral space. Tennis, volleyball, and baseball players may develop symptoms owing to either greater muscular development of the dominant arm, increased scapular depression as a result of failure to maintain adequate scapular stabilization with repetitive motions (e.g., fatigue or weakness in the scapular muscles), or repetitive elevation of the upper extremity.[31,48] Prolonged keyboard use and reaching for a computer mouse can also provoke symptoms.

Because the exact diagnosis of TOS is difficult to confirm, symptoms in the upper extremity should always be evaluated carefully to differentiate true TOS from shoulder instabilities, cervical radiculopathies, and other peripheral nerve injuries. Treatment is directed at restoring posture of the spine and scapulae and muscle balance of trunk, shoulder, and shoulder girdle musculature to correct chronic scapular depression[49]; restoring diaphragmatic breathing patterns to reduce recruitment of the scalene muscles; and reducing sensitivity to neurodynamic tests in the upper extremity. Modification of technique or avoidance of some activities may be necessary to prevent recurrence of symptoms.[21,50]

Spinal Accessory Nerve Injury

The spinal accessory nerve is a motor nerve only and contains the spinal portion of cranial nerve XI. This nerve innervates the sternocleidomastoid and trapezius muscles.

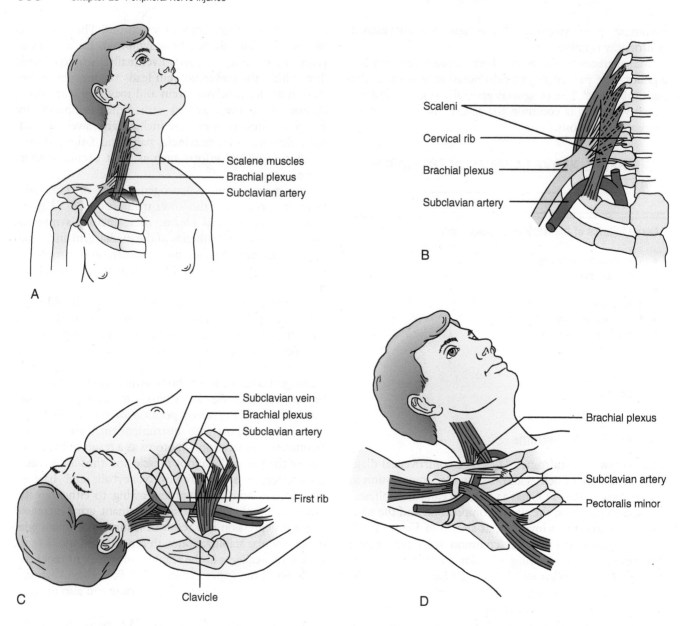

Figure 25-7 Location and causes of thoracic outlet syndrome. **A,** Scalenus anterior syndrome. **B,** Cervical rib syndrome. **C,** Costoclavicular space syndrome. **D,** Hyperabduction syndrome (abduction, extension, and lateral rotation). (From Magee DJ: *Orthopedic physical assessment,* ed 6, p 261, St. Louis, 2014, Saunders/Elsevier.)

It is vulnerable to injury from blunt trauma (e.g., a blow from a hockey stick), radiation, surgical injury,[51] or traction injury.[42] Intracranial tumors can compress the nerve before it exits the jugular foramen. Injury can result in paralysis and atrophy of the trapezius muscle. Weakness usually develops soon after the injury and is accompanied by a persistent ache about the shoulder girdle.[52,53] If the nerve does not recover, scapular stabilizing procedures or transfer of the levator scapulae can be performed surgically. However, the prognosis for full return to athletics or other types of vigorous physical activity is usually poor.[52]

Long Thoracic Nerve Injury (Backpacker's Palsy)

The long thoracic nerve is a motor nerve only that originates from the C5-C7 nerve roots and innervates the serratus anterior muscle, which is essential for scapular stabilization, upward rotation, and protraction. The nerve is vulnerable to blunt trauma as it passes from the brachial plexus across the base of the neck and, more distally, where it lies against the lateral chest wall. For example, during sports, a blow to the ribs underneath an outstretched arm may injure the long thoracic nerve. The nerve may also be entrapped in the scalenus medius or as it runs between the clavicle and second rib[54] or from a traction injury from carrying heavy backpacks for prolonged periods. A traction injury may also occur with combined head flexion, rotation, and lateral (side) flexion away from the involved side and with extreme shoulder flexion.[55] Paralysis of the serratus anterior has also been reported as an overuse injury in sports such as archery, basketball, overhead throwing, bowling, cycling, golf, rope skipping, weight lifting, and tennis.[52] White and Witten[56] reported one incidence of a stretch injury to the long thoracic nerve in a male ballet dancer from aggressive warm-up stretches. In clinical practice, the onset of symptoms has been observed after sleeping in awkward positions, after a viral illness, and with increased exercise in a plank or push-up position. The presenting complaint is often accompanied by aching or burning around the shoulder or scapula.[52] With long thoracic nerve palsy, an individual would have difficulty elevating the arm as a result of winging of the scapula, where the scapular laterally rotates in a transverse plane (i.e., the medial border moves away from the thorax). A simple test for long thoracic nerve palsy is to lean against the wall with outstretched arms (as in performing a wall push-up), causing winging of the involved scapula to become apparent.

The prognosis is good if the injury is the result of overuse. The injury is treated with rest and exercise to maintain range of motion. Closed injuries have a more guarded prognosis; if the injury was caused by compression, the prognosis depends on the duration and the extent of the compression. Taping the scapula can be used to optimize scapular positioning during activities of daily living (ADLs) and exercise.[57] If strength and endurance do not fully recover with conservative management over 24 months, the scapula may have to be stabilized surgically.[52]

Long thoracic nerve injury and thoracic outlet symptoms can be prevented in children who carry backpacks to school. The American Physical Therapy Association suggests that children carry no more than 15% of their body weight. The backpack should fit properly, and both straps should be used. Hip belts and compressive straps help lessen the strain on the upper body.[58]

Axillary Nerve Injury

The axillary nerve is a mixed sensorimotor nerve formed from the C5 and C6 nerve roots and the posterior cord of the brachial plexus. Its motor function innervates the deltoid and teres minor muscles, and it also provides sensory innervation to the glenohumeral joint and a small area of skin over the lower lateral deltoid. After the nerve courses under the axillary recess of the glenohumeral joint, it exits posteriorly along with the posterior humeral circumflex artery, passes through the quadrilateral space (bound by the teres minor superiorly, the teres major inferiorly, the long head of the triceps medially, and the humeral shaft laterally), and then winds around the surgical neck of the humerus.

The most common mechanism of injury is an acute anterior shoulder dislocation or its reduction.[48,50] Other mechanisms of injury include blunt trauma to the shoulder, fracture of the surgical neck of the humerus, compression by a hematoma, irritation by osteophytes of the glenoid margin, compression from a space-occupying lesion (e.g., ganglion cyst), and compression from muscular hypertrophy (e.g., teres minor, teres major, triceps long head) as the nerve passes through the quadrilateral space. The quadrilateral space can be narrowed with shoulder abduction and lateral (external) rotation with accompanying contraction from the teres minor and teres major, such as during overhead throwing, increasing the risk of nerve compression.[52,59,60] Trauma also may occur during many surgical procedures on the shoulder[8,52,61] and poorly placed intramuscular injections in the deltoid.[7]

If EMG findings show incomplete denervation, the prognosis for recovery generally is good, but a long rest from the provoking activity may be necessary.[59] Fortunately, the supraspinatus and infraspinatus muscles can compensate for some of the loss of abduction and lateral (external) rotation after axillary nerve injury, because these muscles assist in both of these shoulder movements.[52]

Butler[62] proposed a test of the sensitivity of the nerve to mechanical loading based on the geography of the nerve relative to the axes of the shoulder joint (Figure 25-8). This test has not been studied to determine whether it provokes symptoms in the distribution of the axillary nerve.

Suprascapular Nerve Injury

The suprascapular nerve is a mixed sensorimotor nerve formed from the upper trunk of the brachial plexus. Its motor function innervates the supraspinatus and infraspinatus muscles. It also provides sensory branches to the

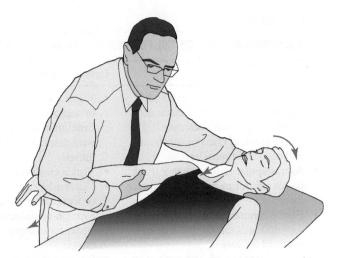

Figure 25-8 Neurodynamic test of the axillary nerve. The test combines medial (internal) rotation of the arm, shoulder girdle depression, and lateral (side) flexion of the cervical spine away from the upper extremity. (Modified from Butler D: *The sensitive nervous system,* p 339, Adelaide, Australia, 2000, Noigroup Publications.)

posterior glenohumeral joint, the acromioclavicular joint, and the subacromial bursa. The five potential sites of trauma along the nerve are outlined in Table 25-3.[52,54,60,63]

The mechanism of injury may be direct trauma, such as a fall on the shoulder or acute dislocation, traction and friction to the nerve as it passes through the suprascapular notch, or compression from a ganglion cyst in the suprascapular notch or the spinoglenoid notch secondary to tears in the shoulder capsule or labrum. The repetitive nature of the overhead throwing motion such as during baseball pitching, the volleyball spike, or the tennis serve can result in superior labrum tears, anterior to posterior in direction (i.e., SLAP lesions), which can lead to the formation of a ganglion cyst. The labral tears occur in part because shoulder lateral (external) rotation during the arm cocking phase of pitching attempts to "peel back" the labrum off the glenoid[64] and via the repetitive force of the long biceps brachii tendon pulling on the posterosuperior labrum as it contracts eccentrically during the arm deceleration phase of pitching to slow down the rapidly extending elbow.[65] These labral tears act as a one-way valve, permitting joint fluid to escape into the ganglion cyst cavity but not allowing the return of the synovial fluid back into the joint.[60] The most common location for labral tears is the superior posterior labrum,[60] which is probably why the most common location for a shoulder ganglion cyst is the spinoglenoid notch. When the ganglion cyst has reached sufficient size to compress the nerve, it leads to isolated denervation of the infraspinatus muscle without pain or other sensory loss.

Rapid stretching of the accompanying suprascapular artery, which travels above the transverse scapular ligament while the suprascapular nerve travels below it, may contribute to ischemic injury of the nerve.[63] Laceration of the nerve during distal clavicle resection has also been reported.[66] Clinically, injury to the nerve has also been seen from prolonged bed rest in left side-lying during a difficult pregnancy with twins.

Volleyball players, swimmers, baseball players, and other individuals who perform repetitive overhead motions are vulnerable to this injury. Suprascapular nerve injury has frequently been reported in baseball pitchers,[52,63,67] owing to the extreme shoulder joint displacements and angular velocities as well as large shoulder joint forces and torques during the arm cocking and arm deceleration phases of pitching or throwing.[63,65,68] These rapid and extreme movements, such as rapid and excessive scapular protraction with glenohumeral horizontal adduction, may, over time, stretch the nerve. A nerve stretched as little as 5% to 10% of its length may result in abnormal function.[60] If the nerve is injured in the suprascapular notch, both motor weakness in the supraspinatus and infraspinatus muscles (resulting in decreased strength in shoulder lateral [external] rotation and possibly abduction) as well as sensory deficits (posterolateral shoulder pain) may result. However, as mentioned previously, if the injury to the nerve is in the spinoglenoid notch, isolated denervation of the infraspinatus muscle is likely with no supraspinatus muscle involvement and no sensory deficits. The atrophy of the infraspinatus muscle may not be easily seen, and a baseball pitcher may have this nerve injury and not even know it. Not limited to baseball, asymptomatic atrophy of the infraspinatus muscle was previously reported in 12 of 96 top-level volleyball players.[69]

The onset of symptoms often is insidious, beginning with a vague shoulder ache and weakness without paresthesia or numbness.[52,63] Visible atrophy and EMG changes may be present without noticeable impairment, even in competitive athletes.[52,67] However, weakness of the supraspinatus and infraspinatus muscles may lead to a loss of functional control of the humeral head and imbalance of force couples around the shoulder, placing other shoulder

TABLE **25-3**

Suprascapular Nerve (C4, C5, C6): Potential Sites of Injury[52,54,60,63]

Site	Signs and Symptoms	Mechanism of Injury
• Spinal roots and upper trunk of brachial plexus between fascia of anterior and middle scalenes • Nerve trunk in fascia of subclavius and omohyoid muscles • Suprascapular notch as nerve trunk passes inferior to transverse scapular ligament • Fascial compartment between supraspinatus muscle and base of coracoid process • Spinoglenoid notch as nerve enters infraspinous fossa	• Vague ache/pain in posterolateral shoulder or weakness in shoulder lateral (external) rotation or abduction secondary to weakness in supraspinatus and infraspinatus muscles • Visible atrophy in infraspinatus muscle • Vague ache/pain in posterolateral shoulder or weakness in shoulder lateral (external) rotation or abduction secondary to weakness in supraspinatus and infraspinatus muscles • Selective atrophy of infraspinatus muscle with injury in spinoglenoid notch; asymptomatic	• Direct trauma from fall or dislocation • Insidious or repetitive nerve injury • Anterior ganglion cyst in suprascapular notch (secondary to tears in the shoulder capsule or labrum) compress suprascapular nerve • Posterior ganglion cyst in spinoglenoid notch (secondary to tears in the shoulder capsule or labrum) compress suprascapular nerve

Modified from Drye C, Zachazewski JE: Peripheral nerve injuries. In Zachazewski JE, Magee DJ, Quillen WS, editors: *Athletic injuries and rehabilitation*, p 448, Philadelphia, 1996, WB Saunders.

structures at risk of impingement, such as the subacromial bursae, supraspinatus muscle, and glenoid labrum. If the nerve lesion fails to recover spontaneously, surgical exploration is indicated to determine whether the nerve is entrapped by ligaments across the suprascapular notch or spinoglenoid notch or whether it is compressed by a lipoma or ganglion cyst.[33,52,60,63,67]

Butler[62] has proposed a test for the sensitivity of the nerve to mechanical loading based on the geography of the nerve relative to the axes of the shoulder joint (Figure 25-9). This test has not been studied to determine whether it provokes symptoms in the distribution of the suprascapular nerve.

Musculocutaneous Nerve Injury

The musculocutaneous nerve is a mixed sensorimotor nerve derived from the C5 and C6 nerve roots and occasionally the C7 nerve root. It arises from the lateral cord of the brachial plexus and provides motor innervation to the biceps, brachialis, and coracobrachialis muscles as it runs between these muscles, and it provides sensory innervation to the radial side of the forearm via the lateral antebrachial cutaneous nerve (i.e., lateral cutaneous nerve of the forearm), which is the continuation of the musculocutaneous nerve after it leaves the arm and enters the forearm. Hypertrophy of the biceps, brachialis, or coracobrachialis muscle can cause compression of the nerve. It can be injured during acute anterior shoulder dislocations[52] or closed clavicle fractures,[70] during a fracture to the humerus, or during any surgical procedure involving the anterior aspect of the shoulder.[8,61] Injury to this nerve rarely occurs in isolation because it is a deep and well-protected nerve.

Several cases in the literature involve injuries to the nerve during athletic activities such as rowing, throwing a foot-

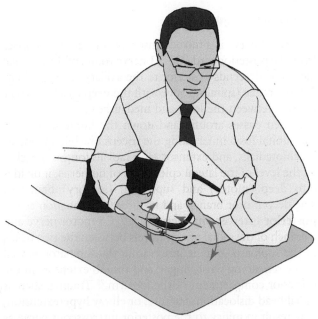

Figure 25-9 Neurodynamic test of the suprascapular nerve. The test combines scapular protraction, depression, and rotation of the scapula medially (internally) or laterally (externally). Note that the examiner uses his chest to assist protraction by applying pressure through the shaft of the humerus. (Modified from Butler D: *The sensitive nervous system,* p 339, Adelaide, Australia 2000, Noigroup Publications.)

ball, throwing a baseball, or lifting weights.[52,71,72] The loss of function of the long head of the biceps may lead to altered shoulder mechanics and may predispose the patient to other shoulder injuries. This is because the long head of the biceps has multiple roles at the shoulder, including acting as a humeral depressor and controlling lateral (external) and medial (internal) rotation.[54] Butler's test for mechanical loading of the musculocutaneous nerve (Figure 25-10) has not been studied to see whether it has diagnostic significance.[62]

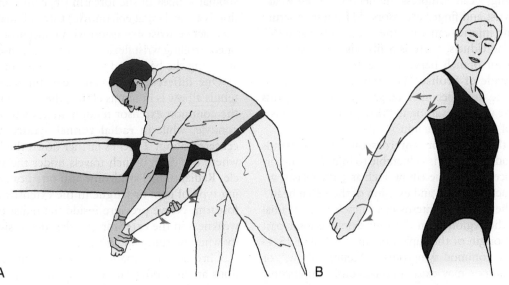

A **B**

Figure 25-10 Neurodynamic test of the musculocutaneous nerve. **A,** The test combines shoulder girdle depression, elbow extension, shoulder extension, and ulnar deviation of the wrist. **B,** The test may also be performed actively. (Modified from Butler D: *The sensitive nervous system,* pp 336, 338, Adelaide, Australia, 2000, Noigroup Publications.)

Radial Nerve Injury

The radial nerve is a mixed sensorimotor nerve that arises from the posterior cord (C5-T1 nerve roots) of the brachial plexus. It descends posterior to the axillary artery and enters the radial (spiral) groove with the deep brachial artery to pass between the long and medial heads of the triceps and then passes around and down the humerus toward the cubital fossa innervating the triceps brachii, anconeus, brachioradialis, and extensor carpi radialis longus muscles. At the level of the lateral epicondyle of humerus, it divides into deep (motor) and superficial (sensory) branches. The deep motor branch and its direct continuation as the **posterior interosseous nerve** (a C7-C8 motor nerve and a branch of the radial nerve) travels between the two heads of the supinator muscle innervating the supinator as well as the remaining wrist, finger, and thumb extensors in the posterior compartment of the forearm.[73] Trauma, such as radial head dislocation, fracture, or elbow hyperextension, may result in injury to the posterior interosseous nerve as it crosses anteriorly to the elbow.[74]

The superficial sensory branch travels deep to the brachioradialis muscle and enters the dorsal web space (between the first and second digits) of the hand, where it provides cutaneous innervation. This **superficial radial nerve** can be compressed proximally as it runs under the brachioradialis, or it can be compressed at the wrist after a fracture or as a result of a tight watchband or bracelet.[75,76]

The radial nerve is injured in one out of every eight humeral shaft fractures.[7,77] It is vulnerable to compression because of poor positioning against rigid structures during surgery.[7] Proximally, as it passes around the radial grove, it is vulnerable to compression as it passes under the lateral head of the triceps in the upper arm, especially in the presence of a fibrous arch.[14,33,75,78] Strong contraction of the triceps muscle, as may occur during throwing or weight training,[33] can compress the nerve, causing weakness in the wrist and finger extensors.[78] Humeral fracture or penetrating injuries can sever the nerve in the arm.[75,79]

In some individuals, there is a fibrous arch overlying the deep motor branch nerve as it enters the supinator called the **arcade of Frohse**. With repetitive and resisted supination, the arch becomes tense and may compress and injure the nerve, resulting in "drop wrist," which is a classic sign of a radial nerve injury.

Because the **posterior interosseous nerve** winds around the radial head, it is vulnerable to injury during orthopedic procedures at the elbow such as arthroplasty, arthroscopy, fracture repair, and excision of the radial head.[7] Lesions of the posterior interosseus branch in the radial tunnel (i.e., the region from the humeroradial joint past the proximal origin of the supinator muscle; Table 25-4) can mimic the common symptoms of "tennis elbow," or the two conditions may exist simultaneously. In chronic presentations of tennis elbow, the pathophysiological process taking place at the common extensor origin is one of

TABLE **25-4**

Radial Nerve (C5-T1): Potential Sites of Injury in the Radial Tunnel[14,82]

Cause/Site	Signs and Symptoms
Anterior to the radial head (as the nerve enters the radial tunnel, it may be tethered by a fibrous band)	Elbow pain reproduced with active supination and elbow flexion
Blood vessels compressing the nerve as they fan across it in the tunnel	Increased symptoms during exercise
The arcade of Frohse (a fibrous band of the superficial head of the proximal supinator muscle; may cause friction or compression against the nerve)	Weakness of finger and wrist extensors (wrist drop); pain with full passive pronation and wrist flexion and resisted supination
The tendinous margins of the extensor carpi radialis longus and brevis muscles of the wrist (may extend medially and compress the nerve)	Pain with full passive pronation and wrist flexion

Modified from Drye C, Zachazewski JE: Peripheral nerve injuries. In Zachazewski JE, Magee DJ, Quillen WS, editors: *Athletic injuries and rehabilitation*, p 449, Philadelphia, 1996, WB Saunders.

tendon degeneration (i.e., tendinitis initially which progresses to the degenerative condition called tendinosis), rather than the active inflammatory process conveyed by the commonly used term **lateral epicondylitis** (also called lateral epicondylalgia or tennis elbow),[80,81] which consists of persistent lateral elbow pain aggravated by palpation of the lateral epicondyle and activation of the extensor/supinator mass of the forearm (its common extensor tendon is at the lateral epicondyle) through manual resistance (i.e., active wrist extension with concentric muscle action, or controlling wrist flexion by eccentric muscle action, such as during the backhand stroke in tennis) or gripping.[80,81]

One difference between radial tunnel syndrome and tennis elbow is in tennis elbow, the pain starts near where the common extensor tendon attaches to the lateral epicondyle, while in **radial tunnel syndrome**, the pain is centered about 2 inches farther down the lateral forearm where the deep branch travels under the supinator muscle. Radial tunnel syndrome also often causes a more aching type of pain or fatigue in the extensor muscles of the forearm. Nerve pressure inside the radial tunnel leads to weakness in the extensor muscles, decreasing wrist stability when grasping and lifting.

Chronic inflammation of the common extensor tendons at the elbow can lead to a reactive synovitis of the annular ligament involving the radial nerve. Fibrosis and local edema from overuse of the tendons may also increase compression on the nerve as it passes under the extensor carpi radialis brevis muscle.[82] Both conditions usually respond to conservative treatment, which includes anti-inflammatory medication, rest, ice, and muscle stretching and strengthening.[14,33,82] In true radial tunnel syndrome, the most effective treatment usually is surgical decompression of the nerve.[14,82]

Differential diagnosis of lesions to this nerve also must include the possibility of cervical radiculopathy. Gunn and Milbrandt[83] examined the cervical spines of individuals with a history of tennis elbow who had failed to respond to treatment directed at the elbow. All 42 patients in their study had EMG findings "consistent with early radiculopathy or neuropathy of the affected myotomes," and all had increased resistance to passive motion of the C5 and C6 apophyseal joints. Treatment was directed to the cervical spine and included spinal mobilization, traction, various treatment modalities, and isometric exercises. This treatment produced good or satisfactory relief of symptoms in 86% of the patients in an average of 5.25 weeks.

Other authors have explored the relationship between lateral epicondylalgia and cervical dysfunction. A retrospective study of patients with lateral epicondylalgia found that adding treatment of the cervical spine to local interventions at the elbow produced successful outcomes in fewer visits (mean, 5.6; standard deviation [SD], 1.7) compared with management directed only at the elbow (mean, 9.7; SD, 2.4).[84]

It also is important to realize that the relationship between lateral epicondylalgia and cervical spine dysfunction may not be consistent across demographic groups. A prospective study by Waugh et al.[85] revealed that the association between lateral epicondylalgia and cervical joint findings is most likely to be present in women working in repetitive jobs and least likely to occur in men employed in nonrepetitive jobs in whom the onset of lateral elbow symptoms was to the result of a sports-related injury.

Clinical Note

When treating patients with lateral epicondylitis (also called lateral epicondylalgia or tennis elbow), the clinician must be sure to clear the cervical spine, especially in patients who are not responding to treatment at the elbow.

The positive response to treatment of the cervical spine in the aforementioned studies does not necessarily indicate that all the symptoms came from a cervical lesion. It is more likely that treatment directed to the cervical spine removed one component of a double crush lesion, which, in theory, occurs when a proximal lesion along an axon predisposes the axons within the nerve to injury at a more distal site along its course through impaired axoplasmic flow involving both the cervical spine and the radial nerve

at the elbow.[86] It may also be that manual therapy treatment of the cervical spine stimulated endogenous descending pain inhibitory systems that result in reduced lateral elbow pain.[80] The interplay of proximal and distal components of nerve irritation, as well as the local effects on the nerve of joint and muscle inflammation, may help explain why the differential diagnosis and treatment of lateral epicondylalgia often are difficult.

Butler[12,62] described this complex interplay between cervical joints and muscle tightness, elbow joint and soft tissue signs, and neural tension tests and neurological findings in the management of a patient with lateral elbow pain. He devised a test known as the **upper limb neurodynamic test 2 (ULNT 2)** with a radial nerve bias, in which mechanical tension is applied to the radial nerve throughout its course. (The text *Orthopedic Physical Assessment* refers to this as the upper limb tension test 3 [ULTT 3].[87]) This test consists of a combination of shoulder depression, elbow extension, shoulder medial (internal) rotation, forearm pronation, wrist flexion and ulnar deviation, and thumb and finger flexion (Figure 25-11). If symptoms have not been provoked by this point in the test, shoulder abduction is performed. Cervical lateral (side) flexion away from the extremity also increases the mechanical load on the brachial plexus,[88] further sensitizing the test. The final forearm position in this test (forearm pronation, wrist flexion and ulnar deviation, and thumb flexion) is a position that is commonly used to test flexibility of the wrist/finger extensor muscles. Pain from muscle stretching in this position can be differentiated from pain from neural structures by the addition of

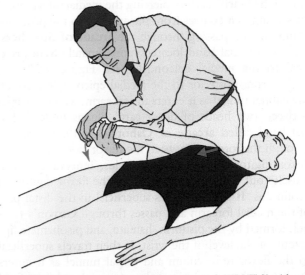

Figure 25-11 The upper limb neurodynamic test 2 (ULNT 2) with a radial nerve bias. The test combines shoulder depression, elbow extension, shoulder medial (internal) rotation, forearm pronation, and wrist and finger flexion. The test is further sensitized with the addition of shoulder depression and abduction and contralateral lateral (side) flexion of the cervical spine. Symptoms are monitored at each position of the test. (Modified from Butler D: *The sensitive nervous system,* p 329, Adelaide, Australia, 2000, Noigroup Publications.)

shoulder abduction or cervical lateral (side) flexion. Both of these maneuvers increase mechanical load through the nerve tract without increasing tension in the extensor muscles.

Yaxley and Jull[89,90] studied the ULNT 2 with a radial nerve bias in 20 subjects with unilateral tennis elbow. Both upper extremities of their subjects had symptoms in the lateral elbow/forearm region, but the symptoms were reported as more intense in the symptomatic elbows/forearms.[90] They observed a statistically significant difference in available range of shoulder abduction in the symptomatic arms of their subjects (12.45° less than the asymptomatic side). They recommended routine inclusion of this test as a part of the differential diagnosis of lateral epicondylalgia. Further support for this recommendation was provided by a prospective case series in which 41% of subjects with lateral epicondylalgia (34 of 83) had their symptoms reproduced during application of the radial bias neurodynamic test.[85]

Clinical Note

The radial nerve biased upper limb neurodynamic test should be used as part of the differential diagnosis process for lateral epicondylalgia.

Ulnar Nerve Injury

The ulnar nerve is a mixed sensorimotor nerve that arises from the medial cord (C8-T1 nerve roots) of the brachial plexus and may also have contributions from the C7 nerve root. It passes down the anteromedial aspect of arm lateral to the brachial artery piercing the medial intermuscular septum as it courses from the anterior to the posterior compartment, passing through the **arcade of Struthers,** a musculofascial band located approximately 8 cm proximal to the medial epicondyle (see Figure 9-22, *C*). It then runs posterior to the medial epicondyle through the cubital tunnel as it enters the forearm, where it passes between two heads of flexor carpi ulnaris under a fascial band called **arcade of Osborne**. It then descends through the forearm between the flexor carpi ulnaris and flexor digitorum profundus muscles, innervating both muscles but only the medial half of the flexor digitorum profundus. It then becomes superficial in the distal part of the medial forearm and passes through **Guyon's tunnel,** formed by the pisiform, hamate, and pisohamate ligament, at the level of the wrist. It then travels superficial to the flexor retinaculum and carpal tunnel as it enters the hand, where it splits into deep (motor) and superficial (sensory) branches. The deep branch innervates most of the intrinsic muscles of the hand including the hypothenar muscles: adductor pollicis, deep portion of flexor pollicis brevis, medial (third and fourth) lumbricals, and dorsal and palmar interossei. The superficial branch supplies the palmaris brevis, skin to the palmar portion of digit 5 (little

finger) and the medial half of digit 4 (ring finger), and the distal medial palm. The dorsal branch of ulnar nerve most commonly supplies skin of the medial aspect of dorsum of hand and dorsal aspects of the little finger and medial half of the ring finger. The palmar cutaneous branch of ulnar nerve supplies skin on the proximal medial palm, overlying the medial carpals.

The ulnar nerve is most vulnerable to injury at two sites: the cubital tunnel at the medial elbow and Guyon's tunnel, or canal, at the wrist.[76,91,92] The cubital retinaculum and arcade of Osborne flatten with elbow flexion, decreasing the volume and increasing pressure within and around the **cubital tunnel**, increasing the likelihood that the ulnar nerve will be compressed. Vigorous and repetitive contraction of the flexor carpi ulnaris muscle over time may also compress the nerve. The four major etiological factors for injury of the nerve at the elbow are presented in Table 25-5.

Injury to the ulnar nerve is common in athletes who perform repeated overhead throwing motions, such as baseball pitching, the volleyball spike, the tennis serve,

TABLE 25-5

Ulnar Nerve (C7-T1): Cubital Tunnel Lesions[91-93]

Cause/Site	Signs and Symptoms
• Traction injuries caused by increased valgus forces: ○ Prior fracture or injury to the growth plate ○ Disruption of the ulnar (medial) collateral ligament (UCL) • Entrapment under: ○ Thickened arcuate ligament ○ Hypertrophic medial head of triceps, anconeus, or flexor carpi ulnaris muscle ○ Postoperative scar or bony osteophyte formation • Irregularities in the ulnar groove (cubital tunnel) caused by osteophytes; may prevent sliding of the ulnar nerve • Subluxation or dislocation of the nerve over the medial epicondyle (usually as a result of laxity of soft tissue restraints) leading to a friction fibrosis	• Medial elbow pain radiating to the medial forearm • Numbness and tingling in the ulnar aspect of the forearm and hand (5th digit and medial 1/2 of 4th digit) • Atrophy in intrinsic muscles of hand • Claw fingers

Modified from Drye C, Zachazewski JE: Peripheral nerve injuries. In Zachazewski JE, Magee DJ, Quillen WS, editors: *Athletic injuries and rehabilitation,* p 450, Philadelphia, 1996, WB Saunders.

and the javelin throw. During overhead throwing, a rise in pressure occurs in the ulnar nerve in the cubital tunnel, as the elbow is flexed in combination with wrist extension, shoulder abduction, trunk lateral (side) flexion, and valgus loading.[65,94-96] Matsuo and Fleisig[96] reported that abnormal pitching mechanics, such as excessive trunk lateral (side) flexion (approximately 40°) and shoulder abduction (approximately 120°) resulted is approximately twice as much varus torque (approximately 125 N·m) that is needed to resist valgus loading during normal pitching mechanics, which may increase the strain on the ulnar nerve.

Muscle imbalance, such as excessive strength in the extensor-supinator forearm musculature, which generates a valgus torque, compared with the flexor-pronator forearm musculature, which generates a varus torque, may increase valgus loading and strain to the ulnar nerve.[97] Weakness or fatigue in the flexor-pronator forearm musculature may also increase valgus loading and ulnar nerve strain. Therefore, with repetitive throwing, it is important to have adequate strength and endurance in the flexor-pronator musculature of the forearm to help control valgus loading and ulnar nerve strain, as well as proper muscle balance between the flexor-pronator and extensor-supinator musculature of the forearm. Over time, excessive ligamentous laxity of the ulnar (medial) collateral ligament at the elbow may also increase valgus mobility and further increase excessive strain on the ulnar nerve in the cubital tunnel. Surgical removal of an excessive posteromedial olecranon osteophyte, which may occur in overhead throwing sports such as baseball, may result in excessive stretch of both the ulnar collateral ligament and the ulnar nerve because of the loss of valgus restraints.[98,99]

In overhead throwing athletes, the ulnar nerve should be evaluated for subluxation during elbow flexion and valgus loading. Pain over the ulnar nerve, a positive Tinel's sign posterior to the medial epicondyle, a positive elbow flexion test (Figure 25-12), as well as ulnar nerve sensory or motor deficits, all may suggest involvement of the ulnar nerve. Most cases of **cubital tunnel syndrome** have an insidious onset of medial elbow pain radiating down the medial forearm and numbness and tingling in the ulnar aspect of the forearm and hand. Symptoms are aggravated by continued use.[91] Symptoms can occur in computer users working in excessive elbow flexion, violinists or violists practicing for long periods, and laborers who perform repeated elbow flexion/extension on the job. Wright et al.[93] reported that the nerve requires 2 cm (1 inch) of unimpeded movement at the elbow and can experience strain values that diminish the circulation to the nerve. Entrapment or inflammation of the nerve lessens the nerve's ability to tolerate movement or changes in intraneural pressure.

Visible signs of ulnar nerve pathology are "**claw hand**," in which the flexor digitorum profundus and extensor digitorum (extrinsic muscles) both pull on the distal phalanx, and without the control of the intrinsic muscles that

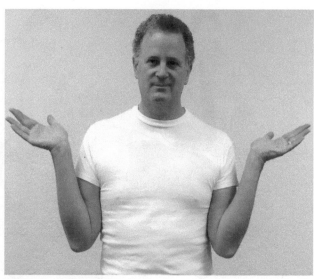

Figure 25-12 The elbow flexion test for ulnar nerve irritation in the cubital tunnel.[100] A positive response is the production of paresthesias along the ulnar border of the forearm and hand. Symptoms should occur in less than 5 seconds but could take several minutes.

attach more proximally, the fingers collapse into the zigzag pattern of metacarpophalangeal hyperextension and proximal interphalangeal and distal interphalangeal flexion. Another visible sign is sunken interosseous spaces in the dorsum of the hand secondary to atrophy of the dorsal interossei muscles. There may also be noticeable atrophy of the hypothenar eminence. Additional signs include an inability to abduct and adduct the fingers or adduct the thumb.

Various tests for lesions along the path of the ulnar nerve have been described in the literature. Buehler and Thayer[100] suggested using the elbow flexion test as a clinical test for cubital tunnel syndrome (see Figure 25-12). A positive response to the test consists of reproduction of paresthesias along the ulnar border of the forearm and hand. Butler's upper limb neurodynamic test with an ulnar nerve bias (ULNT 3; Figure 25-13) is similar but increases the tensile stress on the brachial plexus and proximal portion of the ulnar nerve by adding shoulder girdle depression, glenohumeral abduction, and lateral (external) rotation.[62] (This test has been described as the ULTT 3[47,101] or as ULTT 4 in *Orthopedic Physical Assessment*.[87]) Although the test originally was described with the forearm in supination, pronation of the forearm often makes the test more provocative of symptoms. Cervical lateral (side) flexion away from the extremity being tested can also be added.

Responses to Butler's ULNT 3 (ULTT 4 in *Orthopedic Physical Assessment*[87]) have been studied in healthy patients[101-103] and in symptomatic patients.[101] In most healthy subjects, symptoms of tingling or numbness occurred in the medial forearm and hand. Subjects also frequently reported a sensation of pressure at the medial elbow. Some healthy subjects had no

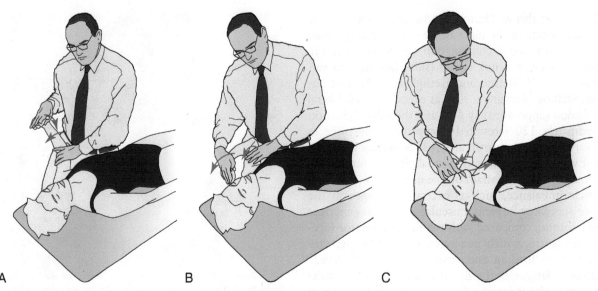

A   **B**   **C**

Figure 25-13 The upper limb neurodynamic test 3 (ULNT 3[62]) was designed to place tensile stress on the ulnar nerve. The test consists of wrist and finger extension and forearm pronation (**A**), elbow flexion and lateral (external) rotation of the arm (**B**), and shoulder abduction and shoulder girdle depression (**C**). Contralateral lateral (side) flexion of the cervical spine further sensitizes the test. (Modified from Butler D: *The sensitive nervous system,* p 334, Adelaide, Australia, 2000, Noigroup Publications.)

symptomatic response to the test. In 18 subjects with a variety of upper extremity or cervical spine symptoms, all subjects had some response to the test. They had more frequent reports of medial upper arm pain (44% versus 18% in healthy subjects) and occasional symptoms in the contralateral extremity.

Clinical Note[87]

A positive neurodynamic test is indicated when:
1. The patient's symptoms are reproduced.
2. There is a difference between right and left arms on testing.
3. A sensitivity test (e.g., cervical side flexion) in the ipsilateral quadrant alters the symptoms.
4. Range of motion is restricted by neurological symptoms.

Twenty-five percent of the subjects tested in the patient group had an onset of symptoms before the addition of shoulder abduction, something that never occurred in asymptomatic subjects. When the range of shoulder abduction at the onset of symptoms in the remaining symptomatic arms was compared with that in healthy subjects, the difference was not statistically significant. Clinically, this seems to indicate that provocation of symptoms in the early stages of the ULNT 3 or with the elbow flexion test is a better measure of the presence of abnormality than the degree of abduction available before the onset of symptoms in the ULNT 3. It should be noted that the sequencing of the components of the test affects the onset of symptoms. In a recent study, when the test was performed with wrist and finger extension followed by forearm pronation, elbow flexion, shoulder lateral (external) rotation, scapular depression, and shoulder abduc-

tion followed by cervical lateral (side) flexion toward the opposite side, 52% of patients felt symptoms with wrist and finger extension alone.[103]

Treatment for cubital tunnel syndrome consists initially of rest, ice, and anti-inflammatory medications. The patient should also be examined for any problems in the cervical spine or shoulder that may be contributing to the symptoms. Altering the mechanics of throwing may help minimize stress on the elbow in the athlete. Where appropriate, computer keyboard height should be adjusted to place the elbow in less than 90° flexion during prolonged computer use. A soft splint worn at night can help symptoms by preventing prolonged elbow flexion during sleep.

If conservative treatment fails, surgical treatment should be considered. Surgical options include (1) release of the ligament at the cubital tunnel, (2) transposition of the ulnar nerve to the anterior surface of the elbow joint, and (3) removal of the medial epicondyle.[76,91,92] Rettig and Ebben[104] retrospectively reviewed the cases of 20 athletes who underwent anterior subcutaneous transfer of the ulnar nerve. The average length of time between surgery and return to sports was 12.6 weeks (range, 6 to 43 weeks), and 19 of 20 athletes returned to their preinjury level of athletic activity.

Injury to the ulnar nerve at the wrist can cause sensory disturbances in the medial hand and motor weakness in the intrinsic muscles of the hand.[76,105] It is vulnerable during surgical procedures on the triangular fibrocartilage complex (TFCC), ulnar styloid, or carpal tunnel.[7] Compression of the ulnar nerve is a common problem for cyclists because of prolonged pressure on the medial hand and wrist.[42,105,106] Fernald[106] studied the incidence of overuse injuries in elite cyclists and found that 21% had sensory changes in the upper extremities. The abnormality may result from acute or chronic compression of the ulnar nerve in Guyon's canal (tunnel) as a result of prolonged weight bearing on the hands or a fall. It also can be caused by traction on the nerve produced by the extended wrist position on the handlebars.[45,105] Normally, cyclists bear approximately 45% of their weight on the upper extremities[106]; therefore the combination of compression and vibration from the road increases the likelihood of neurogenic symptoms.

Strategies to prevent irritation to the nerve at the wrist include changing the position of the hands frequently while riding, using padded gloves and handlebars to increase surface area and decrease pressure, using modified handlebars, and adjusting the overall "fit" of the bike to reduce weight bearing on the hands.[105,106]

Median Nerve Injury

The median nerve is a sensorimotor nerve that arises from the medial and lateral cords of the brachial plexus. The lateral root is a continuation of the lateral cord, receiving fibers from C6 and C7, while the medial root is a continuation of the medial cord receiving fibers from C8 and T1. The nerve enters the cubital fossa medial to brachial artery, passes between the two heads of the pronator teres, descends between the flexor digitorum superficialis and flexor digitorum profundus muscles, and travels under the flexor retinaculum as it passes through carpal tunnel to enter the hand.

The motor component of the nerve innervates most of the flexor/pronator muscles in the anterior compartment of the forearm, the muscles in the thenar region of the hand, and the lateral two lumbricals (first and second). The **anterior interosseous nerve** is a C8-T1 motor nerve that branches off the median nerve in the distal part of the cubital fossa as it emerges from between the two

heads of the pronator teres and then passes inferiorly on the anterior surface of the interosseous membrane. Along its course, it innervates the lateral half of flexor digitorum profundus, the flexor pollicis longus, and the pronator quadratus muscles. These muscles collectively produce the circular **"okay" sign** as the pads of the thumb and index finger come together via interphalangeal joint flexion of the thumb and distal interphalangeal joint flexion of the index finger along with pronation at the distal radioulnar joint.

The sensory component of the nerve supplies skin of the central and lateral palm (**palmar cutaneous branch**), the palmar surfaces of lateral three and a half fingers and the dorsal surface of lateral three and a half distal phalanges via palmar digital branches, and articular branches supply the elbow, wrist, and carpal joints.

Three common compression syndromes affect this nerve: **pronator teres syndrome (PTS), anterior interosseous nerve syndrome (AINS)**, and **carpal tunnel syndrome (CTS).** Common sites, causes, and signs and symptoms of median nerve compression in proximity to the elbow are listed in Table 25-6.[14] Differential diagnostic characteristics of these syndromes are outlined in Table 25-7.[107]

PTS is often secondary to overuse of the pronator teres muscles, and symptoms worsen with elbow flexion and forearm pronation. PTS symptoms may include pain and reduced mobility in forearm pronation and supination; numbness or tingling in the palm, thumb, index finger, or middle finger; and possible weakness and atrophy in the thenar muscles, which is sometimes referred to as **"ape" hand** because of the flattened thenar eminence that resembles an ape's hand. In more severe injuries, the **"hand of benediction"** may be evident. In this case, when the individual starts with all fingers fully extended and then tries to make a fist, the little finger and ring finger partially

TABLE 25-6

Median Nerve (C5-T1): Compression in Proximity to the Elbow[14]

Cause/Site	Signs and Symptoms
Swelling from trauma can compress the nerve in the fibro-osseous tunnel created by the ligament of Struthers as it passes between the supracondylar process and the medial epicondyle	Pain with resisted forearm pronation
Abnormal thickness of the bicipital aponeurosis can compress the nerve during resisted elbow flexion or supination	Pain aggravated by resisted elbow flexion and supination
A fibrous band in the superficial head of the pronator teres muscle may compress the nerve where it passes between the superficial and deep heads, or an inflamed pronator teres secondary to overuse (e.g., hammering, repeatedly using a screwdriver, cleaning fish, or performing any activity that requires repetitive use of the pronator teres, such as overhead throwing)	Pain aggravated by resisted forearm pronation and flexion Atrophy in muscles in thenar eminence
The nerve can be compressed under the fibrous arch on the proximal margin of the flexor digitorum superficialis muscle	Pain in the flexor digitorum superficialis with resisted third finger flexion

Modified from Drye C, Zachazewski JE: Peripheral nerve injuries. In Zachazewski JE, Magee DJ, Quillen WS, editors: *Athletic injuries and rehabilitation*, p 452, Philadelphia, 1996, WB Saunders.

TABLE **25-7**

Differential Diagnostic Characteristics of Carpal Tunnel, Pronator Teres, and Anterior Interosseous Nerve Syndromes

	Paresthesia	Nocturnal Symptoms	Muscle Weakness/ Atrophy	Tinel's Test	Phalen's Test	Direct Compression	Electrodiagnostic Tests
Carpal tunnel syndrome (CTS)	Lateral 3½ digits palmar surface	Yes	Abductor pollicis brevis, opponens pollicis, flexor pollicis brevis	Positive at carpal tunnel	Positive	Positive at carpal tunnel	Diagnostic
Pronator teres syndrome (PTS)	Lateral 3½ digits palmar surface	No	Not a traditional sign but may involve abductor pollicis brevis, opponens pollicis, flexor pollicis brevis, flexor pollicis longus, flexor digitorum profundus (index and middle fingers), pronator quadratus, flexor carpi radialis, palmaris longus	Positive at pronator teres <50%	Negative	Positive at pronator teres, negative at carpal tunnel	Rarely diagnostic
Anterior interosseous nerve syndrome (AINS)	None	No	Flexor pollicis longus, flexor digitorum profundus (index and middle fingers), pronator quadratus	Negative	Negative	Negative	Diagnostic

Modified from Lee MJ, LaStayo PC: Pronator syndrome and other nerve compressions that mimic carpal tunnel syndrome, *J Orthop Sports Phys Ther* 34:601-609, 2004.

flex while the index and middle fingers remain extended. Some PTS symptoms, such as sensory and motor deficits in the hand, may mimic CTS.

CTS symptoms are aggravated by wrist flexion and extension and overuse of the anterior forearm muscles controlling the finger and thumb flexors, because all extrinsic finger and thumb tendons travel with the median nerve through the carpal tunnel. In CTS, more than in PTS, weakness and atrophy of the thenar eminence muscles are observed. A positive Phalen's sign, reverse Phalen's sign, or Tinel's sign over the center of the carpal tunnel may produce tingling and paresthesia in the lateral three and a half fingers, especially the finger pads which have a higher density of sensory receptors compared with other areas of the fingers. In CTS, the palm is usually spared because the palmar branch of the median nerve passes superficial to the flexor retinaculum of the wrist.

If the anterior interosseous nerve is compressed (see Table 25-6), resulting in AINS, it may cause functional weakness in thumb and index finger flexion and weakness in forearm pronation, as well as a weak pinch (i.e., no tip-to-tip pinch). When an individual with anterior in-

terosseous syndrome attempts to make the "okay" sign, a diamond shape forms instead of a circular shape as the pads of the distal phalanx of the thumb and the index finger come together. This is secondary to an inability to flex the interphalangeal joint of the thumb and the distal interphalangeal joint of the index finger. Because the anterior interosseous nerve is primarily a motor nerve, there are typically no sensory symptoms. AINS is rare compared with CTS and pronator syndrome (less than 2%).[107,108]

CTS is by far the most common form of compression of the median nerve (88.2% of median nerve injuries[107,108]). Many activities are considered risk factors, including weight bearing on the hands (with the wrist in end range flexion or extension)[45,105]; repetitive activities such as gripping, typing, throwing, or otherwise engaging in wrist flexion and extension; and the use of vibrating tools. Other physical characteristics linked to a higher incidence of CTS include gender (i.e., more common in females than in males), age, race, and obesity; pregnancy, diabetes, thyroid disease, and connective tissue disorders are also linked to an increased incidence,[109] as is trauma.[110] Splinting in a neutral wrist position may be necessary to facilitate rest because pressure on the nerve increases with wrist flexion or extension. Compliance with splint use has been linked to the fit and comfort of the splint and the ability to continue to work or to sleep while wearing it.[111] Other adjunct procedures include icing, corticosteroid or lidocaine injection, and resection of the transverse retinacular ligament.[105,110] There is a small risk of nerve injury during surgical release or injection in the carpal tunnel, especially if there is variant anatomy.[7]

The differential diagnosis of median nerve compression syndromes includes ruling out cervical radiculopathies. As with radial and ulnar nerve abnormality, the possibility of a mechanical or physiological double crush lesion must always be considered. Murray-Leslie and Wright[112] reported a positive correlation between the incidence of CTS and a decrease in the size of the anteroposterior measurements of the cervical spinal canal at C5 and C6 and a decrease in cervical disc height when subjects were compared with age-matched controls.

The authors' clinical experience has been that symptoms may be present in the median nerve distribution that appear to be caused by adverse mechanics along the course of the nerve, frequently in the absence of EMG abnormalities. A similar observation led Elvey[88] to develop what is currently considered the first upper limb neurodynamic test (ULNT 1; Figure 25-14). His cadaveric studies demonstrated that the C5-C7 nerve roots moved laterally during shoulder abduction. Elbow extension and wrist extension increased the tension on these structures and on the brachial plexus and median nerve. Other studies have confirmed the motion of the median nerve with shoulder abduction, elbow extension, and wrist extension.[19] The response to the end position of the test in asymptomatic subjects is a deep, sometimes painful stretch over the anterior shoulder, elbow, and lateral forearm.[113] It also provokes a mild to moderate amount of tingling in the thumb, index (2nd digit), and middle (3rd digit) finger.

Butler's variation on the ULNT 1 also stresses the median nerve. It uses the same components of motion as Elvey's test but in a different order.[62] Butler developed the ULNT 2 (ULTT 2 in *Orthopedic Physical Assessment*[87]) (Figure 25-15) to replicate more closely the functional movements that reproduced patients' symptoms. The final position of the test is similar to the backswing of a forehand shot in tennis. The response to this test in healthy subjects is similar to that seen in the ULNT 1.[114,115]

All the upper limb neurodynamic tests described are helpful for determining whether abnormal neurobiomechanics are contributing to persistent symptoms. Treatment can then focus on mobilization or release/decompression of the neural tissues involved. Nerve gliding (sometimes called nerve flossing) has been reported to be an effective technique or home exercise for patients with CTS. Seradge et al.[116] used nerve and tendon gliding

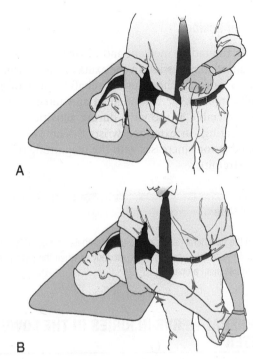

Figure 25-14 The upper limb neurodynamic test 1 (ULNT 1) places tensile stress on the brachial plexus and median nerve throughout its course. The test consists sequentially of shoulder abduction, wrist and finger extension, and forearm supination (**A**) followed by shoulder lateral (external) rotation, elbow extension, and contralateral cervical lateral (side) flexion (**B**). It is essential to maintain shoulder depression when performing the test movements if one hopes to find a positive test. (Modified from Butler D: *The sensitive nervous system*, p 317, Adelaide, Australia, 2000, Noigroup Publications.)

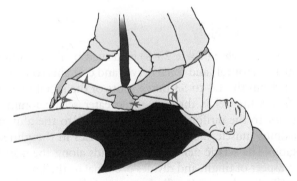

Figure 25-15 The ULNT 2 was developed by Butler[12,62] as an alternative test of the median nerve tract. It consists of shoulder girdle depression, elbow extension, shoulder lateral (external) rotation, supination of the forearm, wrist and finger extension, and shoulder abduction. Contralateral cervical lateral (side) flexion further sensitizes the test. (Modified from Butler D: *The sensitive nervous system*, p 326, Adelaide, Australia, 2000, Noigroup Publications.)

exercises as part of a CTS prevention program in a meat packing plant. They reported a 45% decrease in the incidence of CTS in response to their program.[116,117] Lee and LaStayo[107] and Rozmaryn et al.[118] reported that patients with CTS who performed a home program of nerve gliding exercises had a lower rate of subsequent surgery for CTS (43% versus 71.2% in those who did not perform exercises).

Combined Lesions

Injury to the radial, median, and ulnar nerves can occur as a result of compression in the axilla or upper arm from the misuse of crutches during rehabilitation of lower extremity injuries.[14,76] The median and ulnar nerves are always vulnerable at the wrist during activities requiring weight bearing on extended wrists.[45] The likelihood of combined lesions increases with the magnitude of trauma to the extremity.

Clinical Note

Injury to the peripheral nerves of the upper limb can occur during crutch walking if the crutches are not fitted properly or when the patient is not taught to use them properly.

PERIPHERAL NERVE INJURIES IN THE LOWER QUARTER

Nerve Injuries of the Lumbar Spine and Lower Limb

- Sciatic nerve
- Tibial nerve
- Common fibular (peroneal) nerve
- Femoral nerve
- Obturator nerve

Sciatic Nerve Injury

The sciatic nerve (Table 25-8) is formed by the common fibular (peroneal) and tibial nerves and contains contributions from the L4 to S3 nerve roots of the sacral plexus. It leaves the pelvis through the greater sciatic foramen inferior to the piriformis muscle and deep to the gluteus maximus muscle, but supplies no muscles in the gluteal region. The sciatic nerve then descends along the posterior aspect of thigh, and divides proximal to the knee into the tibial and common fibular (peroneal) nerves. In the thigh, it innervates the adductor magnus (i.e., hamstring portion) and hamstrings (i.e., semimembranosus, semitendinosus, and long head of biceps femoris) by its tibial division. The sciatic nerve also provides articular branches to the hip and knee joints.

The sciatic nerve can be irritated as it passes under or through the piriformis muscle in the buttocks.[119] This is commonly termed **piriformis syndrome**.[120] Pain may be caused by spasm or scarring of the muscle from a muscle strain, trauma, or overuse.[76] Clinically, pain may radiate down the posterior leg with or without dysesthesia[120] with tenderness over the muscle belly. The patient may report pain with prolonged sitting, especially on a hard surface, and resisted hip abduction and lateral (external) rotation. Full passive medial (internal) rotation in flexion and ad-

TABLE 25-8

Sciatic Nerve (L4-S3): Areas of Entrapment or Irritation

Cause/Site	Signs and Symptoms
Compression as nerve runs under or through the piriformis in the buttocks	Tenderness over the piriformis muscle belly; pain with resisted hip abduction and lateral (external) rotation; pain with full passive medial (internal) rotation or hip adduction in hip flexion
Entrapment in the fibers of the origin of the hamstrings at the ischial tuberosity	Pain from ischial tuberosity to posterior thigh; neurological and straight-leg raise tests negative; symptoms provoked by stretching, sitting, and running
In association with hamstring tear	Differentiation: • Hamstring tear alone: pain with palpation of muscle, with or without bruising; slump test negative • Sciatic nerve or nerve root involved; slump test positive (see Figure 25-16)

Modified from Drye C, Zachazewski JE: Peripheral nerve injuries. In Zachazewski JE, Magee DJ, Quillen WS, editors: *Athletic injuries and rehabilitation*, p 454, Philadelphia, 1996, WB Saunders.

duction can also compress the nerve under the piriformis muscle.[120] The pain is not usually associated with neurological loss.[76]

The sciatic nerve is also vulnerable during total hip arthroplasty, especially when a posterolateral approach is used. The risk of injury increases if the surgery involves revising a previous hip replacement, if there was underlying congenital hip dysplasia, or if the surgery results in leg lengthening.[8] There is also the risk of nerve injury during hip arthroscopy because of the traction applied to allow for access to the joint.[8,121]

Hamstring syndrome results from entrapment of the sciatic nerve by tight tendinous bands near the lateral origin of the hamstrings at the ischial tuberosity.[119] It often is found in sprinters and hurdlers. Pain is felt at the ischial tuberosity and may radiate down the posterior thigh to the back of the knee.[122] Symptoms are aggravated by sitting, stretching, or running. There may be hamstring weakness, but the results of neurological and straight-leg raise tests usually are negative.[122] Surgical release of the tendinous bands usually is successful in relieving symptoms.[119]

Pain from a torn (2nd or 3rd degree strain) hamstring muscle must be differentiated from irritation of the lumbar nerve roots and the sciatic nerve. The slump sitting test helps differentiate pain arising from neural or muscular structures (Figure 25-16). The test combines full neck and trunk flexion, knee extension, ankle dorsiflexion, and hip flexion in a sitting position.[12,123] It places tensile stress on the neural tissues throughout the spinal canal and the sciatic nerve. Pain from a stretch on the neural tissue can

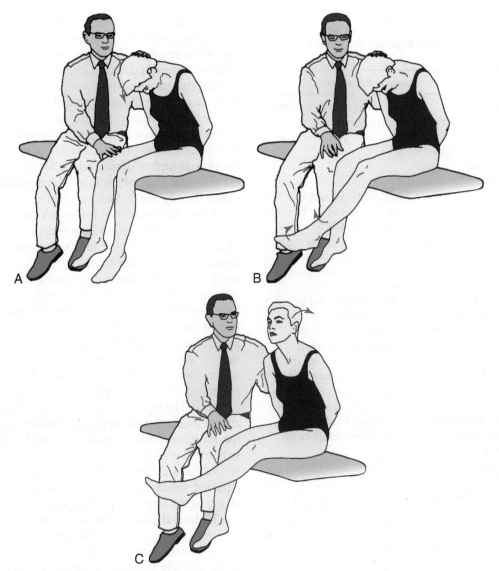

Figure 25-16 The slump test is designed to stress the neural structures in the spinal canal and along the course of the sciatic nerve. The test consists of trunk flexion, neck flexion (**A**), knee extension (**B**), and, as needed, dorsiflexion of the ankle and hip flexion, adduction, or medial (internal) rotation. If knee extension increases or symptoms decrease when the neck flexion component is released (**C**), the test is considered positive. (Modified from Butler D: *The sensitive nervous system,* p 292, Adelaide, Australia, 2000, Noigroup Publications.)

be differentiated from muscular pain from the hamstrings if the leg is maintained in the same degree of knee extension that reproduces the muscle pain and the head and neck are extended. If the pain is decreased, neural structures are implicated, because the muscle length has not been changed, but the tension on the neural tissues has decreased.[124]

Kornberg and Lew[125] demonstrated that use of the slump sitting test as a treatment technique facilitates faster return to play in Australian football players with grade I hamstring tears, indicating that in some cases motion of the sciatic nerve must be impaired as it passes through the muscle either before the tear or from the inflammation and exudate surrounding the nerve after injury. Butler[12,62] advocates early but gentle motion of the muscle and nerve to prevent scarring and adhesion formation between the muscle and nerve.

> **Clinical Note**
>
> With chronic hamstring strains at its insertion, the sciatic nerve should be cleared of any involvement.

Tibial Nerve Injury

The tibial nerve (Table 25-9) is formed from fibers from the L4-S3 nerve roots. It descends vertically through the popliteal space, where it may be vulnerable to compression by trauma to the back of the knee, a **Baker's cyst** (often from chronic knee effusion and concomitant weakening of the posterior capsule), or osteochondroma.[75,76,126] When injured, it can cause paresthesia, pain, and atrophy of the superficial and deep muscles in the posterior compartment of the leg, which includes the gastrocnemius, soleus, plantaris, popliteus,

TABLE **25-9**

Tibial Nerve (L4-S3): Sites of Entrapment or Irritation

Cause/Site	Signs and Symptoms
Popliteal space: • Compression by Baker's cyst • Entrapment in proximal portion of medial gastrocnemius	Posterior knee pain, possibly radiating to calf
Tarsal tunnel: • Space-occupying lesion (e.g., osteophyte, ganglion) • Eversion strain (acute or repetitive)	Pain from medial malleolus to the heel, sole of the foot, and occasionally to the calf Pain worse at night or with walking or running Positive Tinel's test at tarsal tunnel
Medial plantar nerve distal to tarsal tunnel or in hypertrophic abductor muscle of the big toe	Pain and paresthesias in the medial 3½ toes with weight bearing under load or with running
Lateral plantar nerve distal to tarsal tunnel	Pain in the lateral foot and lateral 2 toes; may cause persistent medial heel pain
Interdigital neuromas: • Compression from callus formation under the metatarsal heads • Stretching of nerve under the deep transverse tarsal ligament	Pain and paresthesias at the metatarsal heads that may radiate proximally or to toes Foot drop

Modified from Drye C, Zachazewski JE: Peripheral nerve injuries. In Zachazewski JE, Magee DJ, Quillen WS, editors: *Athletic injuries and rehabilitation,* p 455, Philadelphia, 1996, WB Saunders.

tibialis posterior, flexor digitorum longus, and flexor hallucis longus muscles. The tibial nerve supplies skin on posterolateral leg via its branch, the **medial sural cutaneous nerve**. The tibial nerve also supplies articular branches to the tibiofemoral joint.[127] The calcaneal cutaneous branches of the tibial and sural nerves supply skin to the heel.

Ekelund[128] reported one case of a female athlete who presented with entrapment of the tibial nerve in the proximal portion of the medial gastrocnemius muscle. Her main complaint was posterior knee pain with training. She had tenderness over the nerve on palpation. Surgical release relieved her symptoms completely.

Entrapment of the tibial nerve in the tarsal tunnel (**tarsal tunnel syndrome**) as it passes through the osseofibrous tunnel between the flexor retinaculum and medial malleolus usually occurs as a result of an alteration in the size or shape of the tunnel owing to fracture, dislocation, trauma, lipoma, tendon sheath cyst, acute or chronic hyperpronation during walking or running, or direct pressure.[76,129,130] The classic symptoms include pain and/

or paresthesia at the medial malleolus radiating to the sole of the foot, the heel, and sometimes the calf and worsening of the symptoms at night, with walking or running, with ankle dorsiflexion and eversion, and weakness of toe flexion. Pain or paresthesia is reproduced with Tinel's test over the nerve in the tarsal tunnel.[129]

The tibial nerve splits into medial and lateral plantar nerves in the tarsal tunnel, which innervate (primarily by S2-S3 nerve roots) the four layers of intrinsic muscles in the plantar surface of the foot. It also supplies the skin of the plantar surface of the foot. The **medial plantar nerve** passes distally in the foot between the abductor hallucis and flexor digitorum brevis muscles and divides into motor and sensory branches. Its sensory branch supplies skin of the medial side of the foot and medial portion of the plantar surface of the foot, and the nail beds of medial three and one half digits. Its motor branch innervates the abductor hallucis, flexor digitorum brevis, flexor hallucis brevis, and first lumbrical muscles. Entrapment of the medial plantar nerve usually causes paresthesia or pain in the medial three and one half digits and may also cause weakness or atrophy in the aforementioned intrinsic muscles of the foot.[129,130] The medial plantar nerve can also be entrapped in a hypertrophic or fibrotic abductor hallucis muscle.[76] The repetitive nature of running combined with altered mechanics of the foot and ankle places the nerve at risk for tensile injuries within the tarsal tunnel. Ironically, symptoms may also be provoked by pressure placed on the medial arch by new arch supports.[48] Johnson et al.[131] reported similar problems in a competitive weight lifter owing to the large weight-bearing loads on the foot.

The **lateral plantar nerve** passes laterally in the foot between the quadratus plantae and flexor digitorum brevis muscles and innervates the quadratus plantae and abductor digiti minimi muscles, and then divides into superficial and deep branches. The motor component of the superficial branch innervates the flexor digiti minimi brevis and the fourth plantar and dorsal interossei muscles, while the sensory component supplies skin on the lateral portion of plantar surface of the foot and the skin and nail beds of the lateral one and one half digits. The deep branch (motor only) supplies the first, second, and third plantar and dorsal interossei; the lateral three lumbricals; and the adductor hallucis muscles.

Entrapment of the lateral plantar nerve causes symptoms in the lateral plantar surface of the foot and lateral one and a half digits and may also cause weakness or atrophy in the aforementioned foot intrinsic muscles. Branches of this nerve supply sensation to portions of the medial heel and calcaneus, and the long plantar ligament. Irritation of the calcaneal branch of this nerve is a potential source of persistent heel pain.[129,130]

According to Butler,[12,62] many cases of "plantar fasciitis" may be neurogenic in origin. An important part of the differential diagnosis of neurogenic and fascial pain is the use of tests to detect increased mechanical sensitivity of the tibial nerve. To differentiate the cause of pain, the foot and ankle are positioned in a pain-provoking position for plantar fasciitis (i.e., dorsiflexion of the foot and toes), and movement of a proximal part of the limb (e.g., straight-leg raise) is superimposed, increasing the tension on the tibial nerve and its branches (Figure 25-17). The plantar fascia is not stressed further by a straight-leg raise. Therefore, if symptoms increase in response to the straight-leg raise, there is likely at least a partial neurogenic origin.[12]

Clinical Note

When differentially diagnosing plantar fasciitis, a straight-leg test while maintaining toe extension (and ankle dorsiflexion) will help indicate whether the tibial nerve is involved.

Interdigital neuromas are most common in the second and third and third and fourth intermetatarsal spaces. One common example is **Morton's neuroma** (also called Morton's metatarsalgia), which most commonly involves the second or third plantar intermetatarsal nerve, which are branches of the medial and lateral plantar nerves. This neuroma most often occurs in runners and dancers because of the repetitive dorsiflexion of the metatarsophalangeal joints. It can also result from wearing high-heel shoes or from trauma, callus formation under the metatarsal heads, or inflammatory conditions. Morton's neuroma is most common in females. The nerve is stretched under the deep transverse metatarsal ligament. Pain and paresthesia are felt at the metatarsal heads and may radiate proximally or into the toes.[130] Treatment usually consists of rest, modification of footwear, corticosteroid injection, or surgical excision of the neuroma. Mobilization of the

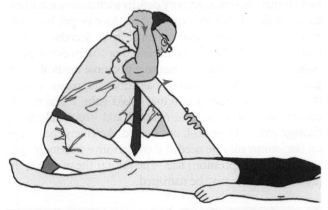

Figure 25-17 Maximum toe extension and dorsiflexion place tensile stress on the plantar fascia. The position shown is maintained while the lower extremity is raised in a straight-leg raise. If symptoms increase with the addition of the straight-leg raise, neural structures are implicated, because the tension on the plantar fascia has not changed. (Modified from Butler D: *The sensitive nervous system*, p 280, Adelaide, Australia, 2000, Noigroup Publications.)

intermetatarsal joints may help alter the mechanical interface among the nerve, the metatarsal heads, and the transverse ligament.[12]

Common Fibular (Peroneal) Nerve Injury

The **common fibular (peroneal) nerve** (Table 25-10) is formed from fibers from the L4-S2 nerve roots. It divides from the sciatic nerve in the upper part of the popliteal space, where it follows the medial border of the biceps femoris and its tendon. The nerve then passes over the posterior aspect of the head of the fibula and winds around the neck of the fibula deep to fibularis (peroneus) longus, where it divides into deep and superficial fibular (peroneal) nerves.

The **superficial fibular (peroneal) nerve** enters the lateral compartment of the leg, where it innervates the fibularis (peroneal) longus and brevis muscles and supplies sensation to the skin on the distal third of the anterior surface of the leg and the dorsum of the foot, except the web space between the first and second toes. The deep fibular (peroneal) nerve enters the anterior compartment

TABLE 25-10

Common Fibular (Peroneal) Nerve (L4-S2): Areas of Entrapment or Irritation

Cause/Site	Signs and Symptoms
Traction injury at bifurcation from sciatic nerve	• Acute onset of severe lateral leg pain from hematoma formation within the nerve after ankle fracture or inversion sprain
Fibular head: compression from a blow or entrapment	• Pain and/or paresthesias of the lateral leg and foot • Electromyogram (EMG) may not be positive in entrapment unless symptoms have been provoked by increased activity
Dorsolateral ankle after a sprain	• Lateral foot and ankle pain/paresthesias; possible EMG findings • Positive straight-leg raise test with plantar flexion/inversion of foot and ankle
Dorsolateral ankle: superficial or deep fibular nerve compressed by fascial bands, swelling, or ill-fitting boots or shoes	• Pain and/or paresthesias in the dorsolateral foot and ankle • Symptoms provoked with palpation of the nerve at the site of the lesion • Positive straight-leg raise test with plantar flexion/inversion of foot and ankle • Drop foot • Paresthesias in cleft between first and second toes (deep fibular compression)

Modified from Drye C, Zachazewski JE: Peripheral nerve injuries. In Zachazewski JE, Magee DJ, Quillen WS, editors: *Athletic injuries and rehabilitation*, p 457, Philadelphia, 1996, WB Saunders.

of the leg, where it innervates the tibialis anterior, extensor digitorum longus, extensor hallucis longus, and fibularis (peroneus) tertius muscles. The deep fibular (peroneal) nerve then enters the dorsum of foot and innervates the extensor digitorum brevis and extensor hallucis brevis muscles. It supplies sensation to the skin over the web space between the first and second toes.

Because the common fibular (peroneal) nerve borders the popliteal fossa, it is susceptible to compression by a Baker's cyst or osteochondroma, although it is affected less often than the tibial nerve.[127] Because of the nerve's proximity to the fibular head, the nerve is vulnerable to compression injuries from a direct blow to the lateral leg, a lower leg cast, or sustained pressure in proximity of the fibular head (e.g., a race car driver leaning his or her leg against a car door or poor positioning during surgery).[33]

Nobel[132] described two patients who developed a hematoma of the common fibular nerve just distal to the bifurcation from the sciatic nerve after an inversion sprain of the ankle or fracture of the lower leg. He hypothesized that the blood vessels supplying the nerve were ruptured by abrupt longitudinal traction on the nerve. Evacuation of the hematoma relieved the patients' discomfort completely.

Clinical Note

During assessment for ankle sprains, the examiner should clear the common fibular (peroneal) nerve and its branches as part of the differential diagnosis.

McMahon and Craig[133] reported a common fibular (peroneal) nerve injury after a severe varus torque caused disruption of the anterior cruciate ligament (ACL), lateral collateral ligament (LCL), iliotibial band, and biceps tendon. Leach et al.[134] found that in runners, the nerve can be entrapped in musculofascial bands at various points around the fibular head. The main symptoms reported were progressive lateral leg and foot pain and paresthesia and weakness of the ankle evertor and toe extensor muscles. Runners seem to be especially vulnerable to irritation at this site because of repetitive stretching of the nerve during inversion and plantar flexion. One other important observation from this study was the fact that many of the patients had normal neurological findings or EMG studies when examined in the physician's office. However, if the patients returned to the office immediately after a long run, the neurological findings and EMG changes were much more pronounced.

Common fibular (peroneal) nerve injury can be a complication of total knee arthroplasty (Incidence: 0% to 9.5%). The risk of injury increases with a preexisting valgus deformity of more than 10°, in patients with rheumatoid arthritis, and with prolonged tourniquet use.[8]

Common fibular nerve injury should also be considered a probable sequela of grade I to III ankle sprains or fractures.[135] Grade III sprains involve disruption of the lateral ligaments, the deltoid ligament, and the distal anterior talofibular ligament. Nitz et al.[136] reported a high incidence of common fibular and tibial nerve injuries in patients with this type of sprain. Of 36 patients, 31 (86%) had evidence of common fibular (peroneal) nerve injuries and 30 (83%) had tibial nerve injuries; 19 patients in this group also had sensory losses. Of 30 patients with grade II sprains (tearing of lateral ligaments and deltoid ligaments), 5 (17%) had common fibular (peroneal) nerve injuries and three had tibial nerve injuries.

Further evidence of possible neural involvement in ankle inversions sprains was provided by Pahor and Toppenberg.[137] These authors explored responses to the slump test with the foot held in plantar flexion and inversion in 18 subjects who had a history of single or multiple ankle inversion injuries (severity not reported), at least 6 months before neurodynamic testing. Subjects experienced greater reductions in knee extension mobility and more widespread symptoms in the distribution of the common fibular (peroneal) nerve on the involved extremities. Releasing cervical flexion reduced symptoms provoked in the slump test position, confirming a neurogenic contribution to the test response and evidence of increased mechanosensitivity in the common fibular (peroneal) branch of the sciatic tract.

A common site of deep fibular (peroneal) nerve compression is **anterior compartment (exertional) syndrome** of the leg resulting from a contusion, fracture, or severe overexertion, which may compress the deep fibular (peroneal) nerve and impede blood flow in the anterior tibial artery that supplies the anterior leg and the dorsal pedal artery that supplies the foot. Anterior compartment syndrome may compromise deep fibular (peroneal) nerve function, resulting in weakness in the dorsiflexor muscles or, in severe cases, drop foot. It may also cause sensory deficits such as abnormal sensation in first dorsal web space of the foot or produce pain as a result of compression ischemia from decreased blood flow to the leg and foot. A diminished or absent dorsal pedal pulse should alert the clinician to a potential medical emergency. Tissues may be hard on palpation, and passive plantar flexion or active dorsiflexion may evoke pain. Initial muscle damage may occur in 4 to 6 hours and irreversible tissue damage within 18 hours if not treated. An emergency surgical fasciotomy may be needed if conservative treatment (i.e., ice without compression) fails. The greater the pressure, the greater the nerve may be damaged.

Red Flag

If one is assessing for or has a high level of suspicion that an anterior compartment syndrome exists, a diminished or absent dorsalis pedis pulse is an indication of a potential medical emergency.

The superficial fibular (peroneal) nerve can be entrapped as it exits from the deep fascia in the lower leg to cross the dorsolateral ankle.[130] Entrapment of this nerve causes numbness or tingling over the dorsum of the foot. The deep fibular (peroneal) nerve can be injured as it crosses the dorsum of the ankle under the extensor retinaculum, where it is vulnerable to compression from ill-fitting boots or shoes or from swelling or osteophytes after a fracture. It also is vulnerable at this site to traction injuries from repetitive ankle sprains.[33] Both sites of injury are more common in runners.[130]

A modification of the straight-leg raise test can be used to differentiate neurogenic causes from ligament or joint causes of persistent dorsolateral foot and ankle pain.[12] The test is similar to the test described earlier for plantar foot pain. In this case the foot and ankle are held in the pain-provoking position of inversion and plantar flexion, and the entire lower extremity is raised into a straight-leg raise (Figure 25-18). Symptoms caused by nerve abnormality along the common fibular (peroneal) nerve tract increase with this test. Symptoms caused by joint and/or ligament abnormality do not change with this test.

Femoral Nerve Injury

The femoral nerve is formed from the L2-L4 nerve roots of the lumbar plexus.[75] It passes deep to the midpoint of inguinal ligament, lateral to the femoral artery and vein, and divides into motor and cutaneous branches as it runs down the anterior compartment of the thigh, innervating the rectus femoris, vastus lateralis, vastus medialis, vastus intermedius, sartorius, pectineus, and iliacus muscles. It also supplies the skin on the anterior thigh and distal medial thigh by the anterior cutaneous nerve of the thigh, and its articular branches supply the hip and knee joints. The **saphenous nerve** branches off the femoral nerve in the proximal thigh and descends down the thigh and medial leg with the great saphenous vein, supplying the skin on the medial leg and foot.

Different mechanisms can cause injury to the femoral nerve. Compression may occur in the iliac compartment as a result of a hematoma, and this possibility should be considered in any patient who is on anticoagulant therapy or who has hemophilia[76] or a history of trauma to the iliacus muscle. Giuliani et al.[138] reported a case of a healthy 14-year-old who developed a hematoma and femoral nerve injury after minor trauma during gymnastics. The nerve is vulnerable to compression as it passes under the inguinal ligament (Figure 25-19) in athletes or workers who must squat for long periods or wear protective clothing that compress this area. It is also vulnerable to injury during gynecological surgery or with anterior or anterolateral approaches to total hip arthroplasty.[8,76]

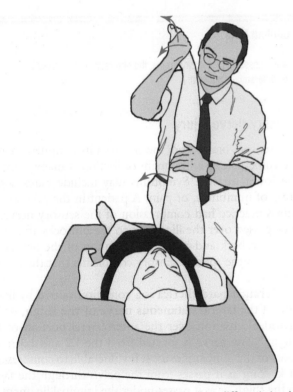

Figure 25-18 The source of lateral ankle pain (i.e., differentiation between a ligament sprain versus nerve irritation) can be differentiated with the following test. The ankle is placed in the pain-provoking position of inversion and plantar flexion. A straight-leg raise is then performed, increasing tensile stresses on the fibular (peroneal) nerve but not on the ankle joint and ligaments. Hip adduction and medial (internal) rotation place further tension on the lumbosacral nerve roots and common fibular (peroneal) nerve. (Modified from Butler D: *The sensitive nervous system*, p 281, Adelaide, Australia, 2000, Noigroup Publications.)

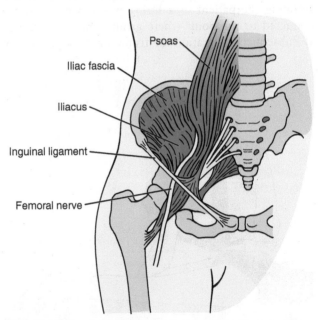

Figure 25-19 Compression of the femoral nerve by an iliacus hematoma. The ballooned right iliacus muscle compresses the femoral nerve against the psoas muscle. (Redrawn from Giuliani G, Poppi M, Acciarri N, Forti A: CT scan and surgical treatment of traumatic iliacus hematoma with femoral neuropathy: case report, *J Trauma* 30:230, 1990.)

Sammarco and Stephens[139] described one case of femoral nerve palsy in a modern dancer. The apparent mechanism of injury was traction from dance positions that required simultaneous hip extension and knee flexion. This position is similar to that used in the prone knee bend test for tension on the femoral nerve and L2-L4 nerve roots (Figure 25-20).[3] Trauma to the groin or proximal anterior thigh regions can also cause injury to the femoral nerve.

Obturator Nerve Injury

The obturator nerve is derived from the L2-L4 nerve roots of the lumbar plexus, travels through the obturator foramen to enter the medial thigh compartment, and then divides into anterior and posterior branches.[75] The anterior branch descends between the adductor longus and adductor brevis muscle and innervates both these muscles as well as the gracilis, and, possibly, the pectineus muscle. The posterior branch descends between adductor brevis and adductor magnus and innervates the obturator externus and the adductor magnus (adductor portion) muscles. The cutaneous branch of the obturator nerve supplies skin on the proximal portion of the medial thigh. Injury can occur from pelvic tumors, obturator hernias, pelvic surgery, or pelvic and proximal femoral fractures.[75]

Butler[12] suggested that entrapment of the obturator nerve may contribute to complaints of persistent groin pain in an athlete with an adductor muscle strain. He suggested modifying the slump sitting test to examine for mechanosensitivity of the obturator nerve by positioning the patient in a sitting position with the leg abducted to the point where groin symptoms are felt. If subsequent alteration of trunk or neck flexion or

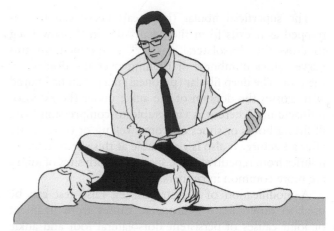

Figure 25-21 This variation of the slump knee bend test increases tensile loading on the obturator nerve by adding hip abduction. (Modified from Butler D: *The sensitive nervous system*, p 306, Adelaide, Australia, 2000, Noigroup Publications.)

lateral (side) flexion alters the groin pain, the disorder may have a neurogenic component. Another neurodynamic test used to evaluate the obturator nerve is the slump knee bend test with the involved leg in abduction (Figure 25-21).[62]

Clinical Note

When assessing for groin strains, the obturator nerve should be cleared for differential diagnosis.

Sensory Nerve Injury

The sensory branches of lower extremity peripheral nerves are vulnerable to entrapment or friction at many points in the lower quarter. Symptoms may include paresthesias, areas of numbness, or pain. A patient in the primary author's practice had compression of the sensory nerves as they passed over the iliac crest to the buttocks after a fall onto the back and buttocks. Palpation of the nerves reproduced the specific sensory complaints that the patient reported.

Meralgia paresthetica is a condition caused by irritation of the **lateral cutaneous nerve of the thigh,** which provides sensation over the anterolateral portion of the thigh.[75] The nerve is formed from the L2 and L3 nerve roots of the lumbar plexus. It is vulnerable to compression or kinking as it passes from the pelvis through the fascia to the thigh or as it passes under the inguinal ligament. It may be compromised by pressure from protective equipment (e.g., a tight belt used to carry tools), from weight belts that are worn too tightly, or by direct trauma.[140] This nerve injury is more common in diabetic, pregnant, and obese patients.[75,76] It also is associated with degeneration of the symphysis pubis in patients older than 40 years of

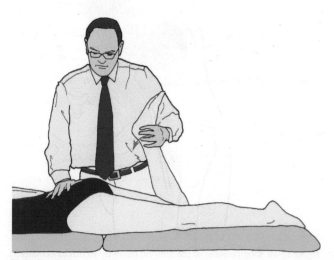

Figure 25-20 Prone knee bending is a common test for tension on the femoral nerve and L3 and L4 nerve roots. (Modified from Butler D: *The sensitive nervous system*, p 302, Adelaide, Australia, 2000, Noigroup Publications.)

age, possibly as a result of increased tension on the ilioinguinal ligament.[141]

The sartorial branch of the saphenous nerve (i.e., the medial crural cutaneous nerve) originates at the medial side of the knee and descends alongside the great saphenous vein to supply skin to the medial aspect of the knee and leg.[75,142] It is vulnerable to injury from valgus stresses at the knee and during surgical procedures on the medial knee.[142]

The **saphenous branch** of the femoral nerve can be entrapped in the adductor (Hunter's) canal of the medial thigh (Figure 25-22). The patient may report medial knee pain or paresthesias in the medial lower leg or medial foot. Compression increases during strong muscular contraction, as seen during squats or knee extension exercises.[48] Pendergrass and Moore[143] reported a case of saphenous nerve injury from a direct blow to the thigh by a heavy truck tire. Release of the resulting fibrotic scar was necessary to resolve the patient's symptoms. Butler[12] has devised a modified femoral nerve stretch test to test for adverse mechanosensitivity along the saphenous portion of the femoral nerve (Figure 25-23).

The **sural nerve,** derived from medial and lateral sural cutaneous branches of the tibial and common fibular (peroneal) nerves, respectively, provides cutaneous innervation to the lateral foot[75]; this nerve should be considered a possible source of lateral foot and calf pain. The nerve emerges through a fibrous arcade approximately 16 cm (6.3

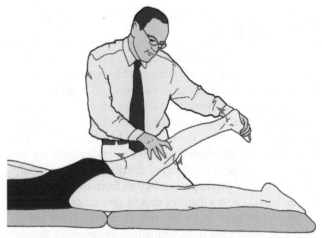

Figure 25-23 Tension can be placed on the saphenous nerve by placing the lower extremity in hip extension, external (lateral) rotation, knee extension, and hip abduction. (Modified from Butler D: *The sensitive nervous system,* p 306, Adelaide, Australia, 2000, Noigroup Publications.)

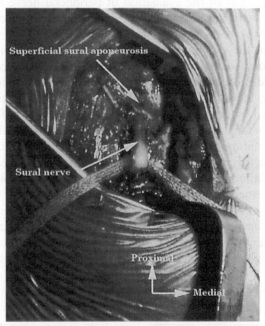

Figure 25-24 The sural nerve can become entrapped in the superficial sural aponeurosis and the fibrous band where the nerve passes through it. (From Fabre T, Montero C, Gaujard E et al: Chronic calf pain in athletes due to sural nerve entrapment, *Am J Sports Med* 28:680, 2000.)

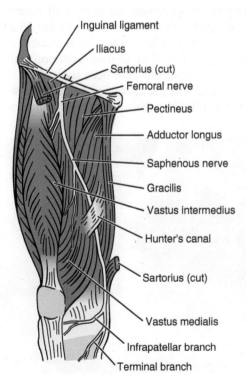

- Inguinal ligament
- Iliacus
- Sartorius (cut)
- Femoral nerve
- Pectineus
- Adductor longus
- Saphenous nerve
- Gracilis
- Vastus intermedius
- Hunter's canal
- Sartorius (cut)
- Vastus medialis
- Infrapatellar branch
- Terminal branch

Figure 25-22 The saphenous nerve is vulnerable to entrapment in the adductor (Hunter's) canal of the thigh.

inches) proximal to the lateral malleolus (Figure 25-24). Fabre et al.[144] found that entrapment at this site was the source of chronic calf pain in 10 runners who failed to respond to conservative treatment. The sural nerve can be palpated in the lateral side of the foot and in the lateral lower leg proximal to the lateral malleolus.[12] Like the common fibular (peroneal) nerve, it is vulnerable to tensile injury from repetitive inversion sprains of the ankle or compressive injuries from ill-fitting shoes.[12,130]

DIFFERENTIAL DIAGNOSIS OF PERIPHERAL NERVE INJURIES

Leffert's advice, "When in doubt, do a history and physical,"[145] is critical in the differential diagnosis of peripheral nerve injuries. The subjective examination must delineate the specific type of symptoms and the area where they are occurring. Paresthesia or sensory losses should be mapped using different sensory devices (e.g., brush, pinwheel, pin, cotton puff) to determine whether the symptoms are in a dermatomal or peripheral nerve distribution.[3] The precipitating injury or predisposing factors from overtraining or biomechanical abnormalities should give clues as to which nerves might have been injured. A nerve injury should always be suspected if an individual experiences sensory changes in addition to weakness or pain.

Important components of objective testing include reflexes, strength, and sensory testing; Tinel's test over the peripheral nerves; and palpation along the course of the nerve (Figure 25-25).[12,62] EMG testing is an important component of the evaluation of peripheral nerve injuries, such as nerve conduction velocity testing and action potential assessment. As mentioned previously, the timing of the examination is crucial. Abnormalities in the **sensory nerve action potentials (SNAPs)** and **combined motor action potentials (CMAPs)** are typically not evident for 7 to 10 days after injury. **Fibrillations** caused by denervation of muscles are not evident for 3 to 5 weeks after injury,[42,145] which makes distinguishing between an axonotmesis and a neurotmesis difficult in the first few days and weeks after an injury. According to Wilbourn,[45] EMG examination is most useful when performed between 3 weeks and 3 to 6 months after injury. In addition to neural conductivity tests, several tests have been described that check for biomechanical sensitivity along nerve trunks. These are useful for identifying the pathomechanics of neural structures and their contribution to symptoms. Butler[12,62] and Shacklock[146] detail the applications and variations of these tests in their texts on mobilization of the nervous system. The tests are thought to be clinically significant when a difference exists in any of the following variables when the symptomatic side is compared with the asymptomatic side:

- available range of motion,
- resistance to motion as perceived by the clinician,
- symptom reproduction, or
- deviation from the established symptomatic responses in normals.

The tests are considered particularly relevant if the exact symptoms of which the patient complains are reproduced during testing.[12,146]

As discussed previously, a compartment (exertional) syndrome may occur when tissue pressures increase within a confined space, compromising circulation and muscle function and possibly injuring the peripheral nerves that traverse the compartment. Expansion of the compartment may be limited by the surrounding fascia or skin or by an external constraint, such as a dressing or cast. The source of increased tissue pressure can be a hematoma that occurs after injury or hypertrophy of the muscles within the compartment, or overexertion.[17] Injury to the nerve can occur as a result of ischemia or direct mechanical compression. Measurement of compartment pressures helps rule out compartment syndromes. Compartment pressures are not elevated in other peripheral nerve entrapment syndromes.[17,136]

Compartment syndromes are commonly traumatic but can be associated with other conditions (Table 25-11).[147,148] Compartment syndromes caused by increased muscular profusion (hypertrophy) are far more common in the lower extremities of athletes but have been reported in the lumbar paraspinals,[149] in the anconeus muscle as a source of lateral elbow pain,[150] in the supraspinatus compartment as

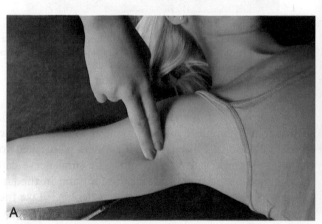
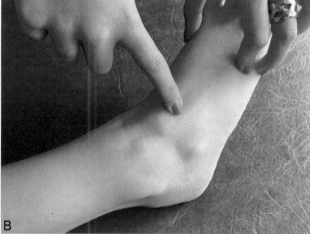

Figure 25-25 Palpation of the nerves is an important part of the examination. Nerves often are tender to the touch at the site of a lesion and palpation may provoke distal pain and paresthesias. **A,** The brachial artery and median and ulnar nerves can be readily palpated in the axilla. **B,** The superficial fibular (peroneal) nerve is visible at the dorsolateral ankle.

TABLE **25-11**

Causes of Compartment Syndrome

Type	Cause
Orthopedic	Fractures
	Fracture surgery
Vascular	Arterial and venous injuries
	Reperfusion injury
	Hemorrhage
	Phlegmasia cerulea dolens
Soft tissue	Crush injury
	Burns
	Prolonged limb compression
Iatrogenic	Puncture in patient undergoing anticoagulation therapy
	Use of pneumatic antishock garment
	External compression:
	• Cast, splint or circular dressing
	• Positioning during surgery or other state of decreased consciousness (e.g., alcohol or drug abuse)
	Pulsatile irrigation
Occasional	Snakebite
	Spider bite[149]
	Overuse of muscles

Modified from Kostler W, Strohm PC, Sudkamp NP: Acute compartment syndrome of the limb, *Injury* 35:1221-1227, 2004.

a source of shoulder pain, and in the 3 forearm compartments and the 10 hand compartments.[151,152] The patient typically reports increased pain and cramping or weakness with increasing activity. Symptoms usually subside when activities stop.[17] If not, surgical decompression is necessary.

MANAGEMENT OF NERVE INJURIES

Management of acute nerve injuries depends on the location and severity of the injury; specific management of several lesions has already been described in this text. Resting the injured part and anti-inflammatory measures (e.g., appropriate medication and icing) may facilitate the initial stages of healing.[14,42,52,92] Corticosteroid or lidocaine injections may be of some use therapeutically and also to confirm the location of the neural lesion.[104]

Butler[12,62] advocated early intervention after injury, beginning with mobilization of the structures surrounding the neural tissue. Gentle mobilization of neural tissues should begin away from the site of the lesion, imparting only gentle movement or tensile loads across the injured nerve. The goal of early mobilization is to prevent scarring between the nerve and the nerve bed or within the connective tissue of the nerve itself as the nerve heals. Care must be taken to avoid tensile loads on a nerve if the patient has acute neurological loss, which suggests the possibility of an axonotmesis or neurotmesis, which are more severe nerve lesions, compared with a mild

neurapraxia lesion. If the symptoms are more chronic in nature, all of the neural tension tests described previously can be used in various ways as mobilization techniques. Some variables that may influence the design of nerve mobilization techniques and interventions include:

- the distance from the moving joint to the site of the lesion,
- the position of adjacent joints, and
- whether joint movement stretches or shortens nerve trunks.

Using these variables while applying nerve mobilization has resulted in up to 12.5 mm of nerve gliding in the median, ulnar, tibial, and sciatic nerves.[153] The goal of this type of treatment is to improve the mobility of the nerve relative to adjacent tissues and to stretch the connective tissue elements of the nerve to improve its tolerance to tensile forces (see texts by Butler[12,62] and Shacklock[146] for guidelines on the use of these techniques in treatment).

Factors to Consider When Doing Neurodynamic Mobilization

- Is injury acute or chronic?
- What is the distance from the moving joint(s) to the site of the injury?
- What is the position of adjacent joints?
- Does the movement stretch or shorten the nerve?

Persistent muscular weakness resulting in nerve injury should be addressed with muscular strength training programs (also muscular endurance training where appropriate) to decrease the risk of nerve injury.[31,32,37,40] For example, with injuries to the brachial plexus, the cervical paraspinal and shoulder musculature must be strengthened to help prevent excessive cervical spine flexion and lateral (side) flexion in high-impact sports such as American football.[30,32] We recommend that an athlete in high-risk sports, such as American football, be able to support the body weight at a 45° angle while maintaining the head and neck in the midline neutral position (Figure 25-26). This may be used as a criterion for preseason physicals and for return to sports participation.

Muscle imbalances, weakness, or fatigue of lower or upper extremity musculature can lead to increases in the tensile or compressive stress or strain on neural tissues as they traverse the upper or lower extremity and cross articulations, which can result in a variety of nerve injuries.[17,52,67,92] Communication among the athletic trainer, physical therapist, and weight-training coaches is important to ensure that compensatory techniques during weight training do not promote further muscle imbalances. Specific examples have been provided in previous sections.

If conservative measures fail to restore normal neurological function, surgery may be indicated to decompress,[17,110,134] transpose,[92,104] or repair a segment

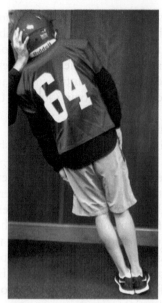

Figure 25-26 To prevent injuries to the cervical spine in sports such as football, the athlete should develop adequate cervical strength to support the body weight in a position at a 30° to 45° angle in the supine, prone, and side-lying positions while maintaining the head and neck in the midline.

of the nerve.[152] The optimal time for repair of most closed nerve injuries is about 3 months after the injury.[152] By that time, it is clear whether the nerve will recover spontaneously (neurapraxia) and, in the case of a more severe injury (axonotmesis), whether swelling has had time to decrease. An interdigital neuroma of the foot often is treated successfully with surgical excision.[130] A laceration of a nerve can be surgically repaired immediately.[154] Factors affecting the prognosis of a surgical repair include the violence of the injury to the nerve, the nerve's vascular supply, and any delay in the repair.[79]

PREVENTION OF NERVE INJURIES

By far, the most important part of the management of peripheral nerve injuries is prevention. Protective equipment and splints used to protect or prevent musculoskeletal in-

juries should be carefully padded to avoid compression over vulnerable nerves such as the lateral femoral cutaneous nerve at the inguinal ligament and the common fibular nerve as it passes around the fibular neck. Careful patient positioning and padding before surgical procedures can prevent many unnecessary intraoperative nerve injuries.

Care must be taken when applying ice over superficial nerves. Bassett et al.[154] reported five cases of cryotherapy-induced nerve injuries. They recommend that ice be applied for no longer than 20 minutes at a time and in a manner that cannot compress a peripheral nerve. Green et al.[155] reported long-term common fibular (peroneal) nerve injury in one patient after icing for only 20 minutes. They hypothesized that the injury, in this case, may have been more severe because of the addition of a compressive wrap over the ice pack and the athlete's ectomorphic body type. They cautioned that the patient should be checked 5 to 10 minutes after the ice is applied for signs of paresthesia or numbness distal to the site of application of the ice and compressive wrap.

SUMMARY

The potential for injury to the nervous system exists with every musculoskeletal injury,[52,125,136] and this possibility should be considered when pain, strength, or sensory deficits fail to resolve in a timely manner. Early recognition of nerve injuries after any trauma helps ensure that the patient receives appropriate acute management, rehabilitation, and advice about continued participation in sports, work, and other activities.

ACKNOWLEDGMENT

The authors wish to thank David Butler, B Phty, GDAMT, M APP SC PT, for generously sharing many of his insights into the intricacies of the nervous system and for stimulating our own clinical practice and research and allowing us to use many drawings from *The Sensitive Nervous System*.[62]

REFERENCES

1. Krivickas LS, Wilbourn AJ: Peripheral nerve injuries in athletes: a case series of over 200 injuries, *Semin Neurol* 20:225–232, 2000.
2. Takazawa H, Sudo N, Akoi K, et al: Statistical observation of nerve injuries in athletes (in Japanese), *Brain Nerve Inj* 3:11–17, 1971.
3. Hirasawa Y, Sakakida K: Sports and peripheral nerve injury, *Am J Sports Med* 11:420–426, 1983.
4. Noble J, Munro CA, Prasad VS, et al: Analysis of upper and lower extremity peripheral nerve injuries in a population of patients with multiple injuries, *J Trauma* 45:116–122, 1998.
5. Birch R, Misra P, Stewart MP, et al: Nerve injuries sustained during warfare: part 1-Epidemiology, *J Bone Joint Surg Br* 94:523–528, 2012.
6. Cheney FW, Domino KB, Posner KL: Nerve injury associated with anesthesia: a closed claims analysis, *Anesthesiology* 90:1062–1069, 1999.
7. Zhang J, Moore AE, Stringer MD: Iatrogenic upper limb nerve injuries: a systematic review, *ANZ J Surg* 81:227–236, 2011.
8. Plastaras CT, Chhatre A, Kotcharian AS: Perioperative lower extremity peripheral nerve traction injuries, *Orthop Clin North Am* 45:47–53, 2014.
9. Topp KS, Boyd BS: Structure and biomechanics of peripheral nerves: nerve responses to physical stresses and implications for physical therapist practice, *Phys Ther* 86:92–109, 2006.
10. Brochwicz P, von Piekartz H, Zalpour C: Sonography assessment of the median nerve during cervical lateral glide and lateral flexion. Is there a difference in neurodynamics of asymptomatic people, *Man Ther* 18:216–219, 2013.
11. Ellis RF, Hing WA, McNair PJ: Comparison of longitudinal sciatic nerve movement with different mobilization exercises: an in vivo study utilizing ultrasound imaging, *J Orthop Sports Phys Ther* 42:667–675, 2012.
12. Butler D: *Mobilisation of the nervous system*, New York, 1991, Churchill Livingstone.
13. Seddon HJ: Three types of nerve injury, *Brain* 66:237, 1943.
14. Posner MA: Compressive neuropathies of the median and radial nerves at the elbow, *Clin Sports Med* 9:343–363, 1990.

15. Lundberg G: *Nerve injury and repair*, Edinburgh, 1988, Churchill Livingstone.

16. Dumitru D: *Electrodiagnostic medicine*, Philadelphia, 1995, Hanley & Belfus.

17. Black KP, Lombardo JA: Suprascapular nerve injuries with isolated paralysis of the infraspinatus, *Am J Sports Med* 18:225–228, 1990.

18. Upton ARM, McComas AJ: The double crush in nerve entrapment syndromes, *Lancet* 2:359–362, 1973.

19. McMellan DL, Swash M: Longitudinal sliding of the median nerve during movements of the upper limb, *J Neurol Neurosurg Psychiatry* 39:566–570, 1976.

20. Rankine JJ: Adult brachial plexus injury, *Clin Radiol* 59:767–774, 2004.

21. Mumenthaler M: Some clinical aspects of peripheral nerve lesions, *Eur Neurol* 2:257–268, 1969.

22. Joiner ER, Andras LM, Skaggs DL: Mechanisms and risk factors of brachial plexus injury in the treatment of early-onset scoliosis with distraction-based growing implants, *J Bone Joint Surg Am* 95:e161, 2013.

23. Lin PY, Luo CY, Kan CD, et al: Brachial plexus injury following coronary artery bypass surgery: a case report, *Kaohsiung J Med Sci* 16:638–642, 2000.

24. Pradat PF, Delanian S: Late radiation injury to peripheral nerves, *Handb Clin Neurol* 115:743–758, 2013.

25. National Collegiate Athletic Association (NCAA): NCAA® Guideline 2h. "Burners" (brachial plexus injuries). In *NCAA Sports Medicine Handbook*, Indianapolis, June 1994, National Collegiate Athletic Association. Revised June 2003.

26. Albright JP, McAuley E, Martin RK, et al: Head and neck injuries in college football: an eight year analysis, *Am J Sports Med* 13:147–152, 1985.

27. Bateman JE: Nerve injuries about the shoulder in sports, *J Bone Joint Surg Am* 49:785–792, 1967.

28. Watkins RG: Neck injuries in football players, *Clin Sports Med* 5:215–246, 1986.

29. Christman OD, Snook GA, Stanitis JM, et al: Lateral flexion neck injuries in athletic competition, *JAMA* 192:613–615, 1965.

30. Speer KP, Bassett FH: The prolonged burner syndrome, *Am J Sports Med* 18:591–594, 1990.

31. Garrick J, Webb D: *Sports injuries: diagnosis and management*, Philadelphia, 1990, WB Saunders.

32. Harrelson GL: Evaluation of brachial plexus injuries, *Sports Med Update* 4:3–8, 1989.

33. Mendell JR: The nervous system. In Strauss RH, editor: *Sports medicine*, Philadelphia, 1989, WB Saunders.

34. Markey KL, Di Benedetto M, Curl WW: Upper trunk brachial plexopathy: the stinger syndrome, *Am J Sports Med* 21:650–655, 1993.

35. Meyer SA, Schulte KR, Callagnan JJ, et al: Cervical spinal stenosis and stingers in college football players, *Am J Sports Med* 22:158–166, 1994.

36. Funk FJ, Wells RE: Injuries of the cervical spine in football, *Clin Orthop* 109:50–58, 1975.

37. Wroble RR, Albright JP: Neck and low back injuries in wrestling, *Clin Sports Med* 5:295–325, 1986.

38. Wroble R, Hoegh J, Albright J: Wrestling in sports medicine. In Reider B, editor: *The school aged athlete*, Philadelphia, 1992, WB Saunders.

39. Charbonneau RM, McVeigh SA, Thompson K: Brachial neuropraxia in Canadian Atlantic University sport football players: what is the incidence of "stingers", *Clin J Sport Med* 22:472–477, 2012.

40. Hershman EB, Wilbourn AJ, Bergfeld JA: Acute brachial neuropathy in athletes, *Am J Sports Med* 17:655–659, 1989.

41. Chuang DC: Management of traumatic brachial plexus injuries in adults, *Hand Clin* 15:737–755, 1999.

42. Hershman EB: Brachial plexus injuries, *Clin Sports Med* 9:311–329, 1990.

43. Gorden JA, Straub SJ, Swanik CB, et al: Effects of football collars on cervical hyperextension and lateral flexion, *J Athl Train* 38:209–215, 2003.

44. Hosey RG, Rodenberg RE: Brachial neuritis: an uncommon cause of shoulder pain, *Orthopedics* 27:833–836, 2004.

45. Wilbourn AJ: Electrodiagnostic testing of neurologic injuries in athletes, *Clin Sports Med* 9:229–245, 1990.

46. Molina JE, D'Cunha J: The vascular component of neurogenic-arterial thoracic outlet syndrome, *Int J Angiol* 17:83–87, 2008.

47. Karas SE: Thoracic outlet syndrome, *Clin Sports Med* 9:297–310, 1990.

48. Bojanic I, Pecina MM, Markiewitz AD: Tunnel syndrome in athletes. In Pecina MM, Krmptoti E, Nemanic JL, Markiewitz AD, editors: *Tunnel syndromes*, Boca Raton, FL, 1991, CRC Press.

49. Watson LA, Pizzari T, Balster S: Thoracic outlet syndrome part 2: conservative management of thoracic outlet, *Man Ther* 15:305–314, 2010.

50. Stockert BW, Kenny L, Edgelow PI: Beyond the central nervous system: neurovascular entrapment syndromes. In Umphred DA, editor: *Neurological rehabilitation*, ed 4, St Louis, 2001, Mosby.

51. Walker HK: Cranial nerve XI: the spinal accessory nerve. In Walker HK, Hall WD, Hurst JW, editors: *Clinical methods: the history, physical, and laboratory examinations*, ed 3, Boston, 1990, Butterworths.

52. Mendoza FX, Main K: Peripheral nerve injuries of the shoulder in the athlete, *Clin Sports Med* 9:331–342, 1990.

53. Vegso JJ, Torg E, Torg JS: Rehabilitation of cervical spine, brachial plexus and peripheral nerve injuries, *Clin Sports Med* 6:135–158, 1987.

54. Miller T: Peripheral nerve injuries at the shoulder, *J Man Manip Ther* 6:170–183, 1998.

55. Martin JT: Postoperative isolated dysfunction of the long thoracic nerve: a rare case of uncertain etiology, *Anesth Analg* 69:614–619, 1989.

56. White SM, Witten CM: Long thoracic nerve palsy in a professional ballet dancer, *Am J Sports Med* 21:626–628, 1993.

57. Dumestre G: Long thoracic nerve palsy, *J Man Manip Ther* 3:44–49, 1995.

58. American Physical Therapy Association: *Is your child's backpack making the grade?* Alexandria, VA, August 1, 2002, American Physical Therapy Association.

59. Paladini D, Dellantonio R, Cinti A, et al: Axillary neuropathy in volleyball players: report of two cases and literature review, *J Neurol Neurosurg Psychiatry* 60:345–347, 1996.

60. Cummins CA, Schneider DS: Peripheral nerve injuries in baseball players, *Phys Med Rehabil Clin N Am* 20:175–193, 2009.

61. Richards RR, Hudson AR, Bertoia JT, et al: Injury to the brachial plexus during Putti-Platt and Bristow procedures, *Am J Sports Med* 15:374–380, 1987.

62. Butler D: *The sensitive nervous system*, Adelaide, Australia, 2000, Noigroup Publications.

63. Ringel SP, Treihaft M, Carry M, et al: Suprascapular neuropathy in pitchers, *Am J Sports Med* 18:80–86, 1990.

64. Burkhart SS, Morgan CD: The peel-back mechanism: its role in producing and extending posterior type II SLAP lesions and its effect on SLAP repair rehabilitation, *Arthroscopy* 14:637–640, 1998.

65. Escamilla RF, Barrentine SW, Fleisig GS, et al: Pitching biomechanics as a pitcher approaches muscular fatigue during a simulated baseball game, *Am J Sports Med* 35:23–33, 2007.

66. Mallon WJ, Bronec PR, Spinner RJ, et al: Suprascapular neuropathy after distal clavicle excision, *Clin Orthop Relat Res* 329:207–211, 1996.

67. Liverson JA, Bronson MJ, Pollack MA: Suprascapular nerve lesions at the spinoglenoid notch: report of three cases and review of the literature, *J Neurol Neurosurg Psychiatry* 54:241–243, 1991.

68. Fleisig GS, Dillman CJ, Andrews JR: A biomechanical description of the shoulder joint during pitching, *Sports Med Update* 10–15, 1991. Fall/Winte.

69. Ferretti A, Cerullo G, Russo G: Suprascapular neuropathy in volleyball players, *J Bone Joint Surg Am* 69:260–263, 1987.

70. Bartosh RA, Dugdale TW, Nielsen R: Isolated musculocutaneous nerve injury complicating closed fracture of the clavicle: a case report, *Am J Sports Med* 20:356–359, 1992.

71. Kim SM, Goodrich JA: Isolated proximal musculocutaneous nerve palsy: case report, *Arch Phys Med Rehabil* 65:735–736, 1984.

72. Stephens L, Kinderknecht JJ, Wen DY: Musculocutaneous nerve injury in a high school pitcher, *Clin J Sport Med* 24:e68–e69, 2014.

73. Chusid JG: *Correlative neuroanatomy and functional neurology*, ed 17, Los Altos, CA, 1979, Lange Medical Publications.

74. Hoffman DF: Elbow dislocations: avoiding complications, *Phys Sports Med* 21:56–67, 1993.

75. Pratt N: Anatomy of nerve entrapment sites in the upper quarter, *J Hand Ther* 18:216–229, 2005.

76. Stewart JD, Aguayo AJ: Compression and entrapment neuropathies. In Dyck PJ, Thomas PK, Lambert EH, Bunge R, editors: *Peripheral neuropathy*, vol 2, Philadelphia, 1984, WB Saunders.

77. Shao Y, Harwood P, Grotz MR, et al: Radial nerve palsy associated with fractures of the shaft of the humerus: a systematic review, *J Bone Joint Surg Br* 87:1647–1652, 2005.

78. Mitsunaga MM, Nakano K: High radial nerve palsy following strenuous muscular activity, *Clin Orthop* 234:39–42, 1988.

79. Shergil G, Bonney G, Munshi P, et al: The radial and posterior interosseous nerves: the results of 260 repairs, *J Bone Joint Surg Br* 83:646–649, 2001.

80. Vicenzino B, Collins D, Wright A: The initial effects of a cervical spine manipulative physiotherapy treatment on the pain and dysfunction of lateral epicondylalgia, *Pain* 68:69–74, 1996.

81. Waugh EJ: Lateral epicondylalgia or epicondylitis: what's in a name? *J Orthop Sports Phys Ther* 35:200–202, 2005.

82. Lutz FR: Radial tunnel syndrome: an etiology of chronic lateral elbow pain, *J Orthop Sports Phys Ther* 14:14–17, 1991.

83. Gunn CC, Milbrandt WE: Tennis elbow and the cervical spine, *Can Med J* 8:803–809, 1976.

84. Cleland JA, Whitman JM, Fritz JM: Effectiveness of manual physical therapy to the cervical spine in the management of lateral epicondylalgia, *J Orthop Sports Phys Ther* 34:713–722, 2004.

85. Waugh EJ, Jaglal SB, Davis AM: Computer use associated with poor long-term prognosis of conservatively managed lateral epicondylalgia, *J Orthop Sports Phys Ther* 34:770–780, 2004.

86. Borgia AV, Hruska JK, Braun K: Double crush syndrome in the lower extremity: a case report, *J Am Podiatr Med Assoc* 102:330–333, 2012.

87. Magee DJ: *Orthopedic physical assessment*, ed 6, St. Louis, 2014, Saunders/Elsevier.

88. Elvey R: *The clinical relevance of signs of adverse brachial plexus tension*, Cambridge, England, 1988, In Proceedings of the International Federation of Manipulative Therapists Congress.

89. Yaxley GA, Jull GA: A modified upper limb tension test: an investigation of responses in normal subjects, *Aust J Physiother* 37:143–152, 1991.

90. Yaxley GA, Jull GA: Adverse tension in the neural system: a preliminary study of tennis elbow, *Aust J Physiother* 39:15–22, 1993.

91. Allman FL: Overuse injury in the throwing sports. In Torg J, Welsh RP, Shepherd RJ, editors: *Current*

therapy and sports medicine, vol 2, Philadelphia, 1985, BC Decker.

92. Glousman RE: Ulnar nerve problems in the athlete's elbow, *Clin Sports Med* 9:365–377, 1990.

93. Wright TW, Glowczewskie BA, Cowin D, et al: Ulnar nerve excursion and strain at the elbow and wrist associated with upper extremity motion, *J Hand Surg [Am]* 26:655–662, 2001.

94. Pechan J, Julis I: The pressure measurement in the ulnar nerve: a contribution to the pathophysiology of the cubital tunnel syndrome, *J Biomech* 8:75–79, 1975.

95. Escamilla RF, Fleisig GS, Barrentine S, et al: Kinematic and Kinetic Comparisons between American and Korean Professional Baseball Pitchers, *Sports Biomech* 1:213–228, 2002.

96. Matsuo T, Fleisig GS: Influence of shoulder abduction and lateral trunk tilt on peak elbow varus torque for college baseball pitchers during simulated pitching, *J Appl Biomech* 22:93–102, 2006.

97. Buchanan TS, Delp SL, Solbeck JA: Muscular resistance to varus and valgus loads at the elbow, *J Biomech Eng* 120:634–639, 1998.

98. Cain EL, Andrews JR, Dugas JR: Outcome of ulnar collateral ligament reconstruction of the elbow in 1281 athletes: results in 743 athletes with minimum 2-year follow-up, *Am J Sports Med* 38:2426–2434, 2010.

99. Levin JS, Zheng N, Dugas J: Posterior olecranon resection and ulnar collateral ligament strain, *J Shoulder Elbow Surg* 13:66–71, 2004.

100. Buehler MJ, Thayer DT: The elbow flexion test: a clinical test for the cubital tunnel syndrome, *Clin Orthop* 233:213–216, 1988.

101. Drye C: *The upper limb tension test 3: an investigation of the intrarater and interrater reliability and the subjective response to the test*, Unpublished master's thesis, Boston, 1993, MGH Institute of Health Professions.

102. Flanagan M, Bell A: *The normal response to the ulnar nerve bias upper limb tension test, Poster presentation at the Manipulative Physiotherapy Association of Australia Eighth Biennial Conference*, West Australia, 1993, Perth.

103. Martínez MD, Cubas CL, Girbés EL: Ulnar nerve neurodynamic test: study of the normal sensory response in asymptomatic individuals, *J Orthop Sports Phys Ther* 44:450–456, 2014.

104. Rettig AC, Ebben JR: Anterior subcutaneous transfer of the ulnar nerve in the athlete, *Am J Sports Med* 21:836–840, 1993.

105. Mellion MB: Common cycling injuries: management and prevention, *Sports Med* 11:52–70, 1991.

106. Fernald D: *Incidence of upper extremity "overuse" injuries in elite cyclists, Unpublished master's thesis*, Boston, 1988, MGH Institute of Health Professions.

107. Lee MJ, LaStayo PC: Pronator syndrome and other nerve compressions that mimic carpal tunnel syndrome, *J Orthop Sports Phys Ther* 34:601–609, 2004.

108. Gessini L, Jandolo B, Pietrangeli A: Entrapment neuropathies of the median nerve at and above the elbow, *Surg Neurol* 19:112–116, 1983.

109. Boz C, Mehmet O, Vildan A, et al: Individual risk factors for carpal tunnel syndrome: an evaluation of body mass index, wrist index and hand anthropometric measurements, *Clin Neurol Neurosurg* 106:294–299, 2004.

110. Rettig AC: Neurovascular injuries in the wrists and hands of athletes, *Clin Sports Med* 9:389–417, 1990.

111. Walker CW, Metzler M, Cifu DX, et al: Neutral wrist splinting in carpal tunnel syndrome: a comparison of night-only versus full-time wear instructions, *Arch Phys Med Rehabil* 81:424–429, 2000.

112. Murray-Leslie CF, Wright V: Carpal tunnel syndrome, humeral epicondylitis, and the cervical spine: a study of clinical and dimensional relations, *Br Med J* 1:1439–1442, 1976.

113. Kenneally M, Rubenach H, Elvey R: The upper limb tension test: the SLR test of the arm, *Clin Phys Ther* 17:167–194, 1988.

114. Richards J: *The upper limb tension test 2: An investigation of the responses and reliability in testing asymptomatic subjects*, Birmingham, AL, 1991, University of Alabama. Unpublished Masters Thesis.

115. Reisch R, Williams K, Nee RJ, et al: ULNT2: a median nerve bias—examiner reliability and sensory responses in asymptomatic subjects, *J Man Manip Ther* 13:44–55, 2005.

116. Seradge H, Parker W, Baer C, et al: Conservative treatment of carpal tunnel syndrome: an outcome study of adjunct exercises, *J Okla State Med Assoc* 95:7–14, 2002.

117. Michlovitz SL: Conservative interventions for carpal tunnel syndrome, *J Orthop Sports Phys Ther* 34:589–600, 2004.

118. Rozmaryn LM, Dovelle S, Rothman ER, et al: Nerve and tendon gliding exercises and the conservative management of carpal tunnel syndrome, *J Hand Ther* 11:171–179, 1998.

119. Puranen J, Orava S: The hamstring syndrome, *Am J Sports Med* 16:517–521, 1988.

120. Cassidy L, Walters A, Bubb K, et al: Piriformis syndrome: implications of anatomical variations, diagnostic techniques, and treatment options, *Surg Radiol Anat* 34:479–486, 2012.

121. Wolf M, Bäumer P, Pedro M, et al: Sciatic nerve injury related to hip replacement surgery: imaging detection by MR neurography despite susceptibility artifacts, *PLoS One* 9:2014. e89154.

122. Young IJ, van Riet RP, Bell SN: Surgical release for proximal hamstring syndrome, *Am J Sports Med* 36:2372–2378, 2008.

123. Maitland GD: The slump test: examination and treatment, *Aust J Physiother* 31:215–219, 1985.

124. Lew P, Briggs CA: Relationship between the cervical component of the slump test and change in hamstring muscle tension, *Man Ther* 2:98–105, 1997.

125. Kornberg C, Lew P: The effect of stretching neural structures on grade I hamstring injuries, *J Orthop Sports Phys Ther* 13:481–487, 1989.

126. Goçmen S, Topuz AK, Atabey C, et al: Peripheral nerve injuries due to osteochondromas: analysis of 20 cases and review of the literature, *J Neurosurg* 120:1105–1112, 2014.

127. Sanchez JE, Conkling N, Labropoulos N: Compression syndromes of the popliteal neurovascular bundle due to Baker cyst, *J Vasc Surg* 54:1821–1829, 2011.

128. Ekelund AL: Bilateral nerve entrapment in the popliteal space, *Am J Sports Med* 18:108, 1990.

129. Jackson DL, Haglund B: Tarsal tunnel syndrome in athletes, *Am J Sports Med* 19:61–65, 1991.

130. Schon LC, Baxter DE: Neuropathies of the foot and ankle in athletes, *Clin Sports Med* 9:489–509, 1990.

131. Johnson ER, Kirby K, Lieberman JS: Lateral plantar nerve entrapment: foot pain in a power lifter, *Am J Sports Med* 20:619–620, 1992.

132. Nobel W: Peroneal palsy due to hematoma in the common peroneal nerve sheath after distal torsional fractures and inversion ankle sprains, *J Bone Joint Surg Am* 48:1484–1495, 1966.

133. McMahon MS, Craig SM: Interfascicular reconstruction of the peroneal nerve after knee ligament injury, *Ann Plast Surg* 32:642–644, 1994.

134. Leach RE, Purnell MB, Saito A: Peroneal nerve entrapment in runners, *Am J Sports Med* 17:287–291, 1989.

135. Mitsiokapa EA, Mavrogenis AF, Antonopoulos D, et al: Common peroneal nerve palsy after grade I inversion ankle sprain, *J Surg Orthop Adv* 21:261–265, 2012.

136. Nitz AJ, Dobner JJ, Kersey D: Nerve injury and grades II and III ankle sprains, *Am J Sports Med* 13:177–182, 1985.

137. Pahor S, Toppenberg R: An investigation of neural tissue involvement in ankle inversion sprains, *Man Ther* 1:192–197, 1996.

138. Giuliani G, Poppi M, Acciarri N, et al: CT scan and surgical treatment of traumatic iliacus hematoma with femoral neuropathy: case report, *J Trauma* 30:229–231, 1990.

139. Sammarco GJ, Stephens MM: Neuropraxia of the femoral nerve in a modern dancer, *Am J Sports Med* 19:413–414, 1991.

140. Ulkar B, Yildiz Y, Kunduraciouglu B: Meralgia paresthetica: a long-standing performance-limiting cause of anterior thigh pain in a soccer player, *Am J Sports Med* 31:787–789, 2003.

141. Bierma-Zeinstra S, Ginai A, Prins A, et al: Meralgia paresthetica is related to degenerative pubic symphysis, *J Rheumatol* 27:2242–2245, 2000.

142. Arthornthurasook A, Gaew-Im K: The sartorial nerve: its relationships to the medial aspect of the knee, *Am J Sports Med* 18:41–42, 1990.

143. Pendergrass TL, Moore JH: Saphenous neuropathy following medial knee trauma, *J Orthop Sports Phys Ther* 34:328–334, 2004.

144. Fabre T, Montero C, Gaujard E, et al: Chronic calf pain in athletes due to sural nerve entrapment, *Am J Sports Med* 28:679–682, 2000.

145. Leffert R: Clinical diagnosis, testing, and electromyographic study in brachial plexus traction injuries, *Clin Orthop* 237:24–31, 1988.

146. Shacklock MO: *Clinical neurodynamics: a new system of musculoskeletal treatment*, Edinburgh, 2005, Elsevier Butterworth Heinemann.

147. Kostler W, Strohm PC, Sudkamp NP: Acute compartment syndrome of the limb, *Injury* 35:1221–1227, 2004.

148. Cohen J, Bush S: Case report: compartment syndrome after a suspected black widow spider bite, *Ann Emerg Med* 45:414–416, 2005.

149. Khan RJK, Fick DP, Guier CA, et al: Acute paraspinal compartment syndrome: a case report, *J Bone Joint Surg Am* 87:1126–1128, 2005.

150. Steinman SP, Bishop AT: Chronic anconeus compartment syndrome: a case report, *J Hand Surg [Am]* 25:959–961, 2000.

151. Stahlfield KR, Parker JE, McClain EJ: Supraspinatus compartment syndrome, *Am J Orthop* 33:615–617, 2004.

152. Ehni BL: Treatment of traumatic peripheral nerve injuries, *Am Fam Pract* 43:897–905, 1991.

153. Silva A, Manso A, Andrade R: Quantitative in vivo longitudinal nerve excursion and strain in response to joint movement: a systematic literature review, *Clin Biomech (Bristol, Avon)* 29:839–847, 2014.

154. Bassett FH, Kirkpatrick JS, Engelhardt DL, et al: Cryotherapy-induced nerve injury, *Am J Sports Med* 20:516–518, 1992.

155. Green GA, Zachazewski JE, Jordan SE: Peroneal nerve palsy induced by cryotherapy, *Phys Sports Med* 17:66–70, 1989.

CHAPTER 26

Repetitive Stress Pathology: Bone

ROBERT C. MANSKE, ANDREW PORTER, DANIEL QUILLIN, STUART J. WARDEN, DAVID B. BURR, PETER D. BRUKNER

INTRODUCTION

Repetitive stress pathology in bone manifests clinically in the form of stress reactions and typically as stress fractures. A stress fracture is a common injury that begins with repetitive and excessive stress on the bone and represents the inability of a bone to withstand repetitive bouts of mechanical loading, which results in structural fatigue and resultant signs and symptoms of localized pain and tenderness. This results in acceleration of normal bone remodeling, the production of microfractures (caused by insufficient time for the bone to repair), the creation of a bone stress injury (stress reaction), and eventually a stress fracture.[1] This chapter discusses prevention and treatment options for stress fractures. In doing so it also discusses stress reactions because these can present clinically and are part of a pathology continuum that can progress to stress fracture and in some cases complete bone fracture. To enable the clinician to appreciate the prevention and treatment options for stress fractures, necessary precursory background information is provided on pathophysiology, epidemiology, and risk factors. The chapter concludes by discussing the management of low-risk and high-risk stress fractures.

PATHOPHYSIOLOGY OF STRESS FRACTURES

The proposed pathophysiology for stress fractures is presented in Figure 26-1. A major role of the skeleton is to provide internal support to enable the force of gravity to be countered. In fulfilling this role, bones are exposed to repetitive bouts of mechanical loading. When a bone is mechanically loaded, it experiences internal strain. **Strain** refers to the change in length per unit length of a bone; it is a unitless value, but because it is very small for bone, it often is expressed in terms of *microstrain (με)*. One thousand microstrain is equivalent to 0.1% of deformation or in other words a deformation of 0.1 mm for a 10-cm (3.9-inch) long bone. Bone strains typically range from 400 to 1500 με during usual activities of daily living, although

activities that involve high-impact loads result in higher bone strains and strain rates.[2] The **strain rate** is how fast the strain is introduced; together with the absolute strain magnitude, it has important implications for the risk of stress fractures.

Complete bone fractures typically are caused by single loads that generate strains on the order of 10,000 με; therefore the safety factor between usual and failure strains is large. However, strains below this level are capable of causing damage when introduced repetitively. As with other structural materials, a natural phenomenon associated with repetitive strain in bone is the generation of damage (often called **microdamage**) (Figure 26-2).[3-5] In most instances this damage is of little consequence because bone is different from nonbiological materials and is capable of self-repair through targeted remodeling.[6] **Remodeling** is the removal of damaged bone by osteoclastic cells and its subsequent replacement with new bone by osteoblastic cells. Bone is capable of adapting to its mechanical environment by means of this mechanism. However, under certain conditions, imbalances can develop between the generation of damaged bone and its removal. The subsequent accumulation of damage is the start of a pathological continuum that can result clinically in stress reactions, stress fractures, and ultimately complete bone fractures (see Figure 26-1).[3,7,8]

The magnitude and rate of introduction of an applied load influence whether damage is generated by strain. Damage is a threshold-related phenomenon, which means that strain magnitudes above a certain level cause damage.[9] With increasing strain, damage increases.[10] The rate at which the strain is introduced influences damage formation. Strains introduced over shorter periods result in significantly greater damage formation.[11] The interaction between the strain magnitude and the strain rate ultimately reduces the number of loading cycles a bone can withstand before fatigue failure. Clinically this means that any activities that increase the magnitude or rate (or both) of

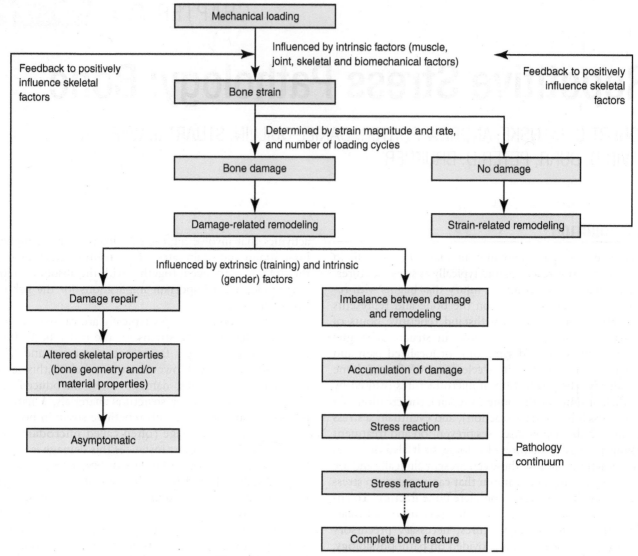

Figure 26-1 Pathophysiology of stress fractures.

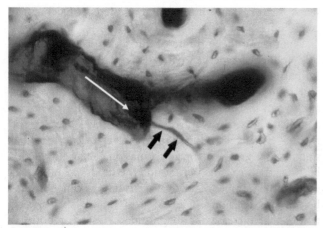

Figure 26-2 Bone microdamage viewed microscopically. The *black arrows* indicate a microcrack, and the *white arrow* indicates a resorption space associated with the targeted remodeling of the microcrack.

bone loading may contribute to damage formation, with subsequent progression to a stress fracture. These activities typically involve some form of impact loading in which high loads are introduced over short periods. Similarly damage accumulation and stress fracture may result from pure cyclic overloading.[12] This occurs when remodeling is given insufficient time to repair damage, and additional loading cycles cause damage to accumulate. Therefore factors that increase the number of loading cycles also may contribute to the development of a stress fracture.

EPIDEMIOLOGY OF STRESS FRACTURES

Because the pathophysiology of stress fractures involves repetitive mechanical loading, it is not surprising that they occur predominantly in athletes and military recruits. In both of these populations, stress fractures appear to be a common overuse injury; however, the precise incidence is difficult to ascertain.[13] Retrospective studies have found that 8.3% to 52% of runners have had a history of stress fracture,[14,15] and the incidence in a 12-month prospective study of track and field athletes was 21.1%.[16,17] Expressed as a percentage of all injuries, stress fractures have been reported to account for 0.7% to 20% of all injuries sustained by athletic populations.[13,17] Prospective data in recruits undergoing basic training indicate a stress fracture incidence rate of 3.3% to 8.5% in the U.S. military[18-21] and 3.6% to 28.9% in the Israeli military.[22,23]

Stress fractures are site specific, which means that they occur at sites exposed to repetitive mechanical loading. Given their association with mechanical loading, stress fractures predominantly occur at weight-bearing sites, and the most common sites are the tibia, metatarsals, and fibula.[24] The exact location depends on the way the skeleton is loaded; different activities result in different loading patterns in different bones. For example, power athletes (sprinters) load the bones of their feet relatively more than endurance athletes (distance runners).[25] Consequently the former are at greater risk of tarsal and metatarsal stress fractures.[17]

Although stress fractures predominantly occur at weight-bearing sites, they also occur in response to repetitive loading at non–weight-bearing sites. Rowers repetitively load the rib cage during the drive phase of the rowing stroke.[26] Consequently they are at greater risk of generating rib stress fractures.[27] Because stress fractures can occur at both weight-bearing and non–weight-bearing sites, they can occur in virtually any bone in the body (Table 26-1).[8] They therefore need to be considered in the differential diagnosis of all presenting injuries.

The most common locations for stress fractures are the tibia (23.6%), tarsal navicular (17.6%), metatarsal (16.2%), fibula (15.5%), femur (6.6%), pelvis (1.6%), and spine (0.6%).[1,24,28] Much less common are upper extremity stress fractures that occur in athletes who are involved in throwing sports or those with overhead motions.[29]

RISK FACTORS FOR STRESS FRACTURES

An understanding of the risk factors that contribute to stress fractures is necessary to prevent them and also to develop appropriate management strategies when they occur. As with most overuse conditions, the development of a stress fracture is likely due to a range of factors, with the relative contribution of each factor varying among individuals. These factors can be grouped into two categories: extrinsic and intrinsic factors (Table 26-2).

TABLE **26-1**

Sites of Stress Fractures and Commonly Associated Activities

Skeletal Site	Stress Fracture Site	Commonly Associated Sport or Activity
Scapula	Coracoid process	Trapshooting
	Body	Running with handheld weights
Humerus	Diaphysis	Throwing, racquet sports
Ulna	Diaphysis	Racquet sports (especially tennis), gymnastics, volleyball, weight lifting
	Olecranon	Throwing/pitching
Ribs	First rib	Throwing/pitching
	Second to tenth ribs	Rowing, kayaking, golfing
Lumbar spine	Pars interarticularis	Gymnastics, ballet, cricket fast bowling, volleyball, springboard diving
Pelvis	Pubic ramus	Distance running, ballet
Femur	Neck	Distance running, jumping, ballet
	Diaphysis	Distance running
Patella		Running, hurdling
Tibia	Plateau	Running
	Diaphysis	Running, ballet
	Medial malleolus	Basketball, running
Fibula		Running, aerobics, race walking, ballet
Talus	Lateral process	Pole vaulting
Navicular		Sprinting, middle-distance running, hurdling, long/triple jump, football
Metatarsals	General	Running, ballet, marching
	Base of the second metatarsal	Ballet
	Fifth metatarsal	Tennis, ballet
Sesamoid bones of the foot		Running, ballet, basketball, skating

TABLE 26-2

Extrinsic and Intrinsic Risk Factors for Stress Fractures

Type of Risk Factor	Subcategories
Extrinsic factors	• Type of activity or sport • Training program factors • Equipment factors • Environmental factors
Intrinsic factors	• Skeletal factors • Muscle factors • Joint factors • Biomechanical factors • Physical fitness factors • Nutritional factors • Gender factors

Extrinsic Risk Factors

Extrinsic risk factors are factors in the environment or external to the individual that influence the likelihood of an injury occurring. In terms of stress fractures, these include the type of activity or sport, training factors, equipment factors, and environmental factors.

Type of Activity or Sport

The type of activity or sport in which an individual participates is a risk factor for the generation of stress fractures. As mentioned, the pathophysiology of stress fractures involves mechanical loading. Because most sports involve some form of mechanical loading, participation in a sport by itself raises the risk of stress fracture. This is reflected in the high incidence of stress fractures in athletes compared with sedentary controls. However, individuals in different sports are at varying risk of developing a stress fracture based on the sport or sports in which they participate.[30] Different sports expose the skeleton to different loads. Damage generation in bone and its progression to stress fracture depends on both the magnitude and the rate of introduction of an applied load. Individuals who participate in sports that involve high-magnitude loads that are introduced over short periods have a greater risk of developing a stress fracture. These sports, which typically involve some form of ground impact, include jogging, running, or sprinting.

Another contributing factor to stress fracture generation is the number of loading cycles to which the skeleton is exposed. Individuals who participate in sports that involve high numbers of load repetitions are at greater risk. Such sports include rowing, throwing, and long-distance running. Because different sports load different parts of the skeleton, the sport in which individuals participate influences their susceptibility to a stress fracture at particular skeletal sites (see Table 26-1). It is important that clinicians remember this association of different sports with different stress fracture locations when presented with an athlete who participates in a particular sport.

Training Factors

Training program factors appear to be critical in the development of stress fractures. Depending on the characteristics of the loading stimulus, bone loading can cause damage generation. Damage serves as a stimulus that activates bone remodeling, a sequential process involving cellular activation, bone resorption, and finally bone formation. The remodeling response ensures relative homeostasis between damage formation and its repair and maintains the mechanical competence of the skeleton. It also enables a bone to adapt over time to its mechanical environment so that it can meet increasing levels of loading. Modification of a training routine can disturb this homeostasis.

Remodeling normally removes damage approximately as fast as it occurs. However, remodeling is time dependent. The remodeling time required to reach a new equilibrium after a disturbance is about one remodeling period, or approximately 3 to 4 months.[31,32] If insufficient time is allowed for adaptation to a change in the training routine, additional damage may occur. Although a remodeling reserve exists that allows increased activation of remodeling units in response to increases in damage formation, an increase in the number of active remodeling units removes bone temporarily, reducing bone mass and potentially increasing the chance for damage initiation when loading is continued. This feedforward occurs because resorption precedes formation in the remodeling process, and an increase in the number of currently active remodeling units is associated with an increase in bone porosity. This reduces the elastic modulus of the bone, which in turn increases strain and subsequently the rate of damage formation. The accumulation of damage may progress into a stress fracture. Therefore from a biological perspective, an alteration in the local mechanical environment of a bone through a change in the training routine has the potential to contribute to the development of stress fractures.

Remodeling Time

- Normal remodeling takes up to 3 to 4 months to replace damaged bone
- Damage may accumulate or enlarge if loading exceeds the rate at which bone is replaced

---

Changes in a training routine that may contribute to the development of stress fractures include any changes that alter the magnitude or rate of bone strain at a particular site, such as a change in training intensity. Increasing training intensity (e.g., increasing speed) may increase the magnitude or rate of bone strain at a particular site. Similarly, a change in training, such as an increase in the number or duration of training sessions, may also contribute to stress fracture generation. This increases the number of bone loading cycles, a factor that reduces bone fatigue life. These training changes may disturb the balance between damage formation and remodeling. Surveys showed that up to 86% of injured athletes could identify some change in their training before they developed a stress fracture.[30,33] However, it has not been established how many athletes do not develop a stress fracture after a change in their training program. This is important because athletes frequently alter the characteristics of their training program without pathological consequences.

Equipment Factors

Equipment factors can influence the risk of stress fractures by altering the loading environment of the skeleton, whether by increasing bone strain or by redistributing strain so that it occurs at less accustomed locations in a bone. The most commonly implicated pieces of equipment in stress fracture development are shoes and inserts (insoles and orthotics). Located at the foot-ground interface, shoes and inserts act as filters that theoretically attenuate ground impact forces. In addition, they have the potential to influence the motion of the foot and ankle and the subsequent mechanics proximally in the kinetic chain. Through these two mechanisms, shoes and inserts may influence bone strain and subsequently affect the risk of stress fracture. Gardner et al.[34] found that military recruits who started training in shoes of advanced age (an indicator of possible reduced shock absorptive capacity) were at greater risk of developing a stress fracture. (Because most studies of the role of shoes and inserts in stress fracture risk have involved intervention trials, their role is discussed further in the section, Prevention and Management Options for Stress Fractures.)

Rowers provide further evidence of the role of equipment factors in the risk of stress fracture. In the early 1990s the incidence of rib stress fractures appeared to increase among rowers.[35] This coincided with the introduction of a new blade shape for the oar; the blade was changed from narrow and long to broader, shorter, and more rectangular. These changes made the oar easier to handle, gave it greater stability in the water, and prevented backwatering at the shaft end.[36] In addition, the oar shaft was converted from wood to carbon fiber. This made the oar stiffer, allowing the force developed by the rower to be transmitted more efficiently to the blade. These changes in construction made for a more efficient rowing stroke. However, they also resulted in the generation of a greater force at the handle when the same load was applied. This increased the magnitude of loading, theoretically exposing the ribs to higher levels of strain and potentiating the development of stress fractures.[27] Therefore, equipment and changes in equipment may contribute to the risk of stress fractures.

Environmental Factors

The primary environmental factor in the etiology of stress fractures is the training surface, which has long been considered a contributor to the development of these fractures.[37] Running on cambered or uneven surfaces may accentuate biomechanical problems, and running on less compliant surfaces can increase impact forces and the subsequent magnitude and rate of bone loading.[38,39] Confirming the influence of training surface compliance on bone loading, Milgrom et al.[40] showed that running on a treadmill resulted in significantly lower tibial bone strain than running over ground. Although this suggests that running on softer, more compliant surfaces may reduce the risk of stress fracture, the issue may be influenced by muscle fatigue. Running on compliant surfaces (i.e., sand, dirt, gravel) requires a greater expenditure of energy and may hasten muscle fatigue.[41] This has the potential to influence bone loading (see the Muscle Factors section).

Although the training surface anecdotally has been associated with stress fractures, large epidemiological studies of running injuries have failed to show an association between injuries and training surface or terrain after controlling for weekly running distance.[42,43] However, this may be related to difficulty in quantifying running surface parameters accurately and to sampling bias.[41] One investigation of stress fractures in female military recruits found an increase in the incidence of stress fractures when training was changed from a usual flat, predictable terrain to a hilly, rocky terrain.[44]

Intrinsic Risk Factors

Extrinsic risk factors are critical to the development of stress fractures because some form of loading must be placed on a bone to generate damage and enable the stress to cause pathology. However, stress fracture development also is influenced by the body's ability to respond to applied loads. **Intrinsic risk factors** are characteristics within individuals themselves and the way their bodies respond to mechanical loading and the damage it may generate. The contribution of intrinsic risk factors is indicated by the fact that not all individuals exposed to an equivalent loading regimen develop a stress fracture. Intrinsic risk factors include skeletal, muscle, joint, biomechanical, physical fitness, nutritional, and gender factors.

Skeletal Factors

The contribution of skeletal factors to the risk of stress fracture has been well established. Seminal work by Carter and Hayes[45,46] demonstrated that a bone's ability to withstand repetitive low-magnitude loads depends on how much bone is present (mass) and the distribution of this bone (structure). Warden et al.[47] demonstrated that skeletal fatigue resistance significantly correlates with measures of both bone mass and structure. Although these findings have gained variable clinical support from numerous cross-sectional studies,[14,18,48-52] statistically more powerful prospective studies have confirmed that susceptibility to stress fractures is directly related to skeletal properties.[16,19,20]

Specifically, Bennell et al.[16] showed that female athletes who sustained a tibial stress fracture had lower generalized (whole body) bone mineral content and localized (tibial and fibular) bone mineral density than those who did not sustain a stress fracture. Meanwhile, Beck et al.[19] found that tibial stress fractures occur in individuals with smaller cross-sectional areas, section moduli, and widths. These structural properties are important because they reflect the ability of a bone to resist bending.

Muscle Factors

An intimate mechanical relationship exists between muscle and bone. Therefore muscles have the potential to influence bone loading and consequently may have a role in the etiology of stress fractures. Some suggest that stress fractures are initiated by excessive repetitive muscular forces,[53] but the consensus is that muscle is protective against rather than a cause of stress fractures.[54-57]

During impact loading, muscle is believed to serve as an active shock absorber, helping to attenuate loads as they are transmitted proximally along the kinetic chain. When muscles are dysfunctional (i.e., weakened, fatigued, or altered in their activation patterns), their ability to absorb loads becomes compromised, potentially leading to increased loading on the skeleton. Laboratory-based studies show that muscle fatigue causes an increase in both the magnitude and rate of bone strain.[58-61] Further support for a protective role for muscle in the development of stress fractures comes from prospective clinical studies, which have demonstrated that susceptibility to stress fractures is directly related to muscle factors (as indicated by measures of thigh and calf girth).[16,18,62]

Joint Factors

Joints and their associated structures (e.g., capsules, ligaments, and menisci) are important mediators in the transmission of applied loads; consequently, joint factors may contribute to the risk of stress fractures. During impact loading, joints typically are in an open-packed position and move through a certain range of motion. This arrangement is primarily to protect articular cartilage from excessive axial loads; however, it also functions to propagate forces away from the skeleton and to nonarticular structures (i.e., muscle). The best example of this is in the lower extremity, where knee and ankle flexion during landing from a jump are believed to reduce the magnitude of skeletal loading and thus protect against the development of stress fractures.[63,64] When joint motion is restricted, the consequence may be an increased magnitude of bone strain and an altered rate of bone loading.[65] Given the role of these load characteristics in microdamage formation, joint restriction may potentiate the formation of a stress fracture. Hughes[66] found a decrease in ankle dorsiflexion to be associated with the development of stress fractures, although subsequent research has failed to validate this finding.[16,67]

Biomechanical Factors

Muscle, joint, and bone factors by themselves may contribute to the intrinsic risk of stress fractures, but the way these factors work together as a functional unit also is important. Biomechanics are believed to influence the risk of stress fracture by influencing the magnitude, rate, and distribution of loads applied to the skeleton. However, establishing the relationship between individual biomechanical features and the risk of stress fractures is very difficult. Two primary reasons account for this: (1) assessment of dynamic biomechanical features typically requires complicated measurement tools that frequently are not readily available and that are time-consuming to use, and (2) a prospective study of risk factors for stress fractures requires the study of large numbers of individuals over long periods to generate sufficient statistical power. Consequently, few prospective studies have been done on the influence of specific biomechanical features on the risk of stress fractures.

According to the available literature, biomechanical factors that may predispose individuals to stress fracture are a high degree of external rotation of the hip,[68-70] leg length discrepancy,[16,71] and pes planus[33,67] and pes cavus.[28,72-74] Of these, the structure of the foot (pes planus or pes cavus) has received the most attention. A foot with a high longitudinal arch (pes cavus) is more rigid and has a reduced shock-absorbing capacity; this may allow more force to be transmitted proximally. A more flexible type of foot (pes planus) may attenuate more force, allowing less to be propagated proximally. This hypothesis is supported by the findings of Simkin et al.[74] who demonstrated that the foot arch structure influenced the location of stress fractures. Femoral and tibial stress fractures were more common in subjects with high-arched feet, whereas metatarsal stress fractures were more common in low-arched feet.

However, studies investigating the role of these foot types frequently assess the foot statically or when it is in a nonfunctional position. Clinically, what appears to be more important is the amount and duration of foot motion during dynamic loading. Static measurements do not necessarily correlate with the dynamic situation.[75] Prolonged pronation or hyperpronation during loading may lead to excessive torsion on the tibia, whereas limited pronation may reduce force attenuation by the foot and result in its subsequent proximal propagation.[41]

Lower Limb and Repetitive Stress

- The amount and duration of foot motion, rather than the type of foot (i.e., high arch or low arch), are most important in the development of repetitive stress injuries
- Leg length discrepancy plays a role in stress fractures

Although the structure of the foot has received the most attention, leg length discrepancy provides the most conclusive evidence for a biomechanical risk factor for stress fractures. A leg length discrepancy has been postulated as a risk factor for stress fracture because of its effect on skeletal alignment and loading symmetries. In their prospective study, Bennell et al.[16] found that a difference in leg length of more than 0.5 cm (0.2 inch) was more common in women who developed stress fractures than in those who did not. Stress fractures in these individuals occurred with equal frequency in the shorter and longer limbs; however, they were more likely to occur in the dominant limb.

Physical Fitness Factors

Physical fitness appears to be a predictor of the risk of stress fracture.[76] Studies in the military consistently have shown significant associations between low aerobic fitness levels and a higher risk of stress fracture during basic training.[77,78] Milgrom et al.[23] demonstrated in three prospective epidemiological studies that military recruits who played ball sports regularly for at least 2 years before basic training had less than half the risk of developing a stress fracture than recruits who did not play ball sports. Similarly, Lappe et al.[21] demonstrated that a history of regular exercise in military recruits was protective against stress fracture and that a longer history of exercise further reduced the relative risk. The reason for these differences has not been established; however, physical activity may cause beneficial changes in other intrinsic risk factors, such as skeletal, muscle, and joint factors. Although the risk factor of poor physical conditioning does not seem to apply to athletes because stress fractures often occur in well-conditioned individuals who have been training for years,[41] maintaining physical fitness after diagnosis of a stress fracture may be important for future risk.

Nutritional Factors

Four nutritional or dietary factors have been linked with stress fractures. The first relates to the dietary intake of calcium. Calcium deficiencies may contribute to the development of stress fractures by influencing bone density and remodeling. However, calcium appears to be important primarily during growth, when calcium intake influences bone accrual,[79] and after menopause, when calcium supplementation can reduce bone turnover and loss.[80,81] Lappe et al.[82] in a study of female Navy recruits showed reduction in stress fractures in those consuming 2000 mg of calcium and 800 International Units of vitamin D daily either as a supplement or through intake of dairy products.

The second dietary factor linked to the risk of stress fractures involves dietary behaviors and eating patterns. Stress fractures have been found to be more likely to occur in individuals who restrict caloric intake, avoid high-fat dairy foods, consume low-calorie products, have a self-reported history of an eating disorder, and have a lower percentage of ideal body weight.[83] In a cross-sectional study of young adult female track and field athletes, those with a history of stress fractures scored significantly higher on the **Eating Attitudes Test (EAT)-40** (a validated test relating to dieting, bulimia, and food preoccupation) and were more likely to engage in restrictive eating patterns and dieting.[14] Whether this association of stress fractures with dietary behaviors and eating patterns is causal or is due to some other factor is not clear.[41]

Third, lower levels of 25-hydroxyvitamin D may place men at risk for development of stress fractures. A study found that Finnish male military recruits who developed stress fractures were more likely to have lower levels of 25-hydroxyvitamin D.[84]

Lastly, a study of female military recruits demonstrated an increased risk of stress fracture with a history of smoking, exercising less than 3 times per week, and consuming more than 10 alcoholic drinks per week before the start of basic training.[20]

Stress Fractures are More Likely to Occur in Individuals Who:

- Restrict calorie intake
- Avoid high-fat dairy foods
- Consume low-calorie products
- Have a self-reported history of an eating disorder
- Have a lower percentage of ideal body weight
- Have a history of smoking
- Drink more than 10 alcoholic drinks per week

Gender Factors

Gender factors appear to contribute to susceptibility to stress fractures, and females are at greater risk.[41,76,85] A number of military studies have shown that women performing the same prescribed physical activities as men incur stress fractures at incidences 2 to 10 times higher than those for men.[77,86-89] This gender difference is not as evident in sports participation populations; studies in male and female athletes show either no difference or only a slightly increased risk for women.[15,17,30] However, the latter studies are somewhat limited because they were not able to control for differences in the amount or intensity of activity between genders.

The cause of the apparent higher incidence of stress fractures in females is not known. A possible cause may relate to gender-specific differences in endocrine factors. Physically active females have a higher prevalence of menstrual disturbances compared with the general female population.[90,91] Menstrual disturbance is a risk factor for stress fracture; the relative risk for stress fracture in amenorrheic female athletes is 2 to 4 times greater than in their eumenorrheic counterparts.[90] The mechanism by which endocrine disturbances in female athletes potentiate the development of stress fractures is not clear; however, they may alter the repair response to microdamage. Amenorrhea is associated with a reduction in bone turnover, particularly bone formation,[92,93] and a reduction in bone formation reduces the bones' ability to repair loading-induced microdamage. The net result is microdamage accumulation and potential progression to stress fracture.

CLINICAL DIAGNOSIS OF STRESS FRACTURES

Stress fractures typically present with a history consistent with an overuse injury—the gradual onset of activity-related pain. Because they occur along a continuum of pathology, signs and symptoms may vary, depending on the point along the continuum at which the patient presents. The stage along the continuum can be assigned clinically (Table 26-3).[94-96] An astute clinician can diagnose the pathology at the stress reaction stage. However, some patients may not present until the pathology has progressed

to a stress fracture, in which the bony cortices have actually been disrupted. The earlier in the continuum a diagnosis is made, the more likely it is that the pathology will respond quickly and favorably to treatment. Conversely, a delay in diagnosis potentially increases morbidity, which may influence the individual's long-term participation in the chosen activity. Therefore a certain level of suspicion must be maintained at all times in appropriately presenting patients to ensure prompt diagnosis.

A didactic history is the first step in the diagnosis of a stress fracture. In many cases individuals with stress fractures have a consistent, predictable history that typically centers around pain. At the start of the pathology continuum, pain usually is described as a mild ache that occurs after a specific amount of exercise. Because this initial pain typically subsides soon after exercise is completed and it is not present during rest, it often is ignored at first.

TABLE 26-3

Clinical and Radiographic Staging and Grading of Repetitive Stress Injuries to Bone

	STAGE OR GRADE				
	0	1	2	3	4
Pathology	None (normal remodeling)	Mild stress reaction	Moderate stress reaction	Severe stress reaction	Stress fracture
Signs and symptoms	Asymptomatic Can perform normal activity without symptoms	Local pain toward end of activity No resting pain	Local pain earlier during activity Tender on palpation	Significant pain during activity that does not abate after cessation of activity	Pain with everyday activities, at rest, and/or night pain
Radiography	Normal	Normal	Normal	Possible visible sclerosis and/or periosteal bone formation	Possible visible fracture line
Bone scintigraphy	Normal	Poorly defined area of increased uptake	More intense uptake but still poorly defined	Sharply marginated area of focal or fusiform increased activity	More intense, transcortical, localized uptake
CT	Normal	Normal	Normal	Focal cortical lucency, periosteal new bone, cortical bridging or focal stenosis	Visible cortical defect
MRI	Normal	Positive STIR image	Positive STIR and T_2 image	Positive T_1 and T_2 images but without definite cortical defect	Positive T_1 and T_2 images with definite cortical fracture line
Time course for recovery					

CT, computed tomography; *MRI*, magnetic resonance imaging; *STIR*, short T1 inversion recovery.

However, with continued exercise and progression of the pathology, the pain may become more severe or occur at an earlier stage, or both. It also may persist for longer periods after exercise is finished, and it may manifest during activities that involve lower levels of bone loading, such as walking. Ultimately, the pain can result in exercise restriction or the need to stop training completely. At this more advanced stage, the associated inflammatory response to the injury may occasionally contribute to resting and night pain.

On physical examination, the most obvious feature of a stress fracture is localized bony tenderness. This obviously is easier to establish in bones that are relatively superficial, and it may be absent with stress fractures in deep-seated bones, such as those in the shaft or neck of the femur. It is important to be precise in the palpation of the affected areas, particularly in regions such as the foot, where a number of bones and joints are located in a relatively small area. Because stress fractures are associated with an inflammatory reaction, localized redness, swelling, and warmth occasionally may be seen. In longer-standing conditions, periosteal thickening and callus formation may be felt.

The application of percussion, a vibrating tuning fork, or ultrasound have all been suggested as potential clinical tools for diagnosing stress fractures, but the sensitivity of each of these methods has been found to be low, and each is associated with high rates of false-negative findings.[97-99] In addition, a single leg hop test that produces severe localized pain in lower extremities has been reported as a method to help diagnose, although no recent literature supports this idea.[1] A fulcrum test can be used to assess for stress fractures of the femoral shaft. The patient will have pain at the fracture site when the clinician applies a bending force (e.g., over the exam table) to the distal femur.[100] A similar maneuver may be applied to any long bone although there is no supporting literature.

Besides obtaining a history of the pain and its relation to exercise, the clinician must determine whether any of the previously discussed risk factors is present. This is crucial because a history of a stress fracture is a significant risk factor for subsequent stress fractures.[101] By establishing potential risk factors during healing and intervening, it may be possible to influence future susceptibility. With all stress fractures involving the lower limb, a full biomechanical examination must be performed. Any evidence of leg length discrepancy, malalignment, muscle imbalance, weakness, or lack of flexibility or control should be noted.

A training or activity history also is essential. The clinician should note any recent changes in the patient's activity level, such as an increased amount or intensity of training, as well as any changes in surface, equipment, or technique; this information may need to be obtained from the patient's coach or trainer. A full dietary history should be taken, and particular attention should be paid to the possible presence of eating disorders. A menstrual history should be taken with female patients, including

the age of menarche and subsequent menstrual status. A history of previous similar injury or any other musculoskeletal injury should be obtained.

It is essential to obtain a brief history of the patient's general health, medications, and personal habits to ensure that none of these include factors that may influence bone health.

Factors to Consider in Assessing for Stress Fracture

- Pain
- Localized bone tenderness
- Level of activity and any changes to activity level
- Risk factors
- Leg length discrepancy (lower limb)
- Muscle imbalance
- Lack of flexibility
- Lack of movement control
- Dietary history
- Menstrual history (in females)
- History of stress fractures
- General health

DIAGNOSTIC IMAGING OF STRESS FRACTURES

Given its sensitivity in the diagnosis of stress fracture, clinical examination is sufficient in many cases. However, imaging can play an important supplementary role when the diagnosis is uncertain or when more specific knowledge is desired. A number of imaging techniques can be used for this purpose, but those most commonly used are radiography, bone scintigraphy, computed tomography (CT), and magnetic resonance imaging (MRI).

Radiography

Plain radiography (x-ray) typically is the most accessible imaging tool; however, it is the least useful for confirming a stress fracture because of its poor sensitivity. Although radiography primarily images the skeletal system and is useful for frank bone fractures, it is inherently planar in nature and has relatively low spatial resolution. These features do not allow radiography to detect the small defects associated with stress fractures; therefore radiography is associated with a high incidence of false-negative findings.[102]

X-rays may be able to demonstrate a stress fracture at later stages in the pathological process. Healing of a stress fracture typically involves initial resorption and subsequent formation of bone at the injured site, as well as callus formation periosteally. This may make the stress fracture site visible on radiography; the classic radiographic abnormalities are new periosteal bone formation, a visible area of sclerosis, the presence of callus, or a visible fracture line (Figure 26-3). These features, which typically are seen no earlier than 2 to 3 weeks after the onset of symptoms, are indicators of the reparative process. If any of these

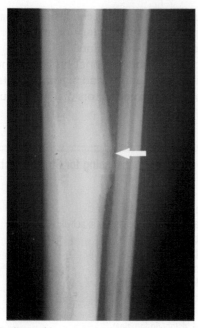

Figure 26-3 Radiographic appearance of a tibial stress fracture. The white arrow indicates a visible fracture line. Note the presence of new periosteal bone formation (callus).

radiographic signs are present, the diagnosis of stress fracture can be confirmed. However, in many cases of stress fracture, obvious radiographic abnormalities are not seen at any stage. Consequently, radiography is not considered a particularly useful tool for confirming a stress fracture. That being said, plain radiography is the best imaging modality to begin with.

Bone Scintigraphy

If plain radiography shows a stress fracture, further investigations may still be required. However, with high clinical suspicion of a stress fracture but a negative radiograph, bone scintigraphy is a frequent mode of investigation. Because of its nearly 100% sensitivity in the detection of stress fractures and its ability to indicate changes as early as 48 to 72 hours after the onset of symptoms, scintigraphy is frequently used.

Bone scintigraphy often is performed in the form of a triple-phase bone scan. This involves intravenous injection of a radiopharmaceutical marker, commonly a ^{99m}Tc-phosphate analogue. Three phases of marker uptake subsequently are assessed to determine the differential uptake of the marker. The initial phase (blood flow and angiogram phase) consists of serial images that are obtained during injection of the marker. This phase is used to demonstrate perfusion of the marker within the circulatory system, indicating areas of hyperperfusion. The second phase (blood pool phase) is imaged within 5 to 10 minutes after injection of the marker; this phase is used to indicate the extent of the extracellular fluid volume, thereby demonstrating areas of tissue hyperemia. The final phase (delayed phase) consists of images taken

2 to 4 hours after injection of the marker. By this time, urinary excretion of the marker has reduced the amount of marker present in soft tissues. The delayed phase therefore demonstrates uptake only in the osseous structures.

Because the delayed scan demonstrates uptake only in osseous structures, a conventional single-phase bone scan may be used to diagnose a stress fracture. On these and the delayed phase of the triple-phase bone scans, a stress fracture is characterized by a sharply marginated or fusiform area of increased local uptake involving one cortex or occasionally extending the width of the bone (Figure 26-4).[103] Based on the intensity of this uptake, the stage in the pathology continuum can be estimated (see Table 26-3)[103–105]; however, the grading systems for bone scintigraphy are not widely accepted.

Although bone scintigraphy has virtually 100% sensitivity, it is not without limitations. False-positive findings can occur, because other nontraumatic lesions (e.g., tumors, infections, and bone infarctions) can also cause localized increased uptake of the marker.[102,106] Therefore, bone scintigraphy lacks specificity.[107] Specificity can be increased somewhat by using a triple-phase rather than a single-phase bone scan because the former allows differentiation between soft tissue and osseous pathology.

A stress injury to bone is identified by localized increased uptake of the radiopharmaceutical marker in all three phases of the scan.[108,109] This is not the case with other bony abnormalities (e.g., periostitis), which are only positive on delayed images,[109,110] or with soft tissue injuries, which are positive only in the blood flow and blood pool phases.[111] Even with this approach, the specificity of bone scintigraphy is limited because it does not allow direct visualization of the fracture itself, and precisely

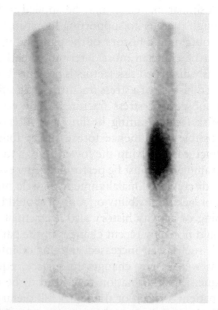

Figure 26-4 Bone scintigraphy (scintigram) of a tibial stress fracture. The stress fracture is revealed by the fusiform area of increased uptake of the radiopharmaceutical marker.

locating the site, especially in the foot, can be difficult. This may be important for management considerations. An additional limitation for the use of bone scintigraphy is the level of ionizing radiation associated with the test.

Computed Tomography

CT can be useful for diagnosing the more advanced stages on the pathology continuum (i.e., stress fractures); it has a high specificity because of its ability to image bone with good spatial resolution. However, it does not appear particularly useful for diagnosing stress reactions in which a cortical defect does not exist. In addition, the role of CT is mainly limited to differentiating causes of increased uptake on bone scan that may mimic stress fracture. These include osteoid osteoma, osteomyelitis with a Brodie's abscess, and other malignancies.[111] A stress fracture on CT is identified by a combination of a visible cortical defect, focal cortical lucency, periosteal new bone, and cortical bridging (Figure 26-5).[112-114] Although CT is used primarily in differential diagnosis, it can also be useful in cases in which plain radiography is normal, the isotope bone scan shows increased uptake, and demonstration of a fracture line may affect treatment.[85,111] Such a scenario occurs with stress fractures of the navicular[112,115] and longitudinal stress fractures of the tibia and femur.[116,117]

Magnetic Resonance Imaging

Of all the imaging techniques for stress fractures, MRI has emerged as the premier technique. Although MRI does not image cortical bone as well as CT and its sensitivity is comparable to that of bone scintigraphy, it has surpassed these techniques in the detection of stress fractures because it has much greater specificity as a result of its wide contrast resolution and high spatial resolution.[107,118,119] In addition, the patient is not exposed to radiation. MRI is able to image osseous tissues and provides simultaneous excellent representation of soft tissues and

associated processes, thereby providing greater diagnostic information than can be obtained from other imaging techniques. This includes depiction of the extent and orientation of a stress fracture, factors that may influence management.[120]

MRI can be performed on a wide array of equipment and using a variety of pulse sequences. The best equipment for imaging stress fractures is that which provides the optimum contrast and spatial resolution. In terms of sequences, those most commonly used are T_1- and T_2-weighted images and fat-suppression techniques, such as short T_1 inversion recovery (STIR) and T_2 fat saturation views. Specific MRI characteristics of stress fractures, which depend on the sequence used, include (1) a fracture line that appears on all sequences as a very low signal medullary band contiguous with the cortex; (2) surrounding marrow hemorrhage and edema, seen as low signal intensity on T_1-weighted images and as high signal on T_2-weighted and STIR images; and (3) periosteal edema and hemorrhage, which appear as high signal intensity on T_2-weighted and STIR images and low signal intensity on T_1-weighted images (Figure 26-6).[121] The stage in the pathology continuum can be estimated based on the findings with each sequence (see Table 26-3).

MRI can image bone edema and can be used to depict a bone stress reaction. This is considered a precursor to a stress fracture, and it shows on MRI as an area of altered intensity signal (increased signal on T_2-weighted and STIR images, decreased signal on T_1-weighted images) without the presence of a fracture line. However, the finding of stress reactions on MRI in asymptomatic individuals does not appear to be of clinical significance.[122] Stress reactions are common in individuals who take part in intensive physical activity, and they commonly heal or remain asymptomatic, even if

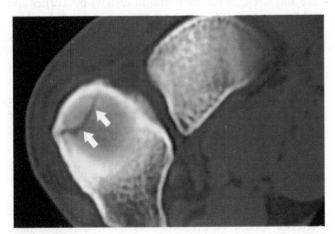

Figure 26-5 CT (tomogram) of a navicular stress fracture. The arrows indicate a visible cortical defect.

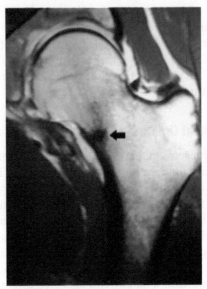

Figure 26-6 MRI scan of a femoral neck stress fracture. The arrow indicates a region of altered signal intensity.

the intensive physical activity continues.[120,122] Therefore the use of MRI to detect areas of stress reactions in asymptomatic individuals does not appear to be warranted.

False-negative MRI findings in the assessment of stress fractures do occur; however, they typically are due to reader error, suboptimum choice of imaging planes and sequences, inhomogeneities in fat suppression, and partial volume effects.[118,123] For this reason, MRI operators and readers experienced in the imaging of stress fractures are critical to an accurate diagnosis.

PREVENTION AND MANAGEMENT OPTIONS FOR STRESS FRACTURES

Prevention

Despite the clinical significance of stress fractures, currently only limited prevention strategies are available.[124] The primary reason for this is the apparent multifactorial etiology of the condition. Stress fractures appear to occur in different people as a result of different factors. Consequently there is no single factor that can be modified to prevent stress fractures. However, because stress fractures result from the accumulation of loading-induced damage, preventive strategies typically focus on controlling the strain experienced by the skeleton. By reducing the magnitude and rate of strain within a bone and the absolute number of loading cycles, the amount of damage and the consequent risk for stress fracture may be positively influenced.

It seems reasonably safe to assume that modification of training schedules is a good way to start reducing the incidence of stress fractures. Decreasing either the intensity or volume of training may benefit the system by allowing much needed recovery time between activity bouts.

Orthotic inserts, such as those that cushion a supinated foot, may be helpful in preventing lower limb stress fractures. Shock-absorbing shoe inserts have been proven to be effective in reducing the occurrence of lower extremity stress injury in military recruits.[125]

Consuming 2000 mg of calcium and 800 International Units of vitamin D daily either as a supplement or through intake of dairy products will help decrease the chance of stress fractures as well.[82]

Management Options

As with prevention, few established intervention techniques exist for treating a stress fracture.[124] The major goal for clinicians in managing acute musculoskeletal injuries is to return the individual to the preinjury level of function, ideally in the shortest time possible and without compromising healing at the tissue level. One method of accomplishing this is to accelerate the rate of tissue repair. Unfortunately, limited interventions are capable of achieving this. The current, accepted alternative is to facilitate rehabilitation and return the patient to activity

while ensuring that tissue healing is not overtly compromised.[126] The following sections discuss different options in the prevention and management of stress fractures and when available the scientific evidence behind their use.

Exercise

Exercise has important roles in both the prevention and treatment of stress fractures through its effects on intrinsic risk factors, including skeletal, muscle, and joint factors. Because the risk of stress fractures is directly influenced by bone factors, it has been hypothesized that modification of these properties through an exercise program may be a means of preventing stress fractures.[19,22,23,47,127]

Although an exercise program that incorporates mechanical loading can lead to skeletal fatigue, it also can act as a potent anabolic stimulus.[128] Bone is inherently mechanosensitive and responds and adapts to its mechanical environment. Warden et al.[47] demonstrated that bone structural changes induced by a mechanical loading program cause an exponential increase in fatigue resistance; this occurs as new bone formation in response to loading at biomechanically relevant sites. This enables a bone to better resist applied loads, which subsequently reduces the magnitude of strain the bone experiences.

An exercise program that incorporates mechanical loading may be used to positively modify skeletal risk factors in sedentary individuals before a training program is started (such as in military recruits). However, those who design exercise programs to influence the risk of stress fractures must keep in mind that although repetitive mechanical loading can act as a potent anabolic stimulus, it also can lead to skeletal fatigue. Therefore exercise programs need to be designed to induce the desired changes in bone structure without inflicting harm in the form of generated damage and its accumulation. One method of achieving this is to ensure that the duration of exercise (and therefore the number of loading cycles to which a bone is exposed) is restricted. Further details on designing an exercise program to enhance bone structure and strength can be found in reviews by Turner and Robling[129,130] and Warden et al.[128]

Although an exercise program may positively influence skeletal risk factors for stress fractures in sedentary individuals, its potential to reduce the risk of stress fractures in athletes is debatable. Studies consistently have demonstrated that athletes have increased bone mass and size compared with controls.[25,131-133] The ability of an exercise program to further modify bone material and structural properties in these individuals is questionable. However, an exercise program in athletes can be used to modify muscle and joint risk factors. Athletes should be regularly screened for muscle activation patterns, strength, and endurance. Preventive muscle strengthening and endurance exercises should be prescribed to individuals who have had a stress fracture.

The use of exercise as a possible prevention strategy for stress fractures has previously been hypothesized[19,22,23,127] and has initial clinical support.[21-23,134] Milgrom et al.[23] demonstrated in three prospective epidemiological studies that military recruits who played ball sports regularly for at least 2 years before basic training had less than half the risk of developing a stress fracture than recruits who did not play ball sports. Similarly, Lappe et al.[21] demonstrated that a history of regular exercise in military recruits was protective against stress fracture and that a longer history of exercise further reduced the relative risk.

Shoes and Inserts

Shoes and inserts (i.e., orthotics and insoles) have been suggested as potential means of modifying the risk of stress fractures during weight-bearing activities. Located at the foot-ground interface, shoes and inserts act as filters that theoretically attenuate ground impact forces. In addition, they have the potential to influence the motion of the foot and ankle and the subsequent mechanics proximally in the kinetic chain. Through these two mechanisms, shoes and inserts may lower bone strain, which may reduce the risk of stress fractures.

The evidence on the ability of shoes and inserts to prevent stress fractures is contradictory, and most of these data are generated in military studies. Initial studies failed to find any benefit in preventing stress fractures from placing a shock-absorbing insole in a standard military boot.[34,135] A more recent prospective, randomized controlled trial demonstrated a statistically significant difference in the incidence of stress fractures between recruits who trained with custom orthoses and those who trained without such devices; the incidence was double among nonusers of the orthoses.[68] However, this finding was not confirmed in a subsequent study by the same research group, who found no significant differences between recruits wearing either soft or semirigid prefabricated or custom orthoses.[136] Combining the findings of four trials, a Cochrane review suggested that the use of shock-absorbing insoles may prevent stress fractures of the lower extremities.[124]

For shoes, the evidence is similarly contradictory. Although recruits who trained in a modified basketball shoe had a lower incidence of metatarsal stress fractures compared with those who trained in a standard infantry boot, no differences were seen in the incidence of tibial or femoral stress fractures.[137] No differences were also noted in the total number of stress fractures between the two groups. In contrast, Gardner et al.[34] found that the shock absorption provided by shoes may be important in preventing stress fractures. This was indicated by the fact that the risk of stress fracture increased when military training was started with a shoe of advanced age.

If shoes and inserts potentially are able to influence bone strain and therefore the risk of stress fracture, the question remains as to how to apply this information to individual patients. Shoes and inserts reportedly are used to prevent stress fractures by improving cushioning (i.e., reducing bone strain) and aligning the skeleton (i.e., changing mechanics). Although these mechanisms seem logical, supportive scientific evidence is lacking. In one study, when soft or semirigid orthoses were worn with running shoes, neither significantly influenced tibial peak strain or strain rates during running.[138] Similarly, studies have been unable to find significant differences between shoes of differing shock absorptive capacity in tibial peak strain or strain rates during running.[139-141]

In terms of the ability of shoes and inserts to influence skeletal alignment, studies using bone pin markers have shown that the differences in bone movements between barefoot and shod running are small and unsystematic (mean effects were less than 2) compared with differences between subjects (up to 10).[142,143] Similarly, inserts do not appear to alter rear foot and tibial joint coupling substantially during running.[144,145] What can be gathered from this is that bone strains and skeletal kinematics during running appear to be unique to each individual, and shoe and insert modifications do not seem to be able to change them substantially.

Because shoes and inserts do not appear to be able to reduce bone strain or change skeletal mechanics substantially, other mechanisms need to be considered to guide their clinical prescription. A growing concept is the effect of shoes and inserts on muscle activity.[146,147] Muscle activity in the leg is tuned in response to impact force characteristics.[148,149] This activity is influenced by running in shoes of differing material characteristics.[150,151] Whether this tuning affects the risk of stress fracture has not been established; however, with shoe and insert prescription, the paramount issue appears to be comfort. This is important both for adherence and for potential benefit. If a shoe or insert is not comfortable, it will not be used, and any potential benefit will not be gained. Also, the comfort of inserts has been found to influence the kinematics, kinetics, and muscle activity in the lower extremity during running.[152] Therefore from a practical perspective, shoes and inserts should be chosen based on their comfort to the individual. Typically this is a shoe or insert that is appropriate for the individual's foot structure and mechanics.

Pneumatic Leg Braces

Pneumatic leg braces are frequently used in the management of stress fractures, primarily stress fractures of the tibial diaphysis.[153-160] The most commonly used brace is the Aircast leg brace (Aircast Corp., Summit, NJ) (Figure 26-7). Although pneumatic leg braces are not believed to influence the rate of tissue healing directly, they appear to function as stress sharing devices that help redistribute and attenuate ground impact forces. This, combined with the application of pressure to the injured limb, appears to help reduce the pain associated with stress fractures and

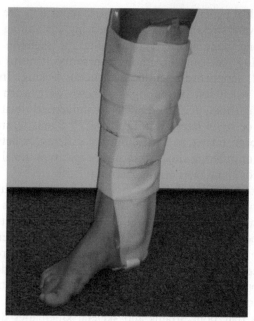

Figure 26-7 Aircast leg brace. (From Magee DJ, Zachazewski JE, Quillen WS, editors: *Scientific foundations and principles of practice in musculoskeletal rehabilitation,* p 612, St Louis, 2007, WB Saunders.)

allows an earlier return to function, apparently without detriment to the healing tissues.

Preliminary evidence indicates the efficacy of pneumatic leg braces in the management of stress fractures.[154-157,159,160] The most convincing evidence was provided by Swenson et al.[159] In a randomized, prospective study of 18 competitive and recreational athletes, they found that use of the Aircast allowed earlier return to light and full activity after a tibial diaphyseal stress fracture. Furthermore, they noted that athletes who used the brace became pain free at a median of 14±6 days after initiation of treatment, compared with 45±9 days in athletes who did not use the brace. A subsequent study attempted to replicate this finding in a military population.[153] However, this study suffered severely from a large dropout rate (35%) and an inappropriate study design, which compromised the researchers' ability to detect a significant difference between groups. Supporting the use of pneumatic air braces, a Cochrane review indicated a likely benefit of such braces for a faster return to sports.[124]

A Cochrane review pooling data from three small studies suggested that patients with a tibial stress fracture who used a pneumatic brace (e.g., a stirrup leg brace) showed a significant reduction in time to recommencing full activity; however, more evidence is needed because the information is based on a small number of subjects.[125]

Training Program Design

If stress fractures are to be prevented, training programs need to be designed with consideration given to their effects on the skeleton. Although individuals need to progress their training or activity programs to induce adaptation in desired systems and improve performance, this can have adverse effects on the skeleton. Changes in training or activity, intensity, duration, frequency, type, surface, technique, and equipment all can affect the generation of damage and its accumulation in bone. A training or activity program that introduces multiple, simultaneous changes in training may lead to the development of a stress fracture. For example, military studies have shown that those who experience a significant change in a training program (e.g., recruits with no history of physical activity before starting intense infantry training) are at greater risk of a stress fracture.[22,24] Therefore changes in a training or activity program should be made progressively, and limited variables should be changed at a given time.

In addition, the use of cyclical training methods should be explored, particularly in those prone to stress fractures as indicated by a past history of such injuries. Cyclical training may involve the introduction of rest periods into a training program or the replacement of high bone-loading activities, such as running, with low bone-loading activities, such as cycling, swimming, or water running. This may involve a monthly regimen of 3 weeks of high-load activities and 1 week of no load or low-load activities. Such a program has been shown to reduce the incidence of stress fracture in military populations.[161]

Training and Activity Programs and Stress Reduction

- Changes should be progressive
- Variables should be limited
- Time should be allowed between changes
- Cyclic training methods with rest periods should be used
- Both high-load and low-load activities should be included

Pharmacological Intervention

Bisphosphonates

Bisphosphonates cause osteoclast apoptosis[162] and are traditionally prescribed to prevent the loss of bone associated with aging. However, bisphosphonates also have been suggested as a means of preventing stress fractures.[163] Osteoclasts participate in targeted remodeling by resorbing bone to remove areas of damage.[164] Although this removal of damage is important, an increase in the number and activity of osteoclasts augments damage formation by increasing bone porosity. This feedforward reduces the elastic modulus of the bone, which in turn increases strain and subsequently the rate of damage formation. Therefore short-term suppression of bone turnover with bisphosphonates may prevent the initial loss of bone during the remodeling response to damage and may prevent progression to stress fracture.[163] However, evidence for this hypothesis is scarce, and the only currently available clinical trial demonstrated that one bisphosphonate (i.e., risedronate) did not influence the incidence of stress fractures in military recruits.[22]

Nonsteroidal Anti-inflammatory Drugs

Nonsteroidal anti-inflammatory drugs (NSAIDs) frequently are used as adjunct therapies in the treatment of stress fractures,[165,166] in which the basic tenet for their use is to treat symptoms related to inflammation (i.e., pain). Although these drugs are effective pain relievers, their role during the repair of stress fractures has been questioned.[167-169] Pain is an important indicator of the pathology in stress fractures, one that is used not only for diagnosis but also to determine the progression of treatment and the patient's eventual return to full activity. Inhibiting this pain may mask possible progression of symptoms and the pathology.

In addition to masking symptoms, NSAIDs also may delay tissue-level healing at the stress fracture site.[168,169] NSAIDs exert their predominant effects by inhibiting cyclooxygenase (COX) enzyme activity. The COX isozymes catalyze the rate-limiting step in the formation of prostaglandins (PGs) from arachidonic acid. PGs synthesized after injury participate in inflammation by causing vasodilation and increasing local vascular permeability.[170] Although limiting this response may appear advantageous, the PGs synthesized after injury are crucial to the repair of injured bone. PGs affect bone formation and resorption, which are mediated through the proliferation and differentiation of osteoblasts and the regulation of osteoclast differentiation.[171] In animal models, removal of these effects through NSAID inhibition of the COX enzymes appears to be detrimental to the repair process.[172-175] Although animal studies have limited translation to the clinical setting, NSAIDs should be used sparingly in the management of stress fractures because of their ability to mask symptoms and their potential to influence the rate of tissue-level healing.

Modalities

Therapeutic Ultrasound

Therapeutic ultrasound therapy may represent a unique treatment for stress fractures in that it may accelerate tissue-level repair to facilitate recovery and allow earlier return to activity. Although systematic reviews and meta-analyses repeatedly have concluded that the evidence is insufficient to support current clinical applications of ultrasound,[176-179] research has shown that ultrasound can have clinically significant beneficial effects on injured bone.[180] These benefits were generated using low-intensity (less than $0.1\,W/cm^2$) pulsed ultrasound (LIPUS), a dose alternative to that traditionally used in sports medicine.[181]

LIPUS has developed into an established intervention for bone injuries (for a complete review, see Rubin

et al.[182] and Warden et al.[183,184]). In brief, during fresh fracture repair in three well-designed, randomized controlled trials, LIPUS was shown to accelerate the rate of fresh tibial, radial, and scaphoid fracture repair by 30% to 38%.[185-187] When the results of the 158 fractures investigated were pooled, a weighted average effect size was calculated at 6.41.[188] This converts into a mean difference in healing time of 64 days between the active- and inactive-ultrasound treated groups. In addition to its beneficial effects on fresh fractures, LIPUS has been shown to facilitate healing in fractures with delayed union or nonunion.[189-192] It has been found to stimulate union in 91% of fractures showing delayed union and in 86% of fractures showing nonunion.[190] These fractures covered a range of skeletal sites.

The effect of LIPUS on traditional bone fractures is of interest in the treatment of stress fractures because the latter are believed to heal in stages comparable to those of traditional bone fractures. Previous trials of the effect of LIPUS on fracture repair have shown efficacy for healing of small, undisplaced fractures. This suggests that LIPUS may have beneficial effects on stress fracture repair, a hypothesis that has variable support from preliminary case reports and one clinical trial.[157,193,194]

In seven posteromedial cortex stress fractures of the tibia, introduction of LIPUS enabled continuation of activity and return to competition within 4 weeks.[193] In one tarsal navicular stress fracture, LIPUS reportedly stimulated bony union and allowed return to competition within 5 weeks.[193] In contrast to these case reports, the one available randomized clinical trial (RCT) showed LIPUS to have no effect on tibial stress fracture repair, as assessed by the total number of symptomatic days.[194] Because RCTs are the highest level of evidence, this finding would indicate that LIPUS is not actually beneficial to stress fracture repair. However, the trial was statistically underpowered and could detect only a 36% (20-day) difference in healing time between groups. In contrast to this limited evidence in the treatment of acute stress fractures, LIPUS has been shown to be effective in stress fractures showing delayed union and nonunion; it was found to stimulate union in 98% and 94% of cases, respectively.[190] These findings suggest that LIPUS may have beneficial effects on stress fracture repair; however, this needs to be established through appropriately designed clinical trials.

Electromagnetic Fields

Electromagnetic fields have been considered as a modality that may facilitate stress fracture repair. The use of electromagnetic fields to aid bone healing arose from the discovery that bone tissue generates an internal electrical field when it is deformed by mechanical forces.[195,196] In physiological moist bone, these mechanoelectrical potentials (known as *stress-generated streaming potentials*) are believed to result from the mechanically induced movement of charged particles throughout bone channels.[197]

These streaming potentials are considered to be biologically important, potentially representing an intermediate signal by which bone cells sense functional demands. Therefore it has been hypothesized that the application of electrical fields may be able to stimulate osteogenesis by stimulating the natural endogenous streaming potentials in bone.[198]

Although a rationale exists for the use of electromagnetic fields on damaged bone, strong supportive evidence is lacking. Numerous observational studies have suggested a beneficial role of electromagnetic fields during fracture repair; however, few controlled studies have been performed. The controlled studies that have been performed suggest that electromagnetic fields may be primarily beneficial to fractures that show delayed union or nonunion.[199] Electromagnetic fields do not appear to be beneficial to acute fracture repair processes; however, preliminary evidence has demonstrated that electromagnetic fields may be safely applied to healing stress fractures,[200] although this does not imply efficacy.

Nutrition

Calcium and vitamin D supplementation may help in prevention of stress fractures. A 20% lower incidence of stress fractures compared with a placebo group was seen in female recruits who took a daily calcium supplement (2000 mg) and vitamin D supplement (800 International Units).[82]

MANAGEMENT OF STRESS REACTIONS AND LOW-RISK STRESS FRACTURES

The management of a stress fracture depends on its risk for healing complications.[201] Most stress fractures represent relatively straightforward management problems. These stress fractures are uncomplicated and typically respond to relative rest from the aggravating activity and removal or modification of risk factors.

The major goal for clinicians in managing low-risk stress fractures is to return the patient to the preinjury level of function, ideally in the shortest time possible and without compromising tissue-level healing. To accomplish this, graduated loading programs are commonly used, with pain as the directive variable. Most clinicians agree that pain is a useful guide in assessing the progress of an injury toward healing, particularly stress fractures. In the management of low-risk stress fractures, the objective is to facilitate function while keeping pain below the patient's pain threshold. Because pain is the directive variable, pharmacological manipulation of pain using analgesics or NSAIDs is not advisable. These agents may be used in the initial stages if a patient has resting, night, or severe pain, but they should be withdrawn as soon as possible because they can mask pain and may allow too rapid a progression through a graduated loading program.

A **graduated loading program** is used in the management of low-risk stress fractures to apply controlled loading and to facilitate return to full function in a timely fashion. Although mechanical loading is central to the development of a stress fracture, its complete removal is not necessary or advised during recovery. Bone is mechanosensitive, and removal of all mechanical loading has a negative influence on the skeletal risk factors for stress fractures. In addition, the removal of loading may delay healing, because osteoblasts respond to mechanical loading by increasing necessary reparative bone formation. Therefore the recovery needs of the injured tissue and patient are best met in low-risk stress fractures by a balance of rest from aggravating activities and the performance of appropriate loading. Appropriate loading is defined as loading that does not provoke a patient's signs or symptoms at a rating higher than 2 on a 0 to 10 scale (where 0 is no pain and 10 is the most severe pain the person has ever experienced), either during the activity or after it is completed. Using this definition, individuals can be progressed through a graduated loading program.

Box 26-1 presents an example of a graduated loading program for commonly occurring posteromedial tibial stress fractures. This program consists of a preentry stage and five loading stages. Stage 0, the preentry stage, is the stage in which the patient experiences pain during walking and in normal activities of daily living. During this stage, some patients may require gait aids to facilitate a natural gait pattern; however, these should be removed as soon as possible. Once the patient is completely pain free for 3 consecutive days, the individual can begin stage 1 of the loading program. Stage 1 involves 30-minute exercise sessions of walking and jogging. There are 2 consecutive days of loading, followed by 1 day of rest. On the rest day, the patient should not perform any weight-bearing exercise, including prolonged walking. In stage 2, loading is progressed to solely jogging, which is performed every second day at increasing durations. Jogging duration is further progressed in stage 3 and is performed for 4 days in 1 week. The last two stages incorporate individualized running and activity until return to full activity is achieved.

In each stage of the graduated loading program, successful completion of each level is determined by pain. During each loading session, the patient must stop exercising if the individual experiences pain that he or she would rate higher than 2 on the 0 to 10 scale. If this occurs, the patient must return to the previous loading level for the remainder of the session. If pain rated higher than 2 is still experienced, the patient must stop the loading session. The amount of pain the patient experiences in the last loading session determines the level at which the person will exercise in the next session. If the patient successfully completes a loading session with pain rated below 2 on the 0 to 10 scale and did not experience any pain after completion of loading, the individual can progress to the next level in that stage. When the patient has successfully

BOX 26-1
Graduated Loading Program

Stage 0	**Preentry to graduated loading program**
	Pain during walking in normal activities of daily living

Stage 1	**Walk and jog stage (2 days loading, 1 day rest)**
Level A	Walk 30 min
B	Walk 9 min and jog 1 min (×3)
C	Rest
D	Walk 8 min and jog 2 min (×3)
E	Walk 7 min and jog 3 min (×3)
F	Rest
G	Walk 6 min and jog 4 min (×3)
H	Walk 5 min and jog 5 min (×3)
I	Rest
J	Walk 4 min and jog 6 min (×3)
K	Walk 3 min and jog 7 min (×3)
L	Rest
M	Walk 2 min and jog 8 min (×3)
N	Walk 1 min and jog 9 min (×3)
O	Rest

Stage 2	**Jogging every second day**
Level A	Jog 12 min
B	Rest
C	Jog 15 min
D	Rest
E	Jog 15 min
F	Rest
G	Jog 17 min
H	Rest
I	Jog 17 min
J	Rest
K	Jog 20 min
L	Rest
M	Jog 20 min

Stage 3	**Jogging (4 loading days in 1 week)**
Level A	Jog 25 min
B	Rest
C	Jog 25 min
D	Rest
E	Jog 30 min
F	Jog 30 min
G	Rest

Stage 4	**Individualized running (5 loading days in 1 week)**
Level A	Running
B	Running
C	Rest
D	Running
E	Running
F	Rest
G	Running

Stage 5	**Return to activity (individualized)**

completed each level, he or she can progress to the next stage. However, if the patient is unable to successfully complete a loading session because of pain but can train at the previous loading level for the remainder of the session, then at the next session the patient should reattempt the loading session that could not be completed because of pain. If the patient was unable to successfully complete a loading session because of pain and could not train at the previous loading level because of pain, then at the next loading session the patient should train at the last level he or she successfully attempted.

Using a graduated loading program that is strictly guided by pain to manage low-risk stress fractures, the patient and clinician can facilitate recovery while being relatively confident the pathology is not progressing. Of course, this requires the full understanding of the patient regarding the appropriate progression through the program and adherence to the set pain levels. Patients with lower grade injuries (i.e., stress reactions) may be able to progress more quickly through a graduated loading program, and the total duration of their program may be reduced from that shown in Box 26-1. Program duration should be based on the expected time course for recovery, which in turn depends on the stage of pathology in which the patient presents. Therefore all patients should perform individualized programs.

To further facilitate functional recovery of postero-medial tibial stress fractures, a pneumatic leg brace may be prescribed for wear during waking hours, including during a graduated loading program. In addition, LIPUS may be used to try to accelerate the rate of tissue-level repair. At all times during recovery, patients can maintain fitness by cycling, water running, or working out on exercise machines. In addition, individual risk factors for stress fractures identified during the examination need to be addressed as early as possible during management. The high rate of recurrence of stress fractures is an indication that risk factors are an often neglected component in management programs.

Complete recovery from a stress fracture has occurred when a patient completes the graduated loading program, has no local tenderness, and is able to perform the precipitating activity without pain.[8] This can be achieved with most stress fractures within 6 to 8 weeks of clinical presentation.[8] In most cases attempting to monitor healing radiologically is not useful; the radiological appearance of healing stress fractures can be deceptive, because the fracture still is visible well after clinical healing has occurred.[85,202]

Stress Fractures and Diagnostic Imaging

- Radiographs and bone scans should not be used to monitor the progress of fracture healing because imaging signs of healing lag well behind actual clinical healing.

MANAGEMENT OF *"HIGH-RISK"* STRESS FRACTURES

Most stress fractures heal without complication and have a low risk of complications. However, certain stress fractures present diagnostic and treatment challenges. These include stress fractures that are prone to delayed union or nonunion and/or are at high risk for progression to complete fracture. Specific sites for these stress fractures are the neck of the femur, anterior cortex of the tibia, medial malleolus, talus, navicular, fifth metatarsal, and great toe sesamoids. Stress fractures at these sites require specific management (Table 26-4).

Neck of the Femur

Femoral neck stress fractures are relatively uncommon in athletes (fewer than 5% of all stress fractures),[203] but they can have serious consequences. This stress fracture should be considered in the differential diagnosis when an individual, especially an athlete, presents with a history of gradual or acute-onset anterior hip, groin, or knee pain that is aggravated by exercise.[204-206] The physical examination may also reveal pain and restriction at the end of passive hip range of motion.[205-207] However, early diagnosis can be difficult because these signs are nonspecific; therefore a high level of clinical suspicion is required at all times. Early diagnosis is very important for successful management because delay is not conducive to a good prognosis.[203,208]

Femoral neck stress fractures typically are classified into three categories: *tension, compression,* and *displaced*.[209] Tension femoral neck stress fractures occur on the superior margin of the femoral neck and are radiographically visible as a cortical discontinuity. This type occurs predominantly in older patients, commonly in association with bone disease (osteoporosis), although it has been

---

TABLE 26-4

Common Management Approaches for High-Risk Stress Fractures

Stress Fracture Site	Management
Femoral neck	Initially bed rest and non–weight-bearing crutches, then gradual weight bearing for undisplaced fractures; surgical fixation for displaced fractures
Anterior cortex of the tibia	Rest, non–weight-bearing cast immobilization or surgical intervention (intramedullary rod fixation)
Medial malleolus	Non–weight-bearing cast immobilization for 6 weeks or surgical intervention
Talus (lateral process)	Non–weight-bearing cast immobilization for 6 weeks
Navicular	Non–weight-bearing cast immobilization for 6 weeks
Base of the fifth metatarsal	Cast immobilization or percutaneous screw fixation
Great toe sesamoids	Non–weight-bearing for 4 weeks or surgical intervention

---

reported in active younger patients.[210] Tension stress fractures are at increased risk of progression to complete fracture because they are unstable; therefore management may involve operative stabilization.[206]

Compression femoral neck stress fractures occur on the inferior femoral neck and are characterized radiologically by a periosteal reaction, or callus formation, without evidence of a fracture line.[206] This type typically occurs in younger athletes and has a lower risk of fracture displacement because it is more stable. The typical intervention for these stress fractures and frequently for tension femoral neck stress fractures is conservative, involving rest initially, until passive hip movement is pain free, followed by non-weight bearing on crutches until radiographic evidence of healing is seen.[201] Weight-bearing exercise is resumed gradually and built up to the patient's preinjury level over 6 to 8 weeks.

Displaced femoral neck stress fractures occur with progression of a stress fracture and subsequent displacement of the fractured bones. Displaced stress fractures carry the risk of avascular necrosis of the femoral head and should be treated promptly through surgical fixation.[211,212]

Types of Femoral Neck Stress Fractures

- Tension
- Compression
- Displaced

Anterior Cortex of the Tibia

Most tibial stress fractures occur along the posteromedial aspect of the bone and respond to rest and a gradual return to weight-bearing activity. Less often, stress fractures occur along the anterior tibial cortex; these are a particular concern because they are prone to nonunion and possible progression to complete fracture.[155,213] Nonunion of these stress fractures is demonstrated radiographically by a discontinuity of the anterior part of the cortex (the so-called dreaded black line), which suggests bony resorption at the fracture site (Figure 26-8). At this time, the patient may have been symptomatic for some months, but frequently the symptoms are minimal and the individual has been able to continue activity.[201] This can result in progression to an acute transverse fracture because of the affected tibial mechanics.[214]

The treatment of stress fractures of the anterior cortex of the tibia is aggressive, involving rest, immobilization in a non–weight-bearing cast, or early surgery (insertion of an intramedullary rod).[201,215,216] Each of these methods requires a prolonged recovery period, and return to full activity takes 6 to 12 months.[216,217] An alternative approach may be to use a pneumatic leg brace with an anterior pad for activities of daily living and for free walking once the patient is pain free.[154] However, this approach still requires a lengthy recovery period (7 to 11 months in the reported cases). Other simultaneously introduced interventions may include application of electromagnetic fields and LIPUS therapy.[155,216]

Medial Malleolus

Stress fractures of the medial malleolus occur in distance runners and jumpers (e.g., basketball players and gymnasts).[218–220] These individuals typically present with chronic or acute pain over the medial malleolus, sometimes with an associated ankle effusion.[220,221] On imaging, the stress fractures are identified by focal increased uptake on bone scintigraphy.[218] When observed on radiography, CT, or MRI, the fracture line often is vertical from the tibial plafond and medial malleolus but may arch obliquely from the distal tibial metaphysis.[201,222] Because these stress fractures can develop into a nonunion and progress to complete fracture,[218,219,223] specific management is required.

Several authors have recommended that patients with a visible fracture line on radiography, CT, or MRI undergo open reduction and internal fixation, particularly if they are elite athletes.[219,220] Postoperative management is early range of motion exercises with protected weight bearing.[222] Fractures that are positive on bone scan and negative on more specific forms of imaging (i.e., radiography, CT, and MRI) can be treated with immobilization in a pneumatic brace.[201,220] Whether a conservative or surgical approach is taken, the usual recovery time after the initiation of treatment is 6 to 8 weeks,[220] although it may be extended in some cases (up to 5 months).[221] During recovery, any identifiable risk factors that cause stress overloading of the medial ankle should be addressed.

Talus

Stress fractures of the talus are relatively rare; however, they can occur in multiple locations, the most frequent site being the lateral body of the talus and its lateral process.[224–228] Stress fractures at this site can extend into the subtalar joint and are prone to nonunion.[111] They present with signs and symptoms of severe sinus tarsi syndrome and a gradual onset of lateral ankle pain[225] and demonstrate a characteristic appearance of localized increased uptake of marker on bone scintigraphy. CT and MRI can be useful for imaging the fracture line directly and can aid diagnosis.[225,228] The recommended treatment is immobilization in a non–weight-bearing cast for 4 to 6 weeks if the fracture is diagnosed early.[201,225] Excision of the lateral process of the talus through the fracture line is recommended for long-standing, symptomatic fractures.[201]

Navicular

Stress fractures of the tarsal navicular bone are common, especially among runners, jumpers, hurdlers, and basketball players.[115,229,230] The onset of symptoms usually is insidious, with patients having increased foot pain after sprinting, jumping, or running. These fractures often are poorly recognized, possibly because the patient's symptoms are vague, particularly in the early stages of injury.[231,232] The pain typically radiates along the medial longitudinal arch or along the dorsum of the foot. Symptoms abate rapidly with rest but recur when the patient resumes activity. Examination reveals tenderness over the proximodorsal aspect of the navicular, the so-called **"N spot"** (Figure 26-9),[233] and imaging frequently demonstrates the injury (see Figure 26-5).[112]

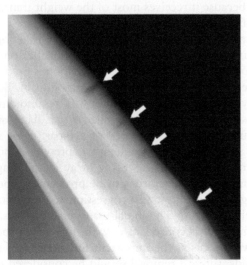

Figure 26-8 Multiple nonunited stress fractures of the anterior cortex of the tibia, as evidenced by the multiple "dreaded black lines" (*arrows*).

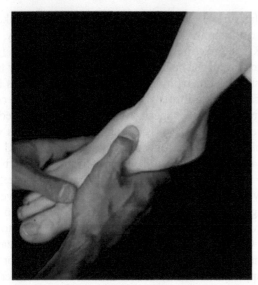

Figure 26-9 Palpation for a navicular stress fracture at the so-called "N spot".

Correct diagnosis and definitive treatment are important in patients with navicular stress fractures because delay in diagnosis can result in prolonged disability. Navicular stress fractures treated with rest and a gradual return to activity have a high incidence of delayed union and nonunion.[115] The recommended treatment for navicular stress fractures is immobilization in a non–weight-bearing cast for at least 6 weeks.[115,233] Even complete navicular stress fractures have been shown to heal with this regimen. After 6 weeks, the patient's cast is removed and healing is assessed by palpation on the "N spot". Radiographs or bone scans should not be used to monitor progress of the fracture because imaging signs of healing lag well behind clinical healing. A 6-week rehabilitation program consisting of joint mobilization, muscle strengthening, and gradual return to activity can begin when the patient has no pain on palpation of the "N spot".[115,233]

Fifth Metatarsal

Stress fractures of the metatarsals most often occur in the second and third metatarsals. A less common yet important variant is a diaphyseal stress fracture of the fifth metatarsal. This type of stress fracture occurs in the proximal 1.5 cm (0.6 inch) of the diaphysis and sometimes is mistaken for a Jones fracture.[234–236] The term *Jones fracture* should be reserved for an acute fracture of the fifth metatarsal, at the level of the articular facet between the fourth and fifth metatarsals, that does not extend distally.[237] Diaphyseal stress fractures of the fifth metatarsal commonly present with localized pain and tenderness near the base of the metatarsal, and dorsal swelling is seen in this area. Diagnosis is important because these fractures have a high potential for delayed union, nonunion, and refracture.[234,238]

The treatment of fifth metatarsal diaphyseal stress fractures depends on their classification. Torg et al.[239] described three subtypes of diaphyseal stress fractures: type I is the

acute or early form, type II is characterized by delayed union, and type III involves nonunion. A type I stress fracture is an early stress fracture with periosteal reaction that represents healing of an incomplete fracture. Radiography confirms the fracture and shows no medullary sclerosis. This subtype has a good prognosis with immobilization in a nonwalking, short leg cast for 6 weeks,[201,235] after which healing is assessed clinically and radiographically. Patients can then gradually resume activity. An alternative management option is to use intramedullary screw fixation; however, the time to union using this technique is identical to that with conservative management.[240]

Type II and type III stress fractures frequently present as an apparent acute fracture, but when questioned, the patient describes a variable history of pain at the fracture site with activity. Radiography shows a fracture line and, depending on the duration of symptoms, may show medullary sclerosis or established nonunion with complete intramedullary obliteration. These subtypes may heal with prolonged cast immobilization (i.e., 3 to 6 months); however, surgical treatment produces more rapid and predictable healing.[241] Intramedullary screw fixation is advocated for type II and type III diaphyseal stress fractures, and bone grafting is variably used for type III stress fractures.[235,240,241] Patients typically return to activity 6 weeks (screw fixation) or 12 weeks (bone grafting) after surgery.[201,222]

Great Toe Sesamoid

The sesamoids of the great toe are embedded in the flexor hallucis brevis and receive fibrous insertions from abductor and adductor brevis muscles. They function to increase the mechanical advantage of the flexor hallucis brevis, assist with weight bearing under the first metatarsal, and elevate the metatarsal head off the ground. As such, they are exposed to repetitive loads and are prone to stress fracture in weight-bearing individuals, especially athletes. Stress fractures most often occur in the tibial sesamoid because it receives most of the weight transmitted by the first metatarsal.[242]

Sesamoid stress fractures typically present as forefoot pain during loading that increases with dorsiflexion of the great toe and decreases with rest. Palpation is used to determine the presence of localized sesamoid pain. Because these symptoms also are consistent with sesamoiditis, the diagnosis often is delayed. Similarly, the diagnosis can be influenced by the presence of a bipartite or multipartite sesamoid, which frequently is present in normal, asymptomatic individuals.[243] Any delay in the diagnosis of sesamoid stress fractures can be problematic, because prolonged morbidity and progression to nonunion are relatively common. The initial management of sesamoid stress fractures is conservative, with non–weight-bearing for 4 weeks. Given the important functional role of the sesamoids, surgical removal should be considered only if conservative management fails.

UNUSUAL STRESS FRACTURES

Scapula

Scapular stress fractures are rare but have been reported in the literature involving the acromial base, the coracoid process, and body of the scapula.[244-247] These injuries, in most cases, occurred following an unusually large increase in activity resulting in repetitive low-to-moderate levels of stress creating the injury. All result in localized painful areas of the scapula.

Humerus

Unlike its lower limb counterpart, the upper limb is relatively shielded from repetitive weight-bearing stress. Despite this, it is well known that the upper arm, including the distal and middle humerus, is prone to injury due to repetitive overhead activity. In skeletally mature patients, humeral shaft fractures can occur owing to generalized and rotational shaft stress.[248] Several papers have reported stress reactions which, if left untreated, can lead to complete stress fractures.[249-252] These humeral injuries can be seen due to the large amount of rotational stress seen during athletic endeavors such as serving in tennis and throwing in baseball, softball, or the javelin.[253] These forces create substantial stress to be placed upon the middle and distal humerus that result in spiral fractures.[254-256] Unfortunately, these injuries may be difficult to diagnose early as they may be characterized as pain in the arm or elbow.[250] If in the elbow, the pain may be initially overlooked as the athlete tries to play though the pain. However, if caught early when symptoms have lasted no more than 2 to 3 weeks, the athlete should be able to rehabilitate and resume play more quickly.

Olecranon

Due to stress similar to those during valgus extension overload, the elbow can incur a transverse or oblique olecranon stress fracture.[257] Throwing can create valgus stress or tensile stress from attachment of the triceps. If triceps tensile traction forces and extension are the primary stress, a transverse type stress fracture occurs. However, when increased valgus stress occurs with extension forces, as is seen in throwing, the injury pattern is that of an oblique stress fracture.[257]

Ribs

Ribs are an uncommon site for stress fractures but have been seen in athletes who use large upper body muscle forces to perform their activity such as rowers and throwers in track and field.[53,258] These injuries have also been seen in golfers.[259] Ribs that may have a stress fracture include the first rib (anterolaterally), the second to fourth ribs (posteromedially), and fourth to ninth ribs (posterolaterally and laterally).[53,258]

SUMMARY

Repetitive stress injuries to bone present along a pathology continuum ranging from stress reactions to complete bone fractures. For this reason, signs and symptoms often vary, depending upon the stage in which a patient presents. Similarly, recovery times also vary. Typically, the earlier an individual is diagnosed, the better and quicker is the response to management. Therefore a certain level of suspicion needs to be maintained at all times in appropriately presenting patients. The diagnosis typically is made clinically by a history consistent with an overuse injury and is confirmed radiographically. In confirmed cases of a repetitive stress injury to bone, management is determined by the risk for healing complications. Low-risk stress injures represent relatively straightforward management problems and typically respond to relative rest from the aggravating activity and removal or modification of risk factors. High-risk stress fractures, on the other hand, are prone to complication and require specific management.

REFERENCES

1. Patel DS, Roth M, Kapil N: Stress fractures: diagnosis, treatment, and prevention, *Am Fam Physician* 83:39–46, 2011.
2. Burr DB, Milgrom C, Fyhrie D, et al: In vivo measurement of human tibial strains during vigorous activity, *Bone* 18:405–410, 1966.
3. Burr DB, Forwood MR, Fyhrie DP, et al: Bone microdamage and skeletal fragility in osteoporotic and stress fractures, *J Bone Miner Res* 12:6–15, 1997.
4. Frost HM: Presence of microscopic cracks in vivo in bone, *Henry Ford Hosp Med Bull* 8:25–35, 1960.
5. Martin RB: Fatigue microdamage as an essential element of bone mechanics and biology, *Calcif Tissue Int* 73:101–107, 2003.
6. Burr DB: Targeted and nontargeted remodeling, *Bone* 30:2–4, 2002.
7. Bennell KL, Malcolm SA, Wark JD, et al: Models for the pathogenesis of stress fractures in athletes, *Br J Sports Med* 30:200–204, 1996.
8. Brukner P, Khan K: Clinical sports medicine, ed 2, Sydney, 2001, McGraw Hill.
9. Burr DB, Turner CH, Naick P, et al: Does microdamage accumulation affect the mechanical properties of bone? *J Biomech* 31:337–345, 1998.
10. Forwood MR, Parker AW: Microdamage in response to repetitive torsional loading in the rat tibia, *Calcif Tissue Int* 45:47–53, 1989.
11. Schaffler MB, Radin EL, Burr DB: Mechanical and morphological effects of strain rate on fatigue of compact bone, *Bone* 10:207–210, 1989.
12. Yerby SA, Carter DR: Bone fatigue and stress fractures. In Burr DB, Milgrom C, editors: *Musculoskeletal fatigue and stress fractures*, Boca Raton, 2001, CRC Press.
13. Bennell KL, Brukner PD: Epidemiology and site specificity of stress fractures, *Clin Sports Med* 16:179–196, 1997.
14. Bennell KL, Malcolm SA, Thomas SA, et al: Risk factors for stress fractures in female track-and-field athletes: a retrospective analysis, *Clin J Sports Med* 5:229–235, 1995.
15. Brunet ME, Cook SD, Brinker MR, et al: A survey of running injuries in 1505 competitive and recreational runners, *J Sports Med Phys Fitness* 30:307–315, 1990.
16. Bennell KL, Malcolm SA, Thomas SA, et al: Risk factors for stress fractures in track and field athletes: a twelve-month prospective study, *Am J Sports Med* 24:810–818, 1996.
17. Bennell KL, Malcolm SA, Thomas SA, et al: The incidence and distribution of stress fractures in competitive track and field athletes: a twelve-month

prospective study, *Am J Sports Med* 24:211–217, 1996.

18. Armstrong III DW, Rue J-PH, Wilckens JH, et al: Stress fracture injury in young military men and women, *Bone* 35:806–816, 2004.

19. Beck TJ, Ruff CB, Mourtada FA, et al: Dual-energy x-ray absorptiometry derived structural geometry for stress fracture prediction in male U.S. Marine Corps recruits, *J Bone Miner Res* 11:645–653, 1996.

20. Lappe J, Davies K, Recker R, et al: Quantitative ultrasound: utility in screening for susceptibility to stress fractures in female Army recruits, *J Bone Miner Res* 20:571–578, 2005.

21. Lappe JM, Stegman MR, Recker RR: The impact of lifestyle factors on stress fractures in female Army recruits, *Osteoporos Int* 12:35–42, 2001.

22. Milgrom C, Finestone A, Novack V, et al: The effect of prophylactic treatment with risedronate on stress fracture incidence among infantry recruits, *Bone* 35:418–424, 2004.

23. Milgrom C, Simkin A, Eldad A, et al: Using bone's adaptation ability to lower the incidence of stress fractures, *Am J Sports Med* 28:245–251, 2000.

24. Brukner P, Bradshaw C, Khan KM, et al: Stress fractures: a review of 180 cases, *Clin J Sports Med* 6:85–89, 1996.

25. Bennell KL, Malcolm SA, Khan KM, et al: Bone mass and bone turnover in power athletes, endurance athletes, and controls: a 12-month longitudinal study, *Bone* 20:477–484, 1997.

26. Warden SJ, Rath DA, Smith M, et al: Rib bone strain and muscle activity in the aetiology of rib stress fractures in rowers, *Med Sci Sports Exerc* 35:S61, 2003.

27. Warden SJ, Gutschlag FR, Wajswelner H, et al: Aetiology of rib stress fractures in rowers, *Sports Med* 32:819–836, 2002.

28. Matheson GO, Clement DB, McKenzie DC, et al: Stress fractures in athletes: a study of 320 cases, *Am J Sports Med* 15:46–58, 1987.

29. Ohta-Fukushima M, Mutoh Y, Takasugi S, et al: Characteristics of stress fractures in young athletes under 20 years, *J Sports Med Phys Fitness* 42:198–206, 2002.

30. Goldberg B, Pecora C: Stress fractures: a risk of increased training in freshman, *Phys SportsMed* 22:68–78, 1994.

31. Frost HM: *Laws of bone structure*, Springfield, 1964, Charles C. Thomas.

32. Parfitt AM: The physiologic and clinical significance of bone histomorphometric data. In Recker RR, editor: *Bone histomorphometry: techniques and interpretation*, Boca Raton, 1983, CRC Press.

33. Sullivan D, Warren RF, Pavlov H, et al: Stress fractures in 51 runners, *Clin Orthop Relat Res* 187:188–192, 1984.

34. Gardner LI, Dziados JE, Jones BH, et al: Prevention of lower extremity stress fractures: a controlled trial of a shock absorbing insole, *Am J Public Health* 78:1563–1567, 1988.

35. Karlson KA: Thoracic region pain in athletes, *Curr Sports Med Rep* 3:53–57, 2004.

36. Christiansen E, Kanstrup I-L: Increased risk of stress fractures of the ribs in elite rowers, *Scand J Med Sci Sports* 7:49–52, 1997.

37. Devas MB, Sweetnam R: Stress fractures of the fibula: a review of fifty cases in athletes, *J Bone Joint Surg* 38:818–829, 1956.

38. McMahon TA, Greene PR: The influence of track compliance on running, *J Biomech* 12:893–904, 1979.

39. Steele JR, Milburn PD: Effect of different synthetic sport surfaces on ground reaction forces at landing in netball, *Int J Sport Biomech* 4:130–145, 1988.

40. Milgrom C, Finestone A, Segev S, et al: Are overground or treadmill runners more likely to sustain tibial stress fracture? *Br J Sports Med* 37:160–163, 2003.

41. Bennell K, Matheson G, Meeuwisse W, et al: Risk factors for stress fractures, *Sports Med* 28:91–122, 1999.

42. Marti B, Vader JP, Minder CE, et al: On the epidemiology of running injuries: the 1984 Bern Grand-Prix study, *Am J Sports Med* 16:285–294, 1988.

43. Walter SD, Hart LE, McIntosh JM, et al: The Ontario Cohort Study of running-related injuries, *Arch Intern Med* 149:2561–2564, 1989.

44. Zahger D, Abramovitz A, Zelikovsky L, et al: Stress fractures in female soldiers: an epidemiological investigation of an outbreak, *Mil Med* 153:448–450, 1988.

45. Carter DR, Hayes WC: Fatigue life of compact bone. I. Effects of stress amplitude, temperature and density, *J Biomech* 9:27–34, 1976.

46. Carter DR, Hayes WC: Fatigue life of compact bone. II Effects of microstructure and densit, *J Biomech* 9:211–218, 1976.

47. Warden SJ, Hurst JA, Sanders MS, et al: Bone adaptation to a mechanical loading program significantly increases skeletal fatigue resistance, *J Bone Miner Res* 20:809–816, 2005.

48. Bennell K, Crossley K, Jayarajan J, et al: Ground reaction forces and bone parameters in females with tibial stress fracture, *Med Sci Sports Exerc* 36:397–404, 2004.

49. Carbon R, Sambrook PN, Deakin V, et al: Bone density of elite female athletes with stress fractures, *Med J Aust* 153:373–376, 1990.

50. Crossley KM, Bennell KL, Wrigley T, et al: Ground reaction forces, bone characteristics, and tibial stress fracture in male runners, *Med Sci Sports Exerc* 31:1088–1093, 1999.

51. Girrbach RT, Flynn TW, Browder DA, et al: Flexural wave propagation velocity and bone mineral density in females with and without tibial bone stress injuries, *J Orthop Sports Phys Ther* 31:54–62, 2001.

52. Lauder TD, Dixit S, Pezzin LE, et al: The relation between stress fractures and bone mineral density: evidence from active-duty Army women, *Arch Phys Med Rehabil* 81:73–79, 2000.

53. Karlson KA: Rib stress fractures in elite rowers: a case series and proposed mechanism, *Am J Sports Med* 26:516–519, 1998.

54. Donahue SW: The role of muscular force and fatigue in stress fractures. In Burr DB, Milgrom C, editors: *Musculoskeletal fatigue and stress fractures*, Boca Raton, 2001, CRC Press.

55. Mizrahi J, Verbitsky O, Isakov E: Fatigue-related loading imbalance on the shank in running: a possible factor in stress fractures, *Ann Biomed Eng* 28:463–469, 2000.

56. Scott SH, Winter DA: Internal forces at chronic running injury sites, *Med Sci Sports Exerc* 22:357–369, 1990.

57. Weist R, Eils E, Rosenbaum D: The influence of muscle fatigue on electrogram and plantar pressure patterns as an explanation for the incidence of metatarsal stress fractures, *Am J Sports Med* 32:1893–1898, 2004.

58. Arndt A, Ekenman I, Westblad P, et al: Effects of fatigue and load variation on metatarsal deformation measured in vivo during barefoot walking, *J Biomech* 35:621–628, 2002.

59. Fyhrie DP, Milgrom C, Hoshaw SJ, et al: Effect of fatiguing exercise on longitudinal bone strain as related to stress fracture in humans, *Ann Biomed Eng* 26:660–665, 1998.

60. Sharkey NA, Ferris L, Smith TS, et al: Strain and loading of the second metatarsal during heel-lift, *J Bone Joint Surg Am* 77:1050–1057, 1995.

61. Yoshikawa T, Mori S, Santiesteban AJ, et al: The effects of muscle fatigue on bone strain, *J Exp Biol* 188:217–233, 1994.

62. Beck TJ, Ruff CB, Shaffer RA, et al: Stress fracture in military recruits: gender differences in muscle and bone susceptibility factors, *Bone* 27:437–444, 2000.

63. McNair PJ, Prapavessis H, Callender K: Decreasing landing forces: effect of instruction, *Br J Sports Med* 34:293–296, 2000.

64. Mizrahi J, Susak Z: In-vivo elastic and damping response of the human leg to impact forces, *J Biomech Eng* 104:63–66, 1982.

65. Seliktar R, Mizrahi J: Partial immobilization of the ankle and talar joints complex and its effect on the ground-foot force characteristics, *Eng Med* 13:5–10, 1984.

66. Hughes LY: Biomechanical analysis of the foot and ankle for predisposition to developing stress fractures, *J Orthop Sports Phys Ther* 7:96–101, 1985.

67. Kaufman KR, Brodine SK, Shaffer RA, et al: The effect of foot structure and range of motion on musculoskeletal overuse injuries, *Am J Sports Med* 27:585–593, 1999.

68. Finestone A, Giladi M, Elad H, et al: Prevention of stress fractures using custom biomechanical shoe orthoses, *Clin Orthop Relat Res* 360:182–190, 1999.

69. Finestone A, Shlamkovitch N, Eldad A, et al: Risk factors for stress fractures among Israeli infantry recruits, *Mil Med* 156:528–530, 1991.

70. Giladi M, Milgrom C, Simkin A, et al: Stress fractures: identifiable risk factors, *Am J Sports Med* 19:647–652, 1991.

71. Friberg O: Leg length asymmetry in stress fractures: a clinical and radiological study, *J Sports Med Phys Fitness* 22:485–488, 1982.

72. Brosh T, Arcan M: Toward early detection of the tendency to stress fractures, *Clin Biomech* 9:111–116, 1994.

73. Giladi M, Milgrom C, Stein M, et al: The low arch, a protective factor in stress fractures: a prospective study of 295 military recruits, *Orthop Rev* 14:709–712, 1985.

74. Simkin A, Leichter I, Giladi M, et al: Combined effect of foot arch structure and an orthotic device on stress fractures, *Foot Ankle* 10:25–29, 1989.

75. Hamill J, Bates BT, Knutzen KM, et al: Relationship between selected static and dynamic lower extremity measures, *Clin Biomech* 4:217–225, 1989.

76. Jones BH, Thacker SB, Gilchrist J, et al: Prevention of lower extremity stress fractures in athletes and soldiers: a systematic review, *Epidemiol Rev* 24:228–247, 2002.

77. Jones BH, Bovee MW, Harris JM, et al: Intrinsic risk factors for exercise-related injuries among male and female Army trainees, *Am J Sports Med* 21:705–710, 1993.

78. Shaffer RA, Brodine SK, Almeida SA, et al: Use of simple measures of physical activity to predict stress fractures in young men undergoing a rigorous physical training program, *Am J Epidemiol* 149:236–242, 1999.

79. Matkovic V, Goel PK, Badenhop-Stevens NE, et al: Calcium supplementation and bone mineral density in females from childhood to young adulthood: a randomized controlled trial, *Am J Clin Nutr* 81:175–188, 2005.

80. Nordin BE, Need AG, Steurer T, et al: Nutrition, osteoporosis, and aging, *Ann N Y Acad Sci* 854:336–351, 1998.

81. Nordin BEC: Calcium and osteoporosis, *Nutrition* 13:664–686, 1997.

82. Lappe J, Cullen D, Haynatzki G, et al: Calcium and Vitamin D supplementation decreases incidence of stress fractures in female navy recruit, *J Bone Miner Res* 23:741–749, 2008.

83. Frusztajer NT, Dhuper S, Warren MP, et al: Nutrition and the incidence of stress fractures in ballet dancers, *Am J Clin Nutr* 51:779–783, 1990.

84. Ruohola JP, Laaksi L, Ylikomi T, et al: Association between serum 25(OH)D concentrations and bone stress fractures in Finnish young men, *J Bone Miner Res* 21:1483–1488, 2006.

85. Brukner P, Bennell K, Matheson G: *Stress fractures*, Melbourne, 1999, Blackwell Scientific.

86. Bijur PE, Horodyski M, Egerton W, et al: Comparison of injury during cadet basic training by gender, *Arch Pediatr Adolesc Med* 151:456–461, 1997.

87. Brudvig TJ, Gudger TD, Obermeyer L: Stress fractures in 295 trainees: a one-year study of incidence as related to age, sex, and race, *Mil Med* 148:666–667, 1983.

88. Protzman RR, Griffis CG: Stress fractures in men and women undergoing military training, *J Bone Joint Surg Am* 59:825, 1977.

89. Reinker KA, Ozburne S: A comparison of male and female orthopaedic pathology in basic training, *Mil Med* 144:532–536, 1977.

90. Bennell K, Grimston S: Factors associated with the development of stress fractures in women. In Burr DB, Milgrom C, editors: *Musculoskeletal fatigue and stress fractures*, Boca Raton, 2001, CRC Press.

91. Papanek PE: The female athlete triad: an emerging role for physical therapy, *J Orthop Sports Phys Ther* 33:594–614, 2003.

92. Zanker CL, Swaine IL: Relation between bone turnover, oestradiol, and energy balance in women distance runners, *Br J Sports Med* 32:167–171, 1998.

93. Zanker CL, Swaine IL: Bone turnover in amenorrhoeic and eumenorrhoeic women distance runners, *Scand J Med Sci Sports* 8:20–26, 1998.

94. Arendt EA, Griffiths HP: The use of MR imaging in the assessment and clinical management of stress reactions of bone in high-performance athletes, *Clin Sports Med* 16:291–306, 1997.

95. Grimston SK, Zernicke RF: Exercise-related stress responses in bone, *J Appl Biomech* 9:2–14, 1993.

96. Jones BH, Harris JM, Vinh TN, et al: Exercise-induced stress fractures and stress reactions of bone: epidemiology, etiology, and classifications, *Exerc Sport Sci Rev* 17:379–422, 1989.

97. Boam WD, Miser WF, Yuill SC, et al: Comparison of ultrasound examination with bone scintiscan in the diagnosis of stress fractures, *J Am Board Fam Pract* 9:414–417, 1996.

98. Lesho EP: Can tuning forks replace bone scans for identification of tibial stress fractures? *Mil Med* 162:802–803, 1997.

99. Romani WA, Perrin DH, Dussault RG, et al: Identification of tibial stress fractures using therapeutic continuous ultrasound, *J Orthop Sports Phys Ther* 30:444–452, 2000.

100. Johnson AW, Weiss CB, Wheeler DL: Stress fractures of the femoral shaft in athletes-more common than expected: A new clinical test, *Am J Sports Med* 22:248–256, 1994.

101. Korpelainen R, Orava S, Karpakka J, et al: Risk factors for recurrent stress fractures in athletes, *Am J Sports Med* 29:304–310, 2001.

102. Prather JL, Nusynowitz ML, Snowdy HA, et al: Scintigraphic findings in stress fractures, *J Bone Joint Surg Am* 59:869–874, 1977.

103. Roub LW, Gumerman LW, Hanley EN, et al: Bone stress: a radionuclide imaging perspective, *Radiology* 132:431–438, 1979.

104. Chisin R, Milgrom C, Stein M, et al: Clinical significance of nonfocal scintigraphic findings in suspected tibial stress fractures, *Clin Orthop Relat Res* 220:200–205, 1987.

105. Floyd WN, Butler JE, Clanton T, et al: Roentgenologic diagnosis of stress fractures and stress reactions, *South Med J* 80:433–439, 1987.

106. Kiuru MJ, Pihlajamaki HK, Ahovuo JA: Bone stress injuries, *Acta Radiol* 45:317–326, 2004.

107. Kiuru MJ, Pihlajamaki HK, Hietanen HJ, et al: MR imaging, bone scintigraphy, and radiography in bone stress injuries of the pelvis and the lower extremity, *Acta Radiol* 43:207–212, 2002.

108. Martire JR: The role of nuclear medicine bone scan in evaluating pain in athletic injuries, *Clin Sports Med* 6:13–37, 1987.

109. Rupani HD, Holder LE, Espinola DA: Three-phase radionuclide bone imaging in sports medicine, *Radiology* 156:187–196, 1985.

110. Sterling JC, Edelstein DW, Calvo RD, et al: Stress fractures in the athlete: diagnosis and management, *Sports Med* 14:336–346, 1992.

111. Brukner P, Bennell K: Stress fractures in female athletes: diagnosis, management and rehabilitation, *Sports Med* 24:419–429, 1997.

112. Kiss ZS, Khan KM, Fuller PJ: Stress fractures of the tarsal navicular bone: CT findings in 55 cases, *Am J Roentgenol* 160:111–115, 1993.

113. Murcia M, Brennan RE, Edeiken J: Computed tomography of stress fracture, *Skeletal Radiol* 8:193–195, 1982.

114. Somer K, Meurman KO: Computed tomography of stress fractures, *J Comput Assist Tomogr* 6:109–115, 1982.

115. Khan KM, Fuller PJ, Brukner PD, et al: Outcome of conservative and surgical management of navicular stress fracture in athletes, *Am J Sports Med* 20:657–666, 1992.

116. Feydy A, Drape J, Beret E, et al: Longitudinal stress fractures of the tibia: comparative study of CT and MR imaging, *Eur Radiol* 8:598–602, 1998.

117. Williams M, Laredo JD, Setbon S, et al: Unusual longitudinal stress fractures of the femoral diaphysis: report of five cases, *Skeletal Radiol* 28:81–85, 1999.

118. Hodler J, Steinert H, Zanetti M, et al: Radiographically negative stress related bone injury: MR imaging versus two-phase bone scintigraphy, *Acta Radiol* 39:416–420, 1998.

119. Ishibashi Y, Okamura Y, Otsuka H, et al: Comparison of scintigraphy and magnetic resonance imaging for stress injuries of bone, *Clin J Sport Med* 12:79–84, 2002.

120. Deutsch AL, Coel MN, Mink JH: Imaging of stress injuries to bone: radiography, scintigraphy, and MR imaging, *Clin Sports Med* 16:275–290, 1997.

121. Tyrrell PN, Davies AM: Magnetic resonance imaging appearances of fatigue fractures of the long bones of the lower limb, *Br J Radiol* 67:332–338, 1994.

122. Kiuru MJ, Niva M, Reponen A, et al: Bone stress injuries in asymptomatic elite athletes: a clinical and magnetic resonance imaging study, *Am J Sports Med* 33:272–276, 2005.

123. Ahovuo JA, Kiuru MJ, Kinnunen JJ, et al: MR imaging of fatigue stress injuries to bones: intra- and interobserver agreement, *Magn Reson Imaging* 20:401–406, 2002.

124. Gillespie WJ, Grant I: Interventions for preventing and treating stress fractures and stress reactions of bone of the lower limbs in young adults, *Cochrane Database Syst Rev* 2000 CD000450.

125. Rome K, Handoll HH, Ashford R: Interventions for preventing and treating stress fractures and stress reactions of bone of the lower limbs in young adults, *Cochrane Database Syst Rev* 2005 CD000450.

126. Kannus P, Parkkari J, Jarvinen TL, et al: Basic science and clinical studies coincide: active treatment approach is needed after a sports injury, *Scand J Med Sci Sports* 13:150–154, 2003.

127. Danova NA, Colopy SA, Radtke CL, et al: Degradation of bone structural properties by accumulation and coalescence of microcracks, *Bone* 33:197–205, 2003.

128. Warden SJ, Fuchs RK, Turner CH: Steps for targeting exercise towards the skeleton to increase bone strength, *Eura Medicophys* 40:223–232, 2004.

129. Turner CH, Robling AG: Designing exercise regimens to increase bone strength, *Exerc Sport Sci Rev* 31:45–50, 2003.

130. Turner CH, Robling AG: Exercise as an anabolic stimulus for bone, *Curr Pharm Des* 10:2629–2641, 2004.

131. Andreoli A, Monteleone M, Van Loan M, et al: Effects of different sports on bone density and muscle mass in highly trained athletes, *Med Sci Sports Exerc* 33:507–511, 2001.

132. Duncan CS, Blimkie CJ, Cowell CT, et al: Bone mineral density in adolescent female athletes: relationship to exercise type and muscle strength, *Med Sci Sports Exerc* 34:286–294, 2002.

133. Karlsson MK, Linden C, Karlsson C, et al: Exercise during growth and bone mineral density and fractures in old age, *Lancet* 355:469–470, 2000.

134. Fredericson M, Ngo J, Cobb K: Effects of ball sports on future risk of stress fracture in runners, *Clin J Sports Med* 15:136–141, 2005.

135. Schwellnus MP, Jordaan G, Noakes TD: Prevention of common overuse injuries by the use of shock absorbing insoles, *Am J Sports Med* 18:636–641, 1990.

136. Finestone A, Novack V, Farfel A, et al: A prospective study of the effect of foot orthoses composition and fabrication on comfort and the incidence of overuse injuries, *Foot Ankle Int* 25:462–466, 2004.

137. Milgrom C, Finestone A, Shlamkovitch N, et al: Prevention of overuse injuries of the foot by improved shoe shock attenuation: a randomized prospective study, *Clin Orthop Relat Res* 281:189–192, 1992.

138. Ekenman I, Milgrom C, Finestone A, et al: The role of biomechanical shoe orthoses in tibial stress fracture prevention, *Am J Sports Med* 30:866–870, 2002.

139. Milgrom C, Burr D, Fyhrie D, et al: The effect of shoe gear on human tibial strains recorded during dynamic loading: a pilot study, *Foot Ankle Int* 17:667–671, 1996.

140. Milgrom C, Burr D, Fyhrie D, et al: A comparison of the effect of shoes on human tibial axial strains recorded during dynamic loading, *Foot Ankle Int* 19:85–90, 1998.

141. Milgrom C, Finestone A, Ekenman I, et al: The effect of shoe sole composition on in vivo tibial strains during walking, *Foot Ankle Int* 22:598–602, 2001.

142. Stacoff A, Nigg BM, Reinschmidt C, et al: Tibiocalcaneal kinematics of barefoot versus shod running, *J Biomech* 33:1387–1395, 2000.

143. Stacoff A, Reinschmidt C, Nigg BM, et al: Effects of shoe sole construction on skeletal motion during running, *Med Sci Sports Exerc* 33:311–319, 2001.

144. Ferber R, McClay Davis I, Williams III DS: Effect of foot orthotics on rearfoot and tibia joint coupling patterns and variability, *J Biomech* 38:477–483, 2005.

145. Stacoff A, Reinschmidt C, Nigg BM, et al: Effects of foot orthoses on skeletal motion during running, *Clin Biomech* 15:54–64, 2000.

146. Nigg BM, Nurse MA, Stefanyshyn DJ: Shoe inserts and orthotics for sport and physical activities, *Med Sci Sports Exerc* 31:S421–S428, 1998.

147. Nigg BM, Wakeling JM: Impact forces and muscle tuning: a new paradigm, *Clin J Sports Med* 11:2–9, 2001.

148. Boyer KA, Nigg BM: Muscle activity in the leg is tuned in response to impact force characteristics, *J Biomech* 37:1583–1588, 2004.

149. Wakeling JM, von Tacharner V, Nigg BM, et al: Muscle activity is tuned in response to ground reaction forces, *J Appl Physiol* 91:1307–1317, 2001.

150. Nigg BM, Stefanyshyn D, Cole G, et al: The effect of material characteristics of shoe soles on muscle activation and energy aspects during running, *J Biomech* 36:569–575, 2003.

151. Wakeling JM, Pascual SA, Nigg BM: Altering muscle activity in the lower extremities by running with different shoes, *Med Sci Sports Exerc* 34:1529–1532, 2002.

152. Mundermann A, Nigg BM, Humble RN, et al: Orthotic comfort is related to kinematics, kinetics, and EMG in recreational runners, *Med Sci Sports Exerc* 35:1710–1719, 2003.

153. Allen CS, Flynn TW, Kardouni JR, et al: The use of a pneumatic leg brace in soldiers with tibial stress fractures: a randomized controlled trial, *Mil Med* 169:880–884, 2004.

154. Batt ME, Kemp S, Kerslake R: Delayed union stress fractures of the anterior tibia: conservative management, *Br J Sports Med* 35:74–77, 2001.

155. Brukner P, Fanton G, Bergman AG, et al: Bilateral stress fractures of the anterior part of the tibial cortex: a case report, *J Bone Joint Surg Am* 82:213–218, 2000.

156. Dickson TB, Kichline PD: Functional management of stress fractures in female athletes using a pneumatic leg brace, *Am J Sports Med* 15:86–89, 1987.

157. Jensen JE: Stress fracture in the world class athlete: a case study, *Med Sci Sports Exerc* 30:783–787, 1998.

158. Matheson GO, Brukner P: Pneumatic leg brace after tibial stress fracture for faster return to play, *Clin J Sports Med* 8:66, 1998.

159. Swenson EJ, DeHaven KE, Sebastianelli WJ, et al: The effect of a pneumatic leg brace on return to play in athletes with tibial stress fractures, *Am J Sports Med* 25:322–328, 1997.

160. Whitelaw GP, Wetzler MJ, Levy AS, et al: A pneumatic leg brace for the treatment of tibial stress fractures, *Clin Orthop Relat Res* 270:301–305, 1991.

161. Scully TJ, Besterman G: Stress fractures: a preventable injury, *Mil Med* 147:285–287, 1992.

162. Reszka AA, Rodan GA: Bisphosphonate mechanism of action, *Curr Rheumatol Rep* 5:65–74, 2003.

163. Burr DB: Pharmaceutical treatments that may prevent or delay the onset stress fractures. In Burr DB, Milgrom C, editors: *Musculoskeletal fatigue and stress fractures*, Boca Raton, 2001, CRC Press.

164. Li J, Mashiba T, Burr DB: Bisphosphonate treatment suppresses not only stochastic remodeling but also the targeted repair of microdamage, *Calcif Tissue Int* 69:281–286, 2001.

165. Sanderlin BW, Raspa RF: Common stress fractures, *Am Fam Physician* 68:1527–1532, 2003.

166. Tuan K, Wu S, Sennett B: Stress fractures in athletes: risk factors, diagnosis, and management, *Orthopedics* 27:583–591, 2004.

167. Stovitz SD, Arendt EA: NSAIDs should not be used in treatment of stress fractures, *Am Fam Physician* 70:1452–1454, 2004.

168. Warden SJ: Cyclooxygenase-2 inhibitors (COXIBs): beneficial or detrimental for athletes with acute musculoskeletal injuries? *Sports Med* 35:271–283, 2005.

169. Wheeler P, Batt ME: Do non-steroidal anti-inflammatory drugs adversely affect stress fracture healing?: a short review, *Br J Sports Med* 39:65–69, 2005.

170. Cirino G: Multiple controls in inflammation: extracellular and intracellular phospholipase A_2, inducible and constitutive cyclooxygenase, and inducible nitric oxide synthase, *Biochem Pharmacol* 55:105–111, 1998.

171. Kawaguchi H, Pilbeam CC, Harrison JR, et al: The role of prostaglandins in the regulation of bone metabolism, *Clin Orthop Relat Res* 313:36–46, 1995.

172. Allen HL, Wase A, Bear WT: Indomethacin and aspirin: effect of nonsteroidal anti-inflammatory agents on the rate of fracture repair in the rat, *Acta Orthop Scand* 51:595–600, 1980.

173. Lindholm TS, Tornkvist H: Inhibitory effect on bone formation and calcification exerted by the anti-inflammatory drug ibuprofen: an experimental study on adult rat with fracture, *Scand J Rheumatol* 10:38–42, 1981.

174. Simon AM, Manigrasso MB, O'Connor JP: Cyclooxygenase 2 function is essential for bone fracture healing, *J Bone Miner Res* 17:963–976, 2002.

175. Zhang X, Schwarz EM, Young DA, et al: Cyclooxygenase-2 regulates mesenchymal cell differentiation into the osteoblast lineage and is critically involved in bone repair, *J Clin Invest* 109:1405–1415, 2002.

176. Bouter LM: Insufficient scientific evidence for efficacy of widely used electrotherapy, laser therapy, and ultrasound treatment in physiotherapy, *Ned Tijdschr Geneeskd* 144:502–505, 2000.

177. Gam AN, Johannsen F: Ultrasound therapy in musculoskeletal disorders: a meta-analysis, *Pain* 63:85–91, 1995.

178. Robertson VJ, Baker KG: A review of therapeutic ultrasound: effectiveness studies, *Phys Ther* 81:1339–1350, 2001.

179. Van der Windt DAWM, van der Heijden GJMG, van den Berg SGM, et al: Ultrasound therapy for musculoskeletal disorders: a systematic review, *Pain* 81:257–271, 1999.

180. Warden SJ: A new direction for ultrasound therapy in sports medicine, *Sports Med* 33:95–107, 2003.

181. Warden SJ, McMeeken JM: Ultrasound usage and dosage in sports physiotherapy, *Ultrasound Med Biol* 28:1075–1080, 2002.

182. Rubin C, Bolander M, Ryaby JP, et al: The use of low-intensity pulsed ultrasound to accelerate the healing of fractures, *J Bone Joint Surg Am* 83:259–270, 2001.

183. Warden SJ, Bennell KL, McMeeken JM, et al: Acceleration of fresh fracture repair using the sonic accelerated fracture healing system (SAFHS): a review, *Calcif Tiss Int* 66:157–163, 2000.

184. Warden SJ, Wong WT, Bennell KL, et al: Facilitation of fracture repair using low-intensity pulsed ultrasound, *Vet Comp Orthop Traumatol* 13:158–164, 2000.

185. Heckman JD, Ryaby JP, McCabe J, et al: Acceleration of tibial fracture-healing by non-invasive, low-intensity pulsed ultrasound, *J Bone Joint Surg Am* 76:26–34, 1994.

186. Kristiansen TK, Ryaby JP, McCabe J, et al: Accelerated healing of distal radius fractures with the use of specific, low-intensity ultrasound, *J Bone Joint Surg Am* 79:961–973, 1997.

187. Mayr E, Rutzki MM, Rutzki M, et al: Beschleunigt niedrig intensiver, gepulster Ultraschall die Heilung von Skaphoidfrakturen? *Handchirurgie, Mikrochirurgie, Plastische Chirurgie* 32:115–122, 2000.

188. Busse JW, Bhandari M, Kulkarni AV, et al: The effect of low-intensity pulsed ultrasound therapy on time to fracture healing: a meta-analysis, *Can Med Assoc J* 166:437–441, 2002.

189. Frankel VH: Results of prescription use of pulse ultrasound therapy in fracture management. In Szabó Z, Lewis JE, Fantini GA, Savalgi RS, editors: *Surgical technology international VII*, San Francisco, 1998, Universal Medical Press.

190. Mayr E, Frankel V, Rüter A: Ultrasound: an alternative healing method for nonunions? *Arch Orthop Trauma Surg* 120:1–8, 2000.

191. Nolte PA, van der Krans A, Patka P, et al: Low-intensity pulsed ultrasound in the treatment of nonunions, *J Trauma* 51:693–702, 2001.

192. Takikawa S, Matsui N, Kokubu T, et al: Low-intensity pulsed ultrasound initiates bone healing in rat nonunion fracture model, *J Ultrasound Med* 20:197–206, 2001.

193. Brand Jr. JC, Brindle T, Nyland J, et al: Does pulsed low intensity ultrasound allow early return to normal activities when treating stress fractures? *Iowa Orthop J* 19:26–30, 1999.

194. Rue JP, Armstrong DW, Frassica FJ, et al: The effect of pulsed ultrasound in the treatment of tibial stress fractures, *Orthopedics* 27:1192–1195, 2004.

195. Bassett CA, Becker R: Generation of electric potentials by bone in response to mechanical stress, *Science* 137:1063–1064, 1962.

196. Bassett CAL: Biologic significance of piezoelectricity, *Calcif Tiss Int* 1:252–272, 1968.

197. Gross D, Williams WS: Streaming potential and the electromechanical response of physiologically-moist bone, *J Biomech* 15:277–295, 1982.

198. Otter MW, McLeod KJ, Rubin CT: Effects of electromagnetic fields in experimental fracture repair, *Clin Orthop Relat Res* 355S:S90–S104, 1998.

199. Aaron RK, Ciombor DM, Simon BJ: Treatment of nonunions with electric and electromagnetic fields, *Clin Orthop Relat Res* 419:21–29, 2004.

200. Benazzo F, Mosconi M, Beccarisi G, et al: Use of capacitive coupled electric fields in stress fractures in athletes, *Clin Orthop Relat Res* 310:145–149, 1995.

201. Brukner P, Bradshaw C, Bennell K: Managing common stress fractures: let risk level guide treatment, *Phys Sportsmed* 26:39–47, 1998.

202. Khan KM, Tress BW, Hare WS, et al: Treat the patient, not the x-ray: advances in diagnostic imaging do not replace the need for clinical interpretation, *Clin J Sport Med* 8:1–4, 1998.

203. Ha KI, Hahn SH, Chung MY: A clinical study of stress fractures in sports activities, *Orthopaedics* 14:1089–1095, 1991.

204. Bailie DS, Lamprecht DE: Bilateral femoral neck stress fractures in an adolescent male runner, *Am J Sports Med* 29:811–813, 2001.

205. Clough TM: Femoral neck stress fracture: the importance of clinical suspicion and early review, *Br J Sports Med* 36:308–309, 2002.

206. Egol KA, Koval KJ, Kummer F, et al: Stress fractures of the femoral neck, *Clin Orthop* 348:72–78, 1998.

207. Devas MB: Stress fractures of the femoral neck, *J Bone Joint Surg Br* 47:728–738, 1965.

208. Johansson C, Ekenman I, Tornkvist H, et al: Stress fractures of the femoral neck in athletes: the consequences of a delay in diagnosis, *Am J Sports Med* 18:524–528, 1990.

209. Fullerton LR, Snowdy HA: Femoral neck stress fractures, *Am J Sports Med* 16:365–377, 1988.

210. Lehman RA, Shah SA: Tension-sided femoral neck stress fracture in a skeletally immature patient: a case report, *J Bone Joint Surg Am* 86:1292–1295, 2004.

211. Lee CH, Huang GS, Chao KH, et al: Surgical treatment of displaced stress fractures of the femoral neck in military recruits: a report of 42 cases, *Arch Orthop Trauma Surg* 123:527–533, 2003.

212. Weistroffer JK, Muldoon MP, Duncan DD, et al: Femoral neck stress fractures: outcome analysis at minimum five-year follow-up, *J Orthop Trauma* 17:334–337, 2003.

213. Brahms MA, Fumich RM, Ippolito VD: A typical stress fracture of the tibia in a professional athlete, *Am J Sports Med* 8:131–132, 1980.

214. Sonoda N, Chosa E, Totoribe K, et al: Biomechanical analysis for stress fractures of the anterior middle third of the tibia in athletes: nonlinear analysis using a three-dimensional finite element model, *J Orthop Sci* 8:505–513, 2003.

215. Chang PS, Harris RM: Intramedullary nailing for chronic tibial stress fractures: a review of five cases, *Am J Sports Med* 24:688–692, 1996.

216. Rettig AC, Shelbourne KD, McCarroll JR, et al: The natural history and treatment of delayed union stress fractures of the anterior cortex of the tibia, *Am J Sports Med* 16:250–255, 1998.

217. Orava S, Karpakka J, Hulkko A, et al: Diagnosis and treatment of stress fractures located at the mid-tibial shaft in athletes, *Int J Sports Med* 12:419–422, 1991.

218. Schils JP, Andrish JT, Piraino DW, et al: Medial malleolar stress fractures in seven patients: review of the clinical and imaging features, *Radiology* 185:219–221, 1992.

219. Shabat S, Sampson KB, Mann G, et al: Stress fractures of the medial malleolus: review of the literature and report of a 15-year-old elite gymnast, *Foot Ankle Int* 23:647–650, 2002.

220. Shelbourne KD, Fisher DA, Rettig AC, et al: Stress fractures of the medial malleolus, *Am J Sports Med* 16:60–63, 1988.

221. Orava S, Karpakka J, Taimela S, et al: Stress fracture of the medial malleolus, *J Bone Joint Surg Am* 77:362–365, 1995.

222. Kaeding CC, Spindler KP, Amendola A: Management of troublesome stress fractures, *Instr Course Lect* 53:455–469, 2004.

223. Reider B, Falconiero R, Yurkofsky J: Nonunion of a medial malleolus stress fracture: a case report, *Am J Sports Med* 21:478–481, 1993.

224. Black KP, Ehlert KJ: A stress fracture of the lateral process of the talus in a runner: a case report, *J Bone Joint Surg Am* 76:441–443, 1994.

225. Bradshaw C, Khan KM, Brukner PD: Stress fracture of the body of the talus in athletes demonstrated with computer tomography, *Clin J Sports Med* 6:48–51, 1996.

226. Haapasaari J, Mäenpää H, Belt EA: Stress fracture of the talar dome, *Clin Rheumatol* 20:385–386, 2001.

227. Motto SG: Stress fracture of the lateral process of the talus: a case report, *Br J Sports Med* 27:275–276, 1993.

228. Umans H, Pavlov H: Insufficiency fracture of the talus: diagnosis with MR imaging, *Radiology* 197:439–442, 1995.

229. Fitch KD, Blackwell JB, Gilmour WN: Operation for non-union of stress fracture of the tarsal navicular, *J Bone Joint Surg Br* 71:105–110, 1989.

230. Torg JS, Pavlov H, Cooley LH, et al: Stress fracture of the tarsal navicular bone, *J Bone Joint Surg Am* 64:700–712, 1982.

231. Coris EE, Lombardo JA: Tarsal navicular stress fractures, *Am Fam Physician* 67:85–90, 2003.

232. Lee S, Anderson RB: Stress fractures of the tarsal navicular, *Foot Ankle Clin* 9:85–104, 2004.

233. Khan KM, Brukner PD, Kearney C, et al: Tarsal navicular stress fracture in athletes, *Sports Med* 17:65–76, 1994.

234. Acker JH, Drez D: Nonoperative treatment of stress fractures of the proximal shaft of the fifth metatarsal (Jones' fracture), *Foot Ankle* 7:152–155, 1986.

235. Hulkko A, Orava S, Nikula P: Stress fracture of the fifth metatarsal in athletes, *Ann Chir Gynaecol* 74:233–238, 1985.

236. Perron AD, Brady WJ, Keats TA: Management of common stress fractures: when to apply conservative therapy, when to take an aggressive approach, *Postgrad Med* 111:95–96, 2002, 99-100, 105-106.

237. Jones R: Fractures of the base of the fifth metatarsal bone by indirect violence, *Ann Surg* 35:697–700, 1902.

238. DeLee JC, Evans JP, Julian J: Stress fracture of the fifth metatarsal, *Am J Sports Med* 11:349–353, 1983.

239. Torg JS, Balduini FC, Zelko RR, et al: Fractures of the base of the fifth metatarsal distal to the tuberosity: classification and guidelines for non-surgical and surgical management, *J Bone Joint Surg Am* 66:209–214, 1984.

240. Portland G, Krelikian A, Kodros S: Acute surgical management of Jones' fractures, *Foot Ankle Int* 24:829–833, 2003.

241. Weinfeld SB, Haddard SL, Myerson MS: Metatarsal stress fractures, *Clin Sports Med* 16:319–338, 1997.

242. Biedert R, Hintermann B: Stress fractures of the medial great toe sesamoids in athletes, *Foot Ankle Int* 24:137–141, 2003.

243. Van Hal ME, Keene JS, Lange TA, et al: Stress fractures of the great toe sesamoids, *Am J Sports Med* 10:122–128, 1982.

244. Sinha AK, Kaeding CC, Wadley GM: Upper extremity stress fractures in athletes: Clinical features of 44 cases, *Clin J Sports Med* 9:199–202, 1999.

245. Veluvolu P, Kolen HS, Guten GN, et al: Unusual stress fracture of the scapula in a jogger, *Clin Nucl Med* 13:531–532, 1998.

246. Ward WG, Bergfeld JA, Carson WG: Stress fracture of the base of the acromial process, *Am J Sports Med* 22:146–147, 1994.

247. Boyer DWJ: Trapshooter's shoulder: stress fracture of the coracoid process. A case report, *J Bone Joint Surg Am* 57:862, 1975.

248. Chang E, Fronek J, Chung C: Medial supracondylar stress fracture in an adolescent pitcher, *Skeletal Radiol* 43:85–88, 2014.

249. Hay G, Wood T, Phillips N, et al: When physiology becomes pathology: the role of magnetic resonance imaging in evaluating bone marrow oedema in the humerus in elite tennis players with an upper limb pain syndrome, *Br J Sports Med* 40:710–713, 2006.

250. Lee JC, Malara FA, Wood T, et al: MRI of stress reaction of the distal humerus in elite tennis players, *Am J Roentgenol* 187:901–904, 2006.

251. Rettig AC, Beltz HF: Stress fracture in the humerus in an adolescent tennis tournament player, *Am J Sport Med* 13:55–58, 1985.

252. Silva RT, Hartmann LG, Laurino CFDS: Stress reaction of the humerus in tennis players, *Br J Sports Med* 41:824–826, 2007.

253. Brukner P: Stress fractures of the upper limb, *Sports Med* 26:415–424, 1998.

254. Polu KR, Schenck RC, Wirth MA, et al: Stress fracture of the humerus in a collegiate baseball pitcher, *Am J Sports Med* 27:813–816, 1999.

255. Herzmark MH, Clune FR: Ball-throwing fracture of the humerus, *Med Ann Dist Columbia* 18:185–187, 1952.

256. Allen ME: Stress fracture of the humerus: a case study, *Am J Sports Med* 12:244–245, 1984.

257. Kancherla VK, Caggiano NM, Matullo KS: Elbow injuries in the throwing athlete, *Orthop Clin North Am* 45:571–585, 2014.

258. Connolly LP, Connolly SA: Rib stress fractures, *Clin Nuclear Med* 29:614–616, 2004.

259. Lord MJ, Ha KI, Song KS: Stress fractures of the ribs in golfers, *Am J Sports Med* 24:118–122, 1996.

CHAPTER 27

Repetitive Stress Pathology: Soft Tissue

NANCY N. BYL, MARY F. BARBE, CAROLYN BYL DOLAN, GRANT GLASS*

INTRODUCTION

The purpose of this chapter is to integrate the basic science of injury, repair, and recovery with patients who have suffered from acute and chronic work-related musculoskeletal trauma related to repetitive overuse in work-related activities. Research findings based on animal and human models can explain the rise in the workplace incidence and prevalence of repetitive strain injuries. The local cellular responses to ongoing repetitive forces are clearly outlined. Peripheralization of the injury is not uncommon when excessive repetitive forces continue too long. Central consequences of overuse, including chronic pain and movement dysfunction (e.g., focal hand dystonia [FHd]), are highlighted, based on laboratory and clinical science research. An etiological model of FHd based on lack of homeostatic plasticity and aberrant learning is proposed as one foundation for effective intervention. The chapter concludes by outlining a comprehensive management strategy for the rehabilitation of patients with occupational hand cramps.

EPIDEMIOLOGY AND MANAGEMENT OF WORK-RELATED MUSCULOSKELETAL DISORDERS OF THE HAND AND WRIST

The Problem

Work-related musculoskeletal disorders (WRMSDs), referred to as work-related repetitive stress (overuse) injuries, have accounted for a significant proportion of work injuries and workers' compensation claims in Western industrialized nations since the late 1980s. The extent to which work is a causal factor in the development of such disorders is still the subject of much controversy. However, recent epidemiological studies have greatly improved methods of distinguishing between the contributions of workplace and nonworkplace risk factors in the development and severity of WRMSDs. The evidence is clear that both workplace and nonworkplace factors can cause or exacerbate WRMSDs, and the key to controlling the impact of such disorders in the workplace is prevention.

Although there is still much to learn about the underlying pathophysiology of work-related repetitive strain disorders, epidemiological research provides information about the scope of the problem and likely causal factors that are being studied in the laboratory and among clinical populations. This section reviews the recent epidemiological literature on WRMSDs of the hand and wrist, with an emphasis on the most prevalent peripheral nerve and musculotendinous disorders.

Definition

Work-Related Musculoskeletal Disorders

The U.S. Department of Labor defines WRMSDs, also known as ergonomic injuries, as injuries or disorders of the muscles, nerves, tendons, joints, cartilage, and spinal discs associated with exposure to risk factors in the workplace. WRMSDs include sprains, strains, tears, edema, fractures, compression, malalignment, disc herniation, and excessive, repetitive movements that challenge the musculoskeletal, connective, or neural tissue reactions (e.g., carpal tunnel syndrome [CTS]) as a result of stressful lifting, bending, climbing, crawling, reaching, twisting, pushing, pulling, poor postural alignment, psychological stress, overexertion, or repetition.[1,2] WRMSDs do not include disorders caused by slips, trips, falls, motor vehicle accidents, or other traumatic injuries.[2] Musculoskeletal disorders (MSDs) also do not generally include Raynaud's phenomenon (although Raynaud's symptoms associated with hand–arm vibration syndrome is a type of WRMSD), tarsal tunnel syndrome, or herniated spinal discs. These types of cases may be related to work stress, but the National Center for Chronic

---

*The authors, editors, and publisher wish to acknowledge Ann Barr for her contributions on this topic in the previous edition.

Diseases considers them separately from musculoskeletal work-related disorders.[1]

Work-Related Musculoskeletal Disorders

Work-related musculoskeletal disorders (WRMSDs) are injuries or disorders of the following:
- Muscles
- Fascia
- Nerves
- Tendons
- Joints
- Cartilage
- Spinal discs

Events or exposures that lead to WRMSDs include the following:
- Bodily reaction/bending
- Climbing
- Crawling
- Reaching
- Twisting
- Lifting
- Pulling
- Poor postural alignment
- Overexertion
- Repetition

WRMSDs include disorders of musculoskeletal, connective, or neural tissues:
- Sprains, strains, tears
- Hurt back
- Pain
- Edema
- Inflammation
- Soreness
- Compression (e.g., carpal tunnel syndrome, neural tension of the brachial plexus or sciatic nerve)
- Hernia
- Musculoskeletal system or connective tissue diseases/disorders
- Biomechanical malalignment
- Psychological stress/anxiety

WRMSDs *do not* include the following:
- Disorders caused by slips, trips, falls, motor vehicle accidents
- Injuries from equipment failures
- Raynaud's phenomenon
- Tarsal tunnel syndrome
- Specific herniated spinal discs

Risk Factors for Work-Related Musculoskeletal Disorders

Certain risk factors are associated with the development or exacerbation of MSDs in the workplace. These risk factors include one or more conditions of physical, biomechanical, environmental, specific job tasks, and/or psychosocial stress in the workplace. In addition, certain worker characteristics, such as obesity, genetics, poor nutrition/hydration, metabolic disease, personality, cumulative exposure, and coping mechanisms, may predispose individuals to MSDs.

Physical and Biomechanical Risk Factors. The primary physical or biomechanical risk factors that contribute to the onset or exacerbation of WRMSDs include the performance of highly repetitive motions and forceful motion.[3-7] The assumption of fixed postures for long periods (particularly when postures place joints in the extremes of physiological range of motion [ROM]), the presence of vibration (e.g., during the operation of handheld power tools), interaction with cold temperatures, or altitude extremes can also increase the risk of repetitive strain injuries.[8-11] There is considerable evidence that the interaction of physical risk factors, such as the combination of high repetition and high force during repetitive power grips or repetitive forceful pinching, disproportionately increases the risk of peripheral neuropathy and musculotendinous disorders of the upper limb.[3-7,12,13] Risks for WRMSDs can also be exacerbated by other medical problems, economic issues, and psychosocial stresses at work and at home, as described in the accompanying textbox.

Risk Factors Contributing to Work-Related Musculoskeletal Disorders

Physical and Biomechanical Risk Factors
- Repetitive movements
- Forceful movements
- Repetitive high-force tasks > either independently
- Fixed postures
- Non-neutral, awkward, or extreme positions
- Vibration
- Cold temperature
- Extreme altitudes

Psychosocial Risk Factors
- High work stress or demands
- Low job security
- Poor job satisfaction
- Low decision control
- Poor workplace social support
- Contentious relationships with supervisors
- Low pay with minimal benefits

Individual Predisposing Risk Factors
- Genetics
- Co-morbid medical conditions
- Physical inactivity
- Physical and psychosocial coping behaviors
- Personality
- Obesity
- Aging
- Female gender
- Life goals and family responsibilities

Psychosocial Risk Factors. Psychosocial risk factors in the workplace, such as job content and demands, job control, and social support, can increase the risk for MSDs.[1,9] Examples of psychosocial factors in the workplace include low worker control over workflow and organization (e.g., assembly line work),[11] contentious relationships with co-workers and supervisors, low decision-making authority, time pressure, low pay and minimal benefits, and excessive employee performance evaluation by management, to name a few.

Individual Predisposing Factors. Nonworkplace factors also can contribute to the development and exacerbation of WRMSDs.[8,14] It is vital that health care providers not only explore such possibilities with workers but also arrange for treatment. These individual predisposing factors not only include physical and psychosocial risk factors (e.g., long hours of practice and performance to maintain a job related skill) but high levels of stress in the home (e.g., partner relationships, adequacy of income, stability of housing, physical, social, educational and psychological challenges of children). Genetics as well as past or current medical conditions also may be co-morbid risk factors for WRMSDs.[9,15,16] Examples include past traumatic injury to the affected body part (e.g., a fracture or sprain), difficulties with digestion, abnormal sleep patterns, obesity, physical inactivity, and systemic diseases (e.g., rheumatoid arthritis, cardiovascular dysfunction, metabolic disorders, diabetes mellitus, celiac disease). Epidemiological studies have linked upper extremity WRMSDs with occupational physical activities involving repetitive arm motions and other risk factors (including force, duration, and female gender).[8,17,18] Advanced age may increase the impact of other risk factors on the severity of MSDs,[19–21] and obesity has been reported to predict the onset of MSDs.[18,22,23]

WRMSDs, therefore, have complex multifactorial causes that contribute to the persistent controversy surrounding governmental regulation of these disorders. Consequently, private industry in the United States addresses these disorders on a voluntary basis, using industry-specific guidelines provided by the Occupational Safety and Health Administration (OSHA) (www.osha.gov).

Clinical Point

When treating patients with WRMSDs, health care providers must bear in mind the complexity of causal factors and attempt to identify and address multifactorial aggravating factors in a comprehensive, holistic approach that emphasizes patient education.

U.S. Department of Labor Survey of Health Statistics

WRMSDs, also known as repetitive strain injuries (RSIs) and work-related overuse injuries, are the most reported types of occupational illnesses. Musculoskeletal conditions, in general, are the second greatest cause of disability globally and have increased 45% worldwide, according to the 2010 Global Burden of Disease Study.[24] WRMSDs are now considered a leading cause of long-term pain and physical disability worldwide,[24–27] with diagnoses including tendinopathies, nerve compression syndromes, and muscular and joint disorders.[28–31]

According to the U.S. Bureau of Labor Statistics reports titled "Nonfatal Occupational Injuries and Illnesses Requiring Days away from Work 2012" and "Workplace Injury and Illness Summary 2012,"[21,32] WRMSDs account for 34% of lost workday injuries and illnesses in the United States and cost on the order of $100 billion annually. The median days away from work—a key measure of severity of injuries and illnesses—was 9 days. Injuries and illnesses resulting from repetitive motion involving microtasks resulted in a median of 23 days away from work to recuperate. Private sector incidence rate for days-away-from-work cases decreased from 105 per 10,000 full-time workers in 2011 to 102 in 2012. Yet, despite this overall decrease, four occupational groups had increases in their incidence rates in 2012: computer and mathematical occupations, community and social service occupations, personal care and service occupations, and transportation and material moving occupations. Seven occupations had rates greater than 375 cases per 10,000 full-time workers: transit and intercity bus drivers; police and sheriff's patrol officers; correctional officers and jailers; firefighters; nursing assistants; laborers and freight, stock, and material movers; and emergency medical technicians and paramedics. Laborers and freight, stock, and material movers had the highest number of days-away-from-work cases in 2012 with 63,690 cases and an incidence rate of 391 (up from 367 in 2011).[21] Overexertion and bodily reaction was the leading event or exposure. Furthermore, because age is a risk factor and the average age of the American and international workforce is rapidly increasing as a result of economic realities, more WRMSDs cases are predicted.[33–35]

Scope of Workplace Musculoskeletal Disorders in U.S. Industry

- WRMSDs accounted for 34% of all injury and illnesses in 2012
- Injuries and illnesses resulting from repetitive motion involving microtasks resulted in a median of 23 days away from work to recuperate
- Overexertion and bodily reaction was the leading event or exposure, with 408,760 cases

Epidemiological Evidence of Work-Related Repetitive Overuse Injuries of the Forearm, Wrist, and Hand

Several comprehensive reviews of the literature concerning WRMSDs have been completed since 1997. A seminal review undertaken by the National Institute for Occupational Safety and Health (NIOSH) included more than 600 epidemiological studies, dating from the 1970s to the mid-1990s, concerning WRMSDs of the neck, upper extremity, and low back.[8] The National Research Council (NRC) and the Institute of Medicine conducted a second, more exclusive review of the WRMSD literature.[36] The NRC review included studies from the late 1970s to the late 1990s that examined tissue pathophysiology; mechanical, organizational, and psychosocial risk factors; and clinical interventions for WRMSDs of the upper extremity and low back. The panel reviewed 42 studies of physical risk factors and 28 studies of psychosocial risk factors. The overall conclusions of both the NIOSH and NRC reviews were that there is evidence supporting associations between workplace physical risk factors and elbow, hand, and wrist WRMSDs and that key risk factors included repetition, force, vibration, gender, age, and others listed earlier. Both reviews identified gaps in the literature in the hope of guiding future research. In subsequent years, investigators began to address some of these issues. Table 27-1 presents a recent update of the epidemiological literature concerning CTS and forearm, hand, and wrist musculoskeletal disorders.

Cumulative Effects of Small Amplitude Forces

MSDs often result from physical demands placed on the musculoskeletal system and peripheral nerves in the workplace.[8,31,36,45] Although acute trauma may be a factor in some cases of MSDs, many WRMSDs are the result of cumulative effects of smaller amplitude forces that occur with overtraining, overexertion, repetitive movements and activities, forceful actions, and prolonged static positioning.[46] The risk for developing lateral epicondylitis (i.e., tennis elbow), for example, is higher with time spent in forearm pronation when combined with increased time in general or increased time spent performing forceful exertions (see Table 27-1).[4] Older age (i.e., 35 to 65 years) is also associated with increased risk for developing lateral epicondylitis[4] (see Table 27-1), perhaps as a consequence of cumulative tissue changes and/or reduced healing as a result of aging. That said, a study examining computer workers found that younger employees were more likely to report hand and wrist symptoms than older workers and postulated that this might have been because the younger employees might have increased hours of computer use as a result of job hierarchy, increased time using computers that was unrelated to work, inappropriate working conditions, first employment, and/or increased awareness of condition, making them more likely to report symptoms (see Table 27-1).[17]

Interaction of Force and Repetition on Tissue Endurance

A recent systematic review of the WRMSD epidemiology literature examined studies that tested for an interaction between two key risk factors: repetition and force (see Table 27-1).[3] Evidence of interaction was found in 10 of 12 epidemiological studies. A consistent pattern of interaction was observed across a number of disorders, including CTS, tendinitis, epicondylitis, and hand pain, with low-force tasks demonstrating a small or modest increase in MSD risk with increased repetition, whereas an escalation in MSD risk was consistently exhibited with high-force tasks, especially when combined with increased repetition.[3] The authors of that review provided a theoretical basis for the interaction between force and repetition, suggesting that this interaction pattern would be anticipated if musculoskeletal tissues incurred damage as

the result of fatigue failure of the tissues with prolonged performance of occupational-related tasks. With fatigue failure, high-force tasks could withstand fewer cycles before failure, but as force was decreased, many more cycles could be tolerated. In addition, there often exists an "endurance limit" below which tissues can be repeatedly loaded without failing (or, at least, tolerate a very large number of repetitions before experiencing failure).[3] This same idea was upheld in a number of other epidemiological studies (see Table 27-1). For example, the risk for arm and wrist tendinosis and epicondylitis increased with increased time spent in forearm pronation performing forceful manual tasks, such as power grip[4] and percentage of time spent in heavy pinch.[6] Recent epidemiological studies clearly showed that the risk for developing CTS was greater with increased repetition, with increased hand force (e.g., high pinch force and power grip), and when performing jobs with forceful hand exertions combined with high repetition.[5,7] Other studies also reported increased prevalence of osteoarthritis in fingers and the thumb in dentists and teachers as a consequence of continued hand joint overloading.[43,44]

Contributions of Posture and Gender

Prolonged static positioning[46] and non-neutral body postures have been identified as key risk factors for WRMSDs.[47] A large cross-sectional study of 2652 subjects (761 males and 1891 females) found that wrist angular velocity was the most consistent physical exposure factor associated with a diagnosis of medial epicondylitis (i.e., golfer's elbow) and CTS and that jobs with high use of wrist flexion were associated with lateral epicondylitis (see Table 27-1).[11] A meta-analysis also showed an increased risk for CTS with increasing hours of exposure to wrist deviation, extension, or flexion.[10] However, a recent prospective study of 2472 employees found no association between wrist posture and risk for developing CTS (finding instead that forceful hand exertion, with or without repetition, was a key factor for incident CTS).[5] Most studies agreed that female gender was a key risk factor associated with development of or a diagnosis of a WRMSD.[6,11] Associated disorders included wrist tendinosis, epicondylitis, CTS, and hand osteoarthritis.

Psychosocial Factors

The 2001 NRC study also examined the importance of psychosocial factors and determined that job content and demands, job control, and social support could increase the risk for MSDs.[1,9] More specifically, psychosocial factors in the workplace included low worker control over workflow and organization (e.g., assembly line work), contentious relationships with co-workers and supervisors, low decision-making authority, time pressure, low pay, minimal benefits, and excessive employee performance evaluation by management. Recent epidemiological studies, such as those shown in Tables 27-1, 27-2 and 27-3, have confirmed that workplace factors, such as low job control,

TABLE 27-1

Selected Recent Epidemiological Studies on Work-Related Musculoskeletal Disorders of the Forearm, Wrist, and Hand

Authors (Country)	Sample	Study Design	Findings	Conclusions
Forearm, Wrist, and Hand Involvement				
Gallagher and Heberger 2013 (USA, Denmark, Finland, and China studies included)[37]	Systematic literature review of 12 epidemiological studies that examined the effects of force and repetition on MSD risk[38-42]	Systematic literature review of 12 cross-sectional studies that allowed statistical evaluation of interaction of force and repetition with respect to MSD risk	10 of 12 studies reported a significant interaction between force and repetition ↑ odds for CTS,[40] hand–wrist tendonitis,[41] LE,[42] prevalent hand pain,[38] and median nerve conduction signal latency[39]	Interdependence of force and repetition with respect to WRMSD risk Repetition = modest ↑ risk for low-force tasks; rapid ↑ for high-force tasks Interaction may be due to fatigue failure thresholds in affected tissues
Forearm Involvement				
Fan et al., 2014 (USA)[4]	611 respondents at risk for LE	Longitudinal–up to 3.5 years Collected information on individual factors (age, gender, race, education), health history, sports, hobbies, job history, and musculoskeletal symptoms to capture work tasks of each worker and to measure quantitative mechanical workload	Adjusted for age and gender: combined effect of forearm pronation ≥45° for ≥40% time and time spent in forceful exertion, including power grip, lifting ≥3% time and duty cycle of forceful exertion ≥10%, = ↑ risk LE Older age (aged 35-64 years) = ↑ risk of developing LE on dominant side	Evidence of etiological role of strenuous manual tasks in occurrence of LE Time spent in pronation, with ↑ time and ↑ forceful exertion = ↑ risk of LE Aging ↑ risk of LE Those reporting good general health had decreased risk of LE on dominant side
Wrist and Hand Involvement				
Harris et al., 2011 (USA)[6]	Workers (413) at four industries employed in hand-intensive work (not office workers)	A prospective study of right wrist tendinosis in blue-collar workers Followed 28 mo, with questionnaires and physical examinations every 4 mo Exposure assessment: repetition rate and percent time (% time) in heavy pinch (>1 kg-force) or power grip (>4 kg-force)	Incidence rate right wrist tendinosis = 5.4/100 person-years Tendinosis of right first dorsal compartment had highest overall incidence (2.7/100 person-years) Adjusting for age, gender, and repetition, wrist tendinosis was associated with % time spent in heavy pinch Being female increased risk	An exposure–response relationship observed for % time spent in heavy pinch for ↑ risk of wrist tendinosis Females have ↑ risk of wrist tendinosis

Authors (Country)	Sample	Study Design	Findings	Conclusions
Nordander et al., 2013 (Sweden)[11]	2652 subjects[17,43]; 8 groups of male workers (761 men) and 19 groups of female workers (1891 women), representing repetitive and/or constrained as well as varied/mobile work	Cross-sectional: occupational groups with high physical exposure and reference groups with low exposure In all groups, prevalence of complaints (Nordic Questionnaire) and diagnoses (physical examination) recorded In 15 groups, psychosocial exposure in terms of job demands, job control, and job support measured	Wrist angular velocity was the most consistent physical exposure factor and associated with one or more diagnosed disorders, including medial epicondylitis and CTS Wrist flexion was associated with lateral epicondylitis Females exhibited higher prevalence of LE Low job control was associated with complaints	Observed an exposure–response relationship between physical workload and elbow/hand disorders Wrist angular velocity was the most consistent risk factor Females have ↑ risk of epicondylitis Low job control = ↑ risk of epicondylitis
Srilatha et al., 2011 (India)[17]	723 subjects (498 men and 225 women)	Cross-sectional survey of computer workers employed at least 6 mo on computer workstations; worked at least 4 hr/day for 5 days/wk Self-administered questionnaire on demographic information and musculoskeletal symptoms in wrist and hand	57.7% reported WRMSD of wrist and hand during the previous 6 mo Women > men (68.9% vs. 52.6%) Computer users ages 21-30 years more likely to report symptoms than subjects ages 40-55 (76.5% vs. 8.5%) Right side > both sides (42% vs. 34%)	Prevalence of WRMSD of wrist and hand is high and dependent on gender and age (Younger employees may have ↑ hours of computer use as a result of job hierarchy; ↑ time with computers unrelated to work; inappropriate working conditions; first employment; and/or ↑ awareness of condition)

Hand Only Involvement

Barcenilla et al., 2012 (Canada, Denmark, Egypt, Finland, France, Hong Kong, China, Iran, Israel, Italy, Korea, Netherlands, Sweden, Taiwan, Thailand, and USA studies included)[7]	Meta-analysis that identified 37 studies examining association between workplace exposure and CTS with respect to exposure to hand force, repetition, vibration, and wrist posture Occupations included industrial plant, forestry, dental office, electronic assembly, grocery store, pork processing workers, and more	Inclusion: Search terms: CTS, carpal tunnel syndrome, median nerve, entrapment, or neuropathy In most studies, the diagnosis of CTS was based on a combination of abnormal nerve conduction findings and a combination of symptoms or signs	When a more conservative definition of CTS was employed to include nerve conduction abnormality with symptoms and/or signs, risk factors significantly associated with an ↑ risk of CTS were vibration, hand force, and repetition	Occupational exposure to excess vibration, increased hand force, and repetition increase risk of developing CTS

(Continued)

TABLE 27-1

Selected Recent Epidemiological Studies on Work-Related Musculoskeletal Disorders of the Forearm, Wrist, and Hand—cont'd

Authors (Country)	Sample	Study Design	Findings	Conclusions
Ding et al., 2010; Solovieva et al., 2005 (Finland)[43,44]	295 dentists and 248 teachers All females, ages 45-63 years, of same socioeconomic level	Cross-sectional study of females in Dental Association and Finnish Teachers' Trade Union First study: investigated association of extensive hand use with radiographic hand joint OA in workers from two occupations with different hand loads[43] Second study: investigated relationship of pinch grip strength with radiographic hand OA and hand joint pain[44]	DIP joints most frequently involved Prevalence of OA in finger and DIP joints in teachers > dentists, especially ring and little OA in right-hand thumb and index and middle fingers in dentists > teachers[43] Symptomatic hand OA (radiological and pain findings) = ↑ risk of low pinch grip strength in both hands, adjusting for age, BMI, hand size, occupation, and hand-loading leisure-time activity[44]	Hand function, specifically continuing hand joint overload, is related to severity of hand OA Finger OA in middle-aged women is highly prevalent, often polyarticular and occupation specific
Harris-Adamson et al., 2014 (USA)[5]	A pooled study cohort from five research groups of 2474 workers (without CTS or possible poly neuropathy at enrollment) employed in hand-intensive work	Longitudinal: followed up to 6.5 years (51,023 person-years) Questionnaires administered to participants at enrollment and during follow-up sessions (work history, demographics, medical history, musculoskeletal symptoms) Individual workplace exposure measures of dominant hand were collected for each task and included force, repetition, duty cycle, and posture Electrodiagnostic studies	7.2% incidence rate of CTS during follow-up period Forceful exertions = those requiring ≥9 N pinch force or ≥45 N of power grip force or a Borg CR-10 ≥2 Biomechanical risk factors associated with ↑ risk of developing CTS include time-weighted average peak hand force, forceful hand exertion repetition rate, and % time of forceful hand exertion Total repetition rate, % time any hand exertion, % time finger pinch or power grip, and wrist posture measures were *not* associated with ↑ CTS risk	Measures of exposure of forceful hand exertion were associated with incident CTS after controlling for important covariates ↑ risk of CTS with ↑ forceful hand exertion repetition rate and ↑ time in forceful hand exertion

Authors (Country)	Sample	Study Design	Findings	Conclusions
You et al., 2014 (USA, Netherlands, United Kingdom studies included)[10]	Meta-analysis that identified six cross-sectional and three case-control design studies that relied on self-report or observer's estimates for wrist posture assessment Occupations included ski industry, industrial plant, electronic assembly, pork processing, and grocery store workers	Inclusion: Search terms: work related, carpal tunnel syndrome, wrist posture, and epidemiology Relative risk of individual studies pooled to evaluate overall risk of wrist posture on CTS Exclusion: office workers because of ↑ risk	The pooled RR of work-related CTS ↑ with increasing hours of exposure to wrist deviation or extension or flexion (RR = 2.01 [1.66-2.43])	Prolonged exposure to non-neutral wrist postures is associated with a twofold increased risk for CTS, compared with low hours of exposure to non-neutral wrist postures

LE, lateral epicondylitis; *MSD*, Musculoskeletal disorder; *CTS*, carpal tunnel syndrome; *WRMSD*, work-related musculoskeletal disorder; *OA*, osteoarthritis; *DIP*, distal interphalangeal; *BMI*, body mass index; *RR*, relative risk; *Borg CR-10*, Borg Category-Ratio Scale of 10 Perceived Exertion Levels; *mo*, month; *hr*, hour; *wk*, week.

TABLE 27-2

Evidence of Multifactorial Etiology

Authors (Country)	Sample	Study Design	Findings	Conclusions
Andersen et al., 2007 (Denmark)[48]	4006 workers from industrial and service companies—quantified contribution of work-related physical and psychosocial, individual, and health-related factors to development of severe musculoskeletal pain (focused on UE here)	Questionnaires completed by 3276 participants (82%) after 24 months follow-up At follow-up, participants with no or minor pain (1513) were included in Cox regression analyses to determine which factors predicted more severe regional pain	Of 4006 baseline respondents, only 7.7% were free of regional pain Of 1513 participants that began with no or minor pain, at 24 months, elbow, forearm, and hand pain associated most with high repetitive work, lifting > 50 kg/hr, fear avoidance for physical activity, low educational status, other chronic disease	More severe regional musculoskeletal pain is multifactorial Physical workplace factors, psychosocial factors, and factors related to health were all associated with more severe regional pain
Ekpenyong and Inyang, 2014 (Nigeria)[49]	1200 males, ages 18-55 years, in construction industry	A cross-sectional site-by-site survey conducted in five existing construction companies Used semistructured Nordic musculoskeletal questionnaire and job content questionnaire on demographics, work and lifestyle characteristics, and workplace risk factors for WRMSDs	WRMSD prevalence = 39.25% Workplace factors with increased odds for WRMSDs = psychological demands, mental workload, age, BMI, low work experience, low education status, awkward movement of head and arms, working against force or vibration, fast work pace	Recorded high prevalence was multifactorial in etiology Multi-intervention strategies are required

UE, Upper extremity; *WRMSD,* work-related musculoskeletal disorder; *BMI,* body mass index; *kg/hr,* kilograms per hour.

TABLE **27-3**

Animal Models of Upper Extremity Work-Related Musculoskeletal Disorders

Authors	Model	Tissue and Functional Changes
Food Retrieval Task (retrieval of a small 45-mg food pellet from a tube within a portal located at shoulder height)		
Elliott et al.[50] Barbe et al.[51] Coq et al.[52]	Young adult rats (2.5 mo of age at onset) LRNF food retrieval task up to 12 wk 3.3 reaches/min, <5% of maximum voluntary grasp force	*Median nerve:* ↑ macrophages and TNF-α in week 12; no neural fibrosis *Forearm flexor muscle/tendons:* No changes *Forearm bones:* No changes *Serum:* Low ↑ MIP2 and MIP3 in weeks 6-8, with LRNF < HRNF *Spinal cord:* ↑ substance P in week 8, and NK-1R in weeks 8-12 in cervical spinal cord segments *Behavior:* No changes in reach rate or task duration; 1.6× ↑ in arm movement reversals in week 8; transient ↓ grip strength week 6
Abdelmagid et al.[53] Al-Shatti et al.[54] Barbe et al.[55] Barbe et al.[51] Barr et al.[56] Clark et al.[57] Coq et al.[52,58] Elliott et al.[59]	Young adult rats (2.5 mo of age at onset) High-repetition, negligible-force (HRNF) food retrieval task up to 12 wk 5 reaches/min, <5% of maximum voluntary grasp force	*Median nerve:* Transient ↑ IL-1α, IL-1β, TNF-α, IL-6 in week 5; ↑ macrophages weeks 8-12; fibrosis by week 12 with 9% ↓ NCV *Forearm flexor muscle and tendons:* Low ↑ IL-1α, IL-1β, IL-10, TNF-α in week 8, with HRNF > LRNF *Forearm bones:* Low ↑ osteoclasts in weeks 4-8, adaptation visible by week 12 *Serum:* Low ↑ IL-1α, MIP2, MIP3, and TNF-α in weeks 6-8, with HRNF > LRNF. *Spinal cord and brain:* ↑ substance P and NK-1R in weeks 6-10 in cervical spinal cord segments; degraded sensorimotor cortical maps *Behavior:* Cyclical task duration, % success after week 3; 2× ↑ arm movement reversals in week 8; ↓ grip strength after 4 wk, with HRNF declines > LRNF and < HRHF (see below)
Handle Pulling Task (reach, grasp, and isometric pull on a stationary handle/lever bar)		
Barbe et al.[13]	Young adult rats (2.5 mo of age at onset) LRLF handle pulling task for 12 wk 2 reaches/min, 15% of maximum voluntary grasp force	*Median nerve:* No changes *Forearm flexor muscle and tendons:* ↓ HSP72 in tendon week 12 = adaptation *Forearm bones and cartilage:* No changes *Serum:* No changes *Spinal cord:* No changes in substance P *Behavior:* Slight ↑ mechanosensitivity
Elliott et al.[60] Barbe et al.[13] Kietrys et al.[61]	Young adult rats (2.5 mo of age at onset) LRHF/MRHF handle pulling task for 12 wk 2 reaches/min, 60% of maximum voluntary grasp force	*Median nerve:* ↑ macrophages, neural fibrosis with 15% ↓ NCV by week 12 *Forearm flexor muscle and tendons:* ↑ macrophages weeks 6-12; transient ↑ IL-1β after training only *Forearm bones and cartilage:* ↑ IL-1α, IL-1β, IL-10, TNF-α by week 12 but < HRHF; ↑ osteoclasts and ↑ osteoblasts = no change in bone volume density *Serum:* Transient ↑ TNF-α in week 6; ↑ MIP3a in weeks 6-12 *Spinal cord:* ↑ substance P and NK-1 in weeks 6-12 *Behavior:* ↓ voluntary reach force and reflexive grip strength in weeks 9-12, ↓ task participation by week 12, ↑ mechanosensitivity (allodynia) in weeks 6-12
Barbe et al.[13,62] Gao et al.[63] Kietrys et al.[64] Xin et al.[65]	Young adult rats (2.5 mo at onset) HRLF handle pulling task for up to 24 wk 5 reaches/min, 15% of maximum voluntary grasp force	*Median nerve:* ↑ TNF-α, macrophages, and neural fibrosis in week 12 *Forearm flexor muscle and tendons:* Transient ↑ TNF-α and IL-1β after training, resolution by week 18; ↓ HSP72 by week 12 = adaptation; ↑ TGF-β 1 and CTGF with tissue fibrosis by week 24 *Forearm bones and cartilage:* ↑ osteoblasts and bone volume density = bone adaptation by week 12; no cartilage changes *Serum:* ↑ MIP2 in week 6; cyclical ↑ TNF-α after training and again week 24; ↑ TGF-β1 in week 18 and CTGF in week 24 with tissue fibrosis *Spinal cord:* ↑ substance P by week 12, with HRLF < LRHF and HRHF *Behavior:* ↑ mechanosensitivity (allodynia) in week 12; progressive ↓ grip strength especially after week 21

(Continued)

TABLE **27-3**

Animal Models of Upper Extremity Work-Related Musculoskeletal Disorders—cont'd

Authors	Model	Tissue and Functional Changes
Elliott et al.[66] Kietrys et al.[64] Xin et al.[65]	Mature rats (14-18 mo of age) vs. young adult rats HRLF handle pulling task for 12 wk 5 reaches/min, 15% of maximum voluntary grasp force	*Median nerve:* Aged rats had ↑T NF-α and fibrosis in week 12 with 23% ↓ NCV *Forearm flexor muscle/tendon:* ↑ IL-1β and IL-6 in aged > young adult in week 12 HRLF rats *Supraspinatus muscle/tendon:* ↑ macrophages in aged > young adult in week 12 HRLF rats *Serum:* ↑ IL-1α and IL-6 in aged > young adult in week 12 HRLF rats *Spinal cord:* ↑ TNF-α in week 12 aged rats *Behavior:* ↓ grip strength and ↑ mechanosensitivity (allodynia) after 4 weeks in aged rats; ↓ grip strength similar in each age group; persistent overhead task avoidance in aged rats
Abdelmagid et al.[53] Barbe et al.[13] Clark et al.[67] Driban et al.[68] Fedorczyk et al.[69] Jain et al.[70] Rani et al.[71-73]	Young adult rats (2.5 mo of age at onset) HRHF handle pulling task for 12 wk 4-8 reaches/min, 60% of maximum voluntary grasp force	*Median nerve:* ↑ TNF-α, macrophages, and neural fibrosis by week 8 with 17% ↓ NCV in week 12 *Forearm flexor muscle/tendons:* ↑ IL-1α, IL-1β, TNF-α after training and through week 12; fibrotic histopathology with progressive ↑ CTGF, collagen 1, TGF-β1, and substance P in weeks 6-12; ↑ HSP72 in each = tissue under stress *Forearm bones and cartilage:* ↑ IL-1α, IL-1β, TNF-α after training and through week 12; ↑ osteoclasts, frank bone loss, and cartilage degradation by week 12 *Serum:* ↑ IL-1α, IL-1β, TNF-α after training and through week 12 *Spinal cord:* ↑ IL-1β and substance P by week 12 *Behavior:* ↓ voluntary reach force and reflexive grip strength in weeks 9-12; ↑ mechanosensitivity (allodynia) by week 12
Barbe et al.[74]	Young adult rats (2.5 mo of age at onset) Compared LRLF, HRLF, LFHF vs. HRHF tasks, performed for 12 wk each	Force × repetition interaction observed, with HRHF > LRHF > HRLF > LRNF in most cases HRHF ↑ risk of musculoskeletal disorder and leads to tissue and behavioral degradation and declines
Blake et al.[75] Byl et al.[76,77] Topp and Byl[78]	Primate model Repetitive, forceful hand squeezing in owl monkeys 15 squeezes/min held 20 msec, against an 80-g force (3-400 trials/ day, training at 80%-90% accuracy) for 2-5 mo	*Tendon:* ↑ hypercellularity and disorganized collagen in digital flexor tendons of 1/3 monkeys; no signs of active inflammation *Brain:* Degraded sensory cortical maps (de-differentiation of normally sharply segregated areas of hand representation); receptive field size, presence of multidigit or hairy glabrous receptive fields, and columnar overlap covaried with animal's ability to use specific digits *Behavior:* Development of focal dystonia

Repetitive Pinching Task

Banks et al.[79] Sommerich et al.[80]	Young adult monkeys (*Macaca fascicularis*) A voluntary, moderately forceful, repetitive pinching task Trained 20 wk to perform a left-handed pad–pad pinch with 60° wrist flexion at a static pinching distance of 3 cm between thumb and fingers	*Median nerve:* ↓ NCV of 25%-31% from baseline in left hand that recovered with several weeks rest; MRI showed enlargement of affected nerves near proximal end of the carpal tunnel, at time of maximal sensory nerve conduction velocity slowing

(Continued)

TABLE **27-3**

Animal Models of Upper Extremity Work-Related Musculoskeletal Disorders—cont'd

Authors	Model	Tissue and Functional Changes
Repetitive Treadmill Running to Load Supraspinatus Muscle		
Carpenter et al.[81] Soslowsky et al.[82]	Rat model Treadmill running loading of supraspinatus tendon ± external compression via Achilles tendon allograft 17 m/min on a decline; 1 hr/day, 5 sessions/wk, up to 16 wk	*Tendon:* Hypercellularity, ↑ tendon cross-sectional area; collagen disorganization, rounded tenocytes; tissue changes ↑ with exposure (compression or time) *Biomechanical testing:* ↓ maximum biomechanical stress
Cyclical Loading of Flexor Digitorum Profundus Muscles		
Nakama et al.[83]	Rabbit model of medial epicondylitis Cyclical loading of flexor digitorum profundus muscles; tendon examined; 2 hr/day, 3 days/wk, for 80 hr total	*Tendon:* ↑ microtear area, ↑ tear densities, and ↑ tear size at medial epicondyle attachment site in loaded limbs; regional differences: outer enthesis > inner enthesis

TNF-α, Tumor necrosis factor alpha; *LR NF,* low-repetition, negligible force; *NK-IR,* neurokinin-IR; *MIP,* macrophage inflammatory protein, a chemotactic molecule; *IL-1,* interleukin-1, a proinflammatory cytokine; *IL-6,* both a proinflammatory and an anti-inflammatory cytokine; *NCV,* nerve conduction velocity; *HR NF,* high-repetition, negligible-force; *IL-10,* anti-inflammatory cytokine; *HSP72,* heat shock protein 72; *LRLF,* low/moderate-repetition, low-force; *LRHF/MRHF,* low/moderate-repetition, high-force; *HRLF,* high-repetition, low-force; *TGF-β1,* transforming growth factor-beta 1; *HRHF,* high repetition, high force; *CTGF,* connective tissue growth factor; *MRI,* magnetic resonance imaging; *mo,* month; *min,* minute; *wk,* weeks; *hr,* hour; *m/min,* meters/minute.

high mental workload, and fast workplace, increased the odds for developing WRMSDs and severe regional musculoskeletal pain.[17,38,48,49] Individual contributing factors include fear avoidance of physical activity, low educational status, low work experience, and presence of other chronic disease.[38,48,49]

Suggested Workplace Strategies

Future workplace strategies should focus on developing the means to avoid overexposure to risk factors, such as high repetition, high force, and prolonged static postures in non-neutral joint positions. One means might be to incorporate more training and engineering interventions that reduce sustained non-neutral wrist postures.[10] Good general health should also be promoted, because it has been shown to decrease some of these risks,[4] whereas the presence of chronic disease increases the risk of developing musculoskeletal pain as a consequence of work. Findings of several workplace and individual psychosocial risk factors indicated that multi-intervention strategies were required to both prevent and treat WRMSDs.

EVIDENCE-BASED REVIEW OF PATHOPHYSIOLOGY OF ACTIVITY-RELATED NEURAL AND MUSCULOSKELETAL DISORDERS

The Problem

Musculoskeletal disorders related to overuse have been associated with a number of changes in neural, muscular, fascial, tendinous, and bony tissues. The following sections review the processes of inflammation and wound healing and factors that affect those processes. Then, current evidence for neural, muscular, and tendinous pathophysiological changes in the development of overuse injuries is presented, as well as possible mechanisms for those changes. A conceptual model for changes in tissue tolerance, with continued tissue loading, that affect inflammation and healing also is presented. This is followed by recommendations for intervention timing as well as for integrating concepts of wellness, physical activity, nutrition, biomechanics, and neural adaptation for effective management of early MSDs.

Review of Wound Healing and Its Relationship to Overuse Injuries

With repetitive forces over time, injuries develop in the local tissues. *Wound healing* is the process by which tissues attempt to restore normal tissue architecture and function after an injury in an effort to restore homeostasis. A complex series of molecular, vascular, and cellular responses are initiated the moment a tissue is injured. Wound healing involves three distinct phases, which develop in an orderly but overlapping manner: hemostasis/acute inflammation, proliferation/fibroplasia, and remodeling/maturation (Figure 27-1).[84,85]

Unfortunately, many factors affect wound healing. For example, if the injury or initiating stimulus is repetitive or chronic, the tissues have little chance to complete the healing process, and either chronic inflammation or fibrosis can result. In these cases, chronic or cyclic release of a

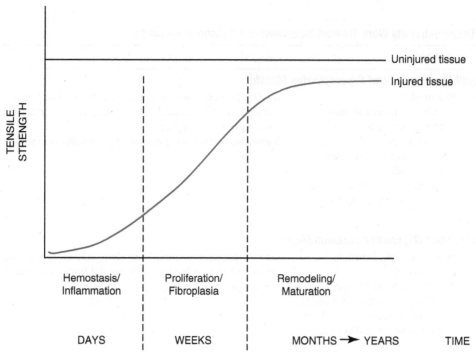

Figure 27-1 Wound healing response in tendons. (From Lin TW, Cardenas L, Soslowsky LJ: Biomechanics of tendon injury and repair, *J Biomech* 37:866, 2004.)

variety of inflammatory or fibrogenic biochemical mediators can perpetuate the inflammatory response or cause excessive proliferation and fibroplasia.[62,63] Some of the inflammatory mediators are cytotoxic at high levels, such as the cytokine tumor necrosis factor-alpha (TNF-α), and can further worsen cellular damage at the injury site. The patient's overall health also must be considered in wound healing. Many metabolic disorders, such as diabetes, can directly affect the success of wound healing, and these disorders therefore must be considered co-morbidities when a treatment plan is designed.[4,48,86]

Acute Inflammatory and Vascular Response

Hemostasis (clotting) and acute inflammation are the tissue's initial responses to acute injury or infection. The hemostasis response causes the wound to be closed by clotting, which occurs through platelet activation. The acute inflammatory response is characterized by infiltration of immune cells and fluid exudate into the affected tissues; it typically lasts 24 to 48 hours and usually is complete in 2 weeks (Figure 27-2). This vascular and immune response is characterized by the cardinal signs of inflammation, which are redness (rubor), swelling (tumor), heat (color), and pain (dolor). The pain (dolor) associated with inflammation usually results from increased pressure on nerves caused by edema. Biochemical mediators, such as histamine, prostaglandin, bradykinin, serotonin, and cytokines (including tumor necrosis factor-alpha [TNF-α] and interleukin-1 [IL-1]), which are released by mast cells, infiltrating immune cells, and injured tissue cells, play crucial roles in the process of vasodilation (Table 27-4; see Figure 27-2).[87-90]

Acute Inflammation

- Vascular reaction
- Cellular reaction (infiltration of platelets, neutrophils, macrophages, and/or lymphocytes)
- Muscle spasm

Cellular Reaction. The migration of cells into the interstitial space is a process called *chemotaxis*. The type of cells that infiltrate depends on the type of stimulus (i.e., injury, infectious, or allergic) and the specific molecules and inflammatory mediators released by the injured cells and tissues. Critical players in this reaction are platelets, mast cells, and leukocytes (including neutrophils and macrophages; see Figure 27-2).

Platelets are anuclear, cytoplasmic fragments derived from megakaryocytes and are the first repair components to appear when a wound is created.[91,92] Their primary function is to initiate the coagulation cascade and form the fibrin plug that fills the tissue gap, a process called *hemostasis*. Platelets release a variety of growth factors and cytokines upon contact with collagen and other extracellular matrix components. For example, they release platelet-derived growth factor (PDGF), which initiates the healing cascade by being chemotactic to neutrophils and monocytes and inducing fibroblast proliferation. Platelets also release transforming growth factor-beta (TGF-β) and proinflammatory cytokines, such as IL-1, IL-6, and TNF-α. These proteins are key mediators of inflammation as well as tissue healing through their ability to induce collagen and fibronectin production by fibroblasts.[91,92]

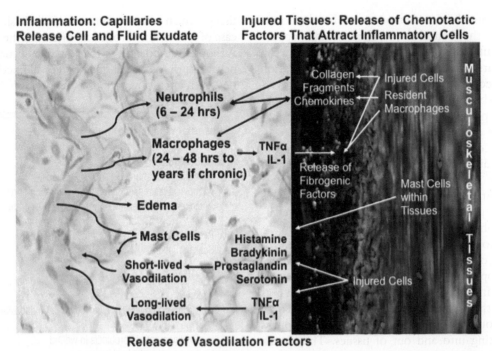

Figure 27-2 Sequence of events in acute inflammation in response to a mechanical injury stimulus. Mechanical injury can damage vascular and musculoskeletal tissues and lead to the mobilization of leukocytes, neutrophils, and macrophages by circulatory distribution and/or by chemotaxis induced by the presence of collagen fragments and other factors at the injury site. Even when the vasculature is spared mechanical injury, the release of inflammatory mediators from tissue mast cells and injured cells release factors (e.g., histamine and bradykinin) that cause vasodilation and leukocyte mobilization. Ideally, acute inflammation resolves, and injured tissue heals either completely or with the formation of a fibrous scar. The latter can occur as a result of release of fibrogenic factors from injured cells, macrophages, or fibroblasts after activation by proinflammatory cytokines, such as tumor necrosis factor-alpha (TNF-α) and interleukin-1 (IL-1). (Modified from Barr AE, Barbe MF: Inflammation reduces physiological tissue tolerance in the development of work-related musculoskeletal disorders, *J Electromyogr Kinesiol* 14:79, 2004.)

TABLE **27-4**

Peptides, Neurotransmitters, and Nerve-Related Proteins Involved in Wound Healing

Analyte	Role in Wound Healing
Bradykinin	An endogenous vasodilator nonapeptide kinin; a very powerful vasodilator that increases capillary permeability; stimulates nociceptors (pain receptors)
Growth-associated protein 43 (GAP43)	High levels in neuronal growth cones during axonal regeneration; a crucial component of an effective peripheral nerve regenerative response
Glutamate	An excitatory neurotransmitter; a key metabolite in cellular metabolism
Kallidin	A decapeptide vasodilator produced by the kallikrein-mediated enzymatic cleavage of kininogen
Nitric oxide (NO)	A free radical; endothelium-derived relaxing factor; an important cellular signaling molecule functioning in vasodilation and neurotransmission
Nerve growth factor receptor P75	Promotes growth cone and neurite formation, elongation, and arborization in regenerating nerve axons
Neuropeptide Y (NPY)	Released from nerves; plays a role in controlling vascular tone, more specifically for thermoregulation
Serotonin (5-HT)	A monoamine neurotransmitter; biochemically derived from tryptophan; a key mediator in the physiology of vascular function, as well as mood
Substance P	Upregulates endothelial cell receptors that promote leukocyte adhesion and migration; chemotactic for neutrophils and macrophages; fibrogenic properties, specifically stimulates the production of collagen by fibroblasts and tenocytes

Neutrophils are the first leukocytes to be chemotactically drawn to the wound site.[84] They typically appear within 1 hour after the wound occurs and peak between 24 and 48 hours after an injury. Neutrophil infiltration can be associated with secondary tissue damage in overloaded muscles because neutrophils release lytic enzymes and produce superoxide free radicals.[93,94] These free radicals, which are antimicrobial, break down injured cells and tissues by disrupting cell membranes, denaturing proteins, and disrupting cell chromosomes. Although neutrophils are short lived, they produce proteinases for debridement and proinflammatory cytokines (e.g., TNF-α) that perpetuate the inflammatory response by attracting macrophages.

In contrast to neutrophils, macrophages are a heterogeneous group of long-lived cells with a myriad of functions.[84,95] Macrophages derive from circulating monocytes, which convert into ameboid, phagocytic cells known as *macrophages* as they invade injured cells and tissues. These cells are voraciously phagocytic and can live for months or years migrating into and out of tissues. They break down necrosed muscle, dead neutrophils, and cell debris through the release of proteolytic enzymes (e.g., collagenase and elastase). Type 1 macrophages (M1) release numerous potentially cytotoxic compounds, including reactive oxygen species and nitric oxide (NO) that can contribute directly to further tissue injury (i.e., secondary tissue injury).[95] Furthermore, activated macrophages secrete proinflammatory cytokines, which act as key mediators of inflammation. In contrast, type 2 macrophages (M2) perform wound-healing functions through their secretion of growth factors (e.g., TGF-β) that stimulate the proliferation of many cell types, leading to tissue repair and healing.[84,95,96] M2 macrophages also secrete anti-inflammatory cytokines (e.g., IL-10) that downregulate the production of proinflammatory mediators and thus promotion of wound healing.[95]

Restorative Repair versus Chronic Inflammation and Fibrosis

Healing and Repair. The process of wound healing is an effort to restore normal tissue function and architecture after injury. Essentially, three primary outcomes are possible with tissue injury: (1) complete resolution with total restoration of normal tissue structure; (2) repair with scar formation of varying degrees, depending on the level of injury; and (3) chronic inflammation. *Complete restoration* is the regeneration or re-creation of the tissue to a state in which it may even be in a better form or condition than before the injury. *Repair* is the process of mending tissue after decay or damage. The mended area may not be complete but may consist of a collagenous scar that fills the damaged tissue region. Substantial tissue injury may also occur in tissues after prolonged edema. The edematous tissue, injury site, or tissue gap then fills with exudate, immune cells, and fibroblasts before converting to fibrotic connective

tissue, which is later remodeled, albeit slowly.[84,97] In the case of tendons, a fibrotic scar often fills the tissue gap.[98–100] Although remodeling of the scar area occurs, tendons may never return to normal structural or biomechanical properties, even after long periods of recovery.[84,100]

Phases of Wound Healing

Repair Phase
- Infiltration of immune cells to clear debris
- Fibroplasia (increased fibroblast proliferation and matrix production)
- Angiogenesis (increased migration and proliferation of endothelial cells)
- Reepithelialization of skin or mucous membrane
- Scar formation

Remodeling Phase
- Remodeling and maturation of tissue toward normal, preinjury structure
  - Collagen conversion: type III (first to be deposited) converted to type I
  - Realignment of fibroblasts in wound
  - Increased mobility of collagen

The repair phase begins once the wound site has been cleared of debris, a process that should occur during the acute inflammatory phase of wound healing (Figure 27-3). The repair phase consists of a proliferation/fibroplasia phase and a remodeling/maturation phase (see Figure 27-1). The proliferative phase is characterized by the migration of fibroblasts into the injury site, which proliferate to fill in the wound site. This phase is also called the granulation tissue formation phase, because microscopically the wound site appears to be filled with many small immune cells and proliferating fibroblasts. The primary function of fibroblasts is to produce new intracellular and extracellular matrix, such as collagen type III.

The remodeling/maturation phase of repair and healing is characterized by collagen conversion, wound contraction, and scar formation.[84] Collagen type III gradually converts to collagen type I, the collagen becomes cross-linked, and fibroblasts realign along the axis of force through the tissue.[84,97] Unfortunately, some tissues, such as tendons, may not recover fully to their original structure and strength because of poor vascularization, insufficient recovery in the damage site (see Figure 27-3), persistent inflammation, or excessive fibrosis/scar formation.

Chronic Inflammation and Fibrosis. Instead of resolving, an acute inflammatory response may be prolonged chronically. Chronic inflammation can be considered an interruption of the normal healing progression and can last for months or years. It is associated with certain conditions that prolong the inflammatory response because of chronic exposure to the initiating stimulus, insufficient repair (see Figure 27-3) or because of a smoldering subacute inflammation or infection. Chronic inflammation

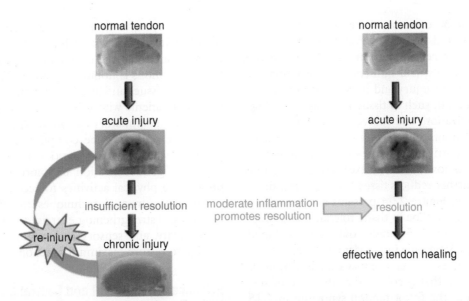

normal tendon

↓

acute injury

insufficient resolution

re-injury

chronic injury

moderate inflammation promotes resolution

resolution

normal tendon

↓

acute injury

↓

effective tendon healing

Figure 27-3 Tendon injury schematic to propose the relationship between inflammation and resolution in the development of tendon injury. **A,** In early-stage injury, inflammation triggers a tendon resolution response, which appears to be transient and reduces with age and time after injury. During the later stages of healing (i.e., chronic injury), it is proposed that insufficient or dysregulated resolution allows low-level inflammation to persist, increasing the propensity for fibrotic healing and reinjury. **B,** To improve the healing response of tendons, a potential therapeutic strategy is to moderate inflammation while simultaneously enhancing the tendon's resolution response. (From Dakin SG, Dudhia J, Smith RK: Resolving an inflammatory concept: the importance of inflammation and resolution in tendinopathy, *Vet Immunol Immunopathol* 158:121-127, 2014.)

is characterized by the prolonged presence of large numbers of mast cells and macrophages in and around the tissues, which contribute to secondary tissue damage through their prolonged phagocytic activity and release of cytotoxic free radicals (see Figure 27-2). Chronic production of inflammatory mediators, such as IL-1 and TNF-α, by macrophages or cells that are injured, irritated, or apoptotic can perpetuate the inflammatory cycle, because these molecules are chemotactic for additional immune cells. Some cytokines released by injured cells and macrophages are fibrogenic mediators, such as connective tissue growth factor (CTGF) and TGF-β. As shown in Figure 27-2, overproduction or chronic production of fibrogenic mediators can lead to excessive fibroblast proliferation and matrix deposition at the wound site, a process called *fibrosis*.[13,62,63,101-104] Several studies support the hypothesis that chronic inflammation generally precedes fibrosis.[62,63] These inflammatory and fibrogenic mediators can enter the bloodstream, circulate, and stimulate systemic inflammatory effects, widespread secondary tissue damage, and widespread fibrosis in healthy tissues.[13,62,63]

Chronic Inflammation

- Perpetuation of inflammatory response
  - Continued presence and activity of macrophages in wound site
  - Continued production of inflammatory mediators by cells in wound site
- Fibrosis
- Either or both of these two components may become widespread or systemic

Factors That Affect Wound Healing. Many diverse factors affect wound healing, including ischemia, scar formation, malnutrition, infection, and stress. Circulating cytokines (discussed previously) can induce bone formation, degradation of cartilage and other connective tissues, and recruitment of leukocytes into widespread tissues areas. As mentioned earlier, invading neutrophils and macrophages lead to secondary tissue damage through phagocytosis, free radical damage, and tissue and protein catabolism. These cells often invade not only the injury site but also nearby healthy tissue and degrade that tissue as well. The overall health of the tissues and of the individual are also key factors in the end success of wound healing.[86]

Other factors in the success of wound healing are neurogenic in origin and arise from a family of biochemical mediators known as *neuropeptides*. Neuropeptides are secreted by autonomic efferent, nociceptive afferent fibers and perivascular terminals of noradrenergic and cholinergic fibers. They have been shown to play a role in all phases of the healing response. Table 27-4 summarizes the primary effects of several neuropeptides as well as several nerve growth factors involved in during wound healing.

Changes in Tissue Tolerance with Continued Tissue Loading

Overexertion is an initiating and a propagating injury stimulus in WRMSDs and overuse injuries. The authors have speculated that the mechanisms leading to tissue repair are prevented by the continued cycle of tissue trauma in repetitive motion injury.[13,105,106] Although cumulative loading of viscoelastic tissues in the short term may increase the likelihood that applied loads will result in tissue injury, it becomes an overexertion event that initiates a cyclical and perhaps persistent inflammatory response. Phagocytic cell infiltration, an increase in the number of free radicals, and induction of inflammatory cytokines by persistent injury and inflammation can lead to tissue degeneration, such as tissue necrosis, pathological tissue reorganization, and subsequent biomechanical failure. Repeated bouts of injury, inflammation, and fibrosis eventually contribute to decreasing tissue tolerance over time, such that lower levels of exertion lead to tissue damage, which further reduces tissue tolerance and functional performance. Figure 27-4 presents a schematic of this dose-dependent decline in tissue tolerance and functional declines. Figure 27-5 shows how these combined tissue responses can combine into a vicious cycle.

Such decreasing tissue tolerance may explain why analyses of human tissue that is collected at the time of surgical repair, such as the flexor tendon synovium in CTS and the extensor carpi radialis brevis tendon in lateral epicondylitis, do not reveal acute inflammatory indicators but instead show tissue degeneration, fibrosis, and/or necrosis.[90,101,102,107–109] The authors postulate that the time of surgery for sensorimotor dysfunction is long after the acute inflammation has resolved.

The authors agree that designating soft tissue injuries as noninflammatory provides important information to clinicians trying to find effective treatments for patients seen late in the process of injury. However, some clinicians disagree that the early pathomechanical initiator of these conditions is noninflammatory. The mere presence of fibrotic tissues and anti-inflammatory mediators in the tissues of patients with overuse injuries strongly suggests earlier proinflammatory episodes. What is clear is that full restorative repair can be complicated, as can best time points in which to intervene (see Figure 27-5). Healthy nutrition, good hydration to improve oxygen delivery, progressive physical activities to accommodate anatomic impairments, manual techniques to release scar tissue, posture and strengthening exercise to improve alignment with gravity, and sensory and motor retraining may be needed to restore maximum function.

Evidence of Peripheral and Central Neural Changes in the Development of Overuse Injuries

Nerve damage can be caused in numerous ways. Typical modes of injury include compression, overstretching, contusion, and frank tears. Compression and overstretching are the most common types of nerve damage associated with repetitive motion.[57,60,66,67,110–113] However, several other modes of nerve injury are not exclusive to overuse injuries; these include crush, immunological causes

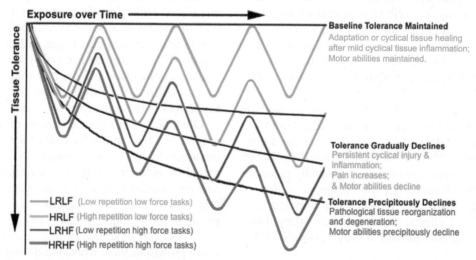

Conceptual Model of Inflammation-Dependent Fluctuation and Decline in Physiological Tissue Tolerance in the Development of MSDs

Exposure over Time

Tissue Tolerance

Baseline Tolerance Maintained
Adaptation or cyclical tissue healing after mild cyclical tissue inflammation; Motor abilities maintained.

Tolerance Gradually Declines
Persistent cyclical injury & inflammation;
Pain increases;
& Motor abilities decline

Tolerance Precipitously Declines
Pathological tissue reorganization and degeneration;
Motor abilities precipitously decline

LRLF (Low repetition low force tasks)
HRLF (High repetition low force tasks)
LRHF (Low repetition high force tasks)
HRHF (High repetition high force tasks)

Figure 27-4 Conceptual model of the hypothesized long-term effects of repeated tissue inflammation on tissue tolerance and underlying mechanisms of tissue responses. This model is consistent with the overexertion theory of the development of work-related musculoskeletal disorders. If tissue exposure levels stay below a critical threshold, inflammation either does not occur or resolves (indicated by the episodic fluctuations of tissue tolerance) and adaptive remodeling to the task occurs (indicated by the return to baseline tissue tolerance of the upper low-repetition, low-force [LRLF] curve between the inflammatory episodes). When tissue exposure exceeds a critical threshold, incomplete healing results (indicated by the lower three lines). Exposure-dependent declines in tissue tolerance lead to persistent injury and inflammation, followed by tissue disorganization, degeneration, or cell death. Depending on the degree of exertion, this decline in tissue tolerance may be gradual (as in the high-repetition, low-force [HRLF] group) or precipitous (as in the high-repetition, high-force [HRHF] group). In addition to the overall decline in tissue tolerance, inflammatory episodes result in transient periods of even lower tissue tolerance, resulting in the fluctuations in tissue tolerance shown. Modification of the tissue exposure level during these transient tissue tolerance episodes may have an important impact on the maximization of tissue tolerance. Furthermore, motor function declines with increasing task demands. (Modified from Barr AE, Barbe MF: Inflammation reduces physiological tissue tolerance in the development of work-related musculoskeletal disorders, *J Electromyogr Kinesiol* 14:83, 2004.)

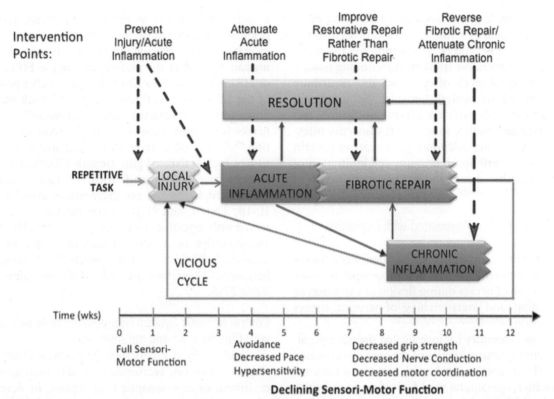

Figure 27-5 Steps in the inflammation-mediated development of work-related musculoskeletal disorders. The timeline at the bottom of the figure relates these inflammatory events to observations of behavioral indicators in a rat model. The three possible exposure-dependent outcomes in this schematic are indicated as follows: (1) acute inflammation followed by resolution and restoration of normal tissue; (2) acute inflammation, which may resolve or may lead to fibrotic repair; and (3) acute inflammation followed by chronic systemic inflammation, with or without fibrotic repair, and initiation of a vicious cycle of further injury and inflammation. At the very bottom of the figure, the physical sign (sensory and/or motor behavior degradation) that reflects underlying pathophysiology is indicated. (Modified from Barr AE, Barbe MF: Inflammation reduces physiological tissue tolerance in the development of work-related musculoskeletal disorders, *J Electromyogr Kinesiol* 14:82, 2004.)

(creating a chronic autoimmune response in the nerve), chronic constriction injury, and vascular disease.[111] Each of these types of injuries can be a compounding factor in a patient with overuse injuries.[39,110–112,114,115]

Clinical, Histological, and Biochemical Signs of Nerve Injury

Clinical signs of nerve damage include acute pain, chronic pain, loss of sensation and discrimination, declines in nerve conduction velocity (NCV), and motor dysfunction. Examples of motor dysfunction include weakness, atrophy, and paralysis of a muscle. Abnormal sensations, such as hyperalgesia (hypersensitivity) and mechanical allodynia (non-noxious pain), may also develop.

Clinical Signs of Nerve Damage

- Acute pain
- Chronic pain state
- Loss of sensation and discrimination
- Reduced nerve conduction velocity
- Numbness and tingling
- Motor dysfunction (weakness, atrophy, or paralysis)

Mechanical disruption of axons and myelin leads to histological signs of nerve damage, such as myelin degradation, Schwann cell necrosis, and axon degeneration. Macrophage infiltration also occurs as a result of disruption of the blood–nerve barrier or injury-induced chemotaxis, or both. The macrophages then add to the loss of Schwann cells and axons by phagocytosing even partly injured cells in an effort to debride the injury site and stimulate repair. Each of these histological changes contributes to the decline in nerve conduction by disrupting the flow of current that would occur after loss of the Schwann cell's myelin sheath or by interfering with axoplasmic flow that would occur after disruption of the axons. Nerve compression, edema, and chronic inflammation also lead to the development of fibrotic tissue in extraneural and intraneural tissues,[57,60,66,67,110] which further contributes to nerve compression if the fibrosed area lies within a constrained space, such as the carpal tunnel.

Biochemical signs of peripheral nerve damage include increased production and release of a variety of mediators of pain, inflammation, and vasodilation by Schwann cells, infiltrating macrophages and mast cells, and the nerve terminal itself.[54,116–119] IL-1, TNF-α, and IL-6 are increased after nerve injury and contribute to further inflammation by recruiting macrophages intraneurally. These same cytokines can enhance pain by sensitizing nociceptors through the activation of the neuron or by lowering the threshold for firing in the larger nerve trunk or surrounding tissues. Increased intraneural levels of cytokines also contribute to hyperalgesia and mechanical allodynia.[60] Schwann cells also produce bradykinin, which results in vasodilation, and the nerve terminals produce substance P, vasoactive intestinal peptide (VIP), and calcitonin gene-reactive protein (CGRP), which contribute to immune cell infiltration of intraneural and other tissues and further sensitization of the nociceptors.[13,50,60,120–124]

Peripheral Nerve Trauma Associated with Repetitive Tasks

In WRMSDs, the primary causes of peripheral nerve trauma are overstretching, increased intracarpal pressure with compression of nerves during flexion or extension or fingertip loading, and overstretching of neuronal tissues during excursion.[5,10,57,60,66,67,110–113,125,126]

The authors' laboratory has investigated the pathophysiology of repetitive motion injuries of the upper limb caused by voluntary high-repetition tasks with or without force using an innovative, operant, rat model of voluntary repetitive and forceful reaching and grasping in order to answer fundamental questions about the effects of such tasks on musculoskeletal tissues. A force training apparatus was designed in which rats can perform at a range of reach rates and force levels. This model has been used to determine the effects on sensorimotor behavior and the pathophysiological outcomes of forelimb tissues that occurred in rats performing tasks at variable force and repetition rates. Some tasks were voluntary low or negligible force tasks (<5%-15% of maximum grip strength) performed at low frequency reach rates (low repetition low force [LRLF] or low repetition negligible force [LRNF]; 2 reaches/min). Others were voluntary low or negligible force tasks performed at high frequency reach rates (high repetitions low force [HRLF] or high repetition negligible force [HRNF]; 8 reaches/min). The remaining two tasks were high force tasks (60% of maximum grip strength) that were performed at either low reach rates (low repetition high force [LRHF]) or high reach rates (high repetition high force [HRHF]). The specific details of these tasks are described and depicted in Barbe et al.[13]

Using this model, the authors examined the median nerve for decreased NCV, a common test used in humans to identify nerve injury. By 10 weeks of an HRNF task, a 9% decrease was seen in NCV, which showed that nerve injury accumulated and led to a clinically relevant loss of function.[57] The decrease in the NCV was even greater (15%) in rats performing the LRHF task for 12 weeks,[60] and was 16% in rats performing the HRHF task for 12 weeks,[13,70] supportive of an exposure response relationship between task exposure level and loss of nerve function. These declines are comparable to the criteria for abnormal median nerve conduction (equivalent to 9% and 24% slowing of NCV) in human studies[127] and

a study in primates by Sommerich et al.[80] (see Table 27-3). Additional findings in the rat overuse injury model included increased myelin degradation and perineural fibrosis in the median nerve after the performance of the HRLF, LRHF, or HRHF tasks for 9 to 12 weeks, but not after performance of the LRNF or LRLF tasks.[13,50,57,60,67,70] Such maladaptive fibrosis in the connective tissue "container" surrounding nerves is thought to be one cause of reduced nerve function,[116,128] as well as reduced physical strength in affected tissues, such as reduced grip strength if forearm muscles and tendons have undergone fibrosis.[63,129] Last, increased M1-type macrophages and proinflammatory cytokines (IL-1α, IL-1β, TNF-α, and IL-6) in the median nerve were observed with repetitive task performance.[54,60,66] These changes are indicative of a nerve inflammatory process, termed *neuritis*,[116,130] which is often associated with increased pain behaviors. These findings and others are summarized in Table 27-3.

Central Nervous System Neuroplasticity Associated with Chronic Pain and Inflammation

Neuroplasticity is a persistent anatomical change occurring in a neuron, recruitment of different neurons, recruitment of new synaptic connections, or development of new neurons (e.g., neurogenesis in the hippocampus) as a result of repeated activity across neural connections. It occurs during development, during regeneration, and within the mature nervous system. Neuroplasticity can occur at any level of the peripheral and central nervous systems, including the spinal cord. Several mechanisms are possible for neuroplasticity. Two of these mechanisms are summarized in Figure 27-6.[131] The different mechanisms increase the efficacy of a synapse, unmask or enhance previously ineffective sites, produce changes in neuronal morphology, prune unused neuronal processes, or create electrophysiological changes in the neuron.

Peripheral nerve injury results in an increased release of excitatory neurotransmitters and neuropeptides (e.g., substance P, glutamate, and CGRP) both peripherally from nociceptor terminals and centrally in a dorsal spinal nerve root or in the dorsal nucleus at the level of the medulla.[132–137] The central release activates postsynaptic receptors for these neurotransmitters, which trigger the release of protein kinases, NO, or both (see Figure 27-6). The molecules then activate intracellular cascades in the postsynaptic neuron. Chronic or repetitive activation of these cascades results in the upregulation of genes, leading to increased production of neuropeptides, hormones, and enzymes, as well as additional receptors. If additional receptors for neurotransmitters/neuropeptides are inserted into the postsynaptic cell membrane, the postsynaptic neuron's ability to bind these molecules is enhanced, which creates a hyperexcitable neuron. Also, as shown in Figure 27-6, NO is a retrograde messenger that can cross cell membranes to the presynaptic cell. It can increase the release of neurotransmitters from

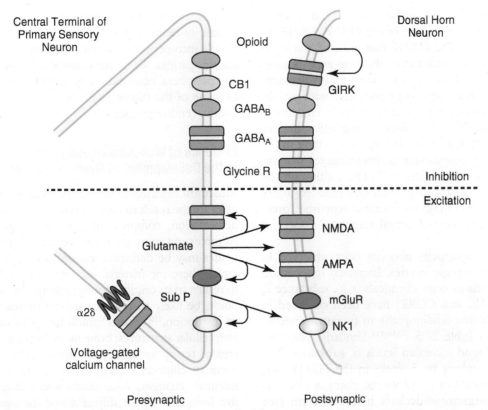

Figure 27-6 Transmission between primary sensory and dorsal horn neurons in the spinal cord is subject to several presynaptic and postsynaptic excitatory and inhibitory influences. *CB1,* cannabinoid receptor type 1; *GABA,* gamma-aminobutyric acid; *Glycine R,* Glycine receptor; *Sub P,* substance P; *GIRK,* G protein-coupled inwardly rectifying potassium channels; *NMDA,* N-methyl-D-aspartate receptor; *AMPA,* α-amino-3-hydroxy-5-methyl-4-isoxazolepropionic acid receptor; *mGluR,* metabotropic glutamate receptor; *NK1,* neurokinin receptor 1; *α2δ,* alpha2delta channel. (Modified from Siegel GJ, Albers RW, Brady ST, Price DL: *Basic neurochemistry: molecular, cellular and medical aspects,* ed 7, p 932, Amsterdam, 2006, Elsevier.)

the presynaptic neuron, which can also lead to hyperexcitability of this synapse.

Chronic pain appears to change the efficacy of a synapse by increasing the release of neuromodulators or neurotransmitters from nociceptor terminals or by increasing the number of synaptic vesicles in the nociceptor terminal.[134,138] Chronic pain also has been reported to alter the enzymatic degradation or reuptake of the neurotransmitter or increase the insertion of receptors into the postsynaptic membrane. Nociceptor hyperexcitability, therefore, may play a role in the pathogenesis of abnormal sensations after peripheral nerve injury. The clinical significance of such neuroplasticity is hyperalgesia, hypersensitivity, and sensory dysfunction.

Abnormal Pain Characteristics

- *Allodynia:* Pain is induced by a normally non-noxious stimulus.
- *Hyperalgesia:* A painful stimulus evokes pain of a greater than normal intensity.
- *Chronic pain:* Pain is of long duration; decreased nociceptor threshold (hyperalgesia).
- *Hypersensitivity:* The autonomic nervous system is operating in a "fight or flight" mode; sensory receptors and nociceptors are overly excitable.

Hypersensitivity and Spinal Cord Neuroplasticity Associated with Repetitive Tasks

The previously discussed studies prompted us to use our model to test sensory function (see Table 27-3). This was done by observing paw withdrawal in response to palmar stimulation using graded von Frey monofilaments. Von Frey monofilaments are calibrated fibers used to test mechanical sensitivity with the application of stimulation to the plantar aspect of the paws. A positive response is defined as immediate withdrawal of the paw from the stimulus and frequently includes licking or shaking of the paw. We observed an exposure–response decrease in the paw withdrawal threshold at 12 weeks in the HRLF, LRHF, and HRHF groups, a change indicative of mechanical allodynia (hypersensitivity to touch).[13,60] Aged HRLF rats showed even greater levels of mechanical allodynia, supporting the contribution of aging to increased regional pain symptoms.[66] The time frame for development of the pain behaviors as well as other behavioral changes, such as motor declines, is indicated in Figure 27-5.

The authors also examined the spinal cord for changes in response to peripheral inflammation induced by each of the four task groups. Dorsal horns in cervical spinal cord segments showed increased substance P and its receptor, neurokinin-1 receptor (NK-1R), as well as increased inflammatory cytokine expression (IL-1β and TNF-α) after 12 weeks of performance of the HRLF, LRHF, or HRHF tasks.[13,50,59,60] The HRHF task induced the highest expression of each substance, showing an exposure-dependent spinal cord response. Evidence for involvement of the spinal cord in the pathology associated with peripheral nerve compression injuries and pain has been demonstrated previously.[123,139] Substance P and inflammatory cytokines play central roles in nociceptor signaling in the spinal cord and in central sensitization changes that are associated with pain behaviors.[123,139] Thus, although the spinal cord is not undergoing direct task-induced injury in this model, these findings indicate that repetitive forceful tasks can induce central neural responses associated with pain behaviors.

Peripheral neuroplasticity also has been observed in conjunction with overuse injuries. Increased innervation and increased levels of neurochemicals (e.g., substance P, glutamate, NK-1R, and CGRP) have been observed in patients with chronic tendinopathy in forearm tendons, as summarized in Table 27-5.[87,140-143] Similarly, using the rat model, we found increased levels of substance P in flexor forelimb tendons by 3 weeks in the HRHF rats, with additional increases by 12 weeks, changes that correlated with sensorimotor declines in the forearm (see Table 27-3).[69] These human and animal findings suggest that increased neuronal innervation, as well as increased release of neurochemicals from activated nociceptor terminals into peripheral tendon tissues, is linked to painful tendinopathies. These data combined suggest that central and peripheral neuroplasticity may be an underlying cause of some of the motor changes observed in patients with painful tendinopathies.

Evidence of Musculoskeletal Injury and Inflammation in the Development of Overuse Injuries

Musculoskeletal injuries caused by repetitive and/or forceful tasks are the result of repeated overstretching, overloading, deformation, compression, friction, or ischemia.[113,152-154] As forces and consequent stress on affected tissues increase, tissues may be deformed enough to reach their "elastic" limit, where the material may start to exhibit an inability to return to its original configuration. This would, at some point, be likely to produce muscle or tendon microtears or disruption,[155-157] mechanical injury of membranes and intracellular structures, bone microscopic damage (e.g., increased resorption spaces and microcracks, which are small linear or elliptical cracks between osteons[158-160]; cartilage tidemark changes, microcracks and subchondral resorptive lesions[161-163]), or diffuse tissue damage when tissues are exposed to additional high-force loading cycles.[3,13] The

TABLE 27-5

Select Human Studies of Overuse Injuries of Hand, Wrist, and Elbow in Which Musculotendinous Tissues or Serum Were Examined

Authors	Description of Patients	Tissue and Functional Changes
Tendon and Tenosynovial Biopsies		
Alfredson et al.[140]	Cases with tennis elbow vs. controls with no history of elbow pain	↑ glutamate in ECRB tendons using microdialysis in cases Long duration of localized pain at the ECRB muscle origin in cases
Ettema et al.[101]	Subsynovial connective tissue biopsies from patients with CTS vs. cadaveric controls	↑ fibroblast density, collagen fiber size, collagen type III fibers, and vascular proliferation in cases
Freeland et al.[144] and Tucci et al.[145]	Flexor tenosynovial biopsies and serum from patients undergoing surgery for CTS vs. volunteers with no evidence of CTS or pain	↑ malondialdehyde in serum and flexor tenosynovium in cases ↑ PGE$_2$ and ↑ IL-6 in flexor tenosynovium in cases
Hirata et al.[90,109]	Flexor tenosynovial biopsies and pain severity testing in patients with CTS; patients divided into symptom duration groups (<4 mo to >12 mo)	↑ PGE$_2$ and VEGF at 4-7 mo of symptom duration ↑ MMP-2 that correlates with pain severity ↑ Synovial fibrosis with disease progression
Ljung et al.[142]	Patients with tennis elbow (lateral epicondylitis) or medial epicondylalgia	↑ Substance P and CGRP in all tendons ↑ NK1-R in lateral epicondyle tendons of patients with epicondylitis
Muscle Biopsies and Muscle Interstitial Fluid (Collected Using Dialysis)		
Ljung et al.[142]	ECRB muscle biopsies from patients with lateral epicondylitis >7 mo	Abnormal muscle NADH staining and muscle necrosis ↑ type IIA fibers and muscle fiber regeneration
Moreno-Torres et al.[146]	Volunteer instrumentalists with nonspecific pain in finger extensor musculature vs. controls	↑ acidic Pi biochemical spectral peaks using P-MRS (phosphorous magnetic resonance spectroscopy) in hand extrinsic extensor muscles

(Continued)

TABLE **27-5**

Select Human Studies of Overuse Injuries of Hand, Wrist, and Elbow in Which Musculotendinous Tissues or Serum Were Examined—cont'd

Authors	Description of Patients	Tissue and Functional Changes
Serum Samples		
Carp et al.[147]	Patients diagnosed with WRMSDs vs. healthy controls; patients divided into groups based on severity of symptoms	↑ IL-6 in mild and moderate WRMSD groups ↑ IL-1α, TNF-α and CRP in severe WRMSD group TNF-α and CRP correlate with symptom severity
Freeland et al.[144]	Patients with idiopathic CTS undergoing carpal tunnel release vs. healthy controls	↑ malondialdehyde in serum of subjects with CTS
Kennedy et al.[148]	Cases of unclear origin with HAVS vs. healthy controls	↑ sICAM-1 and ↓ IL-8 in blood of cases
Lau et al.[149]	Raynaud's clinic patients warranting hospital referral with HAVS vs. general surgical ward patients for minor elective operations	↑ malondialdehyde and PMN activity in blood of subjects with Raynaud's/HAVS
Rechardt et al.[150]	Patients from occupational health units seeking medical advice for specific and nonspecific musculoskeletal disorders, mainly lateral epicondylitis and rotator cuff tendinitis (see paper for complete list), vs. controls	↑ sIL-1RII and ↓ IL-18 in serum of cases
Rechardt et al.[151]	Patients from occupational health care units seeking medical advice for incipient upper extremity pain: shoulder disorders, epicondylitis, wrist tendinitis or CTS, and nonspecific pain	↑ triglyceride and visfatin* in cases with pain ↓ HDL in cases with pain

ECRB, Extensor carpi radialis brevis; *CTS*, carpal tunnel syndrome; *PGE₂*, prostaglandin E_2; *IL-6*, interlukin-6, both a proinflammatory and an anti-inflammatory cytokine; *VEGF*, vascular endothelial growth factor; *MMP-2*, matrix metalloproteinase, a collagenase; *CGRP*, calcitonin gene-reactive protein; *NADH*, nicotine-adenine-dinucleotide reductase; *Pi*, inorganic phosphate, a byproduct of adenosine 5'-triphosphate hydrolysis, released during muscle contraction crossbridge cycle, accumulation during exercise causes a decrement in force production capability; *WRMSDs*, work-related musculoskeletal disorders; *IL-1*, interleukin 1, a proinflammatory cytokine; *TNF-α*, tumor necrosis factor-alpha, a proinflammatory cytokine; *CRP*, C-reactive protein, a nonspecific inflammatory marker; *HAVS*, hand arm vibration syndrome; *sICAM-1*, soluble intercellular adhesion molecule-1; *IL-18*, interlukin-18, also known as interferon-gamma inducing factor, produced by macrophages and other cells; *PMN*, polymorphonuclear cells; *sIL-1RII*, soluble intercellular adhesion molecule 1, facilitates leukocyte adhesion and migration across endothelium and therefore is a biomarker of inflammation; *HDL*, high-density lipoprotein.

*Visfatin is an adipocytokine produced predominantly by human visceral adipose tissue that exerts insulin-mimetic actions through insulin receptors.

authors hypothesize that these injuries first lead to acute inflammatory responses (Figure 27-7). If injury and acute inflammation occur repeatedly, as might be the case with a moderate- to high-demand repetitive task in which the injury cycle overshoots healing, then chronic inflammation, fibrosis, and perhaps even tissue breakdown (disorganization and degeneration) result.

Animal Studies

A number of animal studies have related exercise loading of tendons to early inflammatory changes, as summarized in Table 27-3. In the authors' model of upper extremity overuse injuries in the rat, adaptive-type changes were observed in flexor digitorum muscles and tendons of 12-week HRLF and LRLF rats. These changes included resolution of the inflammatory response and decreased expression of a stress protein, heat shock protein 72 (HSP72).[13,50,64,69] These findings match those from chronic stretch-shortening contractions studies, in which skeletal muscle adaptation can occur if the muscle is able to compensate to the increased demands of an activity.[164-166] In the distal radius and ulna of the reach limbs, signs of bone formation

(including increased osteoblasts and radial trabecular bone volume) were observed in 12-week HRLF and LRHF rats.[13] These findings suggest that the bones were adapting positively to the prolonged loading at LRHF and HRLF levels. These results match findings from other laboratories using involuntary animal loading models showing that bone loaded below the fatigue threshold underwent bone formation.[167-169] These musculoskeletal findings combined suggest that prolonged activity at low-force parameters activates a variety of metabolic and adaptive changes that allow tissues to handle the potentially damaging changes occurring with the tasks more efficiently.

In contrast, continued performance of the HRHF task, and partially the HRLF task, negatively affected flexor digitorum muscles and tendons (see Table 27-3). The greatest inflammatory responses, highest levels of a cell/tissue stress protein (HSP72), and muscle and tendon microdamage were observed in 12-week HRHF rats.[13,60,69] The persistent increases of inflammatory cytokines and macrophages indicate that these tissues were unable to accommodate to this task.[153,170,171] The increased HSP72 in muscles and tendons is consistent with recent findings in

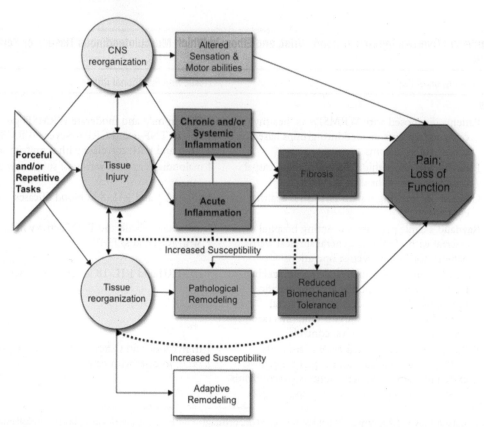

Figure 27-7 Schematic diagram showing three primary pathways hypothesized to lead to work-related musculoskeletal disorders (or adaptive remodeling) caused by repetitive and/or forceful hand-intensive tasks. Interrelationships between components of these pathways are indicated, which illustrates the pathomechanical complexity that may contribute to pain and loss of function. (Modified from Barbe MF, Barr AE: Inflammation and the pathophysiology of work-related musculoskeletal disorders, *Brain Behav Immun* 20:423-429, 2006.)

human subjects by Sjogaard et al.[172] showing that repetitive stressful work increased inducible HSP72 in muscles. Increased fibrogenic proteins (e.g., TGF-β1 and CTGF) and histopathological evidence of fibrosis were also significant in forearm muscles and tendons of 12-week HRHF rats.[53,67,69,71] Fibrogenic changes were prevented in this model if treated early in their development with anti-inflammatory drugs,[53] showing that earlier inflammatory processes are contributing to later developing fibrotic responses. These findings combined indicate that tissue adaptation processes were not keeping pace with tissue injury. Furthermore, fibrotic tissue changes, evident as increased collagen matrix (also known as fascia) within and surrounding muscles, tendons and nerves,[60,66,67,69,71] may distort dynamic biomechanical properties and increase tissue strain even further as a result of adherence to adjacent structures, as postulated by Driscoll and Blyum.[129]

Continued performance of the HRHF task for 12 weeks also negatively affected forearm bones. Increased inflammatory cytokines, increased osteoclasts, decreased trabecular bone volume, thinning of the cortex (i.e., the outer shell) of the bone in the mid-diaphyseal region, and articular cartilage damage was observed in 12-week HRHF rats (see Table 27-3). These changes were indicative of bone and cartilage catabolism and damage as a consequence of this high-demand task. Bone responds to loading along

a continuum ranging from anabolism to catabolism, depending on the magnitude, frequency, and duration of loading.[173-178] Repetitive loading conditions, such as in studies of rats running on treadmills, performing repetitive jumping, and repetitively reaching at high-force loads, also showed that increasing the intensity of weight-bearing or muscle-loading exercise/activities might be associated with diminishing returns in bone morphology, such as declines in bone volume and quality.[72,176,179,180]

Results of other animal models of upper extremity MSDs are also presented in Table 27-3, with similar outcomes. For example, Nakama et al.[83,103,181] found evidence of tendon injury after cyclical loading of the flexor digitorum muscle for 13 weeks at a repetition rate of 2 hours per day, 3 days per week. They observed microscopic microtears in the tendons at their epicondylar attachment to the humerus and increased fibrogenic proteins in the tendon, indicative of repetitive strain–induced tendinopathy.[83,103,181] Carpenter et al.[81] and Soslowsky et al.[82] developed a rat model of running-induced rotator cuff tendinopathy. They found evidence of inflammation and fibrosis (i.e., hypercellularity and tendon thickening) after 4 weeks of running. These tissue changes persisted through 16 weeks. They also found that biomechanical tissue tolerance decreased in the tendons of experimental animals compared with controls.

Human Findings

Human studies examining tendons and tenosynovial biopsies from patients with chronic tendinopathies (e.g., epicondylitis, epicondylalgia, tendinosis, CTS) found evidence of increased levels of injury markers, neurochemicals, inflammatory mediators, angiogenic growth factors, fiber and matrix disorganization, fibrogenic proteins, and fibrosis (see Table 27-5).[87,90,101,109,140,141,143–145,182–184] Furthermore, a study by Hirata et al.[109] showed that the levels of metalloproteinases (MMPs), which are enzymes involved in collagen degradation, correlated with pain severity with tendon synovial fibrosis increasing over time in these patients. It should be noted that not all of the tendon studies in Table 27-5 found each of these tissue changes. Because only a limited amount of tissue could be collected during a biopsy, the number of questions that could be pursued was limited in human studies. Even so, these studies showed that repetitive tasks often lead to fibrotic and degenerative tendon changes and that these changes often are accompanied by localized increases in neurochemicals and their receptors, as well as pain.

Studies also have been performed on muscle tissue biopsied from patients with long-term chronic overuse syndromes (see examples in Table 27-5). These studies showed evidence of muscle tissue changes, including both myopathic changes such as inflammation, muscle fiber necrosis, and cell metabolic changes consistent with injury, denervation, and/or ischemic loss of muscle fibers.[87,185–189] Moreno-Torres et al.[146] examined volunteer instrumentalists with nonspecific pain in finger extensor musculature and observed increased acidic inorganic phosphate biochemical spectral peaks using phosphorous magnetic resonance spectroscopy (P-MRS) in hand extrinsic extensor muscles in instrumentalists with pain versus controls. This is interesting because inorganic phosphate is a byproduct of adenosine 5′-triphosphate hydrolysis and is released during the muscle contraction cross-bridge cycle. Its accumulation causes a decrement in force production capability and would be associated with muscle fatigue.

Serum markers of injury and inflammatory processes have been found in patients with overuse injuries (see Table 27-5). The biomarker malondialdehyde, an indicator of cell stress and therefore injury, has been identified in patients with CTS[144] and in subjects with hand–arm vibration syndrome.[149] Serum from subjects with hand–arm vibration syndrome has increased inflammatory markers, including increased polymorphonuclear cells and levels of soluble intercellular adhesion molecule-1 (*sICAM-1*), a soluble and circulating form of ICAM-1 present on endothelial cells that helps facilitate leukocyte adhesion and migration across endothelium.[148,149]

In patients treated in an outpatient physical therapy clinic for diagnoses related to severe overuse injuries, Carp et al.[190] detected proinflammatory cytokines in serum. The patients were classified into three groups according to symptom severity, as measured by the Upper Body Musculoskeletal Assessment tool (UBMA): mild (UBMA score 51-75; $n=9$), moderate (UBMA score 76-100; $n=9$), and severe (UBMA score >100; $n=9$). A control group consisting of unaffected individuals with an UBMA score below 50 ($n=9$) was used for comparison. The serum results showed significant increases in all proinflammatory cytokines in patients with severe overuse injuries, as well as increases in IL-6 in patients with moderate and mild overuse injuries. Because inclusion in this study required a duration of symptoms no longer than 12 weeks, these findings support the presence of an early inflammatory process in the development of overuse injuries. Another study examining serum from patients seeking medical advice for specific and nonspecific MSDs, mainly lateral epicondylitis and rotator cuff tendinitis, found increased soluble intercellular adhesion molecule 1 (sIL-1RII), a receptor that facilitates leukocyte adhesion and migration across endothelium and is thus a biomarker of inflammation.[191] However, several other inflammatory cytokines were not increased above control subject levels in this same study, and serum levels of IL-18, a member of the IL-1 superfamily, were actually decreased in the MSD cases.[191]

The differences in findings in the aforementioned studies highlight one of the challenges involved in studying workers is the difficulty determining the causality between tissue and behavioral responses. Timing is key. If serum or tissues are examined early in the injury process, injury and/or inflammatory markers are likely to be detected. However, if serum or tissues are examined at the time of surgery, presumably, the initiating injury stimulus is long since passed and the condition of the tissues has been substantially altered from the preinjury state. This means one is likely to detect wound healing or fibrogenic markers instead of inflammatory markers.

Summary

By examining the findings of human and animal studies done on severe overuse injuries, the authors have developed a proposed mechanism of pathophysiological and behavioral changes associated with these injuries.[192] First, repetitive activity leads to injury of cells and tissues (see Figure 27-7). This injury activates the acute inflammatory response: infiltration of immune cells into the injury site and increased production of cytokines by these immune cells and by injured cells and tissues. The acute inflammatory response then activates mechanisms of cell proliferation and matrix production related to wound healing. Unfortunately, the continued cycle of tissue trauma by continued performance of the repetitive task halts the process of tissue repair at this point.[105] Instead, a chronic inflammatory response (with associated secondary tissue damage) is stimulated, along with an excessive fibrogenic response. This postulated mechanism is supported by the many studies, both human and animal, that have found evidence of tendon tissue thickening and fibrosis, nerve and muscle fibrosis, and tissue disorganization and necrosis. Behavior changes related to tissue damage, pain, or both would be clearly apparent at this point as a result of nerve damage, and sensory losses may also be present as a consequence of the nerve damage. Finally, a systemic response is stimulated, apparently by the release of cytokines into the bloodstream from the injured tissues and immune cells still present in the tissues. The circulating cytokines may stimulate several global responses, including widespread stimulation of macrophages and cell proliferation at local and distant tissue sites. The presence of chronic pain and central neuroplasticity stimulates a variety of sensorimotor behavioral consequences that are discussed in detail in the next section.

EVIDENCE-BASED REVIEW OF CENTRAL CONSEQUENCES OF CHRONIC REPETITIVE OVERUSE INJURIES OF THE UPPER LIMB: FOCAL HAND DYSTONIA

The Problem

As reported at the beginning of this chapter, stressful, repetitive use of the upper limb in work or sports can lead to acute pain and loss of function. Rest, anti-inflammatory medications, change in biomechanics, and good ergonomics usually are effective intervention strategies. Unfortunately, some RSIs become chronic. Degenerative changes may be documented in tendons, joints, muscles, and fascia that may limit mobility, compress peripheral nerves, compromise vascular tissues, and lead to chronic pain. However, in some cases, abnormal, involuntary end range twisting postures develop when a person tries to perform a well-learned task. This movement dysfunction is referred to as *occupational hand cramps*.[193] Usually the movements are painless, but in some cases, muscle cramping can be painful.

Dystonia can be general, involving the entire body; focal, involving one body part; segmental, involving multiple adjacent body parts; or task specific, such as golfer's yip (a jerking movement when hitting the ball—usually putting; lack of a smooth stroke) or musician's dystonia or cramp. Focal dystonia involving the hand may be referred to as *hand cramps* or by task specificity (e.g., keyboarder's cramp, writer's cramp). Focal dystonia tends to be primary in adults (e.g., underlying genetic, neurophysiological or sensorimotor integrative dysfunction), whereas in children the problem is more commonly secondary (e.g., cerebral palsy with injury to the basal ganglia).[194,195] The etiology and impact of dystonia are unique in children compared with adults. In children the onset of serious movement dysfunction such as dystonia can significantly disrupt development, independence, and acquisition of motor, sensory, cognitive, and social skills.[196] This section of the chapter focuses on hand dystonia in adults; how-

ever, the information may be applicable to other types of focal dystonias (e.g., cervical, spinal, and leg dystonias).

It is difficult to report the incidence and prevalence of focal dystonia because there are so many different types and different body parts affected. The genetic contribution to focal dystonia in adults has not been widely investigated. Approximately 23% to 30% of those with focal dystonia have a relative with the disorder.[197,198] The incidence of RSIs in performing artists varies from 44% to 84%, with pain, weakness, numbness, or tingling being the most common complaints.[199–201] Approximately 12% of musicians have to take time off work, with nearly 50% returning to performance while still having pain.[200,201] Although the type of dystonia may vary by the instrument played, approximately 1% of professional musicians are affected.[198,202] This is in contrast to the general population, where the prevalence of FHd is estimated as 29.5 per 100,000 in the United States and 61 per 100,000 in Japan.[203,204] In a recent systematic review and meta-analysis including 15 studies (12 service-based and 3 population-based studies), researchers calculated an overall prevalence of primary dystonia as 16.32 per 100,000, with the prevalence higher in the population-based studies than in the service-based studies. The researchers suggested this was probably an underestimate.[205]

Cervical dystonia (i.e., torticollis) is the most common form of adult-onset dystonia. The prevalence of cervical torticollis ranges from 20 to 4100 cases per million. The incidence is estimated at 8 to 12 cases per million person-years.[206]

Etiology of Hand Dystonia (FHd)

Dystonia is a product of genetic factors interacting with physical, psychosocial, and environmental modifiers.[207] When this problem was initially reported in talented musicians, some health care professionals were of the opinion that FHd was a psychological disorder. Today, the etiology of FHd is still considered idiopathic, with a growing body of knowledge supporting a multifactorial etiology for most cases of hand dystonia (Figure 27-8).

Genetics

The risk for FHd can be higher than in age-matched controls if an individual has a familial gene for dystonia.[197,198] A variety of genes are known to cause generalized dystonia, but only a few genes are identified for different types of focal dystonia. For example, the *DYT1* gene has been identified in Ashkenazi Jewish families.[208–211] Not all individuals who carry this gene (genotype) develop clinical dystonia (phenotype).[212,213] The gene is noted to have "low penetrance."[208–211] The clinical phenotype is most likely to develop when multiple aggravating factors are present (e.g., perseverative behavior, phobia, anatomical impairments, stress, traumatic injury, excessive repetition).[208–211] Many genetic studies are currently under way,

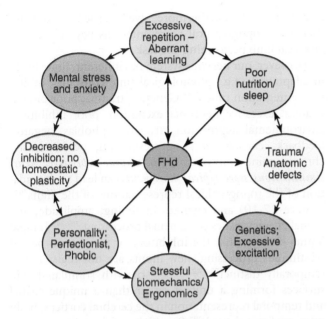

Figure 27-8 The etiology of focal hand dystonia is multifactorial. Multiple risk factors are needed to provide sufficient aggravation to lead to the clinical expression of focal hand dystonia.

and in the future, it is expected that new genes will be identified for both general and focal dystonia.

Musculoskeletal Risk Factors

Individuals performing fast, forceful, accurate, repetitive movements (e.g., typing or programming on a computer, playing a musical instrument, writing, screwing nails) are at risk for developing WRMSDs, including occupational hand cramps.[214] The most common factor contributing to injuries in musicians appears to be excessive practice or performance-related activities.[200,201,215] The musician most likely to develop FHd is the one who is extremely perfectionist, perseverative, persistent, goal oriented, and often phobic.[202]

Researchers report anatomical and musculoskeletal limitations are common in individuals with FHd (e.g., decreased ROM,[216] anatomical variations,[78,217] abnormal kinematics,[218] and excessive use of force[219]). Some clinical researchers report increased neural tension and ulnar nerve subluxation.[220,221]

Some clinical scientists argue that FHd can develop as a consequence of a traumatic injury (e.g., complicated or simple fracture, peripheral nerve entrapment, anatomical restrictions in soft tissue).[222,223] Although the debate about trauma as a cause of hand dystonia has not been resolved, there is some consensus that individuals who develop FHd after trauma to the upper limb are usually at risk for developing dystonia before the injury,[220] with the trauma simply serving as the "last straw."

Neurophysiological Impairments

Impairments in reciprocal and surround inhibition, sensory processing, sensory integration, and maladaptive plasticity are common neurophysiological risk factors for developing occupational hand cramps.[207,224] The imbalance between inhibition and excitation involves the basal ganglia, spinal cord, brain stem, and cortex.[225–228] Inadequate inhibition complemented by lower-than-normal gamma-aminobutyric acid (GABA) levels in the sensorimotor area appear to contribute to excessive plasticity and corticospinal excitability.[229] In addition to inadequate inhibition, impaired neurophysiological processing has been reported in many different areas of the brain. These impairments range from dysfunction in the primary motor cortex,[230–235] degradation in the sensory thalamus,[236,237] disruption in cortical sensory activation, somatosensory representation and spatial perception,[238,239] abnormal gating of somatosensory inputs,[240] abnormal presynaptic synchronization of movement, abnormal muscle spindle afferent firing,[241–243] excessive tendencies to form associations between sensory inputs and motor outputs,[242,244] uncoupling of movements in the primary motor and sensory areas,[245] abnormalities in gray matter,[246] impaired somatosensory function, and difficulty with sensorimotor integration.[247–255] In addition, Siebner et al.[256] reported altered blood flow responses in the premotor areas, putamen, thalamus, and cerebellum (e.g., after repetitive transmagnetic stimulation [rTMS], there was a greater decrease of regional cerebral blood flow (rCBF) in the lateral and medial premotor areas, putamen, and thalamus but a general increased responsiveness of the cerebellum).[256,257]

Neuroplasticity and FHd Etiology

Aberrant Learning. Our hands allow us to perform delicate, complex, individuated, fine motor movements.[258–265] Skilled, well-practiced hand movements represent an interaction of many factors, including orderly, somatotopic, highly differentiated representations of the hand in the thalamus, basal ganglia, and cortex (Figure 27-9).[263,264] Normal primates have a precise somatosensory representation of the hand characterized

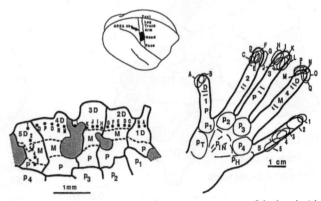

Figure 27-9 Representative normal somatosensory map of the hand with small receptive fields. The digits are organized from distal to proximal. (From Byl NN, Merzenich MM, Cheung S et al: A primate model for studying focal dystonia and repetitive strain injury: effects on the primary somatosensory cortex, *Phys Ther* 77:273, 1997.)

with one receptive field per electrode penetration, small receptive fields (8 μm²) unique to each digit, orderly sequencing of digits from inferior to superior, and orderly representation of the segments from proximal to distal. There is a distinct differentiation of the digits at 100 to 600 μm, and an area of hand representation of 3.2 to 5.1 mm² (see Figure 27-9).[266] With positive learning-based training, the area of representation increases in size, but the receptive fields decrease in size with increased specificity and density.[267-281]

Positive changes in neural adaptive behaviors can be achieved by maturation or by training under conditions of rewarded, spaced, fun, learning-based, goal-directed, task-specific progressive mental and physical practice matched to the interests of the individual.[267-283] Musicians, for example, practice complex fine motor skills to perfect performance (i.e., efficiency, quality, accuracy, control, complexity of decision making, or complexity of movements).[284,285] This practice is associated with improved topographical representation of the hand.[286,287] Thus, it may not be surprising that FHd is reported in

musicians.[288-292] Furthermore, well-learned tasks have their own topographical representations beyond the anatomical limb performing the task.[287]

However, our nervous system has inherent, finite limits in adaptation (e.g., physiological time constants, inhibition, integration time).[234] Genetics, trauma, poor biomechanics, excessive neuronal excitation, poor inhibition, environmental deprivation, drug use, phobias, negative feedback, chronic stress, perseveration, perfectionism, chronic pain, and/or *forceful, rapid, repetitive, near-simultaneous, stereotypical movements* can lead to degradation of the topographical representations of the digits[76,77] (Figure 27-10) and changes in timing, amplitude, and spatial characteristics of neuronal processing.[207,293] If rapid inputs occur within the inhibitory or integration period of stimulus processing, new inputs are not registered as temporally distinct[75-77,232,293-296] or with stimulated skin surfaces forming a unified rather than a unique spatial and temporal representation in the cerebral cortices, brain stem, and spinal cord.[294] Specificity of digital representation is critical to the maintenance of the normal sensory

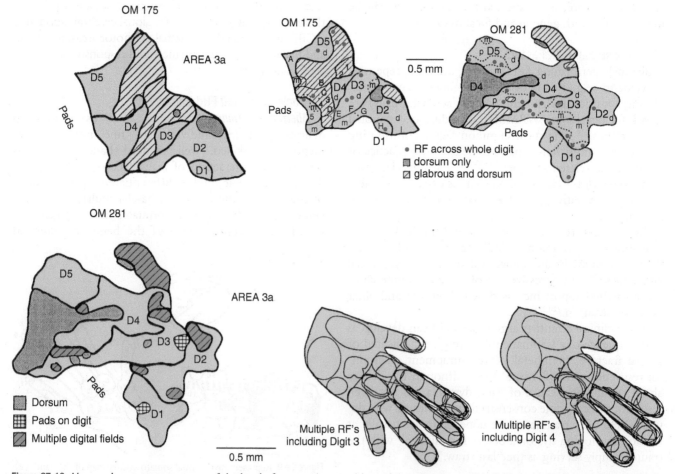

Figure 27-10 Abnormal somatosensory map of the hand after excessive repetitive training. Large receptive fields overlap adjacent digits, adjacent segments, and dorsal and glabrous surfaces. *RF,* receptive fields. (From Byl NN, Merzenich MM, Cheung S et al: A primate genesis model of focal dystonia and repetitive strain injury. I. Learning-induced dedifferentiation of the representation of the hand in the primary somatosensory cortex in adult monkeys, *Neurology* 47:513-515, 1996.)

organization, sensorimotor feedback, and fine motor control.[297,298] These aberrant topographical mappings of somatosensory inputs and motor outputs have been associated with abnormal, involuntary, dystonic motor movements of the hand.[75-77,297,299,300]

With this information, a paradigm shift was developing in the understanding of the etiology of FHd. Based on primate studies of repetitive hand use, Blake et al.[75,296] and Byl et al.[76,77] proposed the "sensorimotor learning hypothesis": repetitive use, near-simultaneous firing, coupling of multiple sensory signals, and voluntary co-activation of flexor and extensor muscles could lead to degradation of the cortical sensory and motor representations of the hand.

In a series of animal research studies based on a repetitive training paradigm, four of six primates developed movement dysfunction consistent with focal dystonia. These primates worked intensively on a daily basis to open and close a hand-piece to release food pellets (e.g., performing 1000 to 2000 repetitions/hour, 2 to 3 hours/day for 1 to 6 months). The two primates who did not develop dystonia trained slowly and casually (closing/opening the hand-piece for 10 minutes and then taking a break, performing fewer than 1000 repetitions in 2 to 3 hours). In addition, these two primates placed the hand on the hand-piece and leaned backward to close the device, minimizing rapid, repetitive, stereotypical, and coincident movements and maintaining normal topographical representation.[76,77]

Both the trained and untrained hands of all the primates were dissected by an anatomist blinded to dystonia status. There were no signs of acute inflammation in any of the animals.[78,291] Interestingly, the monkey who developed the earliest sign of FHd (i.e., hyperextension of D4 after 4 weeks of training) had a congenital defect of the flexor superficialis and flexor profundus tendons on the fourth digit on the trained side and the third finger on the untrained side. The size of the receptive fields of D4 on the trained side were enlarged, overlapping adjacent fingers and dorsal and palmar surfaces. On the untrained side, there were no signs of movement dysfunction even though the receptive fields of D3 were larger than normal. However, the receptive fields on the untrained side did not overlap across adjacent digits or dorsal and glabrous surfaces.[78,291]

On the basis of the sensorimotor hypothesis, Sanger and Merzenich[301] proposed an integrated, multisystem computational model to explain the origin of FHd. If the sensorimotor loop gain and the neural circuitry connecting the deep cortical nuclei, basal ganglia, and thalamus are unstable, a focal or a general dystonia could develop (e.g., depending on the extent of the imbalance across multiple sensory and motor systems).[253,294] The computational model could explain why symptoms (1) develop in otherwise healthy individuals who perform highly attended, repetitive movements; (2) evolve variably in time; (3) appear only during the performance of a target-specific task (i.e., dystonic movements); (4) persist even when the task is no longer performed repetitively; (5) decrease but are not remediated with dopamine-depleting drugs or botulinum toxin; and (6) are associated with abnormalities in somatosensory, sensorimotor, and motor representations of the dystonic limb.

Lack of Homeostatic Plasticity. In the past 10 years, research has provided convincing evidence about excessive brain plasticity in patients with FHd. In a variety of clinical studies, exceptional adaptability of the central nervous system has been reported in patients with focal dystonia.[249,256,302-307] Quartarone and his team hypothesized the degradation in motor control seen in patients with focal dystonia was a consequence of excessive plasticity.[249,256,302,305,306] In other words, there is a lack of homeostatic, associative plasticity in the brain in patients with task-specific dystonia. The brain fails to stop adapting when the most efficient neural firing pattern is achieved. This hypothesis is consistent with the hyperactivity measured in the basal ganglia[249] and the somatosensory, sensorimotor, and motor cortices.[256,302,305,306] This hypothesis is also consistent with recent findings of abnormal synaptic plasticity[308] and defective cerebellar control of plasticity[309] in patients with focal dystonia. Compared with age-matched controls, patients with dystonia have increased neuronal excitation and decreased inhibition with easy modification of the cortical silent period in the premotor and motor cortices following rTMS or anodal and cathodal transcutaneous direct current stimulation (tDCS). These findings suggest the nervous system does not have the usual adaptive mechanisms to limit allowable levels of synaptic potentiation.[302,306]

An Interactive Systems Model

Given the incidence of FHd in musicians, Altenmuller et al.[310] proposed the systems model for understanding the etiology of FHd. This model integrates the task specificity as well as the strength of sensory information to modify the motor dysfunction (i.e., sensory trick). If the sensory stimulus is encoded as a signal vector of a high dimension, then a part of its component directly represents the sensory stimulus while the remaining components describe the context. This etiological model for focal dystonia accounts for the task specificity and the context of the movement dysfunction,[193] while also being consistent with the aberrant topography of the digits,[75-77,267,286,294,296] the lack of homeostatic plasticity,[304,305] and the imbalance of excitation and inhibition.[207] This model explains why weakening dystonic muscles with botulinum toxin does not "cure" FHd.[311] This model also provides a foundation for supporting rehabilitative strategies directed toward stopping the abnormal movements, engaging motivation and commitment to improve biomechanics, reducing unnecessary stressful repetition and creating task-specific, progressive sensory and motor retraining to restore normal motor and somatosensory representations.

History, Clinical Assessment, and Diagnosis of Focal Hand Dystonia

The diagnosis of FHd is made by a careful history and clinical examination.[312–315] Although there may be some common findings among patients with FHd, there are also differences that may be important relative to treatment planning.[316–318] There are no laboratory tests to confirm the diagnosis. The history is begun by inquiring about a genetic workup. The clinician should inquire whether any other family members have dystonia or other types of movement disorders (e.g., Parkinson's disease, essential tremor, neural hyperexcitability [e.g., sensitivity to loud noises], attention-deficit disorders, premature birth, Alzheimer's disease) as well as information about results of imaging and electromyography (EMG).[312]

The clinician should review past or recent traumas to the hand. If there was an injury to the hand, the clinician should determine whether the trauma (1) had a strong temporal-anatomical relationship to the onset of FHd; (2) was severe enough to cause persistent local symptoms and lead to late medical attention; (3) was the same site as the initial anatomical manifestation of the movement disorder; (4) was within days or up to 12 months of the onset of the movement dysfunction; and (5) occurred to the hand or upper limb with preexisting contractures and limitations of passive movement.[222,223] It is essential that the clinician check about levels of stress, periods of intensive repetitive hand use, job instability, application of a new technique, a change in equipment, increased time on task to improve quality of performance, quantity of work expected, or intensity of time involved in performance.[223,319]

The clinician should inquire about the initial onset of signs and symptoms relative to overuse: inflammation, swelling, pain, fatigue, tendinitis, or neuropathy.[319] Some patients report no previous injury, but rather an insidious onset of weakness, incoordination, or involuntary movements when performing a specific task, such as playing the guitar. Still others report a tremor or jerkiness when performing similar tasks, such as typing on the keyboard or playing the piano. The clinician should inquire about stress[217] and assess personality characteristics (e.g., intense, high achiever, perfectionist, impatient, phobic) depression, and emotional stability.[202,320,321]

The clinical examination should include the administration of standardized tests and measurements (Table 27-6).[322–330] A magnetic resonance imaging (MRI) scan may be ordered by the physician to rule out specific brain pathology; however, functional imaging techniques (fMRI, rTMS, repetitive direct current stimulation [rDCS], motor evoked response [MEP], sensory evoked response [SEP]) used in clinical research are not considered a standard part of a FHd examination.[76,77,286,294] The physician may order EMG studies if signs of a peripheral neuropathy are present.[265,292]

TABLE **27-6**

Summary of Clinical Testing Procedures for Examination of Focal Hand Dystonia and Clinical Studies

Measurement Tool	Dependent Variable	Scoring System	Directions	Reliability	Equipment
Graphesthesia (modified subtest of Sensory Integration Praxis Test [SIPT])	Sensory performance	2 = Correct 1 = Partially correct 0 = Incorrect % error calculated	Tip of a paper clip was used to draw designs on subject's fingers while the subject's eyes were closed Subject recreated design with pen with eyes open Two designs per finger pad	Inter-rater = 0.95 Test–retest: $r = 0.91$ (Ayres[331])	Paper clip and design sheet
Kinesthesia (subtest of SIPT)	Sensory performance	Average error (distance from target) in mm	Subject's hand was moved to target and back to start position; subject attempted to relocate digit, eyes were closed Five trials per hand	Inter-rater = 0.95 Test-retest: $r = 0.90$ (Ayres,[331] Byl et al.[251])	Target sheet and ruler
Byl-Cheney-Boczai (BCB) test for stereognosis	Sensory performance	2 = Correct 1 = Partially correct 0 = Incorrect % error calculated	Subject's finger was drawn across the shape twice, eyes were closed Subject attempted to pick correct shape 10 trials for second and fourth finger pads	Inter-rater/ intrarater = 0.995 (ICC) Correlation of $r = 0.60$ between BCB test (Byl et al.[332]) and Purdue Test Lafayette Instruments	20 designs and test sheet of designs

(Continued)

TABLE **27-6**

Summary of Clinical Testing Procedures for Examination of Focal Hand Dystonia and Clinical Studies—cont'd

Measurement Tool	Dependent Variable	Scoring System	Directions	Reliability	Equipment
Digital reaction time	Fine motor performance	Time in msec, average of all trials	Subject turned stopwatch on/off as quickly as possible Three trials per finger	Intrasession reliability ranges from 0.975-0.99 (Bohannon[333])	Stopwatch
Purdue Test	Fine motor performance	Total time to put pegs in and out	Subject put 25 pegs into a board and then removed them	Lafayette Instruments—distributer	Watch, peg board
Manual muscle test (MMT)	Musculoskeletal performance	Kilograms of force: UE and LE Scores total all scores*	Performed per procedures defined by Kendall (Kendall and McCreary[334]) with dynamometers added to increase objectivity used for grip, key, and pinch grip	$R^2 = 0.887$ Multiple correlation with MMT	Jamar, Microfet, and Baseline dynamometers
Range of motion	Musculoskeletal performance	Degrees; sum of active and passive	Performed measurement procedures defined by Norkin and White[335] Arm, wrist, and hand joints summed to an UE score, and joints in the leg summed to a LE score and then totaled	Intratester: $r = 0.91\text{-}0.99$	Goniometer
Posture and balance	Posture and balance	Ordinal scales: 2 = Fully met criteria 1 = Partially met criteria 0 = Did not meet criteria	Posture: Bony landmarks cited for line of gravity (Kendall and McCreary[334]) were coded as 0-2 and summed to a total Balance score summed from feet together (eyes were open and eyes were closed for 20 sec), one foot (eyes were open and eyes were closed for 10 sec), and tandem Romberg (eyes were open and eyes were closed for 10 sec)		
CAFÉ 40	Functional performance	7-point Likert scale: 1 = Least independent 7 = Most independent	Self-scoring of ability to perform functional activities; scores inverted for data analysis	Test–retest: $r = 0.971$ (Fung et al.[330])	Questionnaire-self report

Companies supplying instruments (including administration guidelines): (1) Hoggan Health Industries, Microfet Dynamometer: Medical Products Division, Hoggan Health Industries, Inc., 3653 W 1987 S #7, Salt Lake City, Utah 94014; (2) Jamar Dynamometer: TEC, 60 Page Road, Clifton, New Jersey 07012; (3) Lafayette Instrument Company, Instructions and Normative Data, Purdue Pegboard, P.O. Box 5729, Lafayette, Indiana 47903; and, (4) Finger Tapper, Psychological Assessment Resources Inc., P.O. Box 998, Odessa, Florida 33556.

UE, Upper extremity; *LE,* lower extremity.

*Muscle groups tested: hip flexors and extensors, knee flexors and extensors, ankle dorsiflexors, elbow flexors, shoulder flexors, wrist extensors, lumbricals, grip and pinch (three-jaw chuck and key grip) strength.

Although patients frequently report "weakness," on the clinical musculoskeletal examination, strength is usually normal unless there are clear signs of peripheral nerve compression at the thoracic outlet, cubital tunnel, or carpal tunnel.[265,292,303] However, there may be an imbalance in strength between the extrinsic and intrinsic muscles, with extrinsic muscles exceptionally strong from overuse and the intrinsic muscles disproportionately weak, potentially from limited use.[336] Poor posture (i.e., forward head and shoulders) and poor postural righting are commonly noted.[336] Hypermobility of the interphalangeal and metacarpophalangeal joints in flexion and extension and excessive ulnar deviation of the wrist may be noted. In addition, limitations in finger spread, forearm rotation, and/or shoulder lateral (external) rotation are also commonly measured.[216,284]

The neurological examination is usually considered normal (e.g., reflexes, coordination, gait, light touch, sharp dull). If hyporeflexia or hyperreflexia are noted, then further diagnostic testing may be needed to rule out a peripheral neuropathy or central neural dysfunction. On the other hand, cases of hyperactive dystonia have been reported, primarily in children who have both spasticity and dystonia.[196] Most commonly, the involuntary movements occur primarily when the patient voluntarily performs a target task or a similar task and are usually not present at rest or with sleep.

There may be positive signs of neural tension when the brachial plexus is placed on a stretch for the median or ulnar nerve.[303] In patients with FHd, especially musicians, it is not uncommon to palpate a subluxing ulnar nerve at the elbow.[220,221] If a patient is experiencing pain, ask the patient to rate the pain on a visual analog scale of 1 to 10.[326] Some patients with FHd report a sense of dullness or numbness in the pads of the fingers when they are placed on the target surface. Patients with FHd frequently perform poorly on tasks demanding cortical sensory discrimination, such as stereognosis, graphesthesia, and proprioception.[307-309] It is important to objectively evaluate all motor and sensory skills to establish a foundation for validating change.

The objective validation of FHd is to observe the involuntary movements when the patient is asked to perform the target task. With permission, the patient should be video recorded while performing the target task. Videos can serve as a reference for measuring preintervention and postintervention performance. Traditional dystonia scales should be used to rate the involuntary movements (i.e., quality and severity).[328,329] The Arm Dystonia Scale or the arm component of the Unified Dystonia Rating Scale (UDRS), the Global Dystonia Rating Scale (GDS), or the Fahn Marsden Dystonia Rating Scale (FMDRS) can be used for these ratings (Table 27-7).[302,306,328,329] Some clinicians may have access to motion analysis to more objectively document timing and force abnormalities.[304,327] The Disabilities of the Arm, Shoulder and Hand (DASH) Outcome Measure and Quick DASH are available as applications to the iPad or the iPhone and can be administered to assess general functional limitations in the hand/arm (Institute for Work and Health).[337] It can be helpful to administer a general functional measure (e.g., CAFÉ 40)[330] to document the impact of the hand dystonia on activities of daily living (ADLs) and community participation. The patient should be asked to demonstrate what he or she does to try to control the involuntary movements (i.e., sensory tricks). Based on the underlying neurophysiological findings relative to etiology, is important to examine both the involved and uninvolved limbs.

TABLE **27-7**

Dystonia Scales: Grading Severity of Involuntary Dystonia Movements

Dystonia Scales: Arm/Hand	Area Evaluated	Ordinal Scores
Global Dystonia Rating Scale (GDS)	10 body areas: 1 = Eyes and face 2 = Lower face 3 = Jaw and tongue 4 = Larynx 5 = Neck 6 = Shoulder and proximal arm 7 = Distal arm and hand, including elbow 8 = Pelvis and upper leg 9 = Distal leg and foot 10 = Trunk	Rated on a scale of 0-10: 0 = No dystonia 1 = Minimal dystonia 5 = Moderate dystonia 10 = Most severe dystonia
Unified Dystonia Rating Scale (UDRS)	Rated on an ordinal scale 10 areas of body rated for severity Rating also required for duration	Shoulder and proximal arm (right and left), distal arm and hand (right and left) Score 0-4: 0 = None 1 = Mild; movement <25% of normal 2 = Moderate; movements 25%-50% of range possible 3 = Severe; movements 50%-75% of possible range 4 = Extreme; movements <75% of possible

(Continued)

TABLE **27-7**

Dystonia Scales: Grading Severity of Involuntary Dystonia Movements—cont'd

Dystonia Scales: Arm/ Hand	Area Evaluated	Ordinal Scores
Fahn Marsden Dystonia Rating Scale (FMDRS) (product of symptom frequency and severity)	9 areas of the body evaluated: eyes, mouth, speech, swallowing, neck, trunk, right and left arms, and right and left legs Two clinical rated subscales: movement subscale based on patient examination and disability subscale based on patient's report of disability in activities of daily living (7 areas, including speech, writing, feeding, eating, hygiene, dressing, and walking) The score for eyes, mouth, and neck is multiplied by 0.5 before being entered into the calculation; total movement FMDRS subscore is the sum of the product of provoking, severity, and weighting factors; total maximal score is 120. Training for administration is recommended	Movement scale: 0 = No dystonia present 1 = Slight dystonia; clinically insignificant 2 = Mild: obvious dystonia, but not disabling 3 = Moderate: able to grasp with some manual function 4 = Severe: no useful grasp Disability rated on an ordinal scale of 5 but walking rated on a 7-point scale Provoking factors: 0 = No dystonia at rest or with action 1 = Dystonia only with particular action 2 = Dystonia with many actions 3 = Dystonia on action of distant part of body or intermittently at rest 4 = Dystonia present at rest

Data from www.mdvu.org/library/ratingscales/dystonia/.

Biofeedback can be used to allow the examiner and the patient to observe the onset of involuntary co-contractions of agonists and antagonists, firing patterns, and the ability to turn off a muscle once excited. One characteristic of dystonia is an on/off pattern of muscle firing when the patient recruits a dystonic muscle and tries to hold consistently against resistance. Neural firing can also be "heard" when an EMG injection needle electrode is placed into an overexcited dystonic muscle. EMG monitoring is used to select the muscles to inject with botulinum toxin and monitor an immediate, early quieting after the injection.[311]

The diagnosis of FHd is based on a careful history and clinical examination to try to "rule in" the diagnosis and minimize false-positive and false-negative diagnoses (Figures 27-11 and 27-12).[338] The history

Factors to "Rule in" Diagnosis Focal Hand Dystonia (FHd)

Factors	Yes = 1	No = 0	Comment
1. Normal neurological exam except involuntary movement at target task			
2. Involuntary movement when performing target task			
3. Type A personality (e.g., perfectionist, possibly phobic)			
4. Sensory trick			
5. Under stress, history of high levels of repetitive practice			
6. Abnormal cortical sensory discrimination (e.g., graphesthesia, stereognosis)			
7. Decreased finger spread			
8. Normal magnetic resonance imaging (MRI)			
9. Family history of dystonia or Jewish descent			
Maximum total score	9		

Figure 27-11 Focal hand dystonia is a clinical diagnosis. The diagnosis is ruled in based on the history of onset, signs and symptoms, family history of movement disorders, genetic history, history of high stress, excessive practice or increased work, the presence of involuntary movements when performing a specific well-learned task, the benefit of sensory tricks to temporarily control the involuntary contractions, normal neurological examination, and normal magnetic resonance imaging scans. *Graphesthesia,* ability to recognize writing on skin by sensation of touch; *stereognosis,* the ability to perceive the form of solid objects by touch.

"Ruling in" the Diagnosis of
Focal Hand Dystonia (FHd): Example

Score	Has FHd	Does not have FHd	
9	25	5	30
<9	4	26	30
	29	31	

False positive 4/29 (13.8%)   **False negative** 5/30 (16.7%)

Sensitivity 25/29 = 86%   **Specificity** 26/31 = 84%

Likelihood ratio +(LR+)   **Likelihood ratio −(LR−)**
LR+ = 0.86/0.167 = 5.15   LR− = 0.14/0.84 = 0.17

Figure 27-12 When the clinical criteria are met to rule in the diagnosis of focal hand dystonia (FHd), the objective is to minimize false-positive diagnoses (diagnosed with the disorder when it is not the diagnosis) and false-negative diagnoses (cleared of the diagnosis when the patient does have the disorder). The criteria should lead to a diagnosis that is both sensitive and specific. Here is an example of using the criteria in Figure 27-11 to determine false-positive results, false-negative results, sensitivity, and specificity.

and clinical examination should conclude with a list of impairments and functional limitations that need to be addressed in treatment. Many of these impairments and functional limitations will be consistent across patients with FHd, but it is important to identify impairments that may be unique to each individual patient (Table 27-8).

The prognosis for recovery depends on a variety of factors. These factors range from personal goals, objectives, and commitment to personal and vocational opportunities, access to health care specialists, and community resources for retraining (Table 27-9). The most important factor in recovery is patient motivation and commitment to retraining. The second most important factor is patient access to resources to establish a guided recovery program.

TABLE 27-8

Impairments and Limitations Common in Patients with Focal Hand Dystonia

Anatomic and Neurophysiological Impairments	Functional Limitations
Decrease in range of motion • Finger spread • Forearm pronation/supination • Shoulder external rotation	• Inability to place forearm in full pronation on a keyboard (e.g., playing piano, typing) • Difficulty holding a stringed instrument in full supination (e.g., violin or viola) • Difficulty opening hand on keyboard
Excessive range of motion • Excessive extension of interphalangeal (IP) joints • Excessive extension of the metacarpophalangeal (MP) joints • Excessive wrist ulnar deviation	• Difficulty maintaining stability of the digits on the keyboard • Difficulty controlling coordinated digital movements within an octave • Difficulty writing and typing
Imbalance of strength • Strong extrinsic wrist and finger flexors • Weak intrinsic muscles (interossei and lumbricals)	• Cannot place hand in neutral (e.g., assumes a claw-like position) • Difficult to perform coordinated, controlled fine motor movements
Abnormal sensory processing • Decreased accuracy of spatial/temporal sensory processing • Excessive sensory excitability	• Errors in fine motor movements • Inadequate regulation of velocity and movement force • Disruption of sound quality
Abnormal preparation for movement • Poor sensory gating • Poor motor preparation • Excessive motor firing	• Finger contact with objects produces involuntary, quick, and jerky movements • Quality and efficiency of fine motor control compromised
Lack of inhibition • Involuntary simultaneous contraction of agonists and antagonists • Inability to turn off unwanted firing	• Sensory inputs lead to jerky, quick, forceful, poorly graded movements • Unwanted notes and keys are depressed
Lack of homeostatic plasticity • Hypersensitivity of synaptic connections • Autonomic fight/flight responses (and sometimes hyper-reflexia) • Rapid, high-amplitude response • Difficulty turning off neuronal activation • Prolonged muscle firing	• Light touch leads to reflexive, exaggerated protective motor responses (high-force and amplitude) • Light touch may be painful • Repetitive movements do not get faster despite practice • Difficult to control common digital movements for writing and typing

TABLE **27-9**

Prognosis for Successful Management of Focal Hand Dystonia

Positive Factors	Negative Factors
Expects to get better; motivated to retraining	Feels discouraged about recovery
Positive health and wellness (aerobic exercise, good hydration, good nutrition, adequate sleep)	Has not invested in regular health and wellness program
Not perseverative or phobic but still a perfectionist	Perseverative, perfectionist, phobic
Supportive family; supportive work environment with financial stability	Does not have supportive family, supportive employer, or financial stability
Able to stop abnormal movements (even though needs sensory tricks or modification of surface or position)	Unable to stop abnormal movements
Integrates diaphragmatic breathing; worked through neural tension	Breathes with scalenes; has neural tension and subluxing ulnar nerve and/or carpal tunnel syndrome
Has no numbness or tingling	Has numbness, tingling sensory loss
Has normal reflexes	Has hypoactive or hyperactive reflexes
Has normal range of motion	Has hypermobile metacarpophalangeal (MP) or interphalangeal joints but restricted finger spread
Has good strength of intrinsic hand muscles	Has weakness of intrinsic hand muscles
Manages stress, anxiety, and depression well	Is unusually stressed, tense, and anxious
Has a good coach for task performance (e.g., music teacher)	Does not have a coach for task-specific training
Can take time off from performing task	Financially needs to continue to work at job that creates the dystonia
Sets time for retraining	Cannot find time or retraining; too busy working
Is willing and able to change biomechanics and techniques for performance	Is unable or unwilling to modify biomechanics of upper extremity
Experiences improved sensory discrimination	Has chronic neuropathic pain; neural sensitivity and poor sensory discrimination continues
Is committed to learning something new	Is completely engrained in habitual activities
Progresses practice difficulty; takes frequent breaks	Is unable to space practice; continues with intense practice despite short practice periods
Combines mental imagery and practice with physical practice	Has difficulty performing mental imagery; dependent on excessive physical practice

MANAGEMENT OF WORK-RELATED MUSCULOSKELETAL DISORDERS

Worksite Management

For U.S. employers, the Occupational Safety and Health Administration (OSHA) continued to develop industry-specific and task-specific ergonomic guidelines for voluntary use.[339] Thus far, guidelines have been established for foundries,[340] nursing homes,[341] shipyards,[342] manual materials handling,[343] poultry processing,[344] grocery stores,[345] apparel and footware industries,[346] furniture manufacturing industries,[347] telecommunications industry,[348] farming,[349] baggage handling for the airline industry,[350] construction industries,[351] and more. All of these guidelines embrace the same basic program components of prevention and management, which are set forth, for example, in the OSHA guidelines for nursing homes[341]:

1. *Management support:* Clearly developed program goals, clearly identified program responsibilities for participants, adequate provision of resources, and oversight to ensure the success of the program.

2. *Employee involvement:* Early employee reporting of problems; also, employees provide insight (i.e., suggestions and evaluation) into work design issues and solutions and share responsibility for program development and implementation.

3. *Problem identification:* Systematic procedures using various sources of information, such as OSHA injury and illness logs, data from workers' compensation claims, and surveillance and workplace analysis.

4. *Solution implementation:* Typically involves changes to eliminate or reduce workplace hazards, problematic work practices, or both.

5. *Injury management:* Emphasis on early detection and intervention.

6. *Training of employees and managers:* Training on the risks and detection of MSDs and the procedures required to respond to an MSD incident.

7. *Regular program evaluation:* Determination of quantifiable measures, such as number and severity of MSDs.

The success of such workplace MSD management programs relies on clear communication between workers, managers, and health care providers. Such communication requires an atmosphere of cooperation and mutual trust among all stakeholders. One benefit of establishing such a program is that it often alleviates the impact of psychosocial risk factors by providing employees with an opportunity to contribute directly as members of a cohesive MSD management team.

Essential Components: Workplace Management Program for Musculoskeletal Disorders

- Management support
- Employee involvement
- Problem identification
- Solution implementation
- Injury management
- Training of employees and managers
- Regular program evaluation

Clinical Management

The biopsychosocial model of clinical management has been clearly demonstrated to be the most successful approach to the management of activity-related MSDs. In this model, the interactions of physical impairments, personal psychological factors, and psychosocial factors are recognized and targeted for prevention as well as treatment in a holistic approach to care.[352] Biopsychosocial management programs have several advantages, including the following:

1. Emphasizing prevention and education regarding excessive overuse
2. Addressing the importance of a safe, supportive environment in the workplace
3. Emphasizing the importance of using a multidisciplinary health care team to address the multiple causal factors of activity-related MSDs
4. Illustrating the need for clear communication and cooperation between health care providers, injured workers, and various stakeholders in the workplace
5. Showing that clear communication is greatly enhanced by trained case managers who oversee all aspects of health care and workplace management
6. Demonstrating that effective health care interventions for activity-related MSDs do not necessarily result in a cure but rather lead to long-term worker- and workplace-focused management through effective problem solving by the entire MSD management team

---

Essential Components of a Clinical Management Program for Musculoskeletal Disorders

- Education and prevention
- Holistic approach to care with focus on physical impairments and personal and workplace psychosocial factors

---

- Multidisciplinary health care team
- Communication and cooperation between health care providers, injured workers, and the workplace
- Trained case managers
- Long-term worker- and workplace-focused management

Summary

MSDs account for 34% of lost workday injuries and illnesses in the United States in 2012. The median days away from work—a key measure of severity of injuries and illnesses—was 9 days. Injuries and illnesses resulting from repetitive motion involving microtasks resulted in a median of 23 days away from work to recuperate and increased further in 2012 in four occupational groups: computer and mathematical occupations, community and social service occupations, personal care and service occupations, and transportation and material moving occupations. These disorders have a major effect on workers' compensation costs, absenteeism, and loss of productivity.

Strong epidemiological evidence indicates that risk factors for the development of work-related MSDs of the upper limb include the performance of hand-intensive tasks in a manner that is highly repetitive or forceful (or both) in awkward or sustained postures, with or without vibration and cold temperatures. Psychosocial stress also increases the risk of WRMSDs of the upper limb. Individual predisposing factors that contribute to the risk of upper limb WRMSDs include past or present comorbid medical conditions, female gender, obesity, poor biomechanics, and advanced age.

It is beyond the scope of this chapter to describe in detail MSD clinical management programs for patients with acute MSD injuries. However, several recent examples in the literature can guide the reader.[353–355] The remaining part of this chapter outlines the comprehensive intervention program needed for patients with chronic musculoskeletal disorders that are associated with persistent pain and FHd.

MANAGEMENT OF CHRONIC WORK-RELATED MUSCULOSKELETAL DISORDERS: FOCAL HAND DYSTONIA

General Management

Simultaneous with workplace management, education, ergonomics, facilitation of healing, and clinical problem solving, patients with chronic MSDs must work with a team and engage in a comprehensive rehabilitation program. Rehabilitation must focus on general health and wellness (i.e., exercise, lifestyle modification, improved biomechanics, nutrition) and specific retraining to maximize neural adaptation. The prognosis for functional recovery is affected by a variety of intrinsic and extrinsic factors (see Table 27-9).

The patient and his or her family are critical members of the rehabilitation team. The patient must expect to get better and be willing to invest time and effort in the recovery process. The health care providers on the team include the physician, therapists, psychologist, and nutritionist. Teachers and community movement trainers can support the health care team. The physician should be a specialist in neurology, musculoskeletal disorders, pain management, and/or movement disorders. The physician should be familiar with prescribing systemic drugs as needed for pain, muscle spasm, anxiety, depression, and sleep, as well as with injecting botulinum toxin if needed to decrease muscle cramping. Ideally, the physician should have experience working with a team of nutritionists, physical therapists, occupational therapists, and psychologists experienced in the management of chronic pain, stress, and anxiety. A "coach" (e.g., a music teacher, sports coach, a biomechanist) may be able to suggest new ways to perform job-related tasks without further injury. In addition, relaxation techniques, massage, mindfulness training, meditation, acupuncture, acupressure, and imagery for self-healing along with classes or individual sessions involving movement training (e.g., yoga, tai chi, Ji Gong, Alexander Technique, Feldenkrais Method, Pilates, Nia, tae kwon do, dance) can also be beneficial. The remainder of this chapter describes activities for health and wellness, principles of neural adaptation, and physical and occupational therapy strategies for retraining.

Positive Health Behaviors

Our population is aging. Aging is associated with brain atrophy, memory problems, depression, decreased physical activity, and degenerative disease.[356] In fact, the World Health Organization reports physical inactivity as a primary health problem today.[357] This is the case despite the objectives established in 1979 for *Healthy People 2000*.[358] In fact, physical inactivity is the fourth leading cause of global mortality and is the main cause of approximately 21% to 25% of breast and colon cancer cases, 27% of diabetes cases, and 30% of ischemic heart disease cases. Physically active people have lower rates of coronary heart disease, high blood pressure, stroke, diabetes, colon cancer, and depression. Active people also have a lower risk of falling and hip or vertebral fractures. Young people need a minimum of 60 minutes of intense exercise a week, but those 18 to 65 years and older should have 150 minutes of moderate exercise and 75 minutes of vigorous activity each week.[359]

Longitudinal studies confirm moderate and aerobic exercise complemented with positive lifestyle behaviors is needed to facilitate healthy aging and maintain flexibility, strength, endurance, coordination, posture, balance, and cardiopulmonary function, as well as reduce risks for diabetes, arthritis, and cancer.[360-362] Furthermore, a combination of intense aerobic exercise and cognitive motor training not only may decrease brain atrophy and maintain memory and motor skills but also may potentially be neuroprotective against neurodegenerative disease.[359,363]

Ideally, individuals should walk or ride a bike instead of driving. It is better to walk up or down the stairs instead of taking an elevator. Patients should be encouraged to take daily walks while talking, observing, and learning something new (e.g., noting new activities in the neighborhood and greeting people along the way).

Aerobic exercise should be performed four to five times a week, 30 to 40 minutes per session. In these sessions, each individual should warm up and cool down for 3 to 5 minutes and keep the heart rate at 70% to 80% of maximum ($[220 - \text{age}] \times 80\%$) for approximately 20 to 30 minutes. Patients can chose to run, bike, swim, dance, or practice routines for a sport (e.g., plyometric activities, ball activities, balance). It is important to experience moderate exertion (rated at least 3 out of 10) with associated perspiration and an increase in breathing rate.[364]

All of us, young and old, should participate in learning activities for brain fitness. Focused learning activities drive selective changes in cortical cell differentiation and specialized representations. These changes not only include the expansion of cortical areas of representations, the reduction in the size of receptive fields, and the narrowed columnar spread but also improve co-selection of complementary inputs, increase excitable neurons, enhance salience and specificity of feedback, increase myelination, strengthen synapses between coincident inputs, shorten integration time, and increase complexity of dendritic branching.[266,365-374] The neural adaptation is associated with the emergence of more efficient, accurate, and differentiated behaviors.[268-278,280-283,375]

Learning activities range from simply learning something new each day (e.g., reading, doing crossword puzzles, playing Scrabble, identifying and spelling words, playing card games) to participating in specific, progressive perceptual motor, cognitive, and motor learning activities (e.g., playing games like Wii [wii.com] or Xbox Kinect [www.xbox.com/US/kinect]) or engaging in learning-based exercises from Posit Science (positscience.com) or Lumocity (lumocity.com).[363,364,374,376] In addition to general physical and brain exercises, individuals with FHd must emphasize specific sensory, sensorimotor, motor, and perceptual motor training activities to restore brain topography and function.[363]

Training activities need to take place in a positive environment, with the patient expecting to improve and motivated to engage in attended, goal-directed behavioral activities. The patient must understand the neurophysiology of dystonia and the challenge of inhibiting the involuntary, disruptive movements. The principles of neural retraining (e.g., sensory, sensorimotor, and motor retraining) can be applied across a variety of types of movement dysfunction and pain.

Translation of Principles of Neuroplasticity to Behavioral Training[374]

- "Use it or lose it"
- Remap and improve it; learn something new daily
- Have adequate, repetitive, variable, and progressive repetitions
- Make training intense with learning rather than stress as the focus (2-4 hours/day spread across the day, 4-5 days/week)
- Attend and be focused in practice activities
- Vary training sequences
- Progress difficulty of the tasks
- Be specific (e.g., task training, patient preferences, inspirational, motivational)
- Make learning fun (e.g., laugh, include elements of surprise)
- Spread practice over time (i.e., 8-12 weeks or more)
- Make training salient to each individual
- Make training age and task relevant
- Reinforce learning with feedback/accuracy
- Transfer common learning skills to new tasks
- Strengthen learning with predictable and unpredictable interference

Interestingly, neural learning is significantly affected by sleep. New synaptic networks (engrams) can be refreshed, and poor connections can be erased with not only variation in inputs but also metabolic state, emotions, natural endorphins, and sleep.[377-382] Thus, when retraining, one cannot overlook the importance of making sure patients have enough sleep. Sleep is essential for the nervous system to consolidate learning and recover from stressful life events. Although the number of hours of sleep may vary from individual to individual, everyone needs a comfortable period of deep (rapid eye movement [REM]) sleep. When individuals are stressed, anxious, or depressed, REM sleep may be limited not only by the time in bed but by the amount of worry during sleep.

Although there is no magic to achieve an ideal night of sleep, some behaviors can be helpful. Dinner should occur early, with time to move around and relax before going to bed. Sometimes a warm shower can help relax the muscles before going to sleep. Taking time to review the positive aspects as well as the challenging aspects of the day can be helpful to relax the mind. Thinking ahead to plan for the next day may also help encourage more relaxing sleep.

Current research reports new information about the negative effects of sleep deprivation. Although some individuals claim not to need a lot of sleep, the evidence suggests that a minimum amount of sleep is essential for positive health, learning, and memory.[380-382] On the other hand, sleeping to justify isolation and lack of productivity is not healthy. Further details of the positive and negative effects of sleep are beyond the scope of this chapter.

Nutrition and Healing: Patients with RSI

"Food should be our medicine and our medicine should be our food."
—Hippocrates

The words of Hippocrates have poignant wisdom for every patient with neuromusculoskeletal disorders, including those suffering from RSIs. The purpose of this section is to elaborate on the importance of recovery and how to set the stage for recovery to occur. The authors summarized current nutritional research with findings integrated into management strategies to reduce tissue sensitivity to repetitive force and to maximize and support recovery of patients with chronic musculoskeletal, work-related overuse injuries.

Nutrition affects all of our body systems, including but not limited to, the cardiovascular, neurological, muscular, skeletal, endocrine, pulmonary, dermatological, reproductive, genitourinary, and gastrointestinal (GI) systems. No system operates in isolation. The effects of inflammation from mechanical disruption or physiological processes will produce a response in all systems, albeit with different symptomatology.[13] As a consequence, a multifactorial, or multisystem, intervention strategy is needed to treat patients with overuse disorders. Nutrition fuels all of our body systems, positively or negatively affecting all physiological processes across the spectrum of healing and recovery from overuse injuries. Lack of proper nutrition can lead to chronic inflammatory processes, compromised healing, limited recovery, and reduced potential for rehabilitation.

Impact of Nutrition on Physiological Systems Affecting Healing

Nutritional factors affect the health and injury recovery of the joint, muscle, tendon, and bone. Park et al.[383] reported a link between vitamin D deficiencies in patients with early inflammatory arthritis. Kim et al.[384] reported antioxidants decreased cell death in human rotator cuff tenofibroblasts. Food components, like resveratrol, whey protein, chlorogenic acid, omega-3 fatty acids, and cherry extract, have been linked to increased muscle strength, decreased oxidative stress after exercise, decreased protein cross-linking, and decreased inflammatory markers.[385-388] Tendon healing can be enhanced by nutritional components such as vitamin C[389] and aloe vera.[390] In rat studies, fructose-rich diets have been associated with a metabolic syndrome that may impair bone growth via decreasing osteogenic potentiation.[391] Unfortunately, even medications, intended to improve recovery, may impair musculoskeletal recovery. For example, animal research studies reported nonsteroidal anti-inflammatory drugs (NSAIDs) decreased the biomechanical strength of repaired rat rotator cuff tendons (11 to 20 days after surgery).[392] Statin drugs, common in the treatment of high cholesterol, may produce an imbalance and microdamage of the extracellular matrix of tendons.[393]

The neurological system is also affected by nutritional components. In an obese mouse model, Tucsek et al.[394] reported that a high-fat diet exacerbated systemic inflammation in mice. In addition, there was a disruption in the blood–brain barrier resulting in neuroinflammation and oxidative stress in the hippocampus.[394] In mice,

Baumgarner et al.[395] reported that a high-fat diet produced peripheral cytokines in adipose tissue and the spleen, as well as measurable neuroinflammation and cognitive deficits. In quail embryo, Chen et al.[396] reported gestational diabetes in pregnancy as a result of high glucose and impaired nerve differentiation on the dorsal root ganglion and the developing limb buds. Using a mouse model for asthma, Ramalho et al.[397] reported increased substance P involved in neurogenic inflammation in high fat–induced obesity. Guo et al.[398] reported that older adults who added artificial sweeteners to their coffee or tea had a higher risk of depression than older adults who did not use artificial sweeteners.[398] The **Wahls Protocol**, a new treatment approach for progressive multiple sclerosis (MS), includes nutritional recommendations to assist stabilization, if not reversal, of the disease process, especially in relation to fatigue.[399]

Researchers have also demonstrated that nutrition can directly affect the endocrine system. Diet-induced obesity in rodents results in hepatic inflammation.[400] Interestingly, this inflammation is improved with resveratrol, a whole food nutrient.[400] Increased neutrophils in the mouse liver can be stimulated by high-fructose ingestion.[401] In a longitudinal clinical study, poor glycemic control increased inflammatory markers (insulin-like growth factor [IGF]-1).[402] Additionally, diet had a strong link to insulin sensitivity,[402] a critical physiological hormone that directs many pathways, including inflammation. Both Kanazawa et al.[402] and Young et al.[403] demonstrated that improved glycemic control with dietary factors improved insulin sensitivity and decreased inflammatory markers.

The cardiovascular system is also influenced by nutritional components. Liu et al.[404] evaluated the response of myocardial infarction markers in rats after ingestion of a Chinese herbal formula. Significant improvements in proinflammatory cytokines (TNF, IL-6, IL-1) were found after consuming this Chinese herbal formula.[404] Omega-3 polyunsaturated fatty acid (omega-3 PUFA) supplementation decreased inflammatory cytokines for patients with cardiomyopathy secondary to Chagas disease.[405] Jansen[406] reported that a multinutritional diet had beneficial effects on vascular health in a rat model for atherosclerosis. Supplemental chicken collagen hydrolysate may improve circulation in patients with mild hypertension.[407] A patient's risk of stroke is higher with consumption of sugar-sweetened soda.[408] Proper hydration appears to decrease the risk of a future stroke.[409–412] Ruth et al.[413] reported that a high-fat (60% saturated fat) and low-carbohydrate diet was associated with improvements in blood lipid and systemic inflammation, indicating improved cardiovascular health.

Nutrition has influences on the pulmonary system. For example, a poor dietary inflammatory index has been linked to patients with asthma.[414] Shi et al.[415] reported human consumption of monosodium glutamate (MSG) was positively associated with snoring and a high probability of sleep-disordered breathing (SDB) even if individuals were not overweight. Diet-induced obesity in mice has also been linked to peribronchial inflammation.[397]

There is also a relationship between the GI system and the neurological system, also known as the gut–brains axis. Shulman et al.[416] investigated the relationship between gut permeability and symptoms of life interference and psychological distress symptoms. In this clinical study, GI permeability was assessed using a urinary sucrose and lactulose ratio. In addition, information was collected on ADLs, work, psychological distress, and symptoms. They reported that within the population with irritable bowel syndrome (IBS), there was a distinct group with increased GI permeability who also had dysfunction in daily activities, psychological distress, and IBS symptoms.[416] Dickerson et al.[417] reported that patients with recent-onset psychosis and those with multiepisode schizophrenia have significantly increased levels of immune response to the gluten protein, gliadin, compared with control subjects. This sensitivity to the gluten protein has been associated with acute mania and bipolar disorders, without associated celiac disease (a digestive and autoimmune disorder).[418,419] A randomized, placebo-controlled clinical trial demonstrated that probiotic supplementation (multistrain bacterium) improved a common somatic symptom of bowel difficulty associated with schizophrenia but produced no significant changes in psychiatric symptoms.[420]

There is also evidence that GI health can affect inflammatory disorders. Giardina et al.[421] reported that probiotics of the lactic acid bacteria strain improved inflammatory events associated with oxalate-degrading activity in the intestines in human subjects (e.g., Lactobacillis plantarum, Lactobacillus acidophilus, Bifidobacterium breve, and Bifidobacterium longum). In a randomized, double-blind, placebo-controlled clinical study of patients with rheumatoid arthritis, a significant decrease in disease activity score and a decrease in inflammatory cytokines (e.g., TNF-α, IL-6, IL-10) was reported with probiotic intervention.[422]

These cited research articles are a representative collection to illustrate the association of nutritional components and systemic responses. Many more studies have been published and are worthy of further independent exploration in the fields of cardiology, nutrition, orthopedics, functional medicine, and many others. It will be important for clinicians to keep abreast of nutrition research in the treatment of their patients.

Nutritional Recommendations for the Management of Patient's with Repetitive Strain Injuries

"If we could give every individual the right amount of nourishment and exercise, not too little and not too much, we would have found the safest way to health." —Hippocrates

There is an increasing amount of research associating nutritional factors and their effects on inflammation and healing throughout the body. However, the unanswered question is, what specific nutritional strategies should be integrated with lifestyle changes, stress management, and exercise to decrease inflammation and facilitate healing, remodeling, and recovery from RSIs?[423–426]

One strategy described in the literature is intermittent fasting. *Intermittent fasting* is defined as extending the interval between meals. In particular, intermittent fasting may have a positive effect on inflammation and recovery in the male population. For example, in one study of intermittent fasting following an experimentally induced brain injury in mice, there was a decrease in infarct volume in the mice that were fasted compared with those that ate ad libitum.[427] In another study with neonatal pigs, muscle protein synthesis increased more with intermittent eating versus continuous feeding.[428] In aging men, mood, depression, and nutritional status improved in those who were fasting with calorie restriction.[429] Bahammam et al.[430,431] explored the safety of a fasting strategy in men who followed intermittent fasting during Ramadan, a Muslim annual religious observance. No ill effects were reported. Intermittent calorie restriction has also been used as an effective dietary treatment for drug-resistant epilepsy.[432]

Attenuation of proinflammatory cytokines has been reported following intermittent fasting by healthy subjects.[433] Recent literature reviews concluded that dietary restriction or intermittent fasting could support peripheral nerve health by attenuation of peripheral demyelination, promotion of neurogenesis, and positive health of the peripheral nerve.[434] Thus, calorie restriction or intermittent fasting could be safely tried in males during regeneration and recovery of nerve function following a peripheral neuropathy.

Although intermittent fasting can have positive results for men, one must be cautious to implement this strategy in the female population. Females have a monthly ovulatory cycle that is very sensitive to external stress. Consequently, it is not recommended for females to fast daily without proper monitoring. Month-long fasting for females, as in Ramadan, may adversely affect the reproductive system in irreparable ways. Thus, rather than intermittent fasting, females could implement a narrowed eating window strategy. This might include narrowing the eating window during the hours of 9 AM and 7 PM (10 hours), allowing a natural fasting between 7 PM and 9 AM (14 hours). This fasting would occur more naturally during sleeping hours. Another nutritional management tool involves specific avoidance of inflammatory foods and specific inclusion of anti-inflammatory and nutrient-rich whole foods in the diet.

Based on a review of the literature, there are foods that have been associated with inflammation or inhibition of healing and that should be avoided (Table 27-10). There are also food items that incorporate the nutrients that support health and anti-inflammation (Table 27-11). Dr. Terry Wahls carried out clinical studies integrating the Wahls Protocol with patients with progressive MS. She confirmed not only the safety of a whole foods–type diet but also the

TABLE 27-10

Nutritional Foods Exacerbating Inflammation

Dietary Limitations/ Avoidance	Foods in Which Found
Carbohydrates[396,435–438]	Candies, desserts, flour-derived baked or processed foods, pastas, cereals, granola, fruit juice, beans/legumes, dried fruits (especially if sweetened), anything with added sugars
Fructose[391,401,439]	Agave syrup, honey, dates, raisins, dried fruit, molasses, green grapes, canned fruit in syrup, fruit juice
Aspartame[440]	Nutrasweet, Equal, a potential additive in sweet-tasting "sugar-free" foods
Ethanol[441]	Beer, wine, spirits, mixed adult beverages
Monosodium glutamate (MSG)[442,443]	May be present in an ingredient list as "flavoring," processed packaged foods, restaurant foods
Gliadin (gluten protein)[417,444]	Wheat, oats, barley (anything containing gluten)
Statins[393]	Consult physician about short-term hold of medication during healing of RSI
NSAIDs[392]	Consult physician about short-term hold of medication during healing of RSI, although NSAIDs can protect against cartilage and bone resorption occurring with RSI[70,445]
Trans fats[445]	Vegetable and seed oils (canola, rape seed, soybean, safflower, partially hydrogenated fat/oil)

The foods referenced here can be found on the government website http://ndb.nal.usda.gov/.

RSI, Repetitive strain injury; *NSAIDs,* nonsteroidal anti-inflammatory drugs.

benefits of this type of dieting on neuromuscular function. An important component of the Wahls Protocol diet is the specific exclusion of processed and inflammatory foods and the specific inclusion of nutrient-dense whole foods.[399] The diet not only was safe but was associated with improvement in neuromuscular function.[399]

In summary, a patient recovering from an RSI may improve healing by eating whole foods with high nutrient value. Patients should try to *remove* processed foods (i.e., refined grains, refined sugar, refined vegetable oils, alcohol) and non–nutrient-rich foods (i.e., grains, especially those containing gluten; most dairy; and legumes). The patient should try to *replace* non–nutrient-rich foods with whole organic produce, especially colorful leafy

TABLE **27-11**

Nutritional Components Supporting Healing and/or Anti-Inflammatory Mechanisms

Beneficial Dietary Component	Food in Which Found
Probiotics[421,422,445,446]	Naturally fermented vegetables and dairy (pickles, sauerkraut, kimchi, yogurt, kefir)
Prebiotics[446]	Resistant starch (potato, plantain, inulin)
Leucine-rich diet[447]	Eggs, spirulina, cheese, beef, pork
Olive oil[448,449]	100% pure olive oil
Aloe vera[450]	Aloe vera (juice or capsules)
Gelatin/collagen[450,451]	Pure gelatin or collagen hydrolysate, bone broth
Chinese herbal formula (sini tang)[404]	Recommend consultation with herbalist
Antioxidants[384,452–456]	Anthocyanins (blue, red, and purple berries; cherries; purple grapes; red cabbage), betalains (beets, cactus)
Biotin[457]	Green leafy vegetables, liver
Bovine colostrum[458]	Bovine colostrum
Brazil nuts[459]	Brazil nuts
Green coffee bean extract (chlorogenic acid)[388]	Green coffee bean extract, prunes
Resveratrol[385,400,460–463]	Purple grapes, bilberries, blueberries
Curcumin (turmeric)[464–466]	Turmeric
Docosahexenoic acid (DHA)[405,467–477]	Oily fish (salmon, tuna, sardines, mackerel, and trout)
Cocoa[478,479]	100% chocolate
Glycosaminoglycans (glucosamine)[480,481]	Glucosamine/chondroitin sulfate supplements
Vitamin D[383,482]	Liver, grass-fed dairy, fermented cod liver oil, fish, portabella mushrooms, egg yolk
Spirulina[478,483]	Spirulina, raw or dried
Lean red meat[484]	Lean red meat; beef, wild game
Vitamin C[389,396,485]	Citrus, peppers, kale
Whey protein (if diabetic)[486]	Whey protein powder
Vitamin E[485]	Nuts (almonds, hazelnuts, pine nuts), nut oils
Yeast hydrolysate[487]	Yeast extract

The foods referenced here can be found on the government website http://ndb.nal.usda.gov/.

vegetables and fruits and berries; grass-fed grass-finished organic meats, including organ meats; wild-caught fish; and plenty of healthy fats, such as coconut oil, grass-fed and clarified butter, lard, and unheated olive oil. These nutritional habits should be maintained for 30 to 90 days to *recover* health and see results. These habits of specific avoidance and specific inclusion should be maintained for a lifetime of positive health and healing.

These eating strategies may be daunting to remember for the patient with an RSI. A simple pneumonic can provide some guidance. The *"Triple R" Strategy* (*remove, replace, recover*) can be used as a reminder (Table 27-12). This principle is easily applied in all areas of recovery for the patient with an RSI.

Principles for Recovery from Repetitive Stress Injuries

- Remove the aberrant or inflammatory movement
- Replace it with normal and healthy movement/posture
- Restore function

TABLE **27-12**

"Triple R" Strategy for Nutritional Recovery from Repetitive Stress Disorder

Triple R Strategy	Nutritional Recovery from Repetitive Strain Injury
Remove	Remove refined grains, refined sugars, refined vegetable oils, and processed foods/drinks
Replace	Replace processed foods with whole organic produce, wild-caught fish, grass-fed grass-finished beef, organic meats, healthy fats, and water
Restore	Maintain healthy eating for a minimum of 30 days to restore health and a lifetime for continued health

There is no single nutritional recipe for perfect health that works for every patient with an RSI. There is, however, always a balance and a period of personal and individual trial and error. Should the patient be unable to eat a whole foods diet within these guidelines, demonstrate a lack of progress, or need further help, supplementation should be considered. If needed, further collaboration with functional medicine professionals, specially trained dietitians or nutritionists, and physicians may be warranted.

Clinicians, such as physical therapists, should check with their governing state board and local national chapters to be sure they are in compliance with their state's regulations regarding the scope of practice and making nutritional recommendations along with physical activities to help patients to restore normal healthy pain-free movements, independence, and quality of life.

> *"The natural healing force within each of us is the greatest force in getting well."* —Hippocrates

Clinicians, such as physical therapists, have the opportunity and foundation of knowledge to work with every patient on many levels, with the ultimate goal of facilitating positive health, quality movement, independent function, and prevention of injury or disability. Recent research evidence indicates that physical therapists should help guide the patient to establish a healthy lifestyle to maximize health and restore maximum function after an injury or disease. This lifestyle should include adequate amounts of recovery time, moderate and appropriate exercise, restful sleep, hydration, stress management, and healthy nutrition.

Specific Management Strategies for Patients with Focal Hand Dystonia

Goals for Rehabilitation

Each patient must be treated individually. The patient and the family need to agree on the goals. These goals should be focused on managing the movement dysfunction by reducing risk factors, managing the pain, retraining the brain, and successfully returning to functional activities, work, and quality of life.

Patient Goals for Retraining for Focal Hand Dystonia

- Learn as much as possible about the risk factors, the etiology, and the different approaches to remediate FHd
- Become your own best therapist
- Negotiate a compatible work schedule
- Recruit support of family and friends
- Think positively about recovery
- Maintain self-confidence and self-esteem
- Create a positive environment for learning
- Maximize state of health and wellness

- Stop abnormal movements
- Quiet excessive excitation of muscles
- Restore normal sensory processing
- Restore graded, smooth fine motor movements
- Redifferentiate the sensory, sensorimotor, and motor representations of the hand in cortical and subcortical brain networks
- Relearn how to perform the target task(s)
- Return to preferred work

Medical Management

Successful retraining strategies for FHd are multifactorial. A successful program begins with a good *medical management plan*. The physician will usually assume the responsibility for medications, transmagnetic or direct cutaneous stimulation, and referrals for counseling, surgery, or deep brain stimulation (DBS), as well as referrals for rehabilitation.[292,312,488] It is important for the physician to assess the need for counseling and possibly medications for anxiety, depression, and even more severe psychopathology.[319-321,488,489] It is important that each patient be able to concentrate on retraining.

The most common medical treatment for patients with FHd is the injection of botulinum toxin to reduce the intensity of the dystonic cramping by interfering with neural signals to the muscle.[311,490-492] Baclofen may be helpful when spasticity is present along with dystonia.[493]

Immobilization is another medical management strategy that was initiated in Italy.[494] Based on the possibility that FHd is a consequence of overuse and a change in cortical organization,[75-77,296] immobilization of the hand would discourage use of the hand, decrease the repetition of the abnormal movements, and potentially quiet the overexcitation of the muscles. This could serve as treatment or quiet the neural activity in preparation for retraining. In initial trials this strategy was applied to a small patient group with early-onset dystonia. The hand was immobilized in a cast for 10 days, and decreased dystonia was reported when the cast was removed.[494,495]

Some patients with FHd have clear and objective signs of peripheral nerve compression of the ulnar or the median nerve. These patients may be referred for surgical decompression (e.g., repositioning the ulnar nerve at the elbow).[220,221] Surgical modifications of anatomical variations are sometimes performed.[78,216,217,284]

Repetitive transcranial magnetic stimulation (rTMS) and *transcranial direct current stimulation (tDCS)* are noninvasive techniques used to induce change in corticospinal excitability.[496-498] In the case of FHd, the objective of repetitive stimulation is to improve corticospinal inhibition during stimulation[498] with lasting effects for a short period of time after stimulation.[496,497] For tDCS, depending on the orientation of the cells and the current, cortical membrane potentials may be hyperpolarized or depolarized by a low-voltage current (mV). Although rTMS covers a treatment target area of about 25 mm, tDCS can cover approximately 2500 mm². It can be difficult to be specific with the coils of the TMS. The intensity and the spread of tDCS can be controlled by the size of the electrode (e.g., a smaller electrode would provide more intense coverage in a smaller area).[496] DBS is another possible medical management strategy. However, this surgical procedure is reserved mostly for patients with generalized dystonia. If a focal dystonia is severe and disabling (e.g., cervical dystonia more than hand dystonia), DBS may be considered.[499]

Effectiveness of Medical Management. Generally, medical intervention strategies are effective in terms of management but not in terms of a cure. Botulinum toxin can quiet and weaken overactive muscles.[500-503] The challenge is to inject the correct muscles with the appropriate dose of medication. Unfortunately, the effect is temporary, lasting approximately 3 months. Then another injection is needed. Botulinum toxin does not have a direct effect on remapping the brain; however, the injections may make it easier for patients to participate in retraining. Some patients can become less responsive to the injections with time, resulting in the injections no longer being effective. In general, patients seem to tolerate the botulinum toxin for a long period.[311] In some cases, the patient can develop excessive weakness that does not return to normal when the botulinum toxin wears off.

The initial studies of immobilization with casting were associated with reduction in the severity of the dystonia for patients with early-onset hand dystonia.[494,504,505] A randomized trial was designed to replicate the benefits of immobilization in patients with more established hand dystonia. This trial was terminated early because some patients experienced increased dystonic movements while confined in a cast.

There is some evidence that rTMS, transcutaneous nerve stimulation (tCNS), or computer–brain interface biofeedback can assist inhibition, modify aberrant cortical topography and neurophysiological processing, and improve functional performance. These studies tend to be small pre/post test trials without random assignment, and the amount of repetitive stimulation is short.[496-498,506] In one study, after 1 hour of stimulation to the first dorsal interossei and the abductor pollicis brevis muscles, patients with hand dystonia and control subjects practiced grip-lift handwriting and cyclic drawing tasks. After 1 hour of nonassociative stimulation, the topographical map was reduced in size for both muscles, the center of the digital fields moved farther apart, and there was less movement variability during drawing. In another study, rTMS was administered to age-matched controls and patients with FHd. The effects were measured in terms of blood flow, which lasted approximately 1 hour after stimulation. In patients with FHd compared with age-matched controls, there was a greater decrease of rCBF in lateral and medial premotor areas in the putamen and thalamus, including the stimulated premotor cortex and a larger increase in cerebellar rCBF. This suggests that one session of rTMS can change synaptic activity, with the greatest responsiveness occurring in the

premotor cortex.[257,498] Kimberley et al.[507] and Priori et al.[496] also reported positive changes in cortical responsiveness and topography with rTMS. In addition, anodal tDCS has been associated with decreased cortical excitability.[497]

At this time, treatment of focal dystonia with rTMS, tDCS, and neurobiofeedback with an implanted brain electrode are considered experimental and are not covered by insurance as a medically necessary treatment for FHd. Scientists are still trying to understand how patients with FHd respond differently to rTMS stimulation compared with control subjects.[508] More information is also needed about the intensity and the frequency of the stimulation and how to make the effects longer lasting. On the other hand, minimal risks are associated with this approach to intervention. In the future it is anticipated that physical therapists will have the opportunity to integrate rTMS, tDCS, and/or neurobiofeedback with learning-based training strategies.

Evidence-Based Rehabilitation Strategies for Focal Hand Dystonia

Some patients with hand dystonia chose to change their instrument and even learned to play one handed in order to continue to perform the target task.[509] This is considered a compensatory strategy. However, the neurophysiological evidence regarding aberrant learning, lack of homeostatic plasticity, decreased inhibition, degraded topography, excessive excitation (i.e., magnitude and amplitude of neuronal firing), and poor sensorimotor integration must be translated to rehabilitation strategies that target redifferentiation of cortical and subcortical representations of the hand. This is consistent with the sensorimotor, computational, homeostatic plasticity, and systems etiological hypotheses. Pathological connections must be uncoupled, unwanted movements need to be inhibited, and selective normal movements must be practiced to engage time-relevant, sequenced cognitive, sensory, and motor neuronal networks to restore voluntary movements.

A variety of retraining paradigms have been tried for patients with FHd (Table 27-13).[292,312] These strategies must be supplemented with positive expectations, aerobic exercise, and healthy lifestyle behaviors.[506,510] The retraining paradigms range from kinematic and biomechanical modifications,[511] general strengthening exercises, fatigue training, flexibility training, joint and soft tissue mobilization, neural mobilization/gliding, acupressure, trigger point therapy, dry needling, craniosacral therapy to learning-based training (e.g., biofeedback,[506,510,512] mirror imagery,[513-516] graded motor imagery,[517-521] sensory discrimination training,[522] braille reading,[523-525] fatigue therapy,[519] sensory motor retuning [constraint-induced movement therapy, (CIMT)],[526-534] learning-based sensory motor training,[535-537] cognitive and perceptual motor training,[44,370-373,529] motor retraining,[538-540] performance coaching,[541] hypnosis,[542] or a combination of these strategies[543]).

TABLE **27-13**

Summary of Different Intervention Strategies for Focal Hand Dystonia

Intervention	Strategy
Electrical stimulation	• Stimulation to assist in voluntary contraction of desired muscles (agonists) • Stimulation of forceful repetitive contractions to fatigue muscles • Stimulation of agonists to facilitate strengthening of desired muscles • Stimulation at sensory level to quiet the antagonist or hyperexcitable muscles • Deep brain stimulation • Transcutaneous direct cranial stimulation
Biofeedback	• Quiet overexcited muscles • Inhibit firing of conflicting antagonists • Balance activation and inhibition for stability and mobility • Correct abnormal movements by providing error, visual, or auditory feedback (e.g., feedback from a writing device) • Provide "force reaction information" or kinematic data to improve biomechanics • Guide desired movements with use of a laser pointer and stop abnormal movements or stabilize movements
Exercise	• General moderate flexibility and strengthening exercises • Aerobic exercise • Posture and balance exercises • Strengthening to balance mobility and stability (e.g., intrinsic muscles and extrinsic muscles) • Kinematic training • Fatigue training
Coaching	• Music lessons with exceptional teacher • Guided training and practice, similar to that for competitive sports • Ergonomic modifications at work • Analysis of safe, functional biomechanics needed to perform the target task • Physical training to improve efficiency, effectiveness, endurance, and skill • Anxiety and stress management
Manual techniques	• Joint mobilization • Traction • Soft tissue mobilization • Neural mobilization, nerve gliding • Immobilization with casting • Rocking, vibration
Behavioral retraining	• Sensory retuning (sensory and motor training with splinting following guidelines for constraint induced therapy) • Sensory discrimination training (sensitivity training) • Braille reading • Perceptual motor and cognitive training • Imagery (mental, mirror, graded motor) and virtual reality • Learning-based sensorimotor training
Other holistic strategies	• Movement strategies (Pilates, yoga, Alexander, Ji Gong, tai chi) • Dry needling • Acupressure/acupuncture • Transmagnetic stimulation • Hypnosis • Craniosacral therapy

Biofeedback. Biofeedback can provide auditory, visual, or sensory feedback (e.g., force data) about muscle firing patterns and force dimensions. Patients can concentrate on activating or inhibiting muscle activation or changing the force of the muscle contraction. Error feedback can be used as a method of improving quality of movement. This has been used most frequently with patients having writer's cramp. Patients are directed to use the feedback to decrease the grip force on the pen or the writing pressure.[218,219] Biofeedback is usually combined with other task-specific training techniques such as changing the strategy of gripping the pen[512,544–548] or practicing fine motor movements to improve writing fluency and speed.[248]

Imagery. Mirror imagery, guided mental imagery, and guided imagery for self-healing are helpful strategies to begin retraining, particularly when it is not possible to stop the abnormal movements.[513-516] With imagery, patients can try to quiet overexcitation and enhance inhibition. In addition, patients can integrate mental practice instead of physical practice. Imagery can be associated with changes in brain organization.[513]

Sensory Training (Braille). Sensory stimulation can functionally reorganize the brain.[259] This occurs not only after injury[267] but with heavy hand use like in musicians[250,251] and braille readers.[525] However, cortical de-differentiation is reported in patients with FHd[294] and animals trained intensively until the development of involuntary, uncontrolled hand movements when performing the target task.[75,296,299,300] Improved cortical differentiation is reported in multifinger braille readers.[525] Thus, teaching patients to read braille[523,524] and perform other sensory discrimination activities[522,535,536] has been recommended as a method of driving the reorganization needed to restore motor control in patients with FHd.

Constraint-Induced Movement Therapy (CIMT): Sensory Motor Retuning. CIMT is based on the concept of "forced use" of the paretic upper extremity.[526] It was designed to counter "learned nonuse" most specifically for a patient after stroke and later applied to patients with other movement dysfunction like cerebral palsy and dystonia. CIMT is concentrated and intensive (6 to 8 hours a day over 2 weeks). In CIMT, the unaffected limb is placed in a mitt or a cast for 90% of waking hours to make it difficult to use in daily activities.[527,528,535] Patient-preferred tasks are identified. Then constraint of the unaffected arm/hand is combined with repetitive task-oriented training of the paretic upper extremity for 6 or more hours each day. Derivatives of CIMT have been tried, incorporating shorter periods of training over longer intervention periods, and different variations of progressive and alternating splint immobilization of the digits have been tried for musicians with FHd.[530-534]

Learning-Based Sensorimotor Training (LBSMT). Learning-based sensorimotor training is based on the theoretical constructs of learning and neural adaptation integrated with health and wellness, positive expectations, mental practice, mental imagery, and good biomechanics.[535-537,549] The goal of LBSMT is to match patient needs, preferences, and sensory and motor findings with progressive learning-based target-specific retraining to restore normal topography of the hand, recover target specific function, achieve quality of life, and return to work.

LBSMT training is comprehensive (Table 27-14). This training must be practiced at home as well as in supervised settings where clinicians and coaches can provide guidance concerning progression of activities. Retraining requires time, patient motivation, attention, and progressive learning. Although the training progresses through phases, the early phases will continue to require practice and integration even when behavioral training has progressed to task-specific practice and return to work. Given the neurophysiological challenges of excessive excitation and decreased inhibition, patients must be mindful to minimize the risk factors.

The phases of behavioral retraining in LBSMT are described in Table 27-14. These phases are overlapping with the soft, not rigid boundaries of each phase. The first two phases require modifying lifestyle behaviors to establish a positive foundation of health and wellness.

TABLE **27-14**

Summary of Interactive Phases for Learning-Based Sensorimotor Training

Phase	Description
Phase I: positive health and positive expectations	Expect to get better. Engage in wellness activities and exercise (aerobic, posture, balance, strength, coordination, flexibility). Maintain hydration, good nutrition, and quality sleep. Manage stress and anxiety. Be sure to balance work and play.
Phase II: quieting the nervous system	Stop abnormal movements. Engage in relaxation activities to help quiet the overexcitation of the nervous system. Quiet neural hypersensitivity and pain by rocking, stroking, swinging, swaddling, massage, vibration, and soothing music.
Phase III: sensory discrimination training	Improve accuracy of tactile, auditory, visual, and proprioceptive processing. Think sensory and let sensation of objects open the hand. Strengthen sensory inputs by putting rough surfaces on the instrument to minimize force. Compare and match objects through touch not vision. Locate different stimuli drawn on the skin. Duplicate drawings made on the skin. Have taste and smell contests with flowers, wine, and food. Listen to someone delivering sounds behind you in different locations and point to the location. See Figures 27-13 and 27-14.
Phase IV: imagery and sensorimotor training	Use mental imagery to remind yourself of how it felt to perform the task normally. Mentally practice performing all aspects of the task. Put the unaffected hand in front of mirror and carefully watch the mirror image (looks like affected hand). While positioned with the mirror, perform simple movements and manipulate objects. Try to transfer the mirror image to your affected hand (see Figure 27-15). You can work by yourself or have someone place his or her hands on your hands to help provide more sensory input. You may also improve the sensibility of the hand and motor control by using low-level neuromuscular stimulation on the palm or the dorsum of the hand periodically during the day when you are training.

(Continued)

TABLE 27-14

Summary of Interactive Phases for Learning-Based Sensorimotor Training—cont'd

Phase	Description
Phase V: improve biomechanics and kinematics	Work on integrating normal biomechanics into functional hand use (e.g., keep hand in round comfortable position; especially keep the thumb and index finger round and soft when holding an instrument to play). When dropping the hand on a surface or an instrument, be on your finger pads (middle of finger pad for D2, D3, D4 and lateral surface of pads of D1 and D5). Let the contact surface open the hand. Avoid hyperextension of the interphalangeal joints. Move from the elbow or shoulder and simply drop the hand on a surface. Try to use the aerobic muscles of the hand (e.g., intrinsic hand muscles of lumbricales and interossei and forearm rotators instead of the extrinsic, glycogenic muscles (wrist and finger extensors and flexors). Depress the keys on the piano or computer keyboard or the string on an instrument by moving from the metacarpal phalangeal joint. Practice removing the pressure from the keys by stopping the pressure down rather than lifting up with the extensors. Rather than reaching with excessive finger extension and abduction, rotate the forearm with a fulcrum on the little finger and drop the thumb on the desired key. Then rotate the forearm with the thumb as a fulcrum to drop the little finger down. When doing coordinated movements, let all fingers rest down rather than holding some up; however, put only the necessary pressure on the desired movements. Get a coach to help improve biomechanics of performing with good ergonomics at the target task performance
Phase VI: graded motor training	Practice smooth, graded, nonjerky movements at common daily tasks that balance stability with mobility. Move hand lightly on a moving surface (see Figure 22-16). Find activities that create large slow movements around the shoulder, elbow, and wrist (e.g., yoga, tai chi, Feldenkrais). Gently let different surfaces spread the fingers out (e.g., smooth, rough, powdery, cold, warm surfaces). Make large sweeping brushing or sweeping rhythmical movements of the whole arm. Do large finger painting or try large smooth strokes for water painting with large brushes and large strokes. Practice making designs in shaving cream (see Figure 22-17). Hold a light ball and watch it as you take it to the right, the left, and high and low in front. Purchase a calligraphy board and practice large caligraphy letters that disappear in minutes. Let hand drop on a scale and try to estimate different weights. Then try to pick up objects without increasing the weight on the scale (see Guided Motor Imagery[519]).
Phase VII: task-specific training	Begin process of practicing small parts of the target task in unusual positions and then usual positions. Progress task complexity and difficulty. Use feedback to improve performance (e.g., error feedback, reward feedback, auditory feedback, electrical biofeedback about specific muscle recruitment regarding time to activation and time to turn off muscle firing; see Figure 22-18). Try to improve inhibition (e.g., turning off unwanted contractions). It is essential to spread the practice over time.
Phase VIII: return to work	Return to work (e.g., preferably part-time progressing to full-time). Even when back to work, maintain activities in phases I, II, and III. Schedule more breaks. Learn to manage new stresses related to work. Incorporate mental imagery and practice to supplement physical practice for the job.

Note: Patients may be working in multiple phases simultaneously. This is interactive training not isolated training

Phases III and IV focus on improving sensory discrimination and somatosensory representations while using imagery to practice the target task without creating abnormal movements. Phases V through VIII focus on motor learning, target task practice, and return to work. Lifestyle changes, health and wellness, and behavioral activities initiated in the early phases not only must continue to be practiced throughout the rehabilitation process but must be continued indefinitely. Ideally, retraining progresses without flaring involuntary movements. Figures 27-13 through 27-18 give examples of some of the sensorimotor training strategies. These sensory motor learning-based techniques are frequently complemented with specific coaching from a therapist, teacher, or coach to improve biomechanics and voluntary motor control.[535-537,541,549]

A variety of other general training techniques have been tried with patients with FHd. These strategies range from fatigue therapy for hyperactive muscles (i.e., repetitively, voluntarily performing a maximum contraction of a muscle

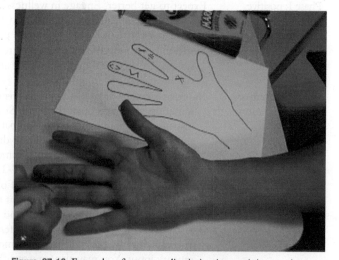

Figure 27-13 Example of sensory discrimination training to improve graphesthesia. Letters, numbers, and designs are written on the skin of the involved hand and digits when the patient with dystonia has the eyes closed; the patient then has to reproduce the stimulus on the exact surface or on a piece of paper.

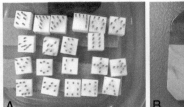
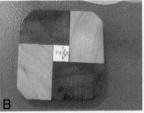
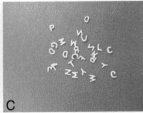

Figure 27-14 Examples of retraining skills at stereognosis. **A,** The Byl-Cheney-Boczai (BCB) test is a test used to evaluate accuracy of stereognosis. Cubes with specific stimuli have been created. **B,** The cube is placed in a holder. The patient has the eyes closed, and the examiner takes the finger across the stimulus twice. Then the cube is covered, and the patient looks at a sheet with all of the different shapes on the cube and tries to identify the correct design. **C,** Alphabet soup letters can be placed on a surface. With the eyes closed, the patient palpates one letter and tries to identify it.

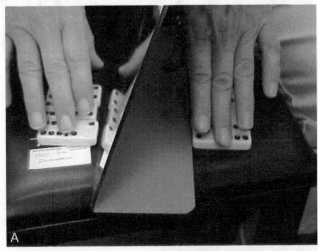
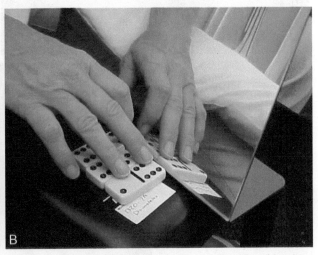

Figure 27-15 A mirror can be used in sensory and perceptual motor learning activities to reinforce normal movement. **A,** The affected hand is put behind the mirror, and the unaffected hand is placed in front of the mirror. The mirror image of the unaffected hand looks like the affected hand. **B,** Watching the mirror image, the patient attempts to manipulate some dominoes placed on both sides of the mirror.

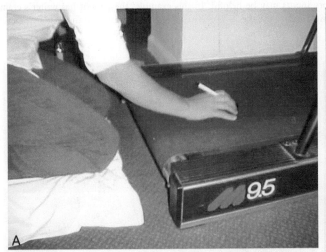
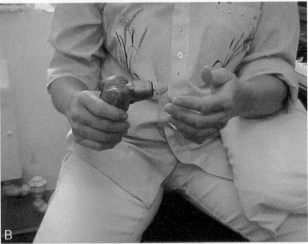

Figure 27-16 Grading movement can be difficult for patients with neural hypersensitivity. When the agonists and antagonists contract simultaneously, performing fine motor tasks is difficult. Creating situations in which a patient has to maintain light contact on a moving object without interfering with the movement of the object can be challenging. **A,** Here a patient is trying to decrease excessive downward pressure and move smoothly by writing while on a moving treadmill. **B,** A patient is trying to lightly touch the plastic fan blades without stopping the blade movement.

until exertion)[526] to general strengthening, flexibility, movement training, and fine motor dexterous skill training.[538] In addition, holistic approaches such as acupressure, acupuncture, dry needling, craniosacral therapy, and hypnosis have also been described, but no specific trials have been reported on using these strategies in isolation with patients with FHd.

Clinical Evidence-Based Research on the Effectiveness of Rehabilitation Strategies for Focal Hand Dystonia

Single-case studies, pre/post test study designs, crossover designs, and small prospective controlled experimental studies have been carried out to evaluate the effectiveness of rehabilitation strategies to enable recovery of task-specific

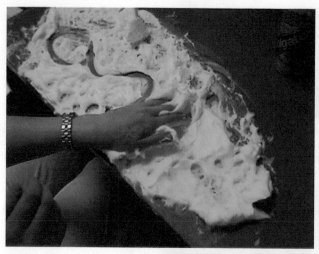

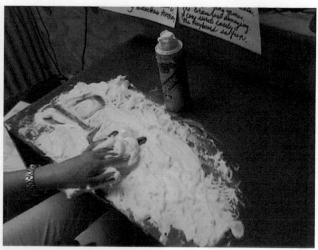

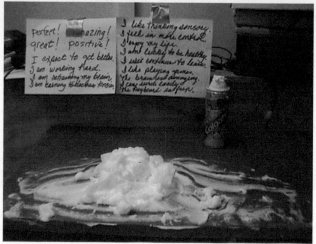

Figure 27-17 When retraining motor skills, increasing or changing sensory inputs may be helpful. In this example, the patient has writer's cramp. She puts shaving cream on a table or a counter and spreads out the shaving cream. First she just practices large movements and then finally practices writing letters and then sentences.

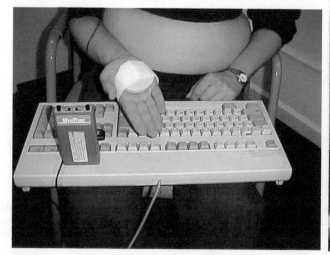

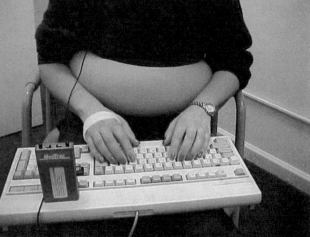

Figure 27-18 Facilitating the functional position of the hand with a palmar pad along with a biofeedback machine with electrodes over the intrinsic muscles helps the patient shape the hand as she begins to retrain her ability to type on a computer keyboard.

function of patients with FHd. Unfortunately, there are no large randomized clinical trials, systematic reviews, or meta-analyses to confirm the efficacy of the results. To date, no intervention strategies have been predicted to be 100% effective to restore normal motor control for patients with FHd. However, there are individuals who describe complete recovery. The strongest measures of validity for learning-based behavioral training are based on the neuroscience evidence of central nervous system plasticity.

Biofeedback: Writer's Cramp. Several controlled studies assessed the effectiveness of biofeedback training for patients with writer's cramp. Patients with writer's cramp heavily grip the pen and push down when writing. The objective was to improve writing frequency and fluency by training patients to reduce grip force and writing pressure, use a modified grip, practice writing,[546,550] and/or combine the strategies.[218,219,544] The research studies confirm that patients can effectively use force biofeedback to reduce grip force and writing pressure.[544,545] The research also confirmed that patients could reduce pen gripping and writing force by using a modified grip and writing practice.[546,547] When combined across studies, the mean effect sizes for improving task performance varied from 2.2 for reducing writing pressure, 2.2 for increasing writing frequency, and 4.52 for improving writing time. The reduction in force could be further enhanced by combining an ergonomic grip with writing practice.[544,545] The improvement in writing could be maintained up to 6 months after training. Interestingly, improvement in fluency and speed of writing was not necessarily specifically correlated with decreased gripping or writing force.[547,548]

In patients with simple and complex writer's cramp, it was assumed that excessive grip force was used in all activities, not just writing.[218,248,548] In a recent well-controlled study by Schneider et al.,[219] the grip force with writing and the dynamic force used when lifting a box were compared between patients with writer's cramp and matched healthy controls. Although the grip force and writing force were significantly greater for patients with writer's cramp, there were no significant differences between the forces used to lift boxes containing different weights.[219] This study raises question about the underlying general state of hyperexcitation with inadequate inhibition in patients with FHd. However, the preservation of the normalcy of the lifting force could also reflect the difference between performing a simple hand task (lifting a box) versus performing precise motor movements.[219]

Imagery. Controlled, randomized trials provide evidence that graded motor imagery can significantly reduce the severity of pathological pain.[517,518,520] Graded motor imagery can also significantly reduce pain associated with an amputation.[522,551] There are no studies confirming graded motor imagery alone significantly improved motor control in patients with FHd. The same is true for mirror imagery. Research using mirror imagery confirms the recruitment of the neurons in the superior parietal lobe during internal representation using a mirror.[514] There is also evidence that mirror training significantly improves function of the upper limb after stroke[515,516] and after amputation in patients with phantom limb pain.[551] Although mirror training is integrated into a variety of learning-based training strategies, no randomized, controlled trials based on mirror training alone were located to confirm effectiveness of restoring voluntary motor control in the case of FHd.

Sensory Training (Braille). In a small pre/post test study, Zeuner et al.[523] provided evidence supporting the benefit of braille reading for patients with writer's cramp. With 10 subjects practicing braille reading daily for 8 weeks, there was a significant improvement in tactile spatial acuity of writing and a decrease in severity of dystonia as measured by the *Fahn dystonia rating scale*. Half of the subjects continued to practice braille reading for up to a year with continued improvement in writing.[524] The patients continued to show improvement and felt their writing was better; however, none achieved full recovery. Sterr et al.[369,525] reported sensory perception changes with braille reading.

CIMT: Sensory Motor Retuning. There is class 1 evidence supporting the efficacy of the original form of CIMT for improving arm–hand activities, the amount of (self-reported) arm–hand use, and the integration of arm–hand movements into functional activities after stroke.[527-530] In general, CIMT improves motor ability and functional use of the affected limb compared with no active therapy or with conventional or dose-matched physical rehabilitation.[526] There is also positive evidence supporting the benefit of this strategy for musicians with dystonia.[531-533] This strategy was found to be more effective with guitarists than with pianists.[532] Sensory motor retuning can also reduce pain in patients with regional pain syndrome.[534] It is important to note that sensory motor retuning, when used for patients with dystonia, integrates a splint for constraint with selective immobilization and release of individual digits instead of a cast.[531-533] The mean effect size of the small studies on sensory motor retuning and reading braille was 1.1 both for improved motor control at the target task and improved fine motor control.

Learning-Based Sensorimotor Training. McKenzie et al.[300] and Byl et al.[336,535-537,549] carried out a series of small clinical studies to gather evidence to confirm the presence of sensorimotor impairments in patients with FHd and to study the effectiveness of LBSMT (i.e., clinical function and cortical remapping). In this series of studies, there was consistency in the eligibility characteristics of the subjects and the LBSMT intervention. The subjects in these clinical studies included controls and patients with FHd (e.g., 20 to 60 years of age, all working in occupations demanding repetitive hand use). The patients with FHd had been diagnosed for at least 6 months and were receiving care from the University of California, San Francisco (UCSF) Peter Ostwald Health Program for Performing Artists or the UCSF Physical Therapy Faculty Practice. Each subject demonstrated (1) observable involuntary twisting movements of the digits and wrist when performing the target or similar task, (2) normal reflexes, and (3) no evidence of objective peripheral neuropathy or central nervous system pathology. None of the subjects had received any injected or systemic drugs to control the dystonia for more than 6 months.

The first two studies were descriptive, with 10 patients with FHd and 10 controls in experiment I and 17 patients with FHd and 15 controls in experiment II. In experiment III (pre/post test design), 12 subjects with FHd received LBSMT twice a week for 3 hours each day for 6 weeks. Gains in performance by patients with FHd were compared with those in 30 controls. Pre/post test experiments IV to VI were intervention studies with one FHd musician with a matched control in experiment IV, 3 FHd cases in experiment V, and 13 subjects (18 hands) with FHd in experiment VI.

All subjects were evaluated at baseline and immediately after treatment by blinded, trained evaluators administering standardized tests (Table 27-15). The outcome variables from the standardized tests[254] were summed into seven dependent variables: (1) physical musculoskeletal performance (i.e., selected ROM, strength, neural tension); (2) sensory discrimination (i.e., graphesthesia, localization, kinesthesia, stereognosis); (3) fine motor efficiency (i.e., Purdue Test time), fine motor skill (i.e., line tracing accuracy and time), and digital reaction time (i.e., averaged across the five digits for each hand); (4) motor control at the target task; (5) posture and balance; (6) functional independence; and (7) pain. In addition, imaging studies were included to understand neurophysiological correlates of clinical performance.

Magnetoencephalography was performed by trained staff in the UCSF Center for Bioimaging and the Department of Radiology.[336] The test–retest value for the magnetic source image (MSI) was high (>0.9).[368] A 37-channel biomagnetometer (Magnes II 4D Neuroimaging, 1.5 fT, San Diego, CA) placed in a magnetically shielded room with two circular sensors (14.4 cm) was used to create a MSI of 1 cm² for 30 milliseconds at 17 to 20 pounds per square inch (PSI) with a pseudorandom interstimulus hold force designed to indent the skin 400 μm. Each digit on each hand was stimulated on the distal pad, the middle segment, and the proximal segment. In addition, a similar stimulus was delivered to each side of the upper lip.

Normal *cutaneous somatosensory evoked field (SEF)* responses were characterized by a peak amplitude at a latency between 30 and 70 msec, subject to a signal-to-noise ratio greater than 4 and goodness of fit (model/data) greater than 0.95, with a minimal confidence volume less than 3000 mm.[336] The dependent variables recorded for each SEF response included latency (in milliseconds); root mean square (rms) amplitude across sensory channels (fT); ratio of amplitude to latency; location of the digits on the *x*-, *y*-, and *z*-axes (in centimeters); spread between digits; order of the digits on the *z*-axis; and volume of the hand representation (4/3*II* times the radius of the spread on the *x*-, *y*-, and *z*-axes).

The results of these studies are summarized in Table 27-15. Descriptively, on both the affected and unaffected arms, subjects with FHd had significantly different neuromusculoskeletal and neurophysiological findings compared with age-matched controls. Clinically, those with dystonic FHd not only had difficulty performing the target task but also had greater problems with balance, postural alignment, finger spread, fine motor control, and sensory discrimination. Compared with controls, the location of the digits on the *x*-axis and the *y*-axis were significantly different in FHd subjects and the digits tended to be clumped in one location rather than sequenced. The ratio of SEF amplitude to latency was higher for FHd subjects compared with controls (Figure 27-19), and the volume of the hand representation was significantly larger on the hemisphere of the unaffected hand compared with the affected dystonic limb. The ratio of the amplitude to latency was positively correlated with the severity of dystonia (i.e., the more severe the dystonia, the higher the ratio). There was a negative correlation between the severity of the dystonia and both fine motor skills and motor control on the target task (i.e., the more severe the dystonia, the greater the compromise of motor skills). A low ratio of amplitude to latency was associated with the worst performance (Figure 27-20). Training was associated with improved amplitude of the somatosensory evoked responses and the sequencing of the digits (Figures 27-21 and 27-22). No changes were reported in the repeated imaging measurements of control subjects.

Attendance at supervised training sessions averaged 85%. No adverse events occurred with training. After LBSMT, subjects significantly improved in clinical performance. In experiment III, significant gains were achieved in motor control, neural tension, and sensory processing but not in strength or ROM. The effect sizes ranged from a mean of 0.72 for motor control to 0.96 for neural tension to 1.03 for sensory processing. In experiment IV, the clinical gains were significant for fine motor control (effect size 0.72), task-specific control (effect size 2.42), and functional independence (effect size 0.38). Posttest musculoskeletal measurements and accuracy of sensory processing were similar to the performance levels of the controls. All but two subjects returned to their previous work. None of the subjects gained 100% of fine motor control of the hand. In the case series in experiment V, the patients with hand dystonia improved the spread of the area of representation on the unaffected side along with improved order of digit and amplitude of magnetic evoked responses for patients with FHd. In experiment VI, subjects performing memory training in addition to supervised LBSMT achieved a higher score on task-specific performance after training (improving from 78.1% to 90%) than subjects performing supervised LBSMT alone (improving from 63.5% to 82%). When followed up 6 months after LBSMT, the subjects maintaining posttreatment skills were those who were partially to fully compliant with home practice.

One-Hand Compensation. The compensatory strategy of playing with one good hand is not uncommon among musicians with focal dystonia, congenital defects, weakness, trauma, or stroke.[509] These adaptations usually

TABLE **27-15**

Summary of Clinical Research Findings on Learning-Based Sensorimotor Training

Parameter	Findings
I. Descriptive Differences: Patients with Focal Hand Dystonia (FHd) and Controls	
A. Neuromusculoskeletal differences (experiment I)[300]	1. In experiment I, subjects with FHd (10) performed significantly worse than healthy controls (10) when using either the affected or unaffected side on musculoskeletal tasks, balance activities, postural alignment, fine motor control, and sensory discrimination.
	2. Subjects with severe dystonia demonstrated the following:
	• Greater restrictions on musculoskeletal skills and target specific motor control
	• Reduced accuracy in sensory discrimination but faster performance than those with mild dystonia
	• Better sensory discrimination accuracy on the unaffected side compared with subjects with mild dystonia
B. Somatosensory evoked field (SEF) responses (experiment I and experiment IV)[254,300]	In experiment I (10 subjects and matched controls):
	1. No significant differences were seen between the mean SEF response latency and the mean amplitude for FHd subjects and reference controls.
	2. The locations of the digits on the x- (bilateral) and y-axes (affected) were significantly different ($p <0.0001$, respectively), and the ratio of SEF mean amplitude to latency was higher for FHd subjects compared with controls ($p <0.05$) (see Figure 27-19).
	3. On the unaffected side, the volume of the hand representation was significantly larger for FHd subjects than for controls ($p <0.05$).
	4. The ratio of SEF amplitude plotted by response latency was significantly lower in the early phase (<100 msec) for the FHd subjects than for controls.
	5. The amplitude was similar for the control subjects and the FHd subjects for the unaffected digits on the affected limb and the digits on the unaffected limb.
	6. There was a bimodal distribution of the mean SEF amplitude plotted by mean latency on the affected side (mean latency ranging from 30-60 msec and the mean amplitude ranging from 20-119 fT).
	7. There was a negative linear trend of amplitude by latency for the digits on the unaffected side for FHd subjects and all of the controls (as the latency increased, the amplitude decreased).
	8. The field evoked firing patterns for controls and those with dystonia (mild and severe) were similar when measured on an unaffected part (i.e., the lip).
	9. Integrating amplitude by latency on the affected limb, those with severe dystonia had a significantly higher amplitude than those with mild dystonia (see Figure 27-20).
	10. Subjects with severe dystonia had a short latency and a high amplitude, and those with mild dystonia had a long latency and a low amplitude (see Figure 27-20).
	11. Bilaterally, the volume of the representation of the hand for those with mild dystonia was larger than the volume for subjects with severe dystonia.
	12. The amplitude of the functional magnetic resonance imaging in the basal ganglia was greater for FHd patients during a motor task than for controls across multiple tasks.
	13. Cortical activity in MI is greater in patients with FHd than in controls.
	14. Cortical activity in the primary motor cortex (PMC) and the supplementary motor area (SMA) is significantly reduced in patients with FHd when performing a manual task with affected hand.
	15. There is hyperactivity in M2 and hypoactivity in PMC/SMA in patients with FHd compared with controls.
	In experiment IV (case-controlled study of a healthy musician and a musician with dystonia):
	1. The magnetic field evoked responses in the primary somatosensory cortex of the musician with dystonia had a disorganized pattern of firing with a short latency, excessive amplitude, but decreased density compared with the musician without dystonia (see Figure 27-19).
	2. The location of the digits on the x-, y-, and z-axes were different, with sequential organization compromised in the musician with dystonia compared with the control musician.

(Continued)

TABLE 27-15

Summary of Clinical Research Findings on Learning-Based Sensorimotor Training—cont'd

Parameter	Findings
C. Correlation of magnetoencephalography (MEG) and clinical performance parameters (experiment II)[336]	In experiment II (17 subjects with FHd [severe and mild] and 15 controls): 1. High, significant correlations were seen (0.9029 affected and 0.8477 unaffected; $p < 0.001$, respectively) between the severity of dystonia and the SEF ratio of amplitude to latency. 2. On the affected side, negative correlations were seen between the SEF ratio and the severity of dystonia with musculoskeletal performance, motor control on the target task, and fine motor skills. 3. FHd subjects with mild dystonia tended to have a low SEF ratio and demonstrated higher performance on these tasks than subjects with severe dystonia. 4. A significantly negative correlation was seen between fine motor skills and the SEF ratio on the affected side; those with a high SEF ratio of amplitude to latency demonstrated greater inaccuracy. 5. On the unaffected side, a significant, moderately positive correlation was seen between the severity of dystonia and performance on the target task; subjects with mild dystonia had lower performance scores on the target task.

II. Effectiveness of Learning-Based Sensorimotor Training (LBSMT) Supervised Programs

Parameter	Findings
A. Patients with musician's cramp (MC) and writer's cramp (WC) experiment (experiment VII)[317]	In a pre/post test design study, 14 with MC and 13 WC participated in 8 weeks of LBSMT. 1. At baseline, MC patients had a higher level of functional independence and better range of motion (ROM) but less strength in affected upper limb compared with those with WC. 2. At baseline, subjects with MC demonstrated greater accuracy on graphesthesia, kinesthesia, and localization at baseline. 3. No differences were noted between groups on motor performance before or after training. 4. After training, both groups improved in musculoskeletal parameters (physical parameters, sensory processing, and motor control) but initial differences in posture, ROM, strength, graphesthesia, and kinesthesia persisted between groups, suggesting LBSMT must be adapted to the individual.
B. Patients with FHd and controls 1. Clinical gains (experiment III)[552]	In experiment III: 1. All subjects (12) improved significantly on all parameters of clinical performance (23%-80%), bringing performance of musculoskeletal parameters (flexibility, strength, postural alignment), sensory discrimination, and fine motor control to the level of healthy controls. 2. After completing LBSMT, the subjects with FHd scored between 80% and 90% on the target task, but none performed at 100%. 3. Motor reaction time was similar to that for controls on both the affected and unaffected sides. 4. Subjects with FHd improved 37%-42% in motor accuracy (performing with the same accuracy as controls but taking more time). 5. Accuracy improved 25%-50% on sensory tests (similar to or better than controls), but subjects with FHd required more time to perform the tests (66-197 sec compared with 37 sec for controls). 6. All but two subjects with FHd returned to their previous work, being careful about ergonomics and taking regular breaks. However, some of the musicians did not return to professional performance in the symphony or orchestra.
2. Change in imaging (experiment I and V)[254,535]	Following training in experiment V 3 case series: 1. Based on repeated magnetic source imaging, there were no changes in the findings for controls, but subjects with FHd improved the topographical somatosensory maps (see Figure 27-21). a. On the affected side, the order of the digits (digits 1 to 5) had an inferior to superior progression, but the order was still less distinct in order than controls (see Figure 27-22). b. On the affected side, the amplitude of the evoked somatosensory potential, integrated over time, was increased and similar to controls on the affected side. 2. There was an increase in the spread of the area of representation on the unaffected side.

Parameter	Findings
III. Effectiveness of Home LBSMT Program	
A. Immediately after training (experiment VI)[549]	Crossover study of home program (8 wk), periodic supervision, cognitive training in 13 subjects (18 hands). 1. Across all subjects, after 8 weeks of task-specific and cognitive training, sensory discrimination and fine motor speed improved 60%-80% ($p < 0.05$). 2. Task-specific performance improved by 12%. 3. Fine motor control time improved by 14.6 sec.
B. Six months later (experiment VI)[549]	Follow-up in 6 months (11 of 13 subjects)" 1. 10/11 returned to work. 2. 9/11 had 85%-90% task-specific performance 3. 34% were fully compliant on home program, 53% partially compliant, and 13% noncompliant. 4. 4%-10% additional improvement in task-specific performance for those fully or partially compliant, but a decrease of 20% score for those noncompliant with home program.

M1, sphenoidal segment; *M2*, part of Sylvian fissure in brain.

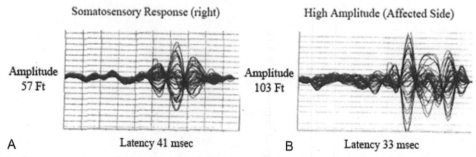

Somatosensory Response (right)

High Amplitude (Affected Side)

Amplitude
57 Ft

Amplitude
103 Ft

A   Latency 41 msec

B   Latency 33 msec

Figure 27-19 Differences in somatosensory evoked responses in a flutist without focal hand dystonia (**A**) and a flutist with focal hand dystonia (**B**). The somatosensory evoked potential for the flutist with focal hand dystonia demonstrates a short latency and a large amplitude compared with the flutist without focal hand dystonia. (From Byl NN, McKenzie A, Nagarajan SS: Differences in somatosensory hand organization in a healthy flutist and a flutist with focal hand dystonia: a case report, *J Hand Ther* 13:302-309, 2000.)

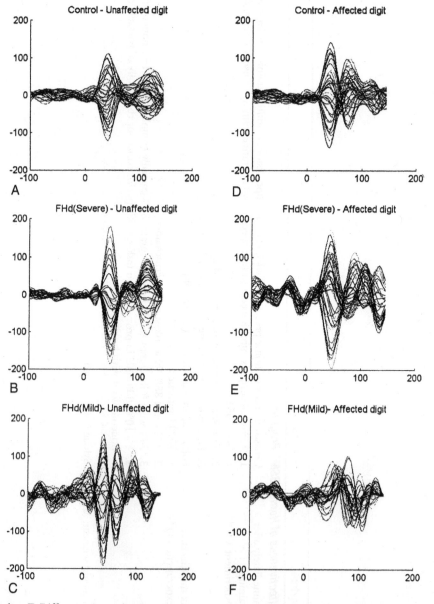

Figure 27-20 **A** to **F**, Differences in amplitude and volume over time for focal hand dystonia (FHd) subjects and controls.

(Continued)

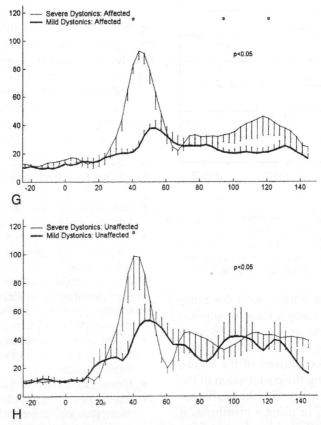

Figure 27-20, Cont'd **G** and **H,** Amplitude integrated by latency for FHd subjects (severe versus mild dystonia). (From Byl NN, Nagarajan SS, Merzenich MM et al: Correlation of clinical neuromusculoskeletal and central somatosensory performance: variability in controls and patients with severe and mild focal hand dystonia, *Neural Plast* 9:190, 193, 2002.)

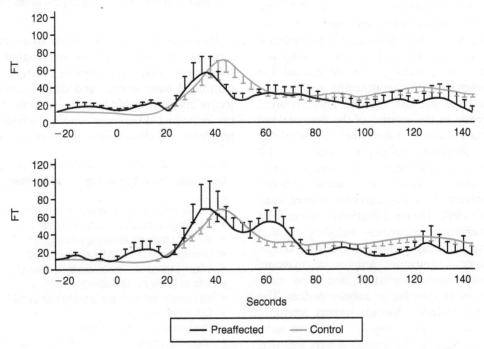

Figure 27-21 After completing a program of learning-based sensorimotor retraining, the amplitude of firing became more like controls; however, there was still a delay in turning off the neurons once they were engaged. *FT,* Fourier transform domain. (From Byl NN, Nagajaran S, McKenzie AL: Effect of sensory discrimination training on structure and function in patients with focal hand dystonia: a case series, *Arch Phys Med Rehabil* 84:1508, 2003.)

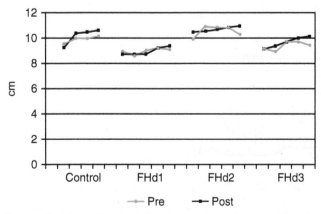

Figure 27-22 After participating in learning-based sensorimotor training, the sequential representation of the digits was improved (four-case series). *FHd*, focal hand dystonia. (From Byl NN, Nagajaran S, McKenzie AL: Effect of sensory discrimination training on structure and function in patients with focal hand dystonia: a case series, *Arch Phys Med Rehabil* 84:1508, 2003.)

require a multidisciplinary team with adaptations ranging from changing the strings, using a stand to support the instrument, using an orthosis to improve stability or assist movement, reconstructing an instrument, using a toggle key system, using the feet instead of the hands, transforming the sound, changing the composition of the piece, adapting the instrument to play with the unaffected side, using a digital instrument, or using a prosthesis. If a patient decides to use the unaffected hand to perform tasks, it is important for the patients to address the same neurophysiological aggravating factors that challenge repetitive use in order to avoid FHd in both limbs.

Motor Retraining. The effect of motor retraining for patients with FHd was studied by Zeuner et al.[538,539] The hand/arm was immobilized before beginning motor retraining. The purpose of immobilization was to minimize the severity of the dystonia and prime the nervous system for learning. Then patients performed general fine motor training exercises and strengthening and flexibility exercises that were not task specific. They reported a significant decrease in the severity of the dystonia and improved voluntary control. Later work by Schabrun et al.[540] confirmed that motor training was associated with normalization of the representation on the motor cortex.

Retraining Musicians. van Vugt et al.[541] carried out a retrospective descriptive study of musicians who received usual care in a musician's clinic. The rehabilitation strategies from one or more intervention strategies—including physical therapy, occupational therapy, movement classes, coaching on performance, acupuncture, acupressure, massage, biofeedback, neuromuscular simulation, and stress management—to the use of splinting or assistive devices. The outcomes measured included dystonia severity, strength, ROM, and performance; some also had objective kinematic examinations. Some of the musicians were followed for up to 4 years. Of those who responded (about 60% of the musicians who initially enrolled in the clinic), subjective feedback was solicited from a nonstandard questionnaire. Objective measurements taken at the beginning of

care were also repeated at follow-up. Only those completing both the initial and follow-up kinematic examination could be included in the analysis of results. The musicians reported significant improvement in motor control and a decrease in the severity of the dystonia. A few musicians claimed they were 100% cured of dystonia. Eighty percent were back to performance but not at the original intensity. Interestingly, the self-reported improvement was not validated by the objective kinematic clinical measurements.[541]

Key Points for Effectiveness of Learning-Based Retraining

- There are no large randomized clinical trials on the effectiveness of behavioral rehabilitative training for FHd.
- Learning-based intervention strategies are effective in improving motor control, with task-specific function recovered to approximately 85% of normal.
- Some patients claim 100% cure, but this is very individual and usually based on testimonials.
- Patients may report greater improvement than documented by standardized, objective kinematic testing.
- Training gains in somatosensory discrimination can bring patients with FHd to a level of performance similar to that of healthy age-matched controls.
- Minimal gains are reported in strength or range of motion.
- Improvement in clinical skills after behavioral training is correlated with neurophysiological improvement as measured by imaging techniques.
- Large, multisite, longitudinal randomized clinical trials are needed to specifically clarify the effectiveness of comprehensive learning-based training strategies (real physical practice and imagery) combined with medications, stress management, positive health behaviors, psychological counseling, biomechanical modifications of practice and performance, and assistive technology.

Patients raise many questions about carrying out behavioral training programs in rehabilitation. At this time, most questions cannot be precisely answered. With continued basic science and clinical research, more objective answers should become available. However, based on individual differences among individuals with FHd, retraining will always need to be matched to each patient.

Questions about Retraining Based on Neuroplasticity

- How long does it take to recover normal movement?
- How long do I need to practice each day?
- How will I know the training is working?
- How many repetitions do I really need to do?
- What if I cannot stop the abnormal movement?
- How do I know if I will recover?
- Do I have to quit doing the target task altogether?
- Can I keep working?
- Do I have to retrain both sides?
- Where can I get more definitive instructions for training?
- How can I find someone in my area to help me?
- Where can I get some resources to help me?

Fortunately, basic science and clinical researchers are trying to provide answers to these questions.

Summary

FHd is a complex movement disorder that affects the hand. This condition may develop as a consequence of genetics, but it can also develop as a consequence of repetitive overuse. This condition may be likely to arise under conditions of stress and repetitive overuse in individuals whose brain is overly adaptive. The condition is associated with overexcitation of some muscles without the ability to inhibit the undesired movements. In both animal and human studies, poor sensorimotor integrative processing has been documented along with a degradation of the somatosensory and motor representations of the hand without signs of local acute inflammation. Clinical studies suggest that patients with FHd have a variety of musculoskeletal and neuromuscular limitations that increase their risks for focal dystonia. Engaging, learning-based behavioral training can lead to objective improvement in clinical function and neural structure. Some researchers also report improved outcomes following general strengthening, flexibility, and ADL training without target specificity. Patients find it difficult to stop the abnormal movements to enable them to focus on retraining. At this time, rehabilitation is rarely 100%. Clinicians do not know whether patients simply cannot stop repeating the abnormal movements, cannot learn to inhibit excessive muscle excitation, or cannot engage sufficient confidence and positive expectations to restore voluntary control. It is also possible that interventions are not adequately adapted to each patient or specific or rigorous enough to fully restore cortical organization and normal voluntary control of movement. Large, longitudinal randomized clinical trials are needed to better define the parameters of intervention and maximize neural adaptation.

Key Points Concerning Focal Hand Dystonia

- There are no clinical tests to rule in or rule out focal hand dystonia (FHd).
- FHd is a multifactorial neurophysiological movement disorder with evidence suggesting aberrant neural learning as a significant risk factor.
- Management is possible; complete recovery is less common.
- Maximizing return of function requires a comprehensive team effort with the patient taking active leadership in learning-based retraining. Randomized trials including neuroimaging and objective clinical performance measurements paired with retraining paradigms will improve our understanding of FHd and effective intervention strategies.

Resources for Patients with Focal Hand Dystonia

A variety of resources are available to help patients who have dystonia. Some organizations have support groups that meet in person. In other cases, it is possible to establish links for online support. In addition, a variety of foundations can help patients find a physician or other team members, including a coach or a teacher (e.g., Dystonia Medical Research Foundation). There are also some Internet-based training opportunities that patients may explore.

Resources for Education and Home Training: Chronic RSI/Focal Hand Dystonia

- Dystonias Fact Sheet: National Institute of Neurological Disorders and Stroke (NINDS): *http://www.ninds.nih.gov/disorders/dystonias/detail_dystonias.htm*
- Foundations:
  - Dystonia Medical Research Foundation: *https://www.dystonia-foundation.org*
  - Bachmann Strauss Dystonia and Parkinson Foundation: *http://www.dystonia-parkinsons.org*
  - National Spasmodic Torticollis Association: *http://www.torticollis.org*
  - Spasmodic Torticollis Dystonia/ST Dystonia: *http://www.spasmodictorticollis.org*
  - American Dystonia Society: *http://www.dystonia.us*
  - NASM-PAMA Advisories on Neuromusculoskeletal and Vocal Health: *http://nasm.arts-accredit.org/index.jsp?page=NASM-PAMA%3A+Neuromuscu loskeletal+and+Vocal+Health*
- *Graded Motor Imagery (GMI) Handbook* by Moseley GL, Butler DS, Beames TB, Giles TJ; PO Box 47009, Minneapolis, MN, 55447-009 USA. The book can purchased on line at *www.optp.com* or *www.gradedmotorimagery.com*. Helpful tools for graded motor imagery training include: 1) mirror (*http://www.optp.com/NOI-Mirror-Box-Triangle#.VhGRkjrqLww*); 2) apps for the iphone "Recognise-Hands", Recognise-Feet" or "Recognise-Back" (*http://www.noigroup.com/en/Product/BTRAPP*); or 3) flash cards: Back (*http://www.optp.com/NOI-Recognise-Back-Flash-Cards#.VhGR8zrqLww*), Hands (*http://www.optp.com/NOI-Recognise-Hand-Flash-Cards#.VhGS7jrqLww*), and Feet (*http://www.optp.com/NOI-Recognise-Foot-Flash-Cards#. VhGSzDrqLww*).
- *Handbook on RSI/Focal Dystonia* by Nancy Byl, PT, MPH, PhD. Available from UCSF Department of Physical Therapy and Rehabilitation Science, School of Medicine, Physical Therapy Health and Wellness Center, 1675 Owens St, SF CA 94158; 415-514-4816 ($20.00), Regents of the University of California.
- Computing Without Pain with the MouseKeyDoTM System, Ergonomic training in mouse and keyboard techniques by Norman J Kahan, MD: *www. mousekeydo.com*
- Sam Brown,[519] musician, with education and training audios for using hypnosis to enhance the recovery of voluntary motor control in musicians with FHd: *www.focaldystoniahypnosis.com*
- Joaquin Farias, PhD, MA, MS: 1) Techniques: *http://www.fariastechnique.com*; 2) Professor and trainer (youtube): https://vimeo. com/41202758; 3) Intertwined - How To Induce Neuroplasticity. A New Approach to Rehabilitating Dystonias: *http://www.fariastechnique.com/ store-books-dvds-joaquin-farias/lmzibcwkffwrauvqhw9z12ygoqbmh2*

- Abigail Brown, Director: Spasmotic Torticollis Recovery Clinic. Inc (STRC., Inc), 5 Bisbee Ct. 109–238, Santa Fe, NM 87508; 1-800-805-9976
- Stress management
  - Mindfulness training
    - 16 exercises: *http://www.practicingmindfulness.com/16-simple-mindfulness-exercises/*
    - Pocket Mindfulness Stop. Breathe. Let Go: *www.pocketmindfulness.com*
    - Effectiveness of Mindfulness training: http://mobile.nytimes.com/blogs/well/2015/09/30/does-mindfulness-make-for-a-better-athlete/
  - Stress and Your Body (Physiology of Stress, volumes 1 and 2), Great Courses Health and Wellness, Professor Robert Sapolsky, Stanford University
- Support Groups for Dystonia (check by State and region):
  - Dystonia Bulletin Boards: www.dystonia-bb.org/
  - Daily Strength: www.dailystrength.org/c/dystonia%20support%20group
  - wow.com/Support+Groups+For+Dystonia
  - Dystonia Support Website: www.caringbridge.org/Dystonia
  - Dystonia Coalition: www.rarediseasesnetwork.org
- Internet Resources
  - Online Dystonia Bulletin Board: http://www.dystonia-bb.org/forums/asd/
  - DMRF's YouTube Channel: http://www.youtube.com/facesofdystonia
  - DMRF on Twitter: https://twitter.com/dmrf
  - DMRF on Facebook: https://www.facebook.com/dystonia
  - Facebook Group: Cervical Dystonia Support Forum: https://www.facebook.com/groups/dmrf.cervical/
- Physical Therapy and Focal Dystonia with Alison McKenzie, PT, PhD: https://www.youtube.com/watch?v=lhew0-BAkC8
- Teachers
  - Guitarist David Leisner in New York: http://davidleisner.com; method: https://www.youtube.com/watch?v=Kqxl4uSkB9w
  - Taubman Tapes and youtube videos for patients with pianist dystonia
    - Tapes (I and II): http://www.taubman-tapes.com/Home.html
    - youtube choreography of the hand: https://www.youtube.com/watch?v=suwdLaYBaAs
    - Piano instruction https://www.youtube.com/watch?v=sgUqBP7kz7s
    - http://www.youtube.com/watch?feature=fvwp&v=66V8AECWOTc&NR=1 (audio only)
    - The story of one pianist: Choreography of the hand: https://www.youtube.com/watch?v=47w_6IKHA1M
    - https://www.youtube.com/watch?v=eevJ937ikGI
    - https://www.youtube.com/watch?v=SSCyb43wQdA
- Stories of patients with focal dystonia:
  - Focal dystonia in a trumpet player - interview: https://www.youtube.com/watch?v=Cp6sw71z_sg
  - Violinist with dystonia: https://www.youtube.com/watch?feature=endscreen&NR=1&v=17oRdtXKcm0
- Patients can search the web for home based movement videos: NIA, Felenkrais, Tai Chi, JiGong, Yoga, Tai Won Do. Below are two Feldenkrais teachers who retrain patients with focal dystonia:
  - Mary Spire (musician) is a Feldenkrais practitioner in Berkeley, California. She works with musicians with RSI, stress and dystonia. She sometimes offers classes in SF: http://optimalmoves.com/
  - Anat Baniel, PhD, Feldenkrais teacher has a focus on improving movement dysfunction. Anat Baniel has a center located at 4330 Redwood Highway, Suite 350, San Rafael, CA 94903, 415-472-6622. She offers individual treatment and classes.

CONCLUSION

In U.S. industry, musculoskeletal disorders account for one in three workdays lost as a result of injuries or illness. Strong epidemiological evidence indicates that a major risk factor for the development of WRMSDs of the upper limb is the performance of hand-intensive, repetitive tasks on an ongoing basis. These tasks are often highly repetitive and forceful and require awkward positions and sustained postures. In addition, the jobs may be performed under poor environmental conditions. These factors interact with psychosocial stress, unhealthy lifestyle, and co-morbid medical conditions.

Most of the overuse impairments develop from local tissue microtrauma and inflammation. The local tissue damage can be treated effectively with anti-inflammatory medications, rest, and work modifications. However, chronic pain and movement dysfunction (e.g., neuropathic pain, FHd) can be secondary, centralized complications of excessive overuse of the hands. These problems are difficult to treat.

In these chronic, complex cases of overuse, the individual must carefully evaluate issues related to goals and objectives, lifestyle behaviors, (e.g., exercise, nutrition, sleep, stress management, mental well-being, and other medical problems), positive expectations, and specific learning-based brain retraining. It is essential to restore healthy biomechanical performance, avoid repetitive abnormal movements, improve the accuracy of sensory processing, and modify timing and amplitude of motor outputs. The retraining activities require attendance and careful grading and must be progressive in difficulty, rewarding, fun, and spaced over time. Computerized instrumentation (e.g., goal-oriented, game-formatted learning paradigms) may enhance the effectiveness of brain retraining. Where possible, training should be supervised and guided but also integrated at home, at work, and in recreational activities.

There is moderately good evidence supporting the effective management of the movement dysfunction in FHd, but only testimonials by a few individuals report a "cure." Given the inherent, neurophysiological risk factors of excessive plasticity, decreased voluntary inhibition, and genetics, the intervention strategies should include a comprehensive, interprofessional team, matching medical management strategies with learning-based training to recover voluntary motor control to enable return to productive performance of target tasks.

REFERENCES

1. National Center for Chronic Disease Prevention and Health Promotion (DoPH): *Work-related musculoskeletal disorders (WMSD) prevention*, 2013. Available at http://www.cdc.gov/workplacehealth-promotion/implementation/topics/disorders.html.

2. Centers for Disease Control and Prevention (CDC): *Work-related musculoskeletal disorders (WMSD) prevention*. Available at http://www.cdc.gov/workplacehealthpromotion/ implementation/topics/disorders.html. Accessed November 16, 2014.

3. Gallagher S, Heberger JR: Examining the interaction of force and repetition on musculoskeletal disorder risk: a systematic literature review, *Hum Factors* 55:108–124, 2013.

4. Fan ZJ, Silverstein BA, Bao S, et al: The association between combination of hand force and forearm posture and incidence of lateral epicondylitis in a working population, *Hum Factors* 56:151–165, 2014.

5. Harris-Adamson C, Eisen EA, Kapellusch J, et al: Biomechanical risk factors for carpal tunnel syndrome: a pooled study of 2474 workers, *Occup Environ Med* 72:33–41, 2015.

6. Harris C, Eisen EA, Goldberg R, et al: 1st place, PREMUS best paper competition: workplace and individual factors in wrist tendinosis among blue-collar workers—the San Francisco study, *Scand J Work Environ Health* 37:85–98, 2011.

7. Barcenilla A, March LM, Chen JS, et al: Carpal tunnel syndrome and its relationship to occupation: a meta-analysis, *Rheumatology (Oxford)* 51:250–261, 2012.

8. Bernard BP: *Musculoskeletal disorders and workplace factors: a critical review of epidemiologic evidence for work-related musculoskeletal disorders of the neck, upper extremity and low back*, DHHS (NIOSH) Publication Number 97-141, Washington, DC, 1997, US Government Printing Office. Available at http://www.cdc.gov/niosh/docs/97-141/.

9. National Research Council & Institute of Medicine (NRC&IOM): *Musculoskeletal disorders and the workplace: low back and upper extremities*, Washington, 2001, The National Academies Press.

10. You D, Smith AH, Rempel D: Meta-analysis: association between wrist posture and carpal tunnel syndrome among workers, *Saf Health Work* 5:27–31, 2014.

11. Nordander C, Ohlsson K, Akesson I, et al: Exposure-response relationships in work-related musculoskeletal disorders in elbows and hands—a synthesis of group-level data on exposure and response obtained using uniform methods of data collection, *Appl Ergon* 44:241–253, 2013.

12. Silverstein BA, Fine LJ, Armstrong TJ: Hand wrist cumulative trauma disorders in industry, *Br J Ind Med* 43(11):779–784, 1986.

13. Barbe MF, Gallagher S, Massicotte VS, et al: The interaction of force and repetition on musculoskeletal and neural tissue responses and sensorimotor behavior in a rat model of work-related musculoskeletal disorders, *BMC Musculoskelet Disord* 14:303, 2013.

14. Barbe MF, Barr AE: Inflammation and the pathophysiology of work-related musculoskeletal disorders, *Brain Behav Immun* 20:423–429, 2006.

15. Roquelaure Y, Ha C, Nicolas G, et al: Attributable risk of carpal tunnel syndrome according to industry and occupation in a general population, *Arthritis Rheum* 59(9):1341–1348, 2008.

16. Leclerc A, Landre MF, Chastang JF, et al: Upper-limb disorders in repetitive work, *Scand J Work Environ Health* 27:268–278, 2001.

17. Srilatha MAG, Bhat V, Sathiakumar N: Prevalence of work-related wrist and hand musculoskeletal disorders (WMSD) among computer users, Karnataka State, India, *J Clin Diagn Res* 5:605–607, 2011.

18. Ratzlaff CR, Gillies JH, Koehoorn MW: Work-related repetitive strain injury and leisure-time physical activity, *Arthritis Rheum* 57:495–500, 2007.

19. Foss L, Gravseth HM, Kristensen P, et al: The impact of workplace risk factors on long-term musculoskeletal sickness absence: a registry-based 5-year follow-up from the Oslo health study, *J Occup Environ Med* 53:1478–1482, 2011.

20. Gerr F, Marcus M, Ensor C, et al: A prospective study of computer users: I. Study design and incidence of musculoskeletal symptoms and disorders, *Am J Ind Med* 41:221–235, 2002.

21. Bureau of Labor Statistics: *Nonfatal occupational injuries and illnesses requiring days away from work 2012*, Washington, DC, November 26, 2013. News Release USDL-13-2257. Available at http://www.bls.gov/news.release/pdf/osh2.pdf.

22. Alavinia SM, van den Berg TI, van Duivenbooden C, et al: Impact of work-related factors, lifestyle, and work ability on sickness absence among Dutch construction workers, *Scand J Work Environ Health* 35:325–333, 2009.

23. van den Berg TI, Elders LA, de Zwart BC, et al: The effects of work-related and individual factors on the Work Ability Index: a systematic review, *Occup Environ Med* 66:211–220, 2009.

24. Horton R: GBD 2010: understanding disease, injury, and risk, *Lancet* 380:2053–2054, 2012.

25. Woolf AD, Pfleger B: Burden of major musculoskeletal conditions, *Bull World Health Organ* 81:646–656, 2003.

26. Bureau of Labor Statistics: *Nonfatal occupational injuries and illnesses requiring days away from work 2011*, Washington, DC November 8, 2012. News Release USDL-12-2204. Available at http://www.bls.gov/news.release/osh2.nr0.htm.

27. Health and Safety Executive: *The Health and Safety Executive Statistics 2010/11*. Available at http://www.hse.gov.uk/statistics/overall/hssh1011.pdf.

28. Piligian G, Herbert R, Hearns M, et al: Evaluation and management of chronic work-related musculoskeletal disorders of the distal upper extremity, *Am J Ind Med* 37:75–93, 2000.

29. Rempel D: Ergonomics—prevention of work-related musculoskeletal disorders, *West J Med* 156:409–410, 1992.

30. Rempel DM, Harrison RJ, Barnhart S: Work-related cumulative trauma disorders of the upper extremity, *JAMA* 267:838–842, 1992.

31. van Rijn RM, Huisstede BM, Koes BW, et al: Associations between work-related factors and the carpal tunnel syndrome—a systematic review, *Scand J Work Environ Health* 35:19–36, 2009.

32. US Bureau of Labor Statistics: Workplace injury and illness summary, *Workplace Injuries and Illnesses 2012*, Washington, DC, 2012, News Release. Available at: http://data.bls.gov/cgi-bin/print.pl/news.release/osh.nr0.htm, Accessed November 7, 2013.

33. Silverstein M: Meeting the challenges of an aging workforce, *Am J Ind Med* 51:269–280, 2008.

34. World Health Organization: US national institute of aging, US national institutes of health, *Global health and aging*, 2011. Available at http://www.who.int/ageing/publications/global_health/en/.

35. Association of Occupational and Environmental Clinics: *Healthy aging for a sustainable workforce*, Silver Spring, MD, 2009, CPWR—The Center for Construction Research and Training.

36. NRC&IOM NRCIoM: *Musculoskeletal disorders and the workplace: low back and upper extremities*, Washington, DC, 2001, The National Academies Press.

37. Gallagher S, Heberger JR: Examining the interaction of force and repetition on musculoskeletal disorder risk: a systematic literature review, *Hum Factors* 55:108–124, 2013.

38. Thomsen JF, Mikkelsen S, Andersen JH, et al: Risk factors for hand-wrist disorders in repetitive work, *Occup Environ Med* 64:527–533, 2007.

39. Nathan PA, Meadows KD, Doyle LS: Occupation as a risk factor for impaired sensory conduction of the median nerve at the carpal tunnel, *J Hand Surg* 13:167–170, 1988.

40. Silverstein BA, Fine LJ, Armstrong TJ: Occupational factors and carpal tunnel syndrome, *Am J Ind Med* 11:343–358, 1987.

41. Armstrong TJ, Fine LJ, Goldstein SA, et al: Ergonomics considerations in hand and wrist tendinitis, *J Hand Surg Am* 12(Pt 2):830–837, 1987.

42. Haahr JP, Andersen JH: Physical and psychosocial risk factors for lateral epicondylitis: a population based case-referent study, *Occup Environ Med* 60:322–329, 2003.

43. Solovieva S, Vehmas T, Riihimaki H, et al: Hand use and patterns of joint involvement in osteoarthritis. A comparison of female dentists and teachers, *Rheumatology (Oxford)* 44:521–528, 2005.

44. Ding H, Solovieva S, Vehmas T, et al: Hand osteoarthritis and pinch grip strength among middle-aged female dentists and teachers, *Scand J Rheumatol* 39:84–87, 2010.

45. van Rijn RM, Huisstede BM, Koes BW, et al: Associations between work-related factors and specific disorders at the elbow: a systematic literature review, *Rheumatology (Oxford)* 48:528–536, 2009.

46. Hauret KG, Jones BH, Bullock SH, et al: Musculoskeletal injuries description of an under-recognized injury problem among military personnel, *Am J Prev Med* 38(Suppl):S61–S70, 2010.

47. Punnett L, Wegman DH: Work-related musculoskeletal disorders: the epidemiologic evidence and the debate, *J Electromyogr Kinesiol* 14:13–23, 2004.

48. Andersen JH, Haahr JP, Frost P: Risk factors for more severe regional musculoskeletal symptoms: a two-year prospective study of a general working population, *Arthritis Rheum* 56:1355–1364, 2007.

49. Ekpenyong CE, Inyang UC: Associations between worker characteristics, workplace factors, and work-related musculoskeletal disorders: a cross-sectional study of male construction workers in Nigeria, *Int J Occup Saf Ergon* 20:447–462, 2014.

50. Elliott MB, Barr AE, Kietrys DM, et al: Peripheral neuritis and increased spinal cord neurochemicals are induced in a model of repetitive motion injury with low force and repetition exposure, *Brain Res* 1218:103–113, 2008.

51. Barbe MF, Elliott MB, Abdelmagid SM, et al: Serum and tissue cytokines and chemokines increase with repetitive upper extremity tasks, *J Orthop Res* 26:1320–1326, 2008.

52. Coq JO, Barbe MF: Peripheral and central changes combined induce movement disorders on the basis of disuse or overuse. In Larsen BJ, editor: *Movement disorders: causes, diagnoses and treatments*, Hauppauge, NY, 2011, Nova Science Publishers.

53. Abdelmagid SM, Barr AE, Rico M, et al: Performance of repetitive tasks induces decreased grip strength and increased fibrogenic proteins in skeletal muscle: role of force and inflammation, *PLoS One* 7:e38359, 2012.

54. Al-Shatti T, Barr AE, Safadi FF, et al: Increase in inflammatory cytokines in median nerves in a rat model of repetitive motion injury, *J Neuroimmunol* 167:13–22, 2005.

55. Barbe MF, Barr AE, Gorzelany I, et al: Chronic repetitive reaching and grasping results in decreased motor performance and widespread tissue responses in a rat model of MSD, *J Orthop Res* 21:167–176, 2003.

56. Barr AE, Safadi FF, Gorzelany I, et al: Repetitive, negligible force reaching in rats induces pathological overloading of upper extremity bones, *J Bone Miner Res* 18:2023–2032, 2003.

57. Clark BD, Barr AE, Safadi FF, et al: Median nerve trauma in a rat model of work-related musculoskeletal disorder, *J Neurotrauma* 20:681–695, 2003.

58. Coq JO, Barr AE, Strata F, et al: Peripheral and central changes combine to induce motor behavioral deficits in a moderate repetition task, *Exp Neurol* 220:234–245, 2009.

59. Elliott MB, Barr AE, Barbe MF: Spinal substance P and neurokinin-1 increase with high repetition reaching, *Neurosci Lett* 454:33–37, 2009.

60. Elliott MB, Barr AE, Clark BD, et al: High force reaching task induces widespread inflammation, increased spinal cord neurochemicals and neuropathic pain, *Neuroscience* 158:922–931, 2009.

61. Kietrys DM, Barr AE, Barbe MF: Exposure to repetitive tasks induces motor changes related to skill acquisition and inflammation in rats, *J Mot Behav* 43:465–476, 2011.

62. Barbe MF, Gallagher S, Popoff SN: Serum biomarkers as predictors of stage of work-related musculoskeletal disorders, *J Am Acad Orthop Surg* 21:644–646, 2013.

63. Gao HG, Fisher PW, Lambi AG, et al: Increased serum and musculotendinous fibrogenic proteins following persistent low-grade inflammation in a rat model of long-term upper extremity overuse, *PLoS One* 8:e71875, 2013.

64. Kietrys DM, Barr-Gillespie AE, Amin M, et al: Aging contributes to inflammation in upper extremity tendons and declines in forelimb agility in a rat model of upper extremity overuse, *PLoS One* 7:e46954, 2012.

65. Xin DL, Harris MY, Wade CK, et al: Aging enhances serum cytokine response but not task-induced grip strength declines in a rat model of work-related musculoskeletal disorders, *BMC Musculoskelet Disord* 12:63, 2011.

66. Elliott MB, Barr AE, Clark BD, et al: Performance of a repetitive task by aged rats leads to median neuropathy and spinal cord inflammation with associated sensorimotor declines, *Neuroscience* 170:929–941, 2010.

67. Clark BD, Al-Shatti TA, Barr AE, et al: Performance of a high-repetition, high-force task induces carpal tunnel syndrome in rats, *J Orthop Sports Phys Ther* 34:244–253, 2004.

68. Driban JB, Barr AE, Amin M, et al: Joint inflammation and early degeneration induced by high-force reaching are attenuated by ibuprofen in an animal model of work-related musculoskeletal disorder, *J Biomed Biotechnol* 2011:691412, 2011.

69. Fedorczyk JM, Barr AE, Rani S, et al: Exposure-dependent increases in IL-1beta, substance P, CTGF, and tendinosis in flexor digitorum tendons with upper extremity repetitive strain injury, *J Orthop Res* 28:298–307, 2010.

70. Jain NX, Barr-Gillespie AE, Clark BD, et al: Bone loss from high repetitive high force loading is prevented by ibuprofen treatment, *J Musculoskelet Neuronal Interact* 14:78–94, 2014.

71. Rani S, Barbe MF, Barr AE, et al: Induction of periostin-like factor and periostin in forearm muscle, tendon, and nerve in an animal model of work-related musculoskeletal disorder, *J Histochem Cytochem* 57:1061–1073, 2009.

72. Rani S, Barbe MF, Barr AE, et al: Periostin-like-factor and Periostin in an animal model of work-related musculoskeletal disorder, *Bone* 44:502–512, 2009.

73. Rani S, Barbe MF, Barr AE, et al: Role of TNF alpha and PLF in bone remodeling in a rat model of repetitive reaching and grasping, *J Cell Physiol* 225:152–167, 2010.

74. Barbe MF, Gallagher S, Massicotte VS, et al: The interaction of force and repetition on musculoskeletal and neural tissue responses and sensorimotor behavior in a rat model of work-related musculoskeletal disorders, *BMC Musculoskelet Disord* 14:303, 2013.

75. Blake DT, Byl NN, Merzenich MM: Representation of the hand in the cerebral cortex, *Behav Brain Res* 135:179–184, 2002.

76. Byl NN, Merzenich MM, Cheung S, et al: A primate model for studying focal dystonia and repetitive strain injury: effects on the primary somatosensory cortex, *Phys Ther* 77:269–284, 1997.

77. Byl NN, Merzenich MM, Jenkins WM: A primate genesis model of focal dystonia and repetitive strain injury: I. Learning-induced dedifferentiation of the representation of the hand in the primary somatosensory cortex in adult monkeys, *Neurology* 47:508–520, 1996.

78. Topp KS, Byl NN: Movement dysfunction following repetitive hand opening and closing: anatomical analysis in Owl monkeys, *Mov Disord* 14:295–306, 1999.

79. Banks JJ, Lavender SA, Buford JA, et al: Measuring pad-pad pinch strength in a non-human primate: Macaca fascicularis, *J Electromyogr Kinesiol* 17:725–730, 2007.

80. Sommerich CM, Lavender SA, Buford JA, et al: Towards development of a nonhuman primate model of carpal tunnel syndrome: performance of a voluntary, repetitive pinching task induces median mononeuropathy in Macaca fascicularis, *J Orthop Res* 25:713–724, 2007.

81. Carpenter JE, Thomopoulos S, Soslowsky LJ: Animal models of tendon and ligament injuries for tissue engineering applications, *Clin Orthop Relat Res* 367(Suppl):S296–S311, 1999.

82. Soslowsky LJ, Thomopoulos S, Tun S, et al: Neer Award 1999. Overuse activity injures the supraspinatus tendon in an animal model: a histologic and biomechanical study, *J Shoulder Elbow Surg* 9:79–84, 2000.

83. Nakama LH, King KB, Abrahamsson S, et al: Evidence of tendon microtears due to cyclical loading in an in vivo tendinopathy model, *J Orthop Res* 23:1199–1205, 2005.

84. Diegelmann RF, Evans MC: Wound healing: an overview of acute, fibrotic and delayed healing, *Front Biosci* 9:283–289, 2004.

85. Lin TW, Cardenas L, Soslowsky LJ: Biomechanics of tendon injury and repair, *J Biomech* 37:865–877, 2004.

86. Atcheson SG, Ward JR, Lowe W: Concurrent medical disease in work-related carpal tunnel syndrome, *Arch Intern Med* 158:1506–1512, 1998.

87. Ljung BO, Forsgren S, Friden J: Substance P and calcitonin gene-related peptide expression at the extensor carpi radialis brevis muscle origin: implications for the etiology of tennis elbow, *J Orthop Res* 17:554–559, 1999.

88. Gerdle B, Hilgenfeldt U, Larsson B, et al: Bradykinin and kallidin levels in the trapezius muscle in patients with work-related trapezius myalgia, in patients with whiplash associated pain, and in healthy controls—A microdialysis study of women, *Pain* 139:578–587, 2008.

89. Ghafouri B, Larsson BK, Sjors A, et al: Interstitial concentration of serotonin is increased in myalgic human trapezius muscle during rest, repetitive work and mental stress—an in vivo microdialysis study, *Scand J Clin Lab Invest* 70:478–486, 2010.

90. Hirata H, Nagakura T, Tsujii M, et al: The relationship of VEGF and PGE2 expression to extracellular matrix remodelling of the tenosynovium in the carpal tunnel syndrome, *J Pathol* 204:605–612, 2004.

91. Sopova K, Tatsidou P, Stellos K: Platelets and platelet interaction with progenitor cells in vascular homeostasis and inflammation, *Curr Vasc Pharmacol* 10:555–562, 2012.

92. Nurden AT, Nurden P, Sanchez M, et al: Platelets and wound healing, *Front Biosci* 13:3532–3548, 2008.

93. Pyne DB: Exercise-induced muscle damage and inflammation: a review, *Austr J Sci Med Sport* 26:49–58, 1994.

94. Clarkson PM, Sayers SP: Etiology of exercise-induced muscle damage, *Can J Appl Physiol* 24:234–248, 1999.

95. Laskin DL: Macrophages and inflammatory mediators in chemical toxicity: a battle of forces, *Chem Res Toxicol* 22:1376–1385, 2009.

96. Dakin SG, Dudhia J, Smith RK: Resolving an inflammatory concept: the importance of inflammation and resolution in tendinopathy, *Vet Immunol Immunopathol* 158:121–127, 2014.

97. Gute DC, Ishida T, Yarimizu K, et al: Inflammatory responses to ischemia and reperfusion in skeletal muscle, *Mol Cell Biochem* 179:169–187, 1998.

98. Lin TW, Cardenas L, Glaser DL, et al: Tendon healing in interleukin-4 and interleukin-6 knockout mice, *J Biomech* 39:61–69, 2006.

99. Lin TW, Cardenas L, Soslowsky LJ: Biomechanics of tendon injury and repair, *J Biomech* 37:865–877, 2004.

100. Voleti PB, Buckley MR, Soslowsky LJ: Tendon healing: repair and regeneration, *Annu Rev Biomed Eng* 14:47–71, 2012.

101. Ettema AM, Amadio PC, Zhao C, et al: A histological and immunohistochemical study of the subsynovial connective tissue in idiopathic carpal tunnel syndrome, *J Bone Joint Surg Am* 86:1458–1466, 2004.

102. Ettema AM, Zhao C, An KN, et al: Comparative anatomy of the subsynovial connective tissue in the carpal tunnel of the rat, rabbit, dog, baboon, and human, *Hand (N Y)* 1:78–84, 2006.

103. Nakama LH, King KB, Abrahamsson S, et al: VEGF, VEGFR-1, and CTGF cell densities in tendon are increased with cyclical loading: an in vivo tendinopathy model, *J Orthop Res* 24:393–400, 2006.

104. Smith CA, Stauber F, Waters C, et al: Transforming growth factor-beta following skeletal muscle strain injury in rats, *J Appl Physiol* 102:755–761, 2007.

105. Barr AE, Barbe MF: Inflammation reduces physiological tissue tolerance in the development of work-related musculoskeletal disorders, *J Electromyogr Kinesiol* 14:77–85, 2004.

106. Barr AE, Barbe MF, Clark BD: Systemic inflammatory mediators contribute to widespread effects in work-related musculoskeletal disorders, *Exerc Sport Sci Rev* 32:135–142, 2004.

107. Fenwick SA, Curry V, Harrall RL, et al: Expression of transforming growth factor-beta isoforms and their receptors in chronic tendinosis, *J Anat* 199(Pt 3):231–240, 2001.

108. Ettema AM, Belohlavek M, Zhao C, et al: High-resolution ultrasound analysis of subsynovial connective tissue in human cadaver carpal tunnel, *J Orthop Res* 4:2011–2020, 2006.

109. Hirata H, Tsujii M, Yoshida T, et al: MMP-2 expression is associated with rapidly proliferative arteriosclerosis in the flexor tenosynovium and pain severity in carpal tunnel syndrome, *J Pathol* 205:443–450, 2005.

110. Novak CB, Mackinnon SE: Repetitive use and static postures: a source of nerve compression and pain, *J Hand Ther* 10:151–159, 1997.

111. Novak CB, Mackinnon SE: Nerve injury in repetitive motion disorders, *Clin Orthop* 351:10–20, 1998.

112. Novak CB, Mackinnon SE: Multiple nerve entrapment syndromes in office workers, *Occup Med* 14:39–59, 1999.

113. Byl C, Puttlitz C, Byl N, et al: Strain in the median and ulnar nerves during upper-extremity positioning, *J Hand Surg Am* 27:1032–1040, 2002.

114. Nathan PA, Meadows KD, Doyle LS: Relationship of age and sex to sensory conduction of the median nerve at the carpal tunnel and association of slowed conduction with symptoms, *Muscle Nerve* 11:1149–1153, 1988.

115. Yoshii Y, Zhao C, Zhao KD, et al: The effect of wrist position on the relative motion of tendon, nerve, and subsynovial connective tissue within the carpal tunnel in a human cadaver model, *J Orthop Res* 26:1153–1158, 2008.

116. Bove GM, Weissner W, Barbe MF: Long lasting recruitment of immune cells and altered epi-perineural thickness in focal nerve inflammation induced by complete Freund's adjuvant, *J Neuroimmunol* 213:26–30, 2009.

117. Ma W, Eisenach JC: Cyclooxygenase 2 in infiltrating inflammatory cells in injured nerve is universally up-regulated following various types of peripheral nerve injury, *Neuroscience* 121:691–704, 2003.

118. Ma W, Eisenach JC: Four PGE2 EP receptors are up-regulated in injured nerve following partial sciatic nerve ligation, *Exp Neurol* 183:581–592, 2003.

119. Sud V, Freeland AE: Biochemistry of carpal tunnel syndrome, *Microsurgery* 25:44–46, 2005.

120. Song Y, Stal PS, Yu J, et al: Marked effects of Tachykinin in myositis both in the experimental side and contralaterally: studies on NK-1 receptor expressions in an animal mode, *ISRN Inflamm* 2013:907821, 2013.

121. Song Y, Stal PS, Yu JG, et al: Bilateral increase in expression and concentration of tachykinin in a unilateral rabbit muscle overuse model that leads to myositis, *BMC Musculoskelet Disord* 14:134, 2013.

122. Danielson P, Alfredson H, Forsgren S: Distribution of general (PGP 9.5) and sensory (substance P/CGRP) innervations in the human patellar tendon, *Knee Surg Sports Traumatol Arthrosc* 14:125–132, 2006.

123. Rothman SM, Kreider RA, Winkelstein BA: Spinal neuropeptide responses in persistent and transient pain following cervical nerve root injury, *Spine* 30:2491–2496, 2005.

124. Hockerfelt U, Franzen L, Norrgard O, et al: Early increase and later decrease in VIP and substance P nerve fiber densities following abdominal radiotherapy: a study on the human colon, *Int J Radiat Biol* 78:1045–1053, 2002.

125. Rempel DM, Diao E: Entrapment neuropathies: pathophysiology and pathogenesis, *J Electromyogr Kinesiol* 14:71–75, 2004.

126. Viikari-Juntura E, Silverstein B: Role of physical load factors in carpal tunnel syndrome, *Scand J Work Environ Health* 25:163–185, 1999.

127. Jablecki CK, Andary MT, So YT, et al: Literature review of the usefulness of nerve conduction studies and electromyography for the evaluation of patients with carpal tunnel syndrome. AAEM Quality Assurance Committee, *Muscle Nerve* 16:1392–1414, 1993.

128. O'Brien JP, Mackinnon SE, MacLean AR, et al: A model of chronic nerve compression in the rat, *Ann Plast Surg* 19:430–435, 1987.

129. Driscoll M, Blyum L: The presence of physiological stress shielding in the degenerative cycle of musculoskeletal disorders, *J Bodyw Mov Ther* 15:335–342, 2011.

130. Leem JG, Bove GM: Mid-axonal tumor necrosis factor-alpha induces ectopic activity in a subset of slowly conducting cutaneous and deep afferent neurons, *J Pain* 3:45–49, 2002.

131. Siegel GJ, Albers RW, Brady ST, et al: *Basic neurochemistry: molecular, cellular and medical aspects*, ed 7, Amsterdam, 2006, Elsevier.

132. Ren K, Dubner R: Inflammatory models of pain and hyperalgesia, *ILAR J* 40:111–118, 1999.

133. Dubner R, Ruda MA: Activity-dependent neuronal plasticity following tissue injury and inflammation, *Trends Neurosci* 15:96–103, 1992.

134. Urban MO, Gebhart GF: Central mechanisms in pain, *Med Clin North Am* 83:585–596, 1999.

135. Zimmermann M, Herdegen T: Plasticity of the nervous system at the systematic, cellular and molecular levels: a mechanism of chronic pain and hyperalgesia, *Prog Brain Res* 110:233–259, 1996.

136. Miclescu A, Gordh T: Nitric oxide and pain: 'something old, something new', *Acta Anaesthesiol Scand* 53:1107–1120, 2009.

137. Falk S, Dickenson AH: Pain and nociception: mechanisms of cancer-induced bone pain, *J Clin Oncol* 32:1647–1654, 2014.

138. Basbaum AI, Bautista DM, Scherrer G, et al: Cellular and molecular mechanisms of pain, *Cell* 139:267–284, 2009.

139. Chao T, Pham K, Steward O, et al: Chronic nerve compression injury induces a phenotypic switch of neurons within the dorsal root ganglia, *J Comp Neurol* 506:180–193, 2008.

140. Alfredson H, Ljung BO, Thorsen K, et al: In vivo investigation of ECRB tendons with microdialysis technique—no signs of inflammation but high amounts of glutamate in tennis elbow, *Acta Orthop Scand* 71:475–479, 2000.

141. Alfredson H, Lorentzon R: Chronic tendon pain: no signs of chemical inflammation but high concentrations of the neurotransmitter glutamate. Implications for treatment? *Curr Drug Targets* 3:43–54, 2002.

142. Ljung BO, Forsgren S, Friden J: Sympathetic and sensory innervations are heterogeneously distributed in relation to the blood vessels at the extensor carpi radialis brevis muscle origin of man, *Cells Tissues Organs* 165:45–54, 1999.

143. Zeisig E, Ljung BO, Alfredson H, et al: Immunohistochemical evidence of local production of catecholamines in cells of the muscle origins at the lateral and medial humeral epicondyles: of importance for the development of tennis and golfer's elbow? *Br J Sports Med* 43:269–275, 2009.

144. Freeland AE, Tucci MA, Barbieri RA, et al: Biochemical evaluation of serum and flexor tenosynovium in carpal tunnel syndrome, *Microsurgery* 22:378–385, 2002.

145. Tucci MA, Barbieri RA, Freeland AE: Biochemical and histological analysis of the flexor tenosynovium in patients with carpal tunnel syndrome, *Biomed Sci Instrum* 33:246–251, 1997.

146. Moreno-Torres A, Rosset-Llobet J, Pujol J, et al: Work-related pain in extrinsic finger extensor musculature of instrumentalists is associated with intracellular pH compartmentation during exercise, *PLoS One* 5:e9091, 2010.

147. Carp SJ, Barbe MF, Winter KA, et al: Inflammatory biomarkers increase with severity of upper-extremity overuse disorders, *Clin Sci (London)* 112:305–314, 2007.

148. Kennedy G, Khan F, McLaren M, et al: Endothelial activation and response in patients with hand arm vibration syndrome, *Eur J Clin Invest* 29:577–581, 1999.

149. Lau CS, Bridges AB, Muir A, et al: Further evidence of increased polymorphonuclear cell activity in patients with Raynaud's phenomenon, *Br J Rheumatol* 31:375–380, 1992.

150. Rechardt M, Shiri R, Matikainen S, et al: Soluble IL-1RII and Il-18 are associated with incipient upper extremity soft tissue disorders, *Cytokine* 54:149–153, 2011.

151. Rechardt M, Shiri R, Lindholm H, et al: Associations of metabolic factors and adipokines with pain in incipient upper extremity soft tissue disorders: a cross-sectional study, *BMJ Open* 3:e003036, 2013.

152. Armstrong RB, Warren GL, Warren JA: Mechanisms of exercise-induced muscle fibre injury, *Sports Med* 12:184–207, 1991.

153. Stauber WT: Factors involved in strain-induced injury in skeletal muscles and outcomes of prolonged exposures, *J Electromyogr Kinesiol* 14:61–70, 2004.

154. Willems ME, Stauber WT: Effect of resistance training on muscle fatigue and recovery in intact rats, *Med Sci Sports Exerc* 32:1887–1893, 2000.

155. Fung DT, Wang VM, Andarawis-Puri N, et al: Early response to tendon fatigue damage accumulation in a novel in vivo model, *J Biomech* 43:274–279, 2010.

156. Neviaser A, Andarawis-Puri N, Flatow E: Basic mechanisms of tendon fatigue damage, *J Shoulder Elbow Surg* 21:158–163, 2012.

157. Perry SM, McIlhenny SE, Hoffman MC, et al: Inflammatory and angiogenic mRNA levels are altered in a supraspinatus tendon overuse animal model, *J Shoulder Elbow Surg* 14(Suppl S):79S–83S, 2005.

158. Colopy SA, Benz-Dean J, Barrett JG, et al: Response of the osteocyte syncytium adjacent to and distant from linear microcracks during adaptation to cyclic fatigue loading, *Bone* 35:881–891, 2004.

159. Kummari SR, Davis AJ, Vega LA, et al: Trabecular microfracture precedes cortical shell failure in the rat caudal vertebra under cyclic overloading, *Calcif Tissue Int* 85:127–133, 2009.

160. O'Brien FJ, Brennan O, Kennedy OD, et al: Microcracks in cortical bone: how do they affect bone biology? *Curr Osteoporos Rep* 3:39–45, 2005.

161. Lacourt M, Gao C, Li A, et al: Relationship between cartilage and subchondral bone lesions in repetitive impact trauma-induced equine osteoarthritis, *Osteoarthritis Cartilage* 20:572–583, 2012.

162. Cattano NM, Barbe MF, Massicotte VS, et al: Joint trauma initiates knee osteoarthritis through biochemical and biomechanical processes and interactions, *OA Musculoskelet Med* 1:2–6, 2013.

163. King KB, Opel CF, Rempel DM: Cyclical articular joint loading leads to cartilage thinning and osteopontin production in a novel in vivo rabbit model of repetitive finger flexion, *Osteoarthritis Cartilage* 13:971–978, 2005.

164. Cutlip RG, Geronilla KB, Baker BA, et al: Impact of stretch-shortening cycle rest interval on in vivo muscle performance, *Med Sci Sports Exerc* 37:1345–1355, 2005.

165. Geronilla KB, Miller GR, Mowrey KF, et al: Dynamic force responses of skeletal muscle during stretch-shortening cycles, *Eur J Appl Physiol* 90:144–153, 2003.

166. Cutlip RG, Baker BA, Geronilla KB, et al: Chronic exposure to stretch-shortening contractions results in skeletal muscle adaptation in young rats and maladaptation in old rats, *Appl Physiol Nutr Metab* 31:573–587, 2006.

167. Hsieh YF, Turner CH: Effects of loading frequency on mechanically induced bone formation, *J Bone Mineral Res* 16:918–924, 2001.

168. Mantila Roosa SM, Turner CH, Liu Y: Regulatory mechanisms in bone following mechanical loading, *Gene Regul Syst Biol* 6:43–53, 2012.

169. Robling AG, Burr DB, Turner CH: Skeletal loading in animals, *J Musculoskelet Neuronal Interact* 1:249–262, 2001.

170. Baker BA, Mercer RR, Geronilla KB, et al: Stereological analysis of muscle morphology following exposure to repetitive stretch-shortening cycles in a rat model, *Appl Physiol Nutr Metab* 31:167–179, 2006.

171. Baker BA, Mercer RR, Geronilla KB, et al: Impact of repetition number on muscle performance and histological response, *Med Sci Sports Exerc* 39:1275–1281, 2007.

172. Sjogaard G, Zebis MK, Kiilerich K, et al: Exercise training and work task induced metabolic and stress-related mRNA and protein responses in myalgic muscles, *Biomed Res Int* 2013:984523, 2013.

173. Rubin C, Turner AS, Muller R, et al: Quantity and quality of trabecular bone in the femur are enhanced by a strongly anabolic, noninvasive mechanical intervention, *J Bone Mineral Res* 17:349–357, 2002.

174. Gross TS, Srinivasan S: Building bone mass through exercise: could less be more? *Br J Sports Med* 40:2–3, 2006. discussion 2-3.

175. Srinivasan S, Weimer DA, Agans SC, et al: Low-magnitude mechanical loading becomes osteogenic when rest is inserted between each load cycle, *J Bone Mineral Res* 17:1613–1620, 2002.

176. Bourrin S, Genty C, Palle S, et al: Adverse effects of strenuous exercise: a densitometric and histomorphometric study in the rat, *J Appl Physiol* 76:1999–2005, 1994.

177. Bentley VA, Sample SJ, Livesey MA, et al: Morphologic changes associated with functional adaptation of the navicular bone of horses, *J Anat* 211:662–672, 2007.

178. Danova NA, Colopy SA, Radtke CL, et al: Degradation of bone structural properties by accumulation and coalescence of microcracks, *Bone* 33:197–205, 2003.

179. Raab DM, Smith EL, Crenshaw TD, et al: Bone mechanical properties after exercise training in young and old rats, *J Appl Physiol* 68:130–134, 1990.

180. Umemura Y, Ishiko T, Yamauchi T, et al: Five jumps per day increase bone mass and breaking force in rats, *J Bone Mineral Res* 12:1480–1485, 1997.

181. Nakama LH, King KB, Abrahamsson S, et al: Effect of repetition rate on the formation of microtears in tendon in an in vivo cyclical loading model, *J Orthop Res* 25:1176–1184, 2007.

182. Pierce CW, Tucci MA, Lindley S, et al: Connective tissue growth factor (CTGF) expression in the tenosynovium of patients with carpal tunnel syndrome—biomed 2009, *Biomed Sci Instrum* 45:30–35, 2009.

183. Chikenji T, Gingery A, Zhao C, et al: Transforming growth factor-beta (TGF-beta) expression is increased in the subsynovial connective tissues of patients with idiopathic carpal tunnel syndrome, *J Orthop Res* 32:116–122, 2014.

184. Oh J, Zhao C, Amadio PC, et al: Immunolocalization of collagen types in the subsynovial connective tissue within the carpal tunnel in humans, *J Orthop Res* 23:1226–1231, 2005.

185. Kadi F, Hagg G, Hakansson R, et al: Structural changes in male trapezius muscle with work-related myalgia, *Acta Neuropathol* 95:352–360, 1998.

186. Larsson SE, Bodegard L, Henriksson KG, et al: Chronic trapezius myalgia. Morphology and blood flow studied in 17 patients, *Acta Orthop Scand* 61:394–398, 1990.

187. Gerdle B, Larsson B: Potential muscle biomarkers of chronic myalgia in humans—a systematic review of microdialysis studies. In Khan T, editor: *Biomarker*, InTech, DOI: 10.5772/38822, 2012. Available at http://www.intechopen.com/books/biomarker.

188. Rosendal L, Kristiansen J, Gerdle B, et al: Increased levels of interstitial potassium but normal levels of muscle IL-6 and LDH in patients with trapezius myalgia, *Pain* 119:201–209, 2005.

189. Ghafouri N, Ghafouri B, Larsson B, et al: Palmitoylethanolamide and stearoylethanolamide levels in the interstitium of the trapezius muscle of women with chronic widespread pain and chronic neck-shoulder pain correlate with pain intensity and sensitivity, *Pain* 154:1649–1658, 2013.

190. Carp SJ, Barbe MF, Winter KA, et al: Inflammatory biomarkers increase with severity of upper-extremity overuse disorders, *Clin Sci (Lond)* 112:305–314, 2007.

191. Rechardt M, Shiri R, Matikainen S, et al: Soluble IL-1RII and IL-18 are associated with incipient upper extremity soft tissue disorders, *Cytokine* 54:149–153, 2011.

192. Barbe MF, Barr AE: Inflammation and the pathophysiology of work-related musculoskeletal disorders, *Brain Behav Immun* 20:423–429, 2006.

193. Cohen L, Hallett M: Hand cramps: clinical features and electromyographic patterns in a focal dystonia, *Neurology* 38:1005–1012, 1988.

194. Kyllerman M: Reduced optimality in pre- and perinatal conditions in dyskinetic cerebral palsy—distribution and comparison to controls, *Neuropediatrics* 14:29–36, 1983.

195. Kyllerman M, Bager B, Bensch J, et al: Dyskinetic cerebral palsy. I. Clinical categories, associated neurological abnormalities and incidences, *Acta Paediatrica Scand* 71:543–550, 1982.

196. Sanger TD: Hypertonia in children: how and when to treat, *Curr Treat Options Neurol* 7:427–439, 2005.

197. Stojanovic M, Cvetkovic D, Kostic VS: A genetic study of idiopathic focal dystonias, *J Neurol* 242:508–511, 1995.

198. Lin PT, Hallett M: The pathophysiology of focal hand dystonia, *J Hand Ther* 22:109–113, 2009. quiz 114.

199. Park KN, Kwon OY, Ha SM, et al: Comparison of electromyographic activity and range of neck motion in violin students with and without neck pain during playing, *Med Probl Perform Art* 27:188–192, 2012.

200. Ackermann B, Driscoll T, Kenny DT: Musculoskeletal pain and injury in professional orchestral musicians in Australia, *Med Probl Perform Art* 27:181–187, 2012.

201. Mehrparvar AH, Mostaghaci M, Gerami RF: Musculoskeletal disorders among Iranian instrumentalists, *Med Probl Perform Art* 27:193–196, 2012.

202. Altenmuller E, Jabusch HC: Focal hand dystonia in musicians: phenomenology, etiology, and psychological trigger factors, *J Hand Ther* 22:144–154, 2009. quiz 155.

203. Nutt JG, Muenter MD, Melton LJ, et al: Epidemiology of dystonia in Rochester, Minnesota, *Adv Neurol* 50:361–365, 1988.

204. Nakashima K, Kusumi M, Inoue Y, et al: Prevalence of focal dystonias in the western area of Tottori Prefecture in Japan, *Mov Disord* 10:440–443, 1995.

205. Steeves TD, Day L, Dykeman J, et al: The prevalence of primary dystonia: a systematic review and meta-analysis, *Mov Disord* 27:1789–1796, 2012.

206. Defazio G, Jankovic J, Giel JL, et al: Descriptive epidemiology of cervical dystonia, *Tremor Other Hyperkinet Mov* 3:2013.

207. Hallett M: Neurophysiology of dystonia: the role of inhibition, *Neurobiol Dis* 42:177–184, 2011.

208. Gasser T, Bove CM, Ozelius LJ, et al: Haplotype analysis at the DYT1 locus in Ashkenazi Jewish patients with occupational hand dystonia, *Mov Disord* 11:163–166, 1996.

209. Illarioshkin SN, Markova ED, Slominsky PA, et al: The GTP cyclohydrolase I gene in Russian families with dopa-responsive dystonia, *Arch Neurol* 55:789–792, 1998.

210. Leube B, Rudnicki D, Ratzlaff T, et al: Idiopathic torsion dystonia: assignment of a gene to chromosome 18p in a German family with adult onset, autosomal dominant inheritance and purely focal distribution, *Hum Mol Genet* 5:1673–1677, 1996.

211. Ozelius L, Hewett JW, Page CE, et al: The early onset of torsion dystonia gene (DYT1) encodes an ATD binding protein nature, *MGenetics* 40:40–48, 1997.

212. Weise D, Schramm A, Beck M, et al: Loss of topographic specificity of LTD-like plasticity is a trait marker in focal dystonia, *Neurobiol Dis* 42:171–176, 2011.

213. Lohmann K, Schmidt A, Schillert A, et al: Genome-wide association study in musician's dystonia: a risk variant at the arylsulfatase G locus? *Mov Disord* 29:921–927, 2014.

214. Fry HJ: Overuse syndrome in musicians—100 years ago. An historical review, *Med J Aust* 145(11-12):620–625, 1986.

215. Salmon PS, Shook CP, Lombart KG, et al: Performance impairments, injuries, and stress tardiness in a sample of keyboard and other instrumentalists, *Med Probl Perform Art* 10:140–146, 1995.

216. Wilson FR, Wagner C, Homberg V: Biomechanical abnormalities in musicians with occupational cramp/focal dystonia, *J Hand Ther* 6:298–307, 1993.

217. Leijnse JN: Anatomical factors predisposing to focal dystonia in the musician's hand—principles, theoretical examples, clinical significance, *J Biomech* 30:659–669, 1997.

218. Hermsdorfer J, Marquardt C, Schneider AS, et al: Significance of finger forces and kinematics during handwriting in writer's cramp, *Hum Mov Sci* 30:807–817, 2011.

219. Schneider AS, Furholzer W, Marquardt C, et al: Task specific grip force control in writer's cramp, *Clin Neurophysiol* 125:786–797, 2014.

220. Charness ME: The relationsip between peripheral nerve injury and focal dystonia in musicians, *Am Acad Neurol* 162:21–27, 1993.

221. Charness ME, Ross MH, Shefner JM: Ulnar neuropathy and dystonic flexion of the fourth and fifth digits: clinical correlation in musicians, *Muscle Nerve* 19:431–437, 1996.

222. Jancovic J: Can peripheral trauma induce dystonia and other movement disorders? Yes!, *Mov Disord* 16:7–11, 2001.

223. Weiner W: Can peripheral trauma induce dystonia? No!, *Mov Disord* 16:13–22, 2001.

224. Neychev VK, Gross RE, Lehericy S, et al: The functional neuroanatomy of dystonia, *Neurobiol Dis* 42:185–201, 2011.

225. Black KJ, Ongur D, Perlmutter JS: Putamen volume in idiopathic focal dystonia, *Neurology* 51:819–824, 1998.

226. DeLong M, Crutcher MD, Georgopoulis AP: Primate globus pallidus and subthalamic nucleus: functional organization, *J Neurophysiol* 53:530–543, 1985.

227. DeLong M: Primate models of movement disorders of basal ganglia origin, *Trends Neurosci* 13:281–285, 1990.

228. Perlmutter JS, Stambuk MK, Markham J, et al: Decreased [18F]spiperone binding in putamen in idiopathic focal dystonia, *J Neurosci* 17:843–850, 1997.

229. Chen RS, Tsai CH, Lu CS: Reciprocal inhibition in writer's cramp, *Mov Disord* 10:556–561, 1995.

230. Chase T, Tamminga C, Burrows H: Positron emission tomography studies of regional cerebral glucose metabolism in idiopathic dystonia, *Adv Neurol* 50:237–241, 1988.

231. Deuschl G, Goddemeier C: Spontaneous and reflex activity of facial muscles in dystonia, Parkinson's disease, and in normal subjects, *J Neurol Neurosurg Psychiatry* 64:320–324, 1998.

232. Toro C, Deuschl G, Hallett M: Movement-related electroencephalographic desynchronization in patients with hand cramps: evidence for motor cortical involvement in focal dystonia, *Ann Neurol* 47:456–461, 2000.

233. Rutledge JN, Hilal SK, Silver AJ, et al: Magnetic resonance imaging of dystonic states, *Adv Neurol* 50:265–275, 1988.

234. Gilman S, Junck L, Young A: Cerebral metabolic activity in diopathic dystonia studies with positron emission tomography, *Adv Neurol* 50:231–236, 1988.

235. Tempel LW, Perlmutter JS: Abnormal cortical responses in patients with writer's cramp, *Neurology* 43:2252–2257, 1993.

236. Lenz FA, Byl NN: Reorganization in the cutaneous core of the human thalamic principal somatic sensory nucleus (ventral caudal) in patients with dystonia, *J Neurophysiol* 82:3204–3212, 1999.

237. Zirh TA, Reich SG, Perry V, et al: Thalamic single neuron and electromyographic activities in patients with dystonia, *Adv Neurol* 78:27–32, 1998.

238. Tinazzi M, Frasson E, Bertolasi L, et al: Temporal discrimination of somesthetic stimuli is impaired in dystonic patients, *Neuroreport* 10:1547–1550, 1999.

239. Tinazzi M, Rosso T, Fiaschi A: Role of the somatosensory system in primary dystonia, *Mov Disord* 18:605–622, 2003.

240. Murase N, Kaji R, Shimazu H, et al: Abnormal premovement gating of somatosensory input in writer's cramp, *Brain* 123:1813–1829, 2000.

241. Grunewald RA, Yoneda Y, Shipman JM, et al: Idiopathic focal dystonia: a disorder of muscle spindle afferent processing? *Brain* 120(Pt 12):2179–2185, 1997.

242. Kaji R, Rothwell JC, Katayama M, et al: Tonic vibration reflex and muscle afferent block in writer's cramp, *Ann Neurol* 38:155–162, 1995.

243. Lourenco G, Meunier S, Vidailhet M, et al: Impaired modulation of motor cortex excitability by homonymous and heteronymous muscle afferents in focal hand dystonia, *Mov Disord* 22:523–527, 2007.

244. Naumann M, Reiners K: Long-latency reflexes of hand muscles in idiopathic focal dystonia and their modification by botulinum toxin, *Brain* 120(Pt 3):409–416, 1997.

245. Melgari JM, Zappasodi F, Porcaro C, et al: Movement-induced uncoupling of primary sensory and motor areas in focal task-specific hand dystonia, *Neuroscience* 250:434–445, 2013.

246. Zheng Z, Pan P, Wang W, et al: Neural network of primary focal dystonia by an anatomic likelihood estimation meta-analysis of gray matter abnormalities, *J Neurol Sci* 316:51–55, 2012.

247. Bertolasi L, Romito S, Tinazzi M, et al: Impaired heteronymous somatosensory motor cortical inhibition in dystonia, *Mov Disord* 18:1367–1373, 2003.

248. Nowak DA, Rosenkranz K, Topka H, et al: Disturbances of grip force behaviour in focal hand dystonia: evidence for a generalised impairment of sensory-motor integration? *J Neurol Neurosurg Psychiatry* 76:953–959, 2005.

249. Peller M, Zeuner KE, Munchau A, et al: The basal ganglia are hyperactive during the discrimination of tactile stimuli in writer's cramp, *Brain* 129(Pt 10):2697–2708, 2006.

250. Rosenkranz K, Seibel J, Kacar A, et al: Sensorimotor deprivation induces interdependent changes in excitability and plasticity of the human hand motor cortex, *J Neurosc* 34:7375–7382, 2014.

251. Byl N, Wilson F, Merzenich M, et al: Sensory dysfunction associated with repetitive strain injuries of tendinitis and focal hand dystonia: a comparative study, *J Orthop Sports Phys Ther* 23:234–244, 1996.

252. Byl N, Hamati D, Melnick M, et al: The sensory consequences of repetitive strain injury in musicians: focal dystonia of the hand, *J Back Musculoskelet Rehabil* 7:27–39, 1996.

253. Bara-Jimenez W, Shelton P, Sanger TD, et al: Sensory discrimination capabilities in patients with focal hand dystonia, *Ann Neurol* 47:377–380, 2000.

254. Byl NN, McKenzie A, Nagarajan SS: Differences in somatosensory hand organization in a healthy flutist and a flutist with focal hand dystonia: a case report, *J Hand Ther* 13:302–309, 2000.

255. Butterworth S, Francis S, Kelly E, et al: Abnormal cortical sensory activation in dystonia: an fMRI study, *Mov Disord* 18:673–682, 2003.

256. Siebner HR, Filipovic SR, Rowe JB, et al: Patients with focal arm dystonia have increased sensitivity to slow-frequency repetitive TMS of the dorsal premotor cortex, *Brain* 126(Pt 12):2710–2725, 2003.

257. Quartarone A, Bagnato S, Rizzo V, et al: Abnormal associative plasticity of the human motor cortex in writer's cramp, *Brain* 126(Pt 12):2586–2596, 2003.

258. Gerloff C, Corwell B, Chen R, et al: The role of the human motor cortex in the control of complex and simple finger movement sequences, *Brain* 121(Pt 9):1695–1709, 1998.

259. Johanson RS: Sensory control of dexterous manipulation in humans. In Wing AM, Haggard P, Flanagan JR, editors: *Hand and brain: the neurophysiology and psychology of hand movements*, San Diego, 1996, Academic Press.

260. Sherrington CS: *The integrative action of the nervous system*, New York, 1906, C. Scribner's sons.

261. Iwamura Y, Tanaka M, Sakamoto M, et al: Functional subdivisions representing different finger regions in area 3 of the first somatosensory cortex of the conscious monkey, *Exp Brain Res* 51:315–326, 1983.

262. Kaas JH: Plasticity of sensory and motor maps in adult mammals, *Annu Rev Neurosci* 14:137–167, 1991.

263. Penfield W, Rasmussen T: *The cerebral cortex of man: a clinical study of localization of function*, New York, 1950, Macmillan.

264. Wang X, Merzenich MM, Sameshima K, et al: Remodelling of hand representation in adult cortex determined by timing of tactile stimulation, *Nature* 378:71–75, 1995.

265. Altenmuller E: Focal dystonia: advances in brain imaging and understanding of fine motor control in musicians, *Hand Clin* 19:523–538, 2003. xi.

266. Jenkins WM, Merzenich MM, Ochs MT, et al: Functional reorganization of primary somatosensory cortex in adult owl monkeys after behaviorally controlled tactile stimulation, *J Neurophysiol* 63:82–104, 1990.

267. Elbert T, Sterr A, Flor H, et al: Input-increase and input-decrease types of cortical reorganization after upper extremity amputation in humans, *Exp Brain Res* 117:161–164, 1997.

268. Jenkins WM, Merzenich MM: Reorganization of neocortical representations after brain injury: a neurophysiological model of the bases of recovery from stroke, *Prog Brain Res* 71:249–266, 1987.

269. Recanzone GH, Jenkins WM, Hradek GT, et al: Progressive improvement in discriminative abilities in adult owl monkeys performing a tactile frequency discrimination task, *J Neurophysiol* 67:1015–1030, 1992.

270. Recanzone GH, Merzenich MM, Dinse HR: Expansion of the cortical representation of a specific skin field in primary somatosensory cortex by intracortical microstimulation, *Cereb Cortex* 2:181–196, 1992.

271. Recanzone GH, Merzenich MM, Jenkins WM: Frequency discrimination training engaging a restricted skin surface results in an emergence of a cutaneous response zone in cortical area 3a, *J Neurophysiol* 67:1057–1070, 1992.

272. Recanzone GH, Merzenich MM, Jenkins WM, et al: Topographic reorganization of the hand representation in cortical area 3b owl monkeys trained in a frequency-discrimination task, *J Neurophysiol* 67:1031–1056, 1992.

273. Recanzone GH, Merzenich MM, Schreiner CE: Changes in the distributed temporal response properties of SI cortical neurons reflect improvements in performance on a temporally based tactile discrimination task, *J Neurophysiol* 67:1071–1091, 1992.

274. Gil Z, Connors BW, Amitai Y: Differential regulation of neocortical synapses by neuromodulators and activity, *Neuron* 19:679–686, 1997.

275. Allard T, Clark SA, Jenkins WM, et al: Reorganization of somatosensory area 3b representations in adult owl monkeys after digital syndactyly, *J Neurophysiol* 66:1048–1058, 1991.

276. Hebb DO: *The organization of behavior: a neuropsychological theory*, New York, 1949, Wiley.

277. Kaas JH, Nelson RJ, Sur M, et al: Multiple representations of the body within the primary somatosensory cortex of primates, *Science* 204:521–523, 1979.

278. Merzenich MM, Kaas JH, Wall J, et al: Topographic reorganization of somatosensory cortical areas 3b and 1 in adult monkeys following restricted deafferentation, *Neuroscience* 8:33–55, 1983.

279. Merzenich MM, Nelson RJ, Stryker MP, et al: Somatosensory cortical map changes following digit amputation in adult monkeys, *J Comp Neurol* 224:591–605, 1984.

280. Nudo RJ: Adaptive plasticity in motor cortex: implications for rehabilitation after brain injury, *J Rehabil Med* (Suppl 41):7–10, 2003.

281. Hebb DO: *The organization of behavior: a neuropsychological theory*, Mahwah, NJ, 2002, L. Erlbaum Associates.

282. Xerri C, Coq JO, Merzenich MM, et al: Experience-induced plasticity of cutaneous maps in the primary somatosensory cortex of adult monkeys and rats, *J Physiol Paris* 90:277–287, 1996.

283. Xerri C, Merzenich MM, Jenkins W, et al: Representational plasticity in cortical area 3b paralleling tactual-motor skill acquisition in adult monkeys, *Cereb Cortex* 9:264–276, 1999.

284. Wilson F, Wagner C, Homberg V, et al: Interaction of biomechanical and training factors in musicians with occupational cramp/focal dystonia, *Neurology* 4(Suppl 1):292–296, 1991.

285. Wilson FR, Omeltschenko L, Yager GG: Coping with test stress: microcomputer software for treatment of test anxiety, *J Behav Ther Exp Psychiatry* 22:131–139, 1991.

286. Elbert T, Pantev C, Wienbruch C, et al: Increased cortical representation of the fingers of the left hand in string players, *Science* 270:305–307, 1995.

287. Rijntjes M, Dettmers C, Buchel C, et al: A blueprint for movement: functional and anatomical representations in the human motor system, *J Neurosci* 19:8043–8048, 1999.

288. Hochberg FH, Harris SU, Blattert TR: Occupational hand cramps: professional disorders of motor control, *Hand Clin* 6:417–428, 1990.

289. Newmark J, Hochberg FH: Isolated painless manual incoordination in 57 musicians, *J Neurol Neurosurg Psychiatry* 50:291–295, 1987.

290. Jankovic J, Shale H: Dystonia in musicians, *Sem Neurol* 9:131–135, 1989.

291. Rothwell JC, Obeso JA, Day BL, et al: Pathophysiology of dystonias, *Adv Neurol* 39:851–863, 1983.

292. Altenmuller E: Causes and cures of focal limb-dystonia in musicians, *Intl Soc Tension Performance* 9:13–17, 1998.

293. Hinkley LB, Webster RL, Byl NN, et al: Neuroimaging characteristics of patients with focal hand dystonia, *J Hand Ther* 22:125–134, 2009. quiz 135.

294. Elbert T, Candia V, Altenmuller E, et al: Alteration of digital representations in somatosensory cortex in focal hand dystonia, *Neuroreport* 9:3571–3575, 1998.

295. Chen R, Hallett M: Focal dystonia and repetitive motion disorders, *Clin Orthop* 351:102–106, 1998.

296. Blake DT, Byl NN, Cheung S, et al: Sensory representation abnormalities that parallel focal hand dystonia in a primate model, *Somatosens Mot Res* 19:347–357, 2002.

297. Pascual-Leone A, Dang N, Cohen LG, et al: Modulation of muscle responses evoked by transcranial magnetic stimulation during the acquisition of new fine motor skills, *J Neurophysiol* 74:1037–1045, 1995.

298. Gelkopf M, Kreitler S, Sigal M: Laughter in a psychiatric ward. Somatic, emotional, social, and clinical influences on schizophrenic patients, *J Nerv Ment Dis* 181:283–289, 1993.

299. Byl NN, Melnick M: The neural consequences of repetition: clinical implications of a learning hypothesis, *J Hand Ther* 10:160–174, 1997.

300. McKenzie AL, Nagarajan SS, Roberts TP, et al: Somatosensory representation of the digits and clinical performance in patients with focal hand dystonia, *Am J Phys Med Rehabil* 82:737–749, 2003.

301. Sanger TD, Merzenich MM: Computational model of the role of sensory disorganization in focal task-specific dystonia, *J Neurophysiol* 84:2458–2464, 2000.

302. Quartarone A, Classen J, Morgante F, et al: Consensus paper: use of transcranial magnetic stimulation to probe motor cortex plasticity in dystonia and levodopa-induced dyskinesia, *Brain Stimul* 2:108–117, 2009.

303. Quartarone A, Girlanda P, Risitano G, et al: Focal hand dystonia in a patient with thoracic outlet syndrome, *J Neurol Neurosurg Psychiatry* 65:272–274, 1998.

304. Quartarone A, Hallett M: Emerging concepts in the physiological basis of dystonia, *Mov Disord* 28:958–967, 2013.

305. Quartarone A, Rizzo V, Bagnato S, et al: Homeostatic-like plasticity of the primary motor hand area is impaired in focal hand dystonia, *Brain* 128(Pt 8):1943–1950, 2005.

306. Quartarone A, Rizzo V, Terranova C, et al: Abnormal sensorimotor plasticity in organic but not in psychogenic dystonia, *Brain* 132(Pt 10):2871–2877, 2009.

307. Quartarone A, Siebner HR, Rothwell JC: Task-specific hand dystonia: can too much plasticity be bad for you? *Trends Neurosci* 29:192–199, 2006.

308. Peterson DA, Sejnowski TJ, Poizner H: Convergent evidence for abnormal striatal synaptic plasticity in dystonia, *Neurobiol Dis* 37:558–573, 2010.

309. Hubsch C, Roze E, Popa T, et al: Defective cerebellar control of cortical plasticity in writer's cramp, *Brain* 136(Pt 7):2050–2062, 2013.

310. Altenmuller E, Ioannou CI, Raab M, et al: Apollo's Curse: causes and cures of motor failures in musicians: a proposal for a new classification, *Adv Exp Med Biol* 826:161–178, 2014.

311. Karp BI, Cole RA, Cohen LG, et al: Long-term botulinum toxin treatment of focal hand dystonia, *Neurology* 44:70–76, 1994.

312. Fahn S, Marsden CD: *The treatment of dystonia*, London, 1987, Butterworths.

313. Dommerholt J: Performing arts medicine in instrumental musicians, Part I—general considerations, *J Bodyw Mov Ther* 13:311–319, 2009.

314. Dommerholt J: Performing arts medicine—instrumentalist musicians, Part II—examination, *J Bodyw Mov Ther* 14:65–72, 2010.

315. Dommerholt J: Performing arts medicine—instrumentalist musicians, Part III—case histories, *J Bodyw Mov Ther* 14:127–138, 2010.

316. Rosenkranz K, Williamon A, Butler K, et al: Pathophysiological differences between musician's dystonia and writer's cramp, *Brain* 128(Pt 4):918–931, 2005.

317. McKenzie AL, Goldman S, Barrango C, et al: Differences in physical characteristics and response to rehabilitation for patients with hand dystonia: musicians' cramp compared to writers' cramp, *J Hand Ther* 22:172–181, 2009. quiz 182.

318. Zeuner KE, Volkmann J: How task specific is task specific dystonia? *Clin Neurophysiol* 125:655–656, 2014.

319. Tubiana R: Musician's focal dystonia, *Hand Clin* 19:303–308, 2003. vii.

320. Altenmuller E, Schurmann K, Lim VK, et al: Hits to the left, flops to the right: different emotions during listening to music are reflected in cortical lateralisation patterns, *Neuropsychologia* 40:2242–2256, 2002.

321. Jabusch HC, Mueller SV, Altenmueller E: *High levels of perfectionism and anxiety in musicians with focal dystonia*. In Paper presented at the International Dystonia Meeting, Atlanta, 2001.

322. Fahn S, Hallett M, DeLong MR: *Rating scales for dystonia: assessment of reliability of three scales*, Philadelphia, 2004, Lippincott Williams & Wilkin.

323. Tubiana R: Focal dystonia. Incidence: classification of severity and results of therapy. In Winspur I, Wynn Parry CB, editors: *The musician's hand: a clinical guide*, London, UK,, 1998, Martin Dunitz.

324. Jabusch HC, Vauth H, Altenmuller E: Quantification of focal dystonia in pianists using scale analysis, *Mov Disord* 19:171–180, 2004.

325. Sanger TD: Toward a definition of childhood dystonia, *Curr Opin Pediatr* 16:623–627, 2004.

326. Lundeberg T, Lund I, Dahlin L, et al: Reliability and responsiveness of three different pain assessments, *J Rehabil Med* 33:279–283, 2001.

327. Zeuner KE, Peller M, Knutzen A, et al: How to assess motor impairment in writer's cramp, *Mov Disord* 22:1102–1109, 2007.

328. Comella CL, Leurgans S, Wuu J, et al: Rating scales for dystonia: a multicenter assessment, *Mov Disord* 18:303–312, 2003.

329. Albanese A, Sorbo FD, Comella C, et al: Dystonia rating scales: critique and recommendations, *Mov Disord* 28:874–883, 2013.

330. Fung S, Byl N, Melnick M, et al: Functional outcomes: the development of a new instrument to monitor the effectiveness of physical therapy, *Eur J Phys Med Rehabil* 7:31–41, 1997.

331. Ayres A: *Sensory integration and praxis tests: SIPT manual*, Los Angeles, CA, 1989, Psychological Services.

332. Byl N, Leano J, Cheney LK: The Byl-Cheney-Boczai Sensory Discriminator: reliability, validity, and responsiveness for testing stereognosis, *J Hand Ther* 15:315–330, 2002.

333. Bohannon RW: Stopwatch for measuring thumb-movement time, *Percept Mot Skills* 81:211–216, 1995.

334. Kendall FP, McCreary EK: *Muscles, testing and function*, ed 3, Baltimore, 1983, Williams & Wilkins.

335. Norkin C, White J: *Measurement of joint motion: a guide to coniometry*, ed 3, Philadelphia, 2003, FA Davis.

336. Byl NN, Nagarajan SS, Merzenich MM, et al: Correlation of clinical neuromusculoskeletal and central somatosensory performance: variability in controls and patients with severe and mild focal hand dystonia, *Neural Plast* 9:177–203, 2002.

337. Institute for Work and Health: *The DASH outcome measure:disabilities of the arm, shoulder and hand*. Available at http://dash.iwh.on.ca/. Accessed November 24 2014.

338. Sackett D, Straus S, Richardson W, et al: *Evidence-based medicine: how to practice and teach EBM*, ed 2, Philadelphia, 2000, Elsevier Churchill Livingstone.

339. United States Department of Labor, Occupational Safety and Health Administration (OSHA): *Back to safety and health topics page*. Available at https://www.osha.gov/SLTC/. Accessed November 24, 2014.

340. United States Department of Labor: Occupational Safety and Health Administration (OSHA), *Guidelines for foundries: solutions for the prevention of musculoskeletal injuries in foundries*, Washington, DC, 2012, OSHA Publication 3465-08, Occupational Safety & Health Administration, United States Department of Labor.

341. United States Department of Labor: Occupational Safety and Health Administration (OSHA), *Guidelines for nursing homes: ergonomics for the prevention of musculoskeletal disorders*, Washington, DC, 2009, OSHA Publication 3182, Occupational Safety and Health Administration, United States Department of Labor.

342. United States Department of Labor: Occupational Safety and Health Administration (OSHA), *Guidelines for Shipyards: ergonomics for the prevention of musculoskeletal disorders*, Washington, DC, 2008, Occupational Safety and Health Administration, United States Department of Labor.

343. United States Department of Labor: Occupational Safety and Health Administration (OSHA), *Ergonomic guidelines for manual material handling*, Cincinnati, OH, 2007, National Institute for Occupational Safety and Health (NIOSH). Available at http://www.cdc.gov/niosh/docs/2007-131/.

344. United States Department of Labor: Occupational Safety and Health Administration (OSHA), *Updated guidelines: prevention of musculoskeletal injuries in poultry processing*, Washington, DC, 2013, OSHA Publication 3213, Occupational Safety and Health Administration, United States Department of Labor.

345. United States Department of Labor: Occupational Safety and Health Administration (OSHA), *Guidelines for retail grocery stores: ergonomics for the prevention of musculoskeletal disorders*, Washington, DC, 2004, OSHA Publication 3192, Occupational Safety and Health Administration, United States Department of Labor.

346. United States Department of Labor, Occupational Safety and Health Administration (OSHA): *American Apparel and Footwear Association (AAFA)—OSHA alliance guidelines. Volume I: An introductory manual for the apparel and footwear industries*. Available at https://http://www.wewear.org/assets/1/7/ErgoManualVol1.pdf.

347. American Furniture Manufacturers Association: *Voluntary ergonomics guideline for the furniture manufacturing industry*. Available at http://digital.nc-dcr.gov/cdm/singleitem/collection/p249901coll22/id/4778/rec/6. Accessed November 24, 2014.

348. National Telecommunications Safety Panel: *Ergonomic guidelines for common job functions within the telecommunications industry*. Available at 2007. http://www.ehscp.org/Documents/Final Version 11-06-07.pdf. Accessed November 24, 2014.

349. United States Department of Health and Human Services (DHHS), National Institute for Occupational Safety and Health (NIOSH): *Simple solutions: ergonomics for farm workers*, Cincinnati, OH, 2004, United States Department of Health and Human Services (DHHS), National Institute for Occupational Safety and Health (NIOSH). Publication No. 2001-111.

350. United States Department of Labor, Occupational Safety and Health Administration (OSHA): *Baggage handling (airline industry) eTool*. Available at https://www.osha.gov/SLTC/etools/baggagehandling/index.html. Accessed November 24, 2014.

351. United States Department of Labor, Occupational Safety and Health Administration (OSHA): *Simple solutions: ergonomics for construction workers*, Cincinnato, OH, Publication No. 2007-122, United States Department of Health and Human Services (DHHS), National Institute for Occupational Safety and Health (NIOSH).

352. Gatchel RJ: Musculoskeletal disorders: primary and secondary interventions, *J Electromyogr Kinesiol* 14:161–170, 2004.

353. Fimland MS, Vasseljen O, Gismervik S, et al: Occupational rehabilitation programs for musculoskeletal pain and common mental health disorders: study protocol of a randomized controlled trial, *BMC Public Health* 14:368, 2014.

354. Esmaeilzadeh S, Ozcan E, Capan N: Effects of ergonomic intervention on work-related upper extremity musculoskeletal disorders among computer workers: a randomized controlled trial, *Int Arch Occup Environ Health* 87:73–83, 2014.

355. Matthias MS, Miech EJ, Myers LJ, et al: An expanded view of self-management: patients' perceptions of education and support in an intervention for chronic musculoskeletal pain, *Pain Med* 13:1018–1028, 2012.

356. Ahlskog JE, Geda YE, Graff-Radford NR, et al: Physical exercise as a preventive or disease-modifying treatment of dementia and brain aging, *Mayo Clin Proc* 86:876–884, 2011.

357. World Health Organization: *Physical inactivity: a global public health problem*. Available at http://www.who.int/dietphysicalactivity/factsheet_inactivity/en/. Accessed October 8, 2014, 2014.

358. Centers for Disease Control and Prevention (CDC): *Health objectives for the nation healthy people 2000: National health promotion and disease prevention objectives for the year 2000*. http://www.cdc.gov/mmwr/preview/mmwrhtml/00001788.htm. Accessed November 24, 2014.

359. Ahlskog JE: Does vigorous exercise have a neuroprotective effect in Parkinson disease? *Neurology* 77:288–294, 2011.

360. McArdle WD, Katch FI, Katch VI: *Exercise physiology: nutrition, energy, and human performance*, Philadelphia, 2014, Lippincott Williams & Wilkins.

361. Ornish D, Lin J, Chan JM, et al: Effect of comprehensive lifestyle changes on telomerase activity and telomere length in men with biopsy-proven low-risk prostate cancer: 5-year follow-up of a descriptive pilot study, *Lancet Oncol* 14:1112–1120, 2013.

362. Needham BL, Mezuk B, Bareis N, et al: Depression, anxiety and telomere length in young adults: evidence from the National Health and Nutrition Examination Survey, *Mol Psychiatry* 20:520–528, 2015.

363. Merzenich M: *Soft-wired: how the new science of brain plasticity can change your life*, San Francisco, 2013, Parnassus Publishing LLC..

364. Green CS, Bavelier D: Exercising your brain: a review of human brain plasticity and training-induced learning, *Psychol Aging* 23:692–701, 2008.

365. Hasselmo ME: Neuromodulation and cortical function: modeling the physiological basis of behavior, *Behav Brain Res* 67:1–27, 1995.

366. Merzenich M, Wright B, Jenkins W, et al: Cortical plasticity underlying perceptual, motor, and cognitive skill development: implications for neurorehabilitation, *Cold Spring Harb Symp Quant Biol* 61:1–8, 1996.

367. Nagarajan SS, Blake DT, Wright BA, et al: Practice-related improvements in somatosensory interval discrimination are temporally specific but generalize across skin location, hemisphere, and modality, *J Neurosci* 18:1559–1570, 1998.

368. Spengler F, Roberts TP, Poeppel D, et al: Learning transfer and neuronal plasticity in humans trained in tactile discrimination, *Neurosci Lett* 232:151–154, 1997.

369. Sterr A, Muller MM, Elbert T, et al: Changed perceptions in Braille readers, *Nature* 391:134–135, 1998.

370. Hikosaka O, Tanaka M, Sakamoto M, et al: Deficits in manipulative behaviors induced by local injections of muscimol in the first somatosensory cortex of the conscious monkey, *Brain Res* 325:375–380, 1985.

371. Merzenich MM, Recanzone GH, Jenkins WM, et al: Adaptive mechanisms in cortical networks underlying cortical contributions to learning and nondeclarative memory, *Cold Spring Harb Symp Quant Biol* 55:873–887, 1990.

372. Nudo RJ, Milliken GW, Jenkins WM, et al: Use-dependent alterations of movement representations in primary motor cortex of adult squirrel monkeys, *J Neurosci* 16:785–807, 1996.

373. Merzenich MM, Tallal P, Peterson B, et al: *Some neurological principles relevant to the origins of—and the cortical plasticity-based remediation of—developmental language impairments*, Berlin, 1999, Springer Verlag.

374. Kleim JA, Jones TA: Principles of experience-dependent neural plasticity: implications for rehabilitation after brain damage, *J Speech Lang Hear Res* 51:S225–S239, 2008.

375. Stryker M, Jenkins WM, Merzenich MM: Anesthetic state does not affect the map of the hand representation within are 3b somatosensory cortex in owl monkeys, *J Comp Neurol* 258:297–303, 1987.

376. Colcombe SJ, Erickson KI, Scalf PE, et al: Aerobic exercise training increases brain volume in aging humans, *J Gerontol A Biol Sci Med Sci* 61:1166–1170, 2006.

377. Gregory MD, Agam Y, Selvadurai C, et al: Resting state connectivity immediately following learning correlates with subsequent sleep-dependent enhancement of motor task performance, *Neuroimage* 102(Pt 2):666–673, 2014.

378. Lin CC, Yang CM: Evidence of sleep-facilitating effect on formation of novel semantic associations: an event-related potential (ERP) study, *Neurobiol Learn Mem* 116:69–78, 2014.

379. Verweij IM, Romeijn N, Smit DJ, et al: Sleep deprivation leads to a loss of functional connectivity in frontal brain regions, *BMC Neurosci* 15:88, 2014.

380. Devore EE, Grodstein F, Duffy JF, et al: Sleep duration in midlife and later life in relation to cognition, *J Am Geriatr Soc* 62:1073–1081, 2014.

381. Acosta-peña E, Camacho-Abrego I, Melgarejo-Gutierrez M, et al: Sleep deprivation induces differential morphological changes in the hippocampus and prefrontal cortex in young and old rats, *Synapse* 69:15–25, 2015.

382. Yaffe K, Falvey CM, Hoang T: Connections between sleep and cognition in older adults, *Lancet Neurol* 13:1017–1028, 2014.

383. Park YE, Kim BH, Lee SG, et al: Vitamin D status of patients with earlinflammatory arthritis, *Clin Rheumatol*, Apr 10 2014.

384. Kim RJ, Hah YS, Sung CM, et al: Do antioxidants inhibit oxidative-stress-induced autophagy of tenofibroblasts? *J Orthop Res* 32:937–943, 2014.

385. Gordon BS, Delgado-Diaz DC, Carson J, et al: Resveratrol improves muscle function but not oxidative capacity in young mdx mice, *Can J Physiol Pharmacol* 92:243–251, 2014.

386. Bell PG, Walshe IH, Davison GW, et al: Montmorency cherries reduce the oxidative stress and inflammatory responses to repeated days high-intensity stochastic cycling, *Nutrients* 6:829–843, 2014.

387. Farup J, Rahbek SK, Vendelbo MH, et al: Whey protein hydrolysate augments tendon and muscle hypertrophy independent of resistance exercise contraction mode, *Scand J Med Sci Sports* 24:788–798, 2014.

388. Kim J, Jeong IH, Kim CS, et al: Chlorogenic acid inhibits the formation of advanced glycation end products and associated protein cross-linking, *Arch Pharmacal Res* 34:495–500, 2011.

389. Hung LK, Fu SC, Lee YW, et al: Local vitamin-C injection reduced tendon adhesion in a chicken model of flexor digitorum profundus tendon injury, *J Bone Joint Surg Am* 95:e41, 2013.

390. Aro AA, Nishan U, Perez MO, et al: Structural and biochemical alterations during the healing process of tendons treated with Aloe vera, *Life Sci* 91(17-18):885–893, 2012.

391. Felice JI, Gangoiti MV, Molinuevo MS, et al: Effects of a metabolic syndrome induced by a fructose-rich diet on bone metabolism in rats, *Metabolism* 63:296–305, 2014.

392. Chechik O, Dolkart O, Mozes G, et al: Timing matters: NSAIDs interfere with the late proliferation stage of a repaired rotator cuff tendon healing in rats, *Arch Orthop Trauma Surg* 134:515–520, 2014.

393. de Oliveira LP, Vieira CP, Da Re Guerra F, et al: Statins induce biochemical changes in the Achilles tendon after chronic treatment, *Toxicology* 311:162–168, 2013.

394. Tucsek Z, Toth P, Sosnowska D, et al: Obesity in aging exacerbates blood-brain barrier disruption, neuroinflammation, and oxidative stress in the mouse hippocampus: effects on expression of genes involved in Beta-amyloid generation and Alzheimer's disease, *J Gerontol A Biol Sci Med Sci* 69:1212–1226, 2014.

395. Baumgarner KM, Setti S, Diaz C, et al: Diet-induced obesity attenuates cytokine production following an immune challenge, *Behav Brain Res* 267:33–41, 2014.

396. Chen Y, Fan JX, Zhang ZL, et al: The negative influence of high-glucose ambience on neurogenesis in developing quail embryos, *PLoS One* 8:e66646, 2013.

397. Ramalho R, Almeida J, Beltrao M, et al: Neurogenic inflammation in allergen-challenged obese mice: a missing link in the obesity-asthma association? *Exp Lung Res* 38:316–324, 2012.

398. Guo X, Park Y, Freedman ND, et al: Sweetened beverages, coffee, and tea and depression risk among older US adults, *PLoS One* 9:e94715, 2014.

399. Bisht B, Darling WG, Grossmann RE, et al: A multimodal intervention for patients with secondary progressive multiple sclerosis: feasibility and effect on fatigue, *J Altern Complement Med* 20:347–355, 2014.

400. Yang SJ, Lim Y: Resveratrol ameliorates hepatic metaflammation and inhibits NLRP3 inflammasome activation, *Metabolism* 63:693–701, 2014.

401. Rodrigues DF, Henriques MC, Oliveira MC, et al: Acute intake of a high-fructose diet alters the balance of adipokine concentrations and induces neutrophil influx in the liver, *J Nutr Biochem* 25:388–394, 2014.

402. Kanazawa I, Yamaguchi T, Sugimoto T: Effects of intensive glycemic control on serum levels of insulin-like growth factor-I and dehydroepiandrosterone sulfate in Type 2 diabetes mellitus, *J Endocrinol Invest* 35:469–472, 2012.

403. Young LR, Kurzer MS, Thomas W, et al: Low-fat diet with omega-3 fatty acids increases plasma insulin-like growth factor concentration in healthy postmenopausal women, *Nutr Res* 33:565–571, 2013.

404. Liu J, Peter K, Shi D, et al: Anti-inflammatory effects of the chinese herbal formula sini tang in myocardial infarction rats, *Evid Based Complement Alternat Med* 2014:309378, 2014.

405. Silva PS, Sperandio da Silva GM, de Souza AP, et al: Effects of omega-3 polyunsaturated fatty acid supplementation in patients with chronic chagasic cardiomyopathy: study protocol for a randomized controlled trial, *Trials* 14:379, 2013.

406. Jansen D, Zerbi V, Janssen CI, et al: Impact of a multinutrient diet on cognition, brain metabolism, hemodynamics, and plasticity in apoE4 carrier and apoE knockout mice, *Brain Struct Funct* 219:1841–1868, 2014.

407. Kouguchi T, Ohmori T, Shimizu M, et al: Effects of a chicken collagen hydrolysate on the circulation system in subjects with mild hypertension or high-normal blood pressure, *Biosci Biotechnol Biochem* 77:691–696, 2013.

408. Larsson SC, Akesson A, Wolk A: Sweetened beverage consumption is associated with increased risk of stroke in women and men, *J Nutrition* 144:856–860, 2014.

409. Faraco G, Wijasa TS, Park L, et al: Water deprivation induces neurovascular and cognitive dysfunction through vasopressin-induced oxidative stress, *J Cereb Blood Flow Metab* 34:852–860, 2014.

410. Crary MA, Humphrey JL, Carnaby-Mann G, et al: Dysphagia, nutrition, and hydration in ischemic stroke patients at admission and discharge from acute care, *Dysphagia* 28:69–76, 2013.

411. Lin LC, Fann WC, Chou MH, et al: Urine specific gravity as a predictor of early neurological deterioration in acute ischemic stroke, *Med Hypotheses* 77:11–14, 2011.

412. Rodriguez GJ, Cordina SM, Vazquez G, et al: The hydration influence on the risk of stroke (THIRST) study, *Neurocrit Care* 10:187–194, 2009.

413. Ruth MR, Port AM, Shah M, et al: Consuming a hypocaloric high fat low carbohydrate diet for 12 weeks lowers C-reactive protein, and raises serum adiponectin and high density lipoprotein-cholesterol in obese subjects, *Metabolism* 62:1779–1787, 2013.

414. Wood LG, Shivappa N, Berthon BS, et al: Dietary inflammatory index is related to asthma risk, lung function and systemic inflammation in asthma, *Clin Exp Allergy* 45:177–183, 2015.

415. Shi Z, Wittert GA, Yuan B, et al: Association between monosodium glutamate intake and sleep-disordered breathing among Chinese adults with normal body weight, *Nutrition* 29:508–513, 2013.

416. Shulman RJ, Jarrett ME, Cain KC, et al: Associations among gut permeability, inflammatory markers, and symptoms in patients with irritable bowel syndrome, *J Gastroenterol* 49:1467–1476, 2014.

417. Dickerson F, Stallings C, Origoni A, et al: Markers of gluten sensitivity and celiac disease in recent-onset psychosis and multi-episode schizophrenia, *Biol Psychiatry* 68:100–104, 2010.

418. Dickerson F, Stallings C, Origoni A, et al: Markers of gluten sensitivity in acute mania: a longitudinal study, *Psychiatry Res* 196:68–71, 2012.

419. Dickerson F, Stallings C, Origoni A, et al: Markers of gluten sensitivity and celiac disease in bipolar disorder, *Bipolar Disord* 13:52–58, 2011.

420. Dickerson FB, Stallings C, Origoni A, et al: Effect of probiotic supplementation on schizophrenia symptoms and association with gastrointestinal functioning: a randomized, placebo-controlled trial, *Primary Care Companion CNS Disord* 16, 2014.

421. Giardina S, Scilironi C, Michelotti A, et al: In vitro anti-inflammatory activity of selected oxalate-degrading probiotic bacteria: potential applications in the prevention and treatment of hyperoxaluria, *J Food Sci* 79:M384–M390, 2014.

422. Vaghef-Mehrabany E, Alipour B, Homayouni-Rad A, et al: Probiotic supplementation improves inflammatory status in patients with rheumatoid arthritis, *Nutrition* 30:430–435, 2014.

423. Szalai Z, Szasz A, Nagy I, et al: Anti-inflammatory effect of recreational exercise in TNBS-induced colitis in rats: role of NOS/HO/MPO system, *Oxid Med Cell Longev* 2014:925981, 2014.

424. Dideriksen K: Muscle and tendon connective tissue adaptation to unloading, exercise and NSAID, *Connect Tissue Res* 55:61–70, 2014.

425. Bower JE, Greendale G, Crosswell AD, et al: Yoga reduces inflammatory signaling in fatigued breast cancer survivors: a randomized controlled trial, *Psychoneuroendocrinology* 43:20–29, 2014.

426. Bhasin MK, Dusek JA, Chang BH, et al: Relaxation response induces temporal transcriptome changes in energy metabolism, insulin secretion and inflammatory pathways, *PLoS One* 8:e62817, 2013.

427. Manzanero S, Erion JR, Santro T, et al: Intermittent fasting attenuates increases in neurogenesis after ischemia and reperfusion and improves recovery, *J Cereb Blood Flow Metab* 34:897–905, 2014.

428. El-Kadi SW, Gazzaneo MC, Suryawan A, et al: Viscera and muscle protein synthesis in neonatal pigs is increased more by intermittent bolus than by continuous feeding, *Pediatric Res* 74:154–162, 2013.

429. Hussin NM, Shahar S, Teng NI, et al: Efficacy of fasting and calorie restriction (FCR) on mood and depression among ageing men, *J Nutr Health Aging* 17:674–680, 2013.

430. Bahammam AS, Almushailhi K, Pandi-Perumal SR, et al: Intermittent fasting during Ramadan: does it affect sleep? *J Sleep Res* 23:35–43, 2014.

431. Bahammam AS, Nashwan S, Hammad O, et al: Objective assessment of drowsiness and reaction time during intermittent Ramadan fasting in young men: a case-crossover study, *Behav Brain Funct* 9:32, 2013.

432. Yuen AW, Sander JW: Rationale for using intermittent calorie restriction as a dietary treatment for drug resistant epilepsy, *Epilepsy Behav* 33:110–114, 2014.

433. Faris MA, Kacimi S, Al-Kurd RA, et al: Intermittent fasting during Ramadan attenuates proinflammatory cytokines and immune cells in healthy subjects, *Nutr Res* 32:947–955, 2012.

434. Lee S, Notterpek L: Dietary restriction supports peripheral nerve health by enhancing endogenous protein quality control mechanisms, *Exp Gerontol* 48:1085–1090, 2013.

435. Lingelbach LB, Mitchell AE, Rucker RB, et al: Accumulation of advanced glycation endproducts in aging male Fischer 344 rats during long-term feeding of various dietary carbohydrates, *J Nutr* 130:1247–1255, 2000.

436. Li Y, Fessel G, Georgiadis M, et al: Advanced glycation end-products diminish tendon collagen fiber sliding, *Matrix Biol* 32:169–177, 2013.

437. Spreadbury I: Comparison with ancestral diets suggests dense acellular carbohydrates promote an inflammatory microbiota, and may be the primary dietary cause of leptin resistance and obesity, *Diabetes Metab Syndr Obes* 5:175–189, 2012.

438. Ruskin DN, Kawamura M, Masino SA: Reduced pain and inflammation in juvenile and adult rats fed a ketogenic diet, *PLoS One* 4:e8349, 2009.

439. Mikulikova K, Eckhardt A, Kunes J, et al: Advanced glycation end-product pentosidine accumulates in various tissues of rats with high fructose intake, *Physiol Res* 57:89–94, 2008.

440. Robbins PI, Raymond L: Aspartame and symptoms of carpal tunnel syndrome, *J Occup Environ Med* 41:418, 1999.

441. Karl JP, Alemany JA, Koenig C, et al: Diet, body composition, and physical fitness influences on IGF-I bioactivity in women, *Growth Horm IGF Res* 19:491–496, 2009.

442. Baad-Hansen L, Cairns B, Ernberg M, et al: Effect of systemic monosodium glutamate (MSG) on headache and pericranial muscle sensitivity, *Cephalalgia* 30:68–76, 2010.

443. Shimada A, Cairns BE, Vad N, et al: Headache and mechanical sensitization of human pericranial muscles after repeated intake of monosodium glutamate (MSG), *J Headache Pain* 14:2, 2013.

444. Bernardo D, Garrote JA, Fernandez-Salazar L, et al: Is gliadin really safe for non-coeliac individuals? Production of interleukin 15 in biopsy culture from non-coeliac individuals challenged with gliadin peptides, *Gut* 56:889–890, 2007.

445. Okada Y, Tsuzuki Y, Ueda T, et al: Trans fatty acids in diets act as a precipitating factor for gut inflammation? *J Gastroenterol Hepatol* 28(Suppl 4):29–32, 2013.

446. Xiao S, Fei N, Pang X, et al: A gut microbiota-targeted dietary intervention for amelioration of chronic inflammation underlying metabolic syndrome, *FEMS Microbiol Ecol* 87:357–367, 2014.

447. Barbosa AW, Benevides GP, Alferes LM, et al: A leucine-rich diet and exercise affect the biomechanical characteristics of the digital flexor tendon in rats after nutritional recovery, *Amino Acids* 42:329–336, 2012.

448. Takeuchi H, Kondo Y, Yanagi M, et al: Accelerative effect of olive oil on adrenal corticosterone secretion in rats loaded with single or repetitive immersion-restraint stress, *J Nutr Sci Vitaminol* 46:158–164, 2000.

449. Takeuchi H, Suzuki N, Tada M, et al: Accelerative effect of olive oil on liver glycogen synthesis in rats subjected to water-immersion restraint stress, *Biosci Biotechnol Biochem* 65:1489–1494, 2001.

450. Atiba A, Nishimura M, Kakinuma S, et al: Aloe vera oral administration accelerates acute radiation-delayed wound healing by stimulating transforming growth factor-beta and fibroblast growth factor production, *Am J Surg* 201:809–818, 2011.

451. Ao J, Li B: Amino acid composition and antioxidant activities of hydrolysates and peptide fractions from porcine collagen, *Food Sci Technol Int* 18:425–434, 2012.

452. San Miguel SM, Opperman LA, Allen EP, et al: Antioxidant combinations protect oral fibroblasts against metal-induced toxicity, *Arch Oral Biol* 58:299–310, 2013.

453. Urios P, Grigorova-Borsos AM, Sternberg M: Flavonoids inhibit the formation of the cross-linking AGE pentosidine in collagen incubated with glucose, according to their structure, *Eur J Nutr* 46:139–146, 2007.

454. Demirkol A, Uludag M, Soran N, et al: Total oxidative stress and antioxidant status in patients with carpal tunnel syndrome, *Redox Rep* 17:234–238, 2012.

455. Park HB, Hah YS, Yang JW, et al: Antiapoptotic effects of anthocyanins on rotator cuff tenofibroblasts, *J Orthop Res* 28:1162–1169, 2010.

456. Grieger JA, Wood LG, Clifton VL: Antioxidant-rich dietary intervention for improving asthma control in pregnancies complicated by asthma: study protocol for a randomized controlled trial, *Trials* 15:108, 2014.

457. Baez-Saldana A, Gutierrez-Ospina G, Chimal-Monroy J, et al: Biotin deficiency in mice is associated with decreased serum availability of insulin-like growth factor-I, *Eur J Nutr* 48:137–144, 2009.

458. Playford RJ, Floyd DN, Macdonald CE, et al: Bovine colostrum is a health food supplement which prevents NSAID induced gut damage, *Gut* 44:653–658, 1999.

459. Colpo E, Dalton DAVC, Reetz LG, et al: Brazilian nut consumption by healthy volunteers improves inflammatory parameters, *Nutrition* 30:459–465, 2014.

460. Busch F, Mobasheri A, Shayan P, et al: Resveratrol modulates interleukin-1beta-induced phosphatidylinositol 3-kinase and nuclear factor kappaB signaling pathways in human tenocytes, *J Biol Chem* 287:38050–38063, 2012.

461. Cho KS, Lee EJ, Kwon KJ, et al: Resveratrol down-regulates a glutamate-induced tissue plasminogen activator via Erk and AMPK/mTOR pathways in rat primary cortical neurons, *Food Funct* 5:951–960, 2014.

462. Lei M, Wang JG, Xiao DM, et al: Resveratrol inhibits interleukin 1beta-mediated inducible nitric oxide synthase expression in articular chondrocytes by activating SIRT1 and thereby suppressing nuclear factor-kappaB activity, *Eur J Pharmacol* 674:73–79, 2012.

463. Liu FC, Hung LF, Wu WL, et al: Chondroprotective effects and mechanisms of resveratrol in advanced glycation end products-stimulated chondrocytes, *Arthritis Res Ther* 12:R167, 2010.

464. Shakibaei M, Mobasheri A, Buhrmann C: Curcumin synergizes with resveratrol to stimulate the MAPK signaling pathway in human articular chondrocytes in vitro, *Genes Nutr* 6:171–179, 2011.

465. Somchit M, Changtam C, Kimseng R, et al: Demethoxycurcumin from Curcuma longa rhizome suppresses iNOS induction in an in vitro inflamed human intestinal mucosa model, *Asian Pac J Cancer Prev* 15:1807–1810, 2014.

466. Ganjali S, Sahebkar A, Mahdipour E, et al: Investigation of the effects of curcumin on serum cytokines in obese individuals: a randomized controlled trial, *ScientificWorldJournal* 2014:898361, 2014.

467. Gomez-Pinilla F, Tyagi E: Diet and cognition: interplay between cell metabolism and neuronal plasticity, *Curr Opin Clin Nutr Metab Care* 16:726–733, 2013.

468. Dawson DR, Branch-Mays G, Gonzalez OA, et al: Dietary modulation of the inflammatory cascade, *Periodontol 2000* 64:161–197, 2014.

469. Kaminski WE, Jendraschak E, Kiefl R, et al: Dietary omega-3 fatty acids lower levels of platelet-derived growth factor mRNA in human mononuclear cells, *Blood* 81:1871–1879, 1993.

470. Passos PP, Borba JM, Rocha-de-Melo AP, et al: Dopaminergic cell populations of the rat substantia nigra are differentially affected by essential fatty acid dietary restriction over two generations, *J Chem Neuroanat* 44:66–75, 2012.

471. Hansen RA, Harris MA, Pluhar GE, et al: Fish oil decreases matrix metalloproteinases in knee synovia of dogs with inflammatory joint disease, *J Nutr Biochem* 19:101–108, 2008.

472. Ahmad SO, Park JH, Radel JD, et al: Reduced numbers of dopamine neurons in the substantia nigra pars compacta and ventral tegmental area of rats fed an n-3 polyunsaturated fatty acid-deficient diet: a stereological study, *Neurosci Lett* 438:303–307, 2008.

473. Lionetti L, Mollica MP, Sica R, et al: Differential effects of high-fish oil and high-lard diets on cells and cytokines involved in the inflammatory process in rat insulin-sensitive tissues, *Int J Molec Sci* 15:3040–3063, 2014.

474. Wei HK, Zhou Y, Jiang S, et al: Feeding a DHA-enriched diet increases skeletal muscle protein synthesis in growing pigs: association with increased skeletal muscle insulin action and local mRNA expression of insulin-like growth factor 1, *Br J Nutr* 110:671–680, 2013.

475. Luo C, Ren H, Wan JB, et al: Enriched endogenous omega-3 fatty acids in mice protect against global ischemia injury, *J Lipid Res* 55:1288–1297, 2014.

476. Cardoso HD, Passos PP, Lagranha CJ, et al: Differential vulnerability of substantia nigra and corpus striatum to oxidative insult induced by reduced dietary levels of essential fatty acids, *Front Human Neurosci* 6:249, 2012.

477. Cardoso HD, dos Santos Junior EF, de Santana DF, et al: Omega-3 deficiency and neurodegeneration in the substantia nigra: involvement of increased nitric oxide production and reduced BDNF expression, *Biochim Biophys Acta* 1840:1902–1912, 2014.

478. McCarty MF, Barroso-Aranda J, Contreras F: Potential complementarity of high-flavanol cocoa powder and spirulina for health protection, *Med Hypotheses* 74:370–373, 2010.

479. Gu Y, Yu S, Park JY, et al: Dietary cocoa reduces metabolic endotoxemia and adipose tissue inflammation in high-fat fed mice, *J Nutr Biochem* 25:439–445, 2014.

480. Laparra JM, Lopez-Rubio A, Lagaron JM, et al: Dietary glycosaminoglycans interfere in bacterial adhesion and gliadin-induced pro-inflammatory response in intestinal epithelial (Caco-2) cells, *Int J Biol Macromol* 47:458–464, 2010.

481. Carames B, Kiosses WB, Akasaki Y, et al: Glucosamine activates autophagy in vitro and in vivo, *Arthritis Rheum* 65:1843–1852, 2013.

482. Angeline ME, Ma R, Pascual-Garrido C, et al: Effect of diet-induced vitamin D deficiency on rotator cuff healing in a rat model, *Am J Sports Med* 42:27–34, 2014.

483. Bachstetter AD, Jernberg J, Schlunk A, et al: Spirulina promotes stem cell genesis and protects against LPS induced declines in neural stem cell proliferation, *PLoS One* 5:e10496, 2010.

484. Daly RM, O'Connell SL, Mundell NL, et al: Protein-enriched diet, with the use of lean red meat, combined with progressive resistance training enhances lean tissue mass and muscle strength and reduces circulating IL-6 concentrations in elderly women: a cluster randomized controlled trial, *Am J Clin Nutr* 99:899–910, 2014.

485. Ryan MJ, Dudash HJ, Docherty M, et al: Vitamin E and C supplementation reduces oxidative stress, improves antioxidant enzymes and positive muscle work in chronically loaded muscles of aged rats, *Exp Gerontol* 45:882–895, 2010.

486. Badr G, Badr BM, Mahmoud MH, et al: Treatment of diabetic mice with undenatured whey protein accelerates the wound healing process by enhancing the expression of MIP-1alpha, MIP-2, KC, CX3CL1 and TGF-beta in wounded tissue, *BMC Immunol* 13:32, 2012.

487. Lee HS, Park SY, Park Y, et al: Yeast hydrolysate protects cartilage via stimulation of type II collagen synthesis and suppression of MMP-13 production, *Phytother Res* 27:1414–1418, 2013.

488. Kolle B: Psychological approach to focal dystonia in musicians. In Tubiana R, Amadio PC, editors: *Medical problems of the instrumentalist musician*, London, 2000, Martin Dunitz.

489. Barahona-Correa B, Bugalho P, Guimaraes J, et al: Obsessive-compulsive symptoms in primary focal dystonia: a controlled study, *Mov Disord* 26:2274–2278, 2011.

490. Pullman SL, Greene P, Fahn S, et al: Approach to the treatment of limb disorders with botulinum toxin A. Experience with 187 patients, *Arch Neurol* 53:617–624, 1996.

491. Brin MF, Fahn S, Moskowitz C, et al: Localized injections of botulinum toxin for the treatment of focal dystonia and hemifacial spasm, *Mov Disord* 2:237–254, 1987.

492. Yoshimura DM, Aminoff MJ, Olney RK: Botulinum toxin therapy for limb dystonias, *Neurology* 42(Pt 1):627–630, 1992.

493. van Hilten BJ, van de Beek WJ, Hoff JI, et al: Intrathecal baclofen for the treatment of dystonia in patients with reflex sympathetic dystrophy, *N Engl J Med* 343:625–630, 2000.

494. Priori A, Pesenti A, Cappellari A, et al: Limb immobilization for the treatment of focal occupational dystonia, *Neurology* 57:405–409, 2001.

495. Priori A: *Immobilization for focal hand dystonia*. In Paper presented at the International Meeting of the French Neurological Society: Dystonia 2003, Paris, France. 2003.

496. Priori A, Hallett M, Rothwell JC: Repetitive transcranial magnetic stimulation or transcranial direct current stimulation? *Brain Stimul* 2:241–245, 2009.

497. Cambieri C, Scelzo E, Li Voti P, et al: Transcranial direct current stimulation modulates motor responses evoked by repetitive transcranial magnetic stimulation, *Neurosci Lett* 522:167–171, 2012.

498. Hoogendam JM, Ramakers GM, Di Lazzaro V: Physiology of repetitive transcranial magnetic stimulation of the human brain, *Brain Stimul* 3:95–118, 2010.

499. Pauls KA, Hammesfahr S, Moro E, et al: Deep brain stimulation in the ventrolateral thalamus/subthalamic area in dystonia with head tremor, *Mov Disord* 29:953–959, 2014.

500. Cole R, Hallett M, Cohen LG: Double-blind trial of botulinum toxin for treatment of focal hand dystonia, *Mov Disord* 10:466–471, 1995.

501. Ceballos-Baumann A, Sheean G, Pasingham RE, et al: Cerebral activation with stereotyped writing in patients with writer's cramp before and after botulinum toxin treatment: a PET study, *Neurology* 45(Suppl):393–396, 1995.

502. Tsui JK, Bhatt M, Calne S, et al: Botulinum toxin in the treatment of writer's cramp: a double-blind study, *Neurology* 43:183–185, 1993.

503. Kruisdijk JJ, Koelman JH, Ongerboer de Visser BW, et al: Botulinum toxin for writer's cramp: a randomised, placebo-controlled trial and 1-year follow-up, *J Neurol Neurosurg Psychiatry* 78:264–270, 2007.

504. Pesenti A, Barbieri S, Priori A: Limb immobilization for occupational dystonia: a possible alternative treatment for selected patients, *Adv Neurol* 94:247–254, 2004.

505. Pesenti A, Priori A, Scarlato G, et al: Transient improvement induced by motor fatigue in focal occupational dystonia: the handgrip test, *Mov Disord* 16:1143–1147, 2001.

506. Liversedge LA, Sylvester JD: *Conditioning techniques in the treatment of writer's cramp*, Oxford, UK, 1960, Pergamon Press.

507. Kimberley TJ, Di Fabio RP: Visualizing the effects of rTMS in a patient sample: small N vs. group level analysis, *PLoS One* 5:e15155, 2010.

508. Stinear CM, Byblow WD: Impaired modulation of corticospinal excitability following subthreshold rTMS in focal hand dystonia, *Hum Mov Sci* 23:527–538, 2004.

509. Woldendorp KH, van Gils W: One-handed musicians-more than a gimmick, *Med Probl Perform Art* 27:231–237, 2012.

510. Mai N, Marquardt C: Treatment of writers cramp. In Faure C, Keuss P, Lorette G, Vinter A, editors: *Advances in handwriting and drawing: a multidisciplinary approach*, Paris, 1994, Europia.

511. Leijnse J: *Finger exercises with anatomical constraints*, Molenaarsgraaf, Netherlands, 1995, Optima Druk.

512. Baur B, Schenk T, Furholzer W, et al: Modified pen grip in the treatment of Writer's Cramp, *Hum Mov Sci* 25:464–473, 2006.

513. Ramachandran VS, Altschuler EL: The use of visual feedback, in particular mirror visual feedback, in restoring brain function, *Brain* 132(Pt 7):1693–1710, 2009.

514. Wolpert DM, Goodbody SJ, Husain M: Maintaining internal representations: the role of the human superior parietal lobe, *Nat Neurosci* 1:529–533, 1998.

515. Altschuler EL, Wisdom SB, Stone L, et al: Rehabilitation of hemiparesis after stroke with a mirror, *Lancet* 353:2035–2036, 1999.

516. Dohle C, Pullen J, Nakaten A, et al: Mirror therapy promotes recovery from severe hemiparesis: a randomized controlled trial, *Neurorehabil Neural Repair* 23:209–217, 2009.

517. Moseley GL: Graded motor imagery is effective for long-standing complex regional pain syndrome: a randomised controlled trial, *Pain* 108:192–198, 2004.

518. Moseley GL: Graded motor imagery for pathologic pain: a randomized controlled trial, *Neurology* 67:2129–2134, 2006.

519. Moseley GL, Butler DS, Beames TB, et al: *The graded motor imagery handbook*, Adelaide, Australia, 2012, Noigroup Publications.

520. Moseley GL, Zalucki N, Birklein F, et al: Thinking about movement hurts: the effect of motor imagery on pain and swelling in people with chronic arm pain, *Arthritis Rheum* 59:623–631, 2008.

521. Priganc VW, Stralka SW: Graded motor imagery, *J Hand Ther* 24:164–168, 2011. quiz 169.

522. Flor H, Denke C, Schaefer M, et al: Effect of sensory discrimination training on cortical reorganisation and phantom limb pain, *Lancet* 357:1763–1764, 2001.

523. Zeuner KE, Bara-Jimenez W, Noguchi P, et al: Sensory training for patients with focal hand dystonia, *Ann Neurol* 51:593–598, 2002.

524. Zeuner KE, Hallett M: Sensory training as treatment for focal hand dystonia: a 1-year follow-up, *Mov Disord* 18:1044–1047, 2003.

525. Sterr A, Muller MM, Elbert T, et al: Perceptual correlates of changes in cortical representation of fingers in blind multifinger Braille readers, *J Neurosci* 18:4417–4423, 1998.

526. Taub E, Morris DM: Constraint-induced movement therapy to enhance recovery after stroke, *Curr Atheroscler Rep* 3:279–286, 2001.

527. Lin KC, Wu CY, Liu JS, et al: Constraint-induced therapy versus dose-matched control intervention to improve motor ability, basic/extended daily functions, and quality of life in stroke, *Neurorehabil Neural Repair* 23:160–165, 2009.

528. Uswatte G, Taub E: Constraint-induced movement therapy: a method for harnessing neuroplasticity to treat motor disorders, *Prog Brain Res* 207:379–401, 2013.

529. Nudo RJ, Milliken GW: Reorganization of movement representations in primary motor cortex following focal ischemic infarcts in adult squirrel monkeys, *J Neurophysiol* 75:2144–2149, 1996.

530. Wolf SL, Winstein CJ, Miller JP, et al: Effect of constraint-induced movement therapy on upper extremity function 3 to 9 months after stroke: the EXCITE randomized clinical trial, *JAMA* 296:2095–2104, 2006.

531. Candia V, Elbert T, Altenmuller E, et al: Constraint-induced movement therapy for focal hand dystonia in musicians, *Lancet* 353:42, 1999.

532. Candia V, Schafer T, Taub E, et al: Sensory motor retuning: a behavioral treatment for focal hand dystonia of pianists and guitarists, *Arch Phys Med Rehabil* 83:1342–1348, 2002.

533. Candia V, Wienbruch C, Elbert T, et al: Effective behavioral treatment of focal hand dystonia in musicians alters somatosensory cortical organization, *Proc Natl Acad Sci U S A* 100:7942–7946, 2003.

534. Pleger B, Tegenthoff M, Ragert P, et al: Sensorimotor retuning in complex regional pain syndrome parallels pain reduction, *Ann Neurol* 57:425–429, 2005.

535. Byl N, McKenzie AA, Nagarajan SS: *Effectiveness of sensory retraining: three case studies of patients with focal hand dystonia*, New Orleans, LA, November 2000, Paper presented at the Society for Neuroscience Annual Meeting.

536. Byl NN, Nagarajan SS, Newton N, et al: Effect of sensory discrimination training of structure and function in a musician with focal hand dystonia, *Phys Ther Case Rep* 3:94–113, 2000.

537. Byl N, Nagarajan SS, McKenzie AA: Effect of sensory discrimination training on structure and function in patients with focal hand dystonia: three case studies, *Arch Phys Med Rehabil* 84:1505–1514, 2003.

538. Zeuner KE, Peller M, Knutzen A, et al: Motor retraining does not need to be task specific to improve writer's cramp, *Mov Disord* 23:2319–2327, 2008.

539. Zeuner KE, Shill HA, Sohn YH, et al: Motor training as treatment in focal hand dystonia, *Mov Disord* 20:335–341, 2005.

540. Schabrun SM, Stinear CM, Byblow WD, et al: Normalizing motor cortex representations in focal hand dystonia, *Cereb Cortex* 19:1968–1977, 2009.

541. van Vugt FT, Boullet L, Jabusch HC, et al: Musician's dystonia in pianists: long-term evaluation of retraining and other therapies, *Parkinsonism Relat Disord* 20:8–12, 2014.

542. Brown S: *Focal dystonia hypnosis*. Available at http://www.focaldystoniahypnosis.com.

543. Farias J: *Intertwined. How to induce neuroplasticity. A new approach to rehabilitating dystonias*, 2012, Galene Editions.

544. Baur B, Furholzer W, Jasper I, et al: Effects of modified pen grip and handwriting training on writer's cramp, *Arch Phys Med Rehabil* 90:867–875, 2009.

545. Baur B, Furholzer W, Marquardt C, et al: Auditory grip force feedback in the treatment of Writer's cramp, *J Hand Ther* 22:163–170, 2009. quiz 171.

546. Mai N, Marquardt C: Treatment of writers cramp. In Faure C, Keuss P, Lorette G, Vinter A, editors: *Advances in handwriting and drawing: a multidisciplinary approach*, Paris, 1994, Europia.

547. Schenk T, Bauer B, Steidle B, et al: Does training improve writer's cramp? An evaluation of a behavioral treatment approach using kinematic analysis, *J Hand Ther* 17:349–363, 2004.

548. Serrien DJ, Burgunder JM, Wiesendanger M: Disturbed sensorimotor processing during control of precision grip in patients with writer's cramp, *Mov Disord* 15:965–972, 2000.

549. Byl NN, Archer ES, McKenzie A: Focal hand dystonia: effectiveness of a home program of fitness and learning-based sensorimotor and memory training, *J Hand Ther* 22:183–197, 2009. quiz 198.

550. Marquardt C, Mai N: A computational procedure for movement analysis in handwriting, *J Neuro Sci Methods* 52:39–45, 1994.

551. Brodie EE, Shyte A, Niven CA: Analgesia through the looking-glass? A randomized controlled trial investigating the effect of viewing a "virtual limb upon phantom limb pain sensation and movement, *Eur J Pain* 22:428–436, 2007.

552. Byl NN, McKenzie A: Treatment effectiveness for patients with a history of repetitive hand use and focal hand dystonia: a planned, prospective follow-up study, *J Hand Ther* 13:289–301, 2000.

CHAPTER 28

Musculoskeletal Developmental Disorders

TOBY LONG, JAMIE HOLLOWAY*

INTRODUCTION

Numerous developmental disorders include musculoskeletal impairments and require the expertise of rehabilitation specialists. Complex musculoskeletal and neurological primary and secondary impairments are present regardless of the pathophysiology. A multidisciplinary team, including the family, coordinates the child's plan of care, with the ultimate goal of maximizing the child's functional potential throughout development. This chapter discusses some of the more common pediatric pathologies and describes the accompanying musculoskeletal impairments.

ARTHROGRYPOSIS MULTIPLEX CONGENITA

Definition and Classification

Arthrogryposis multiplex congenita (AMC), a nonprogressive syndrome present at birth, is characterized by severe joint contractures, muscle weakness, and fibrosis.[1] AMC manifests in various forms, including classic arthrogryposis, or amyoplasia (43%)[2,3]; contracture syndrome (35%); neuromuscular syndrome (7%); distal arthrogryposis (7%); congenital anomalies (6%); and chromosomal abnormalities (2%). Two clinical presentations are seen. In one clinical presentation, the lower extremities are positioned with the hips flexed and dislocated and the knees extended (i.e., jackknifed position) (Figure 28-1), and the child has clubfeet. In the upper extremities, the shoulders are internally (medially) rotated, the elbows are flexed, and the wrists are flexed and ulnarly deviated (Figure 28-2). In the other clinical presentation, the hips are abducted and externally (laterally) rotated, the knees are flexed (i.e., frog-legged), and the child has clubfeet. The upper extremities are positioned in shoulder internal (medial) rotation, elbow extension, and forearm pronation, with the wrists flexed and ulnarly deviated (i.e., waiter's tip) (Figure 28-3).[2]

Etiology, Epidemiology, and Pathophysiology

The reported incidence of AMC is 1 in 3000 to 4000 live births.[2,4,5] Although AMC is nonprogressive, the long-term sequelae are disabling. The exact etiology of AMC is unknown, but it is probably multifactorial. Reported causes include a maternal fever (i.e., greater than 37.8 °C or 100 °F), causing hyperthermia in the fetus; prenatal viral infections; vascular compromise between mother and fetus; and a uterine septum.[2,6] The insult occurs during the first trimester of pregnancy and can result from neurogenic, myopathic, or connective tissue disorders.[6] The neuropathic form of AMC involves degeneration of anterior horn cell causing muscle weakness and consequent periarticular soft tissue fibrosis.[7] Failure of muscle function and joint development in the growing fetus leads to stiffness, joint deformation, and intrauterine joint fixation. The chief pathophysiological mechanism is lack of fetal movement[8]; however, decreased amniotic fluid and intrauterine compression are also cited.[2,5]

Diagnosis and Prognosis

No definitive laboratory studies or procedures, such as amniocentesis or chorionic villous sampling, are available to detect AMC. However, detailed level II ultrasound can identify a decrease in fetal movements, which suggests the diagnosis.

In the embryo, muscle formation proceeds as it typically would; however, during fetal development, fibrous fatty tissue replaces muscle. Histologically, weak muscles show fibrofatty changes. Therefore muscle biopsies and blood tests are done to rule out fatal disorders and to

*The authors, editors, and publisher wish to acknowledge Lorrie Ippensen Vreeman and Zehra H. Habib for their contributions on this topic in the previous edition.

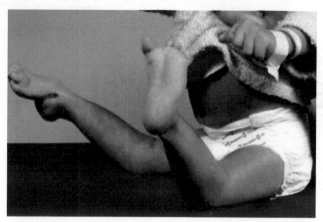

Figure 28-1 Congenital knee dislocation. (From Scott WN: *Insall & Scott surgery of the knee,* ed 5, Philadelphia, 2012, Churchill Livingstone.)

support the diagnosis of AMC. Nerve conduction studies and electromyography (EMG) provide valuable diagnostic information only when the history, examination, and genetic evaluation are unrevealing.[2,9] Children with AMC generally have a positive prognosis. Family support and the severity of the disease, among other factors, however, can influence the prognosis. Sells et al.[10] indicates that by age 5 years, 85% of children with AMC are ambulatory and can perform most of their activities of daily living (ADLs) independently.

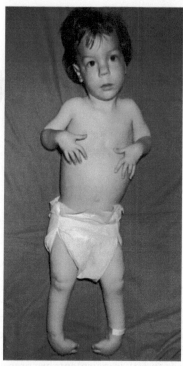

Figure 28-2 This 6-month-old boy has the neurogenic form of arthrogryposis. The marked deformities of the ankles and feet are evident, and the infant has flexion contractures of the wrists, elbows, and knees. (From Swaiman KF, Ashwal S, Ferriero DM: *Pediatric neurology: principles and practice,* ed 5, p 1872, Philadelphia, 2012, Elsevier.)

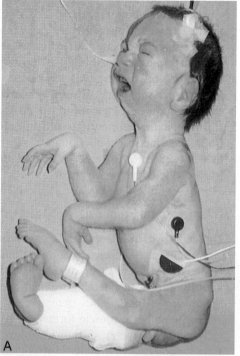

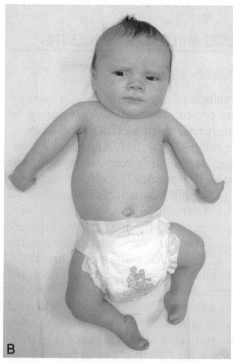

Figure 28-3 **A,** Infant with arthrogryposis multiplex congenita (AMC) with flexed and dislocated hips, extended knees, clubfeet (equinovarus), internally (medially) rotated shoulders, flexed elbows, and flexed and ulnarly deviated wrists. **B,** Infant with AMC with abducted and externally (laterally) rotated hips, flexed knees, clubfeet, internally (medially) rotated shoulders, extended elbows, and flexed and ulnarly deviated wrists. (**A** from Moore KL, Persaud TVN, Torchia MG: *The developing human,* ed 9, Philadelphia, 2013, Saunders. Courtesy of Dr. A.E. Chudley, Section of Genetics and Metabolism, Department of Pediatrics and Child Health, Children's Hospital and University of Manitoba, Winnipeg, Manitoba, Canada. **B** from Bamshad M, Van Heest AE, Pleasure D: Arthrogryposis: a review and update, *J Bone Joint Surg Am* 91[Suppl 4]:40–46, 2009.)

Clinical Manifestations and Primary Impairments

The presentation of AMC varies tremendously. Palmer et al.[11] reported that all four extremities are involved in 90% of all cases.[5] Severely affected body parts include the foot (67%), hip (50%), wrist (43%), knee (41%), elbow (30%), and shoulder (4%).[2] Associated clinical manifestations include hemangiomas, congenital heart disease, absent or decreased finger creases, facial abnormalities, respiratory problems, and abdominal hernias.[2] Additional congenital changes include low-set ears, micrognathia, a high-arched palate, and hypoplastic lungs. Speech and intelligence are unaffected.[5]

Primary Impairments in Arthrogryposis Multiplex Congenita

- Severe joint contractures
- Webbing of the joint
- Decreased muscle bulk and weakness
- Impaired integument
- Diminished deep tendon reflexes
- Clubfeet
- Dislocated hips
- Scoliosis

Medical and Surgical Management

Lower Extremity

The most common foot deformity in the newborn period is clubfoot, the most common form of which is taloequinovarus (TEV). Serial manipulation with casting in this period partially corrects the deformity, but recurrence is common.[2,11] Surgical correction of TEV should be deferred until the child demonstrates pull to stand or ambulatory potential.[2,5] The recommended surgical procedures are posteromedial release (i.e., the lateral border of the foot is shortened, and the medial border is lengthened) combined with elongation of the Achilles tendon.[2,5,12,13] After surgery, mandatory use of ankle–foot orthoses (AFOs) is recommended. In severe cases or if the surgery fails, talectomy may be performed.[14]

Hip subluxation or dislocation can be bilateral or unilateral, and its surgical management is an issue of controversy. The basic premise in surgical correction of dislocated hips is that having mobile, painless dislocated hips is more important than having very stiff located ones.[2] Asif et al.[15] however, suggested that open reduction for bilateral dislocated hips in children with AMC is a suitable option that produces satisfactory results. Along with others, they recommend surgery at an early age for optimum functional outcome.[5] Because high unilateral hip dislocation can lead to severe pelvic obliquity and secondary scoliosis if left untreated, open reduction is essential in these cases.[2,5,16,17]

Knee surgery is reserved for moderate to severe contractures and resistant cases. Posterior capsulotomy and medial and lateral hamstring lengthening are the recommended procedures for young children with a knee flexion deformity of 30° or more.[2,5] Postoperative complications may include posterior subluxation of the tibia and inconsistent muscular response secondary to loss of muscle strength and possible scar tissue formation, both of which may lead to further joint stiffness and recurrence of contracture. A distal femoral osteotomy may be more successful in realigning the knee joint in such cases.[2] Knee extension contractures have a more favorable outcome and are addressed by quadricepsplasty (surgical repair of the quadriceps).[18]

Upper Extremity

If muscle strength and control are adequate, the upper extremities are placed in the optimal position for long-term function and ADLs: one elbow in extension (to reach the perineum), and the other, in flexion (for feeding).[2,5,19] Shoulder range of motion (ROM) usually is adequate for self-care, and surgery is rarely required. The best surgical candidates for tendon transfers of the upper extremity are children older than 4 years of age who have full passive ROM of the elbow in the dominant arm and at least grade 4 muscle strength of the muscle tendons to be transferred.[20] Usually the pectoralis major, triceps brachii, or latissimus dorsi muscle[21] is used in tendon transfers to restore active elbow flexion. Wrist deformities are treated aggressively in infants and young children using passive stretching, serial casting, and custom wrist orthotics.[22] Smith and Drennan,[22] using conservative management, found that children with distal AMC had the greatest improvement in passive ROM, were functionally independent at follow-up, and had no recurrence of deformity. Those with classic AMC had rigid wrist flexion contractures and a 75% incidence of deformity recurrence. Surgical correction of the wrist involves anterior wrist capsulotomy and placement of the wrist in a neutral or slight dorsiflexion position. Long-term protective splinting is required.[5]

Spine

Approximately one-fifth of children and adolescents with AMC have a long C thoracolumbar scoliosis (Figure 28-4).[2] When the curve is less than 30°, the scoliosis is managed conservatively with bracing in ambulators.[23] If the curve progresses, combined anterior and posterior spinal arthrodesis yields the best results.[23]

Rehabilitation Management: Evaluation, Intervention, and Clinical Implications

A multidisciplinary team evaluates a child with AMC. The purpose of the initial evaluation is to determine developmental, musculoskeletal, and functional status of the child

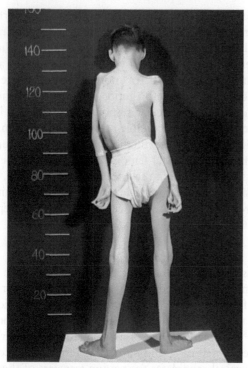

Figure 28-4 This child, who has anterior cell arthrogryposis, has had a number of orthopedic procedures. Marked scoliosis and generalized muscle wasting, particularly of the shoulder girdle, are clearly demonstrated. (From Swaiman KF, Ashwal S, Ferriero DM: *Pediatric neurology: principles and practice,* ed 5, p 1872, Philadelphia, 2012, Elsevier.)

to set realistic goals. Photographs and videos, taken every 2 to 3 months for at least 2 years, could be helpful to show appropriate positioning and stretching of the joint contractures and to provide objective documentation.

Baseline goniometry is necessary, including passive ROM and the resting position of each joint, together with active ROM. Functional ROM (e.g., hand to mouth, hand to the top of the head, hand to forehead, hand to ear, and hand to the back of the neck) also should be assessed.[2] In infants and small children, muscle strength is evaluated by muscle palpation and observation of extremity movement against gravity. Gross motor function and developmental milestones should be evaluated.[2] Formal manual muscle testing (MMT) should begin when appropriate; it is especially important to test the strength of the lower extremity extensor muscles because this determines the appropriate level of lower extremity bracing.

Current and potential gross motor skills and functional mobility, including the use of assistive devices and a manual or power wheelchair, should be evaluated. ADL skills, movement patterns, and muscle substitutions must be assessed to establish an intervention plan with the family and the child as active team members. The ultimate goal of intervention is to maximize the child's independence in ADLs and mobility.

Family education, stretching, positioning, thermoplastic serial splinting, strengthening activities through play, promotion of developmental activities, and teaching of

compensatory strategies (especially in alternative modes of mobility) form the mainstay of physical therapy (PT) in infancy and early childhood. Stretching needs to be incorporated into the daily care of infants. For example, stretching of the lower extremity can be done during diaper changes. During feeding, bathing, and dressing, both the lower and upper extremities can be stretched. The recommended regimen is three to five sets of stretches per day, with three to five repetitions in each set, and each repetition held for 20 to 30 seconds.[2] Low-load, prolonged stretching is preferred over maximum-load stretching for prolonged periods because the latter may cause skin breakdown and intolerance to splints. For infants with the first clinical presentation of AMC described earlier, prone positioning for the first 3 months is essential to stretch the hip flexor muscles. Children with the second clinical presentation of AMC have more positioning options. These children usually are frustrated with prone positioning because they are unable to prop themselves when placed on a wedge or roll. For these children, Velcro straps should be used to position the hips in a neutral position when the child is supine, and a towel roll should be used along the lateral borders of the thigh when the child is sitting (Figure 28-5). Key to positioning is incorporating the activities into daily caregiving as much as possible.

Splints are adjusted for growth and improvement every 4 to 6 weeks. For the newborn, cock-up splints

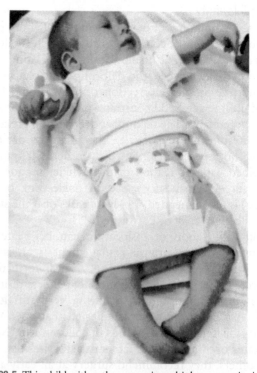

Figure 28-5 This child with arthrogryposis multiplex congenita is wearing a wide Velcro band strapped around the thighs to keep the legs in more neutral alignment. (From Donohoe M: Arthrogryposis multiplex congenita. In Campbell SK, Palisano RJ, Orlin MM, editors: *Physical therapy for children,* ed 4, St. Louis, 2012, Saunders.)

usually are provided 3 months after birth. AFOs to correct clubfeet should be worn 22 hours a day.[2] For the first 3 to 4 months, anterior thermoplastic knee flexion splints for extension contractures or posterior knee extension splints for flexion contractures should be worn 20 hours a day.[2] Knee flexion splints should not be worn at greater than 50° of flexion for sleeping, because this may encourage hip flexion. After 4 months of splinting, knee extension splints can be worn for standing activities and sleeping to help stretch the hip flexors; this encourages optimal lower extremity positioning during independent floor mobility.

Maintaining functional mobility is a major goal of intervention; therefore key functional motor skills, such as rolling, hitching on the buttocks, and standing, should be addressed. Strengthening of muscles that help maintain an upright posture is important during the first 2 to 3 years and can be accomplished through developmental play. For example, dynamic trunk strengthening is promoted by having the child manipulate or reach for toys in various positions of sitting or static standing. Standing is an integral component and should begin by 6 to 9 months of age. Standing is initiated in standing frames with the lower extremities held in as optimally correct position as possible with the help of splints and high-top shoes (Figure 28-6). Advantages of standing include self-stretching of the feet, postural alignment, and commencement of ambulation. Promoting a child's ability

to assume standing from the floor or sitting should be encouraged at about 6 to 8 months of age if the child is strong enough. Limitations in strength and ROM in the lower extremities are addressed through splinting or bracing. If MMT results are less than fair in the hip extensors (3/5), bracing is required above the hip. If MMT results are less than fair in the knee extensors, bracing is required above the knee.[2,4]

In the preschool period, goals should emphasize ability, improvement of the child's function in basic ADLs, and enhancement of independence in mobility and ambulation with minimal bracing and assistive devices. Gait assessment includes evaluating distance, use of assistive devices, speed, symmetry of step length, and any gait deviations. Children with adequate strength and ROM generally require AFOs while walking to prevent recurring clubfeet deformities. Articulating AFOs may be more desirable and appropriate than static AFOs because they provide forefoot control, allow ankle dorsiflexion, and stretch the hindfoot during gait. Ideally, the least amount of bracing should be used; however, if less bracing causes the child to use assistive devices (i.e., walker, crutches, or canes) that previously were not required, then increased bracing is acceptable. Assistive devices can be customized with thermoplastic material to allow for less awkward handgrips. Forearm supports and other modifications can be added to walkers and other assistive devices when required (Figure 28-7).

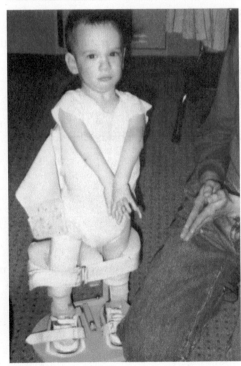

Figure 28-6 Child with arthrogryposis multiplex congenital using a stand frame. (From Donohoe M: Arthrogryposis multiplex congenita. In Campbell SK, Palisano RJ, Orlin MM, editors: *Physical therapy for children,* ed 4, St. Louis, 2012, Saunders.)

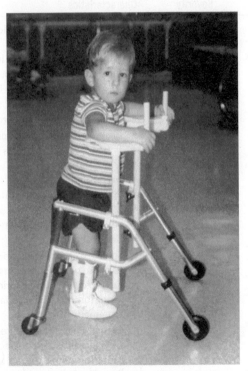

Figure 28-7 Thermoplastic forearm supports can be customized to the walker for a child with arthrogryposis multiplex congenita. (From Donohoe M: Arthrogryposis multiplex congenita. In Campbell SK, Palisano RJ, Orlin MM, editors: *Physical therapy for children,* ed 4, St. Louis, 2012, Saunders.)

Shoes may need external wedges to compensate for hip and knee flexion contractures.[2] Children learning to walk may be limited in their independence if they do not have adequate strength and ROM to manipulate assistive devices. Walkers can be cumbersome and less energy efficient for such children, who typically have inadequate protective responses to falls. Power mobility may be the most energy-efficient means of ambulation for such children. Although walking should be encouraged, it may be more functional to introduce power mobility as soon as possible. Intellectual or learning disabilities are rarely seen in children with AMC, thus, children should be encouraged to interact with their peers as much as possible and participate in community activities. Power mobility may provide a means for independence and socialization.

Families may need assistance in identifying and removing architectural and environmental barriers that impede their child's independence at home. The child should be encouraged to interact with nondisabled peers in school and to participate in extracurricular activities, such as swimming classes. Additional educational and therapy services are essential at this stage to maximize the child's potential.

OSTEOGENESIS IMPERFECTA

Definition and Classification

Osteogenesis imperfecta (OI) is an inherited disorder of connective tissue characterized by increased bone fragility.[24-29] The bone fragility is secondary to decreased bone mass, disturbed organization of bone tissue, and altered bone geometry. OI comprises several distinct syndromes and is genetically heterogeneous with a range of clinical presentations.[30] According to the Osteogenesis Imperfecta Foundation, there are currently eight types of OI. The most severe forms of OI are types II, III, VII, and VIII. People with types IV, V, and VI tend to have more moderate symptoms. People with type I tend to have mild symptoms. The classification system is based on clinical, genetic, and radiological findings.[4,30,31] Table 28-1 differentiates the most common characteristics of the eight types of OI.

Etiology, Epidemiology, and Pathophysiology

In most cases, OI is caused by mutations in one of the two genes encoding type I collagen; the result is a qualitative

TABLE **28-1**

Types of Osteogenesis Imperfecta

Type	Severity	Characteristics
I	Mild	• Most common and mildest type of osteogenesis imperfecta • Few obvious symptoms • Normal or near-normal height; average or slightly shorter than average stature compared with unaffected family members but within the normal range for age
II	Most severe	• Possible infant death within weeks from respiratory or heart complications • Numerous fractures and severe bone deformity at birth • Small stature with underdeveloped lungs and low birth weight
III	Severe	• Progressive bone deformity • Fractures at birth; x-rays may reveal healed fractures that occurred before birth • Short stature • Barrel-shaped rib cage • Spinal curvature and compression fractures of vertebrae
IV	Moderate	• Mild to moderate bone deformity • Spinal curvature and compression fracture of vertebrae • Barrel-shaped rib cage
V	Moderate	• Similar to type IV in appearance and symptoms • Large hypertrophic calluses at fracture or surgical procedure sites • Restricted forearm rotation caused by calcification of the membrane between the radius and ulna • Mutation not in the collagen pathway • Dominant heritance
VI	Moderate	• Extremely rare; similar to type IV in appearance • Distinguished by a characteristic mineralization defect seen in biopsy samples of bone • Mutation not in the collagen pathway • Recessive inheritance
VII	Severe	• Recessive inheritance
VIII	Very severe	• Similar to type II but with recessive inheritance • Severe growth deficiency and under mineralization of the skeleton

and quantitative defect in collagen synthesis.[24,27-29] The incidence of OI is reported to be 1 in 20,000 to 30,000 live births,[4,25,28] and the prevalence is 16 per 1 million.[25] The defect in collagen synthesis results from an abnormality in the processing of procollagen to type I collagen, which leads to brittle bones. It affects the formation of both endochondral and intramembranous bone. The collagen fibers fail to mature beyond the reticular fiber stage.[25] Osteoblasts have normal or increased activity but fail to produce and organize collagen. Osteocytes are relatively abundant, but intracellular matrix is deficient.[25]

Diagnosis and Prognosis

The diagnosis of OI is made primarily from clinical and radiographic findings. No definitive laboratory tests exist to identify OI. In severe OI, the child is born with multiple fractures sustained in utero or during the birth process; these children have a high mortality rate. Infants and children with moderate OI are identified after they experience several fractures from light trauma or a fracture of unknown origin at a young age. In milder forms of OI, pathological fractures occur late in childhood. Joints are hypermobile, and the lower extremities are severely malaligned. Muscle strength is normal in type I OI except in the periarticular muscles of the hip joint; children with type III OI have decreased muscle strength around the hip joint.[25] Developmental progress depends on the type and severity of OI.[4] Milder presentations of OI need to be differentiated from multiple fractures sustained through child abuse.[26,32] Other differential diagnostic conditions include juvenile osteoporosis and rickets.[32]

It is important to note that the classification system does not predict functional outcome, particularly in children with the moderate types of OI (IV, V, and VI). Disuse, weakness, and osteoporosis secondary to immobilization may affect function.[31] Factors that affect independence and mobility include joint contractures, muscle weakness, and endurance capabilities, especially in the child with severe OI.[4]

Clinical Manifestations and Primary Impairments

The clinical features of OI are extremely variable and depend on the type and severity of the disorder. Primary impairments include bone fragility, short stature, scoliosis, defective dentinogenesis, blue sclerae and tympanic membrane, lax ligaments, weak muscles, failure of postnatal growth, and multiple, recurrent fractures sustained from minor or no trauma.[25,32] Bones are diffusely osteoporotic and have thin cortices and an altered trabecular pattern.

Long bones have narrow diaphyses; therefore bowing and resultant deformity are common. Lack of weight bearing in the long bones leads to a honeycomb pattern of ossification. The metaphyseal and epiphyseal areas of long bones show popcorn calcifications secondary to fragmentations of cartilaginous growth plates.[25] The pelvis has a trefoil shape, and protrusio acetabuli (protrusion of the femoral heads through a shallow acetabulum) is common secondary to repeated fractures.[25,32] Osteoporotic vertebrae fracture easily, resulting in a flattened, biconcave shape.[25]

Malformed ribs cause respiratory compromise, and ligamentous laxity results in an increased incidence of joint dislocation. Dentinogenesis imperfecta results in soft, translucent, brownish teeth. Umbilical, inguinal, and diaphragmatic hernias are common.[25,32] Metabolic abnormalities have also been reported in individuals with OI, including increased sweating, heat intolerance, elevated body temperature, and resting tachycardia and tachypnea.[32]

Medical and Surgical Management

Improvements in medical care of respiratory tract infections and orthopedic management have led to better outcomes for children with OI.[25] No effective medications are available to strengthen skeletal structures and reduce or prevent fractures.[25] Recently, the use of bisphosphonates (specifically pamidronate) has been associated with increased bone mineral density and ambulation, decreased bone pain and fracture incidence, improved vertebral shape and mass, greater cortical width, increased cancellous bone volume, and suppressed bone turnover.[24,33,34] Letocha et al.[33] in a randomized, controlled trial of intravenous pamidronate every 3 months in 18 children with OI types III and IV, found a significantly decreased fracture rate in the upper extremities, but not in the lower extremities, during the first year of treatment. Gross motor function, growth improvement, muscle strength, ambulation, and pain did not change significantly. The researchers concluded that for infants with severe OI, cyclical IV pamidronate is beneficial. Munns et al.[34] compared clinical and histomorphometric outcomes between children with OI who had received pamidronate since infancy and age-matched children who had not. They found that cyclical pamidronate treatment started in infancy led to improved bone strength, better gross motor function, and markedly suppressed bone turnover. New areas of research include gene therapy, cell replacement of the mutant gene, bone marrow transplants, and mutant allele suppression.[25]

The major purposes of intervention with children with OI are the treatment of acute fractures and maintenance of mobility and ambulation. Treatment of fractures is difficult because of the structural abnormality of bone and the vicious cycle that occurs with fractures: osteoporosis leads to a fracture, which leads to immobilization, which leads to disuse osteoporosis and further fracture. Therefore every effort is made to limit immobilization to prevent exacerbation of osteopenia. Fractures usually heal within the standard length of time, but the resultant callus is large and of poor quality. Immobilization is necessary for pain relief and proper alignment and can be achieved through the use of splinting, thermoplastic materials or orthoses, a hip spica cast, posterior or anterior shells, or casting.[4,25] Complications of fractures include malunion, angulation and bowing of long bones, and joint contracture and disruption of the physis (i.e., growth plate), leading to asymmetrical growth and deformity. The fracture rate usually declines after puberty.[25]

Multiple corrective osteotomies combined with insertion of intramedullary rods are the most successful means of fixation of long bones in OI.[25,35,36] Advantages of intramedullary fixation include prevention of further fractures through the provision of internal support and prevention of bowing of the long bones. Indications for stabilization with rods include multiple recurring fractures and an increase in long bone deformity that interferes with the fit of orthoses and impairs function.[25] The child's age and the type of bone involved determine the type and timing of surgery.

The type of rod used depends on the type and severity of fractures. Solid rods are not advisable for children with OI because bone growth occurs beyond the ends of the rod, necessitating reoperation, which poses an increased risk of respiratory complications secondary to the use of anesthesia.[25] The extensible intramedullary rod accommodates growth and is the preferred choice. It is used most frequently for the femur but also can be used for the humerus, tibia, and bones of the forearm.[25] The major disadvantage of an extensible intramedullary rod is rotation and migration of the device. Postoperative casting and orthoses may be required.[25]

Spinal deformities, including scoliosis and kyphosis, occur in 50% of people with OI secondary to osteoporosis and vertebral compression fractures.[25] Kyphoscoliosis, present in 20% to 40% of people, can be progressive over the lifetime,[37] further compounding short stature and interfering with function. The most common curve is a thoracic scoliosis. The spinal curves are not amenable to conservative bracing, because the ribs cannot withstand the mechanical forces.[25,32] Spinal stabilization is achieved through early spinal fusion at a 40° curve to halt the progression, maintain function, and prevent respiratory complications.[32]

Bracing allows children to stand and walk earlier than would otherwise be possible.[38] Orthoses usually are used in conjunction with standing frames and parapodiums to increase the child's mobility and ambulation. Children with less severe forms of OI become good household and short distance ambulators with the use of braces.[38] Children usually are fitted with hip–knee–ankle–foot orthoses (HKAFOs) once they begin to develop balance and pull to stand. Children who do not attain independent sitting but have good head control are fitted for standing frames. Children who do not develop independent functional ambulation should be provided with a manual or power wheelchair. As seen with other children with complex motor disabilities, early introduction of power mobility may increase opportunities for mobility, as well as community activities and socialization.

Rehabilitation Management: Evaluation, Intervention, and Clinical Implications

Before starting an examination, clinicians should be knowledgeable about the child's medical history and past and present fractures. They also should know the types of immobilization used. Active ROM at the hips, knees, ankles, and elbows can be measured with a standard goniometer moved through observable ROM. Passive ROM testing is contraindicated, but assessment of functional ROM is recommended. As mentioned previously, muscle strength is assessed in infants by observing the infant's movements against gravity and by palpating contracting muscles. A gross motor developmental evaluation also should be performed to assess delays in motor milestone achievement secondary to frequent fractures and muscular weakness. The parents should be instructed in the use of appropriate equipment for seating and transporting the infant, and independent mobility should be encouraged.

Goals for infants with severe OI are to prevent deformities of the head, spine, and extremities; avert cardiopulmonary compromise by avoiding constant positioning in the supine position; and maximize the child's ability to move actively.[4] Detailed instructions on proper positioning and handling of the child during dressing, bathing, feeding, and playing are a critical component of the home management program for children with OI. An infant with severe OI may be carried and held on a standard-size pillow.[4,25] The head and trunk must be fully supported, with the arms and legs draped across the supporting arm of the caregiver (Figure 28-8).[25] Parents are instructed to avoid overdressing the child to reduce excessive sweating, and they are encouraged to use loose clothing with front and side Velcro closures to facilitate dressing and undressing. For diapering, the infant should be supported through the buttocks and rolled off the diaper rather than lifted by the ankles.[25]

Infant carriers need to be modified to support the head and trunk adequately. Bathing should be done in a padded plastic basin. Supported side-lying with towel rolls or prone positioning on a soft wedge are optimal positions from which to encourage active movements of the child (Figure 28-9). If the child is placed supine, care should be taken to support the arms and keep the hips in a neutral position with the knees over a towel roll. Optimal positioning ensures protection from fractures and minimizes joint malalignment and deformities. The child's position should be changed frequently and should not restrict active spontaneous movements because these movements promote muscle strengthening and bone mineralization.[25]

Promoting sensorimotor development is an ongoing component of the management of infants and children

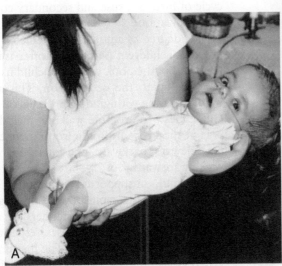
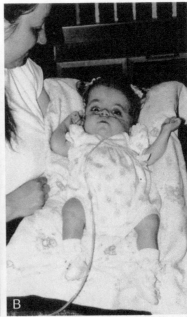

Figure 28-8 A, In handling a young child with osteogenesis imperfecta, support the neck and shoulders and the pelvis with your hands; do not lift the child from under the arm. **B,** Placing the child on a pillow may make lifting and holding easier. (From Myers RS: *Saunders manual of physical therapy practice*, Philadelphia, 1997, Saunders.)

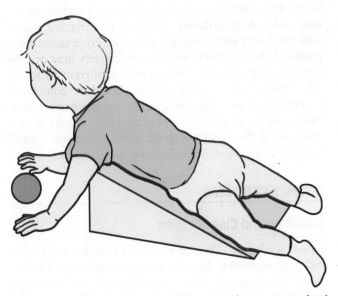

Figure 28-9 Prone positioning of a child on a wedge encourages head and trunk movement and upper extremity weight bearing. (From Martin S, Kessler M: *Neurologic interventions for physical therapy*, ed 2, St. Louis, 2007, Saunders.)

with OI. Comfortable play positions can promote developmental activities; "prone on a roll," for example, allows weight-bearing use of the arms with co-contraction of the shoulder musculature and promotes active control of the neck and the back extensor muscles. Other developmental activities, such as rolling and supported sitting, should be encouraged as tolerated. When the infant attempts to roll over, the arm should be placed alongside the head. Supported sitting is accomplished with seat inserts or corner chairs.[25] Upright supported sitting usually begins on a

parent's lap with a pillow. When head control is achieved, short-sit and straddle activities using a roll, bolster, or caregiver's leg can be started. These activities promote equilibrium responses and protected weight bearing for the lower extremities. A **pull-to-sit maneuver is contraindicated**; instead, the child should be supported around the shoulders when attempting to sit up. Clinicians and parents should support the child through the trunk and pelvis when promoting trunk control.

Pool exercises may begin as early as 6 months. The goal is to promote active movements and weight bearing in the water. Families can be taught pool exercises that can be incorporated into bath time. The child should be supported adequately in a neck and trunk flotation device when in the pool and should wear long-sleeved clothing, because it distributes the absorbed water weight evenly over the length of the limb and thus provides a resistive component to the active movements in water.[25]

An important goal of rehabilitation for the preschool age OI child is preventing or remediating functional limitation and reduced immobility that may have been caused by the initial impairment. Other goals include exploring opportunities for multiple safe modes of mobility, formal gait training in parallel bars with orthoses, and family or parent education. In the preschool period, primary impairments include bone fragility, joint laxity, and decreased muscle strength. Secondary impairments include disuse atrophy and osteoporosis secondary to fracture immobilization.[25] If children walk without adequate support at this stage, further bending or bowing of the long bones will occur, the most common type being femoral anterolateral bowing and tibial anterior bowing. The latter can be controlled with

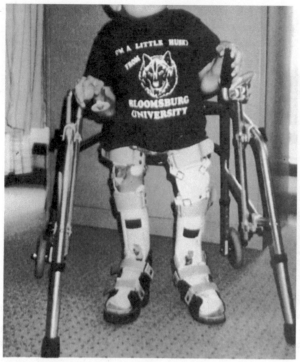

Figure 28-10 Child with osteogenesis imperfecta using long leg braces and a reverse walker. (From Bleakney DA, Donohoe M: Osteogenesis imperfecta. In Campbell SK, Vander Linden DW, Palisano RJ, editors: *Physical therapy for children,* ed 3, Philadelphia, 2006, Saunders.)

appropriate orthoses and assistive devices, such as modified canes, crutches, and walkers (Figure 28-10). Maintaining socialization and participation in activities with peers is crucial, thus, alternative mobility such as powered mobility should be considered as early as possible.

Rehabilitation in the preschool period also emphasizes adequate upright control, protected weight bearing, self-mobility for enhanced independence, and proper positioning, handling, and transferring. The focus eventually shifts to the child's active participation in self-care and safe independence.[25] Active exercise continues to be emphasized to increase muscle strength, especially for the hip extensors and abductors.[4,25] This is achieved through developmental play techniques, such as straddle roll or bolster activity, in which the child attempts sit to stand with the physical therapist supporting the child's pelvis. The activities can be progressed by using a lower roll or bolster.

An aquatic exercise program has excellent therapeutic value because it offers the opportunity to socialize with peers, to improve cardiorespiratory status, and to bear weight in a protected environment. Aquatic therapy is a safe method of strengthening muscles through the resistance and assistance of water.[25] The clinician can grade progression of exercise by using the buoyancy effect of water to assist weak movements. Exercises can be modified with floats. Pool sessions should be limited to 20 to 30 minutes. The water temperature and the child's activity level should be monitored closely, because an elevated water temperature increases body temperature and thus metabolism, which already is elevated at rest in children with OI. Overall, pool therapy may break the cycle of further disuse and secondary complications from immobilization.

The degree of ambulation attainable varies greatly for preschool children. Ambulation often is introduced at the deep end of the pool, where the child usually is immersed in water up to the neck region. This affords protected weight bearing with gradual progression to shallow water. Guidelines[39] to promote walking, include providing support at the pelvis from the front; practicing weight shifting sideways, backward, and forward; and progressing to walking forward.[25]

On land, unsupported standing is not encouraged because it leads to rapid bowing of long bones. Usually, standing frames and prone standers are used in conjunction with splints and orthoses, especially for children with moderate to severe OI. The first brace usually is the HKAFO without the knee joint and with a pelvic band because this helps lock the hips and minimizes femoral rotation.[25] Knee joints may be added later as the child and the limb grow and strength increases. The child graduates from using standing frames to orthoses to ambulating in knee–ankle–foot orthoses (KAFOs) or long leg braces with the knees locked in full extension. Progression from parallel bars to various walkers or crutches may or may not be achievable for children with moderate to severe OI. Customized mobility devices should be considered for children who are unable to ambulate and explore their environment adequately. Power mobility should be encouraged if the child has good head and trunk control and the cognitive ability to operate such devices.[25]

DOWN SYNDROME

Definition and Classification

Down syndrome (DS), or trisomy 21, is the most common chromosomal disorder arising from faulty cell division. This atypical cell division results in 47 chromosomes instead of the usual 46.[40] The three types of DS are nondisjunction, translocation, and mosaicism. Nondisjunction occurs in 91% to 95% of affected children; in this form, an extra small chromosome is present on the twenty-first pair of chromosomes. Translocation occurs in 3% to 4% of affected children; in this type of DS, two nonhomologous chromosomes break, and the broken pieces subsequently reattach to other, intact chromosome pairs. Mosaicism occurs in 1% of affected children; it is a mixed type of DS in which some body cells exhibit trisomy 21 and others are do not.[41] In such cases, physical and cognitive impairments correlate with the percentage of cells that have abnormal chromosomes.[41] DS is characterized by reduced brain volume, increased risk of atypical or abnormality in every body organ, and delays in all developmental areas.[40]

TABLE **28-2**

Neuropathological and Cytological Findings and Physical Characteristics in Down Syndrome

Neuropathological and Cytological Findings	Physical Characteristics
• Decreased weight (76% of normal) • Microcephaly (abnormally small head, underdevelopment of brain) • Decreased anterior-posterior diameter • Microbrachycephaly (small short head, droopy eyelids, cleft lip) • Changed convolutional pattern • Decreased number of secondary sulci • Lack of myelination of nerve fibers in the precentral areas and frontal lobes of the cerebral cortex • Structural abnormalities of the dendritic spine of the pyramidal neurons of the motor cortex • Decreased synaptogenesis (synapse formation) • Decreased number of pyramidal neurons in the hippocampus • Increased neurofibrillary tangles • Increased senile plaques	• Flat contoured face • Depressed nasal bridge with narrow openings • Narrow eyes with slightly slanted eyelids • Epicanthal folds • Micrognathia (underdeveloped jaw) • Narrow palate • Protuberant tongue • Small hands and feet • Inward curved fifth finger • Simian crease across the palm • Short toes and a gap between the first and second toes • Plantar furrows and marmoration of the skin • Short neck • Low-set ears with folded over helices • Down-turned mouth • Lax skin

Pathology

Table 28-2 presents the major neuropathological and cytological findings in the brains of children with DS,[42] as well as common physical characteristics.[40,42]

Etiology, Epidemiology, and Diagnosis

The etiology of DS is unknown, but advanced maternal and paternal age often are cited as a risk factor.[40] The incidence rate is reported to be 1.3 to 1.5 per 1000 live births,[41] and the occurrence is 700 to 800 live births.[41] There are more than 400,000 people living with DS in the United States. DS occurs in people of all races and economic levels. The incidence of births of children with DS increases with the age of the mother. But because of higher fertility rates in younger women, 80% of children with DS are born to women under 35 years of age.

Multiple options are available for prenatal detection of DS, all with varying sensitivity and specificity. First trimester choices include sonographic measurement of nuchal translucency (NT); first trimester serum screening (FSS) for free β-human chorionic gonadotropin (hCG) and pregnancy-associated plasma protein-A (PAPP-A) levels; and combination of serum and sonographic screening (NTSS). Second trimester choices include quadruple serum screening (QUAD), which includes maternal serum α-fetoprotein (AFP), hCG, unconjugated estriol, and dimeric inhibin-A; the integrated combined test (ICS), which includes NTSS and the QUAD screen; integrated serum-only screening (ISS), which includes FSS and QUAD; and sequential screening (SEQ) in which NTSS and QUAD are performed and reported serially.[42,43] Postnatal detection begins with suspected physical findings at birth (see Table 28-2), with follow-up karyotype testing to confirm the diagnosis (Figure 28-11).

Prognosis

Individuals with DS have varying degrees of developmental delays and intellectual disabilities. Most people with DS have a mild to moderate degree of intellectual disabilities. Life expectancy for people with DS has increased dramatically from 25 in 1983 to 60 years of age today.[41]

Musculoskeletal Impairments and Other Impairments

Children with DS experience a wide range of medical problems, such as seizures (5% to 6%), leukemia, thyroid dysfunction, delayed or incomplete sexual development, and intellectual disability.[26,42] Neuromuscular impairments include hypotonia with ligamentous laxity, slow reaction time,[40] and deficits in postural reactions.[44] Cardiopulmonary impairments include congenital heart defects (35% to 50%), most commonly atrioventricular (AV) canal defects and ventriculoseptal (VSD) defects; lung hypoplasia; and pulmonary hypertension.[42] Sensory deficits include hearing loss secondary to narrow eustachian tubes; frequent ear infections; otitis media; and visual defects, such as strabismus, especially esotropia (inward turning of one eye), astigmatism (difficulty focusing the eyes), nystagmus (involuntary rhythmic movement of the eyes), cataracts, myopia (nearsightedness), and Brushfield's spots (pinpoint white or light yellow spots) on the iris.[26,42]

Musculoskeletal impairments include linear growth deficits, joint hypermobility, and ligamentous laxity secondary to hypotonia.[40,45] Ligamentous laxity is a hallmark

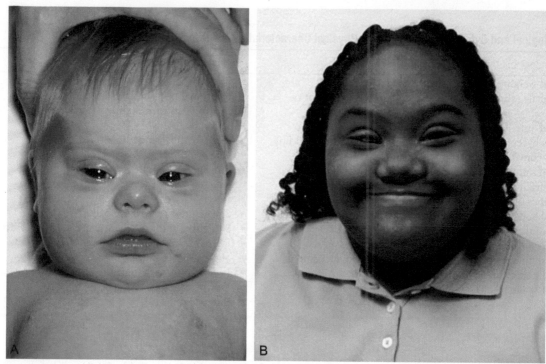

Figure 28-11 A, Newborn with trisomy 21 (Down syndrome). **B,** Adolescent girl with Down syndrome. (**A** from Leifer G: *Maternity nursing,* ed 11, St. Louis, 2012, Saunders. **B** from Rodman R, Pine HS: The otolaryngologist's approach to the patient with Down syndrome, *Otolaryngol Clin North Am* 45:599-629, 2012.)

characteristic of DS and results in orthopedic impairments such as pes planus, scoliosis, patellofemoral instability, and genu valgum, among others.[45] Scoliosis becomes a problem for the older child during growth spurts and usually is treated with Dwyer instrumentation with or without spinal arthrodesis. Knee problems are associated with foot problems and interfere with ambulation.[46] Genu valgum is associated with joint laxity and if persistent can lead to chronic patellar dislocation; the latter, however, does not seem to interfere with function.[46]

Approximately 18% of individuals with DS have atlantoaxial instability (AAI), described as a large space with excessive motion between the atlas (C1 vertebral body) and axis (C2 vertebral body).[47] According to Gajdosik and Ostertag,[48] AAI can be caused by ligamentous laxity (specifically of the transverse odontoid ligament); bony anomalies; trauma, including surgical procedures; and upper respiratory tract infections. Cremers and Beijer[49] assessed general laxity and atlantoaxial distance in 172 children with DS and found no significant correlation between the two measures. Most children with AAI are asymptomatic,[50] and only 1% to 2% have symptoms of spinal cord compression caused by the enlarged space and consequent excessive motion of the atlas on the axis.[50] Many children with DS who have documented AAI also have atlanto-occipital subluxation (AOS), which is associated with AAI and probably results from ligamentous laxity.[51] Therefore radiographs obtained to screen for AAI should be carefully studied for AOS.

Other developmental anomalies of the cervical spine seen in individuals with symptomatic AAI include atlanto-occipital fusion, hemivertebrae, narrowing of the vertebral disc, ossification of atlanto-occipital ligaments, and spondylosis.[48]

Gait abnormalities in children with DS include a wide-based gait with the hips externally (laterally) rotated and the knees in valgus and flexion with the tibias externally (laterally) rotated. The feet are advanced with the medial longitudinal arch leading.[52] Parker and Bronks[53] and Parker et al.[54] reported that children with DS at 5 to 7 years of age exhibited longer stance periods, decreased hip extension, and early hip extension near the end of swing. They also reported decreased ankle sagittal plane rotation and exaggerated abduction of the swing limb for foot clearance in the 7-year-olds. The 5-year-olds showed a longer support phase, shorter step length, greater hip and knee flexion, and a more extended position of the ankle at contact.

Orthopedic concerns include AAI[48]; AOS[51]; foot deformities,[55,56] especially flexible flat foot (pes planus); scoliosis[57]; patellar instability[58,59]; hip subluxation or dislocation[60]; juvenile idiopathic arthritis[58]; and gait abnormalities.[53,54] Clinicians serving children with DS should be aware of the soft neurological signs (e.g., motor control abnormalities, sensory function integration, sensorimotor integration) that may present in children who are symptomatic for AAI.[47,61] If soft neurological signs are noted, immediate referral to a neurologist is mandatory.[50] The role of the clinician in AAI is to serve as a resource for the family regarding education in risk, precautions, and screening recommendations and appropriate medical follow-up.

Soft Neurological Signs of Atlantoaxial Instability

- Areflexia
- Gait changes
- Brisk deep tendon reflexes (hyperreflexia)
- Headaches
- Heel cord tightness
- Incoordination
- Increased muscle tone
- Spasms of neck muscles
- Neck pain
- Neurogenic bladder
- Torticollis
- Scissoring gait
- Reluctance to move the neck
- Progressive myelopathy

Precautionary Measures for Atlantoaxial Instability

- Positions and activities that increase the risk of falling or of trauma to the head and neck should be avoided.
- Exercises that place excessive pressure on the head and neck (e.g., tumbling) should be avoided.
- Exaggerated neck flexion, extension, or rotation should be avoided.
- Caution must be used with joint approximation and compression of the cervical spine.
- Sports such as trampoline jumping and the butterfly stroke in swimming, as well as contact sports, are contraindicated, especially for individuals with documented atlantoaxial instability.

Medical and Surgical Management

Medical management of DS is directed toward specific medical problems (e.g., cardiac problems, infections, thyroid dysfunction) to maximize the child's health. Medical management also focuses on the previously mentioned orthopedic concerns.

Signs and symptoms of spinal cord compression resulting from AAI include changes in gait, torticollis, neck pain, or bowel and bladder incontinence. The American Academy of Pediatrics recommends a cautious sequence of evaluation and treatment when AAI is suspected.[62] The child must be at least 3 years of age to have vertebral mineralization and epiphyseal development for accurate radiographic evaluation of the cervical spine. When a child is symptomatic (e.g., neck pain, gait changes, hyperreflexia), plain cervical spine x-rays are taken in the neutral position. If there are no abnormalities when taken in neutral, measurements from lateral radiographs are taken

in flexion and extension. If abnormalities are present in neutral referral to neurosurgery is immediate.

The use of orthoses is usually successful for children with pes planus.[56] Selby-Silverstein et al.[55] found that a decrease in rear foot eversion was obtained with neutral position orthoses in children 3 to 6 years of age. Compared with children without foot orthoses, children who wore sneakers and foot orthoses showed a decrease in gait angle with greater internal (medial) rotation, which narrowed the base of support and facilitated a more neutral alignment of the hip.

Approximately 30% of children with DS develop spontaneous hip dislocation at 2 to 10 years of age.[63] The hip is retroverted with excessive external (lateral) rotation both in flexion and extension, resulting in an out-toe gait.[63] If left untreated, spontaneous habitual dislocation after age 2, chronic subluxation with acetabular dysplasia, and fixed dislocation follow. Although a standard surgical protocol has not been established, a common surgical choice is pelvic or femoral osteotomy combined with capsular plication carried out during the habitual dislocation phase.[61]

Rehabilitation Management: Evaluation, Intervention, and Clinical Implications

The general goal of rehabilitation is to maintain alignment and encourage movement promoting optimum musculoskeletal development in children with DS. Prevention of anticipated or potential malalignment in the foot and hip region and prevention of instabilities of the atlantoaxial joint are also a focus of intervention. General goals can be achieved through the use of (1) aligned compression or weight-bearing forces to stimulate bone growth longitudinally and promote thickness and density of the bone and shaft; (2) aligned, supported weight bearing to encourage joint stability and formation; and (3) facilitation of co-contraction, force production, and increased muscle tone to support joint integrity.[45]

Clinicians should always monitor the neurological status of children with documented AAI. As recommended by the American Academy of Pediatrics, children with radiological findings indicating neck instability and/or symptomatic subluxation should be surgically fused.[62] The treating clinician, however, is responsible for performing periodic neurological evaluations, paying particular attention to deterioration of gait and fine neuromotor skills and the child's development during high risk periods (e.g., after surgery or during upper respiratory tract or ear infections). Regression in the child's neuromotor skills and the onset of atypical neurological symptoms should be "red flags," and appropriate referral to the neurologist is imperative.

Parent education also is an essential part of intervention. It includes information on symptoms of neurological compromise in AAI, periods of increased risk, and activities to avoid if AAI is identified. When discussing the issues of participation in sports, clinicians should follow the recommendations of the Committee on Sports Medicine and Fitness of the American Academy of Pediatrics.[64]

Some activities may put undue stress on the cervical spine, placing the child at risk for atlantoaxial subluxation. Care must be taken when placing a child in the inverted position or in positions that increase the risk of a fall or trauma to the head. Msall et al.[65] documented developing spinal cord compression over a period of 1 year in a child with DS who received therapy that involved repetitive, vigorous head turning. Therefore exaggerated neck flexion, extension, or rotation movements and repetitive forceful twisting and turning of the head should be avoided.

Screening for scoliosis should be a routine part of life span management for children with DS. Parents should be taught to perform routine screening for scoliosis.[45] Biomechanical assessment of lower extremity and orthotic management, especially for pes planus, should be done on a regular basis. The functionality of the child's shoe can be enhanced by incorporating an orthotic device that is either prefabricated or custom-made to further limit pedal pronation.[46,56]

Promoting a more neutral alignment of the lower extremity during gait is also an intervention focus. Tripping and falling, which may result from a wide-based gait, can be reduced by improving the child's anterior-posterior stability. This can be accomplished by having the child wear high-top sneakers that extend up over the ankle and have rigid, flat soles.[46] Orthopedic assessment of the hip (Ortolani's and Barlow's maneuvers)[26] is a routine part of the clinical evaluation of an infant with DS (see volume 1 of this series, *Orthopedic Physical Assessment*, Chapter 11), and the child should be referred to an orthopedist if hip instability is suspected. Supported standing in a stander is not recommended unless hip stability and proper alignment have been established.[45]

CONGENITAL MUSCULAR TORTICOLLIS

Definition and Classification

Congenital muscular torticollis (CMT) is a postural deformity, usually detected at birth or shortly thereafter, that is caused primarily by unilateral shortening and fibrosis of the sternocleidomastoid (SCM) muscle.[66] The incidence of CMT ranges from 0.3% to 2% of newborns, but it has been reported to be as high as 16%.[67] Although CMT with impairment of the SCM muscle is the most common cause of torticollis in infants, torticollis can also be the result of other underlying disorders. The congenital and developmental causes of torticollis have been classified as osseous, nonosseous, and neurogenic.[68,69] A forceful birth delivery can cause clavicular fracture or brachial plexus injury (BPI), both of which can lead to torticollis.[70]

Pathology

A **pseudotumor** (i.e., a firm, moveable, benign mass) frequently is present in CMT. It is a firm, nontender enlargement of the muscle belly most commonly found in the middle to distal third of the sternal portion of the SCM muscle.[71,72] If the mechanism of injury involves a crush or stretch injury to the SCM muscle, the pathophysiology can include ischemia and reperfusion and possibly hematoma leading to a compartment syndrome. Over time, this can result in the development of scar tissue, leading to muscle shortening and pulling of the head into the typical position (Figure 28-12).[70] Neurological injury to the SCM muscle also is possible, in which damage to nerve fibers causes muscle fiber degeneration and fibrosis of the muscle body.[70] The typical lesion ranges in size from 1 to 3 cm (0.4 to 1.2 inches) in its largest transverse diameter.[73] However, after reaching maximum size, the mass generally recedes at varying rates within the first year, and in most children, resolves slowly over 5 to 21 months.[73,74]

Etiology, Epidemiology, and Diagnosis

The etiology of CMT remains unknown, but many theories have been proposed, including intrauterine crowding,[75,76] muscle trauma during a difficult delivery,[77,78] soft tissue compression that leads to compartment syndrome,[79] and congenital abnormalities of soft tissue differentiation within the SCM muscle.[71,80] The diagnosis usually is made during a physical examination when a palpable, firm,

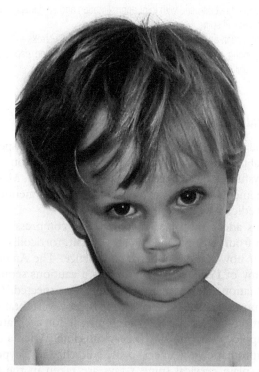

Figure 28-12 Typical appearance of right muscular torticollis in an 18-month-old boy. (From Graham JM: *Smith's recognizable patterns of human deformation*, ed 3, Philadelphia, 2007, Saunders.)

mobile mass[81] is noted in the muscle, along with abnormal head posture, restricted cervical ROM, or plagiocephaly (i.e., malformation of the skull).[66,81] Children with CMT can be assigned to one of three clinical subgroups. **Postural CMT (type 1)** is the mildest form of CMT and presents as an infant's postural preference with no muscle or passive ROM restrictions. With **muscular CMT (type 2)**, SCM muscle tightness and passive ROM restrictions are present. **Type 3 CMT** presents with a fibrotic thickening of the SCM muscle and accompanying passive ROM limitations and is the most severe form.[67,71,82–85]

Prognosis

The chance of full correction with therapy and conservative management is excellent if intervention is initiated within the first 3 months of life, and it remains high if treatment is initiated within the first year of life.[70] When conservative treatment is started before 1 month of age, 98% of children achieve near-normal ROM within 1.5 months; however, waiting until after 1 month of age prolongs intervention to 6 months, and waiting until 6 months of age increases treatment to up to 9 or 10 months.[67] The correction of facial and cranial deformities also is much more successful if the torticollis is corrected before 1 year of age.[70] About 5% of children require surgical intervention, especially if therapy is not initiated early. More invasive procedures are reserved for persistent plagiocephaly and limited ROM after 1 year of age.[70] According to Cheng et al.,[73] predictors of fair to poor outcomes include (1) the presence of a SCM tumor; (2) an initial degree of head rotation greater than 15° from neutral; and (3) age older than 1 year at the time of initial treatment.[81]

Musculoskeletal Impairments and Other Impairments

CMT is characterized by persistent cervical lateral flexion to the involved side with rotation to the opposite side, resulting in limited ROM in lateral flexion toward the uninvolved side and rotation toward the involved side (see Figure 28-12).[26,70] The child has limited muscle extensibility of the shortened and fibrosed SCM muscle and a weakened, overlengthened contralateral SCM muscle.[70] Skewed vertical and midline orientation can result and affect the child's body awareness, midline control, and protective righting reactions, as well as the development of bilateral fine and gross motor skills.[26] The incidence of developmental hip dysplasia associated with CMT is reported to be 2.5% to 17%, and it increases with severity of neck rotation restriction.[67] Secondary impairments can include compensatory cervical and thoracic scoliosis, facial asymmetry, and plagiocephaly. Plagiocephaly is reported in up to 90% of children with CMT and can occur either in conjunction with torticollis at birth or as a result of the torticollis.[85] When plagiocephaly and torticollis coexist in the newborn, limitation of the intrauterine

space is the suspected cause.[86] Plagiocephaly also can result from torticollis, because the unilateral shortening of the SCM muscle causes the infant to position the head consistently on the occiput contralateral to the tight SCM muscle while unloading the occiput on the ipsilateral side when supine. Craniofacial asymmetry also can result from torticollis.[78] These deformities include posterior displacement of the ipsilateral ear, posterior regression of the ipsilateral zygoma and forehead, mandibular deviation toward the affected side, inferior positioning of the affected eye, and deviation of the nasal tip to the affected side.[78] Functionally, the limited ROM may interfere with daily routines of dressing and positioning.[26]

Medical and Surgical Management

The initial examination should begin with a careful history to detect coexisting conditions and rule out other diagnoses, such as congenital cervical vertebral anomalies, infection, inflammation, and neoplasms.[85,87] Recommendations for the use of diagnostic procedures, such as radiographs, vary among authors. Ballock and Song[88] published a useful decision tree for differential diagnosis of young children with torticollis. Clinical practice guidelines for management of positional skull deformities in infants are available in the December 2011 issue of *Pediatrics*.[89] An ultrasound examination of the hips is often performed in the first 4 to 6 weeks of life because of the high incidence of hip dysplasia in children with CMT.

Although surgery is the most recommended treatment for residual torticollis after failure of a conservative stretching program, injections of botulinum toxin (Botox) are becoming a more common treatment.[81] Botox is thought to enhance the effectiveness of stretching on the side of the contracture and allow strengthening of overstretched, weakened muscles on the opposite side of the neck.[81] Oleszek et al.[90] reported that 74% of children had improved cervical rotation or head tilt after Botox injections after initial failure of a conservative stretching program and only 7% experienced transient adverse effects. Although initial studies are favorable, more long-term studies are needed to further examine the effectiveness, side effects, and adverse effects before it can be approved.[67]

Surgical intervention is reserved for children older than 12 months of age who have persistent torticollis and significant deformity despite conservative treatment.[70,91–96] Davids et al.[79] used a criterion of greater than 30° loss in ROM, usually with lateral flexion or significant plagiocephaly.[70] An alternative criterion reported for surgical intervention is the presence of residual deficits in rotational ROM of greater than 15° after at least 6 months of controlled manual exercises.[73,85] Surgical treatments to lengthen tight SCM muscles include unipolar release,[73,85] bipolar release,[68] endoscopic release,[97] and subperiosteal lengthening.[96] Postoperative splinting may be necessary, and PT typically is recommended.[70]

Rehabilitation Management: Evaluation, Intervention, and Clinical Implications

When examining a child diagnosed with CMT, the clinician must be aware of all possible causes and differential diagnoses. A complete history should be documented, including other significant medical information, such as the presence of hip dysplasia, type of delivery, and birth weight and length, as well as records of radiographs and previous interventions.[70] ROM should be assessed, including resting head position, active and passive cervical rotation, and lateral flexion. The primary method of estimating active ROM in young infants is through active head turning during visual tracking as the infant reaches for toys or during head righting reactions.[70,98] The **Muscle Function Scale**[99] is recommended to objectively measure active lateral flexion in infants older than 2 months. The most reliable and valid method for assessing passive cervical ROM in infants involves the use of an arthrodial protractor, as described by Cheng et al.[85] It is suggested that the normal passive range of cervical rotation is up to 110° to each side for infants.[73] Neck flexor and lateral flexor strength can be assessed during pull-to-sit and lateral head righting reactions, respectively, and documented as complete, incomplete, symmetrical, or asymmetrical (Figures 28-13 and 28-14).[70] Inspection of the neck for asymmetrical skin folds and skin condition, as well as palpation of all superficial cervical muscles, is necessary to discover the sources of abnormal head and neck posture.[66] The SCM muscle should be palpated for a lump or tightness, and its size, as well as other physical characteristics, should be documented.[70] Postural assessment should include the entire spine.[74] The hips should be evaluated for any asymmetries or dislocations.[66,70] Any facial asymmetry or plagiocephaly should be documented and described. Photographs are helpful for assessing change over time and for descriptive purposes.[70,72] In addition, pain or discomfort at rest and during active and passive movement should be assessed using the **Face, Legs, Activity, Crying and Consolability (FLACC)** scale.[67] Findings such as suspected hip dysplasia, skull or facial asymmetries, atypical presentations of CMT, abnormal tone, visual abnormalities such as nystagmus, or history of acute onset are considered red flags and warrant consultation with the primary care physician or other appropriate specialists.[67]

Gross and fine motor development should be screened for age appropriateness because underlying impairments of muscle force may be revealed in the assessment of motor skills. Motor skill development should be assessed using age-appropriate, reliable, and valid standardized tools such as the **Test of Infant Motor Performance (TIMP)**[100] through 4 months corrected age and the **Alberta Infant Motor Scale (AIMS)**[101] from 4 to 18 months of age.[67] Challenging the infant in various positions with varying resistance to gravity can reveal muscle weakness. Any problems associated with feeding should be identified and documented, and positioning for feeding should be assessed.[66] The infant should be examined for tolerance to all developmental positions, active movement in these positions, the ability to transition between positions, tolerance to handling, and infant–parent interaction. It also is important to assess family routines and the positions of the infant throughout the day and during all daily activities to plan a therapeutic positioning program.[66]

Intervention is guided by the infant's age, the severity of the torticollis, the parents' ability to perform the exercises and repositioning procedures, the diagnosis of plagiocephaly, and the presence of associated neuromuscular or orthopedic impairments.[70,102] If deformational plagiocephaly (flattening of one side of skull) or torticollis is present, the first priority is to begin an aggressive repositioning program.[66] If facial or cranial deformities are noted but have not been diagnosed, the infant and family should be referred to the pediatrician for evaluation and assessment of treatment, including a helmet, bracing, or surgery.[26]

Conservative management of infants with CMT consists of positioning, gentle ROM, and strengthening through activation of head and trunk muscles as the infant gains control of upright postures.[102,103] Goals of the clinician should include active and passive ROM of the neck and trunk within functional limits, prevention of contractures, craniofacial symmetry, age-appropriate postural reactions, gross motor development, midline head and neck control in the upright position, and family education about home therapy.[103,104]

Families should be educated in handling, stretching, and positioning techniques, as well as activities that encourage midline head and trunk control. The home exercise program of stretching, strengthening, and positioning should be simple and comfortable and should be incorporated into the daily child care routines.[70] Parents should be educated about the importance of their involvement, basic anatomy of the area, kinesiology of the SCM muscle, and avoidance of painful stretching.

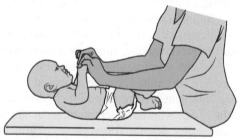

Figure 28-13 Head is kept in line with the body during pull to sit. (Redrawn from Martin S, Kessler M: *Neurological interventions for physical therapy*, ed 2, St. Louis, 2007, Elsevier.)

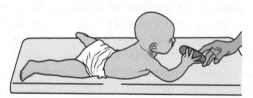

Figure 28-14 Lateral righting reaction. (Redrawn from Martin S, Kessler M: *Neurological interventions for physical therapy*, ed 2, St. Louis, 2007, Elsevier.)

They should be provided with a home program with written instructions and pictures of appropriate exercises.[70]

Manual stretching is the most common form of treatment for CMT and should be performed when the child is relaxed.[71,73,75,85,94,102] Distractors such as toys, music, or pictures can improve the child's tolerance of handling.[26] Although proper stabilization and handling are vital, the stretching program must be modified for family and child comfort to be successful. The method of stretching is determined by the severity of the torticollis, the child's age and tolerance of handling, and the parents' ability to carry out the stretching program.[103] The greatest stretch to the SCM muscle is obtained when the neck is placed in the extended position. Reported stretching protocols vary from a 1-second stretch to a 30-second stretch repeated 5 to 15 times per session and throughout the day. The commonly accepted home stretching program focuses on attaining a sustained stretch into cervical lateral (side) flexion and cervical rotation for at least 30 seconds, repeated 10 to 15 times per session, four to six times per day.[105] A combined stretch of rotating the child's head toward the involved side and tilting away from the involved side also is suggested for the same duration and frequency. Authors agree that *stretches should not be painful* and should be carried out by the parents and caregivers throughout the day.[70,81,92] If necessary, the intensity of the stretch should be reduced to prevent pain and muscle guarding.

Stretching and strengthening exercises should be consistent and age appropriate, and they should be carried out through carrying, holding, and playing with the infant in postures and positions selected to achieve the desired active and passive movements. Strengthening and active motion can be accomplished through postural reactions, visual tracking, and righting reactions as the infant matures and gains better control of the head and trunk.[70] Gravity can be used both to assist weak muscles and to increase resistance as muscles gain strength.[70]

Parents should be given instructions on activities that encourage active ROM on the involved side and facilitate strengthening of the weakened, overlengthened muscles on the opposite side. Activities could include weight-shifting on a ball or lap or using a mobile surface to help the caregiver elicit a combination of lateral cervical flexion and rotation. Another position to elicit head righting is use of the football carry, in which the child is held around the upper trunk and tilted to the side in front of a mirror.[70] The clinician and family must remember that righting reactions can be delayed or incomplete in an infant with CMT. Environmental changes, such as arranging the child's crib and changing table to promote turning of the head to look at caregivers and stimulating active head turning in response to toys or sounds, also can be effective. Towel rolls or small, soft collars can be used to prevent the child's head from falling passively into the shortened direction. Symmetrical head lifting can be encouraged by placing the infant prone on the elbows or over a small towel roll on the caregiver's chest and encouraging the infant to look up at caregiver.[26] Cervical orthoses have been used as treatment adjuncts for children whose lateral head tilt is 6° or greater at 4.5 months of age.[70] A major role of the physical therapist is to support parents and caregivers in performing the exercises, stretching protocols, and positioning.

The most commonly used collar in children with torticollis is the tubular orthosis for torticollis (TOT) collar.[95,102,106] The TOT collar is adjusted to support the neck on the impaired side in the neutral position and is worn only during waking hours. The collar is not used for children younger than 4 months of age.[102,103]

Positioning to create symmetry and prolonged stretching in varying positions provides the opportunity and incentive for the child to perform active ROM. The side-lying position can provide a prolonged cervical stretch. Also, after the child is asleep, the head can be rotated toward the tight SCM muscle by using a towel folded like a wedge to hold the head in place.[70]

Bottle- or breast-feeding can be another preferred time to stretch, and the child can be slowly moved into positions he or she normally may resist. Symmetry of the head, neck, and spine should be achieved in all positioning devices.

Guidelines for monitoring and discharge from therapy are not well defined.[73,81] The clinician should continue to follow up and reexamine, to identify any additional exercises or information that should be given to the family, and to adjust goals appropriately. The family and multidisciplinary team determine the appropriate time for reducing the intensity and frequency of therapy sessions and ultimately for discharge. Caregivers should be informed that the torticollis posture can reappear during periods of growth, illness, teething, and acquisition of new motor functions.[103] Furthermore, the involved SCM muscle may not grow at the same rate as the uninvolved side, creating another risk for the return of contracture.[75]

BRACHIAL PLEXUS INJURY

Definition and Classification

The brachial plexus is a group of nerves that includes the four lower cervical roots, C5-C8, and the first thoracic root, T1. These nerves exit through the anterior vertebral foramen and pass under the clavicle to innervate the upper extremity (Figure 28-15). Any traction of the upper extremity or distraction of the head away from the clavicle can result in a brachial plexus injury (BPI).[107]

In approximately 46% of cases, **Erb's palsy,** a condition involving the upper trunk including the C5 and C6 nerve roots, is at fault.[108] A combination injury of the upper plexus can occur, with injury to the C7 nerve root and occasionally associated damage to the phrenic nerve at the C4 nerve root, which causes ipsilateral hemiparesis of the diaphragm.[109] In about 20% of cases, the entire plexus is injured, including the C5 to T1 nerve roots.[107,109-111] In about 4% of cases, the injury is bilateral, and about 2% of cases show pure lower trunk injury, including the

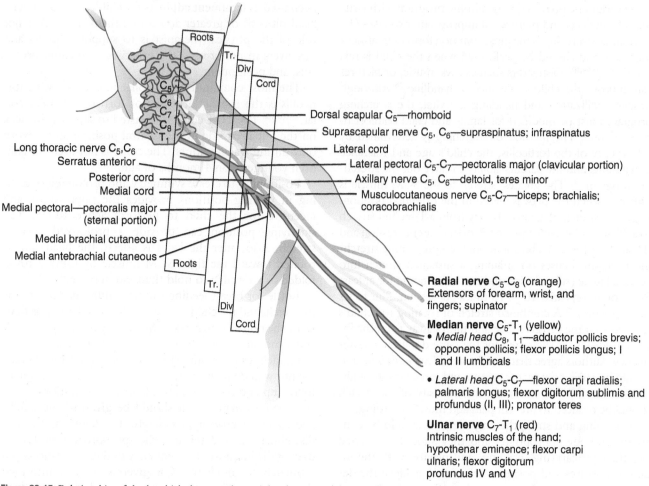

Dorsal scapular C₅—rhomboid

Suprascapular nerve C₅, C₆—supraspinatus; infraspinatus

Lateral cord

Lateral pectoral C₅-C₇—pectoralis major (clavicular portion)

Axillary nerve C₅, C₆—deltoid, teres minor

Musculocutaneous nerve C₅-C₇—biceps; brachialis; coracobrachialis

Dorsal scapular C_5—rhomboid

Long thoracic nerve C_5, C_6
Serratus anterior
Posterior cord
Medial cord
Medial pectoral—pectoralis major (sternal portion)
Medial brachial cutaneous
Medial antebrachial cutaneous

Radial nerve C_5-C_8 (orange)
Extensors of forearm, wrist, and fingers; supinator

Median nerve C_5-T_1 (yellow)
• *Medial head* C_8, T_1—adductor pollicis brevis; opponens pollicis; flexor pollicis longus; I and II lumbricals

• *Lateral head* C_5-C_7—flexor carpi radialis; palmaris longus; flexor digitorum sublimis and profundus (II, III); pronator teres

Ulnar nerve C_7-T_1 (red)
Intrinsic muscles of the hand; hypothenar eminence; flexor carpi ulnaris; flexor digitorum profundus IV and V

Figure 28-15 Relationship of the brachial plexus to the peripheral nerves of the shoulder and arm. Note the formation of the brachial plexus from nerve roots of spinal segments C5-T1. The brachial plexus is divided into roots, trunks, divisions, and cords. The origin of the peripheral nerves and their muscle innervations are listed. The median nerve has a lateral head from the lateral cord (C5, C6, C7) and a medial head from the medial cord (C8, T1). The ulnar nerve also arises from the medial cord, and the radial nerve comes directly from the posterior cord. (From Swaiman KF, Ashwal S, Ferriero DM: *Pediatric neurology: principles and practice,* ed 5, Philadelphia, 2012, Saunders.)

C8 to T1 nerve roots (i.e., **Klumpke's palsy**).[107,109–111] Narakas[112] and others have attempted to categorize this clinical continuum into four categorical groups.[111,113]

Clinical Continuum of Brachial Plexus Injury

Group 1 • Mildest clinical group
• Classic Erb's palsy with involvement of C5-C6 nerve roots
• Initial absence of shoulder abduction and lateral rotation, elbow flexion, and forearm supination

Group 2 • Group 1 impairments with involvement of C7 nerve root
• Absence of wrist and digital extension (classic "waiter's tip" posture)

Group 3 • Flail upper extremity without Horner's syndrome

Group 4 • Most severe clinical group
• Group 3 impairments with Horner's syndrome
• May have associated phrenic nerve palsy, resulting in an elevated hemidiaphragm

---

Pathology

BPI can be described as (1) neuropraxia (Sunderland I), or a stretch injury that results in a temporary nerve conduction block; (2) axonotmesis (Sunderland II-IV), or varying degrees of rupture of the neural axon in which the neural sheath remains intact but internal elements are disrupted; (3) neurotmesis (Sunderland V), or complete rupture of the axon and the encapsulating connective tissue; and (4) avulsion, in which the nerve roots tear away from the spinal cord. The nerve rootlets, mixed nerve roots, trunks, divisions, cords, and peripheral nerves all can be damaged by any of these injuries. A neuroma (a benign, often painful growth of neuron and nerve fibers arising from nervous tissue) may result from a partial or complete rupture.[107,109,110]

Etiology, Epidemiology, and Diagnosis

The incidence of brachial plexus injuries is 1.6 to 3 per 1000 live births. The different rates can be attributed to obstetric care and the average birth weight of infants in different geographical regions. [109,111,114] Numerous risk factors and other complicating factors are associated with BPI.[109] For example, upper trunk ruptures are more common with vertex delivery and dystocia involving the shoulder.[111] C5-C6 nerve root avulsions are common with breech presentations. Entire plexus involvement can result from a combination of stretching, rupture, and avulsion injuries, and this condition generally is more severe.

Risk Factors for Brachial Plexus Injury and Other Complicating Factors

- Large for gestational age
- Multiparous pregnancies
- Previous deliveries resulting in brachial plexus injury
- Prolonged labor
- Vertex delivery
- Assisted and difficult deliveries
- Maternal diabetes
- Sedated, hypotonic infant during delivery
- Shoulder dystocia
- Heavily sedated mother
- Breech delivery and difficult cesarean extraction
- Congenital anomalies (e.g., cervical rib, abnormal thoracic vertebrae, shortened scalenus anticus)

Physical examination of the muscles associated with nerves arising near the ganglion can help determine whether the lesion is preganglionic or postganglionic. A preganglionic lesion is suspected with Horner's syndrome (involvement of the sympathetic nerve chain), an elevated hemidiaphragm (involvement of the phrenic nerve), and the absence of rhomboid (dorsal scapular nerve), rotator cuff (suprascapular nerve,) and latissimus dorsi (thoracodorsal nerve) function.[111] Invasive radiographic studies with myelography, myelography plus computed tomography (CT), and magnetic resonance imaging (MRI) also have been used to distinguish between avulsion and extraforaminal ruptures.[111,115] Although these techniques may improve the quality of preoperative planning, the final diagnosis of avulsion or rupture is still made during surgery.[111] EMG and nerve conduction velocities have been used in an attempt to improve diagnostic accuracy with regard to the severity of the neural lesions.[111,112] Unfortunately, the presence of motor activity in a muscle has not been an accurate predictor of an acceptable level of motor recovery in that muscle.[111] Currently, neurophysiological studies appear to underestimate the severity of the injury and falsely provide optimism about recovery.[111]

Prognosis

It is important to determine whether the level of injury is preganglionic or postganglionic to predict the prognosis and determine the appropriate intervention.[111] Preganglionic lesions are avulsions from the cord that do not spontaneously recover. An infant with a severe avulsion injury probably will have a lifetime of disability despite extensive PT and surgical management.[111] Although recovery usually is limited after ruptures, the prognosis after axonotmesis is better because neurons reconnect more successfully through the intact neural sheath. Axon regrowth proceeds at approximately 1 mm per day, and recovery usually takes 4 to 6 months in the upper arm and 7 to 9 months in the lower arm. Recovery can continue for up to 2 years in the upper arm and up to 4 years in the lower arm.[109] Spontaneous recovery is expected over the first several months of life, and complete recovery is evident by the first year of life with neurapraxic lesions.[109]

The recovery of motor function varies greatly because of the wide variety of lesions. Furthermore, the recovery of sensation can take up to 2 years.[109] The spontaneous recovery rate for brachial plexus injuries in infants has been reported to be from 66%[116,117] to 73%.[118] The prognosis is poorer with C5-C6-C7 involvement.[111] Phrenic nerve involvement increases the likelihood of an avulsion injury and limited spontaneous recovery.[111]

Many studies have reported on the natural history of brachial plexus injuries. It is suggested that infants who recover partial antigravity upper trunk muscle strength during the first 2 months of life should show full recovery over the first 1 to 2 years of life.[108] Microsurgical reconstruction of the brachial plexus is indicated for infants who do not recover antigravity strength by 5 to 6 months of age because successful surgery results in a better outcome than natural history alone. Infants who have partial recovery of C5-C6-C7 antigravity strength at 3 to 6 months of age have permanent, progressive limitations of motion and strength.[108] These infants also are at risk for the development of joint contractures in the affected limb, which can lead to permanent functional limitations.

Musculoskeletal Impairments and Other Impairments

The most common impairments associated with Erb's palsy are paralysis of the rhomboid, levator scapulae, serratus anterior, subscapularis, deltoid, supraspinatus, infraspinatus, teres minor, biceps brachialis, brachioradialis, and supinator muscles. Therefore, the shoulder usually is held in extension, medial (internal) rotation, and adduction with elbow extension and forearm pronation. Although grasp function is intact, sensory loss usually is present.[109] If C7 is involved, impairments include paralysis of the elbow extensors and the long extensors of the wrist, fingers, and thumb, resulting in the classic "waiter's tip" posture described earlier (Figure 28-16).[109,111] Klumpke's palsy involves paralysis of the wrist flexors and extensors and the intrinsic muscles of the wrist and hand. Clinically, hand grasp is poor, although more proximal muscles are intact.[107] Total plexus injuries can be devastating. The infant presents with a clawed hand and a flail and insensate arm.[107,109] BPI frequently results in shoulder weakness,

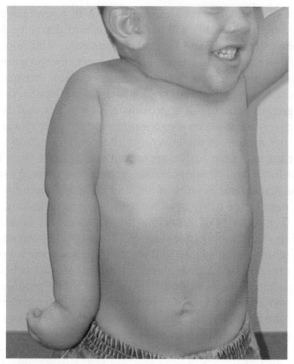

Figure 28-16 Erb's palsy caused by a birth injury. The arm position is characteristic. The arm is adducted, with the humerus internally (medially) rotated, the elbow extended, the forearm pronated, and the wrist flexed. (From Shenaq SM, Bullocks JM, Dhillon G: Management of infant brachial plexus injuries, *Clin Plast Surg* 32:79-98, 2005.)

contracture, and joint deformity. The initial trauma during labor may cause muscular or periarticular injury, leading to myostatic contracture and glenohumeral capsular and ligamentous tightness. Infantile glenohumeral dislocation occasionally occurs during birth trauma.[111]

Commonly, shoulder abduction and lateral (external) rotation weakness from failure of neuromuscular recovery, in conjunction with muscular and periarticular tightness, lead to a medial (internal) rotation and adduction contracture. Abnormal muscle substitutions, muscle imbalance, and persistence of soft tissue contracture during neural regeneration frequently result in progressive abnormal bone growth and glenohumeral joint deformity.[115,119,120] Waters[111] described five grades of deformity progressing from minimal to severe deformity (Table 28-3).

TABLE **28-3**

Five Grades of Brachial Plexus Injury[112]

Class	Description
I	Normal glenohumeral joint: <5° difference in glenoid version compared with contralateral side
II	Increased glenoid retroversion
III	Posterior glenohumeral subluxation with posterior glenoid dysplasia
IV	Development of a false glenoid
V	Flattening of the humeral head and glenoid

These glenohumeral joint deformities complicate the already limited motion, strength, and function of the upper extremity. Other common contractures of the upper extremity include scapular protraction, shoulder extension, and wrist and finger flexion. Additional complications of absent or abnormal sensation may lead to neglect, and injuries to the skin often go unnoticed.[109]

Functional limitations vary greatly, depending on the extent of the initial pathology, nerve regeneration, and resulting secondary impairments.[109] The primary functional limitations involve reaching and grasping, manipulation of objects, and bilateral hand use; all of these affect the child's participation in learning ADLs.[109] Resultant delayed motor activities may include getting into and out of positions over the involved side, protective extension using the involved side, and delayed balance reactions. Creeping may be delayed or replaced by scooting, and some children progress straight into walking at an appropriate age.[109] Significant functional limitations in hand-to-head, hand-to-mouth, and overhead activities may result from persistent shoulder weakness and contracture. As a result of fatigue, the child also may have difficulty placing and maintaining the hand at a desired location in space and therefore, may maintain the affected limb at the side and refrain from using it.[118]

Medical and Surgical Management

Management focuses on maintaining the full passive ROM of the upper extremity to prevent myostatic and periarticular contractures. A gentle home program should begin when the child is 7 to 10 days old, and a formal therapy program should follow. Abduction and lateral (external) rotation splints have been used, but compliance can be poor. Zancolli expressed concern that these splints may increase the risk of injury to the physis and developing joint.[120,121] Botox injections have been used to reduce the contracting muscle forces.[122,123] The use of splints, spica casts, electrical stimulation, and intensified therapy after Botox injection have all been advised; however, currently no evidence is available to guide the clinician on the indications for and expected outcomes of these treatments.[111]

The spectrum of nerve surgery includes neurolysis, neuroma resection with nerve grafting, and nerve transfers.[124] The most recent information suggests that neurolysis alone should be viewed as having little therapeutic benefit.[125,126] The current microsurgical standard of care is resection of the neuroma and nerve grafting in extraforaminal ruptures.[125] Sural nerve grafts are performed in upper trunk ruptures,[127] and nerve transfers in conjunction with nerve grafting are performed using the thoracic intercostals (T2-T4), with or without a band of the spinal accessory nerve (cranial nerve [CN] XI) in the case of segmental avulsions.[112,128] Nerve transfers are the only option in total plexus avulsions and may include the intercostal, spinal accessory, phrenic, cervical plexus, contralateral C7, or hypoglossal nerve.[129-135] In each microsurgical case, the plan is individualized according to the extent of injury and the available reconstructive options.[111]

Although most authors use the timing of specific motor function recovery and the absence of motor recovery as indications for surgical intervention, the timing of microsurgical intervention is very controversial. The most common criterion is the absence of return of biceps muscle function associated with total plexopathy and Horner's syndrome, or an upper trunk lesion. However, shoulder lateral (external) rotation and forearm supination have been reported to be more accurate predictors of full recovery than elbow flexion.[116] Surgical reconstruction of an avulsion is recommended before or at 3 months of age. Reconstruction of extraforaminal ruptures is performed between 3 and 9 months of age; however, the range for repairs cited in the literature is 1 to 24 months.[136,137] It has been suggested that microsurgery improves function and increases the possibility of future secondary tendon transfers that may improve the clinical situation.[111]

Ultimately, the best time for microsurgical intervention is unknown in the case of an extraforaminal rupture, and it often depends on the surgeon's bias toward timing.[111] Regardless of the timing, it is important that the parents understand that microsurgery rarely results in perfect ROM, strength, posture, and function.[111] Most children require secondary shoulder tendon transfers and possibly osteotomies to improve function.[111] Indications for surgical intervention at the shoulder include infantile dislocation, persistent medial (internal) rotation contracture, limitation of abduction and lateral (external) rotation function with plateauing of neural recovery, and progressive glenohumeral deformity.[111] Muscle releases or lengthenings and tendon transfers to improve lateral (external) rotation and abduction have very favorable outcomes when joint deformity is minimal (grades I to III).[115] Arthroscopic surgery also is an option because it allows direct visualization of the joint and assessment of the degree of deformity and soft tissue contractures. Anterior release of thickened middle and inferior glenohumeral ligaments and of the subscapularis can be performed, along with debridement of the joint. With mild deformity, posterior latissimus dorsi and teres major tendon transfers can be performed with excellent results.[111] A humeral lateral (external) rotation osteotomy can improve function when joint deformity is more severe and joint reconstruction is deemed not to be an option.[115]

In a residual C8-T1 neuropathy, an intact biceps muscle with weak or absent triceps, pronator teres, and pronator quadratus muscles can create an elbow flexion and supination deformity. Soft tissue contractures develop, leading to rotation deformities of the radius and ulna and possibly radial dislocation.[138] The biceps tendon can be treated with Z-lengthening and rerouting around the radius to convert it from a supinator to a pronator, thus improving pronation and elbow extension.[111]

Although flail hands and wrists are rare, they can be functionally and cosmetically disruptive to children and families. A flexor carpi ulnaris transfer can be performed to restore active wrist extension. Wrist fusion can provide stability to the flail wrist and improve assistive hand function.[111]

Rehabilitation Management: Evaluation, Intervention, and Clinical Implications

The clinical management of a child with BPI is determined by a multidisciplinary team. The physical therapist should be involved as early as possible and should assess baseline active and passive ROM in the involved upper extremity and cervical spine, being cautious of an insensate extremity and unstable joints. Motor function and active movement of the limb in all developmental positions should be observed and documented, whether spontaneous or facilitated, gravity assisted or gravity dependent. Active muscle contraction also can be assessed when testing reactions and reflexes, such as visual tracking, neck righting, Moro's reflex, Galant's reflex, the parachute reaction, and the hand placing reaction.[109] Asymmetrical abdominal or thoracic movement should be noted, because it may indicate phrenic nerve involvement.[109]

Developmental tests can be used to assess the achievement of developmental milestones. Active muscle strength should be assessed frequently and can be graded by several different methods, including the Medical Research Council grading system, Mallet's classification, or the Hospital for Sick Children scores.[111] In older children, standard manual muscle tests and dynamometers can be used to assess strength. Patterns of movement, abnormal substitutions and compensations, and posturing of the arm should be documented.[109] Muscle tone should be assessed and documented. Spasticity should not be present, and if found, the child should be referred to a neurologist for further examination.[109] Although sensory loss in infants is neither reliable nor sensitive, attempts should be made to identify areas of compromise. Narakas[112] developed a sensory grading system for children with BPI. Temperature, light touch, and two-point discrimination testing is possible in older children.[109] During examination procedures, video recording can be useful for demonstrating change over time.

The ideal outcome for a newborn with BPI is complete return of sensation and motor control. The goals of PT for the first few months are preventive. Achieving and maintaining full ROM, muscle extensibility, normal motor control, strength, functional bilateral activities, and developmental skills are appropriate goals over the first few years of life as neural regeneration continues. Goals should be revised between 9 and 24 months of age, because significant regeneration may no longer be occurring or the child may undergo a variety of orthopedic and neurosurgical procedures.[109] At 2 years of age, goals should include achievement of age-appropriate self-care skills (e.g., dressing and grooming using either extremity) and active participation in age-appropriate movement activities and preschool programs.[109]

The clinician should collaborate with family and caregivers in designing an effective, efficient home exercise program that includes passive ROM exercises and positioning. Home programs should be embedded into the existing daily routines of the family. Education should include the goals of the home program, risk of contractures, importance of joint integrity, precautions to prevent overstretching and joint dislocation, precautions with regard to sensory loss, and how to position the infant for all activities to maintain ROM and regain muscle strength.[109]

Promoting developmental and functional skills should be implemented early and done through therapeutic play activities, such as hand-to-mouth activities; activities that involve reaching, grasping, and manipulating objects or propping on the elbows; use of hands to midline; activities that involve rolling to each side; and bilateral hand activities. Facilitation of a normal scapulothoracic and glenohumeral relationship should be emphasized. A variety of play activities should be used to promote strengthening of weakened muscles. To develop motor control throughout the ROM, the clinician should control time to fatigue, allowing the child to be successful by initially challenging the involved extremity in a gravity neutral position. Activities should involve toys of different sizes, shapes, and textures and should incorporate hand-to-mouth movement, transfer of items from one hand to the other, weight-shifting in prone position, quadruped or sitting, creeping, and reaching for toys at various angles and distances. Constraining the opposite extremity for brief periods or occupying the opposite hand with another object can be extremely helpful in focusing and encouraging the child to use the involved extremity. Transitional movements over the involved extremity, pulling to stand using bilateral hands, challenging balance reactions while sitting on a lap or moveable surface such as a ball or bolster, and performing bilateral upper extremity activities (e.g., catching a large ball, clapping to music, or opening a jar) all are recommended activities for the child with BPI (Figure 28-17). Weight-bearing activities such as wheelbarrow walking, bear crawling, crab walking and wall push-ups are important for the development of shoulder girdle strength and stability as well as to improve proprioception and body awareness.[109]

Intermittent splinting of the wrist and fingers may be indicated to preserve tendon integrity until motor function returns. Functional electrical stimulation (FES) can be used to improve sensory awareness and ROM for functional purposes; however, research on this treatment modality is limited.[109]

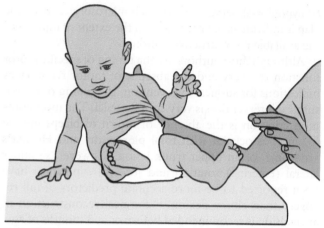

Figure 28-17 Lateral upper extremity protective reaction in response to loss of sitting balance. (Redrawn from Martin S, Kessler M: *Neurological interventions for physical therapy*, ed 2, St. Louis, 2007, Elsevier.)

MYELODYSPLASIA/SPINA BIFIDA

Definition and Classification

Spina bifida results from a neural tube defect in which the spinal column closes imperfectly. This defect can occur anywhere along the spinal column but is most common in the lower segments, where it may allow herniation of spinal membranes, nerves, and meninges. Spina bifida varies in severity with respect to motor and sensory dysfunction and can be associated with a vast number of complex medical complications. Three types of spina bifida have been described. In **spina bifida occulta,** the defect is hidden, and usually no nerve damage is involved. The only evidence of this condition on physical examination may be a tuft of hair or a dimple on the skin overlying the area of the lesion. This is the least severe form of spina bifida, and frequently no evidence of any spinal dysfunction is seen; however, progressive neurological deterioration may become apparent later in childhood or adulthood.[139]

The second form of spina bifida, a **meningocele,** is a skin-covered lesion that protrudes through the spinal defect and usually contains nonfunctional nerves, meninges, and spinal fluid. Meningoceles are not usually associated with paralysis, although some individuals may suffer from minor disabilities and progressive neurological dysfunction later in life.[139-141]

The third type of spina bifida is **myelomeningocele,** which is an open spinal cord defect associated with nerve paralysis and severe disabilities (Figures 28-18 and 28-19). Spinal fluid, nerves, and meninges herniate through the spinal column defect. The extent to which neural elements are involved in the lesion and the level of the spinal column where the lesion occurs determine the clinical severity of motor and sensory deficits, which can vary from asymptomatic to severe.[140]

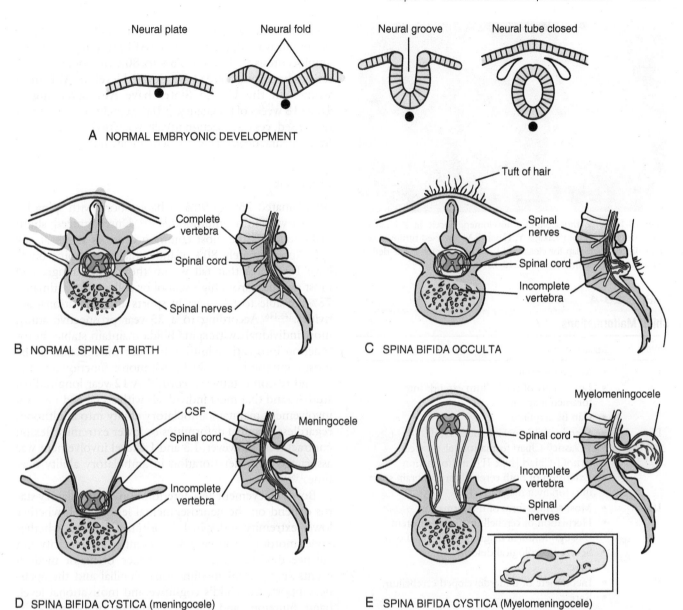

Figure 28-18 Type of spina bifida. **A,** Normal formation of the neural tube during the first month of gestation. **B,** Complete closure with normal development in cross section (*left*) and in longitudinal section (*right*). **C,** Incomplete vertebral closure with no cyst, marked by a tuft of hair. **D,** Incomplete vertebral closure with a cyst of meninges and cerebrospinal fluid (CSF); this is called a *meningocele*. **E,** Incomplete vertebral closure with a cyst containing a malformed spinal cord; this is known as a *myelomeningocele*. (From Martin S, Kessler M: *Neurologic interventions for physical therapy,* ed 2, p 156, St. Louis, 2007, Saunders.)

Pathology

Spina bifida lesions can occur at two different stages in central nervous system (CNS) development: neurulation and canalization. **Neurulation** is the process by which the neuroectoderm cells of the neural plate fold to form the neural tube, which extends from the hindbrain to S2 and gives rise to the CNS. Neurulation begins at the spinal cord level of C1 and progresses simultaneously in both the cephalad and caudal directions until completion by day 28 of gestation.[139] Because the neural tube defect can occur at any location during formation, spina bifida often is associated with other CNS malformations, such as hydrocephalus, Arnold-Chiari type II malformation (a congenital herniation of brain stem and lower cerebellum through foramen magnum into cervical vertebral canal) (Table 28-4), cognitive impairments, and cranial nerve palsies. **Canalization,** the second stage in which spina bifida can develop, is the process by which mesodermal cells distal to the S2 vertebra join to form multiple canals that ultimately fuse and join to the distal end of the spinal cord. Failure of proper canalization can result in skin-covered meningoceles, lipomas, and myelocystoceles, which frequently develop caudal to L3.[139]

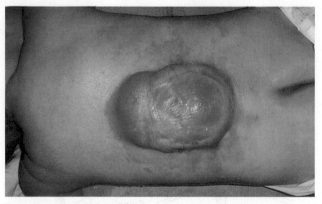

Figure 28-19 Large thoracolumbar myelomeningocele in a 2-day-old female newborn. (From Zakaria Y, Hasan EA: Reversed turnover latissimus dorsi muscle flap for closure of large myelomeningocele defects, *J Plast Reconstr Aesthet Surg* 63: 1513-1518, 2010.)

TABLE **28-4**

Chiari Malformations

Type	Description
I	• Most common • Lower part of cerebellum extends into foramen magnum • Can be acquired
II	• Seen in children with spinal bifida • "Classic" Chiari formation (also called Arnold-Chiari [type II]) malformation • Extension of both cerebellum and brain stem into foramen magnum
III	• Most serious form of malformation • Herniation of cerebellum and brain stem through foramen magnum into spinal cord • Severe neurological defects • Rare
IV	• Incomplete or underdeveloped cerebellum • Rare

Etiology, Epidemiology, and Diagnosis

The etiology of improper canalization is unknown; however, improper neurulation commonly is attributed to a combination of genetics and environmental effects.[139,140] In the United States the risk of neural tube defect in siblings is 2% to 3%.[139,142] Folic acid deficiency, which occurs with maternal alcohol consumption, use of valproic acid, and poor nutrition are associated with an increased risk of myelomeningocele in the developing offspring.[139,140] According to current birth defect surveillance data, 1500 babies are born each year with spina bifida in the United States.[143] Adequate folic acid supplementation during pregnancy could theoretically prevent 50% to 75% of these cases. Women are advised to take 0.4 mg of folic acid per day 3 months before conception and during pregnancy.[139,144] Racial and regional differences are seen in the incidence of spina bifida in the United States.[139]

Spina bifida can be diagnosed prenatally through the use of ultrasound, α-fetoprotein (AFP) serum testing, and amniocentesis.[145] Because 75% to 80% of women whose fetuses have spina bifida have elevated levels of AFP, most women in the United States have AFP screening at 16 to 18 weeks of pregnancy.[145] If the condition is positively diagnosed, cesarean section usually is advised to protect the fragile neural defect from further damage during birth.

Prognosis

An estimated 75% to 90% of babies born with spina bifida survive into adulthood.[145,146] Unrecognized shunt malfunction is the most common cause of death at any age. Approximately 80% of individuals with spina bifida have IQ scores that fall within the average range, and most graduate from high school or college. An estimated 75% are able to take part in sports and recreational activities.[145,146] According to a 25-year prospective study, most individuals with spina bifida maintain stable motor function into early adulthood; shunt malfunction is the most common reason for loss of motor function and the second reason is tethered cord.[146] A 12-year longitudinal study found that most individuals with sacral and L5 level involvement maintain ambulatory ability into adulthood, regardless of spinal deformities or lower extremity flexion contractures. However, L3 and L4 level involvement was associated with deterioration in ambulatory ability over time.[146-148]

Both achievement and deterioration of ambulatory status depend on the neurosegmental lesion level, whether lower extremity and spinal deformities develop, whether upper motor neuron signs are present (e.g., spasticity and balance dysfunction), the occurrence of major medical events (e.g., shunt malfunction), familial and therapeutic support, the child's cognitive and motivational level, hand function, and the development of obesity.[147-154] Medical complications of depression, visual impairments, severe renal disease, obesity, hypertension, and pressure sores all increase with age.[146]

Musculoskeletal Impairments and Other Impairments

Myelomeningocele is associated with numerous musculoskeletal impairments. Table 28-5 presents frequently occurring lower extremity deformities, joint contractures, and postural deviations associated with the lesion level.[139] These complex orthopedic impairments can complicate positioning, energy expenditure, independence with mobility and ADLs, and self-esteem. Factors that contribute to these musculoskeletal impairments include intrauterine positioning, lack of voluntary motor control, impaired or absent sensation and proprioception, coexisting congenital malformations, habitual abnormal posture, weight-bearing and positional deforming forces, muscle imbalance, spasticity, and progressive neurological

TABLE 28-5

Musculoskeletal Impairments Commonly Associated with Meningocele and Myelomeningocele Spina Bifida Lesions

Lesion Level	Lower Extremity Deformities and Joint Contractures	Postural Deviation
High-level lesion (thoracic to L2)	Lateral tibial torsion Knee varus and valgus Knee flexion contractures Ankle plantar flexion contractures	Increased lumbar lordosis
Middle to low-level lumbar lesion (L3-L5)	Hip flexion contractures Knee flexion contractures Genu valgus Calcaneal valgus Pronation of the foot on weight bearing	Increased lumbar lordosis
Low-level lesion (sacral)	Mild hip flexion contractures Mild knee flexion contractures Ankle and foot—either varus combined with pronated forefoot or valgus combined with supinated forefoot	Increased lumbar lordosis

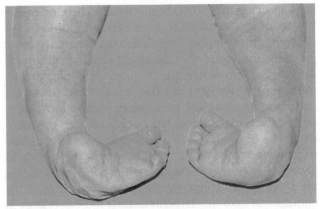

Figure 28-20 Infant with bilateral clubfeet demonstrates the deformities that are part of clubfeet. Note the hyperextension and incurving of the feet. (From Moore KL, Persaud TVN, Torchia MG: *The developing human*, ed 9, Philadelphia, 2013, Saunders. Courtesy of Dr. A.E. Chudley, Section of Genetics and Metabolism, Department of Pediatrics and Child Health, Children's Hospital and University of Manitoba, Winnipeg, Manitoba, Canada.)

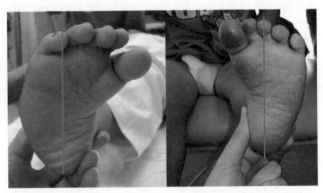

Figure 28-21 Metatarsus adductus; severe *(left)* and mild *(right)*. (From Evans AM: *Pocket podiatry: paediatrics*, Edinburgh, 2010, Churchill Livingstone.)

dysfunction.[139,155,156] Although musculoskeletal disability varies considerably, the level of the lesion can be used to anticipate future impairments and guide interventions to prevent secondary complications.[139,157,158]

Several foot deformities can occur in the various myelomeningocele levels, including ankle equinovarus or clubfoot, forefoot varus or valgus, forefoot supination or pronation, calcaneal varus or valgus, pes cavus or planus, and claw-toe deformities (Figures 28-20 and 28-21).[139,145,156] The most common contracture of the foot and ankle occurs in the ankle plantar flexors.[139,156] Foot and ankle deformities can greatly affect sitting, standing posture, balance, mobility, and shoe fit; therefore proper alignment and plantigrade foot position (walking on sole of foot with heel touching ground) are priorities, regardless of ambulatory status.

The most common knee joint impairment is knee flexion contracture, which occurs most often in children with myelomeningocele of high lumbar or thoracolumbar neurosegmental levels.[148] Knee flexion contractures are observed across all lesion levels and can result from hamstring spasticity, prolonged positioning, and adaptive shortening of muscles secondary to a crouched standing posture and gait.[139,148] Knee extension contractures are also likely, especially after a period of immobilization resulting from surgery or a fracture. According to Shurtleff,[156] knee joint contractures increase in frequency

and severity in all lesion levels from early childhood into adolescence. Genu varus and valgus deformities are also found, along with lateral (external) tibial torsion.

Hip deformities are common and include flexion and extension contractures, subluxation and dislocation, and torsional deformities of anteversion and retroversion. Many individuals with high lumbar lesions experience hip deformities as a result of the unopposed voluntary muscle activity of the hip flexors and adductors.[159] Hip flexion and adduction contractures increase the risk of hip subluxation or dislocation.[148,160] The frequency and severity of hip contractures reportedly is lower with low level lesions.[156]

Spinal deformities, such as scoliosis, kyphosis, and hyperlordosis, also are frequently associated with myelomeningocele. Scoliosis deformities may be congenital (secondary to vertebral anomalies) or acquired (secondary to muscle imbalances and positional deforming forces).[155] According to Trivedi et al.,[161] the prevalence of scoliosis is as high as 90% in children with myelomeningocele, and approximately half of the spinal curves develop before 9 years of age. Scoliosis is more frequently observed in children with a higher level lesion and becomes more prevalent and severe with increasing age in all groups.[155] Trivedi et al.[161] reported that the most useful early predictor of the development of scoliosis is the level of the last posterior arch; thoracic level lesions lead to scoliosis in 89% of cases, high lumbar lesions (L1-L3) lead to scoliosis in 44% of cases, and low lumbar lesions (L4-L5) lead to scoliosis in 12% of cases. Kyphosis may be an isolated abnormality or may occur in conjunction with scoliosis; it may be limited to the lumbar spine or may involve the entire spinal column. Hyperlordosis is more prevalent in higher level lesions of myelomeningocele.

Two of the most obvious primary impairments are motor paralysis and abnormal or complete loss of sensation, especially of proprioception and kinesthetic awareness. The lower extremities are most affected; however, motor weakness in the upper extremities can occur and often is a sign of progressive neurological dysfunction. Osteopenia and the risk of fracture are increased in the lower extremities because of the decreased active muscle contraction forces through the long bones.[139] Sensory loss, which may not correlate with motor level involvement, also is common in the lower extremities, and lack of protective sensation often leads to skin breakdown. According to Shurtleff,[142] by young adulthood, 85% to 95% of children will have had decubitus ulcers or other skin breakdown from tissue ischemia caused by excessive pressure, casts or orthoses, urine and stool soiling, friction and shear forces, and excessive weight bearing over bony prominences.

Many authors have confirmed the presence of abnormal sensory function related to proprioceptive and kinesthetic awareness deficits, which preferentially affect the upper extremity. Fine motor skills are impeded by slowness and inadequate adjustments of manipulative forces, and postural sway is affected by abnormal body position sense, possibly resulting from cerebellar ataxia, motor cortex or pyramidal tract damage, or motor learning deficits.[139,162–165] The motor level is defined as the lowest intact functional neuromuscular segment. Criteria for establishing motor levels were developed by the International Myelodysplasia Study Group using MMT.[139] Sensory levels do not consistently correlate with motor levels; therefore testing of dermatomes is imperative for light touch, pinprick, and vibration sense.[139,166]

Many other impairments or complications are associated with myelomeningocele. About 25% of children with myelomeningocele are born with hydrocephalus, with an additional 60% developing it after surgical closure of their back lesion.[139] From 80% to 90% of children with hydrocephalus require some form of central spinal fluid diversion (Figures 28-22 and 28-23). Shunt malfunction is a common complication caused by mechanical problems or infection, and as Caldarelli et al.[167] reported, almost half of children with myelomeningocele require a shunt

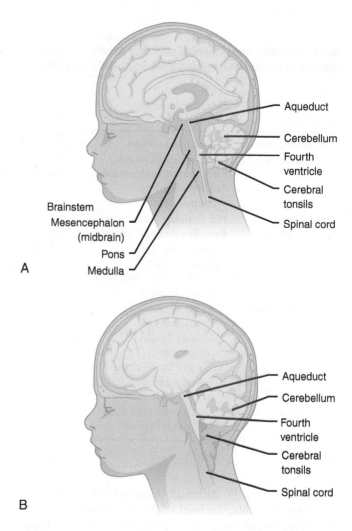

Figure 28-22 A, Normal brain with cerebrospinal fluid (CSF) circulation. **B,** Arnold-Chiari type II malformation with enlarged ventricles; this condition predisposes a child with myelomeningocele to hydrocephalus. The brain stem, the fourth ventricle, part of the cerebellum, and the cerebral tonsils are displaced downward through the foramen magnum, which leads to blockage of CSF flow. Also, pressure on the brain stem, which houses the cranial nerves, may result in nerve palsies. (From Goodman CC, Fuller KS: *Pathology: implications for the physical therapist,* ed 4, St. Louis, 2015, Saunders.)

revision in the first year of life. Early symptoms of shunt complications related to increased intracranial pressure include alterations in the level of consciousness, restlessness, irritability, headache, respiratory changes, fever, and abdominal pain.[145]

Hydrocephalus frequently is associated with Arnold-Chiari type II malformation, characterized by a descent of the cerebellar vermis, fourth ventricle, and brain stem into the cervical spine.[145,167,168] Arnold-Chiari type II malformation is associated with multiple anomalies and may cause depressed respiratory drive (including apneic attacks), caudal cranial nerve palsies, or tetraparesis in the newborn. More often, symptoms arise in infants and children in the form of central apnea, cyanosis, bradycardia, dysphagia, nystagmus, stridor, vocal cord paralysis,

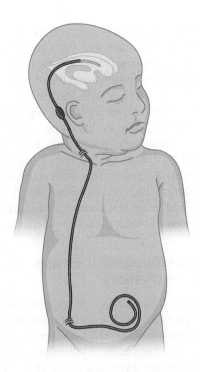

Figure 28-23 Ventriculoperitoneal shunt provides primary drainage of cerebrospinal fluid from the ventricles to an extracranial compartment, usually either the heart or the abdominal or peritoneal cavity, as shown. Extra tubing is left in the extracranial site to uncoil as the child grows. A unidirectional valve designed to open at a predetermined intraventricular pressure and to close when the pressure falls below that level prevents backflow of fluid. (From Goodman CC, Fuller KS: *Pathology: implications for the physical therapist,* ed 4, St. Louis, 2015, Saunders.)

torticollis, opisthotonus (severe muscle spasm), hypotonia, and upper extremity weakness or spasticity.[168–170] Hydromyelia is a complication with symptoms of rapidly progressive scoliosis, weakness of the upper extremities, spasticity, and ascending motor strength changes in the lower extremities.[145]

According to Wagner et al.,[169] tethered cord syndrome results from traction of the cauda equina and occurs in approximately one third of individuals with myelomeningocele. It most commonly presents with progressive scoliosis, gait changes, spasticity, or pain; less commonly, back pain, weakness, contractures of the lower extremities, or changes in bladder function may herald tethered cord syndrome.[146,171] Seizures secondary to brain malformation, cerebrospinal fluid (CSF) shunt malfunction or infection, and residual brain damage from a previous shunt infection or malfunction occur in 10% to 30% of children and adolescents with myelomeningocele.[139]

Other complications include bladder and bowel control difficulties caused by partial or complete denervation of S2 to S4. These complications, which may result from spinal cord tethering, lead to neurogenic bladder.[139,145] Fewer than 5% of children with myelomeningocele develop voluntary control of the urinary or anal sphincter.[139] Urinary tract infections are a common problem.[145]

In a study by Yeates et al.,[172] 50% of individuals with spina bifida had patterns of strengths and difficulties consistent with nonverbal learning disabilities. Dennis and Barnes[173] reported that alterations in functional numeracy, which is predictive of higher social, personal, and community independence, were directly related to the number of shunt revisions. Latex allergies, which are thought to arise from repeated exposure and contact with latex products during both diagnostic and therapeutic interventions, occur in up to 73% of children and adolescents with spina bifida.[145,148,174] Finally, 50% or more of children with spina bifida age 6 years or older are overweight, and more than half of their adolescent and adult counterparts are obese.[145] Obesity leads to the recurrence of spinal deformities, hip and knee flexion contractures, and numerous health problems, including hypertension, skin infections, pressure sores, respiratory disease, heart disease, diabetes, impaired mobility, poor performance of ADLs, and decreased self-esteem.

Medical and Surgical Management

The primary neurosurgical intervention is repair of the open neural tube defect, usually within 48 to 72 hours after birth. The treatment goals are elimination of CSF leakage, preservation of neural function, and prevention of infection and secondary tethering of the spinal cord.[169] In utero repair aims to improve the functional outcome by reducing the exposure of nervous tissue to the amniotic environment and allowing nerve repair to proceed.[149] Two benefits of in utero repair have been found: a reduced need for shunt placement as a result of a reduced incidence of hydrocephalus and reduced or even prenatal reversal of hindbrain herniation.[167,175] Fetal surgery remains controversial because of the high risks to the mother and fetus, and it has not yielded improvements in lower extremity function compared with postnatal closure.[149] Most babies with myelomeningocele are either born with hydrocephalus or develop ventriculomegaly soon after the neural tube defect is repaired. These children undergo ventriculoperitoneal shunting to manage excess CSF accumulation in the ventricles of the brain.[176]

Arnold-Chiari type II malformation, which usually is associated with hydrocephalus, is a significant cause of death and disability for individuals with myelomeningocele; therefore early detection and appropriate management are imperative. Before surgical intervention, the shunt must be evaluated for malfunction, because this may provoke or worsen a Arnold-Chiari malformation.[167] According to Griebel et al.,[177] surgical decompression of the Arnold-Chiari malformation has shown benefit in reducing upper and lower limb spasticity.

Although a goal of myelomeningocele repair is to prevent secondary tethering of the spinal cord, one third of individuals develop symptomatic spinal cord tethering.[169] Phuong et al.[178] reported that the progression of symptoms related to cord tethering was insidious; no effective method is available to prevent retethering, and 90% of individuals eventually undergo surgery to treat recurrent symptoms.[169,178] The surgical goal is to untether the spinal cord by dissecting the encasing arachnoidal adhesions.[169,179]

Most surgeons agree that no intervention is necessary for an individual with myelomeningocele with bilateral hip dislocations; however, whether to intervene with unilateral hip dislocation remains controversial.[149,155] In studying hip dislocation and its relation to functional gait, Gabrieli et al.[180] reported that gait symmetry corresponded to the absence of hip contractures or bilateral symmetrical contractures but showed no relation to the presence of hip dislocation. These authors recommended addressing gait asymmetry by reducing soft tissue contractures rather than by surgically reducing unilateral hip dislocation.[152,180] In contrast, Lorente Moltó and Garrido[150] reported that iliopsoas posterolateral transfer performed on subluxed or dislocated hips was effective in obtaining hip stability in properly selected children with a lesion at level L3. Mayfield[155] stated that a level pelvis and good ROM were more important for function than hip reduction. Furthermore, surgery might be indicated for an individual with a lesion at level L3 or lower if quadriceps function is present and the potential exists for ambulation into adulthood.[139]

Surgical release of hip flexion contractures is frequently required.[160] Complete posterior release and posterior knee capsulotomies often are recommended for individuals with knee flexion contractures of 20° or more. For both knee and hip procedures, upright standing in the early postoperative period and limited immobilization time are recommended for successful outcomes. Knee flexion contractures do recur, usually because of inadequate bracing, postoperative fractures, lack of postoperative PT, obesity, or poor motivation to stand and walk.[181]

Derotational osteotomies for excessive lateral (external) tibial torsion also have been studied. Vankoski et al.[182] reported that children with lateral tibial torsion greater than 20° who failed to exhibit improved knee extension and extension moments in AFOs might benefit from derotational osteotomies.[183]

Numerous foot deformities can occur with all levels of myelomeningocele, leading to an array of surgical corrective procedures. Clubfoot is a deformity consisting of equinus, hindfoot varus, forefoot adductus, and cavus.[183] Treatment of clubfoot in children with myelomeningocele is somewhat controversial and has traditionally consisted of soft tissue release surgery; however, some authors have used the Ponseti serial casting method with good results.[183] Hindfoot valgus is commonly found in low-level myelomeningocele. Medial displacement osteotomy of the calcaneus was reported to be successful in preserving subtalar motion.[184] This procedure is indicated for children with severe hindfoot valgus, associated pain, ulceration, and difficulty wearing a brace.

Surgical treatment is recommended for severe scoliosis. The ideal minimum age for spinal fusion is 10 to 11 years old in girls and 12 to 13 years old in boys.[139,155] Several authors recommend combined anterior and posterior spinal fusion, each with instrumentation for individuals with thoracic level lesions.[148] Nutritional support, use of antibiotics, early mobilization, use of a brace for 1 year, and family education have been stressed.[148,185] The surgical procedure performed to reduce kyphosis is a **kyphectomy.** A kyphectomy with transverse fixation is recommended to improve stability.[149,186] A thorough assessment of the individual's status, including body weight and indications of osteopenia, should also be done.[187]

Rehabilitation Management: Evaluation, Intervention, and Clinical Implications

A child with myelomeningocele requires interdisciplinary care, and special consideration should be given to coordinating goals for the child and providing consistent information to the family. Evaluation and intervention should focus on enhancement of the child's development through management and reduction of impairments and maximization of the child's future functional potential through anticipation of secondary impairments.

After a complete history is obtained, the newborn should be evaluated for motor and sensory function before and after closure of the neural tube defect. This baseline information provides a foundation for planning and prioritizing interventions and family education, anticipating future functional potential and needs, and establishing the newborn's neurological status in order to monitor any changes. The newborn should be examined in the side-lying position to prevent further injury to the lesion.[188] The infant should be in a quiet state when light touch and pinprick sensation are tested, and the testing should begin at the lowest level of sacral innervation and progress to higher levels until a response is elicited. Both deep tendon reflexes and primary reflexes should be examined.

Motor function testing should be done while the infant is in an alert state; these results can be documented as present, weak, or absent. Techniques to elicit voluntary movement include placing the extremity in a gravity-dependent position to see whether the newborn holds the position; placing the extremity in an end-range position to see whether the newborn moves out of the position; tickling; or using a variety of toys to prompt the newborn to move in response to auditory or visual stimuli. Knowledge of motor function can help the clinician predict habitual positioning and joint contractures that may not reduce spontaneously because of decreased active muscle contraction.

The newborn's bilateral upper and lower extremity ROM should be assessed, and the examiner should keep in mind that the observed degree of flexion may be greater than the expected physiological flexion secondary to intrauterine positioning and decreased voluntary movement in the womb. Paralyzed limbs should be moved delicately to prevent factures. Hip adduction should be assessed in the neutral position to prevent hip dislocation or subluxation of an unstable hip.

Baseline muscle tone should be assessed bilaterally in the upper and lower extremities of the newborn. Hypotonia throughout the body is common in neurogenic forms of spina bifida, especially in the neck and trunk; however, hypotonia or hypertonia can be found in the limbs as well. Early bilateral examination of the hips and feet should be performed, because hip and foot deformities are common.

Families should be educated in the handling and positioning of the newborn after closure of the neural tube. They also should be given verbal and written instructions on appropriate ROM, stretching, and soft tissue mobilization techniques, as well as initial developmental activities to facilitate head and trunk control.

During infancy, clinicians should continue to monitor joint alignment, muscle imbalance, and the development of joint contractures. Hip and knee flexion contractures are typical and can be combined with lateral (external) rotation at the hips, especially when hip muscles are very weak or absent. It is imperative to monitor ROM and muscle extensibility closely and to initiate stretching exercises early, with the goal of achieving and maintaining full ROM throughout the lower extremities. Fine and gross motor development should be assessed continually, and intervention should be provided to keep pace with the normal timing of development.[139] Standardized tools, that document attainment of motor skills can be used to monitor acquisition of skills. However, children with spina bifida (unless at a very low level) will not attain gross motor developmental milestones as would be expected. Thus it is important to document functional mobility rather than attainment of milestones. Documenting development in other areas such as cognition, language, and fine motor skills is appropriate using standardized tools. Although motor skills may be delayed because of multiple impairments, infants with spina bifida should be given frequent opportunities to explore the environment to enhance their future motor development. Visual tracking, deep tendon reflexes, and primitive reflexes should also be evaluated.

Muscle strength should be noted in relation to the infant's function, and specific muscle groups can be palpated for contraction while resistance is given in various developmental positions. If an orthosis is indicated to maintain muscle extensibility and joint alignment or to provide stability, the fit of the orthosis should be monitored closely to prevent skin breakdown. The clinician should continue to watch for behavioral changes, a decrease in function, irritability, and other subtle signs of shunt dysfunction.

Along with family education on strategies to challenge their infant's development of upright posture, additional head and trunk support may be necessary using positioning devices to maintain neutral alignment. Assessment of the need for any adaptive equipment should be ongoing. Families should be educated on sensation deficits and instructed to perform regular skin inspection. The family should be taught numerous activities to promote mobility to enhance the infant's development of initiative and independence.[139,188] For children who may not walk as their primary means of mobility, introducing power mobility is critical for environmental exploration, socialization, and independence.[189] Introducing power mobility at about 7 to 12 months of age may be appropriate for children with average cognition.[189,190]

At the toddler through preschool age, joint alignment, muscle imbalance, habitual positioning, contractures, posture, and signs of progressive neurological dysfunction warrant continued monitoring. If a child continues to have limitations in ROM, joint contractures may respond to stretching, and orthoses or positioning splints may be used to maintain alignment.[139] More fixed contractures may respond to serial casting but often require surgical intervention.

Functional muscle testing techniques are useful for assessing strength; these include heel and toe walking, climbing up and down steps, one-legged stance, toe touching, squat to stand, bridging, bicycling while supine, prone kicking, wheelbarrow walking, sit-ups, pull to sit, and standing push-ups.[191] Light touch and position sense can be assessed by eliciting a tickling response or by having the child point to where the examiner or a toy touched him or her.

Assessment of fine and gross motor development should continue, both informally and formally. Table 28-6 lists the typical ambulation prognosis for children based on the level of lesion. Photographs and videos can be helpful for documenting progress over time.

The level of independence in ADLs and mobility should be assessed and appropriate adaptations provided where necessary. If independent mobility is not achieved within the first year, an alternative means must be considered for independence in the home and short distances in the community. A caster cart, Dani stander with wheels,

TABLE **28-6**

Ambulation Potential for Children with Meningomyelocele

Level	Ambulation
High lumbar–thoracic	Early childhood: short distances with long leg braces Adolescents: primarily wheelchair user
Low lumbar	Walk with short leg orthosis and forearm crutches
High sacral	Walk with ankle–foot orthosis and a gluteal lurch

or power or manual wheelchair are all options to consider. Butler et al.[192] reported power drive wheelchairs to be beneficial for children as young as 24 months. More recently, Lynch et al.[190] reported that children as young as 7 months can learn to drive a power drive adapted car, providing increased opportunities for environmental exploration, cognitive development, and socialization. The toddler should learn how to be independent in skin inspection, pressure relief, and joint protection. Creative play activities that promote strengthening and upright posture can involve the entire family. Independence, efficiency, and effectiveness in ADLs should be encouraged throughout preschool.

The need for orthotics to assist with independent standing and walking should be assessed once a child begins to pull to stand. Numerous benefits of encouraging a child with myelomeningocele to walk early include fewer fractures, fewer pressure sores, and greater independence.[157,193] Because bone and joint deformities can develop as a result of unbalanced or abnormal forces, protective stabilization of the lower limb often is required. Orthoses can prevent bone and joint deformities and provide greater independence.[194] Most orthoses for children with myelomeningocele are custom-made AFOs, which are either floor reaction or posterior solid AFOs. Floor reaction AFOs are particularly beneficial because they provide a knee extension force at anterior proximal tibias and a toe lever footplate, which restricts dorsiflexion.[194] Duffy et al.[195] evaluated the effect of AFOs on gait and energy expenditure in children with L4-S1 neurosegmental level conditions and reported that the use of AFOs improved walking speed, stride length, hip flexion at heel strike, oxygen cost, and ankle power generation.

The impact of sensory deficits on functional performance must be kept in mind during gait training and functional tasks. Skin irritation, most common around the medial and lateral malleoli, is reported to be one of the biggest problems associated with unsuccessful use of orthoses.[194] Biped ambulation is feasible for toddlers and preschoolers with a lesion at level L3 and below. When working on upright standing and walking, it is essential that the clinicians maintain ROM and upright posture to evenly distribute weight-bearing forces. Upper limb support may be necessary, and a reverse walker is advised when the child is first learning to stand and walk because it minimizes upper extremity weight bearing and facilitates postural alignment.[196] Once upright gait is established, the child can transition to the use of forearm crutches. Moore et al.[197] evaluated the energy expenditure of reciprocal versus swing-through gait in adolescents with low lumbar myelomeningocele. They found no difference in the rate of oxygen consumption; however, the walking velocity was slower and the oxygen cost was higher for the reciprocal gait pattern. These researchers concluded that the swing-through gait pattern

is more energy efficient and faster than the reciprocal gait pattern.[197]

Children with L5-S1 lesions often abandon upper limb aids when they are young. However, these aids may be necessary, even as the child gets older, for endurance activities and to reduce trunk sway and joint stress for longer distances or rough terrain. Bare et al.[198] concluded that a hip abductor strengthening program to reduce compensatory trunk and pelvic motion may enable a more energy-efficient gait for children with sacral level involvement.[194]

For children with higher level lesions, emphasis should be on preparatory activities for wheelchair mobility, including sitting balance, transfer training, wheelchair propulsion, electrical switch operation, and safety. Children with lesions at the thoracic to L2 levels may use a parapodium, HKAFO, KAFO, or reciprocating gait orthosis for household distance ambulation (Figure 28-24). These orthoses typically require a high energy expenditure; therefore wheelchairs are commonly used for community mobility. When evaluating and teaching functional gait, the clinician must keep in mind that symmetrical alignment of the trunk and extremities is important and extreme ranges of motion, as well as a couch posture, should be avoided. Shoes with nonskid soles for improved traction and long distance capabilities should be considered.

Motor and sensory function should be assessed continually. Education in bowel and bladder management should be provided if necessary, and clinicians must be aware of methods used for bowel and bladder emptying as they relate to toileting, transfer techniques, and orthoses so that assistive devices do not interfere with effective performance. Clinicians must continually assess for signs and symptoms of shunt malfunction and postural deficits of scoliosis and kyphosis. Orthotic intervention for scoliosis and kyphosis may be helpful in maintaining improved trunk position for function; however, it may not prevent progression and sometimes may worsen skin ulcers.[139,188,194] Severe postural deficits can limit chest wall expansion and result in restricted lung ventilation and frequent respiratory infections, which can limit exercise tolerance and also can be life threatening.[139]

Clinicians must be aware of the secondary impairments of upper extremity deformities that result from overuse. Restricted shoulder girdle motion, carpal tunnel syndrome, and pain are common secondary impairments that can be reduced by proper joint alignment, proper fitting of assistive devices, and energy-efficient propulsion mechanisms.[139] Activities emphasizing position sense and body awareness can improve upper extremity coordination. Clinicians should educate families on how to create latex-free environments, and they should provide latex-free environments in the clinic to prevent anaphylactic reactions caused by common latex allergies.

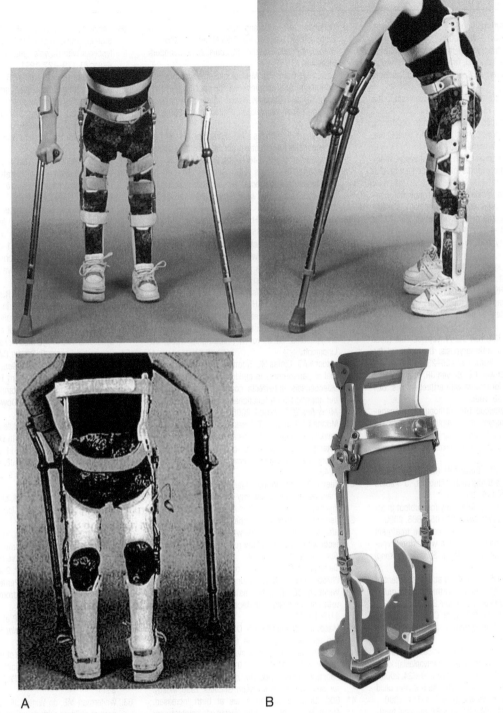

A   B

Figure 28-24 A, Hip guidance orthosis. **B,** Reciprocating gait orthosis (RGO). (**A** from Nawoczenski DA, Epler ME: *Orthotics in functional rehabilitation of the lower limb,* Philadelphia, 1997, Saunders. **B** courtesy Center for Orthotic Design, Redwood City, California.)

SUMMARY

Numerous developmental disabilities have musculoskeletal involvement requiring the consistent and combined efforts of an interdisciplinary team that includes the family and the child. The mainstays of therapeutic management are the promotion and maintenance of joint integrity and ROM, enhancement of functional motor skills, and facilitation of strength and postural control. Prevention of secondary complications and family education and empowerment are essential aspects of intervention of a child with a developmental disability.

REFERENCES

1. O'Flaherty P: Arthrogryposis multiplex congenita, *Neonatal Netw* 20:13–20, 2001.

2. Donohoe M: Arthrogryposis multiplex congenita. In Campbell SK, Palisano RJ, Orlin M, editors: *Physical therapy for children*, ed 4, St. Louis, 2012, Saunders Elsevier.

3. Bernstein RM: Arthrogryposis and amyoplasia, *J Am Acad Orthop Surg* 10:417–424, 2002.

4. Stanger M: Orthopedic management. In Tecklin JS, editor: *Pediatric physical therapy*, ed 4, Philadelphia, 2008, Lippincott Williams & Wilkins.

5. Thompson GH, Bilenker RM: Comprehensive management of arthrogryposis multiplex congenita, *Clin Orthop Relat Res* 194:6–14, 1985.

6. Hall JG: Arthrogryposis (multiple congenital contractures). diagnostic approach to etiology, classification, genetics, and general principles, *Eur J Med Genetics* 57:404–472, 2014.

7. Hall JG: Arthrogryposis, *Am Fam Physician* 39:113–119, 1989.

8. Gordon N: Arthrogryposis multiplex congenita, *Brain Dev* 20:507–511, 1998.

9. Kang PB, Lidov HG, David WS, et al: Diagnostic value of electromyography and muscle biopsy in arthrogryposis multiplex congenita, *Ann Neurol* 54:790–795, 2003.

10. Sells JM, Jaffe KM, Hall JG: Amyoplasia, the most common type of arthrogryposis: the potential for good outcome, *Pediatrics* 97:225–231, 1996.

11. Palmer PM, MacEwen GD, Bowen JR, et al: Passive motion therapy for infants with arthrogryposis, *Clin Orthop* 194:54–59, 1985.

12. Graydon AJ, Eastwood DM: Orthopaedic management of arthrogryposis multiplex congenita. In Bentley G, editor: *European surgical orthopaedics and traumatology: the EFORT textbook*, Philadelphia, 2014, Springer.

13. Widemann RF, Do TT, Burke SW: Radical soft tissue release of the arthrogrypotic clubfoot, *J Pediatr Orthop B* 14:111–115, 2005.

14. Cassis N, Capdevila R: Talectomy for clubfoot in arthrogryposis, *J Pediatr Orthop* 20:652–665, 2000.

15. Asif S, Umer M, Beg R, et al: Operative treatment of bilateral dislocation in children with arthrogryposis multiplex congenita, *J Orthop Surg (Hong Kong)* 12:4–9, 2004.

16. Staheli LT, Chow DE, Elliot JS, et al: Management of hip dislocation in children with arthrogryposis multiplex congenita, *J Pediatr Orthop* 7:681–685, 1987.

17. Sarwak JF, MacEwen GD, Scott CI: Amyoplasia (a common form of arthrogryposis), *J Bone Joint Surg* 72:465–469, 1990.

18. Fucs PM, Suartman C, de Assumcao RM, et al: Quadricepsplasty in arthrogryposis (amyoplasia): long-term follow-up, *J Pediatr Ortho B* 14:219–224, 2005.

19. Ezaki M: Treatment of the upper limb in the child with arthrogryposis, *Hand Clin* 16:703–711, 2000.

20. Van Heest A, Water PM, Simmons BP: Surgical treatment of arthrogryposis of the elbow, *J Hand Surg* 23:1063–1070, 1998.

21. Gagnon E, Fogelson N, Seyfer AE: Use of latissimus dorsi muscle to restore elbow flexion in arthrogryposis, *Plast Reconstr Surg* 106:1582–1585, 2000.

22. Smith DW, Drennan JC: Arthrogryposis wrist deformities: results of infantile serial casting, *J Pediatr Orthop* 22:44–47, 2002.

23. Yingsakmongkol W, Kumar SJ: Scoliosis in arthrogryposis multiplex congenita: results after nonsurgical and surgical treatment, *J Pediatr Orthop* 20:656–661, 2000.

24. Zeitlin L, Frassier F, Glorieux FH: Modern approach to children with osteogenesis imperfecta, *J Pediatr Orthop B* 12:77–87, 2003.

25. Donohoe M: Osteogenesis imperfecta. In Campbell SK, Palisano RJ, Orlin M, editors: *Physical therapy for children*, ed 4, St. Louis, 2012, Saunders Elsevier.

26. Lowes LP, Orlin MN: Musculoskeletal system: considerations and interventions for specific pediatric pathologies. In Effgen K, editor: *Meeting the physical therapy needs of children*, Philadelphia, 2005, FA Davis.

27. Antoniazzi F, Mottes M, Fraschini P, et al: Osteogenesis imperfecta: practical treatment guidelines, *Pediatr Drugs* 2:465–488, 2000.

28. Englebert RH, Prujis HE, Beemer FA, et al: Osteogenesis imperfecta in childhood: treatment strategies, *Arch Phys Med Rehabil* 79:1590–1594, 1998.

29. Rauch F, Glorieux FH: Osteogenesis imperfecta, *Lancet* 363:1377–1385, 2004.

30. Osteogenesis Imperfecta Foundation: Types of OI. Available at http://www.oif.org/site/PageServer?pagename=AOI_Types. Accessed August 21, 2014.

31. Binder H: Rehabilitation of infants with osteogenesis imperfecta, *Connect Tissue Res* 31:S37–S39, 1995.

32. Zaleske DJ, Doppelt SH, Manken HJ: Metabolic and endocrine abnormalities of the immature skeleton. In Morrissy RT, editor: Lovell and Winters pediatric orthopaedics, ed 3, vol 1, Philadelphia, 1990, JB Lippincott.

33. Letocha AD, Cintas HL, Troendle JF, et al: Controlled trial of pamidronate in children with type III and IV osteogenesis imperfecta confirms vertebral gains but not short-term functional improvement, *J Bone Miner Res* 20:977–986, 2005.

34. Munns CF, Rauch F, Travers R, et al: Effects of intravenous pamidronate treatment in infants with osteogenesis imperfecta: clinical and histomorphometric outcome, *J Bone Miner Res* 20:1235–1243, 2005.

35. Tiley F, Albright JA: Osteogenesis imperfecta: treatment by multiple osteotomy and intramedullary rod insertion, *J Bone Joint Surg Am* 55:701, 1973.

36. Jerosch J, Massotti I, Tomasuic M: Complications after treatment of patients with osteogenesis imperfecta with a bailey-dubow rod, *Arch Orthop Trauma Surg* 117:240–245, 1998.

37. Tachdijian MO: In Pediatric orthopedics, ed 2, vol 2, Philadelphia, 1990, WB Saunders.

38. Weintrob JC: Orthotic management for children with osteogenesis imperfecta, *Connect Tissue Res* 31:S41–S43, 1995.

39. Macovei S, Mandache RS: Osteogenesis imperfecta and its consequences on the disabled children's capacity for effort and movement, *Procedia-Social Behavioral Sci* 11:67–73, 2014.

40. Ratliffe KT: *Clinical pediatric physical therapy: a guide for the physical therapy team*, St Louis, 1998, Mosby.

41. CDC: Down syndrome cases at birth increased. Available at http://www.cdc.gov/features/dsdownsyndrome/, 2012. Accessed August 23, 2014.

42. Roizen N: Down syndrome: trisomy 21. In Batshaw ML, Roizen NJ, Lotrechiano GR, editors: *Children with disabilities*, ed 7, Baltimore, 2013, Brookes.

43. Odibo AO, Stamilio DM, Nelson DB, et al: A cost-effectiveness analysis of prenatal screening strategies for Down's syndrome, *Obstet Gynecol* 106:562–568, 2005.

44. Shumway-Cook A, Wollacott MH: Dynamics of postural control in the child with Down's syndrome, *Phys Ther* 65:1315–1322, 1985.

45. Bertoti DB, Smith DE: Mental retardation: focus on down syndrome. In Tecklin JS, editor: *Pediatric physical therapy*, ed 4, Philadelphia, 2008, Lippincott Williams & Wilkins.

46. Caselli MA, Cohen-Sobel E, Thompson J, et al: Biomechanical management of children and adolescents with Down's syndrome, *J Am Podiatr Med Assoc* 81:119–127, 1991.

47. Steingrass KJ, Chicoine B, McGuire D, et al: Developmental disabilities grown up: down syndrome, *J Dev Behav Pediatr* 32:548–558, 2011.

48. Gajdosik CG, Ostertag S: Cervical instability and Down's syndrome: review of the literature and implications for therapists, *Pediatr Phys Ther* 8:31–36, 1996.

49. Cremers MJ, Beijer HJ: No relation between general laxity and atlanto-axial instability in children with Down's syndrome, *J Pediatr Orthop* 13:318–321, 1993.

50. Cohen W: Current dilemmas in down syndrome clinical care: celiac disease, thyroid disorders, and atlanto-axial instability, *Am J Med Genet Part C (Semin Med Genet)* 142C:141–148, 2006.

51. Stein SM, Kirchren SG, Horev G, et al: Atlanto-occipital subluxation in Down's syndrome, *Pediatr Radiol* 21:121–124, 1991.

52. Galli M, Rigoldi C, Brunner R, et al: Joint stiffness and gait pattern evaluation in children with Down syndrome, *Gait Posture* 28:502–506, 2008.

53. Parker AW, Bronks R: Gait of children with Down's syndrome, *Arch Phys Med Rehabil* 61:345, 1980.

54. Parker AW, Bronks R, Synder CW: Walking pattern in Down's syndrome, *J Ment Defic Res* 30:317, 1986.

55. Selby-Silverstein L, Hillstrom HJ, Palisano RJ: The effect of foot orthoses on standing foot posture and gait of young children with Down's syndrome, *Neuro Rehabil* 16:183–193, 2001.

56. Martin K: Effects of supramalleolar orthoses on postural stability in children with Down syndrome, *Dev Med Child Neurol* 46:406–411, 2004.

57. Lerman JA, Emans JB, Hall JE, et al: Spinal arthrodesis for scoliosis in Down's syndrome, *J Pediatr Orthop* 23:159–161, 2003.

58. Mik G, Gholve PA, Scher DM, et al: Down syndrome: orthopedic issues, *Curr Opin Pediatr* 20:30–36, 2008.

59. Merrick J, Ezra E, Josef B, et al: Musculoskeletal problems in down syndrome. European paediatric orthopaedic society survey: the Israeli sample, *J Pediatr Orthop* 9:185–192, 2000.

60. Katz DA, Kim YJ, Millis MB: Periacetabular osteotomy in patients with Down's syndrome, *J Bone Joint Surg Br* 87:544–547, 2005.

61. Bennet GC, Rang M, Roye DP, et al: Dislocation of the hip in trisomy 21, *J Bone Joint Surg Br* 64:289–294, 1982.

62. Bull MJ: American academy of pediatrics committee on genetics: clinic report: health supervision for children with down syndrome, *Pediatrics* 128:393–404, 2011.

63. Weijerman ME, de Winter JP: Clinical practice: the care of children with down syndrome, *Eur J Pediatr* 169:1445–1452, 2010.

64. Committee on Sports Medicine and Fitness: Atlanto-axial instability in Down's syndrome: subject review, *Pediatrics* 96:151–154, 1995.

65. Msall ME, Reese ME, DiGaudio K, et al: Symptomatic atlanto-axial instability associated with medical and rehabilitative procedures in children with Down's syndrome, *Pediatrics* 85:447–449, 1990.

66. Freed SS, Coulter-O'Berry C: Identification and treatment of congenital muscular torticollis in infants, *J Prosthet Orthot* 16:S18–S23, 2004.

67. Kaplan S, Coulter C, Fetters L: Physical therapy management of congenital muscular torticollis: an evidence-based clinical practice guideline, *Pediatr Phys Ther* 25:348–394, 2013.

68. Loder RT: The cervical spine. In Morrissy RT, Weinstein SL, editors: *Lovell and Winters pediatric orthopaedics*, ed 5, Philadelphia, 2001, Lippincott Williams & Wilkins.

69. Berlin H: The differential diagnosis and management of torticollis in children, *Phys Med Rehabil Clin North Am* 14:197–206, 2000.

70. Karmel-Ross K: Congenital muscular torticollis. In Campbell SK, Palisano RJ, Orlin MN, editors: *Physical therapy for children*, ed 4, St Louis, 2012, Elsevier Saunders.

71. Loder RT: Congenital abnormalities of the cervical spine. In Frymoyer JW, Wiesel SW, editors: *The adult and pediatric spine*, ed 3, Philadelphia, 2004, Lippincott Williams & Wilkins.

72. Porter SB, Blount BW: Pseudotumor of infancy and congenital muscular torticollis, *Am Fam Physician* 52(6):1731–1736, 1995.

73. Cheng JC, Wong MW, Tang SP, et al: Clinical determinants of the outcome of manual stretching in the treatment of congenital muscular torticollis in infants: a prospective study of eight hundred and twenty-one cases, *J Bone Joint Surg Am* 83:679–687, 2001.

74. Slate RK, Posnick JC, Armstrong DC, et al: Cervical spine subluxation associated with congenital muscular torticollis and craniofacial asymmetry, *Plast Reconstr Surg* 91:1187–1195, 1993.

75. Ling CM, Low YS: Sternomastoid tumor and muscular torticollis, *Clin Orthop* 86:144–150, 1972.

76. Dunn PM: Congenital postural deformities, *Br Med Bull* 32:71–76, 1976.

77. Canale ST, Griffin DW, Hubbard CN: Congenital muscular torticollis: a long term follow-up, *J Bone Joint Surg Am* 64:810–816, 1982.

78. Hollier L, Kim J, Grayson BH, et al: Congenital muscular torticollis and the associated craniofacial changes, *Plast Reconstr Surg* 105:827–835, 2001.

79. Davids JR, Wenger DR, Mubarek SJ: Congenital muscular torticollis: sequelae of intrauterine or perinatal compartment syndrome, *J Pediatr Orthop* 13:141–147, 1993.

80. Tang S, Liu Z, Quan X, et al: Sternocleidomastoid pseudotumor of infants and congenital muscular torticollis: fine-structure research, *J Pediatr Orthop* 18:214–218, 1998.

81. Luther BL: Congenital muscular torticollis, *Orthop Nurs* 21:21–29, 2002.

82. Macdonald D: Sternomastoid tumour and muscular torticollis, *J Bone Joint Surg Br* 51:432–443, 1969.

83. Hulbert KF: Congenital torticollis, *J Bone Joint Surg Br* 32:50–59, 1950.

84. Dunn PM: Congenital sternomastoid torticollis: an intrauterine postural deformity, *Arch Dis Child* 49:824–825, 1974.

85. Cheng JCY, Tang SP, Chen TMK, et al: The clinical presentation and outcome of treatment of congenital muscular torticollis in infants: a study of 1,086 cases, *J Pediatr Surg* 35:1091–1096, 2000.

86. Gruss J, Ellenbogen RG, Whelan MF: Lambdoid synostosis and posterior plagiocephaly. In Lin KY, Ogle RC, Jane JA, editors: *Craniofacial surgery: science and surgical technique*, Philadelphia, 2002, WB Saunders.

87. Hollier L, Jeong K, Grayson B, et al: Congenital muscular torticollis and this associated craniofacial changes, *Plast Reconstr Surg* 827–834:2000.

88. Ballock RT, Song KM: The prevalence of nonmuscular causes of torticollis in children, *J Pediatr Orthop* 16:500–504, 1996.

89. Laughlin J, Luerssen TG, Dias MS: Prevention and management of positional skull deformities in infants, *Pediatrics* 128:1236–1241, 2011.

90. Oleszek JL, Chang N, Apkon SD, et al: Botulinum toxin type a in the treatment of children with congenital muscular torticollis, *Am J Phys Med Rehabil* 84:813–816, 2005.

91. Wei JL, Schwartz KM, Weaver AL, et al: Pseudotumor of infancy and congenital muscular torticollis: 170 cases, *Laryngoscope* 111:688–695, 2001.

92. Shepherd R: Torticollis. In Shepherd R, editor: *Physiotherapy in pediatrics*, ed 3, Woburn, MA, 1995, Butterworth-Heinemann.

93. Staheli L: *Fundamentals of pediatric orthopedics*, ed 2, Philadelphia, 1998, Lippincott Williams & Wilkins.

94. Lawrence WT, Azizkhan RG: Congenital muscular torticollis: a spectrum of pathology, *Ann Plast Surg* 23:523–530, 1989.

95. Cottrill-Mosterman S, Jacques C, Bartlett O, et al: Orthotic treatment of head tilt in children with congenital muscular torticollis, *J Assoc Child Prosthet Orthot Clin* 1–3:1987.

96. Stassen LF, Kerawala CJ: New surgical technique for the correction of congenital muscular torticollis, *Br J Oral Maxillofac Surg* 38:142–147, 2000.

97. Burstein F, Cohen S: Endoscopic surgical treatment for congenital muscular torticollis, *Plast Reconstr Surg* 101:20–24, 1998.

98. Persing J, James H, Swanson J, et al: Prevention and management of positional skull deformities in infants, *Pediatrics* 112:199–202, 2003.

99. Ohman AM, Nilsson S, Beckung ER: Validity and reliability of the muscle function scale, aimed to assess the lateral flexors of the neck in infants, *Physiother Theory Pract* 25:129–137, 2009.

100. Campbell SK, Kolobe TH, Osten ET, et al: Construct validity of the Test of infant motor performance, *Phys Ther* 75:585–596, 1995.

101. Piper MC, Pinnell LE, Darrah J, et al: Construction and validation of the Alberta infant motor scale (AIMS), *Can J Public Health* 83(Suppl 2):S46–S50, 1992.

102. Emery C: Determinants of treatment duration for congenital muscular torticollis, *Phys Ther* 74:921–929, 1994.

103. Karmel-Ross K: *Torticollis: differential diagnosis, assessment and treatment, surgical management and bracing*, Binghamton, NY, 1997, Haworth Press.

104. Golden KA, Beals SP, Littlefield TR, et al: Sternocleidomastoid imbalance versus congenital muscular torticollis: their relationship to positional plagiocephaly, *Cleft Palate Craniofac J* 36:256–261, 1999.

105. Bandy W, Irion J, Briggler M: The effect of time and frequency of static stretching on flexibility of the hamstring muscles, *Phys Ther* 78:321–322, 1998.

106. Symmetric Designs: TOT collar web page. Available at http://www.symmetric-designs.com/TOT-collar-.html. Accessed December 30, 2005.

107. Dunham EA: Obstetrical brachial plexus palsy, *Orthop Nurs* 22:106–116, 2003.

108. Hale HB, Bae DS, Waters PM: Current concepts in the management of brachial plexus birth palsy, *J Hand Surg Am* 35:322–331, 2010.

109. Vander Linden DW: Brachial plexus injury. In Campbell SK, Palisano RJ, Orlin MN, editors: *Physical therapy for children*, ed 4, St Louis, 2012, Elsevier Saunders.

110. Shen SM, Berzin E, Lee R, et al: Brachial plexus birth injuries and current management, *Clin Plast Surg* 25:527–536, 1998.

111. Waters PM: Update on management of pediatric brachial plexus palsy, *J Pediatr Orthop* 25:116–126, 2005.

112. Narakas AO: Obstetrical brachial plexus injuries. In Lamb DW, editor: *The hand and upper limb, vol 2, The paralyzed hand*, Edinburgh, 1987, Churchill Livingstone.

113. Al-Quattan MM: el-sayed AA, al-kharfy TM et al: obstetrical brachial plexus injury in newborn babies delivered by caesarean section, *J Hand Surg* 21:263–265, 1996.

114. Rouse DJ, Owen J, Goldenberg RL, et al: The effectiveness and costs of elective cesarean delivery for fetal macrosomia diagnosed by ultrasound, *JAMA* 276:1480–1486, 1996.

115. Waters PM, Peljovich AE: Shoulder reconstruction in patients with chronic brachial plexus birth palsy: a case control study, *Acta Orthop Traumatol Turc* 38:161–169, 2004.

116. Hoeksma AF, ter Steeg AM, Nelisson RG, et al: Neurological recover in obstetric brachial plexus injuries: an historical cohort study, *Dev Med Child Neurol* 46:76–83, 2004.

117. Noetzel MJ, Park TS, Robison S, et al: Prospective study of recovery following neonatal brachial plexus injury, *J Child Neurol* 16:488–492, 2001.

118. Hoeksma AF, Wolf H, Oei SL: Obstetrical brachial plexus injuries: incidence, natural course and shoulder contracture, *Clin Rehabil* 14:523–526, 2000.

119. Pearl ML, Edgerton BW: Glenoid deformity secondary to brachial plexus birth palsy, *J Bone Joint Surg Am* 5:659–667, 1998.

120. Zancolli EA, Zancolli ER: Reconstructive surgery in brachial plexus sequelae. In Gupta A, Kay S, Scheker L, editors: *The growing hand*, London, 2000, Mosby.

121. Zancolli E: Classification and management of the shoulder in birth palsy, *Orthop Clin North Am* 12:431–457, 1981.

122. Desiato MT, Risina B: The role of botulinum toxin in the neurorehabilitation of young patients with brachial plexus birth palsy, *Pediatr Rehabil* 4:29–36, 2001.

123. Rollnik JD, Hierner R, Schubert M, et al: Botulinum toxin treatment of contractions after birth-related brachial plexus lesions, *Neurology* 33:1354–1356, 2000.

124. El-Gammal TA, Fathi NA: Outcomes of surgical treatment of brachial plexus injuries using nerve grafting and nerve transfers, *J Reconstr Microsurg* 18:7–15, 2002.

125. Laurent JP, Lee R, Shenaq S, et al: Neurosurgical correction of upper brachial plexus birth injuries, *J Neurosurg* 79:197–203, 1993.

126. Sherburn EW, Kaplan SS, Kaufman BA, et al: Outcome of surgically treated birth-related brachial plexus injuries in twenty cases, *Pediatr Neurosurg* 27:19–27, 1997.

127. Brandt KE, Mackinnon SE: A technique for maximizing biceps recovery in brachial plexus reconstruction, *J Hand Surg Am* 18:726–733, 1993.

128. Oberlin C, Beal D, Leechavengvongs S, et al: Nerve transfers to biceps muscle using a part of the ulnar never for C5-C6 avulsion of the brachial plexus: anatomical study and report of four cases, *J Hand Surg Am* 19:232–237, 1994.

129. Malessy MJ, Thomeer RT: Evaluation of intercostals to musculocutaneous nerve transfer in reconstructive brachial plexus surgery, *J Neurosurg* 88:266–271, 1998.

130. Kawabata H, Kawai H, Masatomi T, et al: Accessory nerve neurotization in infants with brachial plexus birth palsy, *Microsurgery* 15:768–772, 1994.

131. Chaung DC, Cheng SL, Wei FC, et al: Clinical evaluation of C7 spinal nerve transaction: 21 patients with at least 2 years' follow-up, *Br J Plast Surg* 51:285–290, 1998.

132. Gu Y: Distribution of the sensory endings of the C7 nerve root and its clinical significance, *J Hand Surg* 19:67–68, 1994.

133. McGuiness CN, Kay SP: The prespinal route in contralateral C7 nerve root transfer for brachial plexus avulsion injuries, *J Hand Surg Br* 27:159–160, 2002.

134. Nagano A, Tsuyama N, Ochiai N: Direct nerve crossing with the intercostal nerve to treat avulsion injuries of the brachial plexus, *J Hand Surg Am* 14:980–985, 1989.

135. Rutowski R: Neurotizations by means of the cervical plexus in over 100 patients with from one to five root avulsions of the brachial plexus, *Microsurgery* 14:285–288, 1993.

136. Al-Qattan MM: The outcome of Erb's palsy when the decision to operate is made at 4 months of age, *Plast Reconstr Surg* 106:1461–1465, 2000.

137. Birch R, Bonney G, Wynn Parry CB: Birth lesions of the brachial plexus. In Seddon JH, editor: *Surgical disorders of the peripheral nerves*, London, 1998, Churchill Livingstone.

138. Leffert RD: Brachial plexus. In Green DP, Hotchkiss RN, Pederson WC, editors: *Operative hand surgery*, ed 3, New York, 1993, Churchill Livingstone.

139. Hinderer KA, Hinderer SR, Shurtleff DB: Myelodysplasia. In Campbell SK, Palisano RJ, Orlin MN, editors: *Physical therapy for children*, ed 4, St Louis, 2012, Elsevier Saunders.

140. Westcott SL, Goulet C: Neuromuscular system: structures, functions, diagnoses and evaluation. In Effgen K, editor: *Meeting the physical therapy needs of children*, Philadelphia, 2005, FA Davis.

141. Spinal Bifida Association. Available at http://www.sbaa.org. Accessed December 30, 2005.

142. Shurtleff DB: Decubitus formation and skin breakdown. In Shurtleff DB, editor: *Myelodysplasias and exstrophies: significance, prevention, and treatment*, Orlando, FL, 1986, Grune & Stratton.

143. Parker SE, Mai CT, Canfield MA, et al: Updated national birth prevalence estimates for selected birth defects in the United States, 2004-2006, *Birth Defects Res A Clin Mol Teratol* 88:1008–1016, 2010.

144. Centers for Disease Control and Prevention. Available at http://www.cdc.gov/. Accessed December 30, 2005.

145. Barker E, Saulino M, Caristo AM: Spina bifida, *RN* 65:33–39, 2002.

146. Bowman EM, McLone DG, Grant JA, et al: Spina bifida outcome: a 25-year perspective, *Pediatr Neurosurg* 34:114–120, 2001.

147. Bartoneck A, Saraste H, Samuelsson L, et al: Ambulation in patients with myelomeningocele: a 12-year follow-up, *J Pediatr Orthop* 19:202–206, 1999.

148. Segal LS: Advances in myelomeningocele, *Curr Opin Orthop* 12:449–455, 2001.

149. Didelot WP: Current concepts in myelomeningocele, *Curr Opin Orthop* 14:398–402, 2003.

150. Lorente Moltó FJ, Garrido IM: Retrospective review of L3 myelomeningocele in three age groups: should posterolateral iliopsoas transfer still be indicated to stabilize the hip? *J Pediatr Orthop B* 14:177–184, 2005.

151. Asher M, Olson J: Factors affecting the ambulatory status of patients with spina bifida cystica, *J Bone Joint Surg Am* 65:350–356, 1983.

152. Lee EH, Carroll NC: Hip stability and ambulatory status in myelomeningocele, *J Pediatr Orthop* 5:522–527, 1985.

153. Parsch K, Dimeglio A: The hip in children with myelomeningocele, *J Pediatr Orthop B* 1:3–13, 1992.

154. Rendeli C, Salvaggio E, Cannizzaro GS, et al: Does locomotion improve the cognitive profile of children with myelomeningocele? *Childs Nerv Syst* 18:231–234, 2002.

155. Mayfield JK: Comprehensive orthopedic management in myelomeningocele. In Rekate HL, editor: *Comprehensive management of spina bifida*, Boca Raton, FL, 1991, CRC Press.

156. Shurtleff DB: Mobility. In Shurtleff DB, editor: *Myelodysplasias and exstrophies: significance, prevention, and treatment*, Orlando, FL, 1986, Grune & Stratton.

157. Polliack AA, Elliot S, Caves C, et al: Lower extremity orthoses for children with myelomeningocele: user and orthotist perspectives, *J Prosthet Orthot* 13:123–129, 2001.

158. Menelaus MB, editor: *Orthopedic management of spina bifida cystica*, New York, 1980, Churchill Livingstone.

159. Liptak BS, Shurtleff DB, Bloss JW, et al: Mobility aids for children with high-level myelomeningocele: parapodium versus wheelchair, *Dev Med Child Neurol* 34:787–796, 1992.

160. Correll J, Gabler C: The effect with soft tissue release of the hips on walking in myelomeningocele, *J Pediatr Orthop B* 9:148–153, 2000.

161. Trivedi J, Thomson JD, Slakey JB, et al: Clinical and radiographic predictors of scoliosis in patients with myelomeningocele, *J Bone Joint Surg Am* 84:1389–1394, 2002.

162. Hwang R, Kentish M, Burns Y: Hand positioning sense in children with spina bifida myelomeningocele, *Dev Med Child Neurol* 45:249–256, 2003.

163. Norrlin S, Strinnholm M, Carlsson M, et al: Factors of significance for mobility in children with myelomeningocele, *Acta Pediatr* 92:204–210, 2003.

164. Gölge M, Schültz C, Dreesman M, et al: Grip force parameters in precision grip of individuals with myelomeningocele, *Dev Med Child Neurol* 45:249–256, 2003.

165. Shaffer J, Wolfe L, Friedrich W, et al: Developmental expectations: intelligence and fine motor skills. In Shurtleff DB, editor: *Myelodysplasias and exstrophies: significance, prevention, and treatment*, Orlando, FL, 1986, Grune & Stratton.

166. Hinderer SR, Hinderer KA: Sensory examination of individuals with myelodysplasia (abstract), *Arch Phys Med Rehabil* 71:769–770, 1990.

167. Caldarelli M, Di Rocco C, La Marca F: Shunt complications in the first postoperative year in children with meningomyelocele, *Childs Nerv Syst* 12:748–754, 1996.

168. Weprin BE, Oakes WJ: The Chiari malformations and associated syringohydromyelia. In McLone DG, editor: *Pediatric neurosurgery: surgery of the developing nervous system*, Philadelphia, 2001, WB Saunders.

169. Wagner W, Schwarz M, Perneczky A: Primary myelomeningocele closure and consequences, *Curr Opin Urol* 12:465–468, 2002.

170. Cohen AR, Robinson S: Early management of myelomeningocele. In McLone DG, editor: *Pediatric neurosurgery: surgery of the developing nervous system*, Philadelphia, 2001, WB Saunders.

171. Cochrane DD, Rassekh SR, Thiessen PN: Functional deterioration following placode untethering in myelomeningocele, *Pediatr Neurosurg* 28:57–62, 1998.

172. Yeates KO, Loss N, Colvin AN, et al: Do children with myelomeningocele and hydrocephalus display nonverbal learning disabilities? An empirical approach to classification, *J Int Neuropsychol Soc* 9:653–662, 2003.

173. Dennis M, Barnes M: Math and numeracy in young adults with spina bifida and hydrocephalus, *Dev Neuropsychol* 21:141–155, 2002.

174. Gunther K, Nelitz M, Parsch K, et al: Allergic reactions to latex in myelodysplasia: a review in the literature, *J Pediatr Orthop B* 9:180–184, 2000.

175. Hirose S, Meuli-Simmen C, Meuli M: Fetal Surgery for myelomeningocele: panacea or peril? *World J Surg* 27:87–94, 2003.

176. Park TS: Myelomeningocele. In Albright AL, Pollack IF, Adelson PD, editors: *Principles and practice of pediatric neurosurgery*, Stuttgart, 1999, Thieme.

177. Griebel ML, Oakes WJ, Worley G: The Chiari malformation associated with myelomeningocele. In Rekate HL, editor: *Comprehensive management of spina bifida*, Boca Raton, FL, 1991, CRC Press.

178. Phuong LK, Schoeberl KA, Raffel C: Natural history of tethered cord in patients with meningomyelocele, *Neurosurgery* 50:989–995, 2002.

179. Reigel DH: Tethered myelomeningocele. In McLone DG, editor: *Pediatric neurosurgery: surgery of the developing nervous system*, Philadelphia, 2001, WB Saunders.

180. Gabrieli APT, Vankoski SJ, Dias LS, et al: Gait analysis in low lumbar myelomeningocele patients with unilateral hip dislocation or subluxation, *J Pediatr Orthop* 23:330–334, 2003.

181. Snela S, Parsch K: Follow-up study after treatment of knee flexion contractures in spina bifida patients, *J Pediatr Orthop B* 9:154–160, 2000.

182. Vankoski SJ, Michaud S, Dias LS: External tibial torsion and the effectiveness of the solid ankle-foot orthoses, *J Pediatr Orthop* 20:349–355, 2000.

183. Gerlach DJ, Gurnett CA, Limpaphayom N, et al: Early results of the ponseti method for the treatment of clubfoot associated with myelomeningocele, *J Bone Joint Surgery Am* 81:1350–1359, 2009.

184. Torosian CM, Dias LS: Surgical treatment of severe hindfoot valgus by medial displacement osteotomy of the os calcis in children with myelomeningocele, *J Pediatr Orthop* 20:226–229, 2000.

185. Osebold WR: Stability of myelomeningocele spines treated with the Mayfield two-stage anterior and posterior fusion technique, *Spine* 25:1344–1351, 2000.

186. Crawford AH, Strub WM, Lewis R, et al: Neonatal kyphectomy in the child with myelomeningocele, *Spine* 28:260–266, 2003.

187. Thomsen M, Long RD, Carstens C: Results of kyphectomy with the technique of Warner and fackler on children with myelodysplasia, *J Pediatr Orthop B* 9:143–147, 2000.

188. Krosschell K, Pesavento MJ: Congenital spinal cord injury. In Umphred DA, editor: *Neurological rehabilitation*, ed 5, St Louis, 2007, Mosby.

189. Ragonesi CB, Galloway JC: Short-term, early intensive power mobility training: case report of an infant at risk for cerebral palsy, *Pediatr Phys Ther* 24:141–148, 2012.

190. Lynch A, Ryu JC, Agrawal S, et al: Power mobility training for a 7-month old infant with spina bifida, *Pediatr Phys Ther* 21:362–368, 2009.

191. Hinderer KA, Hinderer SR: Muscle strength development and assessment in children and adolescents. In Harms-Ringdahl K, editor: *International perspectives in physical therapy, vol 8, muscle strength*, London, 1993, Churchill Livingstone.

192. Butler C, Okamoto GA, McKay TM: Motorized wheelchair driving by disabled children, *Arch Phys Med Rehabil* 65:95–97, 1984.

193. Liptak GS: Neural tube defects. In Batshaw M, Roizen N, Lotrecchiano G, editors: *Children with disabilities*, ed 7, Baltimore, 2013, Brookes.

194. Tappit-Emas E: Spina bifida. In Tecklin JS, editor: *Pediatric physical therapy*, ed 4, Philadelphia, 2008, Lippincott Williams & Wilkins.

195. Duffy CM, Graham HK, Cosgrove AP: The influence of ankle-foot orthosis on gait and energy expenditure in spina bifida, *J Pediatr Orthop* 20:356–361, 2000.

196. Logan L, Byers-Hinkley K, Ciccone CD: Anterior versus posterior walkers: a gait analysis study, *Dev Med Child Neurol* 32:1044–1048, 1990.

197. Moore CA, Nejad B, Novak RA, et al: Energy cost of walking in low lumbar myelomeningocele, *J Pediatr Orthop* 21:388–391, 2001.

198. Bare A, Vankoski SJ, Dias LS, et al: Independent ambulators with high sacral myelomeningocele: the relation between walking kinematics and energy consumption, *Dev Med Child Neurol* 43:16–21, 2001.

CHAPTER 29

Pediatric and Adolescent Populations: Musculoskeletal Considerations

DONNA L. MERKEL, CAROLE HIGH GROSS, JOSEPH T. MOLONY, JR.*

INTRODUCTION

It is important that physical therapists, along with other health care professionals, parents, teachers, and coaches, understand that children are not small adults.[1-3] Although some aspects of the rehabilitative process may be similar to the adult population, differential diagnosis and the decision-making algorithm of rehabilitation are very different for the skeletally immature individual. As a result, a sound understanding of the immature skeleton and the rapidly maturing and developing body of a child and adolescent allows for accurate diagnosis and management of injuries sustained by this population. This understanding includes recognition of the extremes of overaggressive and improper training of youth athletes as well as childhood obesity and sedentary lifestyles. More than 45 million children and adolescents participate in organized sports in the United States.[2,4]

Benefits of Participation in Sport Include:[2,4-8]

- Regular exercise integrated into lifestyle
- Higher self-esteem
- Improved discipline
- Improved strength and agility
- Enhanced motor skills
- Improved social skills
- Development of healthy nutritional choices (i.e., fruits and vegetables)
- Potentially less interest in taking health risks

Sports participation can assist in reducing the incidence of childhood obesity. Pediatric and adolescent obesity has been increasing since the 1980s, and currently one out of three children in the United States is at risk for obesity. Those at a higher risk of being physically inactive are preadolescent and adolescent children (more often girls) from ethnic minorities, affected by poverty, living in apartments or public housing, or in neighborhoods where outdoor activity is limited due to safety, lack of play areas, and poor climate. This high-risk group also includes children with physical disabilities.[2,9]

Secondary Complications of Obesity Include:[2,3,10]

- Heightened risk of developing
  - Diabetes
  - Heart disease
  - Hypertension
  - Cancer
  - Asthma
  - Sleep apnea
- Low self-esteem
- Musculoskeletal dysfunction
- Pain

On the other side of the spectrum is the culture of intense organized youth sports. In the past, children participated in multiple different sports throughout the year and spent more time with recreational versus organized physical activities. Nowadays, emphasis is placed on single sport participation with year-round seasons.[1,2,4-8] In the United States, 75% of families have at least one child in an organized sport.[2] Many children are participating at earlier ages with sports specialization. Enrolling children in sports that are beyond their developmental ability has

---

*The authors, editors, and publisher acknowledge Jane Gruber, Peter G. Gerbino, Pierre A. d'Hemecourt, and Mychelle L. Shegog for their contributions on this topic in the previous edition.

led to anxiety, stress, frustration, and early dropout and attrition.[2,8,10] Traumatic and overuse sports-related injuries contribute to approximately 25% of all childhood injuries. In the United States, more than 3.5 million children under the age of 14 receive medical care each year, and for those involved in sports, the majority of the injuries occur during practice instead of games.[4,8,9,11]

Sports readiness matches a child's stage of motor development with the requirements of a sport.[2,4–8] It is not until approximately 6 years of age that children have fundamental physical, psychological, and cognitive skills sufficient to allow participation in organized team sports.[2,5,6] Fundamental athletic skills, such as running, jumping, catching, throwing, tumbling, and balance, should be emphasized before the child specializes in a single sport. These skills should also be integrated into a rehabilitation treatment program to improve safety at high activity levels and return to play.[1,2,6]

The American Academy of Pediatrics, Committee on Sports Medicine Recommends That:[2,6,7]

- Weekly training time, number of repetitions, or total distance is not increased by more than 10% per week
- Participation is with only one team per season
- Allowance is made for 1-2 days off per week to recover both physically and psychologically
- 2-3 months of recovery time from a specific sport are provided per year
- The focus of sports participation should be on having fun, acquiring skill, and learning safety and sportsmanship

---

AGE CHANGE ISSUES

The complex and progressive physical, cognitive, and emotional maturity of each individual youth guides and directs sports readiness recommendations. A child's chronological age may differ from a child's skeletal maturity. Skeletal maturity is based on maturation of skeletal bones and may be affected by factors such as gender, environment, genetic influences, and sexual characteristics.[5,12] The **Tanner Stages of Development** (Figures 29-1 to 29-3) describe sexual maturity and physical changes during puberty that relate to skeletal growth and open growth plates (Table 29-1). Two individuals with the same chronological age may have different skeletal maturities.[5,12] The following provides a general summary of chronological development and sports focus.

Clinical Point

A child's chronological age commonly differs from a child's skeletal age.

During **early childhood**, approximately ages 6 to 9 years, increased flexibility and the incidence of hypermobility are evident. Growth plates are open and bones are just beginning to ossify. Children have limited attention spans. Vision is developing, although children may still have difficulty identifying the direction of a moving object. Sport focus should include skill development, fundamental transitional movements, and fun.[2,4–6,9]

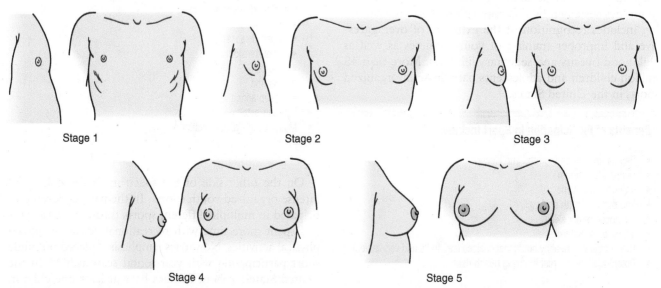

Stage 1   Stage 2   Stage 3

Stage 4   Stage 5

Figure 29-1 Breast development in girls. The development of the mammae can be divided into five stages. In stage 1, only the nipple is raised above the level of the breast (as in the child). In stage 2, the budding stage, there is bud-shaped elevation of the areola. On palpation, a fairly hard button can be felt that is disk or cherry shaped. The areola is increased in diameter, and the surrounding area is slightly elevated. In stage 3, there is further elevation of the mammae; the areolar diameter is further increased, and the shape of mammae is visibly feminine. In stage 4, fat deposits increase, and the areola forms a secondary elevation above that of the breast. This secondary mound occurs in approximately half of all girls and in some cases persists in adulthood. In stage 5, the adult stage, the areola usually subsides to the level of the breast and is strongly pigmented. (Redrawn from Halpern B, Blackburn T, Incremona B et al: Preparticipation sports physicals. In Zachazewski JE, Magee DJ, Quillen WS, editors: *Athletic injuries and rehabilitation*, p 855, Philadelphia, 1996, WB Saunders.)

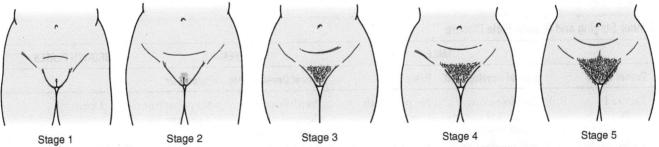

Figure 29-2 Pubic hair development in females. In the development of pubic hair, five stages can be distinguished. In stage 1, there is no growth of pubic hair. In stage 2, initial, scarcely pigmented hair is present, especially along the labia. In stage 3, sparse dark, visibly pigmented, curly pubic hair is present on the labia. In stage 4, hair that is adult in type but not in extent is present. In stage 5, there is lateral spreading (type and spread of hair are adult). (Redrawn from Halpern B, Blackburn T, Incremona B et al: Preparticipation sports physicals. In Zachazewski JE, Magee DJ, Quillen WS, editors: *Athletic injuries and rehabilitation*, p 855, Philadelphia, 1996, WB Saunders.)

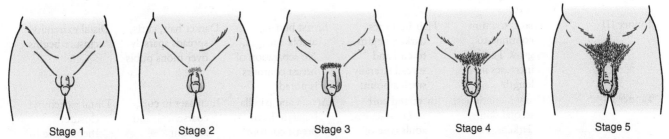

Figure 29-3 Genital and pubic hair development in males. The development of external genitalia and pubic hair can be divided into five stages. In stage 1, the testes, scrotum, and penis are the same size and shape as in the young child, and there is no growth of pubic hair (hair in pubic area is no different from that on the rest of the abdomen). In stage 2, there is enlargement of the scrotum and testes. The skin of the scrotum becomes redder, thinner, and wrinkled. The penis has not grown (or just slightly so). Pubic hair is slightly pigmented. In stage 3, there is enlargement of the penis, especially in length, further enlargement of testes, and descent of scrotum. Dark, definitely pigmented, curly pubic hair is present around the base of penis. In stage 4, there is continued enlargement of the penis and sculpturing of the glans, with increased pigmentation of the scrotum. This stage is sometimes best described as not quite adult. Pubic hair is definitely adult in type but not in extent (no further than the inguinal fold). In stage 5, the adult stage, the scrotum is ample, and the penis reaches almost to the bottom of the scrotum. Pubic hair spreads to the medial surface of the thighs but not upward. In 80% of men, hair spreads along the linea alba. (Redrawn from Halpern B, Blackburn T, Incremona B et al: Preparticipation sports physicals. In Zachazewski JE, Magee DJ, Quillen WS, editors: *Athletic injuries and rehabilitation*, p 855, Philadelphia, 1996, WB Saunders.)

During **late childhood**, from approximately ages 10 to 12 years, positive and negative influences from the emergence of puberty impact the musculoskeletal system, gross motor skills, and overall sports performance. These children are able to perform more complex gross motor skills, attention span widens, and vision and eye-hand coordination improves. However, growth spurts during this time contribute to alteration of length-tension relationships of soft tissues and joint position sensory information as bones grow more quickly than neighboring muscle, tendon, and ligaments. These changes lead to decreased muscular flexibility as well as neuromotor and strength impairments. In girls, menarche is observed approximately 2 years after breast bud appearance and/or 3.3 years after the initial growth spurt. Girls may be taller than boys at this age because puberty typically occurs 1 to 2 years earlier in girls. Distal growth plates may begin to close in both sexes. Sport focus should emphasize tactics and strategies of sport and continued skill development.[2,4-6]

Early adolescence, from approximate ages 13 to 15 years, involves more rapid growth spurts causing further loss of flexibility, predisposition to injury, and maybe even a temporary decline in sport performance.

Adolescence is the time between puberty and adulthood and is a time of physical, cognitive, sex gender, and psychological maturation. Growth plates begin to close distally to proximally, and bones continue to ossify. Growth centers typically close in females 18 to 24 months following menarche. In males, growth plates close later than they do in females. A beard or mustache typically signifies closure of the majority of growth centers in males.[4-6,9] Apophysitis (i.e., irritation of the growth center at the attachment of a tendon) is more evident at this time. Boys begin to become quicker, stronger, and faster. Girls steadily improve on previous skills. The adolescent and coach need to be patient as the emerging individual grows into his or her "new body." Progression from concrete to abstract thinking begins, attention span and memory increases, and the concept of team and sportsmanship expands. The focus of sport should emphasize individual performance of strengths and weaknesses.[2,4-6,9]

Late adolescence, from approximate ages 16 to 18 years, demonstrates a time of skeletal maturity, and injuries will closely mimic those of an adult. Proximal growth plates at the spine and pelvis may still be open; however, the skeleton is maturing rapidly. Males far

TABLE **29-1**

Tanner Staging and Growth Plate Closure

Tanner Stage	MALE Genital Development	MALE Pubic Hair	FEMALE Breast Development	FEMALE Pubic Hair	GROWTH PLATES
Tanner I	Preadolescent: identical to early childhood	No pubic hair present	Preadolescent: elevated papilla, small flat areola	No pubic hair present	Open
Tanner II	Enlargement of testes, scrotum, and penis. Scrotum color becomes a reddish hue, altering its skin texture	Sparse amount of long darker hair at the base of the penis	Breast bud formation. Papilla and areola elevate, areola diameter increases	Sparse amount of long darker hair bilaterally along medial border of the labia majora	Open
Tanner III	Testes, scrotum continue to grow. Penis increases in length	Hair becomes darker, begins to curl and spread laterally, small amount	Breast bud and areola enlarges. No separation of breast contours is noted	Darker hair, curls, spreads sparsely over mons pubis	Distal extremity closure begins
Tanner IV	Growth continues; scrotal skin darkens. Penis grows in width and glans penis develops	Increased curl and coarseness, adult type of distribution but smaller amount	Areola and papilla separate from breast contour to form a secondary mound	Increases in curl, coarseness, and amount	Distal extremity closure. Incomplete proximal physeal closure (pelvis, sternum and spine)
Tanner V	Mature: adult size and shape of testes, scrotum, penis	Mature: with spread to medial thigh. 80% of males have hair grow along the linea alba	Mature: areolar mound recedes into the breast contour, papilla continues to project	Mature: adult female triangular pattern, with spread to surface of medial thigh	Closed

From Merkel DL, Molony JT, eds: *Pediatric and adolescent sports medicine: management and prevention of injuries unique to the young athlete,* American Physical Therapy Association (APTA) Sports Section Home Study Course, 2011.

exceed females in speed, size, strength, power, endurance, and functional testing. Females may have to work harder to make performance gains. The late adolescent individual is more goal oriented and now has the added pressures of attending college and their future. Sport focus should be on promoting enjoyment with achievement of personal and team goals. Typically, athletes will choose a sport at which they are successful and enjoy.[2,4,5,9]

SPECIFIC INJURY CONSIDERATION

Fractures

During the period of skeletal immaturity, bone physiologically differs from the adult in several ways. In general, bone is a viscoelastic material, made up of a mineral-rich matrix, which gives bone rigidity and strength, as well as organic collagen, giving bone flexibility and resilience.

The outer portion of bone is the cortex, and the inner portion (containing the marrow) is made up of cancellous bone (also referred to as spongy or trabecular bone). In a long bone, the central shaft is called the diaphysis, and the area of bone between the diaphysis and the physis (growth plate) is the metaphysis. The area of bone between the physis and the joint space is the epiphysis. During growth the physis expands through the metaphysis (Figure 29-4).

Clinical Point

A fracture in a child is a common occurrence. For the clinician, this provides an opportune "teaching moment" to educate the parents and family or review with them the basics of injury prevention, including the use of seat belts and appropriate protective gear for sports (e.g., helmet, kneepads, wrist guards).

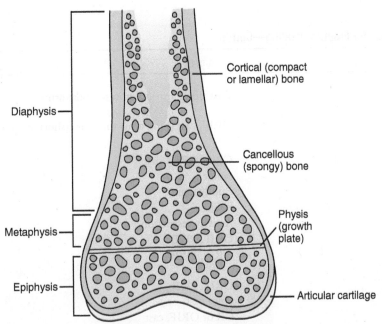

Figure 29-4 Diagram of the immature bone showing different parts of the bone. (From Barr JB, RE Berg: Imaging joints and musculoskeletal tissue: pathoanatomical considerations. In Magee DJ, Zachazewski JE, Quillen WS, editors: *Scientific foundations and principles of practice in musculoskeletal rehabilitation*, p 588, St Louis, 2007, Saunders.)

Healthy bone has the capacity to deform when it is loaded and will return to original shape when unloaded. Children's bones contain more collagen and cartilage than the ossified bones of adults and therefore are much weaker than muscles, tendons, and ligaments. A majority of injuries in children and adolescents occur in the midshaft and at growth centers.[12-14] Immature bone has a faster healing rate (Table 29-2) and better capacity for remodeling due to increased vascularity and thickened periosteum. However, injury to the physis can cause growth disruption.[12-14] Bone growth is critical during adolescence as bone development and formation is greater during puberty than any other

TABLE **29-2**

Treatment and Time Frames for Fracture Healing

Bone	Treatment	Time
Clavicle	Sling	6 wk
Physeal separation	Activity restriction	3-6 wk
Tubercle avulsion	ORIF, sling	3 wk
Humeral shaft	Coaptation splint or functional brace	4-6 wk
Supracondylar fracture, elbow	ORIF, cast	3 wk
T-condylar fracture, elbow	ORIF, cast	6 wk
Medial/lateral epicondyle, elbow	ORIF, cast	6 wk
Olecranon	ORIF, cast	6 wk
Radial head		
Minimally displaced	Sling	1-2 wk
Displaced	ORIF, cast, then sling	2 wk
		2-4 wk
Radial neck		
Minimally displaced	Sling	1-2 wk
Angulation >45°	CR or ORIF, cast, then sling	1-2 wk
		1-3 wk
Radius and ulna (both bones)	CR or ORIF, cast, then splint	6 wk
		3 mo for sports
Distal radius		
Buckle	Cast	3 wk
Displaced, greenstick	CR or ORIF, cast	6 wk

(Continued)

TABLE **29-2**

Treatment and Time Frames for Fracture Healing—Cont'd

Bone	Treatment	Time
Scaphoid		
Nondisplaced	Cast (long arm), then cast (short arm)	4 wk 4-8 wk
Displaced	ORIF, cast (long arm) then cast (short arm)	2 wk 6-8 wk
Metacarpals	CR or ORIF, cast	3-4 wk
Phalanx	Splint	3 wk
	Buddy taping	3 wk
Tuft	Splint	3 wk
Rib	Activity restriction	3-6 wk
Acetabulum	ORIF, PWB	6-10 wk
Femoral head or neck	ORIF, PWB	6-8 wk
Femoral shaft		
Over 6 years old	ORIF, PWB	6 wk
Under 6 years old	Spica cast	6 wk
Distal femoral physis	CR or ORIF, cast	6 wk
Tibial spine	CR, cast	6 wk
	ORIF, brace	6 wk
Tibial plateau		
Minimally displaced	Hinged brace, PWB	6 wk
Displaced	ORIF, hinged brace, PWB	6 wk
Tibial shaft	ORIF, PWB	10 wk
Tibial plafond	ORIF, PWB	6 wk
Lateral malleolus		
Minimally displaced	Cast, PWB	6 wk
Displaced	CR or ORIF, cast	6 wk

CR, Closed reduction; *ORIF,* open reduction and internal fixation; *PWB,* partial weight bearing.

time of life, except infancy. Peak height velocity occurs at approximately 15.8 years for girls and 17.5 years for boys. During this time, teenagers often lack adequate calcium necessary for bone mineralization.[15]

Signs and Symptoms of Children with Fractures

- Tears or crying with movement
- Limp during ambulation (lower limb)
- Decreased weight-bearing ability
- Swelling
- Increased pain with palpation over bone
- Bones close to surface of skin most susceptible

From Merkel DL, Molony JT: Clinical commentary: recognition and management of traumatic sports injuries in the skeletally immature athlete, *Intl J Sports Phys Ther* 7:691-704, 2012.

Stress on bones, cartilage, ligaments, and tendons may produce bone failure and subsequent fractures in children and adolescents. With adults, these same stresses more often develop into soft tissue injury. Underlying pathology may be a contributing factor to fractures when presented in infants less than 12 months of age or with children who acquire multiple fractures over time. Fractures usually present with swelling, deformity, bruising, and positive bone tenderness. Any bone tenderness should be treated as a fracture until proven otherwise. Some physeal fractures may not be evident on plain radiography and therefore absence of a visible fracture line does not disprove the presence of a fracture if tenderness is at a physis. Fractures are described by their location (i.e., diaphyseal, metaphyseal, physeal, or epiphyseal [see Figure 29-4]).[1,12-14]

Immature skeletal fractures can be epiphyseal (i.e., involving epiphysis or part of the bone closest to the joint), physeal (i.e., occurring at the growth plate), metaphyseal (i.e., involving the expanding end of the bone), diaphyseal (i.e., involving central bone shaft), or osteochondral (i.e., including cartilage with involvement of underlying bone).[12,13] Architectural components of the immature skeleton, such as the presence of physes, dense growth lines, secondary centers of ossification and large nutrient foramina, make radiographic diagnosis of bone problems more challenging than in the adult; therefore a comparison of the uninjured extremity may be used to assist in proper diagnosis.[12] It is important to note when viewing a conventional radiograph of the immature skeleton that the cartilaginous physis is radiolucent. Therefore fractures that exist solely within the physis are not visible, unless significant

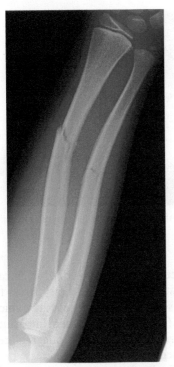

Figure 29-5 Greenstick fractures of the radial and ulnar diaphyses in an 8-year-old boy. The fracture lines only extend through part of the cortex. (From Strouse PJ: Skeletal trauma. In Slovis TL, editor: *Caffey's pediatric diagnostic imaging*, 11 ed, Philadelphia, 2008, Mosby Elsevier.)

displacement has occurred sufficient to identify the physis as widened. As mentioned previously, a comparison view can assist in the determination of physeal widening.

Incomplete fractures occurring in the long bones of children include *Greenstick, Torus or buckle,* and *plastic bowing.* A **Greenstick fracture** (Figure 29-5) occurs when a long bone shaft cortex is fractured on the tension side and the cortex and periosteum remain intact on the compression side of the bone. Plastic bowing or angular deformity may be evident with a Greenstick fracture.[12–14]

A **Torus** or **buckle fracture** (Figure 29-6) is an incomplete, impaction fracture in children that results in buckling of the bony cortex. This fracture typically occurs at the junction of the diaphysis and metaphysis of long bones. This junction is predisposed to failure in the presence of compressive forces because the thicker diaphysis causes disruption of the adjoining metaphysis. This can occur when children fall onto an outstretched hand (FOOSH) or arm. A torus fracture can occasionally be seen in adults with underlying pathology.[12–14]

Plastic bowing (Figure 29-7), often observed in younger children, is an incomplete fracture resulting in a bowing deformity of bone due to excess pressure being placed on the bone. When pressure is released, the bone cannot rebound and remains bowed. This is due to the unique biomechanical nature of developing bone when a longitudinal, compressive force is imposed on a growing bone that is naturally curved. Microscopic fractures and microscopic fatigue lines are evident in deformed bone, and an increase in force can lead to further bone deformation and fracture. Plastic bowing may also be seen with bone pairs, such as the radius and ulna, when a Greenstick fracture is evident in one bone and plastic bowing is evident at the paired bone.[12,13]

Physeal fractures, occurring at the physes or epiphyseal grow plate, account for up to 15% to 30% of all fractures in children. Often children can heal quickly without issue; however, caution must be exercised with growth plate disturbances and resultant partial or complete growth arrest, which occurs in 15% of all physeal injuries.[12–14] Fractures involving the growth plate often increase at the onset of puberty due to biomechanical and structural weaknesses in the physis at this time. Physeal fractures typically heal twice as rapidly as

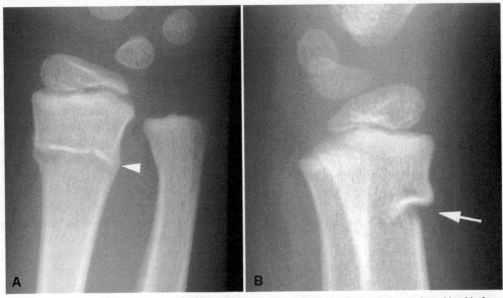

Figure 29-6 Childhood buckle fracture. Posteroanterior (**A**) and lateral (**B**) views show a dorsal distal radial metaphyseal buckle fracture (*arrows*). Note that the epiphysis of the ulna has not yet formed and bony evidence of carpal bones is not complete. (From Manaster BJ, May DA, Disler DG, editors: *Musculoskeletal imaging: the requisites*, ed 4, St. Louis, 2013, Mosby Elsevier.)

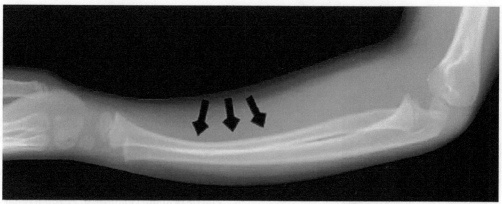

Figure 29-7 Lateral view of a plastic or bowing deformity of the forearm. (From DiFazio R, Atkinson CC: Extremity fractures in children: when is it an emergency? *J Pediatr Nurs* 20:298-304, 2005.)

diaphyseal fractures. The Salter-Harris Classification identifies epiphyseal growth plate fractures according to their fracture line pattern and location (Figure 29-8).[1,12-14] Rang type VI and Ogden VII through IX describe fractures that do not directly involve the physis; however, they describe physeal bridge development as the bone repairs, which may impact bone growth (Figure 29-9).[12,13]

Salter-Harris Classification System for Pediatric Fractures

Type I Fracture lines extend through the physeal plate—*Growth arrest uncommon*

Type II Fracture lines extend through the physeal plate and metaphysis—*May or may not cause growth arrest. Outcomes favorable*

Type III Fracture line extends from the joint surface through the epiphysis and across the physis causing a portion of the epiphysis to become displaced—*Growth arrest likely, often require open reduction internal fixation, an intra-articular injury*

Type IV Fracture line extends from joint surface through the epiphysis, physeal plate, and metaphysis causing a fracture fragment—*Growth arrest likely, almost always require open reduction internal fixation, an intra-articular injury*

Type V Crush injury to the growth plate, not identified until after growth arrest has occurred (6-12 months)—*Rare, growth arrest certain, poor outcomes*

Rang and Ogden classification VI-IX (Expansion of Salter-Harris Classification)

Rang Type VI Injury to perichondral ring or periosteum of the growth plate; little to no direct injury to physis; reparative process may cause osseous bridge; *Possible growth arrest; possible angular deformity; may disrupt physeal blood supply*

Ogden Type VII Osteochondral fracture of epiphysis at articular surface; no injury to physis; *may disrupt physeal blood supply; possible growth disturbance*

Ogden Type VIII Fracture of metaphysis; no injury to physis; *may disrupt physeal blood supply; possible growth disturbance*

Ogden Type IX Avulsion fracture or injury of periosteum; no direct injury to physis; *may disrupt physeal blood supply; possible growth disturbance*

Stress fractures (Figure 29-10), which can be further classified as fatigue and insufficiency stress fractures, are microfractures occurring from repetitive microtrauma to bone. These fractures occur when imbalances exist between bone reabsorption and bone replacement, leading to increased bone weakness, increased stresses, bone fatigue, and finally fracture, and are part of a repetitive injury-overuse syndrome that begins with shin splints (i.e., periostitis) and, if the stress is not relieved, can progress to a stress fracture (see fatigue stress fractures later). Stress fractures commonly occur in the lower extremity; however, they can occur in most bones of the body. Symptoms may begin as dull aching during activity, relieved with rest, progressing to constant pain. Pain may then begin to localize to a specific spot and be reproduced with palpation or the fulcrum test.[1,8,13,14,16] Conventional radiographs are quite commonly negative for stress fracture initially and may continue to not show fracture for several weeks. According to the Academy College of Radiology ACR Appropriate Criteria®, a stress fracture may appear negative on initial radiograph 60% to 82% of the time and remain negative in 40% to 60% of cases.[16] Therefore, magnetic resonance imaging (MRI), due to both its high sensitivity and specificity, may be indicated to confirm if initial radiographs are negative.[1,4] Bone edema and the fracture line can often be identified with MRI.

Fatigue stress fractures involve abnormal activity on bone of normal mineralization or otherwise stated repetitive microtrauma on normal bone. This microtrauma may occur due to a sudden increase in intensity or frequency of activity, change of equipment, malalignment, difference of playing surface or terrain, improper training technique, poor nutrition, inadequate rest, or inappropriate footwear. Young athletes (female more often than male) commonly experience stress fractures from overuse. With the female athlete, additional history needs to be obtained regarding nutrition, menstrual regularity, fatigue and energy level, and activity intensity to address possible additional bone insufficiency.[1,2,13,16]

Insufficiency stress fractures result from normal activity placed on bone deficient of minerals or, as otherwise

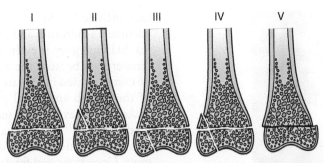

Figure 29-8 Salter-Harris classification of bone fracture in children. Type I: Separation of the epiphysis. Type II: Fracture-separation of the epiphysis. Type III: Fracture of part of the epiphysis. Type IV: Fracture of the epiphysis and the epiphyseal plate; bony union causes premature closure of the plate. Type V: Crushing of the epiphyseal plate; premature closure of the plate on one side with a resultant angular deformity. (Modified from Barr JB, RE Berg: Imaging joints and musculoskeletal tissue: pathoanatomical considerations. In Magee DJ, Zachazewski JE, Quillen WS, editors: *Scientific foundations and principles of practice in musculoskeletal rehabilitation*, p 589, St Louis, 2007, Saunders.)

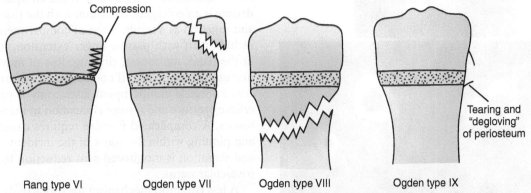

Figure 29-9 Rang-Ogden classification (continuation of the Salter-Harris classification) of bone fracture in children.

stated, normal loading on bone weakened by bone disease or pathology. Some contributing pathologies include osteopenia, rheumatoid arthritis, or metabolic diseases. A differential diagnosis is necessary to ensure proper treatment and to determine the cause of pain. Osteoid osteoma and osteomyelitis may present similarly to a stress fracture, although treatment would be very different.[6,8,12,13]

Risk Factors for Stress Fractures

- Dramatic increase in activity
- Anorexia
- Menstrual irregularity
- Rheumatoid arthritis
- Neuropathy
- Metabolic diseases

Fractures of the clavicle are commonly experienced by those under the age of 25.[17] They represent 4% of all fractures. Ninety percent are caused by a direct blow to the lateral aspect of the shoulder with the arm at the side, with the remaining 10% caused by a FOOSH injury.[18,19] Initial examination indicates pain with overhead and shoulder motions, localized swelling, a palpable defect, and crepitus with movement.[18] Plain radiographs commonly confirm the diagnosis (Figure 29-11). The major-

ity of these fractures occur in the midshaft of the clavicle, are stable, and respond well to conservative nonsurgical treatment. A figure-eight harness or upper extremity sling may be used for 2 to 4 weeks to reduce pain by promoting anatomical alignments. Some athletes report more discomfort when immobilized. In either case, rehabilitation after healing is minimal, and the focus is on posture and restoration of normal motion and strength of the shoulder. Most of these fractures heal with a shortened malunion or enlarged callus, which presents like a bump around the clavicle. The size of the malunion often correlates with the age of the victim, with a younger child having the ability to remodel more quickly and more accurately.[19] Surgery, which is rare especially in this age group, is indicated if there is an open fracture, tenting of the skin over the fracture site, neurovascular compromise, or other surrounding trauma to the area.[19,20]

Supracondylar fractures of the elbow are the most common pediatric elbow fracture in the 5- to 10-year age group due to a thinner cortex and ligament laxity, and these fractures constitute greater than 50% of all elbow fractures.[21] The majority of supracondylar fractures (95%) are caused by a FOOSH injury with a hyperextended elbow that forces the olecranon into the olecranon fossa causing disruption at the anterior cortex.[21] These injuries can be severe and require a thorough neurovascular evaluation and often surgical management.[21] Complications

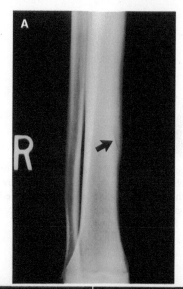

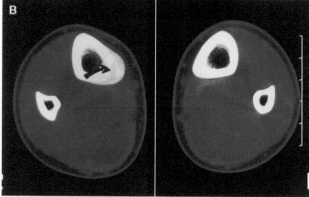

Figure 29-10 Tibial stress fracture. **A,** AP radiograph of the right tibia demonstrates cortical thickening of the tibia medially. There is an oblique fracture line identified in the cortex (*arrow*). **B,** Axial CT scan through both lower legs demonstrates benign periosteal new bone formation along the medial aspect of the right tibia (*curved arrow*). In this patient with an atypical pain pattern for stress fracture, the CT scan was obtained to rule out an osteoid osteoma. There is no radiolucent nidus identified. (From Spitz DJ, Newberg AH: Imaging of stress fractures in the athlete, *Radiol Clin North Am* 40:313-331, 2002.)

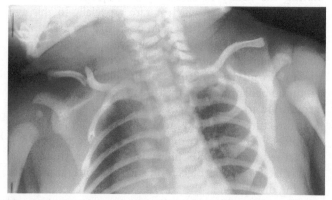

Figure 29-11 Fracture of right clavicle. (From Clark DA: *Atlas of neonatology*, p 8, Philadelphia, 2000, WB Saunders.)

may include loss of motion, neurological deficits, compartment syndrome, and avascular necrosis of the trochlea. Skin integrity is evaluated for color, radial pulse, and temperature because the anterior interosseous nerve may be compromised in 10% to 15% of these fractures. Flexion of the thumb and distal phalanx of the index finger to make the "okay" sign is used to test the integrity of the median nerve.[21] Physical examination reveals swelling, localized tenderness, and a depression over the triceps region. Uncomplicated fractures are immobilized in 70° to 80° of elbow flexion to avoid brachial artery occlusion which may occur if the elbow is maintained in a position of 90°.[21] Excessive swelling and ecchymosis are indicative of extensive soft tissue damage and places the child at risk for compartment syndrome.[22] **Acute compartment syndrome** is an emergent condition with the risk of limb loss and function as a result. Signs of compartment syndrome include pain with passive finger extension, loss of color in the hand, numbness, tingling, loss of movement, and decreased radial pulse. If compartment syndrome is present, a surgical compartment fasciotomy is performed to relieve pressure and restore circulation to the surrounding tissues. A complicated fracture requires closed reduction and pinning within 24 hours of the incident. Hand color and sensation is monitored post reduction to assess neurovascular status.

A less common mechanism for supracondylar fractures occurs if the child falls directly onto the elbow with the arm positioned in flexion. The ulnar nerve is most at risk during this type of fall.

The second most common type of elbow fracture is the distal humerus lateral condyle fracture. It is caused by a FOOSH injury through an avulsion varus force or by a direct blow to the capitellum by the radial head. Treatment consists of closed or open reduction depending on whether the condylar displacement is greater or less than 2 mm. A nonoperative, long arm cast for 4 to 6 weeks is recommended if the displacement is less than 2 mm. Rehabilitation after cast removal may be necessary to restore full elbow and wrist range of motion (ROM) and strength before unrestricted activities.[21]

Avulsion fractures at the elbow (Figure 29-12) are most often seen in teenage boys because the forces generated across the elbow increase with the larger body mass and greater strength of the maturing athlete.[21] The combination of valgus stresses and forceful contraction of the flexor-pronator muscles causes the medial epicondyle to avulse from the underlying bone.[23] A "pop" is often heard or felt at the time of acute onset.[18,21,23] Swelling, ecchymosis, point tenderness, loss of elbow extension, and possible joint instability are present. Anteroposterior (AP) and lateral radiographic views and valgus stress views demonstrate the presence of an avulsion fracture and the amount of displacement.[21,23] Surgical fixation is based on the size and the distance of the displaced fracture

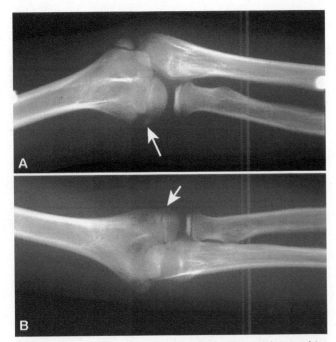

Figure 29-12 A, Oblique projection of a child's elbow with an avulsion fracture of the lateral epicondyle (*arrow*). **B,** Notice that the child's contralateral elbow is normal (*arrow*). Although some advocate taking a radiograph of contralateral anatomy for comparison, it should not be a routine practice in the light of concerns for added cost and radiation exposure. A comparison with an atlas of normal skeletal development would provide the same information without these associated drawbacks. (From Marchiori D: *Clinical imaging*, ed 2, St. Louis, 2005, Mosby Elsevier.)

TABLE 29-3

Common Sites of Avulsion Fractures of the Pelvis, Associated Muscles, and Mechanisms of Injury in the Skeletally Immature

Site	Associated Muscles	Mechanism of Injury
Anterior superior iliac spine	Sartorius	Passive hip extension coupled with knee flexion or active hip flexion coupled with knee extension
Anterior inferior iliac spine	Rectus femoris	Sudden contraction of rectus femoris such as with a vigorous kick
Ischial tuberosity	Hamstrings and adductor magnus	Passive hip flexion coupled with knee extension or active hip extension coupled with knee flexion
Lesser trochanter	Iliopsoas	Sudden active hip flexion
Iliac crest	Abdominal obliques	Sudden contraction of obliques

Modified from Merkel DL, Molony JT: Clinical commentary: recognition and management of traumatic sports injuries in the skeletally immature athlete, *Intl J Sports Phys Ther* 7:691-704, 2012.

(>2 mm), associated joint instability, and the presence of ulnar nerve symptoms. Conservative management with cast immobilization is recommended for 3 weeks for a nondisplaced or minimally displaced fracture of less than 2 mm, as long as there is no nerve involvement or joint instability.[23,24] After cast removal, a hinged brace is worn for 4 to 6 weeks.[23] Gentle ROM exercises begin early to maximize the achievement of terminal elbow extension. Flexor-pronator strengthening is initiated when the athlete is symptom free. A return to throwing program begins when radiographic union is visible.[23]

Avulsion fractures around the hip and pelvis occur at the same six sites as the apophyseal areas.[25,26] The most common sites are the anterior superior iliac spine (ASIS) and the ischial tuberosity. These are acute injuries caused by a sudden powerful contraction of the attached muscles or quick stretch at end ROM that pulls violently on the nonossified apophysis.[25,26] Sports that require running, sprinting, twisting, jumping, cutting, kicking, and lower extremity hyperflexibility have the highest incidence of this type of injury. These injuries are often misrepresented as muscle strains that occur in the adult athlete after the apophysis (secondary growth plate) has closed. A sudden pop is heard or felt followed by pain, swelling, weakness, and possible ecchymosis. Table 29-3 identifies the mechanism of injury at each specific apophysis and

corresponding muscle involvement. Radiographs show gross displacement, and a contralateral comparison view may be necessary to identify subtle changes. Nonoperative treatment includes protected weight bearing, rest, ice, and avoidance of the offending activities. Protective weight bearing lasts until callus formation is noted on the radiographs. Physical therapy begins with symptom resolution. Aquatic therapy may begin early if the child can perform water activities without increasing symptoms. Gentle ROM and active movements with a slow progression to full weight bearing comprise the first phase of rehabilitation. Strengthening of the entire hip area, progression of resisted activities, and unilateral exercises follow. Bilateral and unilateral plyometric and return to sport activities complete the rehabilitation process. Low volumes and decreased intensity and speed are initiated as the child or adolescent returns to activities and sports. Full, symptom-free ROM and the involved extremity displaying 90% of strength compared with the uninvolved side are criteria for return to play.[25-27] Complete resolution of symptoms and full return to play may take up to 3 months. Surgical reattachment of displaced fragment is recommended if the displacement is greater than 3 cm.[28]

In the skeletally immature patient, the tibial spine where the anterior cruciate ligament (ACL) inserts into the tibial plateau is weaker (due to its incomplete ossification) than the ACL and often fails under valgus rotation stresses with the knee extended before rupture of the ACL. **Tibial spine avulsion fractures** are primarily observed in children ages 8 to 14 years and can occur with or without contact.[29-33] Physical findings include pain, rapid onset of effusion, and reduced weight bearing. A positive anterior drawer test may be noted. Extreme ranges of knee motion are limited due to increasing pain. Tibial spine avulsion fractures are best viewed on lateral radiographs. MRI is used to rule out concomitant meniscal tears or other ligamentous injury, which occur in approximately 40% of tibial spine injuries.[30-32] There are four types of tibial spine fractures: type I nondisplaced, type II partially attached, type III displaced, and type IV comminuted.[29,30,32] Acute management involves immobilization and immediate medical evaluation. Minimally displaced fractures are treated with cylinder casting and protective weight bearing for 2 to 6 weeks. Surgical screw fixation is recommended for types III and IV avulsions or when reduction cannot be achieved through casting. Potential complications include loss of ROM, muscle atrophy, nonunion (rare) or malunion, growth disturbance, and residual laxity. Subjective reports of laxity are rare, but positive physical examination findings should be noted.[29,30,32] The residual laxity does not improve with maturation. Loss of knee motion with a tibial spine fracture may be as a result of mechanical impingement of the displaced fracture or arthrofibrosis following immobilization. Early motion after surgery is recommended to prevent stiffness. Rehabilitation goals begin with restoration of ROM, light strengthening exercises, and gradual weight-bearing progression. Intermediate and final phases of rehabilitation follow ACL protocols with a cautious return to sport.

Seventy percent of all carpal bone fractures occur at the scaphoid. A **scaphoid fracture** (Figure 29-13) is often seen in active people between the ages of 15 and 30 years. The scaphoid has a complicated vascular anatomy that impacts healing and therefore treatment decisions.[34] A FOOSH injury is the most common mechanism, with tenderness reproduced in the anatomic snuff box, decreased wrist ROM, as well as swelling and pain with wrist extension. Radiographs may be negative; therefore clinical suspicion of a scaphoid fracture warrants an MRI. Scaphoid fractures are initially treated conservatively to optimize healing and obtain fracture union.[34] In addition to the physical characteristics of the fracture, the sport and position played and goals of the athlete may impact management. The scaphoid fracture is managed initially with casting but some do require surgery. Slow healing or nonunion scaphoid fractures are frequently seen in athletes in which a delay in proper care and diagnosis was evident.[34]

General Management of Scaphoid Fractures

- Cast immobilization for 8-10 weeks without playing
- Cast immobilization and a playing cast for return to sport participation
- Surgical fixation

Chondral (Cartilage) Injuries

Cartilage injuries, occurring in the immature skeleton, may or may not extend to the underlying cancellous bone. If underlying bone is involved, the inflammatory process will assist in healing at the bony level. Cartilage does not have a direct blood or lymphatic circulation or nerve supply; therefore it has minimal ability to self-repair following injury. Generally, bone repair in children is more effective due to increased vascularity to the periosteum and metaphysis. Factors influencing osteochondral lesions are trauma, uneven or excessive pressure, disruption of blood supply to the bone, and genetics.[12,13]

Panner's Disease

Panner's disease (Figure 29-14) is an osteochondrosis of the capitellum at the distal end of the humerus and is often confused with osteochondritis dissecans (OCD) of the same bone. Both diagnoses have similar pathological processes and mechanisms of injury due to repetitive compression forces at the lateral elbow, which compromises blood flow to the capitellum, but differ in stages of development and resultant outcomes.[35,36] Panner's disease is seen in the young athlete (ages 4 to 10 years) who competes in throwing, racquet sports, or gymnastics. A vague description of lateral elbow pain and loss of 10° to 20° extension are classic signs of the condition.[37] Radiographs may show demineralization, fissuring, or fragmentation of the capitellum, avascular necrosis of the ossific nucleus, and flattening of the capitellum.[38] Repeated radiographs are a part of the monitoring process to ensure healing is occurring. Surgery is not indicated unless the condition does not resolve with rest and activity modification. Return to sport usually occurs in the next season without sequelae, and long-term success rates are excellent.[35] Physical therapy prepares the athlete to return to sport

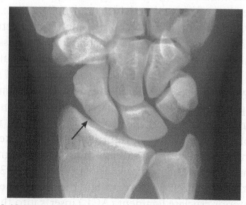

Figure 29-13 Transverse fracture of the scaphoid (*arrow*) in a 16-year-old boy. (From Strouse PJ: Skeletal trauma. In Slovis TL, editor: *Caffey's pediatric diagnostic imaging*, ed 11, Philadelphia, 2008, Mosby Elsevier.)

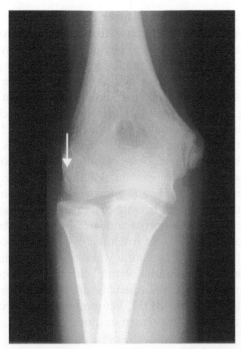

Figure 29-14 Panner's Disease. Note fragmentation of the humeral capitellum and flattening of the articular surface (*arrow*). (From Landry GL: Management of musculoskeletal injury. In Kliegman RM, Behrman RE, Jenson HB, Stanton BF: *Nelson textbook of pediatrics*, ed 18, Philadelphia, 2007, Saunders/Elsevier.)

when sufficient healing has occurred. Reshaping and restoration of the capitellum can take up to 1 to 3 years.

Osteochondritis Dissecans

Osteochondritis dissecans (OCD) of the capitellum occurs in the 10- to 17-year-old athlete, with the median age at 14, when the cartilage separates from the underlying subchondral bone due to vascular compromise from repetitive microtrauma at the lateral elbow.[37,39-41] At this stage of growth, the capitellum is almost fully developed and blood supply is tenuous. High-level athletes who participate in overhead throwing, gymnastics, or weight lifting are at most risk.[42-45] Boys are 2 times as likely as girls to experience this injury; however, gymnasts are at particular risk due to excessive weight bearing with high compressive loads placed across the elbow and are often advised to discontinue gymnastics in the presence of severe OCD injuries. Pain and loss of motion are observed as in Panner's disease, but grinding, clicking, or locking due to fragmentation or loose bodies could be present as well as synovitis. In addition to the extension loss, mild loss in flexion and forearm rotation may also be observed.[40,42,43] MRI is the imaging of choice for full visualization of the OCD lesion, cartilage integrity, and viewing of loose bodies within the joint space.[38] Management of OCD lesions of the capitellum is dependent on the size of the fragment, history of injury, presence of loose bodies, and integrity of the cartilage as well as the age of the patient. Early recognition and appropriate management are

extremely important to produce good results and return the athlete to sport. Younger patients with smaller lesions and an intact articular cartilage have the best outcomes. Older athletes with larger lesions, detached cartilage, and/or loose bodies demonstrate less favorable results and are often unable to return to sports participation at previous level of play because pain and ROM deficits persist.[41,44,45] Surgical interventions depend on the extent of the injury and may constitute loose body removal or refixation, debridement, and/or resurfacing. Techniques to facilitate healing, such as subchondral bone drilling or abrasion chondroplasty, may be used.[40,43,45,46] Postoperative treatment protocols include continuous passive motion (CPM) for 4 to 6 weeks, low-impact physical therapy at 6 weeks, and strenuous exercises and return to sport activities at 6 to 12 months, based on completion of ROM, strength, and symptom goals.

OCD occurs most commonly in the knee, most often on the lateral aspect of the medial femoral condyle. With the condition, there is separation of the articular cartilage from the underlying subchondral bone.[47] OCD lesions are classified in stages I to IV to describe the extent of the lesion and subsequent treatment algorithm. The deformation of the cartilage surface is illustrated in Figure 29-15. Boys ages 5 to 15 years are more susceptible than girls by a 2:1 or 3:1 ratio.[47] The athlete presents with persistent vague knee pain that is worse with activity initially and then the pain becomes constant if ignored.[47] Swelling and stiffness may also be present in the knee. AP, lateral, tunnel, and merchant radiographic views are used for improved viewing of all potential injured structures. MRI is very useful in evaluating the status of the OCD lesion and surrounding structures.[47] Management of OCD lesions depends on the size, fragmentation, and presence of loose bodies in the joint. Small lesions without loose fragments are treated conservatively with several weeks of immobilization and protected weight bearing.[47] Younger

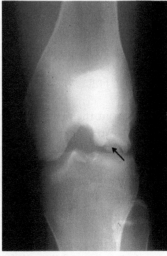

Figure 29-15 Stage III OCD lesion (*arrow*) of the medial femoral condyle.

patients with open growth plates have better outcomes than adolescents with closing growth centers.[47] Surgical intervention is required if conservative treatment (i.e., 3 to 6 months of rest, activity modification and rehabilitation) fails or the presence of large lesions with loose bodies is observed. Surgical approaches include debridement, loose body removal, drilling, or autologous chondrocyte implantation (ACI) transplantation. Rehabilitation focuses on protecting the cartilage while gently reestablishing ROM and strength. Gradual progression of weight bearing occurs as cellular healing is established. Both open- and closed-chain exercises are used in restricted ROM for protection of the healing structures. Initiation of impact activities is delayed for 6 to 9 months, depending on the surgical procedure. Return to sport may take up to a year following surgery.

Growth Plate (Physis) Injuries

Apophysitis

Apophysitis, uniquely seen with the immature skeleton, is the irritation of the apophysis (secondary growth plate). Many of these injuries have been named after individuals (e.g., Sever's) and have been labeled as diseases. However, the pathological process, although it does involve inflammation of a structure (the physis or growth plate), does not follow a disease process. Therefore to call these inflammatory processes a disease is a misnomer. The apophysis is the cartilaginous structure in children, located on a long bone serving as attachment site for the musculotendinous unit. In adults, tendonitis would be experienced because tendons attach directly to bone. Additional stress on the apophysis is most common during times of growth spurts when tendons or ligaments are stronger and muscles are weaker and less flexible. Some examples of apophysitis, which will be covered in detail later in this chapter, are Sever's disease, Osgood-Schlatter syndrome or disease, Sinding-Larsen-Johansson syndrome, and apophysitis occurring in the spine and pelvis. If the traumatic episodes exceed the strength of the apophysis, a child is at risk for an avulsion injury at the apophysis. An avulsion injury occurs when excessive forces separate the apophysis from the underlying bone.[1,8,12,13]

Shoulder Physeal Stress Fracture (Little Leaguer's Shoulder)

The rotational stress about the proximal humerus during repetitive overhead throwing (i.e., pitching) may produce a stress fracture of the humeral physis known as "little leaguer's shoulder."[18,19,23] The throwing athlete (age 11 to 15 years) is most vulnerable, although in general, proximal humeral physeal fractures make up only 3% of all physeal fractures.[19,23] The majority of these fractures (75%) are Salter-Harris type II (see Figure 29-8) and demonstrate excellent nonoperative results if rest and rehabilitation recommendations are followed.[19] Salter-Harris

type I fractures are seen in upper extremity impact sports, such as gymnastics.[23] Because 80% of humeral growth is determined by the humeral physis, early detection is important in prevention of premature closure of the physis, limb shortening, a varus deformity, and possible resultant shoulder impingement. Radiographs are the initial imaging of choice with AP, axillary, stryker notch, and comparison views conducted. Widening of the physis is noted and illustrated in Figure 29-16. Imaging is useful to rule out unicameral bone cysts and bone tumors as a source of pain. Physical examination shows swelling, weakness, decreased ROM, and muscle atrophy around the proximal anterior and lateral humerus. Pain on palpation over the proximal humerus and lateral physis is observed in approximately 70% of patients.[19,23] Treatment consists of rest from throwing and any additional offending activity for 1 to 3 months or until the next season.[19,23,48] Once symptom free, the athlete begins physical therapy to reestablish strength, ROM, neuromuscular control, and gradual symptom-free return to sport.

Little Leaguer's Elbow

The term "Little Leaguer's Elbow" has been discussed and described in the literature, sports medicine offices, and on the field in many different ways. Originally, little leaguer's elbow referred to apophysitis of the medial epicondyle of young baseball pitchers due to the repetitive valgus stresses that occur to the medial elbow during late cocking and the acceleration phase of throwing.[49] Over time, the term has been used to describe many overuse entities around the elbow in the young athlete that occur with lateral compression forces, medial traction stresses, and posterior extension overloads. Panner's disease, OCD of the capitellum, medial epicondyle apophysis, and posterior elbow pain are often grouped together under "little leaguer's elbow" but should be described as separate pathological processes and are observed in gymnasts,

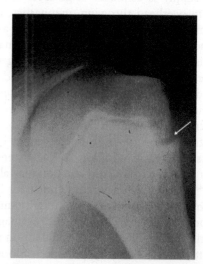

Figure 29-16 AP image of the proximal humerus showing a widened lateral physis (*arrow*), indicative of a stress fracture of the physis.

weight lifters, and other overhead athletes in addition to throwers. A rise in these injuries has been noted with increases in youth sports participation, and it appears contributory factors include early specialization, high activity volumes, participation on multiple same sport teams in a season, attempting or performing sports skills above physical and skeletal readiness, and decreased rest times, with most athletes resting only 1 day a week. Prevention strategies for overuse injuries of the upper extremity are shown in the following textbox.

Upper Extremity Injury Prevention Strategies

- Limit onset of teaching of difficult pitches
- Use of a smaller, youth-sized baseball
- Optimize technique and throwing mechanics
- Insure appropriate strength and conditioning of arms, shoulders, core and legs
- Limit number of pitches
- Recognize total volume of throwing (multiple leagues and teams, free play)
- Recognize that unconditioned athletes tend to have poor mechanics
- Recognize that highly conditioned athletes are predisposed to exceed the limits of the musculoskeletal system

NOTE: Detailed pitching recommendations can be found on the USA Baseball Medical and Safety Advisory Committee Guidelines webpage http://www.asmi.org/asmiweb/usabaseball.htm

From Merkel DL, Molony JT: Clinical Commentary: Recognition and management of traumatic sports injuries in the skeletally immature athlete, *Intl J Sports Phys Ther* 7:691-704, 2012.

Medial epicondyle apophysitis is a traction injury caused by repetitive valgus stresses at the medial elbow and is observed in young athletes (age 8 to 14 years) who exhibit open growth centers. The same mechanism of injury produces ulnar collateral ligament injuries in adult throwers, but because the physis in the young is the "weak link," injury occurs there rather than to the ligament.[50] Symptoms include medial elbow pain, decreased elbow ROM, pain with activity that is initially relieved by rest, and a decrease in performance. Physical examination reveals pain with the following tests: palpation over the medial epicondyle, valgus stress testing, and resisted wrist flexion and pronation.[50,51] Contralateral elbow radiographs assist in depicting widening and fragmentation of the apophysis (Figure 29-17).[50] Rest from offending activities, such as throwing, weight bearing, and sports participation, for 4 to 6 weeks is recommended. Education regarding the risk of continued participation and potential avulsion fracture occurrence is necessary. Physical therapy may begin once symptoms have subsided and the condition is improving. Initially, periscapular, low-resistance exercises and activities below shoulder level are implemented. Gentle stretching to the flexor-pronator mass is performed if the ROM is restricted. Shoulder and core strengthening should also be addressed because proper use of the whole kinetic chain

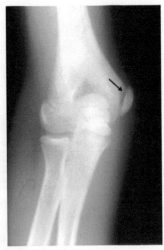

Figure 29-17 AP radiograph showing widening of the medial apophysis (*arrow*).

can decrease the stress on the elbow. Resistance exercises with elastic bands and weights are slowly progressed as tolerated. Good shoulder strength and muscular balance around the entire shoulder complex assists in supporting the elbow during the stresses of throwing. A biomechanical evaluation and gradual return to sport are the focus at the end stages of rehabilitation. The athlete cannot return to sport participation until the highest level skill is practiced and demonstrated in the clinic without symptoms.

Slipped Capital Femoral Epiphysis

Obese, pubescent males are at higher risk for acquiring a slipped capital femoral epiphysis (SCFE). This diagnosis is not sports related but can affect athletes as well. Excessive stresses across the cartilaginous growth plate cause the distal portion of the femoral head, called the epiphysis, to displace from its normal alignment (Figure 29-18).[52] The slippage occurs much like a scoop of melted ice cream falling off its cone. The adolescent presents with pain into the groin, medial thigh, or knee. Limping with the leg positioned in lateral (external) rotation is common. In supine, the patient position of comfort is hip flexion, abduction, and lateral (external) rotation. A loss of medial (internal) rotation and a positive log roll test are characteristic. Surgical pinning of the slipped bony fragment is recommended for best outcomes and to prevent avascular necrosis of the epiphysis.[52] Because the presence of bilateral SCFE occurs in up to 30% of those adolescents affected, monitoring of the unaffected hip is recommended until epiphyseal closure has occurred.[52] Postsurgical physical therapy is recommended following established protocols.

Clinical Point

In children, medial knee pain with no history of trauma should include examination of the hip.

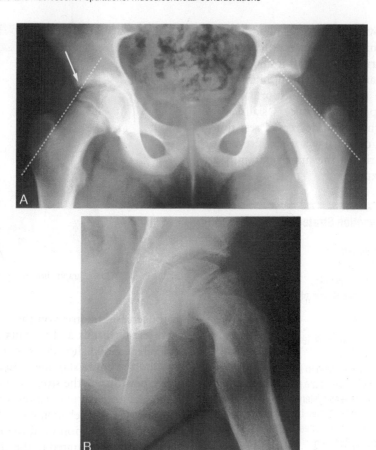

Figure 29-18 A, Right slipped capital femoral epiphysis. Note Klein's line and how epiphysis does not cross line (*arrow*). Compare with normal left hip. **B,** Slipped capital femoral epiphysis in an overweight boy, aged 11. (*A,* from Adam A, Dixon A, Grainger RG, Allison DJ, editors: *Grainger & Allison's diagnostic radiology,* ed 5, Philadelphia, 2008, Churchill Livingstone; *B,* from Long BW, Frank ED, Ehrlich RA: *Radiography essentials for limited practice,* ed 3, St. Louis, 2010, Saunders Elsevier.)

Risk Factors for Slipped Capital Femoral Epiphysis

- Age (adolescence)
- Male
- High activity level
- Obesity

Hip Apophysitis

Apophyseal injuries are more prevalent in the immature skeleton until ossification of the cartilaginous growth centers is complete. Older adolescents and young adults (age 14 through 25 years) commonly experience apophysitis at the remaining open growth centers around the hip and pelvis.[25] The six major sites for apophysitis in this region include the iliac crest, ASIS, anterior inferior iliac spine (AIIS), ischial physis, greater trochanter, and lesser trochanter.[25] The ASIS is the last apophysis to mature, and may remain open until the age of 25. Iliac crest apophysitis is the most frequently observed and often plagues runners, dancers, ice skaters, and football and soccer players. Painful palpation over the iliac crest is noted and pain is reproduced by resisted trunk rotation due to the pull of the abdominal oblique muscles at their insertion on to the pelvis. General treatment for all six sites includes

activity modification or complete rest if symptoms have been prolonged and are constant. Therapeutic exercises include trunk and hip joint ROM as well as flexibility, extensive core and hip strengthening without symptom reproduction, and technique evaluation and adjustment if poor execution of skill is a contributory factor to this overuse syndrome. Biomechanical evaluation of the entire lower kinetic chain is important as weakness or dysfunction away from the site of injury could be problematic.

Distal Femoral Physis Fracture

An adult athlete who sustains a valgus force to a fully extended knee may suffer a medial collateral ligament (MCL) tear. The same mechanism in the immature skeleton of the youth athlete potentially produces a distal femoral physeal fracture due to the origin of the MCL on the femoral epiphysis and the insertion into the stronger tibial metaphysis. Although occurring in less than 1% of pediatric fractures, distal femoral physeal fractures are evaluated thoroughly because growth disturbance at the physis can cause significant angular deformities and leg length discrepancies due to growth centers at the knee that are large and fast growing.[13,30] Acute neurovascular compromise may also be a complication. The young athlete presents with medial knee pain, pain on valgus stress testing, and painful palpation over distal femoral physis with or without tenderness to the MCL. Plain films and MRI are recommended to appropriately view physeal separation and the size of fracture displacement. Salter-Harris fracture classification I through IV (see Figure 29-8) may potentially occur with this mechanism of injury. Salter-Harris I diagnosis is evident with physeal widening without involvement of the epiphysis or metaphysis.[30] Radiographs are usually normal, and the MRI will be positive. Type I injuries are treated conservatively with immobilization for 2 weeks. Fifty-four percent of distal femoral physeal fractures are Salter-Harris type II.[30] The fracture line transverses the physis then exits obliquely across one corner of the metaphysis. If the fracture is nondisplaced, then knee immobilization is initiated for 4 to 6 weeks. A displaced type II fracture requires closed reduction under anesthesia and cast immobilization for 6 to 8 weeks with 2 weeks of non-weight bearing. Salter-Harris type III and type IV often require open reduction and internal fixation. All types of Salter-Harris fractures of the distal femoral physis require long-term monitoring with serial radiographs to identify healing and premature physeal closure.[30]

Apophyseal Injuries of the Knee

Osgood-Schlatter disease or syndrome and **Sinding-Larsen-Johansson** injuries are an inflammation of the apophysis at the tibial tubercle and inferior pole of the patella, respectively. Both of these diagnoses are overuse traction injuries of the anterior knee and are caused by sports that require repetitive running or jumping. Pain occurs during activities and is relieved by rest in the early stages. Preadolescents, both males and females, at the height of their growth spurts are most affected. Osgood-Schlatter disease is painful on palpation of the tibial tubercle and is reproducible with performance of aggravating activities in the clinic. Many athletes acquire a permanent bump on the tibial tubercle. Plain films may show tibial tubercle displacement (Figure 29-19) or avulsion in cases of disease progression. Sinding-Larsen-Johansson shows pain on palpation at the inferior pole of the patella, and

the athlete may demonstrate a quadriceps lag during a straight leg raise. In prolonged cases, the inferior pole of the patella, along with the cartilage and surrounding retinaculum, can avulse and be displaced inferiorly. This is referred to as a **sleeve fracture**.

Athletes with apophysitis are allowed to continue to play with mild pain symptoms, if pain is less than 3 out of 10 on a visual analogue scale (VAS), relieved with rest, and abolished by the next practice session. If the athlete requires pain medication to play or is limping while playing, participation in sport is not advised.

Salter-Harris Fractures of the Distal Fibula

The ankle is a commonly injured body part of athletes of all ages.[21] It is the third most common site of physeal injury in the young athlete.[53] The athlete with an immature skeleton is more likely to suffer a distal fibula growth plate fracture during an ankle inversion injury than an ankle sprain. The presence of a physeal fracture needs to be ruled out in this population. The point of maximal tenderness during palpation is over the physis, which is located one finger width above or proximal to the distal end of the fibula. Ligamentous tenderness on palpation may also be noted. Swelling, ecchymosis, or the ability to weight bear may or may not be present. Plain films may not demonstrate widening of the physis in Salter-Harris type I fractures but palpatory pain over the physis will clinically implicate a fracture. Palpation of the base of the fifth metatarsal and head of the fibula is necessary to identify associated fractures with a lateral ankle injury. Salter-Harris type I and type II fractures of the distal fibular physis most often heal rapidly without sequelae. Cast or boot immobilization for 2 to 4 weeks is commonly implemented.[29] Rehabilitation after immobilization follows treatment protocols for an ankle sprain. Salter-Harris type III and IV are intra-articular, with fracture fragmentation, and required open reduction and internal fixation to restore alignment. Delay in proper diagnosis may create chronic pain, instability, and reduced function.

> **Clinical Point**
>
> In young children, a growth plate fracture due to an ankle inversion injury is more likely than an ankle sprain.

Sever's Disease

Sever's disease (Figure 29-20) is apophysitis of the calcaneus. It is characterized by heel pain, a positive calcaneal squeeze test, and tight gastrocnemius-soleus complex. Sever's disease is typically seen in 8- to 15-year-olds during or just after a rapid growth spurt.[54] Running and jumping activities aggravate the symptoms. Treatment focuses on pain reduction and stretching of the calf muscles. Heel cups and heel lifts which position the foot in slight plantar flexion reduce stress on the calcaneal apophysis.[55,56]

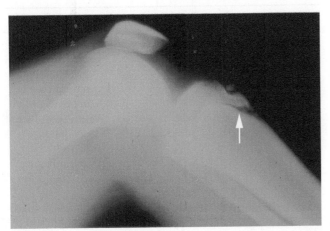

Figure 29-19 Lateral radiograph of showing tibial tubercle fragmentation and physical widening in advanced Osgood-Schlatter disease (*arrow*).

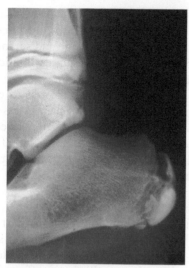

Figure 29-20 Sever's disease in an 11-year-old male with fragmentation of the calcaneal apophysis. (From Macias C, Gabor R: Overuse syndromes and inflammatory conditions. In Baren J, Rothrock S, Brennan J, Brown L editors: *Pediatric emergency medicine*, Philadelphia, 2008, Saunders Elsevier.)

Modification of footwear and orthotics may be indicated. Symptoms typically resolve in a few weeks when early intervention is implemented. Participation in sport is allowed if symptoms are mild and controlled without pain medications. Cast or boot immobilization is indicated for prolonged symptoms, failed conservative methods, and/or a decreased ability to bear weight. *Iselin's disease* is another apophysitis of the foot and is located at the site of attachment of the peroneus brevis muscle on the fifth metatarsal.

Growing Pains

One of the most common complaints of children and adolescents is musculoskeletal pain and in some cases is a cause for missing school and other activities. There can be many contributing overlapping factors to childhood musculoskeletal pain, including night pains, benign hypermobility syndrome, inflammatory conditions, rheumatological conditions, lyme disease, overuse injuries (covered extensively in this chapter), psychogenic factors, or conditions such as osteoid osteoma. A thorough history, observation, and examination are imperative, including overall "ill" versus "well" appearance, school absences, joint pain, muscle atrophy, limitation in extremity, and/or back ROM, tender points, tenderness at apophyses or bony insertion of tendons for older children, swelling, stiffness, weakness, rashes, eye manifestations, and genitourinary or bowel issues.[57,58]

Systemic Musculoskeletal Issues in Children

Anatomical Alignment

Similar to adults, children can develop problems related to variations in their anatomy. Certain malalignment problems tend to be related to particular overuse injuries. Good posture and anatomical alignment are the result of balance in a multisegmental system. Movement takes place at the most flexible segments rather than the area of restrictions. Alterations in the patterns and precision of movement can cause microtrauma, which leads to macrotrauma and pain if not corrected.

Table 29-4 presents a list of some common malalignment conditions, the overuse injury that results, and the means of correction. Historically the grouping of the most common biomechanical features often associated with many overuse injuries (i.e., an increased quadriceps [Q] angle, excessive pronation, increased femoral anteversion, and genu valgum, especially in females) was referred to as *miserable malalignment*. Although this term is rarely used in orthopedics today, it is important that clinicians know its meaning if they encounter it.

Night Pains

Night pains in the lower extremities, of unknown etiology, sometimes occur with children. These pains are not always indicative of serious illness. Toddlers and preadolescent children who sometimes experience thigh and/or calf muscle soreness may respond to anti-inflammatory pain medication, stretching, or vigorous massage before bed. Pain in this age group appears to increase after a busy day. Many young people over age 12 also may complain of leg or foot cramps unrelated to exertion which often interrupts sleep patterns. Stretching is recommended for these adolescents.[1]

Hyperlaxity

Benign hypermobility syndrome is an inherited disease of the connective tissue. It is defined as the presence of joint hypermobility, which is measured using a validated, nine-point scoring system such as the **Beighton-**

TABLE 29-4

Common Malalignments

Malalignment	Injury	Correction
Femoral anteversion	Snapping psoas	Prevention of pelvic rotation by establishing muscle balance in pelvic girdle
Genu valgum	Patella subluxation	Vastus medialis obliquus (VMO) strengthening
Pes planus	Foot pain, knee pain	Orthotic inserts
Medial (internal) tibial torsion	In-toeing, tripping	None, osteotomy

Horan Ligament Laxity Scale (Box 29-1).[59,60] One point is given to each side of the body for items 1 to 4, and a final point is given based on trunk flexion. Benign hypermobility syndrome commonly occurs with children and adolescents, especially females who are involved with activities such as gymnastics. Hyperlaxity in different joints (four out of nine positive sites of laxity) is evident and may be complicated by recurrent sprains, dislocations, or chronic overuse issues. Blood tests are normal and symptoms include diffuse joint pain that worsens at the end of the day and after activity. Children typically do not miss school or activity. Prognosis is excellent with supportive care. Recovery may be gradual because the child's body matures and the child becomes less flexible with age.[57,58]

Hypermobility syndrome is a diagnosis of exclusion, one that is reached after more serious diseases have been ruled out. No widely accepted, effective intervention or physical therapy treatment is available for the condition. Exercise or activity may appear to make the pain worse because a clear link does not always exist between an activity and the onset of pain. The plan for therapy emphasizes joint protection strategies, supportive splints, and avoidance of bringing joints to the end of ROM, as well as stabilization through postural training, strengthening, and proprioception. Children and adolescents with joint laxity or hypermobility should be assessed for preparedness to participate in their desired play and recreational activities.

Growth Spurts

The rapid growth of a child can lead to relative muscle tightness, especially during the adolescent growth surge. This tightness can lead to apophyseal stress or injury. For the extremities, the primary growth centers (i.e., where most growth occurs) for the upper limb are the shoulder and wrist, whereas for the lower limb, it is at the knee.

Inflammatory Disorders

Rheumatic or inflammatory disorders may present with joint pain, swelling, limited ROM, stiffness, and weakness. Rheumatic issues may present with rashes, eye manifestations, genitourinary and bowel symptoms, and the child may not look well. Physicians will be able to assess and order appropriate blood testing and imaging to further determine diagnosis. Some examples of these disorders include spondyloarthropathy syndromes, Reiter's syndrome, seronegative enthesopathy and arthropathy syndrome, spondyloarthritis, and juvenile rheumatoid arthritis.[57,58]

Psychological Considerations

An increasing number of adolescents and preteens appear to experience musculoskeletal symptoms as an emotional defense mechanism to managing pressure for achieving high levels of accomplishment at sports and academics. These children will often miss school or activity time. It is important to promptly provide supportive treatment and to explore the possibility of this phenomenon occurring.[57,58]

Upper Extremity Injuries

Traumatic upper extremity injuries as a result of a FOOSH are common in children because they inadvertently tumble off bikes, scooters, swing sets, and other moving apparatus.[21] These injuries are an inherent risk as youths participate in sports and play, but the risks are well worth taking to combat sedentary lifestyles and childhood obesity. Traumatic injuries of the upper extremity include but are not limited to fractures and dislocations about the shoulder, elbow, wrist, and hand. However, overuse injuries, which can be minimized, are on the rise because early specialization and year-round participation in only one sport is increasingly emphasized. These repetitive stress injuries are preventable, and the trained physical therapist can influence the reduction of these injuries through preventative programs.

Glenohumeral Joint Dislocations

The glenohumeral joint can dislocate both traumatically and atraumatically in three different planes: anterior, posterior, and inferior. Most dislocations occur anteriorly and are more common in adolescents and young adults (Figure 29-21).[19,23,61] Less than 2% of these dislocations occur under the age of 10 years. Most dislocations that do occur in children under the age of 12 are atraumatic, often bilateral, and the result of pathological joint laxity.[23] The most common mechanism of injury for an anterior shoulder dislocation is a blow to the shoulder while positioned in abduction, extension, and lateral (external) rotation.[62] Following anterior dislocation, the affected upper extremity is commonly positioned in slight abduction and medial (internal) rotation.[19] Due to a risk of neurovascular compromise and/or physeal involvement, the adolescent's shoulder reduction is performed in a medical facility where pre and post radiographs and sensation testing are performed to ensure an uncompromised relocation.[63] Immobilization protocols post reduction

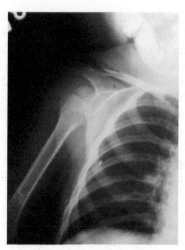

Figure 29-21 An anteroposterior radiograph of right shoulder showing anterior dislocation of the shoulder joint in a 2-year-old child. (From Pawar M, Trikha V, Yadav CS, Rastogi S: Post-traumatic shoulder joint dislocation in a very young child, *Injury Extra* 37:145-146, 2006.)

vary greatly because the literature is inconclusive regarding preferred treatment methods. Many physicians recommend 3 to 6 weeks of immobilization followed by gradual ROM, whereas some physicians advocate early motion within 5 to 7 days of reduction. Conservative management of shoulder dislocations have not shown a difference in re-dislocation rate between shoulder immobilization in lateral (external) versus medial (internal) rotation.[64] Treatment algorithms considering both surgical and nonsurgical interventions for anterior shoulder dislocations are athlete- and surgeon-specific based on presentation, history, sport involved, time of injury (mid-season versus end of season), presence of a Bankart lesion, presence of a Hill-Sachs lesion, amount of pain and dysfunction, and whether physical therapy has been prescribed. A Hill-Sachs lesion is an impaction fracture of the posterior lateral margin of the humeral head as it forcefully contacts the glenoid rim during anterior dislocation.[19,48] Such lesions during dislocation increase shoulder instability if greater than 30% of the humeral articular surface is involved.[19] Detachment of the labrum from the anterior glenoid is called a Bankart lesion and has been shown to occur in 97% of patients who were examined arthroscopically following dislocation.[19,62] Depending on the literature source, a high incidence of reoccurrence (55% to 100%) has been observed for those under the age of 20 years.[19,23,62] Athletes have a 3 times higher rate of redislocation than nonathletes.[62] Intervention for an athlete who sustains a first-time dislocation may include counseling regarding the high incidence of reoccurrence, conservative management after immobilization, and exploration into surgical options, although commonly surgery is not considered unless at least one redislocation has occurred. Shoulder stabilizing braces may be a nonsurgical option for some athletes depending on their sport and position played. There are

numerous braces on the market with both positive and negative aspects.[62] Comfort, ease of application, ROM limitation, impact on athletic performance, and warmth of brace varied among the different types of braces and contribute to the athlete's satisfaction. Some braces may be comfortable and breathable but do not sufficiently restrict motion to prevent instability. Others may adequately prevent instability but negatively impact athletic performance. The main purpose of shoulder brace is to limit shoulder motion to provide stability which may be counterproductive for those sports and positions that require full or extreme ROM for participation.[62] Physical therapy initially consists of gentle motion, periscapular and rotator cuff strengthening, restoration of muscular balance around the glenohumeral joint, and avoidance of provocative positions of abduction and lateral (external) rotation. As healing occurs, pain is reduced, full ROM is achieved, and resistive strengthening in both open- and closed-chain positions is emphasized. Neuromuscular re-education is initially performed in the mid range of ROM, in the plane of the scapula (scaption). As dynamic stabilization improves, these exercises can be progressed toward end range positions, particularly medial (internal) and lateral (external) rotation with the glenohumeral joint elevated to 90° of abduction. As with all upper extremity injuries, core and lower extremity strength and functional deficits are addressed and treated to ensure the whole kinetic chain plays an appropriate role in the child's activities. A gradual return to throwing or sport is initiated with modifications of intensity, frequency, and duration implemented. The player cannot progress to the next phase in rehabilitation unless symptom free at the lower level. Mild symptoms that resolve within 2 hours after exercise and are relieved by cryotherapy are acceptable. Surgery may be indicated for individuals who require full shoulder stabilization to participate in their sport, such as those involved in collision or contact sports or those experiencing recurrent instability in the dominant or throwing arm.[48,65] Postoperative management is often surgeon- or institution-dependent. Preestablished protocol guidelines are usually available from the physician or surgeon. In general, the patient will be placed in an immobilizer for 2 to 4 weeks. Periscapular strengthening and posture begins early and progresses over 12 weeks.[48,65] Active-assisted ROM is initiated approximately 2 to 3 weeks after surgery with limitations on shoulder rotation and end ROM. Return to sport is possible 3 to 4 months after surgery if the following criteria are met: symptom-free full ROM and appropriate strength and endurance for the functional and sport-specific activities the child will return to. Individuals involved in collision or contact sports require longer healing times, and return to sport is not until 4 to 6 months postsurgery.[48,65] Overhead athletes may take as long as 9 months before they are ready to play.[48]

Prevention and Treatment of Overuse Injuries in Throwing Athletes

- Ensure proper conditioning, training practices, and warm-ups
- Keep sessions short
- Limit volume (i.e., innings, number of pitches)
- Ensure 3 to 4 days of rest between games
- Provide coaching in proper techniques
- Discourage pitching at home during and after the season
- Discourage curve balls, sliders, and breaking balls

Multidirectional Shoulder Instability

The majority of multidirectional instability (MDI) or microinstability around the glenohumeral joint is an atraumatic, overuse injury with underlying hypermobility, which occurs in more than one directional plane: anterior, posterior, or inferior.[18,48] The individual often demonstrates MDI in the opposite shoulder and exhibits hyperlaxity of multiple joints in the body.[18,48] A score of greater than 5 may be present on the **Beighton-Horan ligament laxity scale** (see Box 29-1).[66] Erhlos-Danlos or Marfan's syndrome may be present. The individual with congenital ligament laxity can often voluntarily sublux their shoulders and often refer to themselves as "double jointed." The young girl in Figure 29-22 demonstrates bilateral voluntary shoulder inferior subluxation. A positive sulcus sign and apprehension tests are present on examination. Patients will describe diffuse pain, soreness, fatigue, and a decline in performance as symptoms progress.[48] Secondary impingement due to the instability of the glenohumeral joint is often seen in this adolescent and young adult population.[48] Symptoms mimic those of adult rotator cuff pathology with positive Neer and Hawkins impingement signs, pain on palpation over biceps and/or supraspinatus tendons, and restrictions in

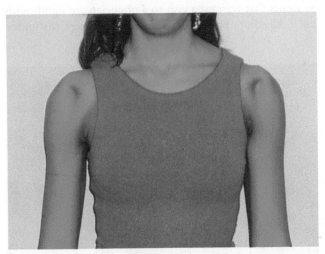

Figure 29-22 Voluntary instability. Note how the patient uses her muscles to sublux the humerus in the glenoid, resulting in an anterior sulcus in each shoulder. (From Magee DJ: *Orthopedic physical assessment*, ed 6, p 259, St. Louis, 2014, Saunders Elsevier.)

medial (internal) rotation. Initial conservative management is treatment of choice with physical therapy lasting 6 months before surgical intervention is considered.[48] Physical therapy intervention for glenohumeral dislocation, MDI, and secondary impingement is similar. Rest, activity modification, and pain-reduction techniques are implemented early. Reestablishing muscular balance around the glenohumeral joint and proper scapular kinematics are crucial. Except for posterior capsular restrictions, ROM is usually not a problem for this population. Caution should be taken to only stretch tissue structures that are restricted and avoid overstretching hypermobile areas. Strengthening of the periscapular and rotator cuff muscles begins below shoulder level and progresses above 90° of shoulder elevation as symptoms subside. Aggressive activities with arms above shoulder level before establishing good strength and scapular control can increase instability and pain. Low-intensity, high-repetition, and multiple sets of one exercise are recommended because many of the muscles that support the glenohumeral joint are postural and need to sustain prolonged activity without fatigue. Technique evaluation by an established expert in each sport for the overhead athlete is important to prevent symptom reoccurrence. In addition, adhering to current recommended pitching guidelines established from the U.S. baseball safety and advisory committee[18] is equally beneficial in prevention of reinjury.

Traumatic Elbow Injuries

Traumatic injuries around the elbow occur less often than at the forearm or wrist.[21] However, due to the superficial location of the neurovascular supply to the upper extremity, aggressive management of elbow injuries is warranted to achieve good results without sequelae. Elbow anatomy of the immature skeleton demonstrates that the physis is weaker than ligaments, the MCL is the primary stabilizer to valgus stress, and bony alignment is the primary stabilizer to varus stress.[67] Acute injuries include avulsion fractures, supracondylar fractures, distal humerus fracture, and elbow dislocations. Painful loss of elbow ROM in either direction compared with the contralateral elbow is a warning sign of elbow pathology. Elevation of the elbow fat pad, known as a positive fat pad sign, has been demonstrated to be indicative of a fracture around the elbow 70% of the time.[21]

Elbow Dislocations

Elbow dislocations are seen in the 13- to 14-year-olds as the physis begins to close. A FOOSH injury produces an axial load, elbow hyperextension, and valgus stress applied to the elbow. It is the common cause of a dislocation or more often a fracture dislocation with the medial epicondyle being the most common site of the fracture. Studies show an associated fracture 75% of the time with elbow dislocations.[68] AP and lateral radiographs are taken to rule out associated fractures. Reduction by conscious sedation is recommended with postreduction radiographs to ensure proper alignment. Neurovascular status is checked throughout the evaluation, paying close attention to the median nerve and brachial artery. Cast immobilization for 2 to 3 weeks with gentle ROM is started immediately after cast removal to prevent flexion contractures. Surgical management is indicated if closed reduction cannot be achieved, an open fracture has occurred, or there is a displaced osteochondral fracture.

Valgus Extension Overload

An increase in forced extension at the olecranon-triceps interface in the posterior elbow may produce olecranon apophysitis via traction of the triceps or mechanical abutment of the olecranon into the olecranon fossa.[69] Loose bodies and osteophytes of the olecranon tip are common. Pain is experienced with forced elbow extension during the acceleration phase of throwing or during upper extremity impact activities, such as gymnastics. Repetitive hyperextension and increased valgus mobility may be contributory to this syndrome.[70] Pain is reproduced at the olecranon with forced extension and valgus stress. Continued sports participation could result in an avulsion fracture of the proximal olecranon. As with medial epicondyle avulsion fractures, the older adolescent is more at risk of suffering an olecranon avulsion. There is an acute onset of posterior elbow pain with throwing. Posterior swelling and ecchymosis with painful palpation over the tip of the olecranon is observed. Tricep weakness and loss of extension are found on examination. In addition to conservative management, treatment may include surgical reattachment of the extensor mechanism.[21]

Wrist and Hand Injuries

Wrist and hand injuries represent some of the most common injuries of all sports.[34] They comprise 3% to 9% of all sports injuries. Fractures of the hand increase rapidly after the age of 8 years and peak around 13 years in boys. Finger dislocations, ligamentous injuries, and nail bed involvement are all very common.[21,34] Hand injuries represent approximately 15% of football injuries. Racquet and batting sports produce both distal ulnar and radial wrist pain. In-depth discussion of hand injuries in athletics is beyond the scope of this chapter, and the more common injuries to the young wrist and hand will be discussed. In the young athlete, wrist sprains are rare, with fractures to the wrist and hand being significantly more common especially in the presence of posttraumatic wrist swelling.

Quick Screen for Hand Injuries

- "Make a fist"
- The fist should close easily without pain
- Nail beds are parallel in the palm
- Finger tips should not overlap
- Finger tips point to the scaphoid tubercle with finger flexion
- Thumb easily crosses the fist and touches the fifth digit

Gymnast's Wrist

Wrist injuries are common in gymnastics and affect 70% to 80% of all gymnasts.[71] Repetitive impact forces placed across the gymnast's wrist during floor, bar, and vault routines compromise the integrity of the distal radial physis. Gymnasts between the ages of 12 and 14 years who participate in gymnastics greater than 35 hours a week are most vulnerable.[72] Dorsal (posterior) wrist pain usually occurs bilaterally but may be seen unilaterally and is exacerbated by wrist extension loading. Radiographic evaluation reveals the extent of physeal involvement.[72] A series of radiographs can be used to identify healing and assist with return to sport recommendations. Treatment consists of rest from offending activities, cross-training, total body strengthening, and interval training to maintain fitness level for return to sport. Modification of upper extremity weight-bearing exercises by keeping the wrist in neutral (resting) position (slight extension) (Figure 29-23) facilitates maintaining strength and stability throughout the upper extremity while decreasing stress at the extremes of ROM. Special wrist splints designed for gymnasts, called Tiger Paws, assist with neutral wrist alignment and load dispersion and can be worn during practices. Continued injury to the physis through reoccurrence or lack of appropriate rest leads to early physeal closure and growth arrest.[71] As the distal radius growth plate closes, the ulna remains open and continues to grow. Depending on the age and Tanner stage of the child, the resultant ulnar variance could be small or large. If the disparity between the ulna and radius becomes too great, ulnar-sided wrist pain may develop as well as injury to the triangular fibrocartilage complex (TFCC). Ulnar shortening surgery may be indicated if this occurs.

Spine Injuries

Unlike adults, complaints of back pain in children and adolescents that warrant a visit to a physician are significantly less.[73] Although back pain incidences are lower, the under-

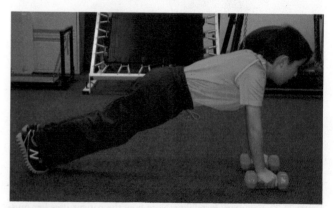

Figure 29-23 Plank exercise performed in neutral wrist position. Dumbbells positioned correctly may help keep the wrists in neutral position to avoid hyperextension overuse injuries while exercises are performed.

lying pathology may be more serious than in adults, requiring a thorough and extensive evaluation. The presence of vertebral fractures, metabolic diseases, neoplastic disorders, and spinal cord involvement produce a heightened concern in the pediatric patient presenting with back pain.[73] Persistent complaints of pain require plain radiographs of AP, lateral, and oblique views followed by MRI or bone scan if initial radiographs are inconclusive.[73-75] Figure 29-24 provides a pictorial representation of the vertebral structures. CT scans are used minimally in the young patient due to the exposure of high levels of radiation.[75]

Spondylolysis

Spondylolysis is a defect in the pars interarticularis, most commonly a stress fracture (Figure 29-25). It occurs in up to 11.5% of the general U.S. population. It is the most

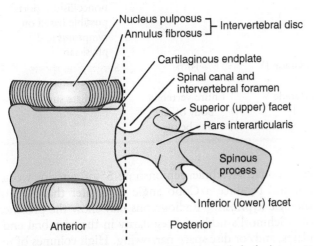

Figure 29-24 The anterior elements of the spine include the intervertebral disc and the vertebral bodies. The posterior elements include the posterior arch with the pedicles, zygapophyseal joints (facets), lamina, spinous process, transverse processes, and attached ligaments.

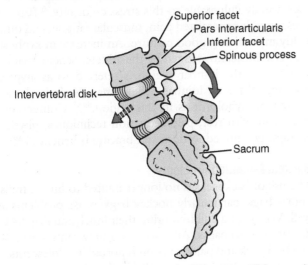

Figure 29-25 The pars interarticularis is the thinnest part of the posterior arch between the facet joints. This is the location of spondylolysis, most commonly a stress fracture, which is caused by overloading with excessive extension and can result in the superior vertebra sliding forward on the inferior vertebra which is called spondylolisthesis.

common cause of low back pain in the young athlete.[76] Young males are twice as likely to sustain this injury compared with females; however, when viewed within individual sports, female athletes who engage in high volumes of lumbar extension activities, such as gymnastics, diving, ice skating, and dancing, have a considerably higher frequency.[77-79] The growing adolescent who participates in activities that require repetitive trunk rotation, lumbar hyperextension, and heavy lifting is most vulnerable. In addition to the previously mentioned sports, football, soccer, and hockey players are also at risk. The majority of fractures or stress reactions occur at the L5 level, with L4 being second most frequent.[76] Symptoms include low back pain with or without buttocks or leg pain, muscle spasm in low back area, and increased pain with trunk rotation, lumbar extension, and end ranges of spinal motions. Standing, walking, and sports participation aggravate the symptoms. Early symptom relief in the presence of mild symptoms includes sitting, slouching, or spinal flexion. As symptoms progress, pain becomes constant and finding a position of comfort becomes more difficult. Physical examination reveals pain on repeated extension and rotation, decreased spine mobility, and lower extremity tightness. Studies show that hamstring tightness is prevalent in the majority of patients with symptomatic spondylolysis.[80] The **one-legged hyperextension test** has been viewed in the literature as both accurate and nonaccurate for the evaluation of spondylolysis in the clinic.[81-83] A positive test reproduces pain on the ipsilateral standing leg when the patient moves into lumbar hyperextension.[82] Due to its potential inaccuracy the interpretation of this special test should be used with caution. Prompt and accurate diagnosis is pertinent for quicker pain-free return to active lifestyle and sport with an average time of 3 to 6 months.[84] A delay in treatment may push the healing time to 1 year. Management of spondylolysis consists of rest and activity modification, symptom-free cross-training and core strengthening. Patients respond well to neutral core principles (i.e., maintenance of a neutral lumbar spine position, primarily avoiding lordosis or kyphosis during exercises and functional activities, from posture through sports participation), spine flexion activities, and avoidance of hyperextension exercises. An isometric hold of a forearm plank activity with lumbar spine in neutral position is an excellent way to facilitate core strength and neuromuscular education (Figure 29-26). When the athlete becomes symptom free, a gradual progression of higher-risk movements, such as lumbar extension and rotation, is implemented to prepare the athlete for return to sport. The achievement of the necessary spinal motion that is required for the athlete to perform his or her sport-specific skill is a prerequisite to return to full, unrestricted sport. For example, a gymnast or dancer needs greater than normal lumbar extension to perform their required skills. The use of a thoracolumbarsacral orthosis (TLSO) is often recommended for symptom relief but is not used

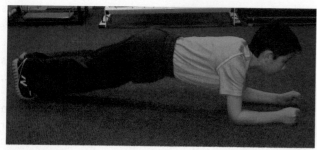

Figure 29-26 Planks are an excellent way to use body weight as resistance. Proper performance requires core strength and stabilization of the scapula.

TABLE 29-5

Spondylolisthesis Grades

Grade	Amount of Slip	Treatment and Return to Sport Recommendations
Grade I	0%-25% of vertebral body	Conservative treatment, return to sport unrestricted
Grade II	25%-50% of vertebral body	Conservative treatment, surgical treatment if failure of conservative treatment, noncontact sports (contact sports ???)
Grade III	50%-75%	Surgical indication, noncontact or noncollision sports possible based on symptoms and physician
Grade IV	75%-100%	Surgery, no sports participation
Grade V	Entire vertebral body off the one below	Immediate surgery

by all physicians.[82,85] Depending on the sport and type of brace (a soft noncustom[85] versus a hard custom clam shell) the athlete may be allowed to return to sport in the brace once symptom free. Eighty-five percent to 90% of young athletes recover within 6 months without the need for surgical intervention. Surgery is usually only recommended when conservative treatment has failed.

Spondylolisthesis

Spondyloisthesis is the forward slippage of the defected, unstable, superior vertebrae on the adjacent inferior vertebrae (see Figure 29-25). Approximately 5% of young athletes with an acquired spondylotic defect will progress to spondylolisthesis.[86] Bilateral pars defects, which compromise the stability of the vertebrae, are at more risk for slippage than unilateral defects. Symptomology for these two conditions is similar and is often treated in the same conservative manner unless the vertebrae slip is too progressive and problematic. A five-level grading system, which represents the severity of the slip, is used in the treatment algorithm. The different grades[87] and subsequent treatment recommendations for spondylolisthesis are outlined in (Table 29-5). The progression of the vertebral slip depends upon the degree and angle of the slip, child's age, gender, and Tanner stage. Younger patients, females, and prepubescents are at most risk for vertebral slip progression.[80]

Schmorl's Nodule

The presence of a Schmorl's nodule in the immature spine may or may not be a significant source for back pain in the young athlete.[88] It is more often seen on MRI than radiographs. A Schmorl's nodule is a vertical disk herniation through the cartilaginous vertebral body endplate referred to as an apophysis at this stage of development.[88] It occurs often in the mid- to low-back region and affects those 14 to 18 years of age. Evidence of Schmorl's nodules exists in both the athlete and nonathlete at the same rates. Surgical intervention is not indicated and conservative treatment which addresses pain and dysfunction is recommended.

Scheuermann's Kyphosis

Scheuermann's kyphosis refers to a structural deformity in the thoracolumbar region where three or more consecutive vertebrae demonstrate 5° of anterior wedging and produce a Cobb angle of greater than 45° of thoracic kyphosis.[89] Radiographs may show the presence of a Schmorl's nodule, irregularity in the vertebral endplates, and/or disc space narrowing. High volumes of repetitive spinal flexion activities during sports may cause deformation of the softer cartilaginous vertebral endplate. Gymnasts, swimmers, and wrestlers who engage in greater than 400 hours a year of sport participation are increasingly vulnerable to this stress deformity.[90] Patients present with generalized pain, muscular fatigue, and difficultly maintaining good posture. An increase in kyphosis may also be acknowledged by the athlete. Scheuermann's kyphosis in the lumbar region is referred to as atypical Scheuermann's or lumbar Scheuermann's. It is characterized by hypolordosis in this region.[89,91] Conservative treatment with rest, pain reduction techniques, physical therapy, posture education, and bracing is beneficial.[89]

Backpack-Related Problems

The use of backpacks is no longer limited to hiking trails. Sports bags, particularly hockey bags, cause problems as well. Very young children bring their lunch and diapers to daycare in backpacks. An association between the weight of a backpack and pain has been reported in adolescents.[92] Adolescents often are seen with a backpack slung over one shoulder or hanging very low on the back.

Prevention first is aimed at choosing a backpack that fits the child or adolescent properly. Shoulder straps should be padded and rest comfortably. The bottom of the pack should rest on the contour of the lower back rather than sagging onto the buttocks. The wearer should distribute the weight evenly by wearing both straps, and the contents of the backpack should be packed evenly, with compression straps adjusted to hold the contents stable. The heaviest items should be placed close to the spine. Students should be taught proper lifting techniques and to limit the weight of the contents. Suggestions for the weight of backpack contents range from 10% to 20% of the body weight.[93-96]

Compensatory Postures When Wearing a Backpack

- Increased forward-leaning trunk
- Increased craniovertebral extension angle
- Increased lumbar lordosis

Some evidence indicates that back pain prevention programs in preadolescents have positive results.[97] Multidisciplinary approaches involving teachers, parents, physicians, physical therapists, and psychologists are encouraged to promote healthy habits in childhood. Working with injured students or students in school prevention programs provides more opportunities for encouraging overall physical fitness. More evidence is needed to confirm the long-term effects of these programs.

Hip Injuries

An acutely limping child or adolescent, either through traumatic or atraumatic means, requires a thorough evaluation of the entire lower extremity, including spine, hip, thigh, knee, lower leg, and ankle. Hip pathology can present as general or localized pain, pain referred to the thigh, groin, or knee and have either gradual or acute onset.[25,98] The seriousness of the underlying pathology varies from minor to life threatening, which warrants the conservative management and evaluation of all lower extremity joints and body systems. Recent illnesses, fever, infections, weight loss, or pain at night are part of the subjective examination. If the patient is unable or having extreme difficulty weight bearing, crutches or a wheelchair is necessary until orthopedic evaluation is completed and definitive diagnosis is established. Clinically, ROM restrictions, joint motion asymmetries both within the same joint and contralaterally, weakness, and painful palpation are evaluated. Radiographs include AP, lateral, and frog views.[29,52,98] The patient's age directly influences differential diagnosis. Table 29-6 outlines presentation and physical examination findings by age group.[52,98]

Legg-Calve-Perthes Disease

Legg-Calve-Perthes disease is a self-limiting avascular necrosis of the femoral head. It appears in children between the ages of 3 and 13 with the majority being present at 5 to 7 years of age. Boys are 3 to 5 times more affected than girls. Clinical presentation includes a limp,

Trendelenburg gait pattern, pain in the groin, thigh, or knee, and loss of hip medial (internal) rotation and abduction.[52,98] Positive log roll test is present, and a hip flexor contracture may be noted as well. Suspicion of Legg-Calve-Perthes disease requires referral to a pediatric orthopedic surgeon for further evaluation and possible surgical intervention. Radiographs show disruption and collapse of the femoral epiphysis.[52] Figure 29-27 illustrates the possible incongruity of the femoral head in Legg-Calve-Perthes disease. Reduction of symptoms and protection of the femoral head in hopes of remodeling are initial treatments. Protective weight bearing is emphasized. If the condition does not improve, surgery may be indicated.

External Snapping Hip or Trochanteric Bursitis or Iliotibial Band Syndrome[99]

The above-mentioned terms all produce lateral hip and thigh pain. Each diagnosis can exist separately but commonly are found overlapping each other. External "snapping hip" occurs as the iliotibial band (ITB) moves over the greater trochanter, often producing an audible or palpable snap.[100] It is often seen in artistic athletes—those who participate in dancing, gymnastics, and ice skating—where repetitive hip rotation and joint hyperflexibility are required.[101] Most athletes can voluntarily reproduce the snap. Runners, football, soccer, and ice hockey players who suffer from a tight ITB and hip abductor and lateral (external) rotation weakness are susceptible as well. Reoccurring "snapping" or rubbing of the ITB over the greater trochanter eventually irritates the underlying bursae which leads to bursitis. Trochanteric bursitis occurs more often in the older athlete and is painful while lying on it. Point tenderness on palpation is noted over the greater trochanter. Lateral hip and thigh pain without snapping which can extend to the lateral knee is indicative of ITB syndrome. A positive Ober test is noted on examination and palpation reveals tenderness along the length of the ITB. Treatment principles for the abovementioned conditions are similar when a conservative approach of rest, ice, activity modification, and physical therapy is implemented.[102-106] Surgical intervention is usually a surgery of last resort if prolonged pain and dysfunction persist. After pain reduction, stretching of ITB and other restricted hip structures begins.[27] Soft tissue massage and self-massage to the ITB may be part of the treatment program.[103] Core and hip strengthening is crucial.[27] Analysis of running gait and dance technique is often necessary to prevent a recurring problem.

Internal Snapping Hip or Iliopsoas Bursitis[99]

Repetitive snapping of the iliospoas muscle over the iliopectineal eminence or femoral neck produces pain in the anterior and medial thigh and groin area.[107,108] Symptoms are reproduced with resisted hip flexion, full passive flexion, and flexion-extension movements of the

TABLE **29-6**

Differential Diagnoses of Hip Pain in the Child and Adolescent

Age (yr)	Diagnosis	History	Physical Examination
4-10	Legg-Calve-Perthes	Limp with hip or knee pain, insidious onset (1-3 mo)	Limited hip abduction, flexion, and internal rotation
	Transient synovitis	Fever, chills, erythema, pain	Trendelenburg gait, stiffness, guarding of movements
11-16	Slipped capital femoral epiphysis (SCFE)	Hip pain, referred pain to anterior thigh or knee. Acute or chronic presentation	Pain, limited internal rotation. Position of comfort hip flexion, abduction and external rotation
	Avascular necrosis of femoral head	Pain in groin, lateral hip and buttock. History of steroid use, prior fracture or SCFE	Pain with ambulation, hip abduction, internal and external rotation
	Femoral neck stress fracture	Endurance athlete, female athlete triad. Pain increases with weight bearing and impact. Groin pain	Pain on palpation over greater trochanter, painful ROM, positive single leg hop test
	Hip pointer	Direct trauma to iliac crest	Pain on palpation, painful ambulation and active hip abduction
	Avulsion fractures	Sudden forceful muscle contraction or stretch. May hear/feel "pop"	Pain over involved apophysis. Pain on PROM or resisted muscle activity.
All ages	Internal snapping hip or iliopsoas bursitis	Pain or snapping in the anterior medial hip and groin area. Can be felt or heard. Excessive snapping irritates the iliopsoas bursae	Pain and snapping occurs when hip is moved from a flexed position into extension. Resisted hip flexion increases pain
	External snapping hip/ greater trochanter bursitis Iliotibial band syndrome (ITB)	Lateral hip or thigh pain, snapping as the ITB moves across the greater trochanter. Excessive snapping irritates the trochanteric bursae. Difficult to lie on involved side. Pain can be local to proximal hip or diffuse along entire ITB.	Tight iliotibial band, pain on palpation over ITB and greater trochanter. History and areas of painful palpation will separate these three overlapping conditions.
	Septic arthritis	Chills, fatigue, fever	Decreased ROM, pain with limb movement and internal rotation, swelling, warmth. Preferred position (flexion, abduction, lateral rotation)
	Osteomyelitis (bone infection)	Fever, chills, irritability, fatigue. Develops rapidly over 7-10 days	Pain/tenderness over hip joint, pain with movement, difficulty weight bearing
	Neoplasms	Night pain, pain that wakes the child up, pain unrelated to activity	Palpable mass, inconsistent musculoskeletal examination findings

PROM, passive range of motion; *ROM*, range of motion.

Modified from Merkel DL, Molony JT: Clinical commentary: recognition and management of traumatic sports injuries in the skeletally immature athlete, *Intl J Sports Phys Ther* 7:691-704, 2012.

hip. The "snap" is felt when the athlete moves the hip from a position of flexion to extension against gravity. Artistic athletes and runners experience this injury. Treatment is conservative as with external snapping hip. Stretching the tight hip iliopsoas muscle is important.[25] Core strengthening and eccentric control of hip flexors help to elevate the tension across the iliopsoas muscle while moving the hip from a flexed to extended position. Imaging is used to rule out intra-articular pathology as a cause for pain and snapping but may fail to identify tendon pathology.[106]

Knee Injuries

Many of the same evaluative procedures and special tests performed on the adult patient experiencing knee problems are used in evaluating the young athlete's knee. Youth athletes, whose growth plates remain open, often encounter different diagnoses than adult athletes when faced with the same mechanism of injury. Pain, limping, decreased weight bearing, effusion, loss of motion, and increased pain on palpation over the bone or physis are indications for knee imaging. Recommended radiographs include AP, lateral, merchant, and notch views.[29-32]

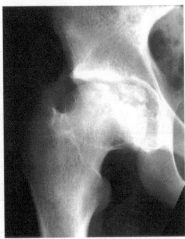

Figure 29-27 Legg-Calvé-Perthes disease, with collapse of the femoral head.

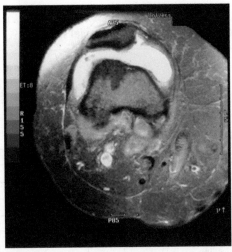

Figure 29-28 MRI scan after dislocation and reduction of the patella showing hemarthrosis, a medial retinaculum tear, and bone bruising to the lateral femoral condyle.

Comparison views are taken if physeal injury is suspected. MRI is indicated in the young athlete if there is suspicion of the following knee injuries: intra-articular, ligamentous, bone contusions, meniscal involvement, and/or physeal injury.[29-32]

Patellar Dislocations

Traumatic patellar dislocations can be suspected with an acute knee injury. Commonly, the dislocation occurs laterally. Recurrent patellar dislocations may occur when athletes, usually females, have an underlying congenital ligament laxity that causes patellar hypermobility or an underdeveloped lateral condyle of the femur. A twisting or pivoting moment at the knee when the foot is planted forces the patella to move laterally. The patella may spontaneously reduce and rarely remains laterally displaced. Subjectively, the athlete may report the knee twisting, feeling or hearing a snap, and a sensation of the knee giving away.[109] Physical examination shows an effused knee, diffuse pain both medial and lateral, positive lateral apprehension test, and decreased ability to bear weight. A hemarthrosis may be present on joint aspiration.[109,110] Merchant view radiographs show the patella position within the femoral groove when the knee is positioned in 30° of flexion. An MRI is used to rule out other injuries, including ACL tears. Figure 29-28 shows a reduced patellar dislocation with hemarthrosis and demonstrates concomitant osteochondral defects and cartilage damage to the patellofemoral joint. Acute patellar dislocations are treated conservatively unless a large osteochondral fracture is present.[109,110] Two to 4 weeks of immobilization followed by physical therapy for quadriceps and hip strengthening is recommended.[29,111] A patellar stabilizing brace is often used for support during jumping, pivoting, and twisting movements. One in six patients who sustains a patellar dislocation will have a recurrence.[29] If repeated patellar dislocations are sustained by the athletes, medial patellar ligament reconstruction may be performed to

stabilize the patella. Rehabilitation for return to sport after this procedure may take up to 6 months.

Knee Overuse Injuries

Overuse injuries of the lower extremity are prolific in the growing young athlete. Repetitive loads, inappropriate training, early specialization, lack of rest, and proper nutrition can all be extrinsic factors that are contributory. Generalized anterior knee pain plagues the young athlete and differential diagnosis includes adult-like pathology and injuries unique to the immature skeleton. Table 29-7 lists special tests and corresponding diagnoses to assist in identifying knee pathologies of the young athlete.

General treatment for overuse injuries of the lower extremity includes rest, ice, activity modification, stretching of tight lower extremity muscles (especially the hamstrings, quadriceps, hip flexors, and ITB), and strengthening throughout the kinetic chain, including core and hip. Analysis of biomechanical alignment both in static stance and during activity is necessary to identify additional areas of dysfunction within the lower extremity. Teaching the athlete proper lower extremity alignment and landing technique has been shown to be beneficial. The use of foot orthotics, either custom made or over the counter, to assist with alignment and reduction of symptoms is conflictual. Analysis and modification of footwear (i.e., sneakers, cleats, turf, and dance shoes) may be necessary for proper fit, support, and performance.

Meniscus Injuries

Menisci can be torn when they are compressed and twisted by the femoral condyles against the tibial plateaus. The blood supply to the menisci is limited to the outer one third but is slightly better in younger children.[112] Few meniscal tears heal on their own, and tears can become enlarged, causing more frequent symptoms, such as pain, swelling, locking, and degeneration.

TABLE **29-7**

Differential Knee Diagnosis and Special Tests

	Osgood Schlatter	Infrapatellar tendonitis	Sinding Larssen Johannson	PFPS	Dislocation/subluxation	OCD	MCL strain	MCL avulsion	ITB syndrome	ACL tear	Tibial spine avulsion	Discoid meniscus	Osteosarcoma
Palpation													
Tibial tuberosity	X												
Infrapatellar tendon		X											
Inerior patellar pole			X										
Medial/Lateral patellar facet				X	X								
Femoral condyles				X	X								
Tibial plateau											X		
Medial joint line							X	X			X		
Lateral joint line						X					X	X	
MCL origin/insertion							X	X					
LCL origin/insertion													
ITB/Gerdy's tubercle									X				
Distal femoral physis								X					
Special tests													
Effusion				X	X	X	X			X	X		
Lachman										X	X		
Anterior drawer										X	X		
Posterior drawer													
Varus													
Valgus							X	X		X	X		
McMurray's												X	
Ober									X				
Seated ITB compression									X				
Patellar grind				X	X								
Patellar apprehension				X	X								
Patellar inhibition				X	X								
Inverted J sign				X	X								

ACL, anterior cruciate ligament; *ITB,* iliotibial band; *LCL,* lateral collateral ligament; *MCL,* medial collateral ligament; *OCD,* osteochondritis dissecans; *PFPS,* patellofemoral pain syndrome.

The history of a meniscal tear is a twisting knee episode followed by gradual synovial swelling over 12 to 24 hours. The child has pain medially or laterally and might report an inability to fully extend the knee (locking). The physical examination may or may not show an effusion. Joint line tenderness is common, but a classic McMurray's test with a painful medial click during extension is found only with large tears. Associated bone bruising or collateral ligament injury can confuse the examination. MRI is definitive but is not necessary to make the diagnosis in most cases (Figure 29-29).

Most meniscal tears, if being repaired, can be addressed operatively within several weeks. Repairs to the outer one third have the best healing potential, but in the young, many surgeons repair any tears in the outer half, because the healing potential is better than in adults.[112] To protect

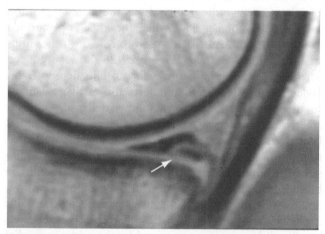

Figure 29-29 MRI scan showing a complex posterior horn medial meniscal tear (*arrow*).

the repair, motion and weight bearing are restricted for 6 to 8 weeks, and sports are allowed at 4 months. No definitive studies suggest that rehabilitation after meniscal repair is different for adults and children.

Discoid Meniscus

A congenital defect of the meniscus, where it is shaped like a disc rather than being semilunar (as is normal), is called a **discoid meniscus**.[113] It occurs primarily in the lateral compartment of the knee and presents as a lateral meniscal tear. The preschool-aged child may complain of snapping during play but does not present with pain until school age, in which an increase in activity occurs.[113] Tenderness along the lateral joint line, along with a positive McMurray test, is found on examination. Diagnosis is confirmed with MRI. Virtually asymptomatic, stable lesions without meniscal degeneration are treated with rehabilitation. Surgical indications include the presentation of pain and dysfunction with a degenerated and/or unstable meniscus.[113] Postsurgical rehabilitation follows the guidelines of meniscal repairs.

Ligament Injuries

The ACL is torn either by a direct blow to the knee that leads to a valgus, varus, hyperflexion, or hyperextension sprain, or by indirect stressing of the knee in those directions with a sudden start, stop, change in direction, or landing from a jump.

When the ACL is torn, the patient often experiences a "pop" and rapid knee swelling within 1 hour, indicating blood swelling (hemarthrosis). The ACL stump, hemarthrosis, and/or a torn meniscus (usually lateral) can block knee extension. An MRI scan shows the ACL tear and any associated meniscal tearing or bone bruising.

Currently, reconstruction is necessary to restore function.[114] Most athletic individuals with an ACL tear require ACL reconstruction to restore knee stability. Surgery can be performed within 48 hours; however, it usually is performed more than 4 weeks after injury to ensure that ROM and swelling have returned to normal, thereby reducing arthrofibrosis postoperatively.[115]

The open physes present a problem for surgeons performing ACL reconstruction in the young. Placing bone or hardware across an open physis can result in premature closure, with subsequent joint deformity or limb shortening. The use of soft tissue through a physis has a much lower rate of problems. In the preadolescent, few surgeons would place any new material through the physis. Current guidelines call for the use of an adult ACL reconstruction technique if less than 2 cm (approximately 1 inch) of growth remains, otherwise adolescents get soft tissue (hamstring or allograft) through the physes, with fixation away from the physes. For preadolescents, hamstring or ITB autograft is used with an intra-articular, extraphyseal technique.

Some authors recommend a slower rehabilitation program for children than adults in an effort to control an overzealous youngster,[116] whereas others advocate programs with similar phasing.[117-119] For the first week, the patient is mostly non-weight bearing, uses ice and compression, and works on ROM and leg control exercises. As ROM is achieved, closed-chain strengthening progresses.

Lower Leg, Ankle, and Foot Injuries

Shin Splints

Shin splints is a lay term for any activity-induced leg pain. It refers to pain from medial tibial periostitis, tibial or fibular stress fractures, exertional compartment syndrome, or vascular pain. Medial periostitis, stress fracture, and compartment syndrome have been described in the child. Medial periostitis is pain along the medial tibial border where the soleus and posteromedial muscles attach. It is thought to occur when shock absorption is poor and the muscle-bone attachment becomes damaged. In reality, it is part of a pathological process that can lead to a stress fracture.

Patients usually report anterior leg pain that begins after several minutes of running and diminishes only after stopping. Radiographic films are negative in many cases. Physical therapy goals include strengthening of the weak lower leg muscles to aid shock absorption. Stretching of the long and short calf muscles is included. Correction of training errors is essential, including running on softer surfaces and cautious changes in training speed, distance, or intensity. Proper footwear is essential to control pronation and increase shock absorption. Orthotics may be used to correct biomechanical faults.

Tarsal Coalition

A congenital malformation in which two or more tarsal bones are fused is referred to as **tarsal coalition** (Figure 29-30). Calcaneonavicular coalition, talocalcaneal coalition, and talonavicular coalition are observed most frequently.[120] Recurrent ankle injuries may be an indicator of this pathology. Symptoms appear between the ages of 8 and 18 years with descriptions of vague pain over the midfoot and hindfoot.[120] The appearance of pain in the foot in this age group corresponds to changes in activity level and intensity, body size, and ossification of the coalition.[121,122] Males are more affected than females. Physical examination reveals a fixed pes planus (flatfoot) deformity, restricted subtalar motion, excessive calcaneal valgus, and pain on inversion.[123-125] Calf muscle tightness may also be present. Treatment recommendations include both surgical and nonsurgical approaches. Conservative management consists of orthotic devices, physical therapy, cortisone injections, and cast immobilization for pain reduction.[123,126] Surgical options include resection of the involved bones or arthrodesis if joint degeneration is problematic.[123,125]

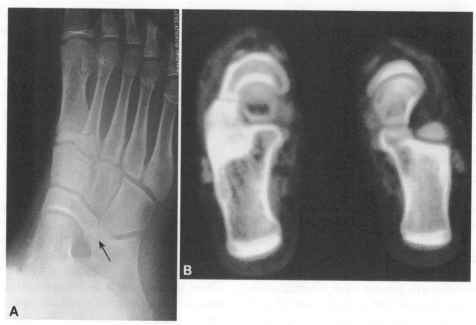

Figure 29-30 Right tarsal (calcaneonavicular) coalition. **A,** Radiograph (*arrow*). **B,** CT scan illustrating bony bridge. (From Blickman JG, Parker BR, Barnes PD: *Pediatric radiology*, ed 3, Philadelphia, 2009, Mosby/Elsevier.)

Accessory Navicular

The accessory navicular is an extra bony ossicle that is present from birth on the medial aspect of the navicular (Figure 29-31).[127] Approximately 12% are embedded in the tibialis posterior tendon. Medial navicular pain, which is aggravated by impact activities, presents around

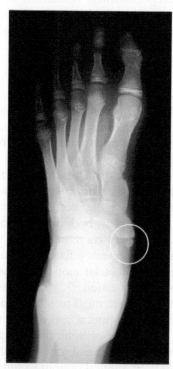

Figure 29-31 Fourteen-year-old dancer with medial foot pain and swelling. An oblique radiograph of the foot demonstrates an accessory navicular bone (*circle*). (From Chambers HG: Ankle and foot disorders in skeletally immature athletes, Orthop Clin North Am 34:445-459, 2003.)

12 years of age with girls 3 times more likely than boys to be afflicted by this condition. The athlete often has a pes planus foot.[127,128] Proper diagnosis is important because an accessory navicular can be confused with posterior tibial tendonitis or a navicular stress fracture. Positive palpation on the medial aspect of the navicular in contrast to pain on the dorsum of the navicular is indicative of an accessory involvement. Conservative treatment of rest, ice, immobilization, foot orthosis, and physical therapy for stretching, balance, and foot intrinsic facilitation is attempted before surgical excision of the ossicle. Surgical excision of the accessory navicular is usually successful and may return the athlete to sport sooner than a trial of conservative management.

TRAINING THE PEDIATRIC AND ADOLESCENT POPULATION

Resistance training has proved safe and effective for the growing child when it is appropriately designed and provided in a supervised environment. Clinicians may need to relieve parents' fears that resistance training is harmful. Questions and concerns often arise about epiphyseal plate injuries, soft tissue injuries, and the potential improbability of strength gains in the absence of testosterone in the young child. Use of the correct terms for different types of training clears up confusion and helps dispel parents' anxieties (Table 29-8).

Whether the setting is a rehabilitation clinic or a fitness gym, the equipment used should fit the child. Some adolescents may be able to use adult-sized equipment. As an alternative, free weights or body weight can be used as resistance to provide a safe, effective program.

TABLE 29-8

Correct Terms for Different Types of Training

Term	Description
Body building	Competitive training that builds up muscle mass symmetry and definition
Body weight	Training using sit ups, push ups, and chin ups
Free weights	Training using dumbbells, barbells, and sandbags
Strength training	Training that uses a systematic method of applying resistance to increase the ability to exert or resist force
Weight lifting	Training involving competitive, Olympic-type lifts
Weight training	Training using free weights or machines

Modified from Vehrs PR: Strength training in children and teens: dispelling misconceptions. Part 1, *ACSM's Health Fit J*, July/August:8-12, 2005.

Readiness for progression to power lifting and weight lifting can be judged by Tanner staging (see Figures 29-1 to 29-3). Power lifting and weight lifting should be restricted to athletes who have reached or passed Tanner stage V. Individuals at Tanner stage IV or lower can safely participate in a strength training program that is specifically and carefully designed for younger athletes. Some authors believe that with proper supervision and cautious progression with quality form, individuals at a lower stage than Tanner stage V can safely participate in weight lifting.[129]

Elements of a Resistance Training Program for Children

- The program should be fun
- Exercises should involve more repetitions with less load
- Child-sized equipment should be used, and free weights or body weight should be used as resistance
- Individual achievement should be encouraged

No conclusive evidence indicates that strength training reduces injury or improves athletic performance in children. Any program designed for this age group, whether a rehabilitation program or a general exercise and strength training program, needs to provide a fun atmosphere to motivate the child to adhere to the program. Identifying the exercises or program with funny or unusual names or making it a game to which the child can relate adds an aspect of fun. Encouraging individual achievement rather than competition among the group provides realistic goals.

The American College of Sports Medicine (ACSM) supports the efficacy and safety of plyometric training for children and adolescents as part of an overall training program. Plyometric exercises use the muscle cycle of stretching and shortening to increase muscle power[130] and enable the muscle to reach maximum strength as quickly as possible.[131] Elements of plyometrics are integral to normal childhood activities, such as jumping, hopping, and skipping. Ball throwing can be added for upper body training beginning with unweighted balls and progressing to medicine balls. These activities and games such as hopscotch and jumping rope can be adjusted for age appropriateness.

CONCLUSION

Musculoskeletal injuries in the active pediatric and adolescent population are an inherent risk with participation in play, recreational activities, and sports. The physical and psychosocial consequences of a sedentary lifestyle make a compelling argument for fostering active lifestyles in the young population. Minimizing sequelae, injury reduction, and keeping youth engaged in physical activities need to be the goals of the health care practitioner who participates in the care of the maturing child. Caring for the young athlete is more dependent on the stage of development than chronological age. The pediatric patient with an immature skeleton sustains different injuries than older mature adolescents.

REFERENCES

1. Gruber J, Gerbino PG, d'Hemecourt PA, et al: Pediatric and adolescent considerations. In Magee DJ, Zachazewski JE, Quillen WS, editors: *Pathology and intervention in musculoskeletal rehabilitation*, ed 1 St. Louis, 2008, Saunders/Elsevier.
2. Merkel DL: Youth sport: positive and negative impact on youth athletes, *J Sports Med* 4:151–160, 2013.
3. Cover K, Grady M, Linton J, et al: Medical conditions which impact youth athletic rehabilitation. In Merkel DL, Molony JT, editors: *Pediatric and adolescent sports medicine: management and prevention of injuries unique to the young athlete*, 2011, American Physical Therapy Association (APTA) Sports Section Home Study Course.
4. Callender SS: The early specialization of youth in sports, *Athl Training Sports Healthcare* 2:255–257, 2010.
5. Purcell L: Sports readiness in child and youth, *Paediatr Child Health* 10:343–344, 2005.
6. American Academy of Pediatrics Committee on Sports Medicine and Fitness and Committee on School Health: Organized sports for children and preadolescents, *Pediatrics* 7:1459–1462, 2001.
7. Brenner J: American Academy of Pediatrics Council on Sports Medicine and Fitness: Overuse injuries, overtraining, and burnout in child and adolescent athletes, *Pediatrics* 119:1242–1245, 2007.
8. Miles C, Merkel DL: Growth and Development. In Merkel DL, Molony JT, editors: *Pediatric and adolescent sports medicine: management and prevention of injuries unique to the young athlete*, 2011, American Physical Therapy Association (APTA) Sports Section Home Study Course.
9. American Academy of Pediatrics: Active healthy living: prevention of childhood obesity through increased physical activity, *Pediatrics* 117:1834–1842, 2006.
10. Stoler F: *Childhood obesity*, 2014. Available at American College of Sports Medicine www.acsm.org.
11. National Center for Sports Safety, 2012. Available at www.sportssafety.org
12. Wolf SL: Radiologic evaluation of fracture. In McKinnis LN, editor: *Fundamentals of musculoskeletal imaging*, ed 4, Philadelphia, 2014, FA Davis Company.
13. Molony JT, Merkel DL: Traumatic disorders and sports injuries. In Tecklin JS, editor: *Pediatric physical therapy*, ed 4 Philadelphia, 2008, Lippincott Williams & Wilkins.

14. Merkel DL, Molony JT: Clinical commentary: recognition and management of traumatic sports injuries in the skeletally immature athlete, *Intl J Sports Phys Ther* 7:691–704, 2012.

15. Greydanus D, Patel D, Pratt H: Essential adolescent medicine. In Sigel EJ, editor: *Adolescent growth and development*, Boston, 2005, McGraw-Hill.

16. American College of Radiology ACR Appropriateness Criteria: Clinical condition: Stress/Insufficiency fracture, 2008.

17. Asher MA: Dislocations of the upper extremity in children, *Orthop Clin North Am* 7:583–591, 1976.

18. Albaugh J, Eckenrode B, Ganley TJ: Upper Extremity Injuries. In Merkel DL, Molony JT, editors: *Pediatric and adolescent sports medicine: management and prevention of injuries unique to the young athlete*, 2011, American Physical Therapy Association (APTA) Sports Section Home Study Course.

19. Patterson PD, Waters PM: Pediatric and adolescent sports injuries, *Clin Sports Med* 19:4, 2000.

20. Pugalte GG, Housner JA: Management of clavicle fractures, *Curr Sports Med Rep* 7:275–280, 2008.

21. Micheli LJ, Purcell L: *The adolescent athlete, a practical approach*, New York, 2007, Springer.

22. Carson S, Woolridge DP, Colletti J, et al: Pediatric upper extremity injuries, *Pediatr Clin North Am* 53:41–67, 2006.

23. Paletta Jr. GA, Meiser K, Matava MJ: Adolescent sports injuries: shoulder and elbow, In 2002 American Orthopaedic Society for Sports Medicine (AOSSM), 28th Annual Meeting.

24. Hugheds PE, Paletta GA: Little Leagues's Elbow, medial epicondyle injury and osteochondritis dissecans, *Sports Med Arthrosc Rev* 11:30–39, 2003.

25. Browning KH: Hip and pelvis injuries in runners: careful evaluation and tailored management, *Phys Sportsmed* 29:23–34, 2001.

26. Jacoby L, Yi-Meng Y, Kocher MS: Hip problems and arthroscopy: adolescent hip as it relates to sports, *Clin Sports Med* 30:435–451, 2011.

27. Nielson J: Pelvic, hip and thigh injuries. In Micheli LJ, Purcell L, editors: *The adolescent athlete, a practical approach*, New York, 2007, Springer.

28. Puranene J, Orava S: The hamstring syndrome: a new diagnosis of gluteal sciatic pain, *Am J Sports Med* 16:517–521, 1988.

29. Ganley TJ, Lou JE, Pryor K, et al: Sports medicine. In Dormans JP, editor: *Pediatric orthopaedics and sports medicine: the requisites in pediatrics*, St. Louis, 2004, Mosby.

30. Horn DB, Wells L, Tamai J: Lower extremity fractures. In Dormans JP, editor: *Pediatric orthopaedics and sports medicine: the requisites in pediatrics*, St. Louis, 2004, Mosby.

31. Chang DS, Mandelbaum BR, Weiss JM: Special considerations in the pediatric and adolescent athlete. In Frontera WR, Herring SA, Micheli LJ, Silver JK, editors: *Clinical sports medicine: medical management and rehabilitation*, Philadelphia, 2007, Saunders Elsevier.

32. McTimoney M: Knee injuries. In Micheli L, Purcell L, editors: *The adolescent athlete*, New York, 2007, Springer.

33. LaFrance RM, Giordano B, Goldblatt J, et al: Pediatric tibial eminence fractures: evaluation and management, *J Acad Orthop Surg* 18:395–405, 2010.

34. Rettig AC: Athletic injuries of the wrist and hand. Part 1: Traumatic injuries of the wrist, *Am J Sports Med* 31:1038–1048, 2003.

35. Kobayashi K, Burton KJ, Rodner C, et al: Lateral compression injuries in the pediatric elbow: Panner's disease and osteochondritis dissecans of the capitellum, *J Am Acad Orthop Surg* 12:246–254, 2004.

36. Kaeding CC, Whitehead R: Musculoskeletal injuries in adolescents, *Prim Care* 25:211–213, 1998.

37. Rudzki JR, Galetta PA: Juvenile and adolescent elbow injuries in sports, *Clin Sports Med* 23:581–608, 2004.

38. Bowen RE, Otsuka NY, Yoon ST, et al: Osteochondral lesions of the capitellum in pediatric patients: role of magnetic resonance imaging, *J Pediatr Orthop* 21:298–301, 2001.

39. Do T, Herrera-Soto J: Elbow injuries in children, *Curr Opin Pediatr* 15:68–73, 2003.

40. Stubbs MJ, Field LD, Savoie FH: Osteochondritis dissecans of the elbow, *Clin Sports Med* 20:1–9, 2001.

41. Chen FS, Diaz VA, Loenbenberg M, et al: Shoulder and elbow injuries in the skeletally immature athlete, *J Am Acad Orthop Surg* 13:172–185, 2005.

42. Busch M: Sports medicine in children and adolescents. In Morrissy RT, Weinstein SW, editors: *Lovell and Winter's pediatric orthopaedics*, Philadelphia, 2001, Lippincott Williams & Wilkins.

43. Ganley TJ, Chan G, Heath AB, Lawrence TRJ:. Elbow arthroscopy for Panner's Disease and osteochondritis dissecans. In Wiesel SW, Flynn JM, editors: ed 1 *Operative techniques in orthopedic surgery*, 2, Philadelphia, 2011, Lippincott Williams & Wilkins.

44. Rusch DS, Cory JW, Poshling GG: The arthroscopic management of osteochondritis dissecans in the adolescent elbow, *Arthroscopy* 14:797–803, 1998.

45. Micheli LJ, Luke AC, Mintzer CM, Waters PM: Elbow arthroscopy in the pediatric and adolescent population, *Athroscopy* 17:694–699, 2001.

46. McManama BG, Micheli LJ, Berry MV, Sohn RS: The surgical treatment of osteochondritis of the capitellum, *Am J Sports Med* 13:11–21, 1985.

47. Ganley TJ, Flynn JM: Osteochondritis dissecans of the knee. In Micheli L, Kocher MS, editors: *The pediatric and adolescent knee*, Philadelphia, 2006, Saunders Elsevier.

48. Guido JA, Brown T: Adolescent shoulder injuries. In Micheli LJ, Purcell L, editors: *The adolescent athlete, a practical approach*, New York, 2007, Springer.

49. Chan KM, Micheli LJ: *Sports and children*, Hong Kong, 1998, Williams and Wilkins Asia.

50. Luke A, Lee M, Safran M: Elbow and forearm injuries. In Micheli LJ, Purcell L, editors: *The adolescent athlete, a practical approach*, New York, 2007, Springer.

51. Wells MJ, Bell GW: Concerns on little league elbow, *J Athl Train* 30:249–253, 1995.

52. Adkins III SB, Figler RA: Hip pain in athletes, *Am Family Phys* 61:2109–2118, 2000.

53. Mizuta T, Benson WM, Foster BK, et al: Statistical analysis of the incidence of physeal injuries, *J Pediatr Orthop* 7:518–523, 1987.

54. Hosgoren B, Koktener A, Dilmen G: Ultrasonography of the calcaneus in Sever's disease, *Indian Pediatr* 42:801–803, 2005.

55. Weiner DS, Morscher M, Dicintio MS: Calcaneal apophysitis: simple diagnosis, simpler treatment, *J Fam Prac* 56:352–355, 2007.

56. Madden CC, Mellion MB: Sever's disease and other causes of heel pain in adolescents, *Am Fam Physician* 54:1995–2000, 1996.

57. Szer IS: Musculoskeletal pain in adolescents: "growing pains" or something else? Part 1, *Consultant* 481, 2000, March.

58. Szer IS: Musculoskeletal pain in adolescents: "growing pains" or something else? Part 2, *Consultant* 1061–1065, 2000, May.

59. Beighton P, Solomon L, Soskolne CL: Articular mobility in an African population, *Ann Rheum Dis* 32:413–418, 1973.

60. Gedalia A, Press J: Articular symptoms in hypermobile schoolchildren: a prospective study, *J Pediatr* 119:944–946, 1991.

61. Kocher MS, Waters PM, Micheli LJ: Upper extremity injuries in the paediatric athlete, *Sports Med* 30:117–135, 2000.

62. Reuss BL, Harding WG, Nowicki KD: Managing anterior shoulder instability with bracing: an expanded update, *Orthopedics* 27:614–618, 2004.

63. Bishop JY, Flatow EL: Pediatric shoulder trauma, *Clin Orthop Relat Res* 4:41–48, 2005.

64. Liu A, Xue X, Chen Y, et al: The external rotation immobilization does not reduce recurrence rates or improve quality of life after primary anterior shoulder dislocation: a systematic review and meta-analysis, *Injury* 45:1842–1848, 2014.

65. Sharkey C, Johnson G: Athletic training and sports medicine, ed 4, Sudbury, 2006, Jones and Bartlett.

66. Beighton P, Grahame R, Bird H: Assessment of hypermobility. In *Hypermobility of joints*, ed 3 London, 1999, Springer Verlag.

67. Hutchinson M: Elbow injuries overuse and traumatic, 2002, American College of Sports Medicine (ACSM) Team Physician Course.

68. Rasool MN: Dislocations of the elbow in children, *J Bone Joint Surg Br* 86:1050–1058, 2004.

69. Wilson FD, Andrews JR, Blackburn TA, McCluskey G: Valgus extension overload in the pitching elbow, *Am J Sports Med* 11:83–88, 1983.

70. Wilk KE, Reinold MM, Andrews JR: Rehabilitation of the thrower's elbow, *Clin Sports Med* 23:765–801, 2004.

71. Keller MS: Gymnastics injuries and imaging in children, *PediatrRadiol* 39:1299–1306, 2009.

72. Patel DR, Nelson TL: Sports injuries in adolescents, *Med Clin North Am* 84:983–1007, 2000.

73. Hosalkar H, Dormans J: Back pain in children requires extensive workup, *Biomechanics* 10:51–58, June 2003.

74. Sundell CG, Jonsson H, Adin L, et al: Clinical examination, spondylolysis and adolescent athletes, *Int J Sports Med* 34:263–267, 2013.

75. Sairyo K, Katoh S, Takata Y et al: MRI signal changes of the pedicle as an indicator for early diagnosis of spondylolysis in children and adolescents. A clinical and biomechanical study, *Spine* 31:206-211, 206.

76. Syrmou E, Tsitsopoulos PP, Marinopoulos D, et al: Spondylolysis: a review and reappraisal, *Hippokratia* 14:17–21, 2010.

77. Micheli LJ, Wood R: Back pain in young athletes. Significant differences from adults in causes and patterns, *Arch Pediatr Adolesc Med* 149:15–18, 1995.

78. Rossi F, Dragoni S: Lumbar spondylolysis: occurrence in competitive athletes. Updated achievements in a series of 390 cases, *J Sports Med Phys Fitness* 30:450–452, 1990.

79. Soler T, Calderon C: The prevalence of spondylolysis in the Spanish elite athlete, *Am J Sports Med* 28:57–62, 2000.

80. Hensinger RN: Spondylolysis and spondylolisthesis in children and adolescents, *J Bone Joint Surg Am* 71:1098–1107, 1989.

81. Masci L, Pike J, Malara F, et al: Use of the one-legged hypersxtension test and magnetic resonance imaging in the diagnosis of active spondylolysis, *Br J Sports Med* 40:940–946, 2006.

82. Bono CM: Low-back pain in athletes, *J Bone Joint Surg Am* 86:382–396, 2004.

83. Jackson DW, Wiltse LL, Dingeman RD, Hayes M: Stress reactions involving the pars interarticularis in young athletes, *Am J Sports Med* 9:304–312, 1981.

84. Sairyo K, Sakai T, Yasui N, et al: Conservative treatment for lumbar spondylosysis to achieve bone healing using a hard brace: what type and how long? *J Neurosurg* 16:610–614, 2012.

85. Litao A, Young CC: Lumbosacral spondylolysis treatment and management, 2013, Medscape Reference Drugs Diseases & Procedures.

86. Blanco S, Green DW, Widmann RF: Spondylolysis and spondylolisthesis in the pediatric patient. In *An interview with HSS surgeon Daniel W*, 2012 Green MD, Hospital for Special Surgery.

87. Tsirikos AI, Garrido EG: Spondylolysis and spondylolisthesis in children and adolescents, *J Bone Joint Surg Br* 92:751–759, 2010.

88. McHorse K, Whitehouse L, Prince M: The management of spinal conditions in the Young Athlete. In Merkel DL, Molony JT, editors: *Pediatric and adolescent sports medicine: management and prevention of injuries unique to the young athlete*, 2011 American Physical Therapy Association (APTA) Sports Section Home Study Course.

89. d'Hemecourt P, Flynn Deede J: Cervical and thoracic spine injuries. In Micheli LJ, Purcell L, editors: *The adolescent athlete, a practical approach*, New York, 2007, Springer.

90. Wojts EEM, Ashton-Miller JA, Husoton LJ, et al: The association between athletic training time and the saggital curvature of the immature spine, *Am J Sports Med* 28:490–498, 2000.

91. Sullivan JA, Anderson SJ: *Care of the young athlete*, Rosemont, 2000, American Academy of Orthopaedic Surgeons/American Academy of Pediatrics.

92. Sheir-Neiss GI, Kruse RW, Rahman T, et al: The association of backpack use and back pain in adolescents, *Spine* 28:922–930, 2003.

93. Brackley HM, Stevenson JM: Are children's backpack weight limits enough?: a critical review of the relevant literature, *Spine* 29:2184–2190, 2004.

94. Grimmer KA, Williams M, Gill T: The relationship between adolescent head on neck posture, backpack weight and anthropometric features, *Spine* 24:2262–2267, 1999.

95. Goodgold SA: Backpack intelligence: implementation of a backpack safety program with fifth grade students, *Orthop Phys Ther Pract* 15:15–20, 2003.

96. American Physical Therapy Association: *Backpack talking points*. (Accessed 06.08.05.) Available at www.apta.org

97. Mendez FJ, Gomez-Conesa A: Postural hygiene program to prevent low back pain, *Spine* 26:1280–1286, 2001.

98. Leet AI, Skaggs DL: Evaluation of the acutely limping child, *Am Family Phys* 61:1011–1018, 2000.

99. Tibor LM, Sekiya JK: Differential diagnosis of pain around the hip joint, *Arthroscopy* 24:1407–1421, 2008.

100. Dobbs MB, Gordon JE, Luhmann SJ, et al: Surgical correction of the snapping iliopsoas tendon in adolescent, *J Bone Joint Surg Am* 84:420–424, 2002.

101. Teitz CC, Garrett WE, Miniaci A, et al: Tendon problems in athletic individuals, *Instr Course Lect* 46:569–582, 1997.

102. Allen WC, Cope R: Coxa saltans: the snapping hip revisited, *J Am Acad Orthop Surg* 3:303–308, 1995.

103. Winston P, Awan R, Cassidy JD, Bleakney RK: Clinical examination and ultrasound of self-reported snapping hip syndrome in elite ballet dancers, *Am J Sports Med* 35:118–126, 2007.

104. Schaberg JE, Harper MC, Allen WC: The snapping hip syndrome, *Am J Sports Med* 12:361–365, 1984.

105. Wahl CJ, Warren RF, Adler RS, et al: Internal coxa saltans (snapping hip) as a result of overtraining: a report of 3 cases in professional athletes with a review of causes and the role of ultrasound in early diagnosis and management, *Am J Sports Med* 32:1302–1309, 2004.

106. Cardinal E, Buckwalter KA, Capello WN, Duval N: US of the snapping iliopsoas tendon, *Radiology* 198:521–522, 1996.

107. Micheli LJ, Solomon R: Treatment of recalcitrant iliopsoas tendonitis in athletes and dancers with corticosteroid injection under fluoroscopy, *J Dance Med* 1:7–10, 1997.

108. Jacobson T, Allen WC: Surgical correction of the snapping iliopsoas tendon, *Am J Sports Med* 18:470–474, 1990.

109. Paolo A, Ciardullo A, Cuomo P: Patellofemoral dysfunction. In Micheli L, Kocher MS, editors: *The pediatric and adolescent knee*, Philadelphia, 2006, Saunders Elsevier.

110. Nomura E, Inouse M, Kurimura M: Chondral and osteochondral injuries associated with acute patellar dislocation, *Arthroscopy* 19:717–721, 2003.

111. d'Hemecourt P, Luke A, Stracciolini A: The child and adolescent knee: primary care perspective. In Micheli L, Kocher MS, editors: *The pediatric and adolescent knee*, Philadelphia, 2006, Saunders Elsevier.

112. Papachristou G, Efstathopoulos N, Plessas S, et al: Isolated meniscal repair in the avascular area, *Acta Orthop Belgica* 69:341–345, 2003.

113. Stanitski CL: Discoid meniscus. In Micheli L, Kocher MS, editors: *The pediatric and adolescent knee*, Philadelphia, 2006, Saunders Elsevier.

114. Murray MM, Spindler KP, Devin C, et al: Use of a collagen-platelet rich plasma scaffold to stimulate healing of a central defect in the canine ACL, *J Orthop Res* 24:820–830, 2006.

115. Petsche TS, Hutchinson MR: Loss of extension after reconstruction of the anterior cruciate ligament, *J Am Acad Orthop Surg* 7:119–127, 1999.

116. Aichroth PM, Patel DV, Zorrilla P: The natural history and treatment of rupture of the anterior cruciate ligament in children and adolescents: a prospective review, *J Bone Joint Surg Br* 84:38–41, 2002.

117. Dorizas CL, Stanitsky CL: Anterior cruciate ligament injury in the skeletally immature, *Orthop Clin North Am* 34:355–363, 2003.

118. Shelbourne KD, Gray T: Results of transphyseal anterior cruciate ligament reconstruction using patellar tendon autograft in Tanner stage 3 or 4 adolescents with clearly open growth plates, *Am J Sports Med* 32:1218–1222, 2004.

119. DeCarlo M, Shelbourne KD, Oneacre K: Rehabilitation program for both knees when the contralateral autogenous patellar tendon graft is used for primary anterior cruciate ligament reconstruction: a case study, *J Orthop Sports Phys Ther* 29:144–159, 1999.

120. Stormont DM, Peterson HA: The relative incidence of tarsal coalition, *Clin Orthop Relat Res* 181:28–36, 1983.

121. Tachdjian MO: The foot and ankle. In Greenfield S, editor: *Clinical pediatric orthopaedics: the art of diagnosis and principles of management*, Stamford, 1997, Appeton & Lange.

122. Korpelainen R: Risk factors for recurrent stress fractures in athletes, *Am J Sports Med* 29:304–310, 2001.

123. Bohne WH: Tarsal coalition, *Curr Opin Pediatr* 13:29–35, 2001.

124. Kelo MJ, Riddle DL: Examination and management of a patient with tarsal coalition, *Phys Ther* 78:518–525, 1998.

125. Saxena A, Erickson S: Tarsal coalitions. Activity levels with and without surgery, *J Am Podiatr Med Assoc* 93:259–263, 2003.

126. Kumar SJ, Guille JT, Lee MS, et al: Osseous and non-osseous coalition of the middle facet of the talocalcaneal joint, *J Bone Joint Surg Am* 74:529–535, 1992.

127. Fredrick LA, Beall DP, Ly JQ, et al: The symptomatic accessory navicular bone: a report and discussion of the clinical presentation, *Curr Probl Diagn Radiol* 34:47–50, 2005.

128. Micheli LJ, Nielson JH, Ascani C, et al: Treatment of painful accessory navicular: a modification to simple excision, *Foot Ankle Spec* 1:214–217, 2008.

129. Benjamin HJ, Glow KM: Strength training for children and adolescents: what can physicians recommend? *Phys Sports Med* 31:19–28, 2003.

130. Potash DH, Chu DA: Plyometrics. In Baechle TR, Earle RW, editors: *Essentials of strength training and conditioning*, ed 2 Lincoln, NE, 2000, National Strength and Conditioning Association.

131. American College of Sports Medicine: Position statement: plyometric training for children and adolescents, December 2001. Available at www.acsm.org.

CHAPTER 30

Management of Osteoarthritis and Rheumatoid Arthritis

MARIE B. CORKERY, MAURA DALY IVERSEN*

INTRODUCTION

The term *arthritis* comprises a complex of diseases that are manifested in more than 100 forms and affect more than 21% adults in the United States.[1] This chapter focuses on **osteoarthritis** (OA) and **rheumatoid arthritis** (RA) and provides analysis and discussion of the rehabilitation management of these two conditions.

OSTEOARTHRITIS

Epidemiology and Pathophysiology

OA involves the entire joint but is primarily a disease of the cartilage (Figure 30-1). Nearly 27 million people in the United States have clinical signs of OA, making it a leading cause of disability.[2] The exact pathogenesis is unknown. The most commonly affected and symptomatic joints are the apophyseal joints of the spine; the distal and proximal interphalangeal joints; the carpometacarpal joints; the first metatarsophalangeal joint; and the knee, hip, and patellofemoral joints.[3] Table 30-1 presents the prevalence rates of each form of OA, stratified by gender.

Risk factors for OA, also referred to as *osteoarthrosis,* can be classified into two major categories: intrinsic and extrinsic. **Intrinsic factors** include knee alignment (a determinant of joint load), muscle strength, obesity, ligament laxity, and proprioception. **Extrinsic factors** include repetitive physical activity and injury.[3] A link between youth sports injury of the knee and ankle and OA has been suggested.[18] Scientists recognize that OA is a slowly progressing, dynamic disease that involves biomechanical, environmental, genetic, and biochemical factors (e.g., cytokines).[19]

Early OA is a focal disease that presents as a distinct lesion of the cartilage.[20,21] Patients with early OA present with joint stiffness and pain on loading of the affected joint. Over time, OA evolves from progressive cartilage destruction to affect the subchondral bone and entire joint. Repeated biomechanical loading, synovial membrane inflammation, and release of cytokines stimulate the production of matrix metalloproteinases, which cause cartilage degradation and loss. Eventually the joint surface is destroyed. The classic appearance of primary OA on radiographs is localized disease with evidence of unequal joint space narrowing, subchondral bone eburnation (i.e., a hard, white appearance), subchondral cysts, and osteophytes (Figure 30-2). These findings increase in frequency after age 50. Only 40% of patients with severe radiographic features present with pain.[22,23]

The Kellgren scale is commonly used to grade the radiographic features of OA (Table 30-2). On radiographs, secondary OA may appear as diffuse or localized disease, depending on the etiology (e.g., RA, diabetes, or trauma). Secondary contractures occur around the involved joint and contiguous joints, altering joint alignment, increasing biomechanical forces on the joint, and accelerating cartilage loss.

> ### Categories of Osteoarthritis
>
> - Primary OA: Results in articular changes, although the etiological basis for the disease is unknown
> - Secondary OA: Caused by underlying factors that accelerate age-related degeneration of cartilage
>   - These factors include inflammatory arthritis (e.g., RA or spondyloarthritis), hypermobility syndromes, metabolic diseases (e.g., diabetes), and congenital and acquired joint surface incongruities, which accelerate damage to the cartilage, as well as trauma or sports-related injuries

*The authors, editors, and publisher wish to acknowledge Linda Steiner for her contributions on this topic in the previous edition.

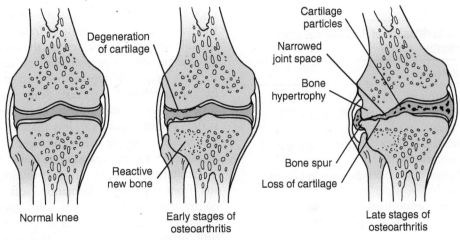

Figure 30-1 Osteoarthritis of the knee.

TABLE **30-1**

Prevalence Rates of Osteoarthritis in Joints

Joints Commonly Affected by Osteoarthritis	Prevalence in Men	Prevalence in Women
Spinal apophyseal	44.7%-74.2% (adults ages 40-60), 69.2%-89% (adults age 60+)[4,5]	
Proximal interphalangeal	4.8%-18.1% (ages 50-65), 20%-29.8% (age 66+)[6-9]	10.2%-29.6% (ages 50-65), 31.6%-35.2% (age 66+)[6-9]
Distal interphalangeal	9.8%-40.5% (ages 50-65), 49.2%-58.8% (age 66+)[6-9]	21.8%-55.5% (ages 50-65), 56.3%-76.0% (age 66+)[6-9]
Carpometacarpal	6%-30.3% (ages 55-65), 23.5%-27% (age 66+)[6-10]	13.5%-34.5% (ages 55-65), 33.9%-46.7% (age 66+)[6-10]
Metatarsophalangeal	5.8%-31.4% (ages 35-60)[6,11,12]	7.9%-43.2% (ages 35-60)[6,11,12]
Hip	0.9%-45%; mean 11.5% (age ≥18)[13]	0.9%-45%; mean 11.5% (ages ≥18.9)[13]
Knee	8%-24% (age 50+)[14,15]	22.3%-47.6% (age 50+)[14-16]
Patellofemoral	13.3%-34.5% (age 55+)[16,17]	24.3%-39.9% (age 55+)[16,17]

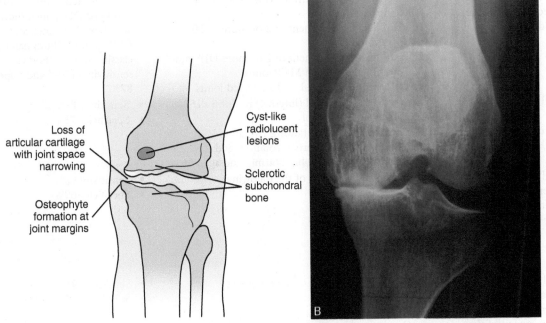

Figure 30-2 **A,** Radiographic hallmarks of osteoarthritis (Kellgren scale). **B,** Radiograph showing the main radiological signs of osteoarthritis. (**A** redrawn from McKinnis LN: *Fundamentals of orthopaedic radiology,* Philadelphia, 2005, FA Davis; **B** from Harris ED, Budd RC, Firestein GS et al: *Kelley's textbook of rheumatology,* ed 7, Philadelphia, 2005, Saunders.)

TABLE **30-2**

Kellgren-Lawrence Classification of Radiological Joint Changes in Osteoarthritis

Classification	Description
Grade 0	No features
Grade 1	Doubtful: Minute osteophyte, doubtful significance
Grade 2	Minimal: Definite osteophyte, unimpaired joint space
Grade 3	Moderate: Moderate diminution of joint space
Grade 4	Severe: Greatly impaired joint space with sclerosis of subchondral bone

Data from Kellgren JH, Lawrence JS: Radiological assessment of osteo-arthrosis, *Ann Rheum Dis* 16:494-501, 1957.

Table 30-3 shows the American College of Rheumatology diagnostic classification criteria for OA of the hand, hip, and knee.

Signs, Symptoms, and Impairments

Joint Pain, Stiffness, Restricted Motion, and Alterations in Alignment

OA causes pain, aching, or stiffness and eventually altered joint alignment. Cartilage does not have nerve endings; therefore OA pain may be caused by stretching of the joint capsule as a result of inflammation, the release of inflammatory cytokines in the synovial fluid, muscle spasm, and/or pressure on the subchondral bone.[27] Patients frequently report that pain increases with activity and is relieved with rest. Some patients have nighttime pain and report stiffness on waking. With OA, the stiffness often resolves in less than an hour and may be present after rest or with prolonged sitting. The clinical features of OA are presented in Table 30-4.

Limitations in joint range of motion (ROM) may result from osteophyte formation, soft tissue and tendon contractures surrounding a joint, periarticular muscle spasm, destruction of joint cartilage, persistent faulty posture, or muscular imbalance. Although a flexed position minimizes intra-articular pressure and reduces pain, maintaining a flexed posture can lead to flexion contractures. Patients may also present with crepitus (a grinding sensation felt under the skin as the joint is passively moved through ROM). This sensation results when irregular opposing cartilage surfaces rub together. In patients with erosive OA, localized joint swelling may also be present.[28]

Pain associated with hip OA may be experienced in the hip, groin, anterior thigh, knee, or buttocks. ROM is often restricted, particularly with medial rotation, and may be accompanied by crepitus. Patients may report difficulties with mobility and personal hygiene, difficulty walking, and experience increased energy expenditure with

TABLE **30-3**

American College of Rheumatology Diagnostic Classification Criteria for Osteoarthritis

Classification Criteria for Osteoarthritis of the Hand[24]	• Hand pain, aching, or stiffness and 3 or 4 of the following features: 1. Hard tissue enlargement of 2 or more of 10 selected joints 2. Hard tissue enlargement of 2 or more DIP joints 3. Fewer than 3 swollen MCP joints 4. Deformity of at least 1 of 10 selected joints	The 10 selected joints are the second and third DIP joints, the second and third PIP joints, and the first CMC joints of both hands. This classification method yields a sensitivity of 94% and a specificity of 87%.
Clinical Classification Criteria for Osteoarthritis of the Hip[25]	• Hip pain and hip medial (internal) rotation <15° and hip flexion ≤115°, or • Hip medial (internal) rotation ≥15°, and • Pain on hip medial (internal) rotation, and • Morning stiffness of the hip ≤60 min and age >50 yr	• Sensitivity 86% • Specificity 75%
Clinical Diagnostic Criteria for Osteoarthritis of the Knee[26]	• Knee pain and at least 3 of the following: 1. Age >50 yr 2. Stiffness <30 min 3. Crepitus 4. Bony tenderness 5. Bony enlargement 6. No palpable warmth	• Sensitivity 95% • Specificity 69%
Clinical and Radiographic Diagnostic Criteria for Osteoarthritis of the Knee[26]	• Knee pain and at least 1 of the following: 1. Age >50 yr 2. Stiffness <30 min 3. Crepitus 4. Osteophytes	• Sensitivity 91% • Specificity 86%

DIP, Distal interphalangeal; *MCP,* metacarpophalangeal; *PIP,* proximal interphalangeal; *CMC,* carpometacarpal.

TABLE **30-4**

Pathology and Clinical Features of Rheumatoid Arthritis and Osteoarthritis

Disease	Tissue Predominantly Involved	Clinical Features	Radiographic Features
Rheumatoid arthritis	Synovium (inflammation)	Symmetrical and bilateral joint involvement Joint pain, swelling, stiffness, and contracture Muscle weakness and fatigue *Acute:* Red, hot, swollen, painful joints; boggy feeling, fatigue, with or without fever; ligamentous laxity; morning stiffness up to a few hours *Subacute:* Effusion, reduced redness and pain *Stable:* Generally no effusion, minimal stiffness	Periarticular swelling, joint effusion, regional osteoporosis, subchondral osteolytic erosions, joint subluxation
Osteoarthritis	Cartilage (degradation)	Affects hips, knees, spine, ankles, distal interphalangeal joints, proximal interphalangeal joints, and metacarpophalangeal joints Joint pain, malalignment Decreased proprioception Muscle weakness *Early:* Focal cartilaginous lesions *End stage:* Loss of cartilage, bone on bone	Osteophytes at joint margins, joint space narrowing, subchondral sclerosis and cysts

Modified from Iversen MD, Liang MH, Bae SC: Exercise therapy in selected arthritides: rheumatoid arthritis, osteoarthritis, systemic lupus erythematosus, systemic sclerosis, and polymyositis/dermatomyositis. In Frontera WR, Dawson DM, Slovik DM, editors: *Exercise in rehabilitation medicine,* Champaign, IL, 2006, Human Kinetics.

activities. Loss of hip range adversely affects the spine and other joints in the kinematic chain. Preventive stretching of soft tissue is important and should be initiated early and often. Functionally based exercises, such as repetitive sit to stand and repeated controlled stepping up and down a stair, can help maintain hip and knee extensor strength. For patients unable to tolerate full gravity exercise, aquatic therapy can be used to allow exercise with reduced load.[27]

The knee is the most commonly affected weight-bearing joint. Knee malalignment, either varus or valgus, may be evident with severe disease (Figure 30-3), although knee varus is the more common presentation. Data indicate that knee varus or valgus is associated with a three-fold to fourfold increase in the odds of OA progression in the medial compartment of the knee.[3] Malalignment and abnormal patella tracking may produce retropatellar pain and chondromalacia patellae. Retropatellar pain often is experienced when the individual walks upstairs or sits for prolonged periods. Despite the location of pain, knee pain can lead to disuse atrophy and deconditioning.[3,29] However, one research study suggested that muscle weakness may be a cause rather than a result of knee OA.[30] Muscle weakness may alter joint biomechanics and produce unequal forces across the joint surface. Joint laxity from muscle inhibition or joint space narrowing unequally distributes the forces across the cartilage surface and can accelerate cartilage degeneration.[27]

Common features of hand OA are Heberden's and/or Bouchard's nodes, which are the result of bony overgrowths (Figure 30-4). Heberden's nodes appear at the

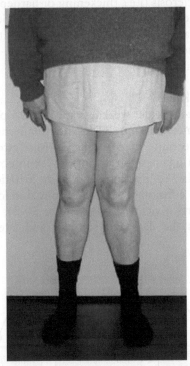

Figure 30-3 Valgus deformity of the knees. This is a common knee deformity that develops in patients with osteoarthritis of the lateral compartment. (From Scott WN: *Insall & Scott surgery of the knee,* ed 5, Philadelphia, 2012, Churchill Livingstone.)

medial and dorsolateral aspects of the distal interphalangeal (DIP) joints, and Bouchard's nodes appear at the proximal interphalangeal (PIP) joints. Finger joints appear bony and become less stable and less functional. Effusions, if present, can over time lead to joint ankylosis.

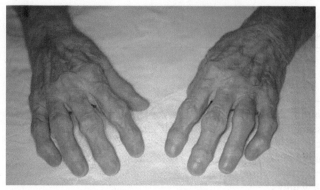

Figure 30-4 Osteoarthritic joint changes of the hand, including Heberden's nodes at the distal interphalangeal joints and Bouchard's nodes at the proximal interphalangeal joints. (From Little JW, Falace D, Miller C, et al: *Little and Falace's dental management of the medically compromised patient,* ed 8, St. Louis, 2013, Mosby.)

These deformities may affect the ability to manipulate small objects or to make a tight fist.

OA of the spine, also known as *spondylosis,* may affect the cervical, thoracic, and/or lumbar regions. Common changes evident on radiographs include osteophytes, which may form adjacent to the end plates and reduce blood supply to the vertebrae; stiffening and bone sclerosis (i.e., thickening or hardening); facet joint degeneration; and disc degeneration. Severe facet joint OA can lead to spinal stenosis. Limited ROM, especially neck rotation pain and stiffness, is evident with cervical OA.[19]

Muscle Weakness

Periarticular muscular weakness adds to OA progression through functional instability and diminished neuromuscular protective mechanisms.[28] Disuse atrophy likely results from ligament stretching, reflex inhibition from pain, capsular contraction, and joint irritation caused by pain and effusion.[27] Muscle atrophy due to reflex inhibition starts a vicious cycle (Figure 30-5), increasing force across the damaged cartilage and altering joint mechanics.

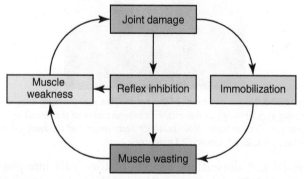

Figure 30-5 Vicious circle of injury. (Redrawn from Stokes M, Young A: The contribution of reflex inhibition to arthrogenous muscle weakness, *Clin Sci* 67:7-14, 1984.)

Proprioceptive Deficits

Proprioception is necessary for appropriate spatial and temporal limb coordination during movement. This increased coordination enhances stability and leads to more normal load distribution, reducing injury risk. Proprioceptive changes occur with age,[31] with sedentary lifestyles and joint instability. Changes in proprioception may result from destructive alterations in the ligaments, cartilage, capsule, or muscle and tendon that alter joint alignment.[22] On examination, reduced joint proprioception may be present along with joint hypermobility. Barrett et al.[32] and Hassan et al.[33] reported that individuals with knee OA have poorer knee proprioception than their healthy age-matched counterparts. In another study designed to assess the impact of OA on joint proprioception,[34] researchers recruited 28 adults with unilateral knee OA (Kellgren scale grade 2 or higher) and 29 adults without knee OA. A computer device and a stepper motor provided angular motion at 0.3°/sec and recorded angular displacement as patients reported the point at which they detected knee joint deflection. Patients with unilateral knee OA demonstrated worse proprioception than their healthy counterparts. Levinger et al.[35] assessed the fall risk of 35 people with knee OA before surgery and at 4 months after surgery and compared this risk to the risk of falls in a control group consisting of 27 asymptomatic age-matched controls. The authors reported that the surgical group exhibited a greater fear of falling and reduced lower limb proprioception and knee extensor strength before and after surgery compared with the control group. Levinger et al.[36] also reported that deficits in lower limb proprioception persisted at 12 months after surgery despite improvements in knee strength and reaction time.

Basic Principles of Rehabilitation and Studies on the Effects of Exercise in Patients with Osteoarthritis

Goals of Rehabilitation and Studies on the Effects of Exercise

The goals of rehabilitation in OA are to maximize function, ROM, and muscle force production and to reduce OA-associated deconditioning of the weight-bearing joints. Studies of regimens to correct or to prevent contractures are almost nonexistent. Heat, followed by passive ROM exercises and joint mobilization, is used clinically to reduce contractures and to improve joint ROM. Proper posture and positioning during extended inactivity or sleep, along with active ROM exercises, are used to maximize functional range and muscle strength. Proprioceptive and balance training are incorporated, particularly for weight-bearing joints to improve functional mobility. In difficult cases, serial casting or splinting can reduce contracture when followed by maintenance exercises.

The American College of Rheumatology (2012) has recommended that nonpharmacological treatment of hip and knee OA include a strong recommendation to participate in cardiovascular and/or resistance, land-based and aquatic exercise, and weight loss (for persons who are overweight).[37] The **Osteoarthritis Research Society International (OARSI) Guidelines** also recommended exercise therapy and weight loss for patients with hip and knee OA.[38] A Cochrane review of land-based therapeutic exercise for knee OA reported that exercise interventions of varying modes yielded small treatment benefits for pain (effect size of 0.4 [95% confidence interval (CI) 0.3 to 0.5]) and physical function (effect size 0.37 [95% CI 0.25 to 0.49]).[39] These effect sizes were comparable with those reported for nonsteroidal anti-inflammatory drugs. The review included a wide range of exercise programs, including individual, class, and home-based modes of delivery, along with aerobic, strengthening, and balance exercises. Studies with exercise programs of fewer than 12 supervised treatments had smaller treatment effects than programs with more than 12 directly supervised sessions.[39] Fransen et al.,[40] in their meta-analysis of land-based therapeutic exercise for hip OA, reported land-based exercise resulted in reduced pain (standardized mean difference [SMD] −0.38, 95% CI −0.55 to −0.20) and improved physical function (SMD −0.38, 95% CI −0.54 to −0.05]. These benefits in decreasing pain and improving function persisted at least 3 to 6 months after monitored treatment ended.[40] Although studies have examined the impact of exercise on function, few investigators have examined the impact of strengthening programs on cartilage.

Evidence suggests that programs incorporating balance and proprioceptive training may be beneficial for patients with lower extremity arthritis.[41,42] However, other studies have reported no additional benefit from adding balance exercises to an impairment-based program for patients with knee OA.[43] Various exercises—such as double-limb stance and single-limb stance activities, weight shifting, walking on toes, standing on unsteady surfaces, and use of boards such as the biomechanical ankle platform system (BAPS) and tilt/rocker boards—were used for balance and proprioception training. Although different underlying mechanisms have been proposed to explain how these interventions affect balance and proprioception, clinicians agree that addressing proprioception is important and may help improve stability during gait and functional activities. Smith et al.[44] conducted a systematic review and meta-analysis to investigate the effectiveness of proprioceptive exercises for patients with knee OA. Clinical outcomes of patients who received an exercise program that included proprioceptive exercises were compared with those without a proprioceptive component or that had a nontreatment control group. Seven randomized, controlled trials (RCTs) involving 560 patients were included in the analysis. Results showed that groups engaged in proprioceptive exercises showed improved joint position sense compared with nonproprioceptive exercise groups (mean difference in joint position angulation error, −2.18; 95% CI −2.7 to 1.66). However, there was no difference in self-reported physical function between groups (mean difference in Western Ontario and McMaster Universities Osteoarthritis Index [WOMAC] physical function score, −12.19; 95% CI −15.67 to −8.71). The authors concluded that, although more evidence was needed, there appeared to be an advantage to adding proprioceptive training to an exercise program for patients with knee OA.

There is evidence that tai chi may be an effective intervention for patients with knee OA. Song et al.[45] examined the effects of a 6-month tai chi program on knee muscle strength, bone mineral density (BMD), and fear of falling in older women with knee OA ($n = 30$) compared with a control group ($n = 35$). Women in the tai chi group had significantly greater knee extensor endurance (mean change, 36.4 for the tai chi group compared with 1.1 watts/kg for the control group), greater BMD in the proximal femoral neck (mean change of 0.09 in T score for the tai chi group compared with −0.1 in the control group), and reported a greater reduction in fear of falling (mean change of −2.4 in the tai chi group compared with 0.66 in the control group). Wang et al.[46] enrolled 40 patients with knee OA in a 12-week tai chi program and compared outcomes to a control group that received a program of stretching and education. The intervention group was highly adherent and reported reduced pain and improved physical function at the end of the trial. This program had the added benefit of improving self-efficacy, depression, and health status for patients with knee OA.

Most studies evaluating the effects of exercise focused on strengthening exercises for patients with mild to moderate OA. A review by Uthman et al.[47] reported that interventions combining strengthening, flexibility, and aerobic conditioning (land or water based) were most effective for patients with hip or knee OA. Table 30-5 presents randomized controlled trials (RCTs) of exercise for hip and knee OA.

Silva et al.[51] compared water and land-based exercises. In their study, 57 patients with knee OA completed an 18-week intensive exercise program, lasting 50 minutes per session. Results demonstrated that patients in both the water- and land-based exercises groups had significant reductions in pain measured by a visual analog scale (VAS) and improved function measured by the WOMAC and Lequesne Index. Reductions in VAS scores of 35.2 mm for the water-based group and 30.9 mm for the land-based group were reported, both exceeding the minimal clinical important difference (MCID) of greater than 17.5 mm, which is considered clinically significant for patients with knee OA. Additionally, patients allocated to the water-based exercise group exhibited significantly greater pain relief before and after completing a 50-feet walk test at week 18 compared with the land-based group. Hinman et al.[49] reported that a 6-week program of aquatic physical therapy resulted in significantly less pain and improved physical function, strength, and quality of life in patients with hip and knee OA compared with a control group who did not receive aquatic therapy. Aquatic

TABLE **30-5**

Randomized, Controlled Trials of Exercise and Manual Therapy in Hip and Knee Osteoarthritis (Since 2005)

Author	Sample	Intervention/Groups	Duration	Study Outcomes
Studies That Included Aerobic Exercise				
Tak et al.[48] (2005)	109 patients with HOA ages 55 yr and older	1. Hop with the Hip program: eight 1-hr weekly sessions of strength training under PT supervision. Also offered home exercise program, personal ergonomics advice from OT, and dietary advice from dietitian 2. Control group: self-initiated standard care	8 wk	The program had a positive effect on pain measured by the pain component of the HHS. Effect size, 0.51 immediately after the intervention program; 0.38 at a 3-mo follow-up. Effects sizes were smaller for VAS pain measurements (effect size, 0.00 after treatment and 0.17 at a 3-mo follow-up). There were improvements in post-test hip function measured by the HHS (effect size, 0.41), self-reported disability, measured by the Sickness Impact Profile at follow-up (effect size 0.29), and the timed up and go test (effect size, 0.35) at follow-up. It did not affect QOL, other measures of observed disability, or BMI.
Hinman et al.[49] (2007)	71 patients with HOA or KOA	1. Treatment group: aquatic physical therapy 2×/wk for 6 wk; program included walking and strengthening exercises 2. No aquatic physical therapy, continued with daily activities	6 wk	For the intervention group, there was increased hip muscle strength, physical function, and QOL, along with decreased pain and joint stiffness. Aquatic therapy participants reported an average reduction in pain of 33% from baseline compared with no change for the control group. Benefits were maintained for 6 wk after completion of therapy.
Lund et al.[50] (2008)	79 patients with KOA	1. Land-based exercise group: warm-up, strengthening/ endurance exercise, balance exercise and stretching exercise 2. Aquatic-based exercise group: warm-up, strengthening/ endurance exercise, balance exercise and stretching exercise 3. Control: interventions consisted of two 50-min sessions per week for 8 wk	8 wk with 3-mo follow-up	No effects observed at 8 wk. At 3-mo follow-up, land-based exercise showed a small improvement of pain and strength compared with the control group. Aquatic exercise group showed no changes compared with the control group but had significantly less adverse effects compared with the land group.
Silva et al.[51] (2008)	57 patients with KOA	1. Water-based exercise group 2. Land-based exercise group Both land and water groups participated in 50-min sessions of lower extremity strengthening, stretching, and gait training, 3×/wk for 18 wk	18 wk	Decrease in pain and improvements in WOMAC and Lequesne index were similar between the two groups. Pain before and after the 50-ft walk test decreased for both groups, but the water-based group experienced a significantly greater decrease in pain after the 50-ft walk test at week 18.
Wang et al.[46] (2009)	40 patients with KOA	1. Exercise group: 60 min of tai chi 2×/wk 2. Attention control (wellness education and stretching): 2×/wk	12 wk with follow-up at 24 and 48 wk	Patients assigned to tai chi exhibited significantly greater improvement in WOMAC pain, patients global VAS, physician global VAS, chair stand time, CES-D index, self-efficacy score, and SF-36 physical component summary.

(Continued)

TABLE **30-5**

Randomized, Controlled Trials of Exercise and Manual Therapy in Hip and Knee Osteoarthritis (Since 2005)—cont'd

Author	Sample	Intervention/Groups	Duration	Study Outcomes
Fernandes et al.[52] (2010)	109 patients with HOA with mild to moderate symptoms	1. Patient education 2. Patient education and supervised exercise The patient education program comprised three group sessions and one individual physical therapy session 2 mo after the group session. The supervised exercise component was 2×/wk for 12 wk. It included warm-up, strengthening, functional, and flexibility exercises.	12 wk with 4-, 10-, 16- mo follow-up	No significant difference was reported in the WOMAC pain score between the two groups. Significant improvements were reported at 10 and 16 months in patients receiving supervised exercise and education compared with patient education alone.
Song et al.[45] (2010)	65 women with KOA	1. Tai chi 2×/wk for 3 wk and then 1×/wk for the remainder of the 6-mo study period 2. Control group received a self-help education program designed for arthritic patients for 2 hr once a month for 6 mo	6 mo	Women in the tai chi group had significantly greater knee extensor endurance and greater bone mineral density in the proximal femoral neck and reported a greater reduction in fear of falling compared with the control group.
Juhakoski et al.[53] (2011)	120 with HOA ages 55-80	1. Combined exercise and general practitioner care group received 12 supervised (1×/wk) and four additional sessions 1 yr later 2. Received general practitioner care only	12 wk; after 1 yr, 4 booster sessions; regular follow-up for 2 yr	No significant difference in self-reported pain scores between the two groups. Patients in the combined exercise group demonstrated significant improvement in WOMAC function after 6 mo and 18 mo, compared with the control group. Shows positive effect of exercise for HOA in the long term. There was no significant difference in health care costs between groups.
Svege et al.[54] (2013)	109 patients with HOA	1. Exercise therapy and patient education[48] 2. Patient education[52]	6 yr cumulatively	22 patients in the group receiving both exercise therapy and patient education and 31 patients in the group receiving patient education only underwent THR during the follow-up period. Median time to THR was 5.4 and 3.5 yr, respectively. The exercise therapy group had better self-reported hip function before THR or end of study, but no significant differences were reported for pain and stiffness.

Studies That Included Manual Therapy Interventions

Author	Sample	Intervention/Groups	Duration	Study Outcomes
Deyle et al.[55] (2005)	134 Patients with KOA	1. Clinical treatment group, supervised exercise, manual therapy, and home exercises for 4 wk 2. Home exercise program	8 wk	Both groups had significantly improved WOMAC scores. The treatment group improvement was 25% more than the home exercise group.

(Continued)

TABLE **30-5**

Randomized, Controlled Trials of Exercise and Manual Therapy in Hip and Knee Osteoarthritis (Since 2005)—cont'd

Author	Sample	Intervention/Groups	Duration	Study Outcomes
Poulsen et al.[56] (2013)	111 patients with HOA	1. Patient education program, 2 individual sessions and 3 group sessions 2. Patient education program plus manual therapy (MT), 2×/wk for a 6-wk intervention period 3. Minimal control intervention (MCI) group	6 wk; follow up at 1 yr	No difference between the patient education and MCI groups. Combined intervention of MT and patient education was more effective than MCI for pain relief, with a clinically relevant reduction in pain score of 1.9 points (effect size, 0.92, 95% CI 0.41-1.42). Patient education alone was not superior to the MCI.
French et al.[57] (2013)	131 Patients with HOA	1. Exercise therapy (ET), 6-8 individual 30-min physiotherapy sessions 2. Exercise therapy and manual therapy (ET and MT), 6-8 individual 45-min physiotherapy sessions, 30 min of exercise therapy, 15 min of manual therapy 3. Waiting list control group; no exercise therapy or manual therapy	8 wk	There was no significant difference in WOMAC physical function between the ET ($n=66$) and ET+MT ($n=65$) groups at 9 wk (mean difference, 0.09; 95% CI −2.93-3.11) or 18 wk (mean difference, 0.42; 95% CI, −4.41-5.25), or between other outcomes, except patient satisfaction with outcomes, which was higher in the ET+MT group. Improvements in WOMAC, hip ROM, and patient-perceived change occurred in both treatment groups compared with the control group. Self-reported function, hip ROM, and patient-perceived improvement occurred after an 8-wk program of exercise for patients with OA of the hip.
Abbott et al.[58] (2013)	193 patients with HOA or KOA	1. Manual therapy procedures including thrust and nonthrust joint mobilization, soft tissue mobilization, and home program of joint range of motion activities 2. Multimodal exercise program 3. Exercise therapy and manual therapy 4. Usual care only, no exercise therapy or manual therapy Intervention groups attended therapy for 50 min 7 times within the first 9 wk, and then 2 more sessions before 16 wk, home exercise program 3×/wk.	16 wk; 1 yr follow-up	Manual therapy provided significant benefits over usual care. Exercise therapy provided significant benefits over usual care. There was no significant benefit in providing manual therapy and exercise therapy together.
Bennell et al.[59] (2014)	102 patients with HOA	1. Active group: consisted of 49 patients. 10 sessions over 12 wk; treatment included education, manual therapy, home exercise, and gait aid if appropriate; continued with unsupervised home exercises for 24 wk after treatment 2. Sham treatment: 53 patients; included inactive ultrasounds and inert gel; applied gel 3×/wk for 24 wk after treatment	12 wk with a 24-wk follow-up	The between-group differences for pain improvements were not significant. The function scores were also not significant between groups. Physical therapy had no significant improvements compared with sham treatment.

HOA, Hip osteoarthritis; *PT,* physical therapist; *OT,* occupational therapist; *HHS,* Harris hip score; *VAS,* visual analog scale; *QOL,* quality of life; *BMI,* body mass index; *KOA,* knee osteoarthritis; *WOMAC,* Western Ontario and McMaster Universities Osteoarthritis Index; *CES-D,* Center for Epidemiology Studies Depression index; *SF-36,* Short Form 36 Health Survey; *THR,* total hip replacement; *ROM,* range of motion.

therapy participants reported an average reduction in pain of 33% from baseline, from an average of 6 to 4 on a 0 to 10 cm VAS scale (effect size, 0.24). Of aquatic therapy participants, 72% reported improvements in pain and 75% reported improvements in function, compared with 17% of the control participants. Lund et al.[50] compared the efficacy of aquatic exercise and a land-based exercise versus control in 79 patients with knee OA. The primary outcome was pain with physical function, quality of life, balance, and knee muscle strength also being assessed. However, Lund et al.[50] reported that patients in the land-based exercise group demonstrated slight improvement of pain and strength compared with the control group, with no significant differences detected between the aquatic exercise and the control group. The authors noted that subjects in the aquatic exercise group reported significantly fewer adverse effects. Thus they recommended a combination of aquatic and land-based exercise as the preferred exercise regimen for patients with knee OA.

Juhakoski et al.[53] enrolled and allocated 120 patients with hip OA either to exercise combined with general practitioner (GP) care or to standard GP care. The combined care group completed a 12-week exercise program administered in weekly sessions at a facility, followed by home-based exercises with four additional sessions 1 year later. Subjects in the combined group demonstrated significant improvements in function (WOMAC scores) at 6 months (mean, −7.5; 95% CI −13.9 to −1.0) and 18 months (mean, −7.9; 95% CI −15.3 to −0.4). compared with the usual care group. These findings suggest some long-term benefits of exercise on function for patients with hip OA. In a study of 109 patients with hip OA, Fernendes et al.[52] reported that adding supervised exercise to a patient education program may improve physical function but not pain over 16 months. The patient education program comprised three group sessions and one individual physical therapy session 2 months after the group session. The supervised exercise component was twice a week for 12 weeks. Significant improvements were reported at 10 and 16 months in patients receiving supervised exercise and education compared with patient education alone. Effect sizes were modest, −0.48 (−0.91 to −0.06,), and −0.47 (−0.93 to −0.02) at 10 and 16 months, respectively. Improvements in WOMAC physical function scores from baseline to 10 and 16 months were 25% and 28%, respectively, indicating a clinically significant change. A long-term follow-up of this randomized trial was conducted to determine the effect of exercise and education on the patients' need for a total hip replacement.[54] Patients were followed up to a duration of 6 years to determine whether they received a total hip replacement. Patients with hip OA who performed supervised exercise in addition to a home exercise program were less likely to have a total hip replacement (THR).[54] Forty percent of patients in the exercise group underwent a THR compared with 57% in the control group. The authors concluded that their findings

supported the use of exercise as a first-line treatment for patients with hip OA. To determine the effects of exercise among older adults with hip OA, Tak et al.[48] conducted an RCT of an 8-week exercise and education program in 109 older adults with hip OA (aged 55 years and older). The intervention consisted of weekly 1-hour strengthening exercises and personalized OA advice on ergonomics and diet ($n = 55$) compared with a control group ($n = 54$). Outcomes were measured at baseline, after completion of the program, and at a 3 month follow-up. Data suggested exercise resulted in a moderate effect on pain relief as measured by the Harris Hip Score (HHS), at posttest, and at follow-up (effect sizes, 0.51 and 0.38, respectively) and resulted in small effects for improvements in hip function as measured by the HHS (effect size, 0.41), in disability as measured by the Sickness Impact Profile (effect size, 0.29), and mobility as measured by the timed up and go test (effect size, 0.35). These findings support the use of exercise for older patients with hip OA.

There is evidence suggesting that combining a weight loss program with exercise is more effective than exercise alone for patients with lower extremity OA.[60,61] Paans et al.[61] reported significant improvements in pain and physical function (including walking) in 35 overweight patients (mean body mass index [BMI] 32 kg/m²±3.9, age 56.9±11.9) with hip OA who completed an 8-month exercise and weight loss program. Messier et al.[60] reported similar improvements in pain and physical function after an 18-month program comparing exercise only, dietary weight loss only, dietary weight loss plus exercise, and usual care healthy lifestyle (control) in 252 older (age 60 years or older), overweight and obese patients with knee OA. The combination of modest weight loss (5.7% of body weight [BW]) combined with moderate exercise provided better overall improvements in function, pain, and mobility in overweight and obese adults ($n = 76$, mean BMI 34±0.7 kg/m²) with knee OA compared with either intervention alone.

A number of studies have examined the effect of manual mobilization techniques combined with exercise in patients with OA. In Table 30-5, RCTs that included manual therapy for hip and knee OA are described. Poulsen et al.,[56] in a study of 111 patients with hip OA, reported that a combined intervention of manual therapy and patient education was more effective than patient education alone or a minimal control intervention of hip stretching. Patients who received manual therapy and patient education exhibited greater pain relief with a clinically relevant reduction in pain score of 1.9 points (effect size, 0.92, 95% CI 0.41 to 1.42) compared with the minimal intervention group. Abbott et al.,[58] investigated the long-term effectiveness of manual physical therapy, multimodal exercise, combined exercise, and manual therapy in patients with hip or knee OA. Patients were randomly allocated to one of the four groups; 193 patients completed the trial, and the primary outcome measure was a change in WOMAC score after 1 year. Patients in the intervention groups received nine 50-minute sessions in the first 7 weeks and two additional sessions at week 16. Adjusted reductions in WOMAC scores at 1 year compared with the usual care group were as follows: usual care plus manual therapy, 28.5 (95% CI 9.2 to 47.8); usual care plus exercise therapy, 16.4 (−3.2 to 35.9); and usual care plus combined exercise therapy and manual therapy, 14.5 (−5.2 to 34.1). All intervention groups improved, but only the usual care plus manual therapy and usual care plus exercise therapy groups achieved clinically significant reductions of greater than 28 WOMAC points from baseline. There was no added benefit reported for combining exercise and manual therapy. The authors theorized that the combined therapy group spent less time on each intervention, thereby decreasing the effectiveness of both.

French et al.[57] conducted an RCT of 9 weeks of exercise therapy compared with exercise combined with manual therapy (and 18-week follow-up) in 131 patients with hip OA. Participants in the exercise group attended six to eight individual 30-minute physical therapy sessions over 8 weeks, which included flexibility and strengthening exercises. The exercise and manual therapy group participants attended six to eight individual 45-minute physical therapy sessions over an 8-week period, which included 30 minutes of exercise and up to 15 minutes of manual therapy. Participants in the control group remained on the wait-list. The researchers reported no significant difference in WOMAC physical function between the exercise ($n=66$) and combined exercise and manual therapy ($n=65$) groups at 9 weeks (mean difference, 0.09; 95% CI −2.93 to 3.11) or 18 weeks (mean difference, 0.42; 95% CI −4.41 to 5.25), nor did they report any significant differences between other outcomes, except patient satisfaction with outcomes, which was higher in the exercise and manual therapy group. Improvements in function (WOMAC), hip ROM, and patient-perceived change occurred in both treatment groups compared with the control group. The mean improvement in the WOMAC physical function at 9 weeks was 6.25 for the exercise and manual therapy group and 4.21 for the exercise group. Improvement for the exercise and manual therapy group exceeded the MCID for the WOMAC physical function, which is 5.4. Self-reported function, hip ROM, and patient-perceived improvement occurred after an 8-week program of exercise for patients with OA of the hip. The authors concluded that manual therapy as an adjunct to exercise provided no further benefit, except for higher patient satisfaction.

Bennell et al.,[59] in a randomized placebo-controlled trial, compared the effects of a 12-week multimodal physical therapy program ($n=49$) with sham physical therapy ($n=53$) in patients with symptomatic hip OA. Participants attended 10 treatment sessions over 12 weeks. Active treatment included education and advice, manual therapy, home exercise, and a gait aid, if appropriate. Sham treatment included inactive ultrasound and inert gel. For 24 weeks after treatment, the active group continued unsupervised home exercise, while the sham group self-applied gel three times weekly. Primary outcome measures were average pain and physical function (WOMAC scores). Interestingly, the authors reported that, although both groups showed improvements in pain and function, there was no significant difference in pain and function scores between groups who received physical therapy consisting of exercise and manual therapy and the group who received a sham treatment.

These mixed findings on the benefits of manual and exercise therapy specifically for patients with hip OA may indicate that there may be a subgroup of patients who might benefit most from manual therapy interventions and that interventions should be specifically selected for patients using a clinical reasoning approach that integrates data from the clinical presentation and stage of pathology. Additionally, interventions may need to be more frequent and intense than those provided in many clinical trials. However, combining interventions such as manual therapy and exercise may result in a reduction in the dose and intensity of both, thereby reducing their effectiveness.

A number of authors have attempted to identify patients with hip OA who were most likely to have a favorable response to physical therapy.[62] Baseline variables that might predict a favorable response to physical therapy include unilateral hip pain, age of 58 years or younger, pain greater than or equal to 6/10 on a numeric pain rating scale, 40-m self-paced walk test time of 25.9 seconds or less, and symptom duration of 1 year or less. However, additional research is needed to validate these findings. The American Physical Therapy Association (APTA) clinical practice guidelines for hip OA recommend that clinicians consider the use of manual therapy procedures to provide short-term pain relief and improve hip mobility and function in patients with mild hip OA.[63]

Variables That May Predict a Favorable Response to Physical Therapy*[62]

- Unilateral hip pain
- Age ≤58 years
- Pain ≥6/10 on numeric pain rating scale
- 40-m self-paced walk test time ≤25.9 seconds
- Symptoms duration ≤1 year

*Based on 90+ subjects.

There appear to be some immediate and long-term benefits from manual therapy in patients with knee OA.[55,64] Moss et al. reported an immediate local and more widespread hypoalgesic effect when patients with knee OA receive joint mobilization. The authors suggested that knee joint mobilization might be an effective method for reducing osteoarthritic pain. Deyle et al.[55] reported that 4 weeks of supervised exercise, manual therapy, and home exercises produced significantly greater improvements in outcomes for adults with knee OA compared with a home exercise program alone. Subjects in the clinic treatment group ($n=66$) received supervised exercise, individualized manual therapy, and a home exercise program over a 4-week period. Subjects in the home exercise group ($n=68$) received the same home exercise program initially, reinforced at a clinic visit 2 weeks later. Outcomes included the distance walked in 6 minutes and the WOMAC Index. Both groups showed clinically and statistically significant improvements in 6-minute walk distances and WOMAC scores at 4 weeks. Improvements were still evident in both groups at 8 weeks, while WOMAC scores at 4 weeks improved by 52% in the clinic treatment group and by 26% in the home exercise group. The average 6-minute walk distances improved by roughly 10% in both groups. The authors concluded that a home exercise program for patients with knee OA provided important benefits and the additional manual therapy and supervised exercise added greater symptomatic relief.

Jansen et al.,[65] in a systematic review and meta-analysis of 12 RCTs of patients with knee OA, reported that the addition of manual mobilization to an exercise program resulted in a superior effect on pain compared with strengthening exercises or a combination of strengthening, ROM, and aerobic exercises alone.

Aerobic walking at moderate intensity appears to improve aerobic capacity by up to 20% without exacerbation of symptoms. In studies by Minor et al.[66] and Kovar et al.,[67] patients with mild to moderate OA of the hips and knees not only improved aerobic capacity but demonstrated improvements in mood when aerobic walking was coupled with supervised stretching and strengthening exercises. Messier et al.[68] showed that aerobic exercise and strengthening programs improved balance and postural control. They enrolled 103 patients with knee OA in an 18-month trial and allocated them to one of three groups: (1) supervised aerobic exercise at 50% to 85% of the maximum heart rate for 50 minutes three times a week for 3 months, followed by a home prescription; (2) supervised upper and lower extremity weight training consisting of 2 sets of 10 repetitions three times a week for 3 months, followed by a home exercise prescription; or (3) monthly educational sessions and scheduled contacts from the research team. At the end of the trial, patients in the exercise groups showed improved balance and postural stability. A meta-analysis by Roddy et al.[69] compared the efficacy of aerobic walking or strengthening exercises for patients with knee OA. The weighted pooled effect size for pain reduction from aerobic walking for the four included studies was 0.52 (98% CI 0.34 to 0.7). An indirect comparison of aerobic walking and quadriceps strengthening showed no advantage of one approach compared with the other with regard to pain and disability.

Conclusions about Exercise, Manual Therapy, and Osteoarthritis

The evidence demonstrates that patients with mild to moderate knee and hip OA can safely engage in effective aerobic, strengthening, aquatic, and tai chi exercise without exacerbating joint symptoms. Improvements in mood, strength, and aerobic capacity are reported, ranging from 15% to 40%, depending on the intensity of the prescribed exercise.[27] Gains in functional performance and reductions in limitations are greatest when the program lasts at least 8 weeks and exercises are performed at least three times a week.[66,67,70-78] As with other populations, compliance with an exercise program is critical to its effectiveness.[69] Efficacy can be improved when home exercise is supplemented with a supervised program. Data also indicate that exercise programs combined with weight loss are more effective than exercise alone in overweight patients with hip and knee OA. Manual therapy interventions in combination with exercise result in improved outcomes in patients with knee OA. Although the evidence to support the use of manual therapy in patients with hip OA is less compelling, it appears to be an effective intervention for appropriately selected patients. The benefits of manual therapy for patients with OA may result in part from pain modulation, which results in improved tolerance to exercise. Additional research is needed to explore the efficacy of balance and proprioceptive training in patients with lower extremity OA and its effect on function and fall prevention.

Clinical Point

- Few studies have addressed the impact of resistance or aerobic exercise on patients with severe osteoarthritis
- The long-term effects of exercise on joint integrity and disability are unknown
- There is growing evidence to support the use of manual therapy combined with exercise to treat patients with knee OA and less so with hip OA

Aerobic exercise improves endurance, reduces fatigue, and has modest effects on muscle strength. With structured exercise (three times a week over 4 months), individuals can improve strength and endurance, leading to decreased dependency and pain and increased functional activity. Some of these benefits continue for up to 8 months after an intense program.[79] The concept that inactivity is a risk factor for OA, rather than just an outcome of the disease, emphasizes the importance of aerobic exercise in disease management.

Achieving a Therapeutic Effect with Exercise. Some evidence indicates that exercises that focus on proprioception and balance may reduce disability and improve strength. However, more research is needed in this area. Despite the evidence that symptoms of hip and knee OA can be improved with exercise and that exercise is recommended in practice guidelines, most patients with OA have not had a prescription for exercise. Even when physicians prescribe exercise, only a small percentage of patients exercise in a manner that can achieve a therapeutic effect.[80] A systematic review and meta-analysis of 48 RCTs by Juhl et al.[81] found that aerobic and knee strength training exercises reduced pain and lowered self-reported disability in patients with knee OA. For best results, exercise programs should be supervised and carried out at least three times per week and consist of at least 12 sessions.

Certain patients with hip OA can exercise at home just as effectively as with outpatient hydrotherapy to improve joint mobility and increase muscle strength.[82] Including manual therapy with exercise appears to provide added benefits. With respect to exercise in adults with knee osteoarthritis (KOA), *caution needs to be applied in patients with lax or malaligned knees, especially with tibiofemoral OA, in which quadriceps strengthening may exacerbate symptoms.* Table 30-6 summarizes the exercise recommendations for OA based on pain level and pathology.

Gait Problems and Use of Assistive Devices

Patients with hip and knee OA exhibit gait adaptations including reduced gait speed.[83] Patients describe difficulty and pain when walking or climbing stairs and reduced functional independence. Decreased muscle strength and reduced joint proprioception also are associated with an increased incidence of falls.[84]

In one study,[79] an exercise program consisting of individualized progressive training, including isometric and dynamic exercises for patients with knee OA, significantly improved muscle function, functional capacity, and walking time (as much as 21%) and reduced self-reported difficulty with walking and pain. Stationary cycling also has demonstrated improvements in walking speed, aerobic capacity, and pain.[85]

Studies have also reported improved rates of recovery in patients with end-stage hip arthritis after preoperative and perioperative exercise programs for total hip arthroplasty (THA).[86,87] Assistive devices are recommended as needed for patients with hip and knee OA.[37] An RTC by Jones et al.[88] found that patients with knee OA, who used a cane daily for 2 months, reported reduced pain and improved function compared with patients who did not use a cane. Gait modification strategies have also been suggested to offload the medial compartment of the knee and further research is needed in this area.[89]

TABLE 30-6

Summary of Rehabilitation Interventions for Osteoarthritis

Type of Osteoarthritis (OA)	Recommendations
OA of the hip and knee	
Mild pain	• AROM exercises (10 repetitions), 3-5 repetitions of flexibility and static exercises (8-10 repetitions of 6 seconds' duration) • Dynamic exercises, especially of the quadriceps and hamstrings (8-10 repetitions) • Low-impact aerobic activities (pool, bicycling) 20 min 3×/wk • Balance activities (BAPS and tilt boards), single-limb stance
Moderate pain	• Static and dynamic exercises—reduce to 5 repetitions • Flexibility exercises, 3-5 repetitions • Low-impact aerobic exercises (pool, bicycling) for 20 min 3×/wk • Balance and proprioception activities—bilateral • Use of cane or lateral heel wedge foot orthosis, neoprene knee sleeve
Severe pain	• Static and dynamic exercises (no resistance), 3-5 repetitions except with internal joint derangement • Low- or no-impact aerobic exercises (pool) • *Note: Advise functional activities to keep moving*
Bone on bone	• Same as for severe form but few or no repetitions of dynamic exercises; patient education is important • *Note: Caution should be used in prescribing quadriceps strengthening exercises for patients with ligamentous laxity and malalignment.* • Orthosis: Varus unloader-type knee orthosis; may need crutches or walker
OA of the hand	• Active movements, few repetitions, low resistance • Teach home exercises, which the patient should repeat daily • Aim to maintain full range of motion of MCP, PIP, and DIP joints

AROM, Active range of motion; *BAPS,* biomechanical ankle platform system; *MCP,* metacarpophalangeal; *PIP,* proximal interphalangeal; *DIP,* distal interphalangeal.

Modified from Iversen MD, Liang MH, Bae SC: Exercise therapy in selected arthritides: rheumatoid arthritis, osteoarthritis, systemic lupus erythematosus, systemic sclerosis and polymyositis/dermatomyositis. In Frontera WR, Dawson DM, Slovik DM, editors: *Exercise in rehabilitation medicine,* Champaign, IL, 2006, Human Kinetics.

Gait problems are common in patients with OA of any of the weight-bearing joints and are a clue to underlying pathology of the soft tissues or the joints themselves. Left untreated, they can cause problems. Clinicians should be attentive to this diagnosis and design treatments that maximize joint function.

Orthoses for Osteoarthritis

Much of the research examining the effects of bracing for OA has concentrated on devices to relieve knee pain and disability. In OA, the knee is subjected to increased medial compartment pressures secondary to varus loading during gait. Two techniques have been used to decrease these excessive forces: unloader-type knee orthoses (KOs) and lateral wedge insoles at the foot. An unloader KO for varus gonarthrosis, or knee varus (genu varum), can be either a thrust-type (Figure 30-6) or prestressed brace. The thrust-type, hinged KO has a single upright designed to create a valgus-correcting force at the knee to unload the medial compartment.[90] Kirkley et al.[91] compared the use of a varus unloader KO with a neoprene sleeve or with medical treatment alone in a group of 119 subjects with OA. After 6 months, the subjects who wore the unloader KO showed a significant difference in pain relief with functional tasks (i.e., a 6-minute walk and a 3-minute stairclimb) compared with the group that wore the neoprene sleeve. Both groups performed better than the nonbrace group. Brouwer et al.[92] studied the additive effect of a valgus brace on medial knee OA and a varus brace on lateral knee OA on conservative care. At a 12-month follow-up, patients who wore a brace reported less knee pain than patients in the control group. However, treatment effects

were small, and adherence to the brace was poor. A subgroup analysis indicated that patients with medial compartment knee OA who were younger than 60 years of age had a better therapeutic response to a valgus brace. Lindenfeld et al.[93] assessed biomechanical properties of the brace to reduce the varus forces as well as pain. The authors compared 11 subjects with OA before and after 4 weeks of brace wear and then compared them with 11 healthy controls. As measured on the Cincinnati Knee Rating System, pain, function, and biomechanical alignment all improved in the brace group. Alignment levels were reported to approach that of the normal control group.

Lateral wedge insoles or a variant, subtalar strapped insoles, are prescribed to make use of the closed chain properties of a foot orthosis (FO) to reducing compressive forces on the medial tibiofemoral joint compartment. Brouwer et al.[94] reported that some limited evidence indicated that lateral wedges reduced the use of pain medication by patients with OA when compared those who wore a neutral insole. However, function, as measured by the WOMAC functional scale, was not improved in the group that used neutral insoles after 6 months of wear. These researchers also reported that a lateral wedge insole with strapping for the subtalar joint demonstrated a biomechanical realignment effect, as measured by the femorotibial angle (FTA), but that those wearing these insoles reported more low back and foot pain. In contrast with these findings, Bennell et al.,[95] in an RCT of 200 patients with medial knee OA, reported no benefit to wearing lateral wedge insoles compared with flat insoles. Van Raaij et al.[96] compared the use of a lateral wedge insole with use of a valgus brace in 91 patients with medial compartmental knee OA and reported no difference in pain or WOMAC scores between groups after 6 months. Patients wearing the insole were more adherent and responded slightly better than the patients wearing the brace. These authors suggested that a lateral insole might be an alternative to valgus bracing. Arazpour et al.[97] compared the use of an unloader KO with the use of a lateral wedge insole in 56 patients with medial compartment knee OA. The Knee Injury and Osteoarthritis Outcome Score (KOOS) was used to assess status at baseline and 6 months after intervention. There were significant decreases in pain and increases in daily living activities, recreational and sport function, and quality of life with each intervention. The knee unloader orthoses were more effective than lateral wedge insoles in reducing pain levels. However, the lateral wedge insoles were more effective at improving quality of life as measured by the KOOS quality of life subscale. The authors concluded that lateral wedges were a suitable alternative to knee unloader orthoses for patients with medial compartment knee OA. There is some preliminary evidence that the use of a medial wedge orthosis is helpful in reducing knee pain in patients with valgus knee OA[98]; however, additional research is needed in this area. There is also evidence to support the use of medially directed knee taping to reduce pain in patients with knee OA.[99]

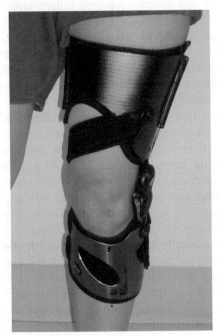

Figure 30-6 A thrust-type varus unloader knee brace. Note single lateral hinge.

The clinical decision to use these devices should be based on current research findings, the patient's degree of disability, the potential for compliance with an orthosis, and the cost of the device.

Case Study in Osteoarthritis

John is a 77-year-old male who presents with a diagnosis of right hip OA. His radiographic findings suggest decreased joint space with small acetabular osteophytes off the anterior aspect of the joint. He has opted to delay surgical intervention and wants to use physical therapy to enhance his overall physical status. He reports minimal difficulty with activities of daily living (ADLs) and instrumental activities of daily living (IADLs) (see Volume 1 of this series, *Orthopedic Physical Assessment*, Chapter 1). However, he has been increasingly sedentary since retiring from the post office 10 years ago. Currently, he reports late afternoon soreness on the anterior aspect of the leg and along the groin to his medial thigh, especially after doing a lot of walking.

On examination, John walks with a slow, deliberate gait pattern. He demonstrates decreased stance time on the right leg, and his right hip is maintained in flexion throughout the gait cycle. Decreased step length is noted on the left, and a positive Trendelenburg's sign is noted on the right. Right hip flexion ROM is 20° to 100° with a firm, unyielding end feel and restricted extension ROM; medial (internal) rotation and abduction is 0° to 20° with a firm end feel; and lateral (external) rotation is 0° to 35°. Left hip ROM is within normal limits (WNL). Right hip muscle strength is in the fair range. Lower abdominal strength is poor. Knee strength is good, and ankle strength is WNL. The patient has a positive Thomas test (20°) on the right. He demonstrates an inability to squat without visible muscle shaking and altered posture, a positive Trendelenburg's sign with unilateral squat, and increased trunk flexion with bilateral squat. Sensation is intact to light touch, but right hip kinesthesia and proprioception are reduced. He is able to maintain single-limb stance for approximately 5 seconds with eyes open. His past medical history is significant for coronary artery disease (no history of myocardial infarction), hypercholesteremia, gastroesophageal reflux disease, and a weight gain of 13.6 kg (30 lb) over the past 10 years. His BMI is 27 kg/m². He currently is taking the following medications: Zestril, Lipitor, and Prilosec.

1. *What rehabilitation program would you advise?*
2. *What education about restrictions to his activities would you recommend?*
3. *What type of exercise would you recommend?*
4. *Do you think an assistive device would be useful?*

Case Discussion

The patient's impairments of decreased hip muscle flexibility, poor muscle performance of the hip and trunk,

poor motor control, pain, joint mobility, and diminished proprioception contribute to his altered gait and should be addressed in the rehabilitation program. Flexibility exercises and joint mobilization, including hip distraction techniques, will help restore mobility and unload the hip joint while allowing a more normal gait pattern. Depending on the degree of pain, short-term use of a straight cane can further unload the joint for long-distance walking. He will benefit from an exercise program that emphasizes strengthening of the proximal musculature of the hip, especially the weak gluteus medius. An exercise program should be started that incorporates stability exercises in weight bearing, such as rhythmic stabilization in standing, and progresses to unilateral static and dynamic control. The progression should take place as pain diminishes and proximal motor control improves. These activities not only improve motor coordination and strength but also enhance proprioception. Aerobic exercise, such as aquatic classes and/or elliptical training, performed at 60% to 80% of his maximum heart rate, three times per week, should be incorporated into his program. The patient needs to learn how to modify his exercise regimen to adjust for his level of pain and to progress his exercises over time. Because his BMI is in the overweight range, research indicates that his exercise program will be more effective if combined with weight loss. A consultation with a nutritionist may be indicated to provide assistance with dietary modification to assist with this process.

RHEUMATOID ARTHRITIS

Epidemiology and Pathophysiology

Classic RA is a chronic systemic inflammatory disorder that not only affects joints but also has multiple systemic manifestations. RA affects approximately 1.3 million adults in the United States[1] and shortens life expectancy by about 10 years.[100] RA begins in early to middle life and affects women more often than men, and its incidence increases with age.

Inflammation of the synovium of diarthrodial joints is the predominant pathology, leading to a state of chronic synovitis. Synovitis that goes uncontrolled can lead to joint destruction (see Table 30-4). The chronic fluctuating course of RA can follow various patterns of exacerbation and remission. Patients may experience a continuous, low-grade exacerbation or have periods of remission followed by exacerbations of various intensities. Although exacerbations are a feature of the disease, they can be triggered by infection or trauma or can occur after medications have been stopped. Fewer than 10% of patients with RA go into prolonged remissions.[101]

The pattern of joint involvement is typically symmetrical and polyarticular. Nearly 10% of those affected develop some joint deformities within 2 years of diagnosis. Radiological changes often are seen first in the feet and hands. The Sharp score, as modified by van der Heijde,[102] is a method of documenting the disease progression. Radiologists score the number of bony erosions and areas of joint space narrowing in 30 to 32 joints of the hand and 12 joints in the feet. The total score is recorded (maximum involvement equals 448 points) and monitored on successive radiographs to track progression.

Although RA can affect any area, the most commonly affected joints are the wrists, metacarpophalangeal (MCP) joints, and PIP joints in the upper extremity (Figure 30-7) and the ankle and foot (Figure 30-8) in the lower extremity. In the spine, RA is more common in the cervical area but can involve all segments. Because this is a systemic disease, extra-articular clinical symptoms may involve the cardiovascular system, pulmonary system, integumentary, and/or nervous system. Pleurisy, often presenting as shortness of breath or dyspnea on exertion, has been reported in up to 70% of patients with RA. Pericarditis,

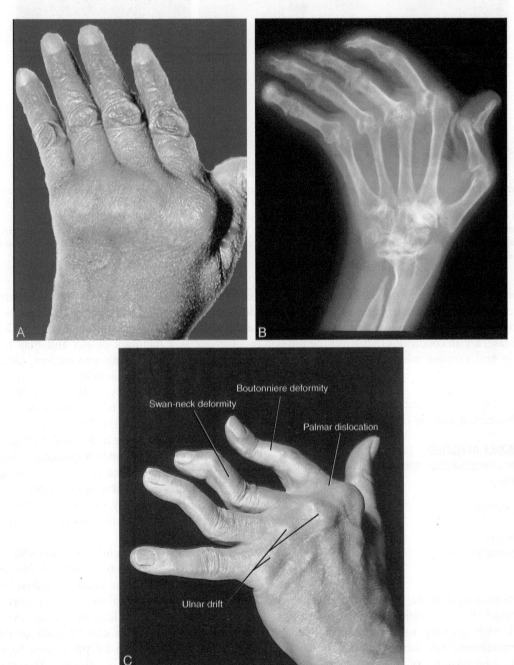

Figure 30-7 A, Swelling and capsular injury at the metacarpophalangeal (MCP) joint, resulting in lateral slippage of the extensor tendon and ulnar deviation of the fingers in a patient with rheumatoid arthritis. **B,** Radiograph showing the destructive changes associated with advanced rheumatoid arthritis. Note especially the marked bone destruction at the wrist, the subluxation and ulnar deviation at the MCP joints, and the dislocation of the interphalangeal joint of the thumb. **C,** Rheumatoid arthritis of the hand, showing advanced changes with ulnar drift and palmar subluxation at the MCP joints and swan neck and boutonniere deformities in the fingers. (From Harris ED, Budd RC, Firestein GS et al.: *Kelley's textbook of rheumatology,* ed 7, Philadelphia, 2005, WB Saunders.)

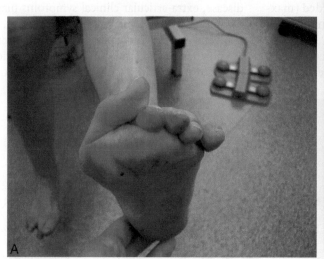
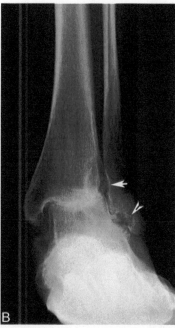

Figure 30-8 A, Advanced rheumatoid foot showing severe hallux valgus deformity, dorsal subluxation of lesser toes and consequent metatarsalgia, with keratotic skin noted under the metatarsal heads. **B,** Rheumatoid arthritis of the ankle, showing diffuse loss of cartilage space with erosions of the fibula *(arrow and arrowhead)*. The scalloping along the medial border of the distal fibula *(arrow)* is called the fibular notch sign and is a characteristic finding in rheumatoid arthritis. The hindfoot is in valgus alignment. (**A** from Walker R, Redfern D: The foot in systemic disease: management of the rheumatoid or diabetic patient, *Orthopaed Trauma* 25:241-252, 2011. **B** from Firestein GS, Budd RC, Harris ED, et al: *Kelley's textbook of rheumatology*, ed 8, Philadelphia, 2009, Saunders.)

myocarditis, and vasculitis, which may affect as many as 30% of patients, as well as renal effects secondary to vasculitis or to the toxic effects of long-term drugs used to control the disease, are all conditions that affect the physical functioning and exercise tolerance of patients with RA.[100,101,103]

Features of Rheumatoid Arthritis

JOINTS COMMONLY AFFECTED
- Wrist, metacarpophalangeal joints, proximal interphalangeal joints, foot, ankle, knee

SYSTEMIC FEATURES
- Pleurisy
- Pericarditis, myocarditis
- Vasculitis and renal disease

In RA, osteoporosis is more prevalent than in age-matched cohorts.[104,105] In addition to the risk factors normally seen with primary osteoporosis, individuals with RA have additional risk factors such as periods of immobilization, long-term use of corticosteroids, and use of disease-modifying antirheumatic drugs (DMARDs) (see Volume 2 of this series, *Scientific Foundations and Principles of Practice in Musculoskeletal Rehabilitation*, Chapter 12). Patients with RA have a 1.5 times greater risk of osteoporotic fracture than patients who do not have RA.[106] However, Haugeberg et al.[107] reported that

even with the use of DMARDs and corticosteroids, bone loss can be mitigated if the patient with RA is treated with antiresorptive drugs, calcium, and vitamin D.

Fatigue is a hallmark of RA and may result from a combination of cytokine production, deconditioning from lack of exercise or activity, and altered biomechanics of involved joints. As with many chronic diseases, patients with RA have a higher risk of depression, which may also contribute to the fatigue. This factor coupled with the systemic nature of RA and increased metabolic cost of daily activities may significantly limit function and restrict independence as the disease progresses. The American College of Rheumatology provides guidelines to help clinicians classify the effect of the multiple impairments on the patient's global functional capacity (Table 30-7).[108]

RA may also affect children. **Juvenile rheumatoid arthritis** (JRA; referred to as *juvenile idiopathic arthritis* [JIA] by the European League Against Rheumatism) is diagnosed when symptoms occur before 16 years of age and persist for at least 6 consecutive weeks. No specific diagnostic tests can be used to confirm JIA; rather, several tests can be performed to support the clinical impression of the disease. The three primary subtypes of JIA established by the American College of Rheumatology are pauciarticular JIA, polyarticular JIA, and systemic JIA. These subtypes are based on the number of joints involved, the presence or absence of systemic features, and in some cases, the age of onset.[109] Because these classifications are based on

TABLE 30-7

American College of Rheumatology's Classification of Global Functional Status in Rheumatoid Arthritis

Classification	Description
Class I	Completely able to perform usual activities of daily living (self-care, vocational, and avocational*)
Class II	Able to perform usual self-care and vocational activities but limited in avocational activities
Class III	Able to perform usual self-care activities but limited in vocational or avocational activities
Class IV	Limited in ability to perform usual self-care, vocational, and avocational activities

* Self-care activities include dressing, feeding, bathing, grooming, and toileting; avocational activities (recreational and/or leisure activities) and vocational activities (work, school, homemaking) are patient desired and age and gender specific.

From Hochberg MC, Chang RW, Dwosh I et al: The American College of Rheumatology 1991 revised criteria for the classification of global functional status in rheumatoid arthritis, *Arthritis Rheum* 35:498, 1992.

the characteristics of the disease at onset, they may not indicate its course over time.[110]

Pauciarticular JIA is defined as synovitis in four or fewer joints, usually the elbows, knees, and ankles, and is most often asymmetrical and nonsystemic. In pauciarticular JIA, the rheumatoid factor usually is negative. Pauciarticular JIA has two subtypes, based on the onset of disease and the clinical presentation. Early-onset pauciarticular disease often occurs in girls before the age of 5. Late-onset pauciarticular disease occurs around the ages of 10 to 12 years and most often affects the large weight-bearing joints (i.e., hips and knees) and entheses (muscle insertions). Stiffness and pain are the predominant complaints.[109]

Classification of Rheumatoid Arthritis in Children

- Pauciarticular (≤4 joints)
  o Early onset
  o Late onset
- Polyarticular (≥5 joints)
- Systemic

Polyarticular JIA affects girls more often than boys. It is characterized by synovitis in five or more joints, often symmetrical. Patients may present with systemic features. Although polyarticular JIA may involve any joint, the cervical spine frequently is affected. It is important to note that polyarticular JIA also affects normal growth and development.[109]

Systemic JIA can occur at any age and may occur in boys or girls. It is characterized by high, spiking fevers; a classic rash (pink to salmon colored) that often occurs on the trunk and proximal extremities; and synovitis in one or more joints. The fever generally is the first symptom and may precede other symptoms within months. Malaise, anemia, pericarditis, thrombocytopenia, lymphadenopathy, hepatomegaly, and other systemic features evident with adult RA may be present. These children are so ill that they often present with severe functional limitations and growth retardation (below the 5th percentile).[109]

Signs, Symptoms, and Impairments

Pain, Stiffness, and Swelling

RA can cause adaptive shortening of the soft tissues, tendons, and joint capsules. Bone erosion and cartilage loss reduce joint space and may contribute to subluxation, limiting joint motion. Swelling associated with joint effusion and extra-articular edema further reduces mobility. These changes result in significant mobility impairments and pain, especially during exacerbations. Analgesic and anti-inflammatory medications are the mainstays of medical management for these patients (see Volume 2 of this series, *Scientific Foundations and Principles of Practice in Musculoskeletal Rehabilitation*, Chapter 12). However, physical modalities and exercise play an important role in reducing functional loss.

Signs and Symptoms of Rheumatoid Arthritis

- Chronic inflammation
- Exacerbations and remissions
- Symmetrical, polyarticular joint involvement
- Osteoporosis
- Fatigue
- Pain
- Deformity (subluxations)
- Mobility impairment
- Muscle weakness
- Depression

Studies That Address Pain, Stiffness, and Swelling. Cold helps reduce inflammation and pain when the joints are acutely inflamed. Heat should be avoided at this time because heat may exacerbate the inflammatory process.[111] When the inflammation resolves, either heat or cold can be used to relieve pain.[112] Local heat may be preferred before gentle exercise to reduce joint stiffness. In general, few studies examine the effectiveness of modalities. An Ottawa Panel[113] concluded that some (but limited) evidence supported the use of ultrasound, paraffin, transcutaneous electrical nerve stimulation (TENS), and low-level laser therapy in the management of pain and flexibility. The panel's guideline further stated that evidence for including or excluding electrotherapy modalities is inconclusive at this time.

Exercise stimulates endogenous opiates and may be used to reduce joint pain and stiffness. Ekdahl et al.[114] studied endorphin levels in patients with RA during exercise. Serum levels of internal opiates were directly related to the intensity and frequency of active exercise. Numerous research studies have reported that ROM exercises safely and efficiently maximize joint motion in patients with RA even when performed for long periods.[115–119] Lee et al.[120] and Wang et al.[121] reported physical and psychological benefits from tai chi exercise in patients with RA. Patients with early or stage I disease can safely perform daily exercise, including active flexibility and ROM, doing a few repetitions at each joint. Passive stretching should be deferred until the joints are not in an active exacerbation.[27]

Muscle Weakness

Muscle weakness is common with RA.[110,122] Weakness may be attributable muscle fiber atrophy. Myositis, characterized by inflammation within the muscle itself, is not always present or apparent but can be assessed through muscle enzyme testing. If myositis is not present or is minimal, muscles can be exercised sufficiently so that training effects for muscle strengthening can be achieved.[123] Atrophy has been shown to occur in both type I and type II muscle fibers and may stem either from disuse or from changes to the muscle tissue itself.[124]

Studies of Strength Training. Studies of strength training for patients with RA have focused on effectiveness and safety.[125–127] Early studies of strength training focused on the impact of low-intensity training, such as active ROM, isometric, or low load-resistance exercise programs.[124] These studies incorporated exercise of varying intensity, frequency, and duration to avoid exacerbation of symptoms. More recent investigations studied moderate- to high-intensity strength training programs, which are defined as 50% or greater of maximum voluntary contraction (MVC). Considerable emphasis was placed on determining whether patients with RA could tolerate higher loads without sacrificing joint integrity. The RCTs of exercise in patients with RA are reviewed in Table 30-8.

TABLE **30-8**

Randomized, Controlled Trials of Exercise in Rheumatoid Arthritis (Since 2005)

Author	Sample	Intervention/Groups	Duration	Study Outcomes
Studies That Included Aerobic Exercise				
Bilberg et al.[128] (2005)	46 patients with class I, III disease; stable medications	1. Group pool exercise, moderate-intensity aerobic and strength exercise 2×/wk 2. Home exercise	12 wk	Moderate pool exercise resulted in significant improvement in muscle endurance and vitality score on SF-36. No significant difference was seen in aerobic capacity measured by submaximum cycle ergometer.
Neuberger et al.[129] (2007)	220 adults with RA	1. Low-impact aerobic exercise class, 1 hr 3×/wk for 12 wk 2. Video recorded home-based exercise, 1 hr 3×/wk for 12 wk 3. Control group: exercised at baseline amounts	12 wk	Overall symptoms (pain, fatigue, and depression) decreased significantly at 12 wk for the class exercise group compared with the control group. Walk time and grip strength were significantly improved in both treatment groups compared with the control group. Disease activity was unchanged in all groups compared with baseline.
Breedland et al[130] (2011)	34 patients with RA	1. Intervention group: physical exercise (circuits, bike training, sports, aqua jogging) and an educational component 2. Control group	8 wk with 22-wk follow-up	Intervention group showed a significant improvement in VO_2max (12.1%), muscle strength (elbow and knee flexors and extensors), health status, and perceived self-efficacy.

(Continued)

TABLE **30-8**

Randomized, Controlled Trials of Exercise in Rheumatoid Arthritis (Since 2005)—cont'd

Author	Sample	Intervention/Groups	Duration	Study Outcomes
Stavropoulos-Kalinoglou et al.[131] (2013)	40 patients with RA	1. Exercise group: 6-mo individualized aerobic and resistance high-intensity exercise intervention, 3×/wk, two supervised, one unsupervised 2. Control: received advice on exercise benefits and lifestyle changes	6 m	Participants in the exercise group demonstrated significant improvements in VO_2max, blood pressure, triglycerides, high-density lipoprotein (HDL), total cholesterol-to-HDL ratio), BMI, body fat, 10-year CVD event probability, CRP, DAS28, and HAQ compared with those in the control group.

Studies of Strengthening Exercises, Flexibility, and Other Interventions

Author	Sample	Intervention/Groups	Duration	Study Outcomes
Lee et al.[120] (2012)	21 patients with RA	1. Tai chi exercise program 2×/wk for 12 wk 2. Tai chi exercise program 2×/wk for 12 wk and auricular acupressure	12 wk	Tai chi exercise improved balance, grip strength, pinch strength, self-efficacy in relation to pain control, etc. Tai chi exercises appeared to be helpful both mentally and physically. No evidence suggested that auricular acupressure enhanced Tai chi.
Cima et al.[132] (2013)	20 women with RA	1. Patients participated in exercise program that targeted hand grip strength, pinch strength, and motor coordination of the hand, 20 sessions 2×/wk for 10 wk 2. No hand treatment	10 wk	Exercise group had significant gains in hand grip strength and pinch strength as well as functionality.
Manning et al.[133] (2014)	108 patients with RA of <5 years	1. Usual care 2. EXTRA program: 4 (1-hr) group education, self-management, and global upper extremity exercise training sessions supplementing the first 2 wk of a 12-wk individualized, functional home exercise regimen in addition to usual care	12 wk	EXTRA program improved upper extremity disability, function, hand grip strength, and self-efficacy for pain, symptoms, and disease activity.

SF-36, Short Form SF-36; *RA*, rheumatoid arthritis; *VO₂max*, maximum amount of oxygen in milliliters; *BMI*, body mass index; *CVD*, cardiovascular disease; *CRP*, C-reactive protein; *DAS28*, Disease Activity Score-28; *HAQ*, Health Assessment Questionnaire.

In the aggregate, studies demonstrate that both static and dynamic strengthening programs improved strength and function in patients with RA in the range of 15% to 50%. Most studies included exercise at a frequency of two to three times a week. Studies of low to moderate intensity (25% to 50% MVC) demonstrated improvements in strength of approximately 15% to 30%; those of higher intensity showed greater gains. For example, McMeekan et al.[134] assigned 36 patients with nonactive RA either to a control group or to a group that performed knee flexor/extensor strengthening exercises at 70% MVC for 45 minutes, two to three times a week, for 6 weeks. At the 6-week follow-up, patients in the exercise group were able to generate significantly greater isokinetic torque than the control group. In addition, the exercise group reported less pain and greater function and mobility on a health assessment questionnaire (HAQ).

Hakkinen et al.[135] compared the effect of a home strength training program performed at 50% to 70% maximal repetitions for upper extremity and lower extremity muscle groups with a home program of ROM exercises with both groups exercising twice weekly. Both groups also performed an aerobic exercise program three times a week. Variables studied included knee extension and hand grip strength, BMD of the femoral neck and lumbar spine, and radiographic joint changes. At the 2-year point, 62 patients had completed the program. The exercise group demonstrated significant gains in maximum strength on a dynamometer and little joint damage. BMD showed little or no change. Subjects continued the exercise program on a self-monitored basis for 3 years. At the end of 3 years (i.e., 5 years total of exercise), 59 of the original 62 patients were evaluated again. Strength gains were maintained for the resistance-trained groups through the subsequent 3-year self-monitored phase. BMD was unchanged, and radiographic evidence of joint damage continued to be low. Cima et al.[132] reported on the effects of an exercise program aimed at improving handgrip strength (HS), pinch strength (PS), and motor coordination of the hand in patients with hand RA. Twenty women with hand RA were randomly allocated to an exercise group ($n = 13$) and a control group ($n = 7$) that received no treatment. Patients in the exercise group completed a hand exercise program for 20 visits over 10 weeks and exercises at home. The exercise group reported improvements in HS, PS, and functionality. Manning et al.[133] compared the effectiveness of usual care to a program consisting of group education, self-management, and global upper extremity exercise training sessions, supplementing a 12-week individualized, functional home exercise regimen (EXTRA program). One hundred and eight patients with RA of 5 years' or less duration were randomly allocated to either group. Outcome measures included the Disabilities of the Arm, Shoulder and Hand questionnaire (primary outcome measure), the Grip Ability Test, HS, the Arthritis Self-Efficacy Scale (pain, function, and symptoms subscales), and the 28-joint Disease Activity

Score and were assessed at baseline, 12 weeks (primary end point), and 36 weeks. Results indicated a significant ($p < 0.05$) between-group difference at 12 weeks, in the mean change in disability (−6.8 [95% CI −12.6, −1.0]), function (−3.0 [95% CI −5.0, −0.5]), nondominant HS (31.3 N [95% CI 9.8, 52.8]), self-efficacy (10.5 [95% CI 1.6, 19.5] for pain and 9.3 [95% CI 0.5, 18.2] for symptoms), and disease activity (−0.7 [95% CI −1.4, 0.0]), all favoring the EXTRA program.

Hurkmans et al.,[136] in their review of eight RCTs, reported that short-term (pooled effect size 0.47 [95% CI 0.01 to 0.93]) and long-term land-based aerobic capacity and muscle strength training showed moderate evidence for a positive effect on aerobic capacity and muscle strength in patients with RA.

Fatigue and Endurance

Studies have reported that aerobic capacity is diminished in patients with RA compared with healthy subjects. Physical inactivity and/or pain combined with direct effects of the disease on the cardiovascular or pulmonary systems may contribute to reduced aerobic capacity. However, physical function can increase and cardiovascular fitness can be improved by 20%, as measured by VO_2max with short-term cardiovascular programs.[116,119] The greatest improvements in aerobic capacity are gained with exercise regimens at 50% to 80% of VO_2max.[27]

Aerobic exercise programs for patients with RA should be designed to accommodate the patient's functional limitations and degree of joint involvement. Non–impact-loading forms of land exercise, such as walking or cycling, reduce stress to joints. Swimming and other aquatic exercise regimens have the advantage of using the buoyancy of water to reduce load. The recommended water temperature for patients with arthritis is 37° to 40°C (98.6° to 104°F), warm enough to help control pain and reduce muscle tension and joint stiffness.[122]

Studies of Aerobic Exercise. Initial studies of aerobic exercise enrolled patients with nonactive disease and used bicycle ergometry. In these earlier trials, exercise prescriptions were maintained at a relatively low intensity. Neuberger et al.[129] studied 220 adults with RA who completed a 12-week program of class exercise or home exercise and a control group who exercised at baseline. The exercise class was 1 hour, three times weekly, and consisted of four phases: warm-up exercises, strengthening exercises, low-impact aerobic exercises, and cool-down exercises. Participants in the home exercise group exercised at home using a videotape of the same exercise program. Significant improvements were reported in overall symptoms (i.e., fatigue measured with the 14-item Global Fatigue Index of the Multidimensional Assessment of Fatigue questionnaire; pain measured with the Short Form of the McGill Pain Questionnaire, and depression measured with the Center for Epidemiologic Studies Depression Scale) in the class group compared with the control group. Walk time and grip strength were significantly improved in both treatment groups compared with the control group.

Van Ende et al.[137] studied 100 patients with RA in a 12-week program of high-intensity exercise versus ROM and isometric exercises. The high-intensity program included weight-bearing exercises and bicycling at 70% to 85% of the patient's age-predicted maximum heart rate. The low-intensity groups did ROM and static strengthening exercises for the trunk and lower extremity, or an individual low-intensity ROM and static exercise program, with instruction from a physical therapist, or a written home program of ROM and static exercises. At the end of 12 weeks, those exercising at the higher intensities showed significant improvement in aerobic capacity and knee muscle strength and mobility. An important find was that no exacerbation of joint symptoms was seen in any group, and joint symptoms actually decreased among the high-intensity exercisers. Muscle strength gains were maintained, but aerobic gains were lost at a follow-up 12 weeks after the program ended.

Research on alternative forms of aerobic exercise, such as aquatic programs, have demonstrated mixed results. A study by Bilberg et al.[128] assigned 46 subjects with class I to class III RA to either a treatment group, which participated in supervised aquatic therapy two times a week for 12 weeks, or to a control group, which continued with their regular activities. These authors reported no significant aerobic effect from water exercise, as measured by cycle ergometry. However, they did report improved muscle endurance for both upper and lower extremity muscle groups, as measured by isometric grip strength and a functional chair rise test. A Cochrane Review by Hurkmans et al.,[136] which included eight RCTs, reported that short-term, land-based aerobic capacity training showed moderate evidence for a positive effect for aerobic capacity (pooled effect size 0.99 [95% CI 0.29] to 1.68) and short-term, water-based aerobic capacity training showed limited evidence of a positive effect on functional ability and aerobic capacity in patients with RA. An RCT by Breedland et al.[130] reported on the effects of a group-based exercise and educational program on the physical performance and disease self-management of patients with RA. A total of 34 patients diagnosed with RA were randomly assigned to either an intervention group ($n = 19$) or a waiting list control group ($n = 15$). The intervention was an 8-week, multidisciplinary, group therapy program consisting of physical exercise designed to increase aerobic capacity and muscle strength together with an educational program to improve health status and self-efficacy for disease self-management. The physical exercise component was conducted in group sessions and consisted of a muscle exercise circuit and bicycle training once a week for 60 minutes, sports once a week for 60 minutes, and aqua jogging twice a week for 30 minutes. Each participant

exercised for a total of 3 hours per week on two separate days. Main outcome measures were maximum oxygen uptake (VO_2max), elbow and knee flexors and extensors muscle strength, health status, and perceived self-efficacy. All data were recorded at baseline, after 9 weeks, and at follow-up in week 22. The intervention group showed significant improvement (12.1%) in VO_2max at week 9 compared with the control group (−1.7%). Significant within-group changes were reported over time for muscle strength of the upper and lower extremities and health status that favored the intervention group. However, no between-group changes were reported regarding these outcomes.

There is some evidence that individualized aerobic and resistance exercise intervention can improve cardiorespiratory fitness (CRF), cardiovascular disease (CVD) risk factors, and physical function in patients with RA. A case control study by Stavropoulos-Kalinoglou at al.[131] matched 40 patients with RA to a control group. Patients were allocated to either an exercise program (receiving 6 months individualized aerobic and resistance high-intensity exercise intervention three times per week) or a control group (receiving advice on exercise benefits and lifestyle changes). Participants were assessed at baseline, 3 months, and 6 months for aerobic capacity (VO_2max), individual CVD risk factors (i.e., blood pressure, lipids, insulin resistance, body composition), 10-year CVD event probability, and RA characteristics (i.e., C-reactive protein [CRP]), Disease Activity Score 28 (DAS28), and HAQ. Participants in the exercise group demonstrated significant improvements in VO_2max, blood pressure, triglycerides, high-density lipoprotein (HDL), total cholesterol-to-HDL ratio, BMI, body fat, 10-year CVD event probability, CRP, DAS28, and HAQ compared with those in the control group.

Articular Changes

The effect of moderate to high-intensity exercise on joint integrity has been examined. De Jong et al.[125,126,138,139] reported on a series of studies in which patients with stable class I to class III RA who participated in higher levels of exercise were monitored over 2 years. In one study, 309 patients with stable RA who were enrolled in the Rheumatoid Arthritis Patients in Training (RAPIT) program were randomly assigned either to a usual care group or to an intensive supervised exercise group. The exercise group met for 75 minutes two times a week for 2 years. The exercise program was threefold: bicycle aerobic training for 20 minutes, a 20-minute exercise circuit consisting of 8 to 10 exercises, and a sport or game for 20 minutes. The exercise session also included warm-up and cool-down periods. Impact loading for joints included jumping during the warm-up and the selection of sports such as basketball, volleyball, indoor soccer, and badminton (281 subjects finished the study). Researchers assessed the effect of high-intensity impact-generating exercise on the small joints of the feet and hands of 136 participants (145 subjects had usual care). After 2 years, not only did the rate of joint changes for the small joints not increase, the exercisers' feet showed less progression. In the larger weight-bearing joints (i.e., the knee and hip), the mean radiographic change was not significant for the whole group. However, participants who began the study with more radiological evidence of changes in the larger weight-bearing joints did show a progression of changes.[125,138] The researchers also reported improved aerobic capacity for the exercise group. These studies suggest caution in prescribing exercise to patients who already have significant joint damage, especially in the large weight-bearing joints; however, they also support the use of such exercise in the small joints of the hands and feet.[126]

Basic Principles of Rehabilitation and Studies on the Effects of Exercise in Patients with Rheumatoid Arthritis

The goals of rehabilitation in the management of RA are to maximize strength, flexibility, endurance, and mobility and to promote independence while minimizing the potential for further joint destruction and deformity. A well-designed intervention program incorporates information about the extent of the joint impairments, as well as the patient's stage of disease, motivation, and adherence to therapy.[27] It is also important to consider the patient's psychological state and motivation for rehabilitation. Depression and reduced self-efficacy are common in a chronic disease such as RA.[140,141] Interventions used

in the management of RA include various forms of exercise, orthoses, adapted ambulatory aids, modalities, and patient education in energy-conservation techniques.

Physical activity levels are low in patients with RA. A study on physical fitness and health perceptions of individuals with RA indicated that 47% of 298 participants reported low to fair levels of activity on a regular basis.[142] Patients with a chronic disease such as RA have to incorporate exercise and physical activity into their daily lives. A trial by Munneke et al.,[143] which examined exercise adherence in 146 patients with RA, reported that 81% of the participants were still engaged in the supervised exercise program after 2 years. Patients with high disease activity and low functional ability at baseline were slightly more likely to drop out of the trial. However, strategies can be used to enhance adherence. Iversen et al.[144] reported that a positive social support system can improve the adherence rate by 300%. It also is important to recognize the impact of the clinicians' own beliefs and expectations on the patient's adherence to therapy. Provider expectations and beliefs about various modes of exercise have been shown to affect patient adherence to exercise prescriptions.[145,146]

Summary of Exercise Recommendations for the Patient with Rheumatoid Arthritis

Exercise should be considered an important, lifelong component in the management of RA. Exercise improves mobility, strength, endurance, daily function, and mood in patients with RA. Table 30-9 summarizes the exercise recommendations at various levels of disease presentation

TABLE **30-9**

Summary of Rehabilitation Interventions for Rheumatoid Arthritis

Form of Rheumatoid Arthritis	Recommendations
Acute flare (hot joint)	AROM exercises for involved joints, 2 repetitions/joint/day Resting orthoses and assistive devices with built-up handles or platform attachments
Subacute	AROM exercises, 8-10 repetitions/joint/day Static exercises, 4-6 contractions lasting 6 seconds each Isotonic exercises with light resistance (avoid if joints are unstable or with tense popliteal cysts or internal joint derangement) Aerobic training, 15-20 min 3×/wk; cardiac evaluation recommended for men >35 yr and women >45 yr; establish heart rate parameters and use perceived rating of exertion scale (e.g., Borg scale of perceived exertion)
Stable or inactive	AROM and flexibility exercises Static and dynamic strength training (avoid dynamic exercises if joints are unstable or with tense popliteal cysts) Aerobic training, 15-20 min 3×/wk; cardiac evaluation recommended for men >35 yr and women >45 yr; establish heart rate parameters and use perceived rating of exertion scale Orthoses: lower extremity—accommodative or custom foot orthoses in extra-depth shoes or moldable shoes; upper extremity—consider working wrist/hand support

AROM, Active range of motion.

Modified from Iversen MD, Liang MH, Bae SC: Exercise therapy in selected arthritides: rheumatoid arthritis, osteoarthritis, systemic lupus erythematosus, systemic sclerosis and polymyositis/dermatomyositis. In Frontera WR, Dawson DM, Slovik DM, editors: *Exercise in rehabilitation medicine,* Champaign, IL, 2006, Human Kinetics.

for RA. ROM exercises, incorporated into daily routines, should be performed on affected joints to maintain mobility and prevent contractures. During an exacerbation, two to three repetitions of active range of motion (AROM) exercises can be performed without unduly stressing the joints. Byers[147] recommends that patients exercise in the evening to help reduce the morning stiffness associated with RA. When the disease is in remission, ROM exercises can be increased to 8 to 10 repetitions a day for each involved joint.

Strengthening programs can incorporate isometric or active exercises with resistance when the patient is not experiencing an active flare-up (also called a *flare*), or exacerbation. Isometric exercise generally results in less inflammation, less of an increase in intra-articular pressure, and less shear.[110,148] The clinician must keep in mind, however, that sustained exercises of large muscle groups may put an increased load on the cardiovascular system and may be contraindicated in patients with RA who have cardiac problems.

Clearly, aerobic exercise programs, including those with weight-bearing components, appear to be better tolerated than previously thought, at least in patients with stable disease (i.e., disease that is not in a period of active flare-up). The effect of more intensive exercise on patients with a more aggressive disease process is not yet clear, but the most recent studies recommend caution with high intensity or impact loading on the larger weight-bearing joints if the patient shows significant radiological joint changes. In addition to other signs of inflammation, pain should be a guide to determining the appropriate intensity of the program. Acute pain during exercise indicates a need to modify the program; vague, diffuse pain that resolves in less than 2 hours does not indicate a need for program modification.[112] Patients must recognize the signs of an acute flare (i.e., redness, inflammation, pain, and stiffness) and reduce the frequency and intensity of exercise. Exercise prescriptions should include the intensity, frequency, and duration at which each exercise should be performed and take into account the current stage of the disease.

Orthoses for Rheumatoid Arthritis

Orthoses, splints, and special shoes often are recommended, with the stated goals of relieving pain, reducing edema, providing increased joint stability, and thereby improving overall function. The most commonly prescribed devices are wrist and hand splints, extra-depth shoes, and custom or prefabricated insole or foot orthoses.

Wrist and hand splints are categorized as resting splints and working splints (i.e., those designed to be worn for functional activities). Such splints can be custom-made for the individual or purchased over the counter. Janssen et al.[149] evaluated the effect of using a resting splint on pain, grip strength, and swollen joints and reported no difference between use and nonuse. Similarly, Kjeken et al.[150]

reported no differences in pain, stiffness, grip strength, or self-reported quality of life between patients who used a working splint and those who did not. However, they did find evidence of some loss of motion while the splint was worn for work tasks. Stern et al.,[151] on the other hand, evaluated three common commercial elastic working splints and reported no difference in dexterity with or without the splints in any of the ones used. Egan et al.,[152] in a Cochrane review, concluded that, because working wrist splints do not appear to be detrimental in terms of motion, they might be useful for a degree of pain relief in some patients. The authors further concluded that the evidence currently is insufficient to support the use of resting splints, although the authors acknowledged that some patients report a preference for wearing them for comfort reasons during acute exacerbations.

In the foot, thinning of plantar fat pads and interossei muscle atrophy are often seen. Along with subluxation of tendons, these changes can lead to deformities, especially of the forefoot, such as hammer toes and metatarsal subluxation.[153] Loss of medial arch support from overstretching of repetitively inflamed soft tissues may lead to significant overpronation. Extra-depth shoes and shoes made of heat-moldable material are commonly prescribed footwear.[154] The extra-depth shoe has an additional 0.64 to 0.95 cm (0.25 to 0.38 inch) of volume to accommodate any foot deformities and to allow use of an insert or FO (Figure 30-9). Inserts in the form of both accommodative and custom posting often are prescribed. In one study, patients who wore extra-depth shoes with a semirigid orthotic for 12 weeks reported less pain than when they wore just an extra-depth shoe.[155] Soft inserts were not reported to provide any further pain relief over just wearing the extra-depth shoe alone. However, in another study, use of a functionally posted, semirigid FO alone did not appear to make a difference in pain or disability measures compared with a placebo insert.[156]

Ambulatory Aids and Adaptive Equipment

Many patients with RA have significant upper extremity joint dysfunction, especially of the hands and wrists,

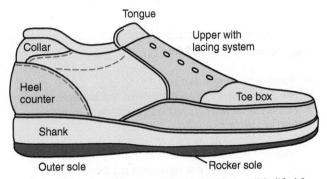

Figure 30-9 Extra-depth foot segments and shoe design. (Modified from the Association of Rheumatology Health Professionals: *Clinical care in the rheumatic diseases,* ed 3, p 268, Atlanta, 2007, The Association.)

which makes use of a cane, crutch, or walker difficult or painful. The use of platform attachments that distribute weight-bearing forces over the forearm may reduce stress on the hands and wrists. Devices with wider, flatter handgrips often are more comfortable than the standard grip. Cone-type handgrips are designed so that the ulnar side of the hand is on the wider part of the cone; this improves grip strength and resists the tendency for ulnar drift or deviation. A low-cost alternative is to build up the handgrip of ambulatory aids or utensils and writing implements with moldable foam, which helps prevent compression on vulnerable joints while improving the ability to grip.

Energy Conservation Techniques

Because RA is a systemic disease, patients can easily become fatigued. Although all patients should be encouraged to participate in exercise programs as appropriate, educating patients in strategies for conserving energy while performing routine ADLs is equally important.[157] This becomes imperative during periods of exacerbation.

Energy Conservation Strategies[155]

- Schedule activities so that demanding physical tasks are alternated with less strenuous ones
- Sit to perform tasks when possible
- Gather all necessary supplies before a task
- Limit trips, especially up and down stairs
- Schedule adequate rest periods

In addition, patients should be taught to avoid positions and activities that perpetuate joint deformity. Squeezing a ball for hand exercise should be avoided because it may contribute to subluxation at the MCP and interphalangeal (IP) joints as a result of excessive force on the ulnar side of the joints. Prolonged flexed positions of the hands and other extremity joints may shorten soft tissue and contribute to contractures.

Suggestions for Patient Education

- Provide simple, clear instructions
- Link the exercise or modality to a clear outcome and explain its use
- Provide patients with key symptoms that indicate a flare and the need for exercise modification
- Provide guidelines for modifying an exercise
- Encourage social support for exercise
- Ask patients to explain their expectations and attitudes toward exercise to help determine their willingness to exercise and perceived barriers to exercise

---

Case Study in Rheumatoid Arthritis

Holly is a 38-year-old female who presents with 5 months of bilateral knee, wrist, and hand pain. Upon examination, she exhibits pain (VAS score, 6/10) and 2+ swelling in the PIP joints, MCP joints, and wrist, with limited ROM. Several PIP joints exhibit 15° hypertension, and subcutaneous nodules are evident on the right fourth and fifth PIP joints. Slight ulnar deviation of the MCP joints is seen, left greater than right. Her knees are warm, painful, and swollen, and these symptoms are greater on the left than the right. The patella ballottement test is positive bilaterally. She has restricted ROM in her left knee of 10°. Both feet show hallux valgus and hammer toe deformities. The stiffness and swelling in her fingers, wrists, feet, and knees are worse in the morning, lasting up to 3 hours. By late afternoon, her hands, wrists, feet, and knees are aching, and she states that aspirin does not alleviate her pain. She is having difficulty performing her job as a university professor. Her typing is labored, and she has trouble demonstrating manual skills that require hand dexterity; she also has trouble with prolonged standing while conducting her laboratory courses. She saw her rheumatologist, who prescribed prednisone (10 mg), methotrexate, folic acid, and a multivitamin and referred her to physical therapy.

Case Discussion

This patient is in a "flare". The prescribed medical therapy—a fast-acting pharmaceutical agent (i.e., prednisone) combined with a slow-acting disease-modifying drug (i.e., methotrexate)—hopefully will bring the disease under control. Her rehabilitation program should include gentle ROM exercises for the whole body, with special emphasis on her wrists, hands, fingers, knees, and feet. The synovitis evident in her hands and knees can lead to stretching of the joint capsule and ligaments. With synovitis, biomechanical forces across the joint are increased, and ligaments and tendons can become involved, leading to joint instability. Common changes evident in the hands (the joints commonly involved first) are radial deviation of the wrist, subluxation of the proximal carpal row, and radial rotation of the distal carpal bones. Therefore it is important to check for volar drop of the MCP joints by palpating the heads of these joints in relation to the extended first phalanx. Although flexed posturing generally is more comfortable, flexion can lead to intrinsic tightness. Resting splints for evening and dynamic splints may help maintain alignment during physical activities. Resistive dynamic exercises should be avoided with synovitis. In the hand, forceful squeezing results in joint deformities and may result in pathomechanical changes. ROM and isometric exercises are preferred, along with the use of ice to reduce swelling. A can of food or a cylinder can be used to perform isometric grasping and is preferred to ball squeezing, which can lead to ulnar drift.

Proper footwear that provides adequate support and allows accommodation of her foot deformities should be recommended. An extra-depth shoe allows for use of a soft insole with enough room to accommodate the foot deformities. An ergonomic evaluation of her work space and home environment should be done so that recommendations can be made for individualized energy-conserving techniques. She may benefit from an ergonomically designed computer keyboard and/or mouse that minimizes ulnar drift and allows an easier grasp. Because prolonged standing is fatiguing, an appropriate supportive chair should be sought. Frequent monitoring of blood pressure is required with the use of steroids because these drugs can lead to weight gain and subsequent hypertension.

SUMMARY

This chapter discussed the roles of exercise therapy, ambulatory aids, modalities, and orthoses in addressing OA and RA. The evidence supporting the use of various types of exercise, the strengths and limitations of these studies, and new recommendations were presented. The importance of prescribing the correct frequency, duration, intensity, and type of exercise for the various stages of disease was highlighted, as was the current data on the use of orthoses and appropriately adapted aids and assistive devices. Suggestions were presented for important patient educational material that can be included in the intervention plan.

REFERENCES

1. Helmick CG, Felson DT, Lawrence RC, et al: Estimates of the prevalence of arthritis and other rheumatic conditions in the United States, Part I, *Arthritis Rheum* 58:15–25, 2008.
2. Lawrence RC, Felson DT, Helmick CG, et al: Estimates of the prevalence of arthritis and other rheumatic conditions in the United States, Part II, *Arthritis Rheum* 58:26–35, 2008.
3. Sharma L: Local factors in osteoarthritis, *Curr Opin Rheumatol* 13:441–446, 2001.
4. Kalichman L, Li L, Kim D, et al: Facet joint osteoarthritis and low back pain in the community-based population, *Spine* 33:2560, 2008.
5. Gellhorn AC, Katz JN, Suri P: Osteoarthritis of the spine: the facet joints, *Nat Rev Rheumatol* 9:216–224, 2012.
6. Van Saase JL, Van Romunde LK, Cats A, et al: Epidemiology of osteoarthritis: Zoetermeer survey. Comparison of radiological osteoarthritis in a Dutch population with that in 10 other populations, *Ann Rheum Dis* 48:271–280, 1989.
7. Butler WJ, Hawthorne VM, Mikkelsen WM, et al: Prevalence of radiologically defined osteoarthritis in the finger and wrist joints of adult residents of Tecumseh, Michigan, 1962-65, *J Clin Epidemiol* 41:467–473, 1988.
8. Haugen IK, Englund M, Aliabadi P, et al: Prevalence, incidence and progression of hand osteoarthritis in the general population: the Framingham Osteoarthritis Study, *Ann Rheum Dis* 70:1581–1586, 2011.
9. Wilder FV, Barrett JP, Farina EJ: Joint-specific prevalence of osteoarthritis of the hand, *Osteoarthritis Cartilage* 14:953–957, 2006.
10. Haara M, Kröger H, Arokoski J, et al: 01105 Osteoarthritis of carpometacarpal joint in finns aged 30 years or over: prevalence, determinants and association with mortality, *J Bone Joint Surg Br* 86:238, 2004.
11. Munteanu SE, Zammit GV, Menz HB: Factors associated with foot pain severity and foot-related disability in individuals with first metatarsophalangeal joint OA, *Rheumatology* 51:176–183, 2012.
12. Roddy E, Thomas MJ, Marshall M, et al: The population prevalence of symptomatic radiographic foot osteoarthritis in community-dwelling older adults: cross-sectional findings from the clinical assessment study of the foot, *Ann Rheum Dis* 74:156–163, 2013.
13. Pereira D, Peleteiro B, Araujo J, et al: The effect of osteoarthritis definition on prevalence and incidence estimates: a systematic review, *Osteoarthritis Cartilage* 19:1270–1285, 2011.
14. Kacar C, Gilgil E, Urhan S, et al: The prevalence of symptomatic knee and distal interphalangeal joint osteoarthritis in the urban population of Antalya, Turkey, *Rheumatol Int* 25:201–204, 2005.
15. Duncan RC, Hay EM, Saklatvala J, et al: Prevalence of radiographic osteoarthritis--it all depends on your point of view, *Rheumatology* 45:757–760, 2006.
16. Davies AP, Vince AS, Shepstone L, et al: The radiologic prevalence of patellofemoral osteoarthritis, *Clin Orthop Relat Res* 402:206–212, 2002.
17. Driban JB, Eaton CB, Lo GH, et al: Association of knee injuries with accelerated knee osteoarthritis progression: data from the Osteoarthritis Initiative, *Arthritis Care Res (Hoboken)* 66:1673–1679, 2014.
18. Caine DJ, Golightly YM: Osteoarthritis as an outcome of pediatric sport: an epidemiological perspective, *Br J Sports Med* 45:298–303, 2011.
19. Lozada CJ, Altman RD: Osteoarthritis. In Robbins L, Burckhardt CS, Hannan MT, DeHoratius RJ, editors: *Clinical care in the rheumatic diseases*, 2 ed., Atlanta, 2001, Association of Rheumatology Health Professionals.
20. Yoshioka H, Alley M, Steines D, et al: Imaging of the articular cartilage in osteoarthritis of the knee joint: 3D spatial-spectral spoiled gradient–echo vs. fat-suppressed 3D spoiled gradient–echo MR imaging, *J Magn Reson Imaging* 18:66–71, 2003.
21. Gandy SJ, Dieppe PA, Keen MC, et al: No loss of cartilage volume over three years in patients with knee osteoarthritis as assessed by magnetic resonance imaging, *Osteoarthritis Cartilage* 10:929–937, 2002.
22. Hochberg MC: Radiographic features and functional status in rheumatoid arthritis, *Arthritis Rheum* 32:1340–1341, 1989.
23. Kellgren JH, Lawrence JS: Radiological assessment of osteoarthritis, *Ann Rheum Dis* 16:494–502, 1957.
24. Altman R, Alarcón G, Appelrouth D, et al: The American College of Rheumatology criteria for the classification and reporting of osteoarthritis of the hand, *Arthritis Rheum* 33:1601–1610, 1990.
25. Altman R, Alarcón G, Appelrouth D, et al: The American College of Rheumatology criteria for the classification and reporting of osteoarthritis of the hip, *Arthritis Rheum* 34:505–514, 1991.
26. Altman R, Asch E, Bloch D, et al: The American College of Rheumatology criteria for the classification and reporting of osteoarthritis of the knee, *Arthritis Rheum* 29:1039–1049, 1986.
27. Iversen MD, Liang MH, Bae S: Selected arthritides: rheumatoid arthritis, osteoarthritis, spondyloarthropathies, systemic lupus erythematosus, polymyositis/dermatomyositis, and systemic sclerosis. In Frontera WR, Dawson DM, Slovik DM, editors: *Exercise in rehabilitation medicine*, Champaign, IL, 2006, Human Kinetics.
28. Klippel JH, et al: Osteoarthritis. In Klippel JH, Crofford LJ, Stone JH, Weyand CM, editors: *Primer on rheumatic diseases*, 12 ed., Atlanta, 2001, Arthritis Foundation.
29. Steultjens MP, Dekker J, Bijlsma JW: Avoidance of activity and disability in patients with osteoarthritis of the knee: the mediating role of muscle strength, *Arthritis Rheum* 46:1784–1788, 2001.
30. Slemenda C, Brandt KD, Heilman DK, et al: Quadriceps weakness and osteoarthritis of the knee, *Ann Intern Med* 127:97–104, 1997.
31. Pai YC, Rymer WZ, Chang RW, et al: Effect of age and osteoarthritis on knee proprioception, *Arthritis Rheum* 40:2260–2265, 1997.
32. Barrett DS, Cobb AG, Bentley G: Joint proprioception in normal, osteoarthritic and replaced knees, *J Bone Joint Surg Br* 73:53–56, 1991.
33. Hassan BS, Mockett S, Doherty M: Static postural sway, proprioception, and maximal voluntary quadriceps contraction in patients with knee osteoarthritis and normal control subjects, *Ann Rheumatic Dis* 60:612–618, 2001.
34. Sharma L, Dunlop DD, Cahue S, et al: Quadriceps strength and osteoarthritis progression in malaligned and lax knees, *Ann Intern Med* 138:613–619, 2003.
35. Levinger P, Menz HB, Wee E, et al: Physiological risk factors for falls in people with knee osteoarthritis before and early after knee replacement surgery, *Knee Surg Sports Traumatol Arthrosc* 19:1082–1089, 2011.
36. Levinger P, Menz HB, Morrow AD, et al: Lower limb proprioception deficits persist following knee replacement surgery despite improvements in knee extension strength, *Knee Surg Sports Traumatol Arthrosc* 20:1097–1103, 2012.
37. Hochberg MC, Altman RD, April KT, et al: American College of Rheumatology 2012 recommendations for the use of nonpharmacologic and pharmacologic therapies in osteoarthritis of the hand, hip, and knee, *Arthritis Care Res (Hoboken)* 64:465–474, 2012.
38. Zhang W, Moskowitz RW, Nuki G, et al: OARSI recommendations for the management of hip and knee osteoarthritis, Part II: OARSI evidence-based, expert consensus guidelines, *Osteoarthritis Cartilage* 16:137–162, 2008.
39. Fransen M, McConnell S: Exercise for osteoarthritis of the knee (Review), *Cochrane Database Syst Rev*, 2008. Oct 8: CD004376.
40. Fransen M, McConnell S, Hernandez-Molina G, et al: Exercise for osteoarthritis of the hip, *Cochrane Database of Syst Rev*, 2014. Apr 22: CD007912.
41. Williams SB, Brand CA, Hill KD, et al: Feasibility and outcomes of a home-based exercise pro-gram on

improving balance and gait stability in women with lower-limb osteoarthritis or rheumatoid arthritis: a pilot study, *Arch Phys Med Rehabil* 91:106–114, 2010.

42. Diracoglu D, Aydin R, Baskent A, et al: Effects of kinesthesia and balance exercises in knee osteoarthritis, *J Clin Rheumatol* 11:303–310, 2005.

43. Fitzgerald KG, Piva SR, Gil AB, et al: Agility and perturbation training techniques in exercise therapy for reducing pain and improving function in people with knee osteoarthritis: a randomized clinical trial, *Phys Ther* 91:452–469, 2011.

44. Smith TO, King JJ, Hing CB: The effectiveness of proprioceptive-based exercise for osteoarthritis of the knee: a systematic review and meta-analysis, *Rheumatol Int* 32:3339–3351, 2012.

45. Song R, Roberts BL, Lee E, et al: A randomized study of the effects of tai chi on muscle strength, bone mineral density, and fear of falling in women with osteoarthritis, *J Altern Complement Med* 16:227–233, 2010.

46. Wang C, Schmid CH, Hibberd P, et al: Tai chi is effective in treating knee osteoarthritis: a randomized controlled trial, *Arthritis Rheum (Hoboken)* 61:1545–1553, 2009.

47. Uthman OA, van der Windt DA, Jordan JL, et al: Exercise for lower limb osteoarthritis: systematic review incorporating trial sequential analysis and network meta-analysis, *BMJ* 347:f5555, 2013.

48. Tak E, Staats P, Van HA, et al: The effects of an exercise program for older adults with osteoarthritis of the hip, *J Rheumatol* 32:1106–1113, 2005.

49. Hinman RS, Heywood SE, Day AR: Aquatic physical therapy for hip and knee osteoarthritis: results of single-blind randomized controlled trial, *Phys Ther* 87:32–43, 2007.

50. Lund H, Weile U, Christensen R, et al: A randomized controlled trial of aquatic and land-based exercise in patients with knee osteoarthritis, *J Rehab Med* 40:137–144, 2008.

51. Silva LE, Valim V, Pessanha APC, et al: Hydrotherapy versus conventional land-based exercise for the management of patients with osteoarthritis of the knee: a randomized clinical trial, *Phys Ther* 88:12–21, 2008.

52. Fernandes L, Storheim K, Sandvik L, et al: Efficacy of patient education and supervised exercise vs patient education alone in patients with hip osteoarthritis: a single blind randomized clinical trial, *Osteoarthritis Cartilage* 18:1237–1243, 2010.

53. Juhakoski R, Tenhonen S, Malmivaara A, et al: A pragmatic randomized controlled study of the effectiveness and cost consequences of exercise therapy in hip osteoarthritis, *Clin Rehabil* 25:370–383, 2011.

54. Svege I, Nordsletten L, Fernandes L, et al: Exercise therapy may postpone total hip replacement surgery in patients with hip osteoarthritis: a long-term follow-up of a randomised trial, *Ann Rheum Dis* 74:164–169, 2013.

55. Deyle GD, Allison SC, Matekel RL, et al: Research report effectiveness for osteoarthritis of the knee: a randomized comparison of supervised clinical exercise and manual therapy procedures, *Phys Ther* 85:1301–1317, 2005.

56. Poulsen E, Hartvigsen J, Christensen HW, et al: Patient education with or without manual therapy compared to a control group in patients with osteoarthritis of the hip. A proof-of principle three-arm parallel group randomized clinical trial, *Osteoarthritis Cartilage* 21:1494–1503, 2013.

57. French HP, Cusack T, Brennan A, et al: Exercise and manual physiotherapy arthritis research trial (EMPART) for osteoarthritis of the hip: a multicenter randomized controlled trial, *Arch Phys Med Rehabil* 94:302–314, 2013.

58. Abbott JH, Robertson MC, Chapple C, et al: Manual therapy, exercise therapy, or both, in addition to usual care, for osteoarthritis of the hip or knee: a randomized controlled trial. 1: clinical effectiveness, *Osteoarthritis Cartilage* 21:525–534, 2013.

59. Bennell K, Egerton T, Martin J, et al: Effects of physical therapy on pain and function in patients with hip osteoarthritis, *JAMA* 311:1987–1997, 2014.

60. Messier SP, Loeser RF, Miller GD, et al: Exercise and dietary weight loss in overweight and obese older adults with knee osteoarthritis: the Arthritis, Diet, and Activity Promotion Trial, *Arthritis Rheum* 50:1501–1510, 2004.

61. Paans N, Akker-Scheek I, Diling RG, et al: Effect of exercise and weight loss in people who have hip osteoarthritis and are overweight or obese: a prospective cohort study, *Phys Ther* 93:137–146, 2013.

62. Wright A, Cook CE, Flynn TW, et al: Predictors of response to physical therapy intervention in patients with primary hip osteoarthritis, *Phys Ther* 91:510–524, 2011.

63. Cibulka MT, White DM, Woehrle J, et al: Hip pain and mobility deficits—hip osteoarthritis: clinical practice guidelines linked to the international classification of functioning, disability, and health from the orthopaedic section of the American Physical Therapy Association, *J Orthop Sports Phys Ther* 39:A1–A25, 2009.

64. Moss P, Sluka K, Wright A: The initial effects of knee joint mobilization on osteoarthritis hyperalgesia, *Manual Ther* 12:109–118, 2007.

65. Jansen MJ, Viechtbauer W, Lenssen AF, et al: Strength training alone, exercise therapy alone, and exercise therapy with passive manual mobilisation each reduce pain and disability in people with knee osteoarthritis: a systematic review, *J Physiother* 57:11–20, 2011.

66. Minor MA, Hewett JE, Webel RR, et al: Efficacy of physical conditioning exercise in patients with rheumatoid arthritis and osteoarthritis, *Arthritis Rheum* 32:1396–1405, 1989.

67. Kovar PA, Allegrante JP, MacKenzie CR, et al: Supervised fitness walking in patients with osteoarthritis of the knee: a randomized, controlled trial, *Ann Intern Med* 116:529–534, 1992.

68. Messier SP, Royer TD, Craven TE, et al: Long-term exercise and its effect on balance in older, osteoarthritic adults: results from the Fitness, Arthritis, and Seniors Trial (FAST), *J Am Geriatr Soc* 48:131–138, 2000.

69. Roddy E, Zhang W, Doherty M, et al: Evidence-based recommendations for the role of exercise in the management of osteoarthritis of the hip or knee—the MOVE consensus, *Rheumatology (Oxford)* 44:67–73, 2005.

70. Foley A, Halbert J, Hewitt T, et al: Does hydrotherapy improve strength and physical function in patients with osteoarthritis? A randomised controlled trial comparing a gym based and a hydrotherapy based strengthening programme, *Ann Rheum Dis* 62:1162–1167, 2003.

71. Messier SP, Royer TD, Craven TE, et al: Long-term exercise and its effect on balance in older, osteoarthritic adults: results from the Fitness, Arthritis, and Seniors Trial (FAST), *J Am Geriatr Soc* 48:131–138, 2000.

72. Bautch JC, Malone DG, Vailas AC: Effects of exercise on knee joints with osteoarthritis: a pilot study of biologic markers, *Arthritis Care Res* 10:48–55, 1997.

73. Penninx BW, Messier SP, Rejeski WJ, et al: Physical exercise and the prevention of disability in activities of daily living in older persons with osteoarthritis, *Arch Intern Med* 161:2309–2316, 2001.

74. Callaghan MJ, Oldham J, Hunt J: An evaluation of exercise regimes for patients with osteoarthritis of the knee: a single-blind randomized controlled trial, *Clin Rehabil* 9:213, 1995.

75. Borjesson M, Robertson E, Weidenhielm L, et al: Physiotherapy in knee osteoarthrosis: effect on pain and walking, *Physiother Res Int* 1:89–97, 1996.

76. Van Baar ME, Dekker J, Oostendorp RA, et al: The effectiveness of exercise therapy in patients with osteoarthritis of the hip or knee: a randomized clinical trial, *J Rheumatol* 25:2432–2439, 1998.

77. Gur H, Cakin N, Akova B, et al: Concentric versus combined concentric-eccentric isokinetic training: effects on functional capacity and symptoms in patients with osteoarthrosis of the knee, *Arch Phys Med Rehabil* 83:308–316, 2002.

78. Topp R, Woolley S, Hornyak J, et al: The effect of dynamic versus isometric resistance training on pain and functioning among adults with osteoarthritis of the knee, *Arch Phys Med Rehabil* 83:1187–1195, 2002.

79. Fisher NM, Pendergast DR, Gresham GE, et al: Muscle rehabilitation: its effect on muscular and functional performance of patients with knee osteoarthritis, *Arch Phys Med Rehabil* 72:367–374, 1991.

80. Dexter PA: Joint exercises in elderly persons with symptomatic osteoarthritis of the hip or knee: performance patterns, medical support patterns, and the relationship between exercising and medical care, *Arthritis Care Res* 5:36–41, 1992.

81. Juhl C, Christensen R, Roos EM, Zhang W, et al: Impact of exercise type and dose on pain and disability in knee osteoarthritis: a systematic review and meta-regression analysis of randomized controlled trials, *Arthritis Rheum* 66:622–636, 2014.

82. Green J, McKenna F, Redfern EJ, et al: Home exercises are as effective as outpatient hydrotherapy for osteoarthritis of the hip, *Br J Rheumatol* 32:812–815, 1993.

83. Constantinou M, Barrett R, Brown M, et al: Spatial-temporal gait characteristics in individuals with hip osteoarthritis: a systematic literature review and meta-analysis, *J Orthop Sports Phys Ther* 44,2014. 291-B7.

84. Wegener L, Kisner C, Nichols D: Static and dynamic balance responses in persons with bilateral knee osteoarthritis, *J Orthop Sports Phys Ther* 25:13–18, 1997.

85. Mangione KK, McCully K, Gloviak A, et al: The effects of high-intensity and low-intensity cycle ergometry in older adults with knee osteoarthritis, *J Gerontol A Biol Sci Med Sci* 54:M184–M190, 1999.

86. Crowe J, Henderson J: Pre-arthroplasty rehabilitation is effective in reducing hospital stay, *Can J Occup Ther* 70:88–96, 2003.

87. Wang C, Collet JP, Lau J: The effect of tai chi on health outcomes in patients with chronic conditions: a systematic review, *Arch Intern Med* 164:493–501, 2004.

88. Jones A, Silva PG, Silva AC, et al: Impact of cane use on pain, function, general health and energy expenditure during gait in patients with knee osteoarthritis: a randomised controlled trial, *Ann Rheum Dis* 71:172–179, 2012.

89. Farrokhi S, Voycheck CA, Tashman S, et al: A biomechanical perspective on physical therapy management of knee osteoarthritis, *J Orthop Sports Phys Ther* 43:600–619, 2013.

90. Matsuno H, Kadowaki KM, Tsuji H: Generation II knee bracing for severe medial compartment osteoarthritis of the knee, *Arch Phys Med Rehabil* 78:745–749, 1997.

91. Kirkley A, Webster-Bogaert S, Litchfield R, et al: The effect of bracing on varus gonarthrosis, *J Bone Joint Surg Am* 81:539–548, 1999.

92. Brouwer RW, van Raaij TM, Verhaar JN, et al: Brace treatment for osteoarthritis of the knee: a prospective randomized multi-centre trial, *Osteoarthritis Cartilage* 14:777–783, 2006.

93. Lindenfeld TN, Hewett TE, Andriacchi TP: Joint loading with valgus bracing in patients with varus gonarthrosis, *Clin Orthop Relat Res* 244:290–297, 1997.

94. Brouwer RW, Jakma TSC, Verhagen AP, et al: Braces and orthoses for treating osteoarthritis of the knee, *Cochrane Database Syst Rev.* 2005, Jan 25:CD004020.

95. Bennell KL, Bowles K, Payne C, et al: Lateral wedge insoles for medial knee osteoarthritis: 12 month randomised controlled trial, *BMJ* 342:d2912, 2011.

96. Van Raaij TM, Reijman M, Brouwer RW, et al: Medial knee osteoarthritis treated by insoles or braces: a randomized trial, *Clin Orthop Relat Res* 468:1926–1932, 2010.

97. Arazpour M, Zarezadeh F, Bani MA: The effects of unloader knee orthosis and lateral wedge insole in patients with mild and moderate knee osteoarthritis, *Iranian Rehabilitation Journal* 10:60–65, 2012.

98. Rodrigues PT, Ferreira AF, Pereira RMR, et al: Effectiveness of medial-wedge insole treatment for valgus knee osteoarthritis, *Arthritis Rheum* 59:603–608, 2008.

99. Warden SJ, Hinman RS, Watson MA, et al: Patellar taping and bracing for the treatment of chronic knee pain: a systematic review and meta-analysis, *Arthritis Rheum* 59:73–83, 2008.

100. Harris ED: Rheumatoid arthritis: pathophysiology and implications for therapy, *N Engl J Med* 322:1277–1289, 1990.

101. Gornisiewicz M, Moreland LW: Rheumatoid arthritis. In Robbins L, Burckhardt CS, Hannan MT, DeHoratius RJ, editors: *Clinical care in the rheumatic diseases*, 2 ed., Atlanta, 2001, Association of Rheumatology Health Professionals.

102. van der Heijde D: How to read radiographs according to the Sharp/van der Heijde method, *J Rheumatol* 27:261–263, 2000.

103. Panel Ottawa: Evidence-based clinical practice guidelines for therapeutic exercises in the management of rheumatoid arthritis in adults, *Phys Ther* 84:934–972, 2004.

104. Haugeberg G, Uhlig T, Falch JA, et al: Bone mineral density and frequency of osteoporosis in female patients with rheumatoid arthritis: results from 394 patients in the Oslo County rheumatoid arthritis register, *Arthritis Rheum* 43:522–530, 2000.

105. Haugeberg G, Orstavik RE, Kvien TK: Effects of rheumatoid arthritis on bone, *Curr Opin Rheumatol* 15:469–475, 2003.

106. Kim SY, Schneeweiss S, Liu J, et al: Risk of osteoporotic fracture in a large population-based cohort of patients with rheumatoid arthritis, *Arthritis Res Ther* 12:R154, 2010.

107. Haugeberg G, Orstavik RE, Uhlig T, et al: Bone loss in patients with rheumatoid arthritis: results from a population-based cohort of 366 patients followed up for two years, *Arthritis Rheum* 46:1720–1728, 2002.

108. Hochberg MC, Chang RW, Dwosh I, et al: The American College of Rheumatology 1991 revised criteria for the classification of global functional status in rheumatoid arthritis, *Arthritis Rheum* 35:498–502, 1992.

109. Klippel JH, Crofford LJ, Stone JH, et al: Appendix I: criteria for the diagnosis of juvenile arthritis. In Klippel JH, Crofford LJ, Stone JH, Weyand CM, editors: *Primer on the rheumatic diseases*, 12 ed., Atlanta, 2001, Arthritis Foundation.

110. Taylor J, Erlandson DM: Pediatric rheumatic diseases. In Robbins L, Burckhardt CS, Hannan MT, DeHoratius RJ, editors: *Clinical care in the rheumatic diseases*, 2 ed., Atlanta, 2001, Association of Rheumatology Health Professionals.

111. Hicks JE: Exercise in rheumatoid arthritis, *Phys Med Rehabil Clin North Am* 5:701, 1994.

112. Hayes KW: Heat and cold in the management of rheumatoid arthritis. In Chang RW, editor: *Rehabilitation of persons with rheumatoid arthritis*, Gaithersburg, MD, 1996, Aspen.

113. Panel Ottawa: Evidence-based clinical practice guidelines for electrotherapy and thermotherapy interventions in the management of rheumatoid arthritis in adults, *Phys Ther* 84:1016–1043, 2004.

114. Ekdahl C, Andersson SI, Moritz U, et al: Dynamic versus static training in patients with rheumatoid arthritis, *Scand J Rheumatol* 19:17–26, 1990.

115. Brighton SW, Lubbe JE, van der Merwe CA: The effect of a long-term exercise programme on the rheumatoid hand, *Br J Rheumatol* 32:392–395, 1993.

116. Ekblom B, Lovgren O, Alderin M, et al: Effect of short-term physical training on patients with rheumatoid arthritis: a six-month follow-up study, *Scand J Rheumatol* 4:87–91, 1975.

117. Lyngberg K, Danneskiold-Samsoe B, Halskov O: The effect of physical training on patients with rheumatoid arthritis: changes in disease activity, muscle strength and aerobic capacity—a clinically controlled minimized cross-over study, *Clin Exp Rheumatol* 6:253–260, 1988.

118. Perlman SG, Connell KJ, Clark A, et al: Dance-based aerobic exercise for rheumatoid arthritis, *Arthritis Care Res* 3:29–35, 1990.

119. Van den Ende CH, Hazes JM, le Cessie S, et al: Comparison of high and low intensity training in well controlled rheumatoid arthritis: results of a randomised clinical trial, *Ann Rheum Dis* 55:798–805, 1996.

120. Lee HY, Hale CA, Hemingway B, et al: Tai chi exercise and auricular acupressure for people with rheumatoid arthritis: an evaluation study, *J Clin Nurs* 21:2812–2822, 2012.

121. Wang C, Roubenoff R, Lau J, et al: Effect of tai chi in adults with rheumatoid arthritis, *Rheumatology (Oxford)* 44:685–687, 2005.

122. Hicks JE: Compliance: a major factor in the successful treatment of rheumatic disease, *Compr Ther* 11:31–37, 1985.

123. Gerber LH: Exercise and arthritis, *Bull Rheum Dis* 39:1–9, 1990.

124. Semble EL, Loeser RF, Wise CM: Therapeutic exercise for rheumatoid arthritis and osteoarthritis, *Semin Arthritis Rheum* 20:32–40, 1990.

125. Stenstrom CH, Minor MA: Evidence for the benefit of aerobic and strengthening exercise in rheumatoid arthritis, *Arthritis Rheum* 49:428–434, 2003.

126. De Jong Z, Munneke M, Zwinderman AH, et al: Is a long-term high-intensity exercise program effective and safe in patients with rheumatoid arthritis? Results of a randomized controlled trial, *Arthritis Rheum* 48:2415–2424, 2003.

127. De Jong Z, Vlieland TP: Safety of exercise in patients with rheumatoid arthritis, *Curr Opin Rheumatol* 17:177–182, 2005.

128. Bilberg A, Ahlmen M, Mannerkorpi K: Moderately intensive exercise in a temperate pool for patients with rheumatoid arthritis: a randomized controlled study, *Rheumatology* 44:502–508, 2005.

129. Neuberger GB, Press AN, Lindsley HB, et al: Effects of exercise on fatigue, aerobic fitness, and disease activity measures in persons with rheumatoid arthritis, *Res Nursing Health* 20:195–204, 1997.

130. Breedland I, van Scheppingen C, Leijsma M, et al: Effects of a group-based exercise and educational program on physical performance and disease self-management in rheumatoid arthritis: a randomized controlled study, *Phys Ther* 91:879–893, 2011.

131. Stavropoulos-Kalinoglou A, Metsios G, Veldhuijzen van Zanten J, et al: Veldhuijzen van Zanten J et al: Individualised aerobic and resistance exercise training improves cardiorespiratory fitness and reduces cardiovascular risk in patients with rheumatoid arthritis, *Ann Rheum Dis* 72:1819–1825, 2013.

132. Cima SR, Barone A, Porto JM, et al: Strengthening exercises to improve hand strength and functionality in rheumatoid arthritis with hand deformities: a randomized, controlled trial, *Rheumtol Int* 33:725–732, 2013.

133. Manning VL, Hurley MV, Scott DL, et al: Education, self-management, and upper extremity exercise training in people with rheumatoid arthritis: a randomized controlled trial, *Arthritis Care Res* 66:217–227, 2014.

134. McMeeken J, Stillman B, Story I, et al: The effects of knee extensor and flexor muscle training on the timed-up-and-go test in individuals with rheumatoid arthritis, *Physiother Res Int* 4:55–67, 1999.

135. Hakkinen A, Sokka T, Hannonen P: A home-based two-year strength training period in early rheumatoid arthritis led to good long-term compliance: a five-year follow-up, *Arthritis Rheum* 51:56–62, 2004.

136. Hurkmans E, van der Giesen FJ, Vliet Vlieland TP, et al: Dynamic exercise programs (aerobic capacity and/or muscle strength training) in patients with rheumatoid arthritis (Review), *Cochrane Database Syst Rev*, 2009. Oct 7:CD006853.

137. van den Ende CH, Breedveld FC, le Cessie S, et al: Effect of intensive exercise on patients with active rheumatoid arthritis: a randomised clinical trial, *Ann Rheum Dis* 59:615–621, 2000.

138. De Jong Z, Munneke M, Zwinderman AH, et al: Long term high intensity exercise and damage of small joints in rheumatoid arthritis, *Ann Rheum Dis* 63:1399–1405, 2004.

139. De Jong Z, Munneke M, Jansen LM, et al: Differences between participants and nonparticipants in an exercise trial for adults with rheumatoid arthritis, *Arthritis Rheum* 51:593–600, 2004.

140. Stenstrom CH: Therapeutic exercise in rheumatoid arthritis, *Arthritis Care Res* 7:190–197, 1994.

141. Smestad MV, Liang LH: Psychosocial management of rheumatic diseases. In Kelley WN, Harris TN, Ruddy S, Sledge CB, editors: *Textbook of rheumatology*, Philadelphia, 1997, WB Saunders.

142. Eurenius E, Stenstrom CH: Physical activity, physical fitness, and general health perception among individuals with rheumatoid arthritis, *Arthritis Rheum* 53:48–55, 2005.

143. Munneke M, de Jong Z, Zwinderman AH, et al: Adherence and satisfaction of rheumatoid arthritis patients with a long-term intensive dynamic exercise program (RAPIT program), *Arthritis Rheum* 49:665–672, 2003.

144. Iversen MD, Fossel AH, Daltroy LH: Rheumatologist-patient communication about exercise and physical therapy in the management of rheumatoid arthritis, *Arthritis Care Res* 12:180–192, 1999.

145. Iversen MD, Fossel AH, Ayers K, et al: Predictors of exercise behavior in patients with rheumatoid arthritis 6 months following a visit with their rheumatologist, *Phys Ther* 84:706–716, 2004.

146. Munneke M, de Jong Z, Zwinderman AH, et al: High intensity exercise or conventional exercise for patients with rheumatoid arthritis? Outcome expectations of patients, rheumatologists, and physiotherapists, *Ann Rheum Dis* 63:804–808, 2004.

147. Byers PH: Effect of exercise on morning stiffness and mobility in patients with rheumatoid arthritis, *Res Nurs Health* 8:275–281, 1985.

148. Semble EL: Rheumatoid arthritis: new approaches for its evaluation and management, *Arch Phys Med Rehabil* 76:190–201, 1995.

149. Janssen M, Phiferons JPWM, van den Velde EA: The prevention of hand deformities with resting splints in rheumatoid arthritis: a randomized single blind one year follow-up study, *Arthritis Rheum* 33:123, 1990.

150. Kjeken I, Moller G, Kvien TK: Use of commercially produced elastic wrist orthoses in chronic arthritis: a controlled study, *Arthritis Care Res* 8:108–113, 1995.

151. Stern EB, Ytterberg SR, Krug HE, et al: Immediate and short-term effects of three commercial wrist extensor orthoses on grip strength and function in patients with rheumatoid arthritis, *Arthritis Care Res* 9:42–50, 1996.

152. Egan M, Brosseau L, Farmer M, et al: Splints/orthoses in the treatment of rheumatoid arthritis, *Cochrane Database Syst Rev*, 2003. CD004018.

153. Hillstrom HJ, Whitney K, McGuire J, et al: Evaluation and management of the foot and ankle. In Robbins L, Burckhardt CS, Hannan MT, DeHoratius RJ, editors: *Clinical care in the rheumatic diseases*, 2 ed., Atlanta, 2001, Association of Rheumatology Professionals.

154. Janisse DJ: Prescription footwear for arthritis of the foot and ankle, *Clin Orthop Relat Res* 349:100–107, 1998.

155. Chalmers AC, Busby C, Goyert J, et al: Metatarsalgia and rheumatoid arthritis: a randomized, single blind, sequential trial comparing 2 types of foot orthoses and supportive shoes, *J Rheumatol* 27:1643–1647, 2000.

156. Conrad KJ, Budiman-Mak E, Roach KE, et al: Impacts of foot orthoses on pain and disability in rheumatoid arthritics, *J Clin Epidemiol* 49:1–7, 1996.

157. Luck J: Enhancing functional ability. In Robbins L, Burckhardt CS, Hannan MT, DeHoratius RJ, editors: *Clinical care in the rheumatic diseases*, 2 ed., Atlanta, 2001, American College of Rheumatology.

CHAPTER 31

Systemic Bone Diseases: Medical and Rehabilitation Intervention

PART **A** | Medical Intervention

ASHLEY G. STERRETT, ALEJANDRO RAMIREZ, HELEN E. BATEMAN*

INTRODUCTION

Systemic bone disease, also known as **metabolic bone disease**, refers to a heterogeneous group of disorders affecting the skeletal system. Disorders of the skeletal system may affect ambulation, protection of vital soft tissues, and calcium and other mineral homeostatic metabolic processes.

This chapter addresses three common systemic bone diseases: osteoporosis, primary hyperparathyroidism (PHPT), and Paget's disease of bone (PDB), which are all affected by changes in bone turnover and remodeling. Other, less prevalent bone diseases are described elsewhere.[1]

OSTEOPOROSIS

Introduction

Osteoporosis, the most common metabolic bone disease, is a systemic skeletal disorder characterized by low bone mass and microarchitectural deterioration of bone. The most important sequelae of osteoporosis is a **fragility fracture**, which is defined as a fracture that occurs when falling from equal to or less than standing height.[2] Low bone mass (also known as **osteopenia**) is the stage before osteoporosis, and its recognition is key to prevent progression to osteoporosis and fractures.

Epidemiology

Fifty-four million Americans have either osteoporosis or low bone mass. Studies suggest one in two women and one in four men over the age of 50 will have a fragility fracture (i.e., osteoporotic fracture). More than 2 million osteoporotic fractures occur in the United States each year, resulting in $19 billion in related costs. The most common sites for osteoporotic fractures are the spine (Figure 31-1), wrist, and hip.[2,3]

Pathogenesis and Etiology

To understand osteoporosis and systemic bone disease, a basic understanding of the bone turnover process is necessary. Disruption in bone turnover can lead to a reduction in bone strength and ultimately osteoporosis. The mature skeleton uses a regenerative process called **bone remodeling** to repair damage that occurs during daily activities. Remodeling preserves skeletal strength using intrinsic bone cells called **osteoclasts** to remove bone. **Osteoblasts**, the "bone builders," subsequently replace localized areas of removed skeleton.[4] The bone remodeling cycle is divided into four phases: activation, resorption, reversal, and formation.

Phases of the Bone Remodeling Cycle[4]

1. Activation: osteoclasts stimulated
2. Resorption: microtrench formed
3. Reversal: osteoblasts stimulated
4. Formation of new bone

Within activation, osteoclasts are stimulated to remove localized packets of bone. Both the mineralized and the organic components of the skeleton are removed. Over several days, osteoclasts excavate a "microtrench" on the surface of the skeleton. In reversal, osteoclastic bone resorption abates, the osteoclasts leave, and osteoblasts are stimulated to migrate onto the surface of the resorption cavity (i.e., in the microtrench), where the organic components (i.e., calcium and phosphorus) of the skeleton are laid down and subsequently mineralized, leading to bone formation.[4] In healthy individuals the amount of resorbed skeleton is replaced by normal bone. As people age, the balance between osteoblasts and osteoclasts is disrupted, which can induce

---

*The authors, editors and publisher acknowledge James W. Edmondson and Emily Veeneman for their contributions on this topic in the previous edition.

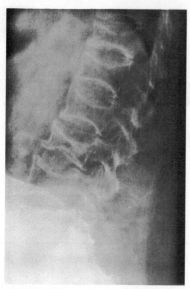

Figure 31-1 Lateral radiograph of the lumbar spine showing the biconcave appearance and compression of vertebral bodies seen in senile osteoporosis. (From Gartland JJ: *Fundamentals of orthopedics*, p 120, Philadelphia, 1979, WB Saunders.)

loss of bone mass and ultimately osteoporosis. Other factors can also influence the bone remodeling cycle, including parathyroid hormone (PTH) and serum vitamin D.

An understanding of the importance of vitamin D in the pathophysiology of osteoporosis requires a review of the feedback loop involving PTH, calcium, and phosphorus. Vitamin D is obtained from two main sources: diet and the conversion of 7-dehydrocholesterol to cholecalciferol through ultraviolet sunlight in the skin.

Although osteoporosis is considered a disease of the elderly, the foundation for good bone health starts early in life. Bone mass steadily increases from birth and reaches its peak early in the third decade of life.[5] Peak bone mass is affected by gender, race, and heredity, along with diet and activity level. Osteoporosis may be primary or secondary. **Primary osteoporosis** is the most common, due to both age (known as **senile or type II osteoporosis**) and declining hormonal levels (also known as **postmenopausal or type I osteoporosis**), leading to a rate of bone resorption that exceeds the rate of formation resulting in a net loss of bone. Bone density testing via dual-energy x-ray absorptiometry (DXA) is usually considered in postmenopausal women and men over age 70.[2]

Secondary osteoporosis can be seen with various other etiologies (Table 31-1). With regard to medications and conditions listed in Table 31-1, a baseline DXA at a younger age may be considered to assess for iatrogenic low bone mass or osteoporosis.

Additional risk factors for osteoporosis include a family history of osteoporosis, patients of Asian or Caucasian descent, and lifestyle factors, including excessive alcohol intake, smoking, and extreme weight loss. Marfan's disease, Ehler Danlos syndrome, and osteogenesis imperfecta are inherited connective tissue disorders that carry additional risks for osteoporosis.

Finally, a history of prior fragility fracture significantly increases the risk of future fractures as highlighted by important studies by Wasnich et al.[6] and Davis et al.[7] Furthermore, data from the Study of Osteoporotic Fractures also illustrated that women with a history of a premenopausal fragility fracture are 35% more likely to suffer a subsequent fracture once they are postmenopausal.[8] Lindsey et al.[9] showed that the risk of repeat fracture is greatest 1 year after the first fragility fracture. A subsequent study has supported this: one in four postmenopausal women with incident vertebral fractures has an osteoporotic fracture again within 2 years.[10]

Osteoporosis in Men

Although osteoporosis is less common in men than women, it is still underappreciated and underdiagnosed. Approximately 1.5 million U.S. men have osteoporosis and another 3.5 million are at risk (with low bone mass).[2] A 60-year-old man has a 25% chance of having an osteoporotic fracture. The prevalence of vertebral and hip fractures in men is one third that of women, and the prevalence of a Colles fracture is one sixth as common.[11] However, the morbidity and mortality associated with

TABLE 31-1

Secondary Causes of Osteoporosis[2]

Medications	Lifestyle	Medical Conditions
• Steroids • Antiandrogens and antiestrogens • Anticonvulsants • Heparin • HIV medications • Chemotherapy • Lithium • High-dose thyroid replacement • Pioglitazone • Proton pump inhibitors	• Female athlete triad (i.e., eating disorder, amenorrhea, osteoporosis) • Thin body habitus: women less than or equal to 57.6 kg (127 pounds) • Smoking and/or alcohol abuse (more than three drinks per day)	• Endocrine: hyperthyroidism, hyperparathyroidism, Cushing's disease, hypogonadism • Malignancy, such as multiple myeloma • Surgical menopause • Vitamin D deficiency • Malabsorption syndromes (e.g., celiac disease, bariatric surgery, inflammatory bowel disease) • Decreased weight bearing (e.g., severe complex regional pain syndrome, stroke, spinal cord injury, multiple sclerosis)

osteoporotic fractures in men are higher, and men are less likely to be screened and treated appropriately for osteoporosis.[12,13] Therefore education about screening of men is important and more understanding about the pathogenesis of osteoporosis in men is needed.

Clinical Features and Assessment

Osteoporosis is typically a silent, slowly progressive disease but may present with kyphosis, which is excessive curvature of thoracic spine also known as "Dowager's hump" (Figure 31-2) due to spontaneous vertebral compression fracture in postmenopausal women. Vertebral compression fractures may be asymptomatic or significantly painful. Other fragility fractures include Colles fracture of the radius and femoral neck fractures. The presence of these fractures, in the absence of trauma or other underlying causes, indicates clinical osteoporosis.

According to the Centers for Disease Control and Prevention (CDC), approximately 300,000 patients are admitted for hip fractures in the United States each year. Age and bone density are independent risk factors for hip fractures (Figure 31-3). Hip fractures carry a significant increase in morbidity and mortality—in-hospital mortality rates range from approximately 1% to 10%, varying upon the location of the fracture and patient characteristics, and 1-year post hip-fracture mortality rates range from 12% to 37%.[14,15] Nearly half of patients are unable to live independently after a hip fracture.[16] Therefore prevention of hip fractures can significantly reduce morbidity and mortality.

The gold standard for diagnosis of osteoporosis before fragility fracture is by central bone densitometry (DXA) testing. In 2004, a World Health Organization (WHO)

expert panel refined the original diagnostic criterion for normal and low bone mass and osteoporosis based on bone mineral density (BMD) (Figure 31-4).[17] The WHO international reference standard for the diagnosis of osteoporosis by DXA is a T-score of −2.5 or less at one of the following regions: the total lumbar spine (L1-L4), femoral neck, or total hip.[2] The reference standard from which the T-score is calculated is the Caucasian female (National Health and Nutrition Examination Survey [NHANES] III database).[2] When one of the standard sites (i.e., total spine, total hip, or femoral neck) is unable to be used, the distal 33% radius (also called one-third radius) may be used applying the International Society for Clinical Densitometry (ISCD) guidelines.

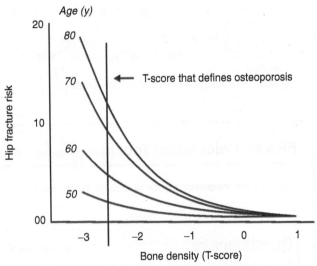

Figure 31-3 Age and bone density are independent predictors of the risk of hip fracture. (Data from De Laet C, Kanis JA, Oden A et al: Body mass index as a predictor of fracture risk: a meta-analysis, *Osteoporos Int* 16:1330-1338, 2005.)

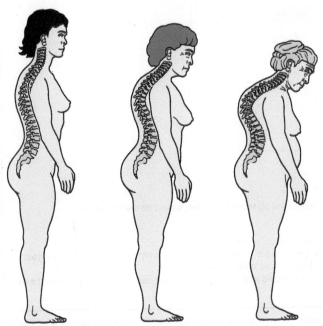

Figure 31-2 Progressive thoracic kyphosis with advancing age and vertebral compression fracture. "Dowager's hump" is illustrated on the right.

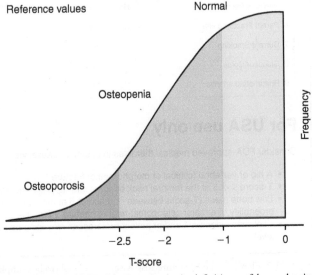

Figure 31-4 World Health Organization's definitions of bone density classification.

The application of T-score is used to diagnose osteoporosis in postmenopausal women or men over the age of 50. Bone density cannot diagnose osteoporosis in premenopausal women or men under the age of 50. In those patients a Z-score is used to compare the patient's BMD to age-, sex-, and ethnicity-matched individuals, and the BMD is reported as normal or lower than expected for the patient's age. The Z-score is also used in children.[2] The indications for DXA screening are listed in the following textbox.

Many of the current preventive goals have been directed toward individuals with significantly low bone density. However, data from the National Osteoporosis Risk Assessment (NORA) study and other studies indicate that 50% of osteoporotic fractures occur in those whose BMD has not reached the osteoporotic range.[3] It is currently believed that BMD and age contribute only approximately half of the risk to osteoporotic fractures. Given this disparity, an additional tool, FRAX, was developed to further identify patients at risk.

Considerations for DXA Screening[2]

- All women aged 65 and older or women who are at risk for low bone mass, including postmenopausal women
- All men age 70 and older or men aged 50 and older who are at risk for low bone mass
- Previous fragility fracture
- Starting a medication, such as steroids, that increases risk for low bone mass
- Patients with a disease that could affect bone density

FRAX®: World Health Organization Fracture Risk Assessment Tool

Developed by the WHO as a tool for underdeveloped countries without access to DXA (the calculation can be performed without a prior bone density), the FRAX® assesses osteoporotic fracture risk over the next 10 years. It is a web-based calculator (www.shef.ac.uk/FRAX) in which a patient's unique characteristics such as race, gender, previous fragility fracture, as well as femoral neck BMD (if available) are entered into a program (Figure 31-5).

FRAX® Calculation Tool (to be completed online at: www.shef.ac.uk/FRAX/tool.jsp)

Please answer the questions below to calculate the ten year probability of fracture with BMD.

Country: US (Caucasian)   Name/ID: _____

Questionnaire:

1. Age (between 40 and 90 years) or Date of Birth
   Age: _____   Date of Birth: Y: ____ M: ____ D: ____

2. Sex   ○ Male ○ Female

3. Weight (kg) _____

4. Height (cm) _____

5. Previous Fracture   ○ No ○ Yes

6. Parent Fractured Hip   ○ No ○ Yes

7. Current Smoking   ○ No ○ Yes

8. Glucocorticoids   ○ No ○ Yes

9. Rheumatoid arthritis   ○ No ○ Yes

10. Secondary osteoporosis   ○ No ○ Yes

11. Alcohol 3 or more units/day   ○ No ○ Yes

12. Femoral neck BMD (g/cm²)

Select BMD ▼

[Clear] [Calculate]

For USA use only

Consider FDA-approved medical therapies in postmenopausal women and men aged 50 years and older, based on the following:

- A hip or vertebral (clinical or morphometric) fracture
- T-score ≤ -2.5 at the femoral neck or spine after appropriate evaluation to exclude secondary causes
- Low bone mass (T-score between -1.0 and -2.5 at the femoral neck or spine) and a 10-year probability of a hip fracture ≥ 3% or a 10-year probability of a major osteoporosi-related fracture ≥ 20% based on the US-adapted WHO algorithm
- Clinicians judgement and/or patient preferences may indicate treatment for people with 10-year fracture probabilities above or below these levels

Figure 31-5 FRAX®: WHO Fracture Risk Assessment Tool (to be completed online at: www.shef.ac.uk/FRAX/tool.jsp). WHO Collaborating Centre for Metabolic Bone Diseases, University of Sheffield, UK.

(Continued)

Risk factors

For the clinical risk factors a yes or no response is asked for. If the field is left blank, then a "no" response is assumed. See also notes on risk factors.

The risk factors used are the following:

Age	The model accepts ages between 40 and 90 years. If ages below or above are entered, the programme will compute probabilities at 40 and 90 year, respectively.
Sex	Male or female. Enter as appropriate.
Weight	This should be entered in kg.
Height	This should be entered in cm.
Previous fracture	A previous fracture denotes more accurately a previous fracture in adult life occurring spontaneously, or a fracture arising from trauma which, in a healthy individual, would not have resulted in a fracture. Enter yes or no (see also notes on risk factors).
Parent fractured hip	This enquires for a history of hip fracture in the patient's mother or father. Enter yes or no.
Current smoking	Enter yes or no depending on whether the patient currently smokes tobacco (see also notes on risk factors).
Glucocorticoids	Enter yes if the patient is currently exposed to oral glucocorticoids or has been exposed to oral glucocorticoids for more than 3 months at a dose of prednisolone of 5mg daily or more (or equivalent doses of other glucocorticoids) (see also notes on risk factors).
Rheumatoid arthritis	Enter yes where the patient has a confirmed diagnosis of rheumatoid arthritis. Otherwise enter no (see also notes on risk factors).
Secondary osteoporosis	Enter yes if the patient has a disorder strongly associated with osteoporosis. These include type I (insulin dependent) diabetes, osteogenesis imperfecta in adults, untreated long-standing hyperthyroidism, hypogonadism or premature menopause (<45 years), chronic malnutrition, or malabsorption and chronic liver disease
Alcohol 3 or more units/day	Enter yes if the patient takes 3 or more units of alcohol daily. A unit of alcohol varies slightly in different countries from 8-10g of alcohol. This is equivalent to a standard glass of beer (285ml), a single measure of spirits (30ml), a medium-sized glass of wine (120ml), or 1 measure of an aperitif (60ml) (see also notes on risk factors).
Bone mineral density (BMD)	(BMD) Please select the make of DXA scanning equipment used and then enter the actual femoral neck BMD (in g/cm2). Alternatively, enter the T-score based on the NHANES III female reference data. In patients without a BMD test, the field should be left blank (see also notes on risk factors) (provided by Oregon Osteoporosis Center).

Notes on risk factors

Previous fracture

A special situation pertains to a prior history of vertebral fracture. A fracture detected as a radiographic observation alone (a morphometric vertebral fracture) counts as a previous fracture. A prior clinical vertebral fracture or a hip fracture is an especially strong risk factor. The probability of fracture computed may therefore be underestimated. Fracture probability is also underestimated with multiple fractures.

Smoking, alcohol, glucocorticoids

These risk factors appear to have a dose-dependent effect, i.e. the higher the exposure, the greater the risk. This is not taken into account and the computations assume average exposure. Clinical judgment should be used for low or high exposures.

Rheumatoid arthritis (RA)

RA is a risk factor for fracture. However, osteoarthritis is, if anything, protective. For this reason reliance should not be placed on a patient's report of 'arthritis' unless there is clinical or laboratory evidence to support the diagnosis.

Bone mineral density (BMD)

The site and reference technology is DXA at the femoral neck. T-scores are based on the NHANES reference values for women aged 20-29 years. The same absolute values are used in men.

Figure 31-5, Cont'd

The tool then calculates the patient's risk of fracture for both major osteoporotic fracture and hip fracture. Currently the National Osteoporosis Foundation (NOF) recommends that any patient with a major osteoporotic fracture risk of 20% or greater in the next 10 years or a risk of hip fracture of 3% or greater in the next 10 years (based on the FRAX® tool calculation) be considered for treatment with osteoporosis medication (based on clinical judgment).[18]

When evaluating a patient with osteoporosis or low bone mass, it is important to consider secondary causes (see Table 31-1) through a careful history and physical examination. Initial basic laboratory evaluation may include serum testing of 25-hydroxyvitamin D, thyroid-stimulating hormone (TSH), PTH, renal function, phosphorus, magnesium, serum protein electrophoresis, and in males, testosterone levels. If a malabsorption syndrome is suspected, a celiac disease screen is recommended. Additional testing should be guided by a patient's clinical presentation.

Prevention and Management of Low Bone Mass and Osteoporosis

Diet

Adequate daily calcium and vitamin D, either by diet or by supplemental intake, are essential to good bone health. For those living in well-developed countries, foods such as fortified milk, bread, and cereal, as well as fatty fish, provide much of the dietary source of vitamin D. Table 31-2 lists the age-specific recommendations for vitamin D daily intake.

Elderly patients have the highest incidence of vitamin D deficiency for several reasons: poor diet, malabsorption, and reduced sunlight exposure from increased time indoors. For all ages, risk factors for vitamin D deficiency include: bariatric surgery and post-gastrectomy, pancreatic insufficiency, and small bowel disease, including celiac disease or inflammatory bowel disease. Although deficiency of vitamin D has traditionally been considered in locations further from the equator, it has also been reported in southern states, such as Florida.[19-21]

Renal failure, nephrotic syndrome, and obesity cause vitamin D deficiency. In addition, as people age, liver and kidney functions tend to decline, which can lead to problems with hydroxylation of vitamin D. Medications, such as anticonvulsants that increase P-450 enzymatic activity, can also result in the inactivation of vitamin D and reduce hepatic conversion of 25-hydroxyvitamin D.

Severe, chronic vitamin D deficiency ultimately can result in myopathy, osteomalacia, weakness including loss of muscle mass (i.e., sarcopenia), and osteoporosis.[22] There is some suggestion of a link between low vitamin D and an increased fall risk.[23,24] Although studies have not supported the reduction in fractures, vitamin D supplementation in nursing home populations did reduce the risk of falls, but the mechanism is unclear.[24] In addition, a study by the NHANES III found that postmenopausal women with low levels of 25-hydroxyvitamin D stores have lower DXA scores.[21]

Exercise

Moderate exercise of 30 minutes 3 times per week has been shown to reduce the incidence of osteoporotic fractures in older adults by meta-analysis of 10 trials.[25] The effects were statistically significant for hip but not vertebral fractures. Exercise has also been shown to improve BMD by another systematic review of 43 prospective trials.[26] Non–weight-bearing exercise, such as resistance strength training, was most effective for improving femoral neck BMD, whereas a mixed exercise program was more effective for improving lumbar spine BMD. There is no evidence that high-intensity exercise, such as running, is superior to low-intensity exercise, such as walking.[27]

Lifestyle

Patients should be counseled to stop smoking and reduce alcohol intake. A meta-analysis in 2005 linked an increased risk of hip fractures with smoking (Figure 31-6).[28] Although there is more evidence and known association of alcoholism and bone loss in men, alcohol abuse has been shown to increase the rate of hip fractures and osteoporosis and lead to more falls.[29]

TABLE **31-2**

Recommended Dietary Allowances (RDAs) for Vitamin D

Age	Male	Female	Pregnancy	Lactation
0-12 mo*	400 IU (10 mcg)	400 IU (10 mcg)	—	—
1-13 yr	600 IU (15 mcg)	600 IU (15 mcg)	—	—
14-18 yr	600 IU (15 mcg)	600 IU (15 mcg)	600 IU (15 mcg)	600 IU (15 mcg)
19-50 yr	600 IU (15 mcg)	600 IU (15 mcg)	600 IU (15 mcg)	600 IU (15 mcg)
51-70 yr	600 IU (15 mcg)	600 IU (15 mcg)	—	—
>70 yr	800 IU (20 mcg)	800 IU (20 mcg)	—	—

IU, International units; *mcg*, micrograms.

*Adequate intake (AI).

From Institute of Medicine, Food and Nutrition Board: *Dietary reference intakes for calcium and vitamin D*, Washington, DC, 2010, National Academy Press.

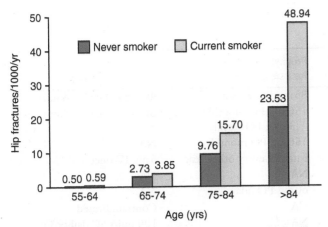

Figure 31-6 Effect of smoking on hip fractures in 11,861 subjects. (Data from Law MR, Hackshaw AK: A meta-analysis of cigarette smoking, bone mineral density and risk of hip fracture: recognition of a major effect, *Br Med J* 315:841-846, 1997.)

Osteoporosis Pharmacotherapy

The NOF recommends treatment for patients based on one of the following criteria: (1) fragility (osteoporotic) fracture, (2) T-score of −2.5 or less at the hip or spine, or (3) high 10-year risk of fracture based on FRAX® calculation (see the FRAX® section). Response to therapies can be monitored by scanning with bone densitometry (frequency of scanning is determined by individual patient risk).

Therapy is mediated via two mechanisms: (1) osteoclast inhibition or (2) osteoblast activation. The following textboxes summarize these mechanisms along with first- and second-line therapy.

Calcium and Vitamin D. Calcium and vitamin D are essential for the bone matrix. In order to enhance intestinal calcium intake and skeletal mineralization, optimum daily elemental calcium intake for adult men and women is thought to be approximately 1000 to 1200mg, plus 800 International Units of vitamin D (see Table 31-2 for age-specific recommendations). The metabolite 25-hydroxyvitamin D is used as a marker of vitamin D adequacy. The optimum serum range is 30 to 50ng/mL, vitamin D insufficiency is 20 to 30ng/mL, and vitamin D deficiency is less than 20ng/mL. Vitamin supplements are available as a combination tablet with both calcium

---

Bone Resorption Inhibitors

- Bisphosphonates: first line of defense
- Denusumab: second line of defense
- SERMs: second line of defense
- Calcitonin: second line of defense

Bone Formation Stimulators

- Teriparatide: second line of defense
- Strontium: not available in the United States

---

and vitamin D for patient convenience. For patients with significant vitamin D deficiency (e.g., levels under 20ng/mL), higher supplementation of vitamin D, on the order of 50,000 International Units per week for 8 to 12 weeks, may be needed to replenish the vitamin D stores.

Bisphosphonates: Antiresorptives.

Formulations and Mechanism of Action. Bisphosphonates have emerged as the first-line therapy for both the prevention and treatment of osteoporosis for several reasons. First and foremost, the clinical literature demonstrates the efficacy of bisphosphonates in the prevention of vertebral and nonvertebral fractures. Their efficacy has also been shown in postmenopausal women, males with osteoporosis, and patients of both genders with glucocorticoid-induced osteoporosis in preventing further bone loss and fracture.

Before the results of the Women's Health Initiative (WHI), hormone replacement therapy (HRT) was often used for the prevention and treatment of osteoporosis in postmenopausal women. However, the WHI raised concerns about the increased risk of thromboembolic and cardiovascular disease and breast cancer with HRT.[30] Consequently, HRT is not used as a treatment for osteoporosis but may be used for prevention of the problem in certain patient populations.

Several different bisphosphonates are available in the United States. Oral preparations include alendronate and risedronate, zolendronate is given intravenously, and ibandronate is available in both oral and intravenous (IV) forms. All are used routinely in the prevention and treatment of osteoporosis; however, ibandronate does not have data supporting reduction in the rate of hip fractures. All bisphosphonates inhibit osteoclastic bone reabsorption, and this antiresorptive action is especially pronounced at sites of increased active absorption. Therefore, bisphosphonates have a potent ability to help counterbalance the increase in the resorption:formation ratio characteristically seen in osteoporotic bone. Pamidronate, etidronate, and tiludronate are no longer used for the prevention or treatment of osteoporosis given the newer, more effective nitrogen-containing bisphosphonates now available. These older bisphosphonates can still be used in the treatment of Paget's disease (see later in chapter).

The American College of Rheumatology (ACR) and the American College of Endocrinology also recommend consideration of bisphosphonate treatment for patients on prolonged oral steroids, which can accelerate bone loss; thus these patients are at risk for osteoporosis. If a postmenopausal woman or man over age 50 who is considered at risk for osteoporotic fractures (FRAX calculation recommended) is expected to be on a steroid dosage greater than 7.5mg per day for more than 3 months, the ACR recommends consideration for treatment with a bisphosphonate as well for at least the duration of corticosteroid therapy.[31]

Dosages and Administration. The bisphosphonate agents most commonly used for osteoporosis and their doses are listed in Table 31-3. The absorption of

TABLE **31-3**

Therapies for Osteoporosis and Paget's Disease of the Bone

Drug	Treatment Dosage for Osteoporosis	Prophylaxis Dosage for Osteoporosis	Paget's Treatment
Alendronate	70 mg PO weekly; 10 mg PO daily	35 mg PO weekly	40 mg PO daily × 6 mo
Risedronate	150 mg PO monthly; 35 mg PO weekly; 5 mg PO daily	150 mg PO monthly; 35 mg PO weekly	30 mg PO daily × 2 mo
Ibandronate	150 mg PO monthly; 3 mg IV every 3 mo	150 mg PO monthly	NA
Zolendronate	5 mg IV yearly	5 mg IV every other year	5 mg IV once
Denosumab	60 mg SC every 6 mo	NA	NA
Raloxifine	60 mg PO qday	60 mg PO qday	NA
Teriparatide	20 mcg SC daily	NA	Contraindicated
Calcitonin	200 units intranasal or IM daily; or 100 units SC daily × 6 mo	NA	100 units SC daily × 3 mo
Etidronate	Not used	NA	5 mg/kg PO × 6 mo
Pamidronate	Not used	NA	30 mg IV given over 3 days q 3 mo
Tiludronate	Not used	NA	400 mg PO daily × 3 mo
Clodronate	Not approved for use in the United States	—	PO/IV
Neridronate	Not approved for use in the United States	—	IV/IM
Strontium	Not approved for use in the United States	—	NA

PO, By mouth; *IV*, intravenous; *SC*, subcutaneous; *qday*, 4 times per day; *IM*, intramuscular; *NA*, not applicable.

Data from Crandall C, Newberry S, Diamant A et al: Comparative effectiveness of pharmacologic treatments to prevent fractures: an updated systematic review, *Ann Intern Med* 161:711-723, 2014.

oral bisphosphonates is 1% to 5% of the total dose.[32] Approximately 30% of the medicine is expected to be taken up by the bone, and the remainder of the drug is excreted by the renal system.[32] The antiresorptive effects of bisphosphonates continue long after a patient has finished taking them—in terms of oral bisphosphonates, BMD can be stable for over 1 year; with zolendronate the effects of one dose can be seen for more than 5 years.[33]

Side Effects and Precautions. The main concerns with bisphosphonate therapy are the gastrointestinal (GI) side effects, such as pill-induced esophagitis, esophageal ulcers, gastroesophageal reflux disease (GERD) symptoms, and esophageal stricture. GI side effects are more common in patients who do not properly follow precautions for taking the medication.

Because of the high renal clearance of bisphosphonates, caution should be used in patients with renal insufficiency (testing creatinine level is recommended before each IV bisphosphonate dose).

The risks of several unusual side effects from bisphosphonates must be discussed with patients. For example, osteonecrosis of the jaw (ONJ) has been reported in approximately 1 per 10,000 to 100,000 patient-years.[34] Some risk factors for ONJ are de novo malignancy without bisphosphonate, the use of IV bisphosphonate (particularly in high dosages used for cancer), and radiation therapy as well as dental extractions, dental implants, poorly fitting dentures, use of glucocorticoids, smoking, and preexisting dental disease.[34] There are no data to suggest

that discontinuing bisphosphonates before dental procedures lowers ONJ risk. The task force for the American Society for Bone and Mineral Research recognized that the risk of ONJ is increased with length of therapy and for patients on IV bisphosphonate. Another potential but rare concern is the occurrence of an atypical femur fracture (AFF), which is seen after prolonged duration of treatment with a bisphosphonate (e.g., approximately 10 years of therapy). These fractures occur mid-femur (not typical of an osteoporotic fracture) and can be heralded by thigh pain and cortical thickening (seen on plain x-ray films). A calculated risk based on patients from Kaiser Southern California revealed an incidence of approximately 1.8 per 100,000 patients when on bisphosphonates for 1 to 2 years. That incidence rose to 113 per 100,000 when the patients were on bisphosphonate for 8 to 10 years. The conclusion was that the overall risk of AFF was still significantly lower than that of an osteoporotic fracture but did rise with prolonged use of bisphosphonates.[35] Therefore the current recommendation is to consider not prescribing the drug for a prolonged period of time in patients with stable BMD after 5 to 7 years of bisphosphonate therapy for osteoporosis.[36]

Denosumab (Prolia): Antiresorptive. Denosumab (Prolia) is the first biologic for osteoporosis. It is a fully human monoclonal antibody that binds the cytokine RANKL (receptor activator of NF-κB ligand), an essential factor initiating bone turnover. RANKL inhibition blocks osteoclast maturation, function, and survival, thus reducing bone resorption. Denosumab reduces both hip and vertebral fractures in women[37] but has also been shown to improve bone density in men.[38] Denusumab is used as a second-line agent for the treatment of osteoporosis in patients who fail or are intolerant to bisphosphonates.

Cellulitis has been reported in early studies and therefore it is recommended that denosumab be avoided in immunosuppressed patients or patients on immunosuppressive or biological therapy.[38] Other side effects include back pain and general musculoskeletal pain. There have also been rare cases of ONJ, and atypical fractures have been reported in follow-up studies; therefore it carries similar recommendations to bisphosphonates for routine dental care and consideration of a drug interruption.[39] (For dosage and administration see Table 31-3.)

Teriparatide: Increase Bone Formation. Formulations and Mechanism of Action.

Teriparatide is a recombinant injectable human PTH 1-34 and is the only therapy that stimulates osteoblast function to promote bone formation. It also increases both renal tubular reabsorption and GI absorption of calcium, which improves BMD and prevents fractures. The effects of teriparatide on bone remodeling are transient, peaking at 9 to 12 months, and then begin to decline. Thus treatment duration is limited to 2 years.[40]

Indications. Teriparatide has been shown to be effective in reducing both vertebral and nonvertebral fractures. It is indicated for both men and women at high risk for fractures in whom other therapies have failed. It may also be given to patients who cannot tolerate other osteoporosis therapies (such as bisphosphonates). Trials showed a decreased benefit of combining a bisphosphonate with teriparatide because the effect on BMD was blunted.[41] (For dosage and administration see Table 31-3.)

Side Effects and Precautions. Orthostasis has been described with the initial dose; therefore the first dose usually is given under supervision. Headache is a possible side effect, and nausea and dyspepsia also have been reported (approximately 9% and 5% of patients, respectively). Musculoskeletal side effects include leg cramps and arthralgias. Transient hypercalcemia has been described and occurs most often 4 to 6 hours after administration of the dose.[40]

A theoretical risk of osteosarcoma exists with the use of teriparatide. Studies with rats found an association with osteosarcoma when the rats were exposed to high doses of teriparatide for most of their lifetime. Though no case reports of osteosarcoma in humans undergoing treatment with teriparatide have been described, it should not be used in patients with risk factors for bone cancer or elevated serum alkaline phosphatase due to this potential concern. In addition, because osteosarcoma appears most often in children and young adults, careful consideration and caution should be exercised in the use of teriparatide in young adults. It is not approved for use in pediatric patients.[40] This drug is also not recommended for use in patients with a history of hypercalcemia, hyperparathyroidism, PDB, prior bone radiation, or other skeletal cancer metastases.[40]

Selective Estrogen Receptor Modulators: Antiresorptive.

Raloxifene belongs to the class of antiresorptive agents used for prevention and treatment of osteoporosis as a selective estrogen receptor modulator (SERM). It is unique in that it acts as both an agonist and an antagonist at the site of estrogen receptors, enabling different uses for different SERMs. For example, in bone, SERMs mimic the action of estrogen and prevent bone loss. Studies have shown reloxifene to be effective at reducing the risk of repeat vertebral fractures in women, but they did not reduce the risk of nonvertebral fractures (e.g., hip).[42] Notably trials with other SERMs, bazedoxifene and lasofoxifene, have showed significant promise as a treatment for osteoporosis.[43,44]

Indications. Raloxifene can be taken with or without food at any time of day. Approximately 60% of the drug is absorbed. If used in the United States, bazedoxifene is given with a conjugated estrogen (20 mg/0.45 mg).[44]

Side Effects and Precautions. One of the main concerns with the use of SERMs is the increased risk of superficial thrombophlebitis and deep vein thrombosis (DVT). Studies have found the risk of DVT to be comparable to that seen with the use of estrogen in HRT in postmenopausal women. Therefore, the use of SERMs is not recommended in patients with other risk factors for DVT or pulmonary embolism or a history of either of these conditions. Furthermore, women with a history of uterine or cervical cancer are not good candidates for SERMs given the variable effects of each medication on the endometrial and cervical cells.

The potential cardiovascular effects of SERMs have not been well defined. Data from the WHI study showed an increased risk of cardiovascular events in postmenopausal women with known coronary artery disease (CAD) who were in the hormone replacement group; this has led many clinicians to avoid the use of SERMs in general.

Some women experience significant hot flashes with SERM therapy, which are severe enough to prevent further use of these as antiosteoporotic agents. Other infrequent side effects may include sinusitis and flulike symptoms. Arthralgias have been reported in approximately 10% of patients taking raloxifene.

Calcitonin: Antiresorptive. Formulations and Mechanism of Action.

Calcitonin is a weak antiresorptive agent. Its mechanism of action involves binding to osteoclasts to inhibit bone resorption. Both human and salmon calcitonin are prescribed clinically, but salmon calcitonin is favored because it has a longer half-life and higher affinity for the calcitonin receptor. Nasal calcitonin is the preferred mode of administration, but a randomized controlled study of oral salmon calcitonin use in postmenopausal women showed an increase in lumbar spine BMD with few GI side effects.[45]

Indications. Studies have found calcitonin to be effective for treatment of osteoporotic fractures of the spine but not for nonvertebral fractures, such as hip fractures, which is why the medication is considered second line.[46,47]

One feature that seems to be unique to calcitonin is its ability to reduce pain in patients with an acute vertebral compression fracture.[48] The mechanism of action involved in this analgesic property is not clearly known. Therefore in a patient with significant pain from an osteoporotic vertebral fracture, one choice of therapy is initial treatment with calcitonin and then changing to another, more potent antiresorptive agent once the pain has subsided.

Side Effects and Precautions. The most commonly reported side effects of calcitonin include flushing, nausea and vomiting, anorexia, and diarrhea. These side effects can be minimalized if taken at bedtime. There has been a concern for an association of calcitonin with an increased risk of cancer, although a direct association has not been found. A Food and Drug Administration (FDA) advisory committee concluded that the risks of calcitonin use do not outweigh the potential benefits, but if it is used, the duration should be limited to less than 6 months.[49]

Strontium Ranelate. Strontium is a bone-stimulating agent (anabolic) composed of an organic moiety, ranelic acid, and two atoms of stable strontium. Many patients prefer it over teriparatide because it is taken orally. Data from phase III human studies support the effectiveness of strontium ranelate's mechanism of action in both stimulating bone formation and inhibiting bone resorption. Studies also indicate a significant increase in BMD T-scores at both the lumbar spine and the femoral neck. These studies show a reduction in both vertebral and nonvertebral fracture rates after 1 and 2 years of therapy.[49–51]

Side Effects and Precautions. Although it has been shown to be effective in the treatment of osteoporosis in patients with known osteoporosis, strontium ranelate is not currently available in the United States. The main side effect of strontium ranelate is diarrhea, which typically remits after 3 months. Strontium ranelate offers promise as a future bone-stimulating agent in the therapy of osteoporosis.[50]

Emerging Therapies. There are several new therapies undergoing trial at this time. Odanacatib is an antiresorptive medication that inhibits cathepsin-K. Three anabolic agents (bone-building agents) are also in trial: antisclerostin monoclonal antibodies (i.e., romosozumab and blosozumab) and a PTH-related peptide (i.e., abaloparatide). Ideally these new therapies will provide better efficacy with reduced potential side effects.

Surgical Management of Vertebral Fractures

Kyphoplasty and Vertebroplasty

Kyphoplasty and vertebroplasty are minimally invasive techniques that can be performed in an outpatient setting to treat vertebral compression fractures related to osteoporosis. In kyphoplasty a patient lies prone under local or general anesthesia. The surgeon then inserts a small tube into the collapsed vertebra. A balloon is passed through the tube and is inflated to restore height to the vertebra. Cement is then injected into the vertebral body (Figure 31-7) to maintain the height of the vertebra. Vertebroplasty is a similar procedure in which the cement is injected, but a balloon is not initially used to expand the vertebra. Although there have been past randomized studies that found no difference between surgical intervention and placebo,[52] a more recent study found both procedures to be superior to medical management and reported kyphoplasty superior to vertebroplasty in terms of balance improvement and risk of cement leaking.[53]

A randomized controlled trial, which included 138 patients in the kyphoplasty group and 128 in a control group (i.e., nonsurgical care), found that kyphoplasty was a safe and effective procedure for patients with vertebral fracture.[54] The study was conducted at 21 sites in eight different countries. Patients were eligible if they had one to three vertebral fractures from T5 to L5. At 12 months, 33% of patients in the kyphoplasty group and 25% of the control group had new or worsening radiographic vertebral fractures (7.7% difference, 95% confidence interval [CI] −4.5 to 20.0; $p = 0.220$). However, the authors made note that the study was not powered to detect differences in fractures between the two groups. In a retrospective study of 38 patients, Fribourg et al.[55] found that 10 of these patients

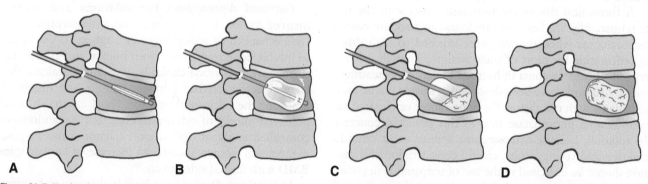

Figure 31-7 Kyphoplasty. **A,** Balloon tamp in place. **B,** Balloon tamp inflated and collapsed vertebral bone restored to near normal height. **C,** Cavity being filled with cement. **D,** Cavity completely filled with cement.

sustained an additional 17 fractures. Eight patients had a second fracture within 2 months of the procedure, and all had at least one fracture at an adjacent level. At this time, more research is needed on the outcomes of this surgical procedure, especially with respect to long-term effect. Because osteoporotic bone is a low-density material, placement of a high-density material, such as cement, adjacent to these vertebrae alters the biomechanical relationship between them and changes the transfer and absorption of forces.

Overall, quick recovery and reduction in pain occur if either procedure is performed early in acute vertebral fractures.[56] However, the procedure is not without potential side effects: osteoporotic bone is a low-density material and placement of a high-density material (cement) adjacent to these vertebrae alters the biomechanical relationship between them and changes the absorption of forces, which can result in fractures above and below "cemented" vertebrae. In a population-based retrospective study of patients with previous vertebral compression fracture, 48 patients who received vertebroplasty or kyphoplasty were compared with 164 patients who did not (comparison group). Treated patients had a significantly greater risk (30%) of subsequent vertebral compression fractures.[57] Extravasation of the cement can also occur into surrounding tissues and rarely can travel in the vasculature tissue post-procedure, resulting in embolization.[58] Subsequent trials have also identified patient age >80 years, cement leakage, vitamin D deficiency, need for procedures at multiple levels, and low BMD as significant risk factors for new vertebral compression fracture following vertebroplasty.[58]

PRIMARY HYPERPARATHYROIDISM

Introduction: Anatomy and Physiology of Parathyroid Glands

Parathyroid hormone (PTH) and vitamin D, which play a key role in bone mineralization, are the most important hormones regulating calcium, phosphate, and magnesium levels in the body. These two hormones act in bone, kidney, and the GI tract to increase serum calcium. PTH is produced by four small parathyroid glands adjacent to the thyroid gland in the lower part of the anterior neck. PTH is responsible for the conversion of inactive vitamin D into its active form 1,25-dihydroxyvitamin D (activated vitamin D).

Extracellular ionized calcium concentrations are closely regulated within a narrow physiological range that is optimal for many processes within cells and organ systems, to play a number of roles as a cofactor for enzymes, secondary messengers, neurotransmitters, and building materials for bone formation. Most of the total body calcium is sequestered in the skeleton (99%), with extracellular and intracellular calcium constituting only 1%. PTH and vitamin D closely regulate these dynamic cal-

cium pools. In addition, their actions over bone-forming osteoblasts and bone-resorbing osteoclasts determine bone density and mineralization.[59,60] Calcitonin (a hormone produced by the thyroid) also decreases bone resorption, playing a minor role in regulation of serum calcium under normal circumstances.[61]

PTH has a very short half-life of 2 to 4 minutes and is secreted constantly to provide immediate and tight regulation to ionized calcium levels.[62] This seemingly instantaneous response is mediated by the calcium-sensing receptor (CaSR), a protein located in the cell membranes of both parathyroid cells and thyroid C cells (which produce calcitonin). CaSR binds to ionized calcium, its main agonist, which activates a cascade of intracellular events leading to the suppression of PTH secretion. PHPT occurs when one or several cells in the parathyroid gland lose their ability to be regulated, developing autonomous excessive release of PTH.

Epidemiology

Primary hyperparathyroidism (PHPT) is the most common cause of hypercalcemia and is associated with long-term complications, such as osteoporosis, disability,[63] hypertension, cardiovascular disease, and cancer.[64] Among ambulatory patients, PHPT accounts for 75% of all causes of hypercalcemia. Figure 31-8 demonstrates some of the typical causes of disorders of calcium homeostasis.

PHPT presents most commonly in women (i.e., 75% of cases) in the sixth and seventh decades of life[63,64] due to a decrease in the restraining effect of estrogen on PTH secretion. The incidence of PHPT has been estimated to be 4 per 100,000 population, a rate lower than before automated laboratory screening panels were introduced.[65]

Etiology

In most patients with PHPT, no clear cause can be identified. Risk factors that have been associated include head and neck irradiation (either by exposure or after radioactive iodine therapy for thyroid diseases) and long-term lithium therapy.[66-68] There are several genes implicated in sporadic and familial PHPT—Cyclin D1 overexpression, a protein of PRAD1/Cyclin D1 gene that has been found in 39% of sporadic parathyroid adenomas.[69] Mutations to multiple endocrine neoplasia type 1 (MEN1), HRPT2, RET, and CDKI have been found in families with familial hyperparathyroidism, and several different germline mutations have been identified. MEN1 is a proto-oncogene implicated in MEN1 syndrome, which is characterized by PHPT, usually starting at an early age (i.e., around the second and third decade of life), as well as other tumors, such as pancreatic and pituitary tumors. Mutations to this gene have been associated with both parathyroid adenoma and hyperplasia development. Presence of acquired somatic MEN1 mutations has been

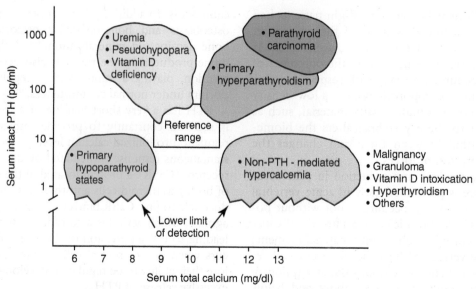

Figure 31-8 Calcium-intact parathyroid hormone (iPTH) relationships.

identified in approximately 30% of sporadic parathyroid tumors.[70] HRPT2 is a tumor suppressor gene associated with the hyperparathyroidism-jaw tumor syndrome and has also been implicated in sporadic parathyroid carcinomas.[71] RET is a proto-oncogene implicated in MEN2A and 2B syndromes, with PHPT reported in 10% to 25% of patients with MEN2A but not in 2B; MEN2A, as well as MEN1, is associated with multigland hyperplasia.[72]

Table 31-4 summarizes the current understanding of the forms of PHPT.

Clinical Features

Advances in modern medicine have made PHPT classic presentation of "stones, bones, moans, and psychic overtones" a rare occurrence thanks to routine calcium measurements that demonstrate hypercalcemia at early stages of disease. This condition is most commonly diagnosed in preclinical stages as asymptomatic PHPT. However, there is evidence that approximately 15% to 20% of

these "asymptomatic" patients will still have chronic complaints, such as anxiety, weakness, depression, fatigue, nephrolithiasis, acid reflux, or bone disease, even when calcium levels are only modestly elevated.[63,73–75] In addition, PHPT is associated with increased insulin resistance, hypertension, and metabolic syndrome. It remains unclear whether surgical cure induces regression to these changes.[76] Bone changes related to PHPT are characterized by loss of mineral density, particularly at sites rich in cortical bone, such as the radius. The more severe form of this type of bone loss is osteitis fibrosa cystica, which currently is almost exclusively seen in developing countries or as part of the metabolic bone disease related to chronic kidney disease (i.e., secondary hyperparathyroidism). Cross-sectional studies show an increased rate of fractures among persons with PHPT, with fracture risk not returning to normal until years after surgical cure.[77] Other abnormalities frequently encountered in patients with PHPT are hypophosphatemia (due to renal losses), normal or low 25-hydroxyvitamin

TABLE 31-4

Genes and Syndromes Associated with Familial Hyperparathyroidism

Gene	Pathology Associations	Clinical Features
MEN1	MEN1 syndrome	Pituitary, pancreatic tumors, Zollinger-Ellison syndrome, VIPoma, carcinoid, angiofibromas
HRPT2	Hyperparathyroidism-jaw tumor syndrome	Parathyroid adenoma and parathyroid carcinoma (HRPT)
RET	MEN2A MEN2B (PHPT is not associated)	MEN2A: Familial medullary thyroid carcinoma (FMTC), pheochromocytoma MEN2B: FMTC, Mucosal neuromas, Marfanoid habitus
CDKI	Sporadic parathyroid adenoma	PHPT
PRAD1/Cyclin D1	Sporadic parathyroid adenoma	PHPT

MEN1, multiple endocrine neoplasm, type 1; *HRPT2*, hyperparathyroidism 2; *RET*, ret proto-oncogene; *CDKI*, cyclin-dependent kinase inhibitor gene; *PRAD1*, parathyroid neoplasm gene

D (a higher PTH correlates with lower vitamin levels), and hypercalciuria.[78]

During a study of patients with fragility fractures or osteoporosis by DXA, PTH levels are frequently measured, and as a consequence a variant of PHPT known as normocalcemic PHPT has been identified. This is characterized by normal calcium but persistently elevated PTH levels. This diagnosis should be made only after all causes of secondary hyperparathyroidism have been ruled out.[79,80] Its prognosis and indications for treatment are the focus of current and future research.

Diagnosis

The classic features of PHPT are an elevated serum calcium level (i.e., hypercalcemia) and an elevated or inappropriately normal (for the level of serum calcium) intact parathyroid hormone (iPTH) level. In the evaluation of suspected PHPT, a 25-hydroxyvitamin D level should be obtained and any deficiency corrected.[78] When PHPT is determined, a biochemistry panel is recommended, including blood urea nitrogen, creatinine, phosphate, and alkaline phosphatase levels. A 24-hour urine calcium excretion should be obtained as well. If patients have a history of nephrolithiasis (i.e., process of morning a kidney stone) or if initial results show hypercalciuria (i.e., elevated calcium in the urine), patients should have a 24-hour urine biochemical stone profile, which helps to determine the risk of future stone formation. Surgery is recommended for asymptomatic patients with estimated glomerular filtration rates below 60 mL/min or high risk of nephrolithiasis.[81] An elevated alkaline phosphatase level is a risk factor for postoperative hypocalcemia, also known as hungry bone syndrome.[82]

BMD should be obtained at the time of diagnosis of PHPT by central DXA using spine, hip, and in addition, distal third of radius scanning for higher sensitivity to detect cortical bone loss.[83] When clinically indicated, useful additional studies are vertebral x-rays and vertebral fracture assessment by DXA.[81]

Because approximately 30% of circulating calcium is bound to albumin, the total serum calcium levels should be adjusted with albumin concentrations using the following formula:

$$\text{Corrected total calcium} = \left(\begin{array}{c} \text{measured total calcium} \\ \text{in mg per deciliter} \end{array} \right) + \left[0.8 \times \left(\begin{array}{c} 4.0 - \text{patient's} \\ \text{serum albumin} \\ \text{concentration in} \\ \text{g per deciliter} \end{array} \right) \right]$$

Hyperalbuminemia (i.e., increased concentration of albumin in the blood) occasionally results in artifactual hypercalcemia; therefore measurement of ionized calcium levels may be useful in these circumstances.[80]

iPTH values more than 40 pg/mL accompanied by hypercalcemia strongly point to a diagnosis of PHPT. Similarly hypercalcemia with low or low-normal iPTH levels usually suggests another etiology, such as malignancy-associated hypercalcemia (the second most common cause of elevated calcium levels).

Mild hypercalcemia associated with normal or unsuppressed PTH levels is commonly seen in patients taking thiazide diuretics or lithium, as well as in a rare condition called familial hypocalciuric hypercalcemia (FHH). The differential diagnosis is summarized in Table 31-5. Lithium can induce multigland hyperplasia or adenoma as documented in multiple case series with persistent hypercalcemia after withdrawal.[68] Whenever possible, discontinuation of thiazides and lithium is recommended with hypercalcemia. Early or mild PHPT is thought to be unmasked by these agents, for which monitoring of calcium and PTH levels is recommended after cessation of thiazides and lithium. FHH is caused by an inactivating mutation in the gene encoding the CaSR protein. It leads to an upward shift in the threshold for suppression of PTH secretion and consequent mild, asymptomatic hypercalcemia starting in childhood. This condition is inherited in an autosomal dominant pattern with high penetrance. Obtaining calcium levels from first-degree relatives (i.e., parents) helps clarify the diagnosis. A 24-hour urine calcium to creatinine ratio is recommended, and results of less than 0.01 (during normal calcium consumption and off any diuretics) can confirm the diagnosis. Treatment is not indicated for FHH because of its benign prognosis.[84]

Familial PHPT accounts for approximately 5% of cases and should be considered in patients younger than 30 years, those with family history of hypercalcemia, and/or other neuroendocrine tumors (Table 31-5). When suspicion is high, serum calcium should be measured in all first-degree relatives. This may help to support the diagnosis and offer early diagnosis and counseling to affected relatives. Genetic testing is available and may be offered in cases of familial forms of PHPT and FHH.[83]

Localization of an adenoma (or hyperplasia) can also be attempted by means of parathyroid scintigraphy or diagnostic ultrasound, but studies[85,86] have demonstrated a variable sensitivity. Imaging studies are not required for diagnosis. These tests are usually reserved for patients who meet criteria for surgery. In one study, the use of planar sestamibi scanning performed the morning of the operation was sufficient to assist the surgeons achieve a surgical cure rate of approximately 95%.[64]

Ultrasonography and spiral computed tomography of the kidneys are useful to quantify nephrolithiasis, hydronephrosis, and nephrocalcinosis, and screening in asymptomatic patients without a history of stones is recommended.[81] Parathyroid carcinoma, which is very rare, should be suspected in patients with extremely elevated PTH levels (i.e., greater than threefold above normal), severe hypercalcemia (i.e., greater than 14 mg/dL), and those with a neck mass.

TABLE 31-5

Differential Diagnosis of Common Causes of Hypercalcemia

	Calcium Elevation	25-(OH) D	Phosphorus	iPTH	Improves with Medication Withdrawal	Age	Urine Calcium
PHPT	+/+++	Normal/low	Low	High	No*	6th-7th decade	+++
Familial hypocalciuric hypercalcemia (FHH)	+	Normal	Normal†	Normal/ mildly high	No	All ages	—
Cancer-Associated Hypercalcemia	+++	Normal	Normal	Low‡	No	Usually elderly	+++
Thiazide	+	Normal	Normal	Normal	Yes	Middle-age adult	—
Lithium	+/++	Normal/low	Normal/low	High	Yes	Middle-age adult	++
Artifactual Hypercalcemia	+/Corrects to normal	Normal	Normal	Normal	N/A	All ages	Normal

iPTH, Intact parathyroid hormone. *PHPT*, primary hyperparathyroidism; *25-(OH) D*, 25-hydroxyvitamin D

* Thiazides and lithium have the potential to worsen hypercalcemia in patients with PHPT.

† Magnesium levels are typically elevated in FHH.

‡ Commonly mediated by parathyroid hormone related-protein (PTHrp).

Treatment of Primary Hyperparathyroidism

Greater than average fluid intake is recommended to all patients with PHPT and emphasized on those who do not undergo surgery. Acute hypercalcemia due to PHPT may require hospitalization, especially when calcium levels are severely elevated or when symptomatic. For patients with severe hypercalcemia (>12 mg/dL), IV hydration is recommended. Use of loop diuretics (i.e., diuretics that act in the loop of Henle in the kidneys) can be added later to prevent fluid overload and support calciuria. IV bisphosphonates and denosumab have been demonstrated to produce significant reductions in calcium levels, usually after 36 to 72 hours of administration.[87,88] These drugs are usually reserved for more severe cases.

Parathyroid Surgery

Surgery remains the mainstay of treatment of PHPT and reported cure rates are as high as 95% after 10 years. Surgery is recommended for all symptomatic patients with PHPT, and remains an option for all asymptomatic patients as the only curative treatment available.

Guidelines from the fourth international workshop on hyperparathyroidism, published in 2014, recommend surgery for asymptomatic patients who are younger than 50 years of age, have moderate-to-severe hypercalcemia (i.e., >1 mg/dL above normal), have reduced renal function glomerular filtration rate (i.e., <60 mL/min), or renal changes (i.e., high risk of stone formation, nephrolithiasis, or nephrocalcinosis) detected by screening studies, or are complicated by osteoporosis. Asymptomatic patients in whom long-term follow-up is not possible should also be referred for surgery. Table 31-6 summarizes current indications for surgery.

Multiple approaches and surgical techniques have been developed, including a minimally invasive approach. Many centers prefer a unilateral or single gland approach,[89] whereas others have adopted four parathyroid gland explorations.[64,90] Parathyroidectomies should be performed by experienced surgeons to maintain complication risks under 1% to 3%.[91] Intraoperative PTH has been used as a marker of success during surgery.[62] A drop of 50% in PTH levels has been associated to a cure rate of greater than 90% to 95% at 1 year. However, others argue that multiple gland explorations are required to provide a long-term cure because multiple adenomas or hyperplasia are present in up to 25% of cases.[64,90] This latter technique does not rely on intraoperative PTH.

Medical Therapy for Primary Hyperparathyroidism

Patients who cannot undergo surgery but present with symptomatic hypercalcemia may benefit from cinacalcet.[88] This agent is commonly used for secondary hyperparathyroidism secondary to renal failure, and the FDA has approved its use in PHPT with severe hypercalcemia. It increases sensitivity in the CaSR of the parathyroid glands, thereby decreasing PTH secretion. Doses of 60 to 120 mg divided twice per day help to normalize calcium

TABLE 31-6

Indications for Parathyroid Surgery

Variable	Criterion for Surgery	Suggested Following without Surgery
Age	Younger than 50	—
Calcium (serum)	>1.0 mg/dL above upper range	Once yearly
Kidney	GFR <60 mL/min × 1.73 m² Urine calcium >400 mg/day/biochemical stone profile Renal imaging (ultrasound, CT scan, or x-ray)	Once yearly
Bone disease	T-score < −2.5 at any site* and/or previous fracture fragility* by central DXA; VFA, CT scan, MRI, or vertebral x-ray Pathological fractures	Every 1-2 years (include distal one-third radius)†

mg, milligrams; *dL*, decaliter; *GFR*, glomerular filtration rate; *CT*, computed tomography; *DXA*, dual-energy x-ray absorptiometry; *VFA*, vertebral fracture assessment; *MRI*, magnetic resonance imaging.

*ISCD recommends use of Z-scores instead of T-scores when evaluating BMD in premenopausal women and men younger than 50 yr.

†Lumbar spine, total hip, femoral neck, or distal third of radius. There may be different time frame recommendations according to specific countries.

levels in most cases, although PTH reductions are usually more modest. It has been studied in a wide range of stages of PHPT with consistent success and tolerability.[92] The effects are short lived and patients must remain under treatment to avoid recurrence. BMD remained stable for up to 5 years in one study with this agent.[93]

PAGET'S DISEASE OF BONE (OSTEITIS DEFORMANS)

Introduction

PDB (also known as osteitis deformans) was first described by Sir James Paget in 1877. Although it is considered a systemic bone disease, it is more accurately described as a localized disorder of bone remodeling that may occur at multiple sites.[94] The most commonly affected sites of the skeleton are the skull, femur, pelvis, vertebra, and tibia. One skeletal site (monostotic) or multiple sites (polyostotic) may be involved.

Paget's disease affects approximately 3% of people in the United States over age 50 and 10% of those over age 80.[95] Men and women are affected with nearly equal frequency, but it is relatively uncommon before age 25. It is most common in the United Kingdom and in those of northern European descent, and it is uncommon in Africans and Asians. The disease is often asymptomatic and is usually discovered incidentally through radiographs or by an increase in serum alkaline phosphatase activity.

Pathogenesis and Etiology

Although the etiology of Paget's disease is incompletely understood, both genetic and environmental pathogenesis have gained strong research support.[96] In the past, several pedigrees of families with several afflicted individuals have been described, thus providing a strong basis for a genetic cause of the disease. Paget's disease has since been linked to chromosome 18q and other loci with mutations in the coding of the ubiquitin-associated (UBA) domain of the sequestosome-1 (SQSTM1) gene, which encodes the p62 protein, leading to elevated NF-κB in osteoclasts.[95,96] However, when bone from patients with this mutation is examined microscopically, the osteoclasts do not appear to be "pagetic" (see later), and therefore an environmental factor is suspected to be necessary to induce the expression of Paget's disease. Chronic measles infection has been the most suspected and thus the most studied, but other viral mechanisms could be responsible.[95]

In Paget's disease there are a disproportionate number of osteoclasts compared with osteoblasts. These osteoclasts have abnormal nucleoli along with hypersensitivity to vitamin D. This combination results in accelerated bone turnover leading to abnormal deposition of lamellar bone. The "new" bone is disorganized in appearance, with thickened trabeculae rimmed by numerous osteoblasts. This characteristically mosaic pattern is formed by randomly arrayed units of lamellar bone delineated by irregular "cement lines." The disorganized bone increases the bone volume but not the strength, and the bone marrow is replaced by highly vascular stromal (connective) tissue. The pagetic bone is mechanically weaker and more susceptible to fractures despite its sclerotic appearance and a higher density by DXA.

Clinical Features

Although the disease is commonly asymptomatic, the most common symptom in Paget's disease is bone pain. Fractures may also occur from Paget's disease and healing is slow because of the altered mechanical structure of the bone itself. The incidence of nonunion fractures has been reported as high as 40%, especially when the fracture involves the proximal femur.[97] In addition, increased weight bearing, which stimulates bone growth and remodeling in normal bone, is a less effective means of fracture prevention in individuals with Paget's disease.[95,97] Osteoarthritis secondary to Paget's disease, when affecting bones adjacent to joints, may eventually require a total joint replacement.

When Paget's disease is suspected, a careful history and physical examination should be performed to look for skeletal deformity, pain, and a temperature change over the affected areas of bone. Pagetic bone may have an increased vasculature supply with increased warmth and occasionally a bruit (i.e., abnormal sound of blood indicating increased turbulence to blood flow) can be heard (by stethoscope). Rarely patients with polyostotic Paget's disease may have congestive heart failure, particularly if they become inactive or suffer fracture of the affected bone. Patients with Paget's disease of the basilar skull may have sensorineural hearing loss due to entrapment of the eighth cranial nerve.[97]

Symptoms of Paget's Disease[97]

- Bone pain from microfractures or osteoarthritis
- Bowing of a limb
- Thoracic kyphosis and compression fracture
- Loss of hearing—when skull is involved
- Neurological symptoms from nerve compression caused by bone growth (spine, skull, limbs)
- Spinal stenosis
- Heart failure if active polyostic involvement and patient is suddenly immobile
- Hypercalcemia if significant bone involvement and patient is immobile and/or fractures

---

Diagnosis

The diagnosis of Paget's disease is typically made radiographically by the characteristic localized disruption of skeletal architecture (Figure 31-9), although pagetic bone can also be recognized on scintigraphic bone scans. Most often the differential diagnosis includes Paget's disease, osteoblastic malignancy (e.g., prostate cancer, thyroid cancer, osteosarcoma), hyperparathyroidism, and severe vitamin D deficiency. Occasionally a bone biopsy is required to establish a specific diagnosis but more importantly to exclude malignancy, particularly osteosarcoma.

The biochemical features of Paget's disease are those of increased skeletal turnover. They include an elevated serum level of alkaline phosphatase or bone-specific alkaline phosphatase and increased urinary resorption markers (N-telo-peptide and CTX).[4,95] With active polyostotic Paget's disease, the serum alkaline phosphatase may exceed the upper end of the reference range by 10-fold.

Treatment of Paget's Disease of the Bone

The decision to treat symptomatic patients with Paget's disease is based on several factors:
1. Pain from the bony involvement
2. Location: skull involvement with eighth cranial nerve entrapment causing hearing loss and headaches

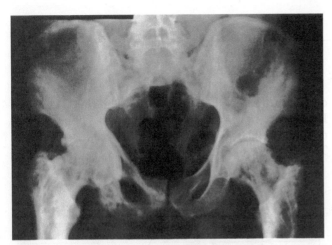

Figure 31-9 Radiograph of a pelvis affected by Paget's disease showing concentric-type Paget's arthritis of the right hip. (From Merkow RL, Lane JM: Current concepts of Paget's disease of bone, *Orthop Clin North Am* 15:747-763, 1984.)

3. If plan for surgery on the affected bone: preoperative treatment to prevent hypercalcemia, if patient is immobile
4. Polyostic involvement, which increases the risk of fractures and heart failure

Pharmacotherapy may improve symptoms of bone pain if related to Paget's disease, but braces and other devices may also be needed. Treatment for asymptomatic patients is indicated when the involved bone has the potential for complication:
1. Weight-bearing bones (to prevent bowing)
2. Bones adjacent to a joint (to prevent advanced degenerative joint disease [DJD])
3. Spine (to prevent vertebral fractures and spinal stenosis)
4. Skull (to prevent hearing loss and headaches)

In addition, in asymptomatic patients with pagetic bone not at a concerning site, it is reasonable to consider therapy if the serum alkaline phosphatase is more than 2 to 4 times the upper limit of normal.

The mainstays of treatment for Paget's disease are the bone resorption inhibitors (i.e., bisphosphonates), which may be administered orally or intravenously. For Paget's disease, the total dosage of oral bisphosphonates (see Table 31-3) is much higher than that taken for osteoporosis (i.e., taken daily for 3 to 6 months), depending upon the agent selected. IV bisphosphonates are most often used in patients with refractory Paget's disease or those with contraindications to oral medications.

SUMMARY

Systemic bone disease (i.e., metabolic bone disease) encompasses a spectrum of medical conditions that may have a major effect on bone by differing mechanisms. Osteoporosis affects men and women at different rates and for various reasons, but the resulting outcome is similar. Osteoporosis is a focus of ongoing research for prevention of fractures through medications[98] as well as other modalities, with a goal of reduction of morbidity and mortality among the elderly. Hyperparathyroidism is another common systemic bone disease and is interrelated with osteoporosis as a risk factor for fractures if uncontrolled. Finally, although less common, PDB can lead to disability and fractures if unrecognized. This chapter highlights the importance of recognition as well as some basic management of these conditions.

PART B | Rehabilitation Intervention

HOLLIE KIRWAN, JENNIFER BESSIRE

OSTEOPOROSIS

It is estimated that 54 million Americans have osteoporosis or low bone mass and that more than 2 million osteoporosis-related fractures result in medical costs amounting to U.S. $17 billion. By 2025, annual fractures and costs are expected to increase to more than 3 million and U.S. $25 billion, respectively.[99] Typically patients referred to physical therapy are not referred with a primary diagnosis of osteoporosis. Referrals are more likely to be received for individuals who have sustained a fracture as a result of this underlying condition or who are referred for unrelated diagnoses. A knowledge of the impact and possible physical consequences of osteoporosis, and of ways of developing a treatment plan for patients who have this condition regardless of the referral diagnosis, is paramount. Nonvertebral fractures account for 73% of the reported fractures, with nontypical osteoporosis-related sites (i.e., pelvis and areas other than wrist, hip, or vertebra) accounting for 40% of fractures. With this in mind, physical therapists should focus treatment on all skeletal sites and avoid focusing on the spine and hip when treating patients with osteoporosis.

Osteoporosis can be defined as a disease characterized by low bone mass and structural deterioration of bone tissue, leading to bone fragility and increased risk of fracture (Figure 31-10).[100] A bone mineral density (BMD) test can be performed to clinically define osteoporosis or osteopenia (i.e., low bone mass) (Figure 31-11). The BMD refers to the relative fracture risk of a bone and the test used to classify bone health; the result is given as a T-score of the hip BMD.

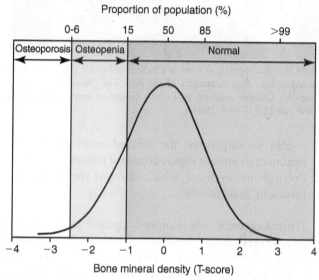

Figure 31-11 Normal distribution of BMD scores, represented as T-scores. Note that a score of −1 to −2.5 represents osteopenia, and a score of −2.5 or lower indicates osteoporosis. (Redrawn from Kanis JA: Osteoporosis III: diagnosis of osteoporosis and assessment of fracture risk, *Lancet* 359:1929-1936, 2002.)

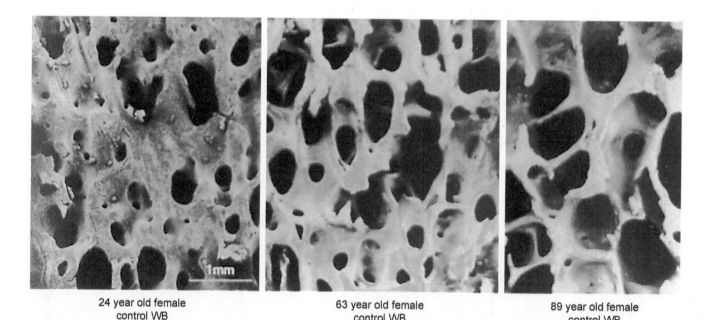

24 year old female
control WB

63 year old female
control WB

89 year old female
control WB

Figure 31-10 Age-related changes in apparent density and architecture of human trabecular bone from the lumbar spine. (Courtesy Marc D. Grynpas. In Buchwalter JA et al: *Orthopaedic basic science*, ed 2, Rosemont, 2000, American Academy of Orthopaedic Surgeons.)

From an epidemiological perspective, approximately 10 million individuals in the United States have osteoporosis, and an additional 34 million have osteopenia. One in two women and one in four men over age 50 will have an osteoporosis-related fracture at some time in their life.[101] This means that clinicians working with those over age 50 are very likely to have patients with osteoporosis or osteopenia, and these patients therefore are at greater risk of injury or impairment related to these disease processes. For these reasons, consideration of the patient's bone status is vital, regardless of the referral diagnosis.

With the high incidence of fracture rates in patients with osteoporosis, fractures are often the reason for their encounters with clinicians. Fractures of the hip, spine, wrist, arm, and leg may occur as a result of a fall. However, simple household tasks can result in vertebral fractures that can often go undiagnosed.[100] The primary symptom of these fractures, back pain, often is attributed to "arthritis" or is thought to be a normal part of aging. The most serious and debilitating fracture is a hip fracture, and these patients often are referred for rehabilitation after surgery.

Clinicians must base their intervention not on the medical diagnosis, but on the resultant impairments and functional limitations that impact the patient that are found during their initial evaluation. Treatment of individuals with osteoporosis is no different. Therefore this section covers the past medical history, assessment, primary prevention, treatment of common impairments, effects of exercise on the skeleton, and kyphoplasty. The overriding objective for these patients is to improve functional ability and prevent fractures, which can lead to further significant declines in function. To this end, the goals of treatment include increasing strength, flexibility, and range of motion (ROM); improving balance (90% of hip fractures are the result of a fall)[102]; correcting posture when possible; modulating pain; and educating the patient about lifestyle adaptations.

Spinal Biomechanics

During upright standing in a person with normal spinal curvature, there is minimal spinal muscle involvement to maintain static equilibrium. However, if there is a change to the normal spinal curvature, such as that seen in patients with thoracic kyphosis, this muscle balance will be disrupted and cause alterations in the physiological loading of the spine as a consequence of the forward shift of body mass. Untreated vertebral fractures can result in increased kyphosis, which leads to changes in the postural position of the patient's cervical spine and head, bringing the center of mass further anterior to the spine (see Figure 31-2). This postural alteration can result in a vicious cycle, causing a further increase in kyphosis. The kyphosis compresses the lungs and abdominal organs, making breathing and even eating difficult. These postural changes may also lead to a decrease in upper extremity function, especially with reaching, whereas increases in cervical lordosis lead to decreased cervical flexibility and ultimately affect visual navigation of the environment.

Any assessment or intervention for patients with or at risk for osteoporosis must take into consideration spinal biomechanics and safety. Spinal flexion requires a balance between flexor and extensor forces (Figure 31-12) (*force* is the capacity to do work; *work* is force exerted over a distance).

Any force that falls anterior to the spine exerts a *flexion moment* (i.e., force acting at a distance perpendicular to a point) on the spine; any force that is posterior to the spine exerts an *extension moment* (Figure 31-13). Flexion moments include the *center of gravity* (i.e., the vertical displacement of the center of mass onto the ground). In older adults, this flexion moment often is increased because of the flexed posture they assume (see Figure 31-12, *B*). An increase in thoracic kyphosis (i.e., spinal flexion) increases the distance that the force acts on the spine and thus increases the flexion moment, leading to greater compression and shear forces on the spinal segments.

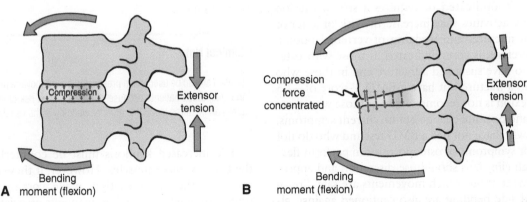

Figure 31-12 A, State of balance between flexors and extensors and the resulting biomechanics. **B,** State of increased flexor force and insufficient extensor force, resulting in compression on the anterior part of the vertebral body and the intervertebral disc. (Redrawn from Carlson JM: Clinical biomechanics of orthotic treatment of thoracic hyperkyphosis, *J Prosthet Orthot* 15: 31-35, 2003.)

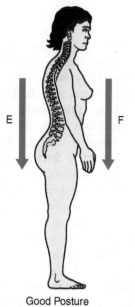
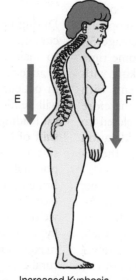
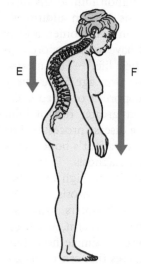

Good Posture
Flexion moment = Extension moment

Increased Kyphosis
Flexion moment > Extension moment

Significantly Increased Kyphosis
Flexion moment >> Extension moment

Figure 31-13 Changes in flexor and extensor moments of the thoracic spine with progressive increases in thoracic kyphosis. As the kyphosis increases, the flexor moment increases. The increase in flexor moment requires an equally large extensor moment to reduce force through the anterior part of the vertebral bodies. *E,* Extensor moment; *F,* flexor moment.

Thoracic kyphosis can increase the risk of vertebral fractures and intervertebral disc degeneration, cause loss of spinal muscle strength, and result in degeneration of intervertebral ligaments.

The extensor muscles counteract the flexion moment. However, the back extensors and paraspinal musculature can often be compromised in patients with a kyphosis due to alterations in the length-tension relationships, moment arm lengths, and force vector orientations.[103] Patients with weak extensors will have difficulty counteracting the flexion and so the kyphosis remains or will gradually worsen unless treated appropriately.

Additional *stress* (i.e., a force exerted when one body or body part presses on, pulls on, pushes against, or tends to compress or twist another body or body part) or an increase in the flexor moment caused by asking these patients to participate in physical activities that increase flexion is **contraindicated** or requires a strong caution because these activities may increase the risk of anterior compression fractures and wedging of vertebral bodies. Flexion, therefore, is contraindicated in those with osteoporosis who have sustained a fracture and in those who have not had a fracture but have a BMD T-score of −2.5 or lower. Flexion is not recommended in those who show height loss and postural change but no current symptoms. Individuals who have not had a BMD test and who do not have signs or symptoms of osteoporosis can perform flexion, although clinicians should use discretion and appropriate judgment about which movements are safe. Spinal rotation and side bending are also cautioned against, although not as strongly as flexion, for the same groupings (Table 31-7).[104–106] These motions are not advised due to

TABLE 31-7

Contraindications to Spinal Flexion Based on Bone Mineral Density (BMD) Score

BMD Score	Spinal Flexion
T score of −2.5 or lower	Contraindicated
T score of −1 to −2.5	Not recommended; clinical judgment required
No BMD results available, but height loss, vertebral fracture, and kyphosis are present	Contraindicated

the compressive forces they place on the vertebral bodies. This can lead to a vertebral compression fracture, especially if the motions of flexion, rotation, and side bending are combined.

Clinical Note

Caution should be used when prescribing flexion movements or exercises to osteoporotic patients because of the increased risk of vertebral compression fractures leading to anterior wedging of the vertebral bodies.

The increased kyphosis must be counterbalanced by the back extensor muscles. However, if these muscles are too weak, they quickly fatigue while working to keep the spine extended. Postural adjustments associated with increased kyphosis include posterior tilt or translation of the pelvis, hip extension, knee flexion, and ankle dorsiflexion to counter the anterior shift of the body mass.[107] Each of these adjustments will affect the biomechanical environment of the spine. Clinicians responsible for the rehabilitative management of patients with these types of problems must consider all these factors in designing a program to minimize kyphosis. The program must include education and counseling to make patients aware of the effects of inappropriate posture on their condition, bracing if appropriate, and improving the strength and endurance of the thoracic extensor and scapula retractor muscles.

Primary Prevention

The ability of the skeleton to respond to mechanical loading is greatest during childhood and decreases with age. Weight-bearing exercise when young has been found to have lasting effects on bone mass and structure following cessation of exercise.[108] **Peak bone mass** is defined as the highest level of bone mass achieved as a result of normal growth.[109] Once bone mass peaks during adolescence, it cannot be effectively altered during later years. However, the consequences of insufficient bone mass are not seen until old age, when levels become so low as to result in fractures. Consequently, osteoporosis is not a disease of old age, but a pediatric disease that does not manifest itself until old age.[110] Therefore, the target population for prevention should be premenarcheal and young premenopausal women and young boys. There is no cure for osteoporosis, so the most effective management is prevention. The goal of prevention is to maximize bone mass and BMD. (Although density is "the mass of a substance per unit volume," [Merriam-Webster] and mass is "a measure of the amount of a material," the terms *bone mass* and *bone mineral density* often are used interchangeably.) Addressing prevention through education of adolescents about bone density development and bone density risk behaviors is advocated by the International Osteoporosis Foundation.[111] They have called for a national effort to educate the youth about osteoporosis. This will allow adolescents to understand the importance of achieving and maintaining optimal peak bone mass and how to reduce the risk of osteoporosis in later life. However, several studies have reported on the lack of knowledge surrounding risk factors and preventative techniques in adolescent populations. One study investigating knowledge of bone health in female adolescents reported that the students performed poorly in osteoporosis knowledge pretests and this was improved following an educational in-service program.[112] Another study investigated gender differences in osteoporosis health beliefs and knowledge in a group of collegiate students and concluded that there are definite limitations in college student's knowledge and health beliefs associated with osteoporosis. Women had higher perceptions of threat of osteoporosis and less confidence in their ability to be physically active. The authors

advised that education and prevention targeting men and women may be beneficial to offset the development of osteoporosis in later life.

Clinical Note

The goal for preventing osteoporosis is to maximize bone mass and bone mineral density (BMD); this must begin in adolescence.

Exactly when bone mass peaks is the subject of debate, the suggested age ranges from middle to late teens[113-115] to the 20s.[116-118] However, according to Huijbregts et al.,[104] by the time girls are 12 years old, they have already achieved 80% of their adult BMD, and by the time boys have reached age 19 to 20, they have acquired 95% of their peak bone mass. Regardless of when peak bone mass is reached, it generally is agreed that the key ages for laying down bone mass are 11 to 16 in girls and a few years later in boys.[119] Genetics accounts for 70% of the variation seen in peak bone mass. However, strong support exists for the effect of three environmental factors on bone mass: habitual physical exercise, nutrition, and reproductive hormone status.[120] With rapid skeletal model mineral acquisition occurring in adolescence, the exogenous factors that can help to optimize peak bone mass need to be precisely identified and characterized within the scope of primary prevention.[108]

Key Ages for Laying Down Bone Mass

- Girls: 11 to 16 years
- Boys: 13 to 20 years

Factors that Affect Bone Mass in Youth

- Physical activity
- Nutrition
- Reproductive hormone status
- Genetics

What are the roles of the various clinicians who focus on rehabilitation? A critical primary consideration is to educate patients and the public about the importance of exercise and appropriate nutrition for young children and adolescents. Research shows that in both children and adolescents, regular physical activity is directly related to increases in BMD[121-125] and to permanent increases in cross-sectional areas of trained skeletal regions.[126,127] Exercise during growth adds extra material to loaded sites to increase the quantity of bone present as displayed in Figure 31-14. Bone formation in response to loading occurs in a site-specific manner,

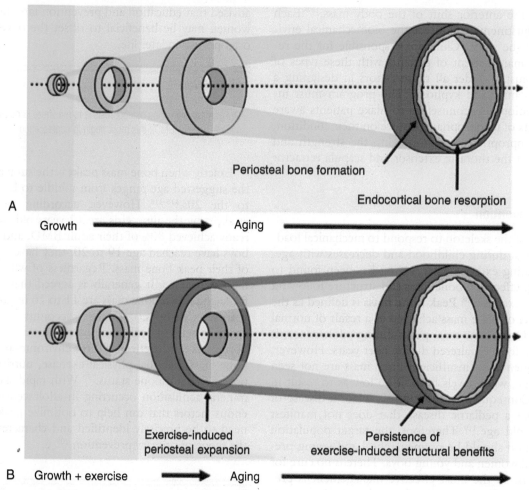

Periosteal bone formation

Endocortical bone resorption

A

Growth ➔ Aging ➔

Exercise-induced
periosteal expansion

Persistence of
exercise-induced structural benefits

B   Growth + exercise ➔ Aging ➔

Figure 31-14 Bone structural adaptations associated with aging (**A**) and exercise (**B**). **A,** Bone loss during aging occurs primarily via bone resorption on the endocortical surface. There is concomitant bone formation on the periosteal surface, which assists in maintaining bone structure, but this can be insufficient to maintain bone mass. **B,** Exercise during growth will facilitate periosteal bone formation, which optimizes bone structure. Bone loss during aging occurs from the inside out, so the enhanced structure achieved through exercise during growth has the potential to remain intact regardless of age-related changes to bone mass. (From Warden SJ, Fuchs RK: Exercise and bone health: optimizing bone structure during growth is key, but all is not in vain during ageing, *Br J Sports Med* 43:885-887, 2009.)

where the mechanical demands are highest. This leads to optimization of the skeletal structure, with greater bone material being positioned to resist external forces and load. This explains why new bone is preferentially laid down on the periosteal surface of loaded bones and why mechanical loading associated with weight-bearing activities generates large increases in bone strength without similar increases in bone quantity.[128] During early life, exercises that include high-impact activities and loads in multiple directions, such as gymnastics and basketball, are most beneficial. The only caveat is that the intensity of the exercise must not be so high as to cause the cessation of menses in females, which can lead to a decrease in BMD.

The female athlete triad has garnered more attention in recent years. It has been shown that up to 78% of high school varsity female athletes have one or more components of the triad.[129] The components of the triad are low energy availability with or without disordered eating, menstrual dysfunction, and low BMD, as displayed in Figure 31-15. Female athletes may present with one or more of the three triad components, and early intervention is essential to prevent progression to clinical eating disorders, amenorrhea, and osteoporosis. It has been reported that up to 62% of female collegiate level athletes have disordered eating, 66% of female athletes are amenorrhic, and 78% of recreational runners have had one or more irregular menstrual cycles when monitored over a 3-month period.[130] Low BMD was reported in 38% of amenorrhic adolescent athletes.[131] These three symptoms can lead to stress fractures caused by the premature bone loss and the low energy availability can negatively impact bone formation and increase bone resorption through suppression of metabolic and reproductive hormones. Bone stress injuries including stress reactions and stress fractures are more common in female athletes with menstrual irregularities or low BMD.[130]

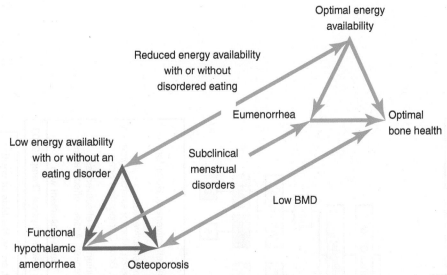

Figure 31-15 Spectra of female athlete triad. The three interrelated components are energy availability, menstrual status, and bone health. The availability of energy will affect menstrual status, and in turn menstrual status and energy availability will impact bone health. Optimal energy availability, eumenorrhea (normal menstruation), and optimal bone health will help the body to achieve optimal health and at the other end of the spectrum, the most severe presentation of the female athlete triad, which includes low energy availability, with or without disordered eating, functional hypothalamic amenorrhea, and osteoporosis. *BMD*, body mass density. (From De Souza MJ, Nattiv A, Joy E et al: 2014 Female athlete triad coalition consensus statement on treatment and return to play of the female athlete triad: 1st international conference held in San Francisco, California, May 2012 and 2nd International Conference held in Indianapolis, Indiana, May 2013, *Br J Sports Med* 48:289, 2014 adapted with permission from Nattiv A, Loucks AB, Manore MM et al: American College of Sports Medicine position stand. The female athlete triad, *Med Sci Sports Exerc* 39:1867-1882, 2007.)

Female Athlete Triad

- Low energy availability with or without disordered eating
- Menstrual dysfunction
- Low bone mineral density (BMD)

Appropriate nutrition also is vital; regular exercise combined with a sufficient intake of calcium can increase bone mass in adolescents.[121,132] Exercise and diet from the age of 4 have been shown to influence BMD.[133]

Investigators found that in a free-living population, cohort levels of daily moderate to very vigorous physical activity were associated with hip size and density at 4 years of age and that those associations were more marked in children consuming more than the median daily intake of calcium.[133] The authors suggested this finding confirms the notion that adequate dietary intake of calcium may be necessary for optimal action of physical activity on bone development. In addition to calcium intake, a positive relationship exists between protein intake and bone mass gained during pubertal maturation.[113] Carbonated drinks are a significant risk factor for bone fractures, even after adjustments for age, weight, height, activity level, and total caloric intake in adults age 21 to 80.[134,135]

These nutritional factors can be discussed directly with children and adolescents and their parents, regardless of the reason the patient seeks therapy. Clinicians also should consider discussing the topic with any adult patient who has children or grandchildren. To be effective, education needs to be ongoing and aimed at various audiences.

The settings and possibilities for education are many and varied.

Assessment of the Adult with Osteoporosis

Current and Past Medical History

Various factors that increase an individual's risk for osteoporosis were outlined in the previous section. Questions concerning these factors should be included in the past medical history form and discussed during the patient interview. Results of a BMD test are extremely helpful in guiding treatment. Clinicians also should keep in mind that a family history of a maternal hip fracture doubles the patient's risk for a hip fracture, regardless of current BMD levels.[126] Individuals with a vertebral compression fracture have a 15% higher mortality rate than those who do not experience fractures, and most compression fractures occur at T8-T12, L1, and L4.[100] Figure 31-16 presents a decision tree to help guide intervention.[136]

Examination. The objective examination can include tests and measures of height and weight, vision, cognition, posture, ROM, strength, flexibility, balance, gait, and sensation, depending on the specific diagnosis. All these factors have the potential to contribute to falls; the findings also provide a baseline measure before therapy is started and help guide the treatment plan. The following list is intended to guide the selection of specific tests and measures for patients with osteoporosis or to alert the clinician to factors to consider if these tests and measures are administered to individuals who may have osteoporosis or osteopenia but have been referred for an unrelated diagnosis. All measures should be as objective as possible.

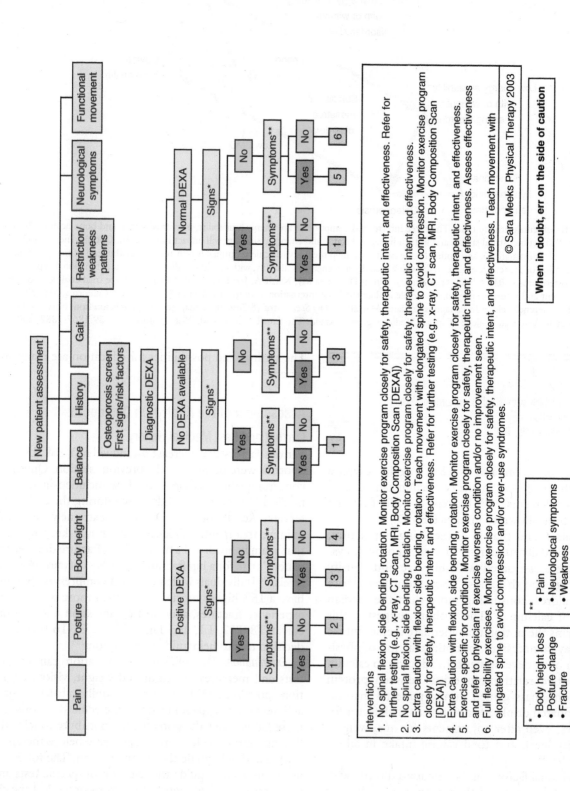

Interventions

1. No spinal flexion, side bending, rotation. Monitor exercise program closely for safety, therapeutic intent, and effectiveness. Refer for further testing (e.g., x-ray, CT scan, MRI, Body Composition Scan [DEXA])
2. No spinal flexion, side bending, rotation. Monitor exercise program closely for safety, therapeutic intent, and effectiveness.
3. Extra caution with flexion, side bending, rotation. Teach movement with elongated spine to avoid compression. Monitor exercise program closely for safety, therapeutic intent, and effectiveness. Refer for further testing (e.g., x-ray, CT scan, MRI, Body Composition Scan [DEXA])
4. Extra caution with flexion, side bending, rotation. Monitor exercise program closely for safety, therapeutic intent, and effectiveness.
5. Exercise specific for condition. Monitor exercise program closely for safety, therapeutic intent, and effectiveness. Assess effectiveness and refer to physician if exercise worsens condition and/or no improvement seen.
6. Full flexibility exercises. Monitor exercise program closely for safety, therapeutic intent, and effectiveness. Teach movement with elongated spine to avoid compression and/or over-use syndromes.

© Sara Meeks Physical Therapy 2003

When in doubt, err on the side of caution

* • Body height loss
  • Posture change
  • Fracture

** • Pain
   • Neurological symptoms
   • Weakness

Figure 31-16 Decision tree for improved screening of patients for osteoporosis. (Modified from Meeks SM: The role of the physical therapist in the recognition, assessment, and exercise intervention in persons with, or at risk for, osteoporosis, *Topics Geriatr Rehab* 21:42-56, 2005.)

Height and Weight. Patients should be assessed standing without shoes. Regular measurement of height is important because loss of height is one of the first signs of osteoporosis. A loss greater than 6 cm (2.4 inches) in those over age 60 and greater than 4 cm (1.6 inches) in those under age 60 suggests a vertebral fracture.[137] The current measurement is compared with the patient's recall of his or her tallest height.

Vision. Poor vision or visual field deficits can contribute to falls. Patients should be instructed to track the clinician's finger in all directions without moving the head to check for visual field deficits.

Cognition. The **Beck Depression Inventory**[138] can alert the clinician to possible depression, which may lead to decreased social interaction and physical activity, which can contribute to falls. Checking for orientation to time, place, and year can alert the clinician to overall cognitive status; if decreased, the patient may have difficulty following directions or in performing a home exercise program.

Posture. A photograph of the patient taken from the side and front (after receiving signed consent) allows the clinician to educate the patient about posture and demonstrate changes between specific follow-up evaluations and sessions. For repeatability, the patient should wear the same clothes each time a photograph is taken. A flexicurve ruler can be used to measure the curves of the spine (http://www.umshp.org/pt/geritool). For cervical or thoracic deformity, the patient should be instructed to stand with the heels and buttocks against the wall, the head level, and the distance between the mastoid process and the wall should be measured in centimeters.[139] Posture in osteoporotic patients is classified into five types: normal, round back, hollow round back, lower acute kyphosis, and whole kyphosis.

Range of Motion. Regardless of which joints need to be measured, precautions for spinal motion should be followed, depending on the patient's BMD test results and/or clinical presentation, as outlined previously under *Spinal Biomechanics*.

Strength. Key muscles include the trunk extensors, hip abductors (crucial to lateral balance control), and the gastrocsoleus complex (important for balance reactions). For very frail patients, the clinician must keep in mind that traditional manual muscle testing of the extremities requires stabilization at the trunk, which may be difficult or painful. For patients who can lie prone, trunk extensor endurance can be measured by placing a pillow under the pelvis and having the patient hold the sternum off a plinth for up to 20 seconds.[140] A 1 repetition maximum (1 RM) or 10 RM is another option for those who are not as frail. Trunk extensor endurance is more important than pure strength because these muscles are used for maintaining upright posture. Timed, loaded standing has been identified as a measure of combined trunk and arm endurance that is suitable for use in people with vertebral osteoporosis.[141] This test measures the time a person can stand while holding a 2-lb (1-kg) dumbbell in each hand with the arms held in 90° shoulder flexion, elbows extended and wrists in a neutral position.

Balance and Gait. A standardized assessment, such as the **Berg Balance Scale**,[142,143] **Tinetti Performance Oriented Mobility Assessment**,[144] **Activities-Specific Balance Scale**,[145] or **Dynamic Gait Index**,[146,147] can be used to determine the fall risk and specific activities that are difficult for the patient.

Sensation. Tests of sensation, especially of the feet, may reveal changes in perception that can contribute to falls. These could include sharp or blunt discrimination, tactile (detecting and localizing touch), temperature discrimination, proprioception, and two-point discrimination.

Functional Assessment. The **Osteoporosis Functional Disability Questionnaire**[148] can be used to establish the level of disability, which can aid goal setting. The **Osteoporosis Assessment Questionnaire—Physical Functioning (OPAQ-PF)** is a 15-item, patient-reported outcome measure developed to meet the requirements of evaluating osteoporosis treatment effectiveness. It captures the impact of osteoporosis on patients' ability to perform activities of daily living requiring physical function and was adapted from the OPAQ version 2.0.[149] This measure has been found to be suitable in detecting change in daily activities of physical function of osteoporosis patients, whether they have or have not sustained a recent fracture. Pain can be assessed with the **Visual Analog Scale**. Repeating these tests and measures during reassessments provides solid, objective documentation of the patient's progress and response to the intervention program.

Intervention

Physical therapy intervention will often focus on patient education, pain management, reducing risk of falls and fear of falling, and remodeling bone tissue. Intervention for patients who have sustained a hip fracture or Colles fracture of the wrist as a result of a fall will differ from those who have sustained vertebral fractures. Rehabilitation after a hip fracture or Colles fracture should address impairments in lower or upper extremity strength and endurance, disturbances in balance, and gait impairments. Additional emphasis should be placed on education aimed at preventing further falls and establishing an appropriate exercise program for the patient to follow after discharge from physical therapy.

How do clinicians know that weight-bearing exercises are effective for adults with osteoporosis? This knowledge is based on the substantial evidence that elite athletes and long-term exercisers have greater bone mass and BMD at sites that undergo mechanical loading during exercise than age-matched sedentary individuals.[150-152]

For example, runners age 50 to 72 have approximately 40% greater vertebral trabecular bone density than nonrunners.[151] Both male and female recreational and world-class weight lifters age 20 to 40 have 10% to 35% greater lumbar spine BMD[153-155] and vertebral trabecular bone density than controls.[156,157] Heinonen et al.[158] investigated the effects of high-impact training and detraining on femoral neck structure in a group of 98 premenopausal women by applying an 18-month high-impact exercise program which involved supervised 60-minute training sessions 3 times per week. Forty-nine women were assigned to the intervention, and 49 were instructed to maintain their normal level of activity. Results from DXA scans, which are used to diagnose and follow osteoporosis, revealed increased femoral neck strength in the intervention group after 18 months. At a 3.5-year follow-up point, the exercise-induced benefits had diminished. However, the exercise benefits for physical performance, measured by lower limb power generation, were maintained 3.5 years after intervention.

Reviews of the association between physical activity and the risk of osteoporotic fractures have shown that maintaining a physically active lifestyle reduces the risk of hip fracture, although most of the evidence is based on observational studies. Despite there being a lack of evidence from randomized controlled trials, there is evidence from cohort studies that suggests older adults should be encouraged to maintain a physically active lifestyle.[159] Whether this affects all osteoporotic fracture sites or just those at the hip remains unknown.

Based on the impairments uncovered, intervention for those who have sustained a vertebral fracture can be directed at reducing pain; improving posture, balance, strength, and flexibility and ROM; and patient education.

Most of these interventions can be addressed by designing a comprehensive exercise program for the patient. A significant amount of research supports the use of weight-bearing and resistance exercise programs in older adults and those with osteoporosis to assist in preventing BMD loss, to improve balance and reduce the risk of falls.[160-165]

Principles of Exercise Intervention and Effects of Exercise on the Skeleton

Bone responds to force in a predictable manner described by Wolff's law. *Wolff's law states that every change in the form and function of a bone or in the function of the bone alone leads to changes in its internal architecture and in its external form.* Bone is deposited and resorbed in accordance with the stresses placed upon it. Wolff's law works not only through weight bearing through gravity (e.g., walking or running transmits forces through the limbs and results in increased BMD in the hip and lumbar spine) but also through the pull from tendons on bones that occurs when a muscle produces force. Hence increases in strength through weight training or muscle contractions that are not directly in a weight-bearing position or are in a gravity-reduced or gravity-eliminated position (e.g., supine scapular retraction) cause increased force on the bone and result in increases in bone modeling. However, this law works both ways; for example, in response to increased loads through weight training, the bone responds by increasing its mass. However, once the exercise is stopped, the bone responds again by decreasing its mass because the stress is no longer being applied. Therefore an exercise intervention program must be continuous for the effects to be maintained.

Nikander et al.[162] conducted a meta-analysis of the effect of long-term exercise on bone strength at different stages of life. Bone strength was measured by peripheral quantitative computer tomography-, magnetic resonance imaging (MRI)-, and DXA scan-based structural hip analysis. The intervention was composed of weight-bearing impact training, resistance or endurance training, or a combination of all three. The results demonstrated that there was a significant, albeit small, effect on lower extremity bone strength in prepubertal boys but no significant effect on prepubertal girls and premenopausal and postmenopausal women. However, the authors acknowledge that these disappointing results could be a consequence of the short duration and inadequate power of the trials.

The acronym of **FITTE** should be considered for all patients encountered. This means planning and progressing *F*requency, *I*ntensity, *T*ime, *T*ype, and *E*njoyment. The American College of Sports Medicine (ACSM) emphasizes the importance of strength training for older adults to assist in prevention of loss of muscle mass and bone density.[166]

American College of Sports Medicine Exercise Recommendations for Adults over the Age of 65 Years (or Adults with Chronic Conditions, such as Arthritis)[166]

- Do moderately intense aerobic exercise 30 minutes a day/5 times per week

or

- Do vigorously intense aerobic exercise 20 minutes a day/3 times per week

and

- Do 8 to 10 strengthening exercises, with 10 to 15 reps/exercise, 2 to 3 times per week

and

- Have a physical activity plan

Any exercise must be intense enough to challenge the system to adapt based on Wolff's law but not so intense as to cause a fracture. In old age, the bones' responsiveness to mechanical loading has been reported to decline, peak strains and strain rates become lower, and the range of loading configurations is more limited.[136] Unfortunately, there is no research to call upon regarding dose-response relationships to exercise; therefore no easy method is available to make this determination except clinical judgment. The fracture point of any bone is determined by its current BMD, the forces applied to the bone, and the moment caused by that force (i.e., the location of the application of the force; e.g., 2.3 kg [5 lbs] in the hand creates a greater moment at the shoulder than 2.3 kg [5 lbs] at the elbow). An adult with good posture who has a normal BMD can perform exercises that increase the flexion force on the spine, such as abdominal crunches, without risk of vertebral fracture. This is because the moment arm is small (see Figure 31-13), and the force is at a level the normal bone can tolerate. However, if a patient has osteoporosis and presents with a significant kyphosis (see Figure 31-13), the same exercise could result in an anterior vertebral fracture. In this case, the moment is much larger and the bones lack the BMD to withstand this amount of force. Clinicians should be aware that the resultant forces on bone are those arising from muscle contraction and should consider the effect of positioning of the patient during exercise to maximize the forces on bone without causing injury to the bone.

The exercise intervention must also be specific to the anatomical site and varied so that the system continues to adapt and improve. If strengthening the back extensors is the goal, the clinician must ensure that the exercises prescribed specifically strengthen the extensors. In addition, the frequency and intensity of the exercise, as well as the manner in which the bone and muscle are used, must be varied so that they can adapt appropriately. For example, performing 10 repetitions of standing hip abduction against the resistance of light elastic bands or tubing 3 times a week for an entire month is not enough of a varied

stimulus to achieve gains in bone or muscle. The intensity and/or frequency must be increased, and other exercises aimed at strengthening the same muscle must be incorporated into the treatment program. A meta-analysis showed that programs combining random or high-impact exercise with resistance training increased bone mass at the hip and lumbar spine.[161] High-impact activity alone only promoted increased hip bone density. A high-intensity multipurpose exercise program has also been found to have more beneficial effects, including BMD gains in the femoral neck and lumbar spine in addition to a reduced falls rate when compared with a low-intensity, low-frequency program.[167] The multipurpose exercise program included an aerobic warm-up, static and dynamic balance training, functional gymnastics, isometric strength training and stretching sequences, upper body strength exercises, and a home exercise program emphasizing strength and flexibility.

Basic Principles of Osteoporosis Exercise Training

- Intensity must be sufficient to challenge the system
- Exercise must be specific to the anatomical site
- Exercise must be varied so that the system can continue to adapt

Exercise in Postmenopausal Women and Osteoporosis

Many national and international organizations, such as the International Osteoporosis Foundation, advocate the use of physical activity or exercise for the prevention of bone loss, falls, and fractures. Considerations that must be taken into account when prescribing exercise to osteoporotic patients include how to safely modify exercises when mobility or posture is altered and will exercise increase the risk of falls or fractures.

Because women are much more likely to develop osteoporosis than men, most of the research on the effects of exercise in osteoporosis have included only women. In addition, much more research has been conducted on postmenopausal women than on postmenopausal women with osteoporosis. Studies have shown that structured exercise programs that use a combination of odd- and high-impact loading with resistance training significantly improve BMD in the femoral neck and lumbar spine in postmenopausal women.[168] High-impact loading refers to vertical jumps, rope jumps, and running. Odd-impact loading refers to aerobic and step classes, bounding activities, agility exercises, and games that require movement in directions to which the body is not accustomed. Weight-bearing exercises such as walking are important for BMD of the hips and lower extremities. In postmenopausal women, Nelson et al.[169] found a reduced loss of trabecular bone density in the lumbar spine after a 1-year walking program. In their study, Chow et al.[170] used a control group, an aerobic exercise group, and an aerobic exercise plus weight-training group. The two exercise groups were followed 3 times a week for 1 year. At the end of the study, both groups demonstrated a 4% to 8% increase in bone mass, whereas the control group had a 1.1% loss. In addition to strength training, tai chi may improve coordination, equilibrium, and flexibility, and lead to fall reduction. Its effect on bone mass has been comparable to moderate-speed or slow walking exercises.[171] More evidence is required to confirm whether tai chi has a role in the prevention or treatment of osteoporosis.

A study by Bergstrom et al. included 121 women 45 to 65 years of age, with forearm fractures and a T-score of −1.0 to −3.0.[160] The women were separated into an exercise group and a control group. The exercise group completed 30 minutes of fast walking 3 times a week in addition to one or two sessions in a gym. The gym routine included a 5-minute warm-up, 25 minutes of strength work, 25 minutes of aerobic work, and 5 minutes of stretching. The women in the control group were not given any intervention but were free to participate in physical activity if they chose. BMD was measured at baseline and after 1 year of intervention. The total hip BMD in the exercise group increased 0.58% and in the control group decreased 0.36%. No significant effects of training were seen in the lumbar spine. These results indicate a small but positive effect of the exercise intervention on hip BMD in this group of postmenopausal women with low BMD. In a study involving postmenopausal women with osteoporosis, Krolner et al.[172] had women age 50 to 73 who had had a previous Colles' fracture participate in 8 months of aerobic exercise. The exercise group showed a 3.5% increase in lumbar BMD, whereas the control group, who performed no specific exercise program, showed a 2.5% decrease. Chow et al.[173] designed an exercise program to improve functional capacity and to provide social interaction through 30 minutes of aerobic exercise, such as dance or walking, and 30 minutes of strength training performed at low loads with high (10 to 30) repetitions. The results were compared with a control group of individuals who did not exercise and had no improvement in maximum oxygen volume (VO_2 max) from baseline testing and 2 years later. After 2 years of 3 times weekly exercise, the exercise group demonstrated significantly fewer vertebral fractures than the control group: 3 of 53 women in the exercise group suffered fractures, compared with 7 of 37 women in the control group.

Exercise has also been shown to be effective in the treatment of vertebral fractures and in increasing back extensor strength. Bennell et al.[168] investigated the efficacy of a physical therapy program incorporating manual therapy techniques, clinician-led exercises, and home exercises designed to reduce back pain, increase back extensor strength and lower limb muscle strength, and improve posture, trunk stability, and trunk mobility in adults with osteoporosis. There were 11 participants in the intervention group and 9 in the control group. Subjects were aged 53 to 90 years, and 17 were female. Participants had sus-

tained at least one vertebral compression fracture between 3 months and 2 years previously. The intervention group attended 10 weekly sessions following a standardized progressive treatment protocol, which included postural taping, soft tissue massage, mobilizations, postural exercises, and resistance and weighted exercises. They were also given a home exercise program to follow, which included daily exercises for posture and ROM in addition to strength and control exercises to be performed 3 times a week. The control group did not receive any additional intervention or complete any home exercises during the 10-week study. Results demonstrated a significant reduction in pain during movement and at rest in addition to greater improvements in timed loaded standing, perceived change in back pain, and **Qualeffo physical function scores**. The Qualeffo is a quality of life questionnaire especially developed for patients with osteoporotic vertebral deformities.[174,175] Sinaki and Mikkelsen[105] studied women who had sustained a vertebral compression fracture. They found that resistance exercises to strengthen the back extensors led to a reduction in new fractures compared with controls, whereas exercises that strengthened the back flexors led to an increase in vertebral deformities.

An expert panel was formed by the International Osteoporosis Foundation and NOF with the mission of providing exercise recommendations for individuals with osteoporosis with no fracture history and individuals with a history of osteoporotic vertebral fracture. Their recommendations are shown in the accompanying textbox.

International Osteoporotic Association Exercise Prescription

For older adults with osteoporosis:
- Strongly recommend engagement in a multicomponent exercise program that includes resistance training in combination with balance training.
- Recommend that these individuals do not engage in aerobic exercise to the exclusion of resistance or balance training.

For older adults with osteoporotic vertebral fracture:
- Strongly recommend engagement in a multicomponent exercise program that includes resistance training in combination with balance training. Consultation with a physical therapist is advised to ensure safe and appropriate exercise.
- Recommend individuals do not engage in aerobic exercise to the exclusion of resistance or balance training.

Some of the most compelling research on the importance of back extensor strength was performed by Sinaki et al.[106] who performed a 10-year prospective study of the effects of back extensor strengthening on postmenopausal women. In their study, 65 women age 48 to 65 years who were healthy, nonsmoking, and Caucasian and who did not participate in HRT were randomized into a back exercise or control group. The exercise group wore a backpack containing weight equal to 30% of their maximum isometric back extensor strength and lifted the weight 10 times while prone. This was performed daily, 5 days a week. The weight was increased, but not to more than 22.7 kg (50 lbs). Every 4 weeks, muscle strength and physical activity were assessed, and proper lifting and good posture were reviewed with the subjects. After 2 years, the exercise group discontinued the exercise, and the subjects were not monitored. Eight years later, the subjects were reevaluated; 27 of the exercise group and 23 of the control group returned. Follow-up testing revealed more vertebral fractures in the control group than in the exercise group (30% vs. 11% of subjects), a decrease in back extensor strength from baseline in both groups (16.5% in the exercise group and 27% in the controls), and significantly greater BMD of the spine in the exercise group. The author of this study acknowledged that the muscle resistance with a heavy backpack could be too strenuous for fragile women with osteoporosis. In this case, low-intensity back strengthening without a backpack can improve back extensor strength and quality of life.[176]

Clinical Note

Studies have shown that an increase in relative spinal extensor strength can lead to reduced thoracic kyphosis, fewer vertebral fractures, and less loss of height and anterior rib cage pain,[177–179] as well as to decreased pain, increased mobility, and overall improvement of quality of life.[180]

Key Points in the Treatment of Osteoporosis

- Exercise intervention in older adults with osteoporosis may not increase BMD, but it can slow age-related loss of BMD
- Flexion exercises are **contraindicated** in adults with osteoporosis and a low BMD score
- Strengthening of the back extensor muscles is critical
- Osteoporosis is a childhood disease that does not manifest until old age; *prevention is paramount*

Even in light of the convincing evidence of the positive effects of increased trunk extensor strength, implementing extensor strengthening can be difficult in older adults. It requires implementation of exercises that can increase axial stability without causing vertebral wedging or fracture. By the time they are seen for treatment, many of these patients have an increased thoracic kyphosis and a forward head posture that makes even lying supine difficult. These postural deviations, along with decreased shoulder flexibility and decreased cervical rotation, can also make lying prone difficult, if not impossible. If the patient cannot tolerate supine or prone lying, he or she may start in a seated position to perform back extension exercises and progress to prone. The supine position can be modified with pillows used as needed to support the flexed spine. Initial treatments may be as basic as emphasizing attempts at lying supine with slowly decreasing support as the spine gently lengthens and extends so that the patient can eventually lie with one or no pillows under the head. This may not be a possibility for some patients because of long-standing bony deformities. A comprehensive extension and postural reeducation program designed specifically for this population is presented in *Walk Tall!* by Sara Meeks.[181] The book includes diagrams for each exercise and is spiral bound, making it easy to follow. As aforementioned, sitting is also a good option if the patient cannot tolerate the supine position. However, the proprioceptive feedback from the plinth can help the patient maintain elongation of the spine, as opposed to tilting the head up, and also lets the person know how far forward the head and/or shoulders are. Once a comfortable, lengthened, and extended supine position has been achieved, gentle cervical and thoracic extension can be initiated through isometrics, such as pushing the back of the head and the shoulders into a plinth. Progressions from here include extending one leg along the surface of the plinth keeping the leg in alignment with the hip and pulling the toes toward the knee, extending the heel. This will assist in lengthening the quadratus lumborum and hip flexors while strengthening the quadriceps and ankle dorsiflexor muscles. This can be progressed to actively pushing the outstretched leg into the plinth, which will engage the hip extensors, lower erector spinae, and the ankle dorsiflexor muscles. The last two progressions not only assist in back alignment and strengthening, but will also improve hip alignment and strength.[136] Older adults who tend toward a flexed posture will likely have tight hip flexors, hamstrings, quadriceps, and calf muscles. These muscles all need to be stretched as the clinician works on gaining extension and length throughout the spine. The same difficulties in positioning need to be addressed to stretch the lower extremities as those addressed in working on spinal extension (e.g., supine with pillows under the head and progressing to fewer or no pillows). Positioning in side lying can be a good way for the clinician to stretch the quadriceps and hip flexors manually.

If the patient can tolerate lying prone, various extension exercises can be performed (Figure 31-17). These include arm and leg lifts, with the arms at the side, out to the side, or overhead. Combinations of arms only, legs only, or ipsilateral and contralateral arm and leg can all be used. Because these exercises can be difficult, the clinician should start with one extremity only and progress to alternating the same extremity. The last step in the progression should be extension of all four extremities together or alternating arm and leg extension, which can be difficult for patients to coordinate. For those who are familiar with yoga and have patients who practice it, poses such as the cobra and locust may be familiar (Figure 31-18). Patients are instructed to think of extending and

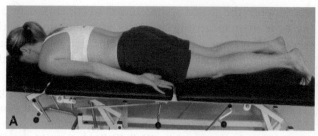
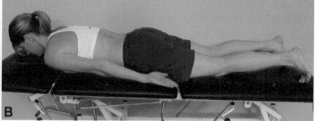

Figure 31-17 Upper back lift. This intermediate exercise strengthens the back muscles. **A,** The patient lies face down on the plinth with a pillow under the hips and lower part of the abdomen. A rolled towel may be used to cushion the forehead. Keeping the arms at the sides and the head in line with the neck and torso, the patient tightens the abdominal muscles. The individual must focus on keeping the shoulders down so that they do not shrug up toward the ears. **B,** The patient inhales and raises the head and chest a few inches off the plinth. Breathing normally, the patient holds this position for 5 seconds and then returns to the starting position. The patient rests for a few seconds and then repeats this exercise 5 to 10 times, as the person is able.

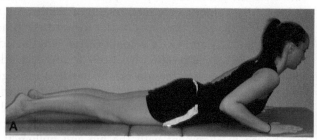
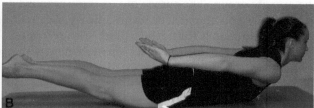

Figure 31-18 Yoga poses. **A,** Cobra pose. **B,** Locust pose.

lengthening through the extremities as they lift to promote elongation of the spine and to avoid compressing the back. However, Sinaki[182] discusses a case series to raise awareness of the effect of strenuous yoga flexion exercises on the spines of patients with osteoporosis or osteopenia. The case series described three females who were previously healthy, physically active, and had low BMD. These patients experienced new pain and fracture areas following participation in yoga flexion exercises. Clinicians should educate patients on the merits and dangers of poses involving flexion. Although yoga can be a beneficial exercise for improving balance, posture, and flexibility, some of the poses may exceed the biomechanical limits of the spine. In her paper, Sinaki explained that compressive forces of the spine during flexion exercises are increased in yoga because of the contraction of the spinal flexor muscles and the strain of the longitudinal ligaments of the spine in a position in which ability of the discs to absorb shock is reduced.[182]

Manual therapy can also be an effective treatment intervention to address back pain in adults with osteoporosis. Bautmans et al.[183] investigated thoracic spine mobilization in a group of 48 postmenopausal females with osteoporosis. The subjects were divided into a control group ($n = 19$) and an intervention group ($n = 29$). The intervention group participated in 18 sessions of spinal rehabilitation with a physical therapist. Sessions were designed to correct the posture of the thoracic spine by gentle mobilizations using manual techniques, taping, and exercises for postural correction. The control group did not receive physical therapy treatment

until the conclusion of the study. Thoracic kyphosis was measured at baseline and after 3 months using a Spinal Mouse device, which is a handheld inclinometer connected to a computer that provided data on the inclination angles at each vertebral segment. Of the 21 subjects who completed the intervention, 15 attended more than 50% of the sessions. The results showed that thoracic kyphosis significantly improved in the intervention group. However, due to study design, it is not possible to determine which mechanism leads to thoracic kyphosis improvement. A further limitation was the relatively poor compliance to rehabilitation. The impact of manual mobilizations to the thoracic spine needs further investigation before recommendations can be made on whether it is beneficial to include the technique in treatment programs for osteoporotic patients with thoracic kyphosis.

Aquatic therapy has garnered more research attention in recent years. It can provide a useful alternative to land training in patients who have fear of falls, poor balance, pain, or lack of motivation. Arnold et al.[184] compared an aquatic exercise program with land exercise and a sedentary control in a group of 68 women with osteoporosis. The interventions were standardized for time and frequency, each lasting 50 minutes, 3 times a week for 20 weeks. The women in the control group were instructed to not change their activity level or participate in any new exercise programs for the 20-week period. Only one balance measure, the backward tandem walk, significantly improved in the aquatic exercise group compared with the land training group. Function and quality of life did not significantly differ compared with the control group at follow-up testing. The authors concluded that the improvement in balance and global change suggested aquatic training could be a viable alternative for those who have difficulty exercising on land. A group in Brazil has investigated the benefits of high-intensity aquatic exercises on BMD, bone metabolism, and bone mass in postmenopausal women.[185,186] The intervention consisted of a 24-week aquatic program, lasting 50 minutes, 3 days per week. The control group was sedentary for the 24-week period. Measures were taken at baseline and after 24 weeks. The results of these studies showed a reduction in pain, number of falls, and an increase in physical fitness. Regarding effects on the skeleton, there was an attenuation of bone resorption and enhanced bone formation, which prevented a reduction in the BMD of the greater trochanter. In women with vertebral fractures, there was an incremental rise in BMD and T-score of the femoral head.

Compression Fractures

The primary goal of treatment for patients with vertebral fractures is the same for those without fractures: getting to a point where the patient can tolerate extension exercises. Initially, intervention is likely to focus on addressing pain, instructing the patient in proper body mechanics for transfers, and perhaps fitting the patient with a corset or lumbosacral orthosis.[187,188]

Fall Prevention

Because more than 90% of hip fractures occur as a direct result of a fall,[120] and two thirds of those who sustain a hip fracture do not return to their premorbid functional level,[189] a comprehensive treatment program for patients with osteopenia or osteoporosis must include interventions designed to prevent or reduce the likelihood of falling. Functional decline and fear of falling are severe threats to independence and quality of life in older individuals. Inactivity and low physical activity levels, reduced muscle strength, and hyperkyphosis all have been shown to be risk factors for falling and hip fracture.[102,190-196] Conversely, a large body of research has shown that higher physical activity levels and greater strength lower the risk of falling and subsequent fractures in both women and men. Clinicians can best address the risk of falling by stressing the importance of increased physical activity, even if the activity is not enough to increase strength in a very frail individual; they also can emphasize strengthening exercises for the muscle groups most likely to help improve balance, such as the hip abductors, hip extensors, and calf musculature, which are important in righting reactions. The most important elements of the exercise program are balance and strength training, and secondarily flexibility and endurance training.[197] A meta-analysis has shown that physically challenging balance training and a high amount and frequency of exercise are the components of the most successful programs in reducing falls.[198] Walking or resistance training alone may not have a significant effect on falls and if used for falls, prevention should be combined with some type of three-dimensional balance training.[164] Three-dimensional training is described as constant movement in a controlled, fluid, repetitive way through all three spatial planes and can include tai chi or dance. Clinicians should search for group or community programs in which patients can enroll for multicomponent exercise programs. This type of community and peer support may increase the likelihood of follow-through after discharge, as well as improve the patient's social interactions, which also makes carryover more probable. Clinicians must keep in mind that strengthening exercises need to be of sufficient intensity to achieve strength gains. Performing a 1-RM or a 10-RM test for lower extremity muscles can guide selection of the appropriate weight. Strength gains have been found in older adults with either increases in resistance or increases in repetitions.[199,200] Gains in functional abilities have also been found with regimens that vary from 1 to 3 times a week.[200]

Other areas that must be addressed to reduce the risk of falls include vision, ROM limitations, the home setting (e.g., lighting, throw rugs, small pets underfoot), cognition, a previous history of falling, which may lead to fear of falls, co-morbidities, provision of assistive devices, footwear, provision of hip protectors, and medication use.

Osteoporosis in Men

Osteoporosis has traditionally been thought of as a women's disease but in recent years, the idea that bone loss is an inevitable part of aging in men has stimulated more discussion of this issue. Men in their 50s do not experience the rapid loss of bone that women do in the time following menopause. Because men have larger skeletons, their bone loss starts later and progresses more slowly than in females. However, by the time men reach the age of 65 to 70, they lose bone mass at the same rate as women and the absorption of calcium, an essential nutrient for bone health, decreases in both males and females.[201] The NOF recommends men take part in weight-bearing exercises, such as hiking, jogging, brisk walking, racquet sports, basketball, or soccer for 30 minutes on most days of the week.[202] NOF also recommends muscle strengthening or resistance exercises, such as lifting weights, using elastic exercise bands, weight machines, or body weight exercises 2 to 3 times per week. Clinicians must remember when treating male patients that osteoporosis and fractures also occur in men and that investigation and treatment are needed alongside educating male patients on bone health measures.[203]

Risk Factors for Osteoporosis in Men

- Chronic diseases that affect the kidneys, lungs, stomach, and intestines or alter hormone levels
- Regular use of certain medications, such as immunosuppressive drugs
- Undiagnosed low testosterone levels
- Unhealthy lifestyle habits, such as excessive alcohol consumption, low calcium intake, and inadequate physical activity
- Age—older men are at greater risk
- Race—Caucasian men are at higher risk

Osteoporosis in the Young and Physically Disabled

Osteoporosis is often associated with older people, but it can affect children. In very young children, it can be caused by underlying diseases, such as osteogenesis imperfecta. In addition, in young people with complex disease or disability, the effects of medication and reduced mobility can lead to an increased risk of developing osteoporosis. Percutaneous endoscopic gastrostomy (PEG) feeding is sometimes used to supplement the diets of those at risk of developing aspirational pneumonia or with an inability to eat sufficient quantities of food, both of which can be common problems in young adults with complex care needs. Studies have shown that PEG feeding over time can result in malabsorption of nutritional components, such as calcium in the duodenum, which can lead to inadequate intake of crucial vitamins and minerals.[204,205] The reduced muscle activity and thus reduced physical activity seen in conditions such as cerebral palsy can lead to reduced bone size and reduced BMD. The effect of reduced physical activity levels was studied in a group of 38 subjects (under 40 years of age) with varying levels of physical disability.[206] Bone scans of the radius were performed using a bone sonometer. Results confirmed that immobility is associated with bone loss and that subjects who were PEG-fed were at a higher risk of diminished BMD. Clinicians should be cognizant of this when treating patients with complex physical disabilities, especially if teaching manual handling techniques to family or caregivers and when providing therapeutic exercise programs.

Postsurgical Management of Vertebral Fractures

Kyphoplasty

Although rehabilitation is not needed to help patients to recover from kyphoplasty, these individuals do benefit from treatment to address other issues related to the fracture. They may need to be seen for the same issues that a person without a fracture would require rehabilitation: abnormal posture (i.e., increased kyphosis), weakness of the back extensors and lower extremity muscles required for balance, fall prevention and balance training, and education about lifestyle modifications.

PAGET'S DISEASE OF BONE AND PRIMARY HYPERPARATHYROIDISM

Clinicians are extremely unlikely to see patients referred with either PDB or PHPT as a primary diagnosis. However, both conditions can result in osteopenia and osteoporosis and therefore are included to alert the clinician to other diagnoses that must be considered in the overall treatment of patients and to present some basic information about epidemiology, signs, and symptoms to facilitate proper diagnosis.

Paget's Disease of Bone (PDB)

PDB is the most common bone disorder after osteoporosis. It affects approximately 3% of people in the United States over age 50 and 10% of those over age 80; however, its incidence appears to be decreasing.[207] PDB is most common in the United Kingdom and in those of European descent. It is uncommon in Africans and Asians. This disease is often asymptomatic and is discovered incidentally through radiographs or an increase in serum alkaline phosphatase activity.[208] Bone pain is the most common symptom of the disease. It involves accelerated bone resorption followed by deposition of a dense and disorganized bone matrix.[209] Physical therapists may never see these patients because medical intervention (e.g., a course of bisphosphonates) is very effective in reducing the bone pain, and this reduction can last for years after cessation of the medication.[207]

Because of the structural weakness of pagetic bone, the most common complications are pain, structural deformity, and fracture. If a diagnosis of PDB has not been made in an individual presenting for rehabilitation, specific physical symptoms can alert the clinician to this diagnosis (see textbox in Part A, p 1116).

The bone pain reported by patients with PDB can be distinguished from pain caused by osteoarthritis because the pain increases with rest, with weight bearing, when the limbs are warm, and at night. It is continuous and reported to be a dull, boring pain.[207] Rehabilitation is aimed primarily at reducing pain through the use of acupuncture, transcutaneous electrical nerve stimulation, or other physical agents, aquatic exercise, or land-based exercises that do not put stress on the affected bone or bones.[210-212] Orthotic devices, such as walking aids, can help with specific problems, such as limb shortening, in addition to reducing pain caused by musculoskeletal changes and deformities.[212] Other potential rehabilitation interventions include bracing for structural abnormalities (e.g., bowing of the lower limb) in an attempt to realign the bones to provide for proper weight bearing; correction for leg length differences that may also result from bony deformities; and bracing for the spine in the case of spontaneous compression fractures resulting from unstable bone.

The brittleness of pagetic bone can lead to spontaneous fracture, and these occur most commonly in the femur, tibia, humerus, and forearm.[213] In the case of fracture resulting from PDB, healing is slow because of the altered mechanical structure of the bone itself. Nonunion of fractures in PDB has been reported to be as high as 40%, especially when the fracture involves the proximal femur.[214,215] In addition, increased weight bearing through the bone, which stimulates bone growth and remodeling in healthy individuals, is a less effective process in individuals with PDB. Osteoarthritis secondary to Paget's disease eventually may require a total joint replacement or tibial osteotomy. Exercise intervention for those requiring joint replacement should take into consideration other lesions or areas affected by the disease that may require modification of traditional intervention so as to not cause fracture at another site. In addition, as with fractures that are not treated surgically, rehabilitation will be extended because of the abnormalities of the bone structure.

The key point that clinicians should remember with individuals with PDB, whether they are being treated for complications of the disease or for other diagnoses, is that the bone remodeling process in the affected areas is abnormal and produces a weak bone structure that is susceptible to fracture. Treatment of those who have undergone orthopedic surgery to repair fractures will likely be extended compared with those with normal bone status.

Primary Hyperparathyroidism

The function of the parathyroid glands is to maintain serum calcium concentrations and to regulate bone metabolism. In PHPT, overproduction of PTH results in an increase in the release of calcium from the bones and into the blood. Hyperparathyroidism increases bone breakdown and replaces bone with fibrous tissue, resulting in generalized bone demineralization, resorption, and pathological fractures. Women are affected 2 to 3 times more often than men, and the average age at diagnosis is 55 years. Over 15 years, 60% of untreated asymptomatic patients will lose >10% of their bone density.[216] BMD loss is greater in cortical bone (e.g., the forearm) than in trabecular bone (e.g., the spine) or in mixed cortical and trabecular bone (e.g., the hip).

Other than bone pain, symptoms can include thirst, generalized weakness, osteoporosis, kidney stones, polyuria, and constipation. In its severest form, pathological fractures occur as a result of advanced osteoporosis. However, it is now extremely uncommon for the disease to progress to an advanced stage without being recognized during routine laboratory work.

For clinicians, the primary consideration in hyperparathyroidism is that osteoporosis at a relatively young age (i.e., approximately 55 years) should serve as a warning of the possibility of this condition.

REFERENCES

1. Favus MJ, editor: *Primer on the Metabolic Bone Diseases and Disorders of Mineral Metabolism*, Philadelphia, 2003, Lippincott Williams & Wilkins.
2. Cosman F, de Beur S, LeBoff M, et al: Clinician's guide to prevention and treatment of osteoporosis, *Osteoporos Int* 25:2359–2381, 2014.
3. Siris E, Brenneman S, Barrett-Connor E, et al: The effect of age and bone mineral density on the absolute, excess, and relative risk of fracture in postmenopausal women aged 50-99: results from the National Osteoporosis Risk Assessment (NORA), *Osteoporos Int* 17:565–574, 2006.
4. Robling A, Castillo A, Turner C: Biomechanical and molecular regulation of bone remodeling, *Ann Rev Biomed Eng* 8:455–498, 2006.
5. Sundberg M, Gardsell P, Johnell O, et al: Physical activity increases bone size in prepubertal boys and bone mass in prepubertal girls: a combined cross-sectional and 3-year longitudinal study, *Calcif Tissue Int* 71:406–415, 2002.
6. Wasnich R, Davis J, Ross P: Spine fracture risk is predicted by non-spine fractures, *Osteoporos Int* 4:1–5, 1994.
7. Davis J, Grove J, Wasnich R, et al: Spatial relationships between prevalent and incident spine fractures, *Bone* 24:261–264, 1999.
8. Hosmer W, Genant H, Browner W: Fractures before menopause: a red flag for physicians, *Osteoporos Int* 13:337–341, 2002.
9. Lindsay R, Silverman S, Cooper C, et al: Risk of new vertebral fracture in the year following a fracture, *JAMA* 285:320–323, 2001.
10. Roux C, Fechtenbaum J, Kolta S, et al: Mild prevalent and incident vertebral fractures are risk factors for new fractures, *Osteoporos Int* 18:1617–1624, 2007.
11. Melton L, Chrischilles E, Cooper C, et al: How many women have osteoporosis? *J Bone Miner Res* 7:1005–1010, 1992.
12. Trombetti A, Herrmann F, Hoffmeyer P, et al: Survival and potential years of life lost after hip fracture in men and age-matched women, *Osteoporos Int* 13:731–737, 2002.
13. Kiebzak G, Beinart G, Perser K, et al: Undertreatment of osteoporosis in men with hip fracture, *Arch Intern Med* 162:2217–2222, 2002.
14. Panula J, Pihlajamäki H, Mattila V, et al: Mortality and cause of death in hip fracture patients aged 65 or older: a population-based study, *BMC Musculoskelet Disord* 12:105, 2011.
15. LeBlanc E, Hillier T, Pedula K, et al: Hip fracture and increased short-term but not long-term mortality in healthy older women, *Arch Intern Med* 171:1831–1837, 2011.
16. Morrison R, Chassin M, Siu A: The medical consultant's role in caring for patients with hip fracture, *Ann Intern Med* 128:1010–1020, 1998.
17. World Health Organization (WHO): Assessment of fracture risk and its application to screening for postmenopausal osteoporosis: report of a WHO Study Group, *World Health Organ Tech Rep Ser* 843:1–129, 1994.
18. Kanis J, Oden A, Johansson H, et al: FRAX® and its applications to clinical practice, *Bone* 44:734–743, 2009.
19. Thomas M, Lloyd-Jones D, Thadhani R: Hypovitaminosis D in medical inpatients, *N Engl J Med* 338:777–783, 1998.
20. Harris S, Soteriades E, Coolidge J, et al: Vitamin D insufficiency and hyperparathyroidism in a low income, multiracial, elderly population, *J Clin Endocrinol Metab* 85:4125–4130, 2000.
21. Zadshir A, Tareen N, Pan D, et al: The prevalence of hypovitaminosis D among US adults: data from the NHANES III, *Ethn Dis* 15(suppl 5):S5–S97, 2005.
22. Pfeifer M, Begerow B, Minne H: Vitamin D and muscle function, *Osteoporos Int* 13:187–194, 2002.
23. Cauley J, Lacroix A, Wu L, et al: Serum 25-hydroxyvitamin D concentrations and risk for hip fractures, *Ann Intern Med* 149:242–250, 2008.
24. Murad M, Elamin K, Abu Elnour N, et al: Clinical review: the effect of vitamin D on falls: a systematic review and meta-analysis, *J Clin Endocrinol Metab* 96:2997–3006, 2011.
25. Kemmler W, Häberle L, von Stengel S: Effects of exercise on fracture reduction in older adults: a systematic review and meta-analysis, *Osteoporos Int* 24:1937–1950, 2013.
26. Howe T, Shea B, Dawson L, et al: Exercise for preventing and treating osteoporosis in postmenopausal women, *Cochrane Database Syst Rev* (7),2011, CD000333.
27. Dalsky G, Stocke K, Ehsani A, et al: Weight-bearing exercise training and lumbar bone mineral content in postmenopausal women, *Ann Intern Med* 108:824–828, 1988.

28. Kanis J, Johnell O, Oden A, et al: Smoking and fracture risk: a meta-analysis, *Osteoporos Int* 16:155–162, 2005.

29. Spencer H, Rubio N, Rubio E, et al: Chronic alcoholism. Frequently overlooked cause of osteoporosis in men, *Am J Med* 80:393–397, 1986.

30. Hsia J, Langer R, Manson J, et al: Conjugated equine estrogens and coronary heart disease: the Women's Health Initiative, *Arch Intern Med* 166:357–365, 2006.

31. Grossman J, Gordon R, Ranganath V, et al: American College of Rheumatology 2010 Recommendations for the Prevention and treatment of Glucocorticoid-induced osteoporosis, *Arthritis Care Res* 62:1515–1526, 2010.

32. Fleisch H: Pharmacokinetics. In *Bisphosphonates in bone disease: from the laboratory to the patient*, Berne, 1993, University of Berne.

33. Grey A, Bolland M, Horne A, et al: Five years of anti-resorptive activity after a single dose of zoledronate–results from a randomized double-blind placebo-controlled trial, *Bone* 50:1389–1393, 2012.

34. Khosla S, Burr D, Cauley J, et al: Bisphosphonate-associated osteonecrosis of the jaw: report of a task force of the American Society for Bone and Mineral Research, *J Bone Miner Res* 22:1479–1491, 2007.

35. Dell R, Adams A, Greene D, et al: Incidence of atypical nontraumatic diaphyseal fractures of the femur, *J Bone Miner Res* 27:2544–2550, 2012.

36. McClung M, Harris S, Miller P, et al: Bisphosphonate therapy for osteoporosis: benefits, risks, and drug holiday, *Am J Med* 126:13–20, 2013.

37. Cummings S, San Martin J, McClung M, et al: Denosumab for prevention of fractures in postmenopausal women with osteoporosis, *N Engl J Med* 361:756–765, 2009.

38. Orwoll E, Teglbjærg C, Langdahl B, et al: A randomized, placebo-controlled study of the effects of denosumab for the treatment of men with low bone mineral density, *J Clin Endocrinol Metab* 97:3161–3169, 2012.

39. Bone H, Chapurlat R, Brandi M, et al: The effect of three or six years of denosumab exposure in women with postmenopausal osteoporosis: results from the FREEDOM extension, *J Clin Endocrinol Metab* 98:4483–4492, 2013.

40. Hodsman A, Bauer D, Dempster D, et al: Parathyroid hormone and teriparatide for the treatment of osteoporosis: a review of the evidence and suggested guidelines for its use, *Endocr Rev* 26:688–703, 2005.

41. Black D, Greenspan S, Ensrud D, et al: The effects of parathyroid hormone and alendronate alone and in combination in post-menopausal osteoporosis, *N Engl J Med* 349:1207–1215, 2003.

42. Cummings S, Eckert S, Krueger K, et al: The effect of raloxifene on risk of breast cancer in postmenopausal women: results from the MORE randomized trial. Multiple outcomes of Raloxifene evaluation, *JAMA* 281:2189–2197, 1999.

43. Cummings S, Ensrud K, Delmas P, et al: Lasofoxifene in postmenopausal women with osteoporosis, *N Engl J Med* 362:686–696, 2010.

44. Silverman S, Christiansen C, Genant H, et al: Efficacy of bazedoxifene in reducing new vertebral fracture risk in postmenopausal women with osteoporosis: results from a 3-year, randomized, placebo-, and active-controlled clinical trial, *J Bone Miner Res* 23:1923–1934, 2008.

45. Binkley N, Bone H, Gilligan J, et al: Efficacy and safety of oral recombinant calcitonin tablets in postmenopausal women with low bone mass and increased fracture risk: a randomized, placebo-controlled trial, *Osteoporos Int* 25:2649–2656, 2014.

46. Chesnut CI, Silverman S, Andriano K, et al: A randomized trial of nasal spray salmon calcitonin in postmenopausal women with established osteoporosis: the Prevent Recurrence of Osteoporosis Fracture Study, *Am J Med* 109:267–276, 2000.

47. MacIntyre I, Stevenson J, Whitehead M, et al: Calcitonin for prevention of post-menopausal bone loss, *Lancet* 1:900–902, 1988.

48. Knopp-Sihota J, Newburn-Cook C, Homik J, et al: Calcitonin for treating acute and chronic pain of recent and remote osteoporotic vertebral compression fractures: a systematic review and meta-analysis, *Osteoporos Int* 23:17–38, 2012.

49. Seeman E: Strontium ranelate: vertebral and non-vertebral fracture risk reduction, *Curr Opin Rheumatol* 18:S17–S20, 2006.

50. Meunier P, Slosman D, Delmas P, et al: Strontium ranelate: dose-dependent effects in established post-menopausal vertebral osteoporosis: two year randomized, placebo controlled trial, *J Clin Endocrinol Metab* 87:2060–2066, 2002.

51. Anonymous: Strontium ranelate for osteoporosis? *Drug Ther Bull* 44:29–32, 2006.

52. Papanastassiou I, Phillips F, Van Meirhaeghe J, et al: Comparing effects of kyphoplasty, vertebroplasty, and non-surgical management in a systematic review of randomized and non-randomized controlled studies, *Eur Spine J* 21:1826–1843, 2012.

53. Papanastassiou I, Filis A, Gerochristou M, et al: Controversial issues in kyphoplasty and vertebroplasty in osteoporotic vertebral fractures, *Biomed Res Int* 2014:934206, 2014.

54. Wardlaw D, Cummings SR, Van Meirhaeghe J, et al: Efficacy and safety of balloon kyphoplasty compared with non-surgical care for vertebral compression fracture (FREE): a randomised controlled trial, *The Lancet* 373:1016–1024, 2009.

55. Fribourg D, Tang C, Sra P, et al: Incidence of subsequent vertebral fracture after kyphoplasty, *Spine* 29:2270–2276, 2004.

56. Boonen S, Van Meirhaeghe J, Bastian L, et al: Balloon kyphoplasty for the treatment of acute vertebral compression fractures: 2-year results from a randomized trial, *J Bone Miner Res* 26:1627–1637, 2011.

57. Mudano A, Bian J, Cope J, et al: Vertebroplasty and kyphoplasty are associated with an increased risk of secondary vertebral compression fractures: a population-based cohort study, *Osteoporos Int* 20:819–826, 2009.

58. Martinez-Ferrer A, Blasco J, Carrasco J, et al: Risk factors for the development of vertebral fractures after percutaneous vertebroplasty, *J Bone Miner Res* 28:1821–1829, 2013.

59. Shaker J, Deftos L: *Calcium and phosphate homeostasis.* In: Endotext. www.endotext.org, (Accessed 26.08.14.).

60. Brown E: Physiology of calcium homeostasis. In Bilezikian P, Marcus R, Levine A, editors: *The parathyroids: basic and clinical concepts*, San Diego, 2001, Academic Press.

61. Watts N: Estrogens, estrogen agonists/antagonists, and calcitonin. In Rosen CJ, Bouillon R, Compston JE, Rosen V, editors: *Primer on the metabolic bone diseases and disorders of mineral metabolism*, 8 ed, Chichester, 2013, Wiley-Blackwell.

62. Leiker A, Yen T, Eastwood D, et al: Factors that influence parathyroid hormone half-life: determining if new intraoperative criteria are needed, *JAMA Surg* 148:602–606, 2013.

63. Oltmann S, Rajaei M, Sippel R, et al: Primary hyperparathyroidism across the ages: presentation and outcomes, *J Surg Res* 190:185–190, 2014.

64. Norman J, Lopez J, Politz D: Abandoning unilateral parathyroidectomy: why we reversed our position after 15000 parathyroid operations, *J Am Coll Surg* 214:260–269, 2012.

65. Wermers R, Khosla S, Atkinson E, et al: Incidence of primary hyperparathyroidism in Rochester, Minnesota, 1993-2001: an update on the changing epidemiology of the disease, *J Bone Miner Res* 21:171–177, 2006.

66. Cohen J, Gierlowsky T, Schneider A: A prospective study of hyperparathyroidism in individuals exposed to radiation in childhood, *JAMA* 264:581–584, 1990.

67. Colaço S, Si M, Reiff E, Clark O: Hyperparathyroidism after radioactive iodine therapy, *Am J Surg* 194:323–327, 2007.

68. Szalat A, Mazeh H, Freund H: Lithium-associated hyperparathyroidism: report of four cases and review of the literature, *Eur J Endocrinol* 160:317–323, 2009.

69. Vasef M, Brynes R, Sturm M, et al: Expression of cyclin D1 in parathyroid carcinomas, adenomas, and hyperplasias: a paraffin immunohistochemical study, *Mod Pathol* 12:412–416, 1999.

70. Heppner C, Kester M, Agarwal S, et al: Somatic mutation of the MEN1 gene in parathyroid tumours, *Nat Genet* 16:375–378, 1997.

71. Krebs L, Shattuck T, Arnold A: HRPT2 mutational analysis of typical sporadic parathyroid adenomas, *J Clin Endocrinol Metab* 90:5015–5017, 2005.

72. Schuffenecker I, Virally-Monod M, Brohet R, et al: Risk and penetrance of primary hyperparathyroidism in multiple endocrine neoplasia type 2A families with mutations at codon 634 of the RET proto-oncogene. Groupe D'etude des Tumeurs à Calcitonine, *J Clin Endocrinol Metab* 83:487, 1998.

73. Adam M, Untch B, Danko M, et al: Severe obesity is associated with symptomatic presentation, higher parathyroid hormone levels, and increased gland weight is primary hyperparathyroidism, *J Clin Endocrinol Metab* 95:4917–4924, 2010.

74. Rejnmark L, Vestergaard P, Mosekilde L: Nephrolithiasis and renal calcifications in primary hyperparathyroidism, *J Clin Endocrinol Metab* 96:2377–2385, 2011.

75. Silverberg S, Lewiecki E, Mosekilde L, et al: Presentation of asymptomatic primary hyperparathyroidism: proceedings of the Third International Workshop, *J Clin Endocrinol Metab* 94:351–365, 2009.

76. Bollerslev J, Rosen T, Mollerup C, et al: Effect of surgery on cardiovascular risk factors in mild primary hyperparathyroidism, *J Clin Endocrinol Metab* 94:2255–2261, 2009.

77. Vestergaard P, Mollerup C, Frokjaer V, et al: Cohort study of risk of fracture before and after surgery for primary hyperparathyroidism, *Br Med J* 321:598–602, 2000.

78. Rolighed L, Rejnmark L, Sikjaer T, et al: Vitamin D treatment in primary hyperparathyroidism: a randomized placebo controlled tiral, *J Clin Endocrinol Metab* 99:1072–1080, 2014.

79. Silverberg S, Bilezikian J: "Incipient" primary hyperparathyroidism: a "forme fruste" of an old disease, *J Clin Endocrinol Metab* 88:5348–5352, 2003.

80. Marcocci C, Cetani F: Primary hyperparathyroidism, *N Engl J Med* 365:2389–2397, 2011.

81. Bilezikian J, Brandi M, Eastell R, et al: Guideline for the management of asymptomatic primary hyperparathyroidism: summary statement from the fourth international workshop, *J Endocrinol Metab* 99:3561–3569, 2014.

82. Brasier A, Nussbaum S: Hungry bone syndrome: clinical and biochemical predictors of its occurrence after parathyroid surgery, *Am J Med* 84:654–660, 1988.

83. Bilezikian J, Khan A, Potts JJ: Guidelines for the management of asymptomatic primary hyperparathyroidism: summary statement from the third international workshop, *J Clin Endocrinol Metab* 94:335–339, 2009.

84. Law WJ, Heath H: Familial benign hypercalcemia (hypocalciuric hypercalcemia). Clinical and pathogenetic studies in 21 families, *Ann Intern Med* 102:511–519, 1985.

85. Aliyev S, Agcaoglu O, Aksoy E, et al: An analysis of whether surgeon-performed neck ultrasound can be used as the main localizing study in primary hyperparathyroidism, *Surgery* 156:1127–1131, 2014.

86. Haber R, Kim C, Inabnet W: Ultrasonography for preoperative localization of enlarged parathyroid glands in primary hyperparathyroidism: comparison with (99 m)technetium sestamibi scintigraphy, *Clin Endocrinol (Oxf)* 57:241–249, 2002.

87. Vellanki P, Lange K, Elaraj D, et al: Denosumab for management of parathyroid carcinoma-mediated hypercalcemia, *J Clin Endocrinol Metab* 99:387–390, 2014.

88. Khan A, Grey A, Shoback D: Medical management of asymptomatic primary hyperparathyroidism: proceedings of the third international workshop, *J Clin Endocrinol Metab* 94:373–381, 2009.

89. Hodin R, Angelos P, Carty S, et al: No need to abandon unilateral, *J Am Coll Surg* 215:297–300, 2012.

90. Stojadinovic A, Pribitkin E, Rosen D, et al: Unilateral vs bilateral parathyroidectomy: a healthy debate, *J Am Coll Surg* 215:300–302, 2012.

91. Abdulla A, Ituarte P, Harari A, et al: Trends in the frequency and quality of parathyroid surgery, analysis of 17082 cases over 10 years, *Ann Surg* 261:746–750, 2014.

92. Peacock M, Bilezikian J, Bolognese M, et al: Cinacalcet HCl reduces hypercalcemia in primary hyperparathyroidism across a wide spectrum of disease severity, *J Clin Endocrinol Metab* 96:E9–E18, 2011.

93. Peacock M, Bolognese M, Borofsky M, et al: Cinacalcet treatment of primary hyperparathyroidism: biochemical and bone densitometric outcomes in a five-year study, *J Clin Endocrinol Metab* 94:4860–4867, 2009.

94. Buchanan W: Sir James Paget (1814-1894), *Rheumatology (Oxford)* 42:1107–1108, 2003.

95. Galson D, Roodman G: Pathobiology of Paget's disease of bone, *J Bone Metab* 21:85–98, 2014.

96. Reddy S: Etiologic factors in Paget's disease of bone, *Cell Mol Life Sci* 63:391–398, 2006.

97. Siris E: Paget's disease of bone, *J Bone Miner Res* 13:1061–1065, 1998.

98. Crandall C, Newberry S, Diamant A, et al: Comparative effectiveness of pharmacologic treatments to prevent fractures: an updated systematic review, *Ann Intern Med* 161:711–723, 2014.

99. Burge R: Dawson-Hughes B, Solomon DH et al: Incidence and economic burden of osteoporosis-related fractures in the United States, 2005–2025, *J Bone Mineral Res* 22:465–475, 2007.

100. Old JL, Calvert M: Vertebral compression fractures in the elderly, *Am Fam Physician* 69:111–116, 2004.

101. National Institutes of Health: *Osteoporosis review,* 2005.

102. Bouxsein ML, Marcus R: Overview of exercise and bone mass, *Rheum Dis Clin North Am* 20:787–802, 1994.

103. Briggs AM, van Dieen JH, Wrigley TV, et al: Thoracic kyphosis affects spinal loads and trunk muscle force, *Phys Ther* 87:595–607, 2007.

104. Huijbregts PA: Osteoporosis: diagnosis and conservative treatment, *J Man Manip Ther* 9:143–153, 2001.

105. Sinaki M, Mikkelsen BA: Postmenopausal spinal osteoporosis: flexion versus extension exercises, *Arch Phys Med Rehabil* 65:593–596, 1984.

106. Sinaki M, Wahner HW, Offord KP, et al: Efficacy of nonloading exercises in prevention of vertebral bone loss in postmenopausal women, *a controlled trial* 64:762–769, 1989.

107. Bruno AG, Anderson DE, D'Agostino J, et al: The effect of thoracic kyphosis and sagittal plane alignment on vertebral compressive loading, *J Bone Mineral Res* 27:2144–2151, 2012.

108. Kato T, Yamashita T, Mizutani S, et al: Adolescent exercise associated with long-term superior measures of bone geometry: a cross-sectional DXA and MRI study, *Br J Sports Med* 43:932–935, 2009.

109. Ilich JZ, Badenhop NE, Matkovic V: Primary prevention of osteoporosis: pediatric approach to disease of the elderly, *Womens Health Issues* 6:194–203, 1996.

110. Dent CE: Osteoporosis in childhood, *Postgrad Med J* 53:450–457, 1977.

111. International Osteoporosis Foundation: *Know and reduce your risk of osteoporosis.* http://www.iofbonehealth.org/sites/default/files/PDFs/know_and_reduce:your_risk_english.pdf. Updated 2007. (Accessed 24.10.14..)

112. Magee JA, Stuberg WA, Schmutte GT: Bone health knowledge, self-efficacy, and behaviors in adolescent females, *Pediatr Phys Ther* 20:160–166, 2008.

113. Bonjour J, Theintz G, Buchs B, et al: Critical years and stages of puberty for spinal and femoral bone mass accumulation during adolescence, *J Clin Endocrinol Metab* 73:555–563, 1991.

114. Lu PW, Briody JN, Ogle GD, et al: Bone mineral density of total body, spine, and femoral neck in children and young adults: a cross-sectional and longitudinal study, *J Bone Miner Res* 9:1451–1458, 1994.

115. Theintz G, Buchs B, Rizzoli R, et al: Longitudinal monitoring of bone mass accumulation in healthy adolescents: evidence for a marked reduction after 16 years of age at the levels of lumbar spine and femoral neck in female subjects, *J Clin Endocrinol Metab* 75:1060–1065, 1992.

116. Geusens P, Dequeker J, Verstraeten A, et al: Age-related, sex-related, and menopause-related changes of vertebral and peripheral bone: population study using dual and single photon absorptiometry and radiogrammetry, *J Nuclear Med* 27:1540–1549, 1986.

117. Recker RR, Davies KM, Hinders SM, et al: Bone gain in young adult women, *JAMA* 268:2403–2408, 1992.

118. Welten D, Kemper H, Post G, et al: Weight-bearing activity during youth is a more important factor for peak bone mass than calcium intake, *J Bone Mineral Res* 9:1089–1096, 1994.

119. Gleeson P: Osteoporosis and the young woman, *Orthop Phys Ther Clin North Am* 7:179–198, 1998.

120. Marcus R: Role of exercise in preventing and treating osteoporosis, *Rheum Dis Clin North Am* 27:131–141, 2001.

121. Anderson J, Metz JA: Contributions of dietary calcium and physical activity to primary prevention of osteoporosis in females, *J Am Coll Nutr* 12:378–383, 1993.

122. Bailey D, McKay H, Mirwald R, et al: A six-year longitudinal study of the relationship of physical activity to bone mineral accrual in growing children: the University of Saskatchewan bone mineral accrual study, *J Bone Mineral Res* 14:1672–1679, 1999.

123. Bass S, Pearce G, Bradney M, et al: Exercise before puberty may confer residual benefits in bone density in adulthood: studies in active prepubertal and retired female gymnasts, *J Bone Mineral Res* 13:500–507, 1998.

124. Inoue T, Kushida K, Kobayashi G, et al: Exercise therapy for osteoporosis, *Osteoporosis Int* 3:166–168, 1993.

125. Ruiz J, Mandel C, Garabedian M: Influence of spontaneous calcium intake and physical exercise on the vertebral and femoral bone mineral density of children and adolescents, *J Bone Mineral Res* 10:675–682, 1995.

126. Bradney M, Pearce G, Naughton G, et al: Moderate exercise during growth in prepubertal boys: changes in bone mass, size, volumetric density, and bone strength: a controlled prospective study, *J Bone Mineral Res* 13:1814–1821, 1998.

127. Morris FL, Naughton GA, Gibbs JL, et al: Prospective ten-month exercise intervention in premenarcheal girls: positive effects on bone and lean mass, *J Bone Mineral Res* 12:1453–1462, 1997.

128. Warden SJ, Fuchs RK: Exercise and bone health: optimising bone structure during growth is key, but all is not in vain during ageing, *Br J Sports Med* 43:885–887, 2009.

129. Hoch AZ, Pajewski NM, Moraski L, et al: Prevalence of the female athlete triad in high school athletes and sedentary students, *Clin J Sport Med* 19:421–428, 2009.

130. De Souza MJ, Nattiv A, Joy E, et al: 2014 female athlete triad coalition consensus statement on treatment and return to play of the female athlete triad: 1st International Conference held in San Francisco, California, May 2012 and 2nd International Conference held in Indianapolis, Indiana, May 2013, *Br J Sports Med* 48:289, 2014.

131. Christo K, Prabhakaran R, Lamparello B, et al: Bone metabolism in adolescent athletes with amenorrhea, athletes with eumenorrhea, and control subjects, *Pediatrics* 121:1127–1136, 2008.

132. Valimaki MJ, Karkkainen M, Lamberg-Allardt C, et al: Exercise, smoking, and calcium intake during adolescence and early adulthood as determinants of peak bone mass. Cardiovascular risk in young Finns study group, *Br Med J* 309:230–235, 1994.

133. Harvey N, Cole Z, Crozier S, et al: Physical activity, calcium intake and childhood bone mineral: a population-based cross-sectional study, *Osteoporosis Int* 23:121–130, 2012.

134. Wyshak G, Frisch RE: Carbonated beverages, dietary calcium, the dietary calcium/phosphorus ratio, and bone fractures in girls and boys, *J Adolescent Health* 15:210–215, 1994.

135. Wyshak G, Frisch RE, Albright TE, et al: Nonalcoholic carbonated beverage consumption and bone fractures among women former college athletes, *J Orthop Res* 7:91–99, 1989.

136. Meeks SM: The role of the physical therapist in the recognition, assessment, and exercise intervention in persons with, or at risk for, osteoporosis, *Topics Geriatr Rehabil* 21:42–56, 2005.

137. Siminoski K: Tools and techniques: Accurate height assessment to detect hidden vertebral fractures, *Osteoporosis Update* 9(2):4, 2005.

138. Beck AT, Ward CH, Mendelson M, et al: An inventory for measuring depression, *Arch Gen Psychiatry* 4:561–571, 1961.

139. Laurent MR, Buchanan WW, Bellamy N: Methods of assessment used in ankylosing spondylitis clinical trials: a review, *Br J Rheumatol* 30:326–329, 1991.

140. Ito T, Shirado O, Suzuki H, et al: Lumbar trunk muscle endurance testing: an inexpensive alternative to a machine for evaluation, *Arch Phys Med Rehabil* 77:75–79, 1996.

141. Shipp K, Purser J, Gold D, et al: Timed loaded standing: a measure of combined trunk and arm endurance suitable for people with vertebral osteoporosis, *Osteoporos Int* 11:914–922, 2000.

142. Berg K: Measuring balance in the elderly: preliminary development of an instrument, *Physiother Can* 41:304–311, 1989.

143. Berg KO, Wood-Dauphinee SL, Williams JI, et al: Measuring balance in the elderly: validation of an instrument, *Can J Public Health* 83(suppl 2):S7–S11, 1992.

144. Tinetti ME: Performance-oriented assessment of mobility problems in elderly patients, *J Am Geriatr Soc* 34:119–126, 1986.

145. Powell LE, Myers AM: The activities-specific balance confidence (ABC) scale, *J Gerontol A Biol Sci Med Sci* 50A:M28–M34, 1995.

146. Shumway-Cook A, Baldwin M, Polissar NL, et al: Predicting the probability for falls in community-dwelling older adults, *Phys Ther* 77:812–819, 1997.

147. Shumway-Cook A, Woollacott M: Motor control: theory and practical applications, Baltimore, 1995, Williams & Wilkins.

148. Helmes E, Hodsman A, Lazowski D, et al: A questionnaire to evaluate disability in osteoporotic patients with vertebral compression fractures, *J Gerontol A Biol Sci Med Sci* 50:M91–M98, 1995.

149. Nixon A, Kerr C, Doll H, et al: Osteoporosis assessment questionnaire-physical function (OPAQ-PF): a psychometrically validated osteoporosis-targeted patient reported outcome measure of daily activities of physical function, *Osteoporosis Int* 25:1775–1784, 2014.

150. Dalén N, Olsson KE: Bone mineral content and physical activity, *Acta Orthop* 45:170–174, 1974.

151. Lane NE, Bloch DA, Jones HH, et al: Long-distance running, bone density, and osteoarthritis, *JAMA* 255:1147–1151, 1986.

152. Marcus R, Cann C, Madvig P, et al: Menstrual function and bone mass in elite women distance RunnersEndocrine and metabolic features, *Ann Intern Med* 102:158–163, 1985.

153. Colletti LA, Edwards J, Gordon L, et al: The effects of muscle-building exercise on bone mineral density of the radius, spine, and hip in young men, *Calcif Tissue Int* 45:12–14, 1989.

154. Granhed H, Jonson R, Hansson T: The loads on the lumbar spine during extreme weight lifting, *Spine* 12:146–149, 1987.

155. Heinrich CH, Going SB, Pamenter RW, et al: Bone mineral content of cyclically menstruating female resistance and endurance trained athletes, *Med Sci Sports Exerc* 22:558–563, 1990.

156. Block JE, Genant HK, Black D: Greater vertebral bone mineral mass in exercising young men, *West J Med* 145:39–42, 1986.

157. Block J, Smith R, Friedlander A, et al: Preventing osteoporosis with exercise: a review with emphasis on methodology, *Med Hypotheses* 30:9–19, 1989.

158. Heinonen A, Mäntynen J, Kannus P, et al: Effects of high-impact training and detraining on femoral neck structure in premenopausal women: a hip structural analysis of an 18-month randomized controlled exercise intervention with 3.5-year follow-up, *Physiother Can* 64:98–105, 2012.

159. Moayyeri A: The association between physical activity and osteoporotic fractures: a review of the evidence and implications for future research, *Ann Epidemiol* 18:827–835, 2008.

160. Bergström I, Landgren B, Brinck J, Freyschuss B: Physical training preserves bone mineral density in postmenopausal women with forearm fractures and low bone mineral density, *Osteoporosis Int* 19:177–183, 2008.

161. Martyn-St James M, Carroll S: Effects of different impact exercise modalities on bone mineral density in premenopausal women: a meta-analysis, *J Bone Miner Metab* 28:251–267, 2010.

162. Nikander R, Sievanen H, Heinonen A, et al: Targeted exercise against osteoporosis: a systematic review and meta-analysis for optimising bone strength throughout life, *BMC Med* 8:47, 2010.

163. Zehnacker CH, Bemis-Dougherty A: Effect of weighted exercises on bone mineral density in post menopausal women. A systematic review, *J Geriatr Phys Ther* 30:79–88, 2007.

164. Giangregorio L, Papaioannou A, MacIntyre N, et al: Too fit to fracture: exercise recommendations for individuals with osteoporosis or osteoporotic vertebral fracture, *Osteoporosis Int* 25:821–835, 2014.

165. Palombaro KM, Black JD, Buchbinder R, et al: Effectiveness of exercise for managing osteoporosis in women postmenopause, *Phys Ther* 93:1021–1025, 2013.

166. Nelson ME, Rejeski WJ, Blair SN, et al: Physical activity and public health in older adults: recommendation from the American College of Sports Medicine and the American Heart Association, *Circulation* 116:1094–1105, 2007.

167. Kemmler W, von Stengel S, Engelke K, et al: Exercise effects on bone mineral density, falls, coronary risk factors, and health care costs in older women: the randomized controlled senior fitness and prevention (SEFIP) study, *Arch Intern Med* 170:179–185, 2010.

168. Bennell KL, Matthews B, Greig A, et al: Effects of an exercise and manual therapy program on physical impairments, function and quality-of-life in people with osteoporotic vertebral fracture: a randomised, single-blind controlled pilot trial, *BMC Musculoskelet Disord* 11:36, 2010.

169. Nelson ME, Fisher EC, Dilmanian FA, et al: A 1-y walking program and increased dietary calcium in postmenopausal women: effects on bone, *Am J Clin Nutr* 53:1304–1311, 1991.

170. Chow R, Harrison JE, Notarius C: Effect of two randomised exercise programmes on bone mass of healthy postmenopausal women, *Br Med J* 295:1441–1444, 1987.

171. Sinaki M, Pfeifer M, Preisinger E, et al: The role of exercise in the treatment of osteoporosis, *Curr Osteoporosis Rep* 8:138–144, 2010.

172. Krolner B, Toft B, Nielsen SP, Tondevold E: Physical exercise as prophylaxis against involutional vertebral bone loss: a controlled trial, *Clin Sci* 64:541–546, 1983.

173. Chow R, Harrison J, Dornan J: Prevention and rehabilitation of osteoporosis program: exercise and osteoporosis, *Int J Rehabil Res* 12:49–56, 1989.

174. Whitfield K, Buchbinder R, Segal L, et al: Parsimonious and efficient assessment of health-related quality of life in osteoarthritis research: validation of the assessment of quality of life (AQoL) instrument, *Health Qual Life Outcomes* 4:19, 2006.

175. Lips P, Cooper C, Agnusdei DF, et al: Quality of life in patients with vertebral fractures: validation of the Quality of Life Questionnaire of the European Foundation for Osteoporosis (QUALEFFO), *Osteoporosis Int* 10:150–160, 1999.

176. Hongo M, Itoi E, Sinaki M, et al: Effect of low-intensity back exercise on quality of life and back extensor strength in patients with osteoporosis: a randomized controlled trial, *Osteoporosis Int* 18:1389–1395, 2007.

177. Itoi E, Sinaki M: Effect of back-strengthening exercise on posture in healthy women 49 to 65 years of age, *Mayo Clin Proc* 69:1054–1059, 1994.

178. Sinaki M, Itoi E, Wahner H, et al: Stronger back muscles reduce the incidence of vertebral fractures: a prospective 10 year follow-up of postmenopausal women, *Bone* 30:836–841, 2002.

179. Sinaki M: Critical appraisal of physical rehabilitation measures after osteoporotic vertebral fracture, *Osteoporosis Int* 14:773–779, 2003.

180. Malmros B, Mortensen L, Jensen MB, et al: Positive effects of physiotherapy on chronic pain and performance in osteoporosis, *Osteoporosis Int* 8:215–221, 1998.

181. Meeks S: *Walk tall! An exercise program for the prevention and treatment of osteoporosis*, Gainesville, 1999, Triad.

182. Sinaki M: Yoga spinal flexion positions and vertebral compression fracture in osteopenia or osteoporosis of spine: case series, *Pain Pract* 13:68–75, 2013.

183. Bautmans I, Van Arken J, Van Mackelenberg M, et al: Rehabilitation using manual mobilization for thoracic kyphosis in elderly postmenopausal patients with osteoporosis, *J Rehabil Med* 42:129–135, 2010.

184. Arnold C, Busch A, Schachter C, et al: A randomized clinical trial of aquatic versus land exercise to improve balance, function, and quality of life in older women with osteoporosis, *Physiother Can* 60:296–306, 2008.

185. Fronza FCAO, Moreira-Pfrimer LDF, dos Santos RN, et al: Effects of high-intensity aquatic exercises on bone mineral density in postmenopausal women with and without vertebral fractures, *Am J Sports Sci* 1:1–6, 2013.

186. Moreira LDF, Fronza FCA, dos Santos RN, et al: The benefits of a high-intensity aquatic exercise program (HydrOS) for bone metabolism and bone mass of postmenopausal women, *J Bone Miner Metab* 32:411–419, 2014.

187. Lord SR, Ward JA, Williams P, et al: The effect of a 12-month exercise trial on balance, strength, and falls in older women: a randomized controlled trial, *J Am Geriatr Soc* 43:1198–1206, 1995.

188. Province MA, Hadley EC, Hornbrook MC, et al: The effects of exercise on falls in elderly patients: a preplanned meta-analysis of the FICSIT trials, *JAMA* 273:1341–1347, 1995.

189. Pfeifer M, Sinaki M, Geusens P, et al: Musculoskeletal rehabilitation in osteoporosis: a review, *J Bone Mineral Res* 19:1208–1214, 2004.

190. Gregg EW, Cauley JA, Seeley DG, et al: Physical activity and osteoporotic fracture risk in older women, *Ann Intern Med* 129:81–88, 1998.

191. Cooper C, Barker DJ, Wickham C: Physical activity, muscle strength, and calcium intake in fracture of the proximal femur in Britain, *Br Med J* 297:1443–1446, 1988.

192. Coupland C, Wood D, Cooper C: Physical inactivity is an independent risk factor for hip fracture in the elderly, *J Epidemiol Community Health* 47:441–443, 1993.

193. Farmer ME, Harris T, Madans JH, et al: Anthropometric indicators and hip fracture. The NHANES I epidemiologic follow-up study, *J Am Geriatr Soc* 37:9–16, 1989.

194. Joakimsen RM, Fønnebø V, Magnus JH, et al: The tromsø study: Physical activity and the incidence of fractures in a Middle-Aged population, *J Bone Mineral Res* 13:1149–1157, 1998.

195. Meyer HE, Tverdal A, Falch JA: Risk factors for hip fracture in middle-aged Norwegian women and men, *Am J Epidemiol* 137:1203–1211, 1993.

196. Silman A, O'Neill T, Cooper C, et al: Influence of physical activity on vertebral deformity in men and women: results from the European Vertebral Osteoporosis Study, *J Bone Mineral Res* 12:813–819, 1997.

197. Gillespie LD, Robertson MC, Gillespie WJ, et al: Interventions for preventing falls in older people living in the community, *Cochrane Database Syst Rev* (2),2009, CD007146.

198. Karinkanta S, Piirtola M, Sievänen H, et al: Physical therapy approaches to reduce fall and fracture risk among older adults, *Nat Rev Endocrinol* 6:396–407, 2010.

199. Pruitt LA, Taaffe DR, Marcus R: Effects of a one-year high-intensity versus low-intensity resistance training program on bone mineral density in older women, *J Bone Mineral Res* 10:1788–1795, 1995.

200. Taaffe DR, Duret C, Wheeler S, et al: Once-weekly resistance exercise improves muscle strength and neuromuscular performance in older adults, *J Am Geriatr Soc* 47:1208–1214, 1999.

201. NIH Osteoporosis and Related Bone Diseases National Resource Center: *Osteoporosis in men.* http://www.niams.nih.gov/Health_Info/Bone/Osteoporosis/men.asp. Updated 2012. (Accessed 17.10.14.).

202. National Osteoporosis Foundation: *The man's guide to osteoporosis.* http://nof.org/files/nof/public/content/file/252/upload/85.pdf. Updated 2011. (Accessed 17.10. 14.).

203. Seeman E: *Invest in your bones - osteoporosis in men: the 'silent epidemic' strikes men too,* 2004, International Osteoporosis Foundation.

204. Duncan B, Barton LL, Lloyd J, et al: Dietary considerations in osteopenia in tube-fed nonambulatory children with cerebral palsy, *Clin Pediatr* 38:133–137, 1999.

205. Cummins A, Chu G, Faust L, et al: Malabsorption and villous atrophy in patients receiving enteral feeding, *J Parenter Enteral Nutr* 19:193–198, 1995.

206. Grainger M, Dilley C, Wood N, et al: Osteoporosis among young adults with complex physical disabilities, *Br J Nursing* 20:171–175, 2011.

207. Schneider D, Hofmann MT, Peterson JA: Diagnosis and treatment of Paget's disease of bone, *Am Fam Physician* 65:2069–2072, 2002.

208. Walsh JP: Paget's disease of bone, *Med J Aust* 181:262–265, 2004.

209. Josse RG, Hanley DA, Kendler D, et al: Diagnosis and treatment of Paget's disease of bone, *Clin Invest Med* 30:E210–E223, 2007.

210. Whyte MP: Paget's disease of bone, *N Engl J Med* 355:593–600, 2006.

211. Sutcliffe A: Paget's: the neglected bone disease, *Int J Orthop Trauma Nurs* 14:142–149, 2010.

212. Ralston SH: Paget's disease of bone, *N Engl J Med* 368:644–650, 2013.

213. Walker J: Pathogenesis, diagnosis and management of Paget's disease of the bone, *Nurs Older People* 26:32–38, 2014.

214. Bradley C, Nade S: Outcome after fractures of the femur in Paget's disease, *Aust N Z J Surg* 62:39–44, 1992.

215. Dove J: Complete fractures of the femur in Paget's disease of bone, *J Bone Joint Surg Br* 62-B:12–17, 1980.

216. Morris LG, Myssiorek D: When is surgery indicated for asymptomatic primary hyperparathyroidism? *Laryngoscope* 119:2291–2292, 2009.

OTHER RESOURCES

International Society of Clinical Densitometry www://.iscd.org.

International Osteoporosis Foundation: http://www.osteofound.org/.

Medline Plus (search for osteoporosis): http://www.nlm.nih.gov/medlineplus/osteoporosis.html.

National Osteoporosis Foundation: www.nof.org.

National Institutes of Health, Milk Matters Campaign aimed at children: http://www.nichd.nih.gov/milk/milk.cfm.

Osteoporosis Canada: http://www.osteoporosis.ca/english/home/default.asp?s=1.

U.S. Bone and Joint Decade: http://www.usbjd.org/index.cfm.

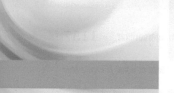

CHAPTER 32

Muscle Disease and Dysfunction

SABRINA PAGANONI, ANNE-MARIE THOMAS, WALTER R. FRONTERA

MUSCULAR DYSTROPHIES

The muscular dystrophies comprise a hereditary group of disorders arising from various genetic defects that alter the structure and function of a range of muscle proteins (Table 32-1).

Dystrophinopathies: Duchenne's Muscular Dystrophy and Becker's Muscular Dystrophy

Genetics/Epidemiology

Duchenne's muscular dystrophy (DMD) and Becker's muscular dystrophy (BMD) share a defect in the muscle protein dystrophin and an X-linked recessive mode of inheritance.[1] DMD is characterized by severely reduced or absent dystrophin, whereas BMD involves a milder dystrophinopathy with decreased or altered dystrophin. Both conditions primarily affect young males. The incidence of DMD is 1 in 3500 male births worldwide, and the incidence of BMD is 5 in 100,000.[2]

Dystrophin is a key component of the sarcolemma of skeletal and cardiac muscles. A deficiency of dystrophin leads to muscle membrane instability during contraction and relaxation (Figure 32-1).

Clinical Features: Duchenne's Muscular Dystrophy

At birth, most boys with DMD appear normal and achieve the milestones of sitting and standing with little or only slight delay. Some affected boys, however, are hypotonic and weak at birth. Subsequently, affected individuals develop a waddling gait and a tendency to walk on the toes and fall. Between the ages of 2 and 6, children with DMD develop difficulties running, jumping, and climbing stairs. The disorder has a characteristic pattern of progressive weakness (i.e., worse in the proximal muscle groups, at least initially) and consequent functional decline. Proximal lower limb muscles, such as the hip extensors, usually are affected earlier than upper extremity and torso muscles; neck flexors are affected more than extensors, and progression is more rapid in the lower extremities than in the upper extremities. Relative preservation of function is seen in the ankle plantar flexors and invertors, levator

ani, external anal sphincter, and cranial nerve–innervated muscles (except for the sternocleidomastoid muscle).[2] By age 2 to 6, most boys develop lumbar lordosis, have difficulties arising from the floor, and use the characteristic **Gower's maneuver** (Figure 32-2) to rise to a standing position.[2,3] By age 5 to 6, hypertrophy develops in certain muscle groups, especially the calves, quadriceps, gluteals, and deltoids. Initially, true hypertrophy of the calf muscle fibers occurs, but later pseudohypertrophy develops because muscle is largely replaced by fat and connective tissue (Figure 32-3).[3] By age 8, the child has difficulty with ambulation and climbing stairs, and by age 10, many patients depend on long leg braces to remain ambulatory; by age 12, most are wheelchair dependent. Bakker et al.[4] identified loss of hip extensor and ankle dorsiflexor strength as primary predictors of loss of ambulation.

Joint contractures and scoliosis occur frequently in DMD. By age 6 to 10, 70% of patients may have contractures of the iliotibial bands, hip flexors, and Achilles tendons. Ankle involvement can lead to toe walking. By age 8, most patients may also have contractures at the knee, elbow, and wrist extensors, which tend to worsen as more time is spent in the wheelchair. Scoliosis may be seen in up to 90% of wheelchair-bound patients with DMD. As paraspinal muscles weaken, kyphoscoliosis worsens. This can complicate activities of daily living (ADLs) and positioning in bed or a wheelchair, and it compounds respiratory impairment. Muscles that support ventilation usually are not significantly involved until the child becomes nonambulatory.[3] Weakness of ventilatory muscles, including the diaphragm and intercostals, is manifested by low maximum inspiratory and expiratory pressures and decreased vital capacity, forced vital capacity, and total lung capacity.[2] A restrictive defect results, with or without the previously mentioned scoliosis, and respiratory function becomes compromised.[5] Ventilatory muscle weakness can also contribute to atelectasis and reduced thoracic compliance. Diaphragmatic weakness can contribute to nocturnal hypoxemia, hypoventilation, and hypercapnic respiratory failure.[5] Without aggressive pulmonary management, respiratory insufficiency, with

TABLE **32-1**

Overview of the Muscular Dystrophies

Type	Mode of Inheritance/ Gene Location/Gene Product	Clinical Presentation	Associated Features	Diagnosis	Treatment
Duchenne's muscular dystrophy (DMD)	XR Xp2I Dystrophin	• Onset: ages 2-6yr • Delayed milestones • Progressive weakness of "girdle" muscles • Calf pseudohypertrophy • Inability to walk after age 12yr • Joint contractures • Scoliosis	• Respiratory failure in 2nd to 3rd decade • Cardiomyopathy • Impaired intellectual function • Gastroparesis	• Clinical • Increased CK • DNA analysis • In some cases, EMG and muscle biopsy	• Pharmacological: steroids • Rehabilitative: PT/ OT, ROM, contracture management, assistive devices, weight control, ambulation, seating, bracing • Pulmonary: assisted ventilation • Surgical: contracture release, spinal stabilization for scoliosis
Becker's muscular dystrophy (BMD)	XR Xp21 Dystrophin	• Onset: variable, but still ambulatory after age 15yr • Progressive weakness of girdle muscles • Calf pseudohypertrophy • Respiratory failure after 4th decade	• Cardiomyopathy • Impaired intellectual function	• As in DMD	• As in DMD
Facioscapulohumeral muscular dystrophy (FSHD)	AD 4q35	• Onset: 1st to 5th decade • Slowly progressive weakness of the face, shoulder girdle and scapular stabilizers, core and pelvic girdle muscles, tibialis anterior	• Pain in the neck, shoulders, posterior chest, lower back • Sensorineural hearing loss and retinal abnormalities in infantile-onset FSHD • Weakness of muscles of ventilation and cardiomyopathy possible in rare cases	• Clinical • CK: normal/ slightly elevated • EMG: myopathic • Muscle bx: myopathic changes • DNA analysis is gold standard for diagnosis	• Pharmacological: none • Rehabilitation: PT, OT, bracing, pain management • Surgical: scapular stabilization

(Continued)

TABLE 32-1

Overview of the Muscular Dystrophies—cont'd

Type	Mode of Inheritance/ Gene Location/Gene Product	Clinical Presentation	Associated Features	Diagnosis	Treatment
Emery-Dreifuss muscular dystrophy (EDMD)	XR Xq28 Emerin AD 1q11 Lamin A/C Mutations in other genes have been identified in selected individuals with an EDMD clinical phenotype	• Triad 1. Early contractures 2. Slowly progressive muscle weakness in humeroperoneal distribution 3. Cardiac abnormalities	• Sudden death from cardiac conduction defects • Gene mutations may manifest as isolated cardiomyopathy	• Clinical • CK: normal/ slightly increased • ECG: conduction abnormalities and arrhythmias • EDX: myopathic • DNA analysis	• Pharmacological: none • Cardiac evaluation, may require pacemaker and or implanted defibrillator • Rehabilitation: contracture management • Surgical: contracture release
Limb-girdle muscular dystrophy	Multiple	• Onset: childhood to adulthood • Slowly progressive muscle weakness in pelvic girdle and shoulder girdle • Cardiac abnormalities (10%) • Onset: late childhood to adolescence	• Respiratory insufficiency	• Clinical, family history • CK: elevated • EDX: myopathic • Muscle bx: necrosis and regeneration, variable fiber size, increased connective tissue • DNA analysis	• Pharmacological: ?Creatine monohydrate • Cardiac monitoring • Rehabilitation: PT, OT to maintain mobility, minimize contractures, provide assistive devices • Ventilatory support
Myotonic muscular dystrophy	AD 19q13 Myotonic dystrophy Protein kinase	• Onset: any age • Slowly progressive muscle weakness in face, distal limb • Percussion myotonia	• Cataracts, cardiac abnormalities, respiratory abnormalities, gastrointestinal abnormalities, CNS abnormalities, endocrine abnormalities	• Clinical • EDX: myotonic discharges • Muscle bx: myopathic • DNA analysis	• Pharmacological: medications for myotonia • Rehabilitation: PT, OT for contracture management, assistive devices, modification of ADLs

XR, X-linked recessive; *CK,* creatine kinase; *DNA,* deoxyribonucleic acid; *EMG,* electromyography; *PT,* physical therapy; *OT,* occupational therapy; *ROM,* range of motion; *AD,* autosomal dominant; *bx,* biopsy; *ECG,* electrocardiography; *EDX,* electrodiagnostics; *CNS,* central nervous system; *ADLs,* activities of daily living.

DMD: Etiology and Pathology

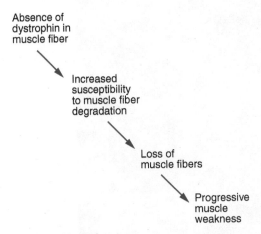

Figure 32-1 Dystrophin dysfunction.

or without pneumonia, may result in death by age 20.[6] The age at which vital capacity falls below 1 L has been reported to be a strong marker of mortality, with a 5-year survival rate of 8%.[7,8]

Dystrophin is also a component of cardiac muscle, smooth muscle, and brain. Therefore the heart, gastrointestinal (GI) tract, and central nervous system (CNS) may manifest abnormalities. Up to 90% of patients with DMD may show characteristic electrocardiographic abnormalities consisting of tall R waves and deep, narrow Q waves in leads I, aV_L, V_5, and V_6, attributable to fibrosis in the posterobasal left ventricle.[2,9] Other patients may show conduction defects, arrhythmias, sinus tachycardia, or cardiomyopathy.[2,9] Up to 40% of patients with DMD may succumb to cardiomyopathy if they also have ventilatory failure and pulmonary hypertension.[2] GI tract manifestations can include vomiting, abdominal pain, and distention caused by acute gastric dilation.[2,9] CNS involvement may include a lower IQ (i.e., below 70-75) in approximately 20% to 30% of patients.[2,9] Bresolin et al.[10] found the mean IQ of patients with DMD to be 82.

Fractures occur in approximately 20% of DMD patients.[11] They can be caused by falls resulting from unsteady gait or by osteoporosis related to disuse in wheelchair-bound patients, and steroid treatment.[3]

Clinical Features: Becker's Muscular Dystrophy
Patients with BMD show a pattern of muscle weakness and atrophy similar to that seen in DMD. Some key differences include a later onset of clinical manifestations (usually after age 5) and the preservation of ambulatory capacity past age 15.[2,3] Unlike with DMD, early in the course of BMD the patient is able to run, hop, lift the head off the bed, and get up from the floor without using Gower's maneuver.[3] Of patients with DMD, 50% may be symptomatic by age 10 and 90% are by age 20.[2] Clinical phenotype can be quite variable even within affected families. Approximately 50% of patients becomes

nonambulatory by the fourth decade.[3] Ventilatory muscle failure usually does not occur until after the fourth decade.[2] Cardiac abnormalities are similar to those seen in DMD.[2,9] Some patients actually manifest only with cardiomyopathy or, with other milder disease phenotypes such as myalgias or asymptomatic elevation in creatine kinase (CK) levels.

Diagnosis of Duchenne's and Becker's Muscular Dystrophies
The presenting clinical features contribute to the diagnosis of DMD and BMD. Laboratory evaluation shows markedly elevated CK levels. In DMD, CK may be elevated as much as 50 to 100 times above normal very early in the course of the disease. It usually peaks by age 3 and falls by approximately 20% each year as a result of muscle loss.[2] In BMD, CK may by elevated 25 to 200 times above normal during the first 10 years of life. Currently, in the appropriate clinical context, the diagnosis is confirmed with genetic testing with no need to perform muscle biopsy or electromyography (EMG).[12] The dystrophin gene, located on chromosome Xp21, is a large gene including 79 exons. The large size of the gene probably accounts for the high spontaneous mutation rate. One third of cases appears as de novo (i.e., first time) mutations. Dystrophin gene analysis can identify large deletions in the majority of patients with dystrophinopathy.[2] The deletions seen in BMD result from in-frame mutations that allow for production of some dystrophin, whereas out-of-frame mutations in DMD result in nearly total loss of dystrophin.[2,9] Duplications and point mutations are responsible for about 5% and 15% of cases, respectively.

EMG may be helpful if there is no family history and in mild forms of BMD, when the differential diagnosis is broader (Table 32-2).[13] Motor and nerve conduction studies usually are normal except in extremely affected muscles, which may show a decrease in the amplitude of the compound motor action potential (CMAP), probably because of the reduction in muscle size.[14] Needle EMG findings show typical myopathic features (see Table 32-2).[13] Muscle biopsy findings for DMD and BMD include necrosis, regeneration, fiber splitting, abnormal fiber size variation, endomysial and perimysial proliferation of connective tissue, and internalized nuclei.[15] Eventually, muscle fibers are replaced by connective tissue and subsequently by adipose tissue.[15] Immunochemistry on muscle tissue shows reduced or absent dystrophin in BMD and DMD, respectively.

Treatment of Duchenne's and Becker's Muscular Dystrophies
The management of muscular dystrophies requires a multidisciplinary, multimodality approach to allow the patient and family the greatest quality of life (Figure 32-4).

Pharmacology. Current standard of care includes treatment with prednisone at a dosage of 0.75 mg/kg/day.[12]

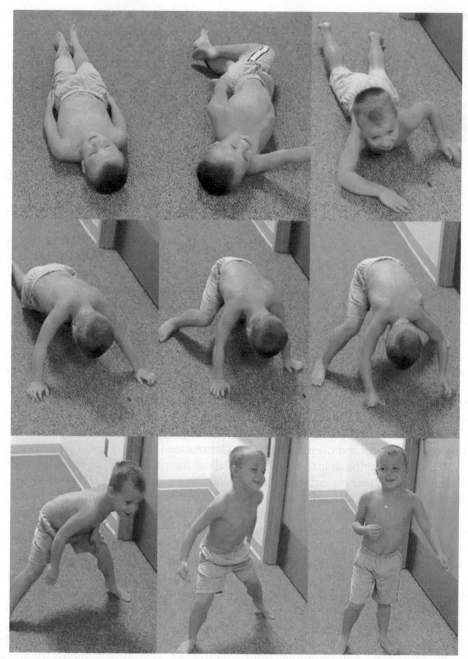

Figure 32-2 A boy with Duchenne's muscular dystrophy showing the typical Gower's maneuver while rising from the floor. (From Rimon DL, Connor MJ, Pyeritz RE, et al: *Emery and Rimoin's principles and practice of medical genetics,* ed 7, Waltham, MA, 2013, Academic Press/Elsevier. Courtesy of Richard S. Finkel, Director of the Neuromuscular Program, The Children's Hospital of Philadelphia.)

This recommendation is based on multiple clinical trials showing slower rates of deterioration and improved function in boys treated with prednisone.[16] Deflazacort (0.9 or 1.2 mg/kg/day), a prednisone derivative with similar effects (not approved by the U.S. Food and Drug Administration [FDA] but used in Europe), produces similar benefits, possibly with fewer side effects such as less weight gain.[2,16,17] Additional controlled trials have confirmed the benefits of prednisone and deflazacort in prolonging ambulation and maintaining pulmonary function.[18]

No clear guideline exists about the best time to initiate corticosteroid treatment.[12] Corticosteroids are generally started between ages 4 and 8, during the plateau phase before clear decline in muscle strength develops.[19] Common side effects, which may limit the dose of steroids, include irritability, weight gain, cushingoid appearance, GI complaints, skin rash, glucose intolerance, hypertension, cataracts, and increased risk for fractures.[16] The patient should be monitored for these side effects, especially with long-term corticosteroid use.[16]

Alternative agents that have been considered to slow disease progression include oxandrolone, an anabolic steroid, as well as creatine and other supplements. Controlled studies of these compounds, however, have failed to show

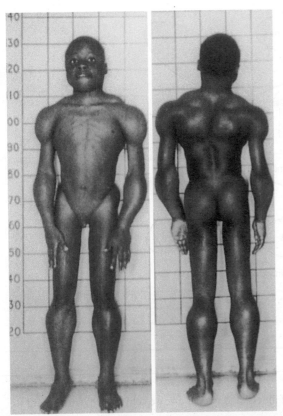

Figure 32-3 Pattern of muscle hypertrophy in Duchenne's dystrophy. (From Emery AEH, Muntoni F: *Duchenne muscular dystrophy*, ed 3, p 31, New York, 2003, Oxford University Press.)

any benefit.[12] More recently, large international efforts have been conducted to improve the design of clinical trials for dystrophinopathies.[20] These efforts are the result of collaboration between multiple stakeholders,[20,21] including patients and their families, who recently developed the first-ever patient-initiated guidance for industry and the FDA to help accelerate development of potential treatments for DMD.[22] An area of focus of these efforts has been the development of biomarkers and more sensitive outcome measures to support the drug development process.[23] These studies led to the validation of the 6-minute walk test (6MWT) as the primary endpoint for clinical trials in ambulatory DMD[24,25] and suggested that the minimal clinically important difference for the 6MWT in DMD boys was about 30 meters. The 6MWT is now included as the primary endpoint in pharmacological trials of novel compounds to slow the progression of DMD.[26,27]

Another important area of current pharmacological research in DMD is how to best manage cardiomyopathy. Recent evidence supports the use of angiotensin-converting enzyme (ACE) inhibitors for the treatment of cardiomyopathy associated with DMD before clinical signs of abnormal heart function develop, although the exact timing and pharmacological agent is still an area of active investigation.[28]

Rehabilitation. Rehabilitation offers multiple approaches in the management of myopathies, as described by Hicks[29] (Table 32-3) and reviewed by Bushby et al.[28]

TABLE **32-2**

Electrodiagnostic Findings in Selected Myopathies

Parameter	Muscular Dystrophy	Congenital	Metabolic	Inflammatory
DL	Normal	Normal	Normal	Normal
NCV	Normal	Normal	Normal	Normal
SNAP amplitude	Normal	Normal	Normal	Normal
CMAP amplitude	Normal*	Normal*	Normal*	Normal*
MUAP analysis	Small-duration, low-amplitude, polyphasic MUAPs†	Either normal or small-duration, low-amplitude, polyphasic MUAPs depending on the specific disease	Either normal or small-duration, low-amplitude, polyphasic MUAPs depending on the specific disease	Small-duration, low-amplitude, polyphasic MUAPs†
Recruitment pattern	Early‡	Either normal or early depending on the specific disease	Either normal or early depending on the specific disease	Early‡
Fibrillation and PSWs	Yes	In some such as myotubular myopathy	In some such as acid maltase deficiency	Yes
Myotonia	In some such as myotonic dystrophy	In some such as myotubular myopathy	In some such as acid maltase deficiency	No

DL, Distal latency; *NCV*, nerve conduction velocity; *SNAP*, sensory nerve action potential; *CMAP*, compound muscle action potential; *MUAP*, motor unit action potential; *PSWs*, positive sharp waves.

*CMAP amplitude may be reduced in long-standing advanced disease.

† In long-standing advanced disease, a few large-duration polyphasic MUAPs may be seen.

‡ In long-standing advanced disease, fast-firing MUAPs may be seen.

Modified from Krivickas L: Myopathies. In Tan FC, editor: *EMG secrets*, p 203, Philadelphia, 2004, Hanley & Belfus.

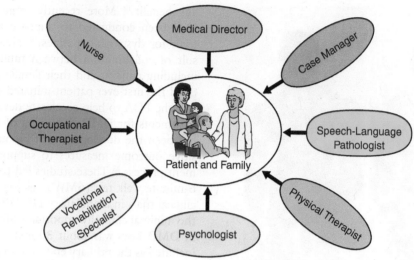

Figure 32-4 Multidisciplinary team.

TABLE **32-3**

Rehabilitation Approaches to the Treatment of Myopathies

Approach	Comments
Patient evaluation	
Initial assessment	Needed to assess impairments, stage of illness, and overall disease activity and damage and to gauge responses to therapy
Function	Needed to assess ability to perform physical tasks, interact psychosocially, and communicate to establish level of disability and to follow outcomes of treatment strategies
Quality of life	Needed to assess overall satisfaction with life activities and make treatment recommendations to improve it
Exercise	
Range of motion and stretching	Needed to preserve, maintain, and increase joint motion
Gentle toning exercises	May be used to maintain muscle strength Avoid overwork, high-resistance and eccentric exercises
Aerobic	Needed to maintain aerobic capacity and improve overall functional level
Recreational	Recommended to improve quality of life and provide socialization and informal exercise
Adaptive thinking	
Educational strategies	Instruction in energy conservation and compliance with exercise is essential
Assistive devices	Assistive devices can raise the individual's functional level from requiring the assistance of a person to independence with assistive devices
Heat and cold	Heat is used to increase collagen extensibility before tight joints are stretched Cold is useful for reducing pain and muscle spasm
Orthoses	Short leg bracing is used to compensate for quadriceps and ankle dorsiflexion weakness Long leg braces may be used to assist with ambulation in select patients

Adapted from Hicks JE: Role of rehabilitation in the management of myopathies, *Curr Opin Rheumatol* 10:551, 1998.

Boys with DMD or BMD should be encouraged to lead active, normal lives during the early stages of the disease, before the onset of difficulties with ambulation. Rehabilitation interventions in DMD focus on prolonging ambulation, preventing or slowing deformities such as joint contractures and scoliosis, and preserving respiratory function. In addition to psychological benefits,[30] the goal of rehabilitation is the highest quality of life for the patient and family. This is accomplished through weight control, passive and active exercises, use of orthoses and assistive devices, and selected surgical interventions.[3]

Preventing obesity is essential for optimal function in patients with DMD. Increased weight can result in greater difficulty with ambulation or elevation activities, such as rising from a chair. Weight control can be accomplished through diet regulation, monitoring weight at every medical visit, and patient and family education

TABLE **32-4**

Prevention of Deformities in Duchenne's Muscular Dystrophy

Intervention	Timing	Comment
Achilles tendon stretching	As soon as possible	Typically already at diagnosis
Night splints	If loss of range of motion is ≥20°	Commonly a few years after diagnosis
Hip stretching	When contractures are detected	Common toward late phases of ambulation
Iliotibial band stretching	When contractures are detected	May occur during late phases of ambulation
Knee stretching	When contractures are detected	Rarely needed; may be found in children with asymmetrical ankle contractures

From Emery AEH, Muntoni F: *Duchenne muscular dystrophy,* ed 3, p 210, New York, 2003, Oxford University Press.

about the importance of weight control in maintaining function. Weight control becomes particularly difficult in patients using a wheelchair.

Passive stretching exercises should be started early to prevent or reduce joint contractures; parents should be trained to carry out these daily stretching exercises.[28] Specific recommendations have been made regarding when to begin stretching various muscle groups (Table 32-4).[3]

Night splints (**ankle–foot orthosis [AFO]**) can be effective in delaying heel cord tightness and should be prescribed when the ankles cannot be dorsiflexed beyond neutral.[3] Passive stretching combined with the use of night splints has been reported to be more effective than stretching alone.[31]

Long leg orthoses can be used to possibly prolong ambulation, but patient compliance is variable because of the discomfort associated with wearing these braces. Once independent ambulation is lost, the patient may use a standing frame (Figure 32-5, *A*). The upright posture provides stretching in lower extremity joints and psychological benefits associated with standing. In a long-term retrospective study, Vignos et al.[32] described an effective contracture management regimen that included daily passive stretching of the hamstrings and Achilles tendons, prescribed standing and walking, Achilles tenotomy, posterior tibial tendon transfer, and **knee–ankle–foot orthoses (KAFOs).** This regimen allowed patients with DMD to continue ambulating to a mean age of 13.6 years. With orthoses they were able to stand for an additional 2 years.

A lightweight plastic or polypropylene knee–ankle foot orthosis (KAFO) with an ischial supporting lip can be considered in early stages to support ambulation (Figure 32-5, *B*). An Achilles tenotomy, performed percutaneously, may be considered to correct an equinovarus deformity and thus allow proper fitting of the orthosis, although no consensus exists on the timing and type of surgical procedures to prolong ambulation in DMD and recommendations for surgery should be based on individual circumstances.[28] A program has been described involving fabrication of the orthosis 1 week before the

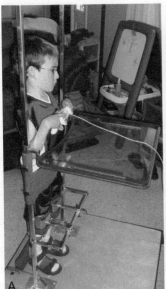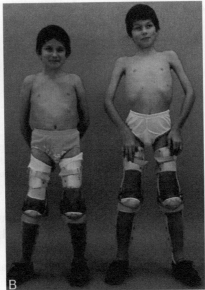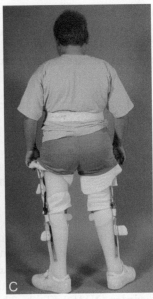

Figure 32-5 A, Standing frame. **B** and **C,** Examples of children standing in knee–ankle–foot orthosis (KAFO). (**A** from Goodman CC, Fuller KS: *Pathology: implications for the physical therapist,* ed 4, St. Louis, 2015, Saunders. **B** from Dubowitz V: Deformities in Duchenne dystrophy, *Neuromuscul Disord* 20:282, 2010. **C** from Herring JA: *Tachdjian's pediatric orthopaedics: from the Texas Scottish Rite Hospital for Children,* ed 5, Philadelphia, 2014, Saunders.)

tenotomy, fitting of the night splint in the operating room, and standing in the KAFOs by the next day.[3] The child is progressed over the next 1 to 1.5 weeks to independent ambulation. Important predictors of loss of ambulation in DMD include loss of hip extensor and ankle dorsiflexor strength.[4]

Scoliosis can be limited or delayed by prolongation of ambulation.[30] Correct seating posture and thoracic orthoses help with comfort, although they cannot prevent the eventual development of scoliosis. The use of custom-molded, lightweight, thoracolumbar orthoses is recommended in patients with DMD who have a curvature greater than 30°.[3] The brace should be worn whenever the patient is seated. An orthopedic surgeon should evaluate patients with DMD who have scoliosis.

Limited evidence on the role of different types of exercise in DMD/BMD is available.[28,33] However, a few general recommendations can be made based on both preclinical and limited clinical studies.[28]

Submaximal, aerobic exercise is encouraged for as long as possible.[28] Swimming makes exercises easier to perform, and young boys with dystrophinopathy are encouraged to engage in gentle, aerobic, community-based recreational activities. During periods of illness or injury, when bed rest may be required, the patient is at risk for disuse atrophy. As soon as the illness allows, return to submaximum aerobic exercise is recommended to minimize the effects of immobilization and deconditioning.[34] Submaximum functional strengthening activities such as gentle toning exercises in the swimming pool and during recreation-based activities are allowed. Light resistance training early on in the disease course is allowed. High-resistance strength training and eccentric exercise, however, are not beneficial in DMD/BMD and should be avoided because of concerns about contraction-induced muscle injury.[28] Muscle pain, delayed-onset muscle soreness, and excessive fatigue interfering with normal activities postexercise should be avoided because they may represent signs of exercise-induced muscle damage.

Clinical Note

Muscle pain, delayed-onset muscle soreness, and excessive fatigue should be avoided during exercise in patients with DMD and BMD because it is a sign of exercise-induced muscle damage.

Respiratory failure caused by progressive weakness of the muscles of ventilation accounts for 90% of the morbidity and mortality in DMD. Respiratory function should be monitored frequently in patients with a neuromuscular disorder (NMD) (Table 32-5),[5] because these diseases produce well-recognized signs and symptoms of hypoventilation (Table 32-6). Respiratory muscle exercises do not prevent the eventual decline in pulmonary

TABLE 32-5

Available Tools for Monitoring and Management of Ventilation in Patients with Neuromuscular Disease

Evaluation	Intervention
History, physical examination/ anthropometrics	Nutritional consultation and guidance on positioning
MIP/MEP	Annual influenza vaccine Chest physiotherapy
PFT (if older than age 5-6 yr)	Respiratory muscle exercises
Polysomnography/sleep oximetry	Insufflator-exsufflator (MIE)
Arterial blood gases	NIV

MIP/MEP, Maximal inspiratory pressure/maximal expiratory pressure; *PFT,* pulmonary function test; *MIE,* mechanical insufflator-exsufflator; *NIV,* noninvasive ventilation.

Modified from Gozal D: Pulmonary manifestations of neuromuscular disease with special reference to Duchenne muscular dystrophy and spinal muscular atrophy, *Pediatr Pulmonol* 29:148, 2000.

TABLE 32-6

Signs and Symptoms of Hypoventilation in Neuromuscular Disease

Signs	Symptoms
Vital signs • Tachypnea **Respiratory** • Use of accessory chest and abdominal muscles • Paradoxical breathing pattern • Diminished chest excursion	**Constitutional** • Generalized fatigue • Weakness **Pulmonary** • Dyspnea • Orthopnea • Secretion/retention **Central nervous system** • Early morning headaches • Daytime hypersomnolence • Mood disturbances **Sleep** • Restless sleep • Nightmares • Enuresis • Frequent arousals

Modified from Perrin C, Unterborn JN, Ambrosio CD, Hill NS: Pulmonary complications of chronic neuromuscular diseases and their management, *Muscle Nerve* 29:15, 2004.

function. Influenza and pneumococcal vaccinations are recommended.

Guidelines have been published regarding the use of mechanical noninvasive positive-pressure ventilation (and, when appropriate, continuous invasive ventilation) in chronic neuromuscular diseases, including DMD.[28,35-37] For patients with an impaired cough, a mechanical insufflator-exsufflator (MIE) can be beneficial for clearing secretions.[28,38]

Surgical Care. Early release of contractures has not been found to be beneficial and is not recommended.[3] In addition to the Achilles tenotomy described previously for correcting an equinovarus deformity, a small percentage of patients with DMD may be considered for release of hip flexion or iliotibial band contractures to allow proper fitting of KAFOs[28]; however, there is no consensus on the use of these procedures.[28] Spinal surgery for scoliosis is recommended when the curvature is greater than 30° and has shown a tendency to deteriorate,[3] especially when the patient starts the pubertal growth spurt. The patient should have a forced vital capacity greater than 25% to 35% of the predicted value before undergoing the procedure. The goals of spinal fusion include prevention of further deformity, pain control, and improved quality of life, as well as slowing of the rate of respiratory decline.[28]

Facioscapulohumeral Muscular Dystrophy

Genetics/Epidemiology

Facioscapulohumeral muscular dystrophy (FSHD) is the third most common muscular dystrophy after DMD and myotonic dystrophy. The onset usually occurs in childhood or young adulthood (range, age 3 to 44), although later onset has been described.[39] The prevalence of FSHD is variable, ranging from 1 in 20,000 to 1 in 455,000, depending on the geographical region.[39,40] The disorder has an autosomal dominant pattern of inheritance linked to chromosome 4q35.[1,41]

Clinical Features

Patients with FSHD usually present in the first to fifth decades with a characteristic pattern of facial muscle weakness. This leads to the appearance of an expressionless face with a decreased ability to smile, whistle, or fully close the eyes because of weakness in the orbicularis oris and orbicularis oculi muscles. The onset usually is insidious. The disorder is slowly progressive and can vary in the location and severity of the weakness.[1,42] Shoulder girdle weakness

may also be noted at presentation.[42] Patients with an earlier onset of symptoms may be more severely affected.[42]

The patient complains of difficulty with activities that require arm elevation, such as combing the hair. Scapular stabilizers are affected in a specific distribution. The serratus anterior, rhomboid, and middle trapezius muscles are characteristically affected early, while the deltoids usually remain strong. This peculiar pattern of weakness leads to scapular winging and a trapezius "hump," with the scapulae laterally deviating on attempted shoulder forward flexion. When the patient attempts to abduct the shoulders, the scapulae ride high (are elevated), interfering with the movement and often restricting shoulder range of motion, preventing the patient from being able to raise the arms overhead despite strong deltoids. Manual stabilization of the shoulder blades, which can be easily performed during examination, allows the patient to increase range of motion when attempting elevation through shoulder abduction. The humeral muscles (i.e., biceps and triceps) are often affected, with sparing of the forearm muscles; this gives the arms a "Popeye" appearance. The sternocostal head of the pectoralis major is also characteristically affected with resulting inversion of the anterior axillary folds which become horizontal. These weaknesses can be asymmetrical.

Lower abdominal muscles can be involved leading to a positive **Beevor sign** with the navel moving up when the patient attempts to flex the neck while supine. In the lower limbs, the tibialis anterior muscle may be affected with possible presence of a foot drop.[42] Prolonged weakness in the ankles may lead to contractures. Gait may be normal initially but often progresses to a waddling gait with hyperlordosis as a result of weakness of the pelvic girdle muscles.

Symptoms usually progress in a descending, stepwise pattern, although clinical presentation can be quite variable. Life expectancy is normal. Only 20% to 25% of patients progress to requiring a wheelchair for mobility.[1,42] Ventilatory muscle weakness that leads to respiratory failure has been reported in rare cases.[43] Cardiac involvement is also rare. Hearing loss and retinal abnormalities are associated with infantile-onset FSHD and requires close monitoring in children with FSHD.

Associated features include pain in the neck, shoulder, posterior chest, and lower back. This pain is musculoskeletal in etiology and is caused by muscle imbalance and strain. It generally responds well to conservative treatment, including physical therapy and bracing.

Diagnosis

CK usually is normal or mildly elevated. EMG shows a typical myopathic pattern in affected muscles. A muscle biopsy shows variation in muscle fiber size, isolated necrotic fibers, and increased connective tissue but is not usually needed because the diagnosis can be confirmed with genetic testing. The genetic basis of FSHD is complex and has been clarified in recent years, with genetic testing now being widely available. From 90% to

95% of affected individuals carry a contracted number of copies of a 3.3-kb DNA repeat unit known as D4Z4 at position q35 on one chromosome 4 (below a threshold of 11 repeats). There is a well-demonstrated correlation between the size of the D4Z4 repeat unit and disease severity.[44] Individuals carrying this genetic mutation are characterized as having FSHD1 or D4Z4 "contraction-dependent" FSHD. The remaining 5% to 10% of cases is "contraction-independent" FSHD, or FSHD2. FSHD2 is not associated with D4Z4 contraction but is characterized by hypomethylation of both 4q35 D4Z4 regions.[45] The genetics of FSHD is still an active area of research, and current studies are likely to clarify genotype–phenotype correlation in the near future.

Treatment

Pharmacology. No effective pharmacological treatments are available for FSHD. A randomized, double-blind, placebo-controlled trial of albuterol in patients with FSHD showed no improvement in global strength or in function and is not currently considered standard of care.[40,46]

Rehabilitation. Rehabilitation plays an important role in patients with FSHD. Features of FSHD amenable to rehabilitative interventions include footdrop, pain, and mobility deficits. A lightweight AFO may be beneficial for footdrop to improve gait and safety. Assistive devices ranging from straight canes to motorized wheelchairs may be needed, depending on the severity of the mobility deficit. For many patients, pain maybe the most debilitating feature of FSHD and is a result of muscle imbalance and fatigue of muscles that support ADLs.[2,47] As an example, shoulder girdle muscles are differentially affected, and patients tend to overuse certain muscles to compensate during activities such as reaching overhead or combing hair. In addition to pharmacological management of pain using nonsteroidal anti-inflammatory agents and acetaminophen, rehabilitation using stretching, light strengthening exercises of the least affected muscles, and bracing to correct postural abnormalities can often have a significant effect on symptoms. Lumbosacral orthoses can help stabilize core muscles and reduce pain associated with hyperlordotic posture. Figure-of-eight bracing may help relieve shoulder pain.

The role of exercise in FSHD has been evaluated in a large randomized trial as well as smaller case series and pilot studies. Based on the limited available evidence, it seems that in moderate-intensity strength training and/or aerobic training in patients with FSHD does not cause harm; however, the evidence is insufficient to establish that exercise offers benefit with respect to muscle strength.[48] A recent study of both aerobic exercise and cognitive-behavioral therapy demonstrated that either intervention can have a significant impact on chronic fatigue, a highly prevalent symptom in this patient population.[49] Therefore it is possible that exercise may be helpful to improve quality of life and overall function.

Surgical Care. Scapular winging may be amenable to surgical fixation of the scapula to the thorax for stabilization.[50] Scapulocostal fixation can afford more than 20° to 30° additional movement, which may improve the patient's ability to lift or carry objects and may help control shoulder pain. Rare complications include brachial plexopathy and frozen shoulder.[51] Unfortunately, the effects may be temporary, and any benefit must be weighed against the risks of surgery and the necessary postoperative immobilization.[39]

Emery-Dreifuss Muscular Dystrophy

Genetics/Epidemiology

Emery-Dreifuss muscular dystrophy (EDMD) is an inherited disorder that is generally caused by either mutations in the *STA* gene, which codes for the key nuclear protein emerin (X-linked EMD) or the *LMNA* gene, which codes for lamins A and C in autosomal dominant EMD.[52] The *STA* gene maps to chromosome Xq28, and the *LMNA* gene, to chromosome 1q21.[53] The X-linked form affects males, but females may present with isolated cardiomyopathy and therefore require cardiac evaluation.[54] The autosomal dominant form affects males and females equally.[54] The underlying pathophysiology is unknown. Mutations in the genes coding for emerin or lamin A/C may be associated with an EDMD phenotype or manifest as isolated cardiomyopathy or other patterns of weakness such as a limb girdle pattern of involvement. In addition, mutations in other genes have recently been reported to be associated with an EDMD phenotype in some individuals who tested negative for mutations in the emerin or lamin A/C genes, highlighting the complexity of the genetics of muscular dystrophy.

Clinical Features

EDMD is characterized by a triad of clinical features: (1) early contractures in the elbows, Achilles tendon, and posterior cervical spinal muscles; (2) slowly progressive muscle weakness, which begins in a humeroperoneal distribution; and (3) cardiac abnormalities such as cardiomyopathy and conduction defects.[55] The muscle weakness and contractures usually present before the cardiac abnormalities. Contractures may precede muscle weakness, are especially common at the elbows and heel cords,[56] and can worsen during the adolescent growth spurt. Late complications of the weakness can include lumbar lordosis and spinal rigidity.

The cardiac abnormalities include conduction defects, atrial and ventricular arrhythmias, and/or dilated cardiomyopathy.[54,55,57-62] In an extensive review, arrhythmias were noted in 92% of patients after age 30, and heart failure was seen in 64% after age 50.[63] The risk of sudden death can be as high as a 46% in patients with EDMD, because many patients are symptom free.[55,58,60,63]

Diagnosis

The diagnosis is based mostly on clinical findings. DNA analysis[59] can confirm the diagnosis.

Treatment

No specific pharmacological therapies are available for EDMD. All patients should have a comprehensive cardiac evaluation and regular follow-up to identify arrhythmias that may be amenable to pacemaker or defibrillator implantation; unfortunately, this is no guarantee that sudden death will be prevented.[63] Anticoagulation may be needed for individuals with atrial flutter or fibrillation or atrial standstill to prevent disabling embolic strokes.[59,60] Diuretics and ACE inhibitors may be beneficial in patients with significant ventricular dysfunction.

Rehabilitative interventions should seek to maintain function and mobility. The contractures usually are not preventable but may be minimized with stretching exercises. Achilles tenotomy may be required to correct an equinus deformity of the foot, and a rigid, hyperextended neck may be improved by orthopedic intervention.

Limb-Girdle Muscular Dystrophies

Genetics/Epidemiology

The limb-girdle muscular dystrophies (LGMDs) constitute a genetically heterogeneous group of disorders with an autosomal dominant (LGMD 1) or autosomal recessive (LGMD 2) mode of inheritance.[1,64] Further alphabetical classification of the LGMDs (e.g., LGMD 1A, LGMD 1B) is based on the underlying genetic mutation and is in constant development as knowledge about these disorders continues to increase. The clinical and laboratory features of the LGMDs are nonspecific; however, some subtypes are characterized by specific findings such as presence of cardiomyopathy, which can help direct genetic testing. The prevalence is approximately 8.1 in 1 million inhabitants.[65] The affected genes code for various muscle proteins associated with sarcolemma, nuclear membrane, contractile apparatus, and enzymatic functions.[66] The exact underlying pathophysiology is unknown.

Clinical Features

Patients with LGMD can present at any age from childhood to adulthood. Common features include preferential proximal lower limb and pelvic girdle weakness, with upper limb weakness and scapular winging occurring later.[66] The weakness is slowly progressive, and some patients become wheelchair users. Facial and extraocular muscles usually are spared. Severe diaphragmatic weakness can result in chronic alveolar hypoventilation and respiratory failure. Elbow, Achilles tendon, and hip flexion contractures may occur in certain subtypes.[64] Cardiac abnormalities have been noted to occur in some LGMDs.[67] In one review of 97 patients with LGMD, 10% were found to have clinically relevant cardiac abnormalities, including conduction defects and dilated cardiomyopathy.[68,69] The wide variability in the clinical findings among the subtypes was extensively described by an international workshop on the LGMDs.[64]

Diagnosis

The diagnosis of LGMD requires a complete physical examination and history, including as complete a family history as possible to identify inheritance patterns. CK levels can be markedly elevated. Genetic analysis and muscle biopsy are important to make the diagnosis and to rule out other myopathies that may present with a limb-girdle distribution of weakness. Muscle biopsy usually reveals necrosis and regeneration, increased internalized nuclei, marked variability of fiber size, increased fibrous and adipose tissue, and fiber hypertrophy.[70] Biopsy may also show many lobulated and moth-eaten fibers.[71]

Treatment

No pharmacological treatment is available for LGMD. Cardiac monitoring throughout the disease is recommended.[66] In the more severe cases, especially when the patient uses a wheelchair for ambulation, respiratory failure may need to be addressed with ventilatory support devices.[37] Rehabilitative efforts should focus on maintaining mobility and minimizing contractures. Stretching exercises are important for maintaining joint range of motion, and AFOs may help compensate for distal lower extremity weakness. The patient's functional status should be monitored closely and can be a more sensitive indicator of disease progression than manual muscle testing.[72]

Myotonic Dystrophy

Genetics/Epidemiology

Myotonic dystrophy type 1 (DM1) is the most common of a heterogeneous group of myotonic disorders. It has an autosomal dominant mode of inheritance mapped to chromosome 19q13,[53] which codes for the myotonic dystrophy protein kinase (DMPK).[73] DM1 is caused by expansion of a trinucleotide repeat. The severity of the myopathy correlates with the size of the repeat, which is unstable and expands from one generation to the next, accounting for anticipation within families. The incidence of myotonic dystrophy is approximately 13.5 in 100,000 live births, and the prevalence is 3 to 5 per 100,000.[14]

Clinical Features

The muscle weakness of DM1 can begin at any age, including the neonatal period (congenital DM1, the most severe form). It is slowly progressive and manifested predominately in the muscles of the face, jaw, and distal (more than proximal) limbs.[73] Frontal baldness, ptosis, and atrophy in the temporalis and masseter muscles result in a characteristic "hatchet-faced" appearance. Dysarthria and dysphagia can result from pharyngeal and lingual muscle weakness. Patients with DM1 often do not report myotonia. **Myotonia** is a delayed relaxation of a contracted muscle that the patient may describe as stiffness and is most often present in the hands. Myotonia can often be easily detected on examination. Action myotonia can be observed as delayed relaxation of the fingers after a forceful hand grip. Percussion myotonia can be elicited by percussion of certain muscle groups such as the thenar eminence or the wrist/finger extensor muscle group in the posterior forearm. It is lessened by repeated activation of the muscle (**warm-up phenomenon**).

Many other systems are involved in DM1; therefore this disease is considered a systemic disorder (Table 32-7).[73] A related disorder is **type 2 myotonic dystrophy (DM2)**, or **proximal myotonic myopathy (PROMM)**. It is also autosomal dominant and shows multisystem involvement (e.g., cataracts, hypogonadism, diabetes mellitus, cardiac conduction defects). Important differences include gene mapping to chromosome 3q, later onset of symptoms, more proximal weakness, minimal or clinically absent myotonia, and higher prevalence of pain in the arms and legs that is not necessarily related to myotonic stiffness.[73]

Diagnosis

The diagnosis is based on a careful history, including family history, physical examination, and commercially available DNA analysis. CK levels may be normal or slightly elevated. Needle EMG shows myotonic discharges with a characteristic pattern of waxing and waning of the frequency and amplitude.[14] A muscle biopsy usually is not needed to make the diagnosis.[73]

Treatment

There are no treatments to improve muscle strength or modify the disease course. Myotonia, if clinically significant and disabling, can be controlled with medications such as mexiletine, and phenytoin. Electrocardiography (ECG) should be monitored frequently when prescribing these medications because of the presence of cardiac conduction defects and arrhythmias in many patients.

Rehabilitation interventions can be important for managing the musculoskeletal complaints. The systemic nature of the disease requires a multidisciplinary approach with many specialists involved to monitor the cardiac, respiratory, endocrine, psychological, and ophthalmological manifestations of the disease (Table 32-8). Distal lower limb weakness or footdrop can be treated with lightweight orthoses, and neck muscle weakness may require a cervical collar or head support. Assistive devices such as canes and

TABLE 32-7

Systemic Involvement in Myotonic Dystrophy

System	Principal Involvement
Smooth muscle	Reduced gastrointestinal motility, constipation, pseudo-obstruction
Heart	Cardiomyopathy and conduction defects, such as heart block, atrial arrhythmias; sudden cardiac death may occur
Lungs	Hypoventilation from and diaphragmatic involvement; sleep apnea; aspiration pneumonia secondary to dysphagia
Brain	Behavioral and cognitive abnormalities common in DM1 and most severe in congenital DM1
Endocrine system	Testicular tubular atrophy; impotence; infertility; diabetes mellitus; hypothyroidism
Eye	Cataracts, ptosis
Skin	Premature balding

Modified from Engel AG, Franzini-Armstrong C, editors: *Myology,* ed 3, vol 2, p 1044, New York, 2004, McGraw-Hill.

TABLE 32-8

Management of Myotonic Dystrophy

Problem	Management
Cardiopulmonary	
Arrhythmias and other heart conduction defects	Regular electrocardiograms and echocardiograms; drug management as appropriate for specific arrhythmia; pacemaker/implanted defibrillator if conduction defect severe or episodes of significant heart block; avoid aggravation by antimyotonic drugs
Hypoventilation	Consider assisted nocturnal ventilation (CPAP, BiPAP)
Central Nervous System	
Somnolence (sleepiness)	Exclude hypoventilation as cause; consider use of modafinil if severe
Depression and behavioral abnormalities	Pharmacological treatment
Gastrointestinal	
Swallowing difficulty	Dysphagia diet and compensatory strategies; feeding tubes may be considered
Constipation	Pharmacological treatment with stool softeners
Endocrine	
Diabetes mellitus type 2	Periodic monitoring of blood glucose and Hb A_{1c}
Other endocrine problems	Periodic monitoring of TSH; endocrine evaluation for infertility/impotence/testicular atrophy if clinically indicated
Ophthalmic	
Cataract	Periodic ophthalmological examination
Surgery and Anesthesia	
	Patients at higher risk for complications from general anesthesia and neuromuscular blocking agents

CPAP, Continuous positive airway pressure; *BiPAP,* bilevel positive airway pressure; *TSH,* thyroid-stimulating hormone; *Hb A$_{1c}$,* glycated hemoglobin.

Modified from Engel AG, Franzini-Armstrong C, editors: *Myology,* ed 3, vol 2, p 1070, New York, 2004, McGraw-Hill.

walkers may prolong mobility. In severe cases, wheelchairs may be prescribed, especially for long distances or outdoor use. Most patients with DM1 remain ambulatory.[73] Dysphagia may be amenable to compensatory strategies to help minimize the risk of aspiration. Feeding tubes may be used with severe dysphagia. Warm-up exercises may result in improved speech production.[45] Pilot studies of moderate resistance and endurance exercise suggested that exercise may be used to maintain function, cardiopulmonary fitness, and quality of life in this patient population, but there is still insufficient evidence of benefit on muscle strength.[74–76]

CONGENITAL MYOPATHIES

The congenital myopathies constitute a heterogeneous group of nonprogressive or slowly progressive muscle disorders that usually present in the neonatal period, although later onset has been described. They are not considered muscular dystrophies because they lack dystrophic changes, such as muscle fiber necrosis and replacement by connective tissue, on muscle biopsy. Rather, congenital myopathies are characterized by distinctive nonprogressive histopathology findings that differ based on the underlying molecular defect. Congenital myopathies share certain clinical features. Usually they present in infancy as generalized weakness and hypotonia (e.g., "floppy baby"). Affected infants may have delayed motor milestones and decreased muscle bulk. Various dysmorphic features may be present depending on the specific myopathy.[77] Some congenital myopathies may present later in childhood or even adulthood. Although these myopathies were historically considered nonprogressive disorders, a clinical characteristic that helped differentiate them from the muscular dystrophies, it is now accepted that some progression of weakness may occur.

Laboratory findings usually include a normal or minimally elevated CK level, which can help distinguish these disorders from the muscular dystrophies. Motor and sensory nerve conduction studies are normal, and needle EMG findings usually are normal or show small, polyphasic motor unit potentials.[14] Myotubular/centronuclear myopathy may have abnormal spontaneous activity on needle EMG (see Table 32-2).

Management options include a multidisciplinary approach to maximize the patient's function and quality of life (Table 32-9). These strategies are highly individualized and depend on the specific clinical presentation, because the degree of weakness, activity limitation, and participation restriction may be quite variable among individuals. As with many other NMDs, coordination of care among different specialists is important because patients may have complex medical needs requiring integration between health care professionals and community resources. Areas of priority include prevention and management of musculoskeletal complications (e.g., scoliosis, contractures, pain) and monitoring of hypoventilation resulting from diaphragmatic weakness.

Some of the better-defined congenital myopathies are discussed in more detail in the following sections; these include central core myopathy, nemaline myopathy, and myotubular/centronuclear myopathy.

Central Core Myopathy

Central core myopathy is a genetic disorder with an autosomal dominant mode of inheritance caused by mutations in the ryanodine receptor gene *(RYR1).*[78] These receptors mediate calcium release from the sarcoplasmic reticulum. The resultant defect in skeletal muscle is thought to be related to abnormalities in calcium ion (Ca^{2+}) regulation.[79] Of note, mutations in *RYR1* are also responsible for familial malignant hyperthermia, which is a potentially fatal inherited disorder usually associated with certain general anesthetics and the drug succinylcholine, resulting in accelerated metabolism in skeletal muscle. Therefore patients with central core myopathy are at higher risk for malignant hyperthermia. One needs to avoid certain anesthetic and neuromuscular blocking agents during anesthesia to minimize the risk of this life-threatening complication. Patients and their families should be aware of the potential for malignant hyperthermia and need to wear medical alert bracelets.

Most patients present at birth or in early childhood with hypotonia, decreased muscle bulk, slender frame, and symmetrical weakness. The degree of weakness can vary even within families and predominantly affects the proximal muscles of the lower limbs, but the face and neck can also be involved.[77] Ptosis (drooping of an eyelid) is not seen, a feature that helps distinguish central core myopathy from nemaline myopathy and myotubular/centronuclear myopathy. Motor milestones are delayed, but most patients are able to walk by age 3 to 4.[77] Muscle weakness may be stable or slowly progressive. Other frequent features include kyphoscoliosis, pes cavus or pes planus, and congenital dislocation of the hip.[77] There are no CNS abnormalities. Mild weakness of the diaphragm with nocturnal hypoventilation may be seen.

Muscle biopsy shows characteristic structural alterations within the center of type 1 muscle fibers known as cores. These cores are single, centrally located, and circular.[77]

Pilot studies have suggested that salbutamol or albuterol may be beneficial for improving muscle strength and functional abilities.[80,81] Larger prospective, randomized, double-blind, placebo-controlled trials are needed to confirm these findings. Lower limb weakness can be treated with appropriate orthotic devices (see Table 32-9).

TABLE **32-9**

Management of Patients with Congenital Myopathies

Problem	Referral	Possible Interventions
Skeletal muscle involvement Hypotonia Weakness Contractures	Physical therapy and occupational therapy	Submaximum aerobic exercise program and gentle toning Active and passive stretching Standing frame Orthoses/splinting (upper and lower limbs) Enhance mobility (walking frames or wheelchair)
Respiratory muscle involvement Nocturnal hypoxia	Physical therapy Lung function tests Sleep study	Chest physiotherapy to clear secretions Nocturnal assisted ventilation
Bulbar involvement Feeding and swallowing difficulties Failure to thrive Excessive drooling	Speech pathologist Dietitian Gastroenterologist	Speech therapy Modified barium swallow Caloric supplementation/thickened feed Feeding tubes Anticholinergic medications
Developmental or psychosocial delay	Occupational therapy Physical therapy Speech pathology Psychologist Developmental physician	Advice about appropriate intervention/liaise with local services Developmental stimulation Home programs Reassessment if deterioration occurs
Scoliosis	Physiotherapy Orthopedic surgeon	Baseline assessment, including spinal radiographs Monitoring of degree of curve Bracing Corrective surgery
Foot deformities	Physical therapy Orthopedic surgeon	Splinting/serial casting Corrective surgery
Cardiac involvement; conduction defects; cardiomyopathy	Cardiologist	Electrocardiogram, Holter monitor, cardiac echocardiogram Medication if indicated
Inability to perform activities of daily living (ADLs); inability to achieve independence with bathing, toileting, dressing, feeding; difficulties with access; handwriting difficulties	Occupational therapy Community nurse	Aids for individual ADLs Wheelchair assessment Home nursing assistance Home visit and modifications School visit and modifications Typing and computer programs Car modifications Liaise with local services
Family support	Social work Muscular Dystrophy Association Government assistance agencies	Disability allowance/pension Caregivers' allowance Support groups Financial assistance with equipment and home modifications Transport and travel assistance
Planning future pregnancies	Genetic counselor	Genetic counseling
Planning surgery	Consult with anesthetist Respiratory physician	Malignant hyperthermia precautions Lung function tests and physiotherapy before surgery
Planning future employment	Vocational counseling service Occupational therapy	Planning school studies Vocational planning Work experience Training, work placement and support
Coordination of care	Pediatrician or subspecialist with an interest Neurologist, geneticist, or rehabilitation specialist	Contact with general practitioner by telephone Liaise with local services Copy of all correspondence to key personnel Arrange case conferences when necessary Determine timing of respiratory, orthopedic, and palliative interventions

Modified from Engel AG, Franzini-Armstrong C, editors: *Myology,* ed 3, vol 2, pp 1521-1522, New York, 2004, McGraw-Hill.

Nemaline Myopathy

Nemaline myopathy is a heterogeneous congenital disorder with an autosomal dominant, recessive, or sporadic mode of inheritance. The disease is caused by mutations in genes that code for proteins that are responsible for the development and function of the Z-disks, including actin, troponin, nebulin, and tropomyosin.[82-88] Patients are classified according to age of onset and clinical severity.[77,89,90] The disease may present as three phenotypes: a severe infantile form, a mild nonprogressive or slowly progressive form with onset in childhood, or a mild adult-onset form.

The most severe phenotype is the infantile onset. Infants often have difficulty with sucking and swallowing and consequently have feeding problems. This form is usually fatal in the first year of life. Mechanical ventilation and feeding tubes may be considered. Contractures and skeletal deformities may develop in these infants.[77]

The most common phenotype is the childhood-onset subtype. This form is characterized by mild, diffuse hypotonia and weakness. Weakness is static or slowly progressive. Gait is often waddling with hyperlordosis. The disease is commonly associated with facial dysmorphic features (i.e., narrow face, high-arched palate) and skeletal abnormalities (e.g., kyphoscoliosis). Facial weakness is common, and ptosis may occasionally be present.

The adult-onset form is not associated with skeletal abnormalities or dysmorphic facies (facial abnormalities). It is characterized by mild diffuse weakness. Ptosis and head drop may be present.

Muscle biopsy reveals characteristic threadlike structures (rods) that consist of Z-disk protein material.[77,91,92] It should be noted that rods are not specific for nemaline myopathy and have been associated with other disorders.[93,94] A predominance of type I fibers muscle fibers is also noted.

No specific pharmacological treatment is available. Rehabilitation should focus on maintaining function and preventing deconditioning through mild exercise and physical therapy. Scoliosis should be monitored and treated. Long periods of immobilization can lead to disuse atrophy with worsening weakness and therefore should be avoided. Pulmonary infections require rapid, aggressive treatment, and breathing function should be monitored regularly for hypoventilation.[95,96] Nocturnal noninvasive assisted ventilation may be needed (see Table 32-9).[97]

Myotubular/Centronuclear Myopathy

Myotubular/centronuclear myopathy is a heterogenous congenital disorder with distinct modes of inheritance. The disease can be X-linked, mapped to chromosome Xq28 at a locus coding for myotubularin. Alternatively, it can have an autosomal dominant or recessive mode of inheritance associated with mutations in the gene coding for dynamin-2.

In the X-linked form, affected males present at birth with severe hypotonia, weakness, feeding difficulties, respiratory distress, bilateral ptosis, limited eye movements, and absent tendon reflexes.[77] Associated features include pectus carinatum ("pigeon chest") and hip and knee contractures.[77] Prognosis is poor, and death usually occurs from pulmonary complications.

The autosomal forms mostly present in early childhood or occasionally early adulthood.[77] Affected children have mild generalized hypotonia and weakness. Gait is waddling and hyperlordotic. As in nemaline myopathy, facial dysmorphic features are often present. In addition, ptosis and ophthalmoparesis (paralysis of one or more of the muscles moving the eye) are common.[77] Muscle biopsy shows myonuclei in the center of the muscle fibers. Treatment for these congenital myopathies requires a multidisciplinary approach that includes various specialties (see Table 32-9). Many interventions are nonspecific and depend on the particular impairment.

INFLAMMATORY MYOPATHIES

Polymyositis and Dermatomyositis

Polymyositis (PM) and dermatomyositis (DM) are idiopathic inflammatory disorders.[98] PM usually presents in those older than age 20, whereas DM has a bimodal age distribution, occurring either in childhood or in adulthood. The female-to-male ratio is approximately 2:1.[99] The underlying etiology remains unknown.[100,101]

Clinical Presentation

Both PM and DM present with a progressive, symmetrical, proximal (i.e., more than distal) pattern of muscle weakness. Patients may report difficulty rising from a seated position or difficulty with overhead activities such as brushing the hair. Muscle pain and tenderness affect approximately one third of these patients and involve the upper limbs more commonly than the lower limbs. Later in the course of the disease, neck, swallowing, and respiratory muscles may become affected, resulting in aspiration pneumonia and respiratory failure.[102] Arthralgia (joint pain) may occur in as many as 50% of patients with PM.[98]

DM is also associated with characteristic erythematous skin lesions, predominantly in the periorbital, perioral, malar, anterior neck, chest, and extensor surfaces of joints.[98] The periorbital rash usually is violaceous (violet) or heliotrope (lilac) in color. **Gottron's rash** is a violaceous, raised, scaly rash over the knuckles. As the disease progresses, scaling, pigmentation, and depigmentation can occur in the area of the rash. The rash sometimes appears before the muscle weakness.[98]

PM and DM are associated with abnormalities in the cardiac and pulmonary systems and may be associated with certain malignancies and connective tissue disorders.[98,103] Cardiomyopathy, pericarditis, left ventricular diastolic dysfunction, atrial arrhythmias, and conduction defects are the most common cardiac abnormalities.[102,104-107]

Interstitial lung disease (ILD) occurs in approximately 30% of patients with PM or DM.[102,108,109] It tends to be more severe and more refractory to corticosteroid treatment in DM.[110] Signs and symptoms suggesting ILD include fever, nonproductive cough, dyspnea, hypoxemia, and lung infiltrates. These signs and symptoms may even precede the skin or muscle abnormalities.[102,111] Patients with PM or DM may have a connective tissue disease, such as rheumatoid arthritis, systemic lupus erythematous, scleroderma, or Sjögren's syndrome. Population-based cohort studies suggest an association with malignancy.[112] Ovarian cancer and lung cancer appear to be more closely associated with DM, and lung cancer and non-Hodgkin's lymphoma are associated with PM.[112] Vasculitis that affects the GI tract may also be seen, especially in children.

Diagnosis

Comprehensive history and physical examination, CK level, EMG, and muscle biopsy findings form the basis of the diagnosis of PM and DM.[113] CK, aldolase, lactate dehydrogenase (LDH), and aspartate aminotransferase (AST) levels all can be elevated with muscle damage. CK levels can be elevated fivefold to fiftyfold in PM and DM. However, in some patients with DM, CK levels may be only mildly elevated, especially in childhood DM and in patients with slow and insidious-onset DM.[98] The erythrocyte sedimentation rate (ESR) usually is normal or mildly elevated and does not accurately reflect disease activity or correlate with the severity of weakness.[98] Antinuclear antibodies may be found in approximately 50% of patients with myositis. Anti-Jo-1 antibodies may be seen in PM more often than in DM and may be associated with ILD.[114] The usefulness of the antinuclear antibody test is limited, because a negative or low titer does not exclude the diagnosis.[98]

On electrodiagnostic testing, sensory and motor nerve conduction studies usually are normal. Needle EMG findings can include positive sharp waves (PSWs) and fibrillation potentials on needle insertion, which suggests muscle membrane instability. This abnormal insertional activity is a good indicator of active disease and may be seen in more than 80% of patients with PM or DM.[115] In chronic disease with significant tissue loss, the PSWs and fibrillation potentials may be decreased; this also may occur after treatment, with resultant stabilization of the muscle membrane.[115] EMG also reveals a decrease in the duration and amplitude of motor unit potentials, reflecting the diminished number of muscle fibers in the motor unit. Increased polyphasia may be seen, reflecting asynchrony in the electrical activity of the remaining fibers as well as early motor unit recruitment. It should be noted that active disease can be present in scattered areas; therefore sufficient time is needed to assess multiple areas of multiple muscles to collect adequate information. Proximal, distal, and paraspinal muscles should be examined. Muscle biopsy findings include necrosis, regeneration, variation in fiber diameter, proliferation of connective tissue, and collections of inflammatory cells.[98]

Treatment

Corticosteroids are an effective first-line treatment in most patients with DM or PM.[98,116] Adults usually require 30 to 40 mg a day initially. In more severe disease, adults may require 1 to 1.5 mg/kg/day, and children may need 1 to 2 mg/kg/day in divided doses. The steroid is given until the serum CK normalizes, which usually takes 6 to 12 weeks. It is then gradually tapered over several months until a maintenance dose is reached in 4 to 6 months.[98] A gradual decline in serum CK usually indicates a favorable response. Improvement in strength can lag behind the normalization of CK levels. Steroid myopathy (discussed later) is a possible complication of long-term use of prednisone. Other side effects of steroids include hypertension, glucose intolerance, weight gain, GI upset, insomnia, mood swings, acne, a cushingoid appearance, cataracts, glaucoma, and osteoporosis. Strategies to minimize these side effects include alternate-day dosing, vitamin D and calcium supplementation, control of food intake, and antacids.

Additional pharmacological agents such as methotrexate should be considered in severe cases.[98] Additional therapies may include azathioprine, cyclosporine, mycophenolate mofetil, cyclophosphamide, intravenous immunoglobulins, or plasma exchange.[98] Refractory ILD may respond to cyclospine[110] or to cyclophosphamide alone or in combination with corticosteroids.[109]

Rehabilitation interventions should focus on maintaining function and maximizing quality of life.[29] Exercises to maintain joint range of motion and flexibility are essential for preventing contractures and should be initiated early in the course of PM or DM. As with other myopathic disorders, assistive devices and mobility aids may become necessary as function declines. Until the 1990s, patients with inflammatory myopathies were asked to not exercise because there was a concern that exercise may exacerbate inflammation. Recent studies, however, have reported that moderate, submaximum aerobic exercise in patients with PM and DM does not result in worsening muscle damage. An aerobic exercise program may actually improve aerobic capacity and overall function.

Outcome of Polymyositis and Dermatomyositis

The outcome in PM and DM is determined by multiple factors. A poor outcome is more likely with older age at presentation; severe disease; delay in diagnosis and treatment; significant cardiac, pulmonary, or GI symptoms; malignancy; and antisynthetase or anti-SRP autoantibodies levels.[103] In one study, 105 patients with DM or PM were reported to have a significantly poorer quality of life than the healthy population as measured by the Short-Form 36-Item Health Status Survey (SF-36); the mortality rate was approximately 14%.[117] In another study the 10-year survival rates were

TABLE **32-10**

Overview of Polymyositis and Dermatomyositis

Disorder	Clinical Presentation	Associated Features	Diagnosis	Treatment
Polymyositis	Symmetrical proximal muscle weakness Muscle pain, tenderness Arthralgias	Interstitial lung disease Cardiac abnormalities Gastrointestinal abnormalities Collagen vascular disease Certain malignancies	Increased creatine kinase EMG Muscle biopsy	Corticosteroids and/or other immunomodulatory agents Range of motion, stretching
Dermatomyositis	As for polymyositis plus rash	Interstitial lung disease Cardiac abnormalities Gastrointestinal abnormalities Collagen vascular disease Certain malignancies	Increased creatine kinase EMG Muscle biopsy	As for polymyositis

EMG, Electromyography.

89.4% for PM and 86.4% for DM, and cardiac muscle involvement was the main predictor of death ($p < 0.01$) (Table 32-10).[118]

METABOLIC MYOPATHIES

The metabolic myopathies constitute a heterogeneous group of disorders caused by genetic defects that compromise muscle energy production. The hydrolysis of adenosine triphosphate (ATP) to adenosine diphosphate (ADP) generates the energy needed for muscle contractions. ATP is used and replenished by key metabolic processes, which require proper functioning of multiple enzymes. Enzyme dysfunction can result in an inadequate supply of ATP. Some important metabolic pathways use glycogen as substrate. At least 14 enzyme defects that affect glycogen synthesis, glycogenolysis, and glycolysis have been described (Figure 32-6).[119] Other metabolic myopathies affect lipid metabolism. The following sections discuss some of the more common metabolic disorders that result in myopathies, including myophosphorylase deficiency, phosphofructokinase (PFK) deficiency, debrancher enzyme deficiency, and acid maltase deficiency (Table 32-11).

Myophosphorylase Deficiency (McArdle's Disease)

During early exercise, energy production in muscles predominantly depends on the metabolism of carbohydrates. Myophosphorylase is the enzyme that initiates the metabolism of glycogen. Myophosphorylase deficiency (also known as glycogenosis type V or McArdle's disease) impedes glycogenolysis in muscles, resulting in low exercise tolerance. This deficiency is the most common disorder of carbohydrate metabolism, with a prevalence

of approximately 1 in 100,000.[119] It has an autosomal recessive mode of inheritance.

The onset usually occurs in childhood or young adulthood. Affected individuals report muscle aches and inability to keep up with peers during play. Most patients are diagnosed by early adulthood. Exercise intolerance is most evident during short bursts of high-intensity activity, such as lifting weights and sprinting, or during sustained moderate intensity activity, such as swimming and jogging. This intolerance can present as myalgia, muscle stiffness, weakness, or early fatigue. Rest usually relieves it. Patients can experience a **"second wind" phenomenon**, which consists of renewed ability to sustain exercise after about 10 minutes of exercise-induced myalgias or cramps. This phenomenon is the result of mobilization of blood-borne glucose. Patients usually are asymptomatic between attacks, and most adapt well and do not lead sedentary lives.[120] Fixed, proximal (greater than distal) weakness can occur in approximately one third of patients, especially older patients.[119,121] A serious complication is muscle necrosis with myoglobinuria and acute renal failure. This can occur in as many as 15% of patients with McArdle's disease.[122-124] Tea-colored urine usually is one of the first clues to myoglobinuria and should spark an aggressive workup.

Diagnosis

Diagnosis of McArdle's disease includes a careful history, including a family history, CK level determination (CK levels are always elevated), EMG (usually normal), forearm exercise test, muscle biopsy, and genetic analysis. In the forearm exercise test, serial lactate and ammonia serum levels are measured after 1 minute of forearm exercise. Both should increase threefold to fourfold. A rise in ammonia, but not lactate, levels points to a disorder

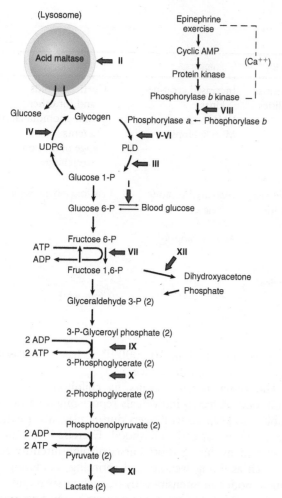

Figure 32-6 Schematic of glycogen metabolism and glycolysis. Roman numerals denote muscle glycogenoses caused by defects in the following enzymes: I, glucose-6-phosphatase; II, acid maltase; III, debranching enzyme; IV, branching enzyme; V, muscle phosphorylase; VI, liver phosphorylase; VII, phosphofructokinase; VIII, phosphorylase b kinase; IX, phosphoglycerate kinase; X, phosphoglycerate mutase; XI, lactate dehydrogenase; XII, aldolase. (Adapted from Dimauro S, Miranda AF, Sakoda S et al: Metabolic myopathies, *Am J Med Genet* 25:635-651,1986.)

of carbohydrate metabolism. Muscle biopsy may reveal nonspecific myopathic changes as well as subsarcolemmal and intermyofibrillar deposits of glycogen that appear as vacuoles. Immunostaining for myophosphorylase and biochemical assays of enzyme activity can be performed on muscle tissue to confirm the diagnosis. Genetic testing for McArdle's disease is now available, obviating the need for muscle biopsy.[125]

Treatment

Dietary changes have been explored in McArdle's disease. Low-dose creatine supplementation has shown modest benefits in a small number of patients.[126] A small, randomized, controlled study suggested that sucrose ingestion before exercise could improve exercise tolerance.[127] A high-carbohydrate diet and vitamin B_6 supplementation may also help.[128] However, none of these interventions

has been confirmed as beneficial, and research is ongoing into what, if any, dietary intervention can ameliorate McArdle's disease.[129]

Certain exercise recommendations may prove useful. Patients should avoid intense weight lifting exercises or maximum aerobic activities such as sprinting. On the other hand, mild-to-moderate exercise may help prevent deconditioning and maintain aerobic fitness. When engaging in exercise, patients should try to leverage the second wind phenomenon by doing a low-intensity warm-up for 10 minutes to promote transition to the second wind before ramping up the exercise.

Phosphofructokinase (PFK) Deficiency

PFK deficiency (also known as glycogenosis type VII or Tarui's disease) has an autosomal recessive mode of inheritance. Clinically, PFK deficiency is similar to McArdle's disease but is less common and less likely to cause myoglobinuria. In addition, the second wind phenomenon does not occur.[119] Jaundice, reflecting hemolytic anemia, and gouty arthritis can further distinguish PFK deficiency from McArdle's disease and result from PFK deficiency in erythrocytes.[130,131]

Diagnosis

CK levels are usually elevated, whereas EMG results are generally normal. Forearm exercise test results in a normal increase in ammonia but blunted rise in lactic acid. Muscle biopsy shows abnormal accumulation of glycogen. PFK immunostaining and enzyme activity in muscle are abnormal.[132] Molecular genetic analysis can provide a definitive diagnosis of PFK deficiency.

Treatment

No specific treatment is available for PFK deficiency. A high-protein diet has been suggested, but its efficacy has not been proved. Unlike in McArdle's disease, glucose or sucrose supplementation before exercise is not effective because it does not bypass the metabolic defect. As previously mentioned, the second wind phenomenon is absent.

Debrancher Deficiency

Debrancher deficiency (DD) (also known as glycogenosis type III, Cori-Forbes disease, or amylo-1,6-glucosidase deficiency) is a genetic disorder of glycogen metabolism that mostly affects the liver and muscle. It has an autosomal recessive mode of inheritance mapped to chromosome 1p21.[133] During normal glycogenolysis, the peripheral chains of glycogen are shortened to a length of four glucosyl units. Further metabolism of glycogen requires the debrancher enzyme to remove these chain remnants. Debrancher enzyme deficiency results in a buildup of glycogen remnant in muscle and liver, leading to myopathy and hepatomegaly.[134]

TABLE 32-11

Metabolic Myopathies Associated with Carbohydrate Metabolism

Glycogenosis/Pattern of Inheritance	Abnormal Enzyme	Clinical Presentation	Diagnosis	Forearm Exercise Test	Treatment
Type V McArdle's disease	Myophosphorylase	Childhood onset Exercise intolerance Myalgias Myoglobinuria (15%)	Increased CK Muscle biopsy DNA analysis	Abnormal	Leverage "second wind" phenomenon Avoid high-intensity exercise
Type VII Tarui's disease	Phosphofructokinase	Exercise intolerance Myalgias Hemolytic anemia arthralgias	Increased CK Muscle biopsy DNA analysis	Abnormal	No specific treatment
Type III Cori-Forbes disease	Debranching enzyme	Exercise intolerance Muscle weakness Cardiomyopathy Hepatomegaly	Increased CK	Abnormal	? High-protein diet
Type II Pompe's disease	α-Glucosidase	Muscle weakness Three variants with different severity: infantile-, childhood-, adult-onset	Increased CK Muscle biopsy Abnormal EMG Dried blood test, followed by DNA confirmation if screening test is positive	Normal	Enzyme replacement

CK, Creatine kinase; *DNA*, deoxyribonucleic acid; *EMG*, electromyography.

DD usually presents in young adulthood. The progression can be variable. As in McArdle's disease and PFK deficiency, many patients with DD complain of exercise intolerance, but some do not.[135] The distal portions of the upper and lower limbs are more commonly affected than the proximal muscles, and myoglobinuria and cramps are much less frequent. A more generalized weakness can include the respiratory muscles and can manifest as respiratory failure.[135,136] Other clinical manifestations usually include hepatomegaly, hypoglycemia, hyperlipidemia, growth retardation, and cardiomyopathy.[137]

Diagnosis

The serum CK usually is elevated in patients with DD. Nerve conduction velocities usually are normal. EMG reveals myopathic features with muscle membrane irritability.[14] No rise in lactate is seen with the forearm exercise test. Cardiac testing may show left ventricular or biventricular hypertrophy. Muscle biopsy reveals glycogen-containing vacuoles in the subsarcolemmal and intermyofibrillar areas. The skin, liver, myocardium, and peripheral nerves may also show glycogen deposits.[119]

Treatment

A high-protein diet during the day, with a high-protein snack at night, has been reported to be beneficial.[135,138,139] The recommended distribution on nutrients is 45% carbohydrates, 25% protein, and 30% fat.[138] In severe cases, liver transplantation may be necessary. Cardiac status should be monitored regularly.

Acid Maltase Deficiency

Acid maltase deficiency (also known as alpha-glucosidase deficiency, glycogenosis type II, or Pompe disease) is a genetic disorder with an autosomal recessive mode of inheritance mapped to chromosome 17q21-23. It results from a deficiency of the lysosomal enzyme acid alpha-1,4-glucosidase, which is required to release glucose from maltose (a disaccharide), oligosaccharides, and glycogen. The enzyme deficiency results in a buildup of glycogen in cardiac and skeletal muscle and the liver. Infantile, childhood, and adult forms have been described.

The infantile form is characterized by hypotonia, cardiomyopathy, hepatomegaly, and rapidly progressive generalized skeletal muscle weakness that starts within months of birth.[140] This is further complicated by feeding and respiratory problems. Without treatment, death usually occurs within 2 years as a result of cardiac or pulmonary failure. The heart, liver, and tongue often are enlarged because of glycogen deposits.

The childhood-onset variant is characterized by slowly progressive muscle weakness and delayed motor milestones. The weakness occurs mostly in the proximal muscles and respiratory muscles; cardiac muscle usually is spared. The adult-onset variant is characterized by the onset of myopathy after age 20. It is slowly progressive and mostly affects the proximal limb and trunk musculature. Respiratory failure may be the initial presentation in approximately one third of cases.[140,141] Obstructive sleep apnea also has been reported in association with macroglossia and tongue weakness.[142] Liver and cardiac enlargement usually is absent in the adult variant.

Diagnosis

Enzyme activity can be assayed in muscle fibers, leukocytes, fibroblasts, and urine.[140] However, false-negative results can occur on the leukocyte assay. Currently, the most sensitive screening test is spot analysis of alpha-glucosidase activity on dried blood.[143] If the dried blood test is positive, confirmatory genetic analysis is performed to finalize the diagnosis. Serum CK levels are always elevated in the early-onset forms but may be normal in adult-onset disease. On electrodiagnostic testing, motor and sensory nerve conduction tests are normal. Needle EMG is characterized by the presence of muscle membrane irritability, including myotonic discharges without clinical myotonia.[14] Motor unit action potentials are small and short and recruit early. Muscle biopsy reveals a vacuolar myopathy in all variants.[140] Cardiac tests may reveal left ventricular hypertrophy and electrocardiographic abnormalities such as left axis deviation, short PR interval, inverted T waves, and large-amplitude QRS complexes.[144] Pulmonary function testing usually reveals a restrictive pattern as a result of diaphragmatic muscle weakness.

Treatment

In the past, no specific treatment existed for Pompe disease. Recently intravenous recombinant acid α-glucosidase (rhGAA) enzyme replacement has become available, revolutionizing the management of Pompe disease.[145] Initially, treatment was approved for patients with the infantile variant. Replacement therapy has now been approved by the FDA in the United States for all variants of Pompe disease.[146,147] The impact of replacement therapy on disease course, survival, and function in the three variants is an active area of research.[147,148]

ENDOCRINE MYOPATHIES

Endocrine disorders frequently manifest with muscular impairment. The features of endocrine myopathies most amenable to rehabilitation intervention include muscle weakness and atrophy. Exercises, orthoses, or assistive devices may be necessary, depending on the severity of the deficits.

The following sections discuss corticosteroid myopathy and the myopathies associated with thyroid abnormalities.

Steroid Myopathy

Steroid myopathy is the most common endocrine myopathy. It may result from excessive endogenous (Cushing's syndrome) or exogenous steroids. Exogenous sources are more common; the incidence is approximately 2.4% to 21% of patients treated with chronic steroids and the risk increases with use of high-dose steroids. Women may be as much as twice as vulnerable as men, and fluorinated corticosteroids (e.g., dexamethasone, beclomethasone, and triamcinolone) are more commonly implicated than nonfluorinated corticosteroids.[149] The severity of the myopathy may also depend on the treatment duration, dosage,[150] and treatment regimen.

Clinical Presentation

Patients with steroid myopathy usually describe an insidious onset of proximal muscle weakness and atrophy, with greater involvement of the lower limbs than the upper limbs. The weakness can develop over weeks to years.

Diagnosis

Laboratory findings usually include normal CK. Muscle biopsy usually shows preferential atrophy of type II fibers. Motor and sensory nerve conduction studies are expected to be normal, because the peripheral nerves are not affected. Needle EMG is also normal.

Treatment

Treatment options include stopping the steroid, switching to alternate-day dosing, reducing the dose, or switching from a fluorinated steroid to an equivalent dose of a nonfluorinated steroid.[149] Endogenous steroid excess is best treated with removal of any glucocorticoid-excreting tumors.[149] The patient may not experience full recovery for several months.

Physical therapy, including strength training exercises, is important for helping the patient overcome the weakness and prevent further muscle wasting that may result from inactivity.

Hyperthyroidism

Varying degrees of weakness may occur in as many as 82% of thyrotoxic patients, and females are affected more frequently than males. The weakness usually is present by the end of the fifth decade, and the incidence appears to correlate with the duration of hyperthyroidism.[149] The pathogenesis is thought to be related to enhanced muscle protein catabolism with increased muscle amino acid release in response to stimulation by the elevated thyroxine (T_4).[151]

Clinical Presentation

The weakness seen in hyperthyroidism is mostly proximal, resulting in difficulty rising from a sitting position or performing overhead activities. It can be associated with muscle atrophy and may be much more severe than the atrophy would suggest. The patient may complain of fatigue, myalgia, and exercise intolerance. Respiratory muscle involvement can be present.[149] Bulbar involvement can result in dysphagia and dysphonia.[115] Tendon reflexes usually are normal or brisk.

Diagnosis

Laboratory testing in primary hyperthyroidism reveals elevated triiodothyronine (T_3) and T_4 and a low thyroid-stimulating hormone (TSH). CK levels usually are normal. Motor and sensory nerve conduction studies are normal.[115] Needle EMG is usually normal, although fasciculations may be present.

Treatment

The myopathy usually improves with treatment of the underlying hyperthyroidism and return to a euthyroid state. It may take several months for strength to improve and even longer for normal muscle bulk to return. Active exercises with physical and occupational therapists can delay or even prevent the development of disuse atrophy. In more severe cases, assistive devices may be required.

Hypothyroidism

The primary myopathic clinical features associated with hypothyroidism are proximal muscle weakness, stiffness, fatigue, and slowed movements. A delay in the relaxation of deep tendon reflexes may also be seen.[149] **Myoedema** refers to painless mounting of muscle tissue and occurs in response to tapping or pinching of the muscle. It can occur in as many as one third of patients with hypothyroidism but is not specific for this disorder.[149] A prospective cohort study in adults newly diagnosed with thyroid disease revealed that neuromuscular complaints were present in 79% of those with hypothyroidism; 38% had clinical weakness in one or more muscle groups on manual muscle testing, 42% had signs of sensorimotor axonal neuropathy, and 29% had carpal tunnel syndrome.[152]

The serum CK usually is elevated, up to 100 times normal, but does not correlate with weakness; it typically normalizes after treatment of symptomatic patients. With primary hypothyroidism, T_3 and T_4 are depressed, whereas TSH is elevated. Nerve conduction studies and needle EMG usually are normal.[115] Myoedema is electrically silent. As in hyperthyroidism, treatment of the underlying thyroid dysfunction significantly improves the clinical findings, and active exercise prevents further weakness from disuse.

TOXIC MYOPATHIES

Table 32-12 summarizes some of the more common toxins that can cause myopathy. Alcoholic myopathy is discussed in more detail.

TABLE **32-12**

Toxic Myopathies Secondary to Medications or Toxins

Myopathy	Medication/Toxin	Clinical Features	Laboratory Findings
Necrotizing	Statins, clofibrate, gemfibrozil Alcohol abuse	Painful proximal myopathy	Increased creatine kinase EMG with muscle membrane irritability Possible myoglobinuria
Hypokalemic	Diuretics Laxatives Alcohol abuse Amphotericin B	Acute-onset weakness Myalgias	Increased creatine kinase Possible myoglobinuria Hypokalemia
Inflammatory	D-Penicillamine Interferon-α	Proximal muscle pain and weakness	Increased creatine kinase EMG with muscle membrane irritability Possible myoglobinuria
Mitochondrial	Zidovudine	Proximal muscle pain and weakness	Normal or increased creatine kinase EMG may be normal or show myopathic units
Focal	Heroin Diazepam Lidocaine	Local pain, swelling Contracture of affected muscle	Normal or increased creatine kinase
Antimicrotubular	Colchicine Vincristine	Proximal muscle weakness Mild peripheral neuropathy	Increased creatine kinase

EMG, Electromyography.

Alcoholic Myopathy

Alcohol can cause neuropathy as well as myopathy. The recognized forms of alcoholic myopathy are acute necrotizing myopathy, hypokalemic myopathy, chronic alcoholic myopathy, and cardiomyopathy.

Acute necrotizing myopathy usually occurs in chronic alcoholics or after particularly heavy bouts of drinking. The patient can present with a weak, swollen, painful, tender limb, which commonly is mistaken for thrombophlebitis.[2] In most cases cessation of alcohol intake results in a full recovery within 2 weeks; severe cases may result in myoglobinuria and acute renal failure.[153] Acute hypokalemic myopathy manifests as isolated acute muscle weakness that evolves over days and is reversible with potassium repletion.[2,154] Chronic alcoholic myopathy may occur in up to two thirds of chronic alcoholics and typically evolves over weeks to months to affect the shoulders and hips equally.[153] Treatment must include alcohol cessation, and even then residual weakness may be present. In severe cases, the patient may require assistive devices and orthoses to maintain function.

SUMMARY

Myopathies constitute a heterogeneous group of disorders with a wide range of etiologies and features. These muscle disorders can be hereditary or acquired. Myopathies can be categorized as muscular dystrophies or as congenital, inflammatory, metabolic, endocrine, or toxic myopathies. A common presenting feature is proximal (greater than distal) weakness. Age of onset, rate of progression, and involvement of other organ systems vary greatly depending on the specific myopathy. Traditionally, diagnosis of muscle disease has relied on a combination of clinical assessment, electrodiagnostic testing and muscle histopathology. Genetic testing has already become commercially available for many hereditary myopathies. Knowledge about the genetics of muscle disease is rapidly accumulating, and it is conceivable that in the near future, genomics techniques such as exome analysis and next-generation sequencing will allow molecular diagnosis for most, if not all, hereditary myopathies. Treatment is supportive. Rehabilitation, with its multidisciplinary approach, is vital to enhance function and quality of life.

REFERENCES

1. Cohn RD, Campbell KP: Molecular basis of muscular dystrophies, *Muscle Nerve* 23:1456–1471, 2000.
2. Engel AG, Ozawa E: Dystrophinopathies. In Engel AG, Franzini-Armstrong C, editors: 3 ed, Myology, vol 2. New York, 2004, McGraw-Hill.
3. Emery AEH, Muntoni F: *Duchenne muscular dystrophy*, ed 3, New York, 2003, Oxford University Press.
4. Bakker JP, De Groot IJ, Beelen A, et al: Predictive factors of cessation of ambulation in patients with duchenne muscular dystrophy, *Am J Phys Med Rehabil* 81:906–912, 2002.
5. Gozal D: Pulmonary manifestations of neuromuscular disease with special reference to duchenne muscular dystrophy and spinal muscular atrophy, *Pediatr Pulmonol* 29:141–150, 2000.
6. Mallory GB: Pulmonary complications of neuromuscular disease, *Pediatr Pulmonol Suppl* 26:138–140, 2004.
7. Phillips MF, Quinlivan RC, Edwards RH, et al: Changes in spirometry over time as a prognostic marker in patients with duchenne muscular dystrophy, *Am J Respir Crit Care Med* 164:2191–2194, 2001.

8. Phillips MF, Smith PE, Carroll N, et al: Nocturnal oxygenation and prognosis in duchenne muscular dystrophy, *Am J Respir Crit Care Med* 160:198–202, 1999.

9. Emery AEH: The muscular dystrophies, *Lancet* 359:687–695, 2002.

10. Bresolin N, Castelli E, Comi GP, et al: Cognitive impairment in duchenne muscular dystrophy, *Neuromuscul Disord* 4:359–369, 1994.

11. McDonald DG, Kinali M, Gallagher AC, et al: Fracture prevalence in duchenne muscular dystrophy, *Dev Med Child Neurol* 44:695–698, 2002.

12. Bushby K, Finkel R, Birnkrant DJ, et al: Diagnosis and management of duchenne muscular dystrophy, part 1: diagnosis, and pharmacological and psychosocial management, *Lancet Neurol* 9:77–93, 2010.

13. Krivickas L: Myopathies. In Tan FC, editor: *EMG secrets*, Philadelphia, 2004, Hanley & Belfus.

14. Amato AA, Dumitru D: Hereditary myopathies. In Dumitru D, Amato AA, Zwarts M, editors: *Electrodiagnostic medicine*, ed 2, Philadelphia, 2002, Hanley & Belfus.

15. Dubowitz V: *Muscle biopsy: a practical approach*, 2 ed, London, 1985, WB Saunders.

16. Moxley RT III, Ashwal S, Pandya S, et al: Practice parameter: corticosteroid treatment of duchenne dystrophy—report of the quality standards subcommittee of the american academy of neurology and the practice committee of the child neurology society, *Neurology* 64:13–20, 2005.

17. Biggar WD, Gingras M, Fehlings DL, et al: Deflazacort treatment of duchenne muscular dystrophy, *J Pediatr* 138:45–50, 2001.

18. Quinlivan R, Roper H, Davie M, et al: Report of a muscular dystrophy campaign funded workshop birmingham, UK, January 16, 2004: osteoporosis in duchenne muscular dystrophy; its prevalence, treatment and prevention, *Neuromuscul Disord* 15:72–79, 2005.

19. Wong BL, Christopher C: Corticosteroids in duchenne muscular dystrophy: a reappraisal, *J Child Neurol* 17:183–190, 2002.

20. Bladen CL, Rafferty K, Straub V, et al: The TREAT-NMD duchenne muscular dystrophy registries: conception, design, and utilization by industry and academia, *Hum Mutat* 34:1449–1457, 2013.

21. Connolly AM, Florence JM, Cradock MM, et al: Motor and cognitive assessment of infants and young boys with duchenne muscular dystrophy: results from the muscular dystrophy association DMD clinical research network, *Neuromuscul Disord* 23:529–539, 2013.

22. *Parent Project Muscular Dystrophy.* Available at http://www.parentprojectmd.org.

23. Lynn S, Aartsma-Rus A, Bushby K, et al: Measuring clinical effectiveness of medicinal products for the treatment of duchenne muscular dystrophy, *Neuromuscul Disord* 25:96–105, 2015.

24. McDonald CM, Henricson EK, Abresch RT, et al: The 6-minute walk test and other endpoints in duchenne muscular dystrophy: longitudinal natural history observations over 48 weeks from a multicenter study, *Muscle Nerve* 48:343–356, 2013.

25. McDonald CM, Henricson EK, Abresch RT, et al: The 6-minute walk test and other clinical endpoints in duchenne muscular dystrophy: reliability, concurrent validity, and minimal clinically important differences from a multicenter study, *Muscle Nerve* 48:357–368, 2013.

26. Mendell JR, Rodino-Klapac LR, Sahenk Z, et al: Eteplirsen for the treatment of duchenne muscular dystrophy, *Ann Neurol* 74:637–647, 2013.

27. Bushby K, Finkel R, Wong B, et al: Ataluren treatment of patients with nonsense mutation dystrophinopathy, *Muscle Nerve* 50:477–487, 2014.

28. Bushby K, Finkel R, Birnkrant DJ, et al: Diagnosis and management of duchenne muscular dystrophy, part 2: implementation of multidisciplinary care, *Lancet Neurol* 9:177–189, 2010.

29. Hicks JE: Role of rehabilitation in the management of myopathies, *Curr Opin Rheumatol* 10:548–555, 1998.

30. Rodillo EB, Fernandez-Bermejo E, Heckmatt JZ, et al: Prevention of rapidly progressive scoliosis in duchenne muscular dystrophy by prolongation of walking with orthoses, *J Child Neurol* 3:269–274, 1988.

31. Hyde SA, Flytrup I, Glent S, et al: A randomized comparative study of two methods for controlling Tendo-Achilles contracture in duchenne muscular dystrophy, *Neuromuscul Disord* 10:257–263, 2000.

32. Vignos PJ, Wagner MB, Karlinchak B, et al: Evaluation of a program for long-term treatment of duchenne muscular dystrophy: experience at the university hospitals of cleveland, *J Bone Joint Surg Am* 78:1844–1852, 1996.

33. Ansved T: Muscle training in muscular dystrophies, *Acta Physiol Scand* 171:359–366, 2001.

34. Vignos PJ: Physical models of rehabilitation in neuromuscular disease, *Muscle Nerve* 6:323–338, 1983.

35. Finder JD, Birnkrant D, Carl J, et al: Respiratory care of the patient with duchenne muscular dystrophy: ATS consensus statement, *Am J Respir Crit Care Med* 170:456–465, 2004.

36. Perrin C, Unterborn JN, Ambrosio CD, et al: Pulmonary complications of chronic neuromuscular diseases and their management, *Muscle Nerve* 29:5–27, 2004.

37. Robertson PL, Roloff DW: Chronic respiratory failure in limb-girdle muscular dystrophy: successful long-term therapy with nasal bilevel positive airway pressure, *Pediatr Neurol* 10:328–331, 1994.

38. Miske LJ, Hickey EM, Kolb SM, et al: Use of the mechanical in-exsufflator in pediatric patients with neuromuscular disease and impaired cough, *Chest* 125:1406–1412, 2004.

39. Flanigan K: Facioscapulohumeral muscular dystrophy and scapuloperoneal disorders. In Engel AG, Franzini-Armstrong C, editors: 3 ed, New York, 2004, McGraw-Hill. Myology, vol 2.

40. Kissel JT, McDermott MP, Mendell JR, et al: Randomized, double-blind, placebo-controlled trial of albuterol in facioscapulohumeral dystrophy, *Neurology* 57:1434–1440, 2001.

41. Tupler R, Gabellini D: Molecular basis of facioscapulohumeral muscular dystrophy, *Cell Mol Life Sci* 61:557–566, 2004.

42. Group TF-D: A prospective, quantitative study of the natural history of facioscapulohumeral muscular dystrophy (FSHD): implications for therapeutic trials—The FSH-DY Group, *Neurology* 48:38–46, 1997.

43. Wohlgemuth M, van der Kooi EL, van Kesteren RG, et al: Ventilatory support in facioscapulohumeral muscular dystrophy, *Neurology* 63:176–178, 2004.

44. Lunt PW, Jardine PE, Koch MC, et al: Correlation between fragment size at D4F104S1 and age at onset or at wheelchair use, with a possible generational effect, accounts for much phenotypic variation in 4q35-facioscapulohumeral muscular dystrophy (FSHD), *Hum Mol Genet* 4:951–958, 1995.

45. Gaillard MC, Roche S, Dion C, et al: Differential DNA methylation of the D4Z4 repeat in patients with FSHD and asymptomatic carriers, *Neurology* 83:733–742, 2014.

46. van der Kooi EL, Vogels OJ, van Asseldonk RJ, et al: Strength training and albuterol in facioscapulohumeral muscular dystrophy, *Neurology* 63:702–708, 2004.

47. Bushby KM, Pollitt C, Johnson MA, et al: Muscle pain as a prominent feature of facioscapulohumeral muscular dystrophy (FSHD): four illustrative case reports, *Neuromuscul Disord* 8:574–579, 1998.

48. van der Kooi EL, Lindeman E, Riphagen I: Strength training and aerobic exercise training for muscle disease, *Cochrane Database Syst Rev*, 2005. CD003907.

49. Voet N, Bleijenberg G, Hendriks J, et al: Both aerobic exercise and cognitive-behavioral therapy reduce chronic fatigue in FSHD: an RCT, *Neurology* 83:1914–1922, 2014.

50. Ketenjian AY: Scapulocostal stabilization for scapular winging in facioscapulohumeral muscular dystrophy, *J Bone Joint Surg Am* 60:476–480, 1978.

51. Bunch WH, Siegel IM: Scapulothoracic arthrodesis in facioscapulohumeral muscular dystrophy: review of seventeen procedures with 3- to 21-year follow-up, *J Bone Joint Surg Am* 75:372–376, 1993.

52. Cenni V, Sabatelli P, Mattioli E, et al: Lamin A N-terminal phosphorylation is associated with myoblast activation: impairment in emery-dreifuss muscular dystrophy, *J Med Genet* 42:214–220, 2005.

53. Cohn RD, Campbell KP: Molecular basis of muscular dystrophies, *Muscle Nerve* 23:1456–1471, 2000.

54. Helbling-Leclerc A, Bonne G, Schwartz K: Emery-Dreifuss muscular dystrophy, *Eur J Hum Genet* 10:157–161, 2002.

55. Maraldi NM, Merlini L: Emery-Dreifuss muscular dystrophy. In Engel AG, Franzini-Armstrong C, editors: ed 3, Myology, vol 2, New York, 2004, McGraw-Hill.

56. Mercuri E, Counsell S, Allsop J, et al: Selective muscle involvement on magnetic resonance imaging in autosomal dominant emery-dreifuss muscular dystrophy, *Neuropediatrics* 33:10–14, 2002.

57. Colomer J, Iturriaga C, Bonne G, et al: Autosomal dominant emery-dreifuss muscular dystrophy: a new family with late diagnosis, *Neuromuscul Disord* 12:19–25, 2002.

58. Becane HM, Bonne G, Varnous S, et al: High incidence of sudden death with conduction system and myocardial disease due to lamins A and C gene mutation, *Pacing Clin Electrophysiol* 23(11 Pt 1):1661–1666, 2000.

59. Bonne G, Yaou RB, Beroud C, et al: 108th ENMC international workshop, third workshop of the MYO-CLUSTER project: EUROMEN, seventh international emery-dreifuss muscular dystrophy (EDMD) workshop, september 13-15, 2002, naarden, the netherlands, *Neuromuscul Disord* 13:508–515, 2003.

60. Boriani G, Gallina M, Merlini L, et al: Clinical relevance of atrial fibrillation/flutter, stroke, pacemaker implant, and heart failure in emery-dreifuss muscular dystrophy: a long-term longitudinal study, *Stroke* 34:901–908, 2003.

61. Ben Yaou R, Becane HM, Demay L, et al: Autosomal dominant limb-girdle muscular dystrophy associated with conduction defects (LGMD1B): a description of 8 new families with the LMNA gene mutations, *Rev Neurol (Paris)* 161:42–54, 2005.

62. Wessely R, Seidl S, Schomig A: Cardiac involvement in Emery-Dreifuss muscular dystrophy, *Clin Genet* 67:220–223, 2005.

63. van Berlo JH, de Voogt WG, van der Kooi AJ, et al: Meta-analysis of clinical characteristics of 299 carriers of LMNA gene mutations: do lamin A/C mutations portend a high risk of sudden death? *J Mol Med* 83:79–83, 2005.

64. Beckmann JS, Brown RH, Muntoni F, et al: 66th/67th ENMC sponsored international workshop: the limb-girdle muscular dystrophies, March, 26-28, 1999, Naarden, The Netherlands, *Neuromuscul Disord* 9:436–445, 1999.

65. van der Kooi AJ, Barth PG, Busch HF, et al: The clinical spectrum of limb-girdle muscular dystrophy: a survey in the netherlands, *Brain* 119(Pt 5): 1471–1480, 1996.

66. Bonnemann C, Bushby K: The limb-girdle muscular dystrophies. In Engel AG, Franzini-Armstrong C, editors: ed 3, Myology, vol 2, New York, 2004, McGraw-Hill.

67. Mascarenhas DA, Spodick DH, Chad DA, et al: Cardiomyopathy of limb-girdle muscular dystrophy, *J Am Coll Cardiol* 24:1328–1333, 1994.

68. van der Kooi AJ, Bonne G, Eymard B, et al: Lamin A/C mutations with lipodystrophy, cardiac abnormalities, and muscular dystrophy, *Neurology* 59:620–623, 2002.

69. van der Kooi AJ, de Voogt WG, Barth PG, et al: The heart in limb-girdle muscular dystrophy, *Heart* 79:73–77, 1998.

70. van der Kooi AJ, Ginjaar HB, Busch HF, et al: Limb girdle muscular dystrophy: a pathological and immunohistochemical reevaluation, *Muscle Nerve* 21:584–590, 1998.

71. Yamanouchi Y, Arikawa E, Arahata K, et al: Limb-girdle muscular dystrophy: clinical and pathologic re-evaluation, *J Neurol Sci* 129:15–20, 1995.

72. Stubgen JP, Stipp A: Limb girdle muscular dystrophy: a prospective follow-up study of functional impairment, *Muscle Nerve* 20:453–460, 1997.

73. Harper PS: Myotonic dystrophy. In Engel AG, Franzini-Armstrong C, editors: ed 3, Myology, vol 2. New York, 2004, McGraw-Hill.

74. Brady LI, MacNeil LG, Tarnopolsky MA: Impact of habitual exercise on the strength of individuals with myotonic dystrophy type 1, *Am J Phys Med Rehabil* 93:739–746, 2014.

75. Voet NB, van der Kooi EL, Riphagen II, et al: Strength training and aerobic exercise training for muscle disease, *Cochrane Database Syst Rev* 7, 2013. CD003907.

76. Kierkegaard M, Harms-Ringdahl K, Edström L, et al: Feasibility and effects of a physical exercise programme in adults with myotonic dystrophy type 1: a randomized controlled pilot study, *J Rehabil Med* 43:695–702, 2011.

77. North KN: Congenital myopathies. In Engel AG, Franzini-Armstrong C, editors: ed 3, Myology, vol 2, New York, 2004, McGraw-Hill.

78. Haan EA, Freemantle CJ, McCure JA, et al: Assignment of the gene for central core disease to chromosome 19, *Hum Genet* 86:187–190, 1990.

79. Du GG, Khanna VK, Guo X, et al: Central core disease mutations R4892W, I4897T and G4898E in the ryanodine receptor isoform 1 reduce the Ca2+ sensitivity and amplitude of Ca2+-dependent Ca2+ release, *Biochem J* 382(Pt 2):557–564, 2004.

80. Messina S, Hartley L, Main M, et al: Pilot trial of salbutamol in central core and multi-minicore diseases, *Neuropediatrics* 35:262–266, 2004.

81. Schreuder LT, Nijhuis-van der Sanden MW, de Hair A, et al: Successful use of albuterol in a patient with central core disease and mitochondrial dysfunction, *J Inherit Metab Dis* 33(Suppl 3):S205–209, 2010.

82. Wang X, Huang QQ, Breckenridge MT, et al: Cellular fate of truncated slow skeletal muscle troponin T produced by Glu180 nonsense mutation in Amish nemaline myopathy, *J Biol Chem* 280: 13241–13249, 2005.

83. Goebel HH: Congenital myopathies in the new millennium, *J Child Neurol* 20:94–101, 2005.

84. Corbett MA, Akkari PA, Domazetovska A, et al: An alpha Tropomyosin mutation alters dimer preference in nemaline myopathy, *Ann Neurol* 57:42–49, 2005.

85. Gomes AV, Barnes JA, Harada K, et al: Role of troponin T in disease, *Mol Cell Biochem* 263:115–129, 2004.

86. Donner K, Sandbacka M, Lehtokari VL, et al: Complete genomic structure of the human nebulin gene and identification of alternatively spliced transcripts, *Eur J Hum Genet* 12:744–751, 2004.

87. Ilkovski B, Nowak KJ, Domazetovska A, et al: Evidence for a dominant-negative effect in ACTA1 nemaline myopathy caused by abnormal folding, aggregation and altered polymerization of mutant actin isoforms *Hum Mol Genet* 13:1727–1743, 2004.

88. Wallgren-Pettersson C, Pelin K, Nowak KJ, et al: Genotype-phenotype correlations in nemaline myopathy caused by mutations in the genes for nebulin and skeletal muscle alpha-actin, *Neuromuscul Disord* 14:461–470, 2004.

89. North KN, Laing NG, Wallgren-Pettersson C: Nemaline myopathy: current concepts—The ENMC International Consortium and Nemaline Myopathy, *J Med Genet* 34:705–713, 1997.

90. Wallgren-Pettersson C, Beggs AH, Laing NG: 51st ENMC International Workshop: nemaline myopathy, June 13-15, 1997, Naarden, The Netherlands, *Neuromuscul Disord* 8:53–56, 1998.

91. Wallgren-Pettersson C, Laing NG: 109th ENMC International Workshop: Fifth Workshop on Nemaline Myopathy, October 11-13, 2002, Naarden, The Netherlands, *Neuromuscul Disord* 13:501–507, 2003.

92. Yamaguchi M, Robson RM, Stromer MH, et al: Nemaline myopathy rod bodies: structure and composition, *J Neurol Sci* 56:35–56, 1982.

93. Lamont PJ, Thorburn DR, Fabian V, et al: Nemaline rods and complex I deficiency in three infants with hypotonia, motor delay and failure to thrive, *Neuropediatrics* 35:302–306, 2004.

94. Tamura Y, Matsui K, Yaguchi H, et al: Nemaline rods in chorea-acanthocytosis, *Muscle Nerve* 31: 516–519, 2005.

95. Wallgren-Pettersson C: Congenital nemaline myopathy: a clinical follow-up of twelve patients, *J Neurol Sci* 89:1–14, 1989.

96. Wallgren-Pettersson C: Nemaline and myotubular myopathies, *Semin Pediatr Neurol* 9:132–144, 2002.

97. Cook BJ, Berkowitz RG: Tracheostomy in children with nemaline core myopathy, *Int J Pediatr Otorhinolaryngol* 69:263–266, 2005.

98. Engel AG, Hohlfeld R: The polymyositis and dermatomyositis syndromes. In Engel AG, Franzini-Armstrong C, editors: ed 3, Myology, vol 2, New York, 2004, McGraw-Hill.

99. Christopher-Stine L, Plotz PH: Adult inflammatory myopathies, *Best Pract Res Clin Rheumatol* 18: 331–344, 2004.

100. Christopher-Stine L, Plotz PH: Myositis: an update on pathogenesis, *Curr Opin Rheumatol* 16:700–706, 2004.

101. Mastaglia FL, Phillips BA: Idiopathic inflammatory myopathies: epidemiology, classification, and diagnostic criteria, *Rheum Dis Clin North Am* 28: 723–741, 2002.

102. Schwarz MI: Pulmonary and cardiac manifestations of polymyositis-dermatomyositis, *J Thorac Imaging* 7:46–54, 1992.

103. Miller FW: Classification and prognosis of inflammatory muscle disease, *Rheum Dis Clin North Am* 20:811–826, 1994.

104. Riemekasten G, Opitz C, Audring H, et al: Beware of the heart: the multiple picture of cardiac involvement in myositis, *Rheumatology (Oxford)* 38:1153–1157, 1999.

105. Gonzalez-Lopez L, Gamez-Nava JI, Sanchez L, et al: Cardiac manifestations in dermatopolymyositis, *Clin Exp Rheumatol* 14:373–379, 1996.

106. Taylor AJ, Wortham DC: Burge JR el al: The heart in polymyositis: a prospective evaluation of 26 patients, *Clin Cardiol* 16:802–808, 1993.

107. Yale SH, Adlakha A, Stanton MS: Dermatomyositis with pericardial tamponade and polymyositis with pericardial effusion, *Am Heart J* 126:997–999, 1993.

108. Schnabel A, Reuter M, Biederer J, et al: Interstitial lung disease in polymyositis and dermatomyositis: clinical course and response to treatment, *Semin Arthritis Rheum* 32:273–284, 2003.

109. Schnabel A, Hellmich B, Gross WL: Interstitial lung disease in polymyositis and dermatomyositis, *Curr Rheumatol Rep* 7:99–105, 2005.

110. Fujisawa T, Suda T, Nakamura Y, et al: Differences in clinical features and prognosis of interstitial lung diseases between polymyositis and dermatomyositis, *J Rheumatol* 32:58–64, 2005.

111. Schwarz MI: The lung in polymyositis, *Clin Chest Med* 19:701–712, 1998.

112. Buchbinder R, Hill CL: Malignancy in patients with inflammatory myopathy, *Curr Rheumatol Rep* 4:415–426, 2002.

113. Nirmalananthan N, Holton JL, Hanna MG: Is it really myositis? A consideration of the differential diagnosis, *Curr Opin Rheumatol* 16:684–691, 2004.

114. Hochberg MC, Feldman D, Stevens MB, et al: Antibody to Jo-1 in polymyositis/dermatomyositis: association with interstitial pulmonary disease, *J Rheumatol* 11:663–665, 1984.

115. Amato AA, Dumitru D: Acquired myopathies. In Dumitru D, Amato AA, Zwarts M, editors: *Electrodiagnostic medicine*, 2 ed, Philadelphia, 2002, Hanley & Belfus.

116. Plotz PH, Dalakas M, Leff RL, et al: Current concepts in the idiopathic inflammatory myopathies: polymyositis, dermatomyositis, and related disorders, *Ann Intern Med* 111:143–157, 1989.

117. Ponyi A, Borgulya G, Constantin T, et al: Functional outcome and quality of life in adult patients with idiopathic inflammatory myositis, *Rheumatology (Oxford)* 44:83–88, 2005.

118. Danko K, Ponyi A, Constantin T, et al: Long-term survival of patients with idiopathic inflammatory myopathies according to clinical features: a longitudinal study of 162 cases, *Medicine (Baltimore)* 83:35–42, 2004.

119. Dimauro S, Hays AP, Tsujino S: Nonlysosomal glycogenoses. In Engel AG, Franzini-Armstrong C, editors: ed 3, Myology, vol 2, New York, 2004, McGraw-Hill.

120. Ollivier K, Hogrel JY, Gomez-Merino D, et al: Exercise tolerance and daily life in McArdle's disease, *Muscle Nerve* 31:637–641, 2005.

121. Wolfe GI, Baker NS, Haller RG, et al: McArdle's disease presenting with asymmetric, late-onset arm weakness, *Muscle Nerve* 23:641–645, 2000.

122. Sauret JM, Marinides G, Wang GK: Rhabdomyolysis, *Am Fam Physician* 65:907–912, 2002.

123. Bonnardeaux A, Querin S, Charron L: McArdle's disease presenting with acute renal failure, *Nephron* 59:696–697, 1991.

124. Mittal SK, Dash SC, Mittal R, et al: McArdle's disease presenting as acute renal failure, *Nephron* 71:109, 1995.

125. Vladutiu GD: Laboratory diagnosis of metabolic myopathies, *Muscle Nerve* 25:649–663, 2002.

126. Quinlivan R, Beynon RJ: Pharmacological and nutritional treatment for McArdle's disease (glycogen storage disease type V), *Cochrane Database Syst Rev*, 2004. CD003458.

127. Vissing J, Haller RG: The effect of oral sucrose on exercise tolerance in patients with McArdle's disease, *N Engl J Med* 349:2503–2509, 2003.

128. Sato S, Ohi T, Nishino I, et al: Confirmation of the efficacy of vitamin B6 supplementation for McArdle disease by follow-up muscle biopsy, *Muscle Nerve* 45:436–440, 2012.

129. Quinlivan R, Martinuzzi A, Schoser B: Pharmacological and nutritional treatment for McArdle disease (Glycogen Storage Disease type V), *Cochrane Database Syst Rev* 11, 2014. CD003458.

130. Mineo I, Kono N, Hara N, et al: Myogenic hyperurice-mia: a common pathophysiologic feature of glycog-enosis types III, V, and VII, *N Engl J Med* 317:75–80, 1987.

131. Kono N, Mineo I, Shimizu T, et al: Increased plasma uric acid after exercise in muscle phosphofructoki-nase deficiency, *Neurology* 36:106–108, 1986.

132. Bonilla E, Schotland DL: Histochemical diagnosis of muscle phosphofructokinase deficiency, *Arch Neurol* 22:8–12, 1970.

133. Yang-Feng TL, Zheng K, Yu J, et al: Assignment of the human glycogen debrancher gene to chromosome 1p21, *Genomics* 13:931–934, 1992.

134. Chen YT, He JK, Ding JH, et al: Glycogen debranching enzyme: purification, antibody characterization, and immunoblot analyses of type III glycogen storage disease, *Am J Hum Genet* 41:1002–1015, 1987.

135. Kiechl S, Kohlendorfer U, Thaler C, et al: Different clinical aspects of debrancher deficiency myopathy, *J Neurol Neurosurg Psychiatry* 67:364–368, 1999.

136. Kiechl S, Willeit J, Vogel W, et al: Reversible severe myopathy of respiratory muscles due to adult-onset type III glycogenosis, *Neuromuscul Disord* 9: 408–410, 1999.

137. Lucchiari S, Fogh I, Prelle A, et al: Clinical and ge-netic variability of glycogen storage disease type IIIa: seven novel AGL gene mutations in the mediterra-nean area, *Am J Med Genet* 109:183–190, 2002.

138. Goldberg T, Slonim AE: Nutrition therapy for he-patic glycogen storage diseases, *J Am Diet Assoc* 93:1423–1430, 1993.

139. Slonim AE, Weisberg C, Benke P, et al: Reversal of debrancher deficiency myopathy by the use of high-protein nutrition, *Ann Neurol* 11:420–422, 1982.

140. Engel AG, Hirschhorn R, Huie M: Acid maltase defi-ciency. In Engel AG, Franzini-Armstrong C, editors: ed 3, Myology, vol 2, New York, 2004, McGraw-Hill.

141. Keunen RW, Lambregts PC, Op de Coul AA, et al: Respiratory failure as initial symptom of acid mal-tase deficiency, *J Neurol Neurosurg Psychiatry* 47:549–552, 1984.

142. Margolis ML, Howlett P, Goldberg R, et al: Obstructive sleep apnea syndrome in acid maltase deficiency, *Chest* 105:947–949, 1994.

143. American Association of Neuromuscular and Electrodiagnostic Medicine, Al-Lozi MT, Amato AA, et al: Diagnostic criteria for late-onset (child-hood and adult) Pompe disease, *Muscle Nerve* 40: 149–160, 2009.

144. Gilbert-Barness E: Review: metabolic cardiomyopa-thy and conduction system defects in children, *Ann Clin Lab Sci* 34:15–34, 2004.

145. Kishnani PS, Beckemeyer AA, Mendelsohn NJ: The new era of Pompe disease: advances in the detec-tion, understanding of the phenotypic spectrum, pathophysiology, and management, *Am J Med Genet C Semin Med Genet* 160C:1–7, 2012.

146. Cupler EJ, Berger KI, Leshner RT, et al: Consensus treatment recommendations for late-onset Pompe disease, *Muscle Nerve* 45:319–333, 2012.

147. Park JS, Kim HG, Shin JH, et al: Effect of enzyme replacement therapy in late onset Pompe disease: open pilot study of 48 weeks follow-up, *Neurol Sci* 36:599–605, 2015.

148. Chien YH, Lee NC, Chen CA, et al: Long-term prog-nosis of patients with infantile-onset Pompe disease diagnosed by newborn screening and treated since birth, *J Pediatr* 166:985–991, 2015.

149. Ubogu E, Ruff R, Kaminski H: Endocrine myopathies. In Engel AG, Franzini-Armstrong C, editors: ed 3, Myology, vol 2, New York, 2004, McGraw-Hill.

150. Amaya-Villar R, Garnacho-Montero J, Garcia-Garmendia JL, et al: Steroid-induced myopathy in patients intubated due to exacerbation of chronic obstructive pulmonary disease, *Intensive Care Med* 31:157–161, 2005.

151. Riis AL, Jorgensen JO, Gjedde S, et al: Whole body and forearm substrate metabolism in hyperthy-roidism: evidence of increased basal muscle pro-tein breakdown, *Am J Physiol Endocrinol Metab* 288:E1067–E1073, 2005.

152. Duyff RF, van den Bosch J, Laman DM, et al: Neuromuscular findings in thyroid dysfunction: a prospective clinical and electrodiagnostic study, *J Neurol Neurosurg Psychiatry* 68:750–755, 2000.

153. Sieb JP: Myopathies due to drugs, toxins and nutri-tional deficiency. In Engel AG, Franzini-Armstrong C, editors: ed 3, Myology, vol 2, New York, 2004, McGraw-Hill.

154. Finsterer J, Hess B, Jarius C, et al: Malnutrition-induced hypokalemic myopathy in chronic alcohol-ism, *J Toxicol Clin Toxicol* 36:369–373, 1998.

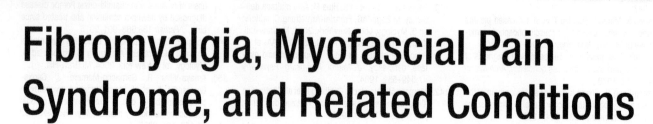

CHAPTER 33

Fibromyalgia, Myofascial Pain Syndrome, and Related Conditions

MELISSA COLBERT, JOANNE BORG-STEIN

Clinicians often encounter patients with a chief complaint of pain or more specifically "muscle pain." It may be regional or diffuse and may be associated with a constellation of other symptoms. When the pain is not explained by soft tissue damage or a clearly defined inflammatory process, patients may be given a diagnosis of **fibromyalgia (FM)** or **myofascial pain syndrome (MPS)**. The purpose of this chapter is to delineate what constitutes these conditions and how they are most appropriately managed.

FM is a disorder defined by pain that is both chronic (i.e., at least 3 months' duration) and widespread, often affecting both sides of the body, above and below the waist. In addition to pain, it is characterized by a constellation of other symptoms, which may include fatigue (almost always), unrefreshing sleep, cognitive dysfunction, mood disturbance, and a variety of somatic symptoms.[1,2]

MPS is a condition in which pain originates from **myofascial trigger points (MTrPs)** in the skeletal muscle, either alone or in combination with other pain generators. MTrPs are discrete areas of focal tenderness in muscle that are characterized by hypersensitive, palpable taut bands of muscle that are painful to palpation. Manual pressure over these points reproduces the patient's presenting pain symptoms and refers pain in characteristic patterns. Some clinicians prefer the designation *regional soft tissue pain* as a term that encompasses pain and localized tenderness not only in muscle but also in contiguous soft tissues, such as ligaments and tendons.[3,4]

There is certainly overlap between FM and MPS, and their distinction remains a topic of debate among clinicians.[5] However, in contrast to FM, MPS is focal (i.e., one particular site) and does not necessarily contain multiple pain generators or somatic symptoms. Furthermore, MPS specifically involves the presence of a taut band, which may or may not be present in a patient with FM.[4] Therefore, understanding these two conditions as discrete entities has significant clinical utility both in terms of approach and treatment.

EPIDEMIOLOGY

FM is present in up to 8% of the population, with similar prevalence among varied countries, cultures, and ethnic groups. It encompasses all ages, including childhood, with increasing prevalence up to age 65. Although FM does have a female predominance, the female to male ratio is now thought to be close to 2:1, which is similar to other chronic pain conditions.[6,7] In addition to female sex, risk factors for widespread pain include increasing age (up to 65 years), low socioeconomic status, high pain severity, previous disabling episode, and somatic symptoms (i.e., physical symptoms but no obvious physical condition present).[1]

A growing body of evidence strongly suggests the presence of genetic risk factors in FM. First-degree relatives of patients with FM are more than 8 times more likely to have FM and other chronic pain.[8] In fact, Arnold's 2013 genome-wide linkage analysis of 116 American families demonstrated that siblings of those with FM have a 13.6-fold greater risk of developing FM compared with the general population. Chromosome 17 was shown to contain a single region that was clearly linked to FM in this population ($P<0.001$).[6,9] Genes affecting several receptors, proteins, and plasma cytokine levels are also implicated in FM.[7,10,11]

MPS has a high prevalence among individuals with regional pain complaints. The prevalence varies, from 21% of patients seen in a general orthopedic clinic, to 30% of patients with regional pain in a general medical clinic, to as high as 85% to 90% of patients presenting to specialty pain management centers. Women and men are affected equally.[12–14]

CLINICAL PRESENTATION

Patients with FM will often state "I hurt all over all the time," or "It feels like I always have the flu." Symptoms consist of diffuse, multifocal pain that waxes and wanes and is often migratory in nature, touch hurts or is tender, dysesthesias (i.e., unpleasant sensation when touched) and paresthesias (i.e., abnormal sensation, burning, tingling), fatigue and sleep disturbance, memory and attention difficulties, mood disturbance, and stiffness upon waking. Symptoms suggestive of sensory hyperresponsiveness, such as sensitivity to bright lights, loud noises, odors, and visceral symptoms, are also often present.[7] Associated conditions, such as migraines, tension headaches, irritable bowel syndrome, tinnitus, restless leg syndrome, and temporomandibular jaw pain, are common.[1,7,15]

The physical examination of a patient with FM should include a thorough medical, neurological, and musculoskeletal examination and will often, but not always, be notable for diffuse soft tissue tenderness, including ligaments and paraspinal muscles. If tenderness is present over only the interphalangeal joints, one should consider a systemic autoimmune disorder. Examination findings for the joints and nervous system are normal, despite commonly reported symptoms of numbness and a swollen feeling in the joints. Range of motion of the cervical and lumbar spine may be slightly restricted due to pain.[1,16]

The characteristic symptoms of MPS may begin after a discrete trauma or injury or may have an insidious onset. Patients note localized or regional deep aching sensations, which can vary from mild to severe.[17] The MTrPs of each muscle have their own characteristic referred pain pattern; therefore the pain distribution can aid in identification of which muscle may contain the MTrP (Figure 33-1).[18] Associated autonomic dysfunction

frequently occurs, including abnormal sweating, lacrimation dermal flushing, and vasomotor and temperature changes.[19] Cervical myofascial pain may be associated with neurotological symptoms, including imbalance, dizziness, and tinnitus.[20] Functional complaints include decreased work tolerance, impaired muscle coordination, stiff joints, fatigue, and weakness. Other associated symptoms may include regional paresthesias or numbness, blurred vision, twitches, and trembling. Later stages may be compounded by sleep disturbance and mood changes.[21-23]

The physical examination of a patient with MPS also begins with a careful medical, neurological, and musculoskeletal examination. Posture, biomechanics, and joint function should be analyzed to identify any underlying factors that may have contributed to the development of the local or regional pain. An active MTrP is typically associated with painful, restricted range of motion. The trigger point should be identified by gentle palpation perpendicular to the direction of the muscle fibers. The examiner should detect a ropelike nodularity within the taut band of muscle. Palpation of this area is exquisitely painful and reproduces the patient's local and referred pain pattern.[21,24]

DIAGNOSTIC STUDIES

Laboratory workup should be normal in both FM and MPS, unless concurrent disease is present. Studies include complete blood count (CBC), basic metabolic panel (BMP), thyroid function tests, vitamin D, erythrocyte sedimentation rate (ESR), and C-reactive protein (CRP), as well as possibly creatinine kinase (CK), iron studies, vitamin B_{12}, and liver transaminases. It is advised to avoid antinuclear antibody (ANA) and rheumatoid factor (RF) unless signs and symptoms are suggestive of an autoimmune disorder because 13% of healthy adults are positive for ANA at a titer of 1:80.[1,6] Diagnostic imaging may reveal coincidental osteoarthritis or discogenic changes. The treating clinician must determine the relevance of these findings based on the specific clinical scenario.[1,21]

Studies currently being investigated as potential tools to better define the scientific underpinnings of FM and or MPS include microdialysis, ultrasound, magnetic resonance elastography, electromyography (EMG), and small fiber nerve biopsy.[5,25,26]

DIAGNOSTIC CRITERIA

According to the 2010 American College of Rheumatology preliminary diagnostic criteria for FM, a patient must have a combination of widespread pain and somatic symptoms to receive the diagnosis[2] (Box 33-1). Somatic symptoms include but are not limited to fatigue, headache, pain and/or cramps in abdomen, numbness

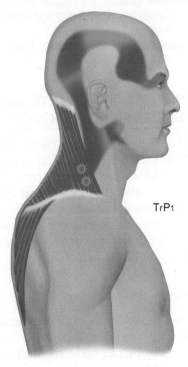

TrP1

Figure 33-1 Referred pain pattern from a trigger point in the upper trapezius muscle. (Adapted from Simon DG, *Travell JG, Simons LS: Travell & Simon's myofascial pain and dysfunction: the trigger point manual*, ed 2, p 279, Baltimore, 1999, Williams & Wilkins, 1999.)

BOX 33-1

Diagnostic Criteria for Fibromyalgia

WIDESPREAD PAIN INDEX (WPI)

Score 0-19, 1 point for each location

Pain in any of the following areas in the last week?

Shoulder girdle (left)	Neck	Upper arm (left)	Upper leg (left)	Hip (left)
Shoulder girdle (right)	Upper back	Upper arm (right)	Upper leg (right)	Hip (right)
Jaw (left)	Chest	Lower arm (left)	Lower leg (left)	Lower back
Jaw (right)	Abdomen	Lower arm (right)	Lower leg (right)	

SYMPTOM SEVERITY SCALE (SSS) SCORE

Score 0-12, severity of specific symptoms (0-9)+general somatic symptoms (0-3)

Severity of each of the following symptoms over the last week?
- Fatigue
- Waking unrefreshed
- Cognitive symptoms

0=no problem
1=slight/mild/intermittent
2=moderate/frequent
3=severe/pervasive/continuous

Number of general somatic symptoms (0=none, 1=few, 2=moderate, 3=many)

FOR A DIAGNOSIS OF FIBROMYALGIA, A PATIENT MUST HAVE THE FOLLOWING:
- WPI of at least 7+SSS of at least 5
  OR
- WPI of at least 3+SSS of at least 9

Data from Wolfe F, Clauw DJ, Fitzcharles M et al: The American College of Rheumatology preliminary diagnostic criteria for fibromyalgia and measurement of symptom severity, *Arthritis Care Res* 62:600-610, 2010.

and/or tingling, dizziness, depression, constipation, nausea, constipation, diarrhea, dry mouth, itching, tinnitus, rash, sun sensitivity, and frequent or painful urination.[2]

MPS, in contrast, is not yet defined by specific criterion. However, in practice the presence of a taut band that, when palpated, reproduces the patient's pain, is adequate to direct treatment.[4,21]

DIFFERENTIAL DIAGNOSIS

In clinical practice the presentations of MPS and FM may overlap. The differential diagnosis is broad. Certain critical questions may be useful for distinguishing contributing factors and can help the clinician develop an appropriate and specific treatment plan.

Differential Diagnosis Should Include but Not Be Limited to the Following Conditions:

- **Joint disorders**: zygapophyseal joint disorder, osteoarthritis, loss of normal joint motion
- **Inflammatory disorders**: polymyositis, polymyalgia rheumatica, rheumatoid arthritis
- **Neurological disorders**: radiculopathy, entrapment neuropathy, metabolic myopathy
- **Regional soft tissue disorders**: bursitis, epicondylitis, tendonitis, cumulative trauma
- **Discogenic disorders**: degenerative disc disease, annular tears, protrusion, herniation
- **Visceral referred pain**: gastrointestinal, cardiac, pulmonary, renal
- **Mechanical stresses**: postural dysfunction, scoliosis, leg length discrepancy
- **Nutritional, metabolic, and endocrine conditions**: deficiency in vitamins B_1, B_{12}, and/or folic acid; alcoholic and toxic myopathy; iron, calcium, or magnesium deficiency; hypothyroidism
- **Psychological disorders**: depression, anxiety, disordered sleep
- **Infectious diseases**: viral illness, chronic hepatitis, bacterial or viral myositis
- **Fibromyalgia or myofascial pain syndrome**

Critical Questions for Development of a Treatment Plan

- Is there regional myofascial pain with trigger points present?
- Is the myofascial pain the primary pain generator or are there other coexisting or underlying structural diagnoses?
- Is there a nutritional, metabolic, psychological, visceral, or inflammatory disorder that may contribute to or cause the myofascial pain or regional muscle pain?
- Is there widespread pain and other associated symptoms?

PATHOPHYSIOLOGY OF FIBROMYALGIA AND MYOFASCIAL PAIN SYNDROME

MPS and FM are situated within a continuum of clinical disorders, with regional, peripherally generated pain (MPS) on one end and widespread, centrally mediated pain (FM) on the other. Both share pathophysiological mechanisms and may coexist in a patient. Although the following discussion is organized by neuroanatomical location, these processes are interrelated and should be considered in an integrated fashion.

Motor End Plate

An important finding in the pathophysiology of myofascial pain is a pathological increase in the release of acetylcholine (Ach) by the nerve terminal of an abnormal motor end plate under resting conditions, an event supported by electrodiagnostic evidence.[21,27,28] This abnormality is considered the primary dysfunction in the integrated hypothesis proposed by Simons et al.[18]

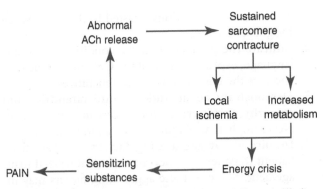

Figure 33-2 Simon's positive feedback loop. *ACh*, acetylcholine. (Modified from Simons DG, Travell JG, Simons LS: *Myofascial pain and dysfunction: the trigger point manual*, vol 1, *Upper half of body*, ed 2, p 71, Baltimore, 1999, Williams & Wilkins.)

and Mense et al.,[24] which postulates a **positive feedback loop** (Figure 33-2).

The concept of the abnormal motor end plate has been supported by electrodiagnostic studies, which have demonstrated end plate noise (EPN) significantly more frequently in MTrPs than in the same end plate zone outside the MTrP.[28,29] Because EPN is characteristic, but not diagnostic, of MTrPs, the significance of these findings is still a matter of debate. Increased EPN has been seen in response to many types of mechanical and chemical stimulation of the end plate structure and does not appear to be specific to myofascial pain.[30,31] However, greater EPN in painful versus latent MTrPs has been demonstrated.[21]

Muscle Fiber

Some researchers hypothesize that increased release of Ach may result in sustained depolarization of the postjunctional membrane of the muscle fiber and produce sustained sarcomere shortening and contracture.[32] Simons referred to this maximally contracted sarcomere in the region of the motor end plate as a **contraction knot** (Figure 33-3).[18] Compelling histological support for this phenomenon is found in canine models of MTrPs: longitudinal sections of dog trigger points demonstrate this sarcomere shortening, and cross sections of dog and human MTrPs strongly suggest it as well.[33,34]

One consequence of chronically sustained sarcomere shortening may be greatly increased local energy consumption and reduction of local circulation, a combination that produces local ischemia and hypoxia.[32] The sustained tension of muscle fibers in the taut band produces an enthesopathy at the myotendinous junction that can be identified as an attachment MTrP. Muscle stretching techniques are effective because they equalize sarcomere length throughout the affected muscle fibers and break the feedback cycle.

Localized muscle ischemias stimulate the release of neurovasoreactive substances, such as prostaglandins,

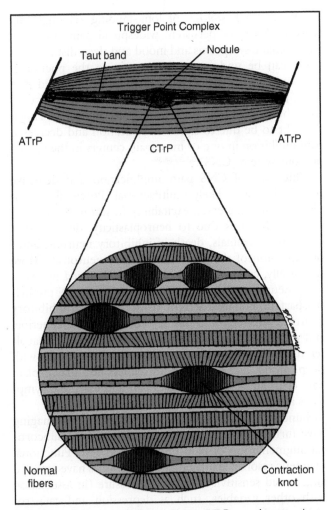

Figure 33-3 Simon's contraction knot. *ATrP*, attachment trigger point; *CTrP*, central trigger point. (From Simons DE, Travell JG, Simons LS: *Myofascial pain and dysfunction: the trigger point manual*, vol 1, *Upper half of body*, ed 2, Philadelphia, 1999, Williams & Wilkins.)

bradykinin, serotonin, and histamine, which sensitize afferent nerve fibers in muscle. These sensitized fibers may account for local muscle tenderness.[24,32]

Central Mechanisms: Spinal and Supraspinal

The local twitch response seen with palpation of MTrPs causes a brief polyphasic, high-amplitude contraction. This response is mediated through the spinal cord, and an intact spinal reflex arc is necessary for this response to occur.[21] In contrast, referred pain associated with MTrPs arises from central convergence and facilitation. Experimental data have shown that under pathological conditions, convergent connections from deep afferent nociceptors to dorsal horn neurons are facilitated and amplified in the spinal cord.[21,24,35] Referral to adjacent myotomes occurs as a result of the spreading and arborization (collection of branches) of first-order, afferent neuronal axons to neighboring spinal segments.[21]

The pathophysiology of longstanding regional pain (chronic MPS) or persistent widespread pain associated with somatic symptoms and mood and sleep disturbances (FM) can be understood by examining the phenomenon known as "**centralized pain.**" In a centralized pain state, patients actually feel more pain than normal controls, based on the level of nociceptive input.[36,37] This is thought to be due to signal amplification and decreased pain inhibition in one or more pain centers in the central nervous system (CNS).[6,7,32,38,39]

This state of CNS pain amplification and defective pain inhibition is likely multifactorial. Potential mechanisms include increased excitability in second order dorsal horn neurons due to neuroplasticity, degeneration of C fiber terminals, death of inhibitory neurons, and/or expansion of the pool of excitatory neurons.[39] More specifically, centralized pain is likely influenced by excitatory neurotransmitters, such as substance P, *N*-methyl-D-aspartate, glutamate, nitric oxide, as well as inhibitory neurotransmitters, such as serotonin, norepinepherine, and γ-aminobutyric acid (GABA). It is well known that altered levels of these neurotransmitters are associated with sleep, mood, and cognition imbalances and may explain why centrally acting analgesics can address these symptoms in addition to pain.[7,39]

Functional, chemical, and structural brain imaging have further characterized the cortical and/or subcortical augmentation of pain processing in FM. Functional magnetic resonance imaging (fMRI) studies have revealed augmented sensitivity to painful pressure (in association with other variables, such as depression and catastrophizing), decreased opioid receptor binding, decreased concentration of neurotransmitters, enhanced intrinsic network connectivity, and decreased regional gray matter in patients with FM. Areas of specific interest include the cingulate cortex, insula, and dorsolateral prefrontal cortex.[37,39–41]

TREATMENT OF FIBROMYALGIA AND MYOFASCIAL PAIN SYNDROME

The following discussion refers to the management of FM and MPS. Much of the research has been done on one or both of these overlapping patient populations. Where clinically relevant, techniques specific to either FM or MPS are noted.

Educational Approach

Treatment should integrate pharmacological and nonpharmacological approaches and, in the setting of chronic, widespread pain, should be multimodal and interdisciplinary. In order to actively engage patients as participants in the process, clinicians should proceed as follows:

1. **Make a firm diagnosis** of FM and/or MPS based on its own characteristics; rule out or identify overlap with potential conditions as listed in the Differential Diagnoses section.
2. **Educate the patient** about the condition. In simple language, explain the role of the CNS in chronic pain and that the condition is nondegenerative.
3. **Demonstrate an attitude of understanding and empathy**; this is crucial for success in management. Never imply that symptoms are "all in your head."
4. **Inquire about aggravating factors** that vary from patient to patient and necessitate individualized management. Some of these aggravating factors may include poor nutrition, poor ergonomics at home or work, poor postural habits, and environmental factors.
5. **Provide an overview of multidisciplinary treatment strategies** and encourage the patient to read information from the Arthritis Foundation.
6. **Recognize and address significant psychosocial factors**, such as depression, anxiety, mental stress (at home or work), and poor coping skills. Explain how they act as aggravating factors regardless of their origin. The physician can use a written questionnaire or interview skills to help identify psychological factors. A minority of patients require referral to a psychiatrist for management of more severe psychiatric disease.
7. **Identify and address any sleep disturbance** through education on normalizing sleep patterns with appropriate sleep hygiene.
8. **Encourage and prescribe a cardiovascular fitness program**. When appropriate, recommend physical therapy for management of regional musculoskeletal disorders and development of a home exercise program. Reassure the patient that even with careful, incremental increases in activity, pain may be worse at first.
9. **Promote behavioral modification** through education, including cognitive behavioral concepts.[15]
10. **Promote stress reduction** through mind-body techniques.

Pharmacological Management

Because of the considerable clinical overlap among MPS and centralized pain disorders, such as FM, chronic tension headache, and temporomandibular dysfunction, agents that are beneficial in one syndrome may be useful in another. In the absence of consistent, controlled data specifically examining drug efficacy in each disorder, clinicians often generalize from these associated disorders. *The goal of pharmacological therapy is improvement in function by addressing mood, sleep, and pain.* A general rule with medications in this population: start low, go slow, and tailor toward the predominant symptom.

Nonsteroidal Anti-inflammatory Drugs

Minimal literature evaluating the use of nonsteroidal anti-inflammatory drugs (NSAIDs) for chronic pain is available. Several studies have found that NSAIDs may have a small benefit in the management of pain in FM if they are used in combination with alprazolam, amitriptyline, or cyclobenzaprine.[42-44] Topical diclofenac may be beneficial for pain reduction in MPS.[45] Despite limited evidence, NSAIDs continue to be popular among patients. A study by Wolfe et al.[46] found that patients with FM considered NSAIDs more effective than acetaminophen for pain management.

Tramadol and Other Opioids

Tramadol is an opioid agonist that also inhibits the reuptake of serotonin and norepinephrine in the dorsal horn. There are no published, controlled trials on the use of tramadol for the treatment of myofascial pain, and limited data in support of its use in FM.[4,7,47] In fact, there is increasing evidence demonstrating that any opioids may do more harm than good in this patient population. Significant adverse affects include addiction, tolerance, and opioid-induced hyperalgesia.[7] There is no evidence to support the use of stronger opioids in FM or MPS.

Antidepressants

Numerous systematic reviews of randomized controlled trials (RCTs) have shown antidepressants to be somewhat effective for the treatment of FM, and an increasing number of studies support their role in MPS.[4,6,7,48] Tricyclic antidepressants (e.g., amitriptyline) have been shown to reduce pain in FM and other pain disorders, including MPS.[4,6,49] Selective serotonin reuptake inhibitors (SSRIs) have been documented in FM for improving pain, sleep, and a global sense of well-being and tend to be most effective when mood is the dominant symptom. Studies support the use of dual reuptake inhibitors (serotonin and norepinephrine inhibitors) in the treatment of FM for pain, sleep, depression, and fatigue.[6,7] Evidence supports the use of amitriptyline, fluoxetine, paroxetine, venlafaxine, and milnacipram.[6,7]

Muscle Relaxants

Tizanidine is an α2-adrenergic agonist that acts centrally at the level of the spinal cord to inhibit spinal polysynaptic pathways and to reduce the release of aspartate, glutamate, and substance P and may be effective in MPS, specifically in reducing pain and disability, as well as improving sleep.[4,50,51]

Anticonvulsants

Several RCTs involving pregabalin (a mixed neurotransmitter inhibitor including glutamate) have demonstrated reduction of pain, disturbed sleep, anxiety, and fatigue compared with placebo.[6,7,52] There is less evidence to support the use of gabapentin (a GABA agonist); however, it is frequently prescribed due to its generic status, lending to greater affordability. Both tend to be better tolerated when most or all of the dose is given at bedtime.[6]

Other Agents

Other pharmaceuticals with potential benefit include low-dose naltrexone in FM and lidocaine patches in MPS; however, both require further study.[4,7]

Nonpharmacological Management

Exercise

Aerobic training and stretching exercises form the basis of treatment for FM and MPS, respectively. The goal of exercise in these populations is decreased pain and increased function (e.g., community, activities of daily living, societal or professional).[4]

For patients with FM, aerobic exercise (e.g., walking, warm water swimming, biking, Nordic walking) that starts at low intensity and progresses over a number of weeks to moderate intensity has shown significant benefit in level of function, as well as pain, mood, and overall quality of life.[53-55] Emerging evidence also indicates that warm aqua therapy decreased pain symptoms in FM, and the effect may be beneficial beyond 20 weeks.[56,57]

The exercise prescription should employ a *"start low, go slow"* approach with an eventual goal of at least 20 minutes of aerobic exercise 2 to 3 times per week.[6,58] It may include walking with a step counter and gradually increasing steps per day in 1000 steps per day increments up to at least 5000 steps per day above baseline.[59] For patients with significant functional limitations, a physical therapy and/or occupational therapy prescription is appropriate because guided physical training may reduce falls and is associated with decreased severity of symptoms.[60]

The exercise prescription for patients with centralized pain states should prioritize aerobic exercises and initially avoid isometric or eccentric muscle work because these may cause CNS hyperexcitation.[61] Some patients with FM may eventually be able to tolerate and will benefit from moderate to high intensity resistance training or moderate strength training.[62,63]

The benefits of exercise in chronic pain are well described.[54] However, patients frequently fail to follow through with suggested regimens or discontinue exercise before seeing a benefit. This may be influenced by the fact that lower thresholds of centralized pain lead to a narrower therapeutic window in this patient population.[61,64] Challenges with patient adherence may explain, but not justify, the infrequency with which physicians provide these patients with an exercise prescription.[55]

For patients with MPS, stretching addresses the muscle tightness and shortening that are closely associated with pain and permits gradual restoration of normal activity. Gentle, sustained stretching throughout the available range of motion is an effective approach.[54] Once muscle pain has decreased and range of motion has been restored, exercise to improve muscle strength and endurance should be instituted to maximize functional outcome. Aerobic exercise should also be included as part of an overall musculoskeletal and cardiovascular fitness program to prevent recurrence.[65]

Importance of Exercise for Myofascial Pain

Exercise is one of the most important aspects of the rehabilitation and management of FM and MPS.[66] The benefits of exercise include:
- Optimization of joint and soft tissue flexibility
- Improved functional status
- Improved mood
- Improved self-efficacy
- Reduction of pain

Postural, Mechanical, and Ergonomic Modifications

Although standard clinical practice and conventional wisdom include efforts to correct postural and ergonomic abnormalities, this approach in treating muscle pain is mainly supported by indirect evidence.[4] A study by Komiyama et al.[67] combined postural training and behavioral therapy in the treatment of myofascial oral pain and found that the subjects receiving the combination therapy were able to regain free, unassisted mouth opening earlier than those treated with behavioral therapy alone; however, the differences in outcome were clinically minor.

The occupational medicine literature provides evidence that injuries are more common when workers are subjected to greater loads and have undesirable postures during work.[68] Occupational MTrPs are theorized to occur as the result of repetitive microtrauma and myofascial shortening. Correction of awkward postures is a standard part of treatment of these disorders, but further long-term efficacy studies are needed.[69]

Stress Reduction

Stress reduction interventions include cognitive behavioral therapy (CBT) and mind-body techniques, such as mindfulness-based stress reduction, yoga, tai chi, and biofeedback. These are often successfully incorporated into chronic pain rehabilitation programs. CBT serves to challenge negative and unhelpful thinking patterns and may enhance the effects of other interventions. There is strong evidence showing its effectiveness in FM in one-on-one, group, or internet settings.[6,7] Mind-body therapies are supported by moderate evidence. A 2010 New England Journal of Medicine RCT showed significant benefit in physical and mental well-being as well as symptoms in patients with FM versus controls at 12 and 24 weeks after a twice weekly, 12-week tai chi class.[70]

Few studies have specifically addressed the efficacy of these techniques for MPS; however, psychological stress has been associated with an increased number of MTrPs.[4]

Acupuncture

Acupuncture is effective for the treatment of MPS.[4] In fact, a remarkably close relationship has been described between acupuncture points and MTrPs; however, specific treatment protocols have yet to be developed.[71]

Evidence supporting the efficacy of acupuncture in FM is mixed. A Cochrane database review of nine trials concluded that the evidence in support of acupuncture in FM was low to moderate.[72] Many of the studies failed to show a significant difference between sham and traditional acupuncture. Interestingly, a 2013 double blinded RCT by Harte et al.[73] demonstrated significant differences in response to sham acupuncture in patients with high pain sensitivity (HPS) and elevated posterior insular glutamate versus those with low pain sensitivity (LPS). The LPS patients had a reduced clinical response to sham acupuncture when compared with those with HPS; however, both treatment groups showed similar and significant responses to traditional acupuncture. Due to these differences in evoked pain sensitivity, further study is certainly required and should take into account the potential analgesic response in some patients but not others to sham acupuncture.[73]

Questions that need to be answered in future RCTs include the true benefit of acupuncture in centralized pain states (which may require differentiating between low and high pain threshold populations), duration of benefit, optimum techniques, and value of booster treatments.

Massage, Electrotherapies, and Ultrasound

Massage combined with stretching exercises has been shown to be effective in reducing the number and intensity of MTrPs.[74,75] Hernandez-Reif et al.[76] found that massage therapy was effective in reducing pain, increasing serotonin and dopamine levels, and reducing symptoms associated with chronic low back pain. Studies validating the use of massage for treatment of myofascial pain are limited, however, and further inquiry is warranted.

Electrotherapies for myofascial pain include transcutaneous electrical nerve stimulation (TENS), electrical muscle stimulation (EMS), electrical twitch-obtaining intramuscular stimulation (ETOIMS), and frequency-modulated neural stimulation (FREMS) therapies. TENS has been shown to be helpful in MPS for several weeks post treatment, whereas the effect of FREMS may persist beyond 3 months.[4,77] Further study is required to determine the efficacy of EMS and ETOIMS in these disorders.

Ultrasound uses alternating compression and rarefaction of sound waves to improve tissue pliability, circulation, and metabolism via the transmission of thermal and mechanical energy. It may be beneficial in MPS alone or in combination with heat and NSAIDs.[4] Trials demonstrating clear efficacy in FM are limited.[7]

Needling Therapy for Myofascial Pain

MTrPs are the hallmark of MPS. Patients with more generalized pain, such as FM, may also have MTrPs. These local areas of painful, shortened muscle can be treated with needling therapy.

It should be noted, however, that stretching and exercise are the mainstays of myofascial pain and that dry needling and trigger point injection (TPI) therapy should be reserved to supplement or augment these exercises.[65] When MTrP needling is used as the primary therapy, patients are at risk of becoming dependent on this treatment for pain relief. Educating patients about the effectiveness of manual stretching techniques and instructing them in these techniques empower patients to self-manage their symptoms effectively. As pain relief and function increase, the patient resumes normal activity, which further helps to inactivate MTrPs. Optimum results are obtained when injections are preceded and immediately followed by manual MTrP release techniques, with the patient learning how to follow a continuing home program.[78]

When needling therapy proves necessary for initiating therapy or for addressing a recalcitrant MFTrP, a series of treatments should be started and the patient should be informed that this treatment has a limited role in the long-term management of myofascial pain. Often, three consecutive weekly visits for dry needling or TPI are recommended for chronic myofascial pain; the patient is reassessed after the third visit to evaluate the efficacy of the injections and to determine whether further injections are necessary. Patients should be informed about potential post-injection soreness, which is expected to resolve.

MTrP therapy may involve the use of dry needling (no medication) or the use of short- or long-acting anesthetics, steroids, or botulinum toxin. A number of techniques may be used, such as slow search,[79] fast in–fast out, superficial dry needling, intramuscular stimulation, twitch-obtaining intramuscular stimulation, and needling and infiltration with preinjection blocks. Several theories have been proposed regarding the mechanism of action of injections for myofascial pain.

Dry needling of MTrPs with acupuncture needles provides as much pain relief as injection of lidocaine but may cause more postinjection soreness.[80] The effectiveness of dry needling depends on the needle eliciting local twitch responses.[81–85] Presumably, the needle mechanically disrupts and terminates the dysfunctional activity of involved motor end plates, with or without injection. TPIs also target the MTrP, with injection of medication after local twitch response is obtained. Longer acting anesthetics (e.g., bupivicane) are more myotoxic and do not show a proven increase in MTrP pain relief over short-acting anesthetic (e.g. lidocaine). The effectiveness of injection steroids in MTrPs is controversial and without a clear evidence of benefit.[4]

In a systematic review article on needling therapies for MTrPs, Cummings and White[86] concluded that based on current medical evidence, the "nature of the injected substance makes no difference to the outcome and that wet needling is not therapeutically superior to dry needling." This is certainly an area in which continued research is needed.

Hong's fast in–fast out technique[80] elicits local twitch responses more quickly than other techniques and presumably reduces needle trauma to muscle fibers from the twitch movement. Baldry et al.[87] recommend superficial dry needling, which they speculate may inactivate MTrPs through stimulation of cutaneous A delta fibers. A study by Chu,[88] based on the work of Gunn,[89] reported a technique in which neurogenically evoked muscle twitches relieved myofascial-type pain. The needling and infiltration technique described by Fischer and Imamura,[90] who used a preinjection block, permits more thorough injection of the trigger point and taut band region with reportedly less patient discomfort.

All of these techniques rely on accurate identification of MTrPs by means of palpation. No definitive evidence indicates that one technique is superior to another in long-term outcome. As Cummings and White[86] remarked, "Because no technique is better than any other, we recommend that the method safest and most comfortable for the patient should be used." Very slim acupuncture needles may have the advantage of minimizing tissue trauma and allowing the practitioner to needle four to six trigger points at one session.

Botulinum Toxin

Botulinum toxin type A (Botox) is FDA approved for treatment of chronic daily headache, and has off-label use in chronic MPSs.[91–93] Both peripheral and central mechanisms may explain the apparent efficacy of botulinum toxin in the treatment of chronic muscle pain. First, blockade of Ach release at the neuromuscular junction reduces muscle hyperactivity, which, in turn, may reduce local ischemia. Second, if, as theorized, trigger points are sustained by excessive release of Ach and sarcomere shortening, botulinum toxin may disrupt the abnormal neurophysiology of the trigger point. Evidence also has been found of retrograde uptake of botulinum toxin into the spinal cord and nucleus raphe, structures that modulate expression of neurotransmitters important in pain perception (e.g., substance P, enkephalins).[94] In addition, Botox inhibits neurotransmitter release from primary sensory neurons in the rat formalin model. Through this mechanism, Botox inhibits peripheral sensitization in these models, which leads to an indirect reduction in central sensitization.[95]

Study results on the use of Botox in myofascial pain are mixed. In fact, a 2012 review by Gerwin on the utility of Botox highlights the variability in study design and numerous pitfalls of studies to date.[96] Therefore, further inquiry with controlled trials is warranted to facilitate the development of appropriate guidelines on its use in myofascial pain.

FUNCTIONAL OUTCOMES IN FIBROMYALGIA AND MYOFASCIAL PAIN SYNDROME

Outcome studies of FM and MPS and their treatments are few. Neither population has increased mortality. In one study of pain, disability, and psychological functioning in chronic low back pain subgroups, patients with low back pain of myofascial origin had outcomes similar to or slightly worse than those with disc herniation, as measured by several standardized questionnaires on pain and disability.[97] Patients with myofascial pain have less accurate beliefs about their pain symptoms, express more dissatisfaction with physician efforts to treat their pain, and report receiving little information from their physicians.[98] A 1998 study by Heikkila et al.[99] investigated the outcome from a multidisciplinary rehabilitation program for patients with whiplash and myofascial pain. After the rehabilitation period, 49% of patients had improved their coping skills for managing chronic pain, and this figure rose to 63% after 2 years. In addition, 46% of patients had increased their life satisfaction. The myofascial pain group also reduced their sick leave time.[99]

In a national six-center longitudinal study, Wolfe et al.[100] determined the intermediate and long-term outcomes of FM in patients seen in rheumatology centers that have a special interest in the syndrome. Although functional disability worsened slightly and health satisfaction improved slightly, measures of pain, global severity, fatigue, sleep disturbance, anxiety, depression, and health status were markedly abnormal at the initiation of the study and were essentially unchanged over the study period.

Poor prognostic factors for chronic widespread pain include behaviors of learned helplessness, poor coping skills, catastrophizing, and a fear that movement will worsen the pain. Most patients with FM have chronic, persistent symptoms; however, most will continue to work (10% to 15% are disabled). Duration of time without a diagnosis adversely affects outcome.[1]

SUMMARY

"Muscle pain" is a common clinical complaint among patients who seek care for musculoskeletal disorders. The clinical presentation covers a spectrum ranging from focal or regional complaints to more widespread pain. Nevertheless, treatment paradigms overlap and are guided by the following major principles[53,101]:

1. Be a sympathetic provider.
2. Make an accurate diagnosis of FM and/or MPS.
3. Educate all patients about the diagnosis and encourage autonomy and self-management.
4. Treat the CNS dysfunction with a balanced, evidence-based approach.
5. Incorporate CBT and mind–body techniques (e.g., meditation, tai chi) to manage chronic pain.
6. Engage all patients with chronic symptoms in a comprehensive exercise and functional restoration program.
7. Treat any associated symptoms (e.g. sleep, mood, headache, bowel, fatigue) or refer the patient to the appropriate provider.
8. Identify and treat any peripheral pain generators (e.g., tendonitis, bursitis, radiculopathy) to reduce the peripheral nociceptive input to the CNS.
9. Judiciously offer needling techniques for local trigger points or other peripheral pain generators to reduce pain and facilitate rehabilitation.

REFERENCES

1. Goldenberg D: Diagnosis and differential diagnosis of fibromyalgia, *Am J Sports Med* 122(12 suppl):S14–S21, 2009.
2. Wolfe F, Clauw D, Fitzcharles MA, et al: The American College of Rheumatology preliminary diagnostic criteria for fibromyalgia and measurement of symptom severity, *Arthritis Care Res* 62(5):600–610, 2010.
3. Borg-Stein J, Simons DG: Myofascial pain, *Arch Phys Med Rehabil* 83(suppl 1):S40–S47, 2002.
4. Borg-Stein J, Iaccarino M: Myofascial pain syndrome treatments, *Phys Med Rehabil Clin North Am* 25(2):357–374, 2014.
5. Bennett R, Goldenberg D: Fibromyalgia, myofascial pain, tender points and trigger points: splitting or lumping? *Arthritis Res Ther* 13(3):117, 2011.
6. Rahman A, Underwood M, Carnes D: Fibromyalgia, *BMJ* 348:g1224, 2014.
7. Clauw D: Fibromyalgia: a clinical review, *JAMA* 311(15):1547–1555, 2014.
8. Arnold L, Hudson J, Hess E, et al: Family study of fibromyalgia, *Arthritis Rheum* 50(3):944–952, 2004.
9. Arnold L, Fan J, Russell I, et al: The fibromyalgia family study: a genome-wide linkage scan study, *Arthritis Rheum* 65(4):1122–1128, 2013.
10. Holliday K, McBeth J: Recent advances in the understanding of genetic susceptibility to chronic pain and somatic symptoms, *Curr Rheumatol Rep* 13:521–527, 2011.
11. Smith S, Maixner D, Fillingim R, et al: Large candidate gene association study reveals genetic risk factors and therapeutic targets for fibromyalgia, *Arthritis Rheum* 64(2):584–593, 2012.
12. Fleckenstein J, Zaps D, Rüger L, et al: Discrepancy between prevalence and perceived effectiveness of treatment methods in myofascial pain syndrome: results of a cross-sectional, nationwide survey, *BMC Musculoskelet Disord* 11(1):32, 2010.
13. Gerwin RD: Classification, epidemiology, and natural history of myofascial pain syndrome, *Curr Pain Headache Rep* 5(5):412–420, 2001.
14. Kaergaard A, Anderson JH: Musculoskeletal disorders of the neck and shoulders in female sewing machine operators: prevalence, incidence, and prognosis, *Occup Environ Med* 57:528–534, 2000.
15. Borg-Stein J, Yunus M: Myofascial and soft tissue causes of low pain. In Cole AJ, Herring SA, editors: *The low back pain handbook*, Philadelphia, 2003, Hanley & Belfus.
16. Henriksson KG: Hypersensitivity in muscle pain syndromes, *Curr Pain Headache Rep* 7:426–432, 2003.
17. Fields HL: Pain, New York, 1987, McGraw-Hill.
18. Simons DG, Travell JG, Simons LS: *Myofascial pain and dysfunction: the trigger point manual, vol 1, Upper half of body*, ed 2, Baltimore, 1999, Williams & Wilkins.
19. Fricton JR, Kroening R, Haley D, et al: *Myofascial pain syndrome of the head and neck: a review of clinical characteristics of 164 patients*, Oral Surg Oral Med Oral Pathol 60:615–623, 1985.
20. Kraybak B, Borg-Stein J, Oas J, et al: Reduced dizziness and pain with treatment of cervical myofascial pain, *Arch Phys Med Rehabil* 77:939–940, 1996.
21. Gerwin R: Diagnosis of myofascial pain syndrome, *Phys Med Rehabil Clin North Am* 25(2):341–355, 2014.
22. Dohrenwend BP, Raphael KG, Marbach JJ, et al: Why is depression comorbid with chronic myofascial face pain?: a family study test of alternative hypotheses, *Pain* 83:183–192, 1999.
23. Schwartz RA, Greene CS, Laskin DM: Personality characteristics of patients with myofascial pain: dysfunction syndrome unresponsive to conventional therapy, *J Dent Res* 58:1435–1439, 1979.

24. Mense S, Simons DG, Russell IJ: Muscle pain: understanding its nature, diagnosis, and treatment, Philadelphia, 2001, Lippincott Williams & Wilkins.

25. Oaklander AL, Herzog ZD, Downs HM, et al: Objective evidence that small-fiber polyneuropathy underlies some illnesses currently labeled as fibromyalgia, *Pain* 154(11):2310–2316, 2013.

26. Giannoccaro M, Donadio V, Incensi A, et al: Small nerve fiber involvement in patients referred for fibromyalgia, *Muscle Nerve* 49(5):757–759, 2014.

27. Mense S: Pathophysiologic basis of muscle pain syndromes, *Phys Med Rehabil Clin North Am* 8:179–196, 1997.

28. Simons DG, Hong CZ, Simons LS: Endplate potentials are common to midfiber myofascial trigger points, *Am J Phys Med Rehabil* 81:212–222, 2002.

29. Couppe C, Midttun A, Hilden J, et al: Spontaneous needle electromyographic activity in myofascial trigger points in the infraspinatus muscle: a blinded assessment, *J Musculoskeletal Pain* 9:7–17, 2001.

30. Liley AW: An investigation of spontaneous activity in the neuromuscular junction of the rat, *J Physiol* 132:650–666, 1956.

31. Heuser J, Miledi R: Effect of lanthanum ions on function and structure of frog neuromuscular junctions, *Proc R Soc Lond Biol Sci* 179:247–260, 1971.

32. Cassisi G, Sarzi-Puttini P, Casale R, et al: Pain in fibromyalgia and related conditions, *Reumatismo* 66(1):72–86, 2014.

33. Simons DG, Stolov WC: Microscopic features and transient contraction of palpable bands in canine muscle, *Am J Phys Med* 55:65–88, 1976.

34. Reitinger A, Radner H, et al: Morphologic studies of trigger points (German), *Manuelle Med* 34:256–262, 1996.

35. Heheisel U, Mense S, Simons DG, et al: Appearance of new receptive fields in rat dorsal horn neurons following noxious stimulation of skeletal muscle: a model for referral of muscle pain? *Neurosci Lett* 153:9–12, 1993.

36. Julien N, Goffaux P, Arsenault P, et al: Widespread pain in fibromyalgia is related to a deficit of endogenous pain inhibition, *Pain* 114(1-2):295–302, 2005.

37. Gracely R, Petzke F, Wolf J, et al: Functional magnetic resonance imaging evidence of augmented pain processing in fibromyalgia, *Arthritis Rheum* 46(5):1333–1343, 2002.

38. Phillips K, Clauw D: Central pain mechanisms in the rheumatic diseases: future directions, *Arthritis Rheum* 65(2):291–302, 2013.

39. Henry D, Chiodo A, Yang W: Central nervous system reorganization in a variety of chronic pain states: a review, *PM R* 3(12):1116–1125, 2011.

40. Harris R, Sundgren P, Craig A, et al: Elevated insular glutamate in fibromyalgia is associated with experimental pain, *Arthritis Rheum* 60(10):3146–3152, 2009.

41. Foerster B, Petrou M, Edden R, et al: Reduced insular γ-aminobutyric acid in fibromyalgia, *Arthritis Rheum* 64(2):579–583, 2012.

42. Goldenberg DL, Felson DT, Dinerman H: A randomized, controlled trial of amitriptyline and naproxen in the treatment of patients with fibromyalgia, *Arthritis Rheum* 29:1371–1377, 1986.

43. Fletcher EM, Michalek JE, McBroom PC, et al: Treatment of primary fibrositis/fibromyalgia syndrome with ibuprofen and alprazolam: a double-blind, placebo controlled study, *Arthritis Rheum* 34:552–560, 1991.

44. Fossaluzza V, DeVita S: Combined therapy with cyclobenzaprine and ibuprofen in primary fibromyalgia syndrome, *Int J Clin Pharmacol Res* 12:99–102, 1992.

45. Hsieh LF, Hong CZ, Chern SH, et al: Efficacy and side effects of diclofenac patch in treatment of patients with myofascial pain syndrome of the upper trapezius, *J Pain Symptom Manage* 39(1):116–125, 2010.

46. Wolfe F, Zhao S, Lane N: Preference for nonsteroidal anti-inflammatory drugs over acetaminophen by rheumatic disease patients: a survey of 1,799 patients with osteoarthritis, rheumatoid arthritis, and fibromyalgia, *Arthritis Rheum* 43:378–385, 2000.

47. Biasi G, Manca S, Manganelli S, et al: Tramadol in the fibromyalgia syndrome: a controlled clinical trial versus placebo, *Int J Clin Pharmacol Res* 18:13–19, 1998.

48. Goldenberg D, Mayskiy M, Mossey C, et al: A randomized, double-blind crossover trial of fluoxetine and amitriptyline in the treatment of fibromyalgia, *Arthritis Rheum* 39:1852–1859, 1996.

49. Goldenberg D: Pharmacological treatment of fibromyalgia and other chronic musculoskeletal pain, *Best Pract Res Clin Rheumatol* 21(3):499–511, 2007.

50. Davies J: Selective depression of synaptic transmission of spinal neurons in the cat by a new centrally acting muscle relaxant, 5-chloro-4-(2-imidazolin-2-yl-amino)-2, 1, 3-bensothiodazole (DS 103-282), *Br J Pharmacol* 76:473–481, 1982.

51. Ono H, Mishima A, Ono S, et al: Inhibitory effects of clonidine and tizanidine on release of substance P from slices of rat spinal cord and antagonism by alpha-adrenergic receptor antagonists, *Neuropharmacology* 30:585–589, 1991.

52. Crofford LJ, Rowbotham MC, Mease PJ, et al: Pregabalin for the treatment of fibromyalgia syndrome: results of a randomized, double-blind, placebo-controlled trial, *Arthritis Rheum* 52:1264–1273, 2005.

53. Häuser W, Bernardy K, Arnold B, et al: Efficacy of multicomponent treatment in fibromyalgia syndrome: a meta-analysis of randomized controlled clinical trials, *Arthritis Rheum* 61(2):216–224, 2009.

54. Thompson J: Exercise in muscle pain disorders, *PM & R: the journal of injury, function, and rehabilitation* 4(11):889–893, 2012.

55. Wilson B, Spencer H, Kortebein P: Exercise recommendations in patients with newly diagnosed fibromyalgia, *PM & R: the journal of injury, function, and rehabilitation* 4(4):252–255, 2012.

56. Lima TB, Dias JM, Mazuquin BF, et al: The effectiveness of aquatic physical therapy in the treatment of fibromyalgia: a systematic review with meta-analysis, *Clin Rehabil* 27(10):892–908, 2013.

57. Tomas-Carus P, Gusi N, Häkkinen A, et al: Eight months of physical training in warm water improves physical and mental health in women with fibromyalgia: a randomized controlled trial, *J Rehabil Med* 40(4):248–252, 2008.

58. Nüesch E, Häuser W, Bernardy K, et al: Comparative efficacy of pharmacological and non-pharmacological interventions in fibromyalgia syndrome: network meta-analysis, *Ann Rheum Dis* 72(6):955–962, 2013.

59. Kaleth AS, Slaven JE, Ang DC: Increasing steps/day predicts improvement in physical function and pain interference in adults with fibromyalgia, *Arthritis Care Res (Hoboken)*, 2014 (Epub ahead of print).

60. Martínez-Amat A, Hita-Contreras F, Latorre-Román PA, et al: Association of the weekly practice of guided physical activity with the reduction of falls and symptoms of fibromyalgia in adult women, *J Strength Cond Res* 28(11):3146–3154, 2014.

61. Daenen L, Varkey E, Kellmann M, et al: Exercise, not to exercise or how to exercise in patients with chronic pain? Applying science to practice, *Clin J Pain* 31(2):108–114, 2015.

62. Busch AJ, Webber SC, Richards RS, et al: Resistance exercise training for fibromyalgia, *Cochrane Database Syst Rev* 12, 2013.

63. Kingsley J, Panton L, Toole T, et al: The effects of a 12-week strength-training program on strength and functionality in women with fibromyalgia, *Arch Phys Med Rehabil* 86(9):1713–1721, 2005.

64. Oh T, Hoskin T, Luedtke C, et al: Predictors of clinical outcome in fibromyalgia after a brief interdisciplinary fibromyalgia treatment program: single center experience, *PM R* 4(4):257–263, 2012.

65. Graff-Radford SB, Reeves JL, Jaeger B: Management of chronic headache and neck pain: effectiveness of altering factors perpetuating myofascial pain, *Headache* 27:186–190, 1987.

66. Mannerkorpi K: Exercise in fibromyalgia, *Curr Opin Rheumatol* 17:190–194, 2005.

67. Komiyama O, Kawara M, Arai M, et al: Posture correction as part of behavioural therapy in treatment of myofascial pain with limited opening, *J Oral Rehabil* 26:428–435, 1999.

68. Edwards RH: Hypotheses of peripheral and central mechanisms underlying occupational muscle pain and injury, *Eur J Appl Physiol Occup Physiol* 57:275–281, 1998.

69. Bhatnager V, Drury CG, Schiro SG: Posture, postural discomfort, and performance, *Hum Factors* 57:189–199, 1985.

70. Wang C: A randomized trial of tai chi for fibromyalgia, *New Engl J Med* 363:743–754, 2010.

71. Melzack R, Stillwell DM, Fox EJ: Trigger points and acupuncture points for pain: correlations and implications, *Pain* 3,3–23, 1997.

72. Deare JC, Zheng Z, Xue CC, et al: Acupuncture for treating fibromyalgia, *Cochrane Database Syst Rev* 5, 2013.

73. Harte S, Clauw D, Napadow V, et al: Pressure pain sensitivity and insular combined glutamate and glutamine (Glx) are associated with subsequent clinical response to sham but not traditional acupuncture in patients who have chronic pain, *Med Acupuncture* 25(2):154–160, 2013.

74. Trampas A, Kitsios A, Sykaras E, et al: Clinical massage and modified proprioceptive neuromuscular facilitation stretching in males with latent myofascial trigger points, *Phys Ther Sport* 11(3):91–98, 2010.

75. Gam AN, Warming S, Larsen LH, et al: Treatment of myofascial trigger points with ultrasound combined with massage and exercise: a randomized controlled trial, *Pain* 77:73–79, 1998.

76. Hernandez-Reif M, Field T, Krasnegor J, et al: Lower back pain is reduced and range of motion increased after massage therapy, *Int J Neurosci* 106:131–145, 2001.

77. Farina S, Casarotto M, Benelle M, et al: A randomized controlled study on the effect of two different treatments (FREMS AND TENS) in myofascial pain syndrome, *Eura Medicophys* 40(4):293–301, 2004.

78. Feinberg BI, Feinberg RA: Persistent pain after total knee arthroplasty: treatment with manual therapy and trigger point injections, *J Musculoskeletal Pain* 6:85–95, 1998.

79. Travell JG, Simons DG: Myofascial pain and dysfunction: the trigger point manual, vol 1, The upper extremities, Baltimore, 1983, Williams & Wilkins.

80. Hong CZ: Lidocaine injection versus dry needling to myofascial trigger points: the importance of the local twitch response, *Am J Phys Med Rehabil* 73:256–263, 1994.

81. Anaswamy TM, De Luigi AJ, O'Neill BJ, et al: Emerging concepts in the treatment of myofascial pain: a review of medications, modalities, and needle-based interventions, *PM R* 3(10):940–961, 2000.

82. Kalichman L, Vulfsons S: Dry needling in the management of musculoskeletal pain, *J Am Board Fam Med* 23(5):640–646, 2010.

83. Tsai CT, Hsieh LF, Kuan TS, et al: Remote effects of dry needling on the irritability of the myofascial trigger point in the upper trapezius muscle, *Am J Phys Med Rhabil* 89(2):133–140, 2010.

84. Tekin L, Akarsu S, Durmus O, et al: The effect of dry needling in the treatment of myofascial pain syndrome: a randomized double-blinded placebo-controlled trial, *Clin Rheumatol* 32(3):309–315, 2013.

85. Kietrys DM, Palombaro KM, Azzaretto E, et al: Effectiveness of dry needling for upper quarter myofascial pain: a systematic review and meta-analysis, *J Orthop Sports Phys Ther* 43(9):620–634, 2013.

86. Cummings TM, White AR: Needling therapies in the management of myofascial trigger point pain: a systematic review, *Arch Phys Med Rehabil* 82:986–992, 2001.

87. Baldry PE, Yunus MB, Inanici F: Myofascial pain and fibromyalgia syndromes: a clinical guide to diagnosis and management, Edinburgh, 2001, Churchill Livingstone.

88. Chu J: Twitch; obtaining intramuscular stimulation: observations in the management of radiculopathic chronic low back pain, *J Musculoskeletal Pain* 7:131–746, 1999.

89. Gunn CC: The Gunn approach to the treatment of chronic pain: intramuscular stimulation for myofascial pain of radiculopathic origin, ed 2, New York, 1996, Churchill Livingstone.

90. Fischer AA, Imamura M: New concepts in the diagnosis and management of musculoskeletal pain.

In Lennard TA, editor: *Pain procedures in clinical practice*, ed 2, Philadelphia, 2002, Hanley & Belfus.

91. Smith HS, Audette J, Royal MA: Botulinum toxin in pain management of soft tissue syndromes, *Clin J Pain* 18(suppl 6):S147–S154, 2002.

92. Dodick DW, Mauskop A, Elkind AH, et al: Botox CDH Study Group: botulinum toxin type A for the prophylaxis of chronic daily headache—subgroup analysis of patients not receiving other prophylactic medications: a randomized double-blind, placebo-controlled study, *Headache* 45:315–324, 2005.

93. Diener HC, Dodick DW, Aurora SK, et al: OnabotulinumtoxinA for treatment of chronic migraine: results from the double-blind, randomized, placebo-controlled phase of the PREEMPT 2 trial, *Cephalgia* 30(7):804–814, 2010.

94. Gobel H, Heinze A, Henize-Kuhn K, et al: Botulinum toxin A for the treatment of headache disorders and pericranial pain syndromes (German), *Nervenarzt* 72:261–274, 2001.

95. Aoki KR: Review of a proposed mechanism for the antinociceptive action of botulinum toxin type A, *Neurotoxicology* 26(5):785–793, 2005.

96. Gerwin R: Botulinum toxin treatment of myofascial pain: a critical review of the literature, *Curr Pain Headache Rep* 16(5):413–422, 2012.

97. Cassisi JE, Sypert GW, Lagana L, et al: Pain, disability, and psychological functioning in chronic low back pain subgroups: myofascial versus herniated disk syndrome, *Neurosurgery* 33:379–386, 1998.

98. Roth RS, Horowitz K, Bachman JE: Chronic myofascial pain: knowledge of diagnosis and satisfaction with treatment, *Arch Phys Med Rehabil* 79:966–970, 1998.

99. Heikkila H, Heikkila E, Eisemann M: Predictive factors for the outcome of a multidisciplinary pain rehabilitation programme on sick-leave and life satisfaction in patients with whiplash trauma and other myofascial pain: a follow-up study, *Clin Rehabil* 12:487–496, 1998.

100. Wolfe F, Anderson J, Harkness D, et al: Health status and disease severity in fibromyalgia: results of a six-center longitudinal study, *Arthritis Rheum* 40:1571–1579, 1997.

101. Amris K, Wæhrens E, Christensen R, et al: Interdisciplinary rehabilitation of patients with chronic widespread pain: primary endpoint of the randomized, nonblinded, parallel-group IMPROvE trial, *Pain* 155:1356–1364, 2014.

CHAPTER 34

Musculoskeletal Bone and Soft Tissue Tumors

ODION BINITIE, CHRISTINE ALVERO, G. DOUGLAS LETSON

INTRODUCTION

The management of musculoskeletal tumors requires a multidisciplinary team from the time of diagnosis through medical treatment, recovery, and rehabilitation. Physical and occupational therapists are an integral part of that team. The optimal goal is to treat the condition conservatively if appropriate and, if not, to resect the malignant tumor and preserve a functional limb. However, there are instances in which an amputation is the only surgical option. Limb-preserving surgery allows patients to retain their limb, allowing for close-to-normal function, ambulation, and appearance. In the pediatric patient, limb-preserving surgeries have to factor in the residual expected growth of the child. Technologies are available that can lengthen the endoprosthesis noninvasively, allowing the limb to "grow" along with the child, without the need for additional surgeries.

Postoperative rehabilitation following any oncologic surgery is one of the most important factors that affects the overall outcome of these patients, and it is even more critical in limb-preserving surgeries. Numerous studies have reported that with standard of care chemotherapy and surgical resection of the tumor with wide margins, limb-preserving surgery, compared with an amputation, results in no difference in local recurrence or overall survival in patients with sarcomas.[1-4]

A sarcoma is a malignant tumor of the mesenchymal cells. In the United States, sarcomas account for about 1% of all cancers diagnosed in adults annually and for about 12% in pediatric patients. About 14,000 new sarcomas are estimated to be diagnosed each year in the United States.[5] Most sarcomas are treated with a combination of chemotherapy, surgical resection of the tumor, and sometimes radiation. Soft tissue sarcomas usually can be resected and the limb preserved; however, in cases in which the tumor also involves the bone, a bony resection and replacement may be necessary. Amputation is sometimes performed for soft tissue sarcomas if a residual function limb cannot be maintained, because of involvement of the neurovascular structures.

COMMON BONE TUMORS

Common Bone Tumors

- Osteosarcoma
- Ewing sarcoma
- Chondrosarcoma

Osteosarcoma

Although **osteosarcoma** is the most common malignant bone tumor in pediatric patients and adults, it is rare, representing less than 1% of cancers diagnosed in the United States.[6] Its highest incidence is in the second decade of life; however, it does have a bimodal distribution, with the second peak occurring in the seventh and eighth decades. There is an incidence of approximately 5.6 per million children younger than 15 years of age.[7] It can occur in any bone in the body, with the most common sites being the distal femur and proximal tibia near the knee and the proximal humerus (Figure 34-1).

The usual presenting signs are pain in the limb that worsens with activity or that occurs at night, swelling, or a mass. X-rays and magnetic resonance imaging (MRI) scans of the limb are used for the initial evaluation. A definitive diagnosis is based on a tissue biopsy. The lungs are the most common site of metastasis (i.e., spread of cancer), with other bones being second; therefore, imaging of the lungs as well as a whole body bone scan are performed to evaluate for metastatic disease. The standard treatment for osteosarcoma is neoadjuvant chemotherapy, followed by resection of the tumor (Figure 34-2) with wide margins and additional adjuvant chemotherapy. Multiple studies have reported no difference in overall survival of patients treated with amputation versus limb-preservation surgery.[1-4] The 5-year survival rate of patients with primary osteosarcoma is 60% to 70%.[8] Most patients can be treated with limb-preservation surgery

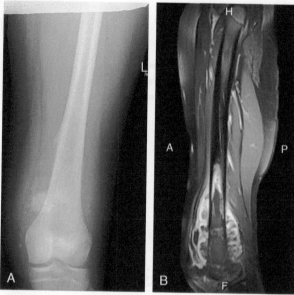

Figure 34-1 **A**, X-ray showing a distal femur osteosarcoma in a 25-year-old. **B**, Sagittal view of a magnetic resonance imaging of the tumor.

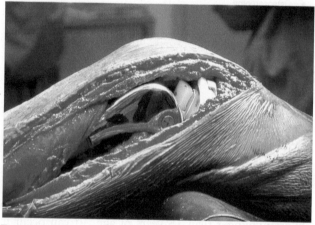

Figure 34-2 Intraoperative view of the lateral approach to the femur with the implanted endoprosthesis.

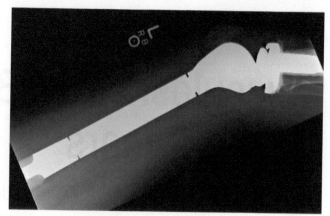

Figure 34-3 Lateral x-ray of the extremity following reconstruction.

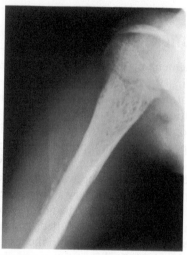

Figure 34-4 Ewing sarcoma of the humerus. Note the mottled areas of rarefaction and subperiosteal reaction. (From Herring JA: *Tachdjian's pediatric orthopaedics*, ed 4, Philadelphia, 2008, Saunders/Elsevier.)

and reconstruction with either an endoprosthesis or an allograft (Figure 34-3). A minority of patients are unsuitable for limb salvage due to extent of the tumor or the desire for high function over cosmesis. Such patients may be treated with an amputation or a rotationplasty. These patients have satisfactory functional and psychological outcomes.[9]

Ewing Sarcoma

Ewing sarcoma is the second most common primary malignancy of bone in young patients. The annual incidence is 2 to 3 per million in the United States. Most patients affected are younger than 21 years of age.[10] Similar to patients with osteosarcoma, patients typically present with pain and sometimes an associated soft tissue mass. Patients

may sometimes present with fever, weight loss, fatigue, and other nonspecific symptoms. The initial workup involves x-rays and advanced imaging of the extremity, as well as a biopsy of the tumor (Figure 34-4). Evaluating for the presence of metastases, with the lung being the most common site, completes staging. Ewing sarcoma is also treated with chemotherapy and surgery. Similar to osteosarcoma, limb salvage can be performed in most patients with Ewing sarcoma in an extremity. Radiation is sometimes used in large unresectable tumors, especially those in the pelvis. The 5-year survival for Ewing sarcoma is about 65% to 75%.[11]

Chondrosarcoma

Chondrosarcoma is a malignant bone tumor typically diagnosed in adults. These tumors have low-, intermediate-, and high-grade variants. The high-grade tumors tend to present with pain and are rapidly fulminant (a process that occurs suddenly and severely, to the point of lethality); however, the lower grade tumors may

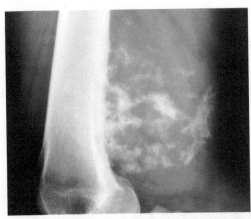

Figure 34-5 Chondrosarcoma. Prominent dense calcification in large neoplastic mass. (From Eisenberg RL, Johnson NM: *Comprehensive radiographic pathology*, ed 4, St. Louis, 2007, Mosby/Elsevier.)

have a slow progression, with a long-standing history of pain, mild swelling, and difficulty with activities.[12] Chondrosarcoma is rare in children and adolescents and is more common in patients in their third through seventh decades.

Like most malignant bone tumors, patients may present with pain. Diagnosis is made with imaging and tissue biopsy (Figure 34-5). These are important in the grading of these tumors, which is a large determinant of prognosis. The prognosis for patients with low- and intermediate-grade tumors is better than that for those with high-grade tumors. The primary treatment of chondrosarcoma is surgery. Chemotherapy and radiation do not play significant roles in the management of this sarcoma.

ANATOMIC CONSIDERATIONS

Distal Femur

This location is the most common site of malignant bone tumors. A distal femoral resection and endoprosthetic reconstruction is one of the more common procedures performed for these tumors (see Figures 34-2 and 34-3). To obtain a good outcome with any limb-preservation procedure, the preservation of blood supply and neural function in the limb is critical. Several approaches have been described for a distal femoral resection—medial, lateral, or anterior, with all sharing the preservation of the popliteal vessels and the tibial and common peroneal nerves. The most common endoprostheses is a rotating hinged prosthesis, allowing the sacrifice of all the stabilizing ligaments about the knee, both cruciates and the collateral ligaments. The extensor mechanism is preserved. An advantage of the lateral approach over the anterior or medial approach is the lack of disruption of the quadriceps, which is thought to allow for quicker recovery. Patients commonly require some form of bracing, typically

a knee immobilizer for several weeks until strength in the quadriceps has returned. However, with resection of the distal femur and some portion of the quadriceps, strength is reduced compared with that of the contralateral limb. Gait training, strengthening, and range of motion are critical to the recovery. Cementation of the endoprosthesis allows for immediate full weight bearing. A press-fit endoprosthesis, which requires bone on-growth onto the stem of the endoprosthesis, requires a period of partial weight bearing until there is evidence of on-growth on radiographs.

Rehabilitation

Although the distal femur replacement does include a total knee replacement, the rehabilitation of this surgery is quite different than a total knee arthroplasty (see Figures 34-2 and 34-3) (Tables 34-1 to 34-4). The physical therapist will need to communicate with the surgeon to discuss the exact surgical approach and the amount of resection. Whether or not the quadriceps muscles have been disrupted or simply moved aside during surgery will create different time frames for returning strength. Regardless of the method of surgical intervention, the patient will be in a knee immobilizer after surgery because of the quadriceps weakness. The purpose of this brace is not to restrict range of motion but simply to support the knee. The patient is prone to knee buckling, and subsequent falls may occur as a result of this initial weakness. The brace is to be worn at all times when out of bed and when performing any mobility activity, transfers, or ambulation. The brace may be removed once the patient is able to perform a straight leg raise without an extensor lag.

Proximal Tibia

The proximal tibia is the second common site of malignant bone tumors and provides its own set of complexities given the anatomy of the tibia and the insertion of the extensor mechanism (Figure 34-6). The preservation of the extensor mechanism is critical in the functioning of the knee after reconstruction. The utilization of a medial gastrocnemius muscle flap allows for soft tissues coverage over the proximal tibia endoprosthesis, reducing the risk of wound breakdown and infection; it also aids in the reattachment of the patellar tendon. The endoprosthesis requires replacement of the distal femoral articular surface (Figure 34-7). A rotating hinge knee replacement is usually used for this, similar to a distal femoral replacement. Following a proximal tibial resection and reconstruction, patients are kept immobilized for at least 6 weeks to allow for healing of the muscle flap and extensor mechanism (Figure 34-8). Range-of-motion exercises do not begin until after that 6-week period. Patients typically have an extensor lag of up to 15° because of the reconstruction (Figure 34-9).

TABLE 34-1

Lower Extremity Limb Rehabilitation After Surgery: Phase I—Acute Phase (Rehabilitation in the Hospital)

Surgery	Estimated Length of Stay	Rehabilitation Focus	Occupational Therapy Consult	Rehabilitation Sessions: Postoperative Day 1	Rehabilitation Sessions: Remainder of Hospital Stay	Discharge Disposition
Distal femur replacement	3 days	• Mobility • Gait training • Stair training (if needed) • Initial ROM • Initial strengthening • Use of knee immobilizer	• Not unless determined by physical therapist that it is needed	• Physical therapy evaluation • Transfer training, bed mobility, gait training—all with immobilizer in place • Start of isometric exercises (glute sets, quad sets), ankle pumps, active assistive heel slides • **Goals:** out of bed, begin ambulation using an assistive device, sitting in chair for several hours, begin ROM, discharge planning	• Therapy sessions daily (twice daily if possible) • Daily improvements in mobility, transfers, ambulation, range of motion • Exercises: hip abduction/adduction, isometric hamstring sets, straight leg raise in immobilizer • Use of the knee immobilizer (taking on/off) • Caregiver training for mobility	• Dependent on resources available at home • Most likely home discharge with home physical therapy
Proximal tibia replacement	2-3 days	• Mobility • Gait training • Stair training (if needed) • Initial strengthening • Use of knee immobilizer	• Not unless determined by therapist that it is needed	• Physical therapy evaluation • Transfer training, bed mobility, gait training—all with immobilizer in place • Start of isometric exercises (glute sets, quad sets), ankle pumps • **Goals:** out of bed, begin ambulation using an assistive device, sitting in chair for several hours, discharge planning	• Therapy sessions daily (twice daily if possible) • Daily improvements in mobility, transfers, ambulation • Exercises: hip abduction/adduction, isometric hamstring sets, straight leg raise in immobilizer • Use of the knee immobilizer (taking on/off) • Caregiver training for mobility	• Dependent on resources available at home • Most likely home discharge with home physical therapy

Proximal femur replacement	3-4 days	• Mobility • Gait training • Stair training (if needed) • Initial strengthening • Education on hip precautions	• Yes, occupational therapy will need to work with the patient on self-care activities while maintaining hip precautions	• Physical therapy evaluation • Transfer training, bed mobility, gait training—all while maintain hip precautions • Start of isometric exercises (glute sets, quad sets), ankle pumps • Education on hip precautions • **Goals:** out of bed, begin ambulation using an assistive device, sitting in chair for several hours, discharge planning	• Therapy sessions daily (twice daily if possible) • Daily improvements in mobility, transfers, ambulation • Exercises: isometric hip abduction/adduction, heel slides • Review of hip precautions • Caregiver training for mobility	• Dependent on resources available at home • Although many will return to home, many others will require a skilled nursing facility or inpatient rehabilitation facility first
Total femur replacement	5-7 days	• Mobility • Gait training • Stair training (if needed) • Initial strengthening • Initial ROM • Education on hip precautions • Education on use of knee immobilizer	• Yes, occupational therapy will need to work with the patient on self-care activities while maintaining hip precautions	• Physical therapy evaluation • Transfer training, bed mobility, gait training—all while maintain hip precautions and wearing the knee immobilizer • Start of isometric exercises (gluteal sets, quadriceps sets), ankle pumps, active assistive heel slides • Education on hip precautions • Education on knee immobilizer • **Goals:** out of bed, begin ambulation using an assistive device, sitting in chair for several hours, discharge planning; begin ROM if pain is controlled	• Therapy sessions daily (twice daily if possible) • Daily improvements in mobility, transfers, ambulation, ROM • Exercises: isometric hip abduction/adduction, active assistive heel slides • Review of hip precautions	• Placement in a skilled nursing facility or preferably inpatient rehabilitation facility

ROM, Range of motion.

TABLE 34-2

Lower Extremity Limb Rehabilitation After Surgery: Phase II—Subacute Phase (May Take Place in a Rehabilitation Facility, Home, or Outpatient Setting)

Surgery	Time Frame	Rehabilitation Goals	Rehabilitation Sessions	Pearls
Distal femur replacement	8-12 weeks	• Progression of ambulation to least restrictive assistive device (or none at all) • Progression to least dependent living situation • Normalized gait pattern • ROM to 120° knee flexion • Return of strength, discontinuation of knee immobilizer	• Begin with gentle AAROM and quad strengthening • PROM may be too aggressive and is not needed • Mobility and gait training • Balance activities	• ROM may return slowly. This is expected; this procedure is not a total knee replacement. • Patient is high risk for falls due to quadriceps weakness. A fall can result in a torn quadriceps tendon. Take the use of the knee immobilizer seriously.
Proximal tibia replacement	6 weeks	• Progression of ambulation to least restrictive assistive device • Progression to least dependent living situation • Quadriceps strengthening in knee immobilizer	• Mobility and gait training • Balance activities • Exercise focused on quadriceps strength	• No knee flexion is allowed. Even minimal ROM (knee flexion) can cause the stitches to break and will cause disruption of the patellar tendon. • Patient may not be involved in skilled PT services throughout this time period. They are often able to continue with a home program.
Proximal femur replacement	12 weeks	• Progression of ambulation to least restrictive assistive device • Progression to least dependent living situation • Normalized gait pattern	• Mobility and gait training • Balance activities	• These patients may need limits set to prevent them from becoming too aggressive in their rehabilitation. Return to recreational activities will come, just not in the first 12 weeks. • Hip precautions are in place for minimum of 3 months.
Total femur replacement	12 weeks	• Progression of ambulation to least restrictive assistive device • Progression to least dependent living situation • ROM to 120° knee flexion • Return of strength, possible discontinuation of knee immobilizer	• Begin with gentle AAROM and quadriceps strengthening • PROM may be too aggressive and is not needed • Mobility and gait training • Balance activities	• ROM may return slowly. This is expected; this procedure is not a total knee replacement. • Patient is high risk for falls due to quadriceps weakness. A fall can result in a torn quad tendon or even hip dislocation. Take the use of the knee immobilizer seriously. • Hip precautions are in place for minimum of 3 months but typically longer after this surgery.

ROM, Range of motion; *AAROM,* active assisted range of motion; *PROM,* passive range of motion; *PT,* physical therapy.

TABLE **34-3**

Lower Extremity Limb Rehabilitation After Surgery: Phase III—Long Term

Surgery	Time Frame	Rehabilitation Goals	Rehabilitation Sessions	Pearls
Distal femur replacement	Up to 6 months after surgery	• Return of strength • Return to recreational activities	• Simulation of motions/activities that the patient would like to return to performing (e.g., golf, hiking)	• Gait speed, oxygen consumption, and strength will be reduced compared with normal controls.[18]
Proximal tibia replacement	Begins 6 weeks after surgery and can extend through 1 year	• Progression of ambulation without assistive device • Return of strength • Return of ROM (knee flexion) to 120° • Eventual return to recreational activities	• AAROM and gentle PROM for knee flexion • Progressive strengthening, gait training, stair training, balance activities • Simulation of motions/activities that the patient would like to return to performing (e.g., golf, hiking)	• This is the most critical point in the rehabilitation of this patient. • Progression of ROM will be *slow.* This is expected. • Full ROM can be attained!
Proximal femur replacement	Up to 6 months after surgery	• Return of strength • Return to recreational activities	• Simulation of motions/activities that the patient would like to return to performing (e.g., golf, hiking)	• Abductor weakness can be a chronic weakness
Total femur replacement	6 months to 1 year after surgery	• Progression of ambulation without assistive device • Return of strength • Return of ROM (knee flexion) to 120° • Eventual return to recreational activities (these will be limited)	• Similar to distal femur and proximal femur	• In the pediatric population, it is quite possible for the patient to return to near-prior functional levels.

ROM, Range of motion; *AAROM,* active assisted range of motion; *PROM,* passive range of motion.

Rehabilitation

Early range of motion, even minimal knee flexion, can cause the sutures used to repair the patellar tendon to break, thereby disrupting the integrity of the extensor mechanism. Only after the 6-week time frame can range-of-motion activities begin, with the patient regaining range of motion through time, effort, and dedication to rehabilitation (see Tables 34-1 to 34-4). These patients return to a high level of function with proper follow-through physical therapy. Patients with a proximal tibia replacement are able to return to an efficient gait and active lifestyle after the surgery and subsequent rehabilitation.[13,14]

Clinical Note

• Maintaining the knee in full extension after a proximal tibial replacement, for at least 6 weeks, is important to allow for healing of the extensor mechanism.

Proximal Femur

Function after a resection of a proximal femur bone sarcoma (Figures 34-10 and 34-11) is affected by the preservation of the muscles that insert onto the femur. A posterior

TABLE **34-4**

Lower Extremity Limb-Preservation Surgeries: Quick Tips

Surgical Procedure	Precautions/Restrictions	Bracing	Weight Bearing
Distal femur replacement	None	Knee immobilizer; can be removed when patient can perform a straight leg raise without extensor lag	As tolerated (cemented) Press fit; partial weight bearing
Proximal tibia replacement	No knee flexion for 6 weeks	Knee immobilizer; remains in place for 6 weeks	As tolerated (cemented) Press fit; partial weight bearing
Proximal femur replacement	Hip precautions	None	As tolerated (cemented) Press fit; partial weight bearing
Total femur replacement	Hip precautions	Knee immobilizer; can be removed when patient can perform a straight leg raise without extensor lag	As tolerated (cemented) Press fit; partial weight bearing

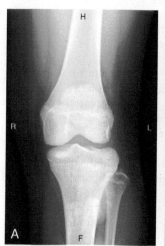
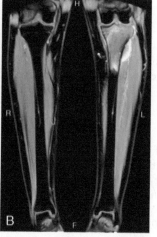

Figure 34-6 A, X-ray of a proximal tibia with an osteosarcoma in a 14-year-old girl. **B,** Magnetic resonance image of the same osteosarcoma.

approach to the hip is the most common surgical approach. Patients usually have a Trendelenburg gait postoperatively. Techniques have been described to aid in the reattachment of these muscles onto the endoprosthesis[15]; however, because of the number of muscular attachments resected, there is commonly residual functional weakness, especially of the abductor muscles. Greater strength deficits and reduced range of motion should be expected in these patients compared with patients undergoing total hip arthroplasties.[13] A bipolar hip component is usually used to reduce the added risk of dislocation of a total hip replacement.

Rehabilitation

The rehabilitation of a proximal femoral replacement is very similar to (and follows the guidelines of) that for a hip replacement that a physical therapist may see in a general orthopedic practice (see Tables 34-1 to 34-4). Typically, the posterior approach to the hip is used; thus,

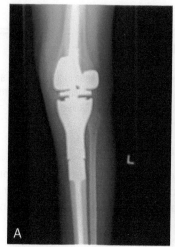
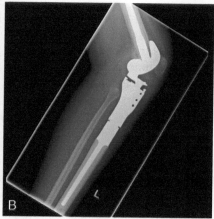

Figure 34-7 X-rays showing a proximal tibial replacement along with a total knee arthroplasty. **A,** Anterior view. **B,** Lateral view.

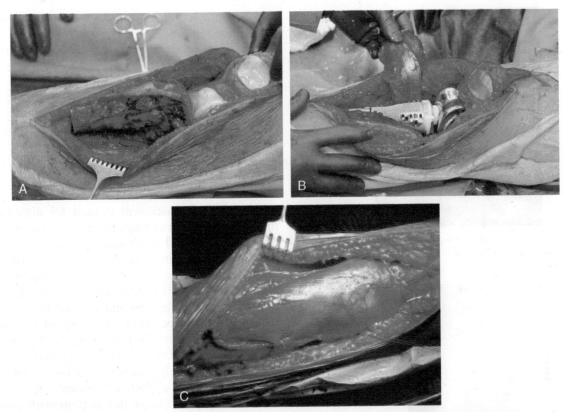

Figure 34-8 A, Resection of a proximal tibia sarcoma with the patella and extensor mechanism preserved. **B,** Medial gastrocnemius rotation flap in the surgeon's hand. **C,** After flap closure, showing coverage of the endoprosthesis.

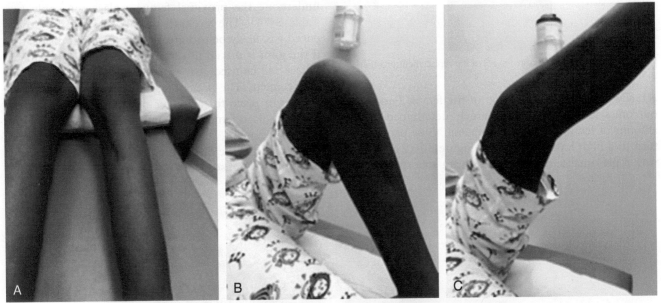

Figure 34-9 Active knee range of motion 1 year after surgery. **A,** Extension. **B,** Flexion. **C,** Quadriceps lag.

posterior hip surgery precautions must be maintained during the rehabilitation phase. These precautions include no hip flexion past 90°, no hip medial (internal) rotation, and no hip adduction past midline. In a typical proximal femoral replacement, it takes at least 3 months to regain strength in order to maintain the integrity of the hip joint and therefore, the clinician must take these

precautions into account when treating the patient. With most proximal femur replacements, the patient will bear weight as tolerated on the operative lower extremity, because these are typically cemented endoprostheses. It is essential that the physical therapist communicate with the surgeon regarding the amount of femur that was removed. Although this surgery is termed proximal, it can

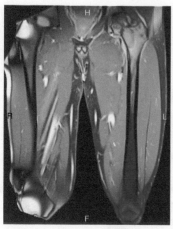

Figure 34-10 Magnetic resonance imaging scan of an osteosarcoma of the proximal femur in a 22-year-old.

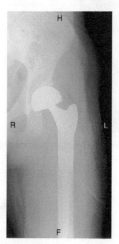

Figure 34-11 Postoperative x-ray images of hip replacement prosthesis.

an efficient gait and active lifestyle after the surgery and subsequent rehabilitation.[13,15]

Posterior Hip Postsurgical Precautions

- No hip flexion past 90°
- No hip medial (internal) rotation
- No hip adduction past the midline

Total Femur Replacement

A total femur replacement is used for diaphyseal tumors that extend proximally to the lesser trochanter and distally to the distal diaphyseal-metaphyseal junction of the tumor. It is unique in that it is composed of a total hip replacement and a total knee replacement (see Figure 34-18). This patient will need extensive education by both the surgeon and physical therapist to establish realistic expectations with regard to functional outcomes (see Tables 34-1 to 34-4).[16,17] A great deal of strength is lost and will never be fully recovered. Thus, the patient will likely always require the use of an assistive device for ambulation. The patient will be required to follow hip precautions, just as those with a proximal femur replacement do, with the caveat that the patient will likely be required to follow these for life or, at a minimum, for much longer than the patient who has undergone the proximal femur replacement only (see Table 34-4). The strength deficits that will be experienced will likely be too great to ever prevent dislocation if the joint is placed in certain positions. A knee immobilizer will be used, just as it is used for the distal femur replacement. The patient should expect that the brace will be in place for a longer period of time compared with the distal femur replacement. As with the distal femur replacement, the patient can discontinue the use of the brace when he or she can perform a straight leg raise without an extensor lag.

actually involve a large portion of the femur. Functional outcomes for the patient are largely determined by the amount of femur replaced. In general, these patients return to a high level of function (Figure 34-12). Patients with a proximal femur replacement are able to return to

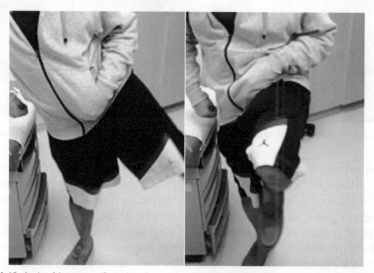

Figure 34-12 Active hip range of motion 2 months postoperatively after surgery for an osteosarcoma.

Clinical Note

- Patients with a total femur replacement will need to maintain posterior hip precautions for life or, at a minimum, much longer than the patient who has undergone only a proximal femur replacement.

Distal Tibia

The distal tibia is a rare site for malignant bone tumors (Figure 34-13). Resection and limb salvage is an option; however, there are complications associated with allograft or endoprosthesis. Range of motion is reduced, making high-impact activities difficult. Below-the-knee amputation is often the best oncologic and functional option in these patients.[12]

Proximal Humerus

Similar to the proximal femur, the preservation and reattachment of any of the rotator cuff muscles, pectoralis, or latissimus dorsi muscles leads to improvement in function postoperatively (Figure 34-14). However, it is common for a large portion of the rotator cuff to be resected along with the tumor. Given this, expectations for range of motion and strength are limited postoperatively. The therapist is indispensable in working to achieve satisfactory results.

Rehabilitation

The proximal humeral replacement is quite different than a general orthopedic shoulder replacement, and the associated outcomes are also very different (Tables 34-5 to 34-8). A hemiarthroplasty is usually performed to

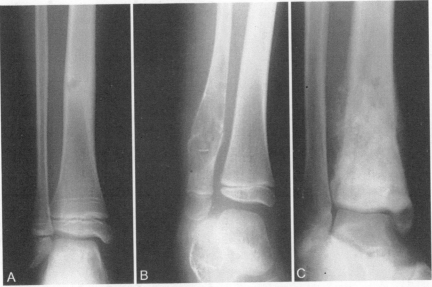

Figure 34-13 Radiographs are essential in evaluating leg pain in an athlete because rare surprises such as these tumors may be discovered. **A,** Radiograph of stress fracture through a benign cartilage tumor of the tibia in a 9-year-old soccer player. **B,** Radiograph of an aneurysmal bone cyst of the fibula in a 7-year-old child. **C,** Radiograph of an osteosarcoma of the distal tibia in an active 16-year-old boy. (Courtesy John Murray, MD. In Coughlin MJ, Mann RA, Saltzman CL: *Surgery of the foot and ankle,* ed 8, St. Louis, 2007, Mosby/Elsevier.)

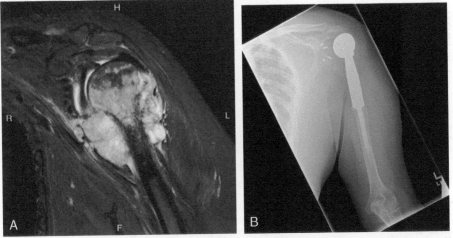

Figure 34-14 A, Magnetic resonance imaging scan of a proximal humerus osteosarcoma. **B,** X-ray showing proximal humeral endoprosthetic reconstruction after resection.

TABLE 34-5

Upper Extremity Limb Rehabilitation After Surgery: Phase I—Acute Phase (Rehabilitation in the Hospital)

Surgery	Estimated Length of Stay	Rehabilitation Focus	Occupational Therapy Consult	Rehabilitation Sessions: Postoperative Day 1	Rehabilitation Sessions: Remainder of Hospital Stay	Discharge Disposition
Proximal humerus replacement	2-3 days	• Initial ROM of elbow, wrist, fingers • Use of shoulder immobilizer	• Yes, in many hospitals, occupational therapists will solely be responsible for these patients	• Occupational therapy evaluation (physical therapy evaluation if needed) • Transfer training, bed mobility with shoulder immobilizer in place • Start of AROM of elbow, wrist, fingers, pendulum exercise • Education in use of the shoulder immobilizer • Education on NWB status of the upper extremity • **Goals:** out of bed, sitting in chair for several hours, begin ROM, discharge planning	• Occupational therapy for one-armed techniques for bathing, dressing, and other self-care activities • Physical therapy involvement if the patient was using an assistive device for ambulation before admission	• Discharge home with an independent home program to continue for 6 weeks
Distal humerus replacement	1-3 days	• Initial ROM of entire upper extremity	• Yes, in many hospitals, occupational therapists will solely be responsible for these patients	• Occupational therapy evaluation (physical therapy evaluation if needed) • Start of AROM of shoulder, elbow, wrist, fingers • Use of shoulder immobilizer for comfort only • **Goals:** out of bed, sitting in chair for several hours, begin ROM, discharge planning	• Progress ROM of elbow joint	• Discharge home with an independent home program or with outpatient therapy
Total humerus replacement	2-3 days	• Initial ROM of elbow, wrist, fingers • Use of shoulder immobilizer	• Yes, in many hospitals, occupational therapists will solely be responsible for these patients	• Occupational therapy evaluation (physical therapy evaluation if needed) • Transfer training, bed mobility with shoulder immobilizer in place • Start of AROM of elbow, wrist, fingers, pendulum exercise • Education in use of the shoulder immobilizer • Education on NWB status of the upper extremity • **Goals:** out of bed, sitting in chair for several hours, begin ROM of elbow, discharge planning	• Occupational therapy for one-armed techniques for bathing, dressing, and other self-care activities • Physical therapy involvement if the patient was using an assistive device for ambulation before admission • Progress elbow ROM	• Discharge home with an independent home program to continue for 6 weeks

ROM, Range of motion; *AROM,* active range of motion; *NWB,* non–weight bearing.

TABLE **34-6**

Upper Extremity Limb Rehabilitation After Surgery: Phase II—Subacute Phase (May Take Place in a Rehabilitation Facility, Home, or Outpatient Setting)

Surgery	Time Frame	Rehabilitation Goals	Rehabilitation Sessions	Pearls
Proximal humerus replacement	6 weeks	• Full elbow, wrist, finger ROM	• Patient will likely be performing a program to include AROM to the elbow, wrist, fingers, shoulder pendulums	• The patient will remain in the shoulder immobilizer during this time with no shoulder ROM. • Beginning ROM too early will result in lack of scar tissue, which is needed for shoulder stability.
Distal humerus replacement	6-12 weeks	• Full ROM • Full strength • Return to full function	• Beginning with AROM and progression to resistive range of motion	
Total humerus replacement	6 weeks	• Full ROM of elbow, wrist, fingers • Full strength of elbow, wrist, fingers	• Beginning with AROM and progression to resistive range of motion of the elbow, wrist, and fingers only	• The patient will remain in the shoulder immobilizer during this time with no shoulder ROM. • Beginning ROM too early will result in lack of scar tissue, which is needed for shoulder stability.

ROM, Range of motion; *AROM,* active range of motion.

TABLE **34-7**

Upper Extremity Limb Rehabilitation After Surgery: Phase III—Long Term

Surgery	Time Frame	Rehabilitation Goals	Rehabilitation Sessions	Pearls
Proximal humerus replacement Total humerus replacement	4-6 months after surgery	• 9° shoulder flexion • Functional use of upper extremity for feeding, grooming, dressing, etc.	• Gentle and relatively pain-free activities • AAROM to the shoulder; PROM not needed • Progression to strengthening activities for the shoulder • Self-care training with use of surgical extremity	• Reliance on scar tissue to maintain shoulder integrity and prevention of subluxation is needed. Aggressive ROM will break the scar tissue, causing instability. • Exercises should continue for life. Regression of attained ROM will occur if the exercises are discontinued.

AAROM, Active assisted range of motion; *PROM,* passive range of motion; *ROM,* range of motion.

TABLE **34-8**

Upper Extremity Limb-Preservation Surgeries: Quick Tips

Surgical Procedure	Precautions/Restrictions	Bracing	Weight Bearing
Proximal humerus replacement	No shoulder range of motion for 6 weeks	Shoulder immobilizer at all times	Partial weight bearing
Distal humerus replacement		Shoulder sling for comfort only	Partial weight bearing
Total humerus replacement	No shoulder range of motion for 6 weeks	Shoulder immobilizer at all times	Partial weight bearing

decrease the risk of instability and dislocation. Given the extent of the surgical resection usually performed in oncologic surgery, the patient will require immobilization for 6 weeks and specialized rehabilitation. Patients should expect to have significant deficits to their functional abilities after this surgery, which is often the only option other than an amputation. Therefore, limited range of motion, strength, and function are all acceptable outcomes of surgery. Long-term goals should include full elbow, wrist, and finger range of motion and strength, as well as active shoulder flexion and abduction to from 60° to 90°. Some of the most prevalent long-term effects include subluxation or instability.

Clinical Note—Caution!

- Upper limb replacement surgery for bone tumors prevents weight bearing (i.e., with crutches or a walker) through the upper limb, until strength has been regained.

Elbow and Forearm

The elbow and forearm are rare sites of malignant tumors (Figure 34-15). Wide resection of the proximal radius or distal ulna can be performed without reconstruction or by the creation of a one-bone forearm by fusion. For the distal humerus or proximal ulna, resection and reconstruction with either an allograft-prosthetic composite (APC) or an endoprosthesis with a total elbow reconstruction can provide favorable outcomes.[18] For tumors of the distal radius, allograft with wrist arthrodesis or an osteoarticular allograft are used after limb-preservation procedures.

Rehabilitation

The distal humeral replacement is a surgery involving a portion of the distal humerus along with an elbow replacement. The results from this procedure are very positive, and the patient is likely to return to full prior level of function, with weight-lifting restrictions (see

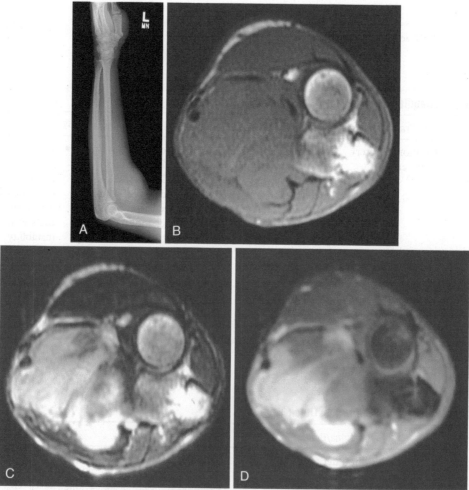

Figure 34-15 Synovial sarcoma in a 24-year-old man. **A,** Lateral radiograph of the left elbow shows a calcified soft tissue mass in the antecubital fossa. **B,** T1-weighted (T1WI) axial magnetic resonance imaging study shows a lobulated isointense soft tissue tumor. **C,** Fat-suppressed T2-weighted (T2WI) axial study with a mildly heterogeneous hyperintense soft tissue tumor with areas of low signal due to intratumoral calcification. **D,** Postcontrast fat-suppressed T1WI axial study shows heterogeneous enhancement of tumor. (From Silverman PM: *Oncologic imaging: a multidisciplinary approach*, Philadelphia, 2012, Saunders/Elsevier.)

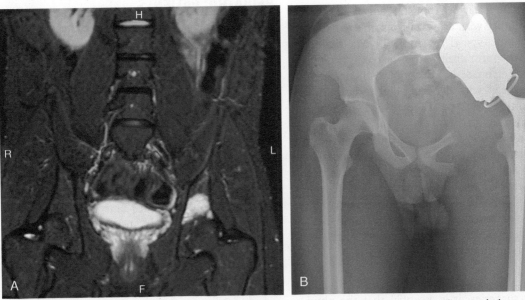

Figure 34-16 **A,** Magnetic resonance imaging scan of the pelvis with a chondrosarcoma involving the ilium and the periacetabular region. **B,** X-ray showing endoprosthetic reconstruction and a total hip arthroplasty after a type II resection.

Tables 34-5 to 34-8). This patient will have few other restrictions and will immediately be allowed to begin fully participating in the rehabilitation process. In contrast to the proximal humeral replacement, this procedure allows for immediate weight bearing through the extremity, as well as immediate elbow range of motion and strengthening.

Total Humeral Replacement

The patient with a total humeral replacement will have components of both a proximal and distal humeral replacement, which includes a total elbow replacement. The patient will have similar restrictions to a proximal humeral endoprosthesis—the shoulder must remain immobilized for 6 weeks postoperatively, and weight bearing through the surgical extremity is not allowed (see Tables 34-5 to 34-8). Patients should expect to have significant deficits in their functional abilities after this surgery, which is often the only option other than an amputation. Therefore, limited range of motion, strength, and function are all acceptable outcomes. Long-term goals should include full elbow, wrist, and finger range of motion and strength, as well as active shoulder flexion and abduction from 60° to 90°.

Clinical Note—Caution!

- Patients who have had a proximal humeral replacement for bone tumors depend on scar tissue to maintain shoulder integrity so any range of motion or stretching activities must be done with extreme caution.

Pelvis

Resection of the pelvis can be broadly categorized into internal hemipelvectomies (resection) and external hemipelvectomies (amputation). The factors that determine limb salvage of a pelvic tumor are the neurovascular structures in the pelvis, the femoral vessels, and adequacy of tissue coverage. After an internal hemipelvectomy, reconstruction may be performed or the limb may be left flail. There are several reconstruction options, including allograft, APC, endoprosthesis (Figure 34-16), and arthrodesis. The Enneking classification[19] of internal hemipelvectomy classifies the resection based on the part of the pelvis resected (Table 34-9). The resection type determines the

TABLE 34-9

Enneking Classification and Reconstruction for Internal Hemipelvectomy[19]

Type	Resection	Reconstruction Options
I	Part or all of the ilium	No reconstruction or sacroiliac fusion with allograft
II	Periacetabular region	Acetabular allograft-prosthetic composite with total hip arthroplasty, iliofemoral arthrodesis, endoprosthesis, or suspension of the femur with no reconstruction (flail limb)
III	Ischiopubic area	No reconstruction
IV	Pelvis with extension into the sacrum	Similar to type II

reconstruction. Type I may be reconstructed should there be pelvic discontinuity with a fusion from the remaining ilium to the sacrum. Type II resections involve the acetabulum and are the most challenging for reconstruction. APCs, iliofemoral arthrodesis, or endoprosthetic reconstructions may be used, with all having high levels of postoperative morbidities.[20-22] Type III resections typically do not require reconstruction.

Depending on the type of pelvic resection, the abductors, adductors, lateral (external) rotators, and hip flexors may be resected and/or removed during the dissection. This leads to limited strength and function of those muscle groups. With normal knee and ankle function, patients are able to ambulate. However, a Trendelenburg gait, a potential leg length discrepancy, and altered mechanics affect ambulation postoperatively (Figure 34-17).

Rehabilitation

For these major surgeries, it is essential that the physical therapist have excellent communication with the surgeon and, if possible, access to postoperative x-rays. Rehabilitation is highly dependent on what portions of the pelvis are resected and how the reconstruction is completed. These patients may be amputees with an external hemipelvectomy, or they may be treated similar to a patient who has undergone total hip arthroplasty, with more strict hip precautions if the resection is a type II. Overall, functional outcome will depend greatly on what was resected and what type of reconstruction, if any, was performed (see Figure 34-16). Patients having an external hemipelvectomy may be fitted for a prosthesis if they are mobile enough; however, given the extensive nature of the amputation, the use of the prosthesis is very challenging, and most patients do not opt for this.

PEDIATRIC PATIENTS

Additional challenges exist with regard to limb preservation in a growing child with a tumor in the extremity, especially the lower extremity; this is because of the expected continued growth of that limb. Endoprosthesis technology has improved from invasive lengthening techniques to noninvasive methods. Currently, several endoprostheses can be gradually lengthened as the child grows. An external revolving magnet slowly lengthens a screw mechanism inside the endoprosthesis (Figure 34-18). The limb is lengthened a few millimeters at a time, typically on a monthly basis (Figure 34-19). Studies have reported good outcomes and patient satisfaction with these techniques.[23,24] In instances in which the child is very young and a large leg length discrepancy is expected, an amputation or rotationplasty may be another viable option.

AMPUTATIONS

When limb salvage cannot be performed or following the failure of a limb-preservation procedure, an amputation may be necessary. Techniques are similar to those used for amputations performed for other diagnoses; however, the primary goal in the presence of cancer is for wide resection of the tumor, so residual limbs may be shorter. The level of the amputation correlates with the amount of energy expenditure when ambulating and walking speed.[25-27] One study compared energy cost during gait in patients with osteosarcoma of the distal femur who underwent an amputation with patients with a distal femoral replacement. Amputees had slower free-walking velocity, higher oxygen consumption per meter traveled, and lower percent maximum aerobic capacity.[28]

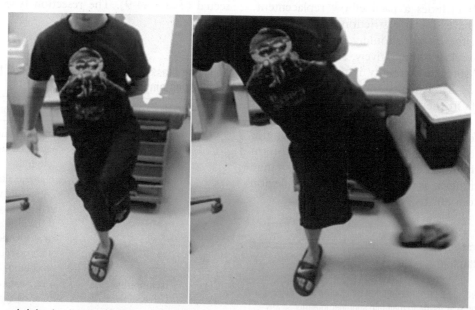

Figure 34-17 Flexion and abduction images of a 23-year-old male who underwent a resection and endoprosthetic reconstruction for an osteosarcoma of the pelvis.

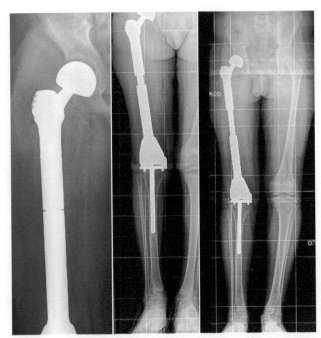

Figure 34-18 X-rays showing a total femur expandable endoprosthesis as it has been lengthened over a 3-year period.

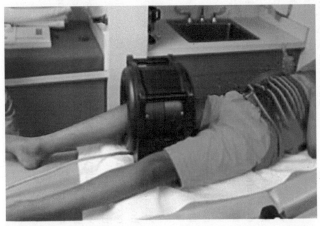

Figure 34-19 A child undergoing a lengthening of a Stanmore noninvasive endoprosthesis with the limb in an external magnet.

Transfemoral amputations lead to an increase in energy expenditure during ambulation. The length of the residual limb affects the prosthetic fit; residual limbs shorter than 5 cm (2 inches) behave functionally as hip disarticulations.[12] A "fish-mouth" incision is typically used. A medial adductor myodesis (i.e., suturing the muscle to the bone) is important to improved adduction power and prevent lateral drift in the prosthetic socket.

Transtibial amputations are a durable option for tumors of the distal tibia, foot, and ankle. The length of the residual limb affects prosthesis fitting and control.

Hip disarticulation is performed for tumors of the proximal femur when limb salvage is not an option. Patients can ambulate with a prosthesis, although they can be cumbersome and require a lot of energy expenditure.[12]

Shoulder disarticulation and forequarter amputations are used when the tumor involves the shoulder girdle and/or proximal humerus and limb salvage and reconstruction or arthrodesis is not a viable option. A forequarter amputation involves resection of the scapula, clavicle, and entire arm. Rotation flaps are typically used for closure. The loss of the shoulder contour does make clothes wearing difficult, and static shoulder pads are sometimes used. Occupation therapy is critical for these patients to help them learn to use their one remaining upper extremity.

Rehabilitation

Regardless of the reason for an amputation (e.g., cancer, infection, trauma), from a physical therapy aspect, the amputee will be treated the same. The patient will have varying needs and expectations, with a prosthesis depending on the size of the residual limb (Figure 34-20). Positioning is an important focus of physical therapy and depends on the portion of the limb that has been amputated (Table 34-10). The patient should be fitted with a shrinker (Figure 34-21) and residual limb (Figure 34-22) protector as soon as possible after surgery (Table 34-11). One of the most important areas to focus on with any amputee is the psychosocial component that comes with this type of surgery—no matter how well prepared the individual may be before surgery. Phantom pains and sensations are real and should be acknowledged; furthermore, the individual should be shown techniques to address these feelings. In an oncology setting, an amputation is rarely an emergency procedure, and the patient has usually had at least a few weeks to begin to process the upcoming surgery and its implications. The hospital's social workers and/or psychologists may be able to lend assistance with the psychosocial component of these surgeries. They also may be accustomed to the extremity lacking in function and do extremely well after surgery.

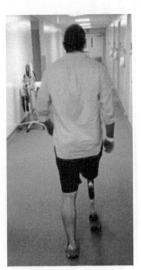

Figure 34-20 A 24-year-old with transtibial amputation, after a local recurrence following a proximal tibial osteosarcoma resection, ambulating with a prosthesis.

TABLE 34-10

Rehabilitation of the Amputee: Acute Phase

Surgery	Estimated Length of Stay	Rehabilitation Focus	Occupational Therapy Consult	Rehabilitation Sessions: Postoperative Day 1	Rehabilitation Sessions: Remainder of Hospital Stay	Discharge Disposition
Transfemoral	2-3 days	• Mobility • Gait training • Stair training (if needed) • Initial ROM • Initial strengthening	• Not unless determined by physical therapist that it is needed	• Physical therapy evaluation • Transfer training, bed mobility, gait training with walker, balance activities • Education on fall risks/fall prevention • Education on proper positioning (hip extension, time spent in prone position), risks for flexion contractures	• Therapy sessions daily • Progression to crutches if appropriate • Daily improvements in mobility, transfers, ambulation, ROM • Start of AROM of the hip • Fitting of shrinker and limb protector	• Dependent on resources at home • Most likely home discharge with home physical therapy (patients will continue this until ready for prosthesis fitting)
Transtibial	2-3 days	• Mobility • Gait training • Stair training (if needed) • Initial ROM • Initial strengthening	• Not unless determined by physical therapist that it is needed	• Physical therapy evaluation • Transfer training, bed mobility, gait training with walker, balance activities • Education on fall risks/fall prevention • Education on proper positioning (knee extension), risks for flexion contractures	• Therapy sessions daily • Progression to crutches if appropriate • Daily improvements in mobility, transfers, ambulation, ROM • Start of AROM of the hip • Fitting of shrinker and limb protector	• Dependent on resources at home • Most likely home discharge with home physical therapy (patients will continue this until ready for prosthesis fitting)
Above elbow	2-3 days	• Initial ROM • Initial strengthening • One-armed functional activities	• Yes, in many hospitals, occupational therapists will be solely responsible for these patients	• Occupational therapy evaluation • AROM of the shoulder • One-armed activities	• Occupational therapy sessions daily • Daily improvements in ROM and strength • Functional tasks with the use of one upper extremity • Fitting of shrinker and limb protector	• Dependent on resources at home • Most likely home discharge with home occupational therapy (patients will continue this until ready for prosthesis fitting)
Below elbow	2-3 days	• Initial ROM • Initial strengthening • One-armed functional activities	• Yes, in many hospitals, occupational therapists will be solely responsible for these patients	• Occupational therapy evaluation • AROM of the shoulder and elbow • One-armed activities • Encouragement of elbow extension positioning	• Occupational therapy sessions daily • Daily improvements in range of motion and strength • Functional tasks with the use of one upper extremity • Fitting of shrinker and limb protector	• Dependent on resources at home • Most likely home discharge with home occupational therapy (patients will continue this until ready for prosthesis fitting)

ROM, Range of motion; *AROM,* active range of motion.

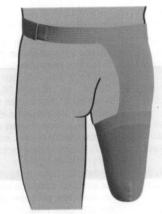

Figure 34-21 Above-the-knee stump shrinker. (Image courtesy of Juzo USA, Cuyahoga Falls, OH.)

If possible, the patient should see the prosthetist before surgery to discuss options for a prosthesis and the patient should try to speak directly to other amputees to visualize what is to come and ask questions of those who have experienced this surgery firsthand. The patient, prosthetist, physical therapist, and occupational therapist should all discuss the available options and what will functionally make the most sense after surgery.

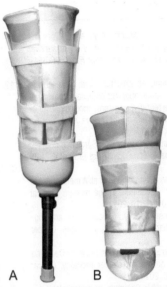

A   B

Figure 34-22 Residual limb protector. **A**, POP-PY (postoperative protector with pylon) System. **B**, POP (postoperative protector). (Image courtesy of Fillauer LLC, Chattanooga, TN.)

TABLE 34-11

Rehabilitation of the Amputee: Final Phase

Surgery	Time Frame	Rehabilitation Goals	Rehabilitation Sessions	Pearls
Transfemoral Transtibial Hip disarticulation Formal hemipelvectomy	• To begin 6 weeks after surgery	• Ambulation with prosthesis using least restrictive device (or no device) • Independent with negotiating stairs with prosthesis • Independent in placing and removing the prosthesis • Independent in skin care	• Gait training, balance activities • Education on fall risks/fall prevention, getting off floor after a fall	• Not all patients will opt for or be appropriate for a prosthesis. • Transfemoral patients will ambulate 43% slower and use 89% more energy than individuals with both limbs. • Transtibial patients will ambulate 36% slower and use 40% more energy than individuals with both limbs.
Above elbow Below elbow Shoulder disarticulation Forequarter amputation	• To begin 6 weeks after surgery	• Independent in use of the prosthesis for functional activities • Independent in placing and removing the prosthesis • Independent in skin care	• Occupational therapy evaluation • AROM of the shoulder • One-armed activities	• An occupational therapist typically works with these patients in conjunction with the prosthesis. • Not all patients will opt for or be appropriate for a prosthesis. • From 70% to 80% of patients with below-the-elbow amputation are able to successfully use a prosthesis.

AROM, Active range of motion.

REFERENCES

1. Ayerza M, Farfalli G, Aponte-Tinao, et al: Does increased rate of limb-sparing surgery affect survival in osteosarcoma? *Clin Orthop Relat Res* 468:1854–2859, 2010.
2. Rougraff BT, Simon MA, Kneisl JS, et al: Limb salvage compared with amputation for osteosarcoma of the distal end of the femur: a long-term oncological, functional and quality-of-life study, *J Bone Joint Surg Am* 76(5):649–656, 1994.
3. Grimer R, Taminiau R, Cannon S: Surgical outcomes in osteosarcoma, *J Bone Joint Surg Br* 84:395–400, 2002.
4. Allison D, Carney S, Ahlmann E, et al: A meta-analysis of osteosarcoma outcomes in the modern medical era, *Sarcoma* 2012:1–10, 2012.
5. American Cancer Society: Cancer facts and figures 2014, Atlanta, GA, 2014, American Cancer Society.
6. Smith MA, Altekruse SF, Adamson PC, et al: Declining childhood and adolescent cancer mortality, *Cancer* 120:2497–2506, 2014.
7. Arndt CA, Crist WM: Common musculoskeletal tumors of childhood and adolescence, *N Engl J Med* 341:342–352, 1999.
8. Mirabello L, Troisi RJ, Savage SA: Osteosarcoma incidence and survival rates from 1973 to 2004: data from the Surveillance, Epidemiology, and End Results Program, *Cancer* 115:1531–1543, 2009.
9. Rödl RW, Pohlmann U, Gosheger G, et al: Rotationplasty—quality of life after 10 years in 22 patients, *Acta Orthop Scand* 73:85–88, 2002.
10. Esiashvili N, Goodman M, Marcus RB: Changes in incidence of Ewing sarcoma patients over the past 3 decades: Surveillance Epidemiology and End results data, *J Pediatr Hematol Oncol* 30:425–430, 2008.
11. Maheshwari AV, Cheng EY: Ewing sarcoma family of tumors, *J Am Acad Orthop Surg* 18:94–107, 2010.
12. Biermann JS, editor: *Orthopaedic knowledge update: musculoskeletal tumors*, Rosemont, IL, 2014, American Academy of Orthopaedic Surgeons.
13. Bernthal NM, Greenberg M, Heberer K, et al: What are the functional outcomes of endoprosthetic reconstructions after tumor resection? *Clin Orthop Relat Res* Apr 2014 [Epub ahead of print].
14. Schwartz A, Kabo M, Eilber F, et al: Cemented endoprosthetic reconstruction of the proximal tibia, *Clin Orthop Relat Res* 468:2875–2884, 2010.
15. Henderson E, Jennings J, Marulanda G, et al: Enhancing soft tissue ingrowth in proximal femoral arthroplasty with aortograft sleeve: a novel technique and early results, *J Arthroplasty* 26:161–163, 2011.
16. Sewell M, Spiegelberg B, Hanna S, et al: Total femoral endoprosthetic replacement following excision of bone tumors, *J Bone Joint Surg Br* 1:1513–1520, 2009.
17. Ruggieri P, Bosco G, Pala E, et al: Local recurrence, survival and function after total femur resection and megaprosthetic reconstruction for bone sarcomas, *Clin Orthop Relat Res* 468:2860–2866, 2010.
18. Funovics P, Schuh R, Adams S, et al: Modular prosthetic reconstruction of major bone defects of the distal end of the humerus, *J Bone Joint Surg Am* 93:1064–1074, 2011.
19. Enneking WF, Dunham WK: Resection and reconstruction for primary neoplasms involving the innominate bone, *J Bone Joint Surg Am* 60:731–746, 1978.
20. Bell RS, Davis AM, Wunder JS, et al: Allograft reconstruction of the acetabulum after resection of stage IIB sarcoma: intermediate-term results, *J Bone Joint Surg Am* 79:1663–1674, 1997.
21. Menedez LR, Ahlmann ER, Falkinstein, et al: Periacetabular reconstruction with a new endoprosthesis, *Clin Orthop Relat Res* 467:2831–2837, 2009.
22. Angelini A, Drago G, Trovarelli G, et al: Infection after surgical resection for pelvic bone tumors: an analysis of 270 patients from one institution, *Clin Orthop Relat Res* 472:349–359, 2014.
23. Henderson E, Pepper A, Marulanda G, et al: What is the emotional acceptance after limb salvage with an expandable prosthesis, *Clin Orthop Relat Res* 468:2933–2938, 2010.
24. Hwang N, Grimer R, Carter S, et al: Early results of a non-invasive extendible prosthesis for limb-salvage surgery in children with bone tumors, *J Bone Joint Surg Br* 94:265–269, 2012.
25. Waters R, Perry J, Antonelli D, et al: Energy cost of amputee: the influence of level of amputation, *J Bone Joint Surg* 58:42–46, 1976.
26. Huang C, Jackson J, Moore N, et al: Amputation: energy cost of ambulation, *Arch Phys Med Rehab* 60:18–24, 1979.
27. Vllasolli T, Zafirova B, Orovcanec N, et al: Energy expenditure and walking speed in lower limb amputees: a cross sectional study, *Orthop Traumatol Rehabil* 16:419–426, 2014.
28. Otis J, Lane J, Kroll M: Energy cost during gait in osteosarcoma patients after resection and knee replacement and after above-the-knee amputation, *J Bone Joint Surg Am* 67:606–611, 1985.

Index

Note: Page numbers followed by *b* indicate boxes, *f* indicate figures and *t* indicate tables.